Hospital Medicine

SECOND EDITION

Hospital Medicine

SECOND EDITION

EDITORS:

▬ ROBERT M. WACHTER, MD

Professor and Associate Chairman
Department of Medicine
University of California, San Francisco School of Medicine
Chief of the Medical Service
UCSF Medical Center
San Francisco, California

▬ LEE GOLDMAN, MD

Julius R. Krevans Distinguished Professor and Chair
Department of Medicine
Associate Dean for Clinical Affairs
University of California, San Francisco School of Medicine
San Francisco, California

▬ HARRY HOLLANDER, MD

Professor
Department of Medicine
Director, Internal Medicine Residency Program
University of California, San Francisco School of Medicine
San Francisco, California

◆ LIPPINCOTT WILLIAMS & WILKINS
A **Wolters Kluwer** Company
Philadelphia • Baltimore • New York • London
Buenos Aires • Hong Kong • Sydney • Tokyo

Acquisitions Editor: Sonya Seigafuse
Developmental Editor: Leah Hayes
Project Manager: Alicia Jackson
Senior Manufacturing Manager: Benjamin Rivera
Marketing Manager: Kathy Neely
Creative Director: Doug Smock
Cover Designer: Teresa Mallon
Production Service: Schawk, Inc.; Publishing Solutions for Retail, Book and Catalog
Printer: Quebecor World-Taunton

© 2005 by LIPPINCOTT WILLIAMS & WILKINS
530 Walnut Street
Philadelphia, PA 19106 USA
LWW.com

Printed in the USA

First Edition, 2000 © Lippincott Williams & Wilkins

Library of Congress Cataloging-in-Publication Data

Hospital medicine / editors, Robert M. Wachter, Lee Goldman, Harry Hollander.—2nd ed.
    p. ; cm.
    Includes bibliographical references and index.
    ISBN 0-7817-4727-9 (alk. paper)
    1. Hospital care. 2. Internal medicine. I. Wachter, Robert M. II. Goldman, Lee, MD. III. Hollander, Harry. [DNLM: 1. Clinical Medicine. 2. Hospitalization. 3. Inpatients.]
RA972.H674 2005
362.11—dc22

2005003522

Care has been taken to confirm the accuracy of the information presented and to describe generally accepted practices. However, the authors, editors, and publisher are not responsible for errors or omissions or for any consequences from application of the information in this book and make no warranty, expressed or implied, with respect to the currency, completeness, or accuracy of the contents of the publication. Application of this information in a particular situation remains the professional responsibility of the practitioner.

The authors, editors, and publisher have exerted every effort to ensure that drug selection and dosage set forth in this text are in accordance with current recommendations and practice at the time of publication. However, in view of ongoing research, changes in government regulations, and the constant flow of information relating to drug therapy and drug reactions, the reader is urged to check the package insert for each drug for any change in indications and dosage and for added warnings and precautions. This is particularly important when the recommended agent is a new or infrequently employed drug.

Some drugs and medical devices presented in the publication have Food and Drug Administration (FDA) clearance for limited use in restricted research settings. It is the responsibility of the health care provider to ascertain the FDA status of each drug or device planned for use in their clinical practice.

10 9 8 7 6 5 4 3 2

About the Cover

An engraving of the Pennsylvania Hospital ("The Building by the Bounty of Government and many Private Persons was proudly founded for the Relief of the Sick and Miserable. Anno 1755"). Artist, William Strickland; Engraver, Samuel Seymour; 1811. The Pennsylvania Hospital is the oldest hospital in the United States. Its first patient was admitted in 1752; its original mission was to care for the "sick poor" and the insane. Benjamin Franklin was co-founder of the hospital (along with Dr. Thomas Bond), and served on its first Board. Reproduced by permission of the American Philosophical Society.

To Our Trainees

Contents

Contributors xi
Preface to the Second Edition xix
Preface to the First Edition xxi

SECTION I: GENERAL ISSUES IN HOSPITAL MEDICINE 1

1 Models of Hospital Care 3
   Robert M. Wachter

2 The Economics of Hospital Medicine 11
   David Meltzer and Chad Whelan

3 Practice Management in Hospital Medicine 17
   John R. Nelson

4 Hospital Interfaces 23
   Winthrop F. Whitcomb and John R. Nelson

5 Hospital Discharge 31
   Preetha Basaviah and Mark V. Williams

6 Bayesian Reasoning and Diagnostic Testing 37
   Warren S. Browner

7 Decision Analysis 43
   Warren S. Browner

8 Evidence-Based Medicine 51
   Holger J. Schünemann and Gordon H. Guyatt

9 Cost-Effectiveness 59
   Joel Tsevat

10 Hospital Information Systems 63
   Saverio M. Maviglia, Gilad J. Kuperman, and Blackford Middleton

11 Effective Clinical Teaching in the Inpatient Setting 71
   Karen E. Hauer and David M. Irby

12 Assessment and Improvement of Quality and Value 79
   Robert M. Wachter and Niraj L. Sehgal

13 Practice Guidelines and Clinical Pathways 87
   Scott Weingarten

14 Patient Satisfaction with Hospital Care 93
   Haya R. Rubin

15 Nutritional Issues in the Hospitalized Patient 99
   Annette Stralovich-Romani and Christopher R. Pennington

16 Approach to the Hospitalized Older Patient 111
   C. Seth Landefeld, C. Bree Johnston, and Mary Anne Johnson

17 Ethical Issues in the Hospitalized Patient 119
   Steven Z. Pantilat and Bernard Lo

18 Pain Management in the Hospitalized Patient 129
   Robert V. Brody

19 End-of-Life Care in the Hospital 139
   Daniel J. Fischberg, Paolo Manfredi, and Diane E. Meier

20 Patient Safety in the Hospital Setting 147
   Kaveh G. Shojania

21 Medication Safety in the Hospital 157
   David W. Bates

SECTION II: CRITICAL CARE MEDICINE 161

22 Approach to the ICU Patient 163
   Neal H. Cohen

23 Ventilator Management 173
   Stephen E. Lapinsky and Arthur S. Slutsky

24 Acute Respiratory Failure 183
   Mark R. Tonelli and Leonard D. Hudson

25 Hypotension, Shock, and Multiple Organ Failure 191
   Bradley D. Freeman and Charles Natanson

26 Sepsis Syndrome 201
   Todd W. Rice and Gordon R. Bernard

27 Procedures in Hospital Medicine 207
   Rachel L. Chin

SECTION III: MEDICAL CONSULTATION 233

28 Medical Consultation 235
   Geno J. Merli and Howard H. Weitz

29 Key Principles of Anesthesiology 241
Neal Cohen

30 Preoperative Evaluation 249
Joshua S. Adler

31 Postoperative Care 261
Richard H. Savel, Jeanine P. Wiener-Kronish, and Michael A. Gropper

32 Medical Complications of Pregnancy 271
Jeffery Pickard, Linda A. Barbour, and Raymond O. Powrie

33 Care of Special Populations: Psychiatry 279
David F. Gitlin and Bernard Vaccaro

34 Trauma 287
Deborah M. Stein, Ronald Rabinowitz, and Ellis Caplan

SECTION IV: CARDIOVASCULAR MEDICINE 295

35 Signs, Symptoms, and Laboratory Abnormalities in Cardiovascular Diseases 297
Randall H. Vagelos, Rachel Marcus, and J. Edwin Atwood

36 Diagnostic Tests in Cardiology 315
Karen P. Alexander and Eric D. Peterson

37 Angina and Unstable Angina 329
Daniel B. Mark

38 Acute Myocardial Infarction 343
Daniel I. Simon, James C. Fang, and Naomi Kenmotsu Rounds

39 Heart Failure 359
Carey D. Kimmelstiel, David DeNofrio, and Marvin A. Konstam

40 Heart Transplantation 373
Maria Ansari and Teresa DeMarco

41 Valvular Heart Disease 381
Richard A. Lange and L. David Hillis

42 Atrial Fibrillation, Atrial Flutter, and Other Supraventricular Tachyarrhythmias 393
Leonard I. Ganz

43 Ventricular Arrhythmias and Cardiac Arrest 409
Graham Gardner, H. Leon Greene, and Peter Zimetbaum

44 Syncope 423
Wishwa N. Kapoor and David J. McAdams

45 Bradycardia and Pacemakers 431
Richard H. Hongo and Nora F. Goldschlager

46 Pericardial Disease 441
Fady Malik and Elyse Foster

SECTION V: VASCULAR MEDICINE 453

47 Signs, Symptoms, and Laboratory Abnormalities in Peripheral Arterial Disease 455
Stanley G. Rockson

48 Urgent and Emergent Hypertension 463
William B. White

49 Aortic Intramural Hematoma and Dissection 471
Lee Goldman

50 Aortic Aneurysm 479
Frank A. Lederle

51 Peripheral Arterial Disease 485
Eric P. Brass, William R. Hiatt, and Mark R. Nehler

52 Deep Venous Thrombosis 495
David A. Garcia and Mark A. Crowther

53 Pulmonary Embolism 505
Thomas M. Hyers

SECTION VI: PULMONARY MEDICINE 515

54 Signs, Symptoms, and Laboratory Abnormalities in Pulmonary Medicine 517
Meshell D. Johnson and Paul G. Brunetta

55 Chronic Obstructive Pulmonary Disease 531
Matthew B. Stanbrook and Kenneth R. Chapman

56 Exacerbations of Asthma 539
Homer A. Boushey

57 Interstitial Lung Disease 549
Talmadge E. King, Jr.

58 Lung Transplantation and Lung Volume Reduction Surgery 561
Steven G. Peters and David E. Midthun

59 Pulmonary Hypertension 569
Lewis J. Rubin

60 Pleural Effusion and Pneumothorax 577
Steven A. Sahn and John E. Heffner

61 Pulmonary Nodules and Mass Lesions 587
Michael K. Gould and Glen A. Lillington

SECTION VII: INFECTIOUS DISEASES 595

62 Signs, Symptoms, and Laboratory Abnormalities in Infectious Diseases 597
Richard A. Jacobs and Karen C. Bloch

63 Infections in Immunocompromised Hosts 613
Nesli Basgoz

64 Parenteral Antibiotics and Antibiotic Resistance 623
Lisa G. Winston and Henry F. Chambers III

65 Community-Acquired Pneumonia 633
Ethan A. Halm and Michael J. Fine

66 Hospital-Acquired Pneumonia 645
Donald E. Craven, Catherine A. Fleming, and Kathleen A. Steger Craven

67 Tuberculosis 655
Charles L. Daley and Phillip C. Hopewell

68 Urinary Tract Infection 667
Thomas M. Hooton

69 Cellulitis and Necrotizing Fasciitis 675
Dennis L. Stevens

70 Meningitis 683
Allan R. Tunkel and W. Michael Scheld

71 Endocarditis 693
Paul M. Sullam

72 Catheter-Associated Infection and Bacteremia 703
Isaam I. Raad and Hend A. Hanna

73 Bioterrorism 711
Thomas E. Terndrup and Sarah D. Nafziger

SECTION VIII: HIV DISEASE 719

74 Signs, Symptoms, and Laboratory Abnormalities in HIV Disease 721
Harry Hollander

75 Pulmonary Manifestations of HIV Infection 729
Laurence Huang and Philip C. Hopewell

76 Neurologic Complications of HIV Disease 739
Christina M. Marra

SECTION IX: GASTROENTEROLOGY 749

77 Signs, Symptoms, and Laboratory Abnormalities in Gastrointestinal Disease 751
Kenneth McQuaid

78 Acute Gastrointestinal Bleeding 767
Jonathan P. Terdiman and Peter K. Lindenauer

79 Esophageal Disorders 781
Asyia Ahmad and James C. Reynolds

80 Peptic Ulcer Disease and Stress-Related Mucosal Disease 789
Brennan M. R. Spiegel and Gareth S. Dulai

81 Inflammatory Bowel Disease 799
Stephen B. Hanauer and Sunanda V. Kane

82 Acute Hepatitis and Liver Failure 809
Marina Berenguer and Teresa L. Wright

83 Cirrhosis and Its Complications 819
Don C. Rockey

84 Disorders of The Biliary System 829
Douglas B. Nelson, Paul Druck, and Martin L. Freeman

85 Liver Transplantation 839
Rapheal B. Merriman

86 Acute Pancreatitis 849
Douglas A. Corley

87 Other Abdominal Emergencies: Appendicitis, Diverticulitis, and Ischemic Bowel 859
Lily C. Chang and E. Patchen Dellinger

88 Ileus and Obstruction of the Gastrointestinal Tract 873
Daniel T. Dempsey and Sean P. Harbison

SECTION X: HEMATOLOGY–ONCOLOGY 883

89 Signs, Symptoms, and Laboratory Abnormalities in Hematology-Oncology 885
Hope S. Rugo

90 Principles of Chemotherapy 897
Robert J. Ignoffo

91 Principles of Transfusion Medicine 907
Susan A. Galel and Edgar G. Engleman

92 Oncologic Emergencies 917
Judith A. Luce

93 Leukemia 929
David A. Rizzieri, Gwynn D. Long, and Nelson J. Chao

94 Lymphoma 937
Ranjana H. Advani, Steven M. Horwitz, and Sandra J. Horning

95 Chronic Myeloproliferative Disorders 947
Ayalew Tefferi

96   Hematopoietic Cell Transplantation 955
Frederick R. Applebaum

97   Sickle Cell Disease 965
Martin H. Steinberg and Harrison W. Farber

98   Hemorrhagic and Thrombotic Disorders 975
Julie Hambleton and Marc Shuman

SECTION XI: RENAL DISEASE 993

99   Signs, Symptoms, and Laboratory Abnormalities in Renal Disease 995
Rudolph A. Rodriguez and Burl R. Don

100   Acute Renal Failure 1007
Ravindra L. Mehta and Frank Liu

101   Management of the Hospitalized Patient on Dialysis 1017
Glenn M. Chertow

102   Renal Transplantation 1027
William J.C. Amend, Jr. and Flavio Vincenti

103   Renal Stone Disease and Obstruction 1037
David S. Goldfarb and Fredric L. Coe

104   Common Electrolyte Disorders 1045
Kerry C. Cho

105   Common Acid-Base Disorders 1055
Orson W. Moe, Daniel Fuster, and Robert J. Alpern

SECTION XII: ENDOCRINOLOGY 1067

106   Signs, Symptoms, and Laboratory Abnormalities in Endocrinology 1069
Kenneth A. Woeber

107   The Management of Hyperglycemia and Diabetes Mellitus in Hospitalized Patients 1079
Harold E. Lebovitz

108   Acute Presentations of Thyroid Disease 1093
Leonard Wartofsky

109   Adrenal Insufficiency and Crisis 1103
David G. Gardner

SECTION XIII: RHEUMATOLOGY 1109

110   Signs, Symptoms, and Laboratory Abnormalities in Rheumatology 1111
Jeffrey Critchfield

111   Vasculitis 1121
Gary S. Hoffman, Carol A. Langford, and Leonard H. Calabrese

112   Acute Presentations of Selected Rheumatic Disorders 1135
Kenneth H. Fye and Kenneth E. Sack

113   Acute Arthritis 1143
John H. Stone and David B. Hellmann

114   Back Pain 1153
Jerry D. Joines and Nortin M. Hadler

SECTION XIV: NEUROLOGY AND PSYCHIATRY 1161

115   Signs, Symptoms, and Diagnostic Tests in Neurology 1163
John W. Engstrom

116   Stroke 1175
Wade S. Smith

117   Central Nervous System Hemorrhage and Increased Intracranial Pressure 1185
Ellen Deibert and Michael N. Diringer

118   Seizures 1199
Paul A. Garcia

119   Depression in the Hospitalized Patient 1209
Richard J. Goldberg

SECTION XV: TOXICOLOGY AND ALLERGY 1219

120   Allergic Reactions and Anaphylaxis 1221
Neil Winawer and Mark V. Williams

121   Drug Overdoses and Dependence 1229
Josef G. Thundiyil, Jon K. Beauchamp, and Kent R. Olson

122   Acute Alcohol Intoxication and Alcohol Withdrawal 1243
Robert H. Lohr

Index 1251

Contributors

JOSHUA S. ADLER, MD Associate Professor of Clinical Medicine, University of California, San Francisco School of Medicine; Medical Director, Ambulatory Care, Department of Medicine, UCSF Medical Center, San Francisco, California

RANJANA H. ADVANI, MD Assistant Professor of Medicine/Oncology, Stanford University School of Medicine, Stanford, California

ASYIA AHMAD, MD Assistant Professor of Medicine, Division of Gastroenterology and Hepatology, Drexel University College of Medicine, Philadelphia, Pennsylvania

KAREN P. ALEXANDER, MD Assistant Professor, Division of Cardiology, Department of Medicine, Duke University School of Medicine, Durham, North Carolina

ROBERT J. ALPERN, MD Ensign Professor of Medicine and Dean, Yale University School of Medicine, New Haven, Connecticut

WILLIAM J.C. AMEND, MD Clinical Professor of Medicine and Surgery, Department of Medicine, University of California, San Francisco School of Medicine, San Francisco, California

MARIA ANSARI, MD Division of Cardiology, Kaiser Permanente, Los Angeles Medical Center, Los Angeles, California

FREDERICK R. APPELBAUM, MD Director, Clinical Research Division, Fred Hutchinson Cancer Research Center; Professor and Head, Division of Medical Oncology, University of Washington School of Medicine, Seattle, Washington

J. EDWIN ATWOOD, MD Professor, Division of Cardiovascular Medicine, Stanford University School of Medicine, Stanford, California

LINDA A. BARBOUR, MD, MSPH Associate Professor and Medical Director of High Risk Obstetrics Clinics, Departments of Medicine and Obstetrics and Gynecology, University of Colorado Health Sciences Center, Aurora, Colorado

PREETHA BASAVIAH, MD Assistant Clinical Professor, Department of Medicine, University of California, San Francisco School of Medicine, San Francisco, California

DAVID W. BATES, MD, MSc Professor of Medicine, Department of Medicine, Harvard Medical School; Chief, Division of General Medicine, Brigham & Women's Hospital, Boston, Massachusetts

NESLI BASGOZ, MD Associate Professor of Medicine, Harvard Medical School; Associate Physician, Infectious Disease Unit, Massachusetts General Hospital, Boston, Massachusetts

JON K. BEAUCHAMP, MD Department of Emergency Medicine, Contra Costa Regional Medical Center, Martinez, California

MARINA BERENGUER, MD Hepatology-Gastroenterology Service, Hospital La FE, Valencia, Spain

GORDON R. BERNARD, MD Director, Division of Allergy, Pulmonary & Critical Care Medicine, Department of Internal Medicine, Vanderbilt University School of Medicine, Nashville, Tennessee

KAREN C. BLOCH, MD, MPH Assistant Professor, Department of Medicine and Infectious Diseases, Vanderbilt University School of Medicine, Nashville, Tennessee

ERIC P. BRASS, MD, PhD Professor, Department of Medicine, David Geffen School of Medicine at UCLA; Director, Department of Medicine, Harbor-UCLA Medical Center, Torrance, California

ROBERT V. BRODY, MD Clinical Professor, Department of Medicine and Department of Family & Community Medicine, University of California, San Francisco School of Medicine; Chief, Pain Consultation Clinic, San Francisco General Hospital, San Francisco, California

HOMER A. BOUSHEY, MD Professor of Medicine, Department of Medicine, University of California, San Francisco School of Medicine; Chief, Asthma Clinical Research Center and Division of Allergy and Immunology, UCSF Medical Center, San Francisco, California

WARREN S. BROWNER, MD, MPH Vice President, Academic Affairs and Scientific Director, Research Institute, California Pacific Medical Center; Adjunct Professor of Medicine and Epidemiology & Biostatistics, University of California, San Francisco School of Medicine, San Francisco, California

PAUL G. BRUNETTA, MD Medical Director, Genentech, Inc., South San Francisco, California

LEONARD H. CALABRESE, MD Vice Chairman, Department of Rheumatic and Immunologic Diseases, Cleveland Clinic Foundation, Cleveland, Ohio

ELLIS S. CAPLAN, MD Associate Professor of Medicine, Section Chief, Infectious Diseases, R. Adams Cowley Shock Trauma Center, University of Maryland Medical Center, Baltimore, Maryland

HENRY F. CHAMBERS III, MD Professor, Department of Medicine, University of California, San Francisco School of Medicine; Chief, Division of Infectious Diseases, San Francisco General Hospital, San Francisco, California

LILY C. CHANG, MD Assistant Professor, Department of Surgery, Boston University School of Medicine, Boston, Massachusetts

NELSON J. CHAO, MD Associate Professor, Department of Medicine, Division of Cellular Therapy, Duke University School of Medicine, Durham, North Carolina

KENNETH R. CHAPMAN, MD, MSc Professor, Department of Medicine, University of Toronto, Toronto, Ontario, Canada

GLENN M. CHERTOW, MD, MPH Associate Professor, Division of Nephrology, Department of Medicine, University of California, San Francisco School of Medicine, San Francisco, California

RACHEL L. CHIN, MD Associate Professor of Clinical Medicine, University of California, San Francisco School of Medicine; Attending Physician, Emergency Services, San Francisco General Hospital, San Francisco, California

KERRY C. CHO, MD Assistant Clinical Professor, Division of Nephrology, University of California, San Francisco School of Medicine, San Francisco, California

FREDRIC L. COE, MD Professor of Medicine and Physiology, Kidney Stone Program, Renal Section, University of Chicago School of Medicine, Chicago, Illinois

NEAL H. COHEN, MD Vice Dean for Academic Affairs and Professor, Anesthesia and Perioperative Care and Medicine, University of California, San Francisco School of Medicine, San Francisco, California

DOUGLAS A. CORLEY, MD, PhD, MPH Assistant Clinical Professor of Medicine, University of California, San Francisco School of Medicine, San Francisco, California; Investigator, Kaiser Permanente Division of Research, Oakland, California

DONALD E. CRAVEN, MD Chairman, Division of Infectious Diseases, Lahey Clinic, Burlington, Massachusetts

KATHLEEN A. STEGER CRAVEN, MD Consultant, Epidemiology and Public Health, Wellesley, Massachusetts

JEFFREY CRITCHFIELD, MD Assistant Clinical Professor, Department of Medicine, University of California, San Francisco School of Medicine; Vice-Chief of Medicine, Clinical Affairs, Department of Medicine, San Francisco General Hospital, San Francisco, California

MARK A. CROWTHER, MD, MSc Associate Professor, Department of Medicine, McMaster University; Head of Section, Division of Hematology, St. Joseph's Hospital, Hamilton, Ontario

CHARLES L. DALEY, MD Professor, Department of Medicine, University of Colorado School of Medicine; Chief, Division of Mycobacterial and Respiratory Infection, National Jewish Medical and Research Center, Denver, Colorado

ELLEN DEIBERT, MD Assistant Professor, Department of Neurology and Neurosurgery, Washington University School of Medicine, St. Louis, Missouri

E. PATCHEN DELLINGER, MD Professor and Vice Chairman, Department of Surgery, University of Washington School of Medicine; Chief, Division of General Surgery, University of Washington Medical Center, Seattle, Washington

TERESA DEMARCO, MD Professor of Clinical Medicine, Heart Failure and Pulmonary Hypertension Program, University of California, San Francisco School of Medicine, San Francisco, California

DANIEL T. DEMPSEY, MD Professor and Chair, Department of Surgery, Temple University School of Medicine, Philadelphia, Pennsylvania

DAVID DENOFRIO, MD Medical Director, Transplantation Program and Cardiology Myopathy Center, Division of Cardiology, Tufts-New England Medical Center, Boston, Massachusetts

MICHAEL N. DIRINGER, MD Associate Professor and Director, Neurology/Neurosurgery Intensive Care Unit, Departments of Neurology, Neurosurgery, and Anesthesiology, Washington University School of Medicine, St. Louis, Missouri

BURL R. DON, MD Associate Professor, Departments of Internal Medicine and Nephrology, University of California, Davis School of Medicine, Sacramento, California

PAUL DRUCK, MD Assistant Professor, Department of Surgery, University of Minnesota Medical School; Staff Surgeon and Medical Director, Minneapolis VA Medical Center, Minneapolis, Minnesota

GARETH S. DULAI, MD, MSHS Assistant Professor of Medicine, David Geffen UCLA School of Medicine and Greater Los Angeles VA Healthcare System; Co-director, Center for the Study of Digestive Healthcare Quality & Outcomes, Los Angeles, California

EDGAR G. ENGLEMAN, MD Professor, Departments of Pathology and Medicine, Stanford University School of Medicine, Palo Alto, California

JOHN W. ENGSTROM, MD Professor and Vice Chairman, Department of Neurology, University of California, San Francisco School of Medicine, San Francisco, California

JAMES C. FANG, MD Associate Professor of Medicine, Cardiovascular Division, Harvard Medical School; Director, Heart Transplant and Circulatory Diseases, Brigham & Women's Hospital, Boston, Massachusetts

HARRISON W. FARBER, MD Professor, Department of Medicine – Pulmonary Critical Care, Boston University School of Medicine; Director, Pulmonary Hypertension Center, Boston Medical Center, Boston, Massachusetts

MICHAEL J. FINE, MD, MSc Professor of Medicine, Division of General Internal Medicine and Center for Research on Healthcare, University of Pittsburgh School of Medicine; Director, VA Center for Health Equity Research and Promotion, VA Pittsburgh Health System, Pittsburgh, Pennsylvania

DANIEL FISCHBERG, MD, PhD Assistant Professor, Department of Geriatric Medicine, The John A. Burns School of Medicine at The University of Hawaii; Medical Director, Pain & Palliative Care Department, The Queen's Medical Center, Honolulu, Hawaii

CATHERINE A. FLEMING, MD Lecturer in Medicine, Department of Medicine, National University, Galway Ireland; Consultant Physician, Department of Medicine, University College Hospital, Galway, Ireland

ELYSE FOSTER, MD Professor, Departments of Medicine and Anesthesia, University of California, San Francisco School of Medicine; Director, Adult Echocardiography Laboratory, UCSF Medical Center, San Francisco, California

BRADLEY D. FREEMAN, MD Associate Professor, Department of Surgery, Washington University School of Medicine; Attending Physician, Department of Surgery, Barnes-Jewish Hospital, St. Louis, Missouri

MARTIN L. FREEMAN, MD Professor of Medicine, Gastroenterology Section, Hennepin County Medical Center and Department of Medicine, University of Minnesota, Minneapolis, Minnesota

DANIEL FUSTER, MD Fellow, Department of Internal Medicine, University of Texas Southwestern Medical Center, Dallas, Texas

KENNETH H. FYE, MD Clinical Professor, Division of Rheumatology, Department of Medicine, University of California, San Francisco School of Medicine, San Francisco, California

SUSAN A. GALEL, MD Associate Professor, Department of Pathology, Stanford University School of Medicine, Stanford, California; Director of Clinical Operations, Stanford Medical School Blood Center, Palo Alto, California

LEONARD I. GANZ, MD Associate Professor, Department of Medicine, University of Pittsburgh School of Medicine; Director of Cardiac Electrophysiology, Cardiovascular Institute, University of Pittsburgh Medical Center, Pittsburgh, Pennsylvania

DAVID A. GARCIA, MD Assistant Professor, Internal Medicine, University of New Mexico; Attending Physician, Internal Medicine, University of New Mexico Health Services Center, Albuquerque, New Mexico

PAUL A. GARCIA, MD Associate Professor, Department of Neurology, University of California, San Francisco School of Medicine, San Francisco, California

DAVID G. GARDNER, MD Professor, Department of Medicine, University of California, San Francisco School of Medicine, San Francisco, California

GRAHAM GARDNER, MD Clinical Fellow, Division of Cardiology, Harvard Medical School and Beth Israel Deaconess Medical Center, Boston, Massachusetts

DAVID F. GITLIN, MD Assistant Professor of Psychiatry, Harvard Medical School; Director, Medical Psychiatry Services, Brigham & Women's / Faulkner Hospitals, Boston, Massachusetts

RICHARD J. GOLDBERG, MD Professor, Department of Psychiatry, Brown University; Psychiatrist-in-Chief, Department of Psychiatry, Rhode Island Hospital and The Miriam Hospital, Providence, Rhode Island

DAVID S. GOLDFARB, MD Professor, Departments of Medicine and Physiology, New York University School of Medicine; Assistant Chief, Nephrology Section, New York Harbor Department of VA Medical Center, New York, New York

LEE GOLDMAN, MD, MPH Julius R. Krevans Distinguished Professor and Chairman, Department of Medicine, University of California, San Francisco School of Medicine, San Francisco, California

NORA F. GOLDSCHLAGER, MD Professor of Clinical Medicine, Department of Medicine, University of California, San Francisco School of Medicine; Director, Coronary Care Unit and ECG Laboratory, San Francisco General Hospital, San Francisco, California

MICHAEL K. GOULD, MD, MS Assistant Professor of Medicine, Division of Pulmonary and Critical Care Medicine, Stanford University School of Medicine, Stanford, California; Research Associate and Staff Physician, Veterans Affairs Palo Alto Health Care System, Palo Alto, California

H. LEON GREENE, MD Professor, Division of Cardiology, University of Washington School of Medicine, Seattle, Washington

MICHAEL A. GROPPER, MD, PhD Professor and Director, Critical Care Medicine, Anesthesia and Perioperative Care, University of California, San Francisco School of Medicine, San Francisco, California

GORDON H. GUYATT, MD Professor, Departments of Medicine and Clinical Epidemiology and Biostatistics, McMaster University, Hamilton, Ontario, Canada

NORTIN M. HADLER, MD Professor, Departments of Medicine and Microbiology/Immunology, University of North Carolina at Chapel Hill School of Medicine, Chapel Hill, North Carolina

ETHAN A. HALM, MD, MPH Associate Chief, Division of Research and Assistant Professor, Health Policy and Medicine, Mount Sinai School of Medicine; Associate Chief, Division of General Internal Medicine, The Mount Sinai Hospital, New York, New York

JULIE HAMBLETON, MD Medical Director, Genentech, Inc., South San Francisco, California

STEPHEN HANAUER, MD Professor and Director, Section of Gastroenterology and Nutrition, Department of Medicine, University of Chicago School of Medicine, Chicago, Illinois

HEND A. HANNA, MD, MPH Assistant Professor, Epidemiologist, Department of Infectious Diseases, Infection Control and Employee Health, University of Texas, MD Anderson Cancer Center, Houston, Texas

SEAN P. HARBISON, MD Associate Professor, Department of Surgery, Temple University School of Medicine, Philadelphia, Pennsylvania

KAREN E. HAUER, MD Associate Professor of Clinical Medicine and Director of Internal Medicine Clerkships, Department of Medicine, University of California, San Francisco School of Medicine, San Francisco, California

JOHN E. HEFFNER, MD Professor of Medicine, Department of Medicine, Medical University of South Carolina; Executive Medical Director, Medical University Hospital, Charleston, South Carolina

DAVID B. HELLMAN, MD Professor of Medicine and Director, Department of Medicine, Johns Hopkins Bayview Medical Center, Johns Hopkins University School of Medicine, Baltimore, Maryland

WILLIAM R. HIATT, MD Professor of Medicine, Chief, Section of Vascular Medicine, Department of Medicine, University of Colorado Health Sciences Center; President, Colorado Prevention Center, Denver, Colorado

L. DAVID HILLIS, MD Professor and Vice-Chairman, James M. Wooten Chair in Cardiology, Department of Internal Medicine, University of Texas Southwestern Medical Center, Dallas, Texas

GARY S. HOFFMAN, MD Chairman, Rheumatic and Immunologic Diseases, Cleveland Clinic Foundation, Cleveland, Ohio

HARRY HOLLANDER, MD Professor and Residency Director, Department of Medicine, University of California, San Francisco School of Medicine, San Francisco, California

RICHARD H. HONGO, MD Staff Electrophysiologist, California Pacific Medical Center, San Francisco, California

THOMAS M. HOOTON, MD Professor, Department of Medicine, University of Washington School of Medicine; Medical Director, HIV AIDS Clinic, Harborview Medical Center, Seattle, Washington

PHILIP C. HOPEWELL, MD Professor of Medicine, University of California, San Francisco School of Medicine, San Francisco, California

SANDRA J. HORNING, MD Professor of Medicine, Division of Blood and Marrow Transplantation, Stanford University School of Medicine, Stanford, California

STEVEN M. HORWITZ, MD Attending Staff Physician, Department of Medicine, Division of Oncology, Memorial Sloan-Kettering Cancer Center, New York, New York

LAURENCE HUANG, MD Associate Professor, Department of Medicine, University of California, San Francisco School of Medicine; Chief, AIDS Chest Clinic, Positive Health Program, San Francisco General Hospital, San Francisco, California

LEONARD D. HUDSON, MD Endowed Chair, Department of Pulmonary Disease Research, University of Washington, Seattle, Washington

THOMAS M. HYERS, MD Clinical Professor, Department of Internal Medicine, St. Louis University School of Medicine; Staff Physician, Department of Pulmonary Diseases, St. Joseph Hospital–Kirkwood, St. Louis, Missouri

ROBERT J. IGNOFFO, PharmD Clinical Professor, Clinical Pharmacy, University of California, San Francisco; Oncology Pharmacist, UCSF Comprehensive Cancer Center, Mt. Zion Hospital, San Francisco, California

DAVID M. IRBY, PhD Professor and Vice Dean for Education, Department of Medicine, University of California, San Francisco School of Medicine, San Francisco, California

RICHARD A. JACOBS, MD, PhD Clinical Professor, Departments of Medicine and Clinical Pharmacy, University of California, San Francisco School of Medicine, San Francisco, California

MARY ANNE JOHNSON, MD Division of Geriatrics, VA Medical Center, San Francisco, California

MESHELL D. JOHNSON, MD Assistant Adjunct Professor, Department of Medicine, University of California, San Francisco School of Medicine, San Francisco, California

C. BREE JOHNSTON, MD Division of Geriatrics, VA Medical Center, San Francisco, California

JERRY D. JOINES, MD, PhD Associate Professor, Department of Medicine, University of North Carolina School of Medicine, Chapel Hill, North Carolina; Faculty Physician, Internal Medicine Program, Moses H. Cone Hospital, Greensboro, North Carolina

SUNANDA V. KANE, MD, MSPH Assistant Professor, Department of Medicine, University of Chicago School of Medicine, Chicago, Illinois

WISHWA N. KAPOOR, MD, MPH Falk Professor of Medicine and Chief, Division of General Internal Medicine, University of Pittsburgh School of Medicine, Pittsburgh, Pennsylvania

CAREY D. KIMMELSTIEL, MD Director, Cardiac Catheterization Laboratory and Interventional Cardiology, Tufts-New England Medical Center Division of Cardiology, Boston, Massachusetts

TALMADGE E. KING, JR., MD Constance B. Wofsy Distinguished Professor and Vice-Chairman, Department of Medicine, University of California, San Francisco School of Medicine; Chief, Medical Service, Department of Medicine, San Francisco General Hospital, San Francisco, California

MARVIN A. KONSTAM, MD Chief, Division of Cardiology, Tufts-New England Medical Center, Boston, Massachusetts

JEANINE P. WIENER-KRONISH, MD Vice-Chairman for Research, Department of Anesthesia, University of California, San Francisco School of Medicine, San Francisco, California

GILAD J. KUPERMAN, MD, PhD Director of Quality Informatics, New York-Presbyterian Hospital, New York, New York

C. SETH LANDEFELD, MD Professor of Medicine, Epidemiology and Biostatistics, Chief, Division of Geriatrics, Department of Medicine, University of California, San Francisco School of Medicine; Associate Chief of Staff, Geriatrics and Extended Care, San Francisco VA Center, San Francisco, California

RICHARD A. LANGE, MD E. Cowles Andrus Professor of Cardiology, Department of Internal Medicine, Johns Hopkins University School of Medicine, Baltimore, Maryland

CAROL A. LANGFORD, MD, MHS Senior Investigator, Immunologic Diseases Section, National Institute of Allergy and Infectious Diseases, Bethesda, Maryland

STEPHEN E. LAPINSKY, MB BCh, MSc Associate Professor, Department of Medicine, University of Toronto School of Medicine; Site Director, Intensive Care Unit, Mount Sinai Hospital, Toronto, Ontario, Canada

HAROLD E. LEBOVITZ, MD Professor, Department of Medicine, State University of New York Health Science Center at Brooklyn, Brooklyn, New York

FRANK A. LEDERLE, MD Professor, Department of Medicine, University of Minnesota School of Medicine; Director, Minneapolis Center for Epidemiological and Clinical Research, VA Medical Center, Minneapolis, Minnesota

GLEN A. LILLINGTON, MD Professor Emeritus of Medicine, Chief, Pulmonary/Critical Care, Department of Medicine, University of California (Davis); Clinical Professor Emeritus, Department of Medicine, Stanford Medical Center, Stanford, California

PETER K. LINDENAUER, MD MSC Assistant Professor of Medicine, Tufts University School of Medicine; Associate Medical Director, Office of Clinical Practice Evaluation and Management, Baystate Medical Center, Springfield, Massachusetts

FRANK LIU, MD Postgraduate researcher, Department of Medicine, University of California, San Diego, Department of Medicine, San Diego, California

BERNARD LO, MD Professor of Medicine and Director, Program in Medical Ethics, Department of Medicine, University of California, San Francisco School of Medicine, San Francisco, California

ROBERT H. LOHR, MD Assistant Professor, Department of Medicine, Mayo Clinic College of Medicine; Consultant, Department of Medicine, St. Mary's Hospital, Rochester, Minnesota

GWYNN D. LONG, MD Associate Professor of Medicine, Department of Medicine, Division of Cellular Therapy, Duke University School of Medicine, Durham, North Carolina

JUDITH A. LUCE, MD Clinical Professor, Department of Medicine, University of California, San Francisco School of Medicine; Director, Oncology Services, San Francisco General Hospital, San Francisco, California

FADY MALIK, MD, PhD Assistant Clinical Professor of Medicine, Division of Cardiology, University of California, San Francisco School of Medicine, San Francisco, California

PAOLO MANFREDI, MD Department of Neurology, Memorial Sloan-Kettering Cancer Center, Pain and Palliative Care Service, New York, New York

RACHEL MARCUS, MD Cardiologist, Washington Hospital Center, Washington, DC

DANIEL B. MARK, MD, MPH Director, Outcomes Research, Duke Clinical Research Institute; Professor of Medicine, Department of Medicine, Duke University School of Medicine, Durham, North Carolina

CHRISTINE M. MARRA, MD Associate Professor, Neurology and Medicine (Infectious Diseases), University of Washington School of Medicine, Seattle, Washington

SAVERIO M. MAVIGLIA, MD, MSc Instructor, Department of Medicine, Harvard Medical School; Department of Clinical Informatics Research & Development, Partners Healthcare System, Wellesley, Massachusetts; Associate Physician, Department of Medicine, Brigham & Women's Hospital, Boston, Massachusetts

DAVID J. MCADAMS, MD, MS Assistant Professor of Medicine, University of Pittsburgh School of Medicine; Co-director, Section of Hospital Medicine, University of Pittsburgh Medical Center, Pittsburgh, Pennsylvania

KENNETH MCQUAID, MD Associate Professor of Clinical Medicine, Department of Medicine, University of California, San Francisco School of Medicine; Director of Endoscopy, VA Medical Center, San Francisco, California

RAVINDRA L. MEHTA, MBBS, MD, DM Associate Professor of Medicine in Residence, Acting Director of Dialysis Programs, Division of Nephrology, University of California, San Diego School of Medicine, San Diego, California

DIANE E. MEIER, MD Professor, Departments of Geriatrics and Medicine and Director, Hertzberg Palliative Care Institute, Mount Sinai School of Medicine, New York, New York

DAVID MELTZER, MD, PhD Associate Professor, Department of Medicine, University of Chicago School of Medicine, Chicago, Illinois

GENO J. MERLI, MD Ludwig A. Kind Professor, Jefferson Medical College; Vice-Chairman of Clinical Affairs and Director, Division of Internal Medicine, Department of Medicine, Thomas Jefferson University Hospital, Philadelphia, Pennsylvania

RAPHAEL B. MERRIMAN, MD, MRCPI Assistant Professor, Department of Medicine, University of California, San Francisco School of Medicine, San Francisco, California

BLACKFORD MIDDLETON, MD, MPH, MSc Assistant Professor of Medicine, Division of General Medicine and Primary Care, Brigham & Women's Hospital and Harvard Medical School, Boston, Massachusetts; Corporate Director, Clinical Informatics Research & Development, Partners Healthcare Systems, Inc., Wellesley, Massachusetts

DAVID E. MIDTHUN, MD Associate Professor of Medicine, Division of Pulmonary and Critical Care Medicine, Mayo Clinic College of Medicine; Staff Consultant, St. Mary's Hospital, Rochester, Minnesota

ORSON W. MOE, MD Professor of Medicine, Division of Nephrology and Chief, Center for Bone and Mineral Metabolism, University of Texas Southwestern School of Medicine, Dallas, Texas

SARAH D. NAFZIGER, MD Instructor, Department of Emergency Medicine, University of Alabama at Birmingham; Chief Resident, Department of Emergency Medicine, University Hospital, Birmingham, Alabama

CHARLES NATANSON, MD Senior Investigator, Department of Critical Care Medicine, National Institutes of Health, Bethesda, Maryland

MARK R. NEHLER, MD Associate Professor, Department of Surgery, University of Colorado Health Science Center, Denver, Colorado

DOUGLAS B. NELSON, MD Staff Physician in Gastroenterology, Department of Medicine, Minneapolis VA Medical Center, University of Minnesota; Associate Professor of Medicine, University of Minnesota School of Medicine, Minneapolis, Minnesota

JOHN R. NELSON, MD Director, Hospitalist Practice, Overlake Hospital Medical Center, Bellevue, Washington

KENT R. OLSON, MD Clinical Professor of Medicine, Pharmacy, and Pediatrics, University of California, San Francisco School of Medicine; Medical Director, San Francisco Division, California Poison Control System, San Francisco, California

STEVEN Z. PANTILAT, MD Associate Professor of Clinical Medicine, Department of Medicine, University of California, San Francisco School of Medicine; Director, Palliative Care Service, UCSF Medical Center, San Francisco, California

STEVEN G. PETERS, MD Professor, Pulmonary, Critical Care, and Internal Medicine, Mayo Clinic College of Medicine; Medical Director, Lung Transplantation, St. Mary's Hospital, Rochester, Minnesota

ERIC D. PETERSON, MD, MPH Associate Professor of Medicine, Division of Cardiology, Associate Vice Chair for Quality, Department of Medicine, Duke University School of Medicine, Durham, North Carolina

JEFFREY PICKARD, MD Associate Professor, Department of Internal Medicine, University of Colorado at Denver, Health Sciences Center; Associate Professor, Department of Internal Medicine, Presbyterian / St. Luke's Medical Center, Denver, Colorado

RAYMOND O. POWRIE, MD Associate Professor, Departments of Medicine and Obstetrics and Gynecology, Brown University Medical School; Director, Division of Obstetric and Consultative Medicine, Department of Medicine, Women and Infants Hospital, Providence, Rhode Island

ISAAM I. RAAD II, MD Professor of Medicine and Chairman, Department of Infectious Diseases, Infection Control and Employee Health, University of Texas, MD Anderson Cancer Center, Houston, Texas

RONALD RABINOWITZ, MD Assistant Professor, R. Adams Cowley Shock Trauma Center, University of Maryland Medical Center, Baltimore, Maryland

JAMES C. REYNOLDS, MD Professor and Chair (Interim), Department of Medicine, Drexel University College of Medicine; Chair of Medicine, Chief of Gastroenterology and Hepatology, Department of Medicine, Hahnemann University Hospital, Philadelphia, Pennsylvania

TODD W. RICE, MD, MSCI Instructor, Division of Allergy, Pulmonary, & Critical Care Medicine, Department of Internal Medicine, Vanderbilt University School of Medicine, Center for Lung Research, Nashville, Tennessee

DAVID A. RIZZIERI, MD Associate Professor, Department of Medicine, Division of Cellular Therapy, Duke University School of Medicine, Durham, North Carolina

DON C. ROCKEY, MD Professor of Medicine, Gastroenterology Division, and Director, Duke Liver Center, Duke University School of Medicine, Durham, North Carolina

STANLEY G. ROCKSON, MD Chief of Consultative Cardiology and Director, Stanford Program for Atherosclerosis and Cardiovascular Therapies; Director, Stanford Center for Lymphatic and Venous Disorders, Falk Cardiovascular Research Center, Stanford University School of Medicine, Stanford, California

RUDOLPH A. RODRIGUEZ, MD Associate Professor of Clinical Medicine, Division of Nephrology, University of California, San Francisco School of Medicine; Director of Clinical Nephrology, San Francisco General Hospital, San Francisco, California

ANNETTE STRALOVICH-ROMANI, RD, CNSD Adult Critical Care Nutritionist, Department of Nutrition and Dietetics, UCSF Medical Center, San Francisco, California

NAOMI KENMOTSU ROUNDS, MD Clinical Cardiologist, South Shore Hospital, South Shore Cardiology, South Weymouth, Massachusetts

HAYA R. RUBIN, MD, PhD HMSA Chair, Healthcare Services and Quality Research, John A. Burns School of Medicine, University of Hawaii, Honolulu, Hawaii

LEWIS J. RUBIN, MD Professor, Department of Medicine and Director, Pulmonary Hypertension Program, University of California, San Diego School of Medicine, La Jolla, California

HOPE S. RUGO, MD Professor of Medicine, Division of Hematology-Oncology, University of California, San Francisco School of Medicine, San Francisco, California

KENNETH E. SACK, MD Professor of Clinical Medicine and Director, Clinical Program in Rheumatology, Department of Medicine, University of California, San Francisco School of Medicine, San Francisco, California

STEVEN A. SAHN, MD Professor of Medicine and Director, Division of Pulmonary and Critical Care Medicine, Medical University of South Carolina, Charleston, South Carolina

RICHARD H. SAVEL, MD Assistant Professor, Department of Medicine, Mt. Sinai School of Medicine, New York, New York; Associate Director, Surgical ICU, Division of Surgical Care, Department of Surgery, Maimonides Medical Center, Brooklyn, New York

MICHAEL SCHELD, MD Professor, Departments of Internal Medicine (Division of Infectious Diseases) and Neurosurgery, University of Virginia, Charlottesville, Virginia

MARC SHUMAN, MD Professor of Medicine, Division of Hematology-Oncology, University of California, San Francisco School of Medicine, San Francisco, California

HOLGER J. SCHÜNEMANN, MD, PhD Associate Professor of Medicine, Preventive Medicine and Clinical Epidemiology & Biostatistics, State University of New York at Buffalo, Buffalo, New York; Department of Clinical Epidemiology and Biostatistics, McMaster University, Hamilton, Ontario, Canada

NIRAJ L. SEHGAL, MD, MPH Assistant Professor, Department of Medicine, Hospitalist Group, University of California, San Francisco School of Medicine, San Francisco, California

KAVEH G. SHOJANIA, MD Assistant Professor, Department of Medicine, University of Ottawa; Attending Physician, Department of Medicine, The Ottawa Hospital-Civic Campus, Ottawa, Ontario, Canada

DANIEL I. SIMON, MD Associate Professor of Medicine, Harvard Medical School; Associate Director, Interventional Cardiology, Brigham & Women's Hospital, Boston, Massachusetts

ARTHUR S. SLUTSKY, MD Professor of Medicine, Surgery and Biomedical Engineering and Director, Interdepartmental Division of Critical Care Medicine, University of Toronto; Vice President (Research), St. Michael's Hospital, Toronto, Ontario, Canada

WADE S. SMITH, MD Associate Professor, Department of Neurology, University of California, San Francisco School of Medicine; Medical Director, Neurovascular Service, USCF Medical Center, San Francisco, California

BRENNAN M.R. SPIEGEL, MD, MSHS Assistant Professor, Department of Medicine, David Geffen School of Medicine at UCLA, Greater Los Angeles VA Healthcare System, Los Angeles, California

MATTHEW B. STANBROOK, MD, PhD Assistant Professor, Department of Medicine, University of Toronto; Staff Physician, Division of Respirology, Department of Medicine, Toronto Western Hospital, University Health Network, Toronto, Ontario, Canada

DEBORAH M. STEIN, MD Assistant Professor of Surgery, R. Adams Cowley Shock Trauma Center, University of Maryland Medical Center, Baltimore, Maryland

MARTIN H. STEINBERG, MD Professor of Medicine, Pediatrics, Pathology and Laboratory Medicine, Department of Medicine and Pediatrics, Boston University School of Medicine; Director, Center of Excellence in Sickle Cell Disease, Boston Medical Center, Boston, Massachusetts

DENNIS L. STEVENS, MD Professor of Medicine, University of Washington School of Medicine, Seattle, Washington; Chief, Infectious Disease Section, Department of Medicine, Veterans Affairs Medical Center, Boise, Idaho

JOHN H. STONE, MD, MPH Associate Professor, Department of Medicine, Johns Hopkins University School of Medicine; Director, The Johns Hopkins Vasculitis Center, Division of Rheumatology, Johns Hopkins Bayview Medical Center, Baltimore, Maryland

PAUL M. SULLAM, MD Associate Professor, Department of Medicine, University of California, San Francisco School of Medicine; Staff Physician, Infectious Disease, VA Medical Center, San Francisco, California

AYALEW TEFFERI, MD Professor of Hematology and Medicine, Division of Hematology and Internal Medicine, Mayo Clinic and Mayo Medical School, Rochester, Minnesota

JONATHAN P. TERDIMAN, MD Associate Professor, Department of Medicine, University of California, San Francisco School of Medicine, San Francisco, California

THOMAS TERNDRUP, MD Professor, Department of Emergency Medicine, University of Alabama at Birmingham; Chair, Department of Emergency Medicine, University Hospital, Birmingham, Alabama

JOSEF G. THUNDIYIL, MD Department of Medicine and Clinical Pharmacology, University of California, San Francisco and San Francisco General Hospital, San Francisco, California

MARK R. TONELLI, MD Associate Professor, Division of Pulmonary and Critical Care Medicine, University of Washington School of Medicine, Seattle, Washington

JOEL TSEVAT, MD Professor of Internal Medicine, Section of Outcomes Research, Division of General Internal Medicine, University of Cincinnati School of Medicine, Cincinnati, Ohio

ALLAN R. TUNKEL, MD, PhD Professor, Department of Medicine, Drexel University College of Medicine, Philadelphia, Pennsylvania

BERNARD VACCARO, MD Instructor in Psychiatry, Harvard Medical School; Associate Director, Medical Psychiatry, Brigham & Women's Hospital, Boston, Massachusetts

RANDALL H. VAGELOS, MD Associate Professor, Division of Cardiovascular Medicine and Medical Director, Cardiac Care Unit, Stanford University School of Medicine, Stanford, California

FLAVIO VINCENTI, MD Professor of Medicine, Division of Nephrology, University of California, San Francisco School of Medicine, San Francisco, California

ROBERT M. WACHTER, MD Professor and Associate Chairman, Department of Medicine, University of California, San Francisco School of Medicine; Chief, Medical Service, UCSF Medical Center, San Francisco, California

LEONARD WARTOFSKY, MD, MPH Professor of Medicine and Physiology, Uniformed Services University of Health Sciences; Chairman, Department of Medicine, Washington Hospital Center, Washington, DC

SCOTT WEINGARTEN, MD, MPH Professor of Medicine, UCLA School of Medicine; President and CEO, Zynx Health Incorporated, Los Angeles, California

HOWARD H. WEITZ, MD Professor of Medicine, Vice Chairman of Education, Department of Medicine, Jefferson Medical College; Co-director, Jefferson Heart Institute, Thomas Jefferson University Hospital, Philadelphia, Pennsylvania

CHAD WHELAN, MD Assistant Professor, Department of Medicine, University of Chicago School of Medicine, Chicago, Illinois

WINTHROP F. WHITCOMB, MD Assistant Professor of Medicine, University of Massachusetts Medical School; Director, Clinical Performance Improvement, Mercy Medical Center, Springfield, Massachusetts

WILLIAM B. WHITE, MD Professor, Department of Medicine, Pat and Jim Calhoun Cardiology Center; Chief and Medical Director, Division of Hypertension and Clinical Pharmacology, University of Connecticut Health Center, Farmington, Connecticut

MARK V. WILLIAMS, MD Professor and Director, Emory Hospital Medicine Unit; Associate Director, Division of General Medicine, Department of Medicine, Emory University School of Medicine, Atlanta, Georgia

NEIL WINAWER, MD Assistant Professor of Medicine, Emory University School of Medicine; Director, Hospital Medicine Unit, Department of Medicine, Grady Memorial Hospital, Atlanta, Georgia

LISA G. WINSTON, MD Assistant Clinical Professor, Department of Medicine, Division of Infectious Diseases, University of California, San Francisco School of Medicine; Hospital Epidemiologist, San Francisco General Hospital, San Francisco, California

KENNETH A. WOEBER, MD Harris M. Fishbon Professor of Clinical Medicine, Department of Medicine, University of California, San Francisco School of Medicine; Clinical Chief, Division of Endocrinology and Metabolism, Department of Medicine, USCF Medical Center at Parnassus and Mount Zion, San Francisco, California

THERESA L. WRIGHT, MD Professor, Department of Medicine, University of California, San Francisco School of Medicine; Chief, Gastroenterology Section, San Francisco VA Medical Center, San Francisco, California

PETER ZIMETBAUM, MD Assistant Professor of Medicine, Department of Medicine, Harvard Medical School; Assistant Professor of Medicine, Cardiology/Medicine, Beth Israel Deaconess Medical Center, Boston, Massachusetts

Preface to the Second Edition

It seems remarkable that a decade has passed since we first described our vision of a generalist physician specializing in hospital care: the *hospitalist* (1). Although a handful of such physicians were scattered around the United States at the time, by 2005 there were more than 10,000. Their ranks are likely to swell to more than 20,000 in the United States in the coming decade (2), and they have linked with similar physicians in Canada, South America, Europe, and even China.

Although we correctly predicted the growth of hospitalists, we (and most other observers) failed to appreciate fully the other winds that would buffet hospital care during the last 10 years. Even though capitation declined in popularity, the mandate for efficiency grew as hospitals filled to the brim, forcing many emergency departments into double duty as mini-wards. A major nursing shortage further constrained hospital capacity, while a shortage of critical care doctors generated a need in many institutions for other physicians who could provide high quality ICU care. And limits on residents' duty hours created the demand for alternative providers in teaching hospitals. All of these forces further promoted the growth of the hospitalist model (3,4).

Meanwhile, the pace of medical progress continued to accelerate. New noninvasive imaging studies and new blood tests, such as troponin, C-reactive protein, BNP, and galactomannan, reshaped our diagnostics strategies for disorders ranging from pulmonary embolism to *Aspergillus* infection. New medications, such as low-molecular-weight heparin and activated protein C, caused us to rethink our management of thrombosis and sepsis, and we also found new uses for old medications, such as spironolactone and N-acetylcysteine. Prevention, once considered the exclusive domain of ambulatory medicine and public health, emerged as a key paradigm in hospital medicine, as the virtues of prophylaxis against thromboembolism, tight glucose control, and strategies to prevent hospital-acquired infections were documented by a steady drumbeat of studies.

Even more striking was the emergence—finally!—of a genuine and sustainable quality movement in health care. Galvanized by two reports from the Institute of Medicine on patient safety (5) and quality (6), patients and payers increasingly demanded that their hospital care be demonstrably safe and effective. In fact, in preparing the second edition of *Hospital Medicine*, we were struck that as much as the clinical chapters had changed, the chapter that changed the most was the one on quality and value (Chapter 12). In the first edition (2000), we described an embryonic movement to measure quality and wondered whether it would ultimately impact inpatient care. At the time, there were only two inpatient quality measures (the use of aspirin and beta blockers in acute myocardial infarction) and only one organization doing the measuring (the National Committee for Quality Assurance). Pay-for-performance ("P4P") was a twinkle in some health economist's eye.

Five years later, scores of inpatient quality measures are being promulgated by organizations ranging from behemoths, such as the Center for Medicare and Medicaid Services (CMS) and the Joint Commission on the Accreditation of Healthcare Organizations (JCAHO), to groups that barely existed in 2000, such as the Leapfrog Group and the National Quality Forum. Not only is hospital care being measured and reported publicly, but early pay-for-performance experiments herald an era in which quality will be demanded, measured, and rewarded. The quality and safety movements are also catalyzing the "wiring" of the American hospital. Because processes of care and outcomes will now be measurable at the click of a button, information technology will increase the pressure on providers to deliver high quality, evidence-based care. Fortunately, the same technology will also facilitate the delivery of such care. Despite a number of tricky learning curves to traverse, it is difficult to view these sea changes as anything but welcome news for patients.

We approached the second edition of *Hospital Medicine* with all of this in mind. The entire book has been updated, and more than 10% of the chapters and 20% of the authors are brand new. More than ever, we emphasize a practical, evidence-based approach to the management of hospitalized patients. Even with all the changes, feedback from readers of the first edition persuaded us to retain the underlying organizing framework of the book: *approaching common hospital disorders and presentations from the perspective of the hospital physician*, with a particular emphasis on the temporal flow of care in the hospital (e.g., "Issues at the Time of Admission," "Issues at the Time of Discharge"). This approach remains unique to *Hospital Medicine*.

Although we expect that many of our readers will be hospitalists, the book remains agnostic regarding who the provider of hospital care is or should be. We were gratified that so many primary care physicians, nurse practitioners, physician's assistants, inpatient pharmacists, residents, and students found the first edition useful, and we prepared this new edition hoping that it would continue to appeal to this broad audience. Regardless of our readers' roles and pedigrees, we hope that *Hospital Medicine* helps them deliver the high quality, evidence-based care that their patients deserve and supports them in their roles as clinicians, teachers, and leaders in making their hospitals safer and better.

Robert M. Wachter, MD
Lee Goldman, MD
Harry Hollander, MD
University of California, San Francisco

REFERENCES

1. Wachter RM, Goldman L. The emerging role of "hospitalists" in the American health care system. *N Engl J Med* 1996;335:514–517.
2. Lurie JD, Miller DP, Lindenauer PK, et al. The potential size of the hospitalist workforce in the United States. *Am J Med* 1999;106:441–415.
3. Wachter RM, Goldman L. The hospitalist movement 5 years later. *JAMA* 2002;282:487–494.
4. Wachter RM. Hospitalists in the United States: mission accomplished or work-in-progress. *N Engl J Med* 2004;350:1935–1936.
5. Kohn L, Corrigan J, Donaldson M. *To Err Is Human: Building a Safer Health System.* Washington, DC: National Academy Press, 2000.
6. Committee on Quality of Health Care in America, Institute of Medicine. *Crossing the Quality Chasm: A New Health System for the 21st Century.* Washington, DC: National Academy Press, 2001.

Preface to the First Edition

As the American healthcare system lurched toward managed care at the close of the twentieth century, there surfaced a prevailing notion that the institution we know as the hospital was a vestige of the old system and was doomed, along with long-playing records and bell-bottom pants, to the wasteheap of history. In the New Medicine, went the mantra, pressures for efficiency would lead to a medley of home care, surgicenters, telemedicine, multispecialty practices, disease management, and mass prevention strategies, all of which would render the hospital an expensive and needless albatross. Those who watched trends in hospital utilization in the late 1980s and early 1990s, particularly in highly managed care markets, had ample evidence to support this scenario.

As the new century dawns, it is clear that this script was wrong. The aging of the population, the growth of new technologies, and the efficiency of having a site for diverse specialists who focus on the care of sick patients, have all led to an *increase* in hospital utilization. With this increase has come a growing recognition that the hospital continues to be the focus of one-third of U.S. health expenditures (accounting for 5% of America's Gross Domestic Product), of the majority of deaths and virtually all births, and of staggering technological innovation and perhaps equally staggering iatrogenesis. In other words, what happens in hospitals matters.

As we began to refocus on hospital care, we were struck by the absence of a clinical textbook that *used the hospital admission as the unit of analysis*. Our goal, therefore, was to produce an authoritative, evidence-based, and practical book that focuses on key issues in the care of the hospitalized adult. In doing so, we cover most of the major issues that arise in inpatients (e.g., end-of-life care, nutritional issues, clinical decision making) as well as 75 of the most common conditions leading to hospital admission. Some signs, symptoms, and laboratory abnormalities are critically important in hospitalized patients, but do not fit into a specific disease framework. We have included these three topics within introductory chapters that precede each of the organ-based specialty sections. Our goal is to be more useful than comprehensive: very unusual diseases or presentations may not be covered in depth, but common ones certainly are. Similarly, fundamental skills such as reading electrocardiograms are not addressed in detail, as we assume a basic level of clinical knowledge and such information can be found in many other sources.

We wrote this book for the physician caring for the hospitalized adult patient. Notwithstanding our interest in the hospitalist model, except for an introductory chapter on "Models of Hospital Care," the book makes no assumptions about who is the inpatient provider, nor judgments about who it should be. Thus, we hope that *Hospital Medicine* will serve the needs not only of practicing hospitalists, but also primary care physicians and specialists caring for inpatients, inpatient nurse practitioners and physician assistants, internal or family medicine residents, and junior or senior medical students on inpatient rotations. There is a strong emphasis on appropriate care and resource use, so *Hospital Medicine* will also be helpful to inpatient case managers and others involved in hospital quality improvement, utilization management, and discharge planning.

We thank our contributors for their superb work and for presenting their information in an evidence-based and practical way. We also are indebted to Mary Whitney, Leah Hayes, Carol Kummer, Amy Markowitz, and Steven Martin for their invaluable assistance in the production of the book. Susan Gay and Tim Hiscock of Lippincott Williams & Wilkins were extremely helpful at all stages of the project. So were our faculty and housestaff colleagues at the University of California, San Francisco, who often found themselves the subjects of impromptu focus groups as we grappled with difficult clinical or organizational questions. Finally, our deepest gratitude goes to our families, who had to tolerate our absences (and sometimes our presence) while we attempted to bring this concept to reality as quickly as possible. We hope that the information contained herein will improve the quality and efficiency of care for an extraordinarily important but vulnerable population, hospitalized adults.

Robert M. Wachter, MD
Lee Goldman, MD
Harry Hollander, MD
San Francisco, California
January, 2000

General Issues in Hospital Medicine

Models of Hospital Care

Robert M. Wachter

INTRODUCTION

The past decade has brought great changes in the organization of hospital care in the United States. Although "inpatient specialists" have long provided inpatient care in Europe and Canada, the United States has only recently considered the potential advantages of a system using dedicated hospital physicians, known as hospitalists. This new model for hospital care has both advantages and disadvantages in comparison with more traditional models of inpatient care.

In the decade since the editors first described the concept of the hospitalist in the medical literature (1), the growth of the model has been remarkable. In many U.S. markets, the majority of hospital care is now delivered by hospital-based physicians. The Society of Hospital Medicine, the professional society for hospitalists, has grown to more than 5,000 members, and published projections point to an ultimate hospitalist workforce of about 20,000, approximately the same size as that of cardiology (2). Although the notion of a site-defined (rather than an organ-, population-, or disease-defined) specialty seems novel, it is not: American medicine embraced the seeming oxymoron of the "generalist specialist" when it codified the specialties of emergency medicine and critical care medicine (Table 1.1) about 40 years ago. What is new, at least in the United States, is the approach of using a site-defined specialist on the main hospital ward.

DEFINITION OF HOSPITALIST

Hospitalists were initially defined as physicians who spend at least 25% of their professional time serving as the physicians of record for inpatients and accepting hand-offs of hospitalized patients from primary care providers; the patients are returned to the care of their primary providers at the time of hospital discharge (3). Although the Society of Hospital Medicine has embraced a more inclusive definition ("physicians whose primary professional focus is the general medical care of hospitalized patients"), focusing on the initial definition allows a discussion of two key elements of the transition from the old model of inpatient care (in which primary care physicians served as the hospital physicians of record) to the hospitalist model. The first is the hand-off—a purposeful discontinuity of care between the outpatient and hospital providers. The second is the notion that some minimum amount of hospital time is necessary for one to meet the spirit of the hospitalist concept.

The hand-off, or referral, is fundamental to the hospitalist model. In fact, the discontinuity is responsible for one of the real strengths of the hospitalist model—the presence of a physician in the hospital throughout the day who is able to coordinate inpatient care and react to clinical data in real time. However, this same discontinuity leads to the two greatest potential liabilities of the model. The first concerns a potential "voltage drop" in information as one moves from office to hospital ward and back to office. The second relates to the potential dissatisfaction of patients associated with the assignment of a new doctor—often a stranger—to care for them at their time of greatest need.

To some extent, the "voltage drop" can be minimized. Computerized or digitized information is easy to transmit from office to hospital and back to office again. This does not mean that this is currently being done in many systems, or that a linked office–hospital information system would entirely solve the problem. A filtering function is needed; otherwise, the vast amounts of computerized data will be simply ignored. Nevertheless, it seems reasonable to posit

TABLE 1.1

EXAMPLES OF SPECIALTIES, DIVIDED BY THEIR ORGANIZING PRINCIPLE

Defined by organ-system	Defined by patient population	Defined by disease	Defined by technical skill	Defined by site of care
Cardiology	Pediatrics	Oncology	Surgery	Hospital medicine
Gastroenterology	Geriatrics	Infectious	Anesthesiology	(Hospitalists)
Rheumatology	Family	diseases	Radiation oncology	Critical care medicine
	medicine			Emergency medicine

that most systems will find ways to successfully transmit computerized data from hospital to outpatient provider over the next decade (although few have done so as of this writing).

However, the hospitalist model is most vulnerable in terms of information that cannot be captured electronically—namely, the patient's life story, values, and preferences regarding end-of-life care. These "soft" data are probably best communicated through personal contact between the hospitalist and the primary physician, at least at the time of admission, discharge, and any important change in patient status. The bottom line is that the hospitalist and the primary physician must act as a team to care for the patient effectively across the continuum of care (Chapter 4).

The other major concern raised by the transfer of care to the hospitalist relates to the potential dissatisfaction of patients when they do not see "their doctor" in the hospital. This legitimate concern has generally been refuted by surveys showing that the level of patient satisfaction under a hospitalist's care is at least as high as that under the old primary physician-based system (4,5). These results indicate that patients may be willing to trade familiarity (of their primary doctor) for availability (of the hospitalist) when it comes to hospital care, particularly if they perceive a strong communication link between the two providers. Some health care systems have also noted that the hospitalist model leads to improvements in outpatients' satisfaction with their primary physicians, who can now be more predictably available to their office patients.

In addition to the purposeful discontinuity, implicit in the hospitalist concept is a minimum time requirement that the physician spends in caring for hospitalized patients. This time commitment has several advantages. First, it should allow the hospitalist to become expert in the care of common inpatient disorders. Next, it should lead to the hospitalist better recognizing outliers and anticipating problems. Third, the hospitalist will become familiar with all key players in the hospital (Chapter 4) and become sufficiently invested in the system to be accountable for its cost and quality. The hospitalist will thus be able to lead quality improvement efforts in this setting (Chapter 12).

STAGES OF HOSPITAL CARE

Four distinct stages of hospital care help explain many of the forces driving the emergence of the hospitalist model (3) (Table 1.2). In stage I, the *primary care provider stage*, all patients admitted to the hospital for nonspecialized medical problems that fall within the usual expertise of an internist (e.g., community-acquired pneumonia or gastrointestinal bleeding) are cared for in the hospital by their own primary care physician. Of course, some patients may be cared for by other physicians for specialized problems during any stage (e.g., an obstetrician during childbirth or a urologist during a prostatectomy). Stage I was the dominant mode of hospital care in the United States until 10 to 20 years ago. It continues to be popular, albeit in a rapidly dwindling number of regions. The system worked best when the primary physician had many patients in the hospital at any given time, when such patients were not terribly ill, when the hospital was next door to the physician's office, and when no one was measuring (or particularly concerned about) hospital or office availability or efficiency. However, the disadvantages of stage I have become evident, particularly in markets with significant cost pressures. In these areas, primary care physicians may have on average only one or two patients in the hospital at any given time, and these patients are likely to be extremely ill and require attention throughout the hospital day. In the meantime, the office is packed with patients to be seen at 15-minute intervals. Interestingly, although primary care physicians were ambivalent (at best) about the hospitalist concept in the early years, many have now recognized the economic inefficiency of providing their own hospital care because revenues from the care of their hospital patients now fail to compensate for the inefficiency of the commute and the disruption to their office practice. In some markets, such physicians have become major supporters of the hospitalist model.

Stage II, the *hospital rotation stage*, attempts to deal with the problem of physician inaccessibility in the hospital by rotating hospital coverage among the members of a medical group. In this model, one member at a time serves as the

TABLE 1.2
ADVANTAGES AND DISADVANTAGES OF VARIOUS MODELS OF HOSPITAL CARE

	Description	Potential advantages	Potential disadvantages
Stage I: Primary care provider stage	Every PCP follows own patients into the hospital.	Inpatient–outpatient continuity. Patient satisfaction from seeing "my doctor." PCPs retain acute care skills and possibly job satisfaction.	PCPs may lack hospital skills and experience to maximize quality and efficiency. PCPs not available throughout hospital day. Hospital care pulls PCPs away from office patients. PCPs unlikely to be accountable for and invested in hospital quality improvement.
Stage II: Hospital rotation stage	Physicians in the group rotate so that members take turns covering the hospitalized patients of the other members.	"Hospital PCP" now available throughout hospital day. Other PCPs freed to be in office all day. Patients may know rotating hospital physician from the office (who may even be the patients' PCP from time to time).	Introduction of an inpatient–outpatient discontinuity. With infrequent rotation intervals (e.g.,1 week in 8), PCPs are still unlikely to develop acute care skills to produce the best outcomes at the lowest cost, or to be invested in improving the hospital system.
Stage III: Voluntary hospitalist stage	Dedicated hospitalists are hired; PCPs may choose to use them or not (there may be incentives to use the hospitalist).	Hospitalist now available throughout hospital day to review results and see patient, family, consultants. Hospitalist hones acute care skills (including communication with PCPs). Hospitalist accountable for hospital quality and cost and is invested in leading improvement.	With outpatient–inpatient discontinuity, potential for information loss. Potential patient dissatisfaction from not seeing "my doctor" in the hospital. Potential PCP loss of acute care skills. Potential hospitalist burnout over time.
Stage IV: Mandatory hospitalist stage	All patients must be handed off by their PCPs to hospitalists for inpatient care.	Same advantages as in moving from stage II to III, except true for all patients. System may now focus on mitigating potential disadvantages by the following: Developing better communication links (both personal and infrastructural). Promoting social visits or calls by PCPs, and other methods to enhance patient satisfaction. Developing CME or other mechanisms to prevent PCPs from losing acute care skills. Developing mechanisms (CME, some outpatient or nonhospitalist work, adequate reimbursement, vacation) to prevent hospitalist burnout.	Same disadvantages as in moving from stage II to III, except true for all patients and providers. Potential decreased incentive for hospitalists to be superb communicators with PCPs (under stage III, PCPs could choose to manage their own inpatients if not completely satisfied with the hospitalist). Potential problems if system has been adopted without buy-in by medical staff. PCP endorsement of both the system and the hospitalists themselves is vital.

CME, continuing medical education; PCP, primary care physician.
Reprinted from Wachter RM. An introduction to the hospitalist model. *Ann Intern Med* 1999;130:338–342, with permission.

physician of record for the inpatients of the others. In many private practice settings, these rotations typically occur at a frequency of about one week per eight-week period (during which time the hospital primary physician—these days, often incorrectly called the "hospitalist of the week"—may be sta-

tioned in the hospital for all or a large part of the day). In the academic setting, it is common for such rotations to take place at a frequency of one month per every 12-month period (the "ward attending" month). In either case, the rotating primary care physician is not in the hospital enough to be a true hospitalist. In comparison with the stage I system, this system has the disadvantage of introducing a new inpatient–outpatient discontinuity, but it does ensure better availability of the rotating physician for inpatients (Table 1.2).

In stage III, the *voluntary hospitalist stage*, a dedicated hospitalist is hired (paid by either the hospital, a medical group, a managed care organization, or a free-standing private practice), but primary physicians retain the option to manage all or some of their own inpatients. The decision by some physicians to continue to manage their hospitalized patients may be influenced by financial incentives. For example, a fee-for-service system may influence primary care physicians to continue to provide hospital care, whereas a capitated system, in which physicians are paid solely based on panel size, may encourage the use of the hospitalist.

Finally, a few systems have moved to stage IV, the *mandatory hospitalist stage*, in which all inpatients must be handed off to hospitalists. Although the advantages of the hospitalist model are now applied to all patients (Table 1.2), political costs may be incurred in moving to this stage. The mandatory hand-off alienates some primary care physicians who want to retain the option to provide hospital care. For this reason, stage IV is most common in systems that have strong institutional control of physician practices, whereas stage III is more prevalent in looser physician–hospital affiliations, such as those in many independent practice associations.

It is important to add a few caveats regarding the four stages. First, the stages *do not* imply a hierarchy of desirability (i.e., that stage IV is necessarily better stage III, which is always better than stage II). Each stage has advantages and disadvantages, and many physicians and health systems will find that a stage III (or II) system serves their needs well. Second, movement up the stages is not inexorable; not all systems ultimately arrive at stage IV, although there is a clear national trend in moving from stage I or II to stage III or IV. Nor will progression necessarily be orderly; some systems, especially those under significant market pressure, have jumped directly from stage I to stage IV.

EVIDENCE REGARDING THE HOSPITALIST MODEL

Early transitions to the hospitalist model were largely driven by the theoretical attractiveness of the concept rather than any specific data addressing the potential advantages and disadvantages. Over the past decade, though, a significant amount of literature has emerged regarding the impact of the hospitalist model on costs and outcomes.

Efficiency

More than 20 studies have compared hospitalist care to that delivered by primary care physicians or traditional academic ward attendings. With few exceptions, the studies have found significant decreases in both length of stay and hospital costs, averaging nearly 15% (5,6). Although concerns have been raised that some of these cost savings are simply transferred to the outpatient setting (7) or consumed by the costs of operating the hospitalist program itself, the magnitude of the savings and the rapid growth of the model nationally (often driven by return-on-investment considerations) argue against this hypothesis. Precisely how hospitalists achieve their efficiencies is not entirely clear. It is probably some combination of anticipating patients' trajectories, better and more rapid deployment of hospital resources, and greater focus on efficiency as an important goal. Some studies have found a learning curve, with hospitalists achieving their ultimate efficiencies only in their second year of practice (8).

Quality

Although it is logical to believe that hospitalists improve the quality of inpatient care (mediated through both "practice makes perfect" and their on-site availability), most studies have found no effect on blunt measures of quality (such as readmissions and mortality rates). Two studies, however, have found significant decreases in inpatient mortality rates associated with hospitalist care (8,9). Another study found lower readmission rates (10), and a fourth found better documentation of end-of-life discussions (11). These studies are promising, but additional research is needed to unequivocally prove a hospitalist quality advantage if, in fact, one exists.

Teaching

Hospitalist programs are now operating in most of the nation's teaching hospitals, driven in part by limitations in resident work-hours implemented in 2003 by the Accreditation Council on Graduate Education. Several studies have compared hospitalist teaching evaluations with those of comparable non-hospitalist ward attendings, and all have found significant advantages for the hospitalists (12–15). Given that many residents were anxious about their potential loss of autonomy under the hospitalist model, these results are reassuring. They support both the hospitalist model itself and the more general premise that additional teaching and oversight should improve, and not harm, medical education (Chapter 11).

ROLES OF THE HOSPITALIST

Under stages III and IV, the hospitalist may begin by caring for some (stage III) or all (stage IV) of the inpatients on a medical service. Additional roles for hospitalists may soon surface (16), depending on the nature of the medical group, the dominant reimbursement methods, and the competitiveness of the market (Table 1.3).

In some settings, the hospitalist will serve as a passive accepter of inpatient admissions from primary care physicians or the emergency department. Such a passive role avoids conflict about the decision to hospitalize and may serve an institution well when most patients are admitted under a payment system utilizing diagnosis-related groups (DRGs). (The main financial incentive of a DRG is to shorten the length of stay rather than decrease the number of hospitalizations.) Under a capitated system or in a hospital operating at full capacity, however, hospitalists may feel pressure to become involved in the *admission decision*, approving outpatients for admission and even evaluating patients in the emergency department and suggesting possible alternatives to acute hospital admission.

Similarly, in an environment in which the system is at risk for the costs of *out-of-network care*, hospitalists may be involved in efforts to transfer such patients back to their home hospitals. These efforts may involve speaking by telephone with the patient's physician at the outlying site, confirming appropriateness of and stability for transport, and organizing the logistics of the transfer. Even in the absence of such managed care-driven arrangements, hospitalists are often engaged in managing interinstitutional transfers, a challenging area that saw little physician involvement in the past.

The interface between the hospital ward and the *intensive care unit* is interesting to consider in light of the hospitalist model. A number of studies have demonstrated the advantages of a closed intensive care unit (in which dedicated critical care specialists are utilized, with patients handed off from the primary physician to the critical care physician at the time of intensive care unit admission), instead of an open unit in terms of outcomes and efficiency (17). The average primary physician's lack of availability and experience in caring for critically ill patients is another example of the advantages of the discontinuity between the hospital ward and the intensive care unit (with separate critical care providers staffing the latter). Under a hospitalist system, the need for this discontinuity may be offset because a competent and busy hospitalist will have a large intensive care unit volume, be available throughout the hospital day, and understand the critical care system well enough to manage it correctly. As a result, the imposition of an outpatient–hospital discontinuity may render a hospital–intensive care unit discontinuity less important and even counterproductive (Figure 1.1). The presence of critical care specialists will remain important, even when hospitalists are admitting to an open unit, when such specialists manage ventilators, perform procedures, and act as consultants on other critical care issues. Nevertheless, the large national shortage of intensive care specialists (18) means that hospitalists will be called upon to perform these complex functions in many institutions. The UCSF Medical Center has a hybrid model, in which hospitalists serve as physicians-of-record for ICU patients but all such patients automatically receive a consultation from an intensive care specialist. The intensivist has the primary role in managing the ventilator and sedation. The model appears to work well but is, as yet, unstudied.

In some institutions, hospitalists are beginning to serve as the *physicians-of-record for surgical patients*. Just as the hospitalists' availability throughout the day enables the primary care physician to manage patients in the office without interruption and provides each patient with a coordinator of hospital care, the hospitalist's involvement in the care of surgical patients during the preoperative and postoperative phases enables the surgeon to be in the operating room all day while ensuring that the floor patient is receiving appropriate care. Only one study has examined the outcomes associated with hospitalist comanagement of surgical patients; it found a modest advantage (19). Clearly, further studies are needed.

Many hospitalists will also choose to have a major role in *hospital quality improvement*, including the development of pathways, guidelines, and reengineering projects (Chapter 12). Hospitalists have already made impressive contributions in patient safety and end-of-life care, areas that clearly benefit from their systems focus, comfort with interdisciplinary collaboration, and alignment with hospital goals. In the same vein, many hospitalists will naturally evolve toward leadership roles in areas related to hospital operation, including the development of hospital policies and procedures, formulary and utilization management, and credentialing.

TABLE 1.3

POTENTIAL ROLES FOR HOSPITAL-BASED PHYSICIANS

Core activities

- Care of medical inpatients
- Traditional medical consultation

Potential additional activities

- Involvement in emergency department triage
- Facilitating transfer of patients from/to other facilities
- Management or comanagement of patients in the intensive care unit[a]
- Management or comanagement of nonmedical patients in the hospital[a]
- Development of palliative care unit and/or consultation service[a]
- Management or comanagement of patients in skilled nursing facilities, hospice, other settings[a]
- Major role in hospital-based quality improvement, patient safety activities[a]
- Major teaching role (in teaching hospitals)[a]
- Research into relevant topics (common inpatient clinical disorders, outcomes, costs, quality, safety, etc.)[a]
- Hospital administration[a]

[a] Hospitalist may benefit from additional training.

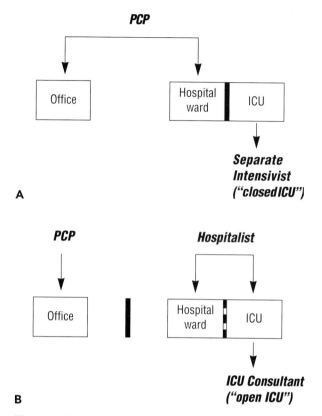

Figure 1.1 Potential impact of a hospitalist on the relative merits of a closed versus an open intensive care unit (*ICU*). **A.** In stage I, the potential lack of ICU expertise and a certain lack of availability of the primary care physician (*PCP*) create advantages for a hospital ward–ICU discontinuity ("closed ICU"). **B.** In stage III or IV, the presence of a hospitalist (and outpatient–hospital discontinuity) may obviate the need for hospital–ICU discontinuity ("open ICU"). Even in this circumstance, an ICU consultant will often considerably enhance patient care.

CONCLUSIONS

The emergence of the hospital model of care has been characterized by rapid growth and accompanied by a reassuring amount of data supporting the premise that hospitalists improve the value (quality divided by cost) of inpatient care. Nevertheless, for the foreseeable future, American hospital care will remain a highly pluralistic system in which the organization of care is determined by quality and cost considerations in the context of local culture and preferences. The method of hospital care chosen by each institution and group of physicians should be the one that promotes the best clinical outcomes and highest patient satisfaction at the lowest costs for both hospitalized and ambulatory patients.

KEY POINTS

- Hospitalists are physicians who accept hand-offs of inpatients from primary care physicians, returning the patients to the primary providers upon hospital discharge.

- Hospital care can be separated into four distinct stages: stage I (primary care providers provide hospital care), stage II (primary care providers rotate responsibility for hospital care), stage III (voluntary hand-offs to hospitalists), and stage IV (mandatory hand-offs to hospitalists).

- Potential advantages of the hospitalist model include increased availability, increased hospital expertise, and increased commitment to hospital quality improvement.

- Published data support the premise that the use of hospitalists leads to lower costs, shorter stays, at least equivalent (and possibly improved) outcomes, and higher teaching evaluations.

- Potential disadvantages of the hospitalist model include an information "voltage drop" when patients move in and out of the hospital, and patient dissatisfaction. The former can be minimized through better personal and computerized communications, and the latter seems not to be a major problem based on emerging data.

REFERENCES

1. Wachter RM, Goldman L. The emerging role of "hospitalists" in the American health care system. *N Engl J Med* 1996;335:514–517.
2. Lurie JD, Miller DP, Lindenauer PK, Wachter RM, Sox HC. The potential size of the hospitalist workforce in the United States. *Am J Med* 1999;106:441–445.
3. Wachter RM. Hospitalists: their role in the American health care system. *Medical Practice Management* November/December 1997:123–126.
4. Wachter RM, Katz P, Showstack J, Bindman AB, Goldman L. Reorganizing an academic medical service: impact on cost, quality, patient satisfaction, and education. *JAMA* 1998;279:1560–1565.
5. Wachter RM, Goldman L. The hospitalist movement 5 years later. *JAMA* 2002;287:487–494.
6. Kaboli PJ, Barnett MJ, Rosenthal GE. Associations with reduced length of stay and costs on an academic hospitalist service. *Am J Managed Care* 2004;10:561–568.
7. Wachter RM. Hospitalists in the United States—mission accomplished or work in progress. *N Engl J Med* 2004;350:1935–1936.
8. Meltzer D, Manning WG, Morrison J, et al. Effects of physician experience on costs and outcomes on an academic general medicine service: results of a trial of hospitalists. *Ann Intern Med* 2002;137:866–874.
9. Auerbach AD, Wachter RM, Katz P, Showstack J, Baron RB, Goldman L. Implementation of a voluntary hospitalist service at a community teaching hospital: improved clinical efficiency and patient outcomes. *Ann Intern Med* 2002;137:859–865.
10. Diamond HS, Goldberg E, Janosky JE. The effect of full-time faculty hospitalists on the efficiency of care at a community teaching hospital. *Ann Intern Med* 1998;129:197–203.
11. Auerbach AD, Pantilat SZ. End-of-life care in a voluntary hospitalist model: effects on communication, processes of care, and patient symptoms. *Am J Med* 2004;116:669–675.
12. Kulaga ME, Charney P, O'Mahony SP, et al. The positive impact of initiation of hospitalist clinician educators. *J Gen Intern Med* 2004;19:293–301.
13. Kripalani S, Pope AC, Rask K, et al. Hospitalists as teachers. *J Gen Intern Med* 2004;19:8–15.
14. Hauer KE, Auerbach AD, McCulloch CM, Woo G, Wachter RM. Effects of hospitalist attendings on trainee satisfaction with attending teaching and internal medicine rotations. *Arch Intern Med* 2004;164:1866–1871.
15. Hunter AJ, Desai SS, Harrison RA, Chan BK. Medical student evaluation of the quality of hospitalist and nonhospitalist teaching faculty on inpatient medicine rotations. *Acad Med* 2004;79:78–82.
16. Lindenauer PK, Pantilat SZ, Katz PP, Wachter RM. Hospitalists and the practice of inpatient medicine. Results of a survey of the

National Association of Inpatient Physicians. *Ann Intern Med* 1999;130:343–349.

17. Pronovost PJ, Angus DC, Dorman T, Robinson KA, Dremsizov TT, Young TL. Physician staffing patterns and clinical outcomes in critically ill patients: a systematic review. *JAMA* 2002;288: 2151–2162.

18. Angus DC, Kelley MA, Schmitz RJ, White A, Popovich J Jr; Committee on Manpower for Pulmonary and Critical Care Societies (COMPACCS). Caring for the critically ill patient. Current and projected workforce requirements for care of the critically ill and patients with pulmonary disease: can we meet the requirements of an aging population? *JAMA* 2000;284:2762–2770.

19. Huddleston JM, Long KH, Naessens JM, et al. Medical and surgical comanagement after elective hip and knee arthroplasty: a randomized controlled trial. *Ann Intern Med* 2004;141:28–38.

ADDITIONAL READING

Auerbach AD, Aronson MD, Davis RB, Phillips RS. How physicians perceive hospitalist services after implementation: anticipation vs. reality. *Arch Intern Med* 2003;163:2330–2336.

Saint S, Flanders SA. Hospitalists in teaching hospitals: opportunities but not without danger. *J Gen Intern Med* 2004;19:382–383.

Wachter RM, Goldmann DR, eds. The hospitalist movement in the United States. *Ann Intern Med* 1999;130, Number 4, Part 2.

Wachter RM, Goldman L. Implications of the hospitalist movement for academic departments of medicine: lessons from the UCSF experience. *Am J Med* 1999;106:127–133.

Wachter RM. The evolution of the hospitalist model in the United States. *Med Clin North Am* 2002;86:687–706.

The Economics of Hospital Medicine

2

David Meltzer   Chad Whelan

INTRODUCTION

Hospital care is expensive and is influenced by complex institutional structures and incentives. In 2003, the United States spent over 14% of gross domestic product—$1.6 trillion—on health care (1). Of that, 32%, or $512 billion, went to hospitals. Moreover, a sizeable fraction of the 22% of total spending on physicians went for hospital care. Given these large expenditures, the federal government and other major payers have enacted policies designed to control hospital expenditures. These policies often create incentives that may lead to conflicts of interest between payers, hospitals, physicians, and patients. Hospital physicians must understand the nature of these incentives and the potential for these conflicting interests in order to be most effective as agents for both their patients and the hospitals in which they work.

The fact that the United States medical economy is complicated and differs in important ways from the traditional market model (2) makes attempts to understand the effects of cost-control policies more difficult. Differences from the traditional model include the multiple organizational forms hospitals take (for-profit, not-for-profit, government-funded), multiple payers and payment systems (direct consumer payment, fee-for-service private insurance, capitated insurance, government insurance), pervasive state and federal regulations, and the complex interactions among these factors (e.g., cost for payers versus health for patients).

HOSPITAL ORGANIZATION AND HOSPITAL–PHYSICIAN RELATIONS

Hospitals are of three major types: not-for-profit, for-profit, and government-funded. All these systems have key components that drive their organizational behavior and influence the behavior of those who regularly interact with the hospital, including physicians. Many of the key stakeholders in each system are similar. They include the hospital leaders, physicians, hospital employees (sometimes including physicians), patients, and payers. Each stakeholder may have different goals—some may hope to increase revenue, and others may hope to decrease costs. These organizational frameworks may differ in how they value the needs and priorities of various stakeholders.

Not-for-profit hospitals are the most common type in the United States. They earn their name because of the requirement that they not distribute profits to shareholders, as would typically happen in a for-profit firm. Although not-for-profit hospitals usually receive the vast majority of their revenue from patient care, they may also receive donations or service in kind from an affiliated organization (e.g., a church) and government subsidies through exemption from corporate taxes. In exchange for subsidies, they must regularly demonstrate evidence of community benefit, such as providing uncompensated care or other programs that benefit the health of the community.

Even not-for-profit hospitals usually aim to have revenues that exceed costs. When they are successful, the excess income is reinvested in the hospital in the form of savings, capital investment, higher payments to physicians and/or employees, or greater spending on uncompensated care, research, or other aspects of the hospital's mission. Physicians may be employees, yet they are generally paid independently (through professional fees) and face different incentives from those of the hospital administration (3). In the not-for-profit system, the hospital administration's goals include increasing revenue, decreasing costs, improving quality of care, having high employee satisfaction, and enhancing the reputation of the hospital. Physicians and other employees may share many of these goals but place different weight on them. For example, hospital administrators may want lower costs, and hospital employees may want higher earnings. Similarly, physicians may want the newest facilities and excess hospital capacity if it benefits them or their patients because the hospital bears the cost of those expenditures. In contrast, hospital administrators may want as little excess capacity as possible.

Because physicians are critical to determining where a patient will be hospitalized and can choose to affiliate themselves with many hospitals, hospitals often compete for physicians. Thus, the relative bargaining power of physicians and hospitals in the not-for-profit setting may have important effects on how care is provided. This bargaining may produce incentives that make care more expensive if hospitals overinvest in infrastructure in an attempt to attract physicians. Efficiency of care may also be impaired by the internal structure of the hospital, which usually includes relatively independent management of services such as nursing, pharmacy, and information services. In the absence of strong central leadership or a culture of cooperation, this can result in a "silo mentality" that complicates efforts for cooperation among these services (Chapter 4).

In *for-profit hospitals*, profits can be returned directly to the stockholders. In theory, this may improve efficiency because stockholders will be less willing to tolerate lost profits than managers will be in a not-for-profit hospital. In practice, however, greater efficiency in for-profit hospitals has not been widely demonstrated (4). There are several reasons for this. Even though profits become an important goal, for-profit hospitals must still compete with not-for-profit hospitals for patients, payers, physicians, and employees. Therefore, they must also respond to the interests of these stakeholders, which leads them to resemble not-for-profit hospitals more than would otherwise be expected. For-profit hospitals are more likely to employ physicians as salaried employees, and so they may have greater power to align physicians' incentives to promote the efficient use of hospital resources, either through exerting influence on individual practice patterns or by increasing the efficiency of hospital infrastructure. However, not-for-profit hospitals are also recognizing that systems and systems improvement are important in optimizing the cost and quality of care. They are also realizing, along with for-profit hospitals, that compensating physicians for these roles and practice patterns can be a critical investment.

Hospitals may also be owned by *federal, state, or local governments*. These hospitals generally receive direct budgetary support that enables them to provide care to patients who would not be covered in other hospitals (such as veterans in the case of VA hospitals or uninsured persons in the case of public hospitals). As a result, these hospitals may not compete as directly with other types of hospitals for patients or payers. Nevertheless, government-owned hospitals may also care for patients with private or other government insurance (such as Medicare), which subjects them to competitive pressures to some degree. Like for-profit hospitals,

government hospitals generally employ physicians as salaried employees. This often gives administrators greater ability (in principle) to direct physician activities, whether with respect to clinical practice or investment in hospital infrastructure. Whether these administrators effectively exercise this ability may be determined by the incentives the administrators face in the organization and the discretion they are given in allocating resources. The size and complexity of bureaucracies in government-funded hospitals may markedly influence the impact of administrators on hospital physicians' activities.

HOSPITAL REIMBURSEMENT

Reimbursement for care in hospitals other than government-owned hospitals has historically been based on a fee-for-service model, in which hospitals bill payers (whether an insurer or the patient) based on the services provided. Except in government-funded and HMO-owned hospitals (where physicians are on salary), physicians generally bill separately, reflecting the historical dominance of the not-for-profit model of care in the United States, with its associated separation of hospital and physician interests. These payment systems are examples of *retrospective reimbursement systems*, which pay based on either the precise services provided or on a proxy for resource use, such as length of stay. Because these systems pay more to hospitals and doctors when resource use is greater, they can provide incentives for greater resource use.

Prospective reimbursement systems contrast with retrospective systems by paying a fixed amount for some episode of care regardless of the amount of care provided. The best example of a pure prospective payment system is a capitated health care system, such as a health maintenance organization, in which a fixed payment is made to provide care for an individual for a given period of time, usually via a monthly or annual premium. In hospital care, prospective payment systems more commonly involve a fixed payment for a single hospitalization for a given cause. Among these systems, the most important is the Medicare prospective payment system, which pays hospitals a fixed amount per episode of hospital care for a specific illness. The diagnosis-related group (DRG) of the patient's primary diagnosis in large part determines the level of compensation. For example, DRG 89 is community-acquired pneumonia.

Hospital reimbursement systems can have important implications for the cost, quality, and organization of care. For example, after the institution of Medicare's prospective payment system, hospital lengths of stay decreased because additional days of hospital care did not yield additional revenue for hospitals. Evidence is reasonably clear that patients were discharged "quicker and sicker," but there is less evidence that outcomes were adversely affected, although some studies suggest small effects on short-term mortality (5,6). Other studies suggest that prospective payment systems may have the largest adverse effects on the sickest patients because these are the least profitable patients under such systems (7). For this reason, it is important that prospective payment systems have reimbursement categories narrow enough to ensure adequate incentives for patients with all diagnoses to receive care. More generally, the concern that prospective payment systems may provide incentives to reduce care makes the ability to measure quality of care especially important in these systems (Chapter 12).

Payment systems also have implications for the organization of care. For example, when hospitals are prospectively paid, the increased incentives for early discharge tend to result in an increase in the use of skilled nursing facilities after discharge (Chapter 4). Likewise, there may be incentives to postpone non-urgent tests, such as endoscopy in patients with stable GI bleeding, until after discharge. Decisions such as these may pit the interests of patients against those of hospitals (Chapter 17). Such conflicts often reflect fundamental tensions that arise because of the need to control health care costs, but they can clearly be exaggerated in systems that do not create incentives to ensure quality while controlling costs. Medical ethics, the threat of malpractice litigation, and circumspect hospital administration can all limit the influence of the lack of cost and quality incentives, but awareness of cost issues is critical to ensuring that they do not harm the quality of care. Integrated health systems, such as HMOs or the VA system, seem to be less likely to suffer from suboptimal incentives, in part because they have strong incentives to focus on integrating services across transitions of care.

Competition among hospitals has the potential to modify many of these relationships among the system of hospital reimbursement and the cost and quality of care. For example, when hospital care is retrospectively reimbursed, having a greater number of hospitals in an area can result in greater competition among hospitals for doctors. This, in turn, can cause hospitals to overinvest in infrastructure, increasing costs in what is sometimes called a "medical arms race" (8). In contrast, greater competition among hospitals under prospective payment generally decreases costs by driving inefficient practices out of the market. Competition under prospective payment may also have a less desirable outcome because it can make it more difficult to cross-subsidize the care of costly patients with payments for the care of less costly patients in the same categories (9). This can happen because hospitals have increased incentives for devoting resources to selectively attracting the healthiest (and most profitable) patients within a diagnostic category. For example, a hospital may decide it is more profitable to redecorate the lobby of the hospital than to modernize the ICU.

HOSPITAL ECONOMICS IN PRACTICE

Because hospitalists can assume important management positions within their hospitals, they are often asked to help their institutions address economic concerns. Such concerns are usually most acute when a hospital's prof-

itability is jeopardized. However, because profits can always be used to meet institutional goals, the pressure to increase profits is ubiquitous. Because profit is defined as revenue minus cost, the essential components of improving profits are increasing revenues and decreasing costs.

Increasing Revenues

Hospital revenues come from patient care, direct government payments (e.g., to VA hospitals), donations, or research support. For all hospitals other than government-owned hospitals, most revenue comes from patient care. Revenue is, therefore, determined primarily by the price and quantity of care provided.

A hospital may receive different prices for the same service from different payers—including sometimes no reimbursement when it is unable to collect on a bill that it issues to a patient or insurer. Therefore, the *payer mix* can have a major effect on revenue. Sixty percent of hospital care is paid for through public funds, mostly through Medicare and Medicaid. Reimbursement rates often vary by hospital, across clinical services, and over time, but public payers tend to reimburse at lower levels than private fee-for-service insurance, with Medicaid paying less than Medicare. The private funding sources are patient self-payment and private insurance. Self-payment is steadily decreasing; it now accounts for less than 20% of all health care costs, down from almost 35% in 1980. Private insurance reimbursement may be fee-for-service or capitated.

Hospitals generally try to develop the best payer mix to maximize revenue. Although simply accepting only the highest-paying private insurance would provide the best payment for a given service, the hospital must also attract enough patients to keep sufficiently busy to cover the costs of running the facility ("covering its fixed costs"). The optimal payer mix for a hospital reflects the available payers, the local environment, the size of the hospital, and more. All these factors must be taken into account when the hospital negotiates contracts.

Billing and collections can significantly affect revenues and are remarkably complex. Rules for billing are highly regulated and increasingly strictly enforced. It is important for a health care organization to bill efficiently and accurately, as this is its major source of funding. Investment in infrastructure to maximize appropriate billing may significantly improve revenues (e.g., assuring that visits that should be reimbursed at a higher level, such as "Pneumonia, pseudomonas" are billed at that level as opposed to being billed at the lower level of, for example, "Pneumonia, not otherwise specified, or NOS").

The quantity of care provided is the other major determinant of revenue. Hospitals influence this by attracting patients, physicians, and payers and by making services available to them when they need them. Quality of care, both actual and perceived, the availability of specialized services, convenience, and amenities such as decor may all be important in attracting patients (Chapters 12 and 14).

Physicians may guide their patients to hospitals based on these same factors but have additional interests relating to their own personal convenience—ranging from the responsiveness of the nursing staff and the availability of clinical services such as radiology to the transit time from their office and the convenience of parking. Hospitals can also increase revenue by adding new resources, such as building a new hospital or more heavily using existing resources. Maintaining a high hospital occupancy rate (e.g., greater than 90%) is the most important factor in assuring high use of existing resources.

Decreasing Costs

The other component of the profit equation is costs. Costs can be conceptualized in several ways, but one of the most important distinctions is between variable and fixed costs. *Variable cost* is the incremental expenditure associated with providing a service, especially in the short run, when basic infrastructure or overall staffing levels are fixed. For example, the variable costs for administering a medication would include the cost of the IV tubing, solution, medication, and gloves worn by the nurse when administering the medication. *Fixed costs* are the remaining portion of the hospital's expenditures after variable costs are removed. These fixed costs are then attributed by an accounting system to the different activities in which the hospital engages. For example, the cost of staffing the pharmacy would be distributed among the number of medication doses provided. Because the vast majority of hospital costs are fixed (more than 80% in some studies (10)), understanding how a cost-saving intervention will affect fixed costs is essential. Assigning costs to a specific activity is often difficult in practice, so hospitals sometimes describe costs in terms of "direct" and "indirect" costs. Direct costs are costs that can be directly identified as being associated with an intervention, for example, the cost of the IV tubing, solution, and medication in the instance noted above. Indirect costs are those costs not identifiable but nevertheless associated with an intervention, for example, the nurse's gloves in the example above (because there is no mechanism to identify that the gloves were used for that particular purpose).

Of particular importance is that fixed costs may become variable costs over a period of time. For example, if more medications are ordered, it may be necessary to hire additional pharmacists. As a result, it can be very difficult to determine the true incremental cost associated with a treatment, and an intervention that reduces costs in one setting may not in another. For example, an intervention that saves pharmacists time may not reduce costs unless pharmacist staffing can be reduced. This may not be possible in a small hospital that has only one person working at a time but might be more likely in a larger hospital that can reduce staffing in proportion to the decrease in workload.

This last example illustrates *economies of scale*, which occur when the cost of producing an output falls as the quantity of outputs provided rises. The most common reason for economies of scale in hospitals is the large component of fixed costs. For example, the fixed-cost component of an MRI scanner that costs $3 million per year to operate while providing 3,000 scans per year is $1,000 per scan. In a smaller hospital in which only 1,000 scans per year are done, the fixed cost would be $3,000 per scan. Even large hospitals often cannot fully exploit economies of scale, providing a major incentive for hospital growth, consolidation, and specialization. Economies of scale can also occur when a larger organization gains experience in providing a given service and that experience results in better outcomes or lower costs (11). Diseconomies of scale can occur as well, as when a hospital becomes too large to manage effectively. Managing such economies of scale is a key part of good hospital leadership. In the earlier pharmacist example, a good manager might recognize that increasing the efficiency of the pharmacist could allow the hospital to implement a more intensive program reviewing medication appropriateness. This manager might also recognize that improving pharmacists' workflow may improve their satisfaction and make it easier to retain excellent pharmacists at more moderate salaries.

Length of Stay

In practice, reducing length of stay (LOS) is often the most significant way in which hospitalists can reduce costs (12,13). The business case for LOS reduction depends on its effects on both revenues and costs, with complex interaction between issues such as reimbursement system and hospital occupancy. For example, under prospective payment, reducing length of stay enables the hospital to obtain added revenue by admitting more patients using the same fixed resources. However, under retrospective per-diem reimbursement, shorter lengths of stay may not translate directly into either added revenue or improved profits. A good example of this is the incentive to discharge patients to a skilled nursing facility at the end of a hospitalization. Under prospective reimbursement, this clearly reduces hospital costs and allows additional revenue to be generated. Under per-diem reimbursement, patients who can be discharged to a skilled nursing facility may be far less expensive to care for than the average hospital patient, making it profitable to keep them in the hospital.

CONCLUSIONS

Hospital economics are influenced by the organizational form of the hospital, the relationship between hospitals and physicians, and complex interactions between reimbursement systems and market competition. In practice, these forces interact with local phenomena relating to reimbursement mechanism, payer mix, and cost structure to determine how changes in hospital operations affect profits through both revenues and costs. Hospitalists (and others) can be most effective when they understand the components of the equation and how to effectively operate within the system.

KEY POINTS

■ Hospital care is expensive and is often reimbursed by prospective payment systems that may create incentives to limit care.

■ Hospitals have different organizational forms, including not-for profit, for-profit, and government-owned.

■ These organizational forms produce incentives that influence both the relationship between physicians and hospitals and the effects of reimbursement systems on the cost of care.

■ In practice, hospitals attempt to increase revenue by improving payer mix and billing practices, by increasing the volume of care provided, and by decreasing costs by identifying variable and fixed costs that can be reduced in the short run or long run.

■ Decreasing length of stay is an important way hospitalists can help hospitals increase revenues and decrease costs.

REFERENCES

1. Levit K, Smith C, Cowan C, Sensenig A, Catlin A. Health Accounts Team. Health spending rebound continues in 2002. *Health Affairs* 2004;23:147–159.
2. Eddy DM. *Clinical Decision Making: From Theory to Practice.* Boston: Jones & Bartlett, 1996.
3. Harris, J. The internal organization of hospitals: some economic implications. *Bell J Economics* 1977;8:467–482.
4. Sloan, F. Not-for-profit ownership and hospital behavior. In: Culyer A, Newhouse J, eds. *Handbook of Health Economics.* Amsterdam: Elsevier Science Press, 2000.
5. Kosecoff J, Kahn KL, Rogers WH, et al. Prospective payment system and impairment at discharge: the 'quicker and sicker' story revisited. *JAMA* 1990;264:1980–1983.
6. Cutler D. The incidence of adverse medical outcomes under prospective payment. *Econometrica* 1995;63:29–50.
7. Ellis R, McGuire T. Provider behavior under prospective reimbursement. *J Health Econ* 1986;5:129–151.
8. Melnick GA, Zwanziger J. State health care expenditures under competition and cost-containment policies. *JAMA* 2002;160:2669–2675.
9. Meltzer D, Chung J, Basu A. Does competition under Medicare prospective payment selectively reduce expenditures on high-cost patients? *RAND J Econ* 2002;33:447–468.
10. Roberts R, Frutos P, Ciavarella G, et al. Distribution of variable and fixed costs of hospital care. *JAMA* 1999;281:644–649.
11. Luft HS. The relationship between surgical volume and mortality: an exploration of causal factors and alternative models. *Medical Care* 1980;18:940–59.
12. Wachter R, Goldman L. The hospitalist movement 5 years later. *JAMA* 2002;287:487–494.
13. Meltzer D, Manning W, Morrison J, et al. Effects of physician experience on costs and outcomes on an academic general medicine service: results of a trial of hospitalists. *Ann Intern Med* 2002;137:866–874.

ADDITIONAL READING

Phelps CE. *Health Economics.* 3rd ed. Boston: Addison Wesley, 2003.

Practice Management in Hospital Medicine

3

John R. Nelson

INTRODUCTION

The increasing pace and complexity of hospital care has led to new approaches to providing that care. This chapter explores these approaches, with a particular emphasis on organizational and financial issues for hospitalist programs.

ISSUES RELATED TO CONTINUITY OF HOSPITAL CARE

The hospitalist model of care involves a discontinuity of care between the primary care physician (PCP) and the hospitalist. Hospitalist groups are thinking carefully about ways to mitigate the potential adverse effects of this discontinuity through effective communication strategies among the PCP, patient, and hospitalist (1). However, an issue often overlooked is the continuity of care between patient and hospitalist during a single hospitalization or across multiple hospitalizations over time. One can speculate that a patient could benefit from seeing the same hospitalist each day of a hospital stay and during future hospitalizations. However, perfect hospitalist–patient continuity, such that the same doctor *always* sees a patient, is unrealistic because it requires that the doctor be constantly available. Thus, it is important for each group to find an appropriate balance between competing needs of continuity and physician lifestyle.

Patient–hospitalist continuity is most often discussed in relation to a single episode of hospital care. Many practices schedule doctors in blocks of days, such that a significant number of hospitalized patients will be cared for by a single physician during the patient's entire stay. The following simple formula offers a way to estimate the optimal length of these blocks:

$$C = \frac{D - (L - 1)}{D} \times 100$$

where C is the percentage of patients having only one hospitalist during a hospitalization ("continuity"), D is the average duration of hospitalist shifts, and L is the average length of stay in days.

For example, the formula tells us that, in a program that uses five-day hospitalist shifts and has a median length of stay of five days, only 20% of patients will see the same hospitalist each day ($C = 20\%$). Increasing the shift length to eight days improves continuity to 50%. The schedule that provides the best continuity (i.e., highest value for C) while still ensuring a reasonable and sustainable lifestyle for the doctor is probably the best choice.

Continuity between patient and hospitalist across multiple hospital stays (admissions) is somewhat more complicated and less often discussed when considering hospitalist schedules. While no data has been published to inform this discussion, it seems reasonable to speculate that having a patient see the same hospitalist during each admission might facilitate a closer bond between patient and physician and reduce the risk of clinical information "falling through the cracks." However, the author's anecdotal experience suggests that most hospitalist practices find this difficult, and typically a patient is assigned to whichever hospitalist is on duty for admissions despite the theoretical benefits of admission-to-admission continuity.

When thinking about how to optimize continuity from one hospital stay to the next, three approaches are attracting interest:

1. For patients readmitted in a short period of time (e.g., less than seven days), have the hospitalist who cared for the patient during the prior stay see the patient again. If that doctor is away at the time of the patient's return, a partner could care for the patient until the original attending hospitalist is back on duty. For patients readmitted after a longer period (and thus somewhat less likely to be returning for the same reason as the original

admission), the attending hospitalist would be the one on duty at the time of the patient's return. Many hospitalist groups take this approach.

2. A patient is paired with a hospitalist at the first admission to the hospitalist practice, and the same doctor sees that patient during every future admission. The only exception would be that a partner hospitalist sees the patient when the patient's main hospitalist is away. Such a system means that each hospitalist essentially builds his or her own patient population in much the same way an office-based doctor does. While this approach may sound ideal, it is unusual because of many complexities. For example, one hospitalist could be extremely busy with patients while a partner hospitalist might have little work to do. This is not a good way to distribute the practice manpower. Additionally, because most hospitalist practices are still relatively new, they are experiencing growth (adding doctors) and turnover. Last, this system is of little value for groups that work a modest number of days per year (e.g., a seven-days-on/seven-days-off schedule) or often use part-time doctors, because there is less chance a given patient's main hospitalist will be working at the time of any future admission.

3. An alternative to the above approach is to pair each hospitalist with an individual referring physician such that any patient referred by that doctor would always see the same hospitalist. This system should have similar advantages and drawbacks to that described above, with one additional advantage. The referring doctor and hospitalist could get to know each other even better and develop a relationship that is close to a true partnership. However, because of the same complexities described above, and because unassigned patient admissions from the emergency department would fall outside this protocol, this approach to continuity is in use in only one practice of which the author is aware.

NIGHT-TIME HOSPITALIST COVERAGE

The ideal system of night coverage for a hospitalist practice varies significantly from one practice to the next. Most small groups of five or fewer doctors use traditional call schedules with one member of the group on call for any night work. However, with larger groups, the burgeoning night work makes it increasingly difficult for a doctor to work the day before and day after being on night call. This leads many to adopt a separate system of night coverage staffed by dedicated doctors who work only at night (colloquially referred to as "nocturnists"), non-hospitalist moonlighters, or members of the hospitalist group rotating responsibility for night coverage for several consecutive nights without accompanying daytime responsibility. In practices with significant amounts of night work, such systems seem likely to provide for more sustainable careers and reduced risk of burnout.

In addition to the potential benefits for physician lifestyle, a system of dedicated night coverage might provide a number of other benefits, including better patient care. It is easy to imagine that an on-call doctor might handle patient care issues differently at night than a dedicated night-shift doctor who is in the hospital and expecting to work rather than worrying about how to get some rest before the next working day. For example, nurses may be more willing to call a night doctor who is awake and in the building than a sleep-deprived on-call physician. Additionally, a dedicated night-shift doctor is likely to form better working relationships with the night nursing staff, and this could translate into improved work satisfaction for all parties. It is possible that dedicated night coverage by hospitalist practices will become one of the key interventions to improve the quality of care and sustainability of the practice.

Successive surveys of hospitalists show that call-based schedules are increasingly being supplanted by shift-based schedules (2). In 2002, 40% of hospitalists responding to a survey reported having no on-call hours (3). Taken together, these results suggest an increasing prevalence of dedicated night coverage. Still, such systems are far from universal, and the barriers to their universal adoption include the following:

- Difficulty in financially supporting the night position
- For small hospitalist groups, a volume of night work that does not justify a dedicated night system
- Difficulty in recruiting doctors willing to work solely or primarily at night

Of these, the issue of financial support for the position can be the most difficult to overcome. The most economically productive time for a hospitalist is daily rounds, and night doctors do not conduct them. At night, the hospitalist might admit several patients, see a few "floor" patients, and field a number of calls from the nursing staff, but these activities seldom generate enough professional fee revenue to provide adequate compensation. Two common solutions can help ensure economic viability of the night system. First, and most commonly, in many health care systems the hospital or a payer (e.g., a managed care organization) sees enough value in a dedicated night system that it provides the funding to make up the difference between collected fees for work at night and the doctor's salary. Second, the night doctor can seek additional revenue sources, such as providing call coverage to doctors outside the hospitalist practice for a fee and then billing for the visits made.

As hospitalist practices mature in the coming years, it appears likely that night on-call systems will be replaced by dedicated systems of night coverage. A number of other specialties—including emergency medicine and hospital-based radiology—have seen a similar evolution or are experiencing it now.

HOSPITALIST CAREER LONGEVITY AND BURNOUT

No clear statistics are available, but anecdotal evidence suggests that physician turnover in hospitalist practice might be higher than in other specialties. A number of organizational and individual characteristics might influence hospitalist career longevity, but one major factor in a higher turnover rate for hospitalists is probably the relatively low barrier to entry to this type of practice. When compared with other generalist careers, hospitalist practice may be an attractive choice because it seems similar to how most residents spent a great part of their training (i.e., caring for hospitalized patients). Moreover, one can join a hospitalist practice and be busy on the first day rather than spend months building a primary care practice. Finally, leaving a hospitalist practice might be less disruptive to colleagues (and patients) because the practice has no regular patients that might leave or need to be reassigned to other doctors. All these factors could increase the chance that doctors might pursue hospitalist practice as a temporary stop before moving on to other training or practice settings.

These factors contribute to physician turnover independent of many other issues related to career longevity, such as professional satisfaction, income, and burnout. Surveys designed to assess these latter features show that most hospitalists are satisfied with their work and intend to remain hospitalists for the foreseeable future (Table 3.1).

TABLE 3.1

HOSPITALIST JOB SATISFACTION

Hospitalist satisfaction, 2000	
Very satisfied	58%
Satisfied	35%
Somewhat dissatisfied	6%
Very dissatisfied	2%

Hospitalist work attitudes, 1999	
Level of job burnout:	
Burned out	12.9%
At risk of burnout	24.9%
No current risk of burnout	62.2%
Years intending to remain a practicing hospitalist	
0–3	17.5%
4–7	18.3%
>7	64.2%

Lindenauer PK, Pantilat SZ, Katz PP, Wachter RM. Hospitalists and the practice of inpatient medicine: results of a survey of the National Association of Inpatient Physicians. *Ann Intern Med* 1999;130:343–349. Hoff TH, Whitcomb WF, Wiliams K, Nelson JR, Cheesman RA. Characteristics and work experiences of hospitalists in the United States. *Arch Intern Med* 2000;161:851–858.

TABLE 3.2

FACTORS ASSOCIATED WITH HOSPITALIST BURNOUT

- Perception of restricted autonomy
- Working for an institution (e.g., hospital or health maintenance organization) rather than self-employed or working in group practice
- Poor "occupational solidarity"
- Poor integration with non-MD co-workers
- Poor recognition by patients/families for job that is done
- Inability to treat entire range of patient problems

Interestingly, the following were not shown to correlate with burnout:
- Number of new patients (admissions and consultations) seen per month
- Portion of compensation linked to financial incentives
- Perceived pressure to contain costs

Hoff TH, Whitcomb WF, Wiliams K, Nelson JR, Cheesman RA. Characteristics and work experiences of hospitalists in the United States. *Arch Intern Med* 2000;161:851–858.

Many remain concerned about the issue of hospitalist burnout. As Table 3.1 shows, 38% of hospitalists were either burned out or at risk of burnout in 1999 (2). These percentages become even more worrisome considering that 85% of survey respondents had been hospitalists five or fewer years (46%, two or fewer years). More research is needed to learn the factors that increase and prevent burnout, but the 1999 survey highlighted several variables associated with burnout (see Table 3.2).

Clearly, more study is needed regarding maximizing satisfaction with the hospitalist career and preventing burnout. The single study in 1999 does not provide enough information to serve as the basis of definitive guidelines for the optimal practice structure. Information from similar specialties such as emergency medicine and critical care medicine may be helpful because they have burnout rates of 40%–60% (4,5). In the absence of definitive guidelines, each practice must carefully consider the available information and the preferences of its doctors to arrive at decisions about operating the practice. It seems clear that such an approach leads many groups to modify their practice schedules frequently.

FINANCIAL VIABILITY OF HOSPITALIST PRACTICE

Survey data from 2002 show that 75% of hospitalists receive some financial support in addition to the collection of professional fees (3). This support usually comes from the hospital served by the hospitalists, but it may come from other sources, such as a managed care organization or a large group medical practice. The median amount of this support was 30% of professional fee revenue for the practice (3). The entity providing this support is usually in the position of benefiting financially from the increased efficiency hospitalists bring about. Hospitalist practices often require this additional support for several reasons, including the following:

- Hospitalists can usually command a salary that is 5%–15% higher than that of doctors with the same training in the same market. For example, an internal medicine-trained hospitalist might make 5%–15% more than an internist in traditional practice in the same area. This is because in most areas the demand for hospitalists exceeds the supply (a situation that may change in a few years as an increasing number of residents seek careers as hospitalists). Additionally, hospitalists usually have more night and weekend responsibilities than PCPs in traditional practice.
- Hospitalists are often asked to care for unassigned patients admitted through the emergency department, a patient population that is usually associated with lower levels of reimbursement.
- The amount of work to be done at night might be such that a traditional on-call schedule is unreasonable and a dedicated system of night coverage is needed. Typically, the night work fails to generate enough professional fee revenue to support the night position, and additional support might be needed.

Despite these factors, the survey indicates that 25% of groups do *not* receive additional financial support (3). However, many of these groups do receive support over and above the prevailing reimbursement rates for the local market. This support comes through a variety of mechanisms, including local payer(s) approving hospitalist fee schedules that are higher than the prevailing rates, or through nonfinancial support (such as a hospital paying for a system of night coverage using moonlighters). Groups that receive such support might indicate on a survey that they receive no money beyond their collected fees, yet they do depend on support beyond prevailing reimbursement rates.

Clearly, some hospitalist practices operate solely with professional fee collections (at the prevailing market rates). The author's experience suggests that these groups either work at a difficult and potentially unsustainable pace, pay salaries below those of hospitalists in other practices, or both.

It is difficult to predict whether support in addition to professional fee revenue will remain a typical part of hospitalist practice in the future, but it does seem unlikely that professional fees (at least those paid via government programs such as Medicare) will increase to make this financial support unnecessary.

HOSPITALISTS AND HEALTH SYSTEM EFFICIENCY

Efficient patient care delivery is one of the most well-studied attributes of hospitalist practice. Nearly all studies that have examined this issue have found that hospitalist care is associated with reductions in length of stay (LOS) and cost per case of about 15%–20% when compared with care delivered by non-hospitalists (6). Data are beginning to accumulate that this improved efficiency does not come at the expense of quality of care; in fact, hospitalist care may be associated with improved patient outcomes (7,8).

Many hospitalist practices carefully measure efficiency-related statistics such as LOS and costs, as well as a number of clinical quality measures. However, these metrics may fail to capture some additional value that the practice might provide to the hospital or health system. For example, a hospitalist practice might increase a hospital's market share of referrals through good relationships with physicians and smaller hospitals in the outlying areas.

Another, and increasingly important, way hospitalists can increase hospital efficiency is by influencing the time of day that a patient is discharged. As hospitals have become increasingly full in the past few years, they have become more dependent on early patient discharges (e.g., approximately 11 AM) so that beds can be made available for scheduled and emergency admissions. Late discharges pose less problems for hospitals that are not full, but those hospitals still incur the cost of needing more nursing staff on the afternoon/evening shift than if patients were discharged early in the day.

The following example illustrates the issue of early discharge and hospital bed availability for full hospitals. Imagine a 100-bed hospital that is full in the morning. Of the 20 discharges that will take place that day, three are delayed until late in the afternoon for nonmedical reasons. That leads to the cancellation of three elective admissions planned for that day. If those delayed patients were discharged early in the day, the hospital might avoid canceling the elective admissions, thereby serving more patients with the same number of beds. In other words, with early discharge, it is as though the hospital has access to three more beds without having to construct them or add new staff to provide care.

Some hospital administrators speak in terms of expediting throughput by reducing LOS and discharging patients earlier in the day. For a 300-bed hospital, a 0.25-day reduction in LOS for all patients would have the effect of making 12 "new" beds available and freeing approximately nine nursing full-time equivalents. Hospitalists are well positioned to address these issues by providing efficient care, by letting patients and families know the anticipated date of discharge as early in the hospital stay as possible, and by visiting patients potentially ready for discharge very early in the day. Of course, the hospital needs to do its part: ensuring that clinical data used to make discharge decisions are made available to the physician early in the day and eliminating hospital-related bottlenecks that lead to the patient remaining in the room unnecessarily after the discharge order is written.

While obvious, it is worth mentioning again that medical issues must take precedence in deciding the day and time of discharge. Some patients cannot be appropriately discharged until late in the day, after their evaluation and treatment is completed. While these patients may first appear to be delayed discharges, they might in fact be very *early* discharges—by being released late in the day rather than the next morning, as might have occurred years ago.

CONCLUSIONS

As the care of hospitalized patients continues to evolve, on-going clinical and economic challenges will require adjustments in the care delivery system to ensure the provision of high-value care. Information from research studies will help determine the most effective ways to improve care delivery, but published research is unlikely to answer all questions about how physicians and hospitals should be organized. Innovation will always be needed in response to local strengths and challenges.

KEY POINTS

- While the hospitalist model of care involves a discontinuity between inpatient and outpatient providers, thoughtful arrangements of the hospitalist's work schedule can maximize patient–hospitalist continuity while preserving a sustainable lifestyle for the doctor.
- The on-site presence of a night hospitalist who does not also work the day before or after the night shift may have important benefits for patient care and hospitalist longevity. However, there are significant challenges to implementing such a system.
- Few data are available to answer questions about hospitalist career longevity and burnout, but they may be similar to what is seen in fields, such as emergency medicine or critical care medicine. Physician turnover in hospitalist practice may be much higher than in other

primary care roles because of the comparatively low barrier of entry to hospitalist practice.
- For many reasons, most hospitalist practices require a source of financial support in addition to the collection of professional fees. This is an area that may see significant changes in the future.
- When medically appropriate, discharge of patients early in the day can have a significant impact on the number of patients that the institution can serve. Discharge early in the day can be valuable to a hospital, but that value does not appear in commonly tracked statistics such as length of stay or cost per case.

REFERENCES

1. Nelson JR, Whitcomb WF. Organizing a hospitalist program: an overview of fundamental concepts. *Med Clin N Am* 2002; 86:887–909.
2. Hoff TH, Whitcomb WF, Wiliams K, Nelson JR, Cheesman RA. Characteristics and work experiences of hospitalists in the United States. *Arch Intern Med* 2001;161:851–858.
3. Society of Hospital Medicine (formerly National Association of Inpatient Physicians). 2002 Survey of Hospitalist Productivity and Compensation.
4. Goldberg R, Boss R, Chan L, et al. Burnout and its correlates in emergency physicians: four years' experience with a wellness booth. *Acad Emerg Med* 1996;3:1156–1164.
5. Gutupalli K, Fromm R. Burnout in the internist-intensivist. *Intensive Care Med* 1996;22:625–630.
6. Wachter RM, Goldman L. The hospitalist movement 5 years later. *JAMA* 2002;287:487–494.
7. Meltzer D, Manning WG, Morrison J, et. al. Effects of physician experience on costs and outcomes on an academic general medicine service: results of a trial of hospitalists. *Ann Intern Med* 2002; 137:866–874.
8. Auerbach AD, Wachter RM, Katz P, Showstack J, Baron RB, Goldman L. Implementation of a voluntary hospitalist service at a community teaching hospital: improved clinical efficiency and patient outcomes. *Ann Intern Med* 2002;137:859–865.

ADDITIONAL READING

Auerbach AD, Aranson MD, Davis RB, Phillips RS. How physicians perceive hospitalist services after implementation: anticipation vs. reality. *Ann Intern Med* 2003;163:2330–2336.
Leigh JP, Kravitz RL, Schembri M, Samuels SJ, Mobley S. Physician career satisfaction across specialties. *Arch Intern Med* 2002; 162:1577–1584.
Pantilat SZ, Wachter RM. The patient-provider relationship and the hospitalist movement. *Am J Med* 2001;111(Suppl).

Hospital Interfaces

4

Winthrop F. Whitcomb   John R. Nelson

INTRODUCTION

In our increasingly complex health care system, patients receive care from a staggering number of providers. This is particularly true in the hospital, where the average patient sees dozens of health care personnel every day. Not surprisingly, fragmentation among various departments and providers is an important obstacle to high-quality and efficient care (1) and has led some to examine how best to manage the myriad hospital interfaces. This chapter explores key physician interfaces, both within the hospital setting and across the care continuum. In addition, the chapter discusses the interactions between physician and nonphysician members of the hospital care team. Specific strategies related to hospital discharge are further considered in Chapter 5.

Rapid advances in information technology aimed at linking the hospital and other care settings will significantly improve the physician's ability to care for patients effectively. However, technology will not diminish the importance of the time spent communicating with and examining the patient, nor will it obviate the need for physicians to properly manage the dozens of personal interactions that frequently determine the outcomes and cost of care.

TERMINOLOGY

As discussed in Chapter 1, a variety of arrangements among physicians are emerging for the provision of hospital care. Whether hospital care is provided under the traditional approach (stage I), a non-hospitalist rounder system (stage II), or a dedicated hospitalist model (stages III and IV), many of the interface issues for the physician in the hospital are the same. Accordingly, this chapter uses the term *hospital physician* regardless of model for hospital care and the term *referring physician* to denote the physician who refers the patient to be cared for by the hospital physician. The referring physician may be a primary care physician or a subspecialist. The hospital physician may be a hospitalist or a traditional physician with significant outpatient responsibilities.

CARE OF THE HOSPITALIZED PATIENT

Physician–Patient Interface

Admission to a hospital can mean that a patient and a physician are meeting each other under stressful circumstances, often for the first time. Hospital physicians should begin by introducing themselves and describing their role, and they should use an empathic interview style to provide both patient and family with a sense of comfort and confidence. An approach to establishing rapport is summed up by the mnemonic PEARLS, for *partnership, empathy, apology, respect, legitimation, and support* (see Table 4.1) (2).

Referring physicians can help build a patient's confidence in a separate hospital physician by explaining the reasons for the referral, letting the patient know that they will be communicating with the hospital physician frequently during the hospitalization, and explaining that they will be the patient's primary doctor after discharge. One Baton Rouge physician captured the essence of the referring physician–hospital physician relationship by using a local metaphor:

> An analogous role [to that of the hospitalist] is performed by Mississippi river pilots. River pilots board all ocean liners as they enter the deceptive and changing currents of the Mississippi River. They guide the vessel safely to and from port, returning the controls to the ship's captain for the homeward voyage. Their collaborative efforts yield navigational quality that neither could attain alone (3).

It is helpful to provide the patient with a written brochure introducing the hospital physician and explaining when the patient can expect to be seen, how the family can contact the hospital physician, and how communication between physicians will occur.

TABLE 4.1

KEY STEPS TOWARD ESTABLISHING RAPPORT (PEARLS)

Element of the approach	Settings and examples
Partnership	*(With a chronically ill patient in the ER about to be admitted for unstable angina)* "We're going to have some difficult decisions to make. I'll need to work with you and your family to provide the best care and the care most consistent with your values and beliefs."
Empathy	*(With an elderly patient traveling alone through your town, admitted with pneumonia)* "You look sad. I can only imagine how hard it must be being ill here, without your family or your own doctor to help you."
Apology	*(With an HMO patient angry about being admitted by the hospitalist, not his or her PCP)* "I'm very sorry that the system doesn't allow your own doctor to care for you here, and that you and I don't have a close relationship. Still, I'd like to try to get to know you, and, after speaking with your doctor on the phone, take as good care of you as I know she would."
Respect	*(With a patient readmitted for COPD, still smoking after many attempts to quit)* "You know, Mr. Jones, I know how hard it is to quit. But even though you're still smoking, you never seem to give up trying to quit."
Legitimation	*(With a patient suspicious of your motives in not consulting a specialist)* "Many people these days are unaware of the skills of internal medicine (family practice, etc.) and have come to equate quality care with subspecialists like cardiologists. I can imagine you'd have some questions about how qualified I am to care for this problem."
Support	*(With a patient about to enroll in hospice)* "Hospice does not mean giving up. The hospice nurses and your family doctor will be with you in the coming months, and if they have questions for me, or if you have questions for me, the hospital operator can page me and I'll call you back as soon as possible."

Adapted from Barnes PB. Rapport and the hospitalist. *Am J Med* 2001;111:31S–35S, with permission.

If meeting the patient for the first time, the hospital physician carries the dual burden of building a relationship with the patient and family and learning the pertinent medical and psychosocial details. The latter task requires a review of prior medical records. In many systems, outpatient records are separate from hospital records, so the hospital physician must request records from outpatient providers and other hospitals. Because this record request is a regular part of the hospital physician's work, it is worth developing a protocol such as the one shown in Figure 4.1 to streamline the process. The hospital physician can complete the form and include it with the admitting orders. Additionally, referring offices should develop similar protocols to provide records to the hospital physician when a patient is admitted. The referring office can send the entire office chart (although transporting it between office and hospital risks losing it), or it can furnish copies of recent records, including (at a minimum) results of the last comprehensive history and physical examination plus medical problem and medication lists.

With medical-surgical lengths of stay averaging less than five days in many regions of the United States, part of the admission process should include initial discharge planning. Early assessment by the physician, nurse, and case manager should elicit the preadmission functional status and social support structure. As the hospital course progresses, new information emerges that can influence the discharge plan, and the patient's need for other services, such as physical and occupational therapy, is frequently revealed. Patient and family satisfaction with the discharge plan has been shown to depend on factors related both to the discharge planning process and to the discharge destination (4).

Hospital discharge is a point at which important communication issues arise for all physicians. The challenge of organizing effective posthospital care is greater for a hospitalist because a different physician provides follow-up with the patient. Detailed conversation between the hospital physician and patient during the final hospital visit, accompanied by written instructions, is helpful (5). For a hospitalist, a phone call to the patient between 24 hours and two weeks after discharge is an excellent opportunity to reinforce discharge instructions, review the results of tests that may have been pending when the patient left the hospital, answer the patient's questions, and remind the patient of the importance of follow-up (6). Follow-up phone calls by nurses, case managers, or clinical pharmacists may also be effective (7). When appropriate, providing the patient and family with a copy of the discharge summary can also serve to reinforce the findings of the hospital stay and the follow-up plans. Finally, some hospitalist programs have established a follow-up service, whereby the patient may be seen once after hospital discharge by the hospital physician before returning to the referring physician (8). Chapter 5 contains further information on hospital discharge.

HOSPITAL MEDICINE SERVICE

Request for Records

Records needed:

☐   All records since _____
                                   Date

☐   Medication list
☐   Most recent history and physical exam
☐   Discharge summaries :   ☐ all since _____
                                                         Date

                                        ☐ most recent

☐   Test reports of particular interest
                          ☐ Cardiac cath   ☐ CBC   ☐ ANA
                          ☐ Echocardiogram   ☐ BUN/Creatinine   ☐ B12
                          ☐ Chest x-ray   ☐ Thyroid tests   ☐ Folate
                          ☐ PT/PTT   ☐ Ferritin
                          ☐ Other _____
                                                  Specify

Records requested from the following institution or office:

_____

_____

_____

_____

Authorization for release of medical information

I, _____ , authorize _____
            Name   Institution, office, or physician

to release to ABC Medical Center any and all of my medical information they possess.
This authorization includes the release of medical records and/or information concerning
drug abuse or drug related conditions and/or alcoholism and/or psychological and/or
psychiatric conditions and/or HIV or other communicable diseases. This will expire sixty
(60) days from the date below.

_____   _____
              Date   Signature of patient

_____   _____
            Witness   Other person legally authorized to give consent

Figure 4.1   A model record request form. A form such as this one can be completed by the admitting physician and included with the admitting orders. It can then be faxed to the office or institution from which records are sought. A section at the bottom documents the patient's consent to provide the records and avoids the need to complete and fax a separate consent form.

Hospital Physician–Referring Physician Interface

Hospital physicians need to establish effective communication links with referring physicians, both to transmit information and to collaborate on inpatient care decisions. They can use each other as telephone consultants in deciding whether to admit or discharge, and they should continually educate each other about the strengths and limitations of care in their respective settings. In this regard, there may be advantages to systems in which the hospital physician maintains some outpatient contact and the referring physician some contact with the inpatient setting.

Situations can arise in which neither physician should make unilateral decisions about the care of a patient, sometimes including the decision to admit or discharge. For example, if a hospital physician decides the patient can be treated with an intravenous antibiotic as an outpatient, the referring physician or another outpatient physician must agree and be ready to assume this responsibility. The list of illnesses once requiring hospitalization that can now be managed in the outpatient setting grows each year, and the hospital physician must involve the referring physician in the decision to employ outpatient treatment.

As a gap between hospital and outpatient care emerges in the United States, concerns have arisen regarding a potential loss of information at the hospital threshold (9). In an Australian survey of 350 outpatient physicians, 84% were not notified of their patients' admission to the hospital; 87% were not notified of major changes in their patients' condition, including death; and 75% were not notified of patient discharge from the hospital (10). Preliminary results from American hospitalists seem more favorable: more than 90% state that they do communicate with referring physicians at discharge (11).

The frequency and nature of contact between the hospital physician and referring physician during the patient's hospital stay can vary a great deal. At a minimum, the hosital physician should notify the referring physician when any significant or unexpected changes in the patient's condition develop and when decisions are made in the hospital that will significantly affect subsequent outpatient care (e.g., starting a complex therapy such as parenteral nutrition that will be continued on an outpatient basis). Additional contact can be tailored to the interests and desires of each physician. Some referring physicians choose to make "continuity visits" to their hospital patients or to contact the patients by telephone. These important contacts, which the hospital physician should encourage, facilitate discussion about psychosocial and ethical issues, assure patients of the referring physician's continued involvement, allow for the referring physician's endorsement of the hospitalist, and bridge the gap in clinical information between hospital and non-hospital settings (12).

At discharge, the hospital physician should give the referring physician a detailed discharge summary that incorporates the usual components of a summary in addition to features commonly found in consultation reports. The summary should include a specific section listing the tests pending at discharge, follow-up studies needed (e.g., repeated chest roentgenogram to follow a lung lesion or coagulation studies to monitor warfarin therapy), a list of medications, and instructions given to the patient. All discharge summaries should have the same format regardless of the physician who prepared them; this ensures that the reader can quickly find pertinent information. Summaries should be provided to the referring physician and other caregivers in a timely manner to help with the transition in care. Many institutions have a summary dictated and transcribed on the day of discharge and faxed to the referring physician the same day. In addition, some referring physicians prefer a phone call from the hospital physician on the day of discharge (13). When patient care is being transferred from hospitalist to primary physician, the principles outlined in Table 4.2 (14) should be kept in mind.

Hospital Physician–Emergency Department Physician Interface

The role of the emergency department (ED) physician is to institute a timely diagnostic and therapeutic plan for patients in the ED. In those who require hospital admission, early involvement of the hospital physician can be an advantage for all parties. Because of their increased or continuous presence in the hospital, hospitalists have the opportunity to become involved in the care of ED patients earlier than primary care physicians can. Early contact with the hospital physician to provide admission services may improve patient flow through the ED, decrease costs, and increase patient satisfaction.

Some patients can be admitted directly to the hospital without involving the ED. Hospital physicians can help facilitate direct admissions by encouraging referring physicians to call them about patients who will require admission rather than send patients to the ED for initial evaluation. Of course, unstable patients should always be seen in the ED first.

Clinical guidelines to coordinate the efforts of ED and hospital physicians are proliferating. By defining each physician's role for a given condition, guidelines can minimize gaps in care and duplication of effort. Creating successful guidelines requires the participation of both ED and hospital physicians on the clinical guideline authoring team. Successful implementation of such guidelines can lead to more rational divisions of labor, with the ED and hospital physicians able to focus on their respective care settings.

TABLE 4.2
SIX PILLARS OF THE HAND-OFF

1. Communicate, but do not irritate.
2. Consult the primary physician.
3. Timeliness is next to godliness.
4. Partner with the patient.
5. Make it clear that you are the patient's advocate.
6. Pass the baton as graciously as you received it (or even better, more graciously).

Reprinted from Goldman L, Pantilat SZ, Whitcomb WF. Passing the clinical baton. *Am J Med* 2001;111:36S–39S, with permission.

Hospital Physician–Intensive Care Unit Physician (Intensivist) Interface

The role of the hospital physician in the ICU is highly variable and depends on hospital size, setting, and organization of care. Evidence suggests that ICUs in which dedicated intensivists play a primary role in patient management outperform ICUs in which primary care physicians play such a role (with no or optional intensivist consultation), with regard to both outcomes and efficiency (15). As a result of caring for many ICU patients, some hospitalists may be more comfortable and competent in ICU procedures than primary physicians with the same training background. This increased skill, along with greater availability during the day, will allow some hospitalists to feel comfortable managing patients both in and out of the ICU. Although hospitalists who are not intensivists will never replace physicians trained in critical care, their presence may result in a decreased need for closed ICUs and their associated discontinuity. Moreover, if the hospital physicians are more readily available than the intensivists, they can provide preliminary critical care services (e.g., airway management or fluid resuscitation) until the intensivists arrive to deliver comprehensive critical care services. Finally, the growing national shortage of intensivists will require that other physicians, usually hospitalists, fill the vacuum (16).

Because hospitalists and non-hospitalist intensivists are readily available within the hospital, both are naturally suited to provide leadership on hospital and medical staff committees concerned with inpatient settings, such as ethics committees, quality improvement committees, and clinical guideline committees. Guidelines developed by members of both disciplines can streamline care (e.g., antibiotic selection) as patients move out of the ICU to a stepdown unit or an acute medical floor. Early transfer of patients out of the ICU can be facilitated by a hospital physician, whose presence and expertise may improve patient flow and bed availability in the ICU.

Hospital Physician–Observation Unit Interface

Observation units are present in many hospitals. They go by a variety of names, including emergency department observation units, clinical decision units, rapid diagnostic and treatment units, or others. These units, commonly located within or near the emergency department (ED), are most often used for ED patients who require diagnostic evaluation or urgent treatment beyond the typical scope of ED care but who do not clearly require hospital admission. Common problems managed this way might be chest pain, asthma, cellulitis, and dehydration. During the patient's time in the observation unit, a decision is made regarding discharge or admission to an inpatient unit of the hospital. Because of their availability, ED physicians most commonly serve as the patient's attending physician during the

observation unit stay, but if the unit is in a location remote from the ED, then hospitalists or other members of the medical staff might serve as attending (17).

For the hospital physician, the presence of an observation unit is likely to significantly decrease the number of inpatient admissions (18). It might also change the nature and acuity of patients admitted after an observation unit stay because they will have undergone more workup and treatment than patients admitted directly from the ED. Physicians in the observation unit and hospital physicians need to work together closely to develop protocols regarding observation unit versus direct hospital admissions from the ED. Both physicians also need to work with hospital administration to correctly designate patients as being on "observation status," per Medicare regulations. Both groups should be comfortable with the time of day that patients are transferred from the observation unit to the inpatient ward and care transferred to the hospital physician. For example, if care is routinely transferred to the hospital physician as the workday begins (e.g., 7 AM), the patient's observation unit attending physician might have left work already, and the hospital physician might be busy discharging patients. A protocol regarding transfer of care should specify that the transfer occur at the optimal time of day for all involved and provide for seamless transfer of the patient's clinical and social history.

Hospital–Skilled Nursing Facility Interface

The hospital–skilled nursing facility interface is a demanding area for practitioners, both in maintaining high-quality care and in preventing loss of pertinent clinical information. Yet physician training in this area has been inadequate. A survey of 389 hospitalists revealed a perception of inadequate residency training in "coordination of care between settings," "prescribing the appropriate level of care," and "knowledge of therapeutic capabilities of nursing homes" (19).

A growing body of literature suggests that hospital physicians can be most effective when discharging patients, including those who will go to a skilled nursing facility, by working with a multidisciplinary team (20). A team approach allows assessment of functional status and evaluation of home supports so that skilled nursing facility transfer can be anticipated early in the hospital course. Upon discharge, the chief concern is the appropriate transmission of patient information across settings. Table 4.3 lists important documents to be sent with the patient at the time of transfer to a skilled nursing facility.

The Hospital Team

The increasing acuity of hospitalized patients requires the hospital physician to carefully orchestrate the delivery of

TABLE 4.3

INFORMATION TO BE SENT TO SKILLED NURSING FACILITY AT TIME OF HOSPITAL DISCHARGE

- Concise yet detailed discharge summary
- Medication and allergy list
- Pertinent doctor, nurse, and therapist progress notes and care plans
- Consultant notes including history and physical exam
- Key diagnostic and lab tests
- Advance directive, including do-not-resuscitate forms
- Fact sheet and demographic information

care. This coordination process applies equally to interactions with both consulting physicians and nonphysician members of the hospital team.

A variety of collaborative initiatives is replacing the traditional fragmentation of hospital disciplines. Many institutions have implemented multidisciplinary patient rounds, integrated medical record documentation, and clinical guidelines involving the entire hospital team. Proponents of such collaborative systems point to the reduced duplication of effort and gaps in care as primary benefits. Lessons from multidisciplinary approaches in ICUs support the hypothesis that this approach improves outcomes (21).

Nursing

The nurse–physician interface is, in many ways, the central relationship affecting the day-in, day-out care of inpatients. The continuous presence of the nurse on the floor provides a comprehensive perspective of the patient's condition, including medical, emotional, and psychosocial concerns. Trust in the hospital team is highly dependent on the physician, who is viewed as its leader, but its foundation is often the patient–nurse relationship because of the close contact between them. Because the physician's time with the patient is limited, the flow of information between nurse and physician must be optimized. Additionally, the physician serves as a vital resource for the nurse in clarifying the care plan and providing important social information about the patient.

This interdependence creates the need for a close working relationship between nurse and physician. The old approach of having the head nurse make rounds with the physician was extremely effective in promoting care that was coordinated and informed and that engendered the trust of the patient, who witnessed and often participated in the exchange of information between the two caregivers. Although this model has been largely abandoned because of the limited availability of both physicians and nurses, the inefficiency of fragmenting care has become apparent, and the idea of coordinated bedside rounds is now regaining favor in some institutions.

The nurse provides the general coordination of patient care from hour to hour, often conveying information from other members of the hospital team to the physician, including consultant recommendations, therapist evaluations, and laboratory or radiographic data. Finally, because of ongoing availability to the patient, the nurse serves as a primary liaison with family members.

Case Management

The hospital physician–case management interface revolves around placing the patient into the appropriate care setting at the appropriate time. The case manager plays a central role in discharge planning. As such, the case manager is usually the first nonphysician to speak with the patient and family about the discharge process, including location (e.g., skilled nursing facility or home), follow-up, and special services needed. Effective models of hospital case management involve regular meetings between the physician and case manager beginning soon after admission to allow for the exchange of important social and medical information, including patient and family needs. These interactions facilitate early involvement of the other members of the hospital team. For example, if a patient with a newly diagnosed stroke has a good family support structure, the patient may be able to go home once physical and occupational therapy, home health care, and transportation services have been arranged.

At or soon after hospital admission, the case manager must often supply payers or the hospital with information regarding the appropriateness of the decision to admit. Case managers obtain this information through physician documentation in the medical record or verbal communication with the physician. In addition, the case manager performs a utilization review function or works closely with the utilization review nurse. In either case, regular determinations of the suitability of a given care setting are made. If the case manager determines that a patient should be moved to a less acute setting, the physician is notified.

Social Services

The work of the social services department complements that of the case manager in many ways. The social worker uses information from the physician to access community resources appropriate for a given patient's needs. Through collaboration, the physician becomes aware of the possibilities for community support for the patient, and the social worker learns of specific medical issues that need to be addressed. Resources that may then be used include medical or psychiatric care, home services, child or adult day care services, post-acute care, support groups, substance abuse programs, public assistance, and protective services.

With the rise of case management as a discipline, social workers in many hospitals are focusing on bedside relations with the patient, fulfilling a critical mental health role. The social worker can provide crisis intervention and counseling to patients and their families during an acute illness. Through an understanding of psychosocial issues, the social worker can assist the physician in dealing effectively with patient–family dynamics.

Pastoral Care

As the emphasis on patient satisfaction grows, the need to understand patients' spiritual and emotional needs has become more apparent. Frequently, the physician is privy to the most telling cues regarding a patient's emotional state. Body language or verbal communication from the patient can alert the physician that a patient is angry, scared, indifferent, or resentful. The role of the pastoral care worker is to assist the patient in exploring personal faith and in managing the gamut of emotions experienced during an acute hospital illness. The physician can most effectively utilize the skills of pastoral care providers by involving them early in the hospital course rather than calling on them only when a patient's demise is imminent.

The physician and pastoral care provider can meet with families to help align disparate views regarding an appropriate course of action in the event the patient has lost decision-making capabilities. In contemplating withdrawal of life support, for example, loved ones must integrate medical with emotional and spiritual information in making a decision. Physician–pastoral care collaboration can most effectively support this process (see Chapter 19).

Pastoral care can also serve the important role of supporting the caregiver. For example, if a patient dies, an event many physicians perceive as professional failure, the pastoral care provider can help explore such feelings and bring them to resolution (22).

Therapy Departments

Departments of physical, occupational, and speech therapy interact with the hospital physician in several important ways. By performing functional assessments, they provide information that is used to determine appropriate acute treatment, timing of patient discharge, and selection of care setting. These departments guide patient recovery through exercise, education, and other measures. The therapist can often detect patient deficits and notify the physician, which allows for timely evaluation and further treatment.

Pharmacists

The role of clinical pharmacists is described in Chapter 21.

CONCLUSIONS

Hospital physicians must establish roles and systems that ensure a good flow of clinical and psychosocial information among all members of the health care team. An examination of the many hospital interfaces sheds light on potential problems and opportunities for improved communication and collaboration. Innovations in computerized real-time and online medical record technologies can assist these efforts, but they will never supplant effective personal interactions among multidisciplinary providers.

KEY POINTS

- The increasing complexity of hospital systems requires careful attention to the management of physician and nonphysician interfaces.
- Communication between the hospital and non-hospital physician depends on the use of existing technologies (telephone, fax, electronic mail) and the development of new ones (e.g., electronic medical record). Protocols for exchanging records between these providers can strengthen this interface.
- Physician leadership of multidisciplinary hospital care teams, including nurses, case managers, social workers, pastoral care providers, pharmacists, therapists, and others, is critical to inpatient care.
- Improving hospitalists' interaction with patients after discharge is likely to improve both quality and patient satisfaction.

REFERENCES

1. Institute of Medicine. *Crossing the Quality Chasm: A New Health System for the 21st Century.* Washington, DC: *National Academy Press,* 2001.
2. Barnett PB. Rapport and the hospitalist. *Am J Med* 2001;111: 31S–35S.
3. Slataper R. Quality of care and the hospitalist. *The Hospitalist* 1997;1:5–6.
4. Procter E, Morrow-Howell N, Albaz R, Weir C. Patient and family satisfaction with discharge plans. *Med Care* 1992;30:262–275.
5. Calkins DR, Davis RB, Reiley P, et al. Patient–physician communication at hospital discharge and patients' understanding of the post-discharge treatment plan. *Arch Intern Med* 1997;157: 1026–1030.
6. Nelson JR. The importance of postdischarge telephone follow-up for hospitalists: a view from the trenches. *Am J Med* 2001;111: 43S–44S.
7. Dudas V, Bookwalter T, Kerr K, Pantilat SZ. The impact of follow-up telephone calls to patients after hospitalization. *Am J Med* 2001;111:26S–30S.
8. Pantilat SZ, Kerr KM, Goldman L, Wachter RM. The follow-up service: easing the transition from the inpatient to the outpatient setting. *J Clin Outcomes Mgmt* 2003;10:257–262.
9. Wachter RM, Goldman L. The emerging role of "hospitalists" in the American health care system. *N Engl J Med* 1996;335: 514–517.
10. Isaac DR, Gijsbers AJ, Wyman KT, Martyres RF, Garrow BA. The GP-hospital interface: attitudes of general practitioners to tertiary teaching hospitals. *Med J Aust* 1997;166:9–12.
11. Lindenauer PK, Pantilat SZ, Katz PP, Wachter RM. Hospitalists and the practice of inpatient medicine: results of a national survey. *Ann Intern Med* 1999;130:343–349.
12. Wachter RM, Pantilat SZ. The "continuity visit" and the hospitalist model of care. *Am J Med* 2001;111:40S–42S.

13. Pantilat SZ, Lindenauer PK, Katz PP, Wachter RM. Primary care physician attitudes regarding communication with hospitalists. *Am J Med* 2001;111:15S–20S.
14. Goldman L, Pantilat SZ, Whitcomb WF. Passing the clinical baton. *Am J Med* 2001;111:36S–39S.
15. Pronovost PJ, Angus DC, Dorman T, Robinson KA, Dremsizov TT, Young TL. Physician staffing patterns and clinical outcomes in critically ill patients: a systematic review. *JAMA* 2002;288:2151–2162.
16. Angus DC, Kelley MA, Schmitz RJ, White A, Popovich J Jr.; Committee on Manpower for Pulmonary and Critical Care Societies (COMPACCS). Caring for the critically ill patient. Current and projected workforce requirements for care of the critically ill and patients with pulmonary disease: can we meet the requirements of an aging population? *JAMA* 2000;284:2762–2770.
17. Ross MA, Graff LG. Principles of observation medicine. *Emerg Med Clin North Am* 2001;19:1–17.
18. Martinez E, Reilly BM, Evans AT, Roberts RR. The observation unit: a new interface between inpatient and outpatient care. *Am J Med* 110:274–277.
19. Plauth WH, Pantilat SZ, Wachter RM, Fenton CL. Hospitalists' perceptions of their residency training needs: results of a national survey. *Am J Med* 2001;111:247–253.
20. Palmer RM. Acute hospital care. In: Cassel CK, Leipzig RM, Cohen HJ, Larson EB, Meier DE, eds. *Geriatric Medicine*. New York: Springer, 2003.
21. Zimmerman JE, Shortell SM, Rousseau DM, et al. Improving intensive care: observations based on organizational case studies in nine intensive care units: a prospective, multicenter study. *Crit Care Med* 1993;21:1443–1451.
22. Lo B, Ruston D, Kates LW, et al. Discussing religious and spiritual issues at the end of life: a practical guide to physicians. *JAMA* 2002;287:749–754.

ADDITIONAL READING

Dichter JR. Teamwork and hospital medicine. A vision for the future. *Crit Care Nurse* 2003;23:8–11.
Pantilat SZ, Wachter RM, eds. The patient-provider relationship and the hospitalist movement. *Am J Med* 2001(suppl); 111.
Siegler EL, Mirafzali S, Foust JB, eds. *An Introduction to Hospitals and Inpatient Care.* New York: Springer, 2003.
[No author listed] Partner with inpatient physicians to achieve your case management goals. *Hosp Case Manag* 2001;9:81–84.

Hospital Discharge

5

Preetha Basaviah   Mark V. Williams

INTRODUCTION

The timing of and events surrounding hospital discharge can have a significant impact on patient satisfaction, patient safety, and the outcomes and cost of care. A growing body of research on optimizing discharge strategies and improving communication at discharge can inform the discharge decision. Several strategies, including structured patient education, predischarge checklists, multidisciplinary discharge planning teams, postdischarge telephone follow-up, and improving communication methods between inpatient and outpatient providers during discharge, have been shown to enhance the discharge process.

With the average day in an American hospital costing from $1,600 to $2,200, there is no doubt that unnecessary hospital days drain health care resources (1,2). However, the motive for timely discharge is not limited to cost considerations. For many patients, the simple unpleasantness of the average hospital room, the lack of privacy, and the human desire to sleep in one's own bed are motivation enough. In addition, patients and families have become aware that the risks of medical errors and nosocomial infections (3) make the hospital a potentially dangerous place.

Of course, discharging patients from the hospital as quickly as possible has its own risks. The subsequent period—from hospital discharge to full recovery—is often traumatic and confusing for both patients and families. After discharge, many patients still feel unwell and yet are expected to follow complex medication regimens and return for follow-up visits and tests. The growth of the hospitalist model means that the inpatient and outpatient providers are often different individuals, which may lead to miscommunication between providers and add to the patient's anxiety over the transition out of the hospital. Finally, for many patients, the costs of hospital care are fully borne by third-party payers, while the costs of skilled nursing or home care must be covered partially or completely with personal resources.

In the past, a physician's decision to discharge a patient was often governed by intuition and experience. In the past decade, high-quality studies have come to provide a scientific basis for many discharge decisions. This chapter illustrates principles of research on the timing and process of hospital discharge, focusing on optimizing the hospital discharge process in four general areas: (1) implementing disease-specific strategies in the form of guidelines or educational initiatives; (2) improving patient safety; (3) enhancing communication and follow-up; and (4) facilitating discharge planning.

EVIDENCE-BASED, DISEASE-SPECIFIC APPROACHES TO DISCHARGE

Community-acquired pneumonia (CAP) probably has the best-elucidated discharge criteria and processes of all the disorders that physicians treat in the hospital (see Chapter 65 for further information on management of CAP). Several studies have tested whether the use of practice guidelines or decision support improves the efficiency and quality of care for patients with CAP (4–6). Most studies show that practice guidelines promoting early identification of low-risk patients and evidence-based choice of antibiotics can lead to earlier discharge with maintained patient outcomes and satisfaction.

Hospitalized patients with CAP can be discharged when they are clinically stable, and the time required to reach clinical stability is more rapid than previously appreciated. Among patients with vital sign abnormalities on presentation, the median time to stabilization of the heart rate (≤ 100 bpm) and systolic blood pressure (≥ 90 mm Hg) is two days (7). The average patient achieves a stable respiratory rate (≤ 24 breaths/min), oxygen saturation ($\geq 92\%$), and temperature ($\leq 99°$ F ($37.2°$ C)) on hospital day three. The time to overall clinical stability, defined as stable vital signs, baseline mental status, and ability to eat, varies depending on the pneumonia severity on presentation: it averages three days for low-risk patients (Pneumonia Severity Index risk class I through III), four days for moderate-risk patients (risk class IV), and six days for high-risk patients (risk class V) (8).

Such explicit criteria defining when a patient is medically stable for discharge may standardize the physician's approach to patients with common medical problems. Evidence-based guidelines and algorithms that help guide the discharge decision are also available for upper gastrointestinal bleeding (9), congestive heart failure (10), asthma (11), and stroke (12). (See also Chapters 78, 39, 56, and 116.)

While such disease-specific discharge criteria and cost effectiveness analyses may help guide lengths of stay, other clinically important factors must be considered. For example, hospitalization beyond three days for patients with uncomplicated myocardial infarction is not cost effective (13). However, when implementing any early discharge guidelines, it is important to measure quality, patient satisfaction, and long-term follow-up to ensure that short-term benefits (in decreased costs caused by shorter lengths of stay) are not associated with detrimental long-term outcomes. In the coming years, clinicians can expect to see more information, much of it computerized, available at the point of care and tailored to their patients' clinical presentation. This information will help inform the discharge process for an array of hospital diagnoses.

PATIENT SAFETY

Hospital discharge is often a chaotic and potentially dangerous time for both patients and providers, ripe with opportunities to improve both patient outcomes and satisfaction. Functional limitations may persist and make patients especially vulnerable to injuries with the increased activity of the peridischarge period. Particularly in hospitalist systems, the transition from inpatient to outpatient care may become fraught with miscommunication and inadequate follow-up.

Many of the adverse events that occur frequently during the post-hospital period are preventable or ameliorable (14). The most common events are adverse drug events, but harm may also come from unaddressed laboratory abnormalities. Changes in system design can improve patient safety during the peridischarge period and should focus on four areas: (1) evaluating patients at the time of discharge; (2) educating patients about drug therapies, side effects, and actions to take if specific problems occur; (3) strengthening monitoring of therapies; and (4) improving monitoring of patients' overall condition.

STRATEGIES FOR EFFECTIVE DISCHARGE

To optimize the effectiveness of the hospital discharge, *communication* at discharge and follow-up must be enhanced. Communication gaps are common at the time of hospital discharge, yet physicians and nurses tend to overestimate patients' comprehension of discharge treatment plans. In one study, physicians believed that 89% of patients understood the potential side effects of their medications, but only 57% of patients confirmed that they understood (15). A similar gap occurred regarding patients' understanding of when to resume normal activities (16).

Although communication is a core skill for physicians, many patients have difficulty understanding what physicians tell them. This is particularly a problem for patients who have inadequate *health literacy*. Health literacy has been defined as the ability to read and comprehend prescription bottles, appointment slips, and written discharge instructions (17). Several strategies, including structured patient education, postdischarge telephone follow-up, communication improvement between inpatient and outpatient providers, and multidisciplinary discharge planning teams, have been shown to improve communication at the time of discharge and may yield more satisfied patients (see Table 5.1).

TABLE 5.1

POTENTIALLY EFFECTIVE DISCHARGE STRATEGIES

Strategy	Comments
Intensive postdischarge care	• Contacting patients after discharge • Improving access • Following up on missed visits (41)
Telephone follow-up	• Substituting for routine clinic follow-up (42) • Using pharmacists/focusing on medication compliance (23)
Patient education and communication	• See Table 5.2
Predischarge checklist	• List of requirements for equipment, services, benefits, and follow-up (43)
Multidisciplinary discharge planning/ discharge coordinator	• Multidisciplinary task force, comprising planner, social worker, nurse, dietician, chaplain, therapist, and utilization review nurse; discusses patients (44)
Home visits	• Collaborative discharge planning and home follow-up (including telephone and home visits by advanced practice nurses for four weeks after discharge) provided to elders hospitalized with common medical and surgical cardiac conditions (45)

Structured Patient Education

Hospital discharge is a critical transition zone, from a time when all care is delivered by hospital staff to one in which the patient, and possibly family, are entirely responsible. Making this transition safely depends on high-quality, structured patient education. Too often, however, such education is neglected, in part because unrecognized barriers interfere. Hospital physicians need to appreciate patients' capability to assimilate discharge instructions. Although providers usually assume patients comprehend their written and oral explanations of illness, several studies have shown that health literacy is often worse than providers think (18). Many health materials, including patient education brochures, discharge instruction sheets, and informed consent documents, are written at levels far exceeding patients' reading abilities. More than one third of patients age 65 and older have inadequate or marginal health literacy (19).

The terminology or language health care providers use in communicating with patients is a significant barrier for patients who have inadequate health literacy. Physicians' facile overuse of medical terms, combined with patients' limited health vocabulary, results in inadequate and even confusing communication. Unfortunately, patients with low health literacy tend to ask fewer questions, even though they may feel overwhelmed with information and lack understanding.

Checking to ensure that the patient's history is accurate and that the patient understands the physician's instructions are the most important interviewing skills. Unfortunately, they are also the least utilized. In one study of audiotaped encounters, primary care physicians assessed patients' understanding only 2% of the time (20). Written materials can be used to augment patient education, but video and computer multimedia programs are even more powerful interventions. Pictographs (simple pictures that represent ideas) markedly enhance recall of spoken medical instructions among all patients. Using pictographs as visual aids (e.g., simply drawing a picture related to what you want the patient to remember) can more than quadruple patients' ability to recall important medical information (21).

Based on published research and the authors' experience in caring for patients, the following six simple steps for structuring patient education are recommended (see Table 5.2) (17). First, slow down and take time to assess patients' health literacy skills. Second, use "living room" language that patients can understand, taking care either to avoid medical terminology or to explain medical terms when they must be used. Third, show or draw pictures to enhance understanding and subsequent recall. Fourth, limit the quantity of information given to patients at each interaction, and repeat instructions several times. Enrolling family members in the process may allow more information to be disseminated and retained. Fifth, use a "teach back" or "show me" approach to confirm comprehension. Ask

---

TABLE 5.2

SIX STEPS TO ENHANCE UNDERSTANDING AMONG PATIENTS WITH LOW HEALTH LITERACY

- Slow down and take time to assess patients' health literacy skills.
- Use "living room" language instead of medical terminology.
- Show or draw pictures to enhance understanding and subsequent recall.
- Limit information given at each interaction, and repeat instructions.
- Use a "teach back" or "show me" approach to confirm understanding.
- Be respectful, caring, and sensitive, thereby empowering patients to participate in their own health care.

---

patients to demonstrate their instructions (i.e., teach back to you how to take their medications or when they should follow up) to ensure that you have done an adequate job of instruction. Never ask, "Do you understand?" because patients will typically acquiesce and say, "Yes." Last, be respectful, caring, and sensitive to the plight of patients who have low health literacy. This six-step approach will enhance patient satisfaction and empower patients to optimize their participation in their health care.

Postdischarge Telephone Follow-Up

Telephone follow-up with discharged patients has been proposed as one way to mitigate discharge communication problems (see Table 5.3). Although this approach is intuitively appealing, surprisingly few studies have been conducted of telephone follow-up at the time of hospital discharge. Telephone follow-up after emergency department visits has improved patient satisfaction and compliance with follow-up instructions and appointments (22). In one small study, a postdischarge follow-up call by a pharmacist involved in the care of hospitalized patients led to enhanced patient satisfaction, fewer returns to the emergency department, and frequent resolution of medication-related issues (23). Postdischarge telephone follow-up may also improve adherence, inform the hospital physician about the results of treatment or of adverse outcomes, and enable hospitalists to receive feedback from the patient and family (24).

Improving Communication Between Inpatient and Outpatient Providers

Appropriate transfer of information at the time of hospital discharge reduces rates of readmission, medication errors, and medical costs (25). Discharge summaries or letters and telephone interchange are the key tools to optimize communication during these hand-offs and to reinforce continuity of care.

TABLE 5.3

STRATEGIES TO IMPROVE COMMUNICATION BETWEEN THE INPATIENT AND OUTPATIENT PHYSICIANS AT DISCHARGE

Intervention	Pros (positive outcomes)	Cons
Telephone follow-up with patients (24)	• Improves adherence • Informs the inpatient physician about the results of treatment or of adverse outcomes • Permits hospitalists to receive feedback from the patient and family	• Time • May interfere with role of PCP • Not reimbursed
Telephone communication between providers (29)	• Provides continuity • Clarifies history or diagnosis • Provides information about chronic problem management • Clarifies psychosocial and cultural factors (30)	• Time • Not reimbursed
Optimization of conventional discharge summaries (26)	• Enhances PCP satisfaction and continuity of care through timely and concise documents • Facilitates follow-up care, especially when focused on relevant discharge-related information	
Discharge information cards/letters (28)	• Draws favorable response from PCPs and patients • Better informs patients about their illnesses and treatments	
Electronic discharge summary (27)	• Enables timeliness, increased PCP satisfaction, cost effectiveness, efficiency, and clinical auditing • Reduces error rates • Increases efficiency, supports continuity of care	• Higher systems costs
Patient-delivered discharge summary (28)	• Compels inpatient physicians to complete summaries early, while information is fresh • Keeps PCPs up to date with discharge details • Saves money on postage costs	• Some patients may have difficulty traveling to hand-deliver their summaries

Despite its documented deficiencies, including delays and inadequacies in information transfer, the discharge summary or discharge letter remains the main means of communication between inpatient physicians and primary care providers. Physicians rate discharge summaries highly if they are timely, concise, and contain focused discharge information. This information includes admission diagnosis, relevant physical examination findings, laboratory results, procedures, hospital complications, discharge diagnoses, discharge medications, active medical problems, and follow-up (26). Using computerized discharge summaries promotes timeliness, increased PCP satisfaction, cost effectiveness, efficiency, reduced error rate, and easier clinical auditing (27). Discharge information cards and associated discharge letters are favorably received by patients and providers, and they better inform patients about their illness and treatment than traditional discharge processes (28).

Interphysician communication by phone can contribute substantially to continuity and quality of patient care during the discharge process. In a survey of family physicians, primary care physicians overwhelmingly stated their preference to communicate with hospitalists by telephone (77%), particularly at admission and discharge (29). Not surprisingly, primary care physicians who are personally contacted are more likely to make hospital visits and help provide continuity, particularly by clarifying history, diagnosis, psychosocial, and cultural factors (30).

Facilitating Discharge Planning

The cumulative impact of communication gaps and other coordination problems leaves patients less satisfied with hospital discharge planning than with any other aspect of hospital care (31). Discharge planning is defined as the development of an individualized discharge plan for a patient in anticipation of leaving the hospital for home or other postdischarge facility. The old adage that discharge planning starts upon admission seems more important today than ever.

Although the concept of advance discharge planning is intuitively attractive, the literature reveals mixed results, possibly reflecting the variable study populations and different means of implementing site-specific interventions. A Cochrane review did not demonstrate that discharge planning was effective in reducing unplanned hospital admissions (32). Yet some evidence suggests that discharge planning may lead to decreased hospital length of stay (33–36) and, in some cases, reduced readmission rates (35,37). Further, discharge planning may improve patient satisfaction (33). Notwithstanding the sparse evidence, the authors believe all hospitalized patients should receive individualized discharge plans in light of the enhanced patient satisfaction and the increasing complexity of treatment regimes.

Disease-specific management teams improve discharge planning, especially among patients with diabetes. Multidisciplinary diabetes teams, typically comprising endocrinologists, nurse-educators, nutritionists, and social workers, bridge the inpatient and outpatient environments, enhance coordination of care, clarify goals of care for patients and team members, provide more consistent patient instructions, and promote involvement of patients and families in their own care (38). Such teams can also reduce hospital length of stay, improve glycemic control, and decrease readmissions. Combining this team approach with a nursing case management model and referral links to podiatry and ophthalmology also reduces length of stay and cost while improving glycemic control and readmission rates (39,40). The applicability of this model to other chronic diseases is under study.

CONCLUSIONS

One of the most important changes in the paradigm of modern medicine is the recognition that high-quality and efficient practice depends as much on the system of care as on the competence of the physicians. This principle is rarely more applicable than at hospital discharge. Patients benefit when discharge planning begins soon after admission, when discharge decisions are informed by evidence, and when patients are cared for in a system that promotes an effective discharge process. Such a system should be designed to make errors less likely, encourage teamwork across disciplines, and facilitate communication across the inpatient-outpatient divide. Improving the discharge process should be an important goal of all health care workers and systems.

KEY POINTS

- Adverse events occur frequently in the peridischarge period, and many can be prevented or ameliorated with simple strategies that improve communication and follow-up at discharge.

- Patient education about conditions, medications, actions to take if symptoms develop, and follow-up care is a critical component of the discharge process.
- Improving communication between inpatient and outpatient providers at the time of hospital discharge is critical to optimizing patient care.

REFERENCES

1. Taheri PA, Butz DA, Greenfield LJ. Length of stay has minimal impact on the cost of hospital admission. *J Am Coll Surg* 2000; 191:123–130.
2. Fine MJ, Pratt HM, Obrosky DS, et al. Relation between length of hospital stay and costs of care for patients with community-acquired pneumonia. *Am J Med* 2000;109:378–385.
3. Rothschild JM, Bates DW, Leape LL. Preventable medical injuries in older patients. *Arch Intern Med* 2000;160:2717–2728.
4. Weingarten SR, Riedinger MS, Hobson P, et al. Evaluation of a pneumonia practice guideline in an interventional trial. *Am J Respir Crit Care Med* 1996;153:1110–1115.
5. Marrie TJ, Lau CY, Wheeler SL, Wong CJ, Vandervoort MK, Feagan BG. A controlled trial of a critical pathway for treatment of community-acquired pneumonia. CAPITAL Study Investigators. Community-Acquired Pneumonia Intervention Trial Assessing Levofloxacin. *JAMA* 2000;283:749–755.
6. Dean NC, Silver MP, Bateman KA, James B, Hadlock CJ, Hale D. Decreased mortality after implementation of a treatment guideline for community-acquired pneumonia. *Am J Med* 2001; 110:451–457.
7. Halm EA, Fine MJ, Marrie TJ, et al. Time to clinical stability in patients hospitalized with community-acquired pneumonia: implications for practice guidelines. *JAMA* 1998;279:1452–1457.
8. Fine MJ, Auble TE, Yealy DM, et al. A prediction rule to identify low-risk patients with community-acquired pneumonia. *N Engl J Med* 1997;336:243–250.
9. Eisen GM, Dominitz JA, Faigel DO, et al. An annotated algorithmic approach to upper gastrointestinal bleeding. *Gastrointest Endosc* 2001;53:853–858.
10. Hunt SA, Baker DW, Chin MH, et al. ACC/AHA Guidelines for the Evaluation and Management of Chronic Heart Failure in the Adult: Executive Summary A Report of the American College of Cardiology/American Heart Association Task Force on Practice Guidelines (Committee to Revise the 1995 Guidelines for the Evaluation and Management of Heart Failure): Developed in Collaboration With the International Society for Heart and Lung Transplantation; Endorsed by the Heart Failure Society of America. *Circulation* 2001;104:2996–3007.
11. National Asthma Education and Prevention Program. Expert panel report: guidelines for the diagnosis and management of asthma update on selected topics—2002. *J Allergy Clin Immunol* 2002;110:S141–S219.
12. Anderson C, Mhurchu CN, Rubenach S, Clark M, Spencer C, Winsor A. Home or hospital for stroke rehabilitation? Results of a randomized controlled trial: II: cost minimization analysis at 6 months. *Stroke* 2000;31:1032–1037.
13. Newby LK, Eisenstein EL, Califf RL, et al. Cost effectiveness of early discharge after uncomplicated acute myocardial infarction. *N Engl J Med* 2000;342:749–755.
14. Forster AJ, Murff HJ, Peterson JF, Gandhi TK, Bates DW. The incidence and severity of adverse events affecting patients after discharge from the hospital. *Ann Intern Med* 2003;138:161–167.
15. Reiley P, Iezzoni LI, Phillips R, Davis RB, Tuchin LI, Calkins D. Discharge planning: comparison of patients and nurses' perceptions of patients following hospital discharge. *Image J Nurs Sch* 1996;28:143–147.
16. Calkins DR, Davis RB, Reiley P, et al. Patient-physician communication at hospital discharge and patients' understanding of the postdischarge treatment plan. *Arch Intern Med* 1997;157:1026–1030.
17. Williams MV, Davis T, Parker RM, Weiss BD. The role of health literacy in patient-physician communication. *Fam Med* 2002;34: 383–389.

18. Health literacy: report of the Council on Scientific Affairs. Ad Hoc Committee on Health Literacy for the Council on Scientific Affairs, American Medical Association. *JAMA* 1999;281:552–557.

19. Gazmararian JA, Baker DW, Williams MV, et al. Health literacy among Medicare enrollees in a managed care organization. *JAMA* 1999;281:545–551.

20. Braddock CH, 3rd, Fihn SD, Levinson W, Jonsen AR, Pearlman RA. How doctors and patients discuss routine clinical decisions. Informed decision making in the outpatient setting. *J Gen Intern Med* 1997;12:339–345.

21. Houts PS, Bachrach R, Witmer JT, Tringali, CA, Bucher JA, Localio RA. Using pictographs to enhance recall of spoken medical instructions. *Patient Educ Couns* 1998;35:83–88.

22. Jones J, Clark W, Bradford J, Dougherty J. Efficacy of a telephone follow-up system in the emergency department. *J Emerg Med* 1988;6:249–254.

23. Dudas V, Bookwalter T, Kerr KM, Pantilat SZ. The impact of follow-up telephone calls to patients after hospitalization. *Dis Mon* 2002;48:239–248.

24. Nelson JR. The importance of postdischarge telephone follow-up for hospitalists: a view from the trenches. *Am J Med* 2001;111: 43S–44S.

25. van Walraven C, Seth R, Austin PC, Laupacis A. Effect of discharge summary availability during post-discharge visits on hospital readmission. *J Gen Intern Med* 2002;17:186–192.

26. van Walraven C, Rokosh E. What is necessary for high-quality discharge summaries? *Am J Med Qual* 1999;14:160–169.

27. Bolton P. A review of the role of information technology in discharge communications in Australia. *Aust Health Rev* 1999;22: 56–64.

28. Sandler DA, Heaton C, Garner ST, Mitchell JR. Patients' and general practitioners' satisfaction with information given on discharge from hospital: audit of a new information card. *BMJ* 1989;299:1511–1513.

29. Pantilat SZ, Lindenauer PK, Katz PP, Wachter RM. Primary care physician attitudes regarding communication with hospitalists. *Am J Med* 2001;111:15S–20S.

30. Ways M, Umali J, Buchwald D. Frequency and impact of housestaff contact with primary care physicians. *J Gen Intern Med* 1995;10:688–690.

31. Hickey ML, Kleefield SF, Pearson SD, et al. Payer-hospital collaboration to improve patient satisfaction with hospital discharge. *Jt Comm J Qual Improv* 1996;22:336–344.

32. Parkes J, Shepperd S. Discharge planning from hospital to home. Cochrane Database Syst Rev 2000:CD000313.

33. Moher D, Weinberg A, Hanlon R, Runnalls K. Effects of a medical team coordinator on length of hospital stay. *CMAJ* 1992;146: 511–515.

34. Naughton BJ, Moran MB, Feinglass J, Falconer J, Williams ME. Reducing hospital costs for the geriatric patient admitted from the emergency department: a randomized trial. *J Am Geriatr Soc* 1994;42:1045–1049.

35. Naylor M, Brooten JD, Jones R, Lavizzo-Mourey R, Mezey M, Pauly M. Comprehensive discharge planning for the hospitalized elderly. A randomized clinical trial. *Ann Intern Med* 1994;120: 999–1006.

36. Parfrey PS, Gardner E, Vavasour H, et al. The feasibility and efficacy of early discharge planning initiated by the admitting department in two acute care hospitals. *Clin Invest Med* 1994;17:88–96.

37. Evans RL, Hendricks RD. Evaluating hospital discharge planning: a randomized clinical trial. *Med Care* 1993;31:358–370.

38. Ellrodt G, Cook DJ, Lee J, Cho M, Hunt D, Weingarten S. Evidence-based disease management. *JAMA* 1997;278:1687–1692.

39. Edelstein EL, Cesta TG. Nursing case management: an innovative model of care for hospitalized patients with diabetes. *Diabetes Educ* 1993;19:517–521.

40. Koproski J, Pretto Z, Poretsky L. Effects of an intervention by a diabetes team in hospitalized patients with diabetes. *Diabetes Care* 1997;20:1553–1555.

41. Weinberger M, Smith DM, Katz BP, Moore PS. The cost-effectiveness of intensive postdischarge care: a randomized trial. *Med Care* 1988;26:1092–1102.

42. Wasson J, Gaudette C, Whaley F, Sauvigne A, Baribeau P, Welch HG. Telephone care as a substitute for routine clinic follow-up. *JAMA* 1992;267:1788–1793.

43. Hunter J, Weir AM, Macpherson K, Mercer S. Is a pre-discharge checklist useful? *J R Coll Physicians Lond* 1996;30:162–163.

44. Pray D, Hoff J. Implementing a multidisciplinary approach to discharge planning. *Nurs Manage* 1992;23:52–53, 56.

45. Naylor MD, McCauley KM. The effects of a discharge planning and home follow-up intervention on elders hospitalized with common medical and surgical cardiac conditions. *J Cardiovasc Nurs* 1999;14:44–54.

ADDITIONAL READING

Forster AJ, Clark HD, Menard A, et al. Adverse events among medical patients after discharge from hospital. *CMAJ* 2004;170:345–349.

van Walraven C, Mamdani M, Fang J, Austin PC. Continuity of care and patient outcomes after hospital discharge. *J Gen Intern Med* 2004;19:624–631.

Bayesian Reasoning and Diagnostic Testing

6

Warren S. Browner

INTRODUCTION

Making clinical decisions often involves using diagnostic tests to determine whether a patient has a particular disease. Some of the best diagnostic tests—such as listening for rales or asking patients whether they have chest pain while walking uphill—are performed during the history and physical examination. The same principles that apply to the interpretation of these customary tests also apply to the interpretation of more sophisticated tests, such as measurement of the serum ceruloplasmin value or ultrasonography to detect an abdominal aortic aneurysm.

Bayesian reasoning is a formal way of doing explicitly what most clinicians do implicitly, that is, interpreting the results of a diagnostic test in light of the clinical situation. The basic paradigm is simple:

> What was thought before the test was done & the test result → what is thought after the test result

The ampersand sign (&) indicates that this is not a simple problem in addition. The mathematics, developed by an 18th-century amateur mathematician, Thomas Bayes, are known as Bayes' theorem.

For example, suppose a clinician believes that a particular disease (e.g., appendicitis in a young man with gastrointestinal symptoms, fever, and right lower quadrant pain) is likely before ordering a diagnostic test. If the test result is positive (say, an abnormal result on an abdominal computed tomogram), the clinician will be almost certain that the patient has appendicitis (Chapter 87). On the other hand, if the clinician thinks that appendicitis is unlikely before ordering the test, and the test result is negative, the clinician will be almost certain that the patient does not have appendicitis. If the clinical impression and the test result differ, or if the clinician was not sure before and the test result is borderline, then the situation remains uncertain.

Clinicians seek the perfect test, or *gold standard*, such that a negative test result rules out the diagnosis and a positive result rules it in. Few tests are perfect, especially because human and machine fallibility mean that even gold standards, such as excisional biopsies, can be tarnished. For nearly all tests, one must be satisfied that a negative result reduces the likelihood of a disease (e.g., normal chest radiographic findings in a case of possible pneumonia), whereas a positive result increases the likelihood of the disease (e.g., a lobar infiltrate on the chest radiogram in a patient with suspected pneumonia).

Many clinicians use time as the gold standard, assuming that all diseases will "declare themselves" given adequate follow-up. Even if this were true, a more efficient diagnostic strategy would involve selecting tests with results sufficiently definitive to affect a patient's management. Not ordering an expensive diagnostic test to save money is rarely an efficient strategy in a hospitalized patient.

A QUALITATIVE APPROACH TO TEST INTERPRETATION

This basic idea can be refined further, as most tests have more than two results. Thus, a highly negative result greatly decreases the probability of a disease, whereas a highly positive result greatly increases the probability. Intermediate results have intermediate effects (see Table 6.1).

Adapted with permission from Guyatt GH, Oxman AD, Ali M, Willan A, McIlroy W, Patterson C. Laboratory diagnosis of iron-deficiency anemia: an overview. *J Gen Intern Med* 1992;7:145–153. (Published erratum in *J Gen Intern Med* 1992;7:423.)

TABLE 6.1

EFFECTS OF A TEST RESULT ON THE PROBABILITY OF A DISEASE

Test results	Example (1)
Very negative, greatly decreases the probability of the disease	Ferritin = 300 mcg/L in the patient in whom iron deficiency anemia is being considered
Slightly negative, slightly decreases the probability of the disease	Ferritin = 100 mcg/L and iron deficiency anemia
Borderline, does not affect the probability of the disease	Ferritin = 30 mcg/L and iron deficiency anemia
Slightly positive, slightly increases the probability of the disease	Ferritin = 20 mcg/L and iron deficiency anemia
Very positive, greatly increases the probability of the disease	Ferritin = 5 mcg/L and iron deficiency anemia

A QUANTITATIVE APPROACH

To express the probability of a disease quantitatively, the elements of the basic paradigm must be converted into numbers:

(*a*)	(*b*)	(*c*)
What was thought before the test was done	& the test result→	what is thought after

The concept of "what was thought before" (*a*) is the *prior probability* of the disease. It estimates how likely it is that the patient has the disease. The prior probability must be estimated before the test result is known. Prior probabilities vary from 0% to 100%. They replace vague terms such as "very unlikely," "probable," and "almost certain." Prior probabilities are sometimes called *pretest probabilities*.

When setting prior probabilities, remember that the patient's problem must have an explanation. Thus, *the sum of all of the prior probabilities for the diagnostic possibilities should be 100%*. It is not adequate to decide—in a patient with dyspnea—that the probability of pneumonia is 1%, of pulmonary embolism 1%, of asthma 2%, of congestive heart failure 3%, and of other conditions even lower percentages.

"The test result" (*b*) is expressed as a *likelihood ratio* (LR). A test does not have a single LR. Rather, each possible result of the test has its own LR for the disease in question. The LR for a test result is between zero and infinity (see Table 6.2). The LRs have been determined for many common diag-

nostic tests and diseases. For coronary artery disease (CAD) (defined as an obstruction of 75% or more in at least one artery), typical angina (exertional substernal chest pressure that is relieved by nitroglycerin or rest within minutes) has an LR of 120! Even atypical angina (in which one of these features is not present) has an LR of about 15 (2). On the other hand, musculoskeletal chest pain (pain that can be reproduced by pressing on the chest) has an LR of about 1. (A more familiar, but less useful, approach expresses the test result in terms of the *sensitivity* and *specificity* of a test; this approach is discussed later.)

"What is thought after" (*c*) is called the *posterior probability*, an estimate of the likelihood that the patient has the disease, made after the test result is known. Posterior probabilities vary from 0% to 100%. They are sometimes called *posttest probabilities*.

If the LR is greater than 1, then the posterior probability is greater than the prior probability. If the LR equals 1, then the posterior probability is the same as the prior probability. And if the LR is less than 1, then the posterior probability is less than the prior probability.

More precisely, Table 6.3 can be used to combine the prior probability with the LR for the test result to estimate the posterior probability. For example, consider a 62-year-old man with hypertension and diabetes who presents with a one-month history of substernal chest pain when climbing hills, relieved in minutes by rest. His serum cholesterol level is 240 mg/dL. Assume that the prior probability of CAD (based on sex, age, and risk factors) is about 20% to 40% (2). The diagnostic test in this case is the history; the result of "typical angina" has an LR greater than 100 for CAD. Use Table 6.3 and look across from the LR of 100; the posterior probability of CAD is between 96% (looking down from a prior probability of 20%) and 99% (looking down from 40%). This example demonstrates that it is

TABLE 6.2

EXAMPLES OF LIKELIHOOD RATIOS AND THEIR EFFECTS ON THE PROBABILITY OF A DISEASE

Likelihood ratio	Effect on probability of the disease
Zero (0)	Test result rules out the disease.
Very small (e.g., 0.01)	Test result greatly decreases the probability of the disease.
<1 (e.g., 0.5)	Test result decreases the probability of the disease.
One (1)	Test result has no effect on the probability of the disease.
>1 (e.g., 2)	Test result increases the probability of the disease.
Very big (e.g., 50)	Test result greatly increases the probability of the disease.
Infinite (∞)	Test result rules in the disease.

TABLE 6.3

CONVERTING PRIOR PROBABILITIES AND LIKELIHOOD RATIOS INTO POSTERIOR PROBABILITIES[a]

Likelihood ratio	Prior probability														
	0.001	0.005	0.01	0.05	0.1	0.2	0.3	0.4	0.5	0.6	0.7	0.8	0.9	0.95	0.99
0.01	0.00001	0.00005	0.0001	0.0005	0.001	0.002	0.004	0.007	0.01	0.01	0.02	0.04	0.08	0.16	0.50
0.02	0.00002	0.0001	0.0002	0.001	0.002	0.005	0.008	0.013	0.02	0.03	0.04	0.07	0.15	0.28	0.66
0.05	0.00005	0.0003	0.0005	0.003	0.006	0.012	0.02	0.03	0.05	0.07	0.10	0.17	0.31	0.49	0.83
0.1	0.0001	0.0005	0.001	0.005	0.01	0.02	0.04	0.06	0.09	0.13	0.19	0.29	0.47	0.66	0.91
0.2	0.0002	0.0010	0.002	0.01	0.02	0.05	0.08	0.12	0.17	0.23	0.32	0.44	0.64	0.79	0.95
0.3	0.0003	0.0015	0.003	0.02	0.03	0.07	0.11	0.17	0.23	0.31	0.41	0.55	0.73	0.85	0.97
0.4	0.0004	0.0020	0.004	0.02	0.04	0.09	0.15	0.21	0.29	0.38	0.48	0.62	0.78	0.88	0.98
0.5	0.0005	0.0025	0.005	0.03	0.05	0.11	0.18	0.25	0.33	0.43	0.54	0.67	0.82	0.90	0.98
0.6	0.0006	0.0030	0.006	0.03	0.06	0.13	0.20	0.29	0.38	0.47	0.58	0.71	0.84	0.92	0.98
0.8	0.0008	0.0040	0.008	0.04	0.08	0.17	0.26	0.35	0.44	0.55	0.65	0.76	0.88	0.94	0.99
1.0	0.0010	0.0050	0.010	0.05	0.10	0.20	0.30	0.40	0.50	0.60	0.70	0.80	0.90	0.95	0.99
1.2	0.0012	0.0060	0.012	0.06	0.12	0.23	0.34	0.44	0.55	0.64	0.74	0.83	0.92	0.96	0.99
1.5	0.0015	0.0075	0.01	0.07	0.14	0.27	0.39	0.50	0.60	0.69	0.78	0.86	0.93	0.97	0.99
2.0	0.0020	0.010	0.02	0.10	0.18	0.33	0.46	0.57	0.67	0.75	0.82	0.89	0.95	0.97	0.99
2.5	0.0025	0.012	0.02	0.12	0.22	0.38	0.52	0.63	0.71	0.79	0.85	0.91	0.96	0.98	0.996
3.0	0.003	0.015	0.03	0.14	0.25	0.43	0.56	0.67	0.75	0.82	0.88	0.92	0.96	0.98	0.997
5	0.005	0.02	0.05	0.21	0.36	0.56	0.68	0.77	0.83	0.88	0.92	0.95	0.98	0.99	0.998
10	0.010	0.05	0.09	0.34	0.53	0.71	0.81	0.87	0.91	0.94	0.96	0.98	0.99	0.99	0.999
20	0.020	0.09	0.17	0.51	0.69	0.83	0.90	0.93	0.95	0.97	0.98	0.99	0.99	0.997	0.999
50	0.048	0.20	0.34	0.72	0.85	0.93	0.96	0.97	0.98	0.99	0.992	0.995	0.998	0.999	0.9998
100	0.091	0.33	0.50	0.84	0.92	0.96	0.98	0.99	0.99	0.993	0.996	0.998	0.999	0.999	0.9999

[a]This table is based on a three-stage process that combines prior probabilities and likelihood ratios to yield posterior probabilities. The mathematics involve converting the prior probability to a prior odds [= Prior Probability ÷ (1 − Prior Probability)], then multiplying the prior odds by the likelihood ratio to obtain the posterior odds, and then converting those posterior odds back to a posterior probability [= Posterior Odds ÷ (1 + Posterior Odds)].

often unnecessary to make a precise estimate of the prior probability. Although there is a twofold difference between 20% and 40%, the posterior probabilities are similar.

On the other hand, suppose that the patient is a 23-year-old woman with a two- to three-week history of left-sided chest pain after swimming that sometimes lasts seconds and sometimes an hour or two. Movement of her arms exacerbates the symptoms. The prior probability of CAD (based on sex and age) is, at most, 0.1%. Because her diagnostic test result (history consistent with musculoskeletal chest pain) has an LR of 1.0 for CAD, her posttest probability is not changed from her pretest value.

WHERE DO LIKELIHOOD RATIOS COME FROM?

The LRs are the ratio of two likelihoods of obtaining a particular test result:

$$\text{LR for a Test Result} = \frac{\textit{Likelihood of Test Result in Patients with Disease}}{\textit{Likelihood of Test Result in Patients without Disease}}$$

(The mnemonic is WOWO, for "with over without.") The LRs are determined by making a column of the number (and percentage) of patients with the disease who have each possible result of a diagnostic test; a similar column is also made for patients without the disease. Table 6.4 shows such results for the exercise stress test (Chapter 36).

For example, the LR for ST segment depression of 2 mm or more is determined as follows:

$$\text{LR } (\geq 2 \text{ mm}) = \frac{\textit{Likelihood of} \geq 2 \text{ mm in CAD}}{\textit{Likelihood of} \geq 2 \text{ mm in no CAD}}$$

$$= \frac{30\%}{1\%}$$

$$= 30$$

In the same way,

$$\text{LR } (1.5 - 1.9 \text{ mm}) = \frac{20\%}{5\%} \qquad \text{LR } (1 - 1.4 \text{ mm}) = \frac{24\%}{10\%}$$

$$= 4 \qquad\qquad = 2.4$$

$$\text{LR (trace)} = \frac{16\%}{24\%} = 0.67 \qquad \text{LR (none)} = \frac{10\%}{60\%} = 0.17$$

TABLE 6.4

CALCULATING LIKELIHOOD RATIOS FOR ST SEGMENT DEPRESSION DURING EXERCISE STRESS TESTING[a]

ST Segment Depression	Coronary artery disease (*N* = 50)		No coronary artery disease (*N* = 200)	
	N	**%**	**N**	**%**
≥2 mm	15	30	2	1
1.5–1.9 mm	10	20	10	5
1–1.4 mm	12	24	20	10
Trace (<1 mm)	8	16	48	24
None	5	10	120	60
Total	50	100	200	100

[a]Simplified for ease of calculation.

USING LIKELIHOOD RATIOS IN SEQUENCE

One attribute of LRs is that they can be used in sequence as long as the test results are independent.[1] That is, one can keep modifying the posterior probability based on a series of results.

Prior & LR Test Result No. 1 →

Posterior & LR Test Result No. 2 →

New Posterior & LR Test Result No. 3 → etc.

For example, consider a 35-year-old man who presents with a chief complaint of dyspnea and pleuritic chest pain. He reports a "vein problem in my legs that was treated with a blood thinner for a few months last year." A chest radiograph shows a patchy infiltrate in the left upper lung field. A room air arterial blood gas specimen has a PO_2 of 92 mm Hg, with a PCO_2 of 38 mm Hg, for an alveolar-to-arterial (A-a) gradient of [147 − (1.25 × 38) − 92] = 7 mm Hg.

You assess the prior probability of pulmonary embolism as the cause of dyspnea in a population of 35-year-old men as about 5%. How helpful are the patient's history and examination and laboratory findings? About 25% of patients with pulmonary embolism have a history of venous throm-

boembolic disease (3), which occurs in about 0.8% of healthy middle-aged men (4), for a likelihood ratio of 25% divided by 0.8%, or about 30. Pleuritic chest pain and abnormal chest radiographic findings are not particularly more common in pulmonary embolism than in other disorders confused with it, so their LRs are about 1 (5). An A-a gradient of 7 mm Hg has an LR of about 0.1 for pulmonary embolism (3).

If you assume that all these test results are independent, then their combined LR is simply the product of the individual LRs, or 30 × 1 × 1 × 0.1 = 3. Thus, if the prior probability that this patient has a pulmonary embolism was about 5%, then the posterior probability is about 15%, according to Table 6.3. This value is in the range that requires an additional diagnostic test, such as a spiral CT scan (6) or a ventilation–perfusion scan (7), before the appropriate treatment can be determined (Chapter 53).

SENSITIVITY AND SPECIFICITY

Sensitivity and specificity are alternate ways to describe the characteristics of a test. The *sensitivity* of a diagnostic test indicates the proportion of persons with a disease who have a positive test result. The *specificity* of a diagnostic test indicates the proportion of persons without a disease who have a negative test result. Returning to the example of the exercise stress test in a patient with chest pain, with a cut-off point of 2 mm or more of ST depression (see Table 6.5), the test would have a sensitivity of only 30% (15/50) but a specificity of 99% (198/200). To improve the sensitivity, one could change the cut-off for a positive test result to 1 mm or more (see Table 6.6). This would improve the sensitivity, but the specificity would decline. The sensitivity and specificity are combined with the prior probability of a disease to estimate the posterior probability. If the test re-

---

[1] Mathematically, independence of test results means that the results of one test convey no meaningful information about the results of another test. Independence may best be understood conversely; totally dependent results convey the same information—for example, measuring someone's temperature with two thermometers, one centigrade and one Fahrenheit, or filling two blood culture vials with blood from the same syringe and needle.

TABLE 6.5

CALCULATING SENSITIVITY AND SPECIFICITY FOR ST SEGMENT DEPRESSION OF 2 MM OR MORE DURING EXERCISE STRESS TESTING (BASED ON TABLE 6.4)

ST Segment Depression	Coronary artery disease (*N* = 50)		No coronary artery disease (*N* = 200)	
	N	**%**	**N**	**%**
≥2 mm	15	30	2	1
<2 mm	35	70	198	99

Sensitivity (positive in disease) = 15 / 50 = 30%.
Specificity (negative in health) = 198 / 200 = 99%.

TABLE 6.6

CALCULATING LIKELIHOOD RATIOS FOR ST SEGMENT DEPRESSION OF 1 MM OR MORE DURING EXERCISE STRESS TESTING (BASED ON TABLE 6.4)

ST Segment Depression	Coronary artery disease (N = 50)		No coronary artery disease (N = 200)	
	N	%	N	%
≥1 mm	37	74	32	16
<1 mm or none	13	26	168	84

Sensitivity (positive in disease) = 37 / 50 = 74%.
Specificity (negative in health) = 168 / 200 = 84%.

sult is positive, then the posterior probability of the disease is determined as follows:

Posterior Probability (positive result)

$$= \frac{\text{Prior Probability} \times \text{Sensitivity}}{}$$

The posterior probability of a disease, given a positive test result, is sometimes called the *predictive value positive*, as it indicates how often someone with a positive test result has the disease.

On the other hand, if the test result is negative, then the posterior probability that the patient has the disease is determined as follows:

Posterior Probability (negative result)

$$= \frac{\text{Prior Probability} \times (1 - \text{Sensitivity})}{[\text{Prior Probability} \times (1 - \text{Sensitivity})] + [(1 - \text{Prior Probability}) \times \text{Specificity}]}$$

The posterior probability of a disease, given a negative test result, measures how often a patient with a negative test has the disease. Subtracting it from 1 yields the *predictive value negative*, which indicates the likelihood that a patient with a negative test does *not* have the disease.

Unfortunately, predictive values, positive and negative, depend on the prior probability of the disease. They are therefore most helpful when the prior probability of the disease is constant, as in the evaluation of tests that are used routinely, such as screening tests.

Sensitivity and specificity are less useful than LRs. They require that test results be either positive or negative, whereas LRs can be used for all sorts of test results. In addition, sensitivity and specificity are not independent terms; you cannot interpret one without knowing the other. By changing the threshold for a positive test result, one can arbitrarily increase the sensitivity of a test and at

the same time reduce its specificity (or vice versa). Finally, the sensitivity and specificity of a diagnostic test may look fine if borderline results are left out, but in actuality, the test may have so many borderline results that it is not of much help.

For a test with only two possible outcomes (positive or negative), a straightforward method can convert sensitivity and specificity to LRs. The LR for a positive test result is determined as follows:

$$\text{LR (positive result)} = \frac{\begin{array}{c}\text{Likelihood of a Positive Result}\\\text{in Someone with the Disease}\end{array}}{\begin{array}{c}\text{Likelihood of Positive Result in}\\\text{Someone without the Disease}\end{array}}$$

$$= \frac{\text{Sensitivity}}{1 - \text{Specificity}}$$

Most tests with a very high specificity will also have a large positive LR because the denominator will be very small. For example, with a sensitivity of 70% and a specificity of 95%, the LR for a positive test result is 14 (70% / 5%).

The LR for a negative test result is determined as follows:

$$\text{LR (negative result)} = \frac{\begin{array}{c}\text{Likelihood of a Negative Result}\\\text{in Someone with the Disease}\end{array}}{\begin{array}{c}\text{Likelihood of Negative Result in}\\\text{Someone without the Disease}\end{array}}$$

$$= \frac{1 - \text{Sensitivity}}{\text{Specificity}}$$

Most tests with a very high sensitivity will also have a small negative LR because the numerator will be very small. For example, with a sensitivity of 98% and a specificity of 70%, the LR for a positive result would be 0.03 (0.02 / 0.70).

LRs, or sensitivity and specificity, are sometimes referred to as the operating characteristics of a test, as in the phrase *receiver–operating characteristic (ROC) curve*. An ROC curve is a pictorial way of representing the changes in sensitivity and specificity of a diagnostic test as the threshold for calling a result "positive" is altered (8).

QUALITY OF THE LABORATORY

When evaluating the results of diagnostic tests, the clinician must also be familiar with the local characteristics of the diagnostic laboratory. Along with the obvious concerns about diagnostic colleagues who "overinterpret" or "underinterpret" abnormalities on subjective tests such as radiographs and nuclear medicine scans, clinicians should be aware that they themselves are the most important laboratory. Clinicians must account for the *precision* and *accuracy* of the diagnostic tests that they perform during the history and physical examination. (*Precision* refers to the reproducibility of a result; *accuracy* refers to whether the result actually measures the phenomenon of interest.) Taking a few extra minutes to verify an important historical detail or to reposition a patient for a better examination of the abdomen, as well as corroborating the accuracy of physical examination findings with more definitive diagnostic tests, may substantially improve the LRs of many findings.

KEY POINTS

- The results of a diagnostic test must be interpreted in the context of the prior probability of the disease.
- Two of the best diagnostic tests are the history and physical examination.
- Likelihood ratios quantify the effect of a test result on the prior probability.
- The likelihood ratios for independent test results can be multiplied together.
- The sum of the probabilities of the various diagnostic possibilities must equal 100%.
- The precision and accuracy of the diagnostic laboratory (including the characteristics of the clinician in the case of the history and physical examination) should always be considered when interpreting the results of a diagnostic test.
- An appreciation of quantitative reasoning and Bayesian analysis allows clinicians to make more rational and ultimately more correct decisions in caring for their patients.

REFERENCES

1. Guyatt GH, Oxman AD, Ali M, Willan A, McIlroy W, Patterson C. Laboratory diagnosis of iron-deficiency anemia: an overview. *J Gen Intern Med* 1992;7:145–153. (Note: Published erratum appears in *J Gen Intern Med* 1992;7:423.)
2. Diamond GA, Forrester JS. Analysis of probability as an aid in the clinical diagnosis of coronary-artery disease. *N Engl J Med* 1979; 300:1350–1358.
3. McFarlane MJ, Imperiale TF. Use of the alveolar-arterial oxygen gradient in the diagnosis of pulmonary embolism. *Am J Med* 1994; 96:57–62.
4. Ridker PM, Hennekens CH, Lindpaintner K, Stampfer MJ, Eisenberg PR, Miletich JP. Mutation in the gene coding for coagulation factor V and the risk of myocardial infarction, stroke, and venous thrombosis in apparently healthy men. *N Engl J Med* 1995;332: 912–917.
5. Stein PD, Saltzman HA, Weg JG. Clinical characteristics of patients with acute pulmonary embolism. *Am J Cardiol* 1991;68:1723–1724.
6. van Strijen MJ, de Monye W, Schiereck J, et al. Advances in New Technologies Evaluating the Localisation of Pulmonary Embolism Study Group. Single-detector helical computed tomography as the primary diagnostic test in suspected pulmonary embolism: a multicenter clinical management study of 510 patients. *Ann Intern Med* 2003;138:307–314. (Erratum in: *Ann Intern Med* 2003;139:387.)
7. The PIOPED Investigators. Value of the ventilation/perfusion scan in acute pulmonary embolism. Results of the prospective investigation of pulmonary embolism diagnosis (PIOPED). *JAMA* 1990;263:2753–2759.
8. Centor RM. Signal detectability: the use of ROC curves and their analyses. *Med Decision Making* 1991;11:102–106.

ADDITIONAL READING

Dawson B, Trapp RG. *Basic and Clinical Biostatistics.* 4th ed. New York: McGraw-Hill, 2004.

Friedland DJ. *Evidence-Based Medicine: A Framework for Clinical Practice.* Stamford, CT: Appleton & Lange, 1998.

Gehlbach SH. *Interpreting the Medical Literature.* 4th ed. New York: McGraw-Hill, 2002.

Greenhalgh T. How to read a paper. Papers that report diagnostic or screening tests. *BMJ* 1997;315:540–543.

Sackett DL, Haynes RB, Guyatt GH, Tugwell P. *Clinical Epidemiology: A Basic Science for Clinical Medicine.* 2nd ed. Boston: Little, Brown, 1991.

Decision Analysis

7

Warren S. Browner

INTRODUCTION

Decision analysis is a formal method to estimate the result of a clinical decision by assigning numeric values to the potential outcomes of that decision and to the probabilities of those outcomes. Analyses of many common clinical problems have been published (1–4). Decision analysis is most useful when uncertainty exists about the best course of action. One does not need a decision analysis to determine whether to obtain blood cultures in a patient with rigors, fever, and a new heart murmur. However, decision analysis would be an appropriate way to determine which antibiotics to use to treat that patient. Indeed, it would be an ideal situation for decision analysis; the clinical scenario is relatively common, and clinical trials have not definitively answered the question.

The process of decision analysis assumes that it is possible to rate the outcomes of a decision on a quantitative scale from best to worst. Thus, decision analysis is sometimes called a *normative process*; given the assumptions in the model, a "best" answer must exist. An analysis can be only as good as the abilities of the decision analyst and the quality of the data used. When little is known about a clinical problem, or when the decision analysis has been prepared by someone who is not familiar with what is known, even the most sophisticated analysis is unlikely to provide much that will be useful in caring for patients.

Although decision analysis is not the only way to approach a clinical problem, it has advantages compared with other methods of decision making under uncertain circumstances, such as dogmatism ("This is the best way to do it."), policy ("This is the way we do it around here."), nihilism ("It doesn't really matter what we do."), deferral to experts or patients ("What do you want us to do?"), and catastrophe avoidance ("Whatever else we do, let's be sure

to not do that."). Especially when the correct decision is too close to call, small changes in one or two assumptions can change the results. The process of creating a decision analysis can often identify key pieces of clinical information that are unknown but essential to determining the best course of action. Decision analysis—because it assigns patient-specific values to the outcomes of clinical decisions—highlights the importance of patient preferences in physician decision making.

BASIC STRUCTURE OF A DECISION TREE

Decision analysis begins with a *clinical decision*, such as whether a patient with chest pain should be admitted to the hospital. The decision, of course, needs analysis only if the course of action is uncertain. Under many circumstances, as when a patient is severely ill, no uncertainty exists: admission to the hospital, not a formal decision analysis, is needed. For certain patients, however, the best decision is not clear.

A decision analysis is usually portrayed as a *tree structure*, progressing from the decision on the left to the outcomes on the right (Figure 7.1).

In general, the *decision* should be framed in terms of the clinical options and the characteristics of the patient and setting. Making a decision about hospitalization for chest pain will be different for a 75-year-old patient with known coronary artery disease than for a 35-year-old patient who runs 3 miles a day without symptoms. Suppose the clinical problem of interest concerns a patient between the ages of 50 and 59 years with new, but resolved, substernal chest pain. This patient has normal electrocardiographic findings and does not live alone. The decision is whether to admit the patient to the hospital or to treat at home with close

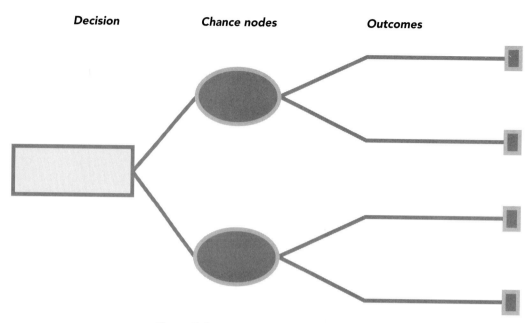

Figure 7.1   Basic structure of a decision tree.

follow-up. The outcome of interest is whether the patient survives the episode. By convention, the decision itself is placed in a rectangle, where each branch represents a different decision. Usually, a decision entails only two options, but additional choices are certainly possible, such as a brief admission to an observation unit. The same principles and techniques would hold.

After the decision node come the *chance nodes*, indicated with circles, which are used whenever clinical uncertainty exists. However, uncertainty from the clinical point of view may not be what matters in a decision analysis. For example, it may seem that the key uncertainty in deciding whether to admit a patient with chest pain is whether the pain is actually cardiac in origin. A more for-

mal approach, though, may indicate that the actual uncertainties that matter are whether the patient has a problem that will get worse with outpatient treatment and how much more likely improvement is to occur with hospital admission.

A simple analysis of this decision (Figure 7.2) might begin with one set of chance nodes—the probability that a life-threatening problem will develop. A decision analysis ends with the *outcomes* of the different possibilities. In this case, four outcomes are possible: admitted and died, admitted and survived, treated at home and died, and treated at home and survived.

This simple tree does not reflect the clinical situation. A more realistic tree (Figure 7.3) needs at least one additional

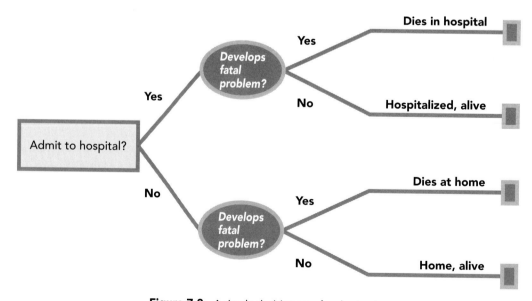

Figure 7.2   A simple decision tree for chest pain.

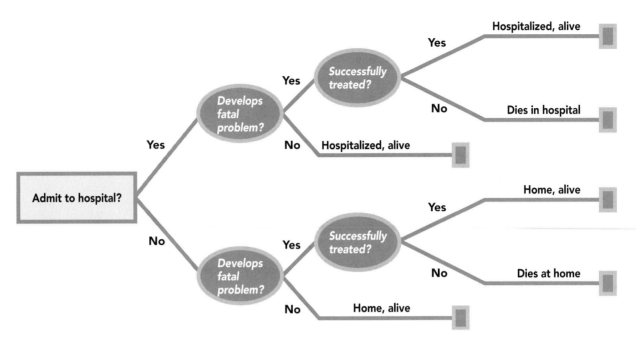

Figure 7.3 A more realistic tree.

layer of complexity—the likelihood that the potentially fatal problem can be prevented by therapy or detected and treated in time to prevent a fatal outcome. That likelihood is presumably greater if the patient is admitted to the hospital; if not, then hospitalization has no benefit, and no uncertainty exists about the right decision, which is to send the patient home.

In this more elaborate tree, the new set of chance nodes reflect the different probabilities. The chance nodes indicate the probability that a potentially fatal complication is destined to develop. This probability is independent of the decision; its likelihood is not influenced by the decision to admit the patient. This concept—that *the decision does not affect the likelihood that a patient already has a particular condition*—is essential to understanding decision analysis. If the patient is not destined to have a life-threatening complication, then the patient will survive whether admitted to the hospital or treated at home.

FILLING IN THE DECISION TREE

After the tree structure has been outlined, the next step in a decision analysis is to assign *probabilities* to the various branches leaving each chance node. The total probability at each chance node must sum to 100%. These probabilities can be obtained by a thorough review of the literature, from original data, or by asking experts. Although the most valid estimates of the effects of treatment are obtained from trials, these are not available for many decisions. Indeed, one of the strengths of formal decision analysis is that it is useful when a randomized trial is not practical or available.

In the example, let us arbitrarily assume that the likelihood that a life-threatening problem would have developed is 5%; thus, the likelihood that such a problem would not have developed is 95%. Next, one must estimate the likelihood of preventing or detecting and successfully treating this problem both at home and in the hospital. Let us assume that this likelihood is 80% if the patient has been hospitalized but only 50% if the patient is at home.

Numeric values must now be assigned to each outcome. These values are called *utilities*. For convenience, the best outcome (in this case, alive and at home) is usually assigned 100 points, and the worst outcome (in this case, dead) is assigned zero points. But how should the utility of the outcome of "alive and in the hospital" be valued? Some "disutility" must be assigned to hospitalization; otherwise, the best decision would be to hospitalize everyone, no matter how small the probability of the development of a life-threatening problem. This disutility results from the cost and inconvenience of hospitalization and from the possibility that the patient will suffer a hospital-related complication. Arbitrarily, let us assume that admission to the hospital for a condition that could have been managed on an outpatient basis has a disutility of two points; thus, the outcome of "alive and admitted" is worth 98 (100 − 2) points.

An important question to ask before assigning utilities is, "Whose utility?" Usually, the perspective for a clinical decision analysis is that of the patient. For example, a physician may view a death that occurs at home as being worse than a death that occurs in the hospital (in the sense that the death at home might have been avoidable had the patient been admitted). From the perspective of the patient, however, it is usually reasonable to assume that a fatal outcome has the same utility whether or not the patient was hospitalized.

ESTIMATING THE UTILITY OF EACH DECISION

After completing the anatomy of the tree and estimating all the probabilities and utilities (Figure 7.4), the decision analyst must determine the expected utility of each alternative decision. The expected utility of a decision is the average utility of all the possible outcomes of that decision, weighted by the likelihood of arriving at each outcome. The decision with the greatest expected utility is the best decision.

This process begins at the most distal nodes of the decision; the expected values at these nodes are determined by multiplying the utility of each outcome by the probability of the twig leading to that outcome. Then one sums the expected values of each twig. For example, a 20% chance of an outcome that is worth zero points and an 80% chance of an outcome that is worth is 100 points has an expected value of 80 points, or (20% × 0) + (80% × 100). This value becomes the expected utility of that chance node, which is then multiplied by the likelihood of arriving at that chance node. The process progresses centrally (from right to left) until the expected values of the original decisions, at the *base case* for the probabilities and utilities, are determined. In this example (see Figure 7.5), the decision to treat the patient at home results in an expected utility of 97.5, whereas admission to the hospital has an expected utility of 97.02 when using the base case assumptions about probabilities and utilities. Thus, the analysis indicates that treating the patient at home

will have a marginally (less than a half point) greater expected utility.

SENSITIVITY ANALYSIS

The decision analyst next varies the assumptions in the model to determine how these changes affect the expected utilities of alternative decisions. This process is known as *sensitivity analysis* because its purpose is to determine whether the value of a decision is sensitive to the assumptions. Decisions that are not greatly affected by a probability or utility are said to be *robust* to that assumption. Sensitivity analyses alter the probabilities at each chance node as well as the utilities through a reasonable range. If only one assumption is varied, the process is known as a one-way sensitivity analysis. If several probabilities and utilities are varied simultaneously, these are called, for example, two-way or three-way analyses. Sensitivity analyses are especially important when the model contains several critical variables and there is disagreement about what the base case values should be.

One potentially confusing aspect of most sensitivity analyses is that the expected utilities of alternative decisions usually decline as the probability of an adverse outcome increases (Figure 7.6). For example, the value of admitting a patient with chest pain and the value of treating the patient at home both decline as the probability increases that a life-threatening complication will develop. That is because complications are usually a result of severe disease; even patients who are hospitalized may have adverse outcomes. However, a comparison of the expected values of the two choices shows that as the likelihood of

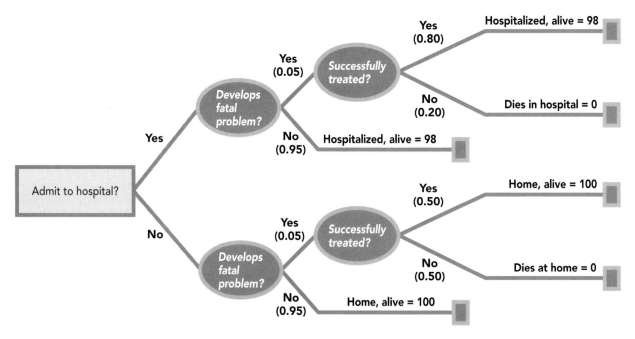

Figure 7.4 The tree with probabilities and utilities added.

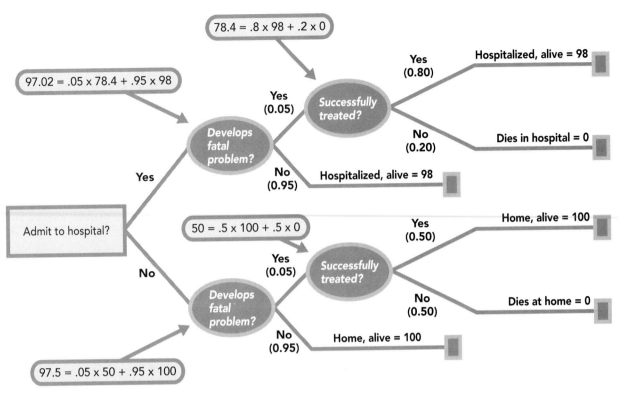

Figure 7.5 The tree with expected utilities *(elongated ovals)* added.

complications increases, the difference between the two therapies becomes more favorable to admission as the two lines diverge.

The point at which the expected values of alternative decisions are identical is the *toss-up* (5). In the example, this occurs when the probability of a complication is 6.6%. When the probability that the patient has a life-threatening condition is less than 6.6% (e.g., a 5% risk, as in the base case assumptions), treatment at home is preferred, albeit not by much. At probabilities greater than 6.6%, hospitalization is the better decision.

SETTING UTILITIES

One of the most difficult aspects of decision analysis is setting the utilities for the expected outcomes (6–9). Sometimes the utilities are obvious—for example, if there are only two of them (such as life and death). At other times, the utilities can be set in years of life expectancy under alternative decisions, such as survival with medical or surgical therapy in patients with left main coronary artery disease. However, for many situations, it is necessary to determine the utilities for one or more intermediate outcomes by using some sort of scale—the higher the utility, the greater the value to the patient.

Consider the following example. You are trying to help a patient determine whether to have femoral–popliteal artery bypass surgery for claudication. The patient is able to walk one block on level ground. The condition has been stable for the past year, during which time the patient has quit smoking. If the surgery is successful, the patient will be able to resume previous activities—walking several blocks a day—without pain. This is the best outcome, and it is assigned 100 points. The main complication of surgery is perioperative death. This is the worst outcome, and it is

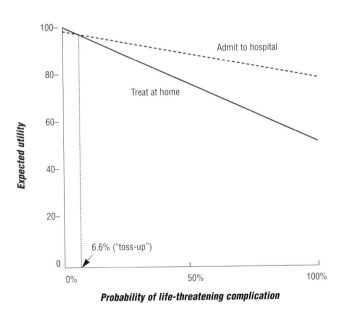

Figure 7.6 One-way sensitivity analysis of expected utilities of treating at home or admitting to the hospital, as a function of probability of life-threatening complication.

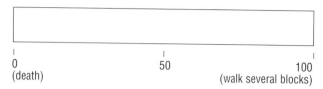

Figure 7.7 The linear utility scale.

assigned zero points. Assume that surgery is otherwise without problems. The utility that needs to be determined is that of the intermediate outcome—being "able to walk one block on the level."

One way to set this utility is to ask the patient, "On a scale of zero (death) to 100 (able to walk without pain for several blocks), how would you rate the current situation, with limited activity? Place a mark on the line that indicates your choice" (Figure 7.7). This is then the patient's utility.

Another way of assessing utilities is known as the *standard gamble* (Figure 7.8), in which the patient is offered two hypothetical scenarios. The first scenario is the intermediate outcome (e.g., living with claudication). The second involves balancing a chance of the best outcome (revascularization and pain-free ambulation) against the alternative of the worst outcome (death). When the chance of the best outcome is low enough that the patient has a difficult time deciding which scenario is more attractive, you have determined the utility of the intermediate outcome. This can be portrayed as a simple decision analysis to determine the probability of surviving a successful procedure that would make the decision a toss-up.

The patient needs to estimate the chance of surviving the procedure that would make the decision a difficult one (a toss-up). At that probability (P), the patient has determined the utility of the intermediate outcome because $P \times 100 + [1 - P] \times 0 =$ claudication utility. One can estimate this probability by beginning with a very high likelihood of surviving surgery and reducing it until the patient no longer

chooses surgery. ("Suppose that surgery could restore your walking back to several blocks without discomfort. Would you choose to undergo surgery if the chance of surviving was 999,999 in a million? 999 in 1,000? 99 in 100? 49 in 50? 1 in 10? 1 in 2?") Alternatively, one can begin with a low surgical risk and increase it. ("Would you choose surgery with a risk for death of 1 in a million? 1 in 1,000? 1 in 100? 1 in 50? 1 in 10? 1 in 2?") If a patient is willing to take no more than a 1 in 20 chance of dying at surgery (at least a 95% chance of a good outcome), that implies that the patient has assigned the value of 0.95 to the utility of living with claudication.

Utilities derived from the standard gamble tend to be greater than those estimated using a linear scale; intermediate outcomes such as claudication tend to cluster close to those for good health. This happens because patients are risk averse and especially because they are death averse. Many are not willing to risk death to improve their current condition.

The standard gamble assumes that patients value a 95% chance of a perfect outcome the same as a 100% chance of an outcome that has a utility of 0.95. Some patients, however, may not like the uncertainty of not knowing and prefer a sure thing, even to the point of overvaluing it.

Often, utilities obtained from a linear scale or the standard gamble combine with life expectancy to yield *quality-adjusted life-years* (QALYs, pronounced "qwallies"). If claudication has a utility of 0.9, then the outcome of "alive for 10 years with claudication" would be equivalent to nine quality-adjusted life-years; so would nine years in perfect health (with a utility of 1.0) or 20 years with a health condition that had a utility of 0.45.

Another way to set utilities is by making time trade-offs to estimate the utility of a year of life in the intermediate state. In this method, the patient is asked to balance time in the current situation with time in a state of perfect health. For example, patients are asked whether they would be

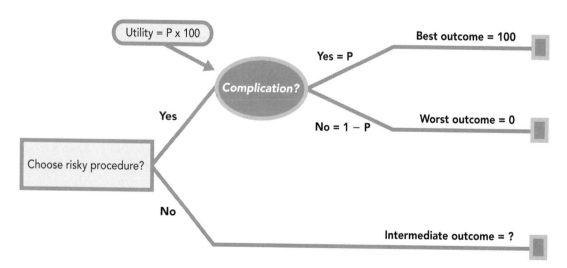

Figure 7.8 The standard gamble.

willing to trade 10 years of life with claudication for *Y* years of "revascularized" life (and death immediately thereafter). In this situation, patients are estimating the quality of life with claudication (e.g., on a scale of 0% to 100%):

$$100\% \times Y \text{ Years}$$
$$= \text{Quality of Life with Claudication} \times 10 \text{ Years}$$

If a patient chooses eight years, this indicates that the current quality of life is 80%:

$$80\% \times 10 \text{ Years} = 100\% \times 8 \text{ Years}$$

In general, time trade-offs give values for utilities that are between those of a linear scale and those of a standard gamble. This occurs because patients, especially young patients, tend to devalue time given away in the future. They are more willing to give some away for the chance of feeling better.

Setting utilities from other perspectives can yield different results in a decision analysis. From the perspective of an insurance company or an overworked physician, admitting a patient to the hospital for five days of treatment for pneumonia has a major disutility, whereas from the patient's perspective, it may have only a minor disutility (or even none at all). Physicians may not value quality of life with a disability, such as the need for long-term dialysis, as highly as patients themselves do.

EVALUATING PUBLISHED DECISION ANALYSES

Before accepting the validity of a decision analysis, one must determine whether it is relevant to the clinical situation. First, are the alternative decisions actually available, or do they involve specialized or unavailable tests or procedures? Second, are the probabilities—both of outcomes and of the effects of treatment—valid in the particular clinical situation in which you find yourself? Were they based on referral populations? Were there other important differences, such as in age, gender, race, or stage of disease, in comparison with patients for whom you care? Were the relevant outcomes considered, and were they valued appropriately?

A well-performed decision analysis should also provide the exact structure of the decision tree that was used. If you cannot re-create the calculations involved in a complex model, then it is difficult to be certain that the authors did them correctly. A decision analysis that is not explicit about the tree structure can hide many branches and may have arrived at the wrong results.

Published analyses should provide the values for each probability for the base case and the ranges of probabilities for the sensitivity analyses, as well as references to the sources of probabilities. More importantly, an analysis should verify their relevance to the clinical situation. A decision analysis, for example, that concludes that anticoagulation is always the best course of action for patients with atrial fibrillation who have a risk for bleeding that varies

between 1% and 10% a year would not be relevant for a patient who has had three gastrointestinal hemorrhages in the previous month.

Utilities should be appropriate. They are often set arbitrarily or by consulting with a few physicians, and thus they bear little resemblance to what patients might say. Bear in mind that most patients value life, even with disability or disease, highly, and that short-lived events (such as hospitalization) have only a minor effect on the quality of life for an entire year.

The advantages of decision analysis—that it requires an explicit structure of the decision, that probabilities and utilities must be estimated, and that a point of view must be adopted—also point to some of its key disadvantages. These requirements are time consuming and often not practical when a decision must be made in real time. However, formal decision analyses are available for many common clinical decisions, and many have been done well (1–4). The process of decision analysis, by highlighting the key uncertainties, may suggest areas in need of research. Many difficult decisions are toss-ups, and the process of decision analysis reminds clinicians of the importance of patient preference in these circumstances. Small changes in the utility of an outcome, such as a preference not to undergo an invasive diagnostic test, may greatly affect the preferred decision.

KEY POINTS

- Decision analysis is a formal method of evaluating clinical decisions made under circumstances of uncertainty.
- The process assumes that it is possible to rank outcomes from best to worst and to assign them numeric values, called utilities.
- The expected utility of a decision is determined by multiplying the utilities of each possible outcome of that decision by the likelihood of reaching that outcome.
- The best decision is the one that leads to the greatest expected utility.
- A decision is a toss-up when the expected utilities of alternative choices are similar.
- Sensitivity analyses determine the effects of changes in the assumptions of a decision analysis on the expected utilities.
- Different methods of setting utilities can result in different values.

REFERENCES

1. Levey AS, Lau J, Pauker SG, Kassirer JP. Idiopathic nephrotic syndrome. Puncturing the biopsy myth. *Ann Intern Med* 1987;107: 697–713.
2. Yock CA, Boothroyd DB, Owens DK, Garber AM, Hlatky MA. Cost-effectiveness of bypass surgery versus stenting in patients with multivessel coronary artery disease. *Am J Med* 2003;115: 382–389.

3. Gould MK, Sanders GD, Barnett PG, et al. Cost-effectiveness of alternative management strategies for patients with solitary pulmonary nodules. *Ann Intern Med* 2003;138:724–735.

4. Hunink MG, Wong JB, Donaldson MC, Meyerovitz MF, de Vries J, Harrington DP. Revascularization for femoropopliteal disease. A decision and cost-effectiveness analysis. *JAMA* 1995;274:165–171.

5. Kassirer JP, Pauker SG. The toss-up. *N Engl J Med* 1981;305: 1467–1469.

6. Hellinger FJ. Expected utility theory and risky choices with health outcomes. *Med Care* 1989;27:273–279.

7. Jensen MP, Karoly P, O'Riordan EF, Bland F Jr, Burns RS. The subjective experience of acute pain. An assessment of the utility of 10 indices. *Clin J Pain* 1989;5:153–159.

8. Nease RF Jr, Kneeland T, O'Connor GT, et al. Variation in patient utilities for outcomes of the management of chronic stable angina. Implications for clinical practice guidelines. Ischemic Heart Disease Patient Outcomes Research Team. *JAMA* 1995;273:1185–1190.

9. Bleichrodt H, Johannesson M. Standard gamble, time trade-off and rating scale: experimental results on the ranking properties of QALYs. *J Health Econ* 1997;16:155–175.

ADDITIONAL READING

McGinn TG, Guyatt GH, Wyer PC, Naylor CD, Stiell IG, Richardson WS. Users' guides to the medical literature: XXII: how to use articles about clinical decision rules. Evidence-Based Medicine Working Group. *JAMA* 2000;284:79–84.

Pauker SG, Kassirer JP. Decision analysis. *N Engl J Med* 1987;316: 250–258.

Petitti DB. *Meta-Analysis, Decision Analysis, and Cost-Effectiveness Analysis: Methods for Quantitative Synthesis in Medicine.* 2nd ed. New York: Oxford University Press, 2000.

Richardson WS, Detsky AS. Users' guides to the medical literature. VII. How to use a clinical decision analysis. A. Are the results of the study valid? Evidence-Based Medicine Working Group. *JAMA* 1995;273:1292–1295. B. What are the results and will they help me in caring for my patients? Evidence-Based Medicine Working Group. *JAMA* 1995;273:1610–1613.

Sox HC Jr. *Medical Decision Making.* Boston: Butterworth–Heineman, 1988.

Evidence-Based Medicine

8

Holger J. Schünemann   *Gordon H. Guyatt*

INTRODUCTION: THE HISTORY AND PHILOSOPHY OF EVIDENCE-BASED MEDICINE

When one of the authors first introduced the term *evidence-based medicine (EBM)* in an informal residency training program document, it was described as "an attitude of enlightened skepticism toward the application of diagnostic, therapeutic, and prognostic technologies in their day-to-day management of patients" (1). In the following years, the term and its philosophy became well known through a series of articles (later published in a collection) by the EBM Working Group (2). A MEDLINE search of the term *EBM* in January 2005 revealed seven citations for the year 1993 and approximately 2,500 citations in 2004.

The need to solve clinical problems has stimulated the evolution of EBM. In contrast to the traditional paradigm of clinical practice, EBM emphasizes that intuition, unsystematic clinical experience, and pathophysiologic rationale are not sufficient for making the best clinical decisions. Although EBM acknowledges the importance of clinical experience, it deems the evaluation of evidence from clinical research as a prerequisite for optimal clinical decision making (3). Moreover, it holds that clinicians must use a formal set of rules to interpret and apply evidence from clinical research results effectively. Another fundamental principle of EBM is the explicit inclusion of patients' and society's values and clinical circumstances in the clinical decision-making process (see Figure 8.1) (4). Patients, their proxies, or (if a parental approach to decision making is desired) the clinician must always weigh the benefits, harms, and costs associated with alternative treatment strategies, and values and preferences always influence those trade-offs.

For clinicians, integrating research evidence in their practice requires an understanding of what constitutes higher-quality versus lower-quality evidence. For instance, a case report describing an "effective" intervention makes one less certain than when evidence about the intervention is summarized in a systematic review of large, randomized controlled trials. EBM teaches that confidence in research results should be greatest when systematic error (bias) is lowest and that confidence should fall when bias is more likely (see Figure 8.2).

SETTING CRITICISM OF EBM STRAIGHT

Although randomized study designs provide the highest-quality evidence, EBM does not neglect other study designs. In fact, EBM acknowledges explicitly that a large body of state-of-the-art evidence comes from observational studies because higher-quality evidence often is unavailable or experimental study designs are infeasible. For instance, consider the role of smoking in the development of lung cancer. Randomizing individuals to smoke or not smoke is infeasible (and unethical), and, thus, the highest-quality evidence comes from observational data. The practice and application of EBM requires an understanding and critical evaluation of all study designs and their appropriateness for specific clinical questions. In addition to study design, rules for formal assessment of evidence allow critical appraisal of whether studies are executed and analyzed correctly. The next sections consider how to develop a clinical question and identify and appraise evidence.

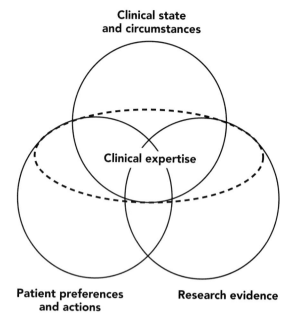

Figure 8.1 Model for Evidence-Based Decision Making. Clinical expertise balances and integrates the "clinical state and circumstances," "patient preferences and actions," and "research evidence," dealing with not only the traditional focus of assessing the patient's state but also the pertinent research evidence and the patient's preferences and actions before recommending a course of action. (Reproduced from Haynes RB, Devereaux PJ, Guyatt GH. Clinical expertise in the era of evidence-based medicine and patient choice. *ACP Journal Club* 2002;136:A11, with permission).

EBM IN ACTION: A CLINICAL SCENARIO

Imagine you are a busy hospitalist in a university-affiliated county hospital, working late at night after admitting several patients over the course of the day. You just admitted a 66-year-old Caucasian man who presented to the emergency room that morning with 15 minutes of left-sided chest pain radiating to his left arm. The pain was severe enough to awaken him, and he reports that he had to sit up in his bed because of difficulties in catching his breath. Finally, his symptoms became so severe that he called an ambulance. A second episode of similar pain in the ambulance was relieved within a few minutes by 0.4 mg nitroglycerin given under his tongue, and he has been free of pain since then. An ECG in the emergency room was unremarkable, and cardiac enzymes drawn at ER arrival were borderline elevated (troponin I 1.0 mcg/l; the hospital's indeterminate range is 0.4–2.0 mcg/l). His chest radiograph was normal.

The patient has a history of hypertension. He takes a diuretic, and his primary care provider had given him 325 mg of aspirin daily to prevent a heart attack. Now, a few hours after his ER arrival, you recheck his laboratory values, and you find that his second troponin I level has risen to 4.8 mcg/l. At this point, you feel that a myocardial infarction without ST segment elevation (a non-ST segment elevation MI) is the most likely diagnosis, and you need to decide what to do after admitting the patient. The patient

Study Design
Randomized controlled trials
Controlled trials (controlled before and
    after studies)
Case-control studies and cohort studies
Cross-sectional studies
Case reports and case series

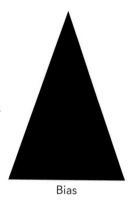

Bias

Figure 8.2 The Hierarchy of Quality of Evidence. As the research design becomes more rigorous (moving from bottom to top), the quality of evidence increases, and the likelihood of bias decreases.

had already received aspirin and low-molecular-weight heparin in the ER, but you wonder about the best action to prevent further cardiovascular events. (The patient refuses any invasive cardiac procedure, including catheterization.) Apart from management of the patient's lipids and lifestyle modifications, you know that cardiologists and neurologists in your hospital often use a second antiplatelet agent (clopidogrel) to prevent further ischemic events. However, you wonder how large the potential benefits and harms are. You are particularly concerned about the risk of bleeding.

You develop the following clinical question according to Table 8.1 (5): *In patients with acute coronary syndromes without ST segment elevation, what is the impact of early and*

TABLE 8.1
FORMULATING THE CLINICAL QUESTION

Component	Explanation
Population	Who are the relevant patients?
Interventions or exposures	What are the management strategies clinicians are interested in (for example, diagnostic tests, drugs, toxins, nutrients, surgical procedures, etc.)?
Comparison (or control) intervention or exposures	What is the comparison, control, or alternative intervention clinicians are interested in? For questions about therapy or harm, there will always be a comparison or control (including doing nothing, placebo, alternative active treatment, or routine care). For questions about diagnosis, there may be a comparison diagnostic strategy (for example, troponin I compared with creatine kinase MB in the diagnosis of myocardial infarction).
Outcome	What are the patient-important consequences of the exposure clinicians are interested in?

long-term use of clopidogrel plus aspirin versus aspirin alone on cardiovascular events and bleeding risk?

While the patient is transferred to the floor, you go to your office and search for appropriate studies. You can find the answer to your question in several ways, including asking a colleague. However, you want to solve this question now because it has come up before but you have always been too busy to answer it.

You consider the resources you have available. First, you could obtain the relevant evidence in the form of published original research and critically appraise these studies yourself. Second, you could rely on prefiltered evidence provided by others with experience in critical appraisal of primary studies. In view of available time and your entirely clinical training, you decide to focus on the latter.

SOURCES OF EVIDENCE

For many hospital-based physicians, the most accessible resources are online. Most resources require use of a computer with a World Wide Web connection, but many have CD-ROM versions available. (For a comprehensive list, see McKibbon et al. (5).) Online or computer-based resources are easy and relatively quick to search. Although there are a number of such resources, no formal comparison in terms of efficiency and patient outcomes exists. This chapter describes some of these resources. The question framed in the previous section is one of therapy, and several sources address questions about therapy.

Prefiltered Medical Information Resources for Hospital-Based Clinicians

The best starting point to look for answers to clinical questions is a systematic review. Systematic reviews are rigorous and all-inclusive summaries of evidence; they often include statistically pooled summary measures of effect called meta-analysis. The best source for systematic reviews and summaries of systematic reviews are the Cochrane Library (6), *ACP Journal Club/Evidence-Based Medicine* (7), and *Clinical Evidence* (8)—all of which are available in CD-ROM versions or on the World Wide Web. The Cochrane Collaboration, an international organization that aims to produce, maintain, and disseminate high-quality systematic reviews of health care interventions, produces the Cochrane Library. *ACP Journal Club* and *Evidence-Based Medicine* contain prefiltered appraisals of primary research and systematic reviews. *Clinical Evidence* provides concise accounts of the current state of knowledge (updated biannually) primarily based on searches for systematic reviews. Another source of prefiltered evidence is *UpToDate* (9), a comprehensive online or electronic textbook updated every four months. The advantages of *UpToDate* include the provision of background knowledge of clinical topics for quick review and its comprehensiveness. Although *UpToDate* does not describe

the methodology used to obtain and appraise the evidence, its editors are working toward being increasingly evidence-based.

Looking for Evidence

You start the search by looking at the OVID collection called "EBM Reviews," which includes *ACP Journal Club* and the Cochrane databases. You know that few studies on clopidogrel exist because of its relatively recent introduction. You type the keyword "clopidogrel" first and then "myocardial infarction OR acute coronary syndrome." You then combine these searches with an "and," yielding a list of 31 references that you review in less than five minutes. Reference number 20 is a *hit* (10), providing an appraised summary of the CURE trial: "Effects of Clopidogrel in Addition to Aspirin in Patients with Acute Coronary Syndromes without ST-Segment Elevation Trial" (11). You decide that you cannot spend the 20–25 minutes reading the primary article, both because you have other patients waiting and because of your limited training in critical appraisal. Just as critically appraising the primary articles addressing a clinical question can be unwieldy, searching for primary evidence using MEDLINE, an electronic database of more than 4,500 biomedical journals, can be inefficient. If searches of preappraised sources prove fruitless, however, one must fall back on MEDLINE.

MEDLINE

MEDLINE is a bibliographic database created and updated by the U.S. National Library of Medicine (NLM). In many hospitals, MEDLINE is available through commercial vendors (such as OVID) that purchase licenses from NLM. Clinicians can also access MEDLINE directly through the NLM PubMed World Wide Web site (http://www.pubmed.org). MEDLINE is helpful in answering focused clinical questions. However, because of its size and complexity, searching MEDLINE can be difficult, time consuming, and frustrating. Using the same keywords described above, your MEDLINE search returns 292 citations. Screening this list of citations will be infeasible for those who need an answer quickly. Therefore, the authors recommend initial use of MEDLINE only when searches of other sources—particularly those that contain prefiltered summaries of evidence—have been unrewarding. In general, for common questions, such as the one in the scenario, the prefiltered databases described above are more useful.

EVIDENCE-BASED CARE FOR THE HOSPITALIZED PATIENT

The *ACP Journal Club* article summarizing the CURE trial provides you with sufficient information about the study to answer typical questions about therapy (see Table 8.2). *ACP Journal Club* provides this assessment for clinicians in

TABLE 8.2

CRITICAL APPRAISAL OF STUDIES ABOUT THERAPY

Question	Therapy or prevention

Study design and execution—evaluation of bias	I. Are the results of the study valid?
	   1. Were patients randomized?
	   2. Was randomization concealed?
	   3. Were patients analyzed in the groups to which they were randomized?
	   4. Were patients in the treatment and control groups similar with respect to known prognostic factors?
	   5. Were patients aware of group allocation?
	   6. Were clinicians aware of group allocation?
	   7. Were outcome assessors aware of group allocation?
	   8. Was follow-up complete?

Results and random error	II. What are the results?
	   1. How large was the treatment effect?
	   2. How precise was the estimate of the treatment effect?

Application and uptake	III. How can I apply the results to my patient care?
	   1. Were the study patients similar to my patients?
	   2. Were all clinically important outcomes considered?
	   3. Are the likely treatment benefits worth the potential harms and costs?

summary format. You learn that the study was a randomized, blind, and placebo-controlled trial with 12 months of follow-up. The investigators randomized patients to clopidogrel or a placebo, but all patients received aspirin as standard therapy. You know that randomized studies have a lower risk of yielding biased outcomes compared with observational studies because known prognostic factors often influence clinicians' or patients' decision about certain therapies. Properly conducted randomized, controlled studies will eliminate the imbalance of known and unknown risk factors. You also know that randomized trials have often led to different results from those of observational studies or commonly held medical opinion. For example, based on a number of observational studies, the use of hormone replacement therapy was thought to prevent coronary heart disease in postmenopausal women, but results of a large randomized controlled trial showed an increased risk for cardiovascular events in patients receiving hormone replacement therapy (12).

EXPRESSING TREATMENT EFFECTS: RELATIVE RISK REDUCTION, ABSOLUTE RISK REDUCTION, AND NUMBER NEEDED TO TREAT

The CURE study included 12,562 patients from 28 countries, and all patients were included in the final analysis. Approximately half the patients received an immediate loading dose of oral clopidogrel, 300 mg, followed by 75 mg daily for 3–12 months; the remaining patients received a placebo resembling clopidogrel; and all patients received aspirin, 75–325 mg daily. Patients were followed for 12 months.

The main outcomes were a composite of death from cardiovascular causes, nonfatal myocardial infarction (MI), or stroke, and a composite of death from cardiovascular causes, nonfatal MI, stroke, or refractory ischemia. Safety outcomes included major and minor bleeding. The focus here is on the latter composite endpoint. Patients in the clopidogrel group had a *relative risk* (RR)—the proportion of the baseline risk in the control group that still is present when patients receive the experimental treatment (in this case, clopidogrel)—of 0.86 (see Table 8.3 for a glossary of key terms in EBM). The easiest measure of risk to understand is the *absolute risk*. In the CURE trial, the absolute risk for the combined primary outcome of recurrent nonfatal myocardial infarction, stroke, death from cardiovascular disease, or refractory ischemia was 16.5%. The absolute risk for this outcome in the control group was 18.8%. One can express treatment effects as the *absolute risk reduction* (ARR) or the risk difference—the difference between the absolute risks in the experimental and control groups. This effect measure represents the proportion of patients spared from the unfavorable outcome if they receive the experimental therapy (clopidogrel) rather than the control therapy (placebo). In the CURE trial, the absolute risk reduction is 2.3% (18.8%–16.5%).

However, the most commonly reported measure of dichotomous treatment effects in clinical studies is the complement of this RR, the *relative risk reduction* (RRR). One can obtain the RRR easily from the RR because it is the proportion of baseline risk that is removed by the experimental therapy, equivalent to $1.0 - RR$. It can be expressed as a percentage: $(1 - RR) \times 100 = (1 - 0.86) \times 100 = 14\%$ for this scenario. A relative risk reduction of 14% means that clopidogrel reduced the risk of the combined outcome by 14% relative to that occurring among control patients. The greater the RRR, the more efficacious the therapy.

Distinguishing between RRR and ARR is important. Assume that the absolute risk of experiencing the combined outcome doubled in both groups in the CURE trial. This could have happened if the investigators had conducted a study in patients at much higher risk of experiencing the endpoint, such as much older patients. In the clopidogrel group, the absolute risk would then become 33% compared with 37.6% in the control group. As a result, the ARR would increase from 2.3%–4.6%, whereas the RR (and therefore the RRR) would remain identical at 0.86 (33% ÷ 37.6% = 0.86), and the RRR would remain approximately 14%. As this example makes clear, doubling of those experiencing the endpoint in both groups leaves the RR (and the RRR) unchanged but increases the ARR by a factor of 2.

Although 14% reduction in the relative risk of the combined endpoint may not sound impressive, its impact on patient groups and practice may be large. The *number needed to treat* (NNT), the number of patients who must receive an intervention during a specific period to prevent

one additional adverse outcome or produce one positive outcome, provides a guide to this impact (13). The NNT is the inverse of the ARR and is calculated as 1 / ARR. Therefore, in the hypothetical example above (with an ARR of 4.6% expressed as a proportion, 0.046), the NNT would be 22 (1 / 0.046%). It was 44 (1 / 0.023%) in the CURE trial.

With this concept in mind, imagine a young patient with no other risk factors for adverse outcomes. Such a patient may carry a much lower baseline risk (say, 4%), and thus the NNT skyrockets to 179 [1 / (0.14 × 4%)]. Given the duration, potential harms (absolute risk increase of 2.7% and 1% for minor and major bleeding, respectively), and cost of treatment with clopidogrel, withholding therapy in this lower-risk patient would be reasonable.

EXPRESSING TREATMENT EFFECTS: CONFIDENCE INTERVALS

Results of any experiment, such as a randomized controlled trial, represent only an estimate of the truth. The true effect of treatment actually may be somewhat smaller or larger than what researchers found. The *confidence interval* (CI) tells, within the bounds of plausibility, how much smaller or greater the true effect is likely to be. The results provided in *ACP Journal Club* show that the CI in the CURE trial around the point estimate of the RRR of 14% ranges from approximately 6%–21%. Both the point estimate and the CI itself help answer two questions. First, what is the single value most likely to represent the true difference between treatment and control; and second, given the difference between treatment and control, what is the plausible range within which the true effect might lie? The smaller the sample size (number of patients in a trial) or the number of events in an experiment, the wider the CI. As the sample size gets larger and the number of events increases, investigators become increasingly certain that the truth is not far from the point estimate calculated from the experiment, and, therefore, the CI is narrower.

One can interpret the 95% CI as the range within which, 95% of the time, the true effect will lie. However, how does the CI facilitate interpretation of the results from the CURE trial? As described above, the CI represents the range of values within which the truth plausibly lies. Accordingly, one way to use CIs is to look at the lower boundary of the interval (the lowest plausible treatment effect) and decide whether the action or recommendation would change compared with assuming that the point estimate represents the truth. The most likely value for the RRR with clopidogrel is 14%, but the true RRR may be as high as 21% or as low as 6%. Values progressively farther from 14% will be less and less likely. One can conclude that patients receiving clopidogrel are less likely to experience the combined endpoint (because even the lower bound of the RRR is greater than zero)—but the magnitude of the difference may be either quite small (and not outweigh the increased

---

TABLE 8.3

GLOSSARY OF KEY TERMS IN EVIDENCE-BASED MEDICINE

Absolute risk increase (ARI): Used as a measure of harm when an investigational therapy causes more harm than good. It is the difference between the absolute risks in the experimental and control groups and represents the proportion of patients that suffer from the unfavorable outcome if they receive the experimental therapy rather than the control/comparison therapy. Conceptually similar to the ARR but indicating an *increase* in risk from the investigational therapy.

Absolute risk reduction (ARR): The difference between the absolute risks in the experimental and control groups. This effect measure represents the proportion of patients spared from the unfavorable outcome if they receive the experimental therapy, compared with those in the control/comparison group.

Confidence interval (CI): The range within which, 95% of the time, the true effect of an intervention will lie.

Evidence-based medicine (EBM): EBM deems the evaluation of evidence from clinical research as a prerequisite for optimal clinical decision making but acknowledges the importance of clinical experience. EBM requires that clinicians use a formal set of rules to interpret and apply evidence from clinical research results effectively. Another fundamental principle of EBM is the explicit inclusion of patients' and society's values and clinical circumstances in the clinical decision-making process.

Number needed to harm (NNH): The number of patients who must receive an intervention during a specific period to cause one additional harmful outcome. Inverse of the ARI.

Number needed to treat (NNT): The number of patients who must receive an intervention during a specific period to prevent one additional adverse outcome or produce one positive outcome during that time period. Inverse of the ARR.

Relative risk reduction (RRR): The proportion of baseline risk that is removed by the experimental therapy, equivalent to 1.0–relative risk (RR).

risk of bleeding and/or the cost) or quite large. This way of understanding the results avoids the yes/no dichotomy of testing a hypothesis.

EXPRESSING HARMS AND TOXICITIES: ABSOLUTE RISK INCREASE AND NUMBER NEEDED TO HARM

The chief toxicity of clopidogrel that concerned the authors of the CURE trial was bleeding. They found that the *absolute risk increase* (ARI) (conceptually similar to the ARR but indicating an *increase* in risk associated with the investigational therapy) for major bleeding was 1% (an increase from 2.7% in the placebo group to 3.7% in the clopidogrel group). The investigators defined major bleeding as substantially disabling bleeding, intraocular bleeding or the loss of vision, or bleeding necessitating the transfusion of at least two units of blood. One can also calculate the number of patients who must receive an intervention during a specific time to cause one additional harmful outcome (analogous to the NNT). The *number needed to harm* (NNH) for major bleeding in the CURE trial is equal to 1 / ARI, or 1 / 0.01 = 100. The authors also provided the information for minor bleeding, which they defined as hemorrhages that led to interruption of the study medication but that did not qualify as major bleeding. The risk for minor bleeding was 5.1% in the clopidogrel group compared with 2.4% in the placebo group. Thus, the NNH for minor bleeding was 1 / 0.027 = 37. Clinicians should keep in mind that estimates of harm also come with uncertainty; therefore, *ACP Journal Club* provides confidence intervals around these harmful effects.

APPLYING EBM PRINCIPLES TO YOUR PATIENT

You now want to know whether you can apply these results to your patient. You examine the study population included in the CURE trial and the associated exclusion criteria. In terms of age, your patient is similar to the study population (66 vs. 64 years), the study included a large proportion of men, and your patient does not fulfill any exclusion criteria. In addition, the study addressed all relevant outcomes. So the study does seem applicable to your situation.

You discuss the option of clopidogrel therapy with your patient, who is now feeling better and appears to have a good understanding of the information you are providing. You explain that—based on your assessment—the benefits and harms of clopidogrel are finely balanced: for every 44 patients treated for one year in the CURE trial, there was one less occurrence of the combined endpoint (the NNT). However, for every 100 patients treated with clopidogrel for one year, one additional patient suffered a

major bleeding episode, and for every 37 patients treated for one year, there was one additional minor bleeding episode (the NNH). You also explain that because these are only estimates, the true benefits and harms might be somewhat smaller or larger. The decision regarding taking clopidogrel thus depends on the patient's values and preferences regarding preventing the combined endpoint vs. incurring additional risk of bleeding (see Figure 8.1). Your patient states that he does not care about the risk for minor bleeding and that he feels the risk for major bleeding is less threatening for him than the risk of the recurrent pain of a heart attack and its subsequent impact on his long-term prognosis. Thus, he would like to use clopidogrel. Uncertain of clopidogrel's cost, you now call the hospital pharmacist. She informs you that the cost is approximately $90 per month and that at least one analysis has suggested the drug is not cost effective (14). The patient tells you that he has a minimal copayment for most medications and remains interested in taking the medication. Thus, you start the patient on a 300 mg loading dose of clopidogrel and continue with 75 mg daily.

CONCLUSIONS

Evidence-based medicine provides an approach to addressing clinical problems. In contrast to the traditional paradigm of clinical practice, EBM emphasizes that intuition, unsystematic clinical experience, and pathophysiologic rationale are not sufficient for making the best clinical decisions. Although EBM acknowledges the importance of clinical experience, EBM's philosophy is that the evaluation of evidence from clinical research provides for the best clinical decision making. Clinicians need to understand a few basic methodological concepts to practice EBM, including developing searching skills and applying the results of clinical studies to their own practice circumstances. A large number of resources facilitate evidence-based clinical practice. Optimal clinical practice includes making the time for obtaining and applying the evidence.

KEY POINTS

- The first step to practicing evidence-based medicine is to develop focused clinical questions.
- Searching for evidence can be simple and efficient.
- A number of electronic and print resources are available for obtaining evidence.
- A basic understanding of risk, measures of effect, and outcomes (both benefits and harms) is necessary to practice or apply EBM (see Table 8.3).
- Patient values and preferences bear on the decision-making process.

REFERENCES

1. Guyatt G. Preface. In: Guyatt G, Rennie D, eds. *Users' Guide to the Medical Literature: A Manual for Evidence-Based Clinical Practice.* Chicago: American Medical Association Press, 2002:xiii.
2. Guyatt G, Rennie D, eds. *Users' Guide to the Medical Literature: A Manual for Evidence-Based Clinical Practice.* Chicago: American Medical Association Press, 2002.
3. Guyatt G. Introduction. In: Guyatt G, Rennie D, eds. *Users' Guide to the Medical Literature: A Manual for Evidence-Based Clinical Practice.* Chicago: American Medical Association Press, 2002:3–13.
4. Haynes RB, Devereaux PJ, Guyatt GH. Clinical expertise in the era of evidence-based medicine and patient choice. *ACP Journal Club* 2002;136:A11.
5. McKibbon A, Hunt D, Richardson SW, et al. Finding the evidence. In: Guyatt G, Rennie D, eds. *Users' Guide to the Medical Literature: A Manual for Evidence-Based Clinical Practice.* Chicago: American Medical Association Press, 2002:16.
6. Available at http://www.cochrane.org. Accessed March 4, 2005.
7. Available at http://www.acpjc.org. Accessed March 4, 2005.
8. Available at http://www.clinicalevidence.org. Accessed March 4, 2005.
9. Available at http://www.uptodate.com. Accessed March 4, 2005.
10. ACP Journal Club. Clopidogrel plus aspirin was effective but increased bleeding in acute coronary syndromes without ST-segment elevation. *ACP Journal Club* March/April, 2002; 136:45.
11. CURE-Investigators. Effects of clopidogrel in addition to aspirin in patients with acute coronary syndromes without ST-segment elevation. *N Engl J Med* 2001;345:494–502.
12. ACP Journal Club. Estrogen plus progestin was not effective for long-term secondary prevention of coronary heart disease in postmenopausal women. *ACP Journal Club* January/February 2003; 138:6.
13. Laupacis A, Sackett DL, Roberts RS. An assessment of clinically useful measures of the consequences of treatment. *N Engl J Med* 1988;318:1728–1733.
14. Gaspoz JM, Coxson PG, Goldman PA, et al. Cost effectiveness of aspirin, clopidogrel, or both for secondary prevention of coronary heart disease. *N Engl J Med* 2002;346:1800–1806.

ADDITIONAL READING

Atkins D, Best D, Briss PA, et al. Grading quality of evidence and strength of recommendations. *BMJ* 2004;328:1490–1494.

Devereaux PJ, Bhandari M, Clarke M, et al. Need for expertise-based randomized controlled trials. *BMJ* 2005;330:88.

Lockwood D, Armstrong M, Grant A. Integrating evidence based medicine into routine clinical practice: seven years' experience at the Hospital for Tropical Diseases, London. *BMJ* 2004;329: 1020–1023.

Montori VM, Jaeschke R, Schünemann HJ, et al. Users' guide to detecting misleading claims in clinical research reports. *BMJ* 2004;329;1093–1096.

Rothwell PM. Treating Individuals 1: External validity of randomised controlled trials: "To whom do the results of this trial apply?" *Lancet* 2005;365;82–93.

Sackett DL, Straus SE, Richardson WS, Rosenberg WMC, Haynes RB, eds. *Evidence-Based Medicine: How to Practice and Teach Evidence-Based Medicine.* 2nd ed. New York: Churchill Livingstone, 2000:233–243.

Straus, SE. What's the E for EBM? *BMJ* 2004;328:535–536.

Cost-Effectiveness

9

Joel Tsevat

INTRODUCTION

Physicians are facing increasing pressures to practice medicine efficiently. To many involved in hospital medicine, efficiency implies avoiding hospitalization when possible, minimizing hospital length of stay for those who need hospitalization, and eschewing expensive tests and treatments. In contrast, the cost-effectiveness paradigm is not to provide as little care as possible but to derive as much value as possible from the limited resources available. Thus, economic analyses in health care often seek to answer the question "How much bang are we getting for our buck?" rather than "How can we spend the fewest bucks possible?"

ECONOMIC ANALYSES

Economic analyses in health care compare two or more diagnostic or treatment modalities. There are several types of economic analyses (1) (Table 9.1). The simplest, *cost-minimization analysis*, assumes that the clinical outcomes of the alternatives under question are equivalent, so the analysis seeks to determine the least costly alternative. For example, one cost-minimization analysis determined the potential savings to a hospital ($2,973 per patient at 12 months) derived from treating patients who have multivessel coronary artery disease by angioplasty and stenting vs. by coronary-artery bypass surgery (2). Cost-minimization analysis is useful for identifying costs but not for evaluating the yield (health benefits) from the expenditures.

A second type, *cost–benefit analysis*, compares the consequences of alternative modalities in common units, usually dollars. For example, cost–benefit analyses of influenza vaccination have found that vaccination and treatment costs were more than offset by savings from reduced morbidity and mortality (3,4). Here, clinical outcomes were expressed in monetary units to compare them directly with the cost of the vaccination program. The principle in cost–benefit analysis is to adopt a program if it is cost-saving, or if it has a more favorable benefit-to-cost ratio than its alternatives.

The most common form of economic analysis is *cost-effectiveness analysis*. Because most choices in health care involve changes in the level or extent of an activity (e.g., ordering an expensive antibiotic vs. a less expensive antibiotic, or ordering computed tomography vs. ultrasonography), cost-effectiveness analysis addresses marginal or incremental changes. Thus, cost-effectiveness analyses examine the net cost (expenditures minus savings) per net unit of effectiveness for one alternative relative to another (5). Effectiveness is usually expressed as *years of life saved*, *quality-adjusted life-years (QALYs) saved*, or *lives saved*. QALYs factor in quality-of-life weights for years of life in various states of health; the weight ranges from zero (representing dead) to 1 (representing full health). The weights are derived by using utility measures, such as (a) the *standard gamble*, which assesses one's willingness to risk a bad outcome, such as death, in exchange for a chance at full health; or (b) the *time trade-off method*, which assesses how much (if any) time a person would be willing to trade in exchange for a shorter but healthy life (6). Cost-effectiveness analyses that express outcomes as the incremental cost per QALY gained are also called cost-utility analyses. Cost-effectiveness ratios can also be expressed in terms of "intermediate outcomes," such as cost per hospital day averted, but use of a "definitive" common denominator such as

TABLE 9.1

COMMON TYPES OF ECONOMIC ANALYSES IN HEALTH CARE

Type	Compares	Expressed In	Comments
Cost-minimization analysis	Costs of alternative strategies	Dollars	Assumes equivalent clinical outcomes
Cost-benefit analysis	Costs and benefits of alternative strategies	Dollars	Benefits converted into dollar savings
Cost-effectiveness analysis	Incremental costs per unit of benefit of alternative strategies	Dollars per year of life saved, per QALY saved, or per life saved	<$50,000 per QALY often considered cost-effective

QALY, quality-adjusted life-year.

QALYs facilitates comparisons among a wider variety of interventions.

Cost-effectiveness analysis is too complex to perform at the bedside, but familiarity with its methods is useful for interpreting published studies. An important distinction is the difference between costs and charges (7). Costs represent the actual consumption of resources that could have been used otherwise, and as such, they are usually the relevant measure. Charges (patient bills), on the other hand, are subject to the vicissitudes of the health care system, such as type (or lack) of insurance, and may bear little resemblance to true resource use (see Chapter 2).

Several types of costs may be germane to an analysis. For example, fixed costs, such as building overhead, do not change during the short term and are thus usually excluded from analyses; on the other hand, variable costs—those directly related to the number of services provided—should be included. In general, costs appropriate to include in the numerator of a cost-effectiveness ratio include the following:

- Costs of health services (so-called direct health care costs, such as medications and laboratory tests)
- Cost of patient time expended while undergoing care (travel time, waiting time, and time actually receiving treatment)
- Costs associated with providing home care for the patient or for obtaining child care while the patient seeks care

In practice, many cost-effectiveness analyses include only direct medical costs. Occasionally, they include income lost because of morbidity or premature death (although such "indirect costs" are more appropriately captured in the denominator of the cost-effectiveness ratio) (8).

Besides which costs are considered, published cost-effectiveness analyses vary in other fundamental areas, such as *perspective* (e.g., that of society, the patient, the hospital, or the insurer), *time horizon*, and *discount rates* (discounting is a method of converting future costs, years of life, or both to their present value). Variability in methodology limits comparison across studies, and this limitation is significant because interventions cannot be considered cost-effective or not cost-effective *per se*—they must be viewed in relation to alternative uses of health care resources. As such, attempts have been made to rank interventions by their cost effectiveness (9,10). Although no official consensus exists regarding an acceptable incremental cost-effectiveness ratio, a *de facto* benchmark of $50,000 per QALY has emerged. Interventions that cost less than $50,000 per QALY are often characterized as worthwhile, whereas those costing more than $50,000 per QALY are often considered to be inefficient.

CARE OF THE HOSPITALIZED PATIENT

Cost-effectiveness analysis is generally regarded as an aid for health policy formulation. Given the premise that we as a society do not have unlimited funds to provide all beneficial health care—no matter how marginally beneficial or how expensive—to everyone, cost-effectiveness analysis can theoretically help to allocate resources to large groups of patients more efficiently.

At the bedside, however, the story may be different. Patients rightfully expect their health care providers to put the patients' own best interests first, not those of society or their insurer. Health care providers often find themselves serving two masters with opposing paradigms.

What then, should a health care provider do? Ubel and Goold (11) contend that bedside rationing of care that is not economically worthwhile does not violate patients' best interests. They argue that physicians should play a role in limiting access to marginally beneficial health care services, especially those that patients would not be willing to pay for themselves in cash or in extra insurance premiums. To do this, they state, physicians need to be trained to identify such marginally beneficial services. If one accepts and extends that viewpoint, then it is probably reasonable for physicians to withhold tests and treatments with incremental cost-effectiveness ratios that greatly exceed accepted benchmarks. Table 9.2 lists the cost-effectiveness ratios of some common inpatient practices.

TABLE 9.2

COST-EFFECTIVENESS RATIOS FOR SOME HOSPITAL-BASED INTERVENTIONS

Problem	Finding	Reference	Comments
Radiofrequency ablation for supraventricular tachycardia	Saves costs and QALYs	13	Comparison is with antiarrhythmic therapy.
Early invasive treatment for unstable angina and non–ST-segment elevation myocardial infarction	$12,739 per year of life saved	14	Comparison is with conservative treatment (catheterization reserved for recurrent ischemia or positive stress test). Productivity costs included.
Gastric bypass for severe obesity (body mass index 40–50 mg/kg^2)	• For women: $5,000–$16,100 per QALY • For men: $10,000–$35,600 per QALY	15	Comparison is with no treatment. Used payer's perspective.
Annual lung cancer screening with helical computed tomography	• For current smokers: $116,300 per QALY • For quitting smokers: $558,600 per QALY • For former smokers: $2,322,700 per QALY	16	Comparison is with no screening.

QALY, quality-adjusted life-year.

CONCLUSIONS

Cost-effective is a buzzword in today's practice of medicine, but the term is often misused and misconstrued (12). Health care practices must be subjected to formal economic analysis before they can be considered to be cost-effective or not cost-effective, and then only when compared with other interventions or consensus standards. When conducted and applied rigorously, cost-effectiveness analysis can aid health care systems in allocating resources as efficiently as possible.

KEY POINTS

- Economic analysis is a tool to allocate limited health care resources efficiently.
- Of the several forms of economic analysis applied in health care, cost-effectiveness analysis is the most commonly used.
- In cost-effectiveness analysis, the relevant evaluation involves the incremental cost per additional benefit received; benefits are usually expressed as years of life or quality-adjusted life-years gained.
- Several types of costs, rather than charges, are germane to cost-effectiveness analysis.
- Published cost-effectiveness analyses may differ with respect to their methodology, which may, in turn, limit comparisons between or among studies.
- Although clinicians have a fiduciary obligation to do what is in their patients' best interests, some argue that withholding marginally beneficial care (or care that is not economically worthwhile) does not violate that obligation.

REFERENCES

1. Eisenberg JM. Clinical economics: a guide to the economic analysis of clinical practices. *JAMA* 1989;262:2879–2886.
2. Serruys PW, Unger F, Sousa JE, et al. Comparison of coronary-artery bypass surgery and stenting for the treatment of multivessel disease. *N Engl J Med* 2001;344:1117–1124.
3. Lee PY, Matchar DB, Clements DA, Huber J, Hamilton JD, Peterson ED. Economic analysis of influenza vaccination and antiviral treatment for healthy working adults. *Ann Intern Med* 2002;137: 225–231.
4. Nichol KL. Cost-benefit analysis of a strategy to vaccinate healthy working adults against influenza. *Arch Intern Med* 2001;161: 749–759.
5. Detsky AS, Naglie IG. A clinician's guide to cost-effectiveness analysis. *Ann Intern Med* 1990;113:147–154.
6. Torrance GW. Measurement of health state utilities for economic appraisal: a review. *J Health Econ* 1986;5:1–30.
7. Finkler SA. The distinction between cost and charges. *Ann Intern Med* 1982;96:102–109.
8. Gold ME, Siegel JE, Russell LB, et al. *Cost-effectiveness in Health and Medicine.* New York: Oxford University Press, 1996.
9. Tengs TO, Adams ME, Pliskin JS, et al. Five-hundred life-saving interventions and their cost-effectiveness. *Risk Anal* 1995;15: 369–390.
10. The CEA registry: standardizing the methods and practices of cost-effectiveness analysis. Available at: http://www.hsph.harvard.edu/cearegistry/. Accessed January 1, 2005.
11. Ubel PA, Goold S. Does bedside rationing violate patients' best interests? An exploration of "moral hazard." *Am J Med* 1998;104: 64–68.
12. Doubilet P, Weinstein MC, McNeil BJ. Use and misuse of the term "cost effective" in medicine. *N Engl J Med* 1986;314:253–256.
13. Cheng CH, Sanders GD, Hlatky MA, et al. Cost-effectiveness of radiofrequency ablation for supraventricular tachycardia. *Ann Intern Med* 2000;133:864–876.
14. Mahoney EM, Jurkovitz CT, Chu H, et al. Cost and cost-effectiveness of an early invasive vs. conservative strategy for the treatment of unstable angina and non–ST-segment elevation myocardial infarction. *JAMA* 2002;288:1851–1858.
15. Craig BM, Tseng DS. Cost-effectiveness of gastric bypass for severe obesity. *Am J Med* 2002;113:491–498.
16. Mahadevia PJ, Fleisher LA, Frick KD, Eng J, Goodman SN, Powe NR. Lung-cancer screening with helical computed tomography in older adult smokers: a decision and cost-effectiveness analysis. *JAMA* 2003;289:313–322.

ADDITIONAL READING

Coast J. Is economic evaluation in touch with society's heatlh values? *BMJ* 2004;329:1233–1236.

Drummond MF, O'Brien B, Stoddart GL, et al. *Methods for the Economic Evaluation of Health Care Programmes.* Oxford, UK: Oxford University Press, 1997.

Drummond MF, McGuire A. *Economic Evaluation in Health Care: Merging Theory with Practice.* Oxford, UK: Oxford University Press, 2002.

Eddy DM. Cost-effectiveness analysis: a conversation with my father. *JAMA* 1992;267:1669–1675.

O'Brien BJ, Heyland D, Richardson WS, et al., for the Evidence-Based Medicine Working Group. Users' guides to the medical literature: XIII. How to use an article on economic analysis of clinical practice: B. What are the results and will they help me in caring for my patients? *JAMA* 1997;277:1802–1806.

Schulman KA, Drummond M, Bootman JL, et al. Health economics: a multimedia computer education program. Sandoz Pharmaceuticals Corporation, East Hanover, NJ, January 19, 1996.

Udvarhelyi IS, Colditz GA, Rai A, et al. Cost-effectiveness and cost-benefit analyses in the medical literature: are the methods being used correctly? *Ann Intern Med* 1992;116:238–244.

Hospital Information Systems

Saverio M. Maviglia   Gilad J. Kuperman   Blackford Middleton

INTRODUCTION

Electronic information systems are critical to the functioning of today's hospitals. Although there is immense heterogeneity in the clinical information systems (CIS) used by hospitals, almost all hospitals use computers to manage financial and patient registration data such as patient demographics and insurance information, to control bed allocation, and to schedule visits, tests, and procedures. While such systems are often implemented as tightly integrated modules, or as independent but cooperative systems, the same cannot be said for the clinical information systems utilized by individual departments within hospitals. Each separate department, such as the laboratory, radiology, pharmacy, and telecommunications, usually has its own system(s) to manage intradepartmental processes and clinical data.

Unfortunately, the rule rather than the exception is that these departmental systems employ different methods to represent clinical data, making information exchange between them difficult. In fact, the institutions with the most advanced information systems are commonly not those with the most computerized processes, but those with computerized processes that are the most integrated, where added value is derived from sharing and cross-referencing data, in order to detect actionable patterns and trends.

This chapter will focus on advances in CIS that are most directly related to providing care to hospitalized patients. These can be broadly classified into two categories, basic and advanced.

BASIC CLINICAL INFORMATION SYSTEMS

Basic clinical information systems are essentially passive tools that increase access to clinically relevant patient information. In the typical hospital, most ancillary departments (such as laboratory, blood-bank, microbiology, radiology, etc.), use their own departmental information systems. These systems manage the local workflow, such as accounting, scheduling, ordering and resulting of tests and procedures performed in the department. Clinical data from these systems are aggregated into a clinical data repository that allows the clinician to have an integrated view of clinical information without the necessity of going to several individual results terminals (Figure 10.1). More sophisticated results viewers augment the informational value of the presented data by co-displaying related results or graphically trending results.

Another example of a basic CIS application is the *report generator*, which is a tool for viewing data across multiple patients. Traditionally utilized by hospital administrators to focus quality improvement or cost reduction efforts, it also is tremendously useful to the rounding physician for keeping track of his or her patients. It can also reduce errors, as demonstrated by one computerized "coverage list" application that standardized the information exchanged between physicians on sign-out, a problem list, medications, and active issues (1, 2). Often, the quality of these reports can make or break a roll-out of a new CIS because, unlike with lab results that

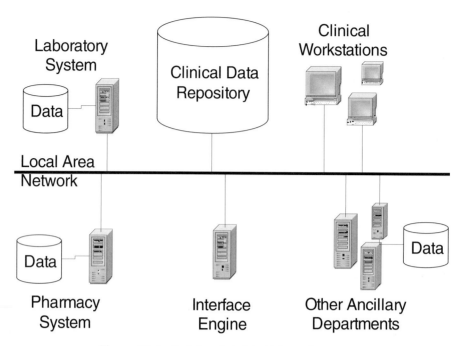

Figure 10.1 Basic hospital clinical information system.

continue to be printed and inserted into the paper chart, there are often no back-up mechanisms to make up for deficiencies in patient tracking. Nothing irritates physicians more than not knowing for which patients they are responsible, where they are located, and what their test results are.

When different types of results viewers are integrated under a single shell, the result begins to form the foundation for an *electronic medical record* (EMR). With an EMR, clinicians can review (to varying degrees), the entire medical history (remote and recent) of the hospitalized patient, along with additional functionality to support clinical decision making. As with hospital information systems in general, the more information that is stored, and the more integrated the data, the more impact an EMR can have on patient care. While typical EMRs record patient allergies, medications, and patient encounter reports (such as consultations, admission history and physicals, discharge summaries, and operative reports), these data elements are usually stored as free-text entries, which restricts how effectively the CIS can impact patient care, as discussed below.

In addition to convenient access to patient information, basic CIS also can provide convenient and quick access to reference information. The Internet has revolutionized the manner by which patients and physicians look up facts, figures, and opinions. As libraries and publishers offer more of their offerings in electronic formats, simply providing terminals with Web access throughout hospitals effectively provides clinicians with a virtual mobile library. Many hospital CIS offer an intranet portal to this material, which can include textbooks, drug information compendiums,

medical journals, medical literature search engines, and locally developed or authored material, such as clinical guidelines, manuals, policies and procedures, forms and formularies, bulletins and newsletters. All members of the hospital staff, not just physicians, commonly and regularly visit these portals (3, 4). Furthermore, such portals have great potential to be unifying forces, especially for integrated delivery networks distributed across multiple institutions and regions.

ADVANCED CLINICAL INFORMATION SYSTEMS

Advanced CIS are characterized by increased interaction with the physician or care provider in return for decision-support, or patient-specific recommendations and guidance about therapy or diagnosis. This usually requires that the clinician contribute data to the system. The most common example of this is computer-based provider order entry, but other advanced CIS include event monitoring, electronic documentation, and barcoding.

Computer-Based Provider Order Entry

With computer-based provider order entry (CPOE), orders for medications, tests, or procedures are entered into the hospital CIS and dispatched to the appropriate departments, either electronically in integrated environments, or printed/faxed. At the least, the computer ensures that orders are legible and complete. Order sets can further simplify and speed up the ordering process for common scenarios (5). The real advantage of computerized orders is that they can be checked against the patient's allergies, current medications, and recent lab results, triggering alerts when a potentially dangerous order has been entered, such as a medication to which a patient is allergic or perhaps cross-sensitive, a medication that has a dangerous drug interaction with another agent that the patient is taking, or a medication whose dose must be adjusted because of impaired renal or hepatic function.

The data on which any computerized decision support intervention runs must be represented in a coded form. This requires that the provider enter allergies, medications, and other data into the system in a computable form, not as free-form text. This can be done in a variety of ways, the most common being a look-up function or "quick-pick" list of one form or another. Although structured data entry is unavoidably time-consuming, many objective studies of well-designed order entry systems show that only a minimal extra time investment is required, and, in the long run, they may in fact be time saving (6,7). But even if they do take a bit more time, this must be balanced against the potential positive impact on patient safety, particularly in the hospital setting (8). For example, one CPOE system, with limited decision support, prevented 55%–86% of serious medication errors that otherwise would have reached the patient (9, 10). Decision support tied to CPOE can also reduce costs (11, 12).

One way that hospitals have tried to ensure successful implementations of computerized order entry is by delegating the time-intensive burden onto clerical staff rather than physicians—physicians write orders by hand in the usual way, and then a unit secretary transcribes the orders into the computer. Although this technique can still prevent errors in the transmission of orders to ancillary departments, decision support is sabotaged because the opportunity to interact with the decision-maker is bypassed.

CPOE is only half the equation when it comes to implementing effective decision support. The other half is crafting, testing, and maintaining the knowledge base of rules that fire and provide corrective recommendations (13,14, Table 10.1). Some rules are readily agreed upon and rarely change (such as *when* to alert on critical lab results), but deciding (and encoding) *who* to alert (physician, nurse, or pharmacist; and which particular one) and *how* (text page, e-mail, or phone call) can be difficult and politically charged (15–17). Even implementing basic drug-allergy checking requires the maintenance of accurate and ever-expanding drug and allergen families (18,19). Even more complicated and labor-intensive is the compilation and maintenance of rules which drive drug-drug (20), drug-disease, and drug-lab interaction checking.

An emerging problem at institutions where extensive rules are implemented is how to reconcile when multiple conflicting rules are triggered—for example, a rule that suggests a formulary change to another medication to which the patient is allergic, or a renal-based dosing rule which suggests a dose that violates an age-based dosing rule. In such cases, more complicated meta-rules must be crafted, tested, and maintained, quickly leading to a situation where the behavior of the CIS system as a whole is difficult to predict and test.

TABLE 10.1

EXAMPLES OF DECISION SUPPORT RULES

Type	Example	References
Drug-allergy	Warn of possible cross-sensitivity when physician orders "Keflex" for patient allergic to "amoxicillin."	19
Drug-drug	Not allow a clinician to concurrently order linezolid and pseudoephedrine because of the risk of severe hypertension.	21, 22
Drug-lab	Warn physician of danger when ordering "digoxin" for patient with a recent potassium level under 3.0.	15, 16, 17
Drug-disease	Warn of a possible adverse event when ordering lovastatin in a patient with cirrhosis.	23
Therapeutic/route substitutions	Suggest switching from intravenous to oral formulation, or from proton-pump inhibitor to an H2 antagonist.	10, 24
Dosing	Suggest lower dose of a drug for patient with renal insufficiency, or an alternative medication in an elderly patient (oxazepam instead of diazepam).	25, 26
Computerized practice guidelines	Suggest appropriate diagnostic or therapeutic steps for a patient admitted with community-acquired or ventilator-associated pneumonia.	27–30

Event Monitoring

An event monitor is a computer program that continually reviews information transactions (or events) that occur within a CIS. As depicted in Figure 10.2, an event monitor or alerting system "listens" for clinical events by monitoring the data transactions occurring across the network. An event that activates a rule is called a *trigger event*. A trigger event may prompt notification of the appropriate clinician with an e-mail or page, depending on the severity of the event. Examples of trigger events are a new lab result for a patient, a new patient registration, a new order, or documentation of a patient encounter. The event monitor examines the new data and decides which, if any, of a database of rules applies to this new piece of data.

A rule usually is encoded as a simple logical statement. For example, "if the patient has a diagnosis of coronary artery disease and the patient is not currently taking aspirin, then remind the physician to order aspirin for the patient," or "if the patient has a new serum potassium result of less than 3.1 meq/liter and the patient is receiving digoxin, then generate an alert notifying the physician about the new lab result." These examples are represented in free text form, but actually must be translated into very precise logical operations on coded concepts in order to have meaning to the CIS.

Rules may require that the event monitor look up other patient-specific data, and so the event monitor must have access to the clinical data repository. When rules are evaluated as "true," some consequent action results. The result of a true rule can be a new monitored event that might trigger another round of rule evaluation, or an unmonitored event, such as the sending of a text message by page or the generation of a report of a possible adverse event (31, 32).

When it comes to impacting patients' care, an event monitor is only as good as the events which can invoke it, the database(s) of rules which it computes, the set of other CIS components with which it can communicate, and the breadth of effects or mechanisms at its disposal (e.g., sending e-mail, paging physicians, generating printed reminders, etc.). However, even simple monitors can be quite effective, especially for critical lab values, for which event monitors have been shown to increase the rate and pace of appropriate care, as well as to reduce morbidity, and even decrease length of stay (33–35).

Electronic Charting and Documentation

Having clinical information in electronic form is valuable for a variety of reasons. Most notably, electronic data can be made available remotely, so the physical limitations of the paper chart are removed. Also, data in coded form are available for clinical decision support (event monitoring). Coded data can also be used for billing, research, management and quality assurance analyses. Clinicians' documentation of the clinical encounter, if represented electronically, could be a boon to quality and safety improvement efforts (see Chapters 12 and 20).

Traditionally, the clinical encounter has been captured on paper, or as transcribed dictation. Although transcription makes the data available for remote viewing (assum-

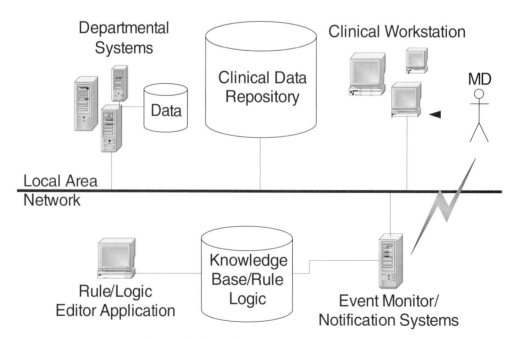

Figure 10.2 Architecture of an event monitor.

ing the appropriate electronic interfaces are in place), the data are not represented in coded form and so are not available for clinical decision support. Many efforts over the last 10–20 years have focused on how to capture encounter information directly from clinicians. As physicians have become increasingly comfortable with typing, many providers now type their encounter notes into the computer themselves. This eliminates the need for transcription (and results in large cost savings); however, it does not result in coded data.

Capturing coded data from clinicians is complex (36). As the requirements for structuring data increase, the flexibility of the data input and expressiveness of the resulting documentation may decrease, thus decreasing physician satisfaction and willingness to use such systems. How best to encode medical concepts involved in documentation (e.g., signs, symptoms, diseases, problems, etc.) is also complex and still lacks a standard solution (37, 38). With the recent free availability of SNOMED (39) (a controlled terminology that attempts to cover these domains), progress towards a more robust and standardized representation of clinical concepts in a computer should proceed more rapidly, which should result in more useful structured physician documentation programs.

Barcoding

Medication errors have been shown to be common (40, 41), and a large proportion (61%) of them occur in the dispensing, transcribing and administering stages (42), after CPOE has had its chance to eliminate them. Barcode technology, in conjunction with an electronic medication administration record system, has been proposed as a promising way to reduce medication errors at these stages (43). However, its efficacy for reducing medication error rates, its acceptance by staff, and its cost-benefit ratio have yet to be evaluated (see Chapter 21).

OTHER CLINICAL INFORMATION SYSTEMS ISSUES

Success Factors for Implementation

The successful implementation of a clinical information system requires more than just a suite of applications that provide the functionality of reviewing test results, entering orders, and guiding decisions. Even systems that perform these functions well may fail to gain the acceptance of their intended users, most notably physicians (44). The problem is that any implementation requires changing practice habits, and such change is difficult even when there is excellent evidence to support the change (45, 46).

There appear to be several factors associated with successful implementation of electronic medical records and decision support. These include both application-dependent characteristics (those that are quick, anticipate the clinician's needs and behaviors, integrate as much as possible into the current workflow, minimize data entry, and guide rather than prevent action) (47) and organization-specific factors (motivation/vision, clinical and administrative leadership, involvement of clinical users, adequate training and support, and responsiveness to user feedback) (48, 49).

Security

All hospital information systems must protect the privacy and confidentiality of clinical information, and the security of their systems. Recent regulations, codified in the Health Insurance Portability and Accountability Act (HIPAA), have defined privacy and security requirements for clinical information systems (50). Typically, hospital information systems operate behind an enterprise "firewall" which guards against intrusions from the outside. Within the hospital environment, access privileges to the information systems are often controlled at the departmental level, or sometimes by the information systems or medical records department. In any case, information security is maintained by requiring users to employ a two-step login procedure (user name and password) to identify themselves and gain permission to use appropriate functions or systems within the environment. Biometric identification (e.g., fingerprint scan) is rarely used today, but may become more common in the future as the reliability of these technologies improves.

Once authenticated into a CIS, a "role-based" security model is often employed to allow users to access information systems applications appropriate for their role. For example, a physician may be permitted to review all clinical data, but a scheduling clerk may be only allowed to access patient demographics and scheduling information. Selected patient-specific information within the CIS environment may also be partitioned off for medical-legal reasons. For example, in some states, HIV test results require special access provisions. Also, in certain settings, mental health-related clinical information might require additional permissions to access. In most settings, however, system designers allow authorized clinical personnel to access any and all clinical information on a patient in an emergency condition, although such access is usually logged.

Hospital Information System Architectures

Most hospital information systems deliver clinical data and functionality to desktop personal computers connected to the hospital network. As depicted in Figure 10.1, ancillary departmental systems communicate via the hospital network to a clinical data repository that aggregates clinical data for presentation to the end user. An interface engine transfers data from one system to another. Additionally, personal computer desktop clinical applications, or Web-based applications, may access the clinical data repository data to present it in useful ways for the end user. For example, as described above, a results viewer application may format clinical laboratory data pooled in the clinical data repository in a way that facilitates rapid review of electrolytes, hematology values, or other data. The most common architecture in use today is a "client-server" architecture that consists of a "back-end" database hosted on a computer (the server), communicating via a secure network to a "front-end" desktop application or Web page (the client), which is viewed by the end user. This approach affords a flexible approach to both front-end and back-end systems design, implementation, and maintenance. Newer approaches may use "application servers" to provide application functionality via Web-based technologies on the client desktop. Additionally, as newer technologies emerge, the front-end may be delivered via wireless network connections that allow the user to access clinical information while mobile, using laptop personal computers, handheld devices, or even cellular phones (51–53).

THE ROLE OF THE HOSPITALIST IN CLINICAL INFORMATION SYSTEMS

The hospitalist can play a unique and pivotal role in the development, implementation, and support of the hospital's clinical information system. First, as a prime consumer of the services provided by CIS, hospitalists are extremely motivated to make sure that the CIS is effective. Because they are at the point of care on a day-to-day and minute-to-minute basis, hospitalists are well positioned to understand the problems of the current health care system and the ways that information technology can help improve matters.

Second, as systems-oriented providers well versed with the processes already at work within the hospital, hospitalists are valuable sources of insight to the developers and implementation team about what will or will not work. They should understand the potential benefits and limitations of information technology to improve care, and mechanisms should be created to regularly elicit their opinions about these matters.

Third, as respected members of the hospital staff and effective communicators, hospitalists can provide leadership in these efforts. One way to promote this is to have hospitalists play an active role in developing and maintaining rules. But, even putting aside specific operational roles,

hospitalists should be advocates for the use of IT as an important way to improve care, and be intimately involved in developing and implementing such systems to ensure that they achieve their intended goals of improving patient care processes, work flow, and outcomes.

CONCLUSIONS

Hospital information systems are critical to the functioning of the modern hospital. They are central to almost all core hospital activities, not just to patient care. Hospital information systems are varied, and the system as a whole can be hampered by the lack of interoperability between subsystems. However, effective hospital information systems can improve patient outcomes, reduce costs, and increase satisfaction among providers. Hospitalists can play a pivotal role in ensuring the success of their hospital's information system.

KEY POINTS

- Hospital information systems are critical to the functioning of today's hospitals, but are limited by poor interoperability and uncoded data entry.
- Effective hospital information systems can improve patient outcomes, reduce costs, and increase satisfaction among providers, largely through clinical decision support provided during order entry, and notification to providers of "panic" or other abnormal test results.
- Successful implementation of advanced hospital information systems requires not just good computer programs, but all the systems, processes, and values that go into changing practice patterns and managing user expectations.
- Hospitalists are uniquely positioned to help develop and implement successful hospital information systems, which can increase their own efficiency and ability to provide high quality care to their patients.

REFERENCES

1. Hiltz FL, Teich JM. Coverage list: a provider-patient database supporting advanced hospital information services. *Proc Annu Symp Comput Appl Med Care* 1994:809–813.
2. Petersen LA, Orav EJ, Teich JM, et al. Using a computerized sign-out program to improve continuity of inpatient care and prevent adverse events. *Jt Comm J Qual Improv* 1998;24:77–87.
3. Barnett GO, Hoffer EP, Schneider E, et al. Distribution of a primary care office information system. *Proc AMIA Symp* 2003: 61–65.
4. Martin MT, Maviglia SM, Kuperman GJ. Handbook: point of care access to clinical knowledge resources. Proceedings of Nursing Informatics, Rio de Janeiro, June 2003.
5. Payne TH, Hoey PJ, Nichol P, Lovis C. Preparation and use of preconstructed orders, order sets, and order menus in a computerized

provider order entry system. *J Am Med Inform Assoc* 2003;10: 322–329.

6. Overhage JM, Perkins S, Tierney WM, McDonald CJ. Controlled trial of direct physician order entry: effects on physicians' time utilization in ambulatory primary care internal medicine practices. *J Am Med Inform Assoc* 2001;8:361–371.

7. Shu K, Boyle D, Spurr C, et al. Comparison of time spent writing orders on paper with computerized physician order entry. *Medinfo* 2001;10(Pt 2):1207–1211.

8. Kuperman GJ, Teich JM, Gandhi TK, Bates DW. Patient safety and computerized medication ordering at Brigham and Women's Hospital. *Jt Comm J Qual Improv* 2001;27:509–521.

9. Bates DW, Leape LL, Cullen DJ, et al. Effect of computerized physician order entry and a team intervention on prevention of serious medication errors. *JAMA* 1998;280:1311–1316.

10. Bates DW, Teich JM, Lee J, et al. The impact of computerized physician order entry on medication error prevention. *J Am Med Inform Assoc* 1999;6:313–321.

11. Tierney WM, Miller ME, McDonald CJ. The effect on test ordering of informing physicians of the charges for outpatient diagnostic tests. *N Engl J Med* 1990;322:1499–1504.

12. Bates DW, Kuperman GJ, Jha A, et al. Does the computerized display of charges affect inpatient ancillary test utilization? *Arch Intern Med* 1997;157:2501–2508.

13. Kuperman GJ, Fiskio JM, Karson A. A process to maintain the quality of a computerized knowledge base. *Proc AMIA Symp* 1999:87–91.

14. Geissbuhler A, Miller RA. Distributing knowledge maintenance for clinical decision-support systems: the "knowledge library" model. *Proc AMIA Symp* 1999:770–774.

15. Kuperman GJ, Teich JM, Bates DW, et al. Detecting alerts, notifying the physician, and offering action items: a comprehensive alerting system. *Proc AMIA Annu Fall Symp* 1996:704–708.

16. Iordache SD, Orso D, Zelingher J. A comprehensive computerized critical laboratory results alerting system for ambulatory and hospitalized patients. *Medinfo* 2001;10(Pt 1):469–473.

17. Raschke RA, Gollihare B, Wunderlich TA, et. al. A computer alert system to prevent injury from adverse drug events: development and evaluation in a community teaching hospital. *JAMA* 1998; 280:1317–1320.

18. Kuperman GJ, Gandhi TK, Bates DW. Effective drug-allergy checking: methodological and operational issues. *J Biomed Inform* 2003;36(1–2):70–79.

19. Kuperman GJ, Marston E, Paterno M, et al. Creating an enterprise-wide allergy repository at Partners HealthCare System. *Proc AMIA Symp* 2003:376–380.

20. Abarca J, Malone DC, Armstrong EP, et al. Concordance of severity ratings provided in four drug interaction compendia. *J Am Pharm Assoc* (Wash DC). 2004;44:136–141.

21. Malone DC, Abarca J, Hansten PD, et al. Identification of serious drug-drug interactions: results of the partnership to prevent drug-drug interactions. *J Am Pharm Assoc* 2004;44: 142–151.

22. Glassman PA, Simon B, Belperio P, Lanto A. Improving recognition of drug interactions: benefits and barriers to using automated drug alerts. *Med Care* 2002;40:1161–1171.

23. Skledar SJ. Hess MM. Implementation of a drug-use and disease-state management program. *Amer J Health-System Pharm* 2000;57 (Suppl 4):S23–29.

24. Teich JM, Merchia PR, Schmiz JL, et. al. Effects of computerized physician order entry on prescribing practices. *Arch Intern Med* 2000;160:2741–2747.

25. Chertow GM, Lee J, Kuperman GJ, et al. Guided medication dosing for inpatients with renal insufficiency. *JAMA* 2001;286: 2839–2844.

26. Oppenheim MI, Vidal C, Velasco FT, Boyer AG, Cooper MR, Hayes JG, Frayer WW. Impact of a computerized alert during physician order entry on medication dosing in patients with renal impairment. *Proc AMIA Symp* 2002:577–581.

27. Sintchenko V, Coiera E, Iredell JR, Gilbert GL. Comparative impact of guidelines, clinical data, and decision support on prescribing decisions: an interactive Web experiment with simulated cases. *J Am Med Inform Assoc* 2004;11:71–77.

28. Evans RS, Pestotnik SL, Classen DC, et al. A computer-assisted management program for antibiotics and other antiinfective agents. *N Engl J Med* 1998;338:232–238.

29. Pestotnik SL, Classen DC, Evans RS, Burke JP. Implementing antibiotic practice guidelines through computer-assisted decision support: clinical and financial outcomes. *Ann Intern Med* 1996; 124:884–890.

30. Maviglia SM, Zielstorff RD, Paterno M, et al. Automating complex guidelines for chronic disease: lessons learned. *J Am Med Inform Assoc* 2003;10:154–165.

31. Jha AK, Kuperman GJ, Rittenberg E, Teich JM, Bates DW. Identifying hospital admissions due to adverse drug events using a computer-based monitor. *Pharmacoepidemiol Drug Saf* 2001;10: 113–119.

32. Classen DC, Pestotnik SL, Evans RS, Burke JP. Computerized surveillance of adverse drug events in hospital patients. *JAMA* 1991;266:2847–2851. Erratum in: *JAMA* 1992;267:1922.

33. Tate KE, Gardner RM, Weaver LK. A computerized laboratory alerting system. *MD Comput* 1990;7:296–301.

34. Rind DM, Safran C, Phillips RS, et al. Effect of computer-based alerts on the treatment and outcomes of hospitalized patients. *Arch Intern Med* 1994;154:1511–1517.

35. Kuperman GJ, Teich JM, Tanasijevic MJ, et al. Improving response to critical laboratory results with automation: results of a randomized controlled trial. *J Am Med Inform Assoc* 1999;6: 512–522.

36. Whiting-O'Keefe QE, Simborg DW, Epstein WV, Warger A. A computerized summary medical record system can provide more information than the standard medical record. *JAMA* 1985; 254:1185–1192.

37. McDonald CJ, Overhage JM, Dexter P, Takesue B, Suico JG. What is done, what is needed and what is realistic to expect from medical informatics standards. *Int J Med Inf* 1998;48:5–12.

38. Rode D. Thompson challenges healthcare industry at first NHII conference. *J AHIMA* 2003;74:14,16–17.

39. Available at http://www.snomed.org. Accessed March 4, 2005.

40. ASHP guidelines on preventing medication errors in hospitals. *Am J Hosp Pharm* 1990;50:305–314.

41. Allan EL, Barker KN. Fundamentals of medication error research. *Am J Hosp Pharm* 1990;47:555–571.

42. Leape, LL, Bates, DW, Cullen DJ, et al. Systems analysis of adverse drug events. ADE Prevention Study Group. *JAMA* 1995;274: 35–43.

43. Bates DW, Cohen M, Leape L, et al. Reducing the frequency of errors in medicine using information technology. *J Am Med Inform Assoc* 2003;8:299–308.

44. Massaro TA. Introducing physician order entry at a major academic medical center: impact on organizational culture and behavior. *Acad Med* 1993:20–25.

45. Cabana MD, Rand CS, Powe NR, et al. Why don't physicians follow clinical practice guidelines? A framework for improvement. *JAMA* 1999;282:1458–1465.

46. Grimshaw JM, Russell IT. Effect of clinical guidelines on medical practice: a systematic review of rigorous evaluations. *Lancet* 1993;342:1317–1322.

47. Bates DW, Kuperman GJ, Wang S, et al. Ten commandments for effective clinical decision support: making the practice of evidence-based medicine a reality. *J Am Med Inform Assoc* 2003: 523–530.

48. Lorenzi NM, Riley RT. Managing change: an overview. *J Am Med Inform Assoc* 2000;7:116–124.

49. Ash JS, Stavri PZ, Kuperman GJ. A consensus statement on considerations for a successful CPOE implementation. *J Am Med Inform Assoc* 2003;10:229–234.

50. Gunn PP, Fremont AM, Bottrell M, Shugarman LR, Galegher J, Bikson T. The Health Insurance Portability and Accountability Act Privacy Rule: a practical guide for researchers. *Medical Care* 2004;42:321–327.

51. Holleran K, Pappas J, Lou H, Rubalcaba P, et al. Mobile technology in a clinical setting. *Proc AMIA Symp* 2003:863.

52. Thomas SM, Overhage JM, Warvel J, McDonald CJ. A comparison of a printed patient summary document with its electronic equivalent: early results. *Proc AMIA Symp* 2001:701–705.

53. Shabot MM, LoBue M. Real-time wireless decision support alerts on a palmtop PDA. *Proc Annu Symp Comput Appl Med Care* 1995;19:174–177.

ADDITIONAL READING

Ash JS, Berg M, Coiera E. Some unintended consequences of information technology in health care: the nature of patient care information system-related errors. *J Am Med Inform Assoc* 2004;11:104–112.

Haux R, et al. *Strategic Information Management in Hospitals: An Introduction to Hospital Information Systems (Health Informatics).* New York: Springer-Verlag, 2004.

Kreider NA, Haselton BJ. *The Systems Challenge: Getting the Clinical Information Support You Need to Improve Patient Care.* Jossey-Bass, 1997.

Shortliffe, EH and Cimino, JJ. *Biomedical Informatics: Computer Applications in Health Care and Biomedicine.* New York: Springer-Verlag, 2004.

Van De Velde R, Degoulet P. *Clinical Information Systems: A Component-Based Approach.* New York: Springer-Verlag, 2003.

Effective Clinical Teaching in the Inpatient Setting

11

Karen E. Hauer   David M. Irby

INTRODUCTION

Inpatient physicians at academic medical centers and teaching hospitals face the opportunity and challenge of combining a busy clinical practice with teaching responsibilities. Attendings can serve as powerful role models and expert instructors of inpatient care for trainees, potentially leading to better future performance and greater interest in internal medicine as a career. Trainees who work with the most highly rated clinical instructors have been shown to perform better on standardized examinations and to be more likely to pursue the specialty of their most valued teacher (1, 2). Highly effective clinical teachers share common traits—they are enthusiastic, they actively involve learners in the educational process, and they plan carefully prior to teaching (3).

In this chapter, we will outline the planning strategies, teaching methods, and reflective practices that inpatient attendings or residents can use to teach and lead a team successfully (Table 11.1). With many academic health centers now employing hospitalists, the inpatient attending role is becoming the responsibility of fewer, more highly experienced physicians (4). Nevertheless, the principles described in this chapter apply to all inpatient team leaders. The *planning* step involves jointly setting expectations with team members, establishing a positive learning climate, and planning for instruction. A variety of *teaching methods* are needed to meet the multiple learning needs of the team in a patient-centered environment. *Reflection* is the process of making sense out of experience and is pro-

moted through thoughtful self-evaluation by learners. This chapter will describe how to apply these three steps with an inpatient team.

PLANNING STRATEGIES

The norms of a group are set at the outset, so attendings should take time to clarify expectations for the team and create a positive learning climate at the start of the rotation. The team will function more effectively and efficiently when responsibilities and roles are clear and consistent.

Jointly Set Expectations

Rounds and Patient Care. Defining expectations at the outset can mitigate later confusion about what was expected or whether a learner has satisfactorily met the requirements of the rotation. Specifically, behaviorally focused expectations are better than generalities. The attending could start this discussion with, "I'm going to share with you the day-to-day expectations I have for all of you to help the team run smoothly; let me know if you have other suggestions." Expectations should be addressed regarding rounds, presentations, workload, communications with the attending, and days off.

Structure of Rounds. Define the relative allocation of time devoted to patient care versus didactics or other teaching. For 90-minute attending rounds, the attending might suggest, "I'd like to devote no more than 30 minutes to

---

TABLE 11.1

STRATEGIES FOR SUCCESSFUL INPATIENT TEACHING

Planning
- Team planning
  - Set clear expectations and provide a rationale for them.
  - Establish learning goals.
  - Create a positive learning climate.
  - Describe the feedback, evaluation, and grading process.
- Plan for teaching

Teaching Methods
- General principles
  - Be learner-centered.
  - Make the same thing count twice by integrating teaching and feedback with patient care.
- Specific methods
  - Teach at the bedside and actively involve the patient and learners.
  - Target teaching to learner needs using the "One Minute Preceptor" model (Table 11.3).
  - Develop and use teaching scripts to address common inpatient illnesses (Table 11.4).
  - Use clinical reasoning in conference room teaching.
  - Promote pattern recognition for classic presentations.

Reflection
- Encourage learners to self-assess and to reflect on their performance.
- Provide frequent, behaviorally focused feedback.
- Include areas for improvement with feedback.
- Schedule periodic meetings for formal feedback.

---

updates on the patients on the service, and leave the last hour for didactic teaching or more in-depth discussion of our toughest case of the day. You can expect that I will have pre-rounded on all the patients, so your presentations can be short and focused."

Presentations. Outline the format and length of presentations for attending rounds and work rounds, and the amount of detail to be provided to the attending versus the resident (Table 11.2). For example, for hospitalists, the traditional model of post-call attending rounds, with the attending first learning about new patients when trainees recite detailed oral presentations, may need to be modified (4). Instead, the attending, who has already seen many of the new patients on call, may prefer to focus on specific teaching points about a case, or on certain patients who raise complex management questions. The resident who leads work rounds should also clarify how much information should be presented for each patient. For example, student presentations can be streamlined with advice such as, "Be sure to update your problem list each day, omitting problems that have been resolved," and "You only need to present labs from the past 24 hours, and only those that are abnormal."

Presentations lasting under 5 minutes are desirable for both trainees and attendings. Trainees may find delivering briefer, more targeted presentations to be challenging, since they lack the background to identify which information to omit after spending hours with the patient and a thick medical record. Learners may be inclined to talk faster or to guess what the attending wants (5). Instead, shorter presentations should prompt the presenter to identify the most pertinent positive and negative data in advance of the assessment. So that trainees are not left guessing what type of presentation the attending will want each post-call day, the attending should state at the start of the month, or on each call day, his/her expectations regarding presentation format. For instance, the attending might say during an on-call phone conversation with the resident, "It looks like we'll cap tonight with 10 new admissions, so please ask each student to be prepared to present a case in no more than 5 minutes, focusing the H & P on the pertinent positives and negatives, and discussing only the main one or two problems in the assessment and plan."

Number and Complexity of Patients To Be Followed. It is particularly important to define this expectation for students.

Communications with the Attending. Tell the team members when to consult or page the attending (such as with critical changes in patient status or possible DNR orders). Explain how best to communicate with the attending (phone versus pager) and the types of clinical situations that warrant immediate communication (versus waiting until rounds). Define regular check-in points throughout the day (e.g., morning rounds with the team and afternoon phone rounds with the resident), and plan for how and when the attending will be involved with new admissions.

TABLE 11.2

GUIDELINES FOR INPATIENT ORAL PRESENTATIONS

- No more than 5 minutes long
- Focus on pertinent positives and negatives—the data that support the differential diagnosis
  - Chief complaint
  - HPI: chronologic, begins with prior medical evaluation and treatment of current problem (if relevant), then current symptoms, then pertinent positive and negative review of symptoms
  - Medical history: major or relevant medical problems
  - Medications: list only without doses
  - Allergies
  - Social history, family history if relevant
  - Exam: vital signs, general appearance, pertinent positives and negatives
  - Laboratory data: abnormal values, pertinent normal values
  - Assessment: differential diagnosis, linking findings above to the most likely diagnoses
  - Plan for each major problem

Adapted from McGee SR, Irby DM. Teaching in the outpatient clinic. Practical tips. *J Gen Intern Med* 2001;16:308–314.

Days Off. Describe the coverage system for team members on days off. For continuity of patient care, it is optimal to have some team members in house every day, by staggering the days off among the team members.

Establish Learning Goals

At the start of the rotation, discuss individual and group learning goals. The attending can initiate this discussion by saying, "I'd like to learn a bit about your interests and goals, so that we can make this month as valuable as possible." Housestaff and students may have initial trouble identifying learning goals—"I'll learn about whatever you want to teach"—but the attending can help team members identify types of learning opportunities in the inpatient setting. For example:

- Clinical skills: physical diagnosis, physical exam of ICU patients, functional assessment of elderly patients
- Diseases and symptoms: evaluation of rash, approach to acute chest pain
- Evidence-based use of diagnostic testing
- End-of-life care
- Role of the physician in the hospital: time management and prioritization, teamwork with ancillary health providers, discharge planning

Create a Positive Learning Climate

The first attending rounds begin with introductions, including interests and goals. In this session, the attending seeks to establish a learning climate that is participatory and respectful of learners at all levels. He or she signals that the team will collaborate in patient care and in the education of one another. He or she role models the enthusiasm, humor, and personal commitment that will support the team's education, motivate performance, and promote teamwork. By inviting questions and suggestions from all team members, the attending also fosters critical thinking and sets the stage for interactive learning, trying to avoid a passive climate in which the attending does most of the talking.

Explain the Process for Feedback, Evaluation, and Grading

Learners should be alerted to the feedback and evaluation process at the start of the rotation. It is important to set a schedule for feedback so that learners will know when to expect feedback and recognize it when they are receiving it. For instance, students will want to know when they will receive feedback on their new patient presentations—immediately after the presentation, later that day, or the next day away from the whole team. The attending might say, "I will plan to give you feedback on your new patient presentations on the post-call day; and if I haven't given

you feedback, it's your job to remind me by the end of the day."

The first attending rounds is also a good opportunity to set a schedule for the three key feedback meetings of the rotation—a first meeting to set expectations and discuss learning goals, a mid-rotation meeting for feedback on progress to date and to decide on priorities for the remainder of the rotation, and a final meeting at the end of the rotation to discuss the evaluation.

For evaluation, the attending should define the attending role: what form or procedure is used, and when it will occur, particularly for students who may be graded on the experience. Students should also be informed of others who may provide input into their final grade.

Plan for Teaching

Attending rounds teaching by necessity is a combination of prepared material and improvised discussion of patients. Attendings who only present prepared didactic material may be perceived as inflexible, and—if their material is only peripherally related to patient care—irrelevant. Alternatively, attending rounds that are focused solely on patient discussions may seem like a disorganized repetition of work rounds. Effective clinical teachers choose one of a number of planning strategies (and often make this choice explicit to the team at the orientation):

- Seeing patients before rounds to expedite presentations and allow for more teaching time
- Reading and preparing handouts before rounds
- Checking in with the resident the day or night before to learn about new patients and solicit topics of interest to the team

Work rounds are the main format for resident teaching and the critical time for most patient care decision-making. To plan for work rounds, the resident should review the patient list each night to identify three to five relevant topics (diagnoses, test results, responses to treatments) to address as teaching points on work rounds the next day. Writing these topics on the patient data cards or in the handheld patient log will remind the resident about these teaching points during discussion of the corresponding patient.

TEACHING METHODS

Highly rated clinical teachers share common characteristics that make their instructional style effective and well received. They are *enthusiastic* about their work and teaching. Inpatient attendings, and hospitalists in particular, have the opportunity to model enthusiasm for inpatient generalism, distinguishing it from ambulatory and subspecialty care. For many housestaff, the presence of dedicated inpatient attendings validates the many months they spend on inpatient rotations by presenting it as a viable and exciting career option. *Flexibility* is a key skill used by effective teachers to adapt their content and teaching style to learners. For instance, a flexible attending will recognize that a post-call intern may not be inclined to generate a long differential diagnosis for chronic abdominal pain, preferring to focus on "what tests do I need to order today." Effective clinical teachers *embed their teaching in the context of cases*, helping learners to retain more information. A particularly powerful learning tool is comparing and contrasting. The attending can stimulate analytic comparisons with questions like, "How does the cardiac exam in this case of shortness of breath differ from the one in the patient we admitted last week with congestive heart failure?" and "What are the key features of each patient's illness?"

Teach at the Bedside and Actively Involve the Patient and Learners

The traditional model of bedside teaching involves the attending shepherding the entire team to the bedside to demonstrate or teach one aspect of physical examination. This process can be quite time-consuming. It can also be difficult to involve all learners actively with one finding or exam technique, often relegating interns or students to the back of the room while others auscultate a murmur. Because many inpatient attendings now aim to see patients on the day of admission, traditional post-call bedside rounds may not synchronize with clinical events, and patient findings may even have resolved.

Attendings who periodically join the team's work rounds (e.g., post call or on the resident's day off) can teach at the bedside while conducting real-time patient care. However, the frequency of such participation in rounds must be carefully planned to maintain the balance between housestaff autonomy and supervision, and the team should be notified in advance of attending participation.

A practical way to implement bedside teaching during the attending's own walk rounds is for the attending to periodically bring one or two learners, particularly students. With the first patient, the learners can observe the attending doing a focused interview and exam. The attending should prepare the learner in advance for what he or she will model at the bedside (6). For example, "I'm going to discuss code status with this patient; watch how the patient responds to my questions," or "My plan is to discuss the risks and benefits of a biopsy versus empiric treatment; see how well you think the patient understands these options." This process can be enhanced by debriefing the learner afterward about general strategies used to address similar problems, or principles the case illustrates. With the next patient, the learner can take the lead, allowing the attending to observe and provide feedback.

For the resident leading work rounds, a major teaching method used at the bedside or in the hallway is *questioning*:

asking interns and students to interpret findings, share their assessment, or suggest a management plan. In general, starting with the junior students and working up to interns allows everyone to participate. Questions should be open-ended to stimulate critical thinking ("How would you put these two findings together?") rather than closed-ended ("What is the most common cause of. . . ? What is the definition of. . . ?"). The other fundamental form of resident teaching is bedside teaching of clinical skills, via modeling of appropriate interaction with patients and verification of clinical findings. The resident should keep in mind that sloppy bedside technique, such as a superficial examination through the patient's gown, while time-efficient, sends a powerful implicit (and unhelpful) message to learners.

Target Teaching to Learner Needs Using the "One Minute Preceptor" for Case Presentations

For daily case presentations, the "One Minute Preceptor" model (Table 11.3) is a useful format that actively involves the learner and incorporates immediate feedback (7). Developed for the ambulatory setting, it can be readily adapted to hospital teaching. After a learner presents the patient data, the model suggests an alternative to a long, meandering discussion of a broad differential diagnosis. Instead, the One Minute Preceptor asks focused questions that help "diagnose" both the patient *and* the learner: "What do you think is going on with this patient?" or "What do you want to do for the patient? What led you to this conclusion?" Based on the answers to these questions, the attending teaches a general point, provides positive feedback, and recommends improvements.

Learners should be advised in advance whether new patient presentations will occur in the hallway or at the bedside. Trainees often prefer conference room or hallway presentations, because bedside presentations may seem intimidating and time-consuming. Bedside presentations nonetheless have advantages: patients may enjoy the attention and information, and bedside presentations ensure some role modeling of bedside care (8). A reasonable balance can be achieved by selecting a few of the most clinically active patients with easily demonstrated physical findings for bedside presentation.

Develop and Use Teaching Scripts to Address Common Inpatient Illnesses

Effective clinical teachers have teaching scripts for common and/or important clinical symptoms and presentations (9). A teaching script is an outline that includes the goals for instruction on a given topic, key teaching points and teaching methods, and learners' typical conceptions and challenges in mastering the topic (Table 11.4). An inpatient attending

TABLE 11.3
THE ONE MINUTE PRECEPTOR—5 EASY STEPS

One minute preceptor steps	Example
The learner presents a case.	*A 40-year-old woman with 3 days of shortness of breath and pleuritic chest pain.*
1. Get a commitment: What do you think is going on with the patient?	*"What do you think is going on with this woman?"*
2. Probe for supporting evidence: What led you to that diagnosis?	*"What led you to think of PE in this case?"*
3. Teach general rules.	*"When clinical suspicion of PE is high, heparin should be started prior to obtaining an imaging study."*
4. Reinforce what is done well: positive feedback.	*"You did a nice job eliciting the potential risk factors for PE."*
5. Correct errors.	*"A normal oxygen saturation does not rule out PE, particularly in a previously healthy patient without underlying cardiopulmonary disease."*

From Furney SL, Orsini AN, Orsetti KE, Stern DT, Gruppen LD, Irby DM. Teaching the one-minute receptor. A randomized controlled trial. *J Gen Intern Med* 2001;16:620–624.

might do well to develop a "toolbox" of 10 to 20 teaching scripts for the most common inpatient symptoms and diagnoses.

Teach Clinical Reasoning in Conference Room Rounds

The explosion of information related to inpatient medicine means that trainees can no longer be expected to have memorized all of the diagnostic criteria and diagnostic steps for every patient presentation. More important than sharing factual knowledge is facilitating the opportunity for critical thinking and self-directed learning. The attending can model critical thinking with every admission. What pertinent information from the history and physical examination led to this diagnostic hypothesis? How were tests interpreted, and how accurate are the tests that were obtained? Although every attending will have his or her

TABLE 11.4
A TEACHING SCRIPT FOR THIRD-YEAR MEDICAL STUDENTS: GI BLEED

- **Goals for instruction:** understand the differential diagnosis and management of a patient with GI bleed
- **Key teaching points:** distinguishing upper from lower GI bleed, identifying the major causes of GI bleed, initiating a diagnostic workup, and stabilizing the patient
- **Teaching methods:** interactive, based on case admitted to the team
- **Knowledge of learners' typical conceptions of and difficulties in mastering specific content:** students typically have difficulty using clues from the history to distinguish causes of GI bleeding, and integrating information to risk-stratify the severity of the bleed

From Irby DM. Three exemplary models of case-based teaching. *Acad Med* 1994;69:947–953.

own style and technique, the most effective inpatient clinical teachers have been shown to use the following principles to promote active learning (10):

First, instruction should be *anchored in clinical cases.* Learner interest and retention will be highest when material is presented in the context of a fascinating or compelling case. The inpatient setting, with the constant stream of new patients, high acuity, and immediately available diagnostic information, provides a rich opportunity for case-based instruction. Adapting teaching scripts can be a very useful strategy here.

Second, *actively involve the learners.* In the conference room, ask each team member to read about a portion of a case (a lab value, physical finding, or item on the differential diagnosis) in advance of the next day's attending rounds. At the bedside, rather than demonstrating a physical finding on a new admission, ask the intern or student to model the exam for the group, and then solicit suggestions from other group members.

Third, *model professional thinking and action.* Although the focus of inpatient teaching is often the didactic attending rounds presentations, much of the teaching and learning occurs in the real-time management of patients. Some of the best teaching comes when the attending talks through a clinical case, sharing the clinical thought process and modeling inpatient expertise. The learner will also then see how the attending deals with uncertainty—how he or she works through different diagnostic possibilities, resolves ambiguous test results, and explains clinical situations to patients and families.

Promoting pattern recognition. Something that looks, sounds, and behaves like your Aunt Minnie is likely to be your Aunt Minnie—there is little need to systematically consider other possibilities (11). In the inpatient setting, where disease often presents in fulminant, dramatic fashion, this teaching principle can be used to highlight classic cases. Instead of asking learners for an extensive case presentation, attendings can request a presentation of the patient's identifying information, chief complaints, or reasons for hospitalization, followed by the working diagnosis. The discussion would then focus on the confirming and disconfirming findings and data.

For example, consider the case of a patient with metastatic cancer who presents with abdominal complaints, altered mental status, dehydration, and worsened bone pain—all hallmarks of hypercalcemia of malignancy (see Chapter 92). Rather than an analytic discussion of differential diagnosis, this method focuses on those key features that learners will remember vividly. Of course, experienced clinicians also expedite their patient assessments by relying on their memory of prototypical case examples, so this method has the additional advantage of introducing trainees to this technique.

REFLECTION

Promoting Reflection in Learners

To encourage self-improvement among trainees, the attending should promote self-assessment and reflection (12). Feedback and evaluation meetings should generally begin with, "I'd like to start by hearing how you think you're doing on the rotation." Rather than telling learners how they've done, or worse yet having them find out the attending's impressions when they read their written evaluation months later, the goal is to create an ongoing dialogue. Although trainees may be reluctant to self-assess, they will feel increasingly comfortable if the attending creates an atmosphere that is collegial and nonjudgmental.

A positive, reflective learning climate is also fostered by allowing for the admission of errors and uncertainty. The attending can model the way in which he or she handles personal limitations—talking at attending rounds about any mistakes that occur in patient management, sharing how to fill in knowledge gaps, and inviting the team to analyze cases with poor outcomes.

To encourage reflection, periodically ask learners to identify one thing they learned from each patient they discharged in the prior week. This strategy is known as "Learning Rounds" (13). It can also be a useful reminder to reflect upon patients who have died, offering trainees the opportunity to learn from deaths on the service and process their emotional reactions to terminal illness (see Chapter 19) (14).

Feedback

Trainees consistently want more feedback and complain that they have not received enough. Feedback provides learners with information about their performance for the purpose of improvement. The attending and resident should create an atmosphere that promotes feedback with careful planning. Residents in particular may not realize that giving feedback is a critical component of effective teaching. Key steps for effective feedback include the following:

- *Set the expectation for feedback* at the start of the rotation. Explicitly state, "Feedback is a priority, and it will occur on a daily basis, with more in-depth feedback meetings midway through the rotation and at the end." Demonstrate an openness to receiving (as well as giving) feedback by soliciting feedback: "I'd like to hear from you how you think I'm doing, teaching at attending rounds, and what I could do to make that time even more useful for you."
- *Immediate feedback* on a daily basis is ideal after hearing a presentation, reading a note, or observing a bedside encounter. Within 5 minutes, give the learner positive feedback to reinforce a specific behavior and make a suggestion for improvement.
- The feedback should be *behaviorally focused*—a description of the specific action performed ("The way that you followed up on the history of alcohol use by quantifying the amount the patient drinks was helpful in revealing the potential impact of alcohol abuse on the cirrhosis") rather than generalizing with adjectives such as "great history" that do not reinforce specific behaviors.
- Feedback should be *based on direct observation* whenever possible. Because residents conduct daily walk rounds

---

TABLE 11.5

GIVING CONSTRUCTIVE FEEDBACK AND MAKING RECOMMENDATIONS FOR IMPROVEMENT

- **Ask the learner to self-assess.** Questions like "How did you feel about your code discussion with the patient?" encourage reflection and often prompt the learner to articulate concerns shared by the attending.
- **Focus on behaviors, not the person.** Instead of saying, "Your presentation style is too slow," feedback could be phrased: "By identifying the pertinent positives and negatives in this patient's physical exam, you can omit the other parts of the exam, like the neurological and skin, to shorten your presentation."
- **Label the feedback "constructive" instead of "negative."** Highly skilled trainees may not have any negative aspects of their performance, but all clinicians at any level of training can make improvements with guidance.
- **Suggest a plan for improvement.** Critical feedback is more readily accepted if it is made as a recommendation for improvement and phrased in the future tense rather than as a reprimand. For example, "Next time you encounter a problem like this, I have found it helpful to do . . . ." This phrasing turns feedback into teaching.
- **Use the feedback sandwich to give frequent feedback that routinely includes reinforcing comments and a suggestion for improvement.** By making constructive comments a regular part of your feedback, you help learners to expect a useful tip along with praise.

TABLE 11.6

GIVING FEEDBACK BASED ON LIMITED INFORMATION

Take the following steps with the learner:

1. Describe the information you received tentatively and avoid drawing conclusions.

   "I heard from Mrs. Jones' daughter that she was frustrated that she wasn't told that her mother was being discharged today, and she was worried it might be too soon for her mom to leave the hospital."

2. Invite joint interpretation of the information.

   "Can you tell me what happened from your perspective? Why do you think her daughter was upset?"

3. Identify areas for positive feedback.

   "You're managing a large service very well, with great attention to detail for each patient."

4. Identify areas of disagreement and develop a plan to collect information to determine if there is really a problem.

   "I understand that you had asked Mrs. Jones' daughter to relay the plans to the family. However, with major changes in the care plan, it's important to make sure the primary spokesperson for the family is fully informed. I have a few suggestions for how you can keep patients and families aware of the plans you're making throughout the day so that they aren't caught by surprise. How about if we start by going to Mrs. Jones' room now and meeting with the family together?"

Gordon MJ. Cutting the Gordian knot: a two-part approach to the evaluation and professional development of residents. *Acad Med* 1995;2:876–880.

with interns and students, residents are ideally situated to observe the team members' clinical skills and critical thinking, following each learner's progress over time. Attendings often hear about and discuss patients in a conference room, and then infer a trainee's history and physical examination skills from the way that findings are presented. By directly observing their interaction with the patient, the resident and attending learn how the information was obtained and can give specific feedback in real time.

- *Frequent feedback* will increase the effectiveness by allowing trainees to quickly modify their behavior before the next observation.

- *Establish a schedule for more formal feedback.* Schedule periodic (e.g., every two weeks or midway through a rotation) longer meetings to give more detailed feedback that serves as a summary of the work to date and an opportunity to set future learning goals. Focus feedback on key objectives of the clerkship or rotation, as well as general areas of inpatient performance. The final feedback meeting doubles as an evaluation of the rotation and feedback for upcoming rotations.

- The *feedback sandwich* is a time-honored format to ensure balanced inclusion of both positive and constructive feedback—begin with positive and reinforcing comments, follow with correction of any errors and sugges-

tions for improvement, and end with praise. It has its place, but effective teachers also find opportunities for unambiguous reinforcing and, when needed, constructive feedback to their trainees (15). Many teachers find it uncomfortable to give constructive feedback. Teachers may feel guilty, or worry that the negative feedback may generate more work in dealing with learner resentment. Steps to make the process of constructive feedback more routine are described in Table 11.5.

- Another challenge confronted by teachers is learning of a trainee's problems second-hand—from another team member, nurse, patient, or family member. The attending may be tempted to dismiss the situation because he or she didn't directly witness it or because it will be uncomfortable to address, thereby missing a key learning moment. The challenge is to use the concern as an opportunity for teaching and feedback without seeming to take sides or misinterpret limited information (Table 11.6).

CONCLUSIONS

The successful inpatient team leader, whether attending or resident, provides a carefully planned experience infused with enthusiasm and active learning. Clarification of expectations at the outset establishes a fair and respectful team dynamic. Highly effective inpatient teaching methods promote critical thinking through bedside interaction and feedback, carefully worded probing questions, and teaching scripts. Self-assessment is a crucial skill that the attending and resident can instill by providing frequent feedback and ensuring that learners reflect on their own performance.

KEY POINTS

- The inpatient attending should set clear expectations with the team at the start of the rotation regarding patient care, learning, and feedback.

- Teaching methods on the inpatient wards should stimulate critical thinking and actively involve learners.

- The attending can promote reflection among learners by prompting self-assessment and by providing frequent, behaviorally focused feedback.

REFERENCES

1. Griffith CH, 3rd, Georgesen JC, Wilson JF. Specialty choices of students who actually have choices: the influence of excellent clinical teachers. *Acad Med* 2000;75:278–282.

2. Griffith CH, 3rd, Georgesen JC, Wilson JF. Six-year documentation of the association between excellent clinical teaching and improved students' examination performances. *Acad Med* 2000; 75:S62–64.

3. Irby DM, Ramsey PG, Gillmore GM, Schaad D. Characteristics of effective clinical teachers of ambulatory care medicine. *Acad Med* 1991;66:54–55.

4. Hauer KE, Wachter RM. Implications of the hospitalist model for medical students' education. *Acad Med* 2001;76:324–330.

5. Haber RJ, Lingard LA. Learning oral presentation skills: a rhetorical analysis with pedagogical and professional implications. *J Gen Intern Med* 2001;16:308–314.

6. McGee SR, Irby DM. Teaching in the outpatient clinic. Practical tips. *J Gen Intern Med* 1997;12 (Suppl 2):S34–40.

7. Furney SL, Orsini AN, Orsetti KE, Stern DT, Gruppen LD, Irby DM. Teaching the one-minute preceptor. A randomized controlled trial. *J Gen Intern Med* 2001;16:620–624.

8. Wang-Cheng RM, Barnas GP, Sigman P, Riendl PA, Young MJ. Bedside case presentations: Why patients like them but learners don't. *J Gen Intern Med* 1989;4:284–287.

9. Irby DM. How attending physicians make instructional decisions when conducting teaching rounds. *Acad Med* 1992;67:630–638.

10. Irby DM. Three exemplary models of case-based teaching. *Acad Med* 1994;69:947–953.

11. Cunningham AS, Blatt SD, Fuller PG, Weinberger HL. The art of precepting: Socrates or Aunt Minnie? *Arch Pediatr Adolesc Med* 1999;153:114–116.

12. Branch WT, Jr., Paranjape A. Feedback and reflection: teaching methods for clinical settings. *Acad Med* 2002;77:1185–1188.

13. Arseneau R. Exit rounds: a reflection exercise. *Acad Med* 1995;70:684–687.

14. Wear D. "Face-to-face with it": medical students' narratives about their end-of-life education. *Acad Med* 2002;77:271–277.

15. Ende J. Feedback in clinical medical education. *JAMA* 1983;250:777–781.

16. Gordon MJ. Cutting the Gordian knot: a two-part approach to the evaluation and professional development of residents. *Acad Med* 1997;2:876–880.

ADDITIONAL READING

Ende, J. What if Osler were one of us? Inpatient teaching today. *J Gen Intern Med* 1997;12(Suppl 2):S41–S48.

Hauer KE, Wachter RM, McCulloch CE, Woo GA, Auerbach AD. Effects of hospitalist attending physicians on trainee satisfaction with teaching and with internal medicine rotations. *Arch Intern Med* 2004;164:1866–1871.

Kroenke K. Attending rounds: guidelines for teaching on the wards. *J Gen Intern Med* 1992;7:68–75.

Assessment and Improvement of Quality and Value

12

Robert M. Wachter   *Niraj L. Sehgal*

INTRODUCTION

The search for value, best described as quality divided by cost, dominates our purchasing decisions. When searching for a car, who would want the cheapest car if there were no guarantee that it was reasonably reliable? Conversely, who could afford the highest quality car if it cost hundreds of thousands of dollars? The goal is to optimize value by weighing quality and cost while being mindful of monetary constraints. The same approach is generally used when planning a vacation, choosing a college, and deciding where to have dinner.

The fact that health care purchasing decisions have not been made on the same basis is an anomaly, primarily explained by the fact that health insurance traditionally insulated both physicians and patients from the cost of care. As a result, it was not until payers—primarily business and government in the United States—decided that health care was too expensive that serious efforts were undertaken to rein in the denominator of the value equation. As for the numerator, the system had neither the tools nor the resources to measure quality effectively. The dominant assumption among patients and purchasers was that all doctors and hospitals provide high quality care, despite the reality that most physicians could easily name colleagues and institutions that they would never consider using, especially if they were sick.

This chapter begins by defining value and its elements, including quality. It highlights problems in health care value, describes how value can be measured, and ends with discussion about how it can be improved.

DEFINING VALUE

One way to consider quality in the context of health care is to separate it into two components—*clinical quality* and *patient satisfaction* (Figure 12.1). This dichotomy produces two entities that are easier to measure and ultimately more amenable to improvement efforts.

The pioneering work of Donabedian (1) on the quality of health care further refined the concept of clinical quality by dividing it into three elements—structure, process, and outcomes. *Structure* refers to *how care is organized*: Does the hospital use hospitalists or primary care physicians to provide inpatient care? Is the intensive care unit open or closed? Is there a designated stroke service? How are the physicians compensated? *Process* refers to *what was done*: Did the patient receive a β-blocker and aspirin after the myocardial infarct? Was the asthma teaching record completed at discharge? *Outcomes* refer to *what happened*: Did the patient live or die? Was the glucose controlled? Did the vessel remain patent? Structure, process, and outcomes are all important in understanding clinical quality, but each has certain advantages and disadvantages when used as a measurement tool (Table 12.1).

The measurement and improvement of patient satisfaction are discussed in Chapter 14. It is worth noting that an assessment of value might consider the satisfaction of "customers" in addition to that of patients. For example, a hospital trying to market its services to a group of primary care physicians would be well advised to survey such physicians. Similarly, a teaching hospital may need to consider how best to optimize not just clinical quality but also education,

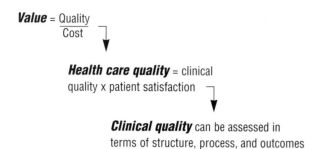

Value = $\frac{Quality}{Cost}$

Health care quality = clinical quality x patient satisfaction

Clinical quality can be assessed in terms of structure, process, and outcomes

Figure 12.1 The health care value cascade.

and so it should survey its trainees regarding their satisfaction (2). Finally, in light of the large national nursing shortage, increasing numbers of hospitals now pay considerable attention to the satisfaction of their nursing workforce (3).

MEASUREMENT OF QUALITY AND VALUE

The innovative studies of Wennberg and Gittelsohn (4), which demonstrated wide and clinically indefensible variations in clinical care, coupled with a breathtaking health care inflation rate throughout the 1970s and 1980s, led many to question the quality and value of health care in the United States. Concerns were further heightened by the publication of data demonstrating a high rate of iatrogenesis and avoidable error in hospital care (5) (Chapter 20). These concerns led to a new emphasis on measuring the elements of value to allow for more informed consumer choice, catalyze quality improvement efforts, and meet regulatory demands. The measurement efforts were given even more urgency by the growth in capitation in the 1990s, a payment model that can provide strong incentives to withhold potentially beneficial care from patients (6).

Prompted by these forces, the health care industry has developed standard "report cards" that measure the elements of value (7). The first influential report card, the Health Plan Employer Data and Information Set (HEDIS), developed by the U.S. National Committee for Quality Assurance, largely focused on process measures in the ambulatory environment (8). The focus on process was understandable: when compared with outcomes, processes are easier to measure, take far less time to develop, and are less demanding of case-mix adjustment (9) (Table 12.1). It is relatively easy to measure whether all diabetics had glycohemoglobin tests and all women had Papanicolaou smears and mammograms at the appropriate ages and intervals. It is far more challenging, costly, and time-consuming to assess the quality of diabetic care by measuring outcomes, such as incidence of renal dysfunction or blindness.

HEDIS's focus on the ambulatory environment was also understandable. In hospitalized patients, even determining what outcomes to measure is problematic. Commonly measured outcomes in complex hospitalized patients, such as mortality and readmission rates, are important but clearly capture only a small part of the picture. Moreover, in the case of mortality, a well-orchestrated death in the hospital may in fact reflect a superb quality of care (Chapter 19).

Over the past few years, a growing number of organizations committed themselves to developing and disseminating quality measures for hospital care. This practice is of particular interest because patients may care more about how a system or physician cares for them when they are sick compared to when they are relatively well (10). The organizations involved in inpatient quality measurement include regulatory agencies [such as the Joint Commission on Accreditation of Healthcare Organizations (JCAHO)], payers [such as the Center for Medicare and Medicaid Services (CMS) and several large private insurers], joint public-

TABLE 12.1

A COMPARISON OF THE THREE TYPES OF CLINICAL QUALITY MEASURES

Measure	Short definition	Advantages	Disadvantages
Structure	How was care organized?	• May be a highly relevant variable in a complex health system	• May fail to capture the quality of care provided by individual physicians • Difficult to determine the "gold standard"
Process	What was done?	• More easily measured and acted on than outcomes • May not require case-mix adjustment • No time lag—can be measured at the time care is provided • May directly reflect quality (if carefully chosen)	• A proxy measure for outcomes • All may not agree on "gold standard" processes • May promote "cookbook" medicine, especially if physicians and systems try to "game" the report card
Outcomes	What happened?	• What we really care about	• May take years to occur • May not reflect quality of care • In need of case-mix and other adjustment

private partnerships [mainly the National Quality Forum (NQF)], and representatives of business coalitions (best illustrated by the "Leapfrog Group," a healthcare advocacy group representing many of the Fortune 500 companies). As one can imagine, although each group shares a commitment to promoting quality, each has a slightly different agenda and a different set of carrots and sticks with which to promote it. For example, while JCAHO measures tend to be process-oriented, emphasize patient safety, and carry the threat of regulatory action for noncompliance, Leapfrog measures tend to be structural (for example, does the hospital have computerized physician order entry?), focus on both safety and quality, and carry little weight of enforcement but the possibility of shifts in market share (and ultimately differential payment) based on performance. Not surprisingly, hospitals that generally lack a tradition of (or infrastructure for) quality measurement and transparency suddenly find themselves struggling to keep up with burgeoning reporting requirements and to prioritize their nascent quality improvement efforts.

Table 12.2 shows some of the existing inpatient quality measures. Although it is a selected list, its scope and breadth reflects how far the inpatient quality initiative has come in a short period. A perusal of the table demonstrates several trends. First, whereas prior quality measures focused on processes, an increasing number of outcome measures are being added. The degree to which such measures reflect true quality will depend on the adequacy of case-mix adjustment. Second, process measures are rapidly being developed for common inpatient diagnoses, building on the successful experience of cardiology (e.g., β-blockers and aspirin in patients with MI) to add process measures for disorders such as pneumonia, stroke, and asthma. Third, the notion of prevention, previously considered exclusively to be an ambulatory issue, is now increasingly being tied to hospital care. Partly because such prevention strategies are easy to understand and do not require case-mix adjustment, many new quality measures seek documentation of smoking cessation counseling, appropriate vaccinations, and prescriptions for preventive medications, such as statins, during a hospital stay. Finally, the list illustrates the chaotic state of quality measurement from the standpoint of the individual hospital, and why many hospitals are reeling trying to keep up with the reporting demands.

The science of *risk adjustment* has advanced to the point that it now adequately accounts for differences in complexity in stereotypic patients undergoing single procedures such as coronary artery bypass grafting (11), although even well-constructed adjusters may be greeted skeptically by clinicians (10). Far more difficult is trying to capture the quality of hospital care for patients with multiple medical disorders, such as those with both diabetic ketoacidosis and community-acquired pneumonia. Although notable progress has been made in the science of risk adjustment and outcomes measurement, much more remains to be done (9). An inadequate methodology of risk adjustment gives hospitals and health systems a potent incentive to recruit healthy patients ("cherry picking") or a ready-made excuse for poor outcomes ("my patients are older and sicker").

The methodologic issues in the measurement of cost and resource use are covered in Chapter 9. Two issues bear emphasis. The discussion of risk adjustment presented above is relevant to the consideration of costs as well as outcomes. A group of physicians caring for sicker patients than another group of comparable quality and efficiency would be expected to have both higher costs and poorer outcomes. An effective adjustment method would be needed to level the playing field in terms of both the numerator and denominator of the value equation. Secondly, the issue of cost shifting needs to be considered in assessing the value of certain services. For example, an intervention that led to shorter hospital stays and lower hospital costs might appear to improve health care value (assuming stable outcomes and satisfaction); however, if the intervention led to costs that were simply displaced to the skilled nursing facility or home, the savings might be illusory. Integrated systems, in which care is delivered across a continuum within the same organization (Chapter 4), may have an advantage in their ability to detect such cost shifting and ensure that overall value has truly been improved.

QUALITY AND VALUE IMPROVEMENT

Changing Physician Behavior

Although physician salaries make up 15% of the American health care dollar, their activities generate 85% of the expenditures, leading to the maxim that "the physician's pen is the most expensive piece of technology in the hospital." Greco and Eisenberg (12) described six ways to change physician behavior: education, feedback, administrative rules, financial incentives, financial penalties, and participation by physicians in efforts to bring about change. All are relevant to efforts to improve value in the hospital.

Educational efforts include continuing medical education, dissemination of practice guidelines, and "academic detailing." In general, studies have shown that continuing medical education leads to no changes in patient outcomes and relatively small changes in practice behavior. Well-designed practice guidelines, especially if locally developed and implemented, can influence physician behavior significantly (Chapter 13). Similarly, academic detailing—in which specific physicians are engaged in the process of educating their peers—can be quite effective, especially when such physicians are opinion leaders in their institutions (13). The degree to which physician participation in continuing education and/or demonstration of up-to-date knowledge (as evidenced by board recertification) reflects

TABLE 12.2

REPRESENTATIVE QUALITY MEASURES ACROSS VARIOUS GROUPS

Clinical condition	Measure	Type of measure	NVHRI[a]	CMS[b]	JCAHO[c]	NQF[d]	Leapfrog[e]
Acute Coronary Syndrome (ACS):	Aspirin at arrival	Process	x	x	x	x	x
	Aspirin at discharge	Process	x	x	x	x	x
	ACE-inhibitor for LVSD	Process	x	x	x	x	x
	β-blocker at arrival	Process	x	x	x	x	x
	β-blocker at discharge	Process	x	x	x	x	x
	Thrombolytic within 30 min of arrival	Process		x	x	x	x
	PCI within 120 min of arrival	Process		x	x	x	x
	Smoking cessation advice/counseling	Process		x	x	x	x
	Inpatient mortality rate	Outcome		x	x	x	x
Coronary Artery Bypass Graft (CABG):	CABG using internal mammary artery	Process				x	x
	CABG volume	Structure				x	x
	CABG mortality	Outcome				x	x
	Prophylactic antibiotic within 1 hr prior to surgical incision	Process			x	x	x
	Prophylactic antibiotic selection for surgical patients	Process		x	x	x	x
	Prophylactic antibiotics discontinued within 24 hrs after surgery	Process		x	x	x	x
	Postoperative hemorrhage or hematoma	Outcome				x	x
	Postoperative physiologic and metabolic derangement	Outcome				x	x
Congestive Heart Failure (CHF):	Left ventricular function assessment	Process	x	x	x	x	x
	Detailed discharge instructions	Process		x	x	x	x
	ACE-inhibitor for LVSD	Process	x	x	x	x	x
	Smoking cessation advice/counseling	Process		x	x	x	x

continued

TABLE 12.2
REPRESENTATIVE QUALITY MEASURES ACROSS VARIOUS GROUPS (continued)

Clinical condition	Measure	Type of measure	NVHRI[a]	CMS[b]	JCAHO[c]	NQF[d]	Leapfrog[e]
Community-Acquired Pneumonia (CAP):							
	Oxygenation assessment within 24 hrs	Process	x	x	x	x	x
	Initial antibiotic selection	Process		x	x	x	x
	Blood culture prior to 1st antibiotic dose	Process		x	x	x	x
	Influenza screening/vaccination	Process		x	x	x	x
	Pneumococcal screening/vaccination	Process	x	x	x	x	x
	Antibiotic timing (1st dose <4 hrs)	Process	x	x	x	x	x
	Smoking cessation advice/counseling	Process			x	x	x
Hip and Knee Replacement:							
	Prophylactic antibiotic within 1 hr prior to surgical incision	Process		x	x	x	x
	Prophylactic antibiotic selection for surgical patients	Process		x	x	x	x
	Prophylactic antibiotics discontinued within 24 hrs after surgery	Process		x	x	x	x
Patient Safety:							
	Catheter-associated UTIs	Outcome				x	x
	Central line-associated infections	Outcome				x	x
	Ventilator-associated pneumonia	Outcome				x	x
	Patient falls	Outcome				x	x
	ICU intensivist	Structure					x
	Computerized provider order entry (CPOE)	Structure				x	x

aThe National Voluntary Hospital Reporting Initiative (Ten Measure Starter Set) sponsored by the American Hospital Association (AHA), Association of American Medical Colleges (AAMC), and Federation of American Hospitals (FAH)
bCenter of Medicare & Medicaid Services (7th Scope of Work Measure)
cJoint Commission on Accreditation of Healthcare Organizations (JCAHO)
dNational Quality Forum (NQF)
eThe Leapfrog Group adopted the 27 safe practices of NQF in addition to their initial endorsements: CPOE, evidence-based hospital referral, and ICU staffing with intensivists
ICU, intensive care unit; PCI, percutaneous coronary intervention; UTI, urinary tract infections.

quality is the subject of ongoing debate; there is little doubt, however, that the public perceives it as such (14).

Feedback involves providing physicians with information about their performance in an effort to improve their performance. Often, there is an implied "gold standard" or "benchmark" against which physicians are compared. The number of national and regional benchmarks related to outcomes and resource utilization that are available for comparison is increasing. Examples include the University HealthSystem Consortium's clinical database, the Centers for Disease Control and Prevention's National Nosocomial Infection Surveillance System (NNIS), and the number of bed-days per thousand population recorded by most managed care organizations. Evidence regarding feedback shows that it can influence practice patterns but its effect is often short-lived. Feedback loops embedded in computerized information systems are likely to have more lasting effects (Chapter 10).

Administrative rules are increasingly being used to influence physician behavior and promote structural changes. Managed care organizations were early adopters of such rules to control costs and decrease variations. As the public became more concerned about the impact of aggressive cost cutting, a spate of governmental regulations emerged covering everything from hospital stays for childbirth to emergency department admissions criteria. Such rules may influence behavior but carry the risk of increasing the "hassle factor" for practicing physicians, and displacing patients from their usual sources of care. Examples of administrative rules include utilizing high-volume providers to perform procedures (15) and reorganizing hospital or critical care services to improve availability and expertise (2,16,17).

Financial incentives and penalties are also used increasingly to modify physician behavior. Although payment methods that motivate physicians to withhold care raise considerable concern (such as capitation arrangements with shared-risk pools), the incentives in fee-for-service arrangements also represent a cause for concern, since physicians are paid more to do more. Controversy continues to exist about whether managed care and capitation harm or improve overall quality and value (6), although it is clear that reimbursement changes do influence practice behavior (18).

Perhaps the most important method of achieving sustainable change in health care practices is to encourage *providers to participate* themselves. This notion was recognized long ago by W. Edward Deming, who promoted the concept of *continuous quality improvement (CQI)*, predicated on a continuous flow of information from the process to the providers. These concepts have been adapted to the health care system during the past decade. In this conceptual model for quality improvement activities, all the participants engage in a continuous cycle of changing, measuring, and changing again (19) (Figure 12.2). In a stunning example of CQI in action, 23 cardio-

thoracic surgeons participated in a three-component intervention that included training in CQI techniques, feedback on outcome data, and site visits to other medical centers. As a result, there were 74 fewer deaths (a 24% reduction) than the expected rate following the intervention period (20).

Pay for Performance

As noted earlier, the last few years have seen an explosion in public quality reporting efforts. Such efforts try to motivate change by dint of transparency: the hope is that by simply reporting comparative performance on quality metrics, organizations and providers will seek to improve their performance. The evidence that this strategy is effective in motivating change is mixed (21, 22).

However, discouraged by the slow pace of change and evidence of poor performance on many quality measures (23), a newer trend goes beyond public reporting to linking compensation to quality performance.(24) As of this writing, an estimated 40 pay-for-performance (PFP) programs have been developed or implemented by health plans and employer coalitions.(25) Most programs involve a "report card" to evaluate providers and groups around designated quality standards, including rates of screening for cervical and breast cancer, markers of management for patients with diabetes and heart disease, and specific patient-satisfaction scores. A number of different incentive strategies have been employed, ranging from paying a "quality bonus" to providers who achieve certain performance goals to linking patients' deductible and copayments to providers' performance (26). Perhaps the most prominent example is Medicare's Premier Hospital Quality demonstration project, in which a group of hospitals are submitting data on patients treated for several conditions, including acute myocardial infarction, community-acquired pneumonia, and coronary artery bypass surgery.(27) Hospitals whose performance

What are we trying to accomplish?
How will we know that a change is an improvement?
What changes can we make that will result in an improvement?

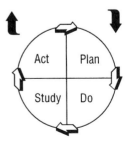

Figure 12.2 Berwick's model for quality improvement, emphasizing the iterative process of change. (From Berwick D, Nolan T. Physicians as leaders in improving health care: a new series in *Annals* of Internal Medicine. *Ann Intern Med* 1998;128:289–292.)

matches evidence-based performance standards will receive an extra 2% in Medicare payments per condition. Many similar programs are under consideration.

The impact of PFP programs is as yet unstudied. We believe that, depending on the extent of their spread and the magnitude of the incentives, they are likely to motivate improved performance by individual providers and systems. The latter issue is extremely important: physicians whose practices are supported by electronic medical records with automatic alerts and robust decision support are likely to perform better, especially on relatively straightforward, algorithmic metrics such as ordering certain tests or medicines at the right time (Chapter 10). Of course, such PFP programs may have the perverse effect of lowering reimbursements to healthcare systems that lack information technology, making it even less likely that the systems will be able to afford the purchase of the needed computers and infrastructure. It will be vital to study the impact of PFP systems to ensure that they are achieving their intended effects.

Other Recent Trends in Quality Improvement

Whether motivated by a professional desire to change, comparative report cards, or pay for performance, hospitals and physicians have come to recognize the inadequacy of traditional, education-based quality improvement strategies. Increasingly, systems are embracing more active and engaging endeavors to impact practice behaviors. Many successful projects have begun by recognizing that reliance on a physician's memory fails to ensure uniform adoption of evidence-based practices. Instead, such projects focus on "hard-wiring" quality improvements. Examples include the use of computer-generated clinical decision-support in antibiotic selection for patients admitted with pneumonia, automatic reminders to provide tobacco cessation counseling and influenza vaccinations, and ventilator management algorithms that are independently executed by respiratory therapists (28). Finding the right balance of "hard wired" approaches to ensure flawless execution of quality strategies while preserving physician autonomy in more complex and less algorithmic situations will be one of medicine's great challenges over the next decade.

CONCLUSIONS

Former *New England Journal of Medicine* editor Arnold Relman (29), writing in 1988, predicted that the American health care system was leaving the eras of expansion of care (1940s to 1970s) and cost containment (1980s) and entering a third era of assessment and accountability. This new era, he wrote, would be one in which measurement of value would become standard practice, and in which patients and purchasers would make their decisions based on such measurements. In this environment, physicians and the systems in which they work would be strongly motivated to assess value continuously and work tirelessly to improve it. Although Relman may have been optimistic in his timing, the activities in the past few years by regulators such as JCAHO, business coalitions such as the Leapfrog Group, and payers such as the Center for Medicare and Medicaid Services (CMS) to measure, promote, and reward quality—and the extent to which hospitals and providers are increasingly participating in activities to improve value—may mean that Relman's vision may finally be realized.

The questions no longer are about whether there will be quality measurement of hospitals and their providers. Rather, they increasingly relate to the methodology of measures (what is the right combination of measures that are evidence-based vs. expert consensus-derived?), the organizational and logistical aspects of measurement (particularly, can measurement sets be consolidated to a manageable group that all stakeholders will accept?), and the appropriate combination of carrots and sticks to promote full implementation. In these chaotic early days, it can be easy to forget that the final outcome of the quality measurement movement will undoubtedly be improved patient care and better outcomes.

KEY POINTS

- Health care purchasing decisions will increasingly be made based on assessments of value, defined as quality divided by cost.
- Quality in health care may be thought of as a product of clinical quality (assessed according to structure, process, or outcomes) and patient satisfaction.
- Although outcome measurements may ultimately be more salient than process measurements, they are more difficult to acquire; furthermore, correct interpretation of outcome measures is highly dependent on adequate case-mix adjustment.
- A number of strategies (including education, feedback, regulation, and incentives) can be used to change physician behavior. Those that actively engage providers themselves in the process of change tend to be the most successful.
- There is a burgeoning trend of public reporting of doctors' and hospitals' quality measures, increasingly accompanied by economic incentives that reflect performance.
- In part to meet these demands, a new trend is to "hard wire" quality improvements by fundamentally altering the processes of care, rather than depending on the physicians' execution of the correct processes.

REFERENCES

1. Donabedian A. The quality of care. How can it be assessed? *JAMA* 1988;260:1743–1748.

2. Wachter RM, Katz P, Showstack J, et al. Reorganizing an academic medical service: impact on cost, quality, patient satisfaction, and education. *JAMA* 1998;279:1560–1565.
3. Berliner HS, Ginzberg E. Why this hospital nursing shortage is different. *JAMA* 2002;288:2742–2744.
4. Wennberg J, Gittelsohn A. Small area variations in health care delivery. *Science* 1973;182:1102–1108.
5. Brennan TA, Leape LL, Laird NM, et al. Incidence of adverse events and negligence in hospitalized patients. Results of the Harvard Medical Practice Study I. *N Engl J Med* 1991;324:370–376.
6. Berwick DM. Payment by capitation and the quality of care: part 5. *N Engl J Med* 1996;335:1227–1231.
7. Epstein A. Performance reports on quality—prototypes, problems, and prospects. *N Engl J Med* 1995;333:57–61.
8. Chassin MR, Hannan EL, DeBuono BA. Benefits and hazards of reporting medical outcomes publicly. *N Engl J Med* 1996;334:394–398.
9. Iezzoni LI, Ash AS, Shwartz M, et al. Predicting who dies depends on how severity is measured: implications for evaluating patient outcomes. *Ann Intern Med* 1995;123:763–770.
10. Angell M, Kassirer JP. Quality and the medical marketplace—following elephants. *N Engl J Med* 1996;335:883–885.
11. Schneider EC, Epstein AM. Influence of cardiac-surgery performance reports on referral practices and access to care—a survey of cardiovascular specialists. *N Engl J Med* 1996;335:251–256.
12. Greco PJ, Eisenberg JM. Changing physicians' practices. *N Engl J Med* 1993;329:1271–1273.
13. Soumerai SB, Avorn J. Principles of educational outreach ("academic detailing") to improve clinical decision making. *JAMA* 1990;263:549–556.
14. Brennan TA, Horwitz RI, Duffy FD, Cassel CK, Goode LD, Lipner RS. The role of physician specialty board certification status in the quality movement. *JAMA* 2004;292:1038–1043.
15. Birkmeyer JD, Dimick JB. Benefits of the new Leapfrog standards: effect of process and outcome measures. *Surgery* 2004;135:569–75.
16. Pronovost PJ, Angus DC, Dorman T, Robinson KA, Dremsizov TT, Young TL. Physician staffing patterns and clinical outcomes in critically ill patients: a systematic review. *JAMA* 2002;288:2151–62.
17. Diez-Tejedor E, Fuentes B. Acute care in stroke: do stroke units make the difference? *Cerebrovasc Dis* 2001;11:31–39.
18. Hillman AL, Pauly MV, Kerstein JJ. How do financial incentives affect physicians' clinical decisions and the financial performance of health maintenance organizations? *N Engl J Med* 1989;321:86–92.
19. Berwick D, Nolan T. Physicians as leaders in improving health care: a new series in *Annals of Internal Medicine. Ann Intern Med* 1998;128:289–292.
20. O'Connor G, Plume S, Olmstead E, et al. A regional intervention to improve the hospital mortality associated with coronary artery bypass graft surgery. *JAMA* 1996;275:841–846.
21. Hannan EL, Kilburn H Jr, O'Donnell JF, Lukacik G, Shields EP. Adult open heart surgery in New York State. An analysis of risk factors and hospital mortality rates. *JAMA* 1990;264:2768–2774.
22. Schneider EC, Epstein AM. Use of public performance reports: a survey of patients undergoing cardiac surgery. *JAMA* 1998;279:1638–1642.
23. McGlynn EA, Asch SM, Adams J, et al. The quality of health care delivered to adults in the United States. *N Engl J Med* 2003;348:2635–2645.
24. Benko LB. A rewarding relationship. Hospitals and docs are seeing more of their pay tied to performance based on quality measures and other contractual objectives. *Mod Healthc* 2003;33:28–30,34–35.
25. Sipkoff M. Will pay for performance programs introduce a new set of problems? *Manag Care* 2004;13:16–17, 21–22.
26. Rewarding for quality: new incentives emerge to improve healthcare and promote best practices. *Qual Lett Healthc Lead* 2002;14:2–5,8–10.
27. Premier Hospital Quality Incentive Demonstration. Center for Medicare and Medicaid Services. Available at http://www.cms.hhs.gov/quality/hospital/PremierFactSheet.pdf. Accessed January 1, 2005.
28. Shojania KG, Duncan BW, McDonald KM, Wachter RM, eds. Making healthcare safer: a critical analysis of patient safety practices. Rockville, MD: Agency for Healthcare Research and Quality; 2001. Evidence Report/Technology Assessment No. 43; AHRQ publication 01-E058.
29. Relman AS. Assessment and accountability: the third revolution in medical care. *N Engl J Med* 1988;319:1220–1222.

ADDITIONAL READING

Berwick DM. Continuous improvement as an ideal in health care. *N Engl J Med* 1989;320:53–56.

Brook RH. Measuring quality of care: part 2. *N Engl J Med* 1996;335:966–970.

Chassin MR. Is health care ready for Six Sigma quality. *Milbank Q* 1998;76:565–591.

Committee on Quality of Health Care in America, IOM. *Crossing the Quality Chasm: S New Health System for the 21st Century.* Washington DC: National Academy Press, 2001.

Deming WE. *Quality, Productivity, and Competitive Position.* Cambridge, MA: Massachusetts Institute of Technology, 1982.

Eddy DM. *Clinical Decision Making: from Theory to Practice.* Sudbury, MA: Jones and Bartlett, 1996.

Hibbard JH, Stockard J, Tusler M. Does publicizing hospital performance stimulate quality improvement efforts? *Health Affairs (Millwood)* 2003;22:84–94.

Kassirer JP. Hospitals, heal yourselves. *N Engl J Med* 1999;340:309–310.

Porter ME, Teisberg EO. Redefining competition in health care. *Harv Bus Rev* 2004;82:64–76,136.

Pronovost PJ, Nolan T, Zeger S, Miller M, Rubin H. How can clinicians measure safety and quality in acute care? *Lancet* 2004;363:1061–1067.

Vips and Med-vantage. Comprehensive study of existing pay-for-performance programs published March 2004. Vips, Inc., Baltimore, MD.

Practice Guidelines and Clinical Pathways

13

Scott Weingarten

INTRODUCTION

Practice guidelines and clinical pathways have been developed by scores of health care and physician organizations in many countries. The dramatic proliferation of guidelines and pathways and the widespread enthusiasm surrounding their development is fueled by the belief that the adoption of guidelines and pathways can lead to a more systematic and consistent approach to the delivery of patient care and result in improved quality and reduced health care costs. Newer approaches to clinical quality improvement, including the use of health care information technology, may be replacing paper-based strategies. Such technology may facilitate the electronic delivery of clinical pathways, practice guidelines, and clinical decision support, creating a more sustainable strategy for improving patient care for diverse populations of patients (1).

VARIATIONS IN MEDICAL CARE

In the past, the strongest influence on medical decisions was the beliefs of individual physicians, formed by their experience, medical training, and understanding of the scientific literature. However, the sheer volume of medical literature has made it virtually impossible for any physician to remain current (2). Currently, physicians spend about one third of their day reviewing, interperting, and integrating clinical information (3). Estimates suggest that more than 100,000 medical research articles are published every month in 20,000 different medical journals, and there are more than 200,000 randomized controlled trials indexed in MEDLINE alone. It is not surprising, then, that individual clinicians are often overwhelmed by the amount of available clinical information.

A variety of studies have demonstrated frequent and unexplained *variations in medical care*. For example, lengths of stay for patients with pneumonia have been shown to vary from one geographic region to another, from hospital to hospital, and even from ward to ward within the same hospital (4). Differences in length of stay have been found to persist even after case complexity and other known patient-related factors are taken into consideration. Many of these variations are believed to result from differences in physician practice style and are unrelated to patients' medical conditions or preferences.

Although some variation in medical care may be desirable, variations can also compromise care, especially when care deviates from the best course of treatment based on the scientific evidence. For example, studies have demonstrated significant interhospital variations in the "door-to-needle" time for the administration of thrombolytic therapy in patients presenting to an emergency department with acute myocardial infarction (5). This variation may reflect differences in approaches to therapy and the time required for informed patient decision making, but delayed administration of thrombolytic therapy can increase mortality rates. Delayed administration of antimicrobial therapy for patients hospitalized with community-acquired pneumonia was associated with increased mortality, and there are wide regional variations in the time to administer antibiotics to such patients (6). Similarly, underutilization of β-blockers and aspirin among selected patients recovering from acute myocardial infarction can result in higher patient mortality. Finally, underuse of angiotensin-converting enzyme inhibitors and angiotensin receptor blockers in appropriate patients with congestive heart failure is associated with reduced survival and increased hospitalization rates. Therefore, variations in medical care can be associated with preventable deaths, and such variations continue to provoke concern in the medical community.

DEVELOPMENT OF PRACTICE GUIDELINES AND CLINICAL PATHWAYS

A variety of approaches have been employed to reduce undesirable variations in medical care and to make medical care more consistent with the published scientific evidence. These approaches have included the creation and dissemination of *practice guidelines, clinical pathways, clinical decision support, protocols,* and *care maps.* Practice guidelines have been defined as "systematically developed statements to assist practitioner and patient decisions about appropriate health care for specific clinical circumstances" (7). Ideally, evidence-based guidelines and clinical pathways would integrate, organize, and summarize the available information for a condition and allow busy clinicians to wade efficiently through it. Additionally, the information would be updated regularly to allow even the busiest of clinicians to remain relatively current. Although the terminology and nomenclature will undoubtedly change, the basic premise of codifying and expressing a somewhat uniform approach to caring for patients that reflects the most up-to-date and relevant scientific evidence should be enduring.

Guidelines and clinical pathways are often developed for high-volume and costly medical and surgical conditions. For example, many institutions have developed guidelines and pathways for conditions such as acute myocardial infarction, congestive heart failure, acute ischemic stroke, total hip replacement, coronary artery bypass graft, and community-acquired pneumonia. The conditions are prioritized because changes in care for the most common conditions carry the greatest potential to improve patient care and reduce health care costs, and are scrutinized by regulatory organizations and payers.

Thousands of guidelines have been funded by subspecialty organizations, such as the American Heart Association and the American College of Cardiology, and countless local organizations. There are probably more than 2,000 published guidelines, and far more have been developed and disseminated within local health care organizations without wider distribution.

Many of these guidelines have been based on study of integrative articles (systematic reviews, meta-analyses, and decision analyses), thorough review of the primary literature, or both (see Chapter 8). Some guidelines rely to a greater extent on *scientific evidence,* others are primarily based on *expert opinion,* and still other guidelines blend these two approaches. Whichever method is used, it can be important to identify explicitly and grade the sources of key recommendations (Table 13.1). Different sources of and approaches to guidelines may engender different levels of confidence. For example, guidelines developed by a trusted subspecialty organization using scientific evidence may be

TABLE 13.1

AN EXAMPLE OF AN EVIDENCE GRADING SYSTEM

Grade A	Randomized, prospective, controlled trials
Grade B	Non-randomized, prospective trial
Grade C	Retrospective analyses
Grade E	Expert opinion unsubstantiated by higher levels of evidence
Grade M	Meta-analyses
Grade Q	Cost-effectiveness/decision analysis
Grade S	Systematic reviews

Adapted from Greengold NL, Weingarten SR. Developing evidence-based practice guidelines and pathways: the experience at the local hospital level. *Jt Comm J Qual Improv* 1996;22:391–402, with permission.

considered more credible by physicians than guidelines developed by a health insurance company or by persons viewed as having a significant financial stake in the course of patient care (8). In any case, guidelines rigorously based on scientific evidence may be considered more credible and less subject to bias than guidelines based solely on expert opinion.

Clinical pathways are management tools that have been used in many industries outside the health care arena (9). Traditionally, they have been employed to describe the goals of work flow processes and the sequencing of events. The perceived success of clinical pathways in these industries has led to the belief that a similar approach could improve patient care. Sometimes, they will embed practice guidelines, which include information about the appropriateness of care in addition to the sequencing of care. Clinical pathways are charted with time displayed along the x-axis. Many guidelines and clinical pathways are developed through a multidisciplinary approach, which includes physicians, nurses, pharmacists, and other ancillary personnel. In many cases, a goal of the clinical pathway is to replace existing documentation, allowing nurses (and sometimes physicians) to document care on the pathway rather than the progress notes. However, many health care providers also believe that the delivery of patient care is unique, complicated, and not readily suited to industrial strategies for automating work flow "processes."

The purchasers of health care (e.g., employer groups) and the payers (e.g., health plans, Center for Medicare and Medicaid Services) are demanding accountability for the quality of care received by patients. Purchaser efforts to document the quality of care and outcomes include the Health Plan Employer Data and Information Set (HEDIS) measures developed by the National Committee on Quality Assurance, and several others. Some payers have asked contracting provider organizations (e.g., hospitals, physician organizations) to document their care in "pay for performance" or incentive-based reimbursement programs (see Chapter 12). It is likely that the use of guidelines and clinical pathways will become even more common as the movement to measure and report quality indicators continues to grow.

EFFECTIVENESS OF PRACTICE GUIDELINES AND CLINICAL PATHWAYS

Although significant effort and resources have been devoted to the creation and dissemination of guidelines, relatively little is known about whether this effort has improved patient care and whether the benefits of these efforts have justified the cost of development and implementation. However, the published literature supports the hypothesis that care can be improved through the use of practice guidelines. A rigorous evaluation of 59 studies on the topic demonstrated that guidelines have led to documented improvements in patient care (10). Of the eleven studies that specifically examined patient outcomes (which reflect what happens to the patient as a result of care), nine demonstrated beneficial effects of guidelines.

There are even fewer published peer-reviewed studies evaluating the effects of clinical pathways on clinical practice or demonstrating a significant improvement in patient outcomes as a result of their implementation. Although some studies have shown reductions in length of stay following the introduction of a clinical pathway, the relative contributions of the pathway and of secular trends that may have been occurring independently of the clinical pathway are not known. Given the dearth of evidence supporting the use of pathways, at present it is unclear whether the cost of developing and implementing them can be justified.

One traditional challenge of implementing practice guidelines and clinical pathways is that paper-based strategies (e.g., paper-based standing orders, paper reminders on the front of charts) are laborious and costly to implement on an ongoing basis. Furthermore, it is difficult to "build" paper-based guidelines and pathways to encompass multiple conditions and procedures across a hospital setting. Also, many hospitalized patients have multiple comorbid conditions, and paper-based guidelines and order sets can potentially oversimplify the care of these complex patients.

One additional problem with evaluating the effects of guidelines and clinical pathways on patient care has to do with the methodologic difficulties associated with conducting scientifically credible studies. Randomized, controlled clinical trials are the "gold standard" for evaluating the safety and efficacy of drugs. Although it would be desirable to test guidelines and clinical pathways in a similarly rigorous manner, the use of clinical trials to assess "systems" of caring for patients poses significant challenges. For example, multiple changes are often instituted simultaneously, which makes it difficult to isolate the impact of guidelines or pathways on patient care. Moreover,

contamination of patient groups may occur, as it is not possible to prevent physicians caring for control patients from familiarizing themselves with the guidelines and applying them to the care of their patients.

CARE OF THE HOSPITALIZED PATIENT

The potential of practice guidelines to improve patient care may depend on whether they are based on firm scientific evidence, are easy to understand, include actionable statements, and are implemented in an effective manner. Because many guidelines express ambiguous statements, their impact on patient care is limited. For example, a guideline that recommends that patients be transferred out of the intensive care unit when they are stable will probably have little effect on patient care.

The key to improving care through the use of guidelines and clinical pathways is *successful implementation*. Many different strategies can be employed to facilitate the widespread dissemination and effective implementation of practice guidelines. For example, continuing medical education is often used to introduce guidelines, although a number of studies suggest that conventional forms of continuing education rarely produce sustained changes in clinical practice. Providing retrospective feedback to physicians, in the form of comparisons with peers or other appropriate benchmarks, may prove more helpful, but most studies demonstrate a modest impact. "Academic detailing," or one-on-one encounters with clinicians, has been shown to change physician behavior, but is costly (11). A strategy that can be effective is when those disseminating the guidelines are regarded as "opinion leaders" by their peers. Guidelines can also be implemented through reminders from case managers or other appropriate non-physician personnel. Hospitalists who are faithfully committed to the use of guidelines and pathways and may have participated in their development can facilitate the successful implementation of guidelines by serving as effective messengers for the rest of the medical staff. Intensivists can serve in comparable roles in the critical care unit.

Many published examples have shown that guidelines, when disseminated and implemented effectively, can improve patient care. For example, a guideline was developed at Cedars-Sinai Medical Center in Los Angeles to risk-stratify patients hospitalized for upper gastrointestinal hemorrhage (12). The guideline was based on patient hemodynamic parameters, endoscopic findings, comorbid conditions, and time elapsed since the initial bleed. A retrospective study found that the guideline accurately identified patients who were at low risk for rebleeding and might not benefit from continued and prolonged hospitalization. Based on the risk information, the guideline prescribed a specific day of discharge for each patient. When tested retrospectively, the guideline would have significantly reduced hospital length of stay while preserving excellent patient outcomes had it been applied to patient care. When the guideline was later applied in clinical practice, hospital length of stay declined from 4.6–2.9 days (mean reduction of 1.7 days per patient, $p < .001$) (12). Moreover, patient outcomes, including hospital readmission rates, emergency department visits, and health-related quality of life, remained unchanged when measured 1 month after discharge from the hospital.

Information technology has great potential to facilitate the implementation of guidelines and clinical pathways, and represents an important aspect of the future of clinical quality improvement. Studies involving computerized clinical decision support have shown important improvements in care (13). When information is made available to physicians while they are caring for patients (at the "point of care"), it becomes easier for them to apply the guidelines in the care of individual patients. Information technology is particularly helpful since most guidelines are too complex to be committed to memory, and effective guidelines undergo frequent revision based on new published evidence and local experience. Computerized entry of provider orders can integrate guidelines and other recommendations into the routine patient care work flow, and can enable deployment of multiple guidelines and pathways at the same time (see Chapters 10 and 12).

Providing *alerts* and *reminders* to physicians while they are caring for patients by using rules-based logic has often proved to be an effective strategy. For example, there is evidence that early antibiotic treatment may be beneficial for patients with community-acquired pneumonia. In the case of a patient presenting to an emergency department, clinical decision support embedded in an information system might notify a physician about the benefits of early antibiotic treatment immediately after a patient with community-acquired pneumonia is hospitalized. A similar intervention in which computer-assisted prescribing of antibiotics was used for intensive care unit patients led to significant reductions in length of stay, costs, and mortality rates (14).

Therefore, as computerized provider order entry and the electronic medical record become more prevalent, they are likely to play an even more substantial role in the implementation of practice guidelines and clinical pathways. The guidelines and pathways may be expressed electronically as clinical decision support, order sets, alerts, reminders, and structured documentation. Published studies are encouraging regarding the impact of health care information technology with clinical decision support on the quality of patient care.

Studies have also explored and demonstrated the potential pitfalls of applying guidelines. For example, if the focus of a guideline or pathway is too narrow, it may not lead to improved outcomes. A study of congestive heart failure patients that focused only on the decision regarding the most appropriate time to transfer them from the intensive care unit or intermediate care unit to an unmonitored bed found little net benefit (15). In fact, while lengths of stay in

monitored settings decreased as a result of an increased emphasis on transferring patients out of the coronary care unit, length of stay in unmonitored settings increased, and total length of stay actually increased. As more rigorous studies of guidelines and clinical pathways are published, we can expect to see more evidence regarding both their benefits and limitations.

Many clinical pathways include information on expected length of stay. However, these figures may be derived from "benchmark" information from other institutions, which may include data on length of stay but no corresponding data on quality or outcomes. For example, if shorter lengths of stay are associated with more patient readmissions, returns to the emergency department, and discharges to skilled nursing facilities rather than home, overall quality of care may have declined and overall costs may have increased (see Chapter 12). To ensure that costs are not simply displaced ("squeezing the balloon") or quality compromised, studies evaluating the impact of guidelines and pathways should generally measure important outcome variables, such as mortality, readmission, and patient satisfaction. They should also make efforts to rule out cost shifting; this is most easily accomplished in integrated systems in which patients can be tracked across the continuum of care.

Another concern about the relevance of clinical pathways or practice guidelines to patient care is that many medical conditions afflict a fairly *heterogeneous population* of patients. For example, it may be difficult to implement guidelines in patients with multiple comorbid conditions. Consider how challenging it would be to develop a standardized course of care for a patient hospitalized with community-acquired pneumonia who also has chronic obstructive pulmonary disease, congestive heart failure, and severe depression.

Finally, there are concerns about the *medicolegal risk* associated with the use of practice guidelines and clinical pathways. The literature is inconclusive on whether guidelines and pathways increase or decrease medicolegal liability (16). One study suggested that guidelines were used more frequently by plaintiff's attorneys against physicians than by attorneys defending physicians. Conversely, it has been difficult to quantify the number of cases in which physician adherence to a guideline resulted in an attorney's declining to take a case. Many believe that the potential medicolegal benefits of guidelines and pathways exceed the risks, but this is an evolving field.

CONCLUSIONS

Many hospitals have supported the development or local adaptation of practice guidelines and clinical pathways. Although relatively little is known about whether clinical pathways have any effect on patient care, a burgeoning literature suggests that carefully implemented practice guidelines can promote high-quality, efficient patient care. For practice guidelines to be beneficial, however, they must be based on sound scientific evidence and implemented in an effective manner. With the introduction of more sophisticated clinical information systems, clinicians will see an expansion in the development and application of systematic approaches to caring for hospitalized patients, including the use of practice guidelines and clinical pathways integrated into information systems.

KEY POINTS

- Practice guidelines, which are "systematically developed statements to assist practitioner and patient decisions about appropriate health care for specific clinical circumstances," have been demonstrated to improve patient outcomes, and lower costs.
- Clinical pathways, which map out the process of work flow over time, have not been convincingly demonstrated to improve patient care.
- A key to improving care with guidelines or pathways is successful implementation.
- Although many strategies have been used to assist in implementation, embedding evidence-based guidelines within clinical information systems used by clinicians at the "point of care" holds the most promise.

REFERENCES

1. Hersh WR. Medical informatics: Improving health care through information. *JAMA* 2002;288:1955–1958.
2. Sim I, Sanders GD, McDonald K. Evidence-based practice for mere mortals: the role of informatics and health services research. *JGIM* 2002;17:302–308.
3. Weiner M, Callahan CM, Tierney W, et al. Using information technology to improve the health care of older adults. *Ann Intern Med* 2003;139:430–436.
4. Weingarten SR, Riedinger MS, Varis G, et al. Identification of low-risk hospitalized patients with pneumonia. Implications for early conversion to oral antimicrobial therapy. *Chest* 1994;105:1109–1115.
5. Gonzalez ER, Jones LA, Ornato JP, et al. Hospital delays and problems with thrombolytic administration in patients receiving thrombolytic therapy: a multicenter prospective assessment. Virginia Thrombolytic Study Group. *Ann Emerg Med* 1992;21:1215–1221.
6. Meehan TP, Fine MF, Krumholz HM, et al. Quality of care, process, and outcomes in elderly patients with pneumonia. *JAMA* 1997;278:2080–2084.
7. Field MJ, Lohr KN, eds. *Clinical Practice Guidelines: Directions for a New Program.* Institute of Medicine. Washington, DC: National Academy Press, 1990:38.
8. Tunis SR, Hayward RSA, Wilson MC, et al. Internists' attitudes about clinical practice guidelines. *Ann Intern Med* 1994;120:956–963.
9. Pearson SD, Goúlart-Fisher D, Lee TH. Critical pathways as a strategy for improving care: problems and potential. *Ann Intern Med* 1995;123:941–948
10. Grimshaw JM, Russell IT. Effect of clinical guidelines on medical practice: a systematic review of rigorous evaluations. *Lancet* 1993;342:1317–1322.
11. Soumerai SB, Avorn J. Principles of educational outreach ("academic detailing") to improve clinical decision making. *JAMA* 1990;263:549–556.
12. Hay JA, Maldonado L, Weingarten SR, et al. Prospective evaluation of a clinical guideline recommending hospital length of stay in upper gastrointestinal tract hemorrhage. *JAMA* 1997;278:2151–2156.
13. Johnston ME, Langton KB, Haynes RB, et al. Effects of computer-based clinical decision support systems on clinician performance and patient outcome. A critical appraisal of research. *Ann Intern Med* 1994;120:135–142.
14. Evans RS, Pestotnik SL, Classen DC, et al. A computer-assisted management program for antibiotics and other antiinfective agents. *N Engl J Med* 1998;338:232–238.
15. Weingarten S, Riedinger M, Conner L, et al. Reducing lengths of stay in the coronary care unit with a practice guideline for patients with congestive heart failure. Insights from a controlled clinical trial. *Med Care* 1994;32:1232–1243.
16. Hyams AL, Brandenburg JA, Lipsitz SR, et al. Practice guidelines and malpractice litigation: a two-way street. *Ann Intern Med* 1995;122:450–455.

ADDITIONAL READING

Shekelle PG, Kravitz RL, Beart J, Marger M, Wang M, Lee M. Are nonspecific practice guidelines potentially harmful? A randomized comparison of the effect of nonspecific versus specific guidelines on physician decision making. *Health Serv Res* 2000;34:1429–1448.
Wallace JF, Weingarten SR, Chiou CF, et al. The limited incorporation of economic analyses in clinical practice guidelines. *J Gen Intern Med* 2002;17:210–220.

Patient Satisfaction with Hospital Care

Haya R. Rubin

INTRODUCTION

Fifteen years ago, many physicians believed that patient satisfaction was of no particular importance, and few hospitals measured it regularly. In this era of increasing competition and patient sophistication, patient satisfaction with medical care has become an important outcome. This transformation has been driven by a number of forces, including (a) competition for market share among hospitals and health systems, especially in markets where employer coalitions are strong and managed care is prevalent; (b) availability to and use of information about patient satisfaction by medical care purchasers; (c) the strong patients' rights movement (evidenced by, among other things, informed consent laws across the nation, the Patient Self-Determination Act, the Patient Bill of Rights, and the Consumer Protection Act), which stresses the philosophical importance of patient satisfaction as an outcome; and (d) our own awareness that physicians' judgments of technical quality of care are sometimes no more informed than our patients' judgments. Because of these factors, regular measurement of patients' experiences with and evaluations of their health care, and efforts to improve care based on the results, are now commonplace among American hospitals' internal quality measures. They have also recently become part of Medicare hospital quality monitoring efforts (1).

What is referred to here as patient satisfaction, out of deference to popular nomenclature, should more properly be called patient evaluation or judgment of hospital care. Patients are usually satisfied with hospital care, but even satisfied patients have various opinions that can be influential when they are deciding between hospitals or recommending hospitals to their friends or family members.

CARE OF THE HOSPITALIZED PATIENT

Studies in the last decade have explored which dimensions of care are most important to hospitalized patients (1–3), and measurement tools reflecting these are both publicly and commercially available. Patients' judgments about nursing care correlate best with their global assessment of their hospital stay and their intentions to recommend the hospital to others (2–4). Of particular importance is how quickly nurses respond when patients call for a bedpan and toileting assistance or for pain medication. The perceived quality of physician care has usually been next, although in other countries that have long traditions of hospital-based physicians, it has sometimes come first (5). In the United States, nursing care probably was given greater weight than physician care because, in the traditional American system, the attending physician in the hospital was usually the patient's outpatient physician. This physician was not present for most of a patient's hospital day, and often was not perceived by patients as being part of the hospital staff. Except in teaching hospitals, physicians were not present enough to figure into patients' opinions about the hospital. Deficiencies in physicians' orders were often interpreted by patients as deficiencies in nursing care. As the hospitalist model grows in popularity (Chapter 1) and hospitalist physicians are available to interact more often with hospitalized patients, their behavior will likely figure more prominently into patient assessments of the hospital. Across all staff groups, sensitive, respectful treatment and clear information are highly prized by hospitalized patients.

Clinicians may be relieved to know that cosmetic changes in the hospital environment do not impress patients in the absence of high quality care. Patients do value restful, clean, attractive environments carefully designed with the needs of physically limited, ill, or postoperative patients in mind. Reflecting this, patients' ratings of noise, cleanliness, appearance of the room and unit, design and condition of the room and bathroom, furnishings, supplies, and equipment are independently associated with their global judgments and their intentions to recommend the hospital to others. Hospitals aiming for high patient satisfaction scores should not ignore these aspects. However, health care environmental factors are more weakly associated with final judgments than are nurse and physician care and information given to patients. Therefore, unless a hospital has a very poor physical plant, *successful efforts to improve care and patient information will yield greater gains in overall satisfaction than will remodeling*. Paint, artwork, and food will not compensate for inconsiderate staff behavior or failure to respond to the call bell, nor for failure to give patients information about their medical condition, treatment, and what they should do when they leave the hospital. In contrast, patients forgive inadequate parking facilities and terrible food in hospitals that get high ratings for physicians' and nurses' skills and caring.

TECHNICAL ASPECTS OF ASSESSING PATIENT SATISFACTION

Patient evaluations of inpatient care can be obtained in a variety of ways. The two most popular are mailing surveys to or calling patients discharged within the last week or two. Surveys can also be conducted by interviewing patients or giving them a questionnaire to complete while in the hospital or at the time of discharge. However, this results in sicker patients not being able to complete the survey, does not allow patients to evaluate the completeness and clarity of instructions they receive about how to care for themselves after discharge, and does not permit an evaluation of billing services. Post-discharge surveys offer these advantages, and provide comparable evaluation results in domains that could be assessed by both methods.

The relationship between survey length and response rate is not linear. Surveys that take more than 15–20 minutes to complete are returned less often than shorter surveys. However, postcards and one-page minimal surveys are also returned less often than more comprehensive surveys because patients believe that they are trivial and do not permit useful and constructive feedback (3). Most commercial surveys obtain a 40%–50% response rate from discharged patients. Although no absolute floor for unacceptable response rates can be specified, patients who are less satisfied with their care are less likely to return their questionnaires, so as the response rate goes down differences among hospitals or units are obscured. Thus, when choosing between surveying a greater number of patients or obtaining a smaller sample and devoting more resources

to follow-up, the latter is preferable as long as at least 100 responses per group will be compared.

Item wording affects results in important ways. Patient satisfaction surveys are highly susceptible to biases created by framing effects and insensitive response scales. Items that ask patients for yes or no answers can obscure areas for improvement if the item is one in which a "no" response still could indicate a serious deficiency with care. In addition, such items are not sensitive to differences across the entire spectrum of quality. It is preferable to use response scales that allow for a wider spectrum of responses, such as one in which answers range from "excellent" to "poor," A to F, or 1 to 10. Double-barreled questions and questions with double negatives are confusing and likely to elicit unreliable and inaccurate responses (Table 14.1). Figure 14.1 gives examples of poorly worded and well-worded questions.

Hospitals that have substantial populations of patients who do not speak English must translate questionnaires into other languages. Competent translations require bilingual translators and back-translation to check accuracy. Because of cultural and language differences in the use of rating scales, ratings obtained in another language should not be directly compared with ratings by speakers of English, but they can be used to track improvements over time for the segment of hospitalized patients who speak the second language.

INTERVENTIONS TO IMPROVE PATIENT SATISFACTION WITH CARE

Clinicians and administrators have numerous opportunities, beginning at the first moment of hospitalization, to influence and improve a patient's experience. Patients value a hospitalization in which they are admitted promptly from the emergency department or the admitting office to the inpatient unit and are treated thereafter with care and respect.

Administrators attempting to improve patient satisfaction throughout a unit or service should focus on training the staff in improving their interpersonal skills and in providing patient education procedures and materials (4). As an example, the Johns Hopkins Department of Medicine implemented a multifaceted program, the Osler Way Project, to increase patient satisfaction with inpatient services. The interventions included institution of joint rounds for nurses and physicians to improve the consistency of information provided to patients; training in interpersonal skills ("service excellence") for nurses' aides, nurses, and house staff physicians; better coordination of the discharge process; putting housekeeping under nursing supervision on individual units; and making physical changes to the environment, such as putting up new wallpaper, adding new artwork, and closing one entry to the unit to reduce noise and improve security. Table 14.2 lists some of the 20 topics included in the "service excellence" training given to all staff categories. The proportion of excellent patient ratings

TABLE 14.1

EXAMPLES OF WORSE AND BETTER ITEMS

Worse	What's wrong	Better
The staff were courteous and respectful. Response choices: Strongly agree, agree, not sure, disagree, strongly disagree	Evaluation is in the stem of the item, allowing for only one cutoff point on the spectrum of opinion. More sensitive items place the evaluation in the response scale rather than asking for agreement.	How courteously and respectfully were you treated by the staff? Response choices: 0 (worst possible) to 10 (best possible), A (best) to F (worst), or excellent to poor
Was the information adequate? Yes/No	Yes/No items create a dichotomy that obscures the full spectrum of possible answers and obscures differences.	Adequacy of the information given (0, worst possible, to 10, best possible)
Please rate the food and how it was served by staff.	Double-barrelled item is difficult to answer if the two items differ.	Separate into two items: 1. Please rate the quality of the food. 2. How was food served by staff?
The doctors did not involve me in decisions. Response choices: Strongly agree, agree, not sure, disagree, strongly disagree	1) Double negative is confusing; 2) value of being involved in decisions is imposed on the patient, not a true patient evaluation item; and 3) agree/disagree scales limit spectrum of possible evaluation.	How much did the doctors involve you in decisions? Response choices: Way too much, somewhat too much, about right, somewhat too little, way too little, or (less informative about patient's expectations but a sound rating item): 0, worst possible, to 10, best possible

of the overall hospital stay doubled after the interventions were implemented, with the greatest improvements in specific ratings corresponding to the areas of intervention (6).

Interpersonal relations can be improved by incorporating interpersonal behavior as a criterion for employee selection and performance evaluation and by providing service excellence training for all types of staff. Patient education can be improved in similar ways, and also by providing patient education materials about common hospital diagnoses, tests, and treatments in a variety of media.

PATIENT CHARACTERISTICS RELATED TO EVALUATIONS OF CARE

Certain types of patients have a greater propensity to find a hospital stay unsatisfactory. Educated patients have higher expectations of care and generally rate their hospital care more unfavorably than do less educated patients. Those who are sicker on admission rate their care less favorably, probably because their needs are greater and therefore staff members are more likely to fail to meet them. Patients with

Poorly worded

I was not told how to take care of myself at home.

Yes

No

Problem: double negative, limited evaluative spectrum

Please rate the privacy and cleanliness of the hospital room.

Problem: double barreled

Well-worded

Please rate the instructions you were given about how to take care of yourself at home:

Excellent   Fair

Very good   Poor

Good

Separate into two items:

1. Please rate the privacy of the hospital room.
2. Please rate the cleanliness of the hospital room.

Figure 14.1   Examples of poorly worded and well-worded rating items.

TABLE 14.2

SOME KEY ELEMENTS OF JOHNS HOPKINS MEDICINE SERVICE EXCELLENCE TRAINING

Module name	Brief description of module
First encounters: Guess who?	Stresses the importance of all staff members introducing themselves and explaining their role; provides examples of good introductions.
First impressions: It's up to you!	Describes what leads to a good first impression, the critical importance of courteous and respectful first contact.
Anticipating customer needs	Encourages staff members to put themselves in patients' shoes and think about what they need.
Dealing with difficult people	Provides some pointers on defusing tension and handling challenging behavior.
Power of nonverbals	Discusses how body language and appearance affect patients' impressions.
How my department conserves cost	Educates staff members about service efficiency.
Moving myself from negative to positive (attitude)	Presents strategies for a constructive and cheerful outlook.
Stages of team development and stress	Gives guidance on how team morale can be improved with respectful interactions.
Choosing the right words	Scripts some common situations and gives tips on avoiding offensive language.
Innovation, my job, and me	Encourages staff members to make suggestions for better care throughout the hospital.

intermediate levels of pain or moderate needs for assistance give lower ratings than do those with the highest and lowest levels. Possibly those with the most pain or disability occupy the staff, and those with little or no pain or disability are not in need, whereas those with moderate pain and disability are more likely to find their needs unmet. Patients who are depressed are more likely to be dissatisfied with care. It is important to identify such patients, especially on medical and surgical wards, and to treat their depression along with their other conditions (Chapter 119). Patients in their twenties and thirties give lower ratings for care than do those in their forties and fifties. Relatively younger patients, especially men, may be less likely than older patients to express their needs because of embarrassment, frustration, and discomfort with revealing disability or vulnerability. It may be necessary for staff members to inquire directly to identify and meet the needs of these patients.

Studies that have examined ratings of care by different racial or ethnic groups have found inconsistent results. However, if large minority populations are present, especially if their race or ethnicity differs from that of most of the hospital care providers, it is important to survey such groups to ascertain whether specific concerns need to be targeted to improve their experiences.

The Elderly Patient

Elderly patients require special sensitivity to toileting needs, and how these are handled can greatly affect their satisfaction with care. To maintain dignity and have the best chance of maintaining continence, elderly patients need to be answered promptly when they call so that they can be taken to the bathroom, placed on a commode, or given a bedpan. When they are incontinent, sheets must be changed promptly. Bedpans are uncomfortable for frail

elderly patients with atrophic skin and should be promptly removed when they are finished using them.

Elderly patients also are more likely than others to become immobile and less physically functional in the hospital because of increased sensitivity to sedatives, opiates, anticholinergic agents, and other commonly used hospital medications. Early ambulation, restraint-free environments, and aggressive physical therapy are very important in preserving independent function. This translates into fewer demands placed on the hospital staff and greater patient satisfaction (Chapter 16).

The Dying Patient

For hospitalized patients at the end of life, patient comfort and patient and family satisfaction are the most important outcomes. Of paramount importance is prompt and effective treatment of the patient's pain and discomfort, emotional support for both patient and family, involvement of both patient and family (as desired by the patient) in treatment decisions, and communication of as much information to patient and family as they desire about the patient's condition and treatment.

Particular care must be taken with families who are unexpectedly faced with the death of a loved one, and those whose relative is receiving mechanical ventilation. Ongoing discussion about the natural history of the patient's condition and treatment options is critical. Treating physicians should set up regular times for communication with the family. One possible mechanism is for the team to designate one physician to be in charge of communicating with the family or the patient's designated advocate. This advocate can then be asked to provide information to other family members.

Family members of dying patients have great emotional needs as they struggle with the imminent loss of a close relative. Small acts on the part of hospital staff members can have powerful long-term comforting effects that assist relatives in adjusting to a death. These may include coming into the patient's room or a family lounge to inquire about the health and emotional state of the family member rather than simply ministering to the patient, providing snacks or juice to family members who are spending many hours by the patient's bedside, communicating regularly about the illness and its treatment, and ensuring that relatives designated by the patient as proxies are involved in treatment decisions. Patients from different backgrounds have widely varied expectations and needs at the time of death, and the staff should attempt to find out early in the hospital stay whether there are any specific issues of concern to individual patients and their family members (Chapter 19).

SYSTEM CHARACTERISTICS RELATED TO PATIENT EVALUATIONS OF CARE

Most studies comparing managed care with fee-for-service care have found a lower rate of satisfaction with care in managed care environments, but these have not concentrated on the hospital environment. However, as cost pressures on hospitals increase under ever more aggressive care management and greater assumption of risk by providers, it will be important to monitor whether patients perceive their hospital stays as too short and feel that not enough instruction and education are provided in preparation for the transition to home.

Patients at large hospitals and teaching hospitals tend to be less satisfied with their care (6). Studies have suggested that this is a consequence of the relatively large number of providers involved with patients, conflicting communications, and the size and complexity of interactions, which lead to a loss of intimacy and caring. To mitigate these effects requires a concerted effort by all providers to keep primary providers and other specialty consultants informed of the care plan and of communications with patients and families, and to keep nurses informed of the care plan so that they can help to convey accurate information to patients and families. A daily goals sheet can alert all personnel to care goals for the day; in one study this simple intervention raised staff awareness of patient care goals from 10%–90% (7). Medical students, residents, fellows, and specialty consultants must be taught to treat patients and families with caring and respect no matter how brief and specialized their interactions with them. Fortunately, the American Council on Graduate Medical Education (ACGME) and several of the Residency Review Committees that accredit residency programs now require competency in communication (see www.acgme.org). Curricula are available for these purposes and are likely in the next few years to become standard parts of house staff and postdoctoral fellowship training (8). These have healthy effects on trainee interactions with patients in teaching hospitals.

CONCLUSIONS

The importance of patient evaluations of hospital care will continue to grow in our environment where hospitals increasingly become cost centers, health plans look for better value (Chapter 12), and consumers become more involved and educated about hospital choice. Hospitalized patients are often too ill to advocate for themselves, and staff members treating them must be particularly sensitive to their needs.

KEY POINTS

- Patient satisfaction is an increasingly important outcome of hospital care.
- Hospital staff can improve patient satisfaction, mostly through improving nursing response to pain and toileting needs, respectful and caring interpersonal treatment, and patient education.
- Systems can improve staff interpersonal and patient education skills by including such skills as criteria for personnel selection and evaluation, providing training in these areas, and offering patient education materials in a variety of different media.
- Family members, especially of dying patients, need a quick response to their relative's pain or discomfort, emotional support, and information, and they should be involved in decisions as appropriate.

REFERENCES

1. Available at http://www.ahrq.gov/qual/cahpsix.htm. Accessed March 8, 2005.
2. Meterko M, Nelson E, Rubin H. Patient judgments of hospital quality: report of a pilot study. *Med Care* 1990;28:S1–S56.
3. Gerteis M, Edgman-Levitan S, Daley J, et al. *Through the Patient's Eyes: Understanding and Promoting Patient-Centered Care.* San Francisco: Jossey-Bass Publishers, 1993.
4. Nelson EC, Larson C, Davies A, et al. The patient comment card: a system to gather customer feedback. *QRB Qual Rev Bull* 1991;17:278–286.
5. Rubin HR. Can patients evaluate the quality of hospital care? *Med Care* 1990;47:267–326.
6. Rubin HR. The Osler way: patients evaluate improvements to the inpatient medical services at the Johns Hopkins hospital. *Eye on Improvement* 1998;V:6.
7. Pronovost P, Berenholtz S, Dorman T, et al. Improving communication in the ICU using daily goals. *J Crit Care* 2003;18:71–75.
8. Roter DL, Larson S, Shinitzky H, et al. Use of an innovative video feedback technique to enhance communication skills training. *Med Educ* 2004;38:145–157.

ADDITIONAL READING

Clark PA, Drain M, Malone MP. Addressing patients' emotional and spiritual needs. *Jt Comm J Qual Saf* 2003;29:659–670.
Fleming GV. Hospital structure and consumer satisfaction. *Health Serv Res* 1981;16:43–63.
Kenagy JW, Berwick DM, Shore MF. Service quality in health care. *JAMA* 1999;281:661–665.

Nutritional Issues in the Hospitalized Patient

15

Annette Stralovich-Romani   *Christopher R. Pennington**

INTRODUCTION

Malnutrition is recognized as a major contributor to morbidity and mortality in hospitalized patients across a spectrum of diagnoses. Many studies of nutritional status in hospital patients, based on anthropometric data, have indicated an incidence of malnutrition of 30%–40% (1). Significant nutritional depletion occurs in the majority of patients during their hospital stay, and those who are already malnourished on admission are the most severely affected. Early identification of patients who will benefit from nutrition intervention can lead to cost-effective and beneficial outcomes. This chapter focuses on the diagnosis, prevention, and management of nutrition depletion in hospitalized patients.

EFFECTS OF STARVATION AND METABOLIC STRESS IN HOSPITALIZED PATIENTS

Food substrates lead to the synthesis of glycogen, lipid, and protein under the influence of insulin. After meals, insulin concentrations are reduced and glycogen is mobilized to supply glucose. During periods of starvation, glycogen stores are rapidly exhausted and fatty acids liberated from tissue stores by lipolysis supply the energy substrate, except

in the central nervous system, which depends on glucose. However, ketones formed in the liver from fatty acids supply some energy to the central nervous system, thus minimizing the requirement for glucose and the catabolism of muscle for gluconeogenesis. This adaptive mechanism is disrupted, however, during periods of acute illness, especially critical illness or injury.

The metabolic response associated with acute stress, critical illness, or injury is often referred to as *hypermetabolism*. Metabolic stress is triggered by the release of the counter-regulatory hormones (catecholamines, glucagon, cortisol), and cytokines (tumor necrosis factor, interleukin-1, interleukin-6). The catabolic hormones stimulate gluconeogenesis, increase net protein catabolism and cause glucose intolerance/insulin resistance. The cytokines produce a spectrum of effects, including skeletal muscle proteolysis, increased metabolic rate, release of acute phase reactants, and depression of hepatic protein synthesis (albumin, prealbumin, transferrin, retinol binding protein).

Stressed starvation has a profound effect on the nutritional status of a patient. Whereas in a previously fit person death from starvation takes about 60 days (depending on initial body stores), the nutritional decline in sick persons is influenced by their disease process and may be much more rapid.

Nutritional intervention is required long before patients become seriously malnourished. One important experiment demonstrated that many weeks are needed to restore lean body tissue, even with nutritional repletion (2). Furthermore, tissue restoration is not attainable in the context of

---

* Deceased.

acute illness, so that minimizing tissue loss is the nutritional objective (3). Impaired organ function can be demonstrated very early in the course of starvation, and reduced muscle strength has been shown after 5 days. Reduced muscle strength may impair mobilization of patients after surgery or illness and may also compromise other important muscle groups, notably the muscles of respiration.

The intestine may be particularly vulnerable to starvation. Besides its role in digestion and absorption, the GI tract has the distinct property of maintaining barrier function and normal bacterial flora of the intestine. Gastrointestinal tissues require direct contact with nutrients to support cell replication and the numerous metabolic and immunologic functions required for successful adaptation to stress (4). Absence of luminal nutrient stimulation, therefore, may lead to gut atrophy, which can result in bacterial translocation. The integrity of intestinal immunity, particularly during a period of physiologic stress, may therefore be helpful in preventing infectious complications and averting the development of multisystem organ failure in the critically ill.

NUTRITIONAL ASSESSMENT

Upon admission to the hospital all patients should undergo nutritional screening to identify those individuals with either pre-existing malnutrition or those who are at risk for nutritional compromise. Many types of hospitalized patients are commonly malnourished. Patients with infectious and inflammatory disorders (e.g., AIDS, cancer) often have cytokine-mediated anorexia. Patients with gastrointestinal disease may be afraid to eat due to abdominal pain or other symptoms, be unable to eat because of dysphagia, or suffer from impaired digestion and absorption resulting from pancreatic and intestinal disease. Elderly patients, those who are depressed, and patients with underlying lung disease (chronic obstructive pulmonary disease, cystic fibrosis) are especially vulnerable to malnutrition. Patients with neurological injury (stroke, subarachnoid hemorrhage, trauma) or other critical illness are also prone to nutritional compromise.

Malnutrition may develop in some patients after admission because of the nature of their illness. Patients unable to swallow as a consequence of cerebrovascular disease, those with intestinal obstruction, and those requiring frequent fasting for investigation or therapeutic intervention will all suffer from starvation unless they receive nutritional therapy.

The evaluation of nutritional staus is a vital step in formulating nutritional care plans for patients. Unfortunately, most markers of malnutrition lack specificity and sensitivity. Therefore, until improved methods of identifying malnutrition are developed, it is necessary to perform a comprehensive assessment which includes carefully selected objective parameters, a nutritionally focused physical exam, and other subjective parameters. However, in daily clinical practice, the nutritional assessment process must center around assessment parameters that are clinically relevant, easy to obtain, and cost-effective (5) (see also Table 16.2).

When evaluating nutritional status, it is important to obtain subjective data from the medical history that may bear relevance on the patient's nutritional well-being. For example, acute or chronic illnesses, medications (immunosuppresive agents, corticosteroids), psychosocial history, diagnostic tests/procedures, surgeries, or other treatment modalities (chemotherapy, radiation therapy) may all significantly influence nutritional status (6). A thorough nutritional history should also be completed and include weight and appetite changes, diet information, bowel habits, chewing and swallowing abilities, and activity level.

Careful observation of physical appearance adds a dimension to the evaluation of nutritional adequacy. Severe wasting of lean body mass and subcutaneous fat stores are signs of frank malnutrition. The physical exam should also focus on edema, dermatitis, and overt signs of vitamin and mineral deficiencies (alopecia, cheilosis, glossitis, stomatitis, bleeding gums, bruising, visual changes, rickets).

Anthropometry can be used to obtain objective parameters for assessment of nutritional status. Body weight—although useful for establishing the diagnosis of malnutrition—provides only a crude evaluation of overall fat and muscle stores. *Body mass index* [weight in kilograms divided by height in meters squared (m^2)], is often used to help determine nutritional status (normal range 20–25). Values below 18 signify important nutritional depletion. Patients with values above 25 and 30 are respectively defined as overweight and obese. Usual body weight, rather than ideal body weight, is a much more useful nutritional assessment parameter in the ill population. Loss of 5% of body weight in one month or greater than 10% of body weight in the 6 months preceding admission signifies nutritional depletion. When assessing the weight status of a critically ill patient, exercise caution as to what weight is being used, for weights are influenced by fluid shifts and therefore are unreliable. Dry weights are more ideal for determining nutritional status, determining nutrient requirements, and monitoring response to nutritional therapy.

Skinfold measurements, although rarely used in the clinical setting, are indirect methods of measuring somatic protein and subcutaneous fat. These measurements have limited utility in the critical care setting due to edema/fluid shifts. Skinfold measurements tend to have more merit in the outpatient arena when nutritional status is being serially evaluated over time or in the pediatric population to assess growth.

Various serum protein levels have been used in assessment of nutritional status. Albumin, transferrin, thyroxine-binding pre-albumin, and retinol-binding protein are most commonly used in the clinical setting. Serum albumin is best evaluated at admission because levels rarely show nutritionally relevant changes during hospitalization due to its long half-life (18–20 days). The advantages of albumin are that it is inexpensive, it is useful with long-term assessments, and it is a valuable prognostic indicator of morbidity and mortality. Serum albumin levels dramatically decrease, however, with metabolic stress and injury. Albumin levels may also change quickly as a result of non-nutritional factors, and respond slowly even with adequate nutrition support. In fact, plasma albumin levels will not increase in stressed patients until the inflammatory response remits. Therefore, little credence should be given to albumin as a marker of nutritional status or response to nutritional therapy during a period of metabolic stress.

Because of their shorter half-lives and smaller protein pools, transferrin, pre-albumin, and retinol-binding protein have been touted as better markers of status. However, like albumin, these constitutive proteins decrease independently of nutritional status during critical illness due to the preferential production of acute phase reactants over the synthesis of visceral proteins. It should not be assumed, therefore, that decreased levels of serum proteins are caused solely by malnutrition. Normal patterns of hepatic protein synthesis and degradation are altered during critical illness, making evaluation difficult (Table 15.1).

NUTRITIONAL REQUIREMENTS

Energy Requirements

The amount of energy required is a function of resting needs (those required to do daily metabolic work), with adjustments added for activity, specific dynamic action of food, healing, repair of nutritional deficits, painful stimuli, and any catabolic insult (such as trauma, sepsis, and surgery). Several methods exist to determine energy requirements. These include predictive equations, nomograms, and indirect calorimetry.

Predictive Equations

Predictive equations are most often estimated using the Harris-Benedict equation (Table 15.2), which estimates resting energy expenditure and then is multiplied by stress factors ranging from 1.2–2.0, depending on the clinical condition of the patient. The utility of this formula in critically ill patients is limited since this equation was developed from data on normal volunteers.

Indirect Calorimetry

A more accurate method to calculate energy expenditure, especially in the complex and rapidly changing setting of critical illness, is indirect calorimetry. This method can be

TABLE 15.1

SERUM PROTEINS FOR NUTRITIONAL ASSESSMENT

Serum protein	Half-life	Normal range	Comments
Albumin	20 days	3.5–5.0 g/dL	Large body pool; reliable predictor of morbidity and mortality; reflects chronic vs. acute protein depletion; responds slowly to changes in nutritional status; decreased levels with fluid overload, malabsorptive states, stress (sepsis, burns, trauma, postoperative states), and certain disease processes (liver failure, congestive heart failure); increased levels with anabolic agents, dehydration, and infusion of albumin, fresh frozen plasma and whole blood
Transferrin	8–10 days	200–400 mg/dL	Smaller body pool; sensitive to changes in nutritional status; calculated from total iron binding capacity; decreased with chronic infection, stress, uremia, iron overdose, overhydration, liver failure; increased with pregnancy, iron deficiency, hypoxia, hepatitis, dehydration, estrogens
Prealbumin (Transthyretin)	2–3 days	15–40 mg/dL	Rapid turnover rate; small body protein pool; quickly changes with changes in nutritional status; decreased levels with stress, inflammation, surgery, liver disease; increased levels with renal dysfunction
Retinol-binding protein	8–10 hours	2.7–7.6 mg/dL	Highly sensitive to changes in nutritional status; decreased levels in same states as pre-albumin, as well as in vitamin A deficiency; increased levels with renal dysfunction and vitamin A supplementation

TABLE 15.2

HARRIS-BENEDICT EQUATION FOR ESTIMATING ENERGY REQUIREMENT

Men: REE = 66.5 + (13.75 × W) +
    (5 × H) − (6.76 × A)
Women: REE = 655 + (9.56 × W) +
    (1.85 × H) − (4.68 × A)
        W = Weight (kg)
        H = Height (cm)
        A = Age (years)

REE, resting energy expenditure, in kcal/day.

carried out at the bedside using portable machines that are costly and require trained personnel to operate. The premise of indirect calorimetry is that it calculates energy expenditure by measurement of respiratory gas exchange (specifically the measurement of oxygen consumption (V02), carbon dioxide production (VCO2), and minute ventilation (VE)), and then applying the Weir equation (7). When measured energy expenditure is obtained from indirect calorimetry, some clinicians add a factor of 10%–20% to account for 24-hour variability.

Protein Requirements

The goal of protein provision is to minimize the degree of net nitrogen loss. Since protein reserves do not exist in the body, protein must be continually replenished. Under normal circumstances the recommended daily intake of protein is approximately 0.8 gm of protein/kg body weight. In critical illness, the proper provision of protein is crucial as it is the most important macronutrient with stress and/or injury. Protein requirements are high with trauma, sepsis, and also go up to meet the demands for healing of burns, necrotizing fasciitis, and other types of large wounds. In some disease states, such as renal failure and hepatic encephalopathy, protein requirements may be reduced (Table 15.3).

Nitrogen Balance

Nitrogen balance, when correctly measured and calculated, remains the best available marker of the effects of acute nutrition intervention, and the best nutritional predictor of outcomes. Urinary nitrogen losses following injury and illness tend to parallel the increased energy expenditure with increased degrees of stress. The magnitude of nitrogen loss varies with the severity of disease (8). Nitrogen balance is equal to nitrogen intake minus urinary nitrogen output plus obligatory losses from skin, stool, and respiration. It ranges from 2–4 grams per day. When there are excessive losses of nitrogen from severe diarrhea, fistula drainage,

burn exudate, ostomy output, or wounds or pleural drainage, total nitrogen content should be determined when practical.

A positive nitrogen balance correlates with net protein synthesis (*anabolic state*) and suggests adequate nutritional support. A negative nitrogen balance, on the other hand, indicates that the rate of protein breakdown exceeds the rate of protein synthesis (*catabolic state*), and therefore indicates the need to adjust the nutritional support regimen. Positive or even neutral nitrogen balance may be difficult to achieve in critically ill patients due to the effects of catabolic hormones, medications, bed rest, fever, and infection. The goal of nutrition support, therefore, is to offset the degree of catabolism rather than to achieve positive balance. Once the source of stress is resolved, an anabolic state should be attainable.

A nitrogen balance study should only be completed after the patient has been on relatively constant protein and energy intake for 3 days, thus allowing the urea cycle and gluconeogenic enzymes to adjust to protein intake. Urine should be kept on ice during the collection and analyzed within 4 hours to prevent loss of urea due to bacterial conversion to ammonia.

The major limitation of using a standard nitrogen balance study in critically ill patients is that a creatinine clearance greater than 50 mL/min is required for accurate interpretation. With liver failure, nitrogen balance studies are usually invalid due to decreased urea production.

TABLE 15.3

ESTIMATING PROTEIN REQUIREMENTS

Normal renal function

Maintenance	0.8–1.2 gm of protein/kg/day
Moderate stress	1.3–1.5 gm of protein/kg/day
Severe stress	1.5–2.0 gm of protein/kg/day

Renal Failure

Non-dialyzed	0.8–1.2 gm of protein/kg/day
Hemodialyzed	1.0–1.4 gm of protein/kg/day (may be adjusted based on frequency of dialysis)
CAPD	1.3–1.5 gm of protein/kg/day
CAVHD/CVVHD	1.6–1.8 gm of protein/kg/day

Hepatic Failure

without encephalopathy	Begin at 1.0 gm of protein/kg/day, increase as tolerated to 1.5–2.0 gm of protein/kg/day
with encephalopathy	0.8–1.0 gm of protein/kg/day (no less than 40 gm/day)

CAPD, continuous ambulatory peritoneal dialysis; CAVHD, continuous arterio-venous hemodialysis; CVVHD, continuous veno-venous hemofiltration dialysis.

NUTRITIONAL SUPPORT FOR PREVENTION OR TREATMENT OF MALNUTRITION

During periods of metabolic stress, tissue wasting should be minimized by the provision of adequate nutrition. This truism is supported by data showing that the use of early enteral feeding in postoperative patients reduces the incidence of infection. There is also abundant evidence that nutritional support and the correction of nutritional depletion, when possible, reduces mortality, morbidity, and length of hospital stay.

Patients with initially normal nutritional status should be considered for nutritional support if they will not be able to eat for more than 5–7 days, or if it is anticipated that their dietary intake will be inadequate for 7–10 days or more. Patients who are malnourished or metabolically stressed should receive nutritional support within 3 days if their oral intake is not satisfactory or if oral feeding cannot be achieved. Significant nutritional depletion should be avoided because of the early effects on organ function, the prolonged period required for nutritional repletion, and the fact that malnutrition cannot be corrected in the stressed patient.

NUTRITION SUPPORT MODALITIES

Enteral Nutrition

Enteral nutrition is the preferred modality of nutrition support because it is cost-effective and has beneficial outcomes. Perhaps the most striking clinical benefit of enteral nutrition is preservation of the gastrointestinal tract. Enteral nutrition is strongly favored over parenteral nutrition because some studies have shown that there is a significantly lower incidence of septic complications in patients fed enterally rather than parenterally.

Liquid oral nutritional supplements in various flavors may be sufficient for some patients with anorexia, failure to thrive, esophageal disease or other disorders associated with malnutrition when the normal diet is inadequate to meet their nutrient needs. Patients with severe impairment of appetite or an inability to eat because of neurologic or oropharyngeal disease will need enteral tube feeding. Tube feeding may also be indicated in patients with intestinal failure, as in Crohn's disease or short bowel syndrome. Critically ill patients will also undoubtedly require enteral nutrition support.

Technological advances in enteral feeding have significantly influenced the practice of enteral support. Improvements in placement procedures, enteral feeding devices, and nutritional products have allowed enteral nutrition to be provided to patients who previously would not have been candidates for it, and would therefore have been on parenteral nutrition.

Newer Clinical Applications for Enteral Nutrition

There are several clinical conditions now deemed appropriate for enteral nutrition support that deserve mentioning (9). The use of enteral feeding in fistula management is becoming more widespread. The ability to enterally feed is contingent upon the site and extent of usable intestine for feeding. To avoid reflux, it is necessary to feed 40 cm distal to the fistula. Spontaneous closure rates comparable to TPN have been reported. In short bowel syndrome, enteral feeding is used in conjunction with parenteral nutrition. Minimal infusion of enteral nutrition has been shown to foster intestinal adaptation/rehabilitation. Utilization of alternative substrates (glutamine, fiber, growth hormone) may promote successful adaptation.

A new alternative for providing nutrition support to the patient with acute pancreatitis has been jejunal feedings placed either nasojejunally or with an operative jejunostomy. Because the cephalic and gastric phases of digestion are bypassed, this method leads to decreased pancreatic stimulation.

Another area in which the efficacy of enteral feeding warrants in-depth investigation is in patients undergoing bone marrow transplantation. There is hope that enteral feeding in this population might help restore the GI mucosa following chemotherapy and radiation therapy, prevent bacterial translocation, maintain normal immune responses, promote smoother transition to oral feeding, and decrease cost.

Timing

Timing may be crucial when it comes to instituting enteral alimentation in critically ill or injured patients. If possible, enteral feeding tubes should be placed within 48 hours of admission to the ICU. Administration of enteral nutrition into the small bowel 8–12 hours following surgery is being practiced widely, and with good success, since peristalsis is often well maintained in the small bowel postoperatively. *Bowel sounds should not be used to indicate feasibility of enteral alimentation, but rather to indicate the adequacy of gastric emptying.* Although gastric and colonic motility are impaired in most critically ill patients, small bowel motility and absorption are usually intact.

Early administration of enteral nutrition appears to minimize gut atrophy, decrease sepsis, enhance immunocompetence, and blunt the hypermetabolic response to stress. The role of pharmacomodulation of the gut has also received increased attention. Pathologic conditions and unavoidable iatrogenic disorders that affect gut function may be able to be managed with drug therapy (octreotide, propofol, 5-hydroxytryptamine-3 receptor antagonists, erythromycin, oral naloxone) to allow enteral feeding to be used (10).

Tube Types and Location

The administration of enteral nutrition is generally accomplished by using nasoenteric feeding tubes inserted into the stomach, duodenum or jejunum. Nasoenteric feeding tubes are the most frequently used because they are easy to place and less costly and risky than tubes requiring surgical insertion. Small bore feeding tubes are preferred over the traditional nasogastric tubes (salem sumps) because there is less risk of tracheoesophageal fistula and aspiration, and they are more comfortable. The downside to using the small feeding tubes is that they are prone to collapse and clogging, making it difficult to check for feeding residuals.

Gastric feeding is suitable for many patients. However, in cases of altered GI motility (gastroparesis, gastric ileus, delayed gastric emptying from opiates, elevated intracranial pressure), the feeding tube should be placed transpylorically. In critically ill or postoperative patients, along with patients who have an absent gag reflex or who are on non-invasive positive pressure ventilation (BiPAP), having the feeding tube in the small bowel is essential. Jejunal feeding tubes are a must when feeding patients with acute pancreatitis.

Many bedside placement techniques for passing weighted tubes beyond the pylorus are available and usually successful. Ascultation while the patient is in the right lateral decubitus position can be used to track the tube into the small intestine. However, if this method is unsuccessful, then endoscopically or fluroscopically guided tube placement may be indicated. Prokinetic drugs can also help facilitate tube positioning. Upon placement of the feeding tube, radiographic confirmation is necessary before initiating the enteral feeding regimen.

Methods of Delivery

Enteral nutrition can be delivered by bolus, intermittent, or continuous feeding. *Bolus feeding* is the rapid infusion of a large volume of enteral formula over a short period of time. GI complications (e.g., diarrhea, nausea, vomiting, aspiration, distention) may result, however. *Intermittent feeding,* using either gravity drip or an infusion pump, can deliver a moderate to large volume of enteral formula over a defined period, usually from 1 to 16 hours. *Continuous tube feeding* is the infusion of a small amount of enteral formula over 24 hours using an infusion pump. *In critically ill patients and with small bowel feedings, the continuous delivery method is essential.* Continuous feedings are better tolerated than bolus or intermittent feedings, and are associated with reduced incidence of high gastric residuals, gastroesophageal reflux, and aspiration.

Formula Composition

There are many commercially available enteral products that differ in composition and proportion of nutrients, as well as cost. All formulas contain carbohydrate, fat, protein, and water, as well as vitamins, minerals, trace elements, and electrolytes (Table 15.4). Polymeric formulas contain intact

---

TABLE 15.4

CLASSIFICATION OF ENTERAL FORMULAS

Category	Subcategory	Comments
Polymeric	Blenderized	Real food; requires normal digestion and absorption; lactose or lactose-free; isotonic; nutritionally complete
	Standard	Intact nutrients; lactose-free; low residue; isotonic; nutritionally complete; requires normal digestion and absorption
	High nitrogen	Intact nutrients; lactose-free; isotonic; protein >15% of total kcal; nutritionally complete; requires normal digestion and absorption
	Fiber-enriched	Intact nutrients; lactose-free; isotonic; soluble and insoluble fiber; regulation of bowel function; nutritionally complete; requires normal digestion and absorption
	Calorically dense	Intact nutrients, 1.5–2.0 kcal/mL; high osmolality; use with fluid restriction; lactose-free; nutritionally complete; requires normal digestion and absorption
	Disease-specific	Intact nutrients; protein, fat, and carbohydrate source varies depending on specific disease-state formula; electrolyte content and osmolality varies; requires normal digestion and absorption; expensive; efficacy controversial
Oligomeric (partially hydrolyzed/ semi-elemental)		Hydrolyzed protein; di-tripeptides, free amino acids; fat content varies (3%–40% of total kcal); lactose-free; osmolality varies (250–700mOsm/kg); nutritionally complete; digestion required; limited absorptive surface of GI tract
Monomeric (elemental/ chemically defined)		Free amino acids; lactose-free; fat varies (1%–15% of total kcal); high osmolality; may include glutamine; nutritionally complete, minimal digestion required; limited absorptive surface of GI tract
Modular		Individual nutrient (carbohydrate, fat, protein) modules; used to modify pre-existing commercial formula to increase nutrient density or to make unique formula; requires normal digestion and absorption

nutrients and require normal digestion and absorption. Lactose-free mixtures are the basic feeding formulation, since most hospitalized patients have genetic or acquired lactase deficiency. These formulas can be isotonic or hypertonic (300–800 mOsm per kg of water). Caloric density varies from 1.0–2.0 kcal/mL, with 40%–55% of total calories from carbohydrate, 12%–20% from protein, and 30%–50% from fat. Fats are provided as long chain triglycerides (LCTs) and medium chain triglycerides (MCTs).

Oligomeric and monomeric formulas are classified as elemental and semi-elemental/peptide-based formulas. They contain one or more partially digested macronutrients and are reserved for patients with compromised GI function (e.g., critical illness, pancreatic or bile salt deficiencies, intestinal atrophy, short bowel syndrome and inflammatory bowel disease). Caloric density is usually 1.0 kcal per mL. Elemental diets have a much higher osmolality than semi-elemental diets. These formulas are considered low fat and may contain a high proportion of fat in the form of MCTs. The efficacy of elemental diets remains controversial.

Widespread use of enteral feeding and an expanding knowledge of specific disease processes has led to an explosion in the development of disease-specific formulas. These formulas have been designed for specific organ failure, metabolic dysfunction, or immunomodulation. Given the cost and questionable efficacy of these specialized formulas, they should be used judiciously. Detailed formula descriptions, clinical indications, and possible benefits are beyond the scope of this chapter.

Formula Selection

Enteral formula selection should be based on the patient's digestive and absorptive capacity, organ function, specific nutrient needs, tolerances, and allergies, and should take into account the formula composition and total calories. Attention must also be given to fluid requirements, vitamin and mineral needs, and osmolality. Most enteral formulas contain water in the general range of 700–900 mL per 1,000 mL of enteral formula. The general rule of thumb is to provide 30 mL water/kg body weight, or as clinical status permits. When provided in sufficient volume, most nutritionally complete products contain adequate vitamins and minerals to meet the U.S. recommended dietary intake (RDI). If necessary, a daily multivitamin and mineral supplement can be added.

Initiation and advancement of enteral feedings will vary with the method of administration. Bolus feedings are generally administered over several minutes and are best tolerated when given at less than 60 mL/min (e.g. 240 mL of formula every 3 hours over at least 3 minutes). Intermittent feedings are generally better received if a maximum of 200–300 mL of formula is delivered over a 30–60 minute period every 4–6 hours. Continuous feedings are introduced at 10–30 mL/hour, and advanced in 10–20 mL increments every 8 to 12 hours until the goal flow rate is attained. For patients who are critically ill, who have not been fed for an extended period of time, and those who are receiving calorie-dense or high osmolality enteral formulas, conservative initiation and advancement rates are highly advised (e.g., 10mL increments every 12–24 hours).

Complications

Complications associated with enteral feeding may be avoided and managed with appropriate monitoring. The major goal of monitoring is to minimize the complications of enteral therapy and to maintain the patency of the small bore feeding tube. An assessment of GI tolerance (i.e., nausea, vomiting, abdominal discomfort/distention, stool pattern) is mandatory when a patient is on enteral nutrition support. Hydration status and laboratory data must also be evaluated when a patient is being enterally fed. Preventive measures should be taken to minimize the risk of aspiration. Keeping the head of the bed elevated at a 30–45 degree angle and checking for tube feeding residuals are recommended to lessen the potential for aspiration. With continuous feeding, residuals should be checked every 4 hours and should not exceed 200 mL. If the patient has a cuffed tracheostomy, the cuff can be deflated 2 hours after bolus feedings; for continuous feeds, the cuff may be deflated only when necessary to prevent tracheal complications. Routine flushing of feeding tubes with 30–60 mL of water every 4–6 hours will help extend the life of the small tubes.

Although enteral nutrition is generally safe, complications may arise. There are three types of complications: mechanical, gastrointestinal, and metabolic. *Mechanical complications* of nasoenteric tube feedings include tube obstruction, displacement, or dislodgement; nasopharyngeal irritation; and gastric rupture. Obstruction or clogging of the tube occurs most frequently from inadequate crushing of medications and from formula residue adhering to the lumen of the tube. Giving liquid medications (elixirs, suspensions) rather than pills or syrups may help to avoid clogging. Flushing with water, as previously described, will help maintain patency of feeding tubes. Following proper procedures for feeding tube placement and verifying tube position will help avoid the complication of tube displacement. Using small soft tubes, lubricating tubes for insertion, and maintaining good hygiene of the mouth and nares improves patient comfort.

The most common complications of tube feedings are *gastrointestinal*, including diarrhea, nausea, vomiting, constipation, delayed gastric emptying, and GI bleeding. The major causes of formula-related diarrhea are rapid infusion rate, formula characteristics (hypertonic, low fiber/residue, high fat), and bacterial contamination. Medications (sorbitol-containing elixirs, antibiotics, laxatives, magnesium and phosphorous supplements), pancreatic insufficiency, fecal impaction, and pathogenic bacteria (*Clostridium difficile*) can all be nonformula–related causes of diarrhea in the tube-fed patient. Treatment of diarrhea is contingent on the etiology. Antimotility agents (lomotil, immodium, paregoric, deodorized tincture of opium) can be used in the treatment of diarrhea, provided stool cultures are negative for an infectious etiology.

High gastric residuals from delayed emptying can result from high fat and fiber formulas, rapid infusion rate, high osmolality formulas, certain disease state (e.g., diabetic gastroparesis), elevated intracranial pressure, sepsis, and certain medications (especially opiates). As previously discussed, checking feeding residuals is an essential component of the monitoring process. If patients have persistently high residuals, giving prokinetic drugs or placing the feeding tube in the small bowel should help alleviate the problem. During small bowel feedings, there should be little or no residuals obtained. If residuals are obtained, then chances are the feeding tube has relocated to the stomach, and verification of tube placement is warranted.

Constipation can result from low fiber/residue formulas, inadequate water/fluid intake, inactivity, decreased bowel motility, and medications such as phosphate binders, opiates, and calcium-channel antagonists. Neuromuscular blocking agents do not paralyze gut smooth muscle but may slow bowel motility via anticholinergic actions (11). Adequate hydration, fiber-enriched formulas, stool softeners, and bowel motility agents are helpful in improving constipation. Monitoring the stool pattern of the patient is also important for prevention of fecal impaction.

Metabolic complications that occur during enteral nutrition therapy are similar to those developed during parenteral nutrition, but are generally less severe. The most common metabolic disturbances are hyperglycemia, dehydration, and electrolyte imbalances (e.g., hyper-hypophosphatemia, hyper-hyponatremia, hyper-hypokalemia). Hyperglycemia is common in patients who are diabetic, who have poor glucose utilization due to insulin resistance from stress (trauma, sepsis), or who are on diabetogenic medications such as corticosteroids. Urine and blood glucose should be monitored at periodic intervals in all patients receiving enteral feeding. For optimal nutrient substrate utilization, blood glucose levels should be ≤150 mg/dL. Insulin administration will be required in patients with persistently elevated blood glucose levels. Subcutaneous administration of insulin is poorly absorbed in critically ill patients; therefore, an insulin infusion is required for the treatment of hyperglycemia. Tight glycemic control (i.e., blood glucose 80–110mg/dL) using an insulin infusion in critically ill patients has been shown to reduce mortality, bacteremia, and the number of days on mechanical ventilation (12) (see Chapter 107).

Repleting malnourished patients can result in the intracellular uptake of phosphorous, potassium, and magnesium as anabolism is stimulated, causing decreased serum levels of these electrolytes. These electrolytes should be closely monitored and replaced as needed. Thiamine supplementation is also needed in the malnourished patient.

Parenteral Nutrition

Parenteral nutrition (PN) is the intravenous administration of a hypertonic solution of carbohydrate, fat, protein, electrolytes, vitamins, minerals, and fluid. Although enteral nutrition support is the preferred modality of nutritional therapy, PN is an important technique in patients who have absolute gut failure, as with short bowel syndrome, small bowel obstruction, ischemia or ileus, severe GI hemorrhage, and fistulas not amenable to enteral feeding. Other patients who might require PN are those with severe mucositis following chemotherapy, or those in whom the use of the intestine is not possible after major excisional surgery. Additionally, PN should be initiated in any patient not tolerating full enteral nutrition support within 5–7 days.

Many patients will require only short-term parenteral nutrition. In these patients, nutrients can be infused via the peripheral veins with conventional cannulae rotated on a daily basis, or ultra–fine-bore 15-cm catheters inserted at the antecubital fossa. For more prolonged treatment, nutrients are infused into central veins through central catheters or peripherally inserted central catheter (PICC) lines. Peripheral access, however, may be limited by the dextrose concentration; a central line is necessary when infusing dextrose concentrations greater than 10%.

Formula Composition

Carbohydrate is the primary energy source in parenteral nutrition solutions. Dextrose monohydrate is the carbohydrate source yielding 3.4 calories per gram, and ranging in concentration from 5%–70%. The most frequently used dextrose concentrations for critically ill patients are 20% and 25%. The quantity of carbohydrate, however, is based on the patient's caloric requirement, optimal fuel balance, and glucose oxidation rate (i.e., hepatic oxidative capacity). Administration of no greater than 4–6 mg dextrose/kg/min per 24-hour period is recommended for optimal oxidation and prevention of fat synthesis (lipogenesis). Excessive carbohydrate provision is also associated with hepatic dysfunction and increased carbon dioxide production.

Crystalline amino acids are the form of protein currently added to PN admixtures. Standard amino acid solutions contain a balance of non-essential and essential amino acids tailored to the normal serum amino acid profile. Concentrations range from 3%–15%; they provide 4.0 calories per gram. Modified amino acid formulas contain a blend of amino acids designed to meet disease or age-specific requirements.

Intravenous fat is an aqueous dispersion containing soybean or safflower oil, egg yolk phospholipid (an emulsifier) and glycerin to achieve isotonicity. Long chain fatty acid emulsions are currently the only commercially available IV fat. They are available as either 10%, 20%, or 30% emulsions. Maintenance essential fatty acids (EFA) requirements can be met by providing 4%–10% of the total calories as fat

(2%–4% as linoleic acid). The 10% lipid emulsion provides 1.1 kcal/mL; 20% provides 2.0 kcal/mL; 30% provides 3.0 kcal/mL. IV fat is contraindicated in patients with disturbances in normal fat metabolism (i.e., triglyceride levels ≥400–500 mg/dL), nephrosis when accompanied by hyperlipidemia, and severe egg allergy. For patients with pancreatitis of etiologies other than hypertriglyceridemia, intravenous fat infusions are not contraindicated. The recommended infusion rate varies depending on the lipid concentrations. For the 10% emulsion, a minimum of 8 hours is suggested. The anesthetic agent propofol is delivered in 10% intravenous fat, providing 1.1 kcal/mL. Attention must therefore be given to those patients who are on PN with lipids and on propofol.

Electrolyte requirements for patients receiving parenteral nutrition are patient-specific and influenced by nutritional status. Organ function, acid-base balance, medications, and gastrointestinal losses will also influence the electrolyte adjustments that will be needed in the PN solution to maintain electrolyte homeostasis. In stable patients, acid-base balance can, for the most part, be maintained by adding equal amounts of chloride and acetate. However, for patients with acid-base disturbances the acetate, which is metabolized to bicarbonate, and the chloride will need to be adjusted in an effort to help correct the abnormality. For example, in patients with severe metabolic acidosis, the chloride would be minimized and the acetate maximized. Vitamins and trace elements are added to PN solutions in doses consistent with the American Medical Association Nutrition Advisory Group's recommendations. Iron is absent in the multi-trace element preparation due to the fear of anaphylaxis, but iron can be given as iron dextran either in the PN formula or intramuscularly. Copper and manganese are excreted via biliary excretion. Consequently, supplementation of copper and manganese should be discontinued if baseline total bilirubin is three times the upper limit of normal or if total bilirubin triples from baseline value.

Initiation and Advancement

Parenteral nutrition therapy should be initiated at a slow rate (e.g., 30–40 mL/hour), using the final concentration planned for therapy and advanced as glucose tolerance permits until the nutrient needs of a patient are met. For critically ill patients, advancement of parenteral nutrition should be conservative (e.g., increased 20 mL every 24 hours until the goal rate is attained). Since dextrose concentration is limited in peripheral parenteral nutrition (5% or 10% dextrose), it may be initiated at the same rate as the usual peripheral IV fluids.

Monitoring

Successful administration of PN requires careful monitoring. Blood glucose monitoring via finger sticks every 4–6 hours (more frequently in the ICU) is indicated until the infusion rate has stabilized. Serum glucose should be main-

tained under 120 mg/dL in ICU patients, and under 150 mg/dL in non-ICU patients. Serum triglycerides should be checked 6 hours after the completion of the intravenous fat infusion to assess the patient's lipid clearing capacity, especially in the face of hyperglycemia and steroid therapy. Serum triglyceride levels should be ≤400 mg/dL. Electrolytes must be followed to assure adequate hydration, renal function and need for supplementation or restriction. Finally, liver function should be periodically monitored.

Complications

Mechanical, metabolic, infectious, and hepatic complications may occur when using parenteral nutrition support. Pneumothorax is the most common mechanical complication. Others include thrombus, catheter occlusion, and air embolus. The infectious complications seen with parenteral nutrition are typically catheter-related (see Chapter 72). Hyperglycemia is the most prevalent metabolic complication. Risk factors for hyperglycemia include metabolic stress, medications, obesity, diabetes, and excess calories and/or carbohydrate. Malnourished patients are prone to refeeding shifts. For an extensive list of the metabolic complications of parenteral nutrition and suggestions for prevention and treatment, the reader is referred to a major text on parenteral nutrition (13).

Hepatobiliary abnormalities have been identified in patients on total parenteral nutrition who have no underlying liver disease. Elevated aminotransferases, alkaline phosphatase, and bilirubin concentrations may occur days to weeks after initiation of parenteral nutrition. Enzyme levels may return to normal while a patient is on PN, but almost always normalize when it is discontinued. Steatosis (fatty liver) is the most frequent hepatic derangement that occurs with PN. High glucose infusions, exceeding 4–6 mg dextrose/kg/min, is the primary etiologic agent in the production of fatty liver. The excessive provision of intravenous fat can also result in fatty infiltration of the liver.

Gallbladder stasis (biliary sludging) is felt to be the primary cause of PN-associated biliary disease. Stimulating gallbladder contractility with enteral feedings usually reverses this process. To manage and prevent PN-induced hepatic dysfunction, use the GI tract whenever possible, avoid overfeeding, provide a well-balanced fuel mix, cycle the PN regimen, consider carnitine and glutamine supplementation, and work up alternative causes such as hepatitis, biliary obstruction, hepatotoxic drugs, and sepsis.

CONCLUSIONS

Malnutrition is common in patients who are admitted to the hospital, and the nutritional status deteriorates during the hospital stay in most patients. Nutrition, therefore, becomes of vital importance in maintaining nutritional status during illness. Fortunately, malnutrition can be prevented or treated in most patients by using nutrition support.

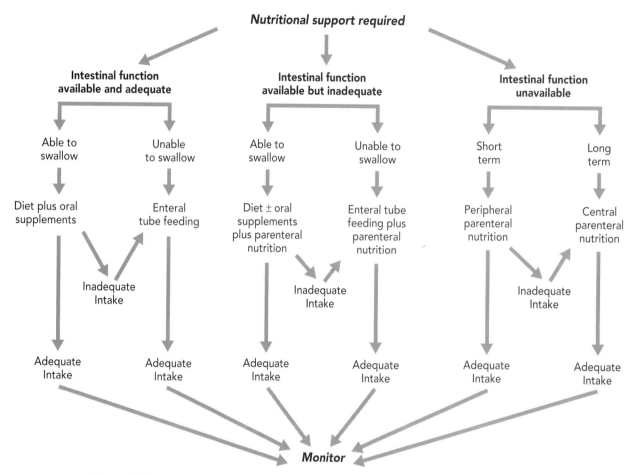

Figure 15.1 Summary of nutritional management in the hospital patient.

Although enteral nourishment is the optimal route of administration, at times it is not medically feasible or well tolerated. Under these circumstances total parenteral nutrition is indicated; however, every effort should be made to switch to enteral feeding when possible (Figure 15.1).

Unfortunately, attempts to improve a patient's prognosis through nutritional intervention can be counterproductive when nutritional therapy is poorly managed. Both enteral and parenteral nutrition (particularly the latter) are associated with serious and sometimes life-threatening complications. Thus, nutritional therapy merits the same high standard of care applied to other therapeutic modalities, and patients who do not need artificial nutrition support should not receive it.

REFERENCES

1. McWhirter JP, Pennington CR. The incidence and recognition of malnutrition in hospitals. *BMJ* 1994;308:945–948.
2. Pennington CR. Disease and malnutrition in British hospitals. *Proc Nutr Soc* 1997;56:1–15.
3. Animashaun A, Hill GL. Body composition research: implications for the practice of clinical nutrition. *J Parent Ent Nutr* 1992; 16:197–218.
4. Lord LM, Sax HC. The role of the gut in critical illness. *AACN Clin Issues* 1994;9:450–458.
5. Shronts EP, Fish JA, Pesce-Hammond K. Nutritional assessment. In Souba WW, Kohn-Keeth C, Mueller C, et al, eds. *The A.S.P.E.N Nutrition Support Practice Manual.* Silver Spring, MD: 1998; A.S.P.E.N.
6. A.S.P.E.N. Standards for nutrition support: hospitalized patients. *Nutr Clin Pract* 1995;10:208–318.

7. McClave SA, Snider HI. Use of indirect calorimetry in clinical nutrition. *Nutr Clin Pract* 1992;7:208–221.
8. Trujillo EB, Robinson MK, Jacobs DO. Critical illness. In Souba WW, Kohn-Keeth C, Mueller C, et al, eds. *The A.S.P.E.N. Nutrition Support Practice Manual.* Silver Spring, MD: 1998;A.S.P.E.N.
9. Stralovich-Romani A, Kees Mahute C, et al. Administrative, nutritional, and ethical prinicples for the management of critically ill patients. In George RB, Light RW, Matthay MA, Matthay RA, eds. *Chest Medicine: Essentials of Pulmonary and Critical Care Medicine,* 4th ed. Philadelphia: Lippincott Williams & Wilkins 2000; 515–560.
10. Bloss CS. Pharmacomodulation of the gut: implications for the enterally fed patient. *Nutr Clin Pract* 1998;231–237.
11. Lord L, Trumbore L, Zaloga G. Enteral nutrition implementation and management. In Souba WW, Kohn-Keeth C, Mueller C, et al, eds. *The A.S.P.E.N. Nutrition Support Practice Manual.* Silver Spring, MD: 1998;A.S.P.E.N.
12. Van Den Berghe G, Wouters P, Weekers F, et al. Intensive insulin therapy in critically ill patients. *N Engl J Med* 2001;345: 1359–1367.
13. Rombeau JL, Rolandelli RR, eds. *Parenteral Nutrition.* Philadelphia: Saunders, 1998.

ADDITIONAL READING

A.S.P.E.N. Board of Directors and The Clinical Guidelines Task Force. Guidelines for the use of parenteral and enteral nutrition in adult and pediatric patients. *J Parenter Enteral Nutr* 2002;26: 1SA–138SA.

Demling RH, DeSanti L. The stress response to injury and infection: Role of nutritional support. *Wounds* 2000;12:3–14.

Fukatsu K, Zarzalur BL, Johnson CD, et al. Enteral nutrition prevents remote organ injury and mortality following a gut ischemic insult. *Ann Surg* 2001;233:660–668.

Heyland DK, Drover JW, MacDonald S, et al. Effect of postpyloric feeding on gastroesophageal regurgitation and pulmonary microaspiration; Results of a randomized controlled trial. *Crit Care Med* 2001;29:1495–1501.

Krystofiak RM, Charney P. Is there a role for specialized enteral nutrition in the intensive care unit? *Nutr Clin Pract* 2000;17: 156–168.

Lobo DN, Memon MA, Allison SP, Rowlands BJ. Evolution of nutritional support in acute pancreatitis. *Br J Surg* 2000;87: 695–707.

Approach to the Hospitalized Older Patient

16

C. Seth Landefeld   C. Bree Johnston   Mary Anne Johnson

INTRODUCTION

Older people are at disproportionate risk of becoming seriously ill and requiring hospital care. Persons 65 years of age or older make up only 13% of the U.S. population but account for 35% of acute-care hospital admissions and 45% of hospital expenditures for adults. The impact of older persons on acute hospital care will increase rapidly with the aging of the population. The number of Americans 65 years of age or older is expected to double to 71 million by 2030, representing 20% of the U.S. population. Particularly striking is the projected growth in the number of persons over age 85, especially in the middle third of the century (Figure 16.1).

Once hospitalized, older patients are at high risk for loss of independence and institutionalization. Among hospitalized medical patients 70 years of age or older, nearly 15% experience a decline in their ability to perform basic self-care activities of daily living (ADL), another 20% are discharged without recovering their baseline abilities, and 15% of those admitted from home are discharged to a nursing home (1). Loss of personal independence is often promoted by the reciprocal effects of the acute illness that led to hospitalization and underlying chronic illnesses and impairments. In addition, many older patients have lost their "bounce"—their ability to recover rapidly and completely from the acute insults of illness and hospitalization to their physiologic, psychological, and social systems. Thus, optimal care for the hospitalized older patient requires the physician to manage acute illness while simultaneously intervening as necessary to promote or maintain independent functioning.

RATIONALE FOR A SYSTEMATIC APPROACH TO HOSPITALIZED OLDER PATIENTS

This chapter outlines an approach to the hospitalized older patient that incorporates systematic assessments at the level of the organ system, the whole person, and the person's environment. This approach can identify areas in which targeted interventions may improve function or reduce risk for adverse outcomes. Although this approach has been designed specifically for older persons, a similar approach may often be appropriate in other patients with complex chronic illness.

Table 16.1 summarizes a suggested approach to the systematic assessment of 10 common problems that are frequently overlooked in hospitalized elders. Seven of these problems are primarily at the level of organ systems, two are at the level of the whole person, and one is at the level of the person's interaction with the environment. These 10 problems were selected on the basis of their relative importance, the quality of relevant evidence, and their specificity to older persons. Other important problems (e.g., use of alcohol or tobacco, pain management, and advance directives) are not specific to older persons, and some problems specific to the elderly (e.g., age-related decline in renal function) are widely recognized.

Although this chapter focuses on addressing these problems in the hospital, it is important to recognize the importance of continuity of care before and after hospitalization. In the care of the hospitalized older patient, initial and ongoing communication between the hospital physician and the primary care physician, if these are two different

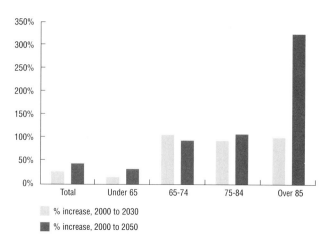

Figure 16.1 The aging of the U.S. population. Projected increase in population cohorts by age between 2000 and 2030 and between 2000 and 2050. (Source: U.S. Bureau of the Census)

persons (Chapter 1), is essential. Knowledge of the patient's prior function, medical and psychosocial history, mental status, and values should inform decisions about acute and post-acute care. Ongoing communication throughout the hospitalization also helps ensure that there will be continuity of care after discharge.

The proposed approach requires the marshaling of resources early in the hospitalization, generally in the form of the time of the physician, nurse, social worker, or other staff. Two types of evidence suggest that these interventions are a good investment. First, for each problem, there is compelling evidence supporting the proposed intervention, either because the efficacy of the intervention is well established (e.g., warfarin to prevent stroke related to atrial fibrillation) or because the associated problem is frequent, often overlooked, and can be relieved with a safe and inexpensive intervention. Second, these types of systematic approaches to the evaluation and management of acutely ill older persons can improve patient outcomes and reduce hospital costs (2).

MANAGEMENT OF THE HOSPITALIZED PATIENT

Assessment at the Level of Organ Systems

Problem 1. Atrial Fibrillation (Cardiovascular Function)

Rationale. Nonvalvular atrial fibrillation is present in 5% or more of hospitalized elders, often found as an incidental finding. Consistent and compelling evidence from randomized trials shows that the risk for stroke in persons with

TABLE 16.1

SYSTEMATIC ASSESSMENT OF HOSPITALIZED OLDER PATIENTS: A FRAMEWORK HIGHLIGHTING 10 COMMON PROBLEMS THAT ARE FREQUENTLY OVERLOOKED

Problem (domain of assessment)	Assessment methods	Illustrative interventions
Assessment at the level of organ systems		
1. Atrial fibrillation (cardiovascular)	Take pulse, ECG	Warfarin, treatment to maintain sinus rhythm
2. Malnutrition (gastrointestinal)	Subjective Global Assessment (Table 16.2)	Supplement water, calorie, protein intake; assess social environment
3. Influenza and pneumococcus (infection)	Ask about vaccination	Vaccination against influenza, pneumococcus
4. Cognitive impairment (neurologic)	Short Portable Mental Status Questionnaire (Table 16.3)	Evaluate for dementia or delirium; assess social environment
5. Immobility and falls (neurologic)	Ask about difficulty walking and falls	Avoid restraints and tethers; prescribe walking and physical therapy
6. Sensory impairment (neurologic)	Assess vision and hearing	Prosthetics (glasses, hearing aids)
7. Depression (psychological)	Depression screen	Attention, cognitive therapy, pharmacotherapy
Assessment at the level of the whole person		
8. Disability (activities of daily living)	Ask about help needed for basic and instrumental activities of daily living	Physical and/or occupational therapy; assess social environment
9. Suboptimal drug use (pharmaceuticals)	Assess indications for therapy, dosing, and potential interactions	Modify prescribing
Assessment at the level of the environment		
10. Maltreatment (social support)	Ask about level of social support and perceived freedom and safety	Early involvement of family and social services in planning to go home

atrial fibrillation can be reduced approximately 75% by treatment with warfarin (e.g., from 4.3% to 0.9% annually). Moreover, the beneficial effect of warfarin is maintained in persons 75 years of age or older and in those with other risk factors for stroke (3). Alternatively, comparable benefits may be attained with cardioversion and pharmacologic maintenance of sinus rhythm. Nonetheless, many older patients with atrial fibrillation are discharged from the hospital without warfarin therapy, even when warfarin is judged to be appropriate (4). Failure to prescribe warfarin is likely a consequence of underestimation of the benefit of therapy, overestimation of its potential risk, and the difficulty of implementing, monitoring, and modifying therapy to minimize adverse effects.

Recommendation. Every hospitalized older patient should be assessed for the presence of chronic nonvalvular atrial fibrillation by examination of the pulse and electrocardiogram. When atrial fibrillation is diagnosed, valvular disease and hyperthyroidism should be ruled out. In the absence of a strong contraindication, treatment should be instituted to prevent stroke, usually with warfarin. A strategy of rate control and anticoagulant therapy may have a lower risk of adverse effects than one focused on attaining and maintaining sinus rhythm (Chapter 42).

Problem 2. Malnutrition (Gastrointestinal Function)

Rationale. Serious deficiencies of macronutrients and micronutrients are common in hospitalized older patients. Key macronutrients are protein, calories, salt, water, and fiber. On admission, severe protein-calorie malnutrition is present in approximately 15% of patients 70 years of age or older, and moderate malnutrition is present in another 25%. Moreover, 25% of older patients suffer further nutritional depletion during hospitalization. Even after the underlying illness, its severity, and comorbid illnesses are controlled for, malnutrition is associated with an increased risk for death, dependence, and institutionalization (5).

In addition to deficiencies of vitamins and electrolytes that may develop with protein-calorie malnutrition,

vitamin D deficiency is especially common among hospitalized elders. In one large hospital, nearly two-thirds of medical inpatients 65 years of age or older were deficient in vitamin D; vitamin D deficiency was nearly as common in inpatients without a risk factor for vitamin D deficiency and in those taking multivitamins (6). These data regarding the high prevalence of vitamin D deficiency in hospitalized elders complement evidence that vitamin D and calcium supplementation reduce by half the frequency of nonvertebral fractures in men and women 65 years of age or older (7).

Recommendation. Assessment of nutritional status is indicated by three considerations: (i) the poor prognosis of patients with malnutrition, (ii) the potential benefit of low-cost, noninvasive interventions, and (iii) increasing evidence of beneficial effects of nutritional supplementation on the outcomes of malnourished patients in other settings (8). The *Subjective Global Assessment* (9) (Table 16.2) is an inexpensive yet accurate method of systematically identifying patients who are moderately or severely malnourished based on weight loss and physical signs of malnutrition. When malnutrition is identified, remediable contributing factors should be sought and corrected, such as difficulty chewing or insufficient time or encouragement to eat. Oral feeding is preferred whenever possible (8). It remains unclear whether the benefits of invasive alimentation (alimentary or parenteral) outweigh their risks, yet they may be beneficial in situations in which prolonging survival is a central goal and the invasive approach will overcome a critical barrier to feeding (Chapter 15). In patients with a progressive terminal illness in whom prolongation of life is not a central goal of care, or in patients who would require long-term restraints for invasive alimentation, the burdens of invasive alimentation are likely to outweigh the benefits. An open and nonjudgmental discussion with the patient or surrogate decision maker can help clarify the role of nutrition within the overall goals of care (Chapters 17 and 19).

Long-term supplementation with vitamin D (1,000 IU daily) and calcium (1,000 mg daily) should be considered for every hospitalized older person.

TABLE 16.2
SUBJECTIVE GLOBAL ASSESSMENT OF NUTRITIONAL STATUS

Nutritional status	Weight loss in past 6 months	Weight loss in past 2 weeks	Physical signs of loss of subcutaneous fat or muscle
Well nourished	<5%	—	None
	>5%	None	None
Moderately malnourished	5–10%	Present	Mild
Severely malnourished	>10%	Present	Severe

From Detsky AS, Smalley PS, Chang J. Is this patient malnourished? *JAMA* 1994;271:54–58, with permission.

Problem 3. Influenza and Pneumococcus (Immune Function)

Rationale. Influenza vaccination reduces hospitalization and mortality in persons 65 years of age or older (10). Pneumococcal vaccination of persons 65 years of age or older reduces serious pneumococcal infections (11). Influenza vaccination should be administered annually in the fall, and pneumococcal vaccination should be administered at least once and probably every 5–10 years. The immune response to vaccination is not seriously compromised by hospitalization or acute illness.

Recommendation. All persons 65 years of age or older should be asked whether they have received influenza or pneumococcal vaccination. Hospitalization provides an opportunity to ensure that these important immunizations are given to those at risk for serious disease. Influenza vaccine should be administered annually in the fall. Pneumococcal vaccine should be administered to all those over 65 who have not previously been vaccinated or whose vaccination status is unknown. Those who have received the vaccine more than 5 years previously and who were under age 65 at the time of vaccination should receive another dose. Delivery of these vaccines to appropriate hospitalized patients is increasingly being assessed in hospital quality report cards, many of which are being made available to the public (see Chapter 12).

Problem 4. Cognitive Impairment (Neurologic Function)

Rationale. Underlying cognitive impairment consistent with dementia is present on admission in 20%–40% of hospitalized elders and frequently goes undetected (12).

Preexisting cognitive impairment is a risk factor for delirium, falls, use of restraints, and lack of adherence to therapy. Also, there is intrinsic value in identifying previously undiagnosed dementia so that appropriate evaluation and management strategies can be implemented after discharge. Tests of mental status are sensitive and specific for dementia. For example, in one study of hospitalized elders, three or more errors on the 10-item Short Portable Mental Status Questionnaire (13) (Table 16.3) was 87% sensitive and 99% specific for a diagnosis of dementia (14).

Delirium is present in 10%–15% of hospitalized elders on admission and develops in up to 30% during the course of hospitalization (15). Delirium is associated with increased rates of in-hospital death, nursing home placement, and prolonged length of stay, and it may worsen chronic cognitive impairment. Roughly one-third of delirium cases are preventable by appropriately managing these six risk factors: cognitive impairment, sleep deprivation, immobility, visual impairment, hearing impairment, and dehydration (16).

Recommendation. Mental status should be assessed by using an established test of cognitive function, such as the Short Portable Mental Status Questionnaire (Table 16.3) or the 30-item Mini-Mental State Exam. The diagnosis of dementia should be considered in those patients with three or more errors on the Short Portable Mental Status Questionnaire or a score of 24 or less on the Mini-Mental State Exam. When dementia is a possibility, the patient should be assessed to rule out reversible causes and to identify those for whom pharmacologic therapy and family oriented interventions are warranted.

The diagnosis of delirium should be considered when any of the following are observed: fluctuation in mental status or behavior, inattention, disorganized thinking, and

---

TABLE 16.3

THE 10 ITEMS OF THE SHORT PORTABLE MENTAL STATUS QUESTIONNAIRE

Item	Correct response
1. What is the date today?	Exact month, date, and year
2. What day of the week is it?	Day of the week
3. What is the name of this place?	Any correct description of the location
4. What is your telephone number?	Correct number, or consistently given number if the correct number is not known to the examiner
5. How old are you?	Stated age corresponds to date of birth
6. When were you born?	Correct month, date, and year
7. Who is the President of the U.S. now?	Last name of the President
8. Who was President just before him?	Last name of the previous President
9. What was your mother's maiden name?	Any female first name, and a last name different from the subject's
10. Subtract 3 from 20 and keep subtracting 3 from each new number, all the way down.	17, 14, 11, 8, 5, 2

From Pfeiffer E. A short portable mental status questionnaire for the assessment of organic brain deficit in elderly patients. *J Am Geriatr Soc* 1975;23:433–441, with permission.

altered consciousness. Prudent measures to prevent or ameliorate delirium include avoiding medicines associated with delirium whenever possible, treating infection and fever, detecting and correcting metabolic abnormalities, frequently orienting patients with cognitive or sensory impairment, and walking.

Problem 5. Immobility and Falls (Neurologic Function)

Rationale. Walking facilitates the performance of virtually all basic and instrumental ADL. The ability to walk briskly and the habit of regularly walking 1 mile or more daily are associated with prolonged survival (17). Immobility during hospitalization, however, leads rapidly to deconditioning and subsequent difficulty walking. The major adverse effect of walking is falling, which can lead to serious injury. Falls and fall-related injuries are associated with cognitive impairment; abnormalities of cognition, gait, balance, and the lower extremities; and multiple chronic medical conditions and depression (18, 19).

Recommendation. The ability to get up from bed, gait, balance, lower extremity strength and anatomy, cognition, and mood should be assessed during the initial physical examination. Persons able to walk independently should be encouraged to do so frequently during hospitalization. The hospital staff should assist those able to walk but unable to do so alone safely several times daily. Formal physical therapy may yield additional benefits. Risk for falls should be assessed by inquiring about a history of falls and by examination. Adopting interventions that reduce falls in other settings may also prevent falls in the hospital (20). Prudent preventive strategies include minimizing bed rest when possible and providing in-bed physical conditioning when bed rest is required, assisting with walking for those who walk with difficulty, and providing physical therapy for those with weakness or gait abnormalities. Soft-tissue and bony abnormalities of the feet should receive appropriate podiatric care. Restraints and tethers have not been shown to reduce fall-related injuries and may result in a variety of untoward consequences, including strangulation. Their use should not generally be considered a strategy to reduce falls.

Problem 6. Sensory Impairment (Neurologic Function)

Rationale. Most hospitalized elders have impaired vision or hearing, and these sensory impairments are risk factors for falls, incontinence, and functional dependence (18). Although most visual and hearing impairments are readily corrected by glasses or hearing aids, these appliances are often not brought to or lost in the hospital. Addressing sensory impairment is part of an effective strategy to prevent delirium (16).

Recommendation. Hospitalized elders should be routinely screened for visual and hearing impairments by asking if they have difficulty with seeing or hearing and whether they use glasses or a hearing aid. Physical examination should include a test of visual acuity (e.g., with a pocket card of the Jaeger eye test) and the whisper test of hearing (in which a short, easily answered question is whispered in each ear) (21). In people with visual or hearing impairments, glasses or a hearing aid should be provided (ideally brought from home), and the staff should be informed that patients may need to use an appliance to communicate effectively. Some hospital units have found it useful to have "pocket amplifiers" and magnification devices on hand to assist in communicating with older persons who lack glasses or hearing aids.

Problem 7. Depression (Psychological Function)

Rationale. Depressive symptoms in hospitalized elders are common and prognostically important, and they can potentially be ameliorated. Major or minor depression occurs in roughly one-third of hospitalized patients age 65 years or older but is often missed. The presence of depressive symptoms is associated with increased risk for dependence in ADL, nursing home placement, and shortened long-term survival, even after baseline function and the severity of acute and chronic illness are controlled for (22).

Recommendation. The possibility of depression should be considered in hospitalized older patients, who should be asked whether they feel down, depressed, or hopeless, or whether they have lost interest or pleasure in doing things (23). A positive response to any one of these questions should trigger a formal assessment for an affective disorder. In hospitalized elders, the presence of three or more of 11 depressive symptoms has been found to be 83% sensitive and 77% specific for a diagnosis of major depression (24).

Detection is the first and most important step in the management of depression, which is frequently missed in hospitalized elders. Psychotherapeutic interventions (environmental, behavioral, cognitive, and family) are safe and often effective, and they should be initiated in all patients with suspected depression. It is rarely necessary to begin pharmacotherapy during hospitalization for a medical or surgical condition, but follow-up shortly after discharge is critical. Strategies incorporating cognitive problem-solving therapy and pharmacotherapy may be most effective (25). If pharmacotherapy is initiated, selective serotonin reuptake inhibitors are often preferred because tricyclic antidepressants are contraindicated in approximately 50% of older hospitalized patients (26). Tricyclic antidepressants are probably more effective in older patients with severe depression; if tricyclic antidepressants are used, desipramine and nortriptyline have fewer anticholinergic and cardiac side effects than do other agents (Chapter 119).

Assessment at the Level of the Whole Person

Problem 8. Disability (Activities of Daily Living)

Rationale. The performance of ADL is necessary to live independently, and dependence in ADL is independently associated with worse quality of life, shortened survival, and increased resource use (27). ADL have traditionally been divided into those performed on a daily basis in the home (e.g., bathing, dressing, using the toilet, transferring from a bed to a chair, eating, and maintaining continence) and those that involve higher levels of integrative function (e.g., cooking, doing household chores, using transportation, and handling financial and medical matters). Although walking is sometimes considered an ADL, it is often considered separately because it facilitates many of the other activities but is not necessary for any one of them.

Recommendation. The ability to perform basic and instrumental ADL should be determined at the time of admission. The etiology of dependence in ADL should be determined (e.g., dependence in instrumental ADL is often associated with dementia), and strategies to maintain and improve functional capacity, such as physical and occupational therapy, should be considered. These strategies may be best implemented by ward staff (i.e., nurses or case managers) without physician consultation or referral (16). Social work consultation and early involvement of family or other caregivers is often necessary to plan post-discharge care for those dependent in ADL (see Chapter 5).

Problem 9. Suboptimal Drug Use (Pharmaceuticals)

Rationale. The number of drugs prescribed to hospitalized patients is directly proportional to their age. Moreover, hospitalization is a period of rapid turnover in drug therapies for elders. In one study, 40% of drugs prescribed before admission were discontinued during hospitalization, and 45% of drugs prescribed at discharge were started during hospitalization (28). Although older patients are at increased risk for inappropriate drug therapy, adverse drug effects, and drug–drug interactions, they may also be undertreated when effective therapies are not used or are used in inadequate doses. Thus, hospitalization is an opportunity for a thorough review of each older patient's medications and to make adjustments as needed. In one study, 88% of older hospitalized patients had one or more clinically significant drug problems, and 22% had at least one potentially serious and life-threatening problem (29). Consultation with clinical pharmacists can lead to more appropriate prescribing and improved adherence (30) in hospitalized elders.

Recommendation. Each patient's medications should be reviewed on admission, and those that are unnecessary or have low therapeutic indices (e.g., sedative–hypnotics) should be discontinued. During hospitalization and discharge, medications should be reviewed in six common categories: inappropriate choice of therapy; dosage; schedule; drug–drug interactions; therapeutic duplication; and allergy. Also, neglected therapies (e.g., vitamin D and calcium) should be considered and instituted if appropriate.

Assessment at the Level of the Environment

Problem 10. Maltreatment (Social Support)

Rationale. Hospitalization of older persons is sometimes precipitated by maltreatment, which includes physical or psychological abuse, neglect, self-neglect, exploitation, and abandonment. Although elder maltreatment was not recognized in the medical literature until 1975, it is now estimated to affect 1 to 2 million Americans annually. In a large, prospective cohort study, the annual incidence of referral to protective services for mistreatment was approximately 1% among persons age 65 years or older (31). Those referred for abuse, neglect, or exploitation had a lower survival rate during 13 years of follow-up (9%) than did those referred for self-neglect (17%) and those not referred (40%). Most older persons referred to protective services because of physical abuse have been seen in hospital emergency departments, and many emergency department visits lead to hospitalization. Sociodemographic factors such as poverty, age greater than 75 years, and nonwhite race are the strongest predictors of elder maltreatment (32).

Recommendation. Universal screening for maltreatment has been recommended and can be implemented by asking each older patient, "Do you feel safe returning where you live?" However, it must be recognized that the sensitivity and specificity of this and other screening approaches are unknown. Further questions can explore the living situation and specific settings or aspects of maltreatment. The diagnosis of maltreatment should be considered when physical or psychological stigmata (e.g., unexplained injury, dehydration, malnutrition, social withdrawal, recalcitrant depression or anxiety) are present. When maltreatment is suspected, Adult Protective Services or the equivalent state agency should be contacted; such contact is required in most states.

KEY POINTS

- Older persons, the fastest-growing segment of the U.S. population, are at disproportionate risk for hospitalization. Once hospitalized, many older patients lose significant functional ability.
- A systematic approach is needed to address the problems of hospitalized older patients.
- Underdiagnosis and undertreatment of common medical problems, such as atrial fibrillation, malnutrition,

delirium, and depression, may contribute to excess mortality and morbidity.

- Efforts should be made to diagnose sensory (such as hearing and vision) and cognitive impairment in elderly inpatients.
- Hospitalization is a good time to review drug use and assess possible toxicity or interactions.
- All hospitalized older patients should be screened for maltreatment.

REFERENCES

1. Covinsky KE, Palmer RM, Fortinsky RH, et al. Loss of independence in activities of daily living in older adults hospitalized with medical illnesses: Increased vulnerability with age. *J Am Geriatr Soc* 2003;51:451–458.
2. Landefeld CS, Palmer RM, Kresevic D, et al. A randomized trial of care in a hospital medical unit especially designed to improve the functional outcomes of acutely ill older patients. *N Engl J Med* 1995;332:1338–1344.
3. Albers GW, Dalen JE, Laupacis A, et al. Antithrombotic therapy in atrial fibrillation. *Chest* 2001;119:194S–206S.
4. Antani MR, Beyth RJ, Covinsky KE, et al. Failure to prescribe warfarin to patients with nonrheumatic atrial fibrillation. *J Gen Intern Med* 1996;11:713–720.
5. Covinsky KE, Martin GE, Beyth RJ, et al. The relationship between clinical assessments of nutritional status and adverse outcomes in older hospitalized medical patients. *J Am Geriatr Soc* 1999;47:532–538.
6. Thomas MK, Lloyd-Jones DM, Thadhani RI, et al. Hypovitaminosis D in medical inpatients. *N Engl J Med* 1998;338:777–783.
7. Dawson-Hughes B, Harris SS, Krall EA, et al. Effect of calcium and vitamin D supplementation on bone density in men and women 65 years of age or older. *N Engl J Med* 1997;337: 660–667.
8. Milne AC, Potter J, Avenell A. Protein and energy supplementation in elderly people at risk from malnutrition (Cochrane Review). In: *The Cochrane Library*, Issue 4, 2003. Chichester, UK: John Wiley & Sons, Ltd.
9. Detsky AS, Smalley PS, Chang J. Is this patient malnourished? *JAMA* 1994;271:54–58.
10. Nichol KL, Nordin J, Mullooly J, et al. Influenza vaccina and reduction in hospitalizations for cardiac disease and stroke among the elderly. *N Engl J Med* 2003;348:1322–1332.
11. Sisk JE, Moskowitz AJ, Whang W, et al. Cost-effectiveness of vaccination against pneumococcal bacteremia among elderly people. *JAMA* 1997;278:1333–1339.
12. Joray S, Wietlisbach V, Bula CJ. Cognitive impairment in elderly medical inpatients. *Am J Geriatr Psychiatry* 2004;12:639–647.
13. Pfeiffer E. A short portable mental status questionnaire for the assessment of organic brain deficit in elderly patients. *J Am Geriatr Soc* 1975;23:433–441.
14. Erkinjuntti T, Sulkava R, Wikstrom J, et al. Short portable mental status questionnaire as a screening test for dementia and delirium among the elderly. *J Am Geriatr Soc* 1987;35:412–416.
15. Cole MG, McCusker J, Bellavance F, et al. Systematic detection and multidisciplinary care of delirium in older medical inpatients: a randomized trial. *CMAJ* 2002;167:753–759.
16. Inouye SK, Bogardus ST Jr, Charpentier PA, et al. A multicomponent intervention to prevent delirium in hospitalized older patients. *N Engl J Med* 1999;340:669–676.
17. Hakim AA, Petrovich H, Burchfiel CM, et al. Effects of walking on mortality among non-smoking retired men. *N Engl J Med* 1998;338:94–99.
18. Tinetti ME, Inouye SK, Gill TM, et al. Shared risk factors for falls, incontinence, and functional dependence. Unifying the approach to geriatric syndromes. *JAMA* 1995;273:1348–1353.
19. Chu LW, Pei CK, Chiu A, et al. Risk factors for falls in hospitalized older medical patients. *J Gerontol A Biol Sci Med Sci* 1999;54: M38–M43.
20. Tinetti ME. Preventing falls in elderly persons. *N Engl J Med* 2003;348:42–49.
21. Macphee GJ, Crowther JA, McAlpine CH. A simple screening test for hearing impairment in elderly patients. *Age Aging* 1988; 17:347–351.
22. Covinsky KE, Fortinsky RH, Palmer RM, et al. The relationship of depressive symptoms to health status outcomes in acutely ill hospitalized elders. *Ann Intern Med* 1997;26:417–425.
23. Whooley MA, Avins AL, Miranda J, et al. Case-finding instruments for depression. Two questions are as good as many. *J Gen Intern Med* 1997;12:439–445.
24. Koenig HG, Pappas P, Holsinger T, et al. Assessing diagnostic approaches to depression in medically ill older adults: how reliably can mental health professionals make judgments about the causes of symptoms? *J Am Geriatr Soc* 1995;43:472–478.
25. Unutzer J, Katon W, Callahan CM, et al. Collaborative care management of late-life depression in the primary care setting. A randomized controlled trial. *JAMA* 2002;288:2836–2845.
26. Koenig HG, Ford SM, Blazer DG. Should physicians screen for depression in elderly medical inpatients? Results of a decision analysis. *Int J Psychiatry Med* 1993;23:239–263.
27. Walter LC, Brand RJ, Counsell SR, et al. Development and validation of a prognostic index for 1-year mortality in older adults after hospitalization. *JAMA* 2001;285:2987–2994.
28. Beers MH, Dang J, Hasegawa J, et al. Influence of hospitalization on drug therapy in the elderly. *J Am Geriatr Soc* 1989;37: 679–683.
29. Lipton HL, Bero LA, Bird JA, et al. The impact of clinical pharmacists' consultations on physicians' geriatric drug prescribing. A randomized controlled trial. *Med Care* 1992;30:646–658.
30. Lipton HL, Bird JA. The impact of clinical pharmacists' consultations on geriatric patients' compliance and medical care use: a randomized controlled trial. *Gerontologist* 1994;34:307–315.
31. Lachs MS, Williams CS, O'Brien S, et al. The mortality of elder mistreatment. *JAMA* 1998;280:428–432.
32. Lachs MS, Williams C, O'Brien S, et al. Older adults. An 11-year longitudinal study of adult protective service use. *Arch Intern Med* 1996;156:449–453.

ADDITIONAL READING

Cassel CK, Cohen HF, Larson EB. *Geriatric Medicine*, 4th ed. New York: Springer-Verlag, 2003.

Courtney C, Farrell D, Gray R, Hills R, et al; AD2000 Collaborative Group. Long-term donepezil treatment in 565 patients with Alzheimer's disease (AD2000): randomised double-blind trial. *Lancet* 2004;363:2105–2115.

Goulding MR. Inappropriate medication prescribing for elderly ambulatory care patients. *Arch Intern Med* 2004;164:305–312.

Lachs MS, Pillemer K. Elder abuse. *Lancet* 2004;364:1263–1272.

Monane M, Matthias DM, Nagle BA, et al. Improving prescribing patterns for the elderly through an online drug utilization review intervention: a system linking the physician, pharmacist, and computer. *JAMA* 1998;280:1249–1252.

Ethical Issues in the Hospitalized Patient

17

Steven Z. Pantilat   *Bernard Lo*

INTRODUCTION

Physicians commonly face ethical dilemmas in the care of inpatients. The family of an elderly Chinese man with newly diagnosed hepatocellular carcinoma asks you not to inform the patient of the diagnosis. The children of a comatose woman with end-stage cirrhosis cannot agree on code status. A patient with end-stage metastatic pancreatic cancer is admitted as a full code. The renal consultant says that it is futile to initiate dialysis on a patient with dementia. A patient who you believe is medically ready for discharge refuses to go home. Such ethical issues can be difficult to resolve, time-consuming, and emotionally draining.

In the ethical arena, primary physicians caring for their own inpatients have an advantage. A hospital physician who is not the primary provider (as in the case of a hospitalist or a house officer on an inpatient rotation) must spend time getting to know the patient and developing a relationship. In such cases, hospital physicians often benefit by learning the patient's goals, values, need for information, and specific preferences for care from the primary care physician.

PRINCIPLES OF MEDICAL ETHICS

In caring for patients, physicians should follow the fundamental ethical principles of *autonomy*, *beneficence*, *non-maleficence*, *justice*, and *confidentiality*.

Autonomy. Physicians must respect a patient's right to make decisions regarding medical care. Competent, informed patients have the right to choose among treatment options and refuse any unwanted medical interventions.

Beneficence. Physicians must act in the best interests of their patients. Patients are vulnerable because of illness and lack of medical expertise. Therefore, they rely on physicians to offer sound advice and act according to patients' best interests. In doing so, physicians must put the interests of their patients ahead of their own interests or those of third parties, such as insurers or managed care organizations. If patients lack decision-making capacity, they need to be protected from making decisions that are contrary to their best interests.

Non-maleficence. The related principle of non-maleficence directs physicians to "do no harm" to patients. Physicians must refrain from providing ineffective treatments or acting with malice toward patients. This principle, however, offers little useful guidance to physicians because many beneficial therapies also have serious risks. The pertinent ethical issue is whether the benefits outweigh the burdens.

Justice. Physicians should treat similarly situated patients similarly and allocate resources fairly. In the face of limited health care resources, physicians should practice cost-effective medicine.

Confidentiality. Physicians must maintain the confidentiality of medical information. Confidentiality respects patient autonomy and encourages patients to seek care and be candid. However, confidentiality can be overridden to protect third parties when there is the potential for serious, foreseeable harm to third parties. Legally-mandated reporting may include certain infectious diseases like tuberculosis, loss of consciousness, child or elder abuse, or domestic violence.

These ethical principles guide and inform the process of gaining consent for or confirming refusal of treatment at every stage of the patient-physician relationship, including times when emotionally charged end-of-life decisions are being considered.

CARE OF THE HOSPITALIZED PATIENT

Decisions for Competent Patients

The centerpiece of ethical delivery of care is informed decision making. Informed, competent patients have the right to choose among, consent to, or refuse medically feasible options for care.

Our understanding of decision making and care for seriously ill hospitalized patients in the United States has been markedly enhanced by the results of the Study to Understand Prognoses and Preferences for Outcomes and Risks of Treatment (SUPPORT) (1). SUPPORT was a large, multicenter, randomized controlled trial designed to study decision making at the end of life. In addition, SUPPORT aimed to facilitate communication between seriously ill patients and physicians regarding prognosis and advance directives, and also to decrease pain and eliminate unwanted interventions at the end of life. Although the intervention improved neither care nor decision making, SUPPORT did provide a wealth of information regarding the treatment of symptoms and the process of communication and decision making for seriously ill patients. Some of its important findings were that physicians are often unaware of their patients' preferences for care; that even when patients preferred to have a "do not resuscitate" (DNR) order written, physicians wrote such orders in only 49% of cases; and that half the patients suffered moderate-to-severe pain in the last 3 days of life.

Decision-Making Capacity

Patients are presumed to have the capacity to make medical decisions unless it is determined otherwise. Decision-making capacity is ascertained by considering the patient's ability to make an informed decision regarding a specific intervention, rather than by a global assessment of mental function (2). Particular diagnoses or medical conditions such as dementia, depression, or hypoxemia do not, *a priori*, mean that a patient lacks decision-making capacity. When in doubt, the physician must assess such capacity formally.

Patients are considered to have adequate decision-making capacity if they can give informed consent for an intervention. Specifically, physicians must ensure the following:

- The patient can make and communicate a choice.
- The choice is stable over time and consistent with the patient's values and goals.
- The patient appreciates the indications, benefits, and risks of the proposed intervention and the alternatives.
- The decision does not result from delusions, psychosis, or mental illness.

Primary care physicians can help assess whether patients are making decisions consistent with their values and goals and

whether their mental status differs substantially from baseline. For example, a patient with severe chronic obstructive pulmonary disease may have indicated a desire for intubation in past office discussions with the primary care physician and family. If the patient refuses intubation at the time of a severe exacerbation characterized by hypoxia and sepsis, but the hospital physician determines that the patient now lacks decision-making capacity, the hospital physician should override the patient's refusal in favor of the one expressed when the patient had full decision-making capacity.

In assessing decision-making capacity, the attending physician should explain the proposed intervention, risks, benefits, and alternatives, including the option to decline treatment. The physician should then ask the patient to paraphrase the information and try to uncover any internal inconsistencies in the patient's reasoning. For example, the physician might say to the patient who is refusing amputation of a gangrenous leg, "Help me understand. You say you want to get rid of the pain and bad smell from your leg but don't want surgery. Could you please explain that to me?" Such probing questions help clarify issues for the patient as well as the physician. Mental status testing can be helpful, but patients who score poorly on a formal mental status exam (such as in Table 16.3) may still be able to give informed consent, and patients who score well may deny their condition or change their minds frequently. In addition, although not required routinely, psychiatric consultation can help determine whether delusions, psychosis, or depression are seriously impairing a patient's capacity to decide.

Although the courts are the ultimate arbiters of whether a patient is competent to refuse medical interventions, physicians routinely assess decision-making capacity at the bedside and turn to surrogates or advance directives if they determine that patients lack this capacity. Nonetheless, it may be necessary and desirable to obtain a court order in rare cases, such as when a patient who lacks decision-making capacity and has no surrogate is actively refusing an invasive procedure or risky treatment designed to save life or function.

Informed Consent

In soliciting informed consent, physicians should provide information about the risks, benefits, and consequences of proposed treatments and alternatives. They should listen more than talk, and use language the patient can understand. Tulsky et al. (3) found that when discussing code status with hospitalized patients, medical house officers spoke more than three-fourths of the time, often used jargon, and frequently missed opportunities for empathic connection. The use of simple statements such as "tell me more about that" or simply "uh huh" may encourage patients to speak more.

Patients' desire for information may depend on their cultural background (4). For example, the family of an elderly Chinese man who has been given a diagnosis of hepatocellular carcinoma may request that the physician not tell the patient the diagnosis. They may believe that speaking of the bad news to the patient will take away all hope and cause a poor outcome. One way of dealing with such family requests is to say to the patient, "I have information about your condition. I generally give this type of information directly to my patients, but some patients prefer that I speak to a family member or friend instead. What would you like me to do?" Even better, ask patients how they would want you to communicate information about the test results before ordering the test.

Refusal of Therapy

Most patients accept treatments recommended by their physician. However, some patients may refuse treatments that the physician believes are highly beneficial (e.g., amputation of a gangrenous leg). In such circumstances, it is appropriate for the physician to try to persuade the patient to accept beneficial treatments, although the physician should not badger the patient or misrepresent the facts. The physician should check that the patient is fully informed of the consequences of the decision and has the capacity to make informed decisions. In the end, the physician must respect a competent, informed patient's right to make decisions about medical care, even if the physician believes a decision is unwise.

Patients Who Lack Decision-Making Capacity

Hospitalized patients may be unable to participate in decision making because of medical illness, psychiatric illness, medications, delirium, or dementia. In such circumstances, the physician's obligation is to protect the patient from the adverse consequences of uninformed decisions. This can be done by consulting an advance directive or an appropriate surrogate.

Advance Directives

Advance directives are oral or written statements, made by patients when competent, to guide care if they lose decision-making capacity. Advance directives may offer substantive directions regarding care, designate a surrogate decision maker, or do both. Physicians must respect advance directives because they promote the patient's autonomy by extending it into the future. The extra effort and consideration required to complete written advance directives give them more weight than oral statements. Nonetheless, in the absence of a written advance directive, clear oral statements of a patient's preferences are ethically acceptable and should be respected. Because some patients fear that in completing an advance directive they relinquish their decision-making authority, it is important to inform them that advance directives take effect only if they lose decision-making capacity. Among the issues commonly addressed in advance directives are the desire for cardiopulmonary resuscitation (CPR), mechanical ventilation, transfer to the intensive care unit, and artificial hydration and nutrition. If the patient with the advance directive shown in Figure 17.1 was admitted with pneumococcal sepsis and was unable to communicate any preferences, the prior written statement would offer guidelines to her surrogate and physician regarding her preferences for care. In

---

I, *Carmen Picatta*, hereby appoint:

Name: Robert Picatta
Address: 123 Main St., San Francisco, CA 94110
Telephone Number: 415/555-1212

As my agent to make health care decisions for me.

If I become ill and need machines to keep me alive, I am willing to have them if there is hope that I will ultimately be able to live independently without them. I do not want to be kept alive on machines indefinitely.

If my heart stops, I want to be allowed to die peacefully. I do not wish to have CPR under any circumstances.

Witness:_____   Signature: *Carmen Picatta*_____

Witness:_____

Figure 17.1   Example of an advance directive.

this case, a trial of mechanical ventilation and a DNR order would be consistent with the patient's wishes and represent the appropriate course of action.

Among the limitations of advance directives are that few people have them, they are usually not available to the hospital physician at the time a decision must be made, and they often fail to address the specific clinical situation at hand (5). When advance directives do provide adequate guidance or designate a surrogate, they must be respected.

Surrogate Decision-Making

If it is feasible, the hospital physician should elicit patient preferences regarding CPR and other aspects of medical care, in addition to the patient's general values, goals, and choice of a surrogate, before this information is actually needed. For example, at the time of admission the physician could say, "There is something I talk about with all the patients I care for in the hospital: Who will help me make decisions about your medical care if you get too sick to tell me directly?" Such a statement serves to normalize the discussion and lessen patient concerns that the physician is raising these issues because of a belief that something bad will happen to the patient. Once the physician

has established the patient's choice of a surrogate, he or she can ask whether the surrogate has been informed of the patient's preferences. The physician can then ask directly about the patient's preferences for CPR. Because patients who have overly optimistic impressions of the outcomes of CPR are less likely to request it after learning of the actual chance of success, physicians should inform patients of the outcomes in addition to the risks and benefits of CPR (6) (Table 17.1). Finally, physicians should remind patients and all members of the health care team that a DNR order itself has no bearing on the provision of any other treatments.

When an advance directive is unavailable and an appropriate surrogate has not been previously designated, it falls to the physician to identify a surrogate for an incompetent patient. In the ideal setting, the surrogate will be someone who knows the patient well, understands the patient's values and goals, has discussed with the patient what he or she would want done in certain circumstances, and is committed to acting in the patient's best interests. The physician needs to probe for statements the patient may have made about values and goals of care, what circumstances the patient had in mind, and whether the patient understood the consequences and alternatives. The goal is to achieve *substituted judgment*, in which decisions are made as

TABLE 17.1

OUTCOMES OF INTERVENTIONS THAT ARE SOMETIMES CALLED "FUTILE"[a]

Study	Patients	Intervention	Outcome	Percentage/(n)
Rubenfeld and Crawford, 1996 (17)	Bone marrow transplant recipients with sepsis or renal and hepatic failure, and respiratory failure	Mechanical ventilation	Survival 30 days after extubation and discharge from the hospital	0 (0/53)
Wachter et al., 1991 (8)	AIDS patients with PCP and respiratory failure	Mechanical ventilation	Survival to hospital discharge	0 (14/35)
Bedell et al., 1983 (9)	All hospitalized patients who suffer cardiac arrest	CPR	Survival to hospital discharge	14 (41/294)
	Subset of patients with pneumonia	CPR	Survival to hospital discharge	0 (0/58)
	Subset of patients with creatinine >2.5 mg/dL	CPR	Survival to hospital discharge	5 (3/64)
Taffet et al., 1988 (10)[b]	Hospitalized patients age 70 or greater who suffer cardiac arrest	CPR	Survival after code	31 (24/77)
			Survival at 24 hours	29 (22/77)
			Survival to hospital discharge	0 (0/77)
	Hospitalized patients less than 70 years of age who suffer cardiac arrest	CPR	Survival after code	43 (137/322)
			Survival at 24 hours	39 (124/322)
			Survival to hospital discharge	7 (22/322)
	Subset of patients with cancer	CPR	Survival to hospital discharge	0 (0/89)
	Subset of patients without cancer	CPR	Survival to hospital discharge	9 (21/240)

[a]Readers may wish to contrast the outcomes with Schneiderman's "zero out of 100" standard in deciding whether the interventions are in fact "futile" (12).
[b]A total of 399 CPR efforts were made for 329 patients. Data for patients over and under age 70 are reported per CPR effort; data for patients with and without cancer are reported per patient.
CPR, cardiopulmonary resuscitation; PCP, *Pneumocystis jirovecii* pneumonia.

patients would make them, not as surrogates want to make them for patients or would want to make them for themselves. Virtually all states allow patients to designate a surrogate or health care proxy. In New York and Missouri, state laws require a high standard of evidence regarding a patient's oral directives and restricts the ability of family members to limit some care in the absence of formal advance directives. Despite such laws, sound clinical and professional ethics advocate respecting a patient's wishes, even if they were orally expressed, and acting in the patient's best interest.

In the absence of a prior designation, it is customary to turn to family. The surrogate hierarchy typically begins with the spouse, then adult children, then other family members, and finally friends. This approach is appropriate because these people are most likely to know the patient's preferences, to the keep the patient's best interests foremost, and to advocate on the patient's behalf. Certain states, such as Illinois, have laws that designate which family members have priority as surrogates. In some cases, it is difficult to determine who the appropriate surrogate should be. For example, an elderly woman who is comatose with end-stage cirrhosis and who gave no advance directive may have two adult children who disagree about her code status. In such circumstances, it is helpful to focus the discussion on what the patient would want in that particular situation. It may require repeated discussions with the patient's children to reach a mutually agreeable decision (12). Other members of the health care team, especially social workers, chaplains, and nurses, may be helpful in talking with the surrogates (Chapter 4).

Realistically, surrogates often do not know what the patient herself would have wanted, and decisions are based on the *best interests* of the patient rather than on substituted judgment. When the physician cannot identify a surrogate for an incompetent patient, it is appropriate for the physician to make decisions based on a perception of the patient's best interests, considering both the quality and duration of life. Quality-of-life considerations must be made with care because of the potential for bias, as physicians and family members tend to underestimate the value that patients place on their quality of life.

DO NOT RESUSCITATE ORDERS AND DECISIONS ABOUT LIFE-SUSTAINING INTERVENTIONS

Decisions about CPR and life-sustaining interventions are very common in the hospital. For example, one study found that decisions to withhold or withdraw life-sustaining interventions accompanied by the writing of DNR orders preceded 90% of deaths in the intensive care units at two teaching hospitals (12). Figure 17.2 provides an algorithm regarding decisions about life-sustaining interventions.

Although DNR orders are common, problems with them remain. First, although physicians may fear that discussing DNR orders will upset patients, studies confirm that the vast majority of patients want to discuss these issues, expect physicians to initiate the discussion, and may be more satisfied with their care after these discussions (13). Second, there are large variations in how often physicians write DNR orders for patients with different diseases but similar prognoses (14), reflecting a potential inequity in treatment. Finally, many physicians fail to write DNR orders for patients who want them (1). Thus, the hospital physician has a responsibility to initiate discussions about DNR orders, to raise the issue equally with all patients, and to write DNR orders when patients request that they do so.

Most patients who ultimately receive DNR orders are competent at the time of admission but not competent when the DNR order is finally written (1). Therefore, *physicians should routinely discuss code status with patients at the time of admission.* In fact, hospital physicians treating a patient for the first time can turn the disadvantage of not knowing the patient into an advantage in discussing code status by honestly saying, "I haven't met you before, and it's important for me to know you as a person and what's important to you about your medical care." Even if the primary care physician has already discussed code status with the patient, the hospital physician can confirm that the patient has made an informed choice and has not had a change of heart.

In the absence of a written DNR order, CPR is initiated for all patients in the hospital who have a cardiopulmonary arrest. This presumption to use CPR is based on the ethical principle of beneficence and the goal of providing a potentially life-saving intervention to patients. In addition, first responders to a cardiac arrest usually do not know the patient. If CPR is not initiated immediately, its effectiveness is reduced. This approach places a responsibility on physicians to establish a code status for each patient early in the hospitalization so that they can respect the wishes of patients who want to forgo CPR.

Do Not Resuscitate Orders in the Operating Room

Occasionally, patients with DNR orders require surgery or an invasive procedure. Some physicians are reluctant to allow a DNR order to remain in effect in the operating room. They argue that general anesthesia and conscious sedation can precipitate the need for more formal resuscitation, and that it is too difficult to operate or administer anesthesia with limitations placed on resuscitative interventions. Despite these arguments, some patients may wish to have

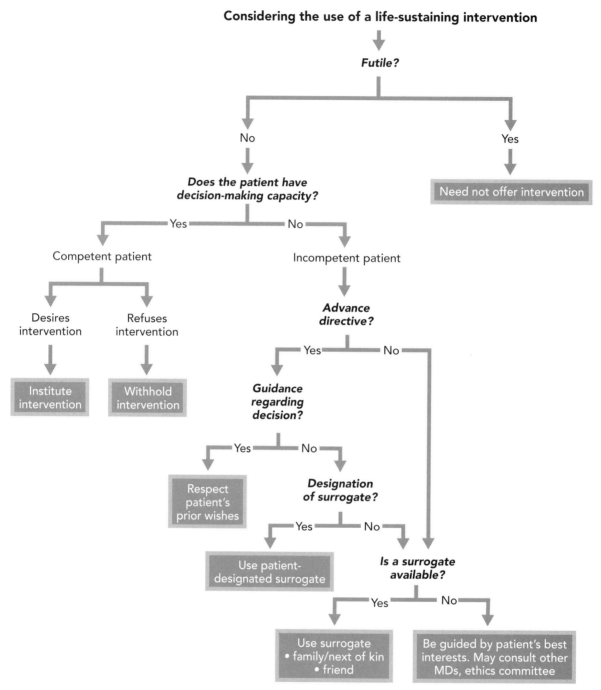

Figure 17.2 Decisions regarding life-sustaining interventions.

surgery to palliate pain or relieve a bowel obstruction yet feel that if they had a cardiopulmonary arrest for any reason in the operating room, they would not want CPR initiated. Physicians should not refuse to perform an operation for a patient simply because the patient insists on forgoing CPR (15). In order to respect patient autonomy, it is best to reconsider code status before surgery and other invasive procedures, to explain how resuscitative efforts work, and to respect the patient's request to keep a DNR order in effect.

Withdrawal and Withholding of Interventions

Withdrawing and withholding life-sustaining interventions are ethically and legally equivalent, although the former is often more emotionally difficult than the latter (16). If interventions could not be withdrawn, patients might be reluctant to attempt them even if potentially beneficial for fear they could not be withdrawn later.

Most often, the physical withdrawal of an intervention falls to nurses or respiratory therapists, not physicians. It is helpful if the attending physician is present or available when care is withdrawn to lend support, respond to problems, and ensure that the patient's suffering is alleviated. The process of withdrawing ventilation ("terminal weaning") is described in Chapter 23, and additional issues in end-of-life care are described in Chapter 19.

Futile Interventions

Occasionally, patients or their surrogates may demand care that the physician believes does not provide any potential medical benefit. Physicians should discuss these situations with patients and surrogates and strongly recommend against such interventions.

Physicians are not obligated to provide an intervention when:

- The intervention has been tried and failed.
- There is no pathophysiologic rationale for the intervention.
- Maximal therapy is failing.
- The intervention cannot achieve the goals of care.

In these situations, interventions are considered futile. The term *futility* is often used by physicians to justify unilateral decisions to withhold certain interventions requested by the patient or surrogate. Such unilateral decisions override the patient's autonomy and the power of surrogates to make decisions for incompetent patients. Hence, unilateral judgments of futility must be made carefully. Schneiderman and colleagues have proposed a "zero out of 100" standard that restricts the use of the term futility to cases in which no successes have been seen in the last 100 similar circumstances (10). Despite seeming objective, such a standard is arbitrary and is not universally accepted by patients or physicians as defining futile care. Still, by this or any comparable standard, it is clear that true futility is rare (Table 17.1) and that physicians often use the term loosely.

In general, it is best to talk about potentially futile situations with patients and their surrogates because an agreement can be reached in almost all circumstances. Even prolonged discussions are preferable to unilateral decisions by the physician that alienate patients and erode trust in the medical care system (17).

Leaving Against Medical Advice

Physicians may encounter a patient who seeks to leave the hospital "against medical advice." In such a case, the physician should explore the reasons for the patient's decision in the hope of uncovering misunderstandings or concerns that can be addressed. If the patient insists on leaving the hospital despite these discussions, the physician should respect the patient's choice by providing the medications, referrals, instructions, home care, and follow-up necessary to maximize the medical outcome. Some physicians are re-

luctant to arrange for such services because they fear they will be liable for providing substandard care. However, the physician's duty to act in the patient's best interest requires that the physician try to optimize a patient's care even if the patient refuses the level of care recommended by the physician.

When patients decide to leave against medical advice, it is helpful, but not absolutely necessary, to have them sign a form stating that they understand and accept the risks associated with leaving. More important than this signature is that a patient be offered services to aid recovery, and that both the patient's understanding of the risks and the attempts to convince the patient to remain in the hospital are carefully documented in the chart.

Emergency Procedures

Occasionally, physicians confront emergency situations in which immediate treatment is necessary to save life or limb, the patient is incapable of giving consent, and a surrogate cannot be located. There is a widespread misconception that in such situations it is necessary to invoke a "two-physician hold," whereby two physicians verify that the patient requires emergency treatment and is incapable of consenting to it. In fact, a determination by one attending physician is sufficient to initiate emergency treatment. In the absence of a DNR order, the presumption is that people would want such care and would not want care delayed by the lack of consent. After the immediate threat is dealt with, the physician should make every effort to discuss ongoing care with the patient or an appropriate surrogate.

ISSUES IN THE CURRENT HEALTH CARE ENVIRONMENT

Ethical challenges arise as a result of the current emphasis on restraining health care inflation. Although controlling costs is important, the mechanisms used to achieve this goal—financial incentives and utilization review, among others—may create conflicts of interest for physicians (18). Nonetheless, physicians have a responsibility to allocate health care resources justly and are not obligated to order an intervention simply because a patient requests it.

Timing of Hospital Discharge

One common situation that exemplifies this issue involves length of stay and the timing of hospital discharge. If a patient with community-acquired pneumonia is clinically stable and medically ready for discharge but refuses to go home, the physician should try to elicit and address the patient's concerns. A patient who is afebrile, breathing room air, and taking oral antibiotics may still feel too weak to go home despite being clinically stable for discharge. Attending to details like social support, transportation, in-home services, rehabilitation, and follow-up may allay a patient's fears about leaving the hospital. If the patient still feels uncomfortable about going home and there is no one at home to care for the patient, short-term placement in a skilled-nursing facility may be appropriate. Patients who still refuse discharge should be informed that they may be at financial risk for subsequent hospital days. Although the patient's request to remain in the hospital is an expression of the patient's autonomy, a physician's responsibility to allocate resources justly means that the patient's request may be rightfully refused.

In some situations, the physician believes that the patient is not quite ready for discharge but the insurer or medical group determines that the patient has exceeded the allocated length of stay. Payers may stop or reduce hospital payments at this point. In such situations, the physician has an obligation to advocate on behalf of the patient. The physician should not misrepresent the patient's condition or institute or continue unnecessary interventions to secure payment, but should make necessary phone calls and write letters to secure additional days. Finally, physicians should keep in mind that length of stay and other guidelines are recommendations, not requirements. A compassionate and effective system will allow for outliers and the use of discretion in individual cases.

Confidentiality and Privacy

Patients expect that their medical information will be kept confidential, and it is this knowledge that helps encourage patients to seek medical care and reveal sensitive information to clinicians. Challenges to confidentiality abound and clinicians must be mindful not to discuss private patient information in public places. The federal government issued new federal privacy regulations under the Health Insurance Portability and Accountability Act (HIPAA) that took effect in April 2003 (19). These regulations cover identifiable health information in electronic, paper, or oral form. Under these regulations, providers and health plans must notify patients about privacy, develop organizational policies and procedures regarding privacy, and educate staff about privacy issues. Despite concerns that the regulations might interfere in the care of patients, they are designed not to. They allow for the use or disclosure of personal patient information without consent for clinical care, treatment, payment, and health care operations. The latter category includes quality assurance and quality improvement programs, accreditation and licensing, training programs, and business planning. Similarly, no patient consent is required for use of or disclosure of patient information for public health, abuse,

neglect, or domestic violence reporting, judicial or administrative proceedings, and law enforcement purposes. Under HIPAA, patients must give specific authorization for use of their personal information for marketing and most clinical research. HIPAA also provides patients with the right to review their medical records and request that corrections be made. States and health care organizations may have confidentiality laws or policies that are stricter than the federal regulations.

In caring for patients in the hospital, these regulations reinforce the ethical principle of confidentiality. Hospital physicians should continue to discuss patients with colleagues involved in a patient's care and obtain help with diagnosis, prognosis, or treatment. However, the HIPAA regulations require clinicians to take reasonable precautions to protect confidentiality. For example, bedside charts in the emergency department or on the wards must be covered or situated in such a way that passersby cannot see the information on the chart. Furthermore, although HIPAA does not forbid physicians from discussing patients at nursing stations, in the hallways, or in semiprivate hospital rooms, physicians should keep their voices down to reduce the possibility that conversations will be overheard. Physicians should continue to discuss their patient's care with people who identify themselves as family members, unless the patient forbids them from doing so or they judge that such discussions would be harmful to the patient. Of particular importance, health care providers must resist the temptation to discuss patient information in public places such as elevators and public cafeterias. Breaches of confidentiality erode trust in physicians and may have adverse economic, social, and psychological consequences for patients. Although the presumption should always be that physicians maintain confidentiality, there are specific circumstances when physicians are required by law to override confidentiality, including child or elder abuse, certain infectious diseases such as tuberculosis and syphilis, and injuries caused by deadly weapons. In these circumstances when confidentiality must be breached, physicians should disclose the least amount of information to the fewest people necessary to fulfill reporting requirements.

Role of Ethics Committees

Ethics committees may provide consultation on difficult cases. The committee typically includes physicians from several clinical departments, nurses, social workers, lawyers, a risk manager, and community members. Although the decisions of the ethics committee are meant to offer guidance and are typically not binding on physicians or patients, the ethics committee can help resolve disagreements among members of the team, among members of the patient's family, or between the health care team and the patient or surrogates. In institutions that lack an active and effective ethics committee, physicians can obtain similar assistance from colleagues.

Ethics and the Hospitalist Model of Care

The traditional relationship between patient and primary care physician provides many ethical protections for patients, including confidentiality, shared decision making, and respect for patient autonomy. Hospitalist models, which introduce a purposeful discontinuity of care, threaten these protections and raise certain ethical concerns (19).

For example, the hospitalist and primary care physician may disagree on the best course of action for an inpatient. In such circumstances, both physicians should be given the opportunity to present the options to the patient clearly and completely to allow the patient to make the final decision. If it can be organized, a joint meeting involving patient, family, and both physicians would provide the patient with the best opportunity to make a truly informed choice.

Ethical issues may also arise during end-of-life decisions. For example, consider a patient with metastatic cancer who prefers to forgo CPR in the event of a cardiac arrest that accompanies a worsening of disease but nevertheless wants CPR for an acute arrest. Or, consider a patient who has a DNR order in the chart but now presents to the emergency department with an anaphylactic reaction that may be easily reversible. Like emergency medicine physicians, the hospitalist is disadvantaged by lacking a prior relationship with a patient who is *in extremis* and unable to communicate the applicability of prior preferences. Hospitalists will need to become expert in discussing advance directives. They will also need to develop systems to involve primary physicians rapidly in these difficult decisions.

As hospitalists assume control of inpatient care, they must also take responsibility for providing ethical protection currently vested in the relationship between the patient and the primary care physician. An approach that keeps the patient's best interests foremost, defines a clear role for the primary physician, and takes advantage of the expertise and availability of hospitalists will best serve both patients and physicians (20).

CONCLUSIONS

In dealing with difficult ethical challenges, physicians need to consult with thoughtful colleagues, be able to tolerate uncertainty, and maintain their own integrity while respecting the opinions of others. By applying basic ethical principles and communicating effectively with patients, surrogates, and other members of the health care team, physicians can resolve nearly all ethical dilemmas that arise in the hospital.

KEY POINTS

- Care should be guided by the ethical principles of autonomy, beneficence, non-maleficence, justice, and confidentiality.
- For patients who lack decision-making capacity and have no advance directive, the physician and surrogate should work together to make decisions to help guide care.
- Hospitalization may be a particularly good time to discuss code status and advance directives.
- The withdrawal and withholding of interventions are ethically and morally equivalent.
- Although physicians need not provide futile interventions, they must be very cautious about using this rationale to deny care because true futility is rare and applying the rationale overrides patient autonomy.
- In emergency situations in which there is an immediate threat to life or limb, the patient lacks decision-making capacity, no surrogate decision maker is available, and there is no indication that the patient would refuse treatment, the presumption is to provide care.
- Ethics committees may provide consultation on difficult cases and can help resolve disagreements.

REFERENCES

1. The SUPPORT Principal Investigators. A controlled trial to improve care for seriously ill hospitalized patients. The study to understand prognoses and preferences for outcomes and risks of treatments (SUPPORT). *JAMA* 1995;274:1591–1598.
2. Larkin GL, Marco CA, Abbott JT. Emergency determination of decision-making capacity: balancing autonomy and beneficence in the emergency department. *Acad Emerg Med* 2001;8:282–284.
3. Tulsky JA, Chesney MA, Lo B. How do medical residents discuss resuscitation with patients? *J Gen Intern Med* 1995;10: 436–442.
4. Kagawa-Singer M, Blackhall LJ. Negotiating cross-cultural issues at the end of life: "You got to go where he lives." *JAMA* 2001;286: 2993–3001.
5. Lynn J, Goldstein NE. Advance care planning for fatal chronic illness: avoiding commonplace errors and unwarranted suffering. *Ann Intern Med* 2003;138:812–818.
6. Murphy DJ, Burrows D, Santilli S, et al. The influence of the probability of survival on patients' preferences regarding cardiopulmonary resuscitation. *N Engl J Med* 1994;330:545–549.
7. Rubenfeld GD, Crawford SW. Withdrawing life support from mechanically ventilated recipients of bone marrow transplants: a case for evidence-based guidelines. *Ann Intern Med* 1996;125: 625–633.
8. Wachter RM, Russi MB, Bloch DA, et al. Pneumocystis carinii pneumonia and respiratory failure in AIDS. Improved outcomes and increased use of intensive care units. *Am Rev Respir Dis* 1991;143: 251–256.
9. Bedell SE, Delbanco TL, Cook EF, et al. Survival after cardiopulmonary resuscitation in the hospital. *N Engl J Med* 1983;309: 569–576.
10. Taffet GE, Teasdale TA, Luchi RJ. In-hospital cardiopulmonary resuscitation. *JAMA* 1988;260:2069–2072.
11. Schneiderman LJ, Jecker NS, Jonsen AR. Medical futility: its meaning and ethical implications. *Ann Intern Med* 1990;112: 949–954.
12. Prendergast TJ, Puntillo KA. Withdrawal of life support: intensive caring at the end of life. *JAMA* 2002;288:2732–2740.

13. Tierney WM, Dexter PR, Gramelspacher GP, et al. The effect of discussions about advance directives on patients' satisfaction with primary care. *J Gen Intern Med* Jan 2001;16:32–40.

14. Wachter RM, Luce JM, Hearst N, et al. Decisions about resuscitation: inequities among patients with different diseases but similar prognoses. *Ann Intern Med* 1989;111:525–532.

15. Craig DB. Do not resuscitate orders in the operating room. *Can J Anaesth* 1996;43:840–851.

16. Meisel A. Legal myths about terminating life support. *Arch Intern Med* 1991;151:1197–1502.

17. Helft PR, Siegler M, Lantos J. The rise and fall of the futility movement. *N Engl J Med* 2000;343:1575–1577.

18. Pantilat SZ, Lo B. Advocates or adversaries: is managed care changing the physician–patient relationship? *Ophthalmol Clin North Am* 1997;10:155–164.

19. Annas GJ. HIPAA regulations—A new era of medical record privacy? *N Engl J Med* 2003;348:1486–1490.

20. Pantilat SZ, Alpers A, Wachter RM. A new doctor in the house: ethical issues in hospitalist systems. *JAMA* 1999;282:171–174.

ADDITIONAL READING

Beauchamp Tl, Childress JF. *Principles of Biomedical Ethics*, 5th ed. New York: Oxford University Press, 2001.

Lo B. *Resolving Ethical Dilemmas: A Guide for Clinicians*, 2nd ed. Philadelphia: Lippincott Williams & Wilkins, 2000.

Pain Management in the Hospitalized Patient

18

Robert V. Brody

INTRODUCTION

There are few symptoms that engender so much patient concern and disability as pain, and few areas in which there is so great a gap between the capabilities of modern medicine and the actual effectiveness of our practice. For more than 25 years, studies have repeatedly documented our failure to manage pain adequately; the more severe the pain, the worse we do at management.

After decades of relative neglect by the medical profession, there is renewed interest in the management of acute and chronic pain. Some of this energy is fueled by a new understanding of the pathophysiology of different types of pain, some by the recent availability of both new medications and more rational strategies for the use of old ones, and much by the increasingly vocal demands of patients and families. Research performed in hospice units has shown satisfaction with pain control in the range of 80%–90%, which leads other patients, particularly those with chronic pain, to ask, "Why do I have to be dying to have my pain controlled?" Increasingly, hospitals, surveyors, and even state medical boards are regarding pain management as a quality-of-care issue (Chapter 12). Nevertheless, studies continue to show a high prevalence of pain in hospitalized patients and significant dissatisfaction with inpatient pain control (1).

This chapter begins by outlining some basic principles of pain assessment and management. Commonly used drugs and other agents are reviewed, and some guiding principles of pharmacologic therapy are developed. Then, common challenges in inpatient pain management are considered: treatment of neuropathic pain, treatment of pain in the patient with a history of substance abuse or HIV infection, and treatment of pain in the older hospitalized patient.

GENERAL PRINCIPLES OF PAIN MANAGEMENT

Nature of Pain

According to the International Association for the Study of Pain, pain is an unpleasant sensory and emotional experience, most often associated with actual or potential tissue damage or described in terms of such damage (2, 3). Pain is not just the unpleasant sensation, not just the perception of the sensation, but also the emotional reaction to or experience of the perceived sensation. As such, *pain is always subjective.* The subjectivity creates a dilemma for the clinician. By virtue of the observations and tests available to clinicians, we know more than a patient does about the structure and function of his or her liver, blood, kidneys, heart, bones, nerves, and even brain. However, no test or observation can accurately tell the clinician whether a patient is in pain. The only "test" the clinician has available is to ask the patient and listen to the answer.

Pain has consequences. In addition to enduring unnecessary suffering, patients with unrelieved pain become

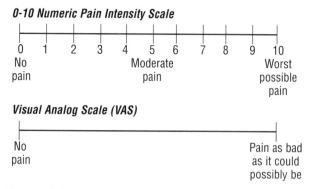

0-10 Numeric Pain Intensity Scale

0   1   2   3   4   5   6   7   8   9   10
No   Moderate   Worst
pain   pain   possible
                                          pain

Visual Analog Scale (VAS)

No   Pain as bad
pain   as it could
                                      possibly be

Figure 18.1 Examples of visual pain intensity assessment scales. (Reprinted from Acute Pain Management Guideline Panel. Acute pain management: operative or medical procedures and trauma. Clinical practice guideline. AHCPR Publication No. 92-002. Rockville, MD: Agency for Health Care Policy and Research, Public Health Service, U.S. Department of Health and Human Services, February 1992, with permission.)

catabolic, respond less well to curative medical or surgical treatments, have a greater complication rate from these therapies, show a higher rate of emotional disturbance, and in some circumstances die sooner.

Cultural and psychological factors influence the expression of and tolerance for pain. Other factors that decrease the pain threshold (i.e., cause the patient to be in more pain) include insomnia, fatigue, nausea, anxiety, fear, misunderstanding, anger, shame, sadness, depression, introversion, any other discomfort, and the memory of past pain and expectation that pain will recur. Conversely, the threshold for pain may be increased (i.e., the patient will be in less pain) with relief of other symptoms, sleep, rest, sympathy, understanding, and diversion, and with the use of anticipatory and around-the-clock dosing of pain medication.

Clinical Assessment and Goals of Pain Management

The approach to the patient in pain begins with a pain history (4). Commonly used tools of pain assessment are shown in Figure 18.1. The patient should be asked to rate the severity of pain on a scale of 0 to 10, with 0 indicating no pain and 10 the worst imaginable pain. Some patients (e.g., children or those with whom it is difficult to communicate) may find it easier to rate their pain by using a picture-based scale (Figure 18.2). After any therapeutic intervention, the provider needs to learn how much relief

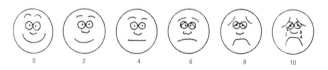

0   2   4   6   8   10

Figure 18.2 An example of a picture-based pain intensity assessment scale.

was achieved; one does so by asking the patient to rate the pain again and recall how long the relief lasted. The dose of the analgesic is adjusted to give the patient adequate pain control; the interval between doses is adjusted so that the analgesic effect is uninterrupted. The goal of pain management is not necessarily "zero" pain; rather, it is the *maximally functional patient*, with the patient ultimately deciding whether the goal has been reached.

Additional questions that should be included in the pain history relate to the following:

- Significant previous or ongoing instances of pain
- Previously used pain control methods and their effect, and the patient's preferences for pain management
- Attitudes of the patient and family toward the use of opioid, anxiolytic, and other medications, and any history of substance abuse
- Typical coping response of the patient for stress or pain, the presence of any psychiatric disorders, and ways that the patient describes or shows pain. A discussion with current or previous providers of outpatient treatment for pain is often enlightening
- The patient's functional status and the contribution of pain to any loss of function
- The meaning the patient ascribes to the pain (e.g., brings back memories of trauma, makes it impossible to support a family, or signifies that death is at hand)

The physician's examination should supplement the history in making as specific a diagnosis of the causes of the pain as possible. Such a diagnosis facilitates treatment of the underlying pathophysiology and allows the symptomatic treatment to be tailored to the specific type of pain. It is common for hospitalized patients to have more than one painful condition. Some patients in significant pain will show evidence of adrenergic stimulation (i.e., sweating, tachycardia), whereas others may be in severe pain and not demonstrate such findings. It cannot be presumed that the patient who dozes off between doses of analgesics is malingering or is being overtreated; such a patient may be making up for a large physiologic sleep deficit, be under the influence of sedatives, or have another cause of altered mental status.

Except when they identify a specific etiology, laboratory tests are unhelpful in the assessment of pain. For example, a bone film or scan may demonstrate a metastatic lesion that would benefit from radiotherapy. An electrocardiogram and measurement of the troponin level may demonstrate that chest or arm pain is caused by myocardial infarction, for which the optimal approach to pain management is rapid reperfusion. However, *there is no blood test or imaging study for pain itself*. Patients in severe pain may have normal white blood cell counts, sedimentation rates, or other markers that have been proposed to help confirm the "reality" of pain. In the end, pain is subjective, and the clinician is left with the patient's assessment as the only test to assess the presence or severity of pain.

Initial Management

There is a tendency to move rapidly toward pharmacologic management of pain, especially in the hospitalized patient, in whom acute pain (which may be self-limited) is likely. It is worth remembering that many patients will benefit from *physical measures*, such as the application of heat or cold, and that *nonpharmacologic approaches*, such as relaxation, distraction, imagery, transcutaneous electrical nerve stimulation, or physical therapy, may also be useful.

Most hospitalized patients in pain, however, will require a pharmacologic agent to help control the symptom. The World Health Organization Committee on Cancer Pain has popularized the concept of an *analgesic ladder*, classifying conventional analgesics into 3 steps: the higher the step, the stronger the agent and the more likely an adverse reaction.

Step 1 agents include aspirin, acetaminophen, nonsteroidal anti-inflammatory drugs (NSAIDs), and propoxyphene. For noninflammatory painful conditions, acetaminophen is usually as effective as an NSAID and lacks the problematic side effects of gastrointestinal bleeding, platelet dysfunction, renal failure, and occasional confusion. For inflammatory conditions, it is useful to remember that there are no data showing greater analgesic or anti-inflammatory efficacy of one NSAID versus another, including parenterally administered ketorolac (5) or COX-2 inhibitors. The latter may cause less gastrointestinal bleeding but have significant rates of other adverse reactions, including GI symptoms, and are expensive. Moreover, the recent findings of increased cardiovascular risk associated with rofecoxib (Vioxx), which led to the drug's withdrawal from the market, have raised concerns about the entire class of COX-2 inhibitors (6).

Step 2 agents include codeine, hydrocodone, tramadol, meperidine, and mixed agonist-antagonists, such as pentazocine. Dose-response curves for these agents reach a plateau, in contrast with the curves of step 3 agents, which have no upper limit in dosing. Because a metabolite of meperidine accumulates and causes irritability and, occasionally, seizures with repeated dosing, the use of meperidine as an analgesic should be limited. However, it remains the best agent for prevention or treatment of rigors and post-anesthesia shivering. Tramadol, a non-opiate with serotonin reuptake inhibiting properties, binds to the μ-opiate receptor; therefore, it has many of the same properties as opiates and, like opiates, can be abused. In addition, it has the potential to cause seizures. Mixed agonist-antagonists, such as pentazocine, cannot be titrated like step 3 agents because of significant psychotomimetic effects. Because of their antagonist properties, they must be allowed to wear off before a stronger, purely agonist opiate can be used.

Step 3 agents that are frequently used include morphine, hydromorphone, oxycodone, fentanyl, methadone, and levorphanol. See Table 18.1 for approximate dose conversions to use when switching from one agent or route of administration to another. *Morphine* is the standard against which other analgesics are measured. Most short-acting preparations give relief for 3–6 hours, whereas the effects of long-acting preparations last 8–12 hours. In general, it is easier to titrate analgesia with short-acting preparations. Once the patient's pain syndrome is stable, the physician can calculate the total 24-hour dose, divide by 2, and administer the equivalent long-acting preparation every 12 hours. Do not allow long-acting tablets to be crushed, because this converts the drugs to short-acting forms.

The dose-response curve of *oxycodone* does not plateau, a similar effect to that of morphine. In the past, oxycodone was usually prescribed in combination with aspirin or acetaminophen; such formulations cannot be titrated above a certain threshold because of the potential toxicity of the second drug. Oxycodone can be prescribed alone in a short-acting form or sustained-release preparations, allowing the clinician to take advantage of oxycodone's lack of a dose-response plateau.

The effects of *fentanyl*, an opiate with a duration of action that is very short when given intravenously, can last as long as 3 days when it is administered by transdermal patch. It takes more than 18 hours for fentanyl to produce a maximum effect when administered in this manner. *The fentanyl patch should be used only to treat stable chronic pain.* Use of the patch is associated with a high incidence of contact dermatitis, which can be prevented by pretreating the skin with several puffs from a metered-dose steroid inhaler.

Although *methadone* is best known for its ability to control the opiate abstinence syndrome, it is also an effective analgesic. Although it is usually given once daily for opiate abstinence, it must be given every 6–8 hours for analgesia. Federal law generally prohibits physicians outside federally licensed methadone programs from prescribing methadone once a day for outpatients but does allow more frequent dosing for pain control. These restrictions do not apply to hospitalized patients.

The following general points about pharmacologic pain management can be made:

■ The biologic half-life of the agent must be taken into account when adjusting dosage and interval. The maximum effect of a given dose may not be seen until the drug has been administered for 4–5 half-lives. In addition, the duration of analgesia may be shorter than the half-life, and the half-life may be prolonged in cases of renal or hepatic failure. In the latter situations, one should use short-acting agents with dosing at longer intervals.

■ Once pain is controlled satisfactorily, the dose of analgesic usually remains stable. An increase in analgesic requirement most often signals disease progression. Tolerance, a poorly understood phenomenon, develops rapidly to the sedative effects of opiates but is much less likely to develop to the analgesic or constipating effects.

■ The onset of analgesia depends on the route of administration. In general, the onset is in 5–10 minutes with

TABLE 18.1

EQUI-ANALGESIC DOSING TABLE FOR OPIOIDS[a]

Drug	Approximate equi-analgesic *oral* dose	Approximate equi-analgesic *parenteral* dose	How supplied (non-parenteral)
Codeine	130 mg q3–4h[b]	75 mg q3–4h[b] (not recommended)	15, 30, 60 mg tablets, as plain codeine or as Tylenol with codeine No. 2, 3, 4, respectively[c]; solution: 5 mL = 12.5 mg codeine + 120 mg acetaminophen or 30 mg codeine + 160 mg acetaminophen
Hydrocodone in Vicodin, Lortab, other	30 mg q3–4h	not available	2.5, 5, 7.5, and 10 mg tablets with 500 mg ASA or 500–750 mg acetaminophen[c]
Oxycodone Roxicodone, Intensol; also in Percocet, Percodan, Tylox, Roxicet, Roxiprin, Endodan, Endocet SR (q8–12h)	20 mg IR q3–4h	not available in U.S.	5 mg per plain or combination tablet;[c] 1 mg/mL, 20 mg/mL solution 10, 20, 40, 80 mg sustained-release tablet
Meperidine (Pethidine) Demerol	300 mg q2–3h (not recommended)	100 mg q2–3h (not recommended for around-the-clock dosing)	50, 100 mg tablets, 10 mg/mL syrup
Morphine MSIR, OMS, Roxanol; MS Contin, Oramorph SR (q 8–12 h)	30 mg IR q3–4h, around the clock: 60 mg single dose or intermittent dosing	10 mg q3–4h	2 mg/mL, 20 mg/mL, and other oral solutions; 15, 30, 60, 100, 200 mg sustained-release tablet[d]
Hydromorphone Dilaudid	7.5 mg q3–4h	1.5 mg q3–4h	1 mg/mL oral solution; 2, 4, 8 mg tablets; 3 mg rectal suppositories[d]; 5 mg rectal suppositories
Oxymorphone Numorphone	not available	1 mg q3–4h	
Methadone Dolophine	60 mg q8h	10 mg q8h	10 mg tablets; 1, 2, and 10 mg/mL solution
Levorphanol Levo-Dromoran	4 mg q8h	2 mg q8h	2 mg tablet
Fentanyl Sublimaze; Duragesic transdermal patch (q 72 h)	not available	2.5 mg/h morphine IV = 30 mg q3h morphine PO = 25 mcg/h fentanyl IV infusion or patch	25, 50, 75, 100 mcg transdermal patch

Use this table for determining approximate dose conversions when changing from one route of administration to another or from one drug to another. The reference dose is morphine 10 mg IV or IM q3-4h. Doses in each column should give about the same amount of pain relief. Use a lower than equi-analgesic dose when changing drugs, then retitrate to the desired clinical response in each patient.

[a] Recommended dosing schedules do not apply to patients with renal and/or hepatic insufficiency or other conditions affecting drug metabolism and kinetics. These dosing recommendations should also be modified for persons weighing less than 50 kg.

[b] Codeine doses more than 120 mg q4h are not useful because of diminishing incremental analgesia but continually increasing constipation and other adverse effects.

[c] Dosing of aspirin or acetaminophen must be considered when combination preparations are titrated.

[d] Rectal administration of morphine and hydromorphone is possible, with dosing approximately the same as the oral route.

ASA, acetylsalicylic acid; IR, immediate-release; SR, sustained release.

From American Pain Society. *Principles of Analgesic Use in the Treatment of Acute Pain and Chronic Cancer Pain: A Concise Guide to Medical Practice*, 2nd ed. Skokie, IL:, 1989. McCaffery M, Beebe A. *Pain: Clinical Manual for Nursing Practice*. St. Louis, MO: Mosby, 1989. World Health Organization. Cancer Pain Relief. Geneva, 1966. Agency for Health Care Policy and Research. *Acute Pain Management: Operative or Medical Procedures and Trauma*. Rockville, MD, 1992.

intravenous administration, 20–40 minutes with subcutaneous or intramuscular administration, and 20–60 minutes for oral administration. With rectal and sublingual administration, the onset may be closer to that with subcutaneous or intramuscular administration because these routes avoid first-pass metabolism in the liver. Intramuscular, intravenous, and subcutaneous doses are considered equi-analgesic for most agents.

■ When possible, treat pain prophylactically. Give analgesics before procedures (including placement and removal of chest tubes and bone marrow biopsies) and dressing changes. *Never rely solely on as-needed medications (PRN) when you know the patient will have significant pain.* In general, for patients with moderate or severe pain, use a long-acting oral or transdermal preparation or a constant intravenous or subcutaneous infusion, plus a shorter-acting agent that may be used as needed for breakthrough pain.

■ Oral administration is preferred over parenteral administration, because it facilitates a more even blood level, is less expensive and less intimidating, does not require special knowledge such as familiarity with infusion pumps, and does not transmit infections the way needles can. Our society needs to relinquish the unscientific expectation that only a "pain shot" can treat severe pain. As soon as patients can take oral liquids, consideration should be given to changing to an oral pain regimen.

■ *Patient-controlled analgesia* (PCA), with doses administered by the patient within professionally established limits, has been shown to lessen postoperative pain, decrease complications, lead to earlier hospital discharge, and lessen the total amount of opiate consumed. Figure 18.3 shows a model PCA order sheet. Although the concept of patient self-administration and control has been applied most frequently to parenteral PCA pumps, it reinforces the desirability of active patient participation in the selection, assessment, and control of analgesic regimens.

■ A *constant opiate infusion* may be indicated for patients with severe stable pain who use a patient-controlled pump. On the other hand, a constant basal infusion is not recommended for patients after simple operative procedures, patients with undiagnosed or changing pain, elderly patients, or patients with hepatic or renal insufficiency.

■ *Intraspinal (epidural or intrathecal) regimens* can provide analgesia at lower dosages and may reduce systemic side effects. This route may be especially useful in acute postoperative pain, particularly after thoracic, abdominal, or pelvic surgery. The equi-analgesic epidural dose of morphine is about one-tenth the parenteral dose, and the intrathecal dose is about one-tenth the epidural dose. Although the combination of dilute concentrations of intraspinal anesthetics and opiates provides some advantages over opiates alone, the use of this strategy is limited by the invasiveness of the intraspinal route,

expense, requirements for close monitoring, and need to involve an anesthesiologist or pain specialist. Recently, many surgeons have been placing local pumps to deliver infusions of anesthetics directly into the incisional site. Emerging evidence is that such infusions decrease the need for systemic opiods (7).

■ Adverse reactions, especially to step 2 and 3 drugs, must be anticipated. *Assume that all patients taking opiates will be constipated.* Stool softeners and propulsant preparations are useful and should be titrated against the consistency of stool and intervals between defecations. Despite the frequency of constipation, prolonged postoperative ileus almost always has a cause other than opiate analgesia. Similarly, when an altered mental status develops in a patient receiving stable opiates, consider other causes before automatically discontinuing the opiate; these include concurrent medications (especially psychoactive medications), sepsis, and stroke. Avoid the use of naloxone (Chapter 121) if at all possible (the patient may wake up screaming) by relying instead on short-term intense observation. Be prepared to use an ambu bag if necessary. If naloxone is used, dilute it (0.4 mg naloxone in 10 mL normal saline solution) and titrate it carefully until the patient's mental status clears.

PAIN MANAGEMENT IN SPECIAL CIRCUMSTANCES

The general principles outlined above are applicable to most hospitalized patients with pain. The following sections focus on patients with special needs. In addition, pain management in the postoperative patient is covered in Chapter 31 (2), and treatment of the patient with sickle cell pain crisis is discussed in Chapter 97 (8).

Patients with Neuropathic Pain

Neuropathic pain (9) is characterized by burning, tingling, numbness, and electrical or pins-and-needles qualities. It accompanies many medical and surgical conditions (HIV disease, diabetes, alcoholism, shingles, amputations and other trauma, and cerebrovascular events) and often goes undiagnosed. Conventional analgesics are most useful for somatic and visceral pain; neuropathic pain, resulting from pathology directly affecting nerves, may respond better to other agents. As hospitalized patients may have multiple pains, each must be individually assessed, and the following algorithm should be considered even if only one pain has neuropathic qualities.

Tricyclic agents have specific analgesic effects in neuropathic pain separate from their antidepressant effect. Analgesia is achieved at lower doses than is relief of depression (e.g., 10–25 mg of desipramine may relieve pain versus 150–300 mg for relief of depression); it also is achieved in less time (e.g., 1–3 days for analgesia versus 3–6 weeks for

Name: _____   DOB: _____   MRN: _____

Diagnosis/Indications: _____   Allergies: _____

Route of administration:_____ IV_____SQ

Morphine
Concentration: ☐ 5.0 mg/mL,or per pharmacy _____ mg/mL.
Patient-controlled dose: _____ mg. Usual range 0.5–2 mg.
Lock out interval: delay _____ minutes between patient-controlled doses. Usual range 5–15 min.
Nurse may bolus with _____ mg q _____ via pump as needed. Usual range 2–5 mg q 15–30 min.
Basal rate: continuous infusion of _____ mg/hr. Usual range 0–2.0 mg/hr.
Naloxone 0.4 mg ampule in medication drawer.

Hydromorphone (1 mg ≅ 5 mg morphine)
Concentration: ☐ 1.0 mg/mL,or per pharmacy _____ mg/mL.
*Patient-controlled dose:*_____ mg. Usual range 0.1–0.4 mg.
Lock out interval: delay _____ minutes between patient-controlled doses. Usual range 5–15 min.
Nurse may bolus with _____ mg q_____ via pump as needed. Usual range 0.2–1.0 mg q 15–30 min.
Basal rate: continuous infusion of _____ mg/hr. Usual range 0–0.4 mg/hr.
Naloxone 0.4 mg ampule in medication drawer.

Fentanyl (50 mcg ≅ 5 mg morphine)
Concentration: ☐ 50 mcg/mL, or per pharmacy _____ mcg/mL.
Patient-controlled dose: _____ mcg. Usual range 5–20 mcg.
Lock out interval: delay _____ minutes between patient-controlled doses. Usual range 5–15 min.
Nurse may bolus with _____ mcg q _____ via pump as needed. Usual range 5–20 mcg q 15–30 min.
Basal rate: continuous infusion of _____ mcg/hr. Usual range 0–20 mcg/hr.
Naloxone 0.4 mg ampule in medication drawer.

Monitor and record respiratory rate, sedation score, pain score, and total patient-controlled analgesia delivered q 2 hrs for the first 8 hrs, then q 4 hrs.
Call M.D. for: _____

Changes in titration parameters for patient-controlled analgesia may be written on the routine order sheet; however, a change in opiate or concentration of opiate requires a new patient-controlled analgesia physician order form.

Physician

_____ am/pm   _____
Date   Time   Print Name   Signature

RN

_____ am/pm   _____
Date   Time   Print Name   Signature

Figure 18.3 A sample patient-controlled analgesia order sheet. In December 2004, JCAHO issued a Sentinel Event Alert regarding "PCA by Proxy": fatalities have resulted when family, friends, or caregivers have given patients extra PCA boluses (10).

depression). Many clinicians avoid amitriptyline because of excessive sedation and anticholinergic adverse effects, instead relying on desipramine, imipramine, or nortriptyline. Note that antidepressants without the tricyclic structure (e.g., selective serotonin reuptake inhibitors; see Chapter 119) lack an analgesic effect, and that tricyclics are useful for neuropathic pain, not somatic or visceral pain. The dose of the tricyclic may be increased as often as every 3 days and titrated to the relief of neuropathic pain or the development of adverse events. The effective analgesic dose may be equal to or even higher than the usual antidepressant dose. If the patient partially responds to a tricyclic agent, it is best to maintain the highest tolerated dose and add an anticonvulsant.

Antiseizure medications (carbamazepine, gabapentin, phenytoin, valproic acid, clonazepam) have been used successfully to treat neuropathic pain. Carbamazepine is generally used at anti-seizure doses. The upper dose limit for gabapentin in the treatment of neuropathic pain has not yet been defined; doses as high as 6 g daily are being used commonly.

Mexiletine, an oral form of lidocaine, has been used to relieve painful diabetic peripheral neuropathy and is effective in other types of neuropathic pain. The usual dose is 150–200 mg 3 times daily, up to a maximum of 1,200 mg daily. All anti-arrhythmics are potentially pro-arrhythmic, so this agent should not be used in patients with known ventricular dysrhythmias or those with a predisposition to dysrhythmias (e.g., severe dilated cardiomyopathy). Up to 20 mg of baclofen 4 times daily may be useful for neuropathic pain as well as for painful muscle spasm. Capsaicin, a topical agent derived from chili peppers, must be applied to painful areas several times per day and may cause burning. Some patients have even responded to analgesic balm. If these modalities, most often used in combination, do not adequately control neuropathic pain, it is reasonable to add opiates to the regimen.

Patients with a History of Substance Abuse

Physical dependence is defined as a condition in which abrupt discontinuation of an agent, after a period of continuous use, causes physical symptoms (withdrawal or abstinence syndrome). It is a common feature of opioid use, as it is also with antihypertensives, benzodiazepines, barbiturates, corticosteroids, and other classes of drugs. It can be easily managed by gradually tapering the medication if it is no longer indicated. Drug abuse is the inappropriate use of a medication for a nonmedical problem (e.g., to escape family, work, and social or financial problems). Taken to extreme, drug abuse becomes drug addiction, a compulsive pattern of drug abuse and socially inappropriate or dangerous behaviors. *The medical use of opioids is not associated with the development of addiction*, with the exception of the patient recovering from opiate addiction, who may be at substantial risk for relapse. Such patients require an open discussion regarding analgesic choices and positive and negative consequences, including the potential relapse of addiction. When opiates are used in these patients, long-acting preparations should be given at scheduled times; needles, an environmental cue for craving, should be avoided (11). Because of physiologic tolerance, regular users of opiates require stronger analgesics and larger doses to achieve the same analgesic effect than do those who are opiate-naïve. It is useful to separate the treatment of addiction from the treatment for pain and establish a dose of methadone sufficient to keep the patient out of withdrawal while using other agents for pain. Buprenor-

phine, a mild opiate agonist that adheres tightly to opiate receptors, is increasingly being used for treatment of addiction; it may have to be discontinued in the hospitalized patient with new significant pain. Consultation with substance abuse experts is often helpful (Chapter 121).

Patients with HIV Disease

Although there are few studies addressing the management of common HIV-related pain syndromes, the approach outlined in this chapter is generally useful in these patients, with several caveats. Neuropathy is very common and causes significant morbidity. It may be caused by antiretroviral therapies, which should be discontinued as soon as this adverse effect is recognized. The algorithm given above for neuropathic pain often must be modified in AIDS patients because of drug interactions; carbamazepine, for example, interacts with many antiretroviral agents; gabapentin appears to be better tolerated. Management of pain in AIDS patients frequently must take into account issues of dementia and substance abuse.

Older Hospitalized Patients

Assessment of pain in the elderly (12) may be complicated by sensory, cognitive, or communication deficits in addition to an attitude among many elders of resignation to pain. Pharmacologic therapy for pain must be administered cautiously in older patients because of several factors. Renal and hepatic function may be compromised, resulting in prolonged effects of usual doses of agents. Marginal brain, bladder, renal, or other organ function may be further compromised by analgesics, including NSAIDs, antineuropathic agents, and opiates; elderly patients are particularly susceptible to medication-induced falls (Chapter 16).

ASSESSING THE RESPONSE TO THERAPY

Successful management of pain in the hospitalized patient requires the active participation of educated nursing and pharmacy staff. Continuous assessment of pain and appropriate titration of pain medication can best be carried out by nurses acting under physician orders that give them a range of options. Nurses can also identify and address common adverse effects of the chosen regimen. Some institutions have advance practice nurses and clinical pharmacists to further the goal of effective pain management. Many have added a pain assessment (0–10) instrument to the vital sign sheet. Pain management is certainly an area in which patients' best interests are served when physicians work closely with nurses and pharmacists, as well as rehabilitation therapists and mental health workers (Chapter 4).

If the patient's pain has not responded to treatment as predicted, several questions should be asked:

- Did the patient in fact receive the ordered medication? "Opiophobia" is so common among patients, family members, and hospital staff that the medication may never have reached the patient.
- Was the patient prescribed PRN dosing when around-the-clock dosing would have been more effective?
- Does the patient have pain that may be relatively resistant to conventional analgesics (e.g., neuropathic pain)?
- Are there additional pathology or complications that have not been diagnosed or fully appreciated? Repeating the history and physical examination along with indicated studies may be revealing. Hospitalized patients often have more than one pain; muscle spasm is common, as is neuropathic pain and flares of gout (the latter often precipitated by surgery, hemorrhage, starvation, or re-feeding). All these entities may respond to specific therapy once diagnosed.

If the patient still has unrelieved pain, consultation with a *pain specialty team* is indicated. Given the high success rates reported in the literature in managing the pain of terminal disease (Chapter 19), and the increasing use of these same techniques in managing nonmalignant, nonterminal pain, patients and providers should expect that pain will be managed. The old notion that the patient "will just have to learn to live with pain" is increasingly unacceptable.

DISCHARGE ISSUES

As the patient progresses toward discharge, the analgesic regimen should be steadily changed toward the least invasive route that still provides adequate control of pain. The analgesics should be switched to the oral route as soon as liquids are tolerated. Ideally, the medication regimen can be stabilized while the patient is in the hospital; this is preferable to discontinuing a parenteral regimen just as the patient is leaving the ward. Careful thought must be given to the patient's need for analgesics at home (including timing of the follow-up visit) so that the patient leaves with enough of the correct medication. Physicians should have no fear of prescribing opiates at discharge if these are indicated by the clinical situation. They should not allow regulatory barriers (e.g., the preprinted prescription forms required for controlled substances in a few states) to distort clinical practice. Regimens should be as simple as possible to promote adherence. Patients who are likely to remain in significant pain after discharge often do best with one long-acting opiate for around-the-clock pain relief plus a short-acting agent for breakthrough pain. Patients with conditions such as sickle cell disease or migraine, which are likely to cause painful flares, should be given the analgesic tools to use at home rather than be required to depend on

drop-in visits for relief. The primary physician can manage most pain satisfactorily if the principles described above are followed. For those with more complicated pain problems, consider referral to a specialty pain clinic.

CONCLUSIONS

The pain of most hospitalized patients can be controlled promptly and safely by taking a careful history, employing rational pharmacologic and nonpharmacologic modalities, and continuously assessing response to initial management and adjusting the approach as needed. The fact that this vision is often unrealized stands as a major flaw in our current practice. It clearly can be improved through clinician education and the use of a multidisciplinary team.

KEY POINTS

- Clinicians cannot determine whether and how much pain is present without asking the patient and listening to the answer.
- Effective pain management depends on initial and ongoing assessment of the type of pain, its severity, and its response to therapy.
- Hospitalized patients often have more than one kind of pain (e.g., both somatic and neuropathic), requiring more than one kind of approach for effective control.
- Anything that influences the patient's emotional state will influence how much pain is experienced, both positively and negatively.
- The goal of pain management is not necessarily the complete absence of pain; rather, it is the maximally functional patient.
- Oral administration is the preferred route for analgesics.
- Knowledge of and comfort with the appropriate use of opiates can overcome our society's "opiophobia."

REFERENCES

1. Whelan CT, Jin L, Meltzer D. Pain and satisfaction with pain control in hospitalized medical patients: no such thing as low risk. *Arch Intern Med* 2004;164:175–180.
2. NIH state-of-the-science statement on symptom management in cancer: pain, depression and fatigue. *NIH Consens State Sci Statements* 2002;19:1–19.
3. Practice guidelines for acute pain management in the perioperative setting: a report by the American Society of Anesthesiologists Task Force on Pain Management, Acute Pain Section. *Anesthesiology* 1995;82:1071–1081.
4. Levy MH. Pharmacologic treatment of cancer pain. *N Engl J Med* 1996;335:1124–1132.
5. Wright J, Price S, Watson W. NSAID use and efficacy in the emergency department: single doses of oral ibuprofen versus intramuscular ketorolac. *Ann Pharmacother* 1994;28:309–312.

6. Bresalier RS, Sandler RS, Quan H, et al. Cardiovascular events associated with Rofecoxib in a colorectal adenoma chemoprevention trial. *N Engl J Med* 2005 Feb 15; [Epub ahead of print].

7. Gupta A, Perniola A, Axelsson K, et al. Postoperative pain after abdominal hysterectomy: a double-blind comparison between placebo and local anesthetic infused intraperitoneally. *Anesth Analg* 2004;99:1173–1179.

8. Brookoff D, Polomano R. Treating sickle cell pain like cancer pain. *Ann Intern Med* 1992;116:364–368.

9. Dworkin R, Backonja M, Rowbotham M, et al. Advances in neuropathic pain: diagnosis, mechanisms, and treatment recommendations. *Ann Neurology* 2003;60:1524–1534.

10. Joint Commission on Accreditation of Healthcare Organizations. Patient-controlled analgesia by proxy. *Sentinal Event Alert* 20 December 2004.

11. Passik SD, Kirsh KL. Opiod therapy in patients with a history of substance abuse. *CNS Drugs* 2004;18:13–25.

12. Young D. *Acute Pain Management.* Iowa City: University of Iowa Gerontological Nursing Interventions Center, 1999.

ADDITIONAL READING

Acute Pain Management Guideline Panel. Acute pain management: operative or medical procedures and trauma: clinical practice guideline. AHCPR Publication No. 92-002. Rockville, MD: Agency for Health Care Policy and Research, Public Health Service, U.S. Department of Health and Human Services, February 1992.

Doyle D, Hanks GWL, Cherny NI, Calman K, eds. *Oxford Textbook of Palliative Medicine,* 3rd ed. New York: Oxford University Press, 2003.

Weiner RS. *Pain Management: A Practical Guide for Clinicians,* 6th ed. Boca Raton, FL: CRC Press, 2002.

End-of-Life Care in the Hospital

19

Daniel Fischberg　　*Paolo Manfredi*　　*Diane E. Meier*

INTRODUCTION

Palliative care is interdisciplinary care aimed at relieving suffering and improving quality of life for patients with advanced illness and their families. Palliative care may be offered simultaneously with appropriate disease-modifying treatments during a chronic illness, or it may become the focus of care near the end of life. Hospitals traditionally have been structured to efficiently treat acute illnesses and exacerbations of chronic illnesses. When prolonging life is no longer the primary goal, hospitals typically fail to provide alternatives, continuing treatment focused on longevity up to the very moment of death (and often beyond that in the form of cardiopulmonary resuscitation). Although the acute-care hospital is usually not the ideal site of death, currently most Americans die in hospitals (1).

Throughout the course of a patient's illness, alleviation of physical and emotional suffering should be the objective of every health care professional. There comes a point in the evolution of many diseases at which the benefits of some or all of the efforts devoted to prolonging life no longer exceed the burden they pose to the patient's quality of life. The timing of this transition varies with the patient's preferences, and it is better thought of as a gradual, iterative process rather than an epiphany. The prompt recognition of the point at which the burden of life-prolonging efforts exceeds their benefit is essential to avoid unnecessary suffering and inappropriate allocation of resources. In this regard, it is important to note that there is never a time at which "there is nothing more that can be done"; every dying patient can benefit from and deserves skilled attention to palliative care issues.

Effective end-of-life care requires consideration of individual preferences (often inferred from the surrogate's perception of the patient's beliefs), integrated with the ability to prognosticate disease courses and to treat symptoms such as pain (see Chapter 18), dyspnea, nausea, delirium, and depression (see Chapter 119). Finally, knowledge of the available support systems inside and outside of the hospital is essential for developing an optimal plan of care for seriously ill and dying patients.

ADVANCE DIRECTIVES AND HEALTH CARE AGENTS

With the introduction of the Patient Self-Determination Act of 1990 (2), the importance of individual preferences has become more prominent in medical decision making. *Advance directives* are crucial for delivery of health care tailored to an individual's needs and preferences (see also Chapter 17). They provide a means by which capable patients can make known their preferences in the event they become unable to speak for themselves. Advance directives may contain specific examples addressing cardiopulmonary resuscitation, artificial nutrition, and hydration. More important in an advance directive, however, is a statement about what quality of life is unacceptable for the paient. For example, many patients say that they would not want continued life-prolonging measures if they were permanently incapable of recognizing and interacting with their loved ones. All patients should be strongly encouraged to designate a health care decision-making agent. Because of the variety and complexity of clinical scenarios, an individual designated by the patient to serve as his or her health care representative in case of lost capacity is critical for real-time decision making. The practical impact of advance directives on the delivery of care in the hospital is still controversial but is likely to increase as their use becomes more prevalent (3).

PROGNOSTICATION

Prognostication for decision-making purposes is the complex task of guessing the duration of life of an individual patient with one disease or, as is more often the case, multiple diseases. The prognosis then is integrated with an understanding of the functional status (quality-adjusted life span) that the patient is likely to achieve and finally with the patient's overall view of his or her own quality of life. The patient's wishes should guide the physician in determining, at any particular moment, the ratio of risk and burden to benefit for each test or treatment (ranging from a finger stick for blood-sugar testing to open-heart surgery). If the patient is unable to express himself, individuals who can speak on behalf of the patient (known as *surrogates* or *proxies*) should be consulted.

Among conditions that cause death in the hospital, the presence of multiorgan failure in patients with metastatic cancer or coma allows for a more accurate prediction of the clinical course than organ-specific processes such as advanced heart or lung disease. According to one study, the median prognoses generated by a statistical model varied substantially among diseases: patients with congestive heart failure were estimated to have about a 40% chance of living 6 months on the day before their actual death; patients with lung cancer were estimated to have about a 5% chance (Figure 19.1). The median prognoses, by physician estimation, were equally inaccurate (4). Another study found that physicians overestimate survival by more than a factor of 5 (5). This lack of precision is inherent to prognostication and highlights the need to begin deliberating about benefits, burdens, and goals of care as soon as a potentially fatal condition is diagnosed.

When trying to prognosticate, it is important to remain mindful of the performance status of the patient, not only at the time of the evaluation but also before the event that prompted hospitalization. For example, consider the case of a 90-year-old patient with a history of dementia who is now in the ICU with respiratory failure after developing aspiration pneumonia while recovering from a fractured hip. In evaluating this patient, the information from the nursing home—that the patient had recently begun to require a

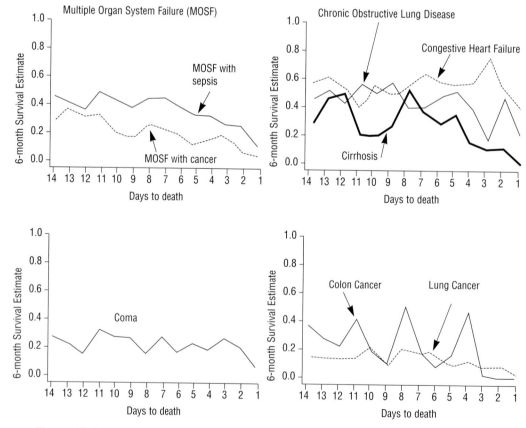

Figure 19.1 Estimates of prognosis in patients near death. Estimates for 6-month survival generated from the model of the Study to Understand Prognoses and Preferences for Outcomes and Risks of Treatment (*y axis*) by days before actual patient death (*x axis*) for patients with various diseases. **Top left.** Multiple organ system failure with sepsis (*solid line*) and with malignancy (*dashed line*). **Top right.** Chronic obstructive lung disease (*solid line*), congestive heart failure (*dashed line*), and cirrhosis (*heavy line*). **Bottom left.** Coma. **Bottom right.** Colon cancer (*solid line*) and lung cancer (*dashed line*).

walker, had frequent falling episodes, and had been losing weight because of refusal to eat—helps the physician determine that, even if weaning from the respirator is possible, at best the patient will be bedridden or chairbound and require a permanent feeding tube.

Another important point, especially for the patient being cared for by an army of specialists, is that there is a general tendency to prognosticate in an organ-specific manner. To continue with the prior example, the surgical wound from the open reduction and internal fixation of the femur appears to be healing, the pneumonia is being treated, the congestive heart failure is mild, the renal function is only moderately compromised, and the nutritional status is fair. Why, then, is the patient still unresponsive and unable to breathe after 10 days of intensive care and ventilatory support? The answer is that the combined impact of multiple insults is more important than the status of single organs and systems.

As often occurs in tertiary-care teaching hospitals, the presence of multiple specialists can be responsible for a fragmentation of care that confuses the clinical picture, especially as the clinical course progressively worsens. This can lead to contradictory and confusing messages about prognosis and goals of care delivered to the patient or the family by different specialists. Regular communication (e.g., through interdisciplinary meetings) with all consultants and family is therefore vital for effective care planning.

INTEGRATION OF PROGNOSIS AND PATIENT'S WISHES

Prognostication is the foundation on which goals of care are established and the plan of care is built. Once it is determined that the elderly woman in our example will not be able to walk or eat even if liberated from the ventilator, the surrogate's knowledge of the patient's wishes under that best-case clinical scenario guides further care. Options at this point include ventilator withdrawal versus continuation of medical care focused on life prolongation, including tracheostomy and gastrostomy for feeding tube placement. From the standpoints of humanitarianism (considering the apparent burden of suffering associated with ongoing aggressive medical care) and economics (in terms of the cost of care and the potential to deploy resources elsewhere) ventilator withdrawal may seem preferable. However, individual (patient or surrogate) preferences continue to strongly influence the goals of care in the United States and often result in the continuation of intensive medical care focused on prolongation of life, regardless of the ultimate quality of the life resulting.

A generation ago, many people separated potentially life-prolonging care into two categories: "heroic" or not. Our more modern understanding has eliminated this false dichotomy, weighing every potential intervention in terms of its benefits and burdens. As such, artificial nutrition

and hydration, antibiotics for infection, diagnostic tests, and rehospitalizations after discharge are all points open for discussion. If the patient is discharged back to the nursing home, it is necessary to clearly communicate the comprehensive plan of care to the receiving institution and medical staff. In discussing goals and options of care with patients and families it is important to emphasize that distressing symptoms (e.g., shortness of breath, pain, fever) can be treated effectively without attempting to reverse or cure the underlying illness, and that withdrawal of artificial nutrition and hydration will not cause suffering (6).

ARTIFICIAL VENTILATION

Artificial ventilation is initiated with the intent to help patients recover from an acute event. Often patients with terminal illnesses or multiorgan failure remain dependent on the ventilator and cannot be weaned. The patient or, if the patient is unable to make his wishes known, the surrogate should be informed about the option of disconnecting the ventilator and the availability of appropriate treatment to prevent and treat dyspnea (see Chapter 23). If, after disconnecting the ventilator, the patient continues to breathe (as may sometimes happen), the most urgent matter is to treat dyspnea (evidenced by tachypnea and use of accessory respiratory muscles) by titrating opioids with or without benzodiazepines or barbiturates until the patient passes away peacefully.

ARTIFICIAL NUTRITION AND HYDRATION

Artificial nutrition and hydration are beneficial for time-limited use while the patient is recovering from an acute event. Their value in treating patients nearing the end of life is controversial (6). Total parenteral nutrition in patients with advanced cancer has not been shown to prolong life.

The provision of nutrients by means of a tube inserted in the gastrointestinal tract or a vein, although clearly a form of medical treatment, carries more emotional weight than other treatments, including artificial ventilation. Even those who wish only comfort measures for their dying relatives often hesitate when asked about withdrawal of artificial nutrition and hydration. It is important to reiterate that artificial feeding is a medical treatment that carries its own burdens, and that dying patients do not suffer if artificial nutrition and hydration are not provided or are discontinued (6). Knowledge of state laws is also important if withdrawal of artificial nutrition and hydration is being considered, especially if the predicted life expectancy of the patient is more than several weeks but the prognosis for any form of functional recovery is dismal (e.g., the patient with advanced dementia).

COMMUNICATING BAD NEWS

Physicians should gather necessary information (e.g., usual prognosis and the pros and cons of treatment alternatives), before meeting with the patient. This may involve team discussions, literature searches, or meetings with consultants. In addition, patients should be asked who they would like to be present during the discussion. Key points are to sit down in a private area, make eye contact, and then start by finding out how much the patient knows—"What is your understanding of the situation at this point?"—and how much he actually wants to know—"Would you like to know all the details of the situation or do you prefer a more general outline? Is there someone else you would like me to speak with?" A substantial minority of patients do not want to be told their diagnoses or prognoses. In this case, the dialogue should continue on more general terms with the patient and on more detailed grounds with a designated health care agent or surrogate. With the majority of patients who *do* want to make informed decisions themselves, the communication of the diagnosis should be followed by a period of silence to allow the patient to register and absorb the information. Subsequently, discuss the treatment alternatives, including palliative care options. It is important to frequently check that the patient is following what the physician is saying, allowing a period of quiet after each question—"Am I making sense? Am I being clear enough?"—and to ask open-ended questions—"How are you doing? Is there anything else that you would like to ask?"

The dialogue then should focus on the available options, including their potential burdens and benefits. Based on the patient's preferences, the goals of care are established and a specific plan of care is outlined. The meeting should end with a clear statement of the plan for the immediate future and reassurance that the physician will stand by the patient throughout the course of the illness (Table 19.1) (7, 8).

EMOTIONAL AND SPIRITUAL CARE

Supportive counseling should be provided by the treating physicians, nurses, and social workers. Patients and families should be given the time and an appropriate place to voice their concerns and have questions answered. Consistency of recommendations and prognostic information is critical. Such consistency requires frequent and regular communication among providers *before* discussion with patients and their families.

More than 80% of Americans claim to be religious, underlining the importance of spirituality, especially nearing the end of life. Facilitating access to religious support for hospitalized patients and families, therefore, should be a priority (Chapter 4). Access to bereavement support groups also should be made available.

TABLE 19.1

COMMUNICATING BAD NEWS: THE SIX-STEP APPROACH

Step 1. Start off well.
  Get the physical context right.
  Silence the pager. Sit down. Arrange at least a 30-minute commitment.
  Decide on the best setting.
  Decide who should be there.
Step 2. Find out how much the patient knows.
  "What have the doctors told you so far?"
Step 3. Find out how much the patient wants to know.
  "Some of my patients want to know all the details and some prefer a more general outline—which kind of person are you?"
Step 4. Share the information (aligning and educating).
  "I'm afraid I have some bad news. The biopsy showed that you have lung cancer." Stop talking and allow some time for silence.
  Proceed with: "We have some decisions to make about what to do next. Would you like to hear about the alternatives?"
  Decide on your agenda (diagnosis, treatment plan, prognosis, support).
  Start from the patient's starting point (aligning).
  Educate: Give information in small chunks.
  Use English, not "medspeak."
  Check reception frequently.
  Reinforce and clarify the information frequently.
  Check your communication level (for example, adult-adult).
  Listen for the patient's agenda.
  Try to blend your agenda with the patient's.
Step 5. Respond to the patient's feelings.
  Identify and acknowledge the patient's reaction.
Step 6. Plan and follow through.
  Organize and plan.
  Make a contract and follow through.
  Give the patient a specific day and time to return to see you. Call to check in on them later that evening.

Adapted from Buckman R. *How to Break the Bad News.* Baltimore: The Johns Hopkins University Press, © 1992, with permission.

PLAN OF CARE

When the goals of care gradually shift from medical treatment focused on prolongation of life to comfort care, efforts should be made to move patients out of the hospital, unless death is imminent. Although some patients die in the hospital while receiving treatments that could have been successful, a more appropriate site of death probably could have been devised for many of the more than 50% of patients who die in hospitals. The odds of dying in an acute-care hospital are directly related to the number of hospital beds per capita in a given area rather than to personal preferences of patients or family members (3). Improving advance-care planning and the support systems for dying patients available outside of the hospital will allow better compliance with the wishes of patients and families.

Hospice refers to both a philosophy of care and an organization that provides care for patients at the end of their life. Although some hospitals and nursing homes have wings devoted to hospice care, most patients receive hospice care at home. Referral to hospice usually involves leaving familiar systems and providers of care to enter a new system. The patient's physician must certify that the patient's life expectancy is less than 6 months, and in most cases there must be a caregiver in the home; the latter requirement is important because a limited number of hours of custodial home-aid services are provided by most hospices (although this varies by hospice and additional short-term help sometimes is added, as the patient's condition progresses).

Through hospice, a team of experts is available to provide nursing, spiritual, and medical care during the dying process. The Medicare program covers both hospice care and the medications used for the treatment of symptoms related to the primary disease. Counseling, support groups, and religious and bereavement services also are provided by hospice.

Although hospice allows the primary care physician to continue in that role, in most cases responsibility for medical care routinely is relinquished to the hospice physician, often leaving the dying patient with a compounded sense of loss and abandonment just as many other serious losses are occurring. This requirement to refer to a separate system of care and caregivers probably explains why only 20% of adult deaths occur in hospice in the United States (9).

If a patient is expected to die within 24–72 hours, it is probably best to continue care in the hospital, unless he or she has expressed clear wishes to die at home. Many hospitals (more than 800 in 2002) have developed palliative-care teams or units to help provide compassionate end-of-life care to inpatients. In addition to home hospices, discharge options for patients receiving terminal care include a nursing home with hospice care and an inpatient hospice. Home health care also can provide medical assistance at home, although, unlike hospice, certified home health agencies are not typically prepared to focus on the care of dying patients. If home care is directed by a team experienced in end-of-life care, it can provide a useful alternative to home hospice, especially because it provides care that remains linked to the hospital setting and does not require separation from familiar professional caregivers and health systems. Increasingly, hospital-hospice partnerships are forming to better reconcile the goals of expertise, availability, and continuity.

SYMPTOM MANAGEMENT AND THE RULE OF DOUBLE EFFECT

The treatment of symptoms at the end of life is characterized by the appropriate use of medications without inappropriate worries about addiction and with reasonable concerns about respiratory depression. According to the "rule of dou-

ble effect," if a desirable effect (symptom relief) is intended, the risk of a foreseen, but not intended, bad effect (hastening death) is acceptable. If the intended good effect is relief of pain or dyspnea and opioids are titrated carefully, the risk of hastening death is very small; therefore, the rule of double effect only rarely applies. While it is widely believed that the use of sedatives to relieve refractory symptoms leads to hastened death, the best evidence suggests that the opposite is true. In a recent study, patients receiving sedation for refractory symptoms actually lived longer than those who did not require sedation (10). Nonetheless, even if hastened death were a risk, as long as the intended effect is relief of suffering, such use of medications is not only acceptable (by the rule of double effect) but *mandatory* to prevent unnecessary distress and suffering.

Neuroleptics, such as haloperidol, chlorpromazine, risperidone, and olanzapine, are very useful in the treatment of preterminal agitation and delirium. All are also very potent antiemetics.

ORCHESTRATING THE "GOOD DEATH"

When patients are moribund, comfort care is the goal and life-prolonging efforts are no longer appropriate or effective. At that point, key steps include:

- Prompt attention to symptoms
- Effective and compassionate communication with and support of family and involved health care staff
- Removal of unnecessary indwelling tubes, catheters, and drains
- Discontinuation of all procedures and medications that are not providing comfort directly

Religious support should be offered to families. Depending on the availability of inpatient and outpatient support, the site of death should be chosen by the family. If death is imminent, it is best to continue care in the hospital. If death is likely in a matter of days, home, nursing home, or inpatient hospice are all reasonable options. If support is available (e.g., through family or home health aides and specialized nurses), home is often the preferred site of death. Family caregivers should be instructed in advance on how to react to common end-of-life symptoms such as pain, shortness of breath, and agitation with as-needed medications and other measures (e.g., upright positioning and a fan can be very helpful for the relief of dyspnea; reassurance from a familiar voice can improve agitation). Medications that should be readily available to a dying patient include morphine sulfate immediate release liquid (20 mg/cc); lorazepam liquid (2 mg/cc); and chlorpromazine liquid concentrate (100 mg/cc). These medications have rapid onset, can be given sublingually or via the buccal mucosa in case of inability to swallow, and will address a wide range of sources of distress including pain, dyspnea, anxiety, agitation, and nausea. A contact nurse or physician should be available at all times and should respond promptly to unforeseen crises (e.g., agitation, a pain crisis, or a seizure). Most crises can be dealt with in the patient's home, and resorting to an ambulance is rarely necessary. A do-not-resuscitate form should be kept in the home to avoid the risk of pointless and burdensome efforts. Arrangements with a funeral home should be made in advance, and, when the patient dies, the funeral director should be called first. He will guide the family through the necessary paperwork and logistical steps.

IMPROVING PALLIATIVE CARE

Widespread access to state-of-the-art palliative care requires a collegial effort to overcome attitudinal, educational, economical, and legal barriers (Table 19.2) (11). The prevalent attitude of health professionals, which stems in part from both fear and denial of death as a natural inevitable process, is that prolongation of life, at all costs, is the primary goal of medicine.

Even among physicians there is considerable confusion about the difference between forgoing medical treatments when they are not benefitting the patient and euthanasia. Until very recently, training in palliative care for physicians and nurses was very limited or nonexistent. Educational and clinical programs to improve the care of dying patients are needed urgently, especially at teaching hospitals. The accrediting authorities for U.S. undergraduate and graduate medical education have recognized this need and have mandated training in palliative and end-of-life care. Data consistently show that well delivered palliative care leads to better clinical outcomes, higher patient and family satisfaction, and more appropriate allocation of resources (12). Modification of state regulations that control and limit the prescription of opioids and other controlled substances also is needed to reduce the worries of prescribing physicians who care for patients at the end of life.

KEY POINTS

- Palliative care, designed to relieve suffering and improve quality of life, should be delivered at the same time as all beneficial and effecive life-prolonging or curative treatments.
- Prognostication—in terms of both expected longevity and function—is a difficult but important task for the physician. A poor prognosis is not a prerequisite for applicability of palliative care.
- The benefits versus burdens of elements of care, including ventilation, nutrition, antibiotics, venipuncture, and diagnostic testing, are worth discussing with terminally ill patients or their surrogates.
- In communicating bad news, provide sufficient time and silence for the information to sink in, a conducive environment, and offers of regular follow-up as well as physical, practical, emotional, and religious support.

TABLE 19.2
APPROACHES TO IMPROVING PALLIATIVE CARE

Improve professional knowledge and skills

Continue faculty development in palliative care
Include palliative care in medical curricula
Include palliative-care topics on board certification examinations
Include palliative-care training in residency review requirements
Include practice guidelines and quality improvement programs in palliative care

Change professional attitudes about care at the end of life

Make a distinction between decisions to discontinue treatment and active euthanasia
Make use of terminal sedation as distinct from euthanasia
Establish standards of futility through consensus by professional organizations
Educate on the limitations of technology and the desirability of a peaceful death
Use advance directives as tools to improve physician-patient communication

Reorganize the health care system

Incorporate the Joint Commission on Accreditation of Healthcare Organizations standards for end-of-life care
Include the International Classification of Diseases, 9th ed., code for terminal care to legitimize hospital palliative care by providing reimbursement
Make use of hospital-based palliative care units and consultation services
Make use of quality standards for end-of-life care in managed-care organizations
Organize formal networks between hospice programs and other health care structures
Modify state regulations that inhibit prescriptions for opioids
Include risk management standards that recognize palliative care and respect patient wishes

From Meier DE, Morrison RM, Cassel CK. Improving palliative care. *Ann Intern Med* 1997;127:225–230, with permission.

- Hospice care, whether in a hospital, nursing home, or home, can help the patient and family achieve a "good death."

REFERENCES

1. Weitzen S, Teno JM, Fennell M, et. al. Factors associated with site of death: a national study of where people die. *Med Care* 2003;41: 323–335.
2. The Patient Self-Determination Act of 1990. 4206, 4751 of the Omnibus Reconciliation Act of 1990. November 5 1990. Pub L No. 101–508.
3. Hammes BJ, Rooney BL. Death and end-of-life planning in one midwestern community. *Arch Intern Med* 1998;158:383–390.
4. Lynn J, Harrell F Jr, Cohen F, et al. Prognoses of seriously ill hospitalized patients on the days before death: implications for patient care and public policy. *New Horiz* 1997;5:56–61.

5. Christakis NA, Lamont EB. Extent and determinants of error in doctors' prognoses in terminally ill patients: prospective cohort study. *BMJ* 2000;320:469–472.
6. Winter SM. Terminal nutrition: framing the debate for the withdrawal of nutritional support in terminally ill patients. *Am J Med* 2000;109:723–726.
7. Baile WF, Buckman R, Lenzi R, et. al. SPIKES—a six-step protocol for delivering bad news: application to the patient with cancer. *The Oncologist* 2000;5:302–311.
8. Buckman R. *How to Break the Bad News.* Baltimore: The Johns Hopkins University Press, 1992:96–97.
9. General Accounting Office, "Medicare: more beneficiaries use hospice but for fewer days of care" (Report GAO/HEHS-001–182, General Accounting Office, Washington, DC, September 2000).
10. Sykes N, Thorns A. Sedative use in the last week of life and the implications for end-of-life decision making. *Arch Intern Med* 2003;163:341–344.
11. Meier DE, Morrison RS, Cassel CK. Improving palliative care. *Ann Intern Med* 1997;127:225–230.
12. Von Gunten CF. Secondary and tertiary palliative care in US hospitals. *JAMA* 2002;287:875–881.

ADDITIONAL READING

Doyle D, Hanks GWC, MacDonald N, eds. *Oxford Textbook of Palliative Medicine,* 2nd ed. New York: Oxford University Press, 1998.
Quill TE. Initiating end-of-life discussions with seriously ill patients: addressing the "elephant in the room." 2000 *JAMA;*284: 2502–2507.
Quill TE. Dying and decision making—evolution of end-of-life options. *N Eng J Med* 2004;350:2029–2032.
Tolstoy L. *The Death of Ivan Ilyich.* New York: Bantam Books, 1987.
Perspectives on care at the close of life (ongoing case-based series). *JAMA;*2001–present.

Patient Safety in the Hospital Setting

20

Kaveh G. Shojania

INTRODUCTION

Long before "medical error" and "patient safety" were commonly used phrases, the medical profession recognized the concept of illness or injury induced by medical care. The term "iatrogenesis" is an ancient word that combines the Greek words *iatros* (healer) and *genesis* (to bring forth) to mean "coming from the healer." Iatrogenesis is particularly common in the hospital. In fact, Florence Nightingale wrote in 1859: "It may seem a strange principle to enunciate as the very first requirement in a hospital that it should do the sick no harm."

In 1999, the Institute of Medicine (IOM) published its now widely known report, *To Err Is Human,* (1) and brought these problems, including the rate at which medical care itself contributes to morbidity and mortality among hospitalized patients, to the attention of the medical community, the media, and the public. The often-quoted estimate produced by the IOM—that medical errors result in 44,000 to 98,000 hospital deaths per year—shocked many Americans. While these figures have been debated, (2,3) the widespread public attention given to them has compelled the health care community to seriously attack a problem that has bedeviled medical care since the time of Hippocrates: how to avoid doing harm to patients.

For physicians practicing in the hospital setting, the current interest in patient safety represents an important opportunity to improve both the care of individual patients and the systems in which they work. This chapter reviews the epidemiology of iatrogenic injury in the hospital setting, the psychological principles that have emerged from the study of human error, and the techniques for responding to adverse events and serious errors. The second half of the chapter discusses specific complications of hospital care and evidence-based practices that reduce their occurrence. Adverse drug events and nosocomial infections, two of the most important categories of hospital-acquired complications, are touched on briefly here and discussed in detail in Chapters 21, 66, 68 and 72.

THE EPIDEMIOLOGY OF ADVERSE EVENTS IN THE HOSPITAL SETTING

Table 20.1 lists studies of iatrogenesis involving general acute hospital care in the United States during the past 40 years. Studies from other countries have produced comparable results, with differences in the rates of adverse events largely due to differences in design and definitions (4).

The two studies that formed the basis of the IOM's widely quoted estimate of 44,000 to 98,000 annual deaths due to medical error were the Harvard Medical Practice (5) and the Utah-Colorado studies (6) (both included in Table 20.1). These studies screened inpatient records for various potential indicators of adverse events, such as death or other undesirable outcome, transfer from a general ward to intensive care, unexpected return to the operating room, and length of hospital stay above 90th percentile for a given diagnosis. Records that met one or more of these criteria were then reviewed independently by at least two board-certified physicians to identify *adverse events*, which were defined as injuries due to medical management rather than underlying illness. These studies had as their goal an assessment of the relationship between iatrogenic injury and malpractice litigation. Thus, both studies identified a subset of *negligent adverse events*, defined as injuries "caused by the failure to meet standards reasonably expected of the average physician."

TABLE 20.1

MAJOR EPIDEMIOLOGIC STUDIES OF ADVERSE EVENTS RELATED TO ACUTE HOSPITAL CARE IN THE UNITED STATES[a]

Study	Setting	Principal findings
Schimmel, 1964 (7)	Medical service of a university-affiliated community hospital in New Haven, CT, from 1960–61	20% of patients experienced a *complication of medical care unrelated to their underlying illness*. 1.6% of hospitalizations involved a *complication regarded as causing or contributing to death*.
California Medical Insurance Feasibility Study (8)	Screening and reviewing charts from 20,864 stays in California hospitals in 1974	4.6% of hospitalizations involved a *potentially compensable event (PCE)*, temporary or permanent disability attributable to health care management. 0.6% of hospitalizations involved a *PCE* that produced death or a major permanent disability.
Steel, 1981 (9)	Two general medical wards, one ICU and one CCU, in a Boston teaching hospital in 1979	36% of patients experienced at least one *iatrogenic illness*. 2% suffered an *iatrogenic illness judged as contributing to death*.
Harvard Medical Practice Study, 1991 (5, 10)	30,121 stays at 51 hospitals in New York State in 1984	3.7% of hospitalizations resulted in an *adverse event*; i.e., an injury caused by medical management. 1% of hospitalizations involved a *negligent adverse event*; i.e., an injury caused by substandard care. 0.6% of hospitalizations resulted in a *fatal or permanently disabling adverse event*.
ADE Prevention Study Group, 1995 (11)	Admissions to 11 medical and surgical units of 2 Boston teaching hospitals in 1993	6.5% of admissions experienced an *adverse drug event (ADE)*. 0.06% of hospitalizations involved a fatal *ADE*. 5.5% of patients experienced a *potential ADE* (serious medication error that produced no injury).
Classen et al., 1997 (12)	Admissions to a teaching hospital in Utah from 1990–1993	6.5% of hospitalized patients experienced an *ADE*. 0.2% of hospitalized involved a fatal *ADE*.
Andrews et al., 1997 (13)	Two intensive care units and one general surgical ward at a Chicago teaching hospital from 1989–1990	17.7% of patients experienced an *adverse event* that produced at least a temporary disability or more serious injury.
Colorado-Utah Study, 2000 (6, 14)	15,000 discharges from 28 hospitals in Colorado and Utah in 1992	2.9% of hospitalizations resulted in an *adverse event*; i.e., an injury caused by medical management. 0.2% of hospitalizations involved an *adverse event* resulting in death. 30% of all *adverse events* were judged as negligent.
Hayward & Hofer, 2001 (3)	111 random cases among all deaths occurring at 7 Veterans Affairs hospitals from 1995–1996	6.0% of deaths rated as "definitely or probably preventable." Reviewers estimated that about 50% of patients would still have died (during this hospitalization). Optimal care for 10,000 patients would result in 1 additional patient living at least 3 additional months in good cognitive health.
Forster et al, 2003 (15)	Consecutive discharges from the medical service of a Boston teaching hospital in 2001	76 patients (19%) experienced *adverse events* after discharge. Adverse events consisted of symptoms reported by patients (65%), symptoms associated with a temporary disability (30%), serious laboratory abnormalities (3%), and permanent disabilities (3%).

[a] Studies included here all reported rates of adverse events and/or errors. Studies without a denominator (e.g., incident reports only) are not included; also excluded from the table are studies with adverse event rates derived primarily from administrative data. The table does not include studies restricted to intensive care units, operating rooms, psychiatric facilities, or nursing homes.
Modified from Shojania KG, Wald H, Gross R. Understanding medical error and improving patient safety in the inpatient setting. *Med Clinic North Am* 2002;86:847–867, with permission.

One criticism of the IOM's estimate of deaths due to medical error is that the details of the calculations were never provided (16). The relevant inputs to the calculation include the percent of hospitalized patients experiencing an adverse event, the proportion of adverse events associated with death, and the proportion of those cases in which death could have been prevented. Figure 20.1 outlines a reasonable scheme (16) for estimating deaths due to med-

ical error. Interestingly, using the same inputs as the IOM report, no combination of these inputs produces the specific estimates of 44,000 or 98,000 deaths.

While the estimates published in *To Err Is Human* are more speculative than generally acknowledged, it is worth noting that these estimates were restricted to deaths, ignoring the many cases of non-fatal iatrogenesis. Even putting aside the debate over the IOM death rates, it is quite sober-

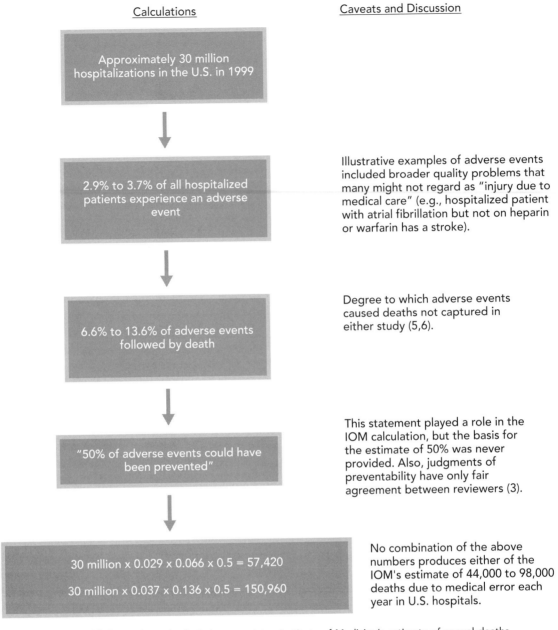

Calculations   Caveats and Discussion

Approximately 30 million hospitalizations in the U.S. in 1999

2.9% to 3.7% of all hospitalized patients experience an adverse event

Illustrative examples of adverse events included broader quality problems that many might not regard as "injury due to medical care" (e.g., hospitalized patient with atrial fibrillation but not on heparin or warfarin has a stroke).

6.6% to 13.6% of adverse events followed by death

Degree to which adverse events caused deaths not captured in either study (5,6).

"50% of adverse events could have been prevented"

This statement played a role in the IOM calculation, but the basis for the estimate of 50% was never provided. Also, judgments of preventability have only fair agreement between reviewers (3).

30 million x 0.029 x 0.066 x 0.5 = 57,420

30 million x 0.037 x 0.136 x 0.5 = 150,960

No combination of the above numbers produces either of the IOM's estimate of 44,000 to 98,000 deaths due to medical error each year in U.S. hospitals.

Figure 20.1 Outline of calculation examining Institute of Medicine's estimate of annual deaths due to medical errors.

ing to compare the adverse event rates in health care with that seen in other hazardous activities and exposures (17, 18). Whereas roughly 1–5 of every hundred hospitalized patients will suffer a major injury from medical care, it takes roughly 8 million enplanements to result in one passenger death. While physicians may balk at the comparison of commercial aviation to the care of complex, acutely ill patients, elective anesthesia in healthy patients probably is a fair comparison. Even in this setting, health care has not achieved a safety record comparable to aviation (19), though anesthesia has been one of the pioneering specialties for patient safety.

Errors vs. Adverse Events

Identifying something as an adverse event does not imply "error" or even poor quality care. It simply implies that an undesirable clinical outcome resulted from some aspect of diagnosis or therapy or even from the mere presence of a patient in the hospital. A large evidence review sponsored by the federal Agency for Healthcare Quality and Research defined a patient safety practice as "any health care structure or process that reduces the probability of adverse events resulting from exposure to the health care system across a range of diseases and procedures" (20, 21).

According to this definition, tracking the rate of falls among hospitalized elders and looking for ways to reduce these rates are patient safety activities, analogous to tracking rates of infection because of resistant nosocomial organisms and developing strategies to reduce these rates. In this broader view of patient safety, errors become the equivalent of intermediate clinical outcomes. Thus, just as we target blood pressure control in order to reduce myocardial infarction and stroke, targeting errors will play a role in preventing many (but not all) adverse events.

Under this view, errors committed by individual health care personnel represent just one element along the causal pathway to adverse events. This perspective serves the immediate purpose of diminishing some of the stigma associated with errors. It also serves the more general constructive purpose of putting individual errors into a broader context of factors contributing to the occurrence of adverse patient outcomes, an approach that has been long used (to great effect) in industries outside of health care.

FRAMEWORK FOR THINKING ABOUT ERRORS

One of the major lessons that health care has had to learn from other safety-conscious industries is that *the pervasive medical culture of individual responsibility and blame stand in the way of efforts to make health care safer.* No amount of individual reprimand will change the fact that all providers will err from time to time. The goal is thus to develop a system that recognizes, and even expects, these occasional human failures and minimizes the chance they will result in patient harm.

The Cognitive Psychology of Errors

The patient safety literature generally defines an error as *an act or omission that leads to an unanticipated, undesirable outcome or to substantial potential for such an outcome* (22, 23). The phrase "act or omission" implies that errors include active behaviors such as prescribing an inappropriate medication dose and passive behaviors such as forgetting to check for allergies prior to prescribing a medication. The term "unanticipated" implies that errors do not include outcomes acknowledged as "acceptable risks" during decision-making processes. For instance, a patient with breast cancer metastatic to brain develops a pulmonary embolism. The treating physicians decide to anticoagulate her after reviewing her most recent head CT scan, which showed no edema, mass effect, or other findings placing the patient at high risk for bleeding. Nonetheless, the patient suffers an intracranial bleed. The decision to administer heparin would not be regarded as an error given that the physicians considered the risk of intracranial hemorrhage from a single metastasis without mass effect and weighed this risk against the expected benefit of anticoagulation for

pulmonary embolism. (On the other hand, this event would still count as an adverse event, since the bleed clearly reflects the impact of medical care and not the patient's medical condition.)

Types of Error

There are two broad categories of error: *slips* and *mistakes* (17). Slips are inadvertent, unconscious lapses in expected behavior or inappropriate persistence of automaticity. They tend to affect schematic (also called "automatic") rather than attentional behaviors. For example, you divide your time between a hospital and a skilled nursing facility and, one morning, you absently drive toward the hospital instead of the nursing facility. Unfortunately, the distraction produced by recognizing one slip may lead to another; so, annoyed with yourself (once you realize your error) and flustered because you are now running late, you drive through a red light. Slips are more frequent in the face of competing sensory or emotional distractions, fatigue, and stress. These factors represent the norm in many health care settings.

Mistakes, by contrast, reflect incorrect choices. Rather than lapses in concentration (as with slips), mistakes typically involve insufficient knowledge, failure to correctly interpret available information, or application of the wrong cognitive "heuristic" or rule. Thus, mistakes are often divided into two types of problems—rule-based and knowledge-based (22). For instance, you admit a 60-year-old diabetic with fever, meningismus, and CSF leukocytosis, but order ceftriaxone by itself (i.e., without including empiric coverage for Listeria with ampicillin or penicillin-resistant pneumococcus with vancomycin). Whereas stress, fatigue, and distraction contribute to slips, mistakes are attributable to insufficient experience or training.

Responses to the Different Types of Errors

Table 20.2 outlines features that distinguish slips from mistakes. One important point is that, while mistakes invade attentional behavior more frequently than slips invade schematic behavior, schematic behavior is the predominant pattern within a health care setting. Consequently, the absolute number of slips far exceeds that of mistakes.

The practical significance of the distinction between slips and mistakes lies in informing the response to a given error. A *mistake* due to incorrect pattern recognition by an inexperienced physician or nurse likely represents insufficient supervision or oversight by the "system" relative to training. By contrast, when a physician forgets to elicit an allergy history or a nurse forgets to check an allergy history that has been elicited, these represent slips that can be expected to occur from time to time. Remedial education and/or increased supervision will generally not help reduce future occurrences of the same error, whereas redesigning the medication system so that no medication can be administered without an

TABLE 20.2

CATEGORIZATION OF HUMAN BEHAVIOR AND ERROR TYPES FROM A COGNITIVE PSYCHOLOGY PERSPECTIVE

Behavior type	Features	Associated error type	Error-inducing conditions	Examples
Attentional	Involves analysis, planning, oversight Generates sense of mental effort, intellectual satisfaction Quite error-prone	Mistakes • Wrong rule applied, pattern recognition failure • Knowledge-based mistakes, wrong judgment	Inexperience relative to supervision Inadequate training Key information presented in ambiguous or inconsistent ways	Physician misinterprets signs of pulmonary embolus for pulmonary edema; physician prescribes antibiotic for sepsis which fails to cover common resistant bacteria.
Schematic	Automated or scripted Repetitive, may be monotonous, unrewarding Usually requires oversight for best performance	Slips more common than mistakes (inappropriate persistence or lapse in automaticity, unconscious "fumbles")	Stress, fatigue, distraction, inadequate oversight, system design insensitive or inflexible to changes in context	Telemetry observer fails to notice frequent premature ventricular contractions; nurse receiving numerous intercom calls gives drug to wrong patient.

allergy check probably would. By contrast, after a patient with meningitis due to *Listeria monocytogenes* dies because of inadequate empiric antibiotic therapy, an in-service on empiric antibiotic therapy would be quite reasonable. An algorithmic decision-aid addressing the treatment of suspected meningitis posted in the emergency department would also be a productive quality improvement response to such an event.

In summary, understanding the difference between slips and mistakes will aid in and developing strategies to reduce the recurrence of specific errors in the future. The current literature does not offer direct supporting evidence for using any particular cognitive theory-based plan for error reduction, but the recommendations shown in Table 20.3 are consistent with relevant cognitive theories for planning error-resistant processes (17).

TABLE 20.3

RECOMMENDED RULES OF THUMB FOR "ERROR-PROOFING" HEALTH CARE PROCESSES

Rule of thumb	Discussion and specific recommendations
Focus on schematic behavior over attentional behavior.	Checklists, standardized order sheets, and protocols reduce opportunities for slips.
Design unambiguous schematic systems, but retain flexibility with respect to operator judgment and experience.	A protocol cannot anticipate all possible clinical scenarios and thus must allow a certain amount of flexibility to avoid endangering patients when unusual situations arise. At the same time, participants should compromise in the interests of reasonable consistency and standardization when necessary.
Enhance attentional behavior through collaboration.	For tasks that must be accomplished with attentional behavior, among the most powerful means for assuring success is collaboration, ranging from informal, "curbside" consultation to formalized team meetings and inclusion of nurses, pharmacists, and various therapists on hospital rounds.
Assume that errors will occur and make their identification and prevention a positive cultural occurrence.	Use the lessons of an error to reduce the likelihood of recurrence. Medical leadership should commend such activities at every opportunity.

Detailed Error Analysis

The above general principles provide a useful framework for thinking about patient safety, but the approach to specific incidents requires detailed analysis of the chronology of events and system factors that contributed to the error or bad outcome. Root cause analysis (RCA) is a retrospective approach to error analysis that was developed to investigate industrial accidents (22) and has more recently been adapted to the investigation of sentinel events in medicine (24). In 1997, the Joint Commission on the Accreditation of Healthcare Organizations (JCAHO) mandated the use of RCA in the investigation of sentinel events in accredited hospitals.

The principles and techniques of RCA are described here using a real case and its discussion (25) presented as the first in a series of case-based conferences focusing on patient safety and quality improvement (26). The salient features of the case are summarized below; the names are pseudonyms.

> Joan Morris is a 67-year-old female who was admitted to the telemetry unit of a teaching hospital for cerebral angiography. Because of bed limitations, Ms. Morris was transferred to the oncology floor after her successful embolization procedure. She remained in stable condition the next morning. Discharge was intended for later that day.
>
> Meanwhile, Jane Morrison was transferred from an outside institution (also to the telemetry unit) for a cardiac electrophysiology (EP) study. This study had been delayed for two days because of scheduling conflicts, with the result that Ms. Morrison was rescheduled as the first case of the morning on the day of Joan Morris' planned discharge from the hospital.
>
> Through a series of miscommunications and misidentifications involving various nurses, physicians, and support staff, Joan Morris was taken to the EP lab instead of Jane Morrison. One hour into the procedure (programmed stimulation of the heart), it became apparent that the wrong patient was on the table. The procedure was aborted, and the patient was returned to her room.

The RCA occurred in two distinct stages. The first was the assembly of a detailed timeline of the events leading up to the recognition of this error through chart review and interviews with involved personnel. This process established the chronology of events and revealed at least 15 distinct "active failures." *Active failures* refer to the errors and violations that occur at the point of direct contact between the patient-system interface (17, 22). The active errors involved in this case included "unsafe acts" and "rule violations" on the parts of various providers involved with the case, such as the following:

- Only the last name was used when the EP nurse phoned the floor to request the patient be sent down for the procedure.
- The floor nurse sent the patient down for the procedure despite no order in the chart and over the objections of the patient.

- The EP fellow obtained informed consent even though the chart contained no information indicating that this patient needed an EP study.
- The EP nurse checked the patient's wrist identification band against the chart that accompanied her, but not against the list of patients scheduled for EP procedures.

Once a critical incident has occurred, active errors are usually quite apparent; hence traditional error investigations tend to focus on them. The RCA aims to uncover the less apparent failures of system design (*latent errors*) that contributed to these active failures or allowed them to cause harm (17, 27). For example, whereas the active failure in a particular adverse event may have been a mistake in programming an intravenous pump, a latent error might be that the institution uses multiple types of infusion pumps, making programming errors more likely. Thus, latent errors are literally "accidents waiting to happen."

The search for active and latent errors forms the second phase of the RCA and is typically guided by a conceptual framework adapted from British psychologist James Reason (22). In this framework, contributory causal factors are categorized as environmental, organizational, process-related, and so on. These categories are depicted in Figure 20.2 in the form of a "fishbone diagram" (common in error analyses), using errors relevant to the example case in this section.

Limitations and Challenges of RCA

Major challenges in the conduct of RCAs include the problems of hindsight bias, the coloring of the analysis by the prevailing concerns of the day (e.g., staffing ratios, inadequate information technology, discontinuities between the inpatient and outpatient settings), medico-legal fears, and the time they take to conduct.

In addition, RCAs are in essence uncontrolled case studies. They are thus best viewed as hypothesis generating; when possible, these hypotheses should be tested. For example, if several RCAs attribute the use of verbal orders as a root cause, one should look to the literature to see if the impact of verbal orders on error rates has ever been assessed. In fact, the one study that conducted such an assessment found that verbal orders were *less* likely to produce an error than were handwritten ones (28).

In industries outside health care, it is clear why RCAs play such an important role, despite the limitations. Major accidents in aviation, nuclear power, and the petrochemical industries are too uncommon to lend themselves to quantitative analysis. Certain adverse events in health care are also uncommon (e.g., wrong site surgery and infant abduction). Well-designed RCAs are therefore reasonable ways to investigate these events. In health care, however, many adverse events occur with sufficient frequency to permit careful study of prevention strategies. The next section addresses the more common situations in which tra-

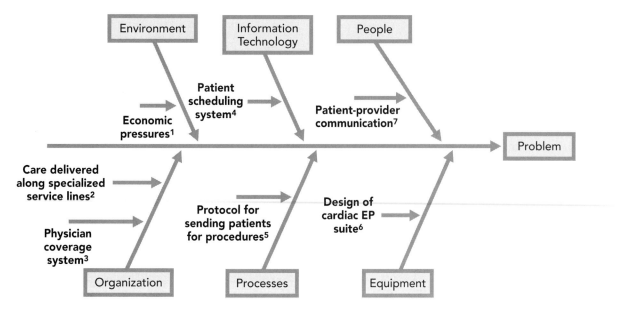

Figure 20.2 Fishbone diagram illustrating categories of latent failures in the "Wrong Patient" case (25).

[1] Economic pressures created some of the organizational strategies (e.g., fragmentation of care along highly specialized "service lines," boarding of patients on floors unfamiliar with that "service line," the physician coverage system, and e-mail scheduling system (all discussed below) that contributed to the errors in this case.

[2] The physicians on the electrophysiology (EP) service at this tertiary referral center had developed a coverage system that allowed them to handle the high volume of consultations from outside hospitals while performing their duties at their own institution. However, this call system meant that the attending and fellow who performed a given EP procedure had often never before met the patient.

[3] The development of specialized services (such as the interventional neuroradiology service that admitted one of the patients and the EP service that admitted the other) increases communication problems and the chance that essential information will slip between the cracks.

[4] The use of an e-mail scheduling system (due to the lack of a systemwide scheduling system) allowed for the occurrence of many minor typographical errors and missing pieces of information (e.g., medical record numbers). Consequently, providers became habituated and indifferent to name discrepancies and did not consistently use patient identification numbers in important communications with other providers.

[5] The hospital had no requirement that an order be present in the chart in order for a patient to be sent off the floor for a test.

[6] The design of the EP suite was such that the attending physician (who in this case had met the correct patient briefly the night before) operated a console behind a window in a room adjacent to the suite, so that the physician could not actually see the patient's face at any time during the procedure.

The patient was taken for the EP procedure despite repeated protests and statements from the patient that she believed there had been a mistake. Physicians and nurses involved in her care assumed she simply did not understand the situation. Routine deficiencies in communication of important issues to patients results in many patients not understanding their medical conditions or plans for their care. As a result, providers expect patients to have misconceptions about tests and procedures, and thus ignore their input, even, as in this case, when the patient is correct.

ditional clinical and epidemiologic research techniques can be applied to improving patient safety.

Evidence-Based Patient Safety Practices

Much of the attention in the literature has focused on large systemwide initiatives, such as acquiring computerized physician order entry or channeling patients to hospitals with high patient volumes. While such initiatives may ultimately prove very powerful quality improvement tools, individual practitioners (or even individual hospitals) will have difficulty implementing sweeping cultural and organizational changes. However, clinicians do have

available to them many evidence-based practices that reduce common complications of hospitalization and do not require major organizational investments (Table 20.4). Other practices related to nosocomial infectious and adverse drug events are discussed in Chapters 21, 66, 68, and 72.

Additional practices and the evidence supporting them are reviewed in *Making Healthcare Safer*, an evidence report sponsored by the federal Agency for Healthcare Quality and Research (20, 21). Readers interested in potential quality improvement activities for their hospital should scan the report's table of contents or the summary chapters listing all of the practices rated by their evidence. The report

TABLE 20.4

SELECTED EVIDENCE-BASED SAFETY PRACTICES CLINICIANS CAN IMPLEMENT WITHOUT LARGE-SCALE INVESTMENTS OF ORGANIZATIONAL RESOURCES

Patient safety target	Patient safety practice
Venous thromboembolism	Appropriate prophylaxis (various strategies) (29)
Perioperative cardiac events in patients undergoing noncardiac surgery	Use of perioperative beta-blockers in selected patients (30)
Mechanical complications from insertion of central venous catheters	Use of real-time ultrasound guidance during central line insertion (31)
Adverse events related to discontinuities in care (15)	Better information transfer between inpatient and outpatient providers (32); follow-up telephone calls after hospital discharge (33)
Radiocontrast-induced nephropathy	Acetylcysteine (plus regular hydration protocol) for diabetics and any patient with chronically elevated Cr (34)
Miscommunication and other problems related to poor teamwork (35)	Teamwork training (e.g., for "code blue" responders) (36)
Unsuspected errors in diagnosis	Obtain more autopsies (37)

covers the complete evidence, implementation issues, potential for harm, and other important aspects of each practice in the specific chapter reviews.

CONCLUSIONS

Improving patient safety incorporates two complementary endeavors. The first, inspired by research in cognitive psychology and the lessons of accident investigation in other industries, provides qualitative methods for anticipating errors, documenting critical incidents, and responding to them in a blame-free and structured manner. Using such qualitative methods, physicians can generate meaningful strategies for preventing similar occurrences in the future. Hospital-based physicians have an important role to play in promoting a culture of safety by championing incident reporting initiatives and participating on multidisciplinary teams that analyze adverse events and promote change.

The second approach involves applying the results of quantitative clinical research to reduce the common hazards of hospitalization. Hospitalists also have an important role to play in this arena because many of these safety targets and the associated clinical practices (especially those that cut across organ-based silos) are not on the radar screens of many hospital-based subspecialists.

In both circumstances, physician collaboration with nurses, pharmacists, nutritionists and other health care professionals would likely produce important improvements in patient care. Moreover, physician involvement in these initiatives will demonstrate visible leadership in promoting a culture of patient safety in hospitals and in health care.

KEY POINTS

- The last few years have seen a new appreciation of the risks of hospitalization, and significant efforts to improve patient safety
- Errors can be classified as slips (inadvertent, unconscious lapses in automatic behaviors) or mistakes (wrong choices). Although the latter may be prevented by education, the former is best addressed by system redesign.
- Detailed error analyses ("Root Cause Analysis") can help identify and help prevent active latent (failures of system design) errors.
- Safety could be markedly improved with widespread implementation of evidence-based safety practices.

REFERENCES

1. Kohn L, Corrigan J, Donaldson M, eds. *To Err Is Human: Building a Safer Health System.* Washington, D.C.: Committee on Quality of Health Care in America, Institute of Medicine. National Academy Press, 2000.
2. McDonald CJ, Weiner M, Hui SL. Deaths due to medical errors are exaggerated in Institute of Medicine report. *JAMA* 2000;284:93–95.
3. Hayward RA, Hofer TP. Estimating hospital deaths due to medical errors: preventability is in the eye of the reviewer. *JAMA* 2001;286:415–420.
4. Thomas EJ, Studdert DM, Runciman WB, et al. A comparison of iatrogenic injury studies in Australia and the USA. I: Context, methods, casemix, population, patient and hospital characteristics. *Int J Qual Health Care* 2000;12:371–378.
5. Brennan TA, Leape LL, Laird NM, et al. Incidence of adverse events and negligence in hospitalized patients. Results of the Harvard Medical Practice Study I. *N Engl J Med* 1991;324:370–376.
6. Thomas EJ, Studdert DM, Burstin HR, et al. Incidence and types of adverse events and negligent care in Utah and Colorado. *Med Care* 2000;38:261–271.
7. Schimmel EM. The hazards of hospitalization. *Ann Intern Med* 1964;60:100–109.

8. Mills DH, ed. *Report on the medical insurance feasibility study / sponsored jointly by California Medical Association and California Hospital Association*. San Francisco: Sutter Publications, Inc., 1977.

9. Steel K, Gertman PM, Crescenzi C, et al. Iatrogenic illness on a general medical service at a university hospital. *N Engl J Med* 1981;304:638–642.

10. Leape LL, Brennan TA, Laird N, et al. The nature of adverse events in hospitalized patients. Results of the Harvard Medical Practice Study II. *N Engl J Med* 1991;324:377–384.

11. Bates DW, Cullen DJ, Laird N, et al. Incidence of adverse drug events and potential adverse drug events. Implications for prevention. ADE Prevention Study Group. *JAMA* 1995;274:29–34.

12. Classen DC, Pestotnik SL, Evans RS, et al. Adverse drug events in hospitalized patients. Excess length of stay, extra costs, and attributable mortality. *JAMA* 1997;277:301–306.

13. Andrews LB, Stocking C, Krizek T, et al. An alternative strategy for studying adverse events in medical care. *Lancet* 1997;349: 309–313.

14. Studdert DM, Thomas EJ, Burstin HR, et al. Negligent care and malpractice claiming behavior in Utah and Colorado. *Med Care* 2000;38:250–260.

15. Forster AJ, Murff HJ, Peterson JF, et al. The incidence and severity of adverse events affecting patients after discharge from the hospital. *Ann Intern Med* 2003;138:161–167.

16. Sox HCJ, Woloshin S. How many deaths are due to medical error? Getting the number right. *Eff Clin Pract* 2000;3:277–283.

17. Shojania KG, Wald H, Gross R. Understanding medical error and improving patient safety in the inpatient setting. *Med Clin North Am* 2002;86:847–867.

18. Chassin MR. Is health care ready for Six Sigma quality? *Milbank Q* 1998;76:565–591, 510.

19. Lagasse RS. Anesthesia safety: model or myth?: a review of the published literature and analysis of current original data. *Anesthesiology* 2002;97:1609–1617.

20. Shojania KG, Duncan BW, McDonald KM, et al., eds. Making health care safer: a critical analysis of patient safety practices. Evidence Report/Technology Assessment No. 43 from the Agency for Healthcare Research and Quality: AHRQ Publication No. 01-E058; 2001.

21. Shojania KG, Duncan BW, McDonald KM, et al. Safe but sound: patient safety meets evidence-based medicine. *JAMA* 2002;288: 508–513.

22. Reason JT. *Human Error*. New York: Cambridge Univ Press, 1990.

23. Leape LL. Error in medicine. *JAMA* 1994;272:1851–1857.

24. Vincent C. Understanding and responding to adverse events. *N Engl J Med* 2003;348:1051–1056.

25. Chassin MR, Becher EC. The wrong patient. *Ann Intern Med* 2002; 136:826–833.

26. Wachter RM, Shojania KG, Saint S, et al. Learning from our mistakes: quality grand rounds, a new case-based series on medical errors and patient safety. *Ann Intern Med* 2002;136:850–852.

27. Rex JH, Turnbull JE, Allen SJ, et al. Systematic root cause analysis of adverse drug events in a tertiary referral hospital. *Jt Comm J Qual Improv* 2000;26:563–575.

28. West DW, Levine S, Magram G, et al. Pediatric medication order error rates related to the mode of order transmission. *Arch Pediatr Adolesc Med* 1994;148:1322–1326.

29. Geerts WH, Heit JA, Clagett GP, et al. Prevention of venous thromboembolism. *Chest* 2001;119(1 Suppl):132S-175S.

30. Auerbach AD, Goldman L. Beta-blockers and reduction of cardiac events in noncardiac surgery: scientific review. *JAMA* 2002;287: 1435–1444.

31. Hind D, Calvert N, McWilliams R, et al. Ultrasonic locating devices for central venous cannulation: meta-analysis. *BMJ* 2003;327:361–360.

32. Cook RI, Render M, Woods DD. Gaps in the continuity of care and progress on patient safety. *BMJ* 2000;320:791–794.

33. Dudas V, Bookwalter T, Kerr KM, et al. The impact of follow-up telephone calls to patients after hospitalization. *Am J Med* 2001;111:26S-30S.

34. Birck R, Krzossok S, Markowetz F, et al. Acetylcysteine for prevention of contrast nephropathy: meta-analysis. *Lancet* 2003;362: 598–603.

35. Sexton JB, Thomas EJ, Helmreich RL. Error, stress, and teamwork in medicine and aviation: cross sectional surveys. *BMJ* 2000;320:745–749.

36. Morey JC, Simon R, Jay GD, et al. Error reduction and performance improvement in the emergency department through formal teamwork training: evaluation results of the MedTeams project. *Health Serv Res* 2002;37:1553–1581.

37. Shojania KG, Burton EC, McDonald KM, et al. Changes in rates of autopsy-detected diagnostic errors over time: a systematic review. *JAMA* 2003;289:2849–2856.

ADDITIONAL READING

Wachter RM, Shojania KG. *Internal Bleeding: The Truth Behind America's Terrifying Epidemic of Medical Mistakes*. New York: Rugged Land, 2004.

Medication Safety in the Hospital

21

David W. Bates

INTRODUCTION

The study that provides the best estimates regarding the risk of hospitalization is the Harvard Medical Practice Study, which evaluated the frequency of iatrogenic injury in patients discharged from hospitals in New York in 1984 (1, 2). Its primary outcome was the "adverse event," defined as an injury caused by medical management that resulted in disability at discharge or a prolonged length of stay. The study found that adverse events occurred in 3.7% of hospitalizations, and 28% of these were judged negligent. The most frequent cause of injury in this study was the adverse drug event, or injury because of a drug, and these accounted for 19% of adverse events.

CARE OF THE HOSPITALIZED PATIENT

Of the main types of adverse events, adverse drug events (ADEs) have received perhaps the most study. In one study, Bates et al. (3) found 6.5 ADEs per 100 admissions in nonobstetric units in a tertiary care hospital; 28% of these were judged preventable. Of the life-threatening and serious ADEs, 42% were preventable, compared with 18% of significant but non-life-threatening ADEs. Errors resulting in a preventable ADE were more likely to be at the ordering (56%) and administration (34%) stages than at the transcription (6%) or dispensing (4%) stages. A key difference between this and previous studies was that all errors that either resulted in or had the potential to result in an ADE were subjected to a systems analysis by multidisciplinary teams (4). These analyses identified 16 major systems failures as the underlying causes of the errors. Seven of these accounted for 78% of the errors; all could have been im-

proved by *better information systems.* The most common defects were in the systems for disseminating knowledge about drugs, and for making drug and patient information available at the time it was needed.

In fact, many of the current "systems" used in medicine were never consciously designed by anyone and, in effect, just evolved in a haphazard and less than rational manner (3). For example, the "allergy detection system" in many hospitals consists of having several people ask patients about their allergies, including the nurse, the attending physician, one or more residents, and sometimes a medical student or pharmacist, although none of these persons is specifically responsible for this issue. Many of them note the allergies in the hospital chart, but such notations are not necessarily recorded in a central location, and there is often no communication with the outpatient record. The pharmacist may check for allergies by reading the physician's order and then visually comparing one list (the ordered medications) with another (the allergy list). Not surprisingly, this highly inefficient system allows a number of orders for drugs to which patients have known allergies to slip through (3). However, this system can be redesigned to put all records of drug allergies in one central electronic location, where they can be mapped by drug family and subsequent orders can be checked for problems. Any allergies detected can be displayed to the ordering clinician.

In addition to studies of adverse drug events, many medication studies have focused on medication errors, defined as an error in ordering, dispensing, administering, or monitoring a drug. These errors are common, making them easier to study than adverse drug events. However, most do not result in injury. For example, one study found that 7 in 100 medication errors had the potential to cause an injury and 1 in 100 actually did so (Figure 21.1) (5). Medication

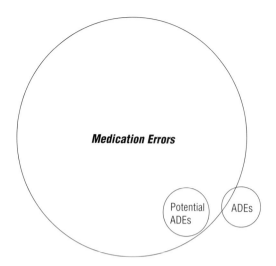

Figure 21.1 Relationships between medication errors, potential adverse drug events (medication errors with the potential to cause injury), and adverse drug events (ADEs). Only a proportion (28% in the Adverse Drug Events Prevention Study) are preventable. (From Bates DW, Boyle DL, Vander Vliet MB, et al. Relationship between medication errors and adverse drug events. *J Gen Intern Med* 1995;10:201, with permission.)

errors almost certainly differ substantially in their propensity to result in injury. For example, a 5-fold overdose may actually be more dangerous than a 100-fold overdose, because it is much more likely to be carried out.

Medication-related risk does not abate when the patient goes home; in fact, the immediate post-discharge period is especially risky. In a recent study, 19% of patients who had just been discharged from a medical service had adverse events, and 66% of these events were adverse drug events (6). Many of these adverse drug events might have been prevented.

MEDICATION SAFETY IMPROVEMENT STRATEGIES

A multidisciplinary panel that included nurses, pharmacists, and physicians made seven key recommendations about actions that organizations could take to reduce the number of ADEs (Table 21.1) (7). Among these, the most powerful is implementation of a systems change: *computerized physician order entry* (CPOE). In two recent studies, such a system prevented 55% to 86% of serious medication errors that otherwise would have reached the patient (8, 9). With CPOE, all orders are legible, and input is structured so that each medication order includes a drug name, dose, route, and frequency. Doses are selected from menus that include only appropriate options, which minimizes the likelihood that too high a dose will be ordered. In addition, orders can be checked for drug allergies, drug-drug interactions, and drug-laboratory interactions. Finally, dosing guidelines for specific drugs, such as aminoglycosides and

heparin, can be displayed, and the computer can calculate doses and recommend monitoring for these agents, which improves outcomes for drugs such as heparin (10) (see also Chapter 10).

When prescriptions are written by hand, the use of abbreviations can cause problems. Although computerization of ordering can minimize many of these issues, most drug orders are still written with the pen. Following the recommendations of the Medication Error and Reporting Program (Table 21.2) (7), which mainly involve avoiding potentially problematic abbreviations, can minimize the likelihood of many such errors.

A variety of additional strategies can improve medication safety. Access to drug knowledge is important, and many applications are now available for handheld devices that can make it easy for physicians to access this information, even if their hospital does not utilize CPOE (11). Bar coding has been used widely in other industries, and, though few published data are available to date regarding its impact in medication dispensing and administration, it is probably beneficial (12, 13). "Smart pumps" are infusion pumps that can be told what medication is being given, and, if too high a dose of medication is entered, the pump can warn the nurse. Importantly, these pumps can also retain a log of what was done, including overrides. Having pharmacists round with the team in the intensive care unit also reduced serious prescribing errors (14). Because a number of these strategies address stages of the medication process other than prescribing, it is likely that to achieve a

TABLE 21.1

TOP-PRIORITY ACTIONS FOR PREVENTING ADVERSE DRUG EVENTS IN HOSPITALS: RECOMMENDATIONS OF AN AMERICAN SOCIETY OF HEALTH SYSTEM PHARMACISTS CONVENED EXPERT PANEL

1. Hospitals should establish processes in which prescribers enter medication orders directly into computer systems.
2. Hospitals should evaluate the use of machine-readable coding (e.g., bar coding) in their medication use processes.
3. Hospitals should develop better systems for monitoring and reporting adverse drug events.
4. Hospitals should use unit dose medication distribution and pharmacy-based intravenous admixture systems.
5. Hospitals should assign pharmacists to work in patient care areas in direct collaboration with prescribers and those administering medications.
6. Hospitals should approach medication errors as systems failures and seek systems solutions for preventing them.
7. Hospitals should ensure that medication orders are routinely reviewed by a pharmacist before first doses and should ensure that prescribers, pharmacists, nurses, and other health workers seek resolution whenever there is any question of safety regarding medication use.

From ASHP guidelines on preventing medication errors in hospitals. *Am J Hosp Pharm* 1993;50:305–314, with permission.

TABLE 21.2

DANGEROUS ABBREVIATIONS AS DEFINED BY THE NATIONAL COORDINATING COUNCIL FOR MEDICATION ERROR REPORTING AND PREVENTION

Abbreviation	Intended meaning[a]	Common error
U	Units	Mistaken for a zero (0) or a four (4), resulting in overdose; also mistaken for "cc" (cubic centimeters) when poorly written.
μg	Micrograms	Mistaken for "mg" (milligrams) resulting in overdose.
Q.D.	Latin abbreviation for daily	The period after the "Q" has sometimes been mistaken for an "I," for every day, and the drug has been given "QID" (four times daily) rather than daily.
Q.O.D.	Latin abbreviation for every other day	Misinterpreted as "QD" (daily) or "QID" (four times daily). If the "O" is poorly written, it looks like a period or an "I."
SC or SQ	Subcutaneous	Mistaken for "SL" (sublingual) when poorly written.
TIW	Three times a week	Misinterpreted as "three times a day" or "twice a week."
D/C	Discharge; also discontinue	Patient's medications have been prematurely discontinued when D/C (intended to mean "discharge") was misinterpreted as "discontinue" because it was followed by a list of drugs.
HS	Half strength	Misinterpreted as the Latin abbreviation "HS" (hour of sleep).
cc	Cubic centimeters	Mistaken as "U" (units) when poorly written.
AU, AS, AD	Latin abbreviation for both ears; left ear; right ear	Misinterpreted as the Latin abbreviation "OU" (both eyes); "OS" (left eye); "OD" (right eye).

[a] In general, these errors can be prevented by spelling out the full word (e.g., "units," "micrograms") instead of using the abbreviation, or by using a computerized order entry.
From U.S. Pharmacopeia. *Drug Information for the Health Care Professional*. Rockville, MD: U.S. Pharmacopeial Convention, 1998, with permission.

large improvement in medication safety it will be important to use many of them simultaneously.

Regarding post-discharge adverse drug events, one study found that a follow-up phone call by a pharmacist involved in the patient's hospitalization was associated with increased patient satisfaction, resolution of medication-related problems, and fewer return visits to the emergency department (15). Scheduling early post-hospital follow-up with the primary care provider or hospitalist is also important.

Monitoring for Adverse Drug Events

Hospitals need to monitor routinely for adverse drug events and use the data to improve quality, without punishing the persons involved unless a repeated pattern of error is identified. Some types of monitoring are required by regulatory agencies, but for adverse drug events, most hospitals rely on spontaneous reporting, an insensitive method that identifies few events (about 1 in 20 ADEs) (16).

A major problem with routine human surveillance is the cost, which is sufficiently high to make it impractical for relatively rare problems like serious adverse drug events. However, computerized searching can be used to look for a variety of events inexpensively by looking for signals, such as use of an antidote (such as Narcan or Flumazemil) or high serum drug levels (17, 18), and it is increasingly available. Computerized adverse drug event monitoring will likely soon become the main strategy for looking for adverse drug events.

Regardless, it is still important for clinicians to report medication safety issues that they identify to their hospital safety program. These reports can be aggregated to help prioritize safety strategies.

Cost Considerations and Resource Use

Adverse drug events are expensive in addition to being harmful to patients. For example, two studies addressing the cost to a hospital of an ADE reached estimates of approximately $2,000 per event (19,20), even though these figures exclude the costs of malpractice, admissions resulting from ADEs, and injuries to patients. In one of the studies, the costs of a preventable ADE were higher, at $4,600 (20). For a 700-bed hospital, the yearly figures are $5.6 million for all ADEs and $2.8 million for the preventable events (20). Nationally, ADEs occurring during hospitalization have been estimated to cost $2 billion per year (17, 21), and admissions caused by ADEs may cost at least as much. Taken together, these data suggest that such events are not only highly undesirable for patients but also extremely costly to the health care system, and they justify investment in strategies for preventing them.

CONCLUSIONS

By judiciously adding the use of technology in the medication process, most hospitals should soon be able to substantially improve medication safety, thereby becoming more rewarding places for physicians to practice. Particularly important prevention strategies include computerized physician order entry, bar coding, "smart" intravenous pumps, and having pharmacists round with care teams.

KEY POINTS

- Adverse drug events are common and costly in both human and economic terms.
- About one-third of adverse drug events are preventable.
- A systems approach that utilizes the theory of error and integrates electronic information tools has the best chance of reducing adverse drug event rates in hospitalized patients.

REFERENCES

1. Brennan TA, Leape LL, Laird N, et al. Incidence of adverse events and negligence in hospitalized patients: results from the Harvard Medical Practice Study I. *N Engl J Med* 1991;324:370–376.
2. Leape LL, Brennan TA, Laird NM, et al. The nature of adverse events in hospitalized patients: results from the Harvard Medical Practice Study II. *N Engl J Med* 1991;324:377–384.
3. Bates DW, Cullen D, Laird N, et al. Incidence of adverse drug events and potential adverse drug events: implications for prevention. *JAMA* 1995;274:29–34.
4. Leape LL, Bates DW, Cullen DJ, et al. Systems analysis of adverse drug events. *JAMA* 1995;274:35–43.
5. Bates DW, Boyle DL, Vander Vliet MB, et al. Relationship between medication errors and adverse drug events. *J Gen Intern Med* 1995;10:199–205.
6. Forster AJ, Murff HJ, Peterson JF, et al. The incidence and severity of adverse events affecting patients after discharge from the hospital. *Ann Intern Med* 2003;138:161–167.
7. ASHP guidelines on preventing medication errors in hospitals. *Am J Hosp Pharm* 1993;50:305–314.
8. Bates DW, Leape LL, Cullen DJ, et al. Effect of computerized physician order entry and a team intervention on prevention of serious medication errors. *JAMA* 1998;280:1311–1316.
9. Bates DW, Teich J, Lee J, et al. The impact of computerized physician order entry on medication error prevention. *J Am Med Inform Assoc* 1999;6:313–321.
10. Raschke RA, Reilly BM, Guidry JR, et al. The weight-based heparin nomogram compared with a "standard care" nomogram. *Ann Intern Med* 1993;119:874–881.
11. Rothschild JM, Lee TH, Bae T, et al. Clinician use of a palmtop drug reference guide. *J Am Med Inform Assoc* 2002;9:223–229.
12. Bates DW. Using information technology to reduce rates of medication errors in hospitals. *BMJ* 2000;320:788–791.
13. Bates DW, Gawande AA. Improving safety with information technology. *N Engl J Med* 2003;348:2526–2534.
14. Leape LL, Cullen DJ, Clapp MD, et al. Pharmacist participation on physician rounds and adverse drug events in the intensive care unit. *JAMA* 1999;282:267–270.
15. Dudas V, Bookwalter T, Kerr KM, et al. The impact of follow-up telephone calls to patients after hospitalization. *Disease-A-Month* 2002;48:239–248.
16. Cullen DJ, Bates DW, Small SD, et al. The incident reporting system does not detect adverse drug events: a problem for quality improvement. *Jt Comm J Qual Improv* 1995;21:541–548.
17. Jha AK, Kuperman GJ, Teich JM, et al. Identifying adverse drug events: development of a computer-based monitor and comparison with chart review and stimulated voluntary report. *J Am Med Inform Assoc* 1998;5:305–314.
18. Classen DC, Pestotnik SL, Evans RS, et al. Computerized surveillance of adverse drug events in hospital patients. *JAMA* 1991;266:2847–2851.
19. Classen DC, Pestotnik SL, Evans RS, et al. Adverse drug events in hospitalized patients. Excess length of stay, extra costs, and attributable mortality. *JAMA* 1997;277:301–306.
20. Bates DW, Spell N, Cullen D, et al. The costs of adverse drug events in hospitalized patients. *JAMA* 1997;227:307–311.
21. Yerdel MA, Karayalcin K, Aras N, et al. Mechanical complications of subclavian vein catheterization. A prospective study. *Int Surg* 1991;76:18–22.

ADDITIONAL READING

Bates DW, O'Neil AC, Petersen LA, et al. Evaluation of screening criteria for adverse events in medical patients. *Med Care* 1995;33:452–462.

Leape LL, Lawthers AG, Brennan TA, et al. Preventing medical injury. *QRB Qual Rev Bull* 1993;19:144–149.

Reason J. *Human Error.* Cambridge, UK: Cambridge University Press, 1990.

Critical Care Medicine

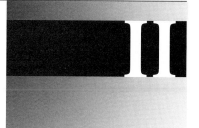

Approach to the ICU Patient

22

Neal H. Cohen

INTRODUCTION

The intensive care unit (ICU) has become one of the major locations for the in-hospital care of both medical and surgical patients. In the United States, approximately 4 million ICU admissions per year cost about $60 billion per year. (1) Equipping and maintaining the technology required to care for critically ill patients is expensive due to both capital costs and the ongoing requirements to maintain the diverse and skilled group of providers needed to deliver the complex care that is required in the ICU setting.

Over the past decade, new pharmacologic agents, different modes of mechanical ventilation, and other new technologies have led to improved outcomes, but mortality remains between about 8% and 19% (2, 3). The variability in the mortality rate is due to many factors, including different patient populations, the skills of the providers, and the degree to which all the critical skills and resources can be brought together to improve clinical management. This variability in outcomes highlights both the economic and ethical dilemmas that must be addressed each time a patient is admitted, as well as the importance of developing administrative and clinical management strategies to optimize care.

This chapter will describe clinical and administrative approaches to the management of the ICU and the care of critically ill patients. It will address some of the challenges and emphasize how problems can be addressed in a cooperative and collaborative manner with a team of providers who bring a broad base of knowledge and skills to the varying needs of ICU patients.

(RE)DEFINING THE CRITICAL CARE UNIT

ICUs were originally created in the 1960s to centralize nursing staff as well as high-cost monitoring and therapeutic equipment in a single environment within the hospital. Although ICUs were originally designed to care for patients who had respiratory failure and also required mechanical ventilatory support, the clinical capabilities and diversity of patients in ICUs have expanded dramatically. At the same time, the definition of an ICU has become more diffuse, and the differentiation between an ICU and other inpatient settings has become less obvious.

Despite this variability, some specific services are available only in the ICU setting. First, the ICU is designed to provide a therapeutic environment that centralizes clinical resources and nursing staff at a higher provider to patient ratio with immediate availability of highly skilled staff. Second, in most hospitals, specific technologies, such as mechanical ventilation for patients with acute respiratory distress, continuous renal replacement therapy, invasive hemodynamic monitoring, and titration of vasopressor and inotropic agents to support hemodynamics and myocardial function, are available only in the ICU environment. Because of the variability in skills required from one ICU to another, and the variability in the patient population from one hospital to another, the approach to each critically ill patient must be flexible enough to take advantage of an institution's capabilities and the skills and training of the staff. Finally, because of the varying capabilities and clinical needs, a given patient might require ICU care in one hospital, but be adequately cared for in a transitional care unit or telemetry unit in another. In larger hospitals and those with specialty services that can support service-specific ICUs, special units have been created to focus care on subsets of patients who have specific physiologic problems (cardiac disease, medical vs. surgical ICUs) or have had certain types of surgical procedures (cardiac surgery, transplant, neurosurgery). For many community hospitals, however, multidisciplinary units remain more common.

One of the biggest challenges for the physician who cares for patients with critical illness is to define each patient's clinical needs and understand how and where best to address them. The hospital-based physician must be knowledgeable about the models of care that are available to the patient, the skill set of the providers, and whether there are dedicated intensive care physicians, respiratory therapists or other staff to assist in patient management. In addition, physicians must understand what services can be provided only in an ICU setting and which ones might be available in a less intensive environment, so that patients can be triaged to optimize the utilization of hospital services. For hospitals with telemetry capability in non-ICU settings, for example, most patients who require cardiac monitoring do not require ICU admission.

ORGANIZATION OF INTENSIVE CARE UNITS

The organization model for the ICU varies from one institution to another—and in many cases within a hospital in units that care for different types of patients. Nevertheless, ceratin principles are fundamental to a successful ICU.

Administrative and Clinical Oversight

Although no single administrative approach is appropriate for every ICU, each unit must have a medical director and a nurse manager. The *medical director* is responsible for setting standards for clinical practice within the ICU and for working with the nurse manager to define staffing patterns, the necessary mix of skills, and the relationships among the physicians, nurses, and other providers. The medical director may be trained in one of many medical specialties, but most commonly the ICU director in medium- and large-size hospitals has specialty training in medicine, pulmonary medicine, cardiology, anesthesiology, or surgery. Critical care medicine, now a recognized subspecialty, crosses multiple medical disciplines. In the United States, critical care medicine training is available as an added qualification after training in internal medicine or its subspecialties, especiallly pulmonary medicine and cardiology. Formal training in critical care medicine can also follow certification in anesthesiology, surgery, or pediatrics.

Many larger hospitals typically have specialty units whose medical directors are trained in the ICU's area of specialized emphasis. Examples include neurologic ICUs (increasingly prevalent as a result of recent advances in the care of patients with acute stroke and neurovascular disease), and perinatal units for hospitals with large obstetric populations. These proliferating models of care create challenges and opportunities, particularly for the hospitalists who will participate in the care of their patients.

As the pool of physicians trained in critical care has expanded and their value documented, the Leapfrog Group has defined standards for critical care coverage in ICUs (Table 22.1) (3, 4). However, many smaller hospitals cannot support an ICU physician, so the skills needed to optimize patient care must be provided by a group of providers who work together to ensure that the patient receives required care.

In smaller hospitals, the ICU census is typically small, the needs of patients are variable, and physicians certified in critical care are infrequently available (5). To overcome this staffing deficit, many hospitalists have acquired skills to provide these critical care needs. In some cases, the hospitalist communicates with and coordinates care with critical care physicians located elsewhere in the community or within the health care system. In other models, "virtual" ICU care is coordinated by remote physicians who monitor patients electronically, review real time clinical data, perform remote clinical examinations, and visually observe patients by video camera. The critical care physician then communicates with the physician or nurse at the bedside and assists with clinical decision-making. Early studies support the premise that this model can help ensure the availability of critical care support to patients who might not otherwise have access to it (6).

ICU care requires participation by a variety of physicians. Some are unit-based (the intensivists), whereas some participate as primary care providers, hospitalists, or consultants. In general, the ICU physician will facilitate

TABLE 22.1

THE LEAPFROG STANDARDS FOR ICUs[a]

ICUs are managed or co-managed by intensivists who:
1. Are present during daytime hours
2. Provide clinical care exclusively in the ICU
3. When not in the ICU, can (at least 95% of the time):
   a. Return ICU pages within 5 minutes, and
   b. Arrange for a FCCS-certified non-physician effector to reach patients within 5 minutes

In addition, partial credit is given to ICUs that do not meet 1–3, but in which:
4. Intensivists lead daily, multidisciplinary rounds or make admission and discharge decisions on weekdays
5. "Teleintensivist" coverage (6) is used

FCCS = Fundamental Critical Care Support course
[a] www.leapfroggroup.org. Accessed January 10, 2005.

coordination of care, although in some settings either the hospitalist or the primary provider will serve in that role. This coordinated model of care (i.e., intensivist and hospitalist) can not only improve management in the ICU, but also foster care throughout the hospital stay and facilitate transition of the patient from the ICU to other settings (transitional care, extended care, skilled nursing care).

In addition to physicians, the ICU must have a *nurse manager* who is responsible for staffing and oversight of the nurses and ancillary personnel. The medical director and nurse manager share responsibility for developing policies and procedures and establishing a quality-assurance program to ensure that care is delivered within accepted standards. As requested by regulatory agencies such as the Joint Commission for Accreditation of Healthcare Organizations (JCAHO), the unit should also have *written policies and procedures for all aspects of care,* including admission and discharge criteria and authority, triage procedures, clinical management procedures, and disaster planning. Because the care provided within the ICU is part of a continuum of care, the quality-assurance activities should be integrated with institutional quality-assurance or quality-improvement programs (see also Chaper 12). The ICU staff should define mechanisms to monitor patient care activity, define the standards of care provided to patients within the ICU, and determine if care is below the standard.

Quality improvement initiatives are most easily integrated into ICUs with a uniform patient population that requires common clinical services. By comparison, multidisciplinary critical care units, which provide care to a wider spectrum of patients, require more complex quality-assessment methods to address the needs of varying patient populations and to assure that the staff has the skills necessary to care for these patients. Nonetheless, these activities are essential if care is to be safe and consistent with the current knowledge.

Quality improvement activities must respond to changes in clinical management and institution of new therapeutic approaches. For example, the introduction of continuous renal replacement therapies has significantly influenced fluid and electrolyte management for some critically ill patients. Reengineering efforts designed to reduce the use of laboratory tests, alter the timing for institution of hyperalimentation, or modify other therapeutic interventions must account for these changes in clinical management.

Because of the interdependent nature of ICU care, all physicians and other key providers must participate in quality improvement and reengineering efforts. For example, the institution of clinical protocols that allow the nurse or respiratory therapist to manage patients more directly can be very effective and appropriate (7, 8). However, these protocols change how and when the providers communicate, and modify the roles and responsibilities of the physicians. Similarly, a decision to change the nursing skill mix can be made only after careful consideration of the impact of the change on physicians' expectations and

interactions. Without this interdisciplinary approach to solving problems, attempts to refine practice will fail, and patient care will suffer.

Morbidity and mortality review is also an essential evaluative tool to assess the quality of care and the outcomes associated with ICU care. Traditional morbidity and mortality reviews typically are conducted on a departmental basis, with evaluation of isolated adverse events. For ICU patients, multidisciplinary morbidity and mortality reviews should include the participation of providers from all departments involved in patient care. The goal of the review is twofold: (1) to assess whether the delivered care was appropriate and (2) to determine if the approaches to care should be modified to improve care for future patients.

The "Open" vs. "Closed" Models of Care: An Arbitrary Distinction

In terms of the roles of physicians, an ICU can be "open" or "closed." In an open unit, the patient has a primary admitting physician who will manage and coordinate care in both the ICU and elsewhere in the hospital before and/or after their stay. This physician may be the patient's outpatient physician, a hospitalist, or a surgeon who performed a procedure. A patient's care may also be transferred to a hospitalist at the time of ICU admission, such as when a surgical patient suffers postoperative complications. In either case, in an open ICU, the primary hospital physician continues to coordinate the care of the patient after transfer to the ICU and to serve as the legally responsible physician. In this model, the ICU physicians and other physicians become consultants to the primary provider. The extent of involvement by the ICU physician varies from one unit to another. In most open units, the ICU physician provides emergency and resuscitative care and may be responsible for airway management, ventilatory support, and emergency care. The extent to which the ICU physician provides more comprehensive care will depend on the skills and availability of the primary physician. Although both the primary care and ICU physicians participate in clinical decision-making, primary responsibility stays with the patient's admitting physician rather than with the ICU consultant (see also Chapter 28).

In the "closed" ICU model, the primary responsibility for the patient's ICU care is assumed by the ICU physician. In this model, ICU physicians are immediately available, often because they are continuously present within the ICU. In closed ICU models, neither the patient's outpatient physician nor any other physician involved (such as a hospitalist or surgeon) makes minute-to-minute clinical decisions or writes routine orders.

The differences between the open and closed models are not as obvious as they might seem. Because of the complexity of ICU care and the diverse clinical needs of ICU patients, care *must* be coordinated. All physicians who have knowledge of the patient's clinical condition (both acute and chronic) should participate in decision-making, even if the ultimate authority for writing orders and making clinical plans rests with one of them, as it must.

Both open and closed models can be successful, but the closed unit has been demonstrated to improve patient care outcomes, and optimize the utilization of resources (3, 9). However, it should be noted that the outcome studies comparing open with closed models were in hospitals in which open models used primary care physicians or traditional (non-hospitalist) ward attendings. To date, there are no studies comparing open model ICUs using hospitalists with closed ICUs, nor studies comparing hybrid models in which intensivists and hospitalists share management responsibilities for patients. Future research in this area will be vitally important (see also Chapter 1).

Whichever model is employed, the key component to providing optimal patient care is ongoing communication among all providers, including critical care physicians, consultants, hospital-based physicians, and the primary care physician. With an ongoing dialogue, all aspects of patient care can be addressed, longstanding relationships with the patient can be maintained, and the transfer of care into and out of the ICU can be achieved without compromising quality.

Key Roles for Non-Physician Staff in the ICU

In addition to physician staffing needs, the ICU requires trained nursing staff, respiratory therapists, and ancillary staff. In some units, only registered nurses are used; in others, the staff includes a combination of registered nurses and licensed vocational nurses. The nurse-to-patient ratio in most ICU settings is either 1:1 or 1:2. Some states mandate ICU nurse-to-patient ratios and the skill mix. In all cases, however, the ratio is dependent on clinical needs and the extent to which ancillary personnel can assume some responsibilities of care.

Staffing patterns have a major impact on the roles and responsibilities of the physicians caring for ICU patients. For example, an experienced ICU nurse often is able to anticipate problems before they occur and notify the physician of subtle changes in the patient's condition. Less skilled personnel may be able to help treat complications when they occur, but be less adept at anticipating them. The relationships among the physicians and the other staff members depend on an understanding of the clinical capabilities and experience of each provider, and a clear delineation of responsibilities.

Other providers are also key to the care of the ICU patient. For example, skilled respiratory therapists can provide a number of diagnostic and therapeutic interventions that can reduce costs, morbidity, and length of ICU stay. Intensive respiratory care, including continuous monitoring of pulmonary function and gas exchange, has allowed early recognition of respiratory failure and rapid institution of interventions (e.g., bronchodilators)

to prevent it. Alternative lung-expansion therapies, including positive expiratory pressure therapy and noninvasive ventilation, also can be provided. In many cases, the expertise of respiratory therapists can prevent the need for tracheal intubation and prolonged mechanical ventilatory support. As ventilator technology has become more sophisticated, the respiratory therapist also often is able to help determine the best mode of ventilation to optimize gas exchange and minimize the complications of positive pressure ventilation.

Emergent airway management is an essential component of ICU care. In most hospitals, tracheal intubation is the responsibility of anesthesiologists, critical care physicians, or emergency-medicine physicians. For hospitals that do not have in-hospital physicians, airway management is usually the responsibility of the respiratory care staff. The physician caring for the ICU patient should understand who is available to provide emergency airway management, their level of skill and experience, and which additional personnel are available to assist if tracheal intubation is difficult or impossible, and if tracheostomy or emergency cricothyroidotomy is necessary.

Physical and rehabilitative therapists, social workers, clinical nurse specialists, pharmacists, and case managers also can significantly improve patient care (see also Chapter 4). For example, the clinical nurse specialist can monitor the quality of care delivered by the nursing staff and teach new skills to improve patient care. Case managers often can help define the appropriate use of clinical resources and facilitate the disposition of the patient when ICU care is no longer required. The physician caring for the ICU patient should interact regularly with these providers and be aware of their skills and experience to maximize the benefit from ICU care and, if appropriate, identify alternatives to the ICU. Most importantly, in all of these examples, the development of clinical protocols that guide management and allow appropriate staff to modify care without waiting for a physician's order will not only minimize delays in care, but also improve care and reduce costs (10).

CARE OF THE CRITICALLY ILL PATIENT

Indications for ICU Admission

New technologies and transitional or intermediate care units have influenced the indications for ICU admission. In some hospitals, services previously restricted to the ICU are now available in other units within the hospital. Furthermore, the indications for ICU admission vary from one institution to another, and often vary from one ICU to another within a hospital. Although the value of the ICU care has traditionally been to optimize nursing care, the need to provide care in an ICU environment is now broader.

With improved understanding of the pathophysiologic mechanisms of critical illness and increased technologic

TABLE 22.2

SOME COMMON INDICATIONS FOR ICU ADMISSION

Acute myocardial infarction
Pericardial tamponade
Cardiogenic pulmonary edema
Hemodynamic instability
  Hypotension, unresponsive to moderate fluid resuscitation or necessitating vasopressor or inotropic therapy
  Hypertensive crisis
Arrhythmias
  Supraventricular arrhythmias associated with hemodynamic instability
  Ventricular arrhythmias
Eclampsia, preeclampsia
Pulmonary disorders
  Compromised gas exchange with superimposed hemodynamic instability
  Acute noncompensated respiratory acidosis
  Hypoxemia, necessitating high flow oxygen therapy
  Respiratory failure necessitating mechanical ventilatory support
  Noncardiogenic pulmonary edema, acute respiratory distress syndrome
Neurologic disorders
  Acute stroke
  Neurologic deficit associated with increased intracranial pressure
  Intracerebral aneurysm with acute bleed
  Acute subarachnoid blood
  Severe traumatic brain injury with Glasgow Coma Scale <9
  Unstable cervical spinal cord injury
  Neuromuscular disease with compromised respiratory status
  External ventricular drainage system
  Status epilepticus
Renal dysfunction
  Acute renal failure necessitating continuous renal replacement therapy
  Life-threatening electrolyte abnormalities
  Metabolic disorder with compromised airway
Gastrointestinal disorders
  Hemorrhage associated with hypotension unresponsive to fluid resuscitation

Acute pancreatitis associated with hemodynamic instability
Liver failure complicated by encephalopathy, renal failure, electrolyte imbalance
Hematologic disorders
  Bleeding disorders necessitating transfusion of large amounts of blood and clotting factors
  Acute leukemia complicated by airway compromise, septic shock, respiratory failure
Infectious disease
  Sepsis and septic shock associated with hypotension, hemodynamic instability
Endocrine diseases
  Diabetic ketoacidosis with hemodynamic instability
  Hyperosmolar coma
  Thyrotoxicosis associated with hemodynamic instability
  Severe myxedema
  Diabetes insipidus associated with severe fluid and electrolyte abnormalities
  Marked hypothermia
Drug ingestion, overdose
  Any overdose or ingestion associated with inability to protect airway
  Ingestion of a drug associated with arrhythmias or hemodynamic instability
Postoperative patients
  Hemodynamic instability, excessive bleeding or coagulopathy following major surgical procedure
  Postoperative patient requiring mechanical ventilatory support, vasopressor or inotropic therapy
  Perioperative myocardial infarction necessitating hemodynamic monitoring or infusion of vasoactive drugs
Miscellaneous
  Severe hypothermia associated with electrocardiographic changes
  Patients at very high risk for airway compromise, respiratory failure, sepsis

capabilities to diagnose and treat complex medical problems, the indications for ICU admission (see Table 22.2) include the need for care by specially trained critical care physicians. Timely observation and assessment for *impending* clinical problems, rather than just treating the problems that have already occurred, has been an increasingly important goal of ICU care.

ICU care is ultimately required for a number of specific clinical indications. For example, patients in need of mechanical ventilatory support for acute respiratory failure require ICU admission. Patients with severe respiratory failure who are not receiving mechanical ventilation also benefit from ICU care, because intensive respiratory care can often prevent progression and avoid the need for tracheal intubation and mechanical ventilation. Respiratory monitoring in the ICU also can more rapidly identify clinical changes that require intervention. In many cases, a care

plan to support the patient with respiratory failure can be initiated in the ICU setting and implemented after transfer from the ICU. Similarly, patients who require invasive hemodynamic monitoring, including arterial lines or pulmonary artery catheters, will generally be managed in an ICU environment capable of providing not only the monitors, but also the staff to interpret the data generated from them and the interventions warranted by that data.

The ICU also remains the preferred location in which to initiate pharmacologic cardiovascular support, including inotropic agents, vasopressors, and intravenous vasodilators. Once a patient is stabilized in an ICU, alternatives to ICU care are available in some hospitals for patients who require continued vasopressor or inotropic therapy but are otherwise stable, without hypotension or arrhythmias. Patients who require invasive therapeutic support, including intraaortic balloon counterpulsation (IABP), a ventricular-assist device (VAD), and extracorporeal membrane oxygenation (ECMO), must be cared for in the ICU. The use of continuous renal replacement therapies (CRRT), such as continuous venovenous hemofiltration, also requires ICU care.

The goal of ICU care, whenever possible, should be to detect potential problems before they occur. In many respects, the most appropriate patients for admission to the ICU are those for whom complications can be avoided by providing greater nursing care or more extensive monitoring. Patients requiring continuous respiratory, cardiovascular, or neurologic monitoring, intensive nursing care, or closer physician observation often can be managed most effectively in an ICU environment. Unfortunately, the justification for ICU admission for these patients is difficult to document, particularly if the ICU care has prevented the clinical problems from occurring. Many payors (and occasionally hospital administrators) cannot understand why ICU care was necessary if no specific intervention was required. As cost-saving strategies mandate a shift of care to less sophisticated environments, outcome studies are needed to demonstrate which patients benefit from ICU care and which clinical services can be provided in alternative sites.

The need for ICU care is also influenced by the availability of transitional or intermediate care units and the capabilities of the other nursing units. In some hospitals, a transitional care unit can provide much of the equipment and clinical capability traditionally delivered in an ICU, especially monitoring to prevent complications or begin to treat them rapidly, if they occur. Using criteria specific to the patient population in the hospital, clinicians can develop strategies for providing graded critical care services that maintain or improve the level of care, while reducing overall costs (11). Some hospitals have increased the nurse-to-patient ratio, added other staff, or modified the skills of the existing staff to expand the clinical capabilities on acute care nursing units so that patients who previously required an ICU can be cared for in a less-intensive environment. For example, cardiac telemetry systems have allowed acute care units to monitor patients at risk for arrhythmias, thereby reducing the need for traditional coronary care unit beds except in the highest risk patients. The use of infusion pumps with fail-safe systems have allowed acute care units to provide safe, continuous infusions of drugs such as dopamine and dobutamine, thereby eliminating the need for transfer to the ICU. Telemetric pulse oximetry and paging devices that notify nursing staff of changes in a patient's condition also allow patients to be "observed" indirectly in traditional acute care nursing units.

Non-ICU facilities also have been developed for patients who are "chronically critically ill" and no longer need the skills and immediate access to critical care providers. For example, the patient who requires long-term ventilatory support can be transferred to a unit or a facility that specializes in the care of ventilator-dependent patients. These settings not only address the specific clinical needs of the patient, but also generally have better rehabilitative and supportive capabilities to facilitate weaning from mechanical ventilation. Although these more focused clinical facilities are valuable additions, access to them varies considerably from one community to another. Physicians caring for critically ill patients should become familiar with these alternatives as well as with the requirements of payors, many of whom limit their reimbursement when patients transition from one unit to another or enter long-term ventilator care facilities.

Coordinating Clinical Management in the Intensive Care Unit

The management of the critically ill patient mandates a thorough understanding of the clinical problems, management options, and goals of therapy. Critical care management frequently requires rapid evaluation of key issues followed by intervention for life-threatening problems before a complete assessment of all underlying medical problems can be accomplished. For example, the causes of septic shock are numerous (see Chapter 26). The patient who is suspected of having pneumonia as the cause of sepsis may require tracheal intubation and institution of mechanical ventilation to improve oxygenation or maintain ventilation to prevent acidemia. For these patients, cultures should be obtained as soon as possible, and broad-spectrum antibiotics should be administered. Once culture results are available, antibiotic management can be more carefully tailored to the specific organisms. Conversely, if the cause for sepsis appears to be an abscess, a drainage procedure might be required at the same time that antibiotics are administered. In other situations, the cause may be unclear, and treatment may be more empiric while diagnostic efforts progress. The inability to provide appropriate intervention quickly can result in further clinical deterioration and development of multisystem failure that requires greater levels of ICU support and increases the likelihood of poor outcome.

The management of the acutely ill patient also often requires that emergent problems be addressed before the physician understands the underlying medical conditions that might influence long-term decision-making or a patient's pre-specified wishes that might affect management. For example, the patient with a terminal illness who has been receiving palliative care may present in acute distress requiring ventilatory support because of respiratory failure. If no prior information is available about the patient's underlying condition, resuscitative efforts should be initiated. If it subsequently becomes clear that continued ICU care is not appropriate, further care can be withheld or care can be withdrawn after discussion with the patient, the patient's family, surrogate decision-makers, and the physician staff (see Chapter 19).

Although chronic medical conditions often are not addressed directly during the management of life-threatening problems, management strategies for the acute problem frequently mandate a thorough knowledge of the underlying medical condition. For instance, the patient with underlying chronic obstructive pulmonary disease (COPD) and hypercapnia may present with acute respiratory failure (see Chapter 55). It is essential for the physician to understand the degree of underlying gas-exchange abnormalities and the degree of respiratory reserve (as evidenced by baseline arterial blood-gas measurements and pulmonary function studies) to determine the most appropriate approach to ventilatory management. For example, in some patients with infection or heart failure, noninvasive ventilation provides sufficient support to allow stabilization and treatment of acute respiratory compromise, and permit the patient to avoid tracheal intubation and prolonged ventilatory support. In other cases, ventilatory management may be dictated by the degree of metabolic compensation for respiratory acidosis. If the patient has a significant compensatory metabolic alkalosis, initial ventilator management should provide a relatively lower minute ventilation, adjusted to correct the pH toward normal, not toward normalizing the partial arterial carbon dioxide pressure. Conversely, if the patient presents with a metabolic and respiratory acidosis, ventilatory management should be aimed at normalizing the pH. Hemodynamic support may be required to improve myocardial function, pulmonary perfusion, and oxygen delivery.

To optimize care within the ICU, professional societies have developed practice guidelines to define management strategies and ensure that care is based on evidence about appropriateness and outcome. Protocols for ventilatory management, weaning, sedation, analgesia, insulin infusions, and antibiotics are now commonly used (see Chapter 23). These protocols are most effectively implemented if they have been developed collaboratively with physicians who participate in the care of ICU patients, knowledgeable consultants, nurses, respiratory therapists, and pharmacists. Although some clinicians have expressed concerns that such protocols undermine their clinical judgment and decision-making, protocols can facilitate patient care and optimize the patient–physician relationship. The protocols must undergo regular review and revision, however, so that they are always based on the most current evidence about clinical management (see Chapter 13).

The optimal model for coordinating care depends on the capabilities and experience of the providers and the organization of the ICU. For example, the ICU physician typically is most knowledgeable about the patient's acute needs, including the need for invasive or noninvasive monitoring, airway protection, and mechanical ventilatory support, and is best able to facilitate care by respiratory therapists, case managers, and clinical specialists. Depending on skills, training, and availability, the intensivist or hospitalist may most effectively coordinate the care provided by consultants and evaluate the need for other interventions, such as circulatory-assistance devices, renal replacement therapies, and so forth. The hospitalist should participate in the decision to admit the patient to the ICU, remain actively involved in clinical decision-making, and manage the transition of care into and out of the ICU. The primary care provider usually has a longstanding relationship with the patient and is knowledgeable about the patient's underlying medical problems, goals for therapy, and important social issues.

The specific roles for the critical care physician and the hospitalist are changing as more critical care services are provided outside of the ICU. The creation of transitional or intermediate care units, expansion of clinical capabilities in other acute care nursing units, and the creation of units to care for chronically critically ill patients have expanded the role for physicians who understand how to treat severely ill patients, prevent deterioration in patients who require monitoring, and help patients transition to less intensive settings. The critical care physician is a valuable resource both for the patient and the hospitalist in defining what care is required throughout the patient's hospitalization, where it can be most effectively provided, and when transfer to or from the ICU is appropriate. For some patients, either the hospitalist or the intensivist may be the most appropriate clinician to coordinate care throughout the patient's hospitalization.

ASSESSING AND ENSURING QUALITY OF CARE IN THE ICU

Evidence-Based Care in the ICU

Clinical medicine has undergone an evolution from primarily experientially based clinical decision-making to evidence-based practice (Chapter 8). Many of the evidence-based practices that are used to optimize perioperative care or medical management of diabetes, hypertension, coronary artery disease, and other conditions, are applicable to the ICU patient and critical care setting. For many patients, the development of evidence-based protocols to facilitate clinical management have been implemented hospital-wide, including in the ICU setting. For example, the use of β-blockers to reduce the incidence of postoperative myocardial ischemia is common in patients requiring postoperative monitoring or ICU care. In some cases, protocols have to be modified or their implementation delayed due to underlying conditions or acute physiologic changes associated with the critical illness. In other cases, the early initiation of evidence-based practices in the ICU setting have been demonstrated to reduce ICU length of stay and improve outcome.

Some examples of evidence-based practices that are now becoming commonly applied in the ICU setting include: respiratory care strategies to reduce ventilator-associated pneumonia, patient positioning and management strategies to reduce the risk of aspiration, prophylaxis of peptic ulcer disease, anticoagulation and other interventions to minimize the risk of deep vein thrombosis in the bed-ridden patient, transfusion therapy, strategies to expedite weaning from ventilators and reduce days of mechanical ventilation, strategies to reduce the risk of ventilator-associated pulmonary complications, and tight control of blood sugar in diabetic patients. Initiation of early feeding in both medical and surgical patients improves outcome by reducing muscle wasting and shortening rehabilitation. The administration of activated protein C to the patient with early sepsis reduces mortality (see Chapter 26) (12). In many situations, the primary care physician and surgeon may not be aware of the evidence upon which the practices are based; the intensivist and hospitalist have key roles in ensuring the use of practices that have been proven to reduce morbidity and mortality.

As evidence-based practices find their way to the ICU setting, the continuous evaluation of the practices and their applicability to the specific patient must be carefully assessed. The impact of underlying diseases, recent surgery, and other potential complicating factors must be taken into account and may mandate that interventions must sometimes be delayed or modified to maximize their benefit and minimize their risks. For example, if a patient has a coagulopathy in the early postoperative period, the use of anticoagulants might have to be delayed or their dose modified; for the septic patient, administration of activated protein C may have to be delayed for 12 to 24 hours because of the risk of bleeding. The upright positioning of the patient with severe acute respiratory distress syndrome (ARDS) may not be possible due to worseing hypoxemia or dead space ventilation. In these cases, even though the evidence-based practices may be temporarily delayed, the patient should be carefully and continuously assessed so evidence-based protocols can be initiated as soon as possible.

Assessing Outcomes in the ICU: Role for ICU Scoring Systems

A number of scoring systems have been developed to guide management in the ICU, to evaluate resource utilization, and to assess potential outcomes of care. For example, the Glasgow Coma Scale (see Table 117.1) assesses the degree of neurologic injury and is often used to estimate the potential for recovery in patients admitted to the ICU with altered neurologic status. The Ranson criteria (Table 86.3) stratify physiologic abnormalities and prognosis associated with acute pancreatitis. Unfortunately, many of these scoring systems were developed prior to advances in clinical management, so their current prognostic value is less clear.

Resource utilization, as a measure of severity of illness, in the ICU can be measured using the Therapeutic Intervention Scoring System (TISS) (Table 22.3). The TISS also can be used to estimate the need for nursing time and the costs of care.

TABLE 22.3

THERAPEUTIC INTERVENTION SCORING SYSTEM (TISS)

4 points
  Pulmonary-artery catheter
  Intraaortic balloon pump
  Controlled mechanical ventilation ($\pm$ positive end-expiratory pressure)
  Vasoactive drug therapy (>1 drug)
3 points
  Chest tube
  Continuous positive airway pressure
  Intermittent mandatory or assisted ventilation
  Arterial catheter
2 points
  Central venous pressure
  Two peripheral intravenous catheters
  Spontaneous ventilation via endotracheal tube or tracheostomy
  Multiple dressing changes
1 point
  Electrocardiographic monitoring
  One peripheral intravenous catheter
  Routine dressing changes
  Urinary catheter

Adapted from Keene AR, Cullen DJ. Therapeutic Intervention Scoring System: Update, 1983. *Crit Care Med* 1983;11:1–3; with permission.

A number of other scoring systems can help compare patients across ICUs or predict outcome of ICU care. Some scoring systems are specific to a single disease or patient population, such as the sequential organ failure assessment (SOFA), whereas others are designed to assess issues such as the level of sedation or pain (13).

The most widely used scoring system is probably the Acute Physiology and Chronic Health Evaluation (APACHE) system (Table 22.4), which considers both the acute physiologic perturbation of critical illness as well as underlying chronic health abnormalities that might influence outcome. The most recent version (APACHE III) has been used to provide benchmarking comparisons among ICUs and to stratify patients for clinical trials. Although less complicated approaches, including the Simplified Acute Physiology Score (SAPS) and the Mortality Probability Model (MPM), have been developed, APACHE remains the most widely-used method for assessing severity and estimating prognosis.

As valuable as these systems may be, it is important to note that none of them can be relied upon to define which individual patient will survive, nor to estimate their quality of life after ICU care.

Transitioning Care

Once a patient has stabilized, the critical illness is controlled, and ICU care is no longer required, an alternative site for care must be identified. Because of the varying

TABLE 22.4

THE ACUTE PHYSIOLOGY AND CHRONIC HEALTH EVALUATION (APACHE III) SCORING SYSTEM

Component	Score
Acute physiology score	
Pulse rate	0–17
Mean blood pressure	0–23
Temperature	0–20
Respiratory rate	0–18
PaO$_2$	0–15
P (A-a)O$_2$	0–14
Hematocrit	0–3
White blood cell count	0–19
Creatinine	0–10
Urine output	0–15
Blood urea nitrogen	0–12
Sodium	0–4
Albumin	0–11
Bilirubin	0–16
Glucose	0–9
Acid–base status	0–12
Neurologic status	0–48
Age <44	0
45–59	5
60–64	11
65–69	13
70–74	16
75–84	17
≥85	24
Comorbid condition[a]	
AIDS	23
Hepatic failure	16
Lymphoma	13
Metastatic cancer	11
Leukemia/multiple myeloma	10
Immunosuppression	10
Cirrhosis	4

[a] Comorbidity is excluded for elective surgery patients.
PaO$_2$, arterial partial pressure of oxygen; P(A-a)O$_2$, alveolar arterial gradient in the partial pressure of oxygen.
Adapted from Knaus WA, Wagner DP, Draper EA, et al. The APACHE III prognostic system: risk prediction of hospital mortality for critically ill hospitalized adults. *Chest* 1991;100:1619–1636, with permission.

clinical needs, different alternative care sites within each community, waiting lists, and differing payor requirements, discharge planning and identification of disposition options should begin at the time of ICU admission, when goals for ICU care should be clarified and the criteria for transfer outlined. A case manager or social worker should be actively involved in discussions about the patient's continued clinical needs and should provide input into alternatives for further care. Goals should be redefined and shared among members of the care team each day (14). For example, if a patient requires ICU admission for ventilatory support for acute respiratory failure and has a high likelihood to need prolonged mechanical ventilatory support, alternative clinical sites capable of providing

the required care should be identified early in the patient's ICU course. By working closely with the staff of the alternative site, care can be coordinated to ensure that the patient is ready for transfer as soon as clinical needs change. If necessary, a tracheostomy and placement of a permanent feeding-tube can be done early enough in the ICU course to prevent a delay in transfer. It is often valuable to allow families an opportunity to visit the facility and participate in planning for transfer.

Addressing Ethical Dilemmas in Intensive Care Management

The increase in clinical capabilities in the hospital in general and the ICU specifically has created many new challenges for physicians caring for critically ill patients. The nature of critical care medicine is to pursue clinical problems aggressively, to address them rapidly, and to resolve them. Many patients, however, now survive for extended periods of time, requiring extensive and aggressive medical management, often with little or no likelihood of meaningful recovery. The patient may "stabilize" but require such extensive care that transition out of an ICU setting becomes difficult. For other patients, the outcome of ICU care is unacceptable, despite initial interventions that were appropriate and timely. In these situations, ICU care, or sometimes any continued medical care, may no longer be appropriate or desired.

As a result, the providers who participate in the care of the ICU patient will be confronted with questions such as these: Should care be provided to the terminally ill patient? When should care be continued for the patient who has little or no likelihood of meaningful recovery, to what end point, and at what cost? Who is the decision-maker for the patient who cannot express her or his own wishes? If care is to be withdrawn, how should it be done? All providers must understand the needs and goals of the patient and family, clarify the expectations of care, and deal with unanticipated consequences. These issues are addressed in Chapter 17.

If and when a joint decision is made to limit care, the clinicians must clarify how it will be limited and whether some interventions will be withdrawn. From an ethical perspective, there is no distinction between withholding and withdrawing care; for patients and families, however, the former may be easier than the latter. When care is limited or withdrawn, routine clinical needs must still be met, and the comfort of the patient must be assured. Some ICU patients who have been receiving analgesics may require large doses of opiates or other medications.

When a decision is made to limit care, the limitations should be documented in the medical record. The discussion with the patient and family should be recorded, and the specific limitations defined in the orders. All providers should be aware of which services will be provided and which will not. If the clinical situation changes and the plans require modification, the changes should similarly be documented in the medical record.

CONCLUSIONS

As the complexity of inpatient care increases, a large percentage of inpatients now receive care in a critical care, or other monitored, environment sometime during their hospital stay. Regardless of whether the ICU is a specialized or general unit, or whether it is open or closed, the safe and appropriate care of the patient necessitates a multidisciplinary, coordinated, and integrated approach to management. Each provider brings different and often important skills, knowledge, and capabilities to the management of the patient. The hospitalist is an integral member of this team, often leading the team in smaller hospitals (without critical care physicians) and participating in decision-making and the transition of the patient from the ICU to other less intensive clinical environments in all intensive care settings.

KEY POINTS

- Both medical and surgical inpatient care is concentrating in critical care environments, necessitating that all hospital-based providers understand the reasons for ICU admission, the capabilities for care within the ICU, and the most effective ways of managing critically ill patients.

- The administrative and clinical models for the ICU vary among hospitals and within a single hospital based on a number of factors, including availability of critical care physicians, patients' needs, and adminstrative organizational factors. ICUs can be managed as either open and closed units, but coordination of care among a variety of providers is essential in either model.

- The clinical capabilities and skills of providers vary both within and among hospitals. Decisions about a patient's location must be based on an understanding of the patient's needs and the capabilities of various units in each hospital.

- Because of the complexity and diversity of clinical needs for ICU patients, care is optimized if it is carefully coordinated among the primary care physician, the ICU physician, and consultants. Protocols that define evidence-based practices and ensure standardization of clinical management reduce morbidity and mortality.

- Since the ICU represents only part of the overall hospital course and care for the critically ill patient, disposition planning should be initiated at the time of admission to the ICU to define long-term needs, desired outcomes of care, and plans for transition to less intensive environments.

REFERENCES

1. Wu AW, Pronovost P, Morlock L. ICU incident reporting systems. *J Crit Care* 2002;17:86–94.
2. Pronovost P, Wu AW, Dorman T, Morlock L. Building safety into ICU care. *J Crit Care* 2002;17:78–85.
3. Young MP, Birkmeyer JD. Potential reduction in mortality rates using an intensivist model to manage intensive care units. *Eff Clin Pract* 2000;3:284–289.
4. Chalfin DB. Implementation of standards for intensivist staffing: is it time to jump aboard the Leapfrog bandwagon? *Crit Care Med* 2004;32:1406–1408.
5. Angus DC, Kelley MA, Schmitz RJ, et al. Committee on Manpower for Pulmonary and Critical Care Societies. Caring for the critically ill patient. Current and projected workforce requirements for care of the critically ill and patients with pulmonary disease: can we meet the requirements of an aging population? *JAMA* 2000; 284:2762–2770.
6. Breslow MJ, Rosenfeld BA, Doerfler M, et al. Effect of a multiple-site intensive care unit telemedicine program on clinical and economic outcomes: an alternative paradigm for intensivist staffing. *Crit Care Med.* 2004;32:31–38. Erratum in: *Crit Care Med* 2004;32:1632.
7. Kollef MH, Shapiro SD, Silver P, et al. A randomized, controlled trial of protocol-directed versus physician-directed weaning from mechanical ventilation. *Crit Care Med* 1997;25:567–574.
8. Rivers E, Nguyen B, Havstad S, et al.; Early Goal-Directed Therapy Collaborative Group. Early goal-directed therapy in the treatment of severe sepsis and septic shock. *N Engl J Med* 2001;345:1368–1377.
9. Baldock G, Foley P, Brett S. The impact of organisational change on outcome in an intensive care unit in the United Kingdom. *Intensive Care Med* 2001;27:865–872.
10. Ely EW, Baker AM, Dunagan DP, et al. Effect on the duration of mechanical ventilation of identifying patients capable of breathing spontaneously. *N Engl J Med* 1996; 335:1864–1869.
11. Beck DH, Smith GB, Taylor B. The impact of low-risk intensive care unit admissions on mortality probabilities by SAPS II, APACHE II and APACHE III. *Anaesthesia* 2002;57:21–26.
12. Liaw PC. Endogenous protein C activation in patients with severe sepsis. *Crit Care Med* 2004;32(5 Suppl):S214–S218.
13. Mondello E, Siliotti R, Noto G, et al. Bispectral Index in ICU: correlation with Ramsay Score on assessment of sedation level. *J Clin Monit Comput* 2002;17:271–277.
14. Pronovost P, Berenholtz S, Dorman T, et al. Improving communication in the ICU using daily goals. *J Crit Care* 2003;18:71–75.

ADDITIONAL READING

Buckley TA, Gomersall CD, Ramsay SJ. Validation of the multiple organ dysfunction (MOD) score in critically ill medical and surgical patients. *Intensive Care Med* 2003;29:2216–2222.

Byers JF, Sole ML. Analysis of factors related to the development of ventilator associated pneumonia: use of existing data bases. *Am J Crit Care* 2000;9:344–351.

Glance LG, Osler TM, Dick A. Rating the quality of intensive care units: is it a function of the intensive care unit scoring system? *Crit Care Med* 2002;30:1976–1982.

Herridge MS. Prognostication and intensive care unit outcome: the evolving role of scoring systems. *Clin Chest Med* 2003;24:751–762.

Higgins TL, McGee WT, Steingrub JS, et al. Early indicators of prolonged intensive care unit stay: impact of illness severity, physician staffing, and pre-intensive care unit length of stay. *Crit Care Med* 2003;31:45–51.

Rosenberg AL. Recent innovations in intensive care unit risk-prediction models. *Curr Opin Crit Care* 2002;8:321–330.

Van den Berghe G, Wouters P, Weekers F, et al. Intensive insulin therapy in the critically ill patients. *N Engl J Med* 2001;345:1359–1367.

Ventilator Management 23

Stephen E. Lapinsky   Arthur S. Slutsky

OBJECTIVES OF MECHANICAL VENTILATION

Mechanical ventilation is a life-saving intervention necessary for the management of respiratory failure complicated by severe hypoxemia or marked hypercapnia. Ventilatory support may result in significant complications, and an important goal should be to minimize or prevent these adverse effects. The first issue to be addressed is whether ventilatory assistance is required and whether intubation is necessary. In many situations in which the patient has severe hypoxemia or cannot protect his or her airway, the decision may be straightforward. However, in some situations the decision requires clinical judgment in which the risks of endotracheal intubation and ventilatory support are weighed against the hazards of not ventilating the patient. Increasing evidence justifies the use of noninvasive ventilation in the cooperative patient.

A major function of ventilatory support is to improve alveolar ventilation. In the patient with hypoventilation, mechanical ventilation corrects hypercapnia and respiratory acidosis. Although the usual goal is to normalize the arterial partial pressure of carbon dioxide (P_aCO_2) and pH, in some situations a P_aCO_2 level higher than normal may be accepted, particularly if high ventilation pressures are required. In the management of severe hypoxemia, ventilation improves oxygenation by the effect of positive pressure on lung volumes and alveolar recruitment, as well as by the ability to deliver a high inspired oxygen fraction. Mechanical ventilation is used to unload the respiratory muscles—an important goal because oxygen consumption by these muscles may account for up to 50% of total oxygen consumption in the patient with acute respiratory failure. This unloading is of particular benefit in the patient with acute myocardial ischemia or reduced oxygen delivery.

BASIC PRINCIPLES

Classification of Ventilators

Ventilation may be achieved by the delivery of either a predetermined volume or pressure to the lungs, on a regular or a demand basis. With *volume-controlled* ventilation, a preset tidal volume is delivered. As a safety feature, a pressure limit is set, which if reached causes pressure to be released and a ventilator alarm to sound. *Pressure-preset* ventilation differs from volume-controlled ventilation in that a level of airway pressure is preset; with this mode, the delivered tidal volume is determined by pulmonary mechanics. For example, a decrease in thoracic compliance results in a proportional decrease in tidal volume. The duration of delivery of the pressure is set as an inspiratory time or as an inspiratory:expiratory ratio and respiratory rate.

Ventilatory Modes

Controlled ventilation, which is the most basic mode of ventilatory support, provides a set tidal volume and rate regardless of the patient's effort or requirements (Table 23.1). A major disadvantage of this mode is the asynchrony that can occur between the patient's spontaneous efforts and the ventilator-generated breaths. *Assisted modes* are triggered by the patient's respiratory efforts and are used to synchronize the patient and the ventilator. In the *assist-control mode*, every patient breath is supported by the ventilator. A minimum rate is set, effectively providing controlled ventilation in the absence of the patient's efforts. This mode is used with volume-preset or pressure-preset ventilation. A disadvantage is that in patients with very high respiratory drives and obstructive airways disease, high minute volumes can produce respiratory alkalosis and/or worsen air trapping.

TABLE 23.1

CLASSIFICATION OF MECHANICAL VENTILATION

Controlled	Assist-control	Synchronized intermittent mandatory ventilation	Support
Pressure or volume preset[a]	Pressure or volume preset[a]	Usually volume preset[a]	Usually pressure preset[a]
Use in the paralyzed patient	Use as an initial ventilatory mode	Use in spontaneously breathing patient	Use only in spontaneously breathing patient with adequate respiratory drive
Patient receives mandatory preset ventilator rate	Patient receives mandatory preset ventilator rate	Patient receives mandatory preset ventilator rate	Patient receives no mandatory ventilator rate
All breaths are ventilator-initiated	Spontaneous breaths are all ventilator-assisted	Spontaneous breaths are not ventilator-assisted	All spontaneous breaths are ventilator-assisted
No spontaneous breathing possible		Can be used as a weaning mode	Can be used as a weaning mode

[a]Pressure-preset ventilation: inspiratory pressure level is set on the ventilator, volume is monitored; volume-preset ventilation: tidal volume and flow rate are set on the ventilator, inspiratory pressures are monitored.

Synchronized intermittent mandatory ventilation (SIMV) combines a preset ventilator rate with spontaneous breathing. As in assist-control modes, the ventilator breaths are patient-triggered and therefore synchronized but are mandatory in the absence of patient effort. However, patient breaths in excess of the preset rate do not receive ventilatory assistance (Figure 23.1). Spontaneous breaths in this mode may require significant patient work because of high circuit or demand-valve resistance. This mode, which has the advantage of allowing the patient to perform a variable amount of respiratory work with the security of a backup rate, also can be used for weaning patients from ventilatory support. SIMV may be performed using volume- or pressure-preset ventilation.

Pressure-support ventilation (PSV) is a pressure-preset, flow-cycled mode in which ventilatory support assists all spontaneous efforts. The delivered pressure is triggered by the patient and is maintained until a specific decrease in inspiratory flow occurs. With PSV, the patient determines both respiratory frequency and inspiratory time, with tidal volume being a function of the set level of pressure, patient effort, and pulmonary mechanics. If appropriately set, this mode may reduce asynchrony and optimize patient control over ventilation. In some patients with severe airways obstruction, however, PSV may lead to patient-ventilator asynchrony, especially at high levels of pressure support. The ability to decrease ventilator support from high pressure to near zero also makes this a useful and effective weaning mode. This mode requires spontaneous respiratory efforts and does not guarantee a minimum tidal volume; an apnea backup capability is therefore necessary.

Ventilator Settings

The respiratory rate may be a function of the ventilator setting, spontaneous breathing, or both, depending on the mode. Synchronization of spontaneous breaths with ventilator breaths is achieved by having the ventilator breath begin when the patient "triggers" the ventilator by generating a small change in airway pressure (e.g., −0.5 to −2 cm H_2O). Insensitive triggering systems may require significant effort from the patient; an oversensitive system may produce spontaneous ventilator cycling. The presence of

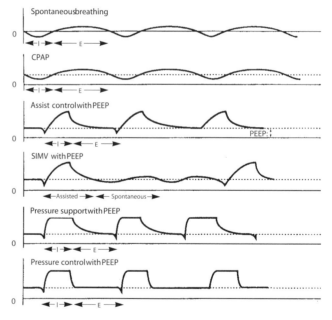

Figure 23.1 Airway pressure tracings during spontaneous respiration and various modes of mechanical ventilation. In the assist-control and pressure-control profiles, the first two breaths are triggered, but the third breath is controlled because no spontaneous effort has occurred. During synchronized intermittent mandatory ventilation *(SIMV)*, spontaneous breathing occurs between ventilator breaths. The pressure-support tracing demonstrates some variation in duration of the inspiratory phase because of flow cycling, compared with the fixed inspiratory period of the time-cycled pressure-control mode. *CPAP,* continuous positive airway pressure; *E,* expiratory phase; *I,* inspiratory phase; *PEEP,* positive end-expiratory pressure. (Adapted from Lapinsky SE, Slutsky AS. Principles of mechanical ventilation and weaning. In: Dantzker DR, Scharf SM, eds. *Cardiopulmonary Critical Care,* 3rd ed. Philadelphia: W.B. Saunders, 1998;253, with permission.)

residual positive alveolar pressure at the end of expiration (auto-PEEP) may inhibit triggering; the patient must create a negative pressure large enough to overcome this positive alveolar pressure before the ventilator senses a change in airway pressure. Flow triggering, using small changes in airway flow, is available on some ventilators and may be more efficient, but clinical benefits have not been demonstrated.

The inspiratory flow rate and pattern of delivery must be set during volume-controlled ventilation but are determined by patient effort and pulmonary mechanics with pressure-preset modes. In the spontaneously breathing patient, the flow rate setting must match the patient's peak inspiratory demands—usually about 40 to 100 L/min in the adult patient. This inspiratory flow may be delivered in a variety of flow patterns (square-wave, sine-wave, or decelerating flow), but no significant benefit has been demonstrated for one flow pattern over another. A decelerating ramp inspiratory flow has the potential advantage of limiting peak pressure and optimizing mean airway pressure.

Inspiratory flow can be terminated by reaching a preset volume (volume-control), time (pressure-control), or flow rate (pressure-support). Volume cycling delivers the preset tidal volume, but additional patient effort does not produce further volume. Pressure-controlled ventilation utilizes time cycling, in which the set airway pressure (and therefore flow) is maintained for a preset inspiratory time. Additional patient effort during this time allows increased tidal volume. Pressure-support ventilation is a preset pressure mode utilizing flow cycling. Airway pressure is maintained until inspiratory flow falls below a certain level (usually 25% of the peak inspiratory flow). This approach increases patient control over the delivered tidal volume and inspiratory time and may improve patient–ventilator synchrony, but care must be taken in patients with airway obstruction.

Maintaining a *positive end-expiratory pressure* (PEEP) is thought to be useful to minimize ventilator-induced lung injury and to improve oxygenation by increasing mean airway pressure, recruiting lung volume, and redistributing lung water from the interstitial space adjacent to the gas-exchanging regions to the compliant perivascular interstitial space. How to determine the appropriate level of PEEP remains controversial; the most popular methods rely on optimizing some desired physiological end point, be it arterial partial pressure of oxygen (P_aO_2), oxygen delivery, or lung compliance. PEEP can have significant deleterious effects, including a decreased cardiac output and hypotension, particularly in the volume-depleted patient.

The lowest inspired oxygen concentration producing an acceptable P_aO_2 should be selected, in order to avoid lung injury induced by a high concentration. Exposure to an inspired oxygen concentration less than 0.5 is probably not of concern. In patients requiring higher concentrations, P_aO_2 sometimes can be raised by manipulating mean airway pressure (by adjusting PEEP, inspiratory:expiratory ratio, or plateau pressure) or improving mixed venous oxygen saturation (by improving cardiac output).

CARE OF THE HOSPITALIZED PATIENT

Noninvasive Ventilation

Ventilatory support traditionally is performed with an endotracheal tube, but intubation is uncomfortable and is associated with significant risks, such as airway damage and nosocomial pneumonia. There has been increasing interest in the noninvasive application of positive pressure ventilation, which may avoid the potential adverse effects and long-term complications of endotracheal intubation.

Noninvasive ventilation is performed using a tight-fitting nasal or oronasal mask attached to a positive pressure ventilator. Although the nasal mask is usually well tolerated, the face mask is becoming a more commonly used interface and is available in a variety of types and sizes. Conventional ventilators may be used to deliver noninvasive ventilation, usually in a pressure-support mode. Several simpler bi-level pressure-support devices are available to ventilate in a pressure-support mode, with or without a backup rate; they have the advantage of low cost and better compensation for air leaks but do not have the monitoring capabilities of most ICU ventilators.

Noninvasive support can be used in the patient who is able to protect his/her airway and who has adequate spontaneous respiratory efforts, but is failing because of respiratory muscle fatigue or progressive hypoxemia. It may be contraindicated in the patient with a decreased level of consciousness, excessive secretions, recent upper-gastrointestinal anastamoses, or hemodynamic instability. An adequate fit for the mask may not be possible in edentulous patients or those with facial injury or deformity. Noninvasive ventilation is most effective in the management of patients with respiratory failure resulting from chronic obstructive pulmonary disease (COPD) (see Chapter 55), in which a mortality benefit has been demonstrated (1). Cardiogenic pulmonary edema (see Chapter 39) can be effectively treated by noninvasive continuous positive airway pressure. Other potential uses of noninvasive ventilation include patients who refuse intubation and those who require short-term support.

Noninvasive ventilation is initiated by gently applying the mask to the patient's face until it is tolerated; then the mask is secured with head straps. The inspiratory pressure and end-expiratory pressure usually are set initially at 8 cm H_2O and 4 cm H_2O respectively; pressures are adjusted to the patient's comfort and later to arterial blood-gas measurements. The acutely distressed patient may require a rapid increase to higher levels of inspiratory pressure (e.g., 16–20 cm H_2O). Most bi-level ventilatory-support devices deliver room-air gas, and oxygen must be titrated into the circuit according to the patient's oxygen saturation. When using conventional ventilators, the pressure support level can be titrated up until the tidal volume reaches about 7 mL/kg. Inspired oxygen concentration can be set on the ventilator to the desired level.

Noninvasive ventilation is most useful for short-term ventilation, although support for several days to a week is feasible. A significant complication of prolonged use is the development of nasal-bridge ulceration. The mask can be removed intermittently for communication, feeding, or patient comfort. The difficult decisions regarding extubation are avoided by the ease of removal and reapplication of the mask. This mode of ventilation is definitely indicated for patients with COPD, but its exact role in other disease states remains to be determined. The success of noninvasive ventilation often depends on the experience and perseverance of the medical personnel. Patients require close monitoring, and facilities for endotracheal intubation and conventional ventilation should be readily available.

Initiating Mechanical Ventilation

Once the decision is made to institute conventional mechanical ventilation, intubation must be performed in a controlled fashion. All necessary equipment must be available including a laryngoscope, suction, resuscitation bag and mask, and endotracheal tubes of different sizes. Electrocardiographic and oxygen saturation monitoring is essential. The method of intubation depends on individual preferences and level of skill; in the acutely ill patient, however, an awake intubation is safest because it allows spontaneous respiration during the procedure and avoids the desaturation that occurs if a patient is rendered apneic by pharmacotherapy. Most patients with acute respiratory failure have an altered level of consciousness, but the procedure should be explained to them. Topical anesthesia can be used, and small doses of a short-acting benzodiazepine may be beneficial. Anesthetic drugs and neuromuscular blocking agents should be available. The patient must be preoxygenated, and oxygen saturation should be monitored during the intubation. For patients who are not fluid-overloaded, a fluid bolus may be initiated to overcome the hypotensive effect of the sedation and positive intrathoracic pressure.

If the patient is fully sedated following intubation, ventilation is commenced in a controlled or assist-control mode. Pressure support may be chosen in the patient with good spontaneous efforts who does not tolerate assist control (Figure 23.2). Inspired oxygen concentration is set initially at 0.80–1.0 and reduced according to oxygen saturation measurements. A tidal volume of 5–10 mL/kg with a rate of 12–16 per minute is adjusted according to the patient's clinical status and initial arterial blood-gas results. A PEEP of 5 cm H_2O often is provided unless contraindicated by hypotension. It is important not to expect to optimize ventilation until the patient has stabilized and the sedative drugs have taken full effect. Fine tuning, including adjustment of inspiratory flow rate, inspiratory:expiratory ratio, PEEP, and triggering sensitivity, then may be appropriate, along with any other necessary troubleshooting (Table 23.2).

Step 1: Ventilatory mode
AC - Initial mode (particularly if patient sedated, limited efforts)
SIMV - consider if some respiratory effort, dysynchrony
Pressure support - only if good patient effort, more comfortable

Step 2: Oxygenation
FiO_2 - Begin with 80–100%, reduce according to SaO_2
PEEP - Begin with 5 cm H_2O, increase according to SaO_2 and hemodynamic effects
Aim for $SaO_2 \geq 90\%$, $FiO_2 \leq 60\%$

Step 3: Ventilation
Tidal volume - begin with 5 to 10 ml/kg
Rate - begin with 12 – 16/min, higher if acidemic
Pressure limit - set at 50 cm H_2O
               - aim for $\leq$35 cm H_2O

Step 4: Fine tuning
Triggering - in spontaneous modes, adjust to minimize effort
Inspiratory flow rate of 40–80 L/min: higher if tachypneic, lower if high pressure is alarming
I:E ratio - 1:2, either set or as function of flow rate
Flow pattern - decelerating ramp reduces peak pressure

Step 5: Monitoring
• Clinical - blood pressure, ECG
• Ventilator - tidal volume, minute ventilation, airway pressures
• Arterial blood gases, pulse oximetry

Figure 23.2 Algorithm for initiating mechanical ventilation. *AC*, assist control; *ECG*, electrocardiogram; *FiO₂*, inspired oxygen fraction; *I:E*, inspiratory:expiratory; *PEEP*, positive end-expiratory pressure; *SaO₂*, arterial oxygen saturation; *SIMV*, synchronized intermittent mandatory ventilation.

Disease-Specific Ventilation

Acute Respiratory Distress Syndrome

Mechanical ventilation with a low tidal volume (6 ml/kg) and plateau pressure less than 30 cm H_2O improves outcome in patients with severe acute respiratory distress syndrome (ARDS) (see Chapter 24) (2). Recognition of the concept of ventilator-induced lung injury has influenced ventilatory strategies. Lung injury in ARDS is not uniform, and the small fraction of uninvolved lung capable of gas exchange should be protected from excessive inflation pressure. In addition to local injury, evidence exists that injurious ventilatory strategies may cause the systemic release of

TABLE 23.2
TROUBLESHOOTING THE VENTILATOR

Problem	Response
Dyssynchrony ("fighting")	Consider synchronized intermittent mandatory ventilation or pressure control or pressure support
	Check trigger sensitivity
	Check inspiratory flow rate
	Check for auto-PEEP
	Consider sedation, neuromuscular blockade
Hypoxemia	Inspired oxygen concentration as high as necessary, but aim for <60%
	Increase PEEP incrementally to 18 cm H_2O
	Consider:
	Recruitment maneuver
	Prone position
	Increasing cardiac output
High-pressure alarm	High peak pressure = airway resistance (e.g., endotracheal tube, bronchospasm)
	High plateau pressure = lung/chest wall compliance (e.g., pulmonary edema, pneumothorax, "fighting")
Low-pressure alarm	Patient disconnected from ventilator
	Inadequate flow rate
Hypotension	Due to volume depletion, sedation, increased intrathoracic pressure
	Initial treatment: fluid bolus
	May need to reduce PEEP, minute volume
	Consider:
	Pneumothorax
	Auto-PEEP
Hypercapnea	Accept moderate hypercapnea (50–80 mm Hg)
	May need bicarbonate for acidosis (controversial)

PEEP, positive end-expiratory pressure.

cytokines (3), potentially resulting in multi-organ failure. For the patient with a noncompliant chest wall (e.g., massive ascites, pleural effusions, pregnancy), higher airway pressures may be accepted. Low tidal volumes may result in alveolar hypoventilation and a rise in P_aCO_2, and this permissive hypercapnia generally is well tolerated (4).

With inadequate PEEP, ARDS may deteriorate because of alveolar damage resulting from repeated opening and closing of alveoli. An adequate level of PEEP is also essential to improve oxygenation and lung compliance. Application of a recruitment maneuver (e.g., 40 cm H_2O continuous positive airway pressure for 40 seconds) may improve oxygenation, particularly in early ARDS (5), but care must be taken to monitor oxygenation and blood pressure during such maneuvers. The utility of these maneuvers in terms of outcome has not been proven. Although the use of the prone position may improve oxygenation by increasing blood flow through well-aerated, previously non-dependent areas and improving pulmonary mechanics, no survival benefit has been noted (6). Nitric oxide may have dramatic effects on oxygenation in a subgroup of patients, but no improvement in any clinically significant end point has been shown in adults.

High frequency oscillation (HFO) is an alternative mode of mechanical ventilation that may be less injurious than conventional ventilation in ARDS. HFO allows delivery of a higher mean airway pressure (improving alveolar recruitment and oxygenation) without high peak pressures. HFO is carried out at a frequency of 3–8 Hz (180–480/min), with initial settings usually at about 6 Hz, and mean airway pressure at 3–5 cm H_2O higher than the mean airway pressure on conventional ventilation. Frequency is adjusted according to $PaCO_2$—lower frequencies produce a higher tidal volume and lower $PaCO_2$. Patients usually require deep sedation or even neuromuscular blockade. There are no data demonstrating a clear outcome benefit over conventional ventilation.

Survivors of ARDS regain their lung volume and spirometric values within 6 months, but carbon monoxide diffusion capacity remains reduced at 12 months. Persistent functional disability relates largely to muscle wasting and weakness (7).

Obstructive Airways Disease

The predominant abnormality in patients with obstructive airways disease is incomplete exhalation due to expiratory airflow limitation, which may produce dynamic hyperinflation or *auto-PEEP*, owing to the residual pressure (and volume) in the alveoli at the end of expiration. Auto-PEEP produces complications such as barotrauma, hemodynamic collapse, and difficulty in triggering the ventilator related to elevated intrathoracic pressure. Auto-PEEP cannot be measured easily in the spontaneously breathing patient, without invasive measurement of pleural or esophageal pressure. The presence of auto-PEEP can be inferred by observing the flow-time tracing—persistent expiratory flow at the onset of the next inspiration suggests that auto-PEEP is present. In the patient on controlled ventilation, auto-PEEP can be estimated by assessing the circuit pressure during brief occlusion of the circuit at the end of expiration. Many modern ventilators perform this measurement automatically. Resistance to inspiratory airflow is increased in asthmatics and results in markedly elevated peak airway pressures (see Chapter 56). A major objective in ventilating patients with obstructive airways disease is to minimize minute ventilation, shorten inspiratory time, and maximize expiratory time, so as to reduce end-expiratory lung volume and auto-PEEP.

Although increasing expiratory time is important, the most important intervention is to reduce minute volume to the lowest acceptable level. In patients with severe airflow limitation, this goal may require controlled hypoventilation with permissive hypercapnia. Heavy sedation or paralysis (see Sedation and Paralysis section on page 179) may be useful to reduce ventilation pressures and to eliminate active expiration in very difficult-to-ventilate patients. The development of hemodynamic compromise resulting from auto-PEEP should be anticipated and managed by a reduction in minute volume and by fluid therapy.

During weaning of the patient with obstructive airways disease, the presence of auto-PEEP may require increased work of breathing to trigger breaths. This problem can be overcome by applying extrinsic PEEP at a level equal to or less than the measured auto-PEEP.

Complications of Mechanical Ventilation

Mechanical ventilation is a life-saving intervention, but it may be associated with significant adverse effects (Table 23.3) related to the endotracheal tube, to ventilator-induced lung injury, to the effects of positive intrathoracic pressure, or to pharmacotherapy necessary to facilitate ventilation.

Endotracheal Intubation

Intubation may produce complications related to local trauma, such as pharyngeal or glottic injury occurring during insertion of the tube, and resulting from prolonged intubation. Cuff inflation pressures greater than 25 cm H_2O may cause ischemic ulceration predisposing to tracheal stenosis. Malpositioning of the endotracheal tube into the right mainstem bronchus produces atelectasis in the other lung and overdistention of the ventilated lung. Inadvertent extubation, a potentially dangerous complication, occurs in the disoriented or uncooperative patient.

TABLE 23.3

COMPLICATIONS OF MECHANICAL VENTILATION

Related to endotracheal intubation
  Pharyngeal and laryngeal injury
  Malpositioning of the endotracheal tube
  Inadvertent extubation
  Nosocomial pneumonia
Related to positive pressure or tidal ventilation
  Hemodynamic (decreased cardiac output)
  Ventilator-induced lung injury:
    Barotrauma (pneumothorax, pneumomediastinum)
    Volutrauma (pulmonary edema)
    Atelectrauma (ventilation at low lung volumes)
    Biotrauma (lung injury by inflammation and mediators)
Related to sedation and neuromuscular blockade
  Hemodynamic (hypotension, tachycardia)
  Skin pressure necrosis
  Deep venous thrombosis
  Muscle weakness (atrophy, myopathy, polyneuropathy)

Nasotracheal intubation improves comfort in some patients, but there is an increased risk of bleeding during insertion of the tube, and sinusitis may occur as a result of ostial occlusion. Nasal tubes are usually narrower, with increased airways resistance. Tracheostomy may provide some protection from glottic injury, but its major benefits are improving patient comfort and secretion clearance as well as allowing oral feeding. Tracheostomy usually is reserved for patients with an expected duration of ventilation of 2–3 weeks, but the optimal timing of tracheostomy is a matter of some debate.

The presence of an endotracheal tube disrupts normal pulmonary protective mechanisms. Coughing and mucociliary transport are impeded, resulting in the retention of secretions. Although gross aspiration is prevented by a cuffed endotracheal tube, pharyngeal secretions nevertheless may enter the trachea and increase the risk for nosocomial pneumonia. Nosocomial pneumonia occurs in about 30% of patients who are mechanically ventilated, and the risk increases with the duration of ventilation (see Chapter 66).

Positive Pressure

High ventilating pressures and high tidal volumes can produce barotrauma, which is manifested as pneumothorax, pneumomediastinum, or subcutaneous emphysema. The critical pressure that likely correlates best with the propensity to develop barotrauma is the transpulmonary pressure (alveolar minus pleural pressure). This pressure usually is not measured clinically—the most commonly monitored pressures are peak inspiratory pressure and plateau pressure. If these values are relatively low, the transpulmonary pressure is likely low, but elevated values may result from increased transpulmonary pressure as well as other causes (e.g., increased airway resistance, decreased chest-wall compliance). Preexisting acute and chronic lung disease predisposes the patient to barotrauma. The clinical picture of sudden respiratory distress associated with increased ventilator pressures should suggest the presence of a pneumothorax, particularly if associated with hemodynamic collapse. The radiographic diagnosis of a pneumothorax may be difficult if the chest radiograph is taken in the supine position. Management involves evacuation of the pneumothorax with a percutaneous chest tube. Healing of injured lung may be compromised, and a persistent bronchopleural fistula may develop.

Overdistention of the lung caused by large tidal volumes or high inflation pressures can produce lung injury. This ventilator-induced lung injury may exacerbate the pulmonary injury in patients with ARDS, where only a small portion of the lung remains aerated, and this portion is overdistended by conventional tidal volumes. Some protection against lung injury may be afforded by the use of pressure-limited ventilatory strategies. PEEP may be beneficial by reducing lung injury caused by the shear stresses associated with repeated opening and closing of alveoli.

Positive pressure ventilation may reduce cardiac output and blood pressure by impairing venous return and right-ventricular filling. This problem is aggravated by associated volume depletion and the use of sedative drugs. The effects are most marked in patients with obstructive airways disease and auto-PEEP. Management involves fluid resuscitation and a reduction in the mean airway pressure and minute ventilation.

Asynchrony

Poor interaction between the preset ventilation pattern and the patient's natural breathing rhythm can result in increased work of breathing, hypoventilation, or barotrauma. This patient–ventilator asynchrony manifests as the patient "fighting" the ventilator; it occurs more commonly with controlled ventilatory modes, high triggering thresholds, and flow capacity insufficient to meet patient requirements. The development of auto-PEEP increases the triggering threshold and the work of breathing.

Patient–ventilator asynchrony may occur if the patient begins expiration before delivery of the preset tidal volume has been completed. Slow inspiratory flow rate may be associated with increased work of breathing resulting from active inspiratory effort by the patient. Pressure-preset ventilatory modes have the advantage of allowing the flow rate to be determined by the patient's requirements. However, a rapid breathing rate in pressure-preset modes can result in a significantly reduced tidal volume.

If ventilator adjustments fail to correct patient–ventilator asynchrony, increased sedation or neuromuscular blockade may be a last resort after all physiological reasons for the asynchrony have been excluded. These interventions eliminate the patient's contribution to ventilation and reduce airway pressures and oxygen consumption.

Sedation and Paralysis

Varying degrees of sedation are necessary during mechanical ventilation to allow for patient comfort. Neuromuscular blockade immobilizes the patient and may be necessary to reduce asynchrony and to facilitate ventilatory strategies such as inverse-ratio ventilation and permissive hypercapnia. Sedative drugs may cause vasodilation and contribute to the hypotension that commonly accompanies positive pressure ventilation. Immobilization puts patients at risk for pressure necrosis of the skin, deep venous thrombosis, retention of secretions, atrophy of the respiratory and peripheral musculature, and atelectasis. If spontaneous respiratory efforts are suppressed, inadvertent disconnection from the ventilator can have disastrous consequences; ventilator alarms require emergent response. Prolonged weakness may occur even after withdrawal of neuromuscular blockade. The depth of paralysis should be limited, and neuromuscular blockade should be withdrawn periodically to assess the neuromuscular status. Daily interruption of sedative drug infusions decreases the duration of mechanical ventilation and the length of ICU stay (8).

Strategies To Reduce Ventilation-Associated Complications

Mechanical ventilation may produce or aggravate lung injury by overdistention of alveoli and by inadequate end-expiratory pressure producing alveolar collapse. Ventilation with low tidal volumes (5–7 mL/kg) to keep plateau airway pressure less than 30 cm H_2O improves outcome, likely by reducing ventilator-induced injury (2). PEEP is protective, reducing the shear stresses associated with repeated opening and closing of alveoli. Similarly, recruitment of previously collapsed lung tissue by periodic sustained inflations (10–40 seconds) at pressures of 30–40 cm H_2O may protect from lung injury as well as improve oxygenation. Pressure-limited ventilation may result in inadequate alveolar ventilation and the development of hypercapnia; this strategy of controlled hypoventilation and permissive hypercapnia is generally well tolerated if the pH is maintained above 7.1. Adequate oxygenation must be ensured, and the patient may require sedation or neuromuscular blockade because of the effects of hypercapnia on respiratory drive.

Standard prophylactic measures often used in the ventilated patient include stress-ulcer prevention with histamine-2 antagonists (see Chapter 80) (9) and low-dosage heparin to reduce the incidence of venous thromboembolism (see Chapter 52). Attention should be paid to providing adequate, preferably enteral, nutrition at the earliest possible time (see Chapter 15).

Weaning and Extubation

Once the underlying cause for acute respiratory failure has resolved, mechanical ventilation can be discontinued. In the patient with a short duration of ventilation and rapidly reversible underlying disease, the ventilator may be disconnected after a trial of spontaneous breathing (see Figure 23.3). After prolonged ventilation, respiratory muscle strength and endurance may be reduced, and a period of progressive withdrawal or "weaning" may be necessary. Different techniques for the gradual withdrawal of ventilatory support have potential advantages and disadvantages. Timing of the removal of the endotracheal tube is important—early extubation may result in respiratory failure and necessitate reintubation, while prolonging unnecessary intubation increases costs and the risk of complications. The most important issue is therefore to have a protocol in which the patient's ability to sustain spontaneous ventilation is assessed on a regular basis (e.g., every 24 hours).

Screening for Weaning

Before mechanical ventilation can be discontinued, both the underlying respiratory problem that required ventilation and any subsequent complications (such as nosoco-

mial pneumonia or atelectasis) must have largely resolved. The patient should be clinically stable, awake, and responsive. The respiratory neuromuscular system must be able to cope with the ventilatory work load, and oxygenation must be adequate at an inspired oxygen concentration less than 50%. Clinical measures that may be used to assess the likelihood of successful weaning include the tidal volume, respiratory rate, spontaneous minute ventilation, vital capacity, and maximum inspiratory force (Figure 23.3). Although these factors are relatively insensitive and nonspecific in predicting weaning success, a low respiratory workload compatible with spontaneous respiration can be indicated by a minute ventilation less than 10 L/min and a respiratory rate of less than 25 per minute. A useful predictor of success is a brief trial of spontaneous breathing while measuring the respiratory rate:tidal volume ratio.

Before removal of the endotracheal tube, the patency of the upper airway and the patient's ability to clear secretions must be assessed by evaluating the level of consciousness, upper-airway edema, the ability to cough, and the quantity of secretions. A *cuff-leak test* is performed by deflating the endotracheal tube cuff and briefly occluding the tube. If the patient can generate airflow around the tube, significant airway obstruction is unlikely after extubation. The inability to move air does not necessarily preclude extubation,

Step 1: Is the patient ready for weaning/extubation?

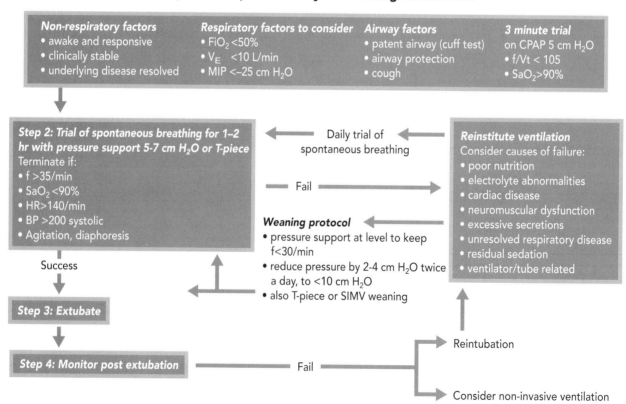

Figure 23.3   Algorithm for weaning and discontinuing mechanical ventilation. *BP*, blood pressure; *CPAP*, continuous positive airway pressure; *f*, respiratory frequency (rate); *FiO₂*, inspired oxygen fraction; *HR*, heart rate; *MIP*, maximal inspiratory pressure; *SₐO₂*, systemic arterial oxygen saturation; *SIMV*, synchronized intermittent mandatory ventilation; *VE*, minute ventilation; *Vt*, tidal volume.

particularly if the endotracheal tube is a large size; however, in such patients, precautions such as preoxygenation and ensuring that personnel and equipment for managing a difficult airway are available must be taken prior to extubation. If mechanical ventilation was initiated to provide an adequate airway because airway patency was compromised, the preexisting airway problem must be alleviated prior to extubation.

For the patient who fails to wean, various factors must be considered. Impaired cardiovascular performance resulting from ischemia or ventricular dysfunction may affect oxygen supply to respiratory muscles or result in pulmonary edema when positive intrathoracic pressure is removed. The presence of electrolyte disturbances (e.g., hypophosphatemia) and poor nutritional status may affect the ability to sustain spontaneous breathing. Residual respiratory disease with excessive secretions and persistent effects of sedation must be considered.

Techniques of Weaning

Following brief ventilation for a reversible condition, ventilatory support may be withdrawn after a trial of spontaneous respiration, which can be performed as a 1- to 2-hour trial on a T-piece or low pressure support (5–10 cm H_2O) while monitoring for signs of fatigue (Figure 23.3). With prolonged ventilation, a period of gradual weaning may be necessary, although daily assessment with a spontaneous breathing trial may suffice. The oxygen concentration often is reduced before weaning from the ventilator is considered; the usual approach is a gradual reduction of the inspired oxygen concentration to a level that can be delivered easily by face mask (e.g., less than 50%). PEEP usually is reduced to a level of about 5 cm H_2O in decrements of 2–3 cm H_2O, while oxygen saturation is monitored. The patient then is weaned gradually from ventilatory support, with monitoring for signs of ventilatory distress or fatigue, such as agitation, tachypnea, diaphoresis, or respiratory acidosis. In recent studies comparing various methods of weaning, weaning failure was less common with a shorter weaning duration using a daily trial of spontaneous breathing than it was with gradual reduction in ventilatory support (10).

As noted above, the critical care unit should have a predefined protocol for daily assessment of spontaneous breathing trials, which can guide the decision of whether to extubate or continue ventilation for another 24 hours (10). Trials in which the patient breathes spontaneously with low-pressure ventilatory support (5–10 cm H_2O) have proved as effective as trials of unaided breathing with a T-piece and have the advantage of overcoming the ventilator-induced work of breathing related to circuit and valve resistance.

Weaning using the T-piece involves gradually increasing periods of spontaneous breathing (e.g., 30 minutes, 60 minutes, etc.), ensuring that the patient does not develop fatigue. Adequate rest periods on ventilatory support between trials of spontaneous breathing are essential. There is little evidence in the literature to guide how long the patient should breathe on the T-piece and how long he or she should rest in the intervening period. The aim is to increase respiratory muscle strength and endurance until the patient tolerates spontaneous breathing without assistance. The T-piece provides no support to overcome ventilator circuit resistance.

Pressure-support weaning is performed by gradually reducing the level of pressure delivered to allow the patient to assume an increasing amount of respiratory work. Pressure support is reduced by 2 cm H_2O several times daily, assessing the patient for signs of fatigue. Once the pressure support is reduced to a level that overcomes the ventilator-induced work of breathing (circuit and valve resistance) but provides no additional support, extubation is considered. This level of pressure support, which varies between about 5 and 12 cm H_2O depending on the ventilator and endotracheal tube size, is difficult to determine in the individual patient.

An alternative weaning approach has used SIMV and gradually reduces the ventilator rate, with the patient increasing the amount of respiratory work performed. However, the SIMV approach to weaning has been documented to be less effective than the use of a T-piece or of pressure-support weaning.

Terminal Weaning

An increasingly common occurrence in the intensive care unit is the decision to withdraw life support. If aggressive life-extending measures have failed, the management goal changes to a comfort-oriented approach that includes withdrawing invasive interventions for which the burdens outweigh the comfort benefits (see Chapters 17 and 19). Compassionate withdrawal of ventilatory support, which is an integral part of this approach, is often more difficult to accept than the withdrawal of other support measures. In this regard, a common and acceptable practice is the discontinuation of other therapies, with the expectation that the patient will die on ventilatory support. Although this approach is effective if the patient is dependent on high-dosage inotropic support, it is important that mechanical ventilation not be continued unnecessarily so the dying process is not inappropriately prolonged.

Terminal withdrawal of mechanical ventilation may be performed rapidly by removing the endotracheal tube or by a more gradual weaning process during which the patient may die with the endotracheal tube in place. Each method has potential advantages and disadvantages, as well as strong proponents and opponents. Of paramount importance is that comfort of the patient be ensured and the family be made aware of the process and expected outcome. Often the decision depends on the perceived comfort of the patient and expressed concerns of the family. Extubation has the advantage of not prolonging the process of withdrawal, but it may be interpreted by some families and staff as being an active intervention with the intent to end the patient's life. Extubation should be preceded by the administration of adequate sedation (usually with benzodiazepines) and opiate analgesics to relieve any sensation of dyspnea. The anticipated outcome should be explained to the family, particularly if demise is expected within minutes, although prediction of the duration of survival is notoriously difficult.

Gradual withdrawal of support may be more comfortable and acceptable but also may prolong the dying process unnecessarily. This approach avoids the very active intervention of extubation. The inspired oxygen saturation may be reduced rapidly to that of room air; ventilatory support (pressure or tidal volume) may be reduced to the minimum; or a T-piece may be used. Adequate sedation and analgesia must be provided to ensure comfort and relief from dyspnea.

CONCLUSIONS

Mechanical ventilation is a necessary intervention to sustain life in the patient with respiratory failure, or to take control of the airway and breathing in the patient with other organ dysfunction. As with any medical intervention, it carries adverse effects, which are related to the presence of an endotracheal tube, the level of pressure delivered, the inspired oxygen concentration, and the duration of ventilatory support. Furthermore, the ventilated patient is at risk for sudden, unexpected catastrophic events such as disconnection from the ventilator or airway obstruction. Close monitoring of even the most stable patient is essential, and the patient should be assessed on a regular basis as to whether continued ventilation is necessary and appropriate.

KEY POINTS

- Correct timing is essential in instituting mechanical ventilation: Too soon or too late exposes the patient to unnecessary hazards.
- Consider noninvasive ventilation in the cooperative patient with an expected short duration of ventilation (e.g., pulmonary edema, exacerbation of chronic obstructive pulmonary disease).

- Prevent ventilator-induced lung injury by avoiding excessive inflation pressures and providing adequate end-expiratory pressure.
- Avoid prolonging ventilation unnecessarily: Assess daily for the ability to wean and discontinue ventilation.

REFERENCES

1. Brochard L, Mancebo J, Wysocki M, et al. Noninvasive ventilation for acute exacerbations of chronic obstructive pulmonary disease. *N Engl J Med* 1995;333:817–822.
2. The Acute Respiratory Distress Syndrome Network. Ventilation with lower tidal volumes as compared with traditional tidal volumes for acute lung injury and the acute respiratory distress syndrome. *N Engl J Med* 2000;342:1301–1308.
3. Ranieri VM, Suter PM, Tortorella C, et al. Effects of mechanical ventilation on inflammatory mediators in patients with acute respiratory distress syndrome: a randomized controlled trial. *JAMA* 1999; 282:54–61.
4. Feihl F, Perret C. Permissive hypercapnia: how permissive should we be? *Am J Respir Crit Care Med* 1994;150:1722–1737.
5. Grasso S, Mascia L, Del Turco M, et al. Effects of recruiting maneuvers in patients with acute respiratory distress syndrome ventilated with protective ventilatory strategy. *Anesthesiology* 2002;96: 795–802.
6. Gattinoni L, Tognoni G, Pesenti A, et al. Effect of prone positioning on the survival of patients with acute respiratory failure. *N Engl J Med* 2001;345:568–573.
7. Herridge MS, Cheung AM, Tansey CM, et al. One-year outcomes in survivors of the acute respiratory distress syndrome. *N Engl J Med* 2003;348:681–693.
8. Kress JP, Pohlman AS, O'Connor MF, Hall JB. Daily interruption of sedative infusions in critically ill patients undergoing mechanical ventilation. *N Engl J Med* 2000;342:1471–1477.
9. Cook D, Guyatt G, Marshall J, et al. A comparison of sucralfate and ranitidine for the prevention of upper gastrointestinal bleeding in patients requiring mechanical ventilation. *N Engl J Med* 1998;338:791–797.
10. MacIntyre NR, Cook DJ, Ely EW, et al. Evidence-based guidelines for weaning and discontinuing ventilatory support. *Chest* 2001; 120(suppl 6):375S–395S.

ADDITIONAL READING

Brochard L. Noninvasive ventilation for acute respiratory failure. *JAMA* 2002;288:932–935.

Brower RG, Ware LB, Berthiaume Y, Matthay MA. Treatment of ARDS. *Chest* 2001;120:1347–1367.

Hogarth DK, Hall J. Management of sedation in mechanically ventilated patients. *Curr Opin Crit Care* 2004;10:40–46.

Pinhu L, Whitehead T, Evans T, Griffiths M. Ventilator-associated lung injury. *Lancet* 2003;361:332–340.

Schumaker GL, Epstein SK. Managing acute respiratory failure during exacerbations of chronic obstructive pulmonary disease. *Respir Care* 2004;49:766–782.

Tobin MJ. Advances in mechanical ventilation. *N Engl J Med* 2001;344:1986–1996.

Acute Respiratory Failure

Mark R. Tonelli   *Leonard D. Hudson*

Any discussion of acute respiratory failure as a clinical entity must begin with the recognition that the disorder varies significantly in presentation and has multiple causes (Table 24.1). Decisions regarding appropriate treatments cannot be made without evaluation of both severity and etiology.

Defining acute respiratory failure has been problematic. Physiologically, respiratory failure can be said to occur if either ventilation or oxygenation is inadequate for optimal function of tissue, organs, or the organism. In this sense, the diagnosis of acute respiratory failure relies on arterial blood-gas measurements demonstrating hypercapnia with acidemia or profound hypoxemia. Clinically, however, the diagnosis of respiratory failure generally is suspected prior to obtaining arterial blood-gas measurements. For example, the patient overdosed on heroin with a respiratory rate of 6 per minute or the tight asthmatic with tachypnea both may be presumed to have an acute change in respiratory status. In such situations, respiratory compromise is clearly present, though respiratory failure is not demonstrated until arterial blood gases are analyzed.

The traditional focus on respiratory physiology and mechanistic distinctions based on classes of gas-exchange abnormalities often obscures more clinically relevant aspects of acute respiratory failure. Although an understanding of pulmonary physiology is important in the assessment of respiratory failure, the clinical evaluation generally begins prior to the measurement of arterial blood gases. Respiratory compromise, evident by physical examination, represents the starting point of evaluation and treatment.

Respiratory compromise may result from intrinsic lung disease, but it also accompanies neurologic injury, upper-airway disorders, heart failure, vascular disease, renal failure, metabolic derangement, and systemic infection or inflammation. Respiratory distress may be a presenting complaint or may develop during the course of another illness. For example, in *acute respiratory distress syndrome* (ARDS), hypoxemic respiratory failure usually develops in patients admitted with another life-threatening illness or injury. However, ARDS sometimes exists on presentation, and virtually any cause of acute respiratory failure can complicate hospitalization. Outcomes research on specific causes of respiratory compromise, such as asthma, chronic obstructive pulmonary disease (COPD), community-acquired pneumonia, pulmonary vascular disease, and heart failure, can guide treatment for those entities.

ACUTE RESPIRATORY COMPROMISE PRESENTING ON ADMISSION

Clinical Presentation

Respiratory compromise should be suspected in any patient presenting complaints of shortness of breath or signs of tachypnea or labored breathing, and it also must be considered in other clinical situations. Neurologic injury or profound central nervous system depression may result in inadequate ventilation as a result of impaired drive or upper-airway compromise without a sensation of dyspnea. Such patients generally are unresponsive and without tachypnea on presentation. Conversely, the patient with inadequate ventilation secondary to other causes may develop neurologic symptoms including agitation, confusion, or depressed level of consciousness.

In the dyspneic and tachypneic patient, other clinical manifestations are dependent on the cause of respiratory compromise. Stridor indicates upper-airway obstruction; audible expiratory wheezing suggests airflow obstruction; and a rapid, shallow breathing pattern often accompanies a restrictive process. The patient with impending respiratory

TABLE 24.1

MAJOR CAUSES OF ACUTE RESPIRATORY FAILURE

Airway/airflow obstruction
  Bronchospasm
    Asthma
    Chronic obstructive pulmonary disease
  Foreign body
  Trauma
  Laryngeal edema
Pulmonary parenchymal
  Infection
    Bacterial
    Viral
  Diffuse lung injury: acute respiratory distress syndrome
Cardiovascular
  Acute myocardial infarction
  Heart failure
  Pulmonary embolism
Neurogenic
  Brainstem injury
    Trauma
    Vascular accident
  Respiratory depression
    Opiates
    Benzodiazepines
    Barbiturates
    Alcohol
  Neuromuscular
    Guillain-Barré syndrome
    Myasthenic crisis
Renal/metabolic
  Volume overload
  Severe metabolic acidosis

struction or heart failure. Acute presentations accompanied by fever, cough, or sputum production suggest infectious etiologies. Sudden onset of dyspnea without systemic symptoms should raise the possibility of airway obstruction, cardiac disease, and pulmonary vascular occlusion. Complaints of chronic and progressive dyspnea with acute worsening most often represent an exacerbation of an underlying pulmonary illness, such as COPD or asthma.

Physical Examination

Initial physical examination should be aimed at both elucidating a cause and assessing the severity of respiratory compromise. Altered mental status without an alternative cause suggests severe respiratory compromise. In patients with airflow obstruction, pulsus paradoxus greater than 20 mm Hg indicates severe obstruction. A respiratory rate greater than 35 per minute in an adult suggests severe respiratory compromise. Estimating the tidal volume by observation and auscultation is an important, but imperfect, measure of severity. Wheezing on auscultation (often both inspiratory and expiratory) usually accompanies severe airflow obstruction, but *wheezing may become inaudible if tidal volume drops low enough*. Rales on examination may accompany heart failure, pneumonia, interstitial lung disease, or diffuse lung injury. Consolidative changes may accompany pneumonia or atelectasis. Normal results of lung examination do not exclude respiratory failure and may accompany some infections (e.g., *Pneumocystis jirovecii* pneumonia), diffuse lung injury, metabolic derangement, and disorders of central respiratory drive.

Laboratory Evaluation

Arterial blood-gas measurement remains the most important laboratory test for determining both the presence and severity of respiratory failure. The hallmark of acute ventilatory failure is the presence of hypercapnia (arterial partial pressure of carbon dioxide [P_aCO_2] >45 mm Hg) along with acidemia (pH <7.35). In acute ventilatory failure, metabolic compensation for hypercapnia has not yet taken place, and the rise in carbon dioxide is directly reflected in a falling pH. In such situations, the base excess remains near zero, and the serum bicarbonate level is close to normal (see Chapter 105). If there has been some time for compensation to occur or if there is an underlying metabolic alkalosis, the bicarbonate level will be high, the base excess will be greater than 2, and the pH will tend toward normal. The presence of a metabolic acidosis (with a base excess of ≤ -2) in the setting of hypercapnia is an ominous sign and should prompt consideration of mechanical ventilation.

Hypoxemia may accompany hypercapneic respiratory failure or may be present if ventilation is adequate. Hypoxemia generally is caused by hypoventilation, by ventilation–perfusion mismatching, or by shunting, often in combination. Low levels (<6 L/min) of supplemental oxygen

failure is usually anxious; somnolence or lethargy should alert the clinician to the possibility that assisted ventilation may be required emergently. It is important to remember that normal oxygen saturations may be present in the setting of significantly impaired ventilation, especially if the patient is breathing supplemental oxygen.

The physician's first task is to ensure that the patient's airway is patent and that breathing is adequate to allow for further evaluation. Supplemental oxygen should be provided to ensure adequate oxygen saturation. The resources necessary to perform rapid endotracheal intubation and assisted ventilation should be available readily (see Chapter 23).

Differential Diagnosis and Initial Evaluation

History

Appropriate therapy cannot be administered without an accurate determination of the cause of respiratory compromise. The medical history should focus on both the pertinent aspects of the present illness, including rapidity of onset and associated symptoms, and the past medical history, especially the presence of previous episodes of airflow ob-

usually correct hypoxemia caused by hypoventilation or ventilation–perfusion mismatch, but significant shunting results in much higher oxygen requirements. Shunting occurs if blood flow in the pulmonary circulation does not pass through areas of ventilated lung en route to the left atrium. In virtually any type of lung disease, large areas of alveolar filling or collapse, radiographically evidenced by increased opacification, produce some degree of shunt. The normal physiologic response of hypoxic vasoconstriction acts to minimize shunting. Clinicians should be aware that vasodilators, including nitrates, can overcome this adaptive response and worsen hypoxemia.

Hypoxemia alone is generally not an indication for mechanical ventilation, as 100% oxygen can be delivered effectively to the spontaneously ventilating patient. In some cases of acute lung injury, however, profound hypoxemia cannot be corrected with supplemental oxygen. In such cases, intubation and mechanical ventilation (see Chapter 23) are indicated to provide positive end-expiratory pressure and other ventilator strategies designed to improve oxygenation.

In the setting of acute-on-chronic respiratory failure, the administration of supplemental oxygen often is accompanied by a rise in P_aCO_2. Although generally attributed to a decreased respiratory drive, the pathophysiology of this phenomenon is more complex (see Chapter 55). For the clinician, *fear of a rising P_aCO_2 should never preclude the administration of enough supplemental oxygen to ensure adequate oxygen delivery*. In general, a target range of 88% to 90% oxygen saturation usually allows for adequate oxygen delivery while minimizing the potential increase in P_aCO_2.

Rapid measurement of B-type natriuretic peptide (BNP) appears to be a useful biochemical adjunct to clinical assessment in determining the cause of acute dyspnea in patients presenting emergently (1). An elevated BNP level is seen almost universally in patients with significant left heart failure; however it is important for clinicians to realize that BNP is often chronically elevated in patients with cor pulmonale and can also rise with acute right ventricular failure, such as might accompany pulmonary embolism. Thus, although BNP is a sensitive indicator of heart failure, it is nonspecific. A thorough clinical assessment for alternative or addtional causes of respiratory failure must still be undertaken even in the presence of an elevated BNP.

The chest radiograph may be particularly helpful in determining the cause of respiratory failure (Figure 24.1). A chest radiograph without parenchymal infiltrates may accompany respiratory failure secondary to respiratory depression, neuromuscular weakness, upper-airway obstruction, pulmonary vascular disease, and airflow obstruction. Respiratory depression and neuromuscular weakness usually are associated with low lung volumes determined radiographically; airflow obstruction caused by COPD or asthma often presents with signs of hyperinflation, including large lung volumes and hyperlucency. Metabolic disturbances such as profound metabolic acidosis and carbon monoxide poisoning present with a normal chest radio-

graph. Pneumonia, particularly *P. jirovecii* pneumonia, may occasionally be radiographically inapparent early in its course. The chest radiograph is diagnostic in cases of respiratory compromise caused by a large pleural effusion or a tension pneumothorax.

Focal infiltrates seen on the chest radiograph suggest bacterial or fungal pneumonia, aspiration, atelectasis, or pulmonary hemorrhage or infarction. Unusual causes of respiratory failure with focal infiltrates include bronchiolitis obliterans with organizing pneumonia (BOOP), vasculitis such as Wegener's granulomatosis, and alveolar proteinosis. Location and character of the infiltrates may suggest specific causes, but radiographic signs are rarely sensitive or specific.

Heart failure generally presents with a diffuse edema pattern with hilar predominance of infiltrates; however, this pattern is nonspecific and can be seen with ARDS and with bacterial, *P. jirovecii*, or viral pneumonia. Respiratory compromise secondary to collagen vascular disease, drug toxicity, and hypersensitivity pneumonitis also generally presents with diffuse infiltrates. In addition, acute eosinophilic pneumonia, acute interstitial pneumonitis, and the fat emboli syndrome all may cause a radiographic pattern of pulmonary edema and hypoxemic respiratory failure indistinguishable from ARDS (Table 24.2).

INDICATIONS FOR HOSPITAL AND INTENSIVE CARE UNIT ADMISSION

After appropriate diagnostic evaluation, admission should be considered if the cause of respiratory compromise remains unclear or if the patient remains refractory to appropriate treatment. New, persistent hypoxemia is generally an indication for hospital admission. Specific criteria and decision rules for admission with asthma or community-acquired pneumonia have been proposed (see Chapters 56 and 65). The need for mechanical ventilation is obviously an absolute indication for admission to the ICU, and this level of careful monitoring is also appropriate for patients in whom noninvasive ventilation has been instituted (see Chapter 23). ICU admission also should be considered for patients at high risk for requiring mechanical ventilation, especially those with increasing oxygen requirements or those requiring nearly continuous nursing or respiratory care, such as for assistance in clearing pulmonary secretions.

INITIAL THERAPIES

Initial therapy for respiratory compromise must be aimed at the underlying condition. The general question in all cases of respiratory compromise is whether invasive mechanical ventilation is required. The quality of explicit data available to aid clinicians in this judgment is poor. Nonetheless, certain criteria and patterns are helpful in determining whether a patient requires mechanical support.

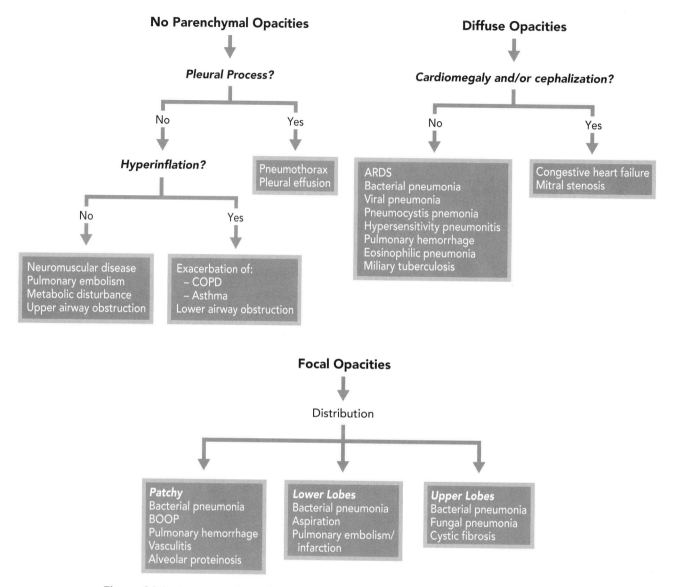

Figure 24.1 Common radiographic manifestations of causes of acute respiratory failure. However, there may be substantial overlap and variation among these patterns. ARDS, acute respiratory distress syndrome; BOOP, bronchiolitis obliterans with organizing pneumonia; COPD, chronic obstructive pulmonary disease.

Indications for endotracheal intubation, with or without mechanical ventilation, include upper-airway injury or inflammation, (e.g., trauma and burns, laryngeal edema, and pharyngeal swelling); and airway compromise, often in the setting of neurologic injury or profound central nervous system depression with loss of protective reflexes, including gag and cough. A patent airway should be guaranteed early, even before the demonstration of attendant hypercapnia. Because intubation is often difficult in patients with anatomic upper-airway obstruction, the assistance of an anesthesiologist or otolaryngologist well trained in airway management is helpful. Intubation over a fiberoptic bronchoscope may also be considered.

Determining whether mechanical ventilation is required in the patient with an exacerbation of airflow obstruction remains problematic. Based on several case series, there is a

concern that mechanical ventilation may worsen outcomes independent of severity of disease, most likely secondary to the hemodynamic consequences of positive pressure ventilation. Hypotension developing after the institution of positive pressure ventilation in the patient with severe airflow obstruction is usually secondary to an intrinsic positive end-expiratory pressure (PEEP) and, if not recognized, may lead to cardiovascular collapse and death (see Chapter 23). Endotracheal intubation also may cause or exacerbate bronchospasm. Generally, it is appropriate to attempt to reverse airflow obstruction aggressively without instituting mechanical ventilation. Because underlying chronic respiratory failure may precede acute decompensation, there is no single level of P_aCO_2 that necessitates mechanical ventilation; the serum pH is generally a better marker of the acute severity of respiratory decompensation. However, se-

TABLE 24.2

CAUSES OF DIFFUSE LUNG INJURY BESIDES ACUTE RESPIRATORY DISTRESS SYNDROME

Acute eosinophilic pneumonia
Bacterial pneumonia
   Mycoplasma
Fungal pneumonia
   Pneumocystis jirovecii
Viral pneumonitis
   Varicella
   Adenovirus
   Respiratory syncitial virus
Drug effect
   Hypersensitivity (e.g., nitrofurantoin)
   Cytotoxic (e.g., busulfan)
Pulmonary hemorrhage
Bronchiolitis obliterans with organizing pneumonia (BOOP)
Collagen–vascular disease
Vasculitis
Fat emboli

rial arterial blood-gas measurements revealing progressive hypercapnia and worsening acidosis are highly predictive of impending respiratory collapse. Physical changes are generally less reliable, as somnolence, decreasing respiratory rate, or a decrease in wheezing may signal either worsening hypercapnia or a positive response to therapy. In the cooperative patient with airflow obstruction, serial measurement of the peak expiratory flow rate is a reasonable noninvasive approach to assessing the effectiveness of therapy (see Chapters 55 and 56).

In the patient with hypoxemia, mechanical ventilation is absolutely required only if 100% inspired oxygen concentration is inadequate to maintain oxygenation (saturations >85%) and there is reason to believe that certain features of positive pressure ventilation, such as PEEP, will improve saturations. For example, abnormal oxygenation in diffuse lung injury is usually responsive to PEEP. If oxygenation is clearly and rapidly worsening in the face of diffuse pulmonary infiltrates, intubation and mechanical ventilation should be considered early in the course, as waiting until saturations are inadequate on 100% oxygen significantly increases the difficulty and risk of intubation. By comparison, large intrapulmonary or intracardiac shunts may result in severe hypoxemia that is minimally responsive to high-flow oxygen but also is unlikely to be improved, and in fact may be worsened, with PEEP.

Given the inherent risks, discomfort, and costs of mechanical ventilation, noninvasive ventilation techniques have become increasingly common over the past decade (see Chapter 23). Noninvasive ventilation may include inspiratory assistance (analogous to pressure-support ventilation), continuous positive airway pressure, or both. Inspiratory assistance is particularly effective if fatigue or neuromuscular weakness is causing or complicating respi-

ratory compromise. Continuous positive airway pressure provides "distending" pressure at end-exhalation, and may both improve ventilation–perfusion matching and increase lung volumes throughout the respiratory cycle, thereby decreasing airway resistance.

There is now good evidence to support the use of noninvasive ventilation for acute exacerbations of COPD, pulmonary edema, and pulmonary contusions (2). Additionally, some reports suggest that this technique may be efficacious in postoperative respiratory insufficiency and acute exacerbations of cystic fibrosis. Weaning mechanically ventilated patients to noninvasive ventilation appears to decrease the incidence of ventilator-associated pneumonia (see Chapter 66) (3). On the other hand, noninvasive mechanical ventilation is not effective in acute hypoxemic respiratory failure (i.e., impending ARDS).

INDICATIONS FOR EARLY CONSULTATION

Because appropriate therapy cannot be provided in the absence of an accurate diagnosis, respiratory failure of unclear cause is an indication for early pulmonary consultation. Respiratory failure associated with diffuse infiltrates seen on chest radiograph without evidence of heart failure has a wide differential diagnosis. Early bronchoscopy may be indicated to exclude viral pneumonitis, *P. jirovecii* pneumonia, pulmonary hemorrhage, hypersensitivity pneumonitis, and acute eosinophilic pneumonia. If bronchoscopy is unrevealing, open lung biopsy is indicated in specific situations (Table 24.3).

In the mechanically ventilated patient, hemodynamic instability may be secondary to ventilator effects, such as intrinsic PEEP and barotrauma. If the treating physician does not have the expertise to detect and deal with these

TABLE 24.3

INDICATIONS FOR BRONCHOSCOPY AND OPEN LUNG BIOPSY IN PATIENTS WITH ACUTE RESPIRATORY FAILURE

Consider fiber-optic bronchoscopy for patients:
  With focal infiltrates and:
    Immunocompromise
    Failure to respond to empiric antibiotics
    Risk or suspicion of endobronchial lesion or foreign body
    Mucus plugging/lobar collapse not responsive to chest physiotherapy
    Hemoptysis
  With diffuse infiltrates and:
    Immunocompromise
    No risk factor for acute respiratory distress syndrome
Consider open lung biopsy in cases in which fiberoptic bronchoscopy is unrevealing

complications directly, then emergent consultation is indicated. Likewise, persistent hypoxemia on high fractions of inspired oxygen (>80%) or high static pressures (>35 cm H_2O) should precipitate a pulmonary consultation, as advanced ventilator strategies likely are required.

ISSUES DURING THE COURSE OF HOSPITALIZATION

The course of acute respiratory failure depends primarily on the underlying etiology. However, several general observations can be made regarding respiratory failure.

If the patient with respiratory compromise fails to improve as expected, evaluation should focus on the likelihood that the presumptive cause of respiratory collapse is in error. For example, the patient with presumed bacterial pneumonia who fails to respond to antibiotics over 72 hours requires a careful evaluation for other possible causes, both infectious and noninfectious, of hypoxemia and a focal infiltrate. Pulmonary consultation, both for an expanded differential diagnosis and for possible bronchoscopy, is generally indicated.

Respiratory failure may also fail to respond to seemingly appropriate therapy because of the development of an additional cause of respiratory compromise. ARDS, for instance, may occur in a significant percentage of patients with bacterial pneumonia and lead to a protracted course of mechanical ventilation. Likewise, both pulmonary embolism and nosocomial pneumonia may complicate the hospital course of any patient.

The conclusion that a protracted course of respiratory failure represents the inexorable progression of a chronic pulmonary disease (such as COPD or cystic fibrosis) is generally a process of excluding other diagnoses. Knowledge of the natural history and outcomes of mechanical ventilation for specific disease states is imperative. Most patients who require mechanical ventilation for even severe COPD can be weaned successfully (4); however the prognosis of patients who require mechanical ventilation for cystic fibrosis is very poor. Respiratory failure in association with hematologic malignancy, and in particular in the course of bone-marrow transplantation, portends a very poor prognosis. Outcomes for many other causes of respiratory failure are less predictable and mortality estimates are often moving targets.

DISCHARGE ISSUES

Guidelines and disease-management strategies have been proposed for specific causes of respiratory failure, including asthma, COPD, and community-acquired pneumonia. In general, discharge should be considered when ventilatory status has returned to near-baseline. Persistent hypoxemia alone does not preclude discharge, as home oxygen therapy is widely available. An oxygen saturation of less than 88%

or an arterial partial pressure of oxygen less than 55 mm Hg, either at rest, nocturnally, or with exercise, is an indication for outpatient oxygen therapy. For all patients with an acute illness, such as pneumonia, and even those with an exacerbation of an underlying illness, such as emphysema, reassessment of oxygen requirements should take place on a regular basis after discharge. Half the patients who require the initiation of oxygen therapy at the time of hospital discharge after an exacerbation of COPD no longer meet criteria for oxygen therapy 1 month later.

Likewise, the need for chest physiotherapy or noninvasive ventilatory assistance does not preclude discharge to home. Multiple devices and techniques are available to enable patients to mobilize secretions, and collaboration with a pulmonologist, nurse, or respiratory therapist familiar with these techniques can facilitate early and safe discharge. Similarly, a variety of ventilatory assist devices, including noninvasive portable ventilators, may allow the patient with chronic respiratory failure, especially that resulting from neuromuscular weakness, to function well at home.

Discharge for patients with prolonged respiratory failure has changed over the past several years. Previously, most mechanically ventilated patients with ongoing medical problems were relegated to the ICUs of acute care hospitals. Largely because of anomalies in Medicare reimbursement, however, facilities specializing in the care of patients undergoing long-term ventilation and other chronically, critically ill patients have arisen in many parts of the United States. Optimally, these facilities provide respiratory care and nursing services similar to ICUs, with an additional emphasis on rehabilitation and the psychological and social needs of patients and families. Quality remains variable, however, and recent revisions in Medicare reimbursement have put economic strains on these institutions. Still, they remain a viable alternative to lengthy stays in the ICU of an acute care hospital.

ACUTE RESPIRATORY FAILURE PRESENTING DURING HOSPITALIZATION

Respiratory compromise may develop in the hospitalized patient because of any of the factors that lead to an initial outpatient presentation with acute respiratory failure. A few causes, however, account for the majority of such cases (Table 24.4). For example, the immobility that often accompanies illness puts patients at significant risk for pulmonary thromboembolic disease, which should be an initial consideration in any inpatient who develops dyspnea, tachypnea, chest pain, or hypoxemia (see Chapter 53).

Inpatients are also at increased risk for developing aspiration, which may precipitate respiratory failure directly or through the development of ARDS or nosocomial pneumonia. The risk factors for aspiration include impaired consciousness, swallowing disorders, and upper-airway in-

TABLE 24.4

COMMON CAUSES OF RESPIRATORY COMPROMISE IN HOSPITALIZED PATIENTS

Pulmonary embolism
Aspiration of gastric contents
Nosocomial/ventilator-associated pneumonia
Acute respiratory distress syndrome
Iatrogenic causes
   Oversedation
   Volume overload
Drug reaction
   Hypersensitivity pneumonitis
   Laryngeal edema
   Anaphylaxis

strumentation, including nasogastric and endotracheal tubes. The intubated patient runs a 1%–3% risk per day of developing ventilator-associated pneumonia (see Chapter 66), which is associated with an increased mortality rate and increased hospital costs. Several maneuvers have been suggested to minimize colonization, aspiration, and ventilator-associated pneumonia, including semirecumbent positioning, early enteral feeding, and the use of sucralfate rather than H_2 antagonists for ulcer prophylaxis, but the available studies have been small and not always well controlled. Various devices that provide suctioning of oropharyngeal contents above the cuff of the endotracheal tube show promise but have not been tested rigorously. Interestingly, frequent changing of the ventilator circuits appears to increase the risk of ventilator-associated pneumonia, and respiratory care protocols that require routine changes more often than every 2 weeks should be reexamined.

A number of iatrogenic causes of respiratory compromise must be considered in hospitalized patients. Opiates are profound respiratory depressants, and injudicious use may lead to respiratory arrest. Laryngeal edema is a rare but life-threatening complication of multiple medications, particularly angiotensin-converting enzyme inhibitors. Anaphylaxis also may be caused by many medications (see Chapter 120). Hypersensitivity pneumonitis caused by medications can develop over several days and result in respiratory compromise and diffuse pulmonary infiltrates.

ARDS is a frequent cause of acute respiratory failure in patients admitted with other serious illnesses or injuries. ARDS represents a diffuse and nonspecific lung-injury pattern, usually developing under the conditions that precipitate a systemic inflammatory response (Table 24.5).

ARDS generally develops within 24–72 hours of the onset of the inciting illness or injury. The clinical presentation is increasing respiratory distress with tachypnea and hypoxemia. The chest radiograph reveals diffuse pulmonary infiltrates, consistent with pulmonary edema, so the presumptive diagnosis of ARDS cannot be made in the setting

of volume overload or left heart failure. Measurement of the pulmonary capillary wedge pressure (see Chapter 25) can help distinguish ARDS from volume overload and cardiogenic pulmonary edema. In patients requiring mechanical ventilation, lung compliance is usually low (<30 mL/cm H_2O) and minute ventilation is usually significantly elevated (>15 L) in ARDS, although these findings are not necessary to make the diagnosis.

Preventing ARDS in individuals at risk has proven elusive, and the management of patients with ARDS remains primarily supportive. A large, multi-centered randomized trial comparing mechanical ventilation with low tidal volumes (6 mL/kg of ideal body weight) versus high tidal volumes (12 mL/kg of ideal body weight) demonstrated a significant (approximately 25%) reduction in mortality in ARDS patients with the low tidal volume stategy (5). Specific therapies to aid in lung healing or function, including exogenous surfactant, inhaled nitric oxide, and the early use of systemic corticosteroids, have not been demonstrated to decrease the mortality rate. Nonetheless, the survival rate for patients with ARDS has improved significantly over the past decade and is currently in the range of 60%–65% (6). The vast majority of patients with ARDS who do not survive die either of their presenting illnesses or after developing sepsis or multiorgan failure. The initial severity of hypoxemia does not predict outcome and, somewhat counterintuitively, the longer a patient remains on mechanical ventilation the higher the survival rate. Thus, the care of the patient with ARDS is aimed primarily at avoiding complications, particularly infection and additional organ failure. Barotrauma is a common complication of ARDS, but the development of pneumothorax or other types of air leaks does not appear to affect the mortality rate significantly.

In general, the long-term prognosis for survivors of ARDS is good. Although initial pulmonary-function testing is likely to reveal some evidence of restrictive physiology (a reduced total lung capacity), recovery of pulmonary function is usually complete, or nearly complete, 6 months after hospital

TABLE 24.5

COMMON RISK FACTORS FOR THE DEVELOPMENT OF ACUTE RESPIRATORY DISTRESS SYNDROME

Infection
   Sepsis
   Pneumonia
Trauma
   Pulmonary contusion
   Multiple fractures
Aspiration
Multiple transfusions (≥10 units)
Near drowning
Pancreatitis

discharge. However, exercise capacity (measured by a 6 minute walk) and health-related quality of life frequently remain diminished for at least 1 year after ICU discharge (7, 8). It has been suggested that the institution of corticosteroids late in the course of severe, persistent ARDS may improve outcome (9) and ameliorate the development of irreversible fibrosis, but this therapy may also increase the likelihood and severity of neuromuscular sequelae, such as critical-illness polyneuropathy and myopathy. We do not presently recommend routine use of corticosteroids in late ARDS.

COST CONSIDERATION AND RESOURCE USE

Although data regarding the costs of acute respiratory failure are limited, several considerations warrant mention. First, the use of noninvasive rather than standard endotracheal mechanical ventilation may not have a profound impact on costs. Because the vast majority of patients on noninvasive positive pressure ventilation (NIPPV) require ICU monitoring, at least initially, physician, nursing, and respiratory care costs are high. Secondly, although patients with persistent respiratory failure (>7 days on mechanical ventilation) represent less than 10% of all ICU patients, they account for one-quarter to one-third of total ICU costs (10). Thus, the prevention of respiratory failure, particularly nosocomial pneumonia and ARDS, will provide significant cost savings.

Considerable interest in weaning from mechanical ventilation also may be driven by cost concerns, although multiple studies suggest that the ventilator mode used during weaning is nearly irrelevant for the vast majority of patients, and that physicians' failure to recognize that patients can be liberated safely from mechanical ventilation is the primary cause of unnecessary days of mechanical ventilation (see Chapter 23). Daily weaning parameters or T-piece trials, undertaken by respiratory therapists according to protocol, on all patients with moderate amounts of supplemental oxygen (<50%), low PEEP ≤5 cm H_2O), and reasonable minute-ventilation requirements (<12 L) may prove to be cost-effective. Weaning certain ventilator-dependent COPD patients to noninvasive ventilation decreases the incidence of ventilator-associated pneumonia and reduces length of stay in the ICU (3). This technique may be applicable to other causes of respiratory failure as well.

KEY POINTS

- Respiratory compromise has myriad causes, and appropriate therapy depends upon the accurate and timely determination of cause and severity.

- Empiric therapy for the most likely cause of respiratory compromise in an individual patient is generally appropriate, but failure to respond as expected should precipitate an evaluation for alternative or contributory causes.

- The incidence of respiratory failure developing in hospitalized patients can be reduced with specific interventions designed to prevent deep venous thrombosis, aspiration, and ventilator-associated pneumonia.

- The survival rate in ARDS is improving, though care remains largely supportive. Lower tidal volumes improve outcome compared with traditional tidal volumes. The avoidance and prompt treatment of complications, particularly secondary infections and additional organ failure, are of paramount importance.

REFERENCES

1. Mueller C, Scholer A, Lanle-Kilian K, et al. Use of B-type natriuretic peptide in the evaluation and management of acute dyspnea. *N Engl J Med* 2004;350:647–654.
2. Peter JV, Moran JL, Phillips-Hughes J, Warn D. Noninvasive ventilation in acute respiratory failure-a meta-analytic update. *Crit Care Med* 2002;30:555–562.
3. Nava S, Ambrosino N, Clini E, et al. Noninvasive mechanical ventilation in the weaning of patients with respiratory failure due to chronic obstructive pulmonary disease. A randomized, controlled trial. *Ann Intern Med* 1998;128:721–728.
4. Breen D, Churches T, Hawker F, Torzillo PJ. Acute respiratory failure secondary to chronic obstructive pulmonary disease treated in the intensive care unit: a long term follow up study. *Thorax* 2002;57:29–33.
5. Acute Respiratory Distress Network. Ventilation with lower tidal volumes as compared with traditional tidal volumes for acute lung injury and the acute respiratory distress syndrome. *N Engl J Med* 2000;342:1301–1308.
6. Milberg JA, Davis DR, Steinberg KP, et al. Improved survival of patients with acute respiratory distress syndrome (ARDS): 1983–1993. *JAMA* 1995;273:306–309.
7. Herridge MS, Cheung AM, Tansey CM, et al. One-year outcomes in survivors of the acute respiratory adult distress syndrome. *N Engl J Med* 2003;348:683–693.
8. Davidson TA, Caldwell ES, Curtis JR, et al. Reduced quality of life in survivors of acute respiratory distress syndrome compared with critically ill control patients. *JAMA* 1999;281:354–360.
9. Meduri GU, Headley AS, Golden E, et al. Effect of prolonged methylprednisolone therapy in unresolving acute respiratory distress syndrome: a randomized controlled trial. *JAMA* 1998;280:159–165.
10. Rubenfeld GD, Caldwell ES, Steinberg KP, et al. Persistent lung injury and ICU resource utilization. *Am J Respir Crit Care Medicine* 1998;157:PA498.

ADDITIONAL READING

Adrogue HJ, Madias NE. Management of life-threatening acid-base disorders: first of two parts. *N Engl J Med* 1998;338:26–34.
Pierson DJ. Indications for mechanical ventilation in adults with respiratory failure. *Respir Care* 2002;47:249–262.
Schmidt GA, Hall JB, Wood LDH. Ventilatory Failure. In Murray JF, Nadel JA, eds. *Textbook of Respiratory Medicine*, 2nd ed. Philadelphia: W.B. Saunders, 2000.

Hypotension, Shock, and Multiple Organ Failure

Bradley D. Freeman   **Charles Natanson**

INTRODUCTION

Hypotension, shock, and multiorgan dysfunction are commonly encountered and potentially lethal clinical problems. This chapter reviews the classification and differential diagnosis of shock, the approach to management of the patient with hemodynamic instability, and recent advances that may decrease morbidity and improve survival in these critically ill patients.

DEFINITION AND CLASSIFICATION OF SHOCK

Though a number of definitions for *shock* are commonly used, the most practical describes an acute syndrome initiated by ineffective perfusion and resulting in severe organ dysfunction. Many conditions can result in shock (Table 25.1). In a given patient, the cause may be apparent (e.g., hypotension in a patient with massive upper-gastrointestinal hemorrhage), unclear (e.g., patients with pulmonary embolism, cardiac tamponade, or adrenal insufficiency), or attributable to multiple factors (e.g., a patient with multiple trauma who develops myocardial ischemia and severe infection). It is useful to classify shock as either *hypovolemic, cardiogenic, extracardiac obstructive,* or *distributive* (Figure 25.1).

Hypovolemic (or *oligemic*) *shock* can occur by any mechanism that decreases intravascular volume, including hemorrhage or fluid loss from the gastrointestinal tract (diar-

rhea, vomiting), urinary tract (diabetic ketoacidosis, diabetes insipidus, excessive diuretic therapy), or skin (burns, extensive desquamation) or into a "third" space (e.g., peritonitis, pancreatitis, postsurgical fluxes). In early stages, compensatory increases in heart rate, peripheral vascular resistance, and myocardial contractility may preserve cardiac and cerebral perfusion. Ultimately, however, the typical hemodynamic picture of shock develops, and is characterized by decreases in mean arterial pressure, stroke volume, and cardiac output (Table 25.2).

Cardiogenic shock is most commonly a consequence of myocardial ischemia or infarction, though other potential causes include cardiomyopathy, arrhythmia, and valvular heart disease. Cardiogenic shock and hypovolemic shock may appear similar hemodynamically, except that cardiogenic shock is associated with elevated central filling pressures and the typical physical findings of jugular venous distention and pulmonary edema. Right-heart catheterization in the setting of cardiogenic shock typically demonstrates a low cardiac index (≤ 2.0 L/min/m^2; normal: 3.0–5.0 L/min/m^2) and elevated pulmonary capillary wedge pressure (17–20 cm H$_2$O; normal: 5–12 cm H$_2$O).

Extracardiac obstructive shock results from physical impairment of adequate forward circulatory flow involving mechanisms other than primary myocardial or valvular apparatus dysfunction. The result is reduced cardiac filling and low cardiac output. Causes include impaired diastolic ventricular filling (e.g., pericardial tamponade, pneumothorax, constrictive pericarditis, extrinsic compression of mediastinal vessels) and increased pulmonary or systemic

TABLE 25.1

DIFFERENTIAL DIAGNOSIS OF SHOCK

Hypovolemic (oligemic)	Extracardiac obstructive	Cardiogenic	Distributive
Hemorrhagic	Extrinsic vascular compression	Myocardial	Infection/inflammatory
Trauma	Mediastinal tumors	Infarction	tissue injury
Gastrointestinal	Increased intrathoracic pressure	Myocarditis	Sepsis
Nonhemorrhagic	Tension pneumothorax	Cardiomyopathy	Pancreatitis
Dehydration	Positive-pressure ventilation	Pharmacologic/toxic	Trauma
Vomiting	Intrinsic vascular flow obstruction	β-blockers, Calcium	Burns
Diarrhea	Pulmonary embolism	channel blockers, etc.	Anaphylactic
Burns	Air embolism	Intrinsic depression	Envenomation, medication
Polyuria	Tumors	SIRS-related, acidosis, etc.	Neurogenic
Diuretic use, diabetes	Aortic dissection	Mechanical	Spinal-cord trauma
insipidus, etc.	Acute pulmonary hypertension	Valvular/dynamic stenosis	Endocrine
Third-space losses	Pericardial tamponade	Valvular regurgitation	Adrenal insufficiency
Peritonitis, ascites	Pericarditis	Ventricular septal defects	
		Ventricular aneurysms	
		Arrhythmias	

SIRS, Systemic Inflammatory Response Syndrome.
Modified from Jiminez EJ. Shock. In: Civetta JM, ed. *Critical Care.* Philadelphia: Lippincott-Raven, 1997:361, with permission.

vascular resistance (e.g., massive pulmonary embolism, acute pulmonary hypertension, aortic dissection).

Distributive shock describes a hemodynamic state caused by loss of vasomotor control resulting in arteriolar and venular dilatation. The hemodynamic profile is typified by an elevated cardiac output, normal to low central venous and pulmonary capillary occlusion pressures, de-

creased systemic vascular resistance, and hypotension. This form of shock is most commonly associated with sepsis, though it also describes the hemodynamic changes resulting from adrenal insufficiency, hyperthyroidism, anaphylaxis, hepatic failure, and neurogenic dysfunction (particularly following spinal or epidural anesthesia, or spinal cord injury).

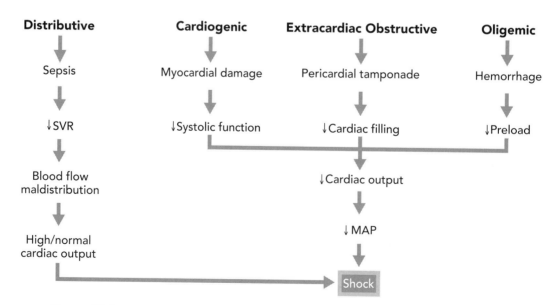

Figure 25.1 The different types of shock. Cardiogenic, extracardiac obstructive, and oligemic shock are characterized by a low cardiac output state causing hypotension. In contrast, in distributive shock, cardiac output usually is preserved or elevated, and hypotension results from a profound decrease in systemic vascular resistance. Myocardial dysfunction is common in sepsis, but cardiac output can be high or normal due to the low SVR. *MAP*, mean arterial pressure; *SVR*, systemic vascular resistance. (Adapted from Natanson C, Hoffman WD. Septic shock and other forms of shock. In: Parrillo JE, ed. *Current Therapy in Critical Care Medicine,* 2nd ed. Philadelphia: B.C. Decker, 1991.)

TABLE 25.2

COMMON HEMODYNAMIC PATTERNS IN SHOCK

Type	Cardiac output[a]	Systemic vascular resistance[b]	Pulmonary capillary wedge pressure[c]	Central venous pressure[d]
Hypovolemic	↓	↑	↓	↓
Cardiogenic				
Left-ventricular myocardial infarction	↓	↑	↑	↔, ↑
Right-ventricular myocardial infarction	↓	↑	↔, ↓	↑
Extracardiac obstructive				
Pericardial tamponade	↓	↑	↑	↑
Massive pulmonary embolism	↓	↑	↔, ↓	↑
Distributive				
Early	↔, ↓, ↑	↔, ↓, ↑	↔	↔, ↑
Late	↓	↑	↔	↔

[a] Normal = 4.0–6.0 L/min.
[b] Normal = 700–1,600 dyne/s/cm^2.
[c] Normal = 3–8 mm Hg.
[d] Normal = 2–5 mm Hg.
Modified from Jiminez EJ. Shock. In: Civetta JM, ed. *Critical Care*. Philadelphia: Lippincott-Raven, 1997:361, with permission.

PRINCIPLES OF INITIAL RESUSCITATION

The patient in shock requires a rapid assessment including a pertinent history and physical examination, adequate intravenous access (such as 2 large bore 14g or 16g peripheral catheters), laboratory studies, an electrocardiogram, a chest radiograph, supplemental oxygen therapy, and usually transfer to either an intensive care or intermediate care ("step down") unit. If substantial hemorrhage is suspected, a blood sample should be obtained for typing and cross-matching of blood for emergent infusion, and the patient's coagulation status should be assessed and corrected as appropriate. In selected settings, such as profound hemorrhagic shock, fluid resuscitation may be most efficiently achieved with the use of a large bore central venous cather (such as a Cordis catheter) and rapid fluid infusion devices. Specific documented or suggested causes must be addressed emergently (see Chapters 26, 38, 43, 53, and 78); empiric antibiotics are critical if sepsis may be a factor. Regardless of etiology, some basic concepts concerning initial shock treatment—including fluid resuscitation, and use of vasoactive drugs, and invasive monitoring devices—are generally applicable to all patients.

FLUID RESUSCITATION

The initial treatment of shock centers on optimizing intravascular volume. Except for cardiogenic shock, in which fluid overload may exist at the time of presentation, fluid administration is the most important initial therapy in shock (Table 25.3). Debate persists regarding the optimal type of fluid for resuscitation (e.g., crystalloids, colloids, or hypertonic solutions).

Crystalloids contain sodium as the major osmotically active particle and have the principal advantage of being readily available and inexpensive. Crystalloids distribute uniformly throughout the extracellular fluid compartment, so that only 25% of the total volume infused remains in the intravascular space. Commonly used crystalloids are lactated Ringer's solution and normal saline (0.9% NaCl). The principal difference is that lactated Ringer's solution contains potassium chloride and a bicarbonate precursor. Ringer's and normal saline may be used interchangeably, except that the latter should be used in patients with significant hyperkalemia or severe metabolic alkalosis. *Hypertonic saline solutions* are appealing for patients with shock or burns because, relative to isotonic crystalloids, smaller quantities are required initially for resuscitation, owing to their ability to expand intravascular volume more rapidly. However, the intravascular hypertonic benefit rapidly dissipates as the fluid redistributes between the intravascular and extravascular spaces. Side effects associated with the use of hypertonic solutions include hypernatremia, hyperosmolality, and hyperchloremia. To date, hypertonic agents have not been demonstrated to have any clear survival advantage over standard intravenous solutions (1).

Hypotonic solutions (D5W, 0.45% NaCl) distribute throughout the total body water compartment and expand the intravascular compartment by as little as 10% of the volume infused. Although these solutions are useful for replacing free-water deficits, they should not be used for fluid resuscitation in shock, because of their negligible effect on intravascular volume.

Colloid solutions (albumin, dextran, hydroxyethyl starch) contain high–molecular-weight substances that do not readily migrate across capillary walls. The use of colloids often is considered if crystalloids fail to sustain plasma

TABLE 25.3

COMPOSITION OF COMMONLY USED PARENTERAL FLUIDS

Solutions	Na$^+$	K$^+$	Ca^{2+}	Mg^{2+}	Cl$^-$	HCO$_3^-$ (as lactate)	Dextrose (g/L)	mOsm/L
Extracellular fluid	142	4	5	3	103	27		280–310
Lactated Ringer's	130	4	3		109	28		273
0.9% NaCl	154				154			308
0.45% NaCl	77				77			154
D$_5$W (5% dextrose in water)							50	252
D$_5$/0.45% NaCl	77				77		50	406
D$_5$LR	130	4	3		109	28	50	525
3% NaCl	513				513			1,026
7.5% NaCl	1,283				1,283			2,567
6% Hetastarch	154				154			310
10% Dextran 40[a]	0/154				0/154			300
6% Dextran 70[a]	0/154				0/154			300
5% Albumin	130–160	<2.5			130–160			330
25% Albumin	130–160	<2.5			130–160			330

Note: Electrolyte concentrations in mmol/L.
[a] Dextran solutions available in 5% dextrose or 0.9% NaCl.
Modified from Freeman BD, Buchman TG. Fluids, electrolytes, and acid–base disorders. In Doherty GM, ed. *Washington Manual of Surgery*. Boston: Little, Brown and Co., 1997, with permission.

volume, potentially because of the low colloid osmotic pressure of crystalloids.

Although *albumin* preparations ultimately distribute throughout the extravascular space, the initial volume of distribution is the vascular compartment. The result can be more rapid restoration of intravascular volume than seen with crystalloid use. Both 25% albumin (100 mL) and 5% albumin (500 mL) preparations expand the intravascular volume by an equivalent amount (450–500 mL). Albumin preparations may offer less benefit to patients with adequate colloid oncotic pressure (serum albumin >2.5 mg/dL, total protein >5 mg/dL). The cost per unit volume of albumin is substantially greater than the cost of the intravascular volume-equivalent amount of crystalloid solutions. Because of cost considerations, albumin preparations should be used judiciously.

A number of synthetic colloid solutions have been developed. *Dextran* is a synthetic glucose polymer that undergoes predominantly renal elimination. Dextran solutions expand the intravascular volume by an amount equal to the volume infused. Side effects include renal failure, osmotic diuresis, coagulopathy, and laboratory abnormalities (i.e., elevations in blood glucose and protein, interference with blood cross-matching). Dextran 40 and Dextran 70 are used most commonly for acute volume expansion. *Hydroxyethyl starch* (hetastarch) is a glycogen-like synthetic molecule that is available as 6% solution in 0.9% NaCl. Infusion of hetastarch, like 5% albumin, increases the intravascular volume by an amount equal to or greater than the volume infused. Whether colloid solutions provide a clinical benefit over crystalloid solutions for resuscitation remains a vigorously debated question (2–5).

Because of the risk of transmission of blood-borne pathogens as well as the logistic problems associated with acquiring, storing, and screening blood products, *blood substitutes*, such as stroma-free hemoglobin, have been developed. At the time of this writing, however, none of these products have been approved by the U.S. Food and Drug Administration for clinical use.

Suggested Approach to the Initial Fluid Management of the Patient with Shock

Initial resuscitation of the patient in noncardiogenic shock begins with rapid fluid infusion. Frequently, it is necessary to infuse a bolus of 2–3 L of crystalloids to restore blood pressure and peripheral perfusion. This aggressive fluid resuscitation supports the patient's blood pressure, cardiac output, and perfusion in the early stages of shock while the underlying cause is sought and more definitive therapy is instituted. The patient with acute blood loss resuscitated without blood replacement requires a volume of crystalloid equivalent to approximately four times the volume of blood lost. For example, approximately 2,000 ml of crystalloid solution is required to compensate for a 500 milliliter blood loss. In the setting of acute massive blood loss, the administration of non-type-specific blood (e.g., type O) should be considered, if type-specific blood is not immediately available. Although the early use of colloids in the resuscitation regimen may result in the more prompt restoration of tissue perfusion and may lessen the total volume of fluid required for resuscitation, no data support any improvement in outcome compared with crystalloid infusion alone.

Patients who receive large volumes of intravenous fluids may develop coagulopathy, due principally to dilution and hypothermia. Accordingly, coagulation profiles and platelet counts should be monitored and corrected as necessary, particularly in patients who have ongoing blood loss or in whom invasive procedures are planned. Similarly, core temperatures should be monitored, and mild degrees of hypothermia (T<36°C) should be treated by external warming and infusion of warm fluids.

VASOPRESSOR THERAPY

In addition to fluid administration, pharmacologic support of blood pressure with vasopressor agents (Table 25.4) is frequently necessary in both the initial resuscitation and subsequent support of patients with shock.

Norepinephrine is a catecholamine vasopressor with both α- and β-adrenergic effects. At low doses, norepinephrine has a positive inotropic effect. However, with increasing doses, its vasoconstrictive effects outweigh its inotropic effects, and cardiac output may decrease as a consequence of increased afterload. A potential adverse effect of norepinephrine is profound vasoconstriction, resulting in hypoperfusion and ischemia. In practical terms, norepinephrine at moderate dosages (1–4 mcg/min) has the ability to increase systemic pressure while maintaining or increasing cardiac performance; because of its marked ability to increase systemic pressure, norepinephrine is becoming the most frequently used pressor for the initial therapy of shock. It is also commonly used as an adjunct to other vasopressors with predominately β-activity, such as dobutamine, in cases of refractory shock. Norepinephrine infusions typically begin at 1 mcg/min and are titrated to the desired effect. The usual dosage range is 2–4 mcg/min, with an upper limit typically of 12 mcg/min.

Dopamine is an endogenous catecholamine and neurotransmitter. When administered intravenously, its cardiovascular effects are dose-dependent and reflect the relative degrees of stimulation of the sympathomimetic (α- and β-) and dopaminergic receptors. At low doses (1–2 mcg/kg/min), dopamine selectively activates dopaminergic receptors in the renal, mesenteric, and cerebral circulations, increasing perfusion to these regions. At intermediate doses (2–10 mcg/kg/min), dopamine stimulates β-receptors in the cardiac and peripheral circulations, producing a modest inotropic effect. At higher doses (>10 mcg/kg/min), dopamine stimulates α-receptors in the systemic circulation, producing vasoconstriction. Dopamine is also commonly used for the initial management of circulatory shock. Of note, clinicians frequently use dopamine at low doses ("renal dose" dopamine, sometimes with other pressors) in an attempt to maintain renal perfusion and promote urine output in patients with (or at risk for) acute tubular necrosis. However, this application has not been prospectively demonstrated to alter renal injury or patient outcome (see Chapter 100).

Dobutamine, a synthetic catecholamine with predominately β1 (inotropic) but also weak β2 (vasodilatation) activity, is often used for the management of low cardiac output states caused by inadequate cardiac systolic function (e.g., low ejection fraction). Because dobutamine does

TABLE 25.4

VASOPRESSORS COMMONLY USED IN THE MANAGEMENT OF SHOCK

Drug	Dosing	Adrenergic effects		Dopaminergic	Indications
		α	β		
Norepinephrine	0.5–80 mcg/min	3+	2+	0	Initial emergency treatment of hypotension (any cause, especially sepsis)
Dopamine	1–2 mcg/kg/min	1+	1+	3+	Oliguria despite normal blood pressure
	2–10 mcg/kg/min	2+	2+	3+	Initial emergency treatment of hypotension
	10–30 mcg/kg/min	3+	2+	3+	(any cause) and alternative treatment for bradycardia
Dobutamine	2–30 mcg/kg/min	1+	3+	0	Cardiogenic shock and cardiogenic pulmonary edema with marginal blood pressure
Epinephrine	0.5–1 mg (1:10,000)	1+	2+	0	Cardiac arrest
	1–200 mcg/min	2+	3+	0	Severe hypotension and bradycardia
	0.3–0.5 mg SQ (1:1,000)				Anaphylaxis
Phenylephrine	20–200 mcg/min	3+	0	0	Distributive shock when no cardiac effect desired
Isoproterenol	2–10 mcg/min	0	3+	0	Refractory bradycardia
Amrinone	Load: 0.75 mcg/kg over 3 min; infuse: 2–15 mcg/kg/min	0	0	0	Cardiogenic shock, usually as a synergistic agent with dobutamine

Modified from Jiminez EJ. Shock. In: Civetta JM, ed. *Critical Care*. Philadelphia: Lippincott-Raven, 1997:363, with permission.

not appreciably increase systolic pressure, it is not indicated as monotherapy for patients with cardiogenic shock. Further, it generally should not be used, even as combination therapy, in patients with cardiac failure secondary to diastolic dysfunction or in patients with hypertrophic obstructive cardiomyopathy, because its β-sympathomimetic effect may exacerbate these conditions. The usual dosage range for dobutamine is 5–15 mcg/kg/min.

Epinephrine is an endogenous catecholamine. Given its potency and potential for untoward effects (myocardial ischemia, tachyarrhythmia, intracranial hemorrhage, etc.), it is not used commonly as initial pharmacologic support for shock in adults. As with dopamine, epinephrine's effects are largely dose-dependent (e.g., primarily a β-agonist at low doses and an α-agonist at higher doses). Epinephrine also inhibits the release of inflammatory mediators from immune cells in response to antigenic challenge, which may partially explain its beneficial effect in the setting of anaphylaxis. Intravenous epinephrine is indicated for the management of cardiac arrest associated with pulseless ventricular tachycardia, ventricular fibrillation, asystole, pulseless electrical activity (initial dose: 1 mg intravenously every 3–5 minutes), and for severe anaphylactic reactions (initial dose: 3–5 mL of 1:10,000 solution [0.1 mg/mL] intravenously) (see also Chapter 120).

Phenylephrine, a catecholamine with pure α-adrenergic activity, is effective in the treatment of distributive shock because it increases systolic blood pressure without producing tachycardia. It should be used with caution in patients with underlying cardiovascular dysfunction, however, because of the risk of precipitating ventricular failure. Typical initial infusion rates are 20–40 mcg/min.

Amrinone is a phosphodiesterase inhibitor that has both vasodilator and inotropic effects. These combined actions produce an increase in cardiac output without an increase in cardiac stroke work, an effect roughly equivalent to dobutamine. Amrinone is indicated as single-agent therapy in the management of low cardiac output states caused by systolic heart failure. It is used most frequently as a second agent that is added to dobutamine in cases of refractory heart failure. Amrinone is given by loading with 0.75–1.5 mg/kg followed by an infusion rate of 5–10 mg/kg/min. Because of excessive vasodilatation, amrinone may cause hypotension, especially in hypovolemic patients.

Vasopressin, which is naturally secreted by the posterior pituitary gland, possesses multiple physiologic effects including vasoconstriction mediated by V1 receptors present in numerous vascular beds. Circulating levels of vasopressin appear to be depressed in shock. When administered exogenously in "physiologic doses" (e.g., 0.01–0.04 units/min), vasopressin is synergistic with exogenous catecholamies, yielding a pressor effect without evidence of organ hypoperfusion. When administered at doses >0.04 units/min, the pressor effect of vasopressin is associated with potentially deleterious renal, mesenteric, and coronary vasoconstriction. Specific recommendations regarding the routine use of this agent for hemodynamic support await more thorough clinical evaluation (6).

Suggested Approach to Initial Vasopressor Therapy

The appropriate use of vasopressors frequently requires accurate assessment of a patient's cardiovascular status by either invasive or noninvasive monitoring. It is not uncommon, however, to institute vasopressor therapy in a patient who remains hypotensive despite rapid fluid infusion and for whom sophisticated monitoring is not immediately available. If hypotension persists (e.g., mean arterial pressure <60 mm Hg) despite aggressive fluid resuscitation, vasopressor therapy may be indicated. The use of an agent with both α- and β-adrenergic activity, such as norepinephrine or dopamine, is an appropriate initial choice: These agents increase systemic pressure via their α-adrenergic effect and augment cardiac output via their β-adrenergic effect. Vasopressors should be started in the therapeutic range and then titrated to the desired hemodynamic effect (e.g., mean arterial pressure ≥60 mm Hg). Empiric vasopressor use is continued until a more detailed assessment of the patients' cardiovascular status and the cause of shock can guide targeted therapy.

INVASIVE MONITORING DEVICES

It is estimated that 1.2 million pulmonary artery catheters are inserted annually in the United States, with an associated cost of $2 billion. Despite this pervasive use, disagreement persists regarding clinical indications for pulmonary artery catheters, the interpretation of data generated by these devices, and the goals of therapy based on these data (7). Randomized trials have shown no benefit for the routine use of pulmonary artery catheters in elderly patients undergoing high-risk surgery (8) or in patients with shock due to sepsis, the acute respiratory distress syndrome, or both (9). In the latter study, only about 5% of patients randomized to initial care without a pulmonary artery catheter later received one for perceived clinical needs. Neither of these studies linked pulmonary artery catheters to specific, protocolized interventions, and earlier randomized trials of goal-oriented hemodynamic therapy in critically ill patients have yielded conflicting results (10). Nevertheless, ongoing trials are evaluating the combination of pulmonary artery catheters with specific therapeutic protocols. Furthermore, no trial has evaluated the utility of pulmonary artery catheterization in shock of unknown cause.

Use of the Echocardiography and/or Pulmonary Artery Catheter to Determine the Type of Shock

If a pulmonary artery catheter and/or echocardiography is needed and used to determine the cause of shock in a patient who otherwise has shock of unknown etiology, it can reveal one of four hemodynamic profiles (Table 25.2).

Oligemic shock is typified by normal cardiac function, a low cardiac output, low pulmonary capillary wedge pressure, and elevated systemic vascular resistance. These findings should prompt the clinician to consider the potential causes of oligemia and to initiate or augment fluid resuscitation.

Cardiogenic shock is indicated by markedly diminished cardiac function and output with elevations in systemic vascular resistance, pulmonary capillary wedge pressure, and central venous pressure. Mixed venous oxygen saturation is typically low. Resuscitation should be directed toward improving cardiac function by optimizing preload and administering potent sympathomimetic agents (e.g., dopamine alone or dopamine and dobutamine in combination). Mechanical cardiac support (e.g., intra-aortic balloon counterpulsation or ventricular-assist device) should be considered in refractory patients. (see Chapter 39).

Extracardiac obstructive shock secondary to cardiac tamponade is evidenced by typical echocardiographic findings, diminished stroke volume with elevation and equalization of cardiac filling pressures (i.e., central venous and pulmonary capillary wedge pressure). Pericardial tamponade requires emergent pericardiocentesis (Chapter 46). Alternatively, extracardiac obstructive shock as a consequence of pulmonary embolism is suggested by diminished cardiac output, elevated central venous and pulmonary artery diastolic pressures, and normal or low pulmonary capillary wedge pressure (Chapter 53). Empiric anticoagulant therapy should be considered pending confirmation by appropriate diagnostic tests.

Distributive shock is suggested by decreased blood pressure and systemic vascular resistance; normal, near-normal, or supra-normal cardiac function, elevations in cardiac output and mixed venous saturation, and normal pulmonary capillary and central venous pressures. Because sepsis is a frequent cause of distributive shock, this hemodynamic profile suggests the need for rapid cultures, broad spectrum antibiotics, and a thorough search for a site of infection (see Chapter 26).

Use of Hemodynamic Endpoints to Guide Fluid Therapy and Vasopressor Use

Patients with normal cardiac function generally should receive intravenous fluids to achieve normal to slightly elevated central venous and pulmonary capillary wedge pressures (12–18 mm Hg). If hypotension persists despite achieving these resuscitation endpoints, vasopressor therapy should be instituted because persistent infusion of fluids alone to reverse shock may increase intravascular pressure and produce complications of volume overload (e.g., pulmonary edema). For patients with poor cardiac performance and low cardiac output (cardiac index <2.5 L/m^2), an agent or agents should be selected to provide both α- and β-adrenergic stimulation (e.g., epinephrine, norepinephrine plus dobutamine, or dopamine plus dobutamine) in an effort to enhance both cardiac contractility and vascular tone. Conversely, for patients with hypotension and preserved cardiac function and output (cardiac index ≥2.5 L/m^2), agents with predominately α-adrenergic activity (e.g., norepinephrine, phenylephrine) should be used to augment blood pressure. These general recommendations may require modification for patients with specific causes such as myocardial infarction (Chapter 38) or pulmonary embolism (Chapter 53). Because the risk:benefit ratio of the pulmonary artery catheter in guiding ongoing management is unclear and because this device has been associated with long-term complications, it should only be used when other methods are insufficient or the patient is unstable hemodynamically. These indications may broaden if ongoing randomized trials demonstrate the catheter's usefulness in other situations.

OTHER INTERVENTIONS THAT MAY BE USEFUL IN PATIENTS WITH SHOCK OF UNKNOWN CAUSE

If easily treatable causes of shock are not apparent, a limited differential diagnosis of potentially life threatening conditions should be entertained. If either anaphylaxis or acute adrenal insufficiency is a diagnostic consideration, corticosteroids should be administered. These agents should be given on a rapidly tapering schedule as the patient stabilizes or as other causes of hemodynamic compromise become apparent. For anaphylaxis, the recommended dose is hydrocortisone 300–500 mg intravenously every 6 hours or methylprednisolone 60–125 mg intravenously every 6 hours, tapering either agent off in 48–72 hours (see Chapter 120). For adrenal insufficiency, the recommended dose is hydrocortisone 100 mg intravenously every 6 hours (although higher doses sometimes are given), tapered according to the patient's response to illness (see Chapter 109).

Timely administration of antibiotics is essential to the successful treatment of septic shock and should be considered whenever there is any suspicion of systemic infection, such as with fever, hyperdynamic cardiac profile, obvious site of infection, or immunocompromise (see

Chapter 26). Anticoagulation is essential in preventing subsequent thromboemboli in patients with pulmonary thromboembolism. Pending definitive diagnosis or exclusion of pulmonary emboli, heparinization should be considered if there is sufficient suspicion based on the presence of predisposing factors or appropriate hemodynamics (see Chapter 53).

Blood products should be administered early if the hematocrit is reduced and occult hemorrhage possibly underlies hemodynamic compromise. If hemodynamic collapse occurs in patients who have undergone recent percutaneous placement of central venous catheters, the diagnosis of tension pneumothorax should be entertained; needle decompression with a large bore (e.g., 14g) catheter followed by tube thoracostomy placement is indicated. If a patient may have pericardial tamponade, due to either recent trauma, an invasive procedure, or preexisting pericardial disease, echocardiography and rapid diagnosis and therapy are lifesaving (Chapter 46).

ENDPOINTS OF RESUSCITATION: CAN OUTCOME FROM SHOCK BE IMPROVED?

One of the principal goals driving the timely resuscitation of the patient with shock is to restore perfusion and prevent organ injury. However, even with extraordinary efforts, organ failure frequently occurs.

One hypothesis suggests that organ failure during critical illness occurs as a consequence of inadequate oxygen delivery. Accordingly, a number of investigators have proposed that patients should be resuscitated to elevated, or supraphysiologic, hemodynamic endpoints so as to prevent organ failure and improve outcome. Several trials testing this hypothesis in patients following ICU admission failed to demonstrate a benefit. A recent study, however, suggests that therapy directed toward achieving *normal* hemodynamic parameters, if implemented early after the diagnosis of shock and prior to ICU admission, may improve survival (11). In this study, patients with severe sepsis or septic shock were randomized immediately following presentation to the emergency department to either conventional therapy or early goal-directed therapy, which included fluid resuscitation to achieve a CVP of 8–12 mm Hg, vasopressor administration titrated to achieve a mean arterial pressure of 65 mm Hg, and blood transfusion to achieve a central venous O_2 saturation of 70%. Patients assigned to standard therapy received significantly less fluid resuscitation and had significantly higher mortality rates. Whether this approach can be generalized to other disease processes remains unstudied, but the findings of this study support appropriate early and aggressive resuscitation of patients with shock.

KEY POINTS

The hemodynamically unstable patient is a challenging clinical problem. The mechanisms by which hypotension and shock ultimately result in organ failure are not fully known. Although the approach to these patients must be individualized based on specific cause, some basic principles apply to all patients:

- The causes of shock can be categorized based on hemodynamic profiles into hypovolemic, cardiac, extracardiac obstructive, and distributive. This framework is particularly helpful in the patient whose cause of shock is unclear or could be attributed to several potential causes.
- The initial resuscitation of the patient with shock should be directed at rapidly restoring circulating intravascular volume through the use of crystalloids, colloids, or blood products. In septic shock, inadequate early fluid resuscitation appears to have an adverse effect on survival.
- The use of vasopressors is essential for restoring systemic perfusion if the patient does not respond quickly to intravenous fluid therapy or is hemodynamically labile. Although therapy must be individualized, norepinephrine and dopamine, individually or in combination, are reasonable empiric choices. The titration of these agents as well as the addition of other agents is based on response to therapy and the acquisition of additional clinical information.
- Echocardiography and/or pulmonary artery catheters can help determine the cause of shock and direct initial therapy. If pulmonary artery catheters are used, the duration of catheterization should be limited to the minimum required time.
- The appropriate endpoints for resuscitation in the critically ill patient are normal values of oxygen delivery and other hemodynamic variables, in conjunction with other clinical evidence of adequate tissue perfusion (e.g., normal mentation, adequate urine production, clearance of acidosis).

REFERENCES

1. Bunn F, Roberts I, Tasker R, Akpa E. Hypertonic versus near isotonic crystalloid for fluid resuscitation in critically ill patients (Cochrane Review). *Cochrane Database Syst Rev* 2004;3:CD002045.
2. Cochrane Injuries Group Albumin Reviewers. Human albumin administration in critically ill patients: systematic review of randomized controlled trials. *BMJ* 1998;317:235–240.
3. Choi PTL, Yip G, Quinonez LG, Cook DJ. Crystalloids versus colloids in fluid resuscitation: a systematic review. *Crit Care Med* 1999;27:200–210.
4. Cook DJ, Guyatt G. Colloid use for fluid resuscitation: evidence and spin. *Ann Intern Med* 2001;135:205–208.
5. Roberts I, Alderson P, Bunn F, et al. Colloids versus crystalloids for fluid resuscitation in critically ill patients. (Cochrane Review). *Cochrane Database Syst Rev* 2004;4:CD000567.
6. Holmes CL, Patel BM, Russell JA, Walley KR. Physiology of

vasopressin relevant to management of septic shock. *Chest* 2001;120:989–1002.

7. Parsons P. Progress in research on pulmonary artery catheters. *N Engl J Med* 2003;348:66–68.

8. Sandham JD, Hull RD, Brant RF, et al. A randomized, controlled trial of the use of pulmonary-artery catheters in high-risk surgical patients. *N Engl J Med* 2003;348:5–14.

9. Richard C, Warszawski J, Anguel N, et al. Early use of the pulmonary artery catheter and outcomes in patients with shock and acute respiratory distress syndrome: a randomized controlled trial. *JAMA* 2003;290:2713–2720.

10. Gattinoni L, Brazzi L, Pelosi P, et al, for SvO2 Collaborative Group. A trial of goal-oriented hemodynamic therapy in critically ill patients. *N Engl J Med* 1995;333:1025–1032.

11. Rivers E, Nguyen B, Havstad S, et al. Early goal-directed therapy in the treatment of severe sepsis and septic shock. *N Engl J Med* 2001; 345:1368–1377.

ADDITIONAL READING

American Society of Anesthesiologists Task Force on Pulmonary Artery Catheterization. Practice guidelines for pulmonary artery catheterization: an updated report by the American Society of Anesthesiologists Task Force on Pulmonary Artery Catheterization. *Anesthesiology* 2003;99:988–1014.

Beale RJ, Hollenberg SM, Vincent JL, Parillo JE. Vasopressor and inotropic support in septic shock: an evidence-based review. *Crit Care Med* 2004;32(11 Suppl):S455–S465.

Dellinger RP. Cardiovascular management of septic shock. *Crit Care Med* 2003;31:946–955.

Landry DW, Oliver JA. The pathogenesis of vasodilatory shock. *N Engl J Med* 2001;345:588–595.

Mullner M, Urbanek B, Havel C, et al. Vasopressors for shock. *Cochrane Database Syst Rev* 2004;3:CD003709.

Sepsis Syndrome

26

Todd W. Rice   Gordon R. Bernard

INTRODUCTION

Sepsis syndrome, the body's systemic response to such disparate infections as pneumonia, peritonitis, pyelonephritis, and meningitis, is the leading cause of death in non-coronary intensive care units and the tenth leading cause of death overall in the United States. Although recent treatment advances have improved outcomes of patients with sepsis, mortality rates still approach 30%–40%. In addition, the incidence of sepsis has steadily increased over the past two decades due to increasing numbers of elderly and immunocompromised patients, increasing use of immunosuppressive therapies, and increasingly widespread use of invasive therapeutic and monitoring devices. Current reports estimate that almost 700,000 cases of sepsis occur in the United States each year (240 cases per 100,000 population) (1,2).

In general, the term sepsis refers to a *systemic inflammatory response syndrome* (sometimes abbreviated as SIRS) resulting from infection. When sepsis causes end-organ dysfunction (renal, cardiovascular, hematologic, neurologic, etc.), it is called *severe sepsis*; and when it causes arterial hypotension and organ hypoperfusion, it is called *septic shock*. Although the phrase "sepsis syndrome" can encompass many different septic conditions, it is routinely used to describe patients with severe sepsis or septic shock. The systemic inflammatory response syndrome is not specific to sepsis and can result from a variety of other pathophysiologic mechanisms, such as hemorrhage, severe dehydration, heart failure, pericardial tamponade, pancreatitis, or trauma, all of which can cause hypotension, shock, and multiorgan system failure. Sepsis produces generalized endothelial dysfunction with resulting inflammation and altered coagulation (3). It is initiated by infection with bacteria or other microorganisms. Then, it is mediated by the effects of their various endo- and exotoxins, and amplified by endogenous inflammatory and coagulation mediators, including leukocytes, macrophages, cytokines (e.g., tumor necrosis factor and interleukins 1, 2, and 6), thromboplastin, and thrombin. These inflammatory and coagulopathic responses, to the extent they serve to eradicate pathogens, are vital. However, these same responses are often nonspecific in their targets and imperfectly regulated, resulting in irreparable damage to normal tissues.

WHEN SEPSIS SYNDROME PRESENTS ON ADMISSION

Issues at the Time of Admission

Clinical Presentation

The spectrum of presenting manifestations of sepsis is extraordinarily broad, ranging from the elderly patient who complains only of weakness and dizziness to the otherwise healthy young adult with overwhelming pneumonia and hypotension. Although signs of a localized infection may be present, patients with sepsis "typically" present with a conglomeration of the signs and symptoms of the systemic inflammatory response syndrome, namely tachycardia, tachypnea, hyperthermia (or hypothermia), and leukocytosis. Tachypnea, which is often the first sign of sepsis, is almost universally present in patients with severe sepsis. Additionally, patients with severe sepsis often demonstrate hypotension, obtundation, oliguria, and a lactic acidosis. Unfortunately, sepsis may present without such typical features, and a high clinical index of suspicion must be maintained whenever a patient (particularly one who is elderly or immunocompromised) presents with nonspecific symptoms.

Initial Evaluation and Differential Diagnosis

The foundation of the initial evaluation is a careful medical history and physical examination. The history should elicit any predisposing factors and possible source of infection to guide the choice of empiric antibiotics. Any immunocompromising conditions (e.g., prior use of corticosteroids, asplenia, radiation or chemotherapy, hematologic malignancy, HIV infection, prior transplantation, alcoholism, or diabetes mellitus) should be noted, along with any unusual recent exposures, such as tuberculosis, meningococcus, influenza, or legionella. Any recent history of procedures (including surgeries, endoscopies, dental work, genitourinary manipulation, intravascular catheters or other indwelling devices) or use of vaginal tampons should be considered. Information about cough or sputum production, headache or neck stiffness, chest or abdominal pain, nausea, vomiting, jaundice, diarrhea, flank pain, dysuria, hematuria, urinary frequency, or skin lesions can help direct further investigation.

The initial physical examination should focus on vital signs including, if possible, supine and standing heart rate and blood pressure, respiratory rate and pattern, and temperature. General attention must be paid to the patient's alertness, orientation, skin temperature, perfusion of hands and feet, skin lesions, and any indwelling catheters. The head and neck should be examined for the presence or absence of scleral icterus, meningismus, and sinus tenderness, as well as for any abnormalities of the tympanic membranes or oropharynx. The lungs should be examined for altered breath sounds, signs of consolidation, rales, rhonchi, wheezes, or pleural rubs. The cardiovascular examination should assess possible jugular venous distention, edema, murmurs, rubs, gallops, peripheral pulses, splinter hemorrhages, Roth spots, Osler's nodes, and Janeway lesions. The abdomen and pelvis must be assessed for tenderness, guarding, rebound, operative scars, the presence and character of bowel sounds, flank tenderness, blood in the stool, and pelvic tenderness or discharge.

In many cases of sepsis, such as a toxic patient with a lobar pneumonia, the diagnosis is readily apparent. In others, a good deal of detective work is needed, and the diagnosis of sepsis is uncertain until results are obtained from blood tests, radiographs, and other investigations (Table 26.1). Non-infectious conditions such as pancreatitis, trauma, severe hemorrhage, myocardial infarction, drug overdoses, and even heat stroke can mimic sepsis and often must be excluded by a thorough history, physical examination, and laboratory testing before the diagnosis of sepsis syndrome can be established.

TABLE 26.1

INITIAL LABORATORY AND RADIOGRAPHIC EVALUATION OF THE PATIENT PRESENTING WITH SUSPECTED SEPSIS SYNDROME

Tests that should be obtained initially in *all* patients:
  Complete blood count with differential and platelet count
  Sodium, potassium, chloride, bicarbonate, blood-urea nitrogen, creatinine, and glucose measurements
  Bilirubin, alkaline phosphatase, and aminotransferase measurements
  Prothrombin time and partial thromboplastin time
  Two sets of blood cultures—at least one drawn from someplace other than an already established IV
  Pulse oximetry
  Chest radiograph (upright preferred if patient is able)
  Urinalysis and urine culture
Tests that should be obtained in *selected* patients:
  Lumbar puncture (in any patient with even a slight suspicion of meningitis)
  12-lead electrocardiogram (in any patient with hypotension, abnormal auscultatory findings, pulse irregularities, chest discomfort, or any history of cardiac disease)
  Echocardiogram (in any patient with suspicion of tamponade, acute cor pulmonale, infective endocarditis, acute valvular regurgitation, or severe left ventricular dysfunction)
  Flat and upright abdominal films (in any patient with worrisome abdominal findings)
  Nasogastric aspiration (in any patient who may be having upper-gastrointestinal hemorrhage)
  Amylase and lipase (in patients with signs and symptoms consistent with pancreatitis)
  Abdominal ultrasound (in patients suspected to have biliary disease or postrenal obstruction)
  Abdominal computed tomography scan (in patients suspected of having pancreatitis, abdominal abscess, or retroperitoneal hemorrhage)
  Urine and serum toxicology screens (in any obtunded patient or patient with possible overdose)
  Arterial blood gases (in patients with tachypnea, decreased oxygen saturation, or acidosis)
  Magnesium, phosphate, and calcium measurements (in patients with renal insufficiency, acid–base disturbances, or other indications)
  Thoracentesis or paracentesis (in patients suspected to have empyema, parapneumonic effusion, or spontaneous bacterial peritonitis)

In the patient with shock, resuscitative efforts must be started immediately, accompanied by an abbreviated, carefully focused initial evaluation. The principal aim of the evaluation is to differentiate septic shock from other forms of shock (e.g., cardiogenic shock, hemorrhagic shock, or pericardial tamponade). Once septic shock is diagnosed, early and aggressive goal-directed resuscitation should be instituted. Aggressive volume repletion with crystalloid, correction of severe anemia with transfusions of packed red blood cells, and support of cardiac function with ionotropic agents help improve the oxygen saturation of mixed-venous blood (4). If the patient is more stable, a more deliberate initial evaluation can be undertaken.

Indications for Hospitalization

All patients with severe sepsis should be hospitalized. Even the patient who "eyeballs well" after hydration and initial antibiotics in the emergency department is at risk for sudden and severe deterioration. Some patients with sepsis improve rapidly with antibiotic therapy, and such patients may only need a day or two of inpatient therapy. Unfortunately, however, the natural history of sepsis is highly variable, and many patients require protracted hospitalization.

Indications for Initial Intensive Care Unit Admission

Many hospitals have well-equipped, well-staffed general medical units or "stepdown" units capable of managing patients with uncomplicated sepsis syndrome. Unfortunately, a large percentage of patients with sepsis syndrome already have, or are at high risk of developing, severe sepsis with organ failure, complications that mandate ICU admission (Table 26.2).

Initial Therapy

As in any life-threatening illness, the hierarchy of therapeutic priorities in sepsis syndrome begins with assuring that the patient has a patent airway, with adequate oxygenation and ventilation. Patients in shock require aggressive resuscitation with crystalloids (often as much as 5–10 liters), combined with transfusions of packed red blood cells and inotropic support to maintain adequate tissue perfusion (4). Beyond the initial stabilization of airway, breathing, and circulation (the "ABCs"), the next priority whenever sepsis syndrome is being considered (even before the diagnosis has been confirmed) is to obtain appropriate culture specimens and then *immediately to begin broad-spectrum antibiotics* directed against all of the likely pathogens, an intervention known to decrease mortality (5). In addition to antibiotic coverage, outcomes are improved when the source of infection is eradicated. Practically, this means that the search for potential sources should begin as

---

TABLE 26.2

SEPSIS SYNDROME: INDICATIONS FOR ICU ADMISSION

Hypotension, and consequent need for vasopressors, if volume resuscitation fails to achieve and maintain a systolic blood pressure of 90 mm Hg or a mean arterial pressure of 65 mm Hg

Hypoxemia, if oxygen by face mask fails to achieve and maintain arterial oxygen saturations above 90% or mechanical ventilation is likely to be needed

Marked metabolic abnormalities (e.g., severe acidosis, uremia, jaundice, or severe electrolyte derangements)

Depressed sensorium, with likely need for endotracheal intubation for airway protection

Oliguria or anuria

Sepsis concomitant with underlying cardiac problems (e.g., arrhythmias, coronary disease, heart failure, or pericardial disease)

Sepsis concomitant with underlying pulmonary problems (e.g., chronic obstructive pulmonary disease)

Desire to utilize invasive monitoring (e.g., arterial cannulation or pulmonary artery catheterization)

---

soon as the hemodynamic and respiratory statuses are stabilized (6). Controlling the source of infection may require percutaneous or surgical drainage of a pocket of pus (e.g., empyema or abscess) (see Chapters 62 and 64), removal of devitalized tissue (e.g., necrotizing fasciitis, necrotic ulcers, or infarcted tissue), or removal of an infected foreign body (intravascular catheter, tampon, or artificial joint). Other elements of initial therapy are tailored to the specific needs of the individual patient (Table 26.3).

ISSUES DURING THE COURSE OF HOSPITALIZATION

Because of the association of sepsis syndrome with multi-organ system dysfunction (see Chapter 25), the problems that arise during its course are legion. As a generalization (and somewhat of an oversimplification), the patient who ultimately succumbs to sepsis has several characteristics. The most important prognostic indicator is the development of organ dysfunction, especially hypotension and acute respiratory distress syndrome (ARDS). Both hypotension, especially septic shock requiring vasopressors for longer than 48 hours, and respiratory failure severe enough to require mechanical ventilation portend a high likelihood of death. Mortality has been estimated to be at least 25% with either, and increases by 15–20% for each additional failing organ (7). In addition, chronic underlying medical co-morbidities and hypothermia further worsen the prognosis (8).

Nonetheless, many septic patients survive despite multi-organ system failure and long, complicated hospital courses. To optimize their chances of survival, with minimal residual

TABLE 26.3

INITIAL THERAPY OF SEPSIS SYNDROME

Assure adequacy of airway patency, oxygeneration, and ventilation.

Assure adequate arterial pressure to maintain cerebral and coronary perfusion; the usual target is a mean arterial pressure of 65 mm Hg or a systolic of 90 mm Hg.

If hypotensive, start with large-volume intravenous fluids.

Fluids may be crystalloid, colloid, or blood products.

Unless pulmonary edema is present, volumes of 5–10 L can be administered.

If arterial pressure does not respond adequately to intravenous fluids, start vasopressors.

Some studies have shown improved outcomes using norepinephrine compared with dopamine (9).

One strategy is to start with norepinephrine at 2 mcg/min, titrate up as needed.

If the patient is still hypotensive on 50 mcg/min of norepinephrine, addition of replacement dose vasopressin (0.04 Units/min) can be considered (10).

If norepinephrine precipitates tachyarrhythmias, switch to phenylephrine, starting at 30 mcg/min.

As soon as culture specimens are obtained, start broad-spectrum parenteral antibiotics (5).

Do not merely write the antibiotic order; *make sure the drug is given immediately.*

Once culture and sensitivity data become available, the spectrum of antibiotic coverage can be narrowed correspondingly.

Call a surgical or interventional consultation if there is undrained pus (e.g., empyema, abscess, etc.) or devitalized tissue needing removal (e.g., necrotizing fasciitis, necrotic ulcers, infarcted tissue, etc.) (6).

Remove any infected foreign bodies (e.g., intravascular catheters, artificial joints, etc.).

If the patient requires ventilatory support for acute lung injury or acute respiratory distress syndrome (ARDS), use a low tidal volume approach (6 cc/kg of ideal body weight, decreased to 4 cc/kg of ideal body weight if needed to keep plateau pressures below 30 cm H_2O) (11).

Address metabolic and hematologic derangements.

Acidosis usually corrects with adequate ventilation and restoration of perfusion; consider bicarbonate administration in extremes (e.g., pH <7.0).

Consider acute hemodialysis for life-threatening hyperkalemia.

Treat hyperglycemia or hypoglycemia.

Correct hypokalemia, hypocalcemia, hypomagnesemia; be cautious if renal function is questionable.

Administer vitamin K and transfuse packed red cells, platelets, or fresh frozen plasma as clinically indicated.

If any question of adrenal impairment, give dexamethasone 10 mg IV.

Dexamethasone does not interfere with an interpretable adrenocorticotrophic hormone (ACTH) stimulation test (see Chapter 109).

Corticosteroids may improve outcome in patients with adrenal insufficiency (12), but are not helpful and may be harmful when patients with sepsis syndrome do not have adrenal impairment.

If febrile, administer acetaminophen and/or ibuprofen.

Start parenteral histamine-2 blockers.

Patients with hemodynamic instability should have arterial cannulas placed:

To facilitate accurate titration of vasopressors.

To facilitate frequent blood sampling.

Start drotrecogin alfa (activated) in patients with severe sepsis and a high-likelihood of death (e.g., APACHE II ≥25; vasopressor requirement) unless contraindicated (3).

Dobutamine and transfusions of packed red blood cells have been advocated to increase cardiac output and oxygen delivery and may improve outcome if used early to correct low mixed-venous oxygen saturation (4).

---

morbidity, clinicians should adhere to a number of important precepts (Table 26.4).

Special Considerations in Selected Populations

Patients with Severe Sepsis (i.e. Organ Dysfunction From Sepsis)

Patients who develop at least one dysfunctional organ from sepsis have severe sepsis. Organ dysfunction occurs because of damage resulting from an over-exuberant systemic inflammatory and thrombotic response to the infection. This response causes endothelial dysfunction and subsequent microthrombi. *Activated protein C,* a protein with anti-inflammatory and anti-thrombotic properties, is reduced in many patients with severe sepsis, and these patients have a poorer prognosis. Recombinant human activated protein C (rhAPC), also known as drotrecogin alfa (activated),

decreases morbidity and mortality in patients with severe sepsis and a high-likelihood of dying (e.g., APACHE II score >25 or need for vasopressors): in a randomized trial, severely septic patients receiving drotrecogin alfa (activated) as a continuous infusion of 24 mcg/kg/min for 96 hours had a 6% absolute reduction and 19% relative reduction in 28-day, all cause mortality (25% mortality in those receiving drotrecogin alfa compared with 31% in those receiving placebo) (3). Overall, one life was saved for every 13 patients receiving drotrecogin alfa treatment, and in the patients with the highest APACHE II scores (i.e. ≥25), one life was saved for every 8 patients treated. The most frequent and concerning adverse event of the drug is bleeding, although only 2% of patients experienced a severe bleed while receiving the drug. The infusion should be held for 2 hours before and 30 minutes after any percutaneous procedure and for 2 hours before and 12 hours after any surgical procedure because of its anticoagulant properties. The mortality benefit of drotrecogin alfa (activated) may not outweigh the risk

TABLE 26.4

THE PATIENT WITH LINGERING SEPSIS AND MULTIORGAN SYSTEM FAILURE: 10 PRECEPTS FOR DAY-TO-DAY MANAGEMENT

1. Examine the patient and listen to the nurses.
2. Review the patient's medications every day, considering dosage adjustments and potential drug interactions.
3. Do not leave hardware in (including central venous catheters, pulmonary artery catheters, bladder catheters, etc.) unless clearly necessary.
4. Obtain and repeat imaging studies whenever substantive questions arise.
5. Ensure the source of infection is controlled (abscess fully drained, all necrotic tissue removed, infected hardware removed, etc.).
6. Prevent complications: ensure acid suppression for ulcer prophylaxis; use heparin (low molecular weight or undifferentiated) or pressure stockings to prevent deep venous thromboses/pulmonary emboli; physical therapy to prevent contractures; good skin care to prevent decubitus ulcers.
7. Prevent secondary infections: insert central lines with sterile technique and maximal barrier protection; wash hands between patients; use gloves and gowns when examining patients with resistant organisms; elevate the head of the bed when giving tube feedings; minimize ventilator tube changes and central venous catheter manipulations; ensure endotracheal and feeding tubes are orally placed.
8. Narrow antibiotic coverage when culture data return; if the patient is not improved after seven days of antibiotics, consider switching or discontinuing them.
9. Individuals vary in their physiologies: If the patient does not mentate or urinate at a mean arterial pressure of 65 mm Hg, push it to 75 mm Hg and see what happens.
10. Be realistic: Experienced clinicians know, with or without help from standardized approaches such as APACHE scores (see Chapter 22), when there is no longer a realistic prospect for survival.

of hemorrhage, specifically intracranial hemorrhage, in patients with severe thrombocytopenia (platelet count <30,000/mL), meningitis, or marked coagulopathy (INR >3), and its use in these patient populations should be undertaken with extreme caution, if at all.

Septic Patients Requiring Mechanical Ventilation

Regardless of the source of the infection, patients with sepsis often develop inflammation in other organs of the body, especially the lungs and kidneys. Acute lung injury, or the acute respiratory distress syndrome (ARDS), occurs in about one of every five patients with sepsis (1), usually resulting in respiratory failure and the need for mechanical ventilation. "Low tidal volumes" (6 mL/kg ideal body weight or less) should be utilized when any patient with ARDS, including those with sepsis, needs mechanical ventilation (11). If plateau pressures exceed 30 cm H_2O when ventilating with tidal volumes of 6 mL/kg ideal body weight (IBW), then the tidal volume should be decreased

(to a minimum of 4 mL/kg IBW) until plateau pressures are below 30 cm H_2O (see Chapter 23).

Persistent Hypotension in Septic Patients

Patients with sepsis typically develop hypotension because of peripheral vasodilation. This hypotension may correct with aggressive fluid resuscitation, but septic patients may require vasopressors to maintain an adequate arterial perfusion pressure. Sometimes, septic patients have refractory hypotension despite the administration of adequate volume and increasing doses or numbers of vasopressors. These patients with refractory hypotension may be either deficient in vasopressin or lack adequate adrenal reserve for their level of illness. Replacement of physiologic doses of vasopressin (i.e., 0.04 units/min) may increase blood pressure and allow weaning of other vasopressors (10). However, the dose of vasopressin should not be escalated as it can result in cardiac and mesenteric ischemia.

Some patients with septic shock have persistent hypotension because of lack of adrenal reserve. A few of these patients meet the traditional criteria for adrenal insufficiency, but more have relative adrenal insufficiency: they possess some adrenal function, but lack the adequate reserve to compensate for their critical illness. These patients have less than a 9 mcg/dL increase over baseline cortisol levels when challenged with a short corticotropin (ACTH) stimulation test and may benefit from glucocorticoid replacement (12). (See also Chapter 109.) However, not all patients with sepsis and persistent hypotension should be treated with exogenous glucocorticoids, since steroids can worsen the outcomes of septic patients with preserved adrenal function.

Discharge Issues

For patients with sepsis syndrome, the principal discharge issue is that of leaving the ICU. It often is difficult to know how to utilize ICUs in the most cost-effective manner, but it clearly is not efficient to discharge patients recovering from sepsis syndrome from the ICU until they have reasonable prospects of not having to be readmitted. In general, this decision implies that patients have been off vasopressors and mechanical ventilation for at least 24 hours and that their renal, hepatic, hematologic, and metabolic parameters are stable or improving. Patients with sepsis syndrome who survive the ICU often experience significant residual weakness and other disability, and many can benefit from a stay in a rehabilitation facility after hospital discharge.

When Sepsis Syndrome Presents During Hospitalization

In most respects, the diagnostic and therapeutic approach to a patient who develops sepsis syndrome during hospitalization is no different than the approach to a patient who presents to the hospital with sepsis syndrome initially. There are, however, a number of additional considerations.

First, the development of sepsis syndrome during hospitalization is much more likely to be related to such iatrogenic factors as surgery, instrumentation, intravascular catheters, Foley catheters, or immunosuppressive therapy. Second, because these are nosocomial infections, there is a much higher likelihood of microorganisms that are relatively resistant to commonly used antibiotics (see Chapter 64). As such, it is prudent to start empiric broader spectrum antibiotics and to consider infectious-diseases consultation sooner rather than later. Third, before developing sepsis syndrome, these patients already had underlying medical or surgical illnesses sufficiently severe to require hospitalization. Thus, their risk of a poor outcome is greater than that of patients who present with sepsis syndrome *de novo*.

Cost Considerations and Resource Use

ICU care consumes enormous personnel, equipment, pharmacy, and blood-bank resources. It is estimated to account for one-third of the overall budget in an average hospital. While a patient with sepsis syndrome is in the ICU, the physician can economize on unnecessary diagnostic tests and may opt for a less expensive antibiotic regimen. However, some expensive treatments, like drotrecogin alfa (activated), should not be withheld simply for financial concerns. In fact, one recent analysis suggested that this expensive therapy may in fact be cost-effective in certain populations (13).

Ultimately, however, there are two promising avenues for significant savings. First, practice diligent, meticulous medicine, avoiding mistakes, minimizing setbacks, preventing complications and secondary infections (see Table 26.4), and recognizing that good medicine might reduce the length of stay of the average patient who survives but paradoxically might increase total costs by extending the length of stay of the person who does not ultimately survive.

Second, be more circumspect in the use of the ICU by uniformly soliciting advance directives from patients who, by virtue of age, illness, debility, or philosophy, might choose to forego aggressive medical care, and more consistently to limit or withdraw care in patients already in the ICU who no longer have realistic prospects for survival (see Chapters 17, 19, and 22).

KEY POINTS

- Sepsis syndrome is the most common cause of death in non-coronary ICUs in the United States and is the tenth most common cause of death overall.
- Despite advances in therapy, the mortality rate of sepsis syndrome remains approximately 30%.
- Resuscitative measures and initiation of antibiotic therapy must occur simultaneous with rapid initial diagnostic evaluation.

- Foci of infection must be sought and eradicated.
- Patients with severe sepsis and most with sepsis syndrome require hospitalization. Most patients with severe sepsis require ICU management.
- As the pathophysiology of sepsis becomes better understood, new specific treatments (e.g., drotrecogin alfa [activated]) can improve outcomes.
- Many patients recover quickly with appropriate antibiotics and hemodynamic support (aggressive fluid resuscitation, with or without vasopressors).
- Unfortunately, many patients with sepsis syndrome develop multiorgan system failure, require costly technology (e.g., mechanical ventilation and hemodialysis), and have lengthy ICU stays.

REFERENCES

1. Martin GS, Mannino DM, Eaton S, et al. The epidemiology of sepsis in the United States from 1979 through 2000. *N Engl J Med* 2003;348:1546–1554.
2. Angus DC, Linde-Zwirble WT, Lidicker J, et al. Epidemiology of severe sepsis in the United States: analysis of incidence, outcome, and associated costs of care. *Crit Care Med* 2001;29:1303–1310.
3. Bernard GR, Vincent J-L, Laterre P-F, et al. Efficacy and safety of recombinant human activated protein C for severe sepsis. *N Engl J Med* 2001;344:699–709.
4. Rivers E, Nguyen B, Havstad S, et al. Early goal-directed therapy in the treatment of severe sepsis and septic shock. *N Engl J Med* 2001;345:1368–1377.
5. Kollef MH, Sherman G, Ward S, et al. Inadequate antimicrobial treatment of infections: risk factor for hospital mortality among critically ill patients. *Chest* 1999;115:462–474.
6. Marshall JC, Maier RV, Jimenez M, Dellinger EP. Source conrol in the management of severe sepsis and septic shock: an evidence-based review. *Crit Care Med* 2004;32 (11 Suppl):S513–S526.
7. Vincent J-L, de Mendeonca A, Cantraine F, et al. Use of the SOFA score to assess the incidence of organ dysfunction/failure in intensive care units: results of a multicenter, prospective study. Working Group on "sepsis-related problems" of the European Society of Intensive Care Medicine. *Crit Care Med* 1998;26:1793–1800.
8. Arons M, Wheeler AP, Bernard GR, et al. Effects of ibuprofen on the physiology and survival of hypothermic sepsis. Ibuprofen in Sepsis Study Group. *Crit Care Med* 1999;27:699–707.
9. Martin C, Viviand X, Leone M, et al. Effect of norepinephrine on the outcome of septic shock. *Crit Care Med* 2000;28:2758–2765.
10. Landry DW, Levin HR, Gallant EM, et al. Vasopressin deficiency contributes to the vasodilation of septic shock. *Circulation* 1997;95:1122–1125.
11. The Acute Respiratory Distress Syndrome Network. Ventilation with lower tidal volumes compared with traditional tidal volumes for acute lung injury and the acute respiratory distress syndrome. *N Engl J Med* 2000;342:1301–1308.
12. Annane D, Sebille V, Charpentier C, et al. Effect of treatment with low doses of hydrocortisone and fludrocortisone on mortality in patients with septic shock. *JAMA* 2002;288:862–871.
13. Angus DC, Linde-Zwirble WT, Clermont G, et al. Cost-effectiveness of drotrecogin alfa (activated) in the treatment of severe sepsis. *Crit Care Med* 2003;31:1–11.

ADDITIONAL READING

Vincent J-L, Abraham E, Annane D, Bernard G, Rivers E, Van den Berghe G. Reducing mortality in sepsis: new directions. *Critical Care* 2002;6(suppl 3):S1–S18.
Wheeler AP, Bernard GR. Current concepts: treating patients with severe sepsis. *N Engl J Med* 1999;340:207–214.

Procedures in Hospital Medicine

27

Rachel L. Chin

INTRODUCTION

Physicians who care for hospitalized patients must commonly perform procedures to facilitate diagnosis and therapy. The risks of such procedures are often increased in hospitalized patients because of comorbid illnesses, poor wound healing, anticoagulation (either therapeutic or caused by the patient's disease state), and the frequent need for haste. It is essential, then, that hospital physicians be skilled in the performance of common procedures and recognize those situations in which a procedure can be done more safely if guided by technology (e.g., ultrasound guidance for thoracentesis or central venous catheterization) or a specialist.

This chapter will review the indications, contraindications, equipment required, and technique of some of the most common procedures performed on hospitalized patients.

ARTERIAL PUNCTURE AND CANNULATION

Introduction

Arterial cannulation is often required in the evaluation of a critically ill patient. Several arteries can be used, but the most common is the radial artery.

Indications

- Arterial pressure monitoring
- Arterial blood gas sampling or blood sampling for any purpose

Contraindications

- Insertion of a needle through an area of cutaneous infection
- Aneurysm with or without a palpable bruit
- Bleeding diathesis or on anticoagulants before correction of the clotting deficits
- Decreased collateral blood flow
- Presence of severe atherosclerosis (a relative contraindication)

Equipment

Positioning

- Armboard
- Folded towel
- Adhesive tape

Skin prep

- Sterile gauze
- Povidone-iodine solution (Betadine®) or prepackaged povidone-iodine sticks
- Alcohol prep pads

Sterile field

- Gloves, mask, sterile drape, local anesthetic

Local anesthetic

- Syringe, 1-mL
- Needle, 25-gauge
- Lidocaine, 1%

Arterial cannulation

■ Angiocath, 20-gauge

or

■ Radial artery catheterization set, 20-gauge (Arrow™), with guidewire

Dressing

■ Antibiotic ointment
■ Sterile gauze

Pressure monitoring

■ Arterial pressure transducer
■ Pressure tubing

Procedure

Before cannulating the radial artery, confirm adequate collateral circulation by performing the Allen test (Figure 27.1). Occlude both the radial and ulnar artery and have the patient pump the blood out of the hand by opening and closing the fist. With the hand open, release one of the occluded arteries and note the return of color to the hand within 5 seconds. Repeat with the other artery. If the circulation is inadequate, do not cannulate the artery.

Position

Place the patient and wrist in supine position with the arm abducted and forearm supinated.

Landmarks

Palpate the radial artery, which is radial to the flexor carpi radialis tendon.

Technique

Dorsiflex the wrist over a folded towel between the wrist and the armboard. Tape the hand to the armboard (Figure 27.2).

Put on a protective mask and gloves. Anesthetize the skin over the site with 1% lidocaine. Be careful not to obscure the artery by injecting too much lidocaine. Prepare and drape the wrist in a normal sterile fashion.

Prepare the catheter by sliding it out, then back in to break the seal. Insert the angiocatheter or radial artery catheterization (Arrow) set with guidewire into the artery at a 45-degree angle to the axis of the vessel (Figures 27.3 and 27.4).

If you see blood flash into the catheter, advance the needle 1–2 mm and then cannulate the artery by sliding the cannula over the needle. If using the Arrow set, first advance the guidewire using the Seldinger technique (see the description under "Central Venous Catheterization," on page 215), and then advance the cannula into the artery over the guidewire (Figure 27.5).

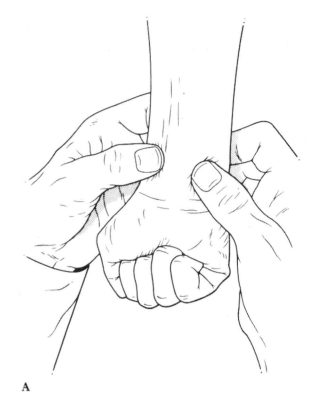

A

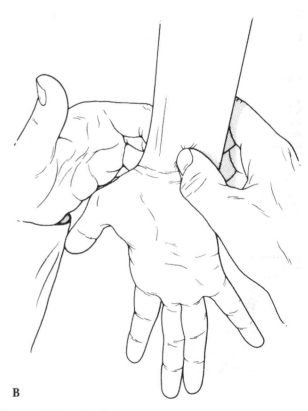

B

Figure 27.1 The Allen test to confirm collateral circulation. **A.** The radial and ulnar arteries are both occluded. **B.** The clinician releases the radial artery to test its patency. The test is then repeated for the ulnar artery. (Reprinted from VanderSalm TJ, Cutler BS, Wheeler HB, eds. *Atlas of Bedside Procedures.* Boston/Toronto: Little, Brown and Company, 1988, with permission.)

Radial artery

Flexor carpi radialis tendon

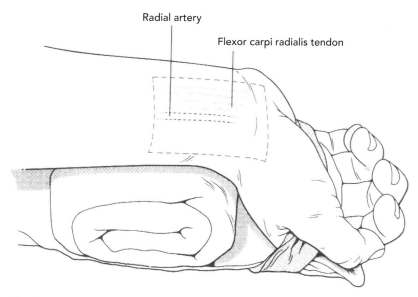

Figure 27.2 Positioning and prepping for arterial cannula insertion. (Reprinted from VanderSalm TJ, Cutler BS, Wheeler HB, eds. *Atlas of Bedside Procedures.* Boston/Toronto: Little, Brown and Company, 1988, with permission.)

Remove the needle while leaving the cannula in place. Strong arterial flow indicates proper positioning.

Attach the cannula to the transducer tubing, and apply dressing. Apply antibiotic ointment to the puncture site, and secure it with sterile dressing.

Remove the towel under the wrist and reapply the armboard securely.

KEY POINTS REGARDING ARTERIAL PUNCTURE AND CANNULATION

- In iodine-allergic patients, pHisoHex® or chlorhexidine gluconate (Hibiclens®) is an acceptable alternative to povidone-iodine (Betadine) solution or prepackaged sticks.
- Avoid tissue necrosis with distal ischemia (typically caused by repeated punctures that result in thrombosis),

especially in patients with poor ulnar arterial flow or patients in shock.

- Apply firm pressure for 5 minutes after puncture and 10 minutes after removal of a peripheral artery catheter, longer if the patient is anticoagulated.
- Retrograde flushing of the cannula can cause retrograde arterial embolism of blood clots.
- The risk of infection increases as the duration of cannulation is prolonged. Arterial catheters should be changed after 4 days if continued monitoring is necessary.
- Avoid catheter embolization by not pulling back the plastic catheter after it has been placed through the needle. The end of the catheter may be sheared off by the sharp needle bevel.

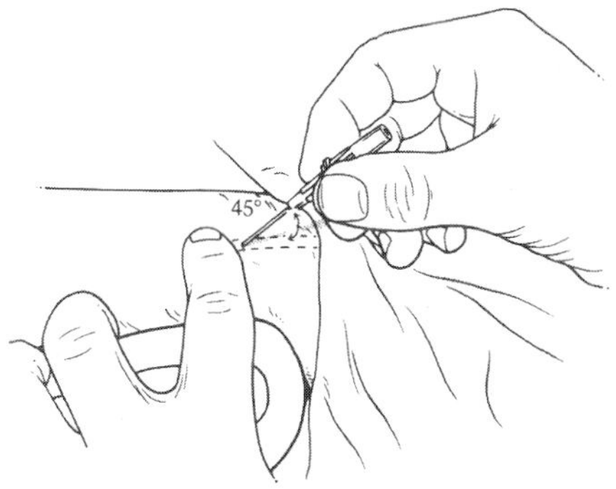

ARTHROCENTESIS

Introduction

Arthrocentesis is both a diagnostic and therapeutic intervention, which commonly is performed at the bedside without complications.

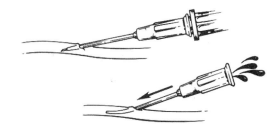

Figure 27.4 Cannulation of the artery is demonstrated by the flash of blood. (Reprinted from VanderSalm TJ, Cutler BS, Wheeler HB, eds. *Atlas of Bedside Procedures.* Boston/ Toronto: Little, Brown and Company, 1988, with permission.)

Figure 27.3 Technique for inserting the angiocatheter through the skin. (Reprinted from VanderSalm TJ, Cutler BS, Wheeler HB, eds. *Atlas of Bedside Procedures.* Boston/Toronto: Little, Brown and Company, 1988, with permission.)

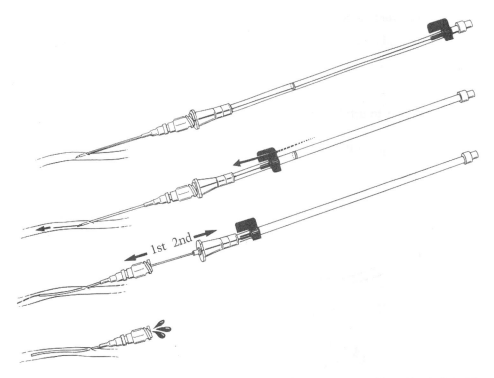

Figure 27.5 Arterial cannulation using the Seldinger technique. (Reprinted from VanderSalm TJ, Cutler BS, Wheeler HB, eds. *Atlas of Bedside Procedures.* Boston/Toronto: Little, Brown and Company, 1988, with permission.)

Indications

- Diagnosis of joint effusions, especially when infectious arthritis is a possibility.
- Traumatic joint effusions such as ligamentous or bony injuries may be confirmed by finding blood in the joint.
- Fat globules in the fluid may diagnose an intra-articular fracture.
- For nontraumatic joint disease, the fluid can be analyzed for a septic joint or crystal-induced arthritis (i.e., gout or pseudogout).
- Arthrocentesis can also provide relief of pain from a tense hemarthrosis or effusion, thereby also enabling the practitioner to examine the joint in question.
- Local instillation of medications such as lidocaine can also provide relief of pain and help in the examination or reduction of a fracture.
- Local instillation of corticosteroids may be appropriate in patients with inflammatory arthritis (such as gout or rheumatoid arthritis) after infection has been excluded.

Contraindications

- Insertion of a needle through an area of infection (cutaneous or osteomyelitis).
- Bleeding diatheses may be a relative contraindication, but arthrocentesis to relieve a tense hemarthrosis in patients with bleeding disorders can be performed if the bleeding disorder is corrected with appropriate clotting factors prior to the procedure (Chapter 98).
- Arthrocentesis of a prosthetic joint should be performed predominantly to exclude an infection, usually by an orthopedic surgeon or rheumatologist unless the procedure is urgent (Chapter 110).

Equipment

Skin prep

- Sterile gauze
- Povidone-iodine solution (Betadine) or prepackaged povidone-iodine sticks
- Alcohol prep pads

Sterile field

- Gloves, mask, sterile drape

Local anesthetic

- Syringe, 5-ml
- Needles, 25- and 22-gauge
- Lidocaine, 1%, 10 mL

Aspiration or injection equipment

- Syringes: 5-, 10-, and 30-mL
- Needles: 22-, 20-, and 18-gauge
- Sterile specimen tubes
- Injectable saline

- Drugs for instillation (i.e., methylene blue, lidocaine, corticosteroids)

Dressing

- Adhesive bandage

General Techniques

1. Define the joint anatomy.
2. Select an approach.
3. Prep and drape.
4. Use universal precautions.
5. Inject local anesthetic along the needle tract.
6. Perform the arthrocentesis.
7. Apply the dressing.

For further information, see specific arthrocentesis techniques below. Use an 18–22 gauge needle of appropriate length. Avoid injury to articular cartilage with the needle by providing traction on the joint, and avoiding "walking" off the bone to find the joint space. Use the largest needle possible to avoid having the lumen become obstructed with blood clots. Send the synovial fluid for studies as indicated (i.e., cell count, microscopic examination, cultures, Gram stain, etc.).

Specific Procedures

Glenohumeral joint (Figure 27.6)

Position: The patient should be sitting upright, arms at the side and hands on lap.

Landmarks: The coracoid process medially and the proximal humerus laterally are palpated anteriorly.

Anterior technique: Insert needle lateral and inferior to coracoid; direct to anterior rim of glenoid.

Posterior technique: Insert needle 2 cm inferior to posterior angle of acromion, direct to posterior rim of glenoid.

Radiohumeral (elbow) joint (Figure 27.7)

Position: The patient should be sitting upright on a gurney with the elbow flexed at 90 degrees. Pronate the forearm, and place the palm flat on the table.

Landmarks: Palpate the lateral epicondyle of the humerus and the head of the radius. To palpate the radial head, pronate and supinate the forearm in a flexed 90-degree angle.

Technique: Place the needle between the lateral epicondyle of the humerus and the radial head. Direct the needle medially.

Radiocarpal (wrist) joint (Figure 27.8)

Position: Flex the wrist to 30 degrees, and apply traction to the hand.

Landmarks: Palpate the bony landmark, the tubercle of Lister. A depression can be palpated just ulnar to the

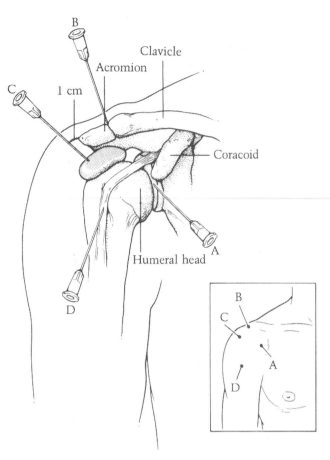

Figure 27.6 Approaches to arthrocentesis of the shoulder. **A.** Glenohumeral joint. **B.** Acromioclavicular joint. **C.** Subacromial bursa. **D.** Bicipital tendon. (Reprinted from VanderSalm TJ, Cutler BS, Wheeler HB, eds. *Atlas of Bedside Procedures.* Boston/Toronto: Little, Brown and Company, 1988, with permission.)

course of the extensor pollicis longus tendon distal and ulnar to Lister's tubercle (Figure 27.9).

Technique: Insert a 22-gauge needle dorsally, distal to tubercle of Lister and medial to extensor pollicis longus tendon.

Interphalangeal and metacarpophalangeal (fingers) joints (Figure 27.10)

Position: Flex the fingers to approximately 15–20 degrees, and apply traction.

Landmarks: On the dorsal surface of the finger, palpate the distal bony prominence of the distal metacarpophalangeal phalanx and proximal end of the proximal phalanx for the metacarpophalangeal joint. For the interphalangeal joints, palpate the distal end of the proximal phalanx and the proximal end of the middle phalanx. The extensor tendon runs down the middle of the digits.

Technique: Insert a 22-gauge needle into the joint space dorsally, medial or lateral to the extensor tendon.

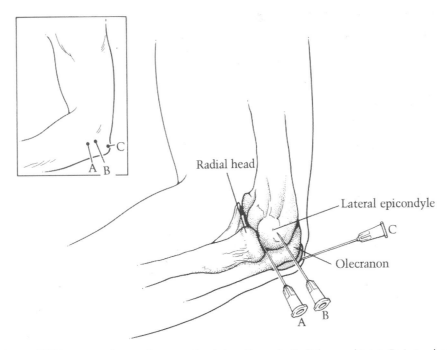

Figure 27.7 Approach to arthrocentesis of the elbow. **A.** Radiohumeral joint. **B.** Lateral epicondyle. **C.** Olecranon bursa. (Reprinted from VanderSalm TJ, Cutler BS, Wheeler HB, eds. *Atlas of Bedside Procedures.* Boston/Toronto: Little, Brown and Company, 1988, with permission.)

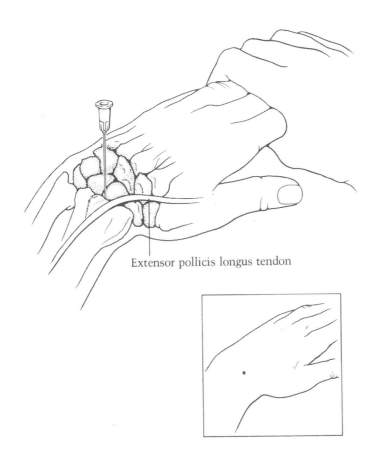

Extensor pollicis longus tendon

Figure 27.8 The wrist (radiocarpal) joint. (Reprinted from VanderSalm TJ, Cutler BS, Wheeler HB, eds. *Atlas of Bedside Procedures.* Boston/Toronto: Little, Brown and Company, 1988, with permission.)

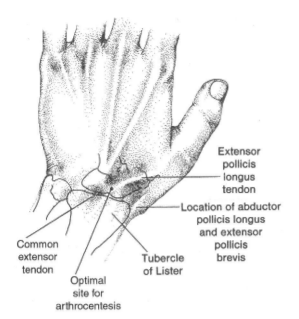

Figure 27.9   The approach to radiocarpal arthrocentesis. The best site of aspiration is through the depression, which can be palpated just ulnar to the course of the extensor pollicis longus tendon, distal and ulnar to Lister's tubercle. (Reprinted from Simon RR, Brenner BE, eds. *Emergency Procedures and Techniques*. 4th ed. Philadelphia: Lippincott, Williams and Wilkins, 2002, with permission.)

Carpometacarpal (thumb) joint (Figure 27.11)

Position: Oppose the thumb to the little finger, and apply traction to the thumb.

Landmarks: Palpate the space between the abductor pollicis longus tendon and the base of the metacarpal, lateral (palmar) to the anatomical "snuff box" (which is dorsal to the abductor pollicis longus). Extend the thumb to palpate the abductor pollicis longus tendon.

Technique: Insert a 22-gauge needle proximal to the prominence of the base of the metacarpal, on the palmar side of the abductor pollicis tendon. Avoid the "snuff box" because it contains the radial artery and superficial radial nerve.

Knee joint (Figure 27.12)

Position: Keep the knee extended and have the leg relaxed.

Landmarks: The medial aspect of the middle/superior portion of the patella.

Technique: Insert an 18-gauge needle 1 cm medial to the patella, and direct it under the patella and into the intercondylar femoral notch. If the patient tenses the quadriceps, the space will be difficult to enter. Be prepared to aspirate 50–70 mL of fluid if there is a large effusion.

Tibiotalar (ankle) joint (Figure 27.13)

Position: Have the patient lie supine on the gurney, and plantar flex the foot.

Landmarks: Palpate the space between the tibialis anterior tendon and the medial malleolus. Dorsiflex the foot to palpate the tibialis anterior tendon.

Technique: Insert a 20-gauge needle 2–3 cm into the space between the tibia and talus. Palpate the anterior tibial tendon, and place the needle medial to it, directed into the hollow at the anterior margin of the medial malleolus.

Interphalangeal and metatarsophalangeal (toe) joints (Figure 27.13)

Position: Have the patient lie supine on the gurney, and flex the toes to 15–20 degrees. Apply traction to the toes.

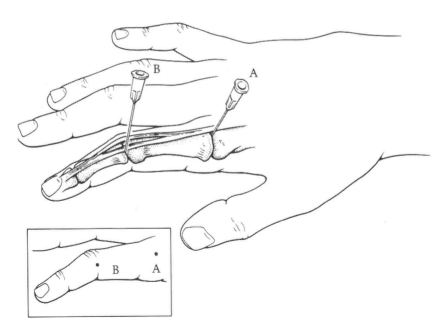

Figure 27.10   The finger joints. **A.** Metacarpophalangeal. **B.** Interphalangeal. (Reprinted from VanderSalm TJ, Cutler BS, Wheeler HB, eds. *Atlas of Bedside Procedures*. Boston/Toronto: Little, Brown and Company, 1988, with permission.)

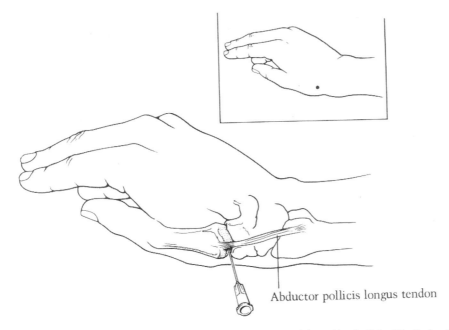

Figure 27.11   The thumb (carpometacarpal) joint. (Reprinted from VanderSalm TJ, Cutler BS, Wheeler HB, eds. *Atlas of Bedside Procedures.* Boston/Toronto: Little, Brown and Company, 1988, with permission.)

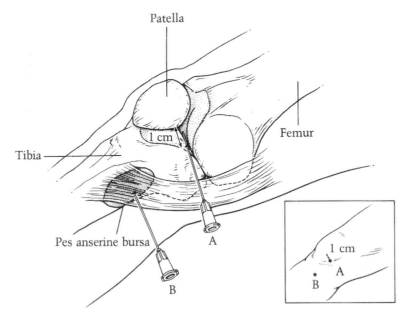

Figure 27.12   The knee. **A.** The knee joint, anteromedial approach. **B.** The pes anserine bursa. (Reprinted from VanderSalm TJ, Cutler BS, Wheeler HB, eds. *Atlas of Bedside Procedures.* Boston/Toronto: Little, Brown and Company, 1988, with permission.)

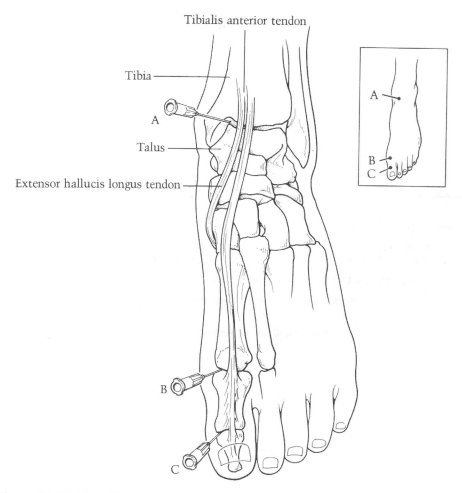

Figure 27.13 The ankle and toe joints. **A.** Tibiotalar (ankle) joint. **B.** Metatarsophalangeal joint. **C.** Interphalangeal joint. (Reprinted from VanderSalm TJ, Cutler BS, Wheeler HB, eds. *Atlas of Bedside Procedures.* Boston/Toronto: Little, Brown and Company, 1988, with permission.)

Landmarks: On the dorsal surface of the toes, palpate the distal bony prominence of the distal metatarsophalangeal phalanx and proximal end of the proximal phalanx for the metatarsophalangeal joint. For the interphalangeal joints, palpate the distal end of the proximal phalanx and the proximal end of the middle phalanx. The extensor tendon runs down the middle of the digits.

Technique: Insert a 22-gauge needle into the joint space dorsal, medial or lateral to the extensor tendon.

KEY POINTS REGARDING ARTHROCENTESIS

- In iodine-allergic patients, pHisoHex® or chlorhexidine gluconate (Hibiclens®) is an acceptable alternative to povidone-iodine (Betadine) solution or prepackaged sticks.
- Use meticulous sterile technique to prevent infection, and never pass the needle through infected skin.
- Take a careful allergy history to avoid a hypersensitivity reaction from an allergy to the medication.

- Clotting abnormalities should be corrected prior to aspirating a hemarthrosis.
- Have the patient in a sitting or lying position to avoid a postprocedural vasovagal episode.
- If you are culturing for *Neisseria gonorrhoeae*, be sure you have the correct culture medium. Store the specimen in an anaerobic environment.
- Be sure to use adequate local anesthesia to keep the procedure relatively painless.

CENTRAL VENOUS CATHETERIZATION

Seldinger Technique

This technique, first described by Sven Ivar Seldinger in 1952, is now the standard approach for the insertion of a catheter into a blood vessel or space. Using the Seldinger technique, the clinician places an introducer needle into the desired blood vessel, next inserts a guidewire *through* the introducer needle, and finally slides the catheter *over* the guidewire (Figure 27.14).

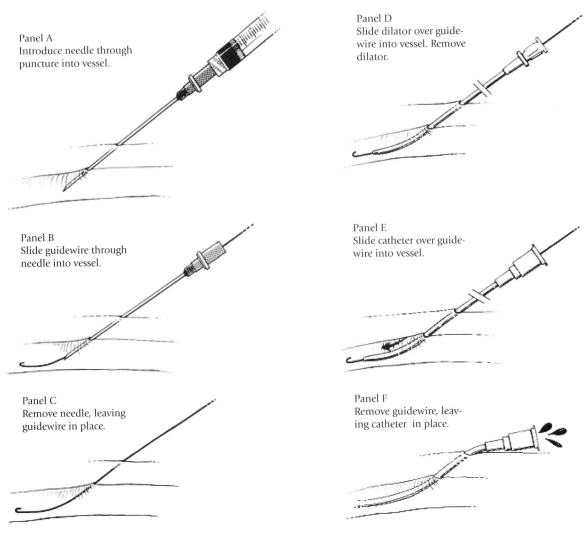

Panel A
Introduce needle through puncture into vessel.

Panel B
Slide guidewire through needle into vessel.

Panel C
Remove needle, leaving guidewire in place.

Panel D
Slide dilator over guidewire into vessel. Remove dilator.

Panel E
Slide catheter over guidewire into vessel.

Panel F
Remove guidewire, leaving catheter in place.

Figure 27.14 The Seldinger technique. **Panel A.** 1. Introduce needle on syringe through puncture wound in skin into the vessel (for arterial cannulation, syringe unnecessary; for venous cannulation, aspirate gently). 2. Remove syringe. **Panel B.** 3. Slide soft-tip of J-tip guidewire through needle into vessel. **Panel C.** 4. Remove needle, leaving guidewire in place. **Panel D.** 5. Insert dilator over guidewire into vessel. 6. Remove dilator. **Panel E.** 7. Slide catheter over guidewire into vessel. **Panel F.** 8. Remove guidewire, leaving catheter in place. (Reprinted from VanderSalm TJ, Cutler BS, Wheeler HB, eds. *Atlas of Bedside Procedures.* Boston/Toronto: Little, Brown and Company, 1988, with permission.)

Indications

- Need for intravenous access in an emergency
- Central venous pressure monitoring (internal jugular or subclavian vein cannulation)
- Hyperalimentation
- Vasopressor administration
- Transvenous pacemaker insertion
- Hemodialysis
- Cardiac catheterization
- Pulmonary angiography

Contraindications

- Insertion of a needle through an area of cutaneous infection
- Patients with distorted local anatomy or landmarks
- Previous radiation therapy to the clavicular area (for subclavian vein cannulation)
- Patients with significant chest wall deformities (for subclavian vein cannulation)
- Bleeding disorders or anticoagulation therapy
- Vasculitis
- Suspected pre-existing injury to the vessel

Equipment

Skin prep

- Sterile sponges, alcohol, povidone-iodine solution

Sterile field

- Mask, gown, gloves, sterile drape

Local anesthetic

- Plastic syringe, 3-ml, with 22-gauge needle
- Lidocaine 1%, 5ml

Cannulation Equipment

- Multilumen (triple-lumen) central venous catheter set with 7 Fr × 6″ (16 cm) radiopaque catheter *or* single-lumen central venous catheter set
- Saline flush
- Suture material in kit
- Scalpel

Dressing

- Antibiotic ointment
- Sponges
- Transparent adhesive film

Infusion

- Intravenous solution, tubing, and IV stand

Technique

Prepare equipment and obtain necessary consent according to hospital policy. Put on a protective mask and gloves. Prepare the insertion area with swab sticks or sterile gauze soaked with the povidone-iodine solution. Warn the patient that the solution will be cold.

Insert the introducer needle into the desired blood vessel as described in the appropriate subsection below. Advance the introducer needle with its cannula into the blood vessel, aspirating gently until there is a flashback of venous blood, usually at a depth of 3–4 cm. For internal jugular or subclavian vein cannulation, keep the needle and syringe almost parallel to the table, at a 20-degree angle. When there is free flow of blood from the open cannula, prepare to slide the guidewire through the blood vessel.

Pulsatile flow identifies an arterial puncture and mandates immediate withdrawal of the needle (1). A single arterial puncture without laceration rarely causes serious harm.

If there is no blood return, aspirate gently to confirm intravenous location. If blood is still not aspirated, remove the needle and start again. Do not reinsert the needle through the *in situ* cannula because of the risk of shearing of the catheter tip.

When it is time to slide the guidewire, occlude the cannula hub with your thumb to prevent bleeding or air embolus. When using a safety syringe and hollow plunger with a guidewire opening, there is no need to remove the needle/cannula from the syringe. For internal jugular or subclavian vein cannulation, ask the patient to exhale, hum, or perform a Valsalva maneuver to raise intrathoracic pressure and reduce the possibility of a pneumothorax. Slide the guidewire through the cannula into the blood vessel. For internal jugular or subclavian vein cannulation, turn the patient's head to the ipsilateral side as the guidewire is advanced to prevent the guidewire from going up the internal jugular vein.

Remove the cannula, holding the guidewire in place. Incise the skin about 1.5 cm with a no. 11 blade over the wire. Pass the vessel dilator over the guidewire, and then remove the dilator while holding the wire in place.

For internal jugular or subclavian vein cannulation, judge the approximate distance from the puncture site to the superior vena cava, and then insert the single- or multilumen central venous catheter over the wire. Thread the catheter over the wire until it protrudes from the infusion port. Hold the wire firmly, and while holding the catheter near the entry, use a twisting motion to push the catheter over the guidewire to the predetermined length, if any.

The guidewire should slide out of the distal infusion port while the catheter is held firmly in place. If the wire does not slide easily, *do not force it in*, but pull the catheter back 1–2 cm and try again. If the wire cannot be removed, both the catheter and wire may have to be removed together.

With the central line catheter in place and the wire removed, draw blood and cultures through the distal port with a vacutainer. After collecting blood, connect this port to the intravenous line or attach the cap.

There should be blood throughout the lumen; if not, aspirate until the lumen is filled with blood, and flush with saline solution to avoid air entrapment. This process should be performed on all the ports.

Secure the catheter to the skin by suturing the catheter clamp or by stapling (some kits have manual staples that fit through the clamp holes) (Figure 27.15). Apply a sterile dressing over the puncture site, and tape securely.

After internal jugular or subclavian vein cannulation, obtain a chest radiograph to confirm placement of the catheter in the superior vena cava and to exclude a pneumothorax or hemothorax.

Internal Jugular Vein Cannulation

The internal jugular vein is the most common site for central venous access. Knowledge of neck anatomy is important.

Procedure

Position

Assure adequate lighting and elevate the bed to a comfortable level. Have the patient in a supine position in Trende-

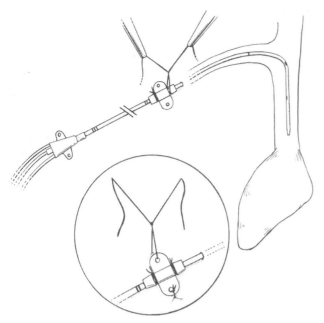

Figure 27.15 Subclavian vein cannulation and the technique of securing the catheter to the skin. (Reprinted from VanderSalm TJ, Cutler BS, Wheeler HB, eds. *Atlas of Bedside Procedures.* Boston/Toronto: Little, Brown and Company, 1988, with permission.)

lenburg 10–20 degrees. Turn the patient's head away from the internal jugular vein site.

Landmarks

The apex of the triangle formed by the two heads of the sternocleidomastoid muscle and the clavicle serves as a landmark. The internal jugular vein runs deep to the sternocleidomastoid muscle and then through this triangle

before it joins the subclavian vein to become the brachiocephalic vein (Figure 27.16).

Technique

After prepping the neck and clavicular area, infiltrate 1% lidocaine anesthetic into the apex of the triangle formed by the two heads of the sternocleidomastoid muscle and the clavicle.

Place the patient in Trendelenburg position with the head rotated 45 degrees away from the site of cannulation. Place the index and middle finger of the nondominant hand on the carotid artery and insert a 22-gauge finder needle through the skin, immediately lateral to the carotid pulse and slightly superior to the apex of the triangle. The needle is advanced past the apex of the triangle, in the direction of the ipsilateral nipple, at an angle of 20 degrees above the plane of the skin, keeping it almost parallel to the bed. The vein is usually located near the surface of the skin and is often cannulated at a depth of less than 1.3 cm. If the first pass is unsuccessful, the needle should be directed slightly more medially on the next attempt.

With the finder needle in place, insert the 18-gauge introducer needle right alongside it and into the vein. Follow the general Seldinger technique as described in Figure 27.14.

Subclavian Vein Cannulation

Procedure

Position

Assure good lighting and elevate the bed to a comfortable level. Have the patient in a supine position in Trendelenburg 10–20 degrees, with the option of placing a roll under the patient's shoulders to accentuate the clavicles. Turn the

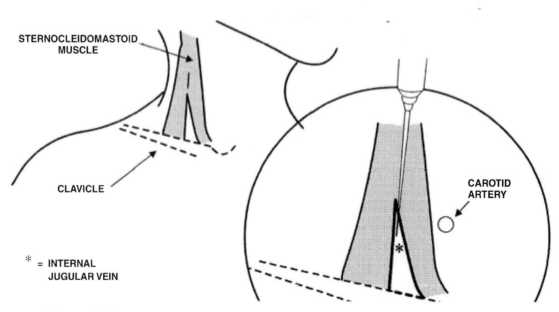

Figure 27.16 Landmarks for internal jugular vein catheterization. (Reprinted from *AHRQ Web M&M*, March 2004: http://webmm.ahrq.gov/spotlightcases.aspx?ic=51, with permission.)

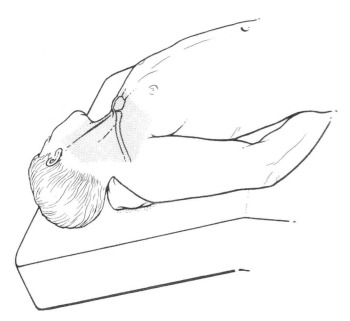

Figure 27.17 Positioning, prepping, and draping for subclavian vein catheterization. (Reprinted from VanderSalm TJ, Cutler BS, Wheeler HB, eds. *Atlas of Bedside Procedures.* Boston/ Toronto: Little, Brown and Company, 1988, with permission.)

patient's head away from the subclavian vein site (Figure 27.17).

Landmarks

The axillary vein, which becomes the subclavian vein as it crosses the first rib, is a 10–20 mm large, valveless vessel. The vein lies posterior to the medial third of the clavicle. It is separated from the subclavian artery by the anterior scalene muscle, which has a thickness of 10–15 mm. Other important structures related to the course of the vein are the vagus and phrenic nerves, which course medially in front of the subclavian artery. The trachea and esophagus lie medial to the vein. No vital structures are crossed in entering the vein at the medial one-third of the clavicle between the subclavian vein and the skin (Figure 27.18).

Technique

After preparing the neck and anterior chest area, infiltrate 1% lidocaine anesthetic into the middle of the clavicle, and insert the needle 2–3 cm caudal under the clavicle (Figure 27.19). If the patient is on mechanical ventilation, the ventilator must be disconnected while performing this maneuver to avoid a pneumothorax from the positive airway pressure.

The left index finger is placed in the suprasternal notch, and the thumb is positioned at the costoclavicular junction. These landmarks serve as the reference points for the direction of the needle as you aim for the suprasternal notch (Figure 27.20).

A finder needle is generally not long enough to locate the subclavian vein and is therefore not used. Insert the 18-gauge introducer needle attached to the syringe through the same anesthetic puncture site into the subclavian vein. Follow the general Seldinger technique as described above.

The correct position of the catheter is in the superior vena cava, not the right atrium or ventricle. The superior vena cava begins at the level of the manubrial-sternal junction and terminates in the right atrium, approxi-

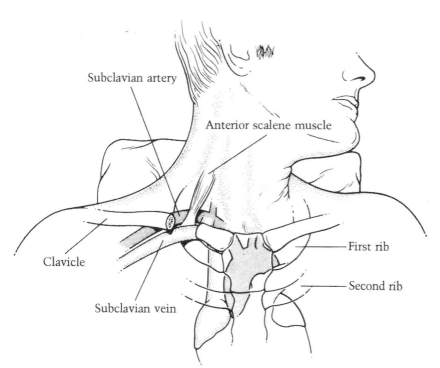

Subclavian artery

Anterior scalene muscle

Clavicle

Subclavian vein

First rib

Second rib

Figure 27.18 Anatomic landmarks for subclavian vein catheterization. (Reprinted from VanderSalm TJ, Cutler BS, Wheeler HB, eds. *Atlas of Bedside Procedures.* Boston/Toronto: Little, Brown and Company, 1988, with permission.)

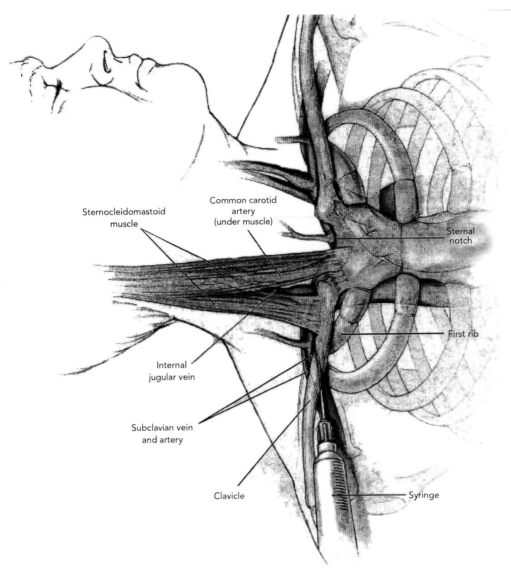

Figure 27.19 Insertion of the catheter into the subclavian vein. (Reprinted from McGee DC, Gould MK. Preventing complications of central venous catheterization. *N Engl J Med* 2003; 348:1123–1133, with permission.)

mately 5 cm lower. Therefore, the catheter should be threaded 2 cm below the manubrial-sternal junction. This distance can be estimated by placing the catheter parallel to the chest wall before insertion. Standard catheters in central line kits are 16 cm long, which is the appropriate length for the average adult. Nevertheless, proper placement is best assessed by a chest radiograph rather than by predetermined measurements.

Femoral Vein Cannulation

The femoral vein is easily located by palpating the femoral artery (the vein is just medial to the artery). Although femoral vein cannulation does not potentially jeopardize critical structures, it carries greater infectious and thrombotic risks than subclavian or internal jugular cannulation. Importantly, complication rates are usually lower when

central lines are placed by experienced physicians ("practice makes perfect"), regardless of the site.

Procedure

Position
Assure good lighting, and elevate the bed to a comfortable level. Have the patient in a supine position. The leg should be slightly abducted and externally rotated to increase exposure of the femoral vein.

Landmarks
Identify the femoral vein by palpating the femoral artery, which is always lateral to the vein in the femoral canal below the inguinal ligament and halfway between the anterior iliac spine and the pubic tubercle. The mnemonic

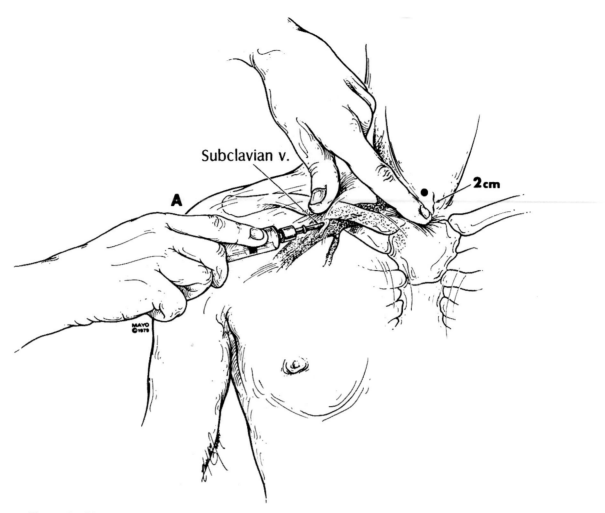

Figure 27.20   Hand positioning during subclavian venipuncture (note that gloves should be worn). (Reprinted from VanderSalm TJ, Cutler BS, Wheeler HB, eds. *Atlas of Bedside Procedures.* Boston/Toronto: Little, Brown and Company, 1988, with permission.)

NAVEL (from lateral to medial: Nerve, Artery, Vein, Empty space, Lymphatics) is a reminder for where the vein is located in relation to the artery. A right-handed physician usually will find it easier to cannulate the right femoral artery.

Technique

After prepping the groin area, infiltrate 1% lidocaine anesthetic medial to the femoral pulse. Aspirate with each change in needle location to avoid injecting directly into a blood vessel.

Place the index and middle finger of the nondominant hand on the femoral artery, and insert a 22-gauge finder needle with a 5-mL syringe through the skin, immediately medial to the femoral pulse and below the inguinal ligament. The needle is advanced at an angle of 45 degrees above the plane of the skin, at a depth of 1–2 cm. If the first pass is unsuccessful, the needle should be directed slightly more medially on the next attempt.

With the finder needle in place, insert the 18-gauge introducer needle right alongside it and into the vein. Follow the general Seldinger technique as described above. Ensure that the patient will not ambulate with the femoral catheter in place. Patients can sit up, but clinicians should be aware that this position may cause discomfort and kinking of the catheter.

Ultrasound Guidance for Central Venous Catheterization

Catheter placement may be assisted by the use of a portable ultrasound device. Real-time ultrasound can provide visualization of the blood vessels and surrounding structures before and during insertion of the catheter and thereby reduce the incidence of complications, especially when the anatomy is difficult to discern by palpation (Figures 27.21 and 27.22). Studies have demonstrated improvements in accuracy and efficiency when internal jugular catheteriza-

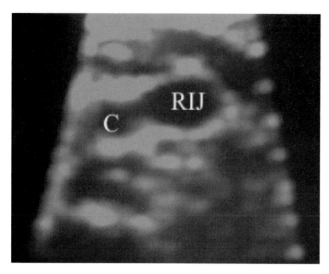

Figure 27.21 Ultrasound guidance for central vein catheterization. Ultrasound image of the right side of the neck. **C.** *carotid artery;* **RIJ.** *right internal jugular vein.* (Reprinted from *AHRQ Web M&M,* March 2004: http://webmm.ahrq.gov/spotlight cases.aspx?ic=51, with permission.)

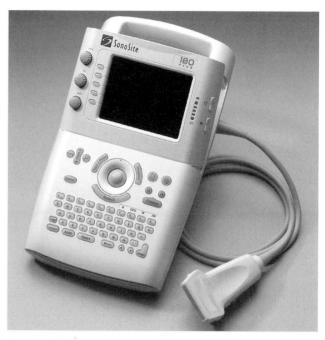

Figure 27.22 Portable ultrasound machine for vascular access procedures. (Reprinted by permission of SonoSite, Inc.)

tion was performed with portable ultrasound; the benefits in subclavian catheterization are less certain (2). However, real-time ultrasound guidance is a relatively new technique and requires sufficient training and experience to achieve competency.

KEY POINTS REGARDING CENTRAL VENOUS CATHETERIZATION

- In iodine-allergic patients, pHisoHex or chlorhexidine gluconate (Hibiclens) is an acceptable alternative to povidone-iodine (Betadine) solution or prepackaged sticks.
- Insert the cannula gently to prevent a hematoma from developing where the venous wall would be injured or traversed.
- Never lose hold of the guidewire, especially when placing the final catheter over the wire.
- Be sure to dilate the soft tissue and vessel by making an adequate scalpel incision and placing the entire dilator into the vessel.
- Do not use the subclavian approach in patients who have coagulation disorders or are receiving full anticoagulation because it is impossible to apply direct pressure to an oozing subclavian vein.
- Subclavian venipuncture is not a good route for rapid volume resuscitation unless no other access is available because very large (i.e., 14-gauge) catheters are best placed in the femoral or a peripheral vein. A peripheral 5 cm, 14-gauge catheter can deliver roughly twice as much fluid as a 20 cm, 16-gauge central venous catheter.

- To avoid a pneumothorax after the cannulation of the internal jugular or subclavian vein, abandon the procedure after two unsuccessful attempts, and keep the syringe on the needle until the needle is in the vein. To avoid air embolism (caused when air enters through the open cannula or needle), maintain the patient in Trendelenburg position, and occlude the open needle hub with a finger. Avoid excessive wire/catheter advancement by premeasuring the length on the patient's chest wall; then confirm the position of the catheter tip on a chest radiograph. After the catheter is placed, raise the head of the bed to reduce venous pressure and thereby prevent a hematoma.
- If a patient with a pre-existing pneumothorax needs central venous access, a vein should be cannulated on the same side as the pneumothorax.
- Remove the catheter as soon as possible to prevent catheter-induced thrombosis.

LUMBAR PUNCTURE

Introduction and Indications

Cerebrospinal fluid (CSF) should be obtained via lumbar puncture in patients with a fever of unknown origin, especially if there is headache, an altered level of consciousness, or suggestion of a stiff neck (Chapter 70). The presence of meningeal signs may not be evident in patients who are old, debilitated, immunosuppressed, or partially treated with antibiotics.

Lumbar puncture should also be performed in patients who are suspected of having subarachnoid hemorrhage despite a normal head CT scan (Chapter 117) because 5%–8% of acute subarachnoid hemorrhages will not be detected by the initial CT scan.

Other uses of the lumbar puncture include injection of anesthetic agents, chemotherapeutic agents, and antibiotics, and drainage of fluids.

Contraindications

- Insertion of a needle through an area of infection (cutaneous or osteomyelitis)
- Bleeding diathesis or anticoagulant therapy
- Papilledema or other signs of increased intracranial pressure
- Focal neurological signs until a space-occupying lesion is excluded

Equipment

Skin prep

- Sterile sponges (usually three swab sticks, or prepackaged povidone-iodine sticks)
- Povidone-iodine (Betadine) solution
- Alcohol prep pads

Sterile field

- Gloves, mask, sterile drape, and towel

Local anesthetic

- Syringe, 3-mL
- Needles, 25- and 22-gauge
- Lidocaine, 1%

Prepackaged lumbar puncture preparation kits, including

- Spinal needle with stylet 20-gauge × 3 1/2 inch
- Four specimen vials with caps, 10 ml

- Manometer with three-way stopcock

Dressing

- Gauze pads
- Bandage

Procedure

Position

The most important step in this procedure is positioning the patient. The lateral decubitus position, with the patient flexed in fetal position, is the most common approach. The back should be at the edge of the bed, and the knees, hips, back, and neck should be maximally flexed. Shoulders and pelvis should be perpendicular to the floor.

Landmarks

Find the midline of L4-L5 or L5-S1, which is an imaginary measured line drawn from the patient's posterior superior iliac crest to the floor (in the lateral decubitus position) (Figure 27.23). The adjacent interspace above or below may be used, depending on which appears to be most open to palpation. The spinal cord ends at the level of L1-L2 in adults.

An alternative is the *sitting-up approach*, which is used for obese patients and patients with lumbar spondylosis, rheumatoid arthritis, scoliosis, or ankylosing spondylitis. Have the patient sit on the edge of the bed, leaning over two pillows or sheets on a bed stand (Figure 27.24). Find the midline of L4-L5 by palpating the posterior superior iliac crest and the spinal interspace.

Technique

Prepare the equipment and obtain necessary consent according to hospital policy. Put on a protective mask and gloves. Prepare the puncture site with swab sticks in the povidone-iodine solution. Warn the patient that the solution will be cold.

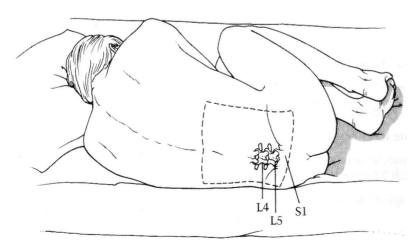

L4
L5
S1

Figure 27.23 Left lateral decubitus position for lumbar puncture. (Reprinted from VanderSalm TJ, Cutler BS, Wheeler HB, eds. *Atlas of Bedside Procedures.* Boston/Toronto: Little, Brown and Company, 1988, with permission.)

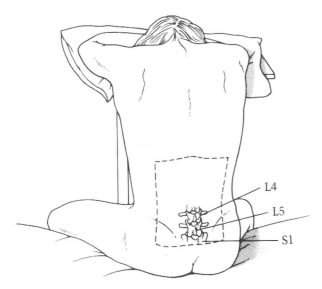

Figure 27.24 The sitting position. (Reprinted from Vander-Salm TJ, Cutler BS, Wheeler HB, eds. *Atlas of Bedside Procedures.* Boston/Toronto: Little, Brown and Company, 1988, with permission.)

microbiologic (Gram stain and cultures) and cytologic studies. Tube 3 is for cell counts and serologic tests for syphilis. In the presence of a traumatic (bloody) spinal tap, cell counts should be performed in tubes 1 and 4—if the source of the blood was tap-related trauma, the red cell count should be markedly lower in tube 4. A traumatic tap is not a particularly dangerous problem, and no specific precautions are needed except that these patients should be observed for signs of cord or spinal nerve compression owing to a hematoma.

Drape the patient. Place a sterile towel between the patient's hip and the bed. Infiltrate a skin wheal with 1% lidocaine anesthetic by using the 25-gauge needle, switching to the 22-gauge needle for deeper infiltration.

Hold the needle between both thumbs and index fingers (Figure 27.25). Insert the spinal needle into the subcutaneous tissue. The needle should have the bevel parallel to the axis of the spine. Some have speculated that pointing the bevel laterally may allow the needle to penetrate the transverse fibers of the dura rather than cut through them, thereby reducing spinal fluid leakage after the needle has been withdrawn.

Angle the needle cephalad, toward the umbilicus. Advance slowly until a very subtle "pop" is felt as the needle passes through the ligamentum flavum dura. The "pop" may not be felt with the very sharp needles in the disposable sets. Accordingly, the operator must remove the stylet frequently and check for flow of cerebrospinal fluid to avoid transgressing the subarachnoid space. If there is no flow, advance the needle with the stylet and check for flow at each 2 mm interval (in adults, the needle should be at a depth of approximately 4 cm, depending on the patient's body habitus).

When the needle is in the subarachnoid space, attach the manometer and three-way stopcock. Normal pressures are 70–180 mm CSF. If the readings are elevated, have the patient relax and extend the legs to decrease intra-abdominal pressure. Avoid having the patient breathe deeply because the resulting hypocapnia induces falsely low pressure readings due to cerebral vasoconstriction.

After measuring the pressure, turn the stopcock and collect the fluid. Tube 1 is used for protein and glucose levels and for electrophoretic studies. Tube 2 is used for

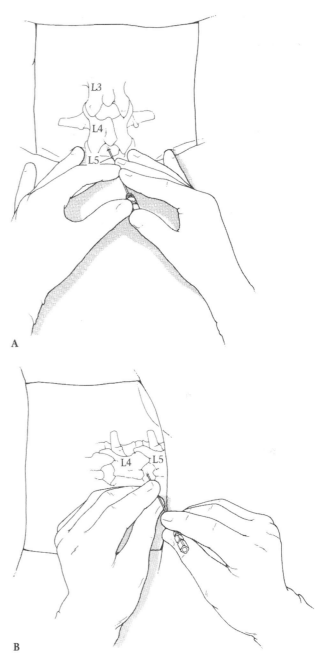

Figure 27.25 Hand position during lumbar puncture, showing the insertion of the spinal needle into the subcutaneous tissue. (Reprinted from VanderSalm TJ, Cutler BS, Wheeler HB, eds. *Atlas of Bedside Procedures.* Boston/Toronto: Little, Brown and Company, 1988, with permission.)

Remove the needle after collection, and apply a dressing. Instruct the patient to remain flat in bed for 1–3 hours.

KEY POINTS REGARDING LUMBAR PUNCTURE

- In iodine-allergic patients, pHisoHex or chlorhexidine gluconate (Hibiclens) is an acceptable alternative to povidone-iodine (Betadine) solution or prepackaged sticks.
- To prevent transtentorial or tonsillar herniation, never perform a lumbar puncture in the presence of papilledema or focal neurological signs unless a mass is excluded.
- Keep stylet in place with the needle. This method prevents viable epithelial cells from entering the spinal canal, where they can form an intraspinal epidermoid cyst.
- Use sterile technique, and avoid performing lumbar puncture through an area of cellulitis to prevent iatrogenic meningitis, epidural empyema, or subdural empyema.
- Remove small volumes of fluid slowly, and prescribe prolonged bedrest (an extra few hours) in elderly patients. The removal of large volumes may result in the tearing or avulsion of perforating veins.
- Avoid excessively lateral or deep penetration so as to keep from lacerating the anterior or lateral epidural venous plexus.
- Transient headache occurs after 5%–30% of all punctures. Headaches usually persist for 1–2 days, but occasionally last up to 10 days. Headaches are usually suboccipital in location. Keep patients well hydrated and remove only the volume of fluid needed for studies.
- Use adequate anesthesia to prevent backaches.
- Insert the spinal needle with the bevel parallel to the axis of the spine to prevent the spinal needle from puncturing or grazing the nerve root and causing transient radicular pain.
- If the opening pressure is unusually high, have the patient straighten the legs, and recheck the pressure.

PARACENTESIS

Introduction

Abdominal paracentesis to remove up to 100 ml of ascites may be performed safely and easily at the bedside with simple needle aspiration. For patients who have reduced respiratory capacity and difficulty breathing, 3–6 liters may be removed slowly, to avoid hypotension and electrolyte disturbances. Large-volume paracentesis (greater than 6

liters) may have an immediate hemodynamic effect, with precipitous hypotension, tachycardia, and oliguric renal failure.

Complications of paracentesis are usually minor and infrequent if appropriate procedure is followed. Procedure-associated risks include a 1% risk of significant abdominal-wall hematoma, a 0.01% risk of hemoperitoneum, and a 0.01% risk of iatrogenic infection. The only absolute contraindications to paracentesis are disseminated intravascular coagulation or recent thrombolytic therapy. Severe coagulopathy and thrombocytopenia (INR >2 or platelet count <50) may need correction prior to the procedure to minimize the risk of bleeding, although there are no data supporting specific cut-offs.

Indications

- Diagnosis of infection or malignancy
- Therapeutic relief of excess peritoneal fluid

Contraindications

- Insertion of a needle through an area of cutaneous infection
- Pregnancy
- Prolonged prothrombin time and a low platelet count (relative contraindications)

Equipment

Commercially prepared thoracentesis/paracentesis kits have most of the equipment, but if a kit is not available, the following equipment can be assembled.

Skin prep
- Sterile gauze
- Povidone-iodine solution or prepackaged povidone-iodine sticks
- Alcohol prep pads

Sterile field
- Gloves, mask, sterile drape

Local anesthetic
- Syringe, 5-ml
- Needles, 25- and 22-gauge
- Lidocaine 1%, 10 mL

Paracentesis
- 50-mL syringe with three-way stopcock
- 14- or 16-gauge angiocatheters or Caldwell paracentesis needle/catheter
- Curved clamps, two
- Sterile connecting tubing (from stopcock to bottle)
- Specimen tubes
- Plasma vacuum bottles

Procedure

Position

The supine position is the most common approach. An alternative approach is the lateral decubitus position.

Landmarks

There are four standard landmarks for paracentesis (Figure 27.26). Most physicians prefer the lower abdominal sites. Others claim that the specific location is not important if the site is lateral to the rectus sheath so that the inferior epigastric artery is avoided.

Technique

Prepare your equipment and obtain necessary consent according to your hospital's policy. Put on a protective mask and gloves. Prepare and drape your patient using sterile technique. Warn the patient that the solution will be cold.

Infiltrate a skin wheal with 1% lidocaine anesthetic by using the 25-gauge needle and switching to the 22-gauge needle for deeper infiltration. For simple diagnostic paracentesis, a 50-mL syringe with a 20- or 22-gauge needle or angiocatheter is sufficient. For removal of large volumes of fluid, insert an 18- or 20-gauge spinal needle or angiocatheter into the subcutaneous tissue.

Insert the needle at an angle, or use the Z-tract technique (retraction of the abdominal skin caudad before inserting the needle). This technique is often used to help seal the needle tract after paracentesis, thereby preventing persistent ascitic fluid drainage.

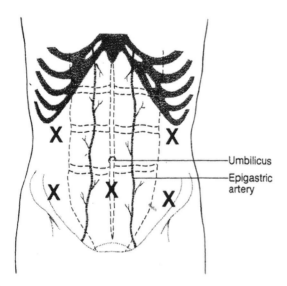

Figure 27.26 Standard landmarks for paracentesis, including the four quadrants lateral to the rectus muscle and a few centimeters below the umbilicus in the middle. (Reprinted from Roberts JR, Hedges JR. *Clinical Procedures in Emergency Medicine.* 3rd ed. Philadelphia: WB Saunders, 1998, with permission.)

A minimum of 50 cc ascitic fluid is required for adequate studies (Chapter 83). In patients with tense ascites that causes respiratory distress, the removal of 1–3 liters will be necessary for symptomatic relief.

Suction should be applied while the needle is advanced and until abdominal fluid is obtained. If the initial fluid stops, the needle or catheter can be rotated or angulated. The catheter should never be withdrawn through the needle, as this may cause shearing of the cannula. Turning the patient to a lateral decubitus position may help if the patient is initially supine.

For removal of large volumes of fluid, attach a 50-ml syringe to a three-way stopcock (optional) and intravenous tubing. Once fluid is aspirated from the syringe, attach the IV tubing to the vacuum bottle, and open the stopcock to the bottle. When the procedure is completed, remove the catheter and needle as a unit in one fast, continuous motion, and apply a sterile occlusive dressing to the site. Published literature supports the use of plasma expanders (particularly albumin) to prevent circulatory dysfunction after large-volume (>5 liters) paracentesis (3).

Commercially prepared thoracentesis/paracentesis kits are another alternative. The catheters in these kits are larger than necessary for paracentesis and can cause leakage at the site after removal.

Patients with definite ascites and no prior surgery can undergo bedside paracentesis safely without radiologic localization. If the fluid level is difficult to detect, or if there are surgical scars, portable ultrasound can be used to help locate the fluid and help visualize the surrounding structures to avoid perforations.

KEY POINTS REGARDING PARACENTESIS

- In iodine-allergic patients, pHisoHex or chlorhexidine gluconate (Hibiclens) is an acceptable alternative to povidone-iodine (Betadine) solution or prepackaged sticks.
- Empty the bladder to prevent puncture of a full bladder.
- Do not insert the needle over sites of surgical scars to prevent bowel perforation resulting from possible intra-abdominal adhesions. In patients with prior surgery, consider the use of ultrasonic guidance.
- Correct clotting abnormalities to avoid serious intraperitoneal or abdominal wall hematoma.
- Avoid the rectus muscle, where the superior and inferior epigastric vessels lie.
- Avoid visible collateral venous channels on the abdominal wall.
- Insertion of the needle through the linea alba (relatively avascular midline) lessens the risk of hemorrhage.
- Persistent fluid leakage may be remedied by placing a purse-string suture around the puncture site and by instructing the patient to lie on the side opposite to the puncture site.

THORACENTESIS

Introduction

Thoracentesis is a method for removing pleural air or pleural fluid for diagnostic or therapeutic purposes. If fluid, blood, or air accumulates in the pleural space, respiration may be compromised. If the accumulation is rapid and progressive (e.g., tension pneumothorax), there may be cardiovascular compromise in addition to severe respiratory effects. The underlying etiology of an effusion will also affect the severity of symptoms.

The pleural space, which is a potential space between the visceral and parietal pleura, normally contains a thin physiologic layer of pleural fluid. With normal inspiration, negative pressure develops within the thorax and is transmitted through the pleural space to the pulmonary parenchyma, thereby allowing the influx of air. During normal expiration, the elasticity of the pulmonary parenchyma and chest wall allows exhalation.

Indications

- Diagnosis of pleural effusion
- Therapeutic removal of pleural air or fluid

Contraindications

- Insertion of a needle through an area of infection
- Bleeding diathesis or anticoagulant treatment without correction of the clotting deficits
- Ipsilateral ruptured diaphragm unless performed under ultrasound or fluoroscopic guidance

Equipment

Commercially prepared thoracentesis needle/catheter kits have most of the equipment, but if a kit not available, the following equipment can be assembled.

Skin prep

- Sterile gauze
- Povidone-iodine solution (Betadine) or prepackaged povidone-iodine sticks
- Alcohol prep pads

Sterile field

- Gloves, mask, sterile drape

Local anesthetic

- Syringe, 5-mL
- Needles, 25- and 22-gauge
- Lidocaine 1%

Thoracentesis

- 50-ml syringe with 3-way stopcock
- 14- or 16-gauge angiocatheters, or 16- or 18-gauge pigtail catheter with a guidewire
- Curved clamps, two
- Sterile connecting tubing (from stopcock to bottle)
- Specimen tubes
- Plasma vacuum bottles

Procedure

Position

Positioning of the patient depends on whether the procedure is intended to remove air or fluid. To evacuate a pneumothorax, the patient should be supine with the head of the bed elevated 30 degrees (Figure 27.27). To drain an

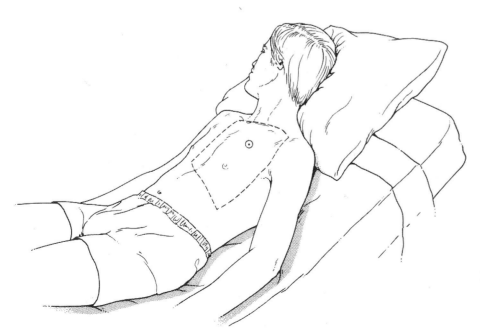

Figure 27.27 Thoracentesis. The position for air removal. (Reprinted from VanderSalm TJ, Cutler BS, Wheeler HB, eds. *Atlas of Bedside Procedures.* Boston/Toronto: Little, Brown and Company, 1988, with permission.)

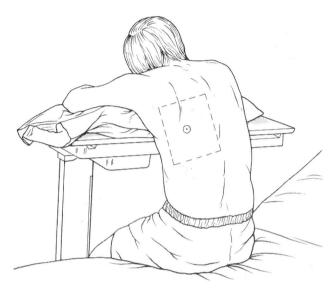

Figure 27.28 Thoracentesis. The position for fluid removal. (Reprinted from VanderSalm TJ, Cutler BS, Wheeler HB, eds. *Atlas of Bedside Procedures.* Boston/Toronto: Little, Brown and Company, 1988, with permission.)

effusion, have the patient sit up and lean forward against a table with a pillow (Figure 27.28).

Landmarks

The site for aspiration of *air* should be the second intercostal space in the midclavicular line unless adhesions are present (Figure 27.29).

The site for aspiration of *fluid* is the midscapular line or the posterior axillary line at a level below the top of the fluid (Figure 27.30). This level is appreciated clinically by the height of dullness to percussion and the decrease in tactile fremitus. Ultrasound guidance should be used, either by the treating physician, if he or she is competent, or by a radiologist, to determine the appropriate level. Radiographic localization (with ultrasound, CT, or fluoroscopy) is also appropriate for small or loculated effusions.

Technique

Prepare the equipment and obtain necessary consent according to hospital policy. Prior to the procedure, place the patient on supplemental oxygen. Hypoxemia invariably follows drainage of a pleural effusion or pneumothorax. The drop in PaO_2 ranges from 5–20 mm Hg and is prevented by oxygen supplementation.

Obtain radiographic studies as needed until you are comfortable with the diagnosis, location, and extent of pleural effusion. Have your current erect chest radiograph at the bedside. Confirm fluid level by percussion and/or by ultrasound. Use the first or second interspace below the fluid level, but not lower than the eighth intercostal space (to prevent intra-abdominal puncture).

Put on a protective mask and gloves. Prep and drape your patient using sterile technique. Infiltrate local anesthetic, and aspirate pleural air or fluid. Advance the needle over the superior edge of the rib and "walk" over

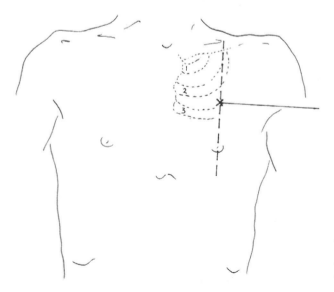

Figure 27.29 The optimal site for needle aspiration of pneumothorax: the second intercostal space at the midclavicular line. (Reprinted from O'Connor RE, Feldstein JS, Bouzoukis JK. Thoracentesis in the emergency department. *J Emerg Med* 1985;2:433–442, with permission.)

withdraw the needle (Figure 27.31). Mark the needle depth with the second clamp to prevent the needle from penetrating too deep and to minimize the possibility of perforating the visceral pleura. Small catheter drainage of pneumothorax has been described but has not gained widespread acceptance. Aspirate to obtain the fluid and confirm placement.

For removal of large volumes of fluid, use a 14-gauge intracath needle on a syringe with a stopcock to the same depth as that marked by the clamp (Figure 27.32). The catheter should never be withdrawn through the needle because shearing of the cannula may result. Once the cannula is in place, remove the clamp, and withdraw the needle stylet as the cannula is advanced. Attach a 50-mL syringe to a three-way stopcock and sterile tubing. After fluid is aspirated from the syringe, attach the tubing to the vacuum bottle, and open the stopcock to the bottle.

Patients may experience severe pleuritic chest pain, dyspnea, or palpitations if large volumes of fluid are removed too rapidly. It is recommended that no more than 1 liter be removed at a time; rarely, removal of large volumes can result in re-expansion pulmonary edema.

Commercially prepared thoracentesis kits are another alternative. Follow the same procedures as above, except use the catheter from the kit (Figure 27.33). Connect the long catheter with a 5-mL syringe and stopcock. Prepare the catheter by sliding it out and then back in to break the seal (Figure 27.34). Insert the needle to the same depth as marked by the clamp. Aspirate to confirm fluid, and advance the catheter into the pleural space. Withdraw the needle from the pleural space while leaving the catheter in the pleural space (Figure 27.35). Attach the tubing in the kit to the vacuum bottle, and remove the effusion.

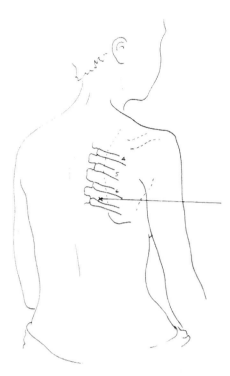

Figure 27.30 The preferred site for thoracentesis: the sixth intercostal space, just medial to the scapula. (Reprinted from O'Connor RE, Feldstein JS, Bouzoukis JK. Thoracentesis in the emergency department. *J Emerg Med* 1985;2:433–442, with permission.)

the rib. The needle is held perpendicularly to the chest and advanced through the intercostal space while the aspiration-infiltration process is continued until the pleura is entered.

Once the presence of air or fluid is confirmed, clamp the needle at the skin level to mark the depth, and then

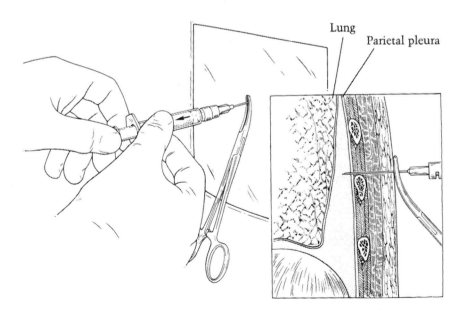

Figure 27.31 The technique of thoracentesis. Infiltration of local anesthesia, then confirming the presence of air or fluid. (Reprinted from VanderSalm TJ, Cutler BS, Wheeler HB, eds. *Atlas of Bedside Procedures.* Boston/Toronto: Little, Brown and Company, 1988, with permission.)

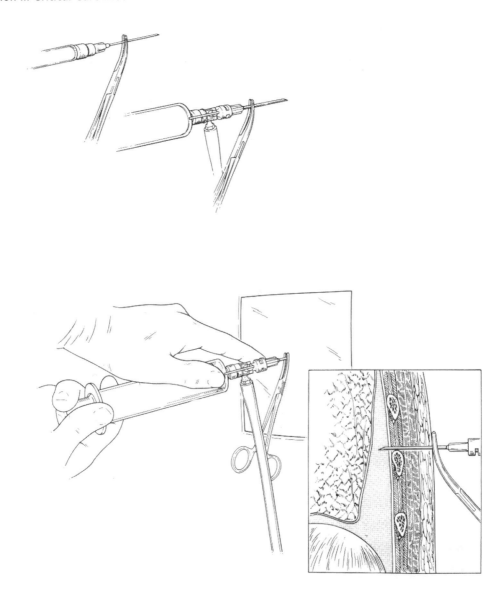

Figure 27.32 Inserting the thoracentesis needle (attached to the syringe) to the same depth as that marked by the clamp. (Reprinted from VanderSalm TJ, Cutler BS, Wheeler HB, eds. *Atlas of Bedside Procedures.* Boston/Toronto: Little, Brown and Company, 1988, with permission.)

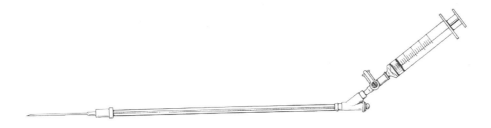

Figure 27.33 An alternative thoracentesis technique, using a catheter with a Y-sidearm. (Reprinted from VanderSalm TJ, Cutler BS, Wheeler HB, eds. *Atlas of Bedside Procedures.* Boston/Toronto: Little, Brown and Company, 1988, with permission.)

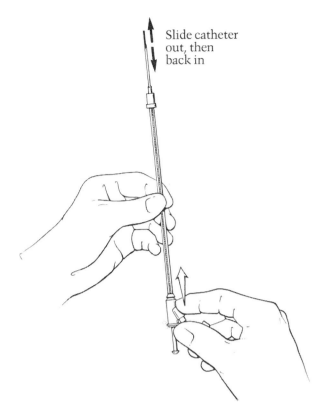

Figure 27.34   Breaking the seal between the Y and the tube. (Reprinted from VanderSalm TJ, Cutler BS, Wheeler HB, eds. *Atlas of Bedside Procedures.* Boston/Toronto: Little, Brown and Company, 1988, with permission.)

When the procedure is completed, remove the catheter and needle as a unit in one fast, continuous motion, and apply a sterile occlusive dressing to the site. Repeat a chest radiograph to ascertain the amount of fluid removed and to check for the possibility of a pneumothorax. Send specimens to the laboratory (Chapter 60).

KEY POINTS REGARDING THORACENTESIS

- In iodine-allergic patients, pHisoHex or chlorhexidine gluconate (Hibiclens) is an acceptable alternative to povidone-iodine (Betadine) solution or prepackaged sticks.
- Be extremely careful when performing thoracentesis in mechanically ventilated patients to prevent tension pneumothorax.
- Use extreme caution in patients with pleural adhesions from conditions such as previous tuberculosis, hemopneumothorax or empyema, because of the danger of piercing the closely approximated visceral pleural and lung.

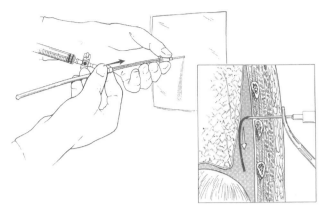

Figure 27.35   Advancing the catheter into the pleural space. (Reprinted from VanderSalm TJ, Cutler BS, Wheeler HB, eds. *Atlas of Bedside Procedures.* Boston/Toronto: Little, Brown and Company, 1988, with permission.)

- Avoid performing thoracentesis lower than the eighth intercostal space posteriorly to avoid a splenic or hepatic puncture.
- Use a short-beveled needle and/or clamp the needle to prevent excessive penetration and to avoid a pneumothorax or organ puncture.
- Insert the needle at the superior margin of the rib to avoid laceration of the intercostal vessels that lie directly under the rib.
- Correct abnormal bleeding prior to procedure.

REFERENCES

1. Feldman JP, Gould MK. Complication after insertion of a central venous catheter. *AHRQ WebM&M*, March 2004. Available at http://webmm.ahrq.gov/spotlightcases.aspx?ic=51.
2. Mansfield PF, Hohn DC, Fornage BD, Gregurich MA, Ota DM. Complications and failures of subclavian-vein catheterization. *N Engl J Med* 1994;331:1735–1738.
3. Ginès P, Cárdenas A, Arroyo V, Rodés J. Management of cirrhosis and ascites. *N Engl J Med* 2004;350:1646–1654.

ADDITIONAL READING

American College of Physicians. *Arthrocentesis and Joint Injection.* Philadelphia: American College of Physicians, 1999.
McGee DC, Gould MK. Preventing complications of central venous catheterization. *N Engl J Med* 2003;348:1123–1133.
Merrer J, De Jongehe B, Golliot F, et al. Complications of femoral and subclavian venous catheterization in critically ill patients: A randomized controlled trial. *JAMA* 2001;286:700–707.
Roberts JR, Hedges JR. *Clinical Procedures in Emergency Medicine.* 3rd Ed. Philadelphia: W.B. Saunders, 1998.
Rothschild JM. Ultrasound guidance of central vein catheterization. In Shojania KG, Duncan BW, McDonald KM, Wachter RM. Evidence Report/Technology Assessment No. 43, Making Health Care Safer: A Critical Analysis of Patient Safety Practices. AHRQ Publication No. 01-E058.
Simon RR, Brenner BE. *Emergency Procedures and Techniques.* Philadelphia: Lippincott Williams & Wilkins, 2002.
VanderSalm TJ, Cutter BS, Wheeler HB. *Atlas of Bedside Procedures.* Boston/Toronto: Little, Brown and Company, 1988.

Medical Consultation

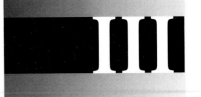

Medical Consultation

28

Geno J. Merli   Howard H. Weitz

INTRODUCTION

Over the past 30 years, the role and responsibilities of the medical consultant have changed. This evolution has resulted, in part, from the availability of consensus and evidence-based guidelines regarding patient evaluation and care as well as from increased social and financial pressures to minimize the length of hospital stay. Traditionally, preoperative assessment and postoperative follow-up of the surgical patient were the predominant roles of the medical consultant. More recently, the medical consultant's role has expanded to include the assessment and care of patients who are hospitalized with medical problems on nonmedical services such as psychiatry, rehabilitation medicine, and obstetrics and gynecology. The medical consultant must possess a broad fund of knowledge and expertise to address an ever-widening scope of responsibility. This chapter introduces fundamental issues of the art and communication of medical consultation.

ORGANIZATIONAL STRUCTURE OF MEDICAL CONSULTATION SERVICES

The structure of medical consultation services varies among institutions, and a range of organizational structures can meet the goal of providing high-quality consultative medicine. The least centralized structure allows or even encourages each generalist and specialist to perform consultations or provide medical comanagement for his or her own patients or the patients of others consistent with any traditional referral patterns at a particular hospital. This approach is analogous to the prehospitalist stage of inpatient medicine. Recently, however, the availability of hospitalists to care for medical inpatients has been transforming practice patterns in inpatient consultative medicine as well. Hospitalists are readily available and should be appropriately skilled to provide timely consul-

tation and needed inpatient follow-up. As a result, the organization of inpatient consultation may well go through stages similar to those for inpatient medical care.

Innovative medical consultation programs have expanded their scope substantially. Instead of a responsive service that provides prompt and efficient consultation on request, these newer services provide routine comanagement of the medical problems of patients hospitalized on nonmedical services [1]. For example, a system may be in place for routine medical consultation whenever a nonmedical attending physician admits a patient with a diagnosis of insulin-dependent diabetes, asthma or chronic obstructive pulmonary disease requiring bronchodilators, prior myocardial infarction, or heart failure [2]. An automatic consultation also may be triggered by the development of a number of in-hospital problems, such as transfer to an intensive care unit, a chest radiograph demonstrating pulmonary edema, a positive ventilation-perfusion scan suggesting pulmonary embolism, or positive blood cultures. In some institutions, these consultations are directed to the relevant medical specialist, but in other settings they initially may generate a consultation with a hospitalist, either because of the hospitalist's ready accessibility or because of multiorgan system disease. In addition, the hospitalist's familiarity with posthospital alternatives, such as skilled nursing facilities and home care, that help explain hospitalists' ability to reduce length of stay, may also be relevant to many nonmedical inpatients.

In the comanagement model, the medical consultant becomes responsible for the patient's nonsurgical issues, either preexisting or newly developed. Comanagement is especially useful in situations in which surgical physicians are not routinely available to deal with postoperative problems because of their heavy commitment in the operating room. Medical expertise is also especially useful for complicated medical problems on services that are less accustomed to dealing with multiorgan system disease, such as orthopedic, urologic, and ear, nose, and throat services. Comanagment is also common on services in which particular types of medical problems are prevalent; examples include cardiologic expertise in patients undergoing vascular surgery and pulmonary expertise in patients undergoing lung surgery. Substantial data indicate that medical comanagement of problems such as insulin-dependent diabetes by an experienced physician can improve the efficiency of inpatient care (2). In these models, the consultant commonly takes delegated responsibility for the medical problem, which generally includes ordering indicated diagnostic tests and therapeutic interventions.

In many institutions, medical physicians may participate in a formal system of preoperative evaluation in a preoperative testing center. Commonly, such units are staffed primarily by anesthesiologists who review the patient's potential anesthetic and surgical risks in the context of the medical history. The ready availability of a medical consultant can increase the efficiency of such units and avoid unnecessary delays in surgery.

TEN COMMANDMENTS OF MEDICAL CONSULTATION

To provide direction for the responsibilities of the medical consultant, 10 "commandments" have been proposed to elevate the art of medical consultation (3). These 10 points, which are not only practical but also appropriate in defining the role of the medical consultant, can be as relevant now as when they were first proposed more than 20 years ago (4).

Once a medical consultant receives a request for a consultation, it is his or her responsibility to complete this request in a timely fashion. If circumstances preclude completion of the consultation, the consultant must notify the requesting physician in ample time for another consultant to complete the task promptly.

The consultant should focus on the issues that the requesting physician has indicated. If the request for consultation is not clear, communication with the requesting physician or house staff is important for defining the reason for consultation.

A complete history, physical examination, assessment of pertinent laboratory tests, and review of appropriate medical records must be provided. The consultant is responsible for acquiring all relevant data that pertain to the request for consultation. This responsibility may require contacting other physicians or hospitals about previous laboratory tests, chest radiographs, cardiac-catheterization results, or electrocardiograms.

The consultant must identify and summarize all the pertinent medical problems with respect to their current status and therapeutic management. This review should be thorough enough for the consultant to be able

to assume responsibility for the patient's care should the need arise.

The management plan should be concise, and the therapeutic regimen should be clearly delineated. Requesting physicians will not read or follow long-winded plans. The consultant always should provide options or alternatives for management to give the requesting physician latitude for care should he or she not be comfortable with a particular form of therapy.

New problems or diagnoses that the consultant discovers must be brought to the attention of the requesting physician. Only if the findings are truly emergent and require immediate intervention should the consultant act on them without prior discussion with the requesting physician.

The consultant must provide appropriate documentation of his or her plan in the chart for the requesting physician. Verbal communication with the physician or house staff increases the likelihood that the therapeutic regimen or diagnostic assessment will be carried out. Comanagers not only provide the consultation but help effect the identified recommendations with the agreement of the requesting physician.

The follow-up care of patients is dictated by the medical problems identified in the initial evaluation. Issues may include the follow-up of abnormal laboratory results, the adjustment of medications, or the evaluation of specific medical problems that are important to the surgeon or postoperative care provider. When the consultant's role in the care of the patient is completed, the consultant should document the termination of care in the medical record.

The consultant must develop a rapport with the requesting physician to define the patient care responsibilities for each physician. This relationship may define the role as pure consultant or as comanager with its associated order writing, test ordering, and day-to-day care.

Requesting physicians will appreciate a consultant who provides insightful information concerning the management of their patient. This teaching function should be done with tact and without condescension.

The primary physician, the consultant, and the patient have a complex relationship. The consultant has responsibilities both to the patient and to the requesting physician. In general, the preferred way for the consultant to maximize the patient's benefit is by acting through the requesting physician. Skilled consultants can resolve any potential differences with the requesting physician and present a unified, easily understandable plan of action to the patient. Although the consultant has a responsibility to the patient to bypass the requesting physician if it is the only way to avoid harm, in practice the two physicians should privately resolve such conflicts to maximize the quality of care and avoid placing patients in a position of grappling with conflicting advice.

FORMAT

The actual documentation of a medical consultation can have many formats. One format is a written document based on the Health Care Financing Agency guideline (5) for appropriate documentation for level of service to assure compliance with established standards for all third-party insurers and a database from which to develop impressions and plans.

The consultation document consists of two pages (Figure 28.1). The front page has the impression and plan of management clearly delineated based on the reason for the consultation and the pertinent findings. The plan is specific with respect to dosing of medications, management strategies for concomitant diseases, and the ordering of additional testing. In the case of surgical patients, this assessment and plan must include cardiac risk stratification, prophylaxis of deep venous thrombosis and pulmonary embolism, and the care of concomitant medical problems.

The second page of the consultation form documents the reason for the consultation, history of the present illness, medical history, surgical history, family history, social history, review of systems, physical examination, and laboratory testing. This detailed database is primarily for the medical consultant's future reference and management planning.

Compliance with consultants' recommendations is more common if the consultant has direct contact with the requesting physician, makes a limited number of recommendations, clearly identifies high-priority recommendations, continues to see the patient after the original consultation, and offers specific recommendations regarding drug dosage, route, and duration (6).

GENERAL INDICATIONS FOR MEDICAL CONSULTATION

Trying to define the indications for a medical consultation is a difficult task. In the case of the surgical patient, the requesting physicians must assess specific diseases for specific surgical procedures. The most practical approach is to assess risk factors based on organ-specific disease and postoperative outcomes. For nonsurgical consultations, the indications are defined by the requesting physician's need for assessment or comanagement of a medical problem. For example, substantial data exist to guide recommendations for patients with cardiovascular disease who undergo noncardiac surgery (5,6), patients with pulmonary disease undergoing surgery (7), and the risk of deep vein thrombosis or pulmonary embolism in the postoperative period (8).

In the case of nonsurgical consultation requests, the requesting physician dictates indications. For example, for a psychiatric patient with anemia and elevated liver enzymes, medical consultation would be requested for evaluation and ongoing care. It is currently difficult to provide specific guidelines for this type of consultation.

INFORMAL CONSULTATION

In addition to formal consultation, informal or "curbside" consultations are a remarkably common component of the medical care system (9,10). Hospital-based physicians are likely to receive many such informal requests because of their high visibility in the hospital corridors and their expertise both with inpatient medical problems and with the interface between the hospital and posthospital care. Informal consultations or requests for targeted advice serve critical roles in medical communication and as ideal mechanisms for assessing the priority and necessity of more formal consultation. By providing useful curbside advice, consultants build trust and camaraderie. The ability to provide useful yet pithy assistance in the curbside mode portends well for a consultant's ability to provide helpful and efficient formal consultation if more detailed evaluation is appropriate. Most consultants believe that responsiveness to curbside questions often can solve a focused problem for the patient at hand and also establish the credibility and hence increase the profile (and ultimately the volume) of medical consultations. However, the consultant must be careful not to make definitive recommendations based on inadequate data. If and when more formal consultation is appropriate, the consultant should make this preference clear. If a consultant feels uncomfortable about giving advice without seeing the patient, it is recommended that the requesting physician be asked a question along the line of, "Do you mind if I see the patient myself before I make a recommendation?"

KEY POINTS

- Medical consultation can be organized in a variety of ways. Innovative services often provide comanagement as well as episodic consultations triggered by particular problems rather than being entirely dependent on requests for consultation.
- General guidelines (e.g., the 10 commandments of consultation) can improve the art and efficiency of consultation.
- The consultant has a complicated tripartite relationship with the requesting physician and the patient.
- Informal "curbside" consultations can be a useful part of the medical care system.
- Compliance with consultative recommendations increases if the consultant directly communicates a limited number of specific, high-priority suggestions guided by continued participation in the patient's ongoing care.

Consultation Request

Date of Request _____

Problem/Reason for Consultation _____

Requesting Physician _____

Consulting Physician or Department _____

Consultation Report

Impressions:

1. _____

2. _____

3. _____

Plan (example):

1. The patient is low risk for postoperative cardiac complications.
2. The patient is very high risk for DVT/PE. Recommend:
   a. Low-molecular-weight heparin (enoxaparin 30 mg SC q12 hrs) beginning 12 to 24 hrs postop for 7 to 10 days.
   b. Extended prophylaxis with either enoxaparin 40 mg SC QD or warfarin with INR goal of 2 to 3. Please refer patient to anticoagulation clinic for follow-up after discharge.
3. The patient's hypertension has been well controlled with atenolol 50 mg QD. Give 50 mg of atenolol by mouth prior to surgery then resume on postop day 1.
4. Hold glyburide the morning of surgery and then resume at 5 mg PO QD on post op day 1. Fingerstick blood sugar checks the evening of surgery and at 8:00, 16:00, 20:00 on postop day 1.

Thank you.

_____
(CONSULTING PHYSICIAN)

Consultation Report (cont.):
Reason for Consultation: <u>Perioperative medical management</u>

History of Present Illness _____

Past Medical History _____

Social History _____

Family History _____

Review of Systems _____

Physical Examination _____

Laboratory Evaluation _____

Figure 28.1 Sample consultation report.

REFERENCES

1. Macpherson DS, Parenti C, Nee J, Petzel RA, Ward H. An internist joins the surgery service: does comanagement make a difference? *J Gen Intern Med* 1994;9:440–444.
2. Levetan CS, Salas JR, Wilets IF, Zumoff B. Impact of endocrine and diabetes team consultant on hospital length of stay for patients with diabetes. *Am J Med* 1995;99:22–28.
3. Goldman L, Lee T, Rudd P. Ten commandments for effective consultation. *Arch Intern Med* 1983;143:1753–1755.
4. Merli G, Weitz H. The role and responsibility of the medical consultant. In: Merli G, Weitz H, eds. *The Medical Management of the Surgical Patient.* 2nd ed. Philadelphia: W.B. Saunders, 1998:1–6.
5. Eagle KA, Berger PB, Calkins H, et al. ACC/AHA guideline update for perioperative cardiovascular evaluation for noncardiac surgery: a report of the American College/American Heart Association Task Force on Practice Guidelines [American College of Cardiology Web site]. Available at: http://www.acc.org/clinical/guidelines/perio/update/periupdate%5Findex.htm Accessed January 14, 2005.
6. American College of Physicians. Guidelines for assessing and managing the perioperative risk from coronary artery disease associated with major noncardiac surgery. *Ann Intern Med* 1997;127:309–312.
7. Arozullah AM, Khuri SF, Henderson WG, Daley J. Development and validation of a multifactorial risk index for predicting postoperative pneumonia after major noncardiac surgery. *Ann Intern Med* 2001;135:847–857.
8. Geerts W, Heit J, Clagett G, et al. Prevention of venous thromboembolism. *Chest* 2001;119:132S–175S.
9. Keating NL, Zaslavsky AM, Ayanian JZ. Physicians' experiences and beliefs regarding informal consultation. *JAMA* 1998;280:900–904.
10. Kuo D, Gifford DR, Stein MD. Curbside consultation practices and attitudes among primary care physicians and medical subspecialists. *JAMA* 1998;280:905–909.

ADDITIONAL READING

Emanuel LL. The consultant and the patient-physician relationship. A trilateral deliberative model. *Arch Intern Med* 1994;154:1785–1790.

Gross R, Caputo G. *Medical Consultation: The Internist on Surgical, Obstetrics, and Psychiatric Services.* 3rd ed. Philadelphia: Williams and Wilkins, 1998.

Huddleston JM, Long KH, Naessens JM, et al. Medical and surgical comanagement after elective hip and knee arthroplasty: a randomized controlled trial. *Ann Intern Med* 2004;14:28–38.

Lubin M, Walker H, Smith R. *Medical Management of the Surgical Patient.* 4th ed. Philadelphia: Lippincott Williams & Wilkins, 2005.

Merli G, Weitz H. *Medical Management of the Surgical Patient.* 3rd ed. Philadelphia: W.B. Saunders, 2005.

Key Principles of Anesthesiology

29

Neal Cohen

INTRODUCTION

The care of the surgical patient has changed significantly over the past 10 years. Advances in anesthesia and surgical practices have reduced the morbidity and mortality rates of surgery. At the same time, a better understanding of the influence of a patient's underlying clinical condition on that patient's surgery has enabled the anesthesiologist to address more effectively the needs of both the patient and the surgeon. The goals for anesthetic management include the following:

- Assessment of the patient's preoperative clinical status
- Preoperative management to address preexisting clinical problems relevant to perioperative care and to optimize the patient's condition prior to surgery
- Development and implementation of a plan for anesthetic management that provides optimal surgical conditions and minimizes physiologic alterations
- Definition of a postoperative management strategy that will ensure the safe transition from the operating room, reduce postoperative pain, minimize the likelihood of complications, and shorten the length of stay

Because of advances in surgical care and anesthetic management options, sicker patients are able to undergo more complex procedures safely—with less pain, shorter recovery periods, and reduced need for inpatient care. Moreover, because of cost pressures, today's patients are rarely admitted to the hospital before surgery, no matter how complex the proposed procedure. In addition, many patients now receive anesthesia, either general or regional, for procedures performed in settings other than the operating room, including endoscopy suites, radiology departments, and physicians' offices. As a result of all these changes in practice, the anes-

thesiologist, primary care provider, and hospital physician must work more closely together than ever before to ensure a thorough preoperative assessment, identify and optimize the management of underlying conditions, and develop a plan of care for intraoperative and postoperative management. Each must have an understanding of the patient's clinical condition and enough knowledge about the surgical procedure and approach to anesthetic management to be able to coordinate care in the perioperative period and beyond.

This discussion reviews some of the most important aspects of the preoperative assessment, defines how decisions are made regarding intraoperative anesthetic management, and describes the major concerns in the early postoperative period.

PREOPERATIVE ASSESSMENT

Improved anesthetic techniques, the expansion of minimally invasive (laparoscopic) surgical procedures, and, perhaps most importantly, a better understanding of the impact of underlying diseases on anesthetic and surgical management have allowed more patients to undergo major surgical procedures more safely than ever before. As a result, the morbidity and mortality associated with anesthesia and surgery are now lower than ever. For many patients with severe chronic illness (i.e., diabetes, coronary artery disease, renal failure), the major risk of complications occurs not while the patient is in the operating room, but a number of days after the procedure. Accordingly, the anesthesiologist, surgeon, and hospitalist must share responsibility for understanding the risks, tailoring perioperative management to minimize them, and developing a strategy that addresses both immediate and longer-term needs.

The initial strategy must include a comprehensive and thoughtful assessment of the patient's underlying physiology and risk, including issues that influence the decision to proceed with surgery or that will alter perioperative care. The first step, therefore, is the preoperative assessment, which should include a number of critical components. First, the potential risks associated with the anesthetic management must be carefully assessed. The American Society of Anesthesiologists (ASA) has developed a physical status classification system that has proved to be a valuable tool for risk stratification (Table 29.1). Although it is not a system that specifically defines anesthetic risk, it has provided a consistent method for evaluating outcome and has been useful in comparing patient populations to modify management strategies based on underlying physiology.

The ASA classification is useful, but it provides only an overview of risk, essentially offering a general assessment that can be used to guide management. Therefore, it must be accompanied by a more specific assessment of the patient's underlying clinical condition and potential risk factors. A thorough history and physical examination continue to be essential components of clinical assessment, although the evaluation is often completed by the primary care provider or anesthesiologist days or weeks prior to surgery. As a result, the evaluation of the patient on the day of surgery can be abbreviated but must include specific assessments that might influence the approach taken in the operating room and thereafter.

For the anesthesiologist, the assessment of the airway is one of the critical components of the preoperative evaluation. For some patients, potential airway problems are apparent based on their history or physical findings. Patients with *obstructive or central sleep apnea* pose significant risks, not only because the airway may be difficult to maintain, but also because of the associated clinical problems, including hypoxemia, hypoventilation, and pulmonary hypertension. In addition, preexisting sleep apnea man-

TABLE 29.1

THE ASA CLASSIFICATION SYSTEM

ASA 1	A normal, healthy patient
ASA 2	A patient with mild systemic disease (e.g., mild diabetes mellitus without complications, controlled hypertension, anemia, chronic bronchitis, morbid obesity without other sequelae)
ASA 3	A patient with severe systemic disease that limits activity (e.g., angina pectoris, obstructive pulmonary disease, prior myocardial infarction)
ASA 4	A patient with an incapacitating disease that is a constant threat to life (e.g., congestive heart failure, renal failure)
ASA 5	A moribund patient not expected to survive longer than 24 hours (e.g., ruptured aortic aneurysm, head trauma with increased intracranial pressure)

TABLE 29.2

THE MALLAMPATI AIRWAY CLASSIFICATION SYSTEM

Class I:	Uvula, faucial pillars, and soft palate are visible
Class II:	Faucial pillars and soft palate are visible
Class III:	Only soft palate is visible
Class IV:	Only the base of the tongue is visible

dates that the anesthesiologist have a plan for ensuring that the patient has the support necessary in the postoperative period to prevent airway obstruction or severe hypoxemia, whether that includes postoperative care in an ICU or requires availability of continuous positive airway pressure (CPAP) or other technologies postoperatively.

Careful assessment of the airway is also essential for every other patient because for most patients, the manifestation of airway problems becomes apparent only after the patient loses normal airway tone and reflexes when fully anesthetized and paralyzed. Nothing is more frightening to the anesthesiologist than to take a perfectly healthy patient to the operating room and have the patient develop serious complications associated with the airway after induction and prior to tracheal intubation.

To minimize the likelihood of airway management problems and to facilitate planning, a number of evaluative methods are used. First, a routine clinical evaluation of the airway is performed. It includes assessment of mouth and jaw mobility, neck mobility, and vocal cord function. In addition, anesthesiologists frequently assess the airway using the technique described by Mallampati (Table 29.2) (1). The classification describes the degree to which, with routine mouth opening, airway structures are visualized.

This classification system, although not perfectly sensitive nor specific, helps alert the anesthesiologist to potential problems during laryngoscopy and tracheal intubation. In doing so, it allows the anesthesiologist to develop contingency plans and consider alternative approaches to the airway, including the use of a laryngeal mask airway, a fiberoptic approach to intubation, or other options. The assessment that airway management may be difficult does not suggest that general anesthesia should be avoided or that regional or local anesthesia should necessarily be considered. In some cases, if airway management is determined to be difficult, elective tracheal intubation becomes even *more* important so that the airway is secured before a problem arises—as can occur even with regional anesthesia (e.g., total spinal anesthesia). For patients known to have a difficult airway or in those situations when tracheal intubation is not straightforward, the ASA has developed a useful algorithm for management of the difficult airway (2).

In addition to airway evaluation, several other critical issues must be clarified before inducing anesthesia. Fluid status and intravascular volume must be optimized prior to induction of anesthesia to minimize the risk of hemodynamic compromise upon administration of anesthetic agents or analgesics or initiation of positive pressure ventilation. The correct evaluation includes assessment of skin turgor, peripheral perfusion, filling pressures, and, indirectly, myocardial function. This assessment is particularly important in patients with congestive heart failure, whether they are receiving diuretics or not, in patients who have had no oral intake for a number of hours prior to induction of anesthesia, in patients who have undergone a bowel prep prior to surgery, and in patients who received intravenous contrast for radiologic studies, particularly because of their risk of renal dysfunction.

Perhaps as important as the usual preoperative evaluation of any patient, additional assessment and often interventions prior to induction of anesthesia are required for patients with underlying conditions. Systemic diseases that compromise cardiac, pulmonary, renal, or hepatic function are of particular concern. Even when the prior medical management has optimized the patient's condition, the anesthesiologist must understand what has been done to improve the patient and how the intraoperative management can maintain that level of support. For example, the patient with severe obstructive pulmonary disease who is receiving bronchodilators and/or steroids may be well controlled preoperatively. The anesthesiologist must understand how acute exacerbations are managed, which drugs most effectively treat the small airway obstruction, and the associated clinical conditions that might influence anesthetic management, such as pulmonary hypertension or hypoxemia associated with gas trapping (Chapters 55 and 59). The same process must be used to assess how best to treat patients with coronary artery disease in the perioperative period, which patients should receive perioperative β-blockers (3), α-blocking agents, or vasodilators, and which patients might benefit from a preoperative coronary angiogram, coronary dilation, or stent (Chapter 30).

For many patients, the management of the underlying disease may not be optimal at the time of presentation for anesthesia and surgery—in some cases because the patient's condition cannot be optimized. One question that is frequently asked of the hospital physician and the anesthesiologist is whether surgery should be postponed and, if so, how the patient's condition can be improved. Although for many of these patients, the intraoperative management may be relatively uncomplicated, the postoperative course will be unstable. For example, the inadequately treated hypertensive patient will have more unstable blood pressure and increased risk of complications in the postoperative period if the blood pressure is not controlled preoperatively. The patient with severe obstructive pulmonary disease may have a complicated perioperative course due to persistent bronchospastic disease in spite of preoperative

treatment because of impaired mucociliary clearance associated with tracheal intubation. As a result, a discussion about the risks and benefits of delaying surgery versus proceeding without better control of underlying medical problems should include the anesthesiologist, primary care provider, and surgeon (Chapter 30).

One of the most difficult clinical problems for which the risk of anesthesia, surgery, and postoperative complications is high is diabetes mellitus. In addition to the problems associated with glucose control, diabetic patients often have a number of complications of their diabetes, including coronary artery disease and renal failure. Each complication makes anesthetic management more challenging. As part of the preoperative evaluation, a thorough assessment for evidence of complications of diabetes is essential so that the patient's physiologic condition can be optimized preoperatively and to provide the information necessary to manage the patient in the perioperative period.

Data now support tight inpatient glucose control to minimize complications of the disease and improve surgical outcomes (4). As a result, the use of insulin infusions preoperatively, intraoperatively, and postoperatively is encouraged (Chapter 107). A glucose-containing intravenous fluid should be started preoperatively at the same time the insulin infusion is started, generally beginning once the patient is not taking anything orally. The infusion will ensure that insulin is administered continuously and that the absorption of the insulin is not compromised by subcutaneous edema or impaired peripheral perfusion. Once the patient begins to take a normal diet, the infusion can be replaced by subcutaneous insulin as needed.

In the operating room, until recently, concerns about hypoglycemia were at least as great as concerns about hyperglycemia. All the usual clinical signs of hypoglycemia are lost in the anesthetized patient, so anesthesiologists were careful not to be too aggressive about glucose control intraoperatively. Recent studies have demonstrated that more rigid control of the blood sugar not only reduces the acute complications of hyperglycemia (including osmotic diuresis that will complicate intraoperative fluid assessment and management), but also improves wound healing. Bedside glucose monitoring devices have made tighter control more feasible.

Many clinicians consider age an independent risk factor for perioperative complications. While elderly patients often have associated clinical problems that affect management and outcome, age alone should not determine whether to proceed with anesthesia and surgery. With improved anesthetic and surgical management, age is no longer an independent predictor of complications for most surgical procedures. In fact, chronologic age is much less important than physiologic abnormalities in predicting outcome after surgery. For the elderly patient, as is true for every other patient, the anesthesiologist and primary care provider or hospitalist must carefully assess the patient to determine what diseases might influence clinical management and optimize them as much as possible. The evaluation must also address assessment of underlying organ function, which may not be apparent based on laboratory data alone. For example, in the elderly patient with little muscle mass, a "normal" or slightly elevated serum creatinine might actually represent a significantly reduced creatinine clearance. In addition, it is important to remember that elderly patients have less physiologic reserve and are more likely to have prolonged hospital stays should complications occur. These patients also tolerate sedatives and analgesics poorly, often becoming disoriented and agitated, which further complicates their management (Chapter 16).

INTRAOPERATIVE MANAGEMENT

The anesthetic plan is based in large part on the patient's underlying clinical condition, although surgical considerations also influence the management alternatives. In addition to addressing maintainance of physiologic control over the patient during the procedure, the plan must address the surgical requirements because one of the goals of good anesthetic management is to create conditions that allow the surgeon to complete the procedure safely and efficiently and to transition the patient from the operating room environment to the postanesthesia care unit (PACU).

Both general and regional anesthesia are reasonable alternatives for most surgical procedures. Some selected cases require one or another anesthetic approach based on specific requirements of either the patient or the surgeon. For example, in brain mapping, as might be required for seizure control, the anesthetic management must ensure that the patient is anesthetized during a portion of the procedure but arousable at the appropriate time. For some cases, a combination of techniques is used to provide optimal surgical conditions, guarantee a secure airway and optimal gas exchange, and reduce the total amount of general anesthesia. Regional anesthesia and analgesia (e.g., epidural analgesics) are often added to general anesthesia to reduce the total amount of systemic opiates as well as to facilitate a smooth transition from surgery to the postoperative period and to provide adequate pain control.

Regional anesthesia is contraindicated in some situations. For patients with neurologic disease, spinal or epidural anesthesia is usually avoided. Although neither are likely to worsen the neurologic deficit, any change in the neurologic disease will be difficult to evaluate, and the effects of the instillation of anesthetic agents into the cerebrospinal fluid or epidural space can be difficult to determine. A more common contraindication to regional anesthesia is systemic anticoagulation. *Regional anesthesia should not be administered to any patient who is receiving heparin or coumadin.* The use of low-molecular-weight heparin contraindicates regional anesthesia even after the drug has been discontinued because the duration of anticoagulation is difficult to monitor (unlike with unfractionated heparin, where a normalization of the partial thromboplastin time indicates the absence of anticoagulant effect).

Anesthetic management has changed significantly over the past decade, in large part due to a broader array of agents, a better understanding of the benefits and physiologic costs associated with them, and, most importantly, a recognition that intraoperative care is only a part of the overall clinical management. Much more attention is now paid to the entire perioperative period, allowing for smoother and safer transition from the operating room to the postoperative period.

Anesthetic induction is usually performed with *intravenous agents* because of their rapidity of onset and ease of administration. Thiopental and propofol are most commonly used. Each produces rapid unconsciousness; for short procedures, propofol is preferred because patients awaken rapidly with little residual effect. For longer cases, the choice of induction agent is less important. Etomidate and ketamine are occasionally used, particularly for patients with unstable blood pressure, because both generally cause less change in hemodynamics.

A variety of *inhalation anesthetic agents* is available. The most commonly used are sevoflurane and desflurane. Both of these agents are well tolerated and have few side effects. Although all inhaled agents affect the cardiovascular system and can alter vascular tone, when used alone or in combination with other agents they can be administered safely with few sequelae and rapid emergence from anesthesia with less nausea, vomiting, or other side effects.

Many patients now receive a combination of agents to provide anesthesia and analgesia, including inhalational anesthetics, intravenous anesthetics, and regional anesthetics and analgesics. The combination of drugs and techniques enables the anesthesiologist to provide effective analgesia, anesthesia, and amnesia to the patient without compromising hemodynamics or gas exchange. The addition of systemic opiates, such as fentanyl, remifentanil, continuous infusions of propofol, and titration of inhaled anesthetics and nitrous oxide, can provide ideal clinical conditions and facilitate the transition from the operating room to the postanesthesia care unit.

Muscle relaxants are also commonly administered intraoperatively, both to facilitate tracheal intubation and to provide optimal conditions for the surgeon. The selection of the muscle relaxant depends on the patient's underlying clinical status and the intraoperative needs. Succinylcholine has historically been used for tracheal intubation. It has a rapid onset and short duration for most patients. It is the only commonly used depolarizing muscle relaxant; it causes fasciculations and raises the serum potassium transiently. It is also associated with malignant hyperthermia.

For the hyperkalemic patient or the patient with severe metabolic acidosis, succinylcholine is usually replaced by a nondepolarizing muscle relaxant. The newer nondepolarizing agents are now most commonly used because the complications associated with their administration are minimal and they have a relatively rapid onset (although not as fast as succinylcholine) and a longer duration of action. The pharmacodynamics of each drug varies; some are cleared primarily by the kidney and should, if possible, be avoided in patients with renal failure. Others are eliminated by a process independent of renal or hepatic clearance.

The choice of the muscle relaxant is not as important as understanding the ramifications of the choice. For some patients, the duration of action can be prolonged and the need for continued ventilatory support critical. All the relaxants have a prolonged duration of action in the acidemic patient (particularly the patient with respiratory acidosis) and the hypothermic patient; many agents have prolonged action in patients with impaired renal function. As a result, every patient who has received a muscle relaxant must be carefully monitored until the effects of the drug on respiratory muscles and upper airway muscles are gone.

Maintenance of *oxygenation* is an essential part of anesthetic management. Although pulse oximetry has improved the ability to monitor oxygenation and minimize the frequency and duration of hypoxemic episodes, adequate oxygen saturation does not ensure adequate ventilation or, more importantly, adequate oxygen delivery. For example, a patient who is anemic or hypovolemic or who has a low cardiac output has impaired delivery of oxygen to peripheral tissues despite a "normal" saturation. To assure adequate delivery, therefore, the anesthesiologist must ensure that intravascular volume is adequate and that oxygen-carrying capacity is ensured by maintaining an adequate hemoglobin and optimizing cardiac output (5). Euvolemic anemia is relatively well tolerated in the patient with good cardiac function; hypovolemic anemia is not.

The amount of *fluids* administered to patients in the operating room can sometimes seem excessive to the nonanesthesiologist. Fluid resuscitation requires an understanding of the preoperative fluid status and must include replacement of the deficit for the patient who has taken nothing by mouth, who may have had limited intake prior to surgery, or who has had excessive extravascular fluid losses (6,7). The administration of bowel preps and fluid extravasation into the bowel, subcutaneous tissues, or other body cavities make assessment of deficit difficult. For some patients, central venous pressure monitoring, assessment of systolic pressure variations with positive pressure ventilation, or other methods may be required to evaluate the intravascular volume. For patients with poor myocardial function, transesophageal echocardiography has become a commonly used and valuable tool for evaluating fluid status, ventricular filling, and myocardial function during surgery (Chapter 36).

In addition to the challenge of evaluating preoperative fluid losses, intraoperative losses are often underestimated. Blood loss is difficult to quantify. Serial hemoglobin and hematocrit levels can provide some guidance as to the adequacy of fluid and blood replacement, although these values may not represent the true blood loss during acute hemorrhage associated with significant fluid shifts. Dilution caused by excessive crystalloid replacement can also affect the accuracy of the hematocrit as a guide to blood requirements. Other sources of fluid loss must also be accounted for and those fluids replaced. Insensible losses can be high in the operating room, particularly when large surfaces are exposed (such as during open exploratory laparotomy). Manipulation of tissues also causes fluid extravasation and necessitates additional fluid administration. It is not unusual for a patient who is undergoing a straightforward but lengthy surgical procedure to require 5–10 liters of fluid in addition to blood products. Such quantities are not necessarily excessive, but their administration requires careful assessment of intravascular volume, urine output, myocardial function, and gas exchange.

Another aspect of intraoperative management that is often underappreciated is the importance of maintaining normal *body temperature*. Patients can lose a great deal of heat when exposed to the cold operating room environment. A number of studies have now confirmed that normothermia is beneficial for several reasons (8). First, normothermia has been demonstrated to reduce the risk of myocardial ischemia. It also appears to improve wound healing and facilitate recovery. Shivering associated with hypothermia is poorly tolerated, not only because it is uncomfortable for the patient, but also because it increases myocardial oxygen consumption. Warming blankets, heated inspired gases, and, for long cases, warming of fluids and blood products will ensure that the patient maintains a normal temperature.

POSTOPERATIVE CARE

The primary goal of the acute recovery period is to manage the transition from surgery with minimal complications. In the first few minutes to hours after surgery, the goals are straightforward. The patient is closely monitored until the effects of the anesthetic, muscle relaxants, and other drugs are no longer present. The patient should be able to maintain a clear airway, have a good cough and gag, and be awake and alert. Hemodynamics are closely monitored to be sure that fluid resuscitation has been adequate, that cardiac function is maintained, and that urine output is satisfactory. In the early postoperative period, the urine output should be at least 0.5 mL/kg/hour. Over the subsequent few days, the urine output should increase as the patient begins to mobilize fluids.

Pain control is also a critical component of postoperative management (9,10). The goal is to provide optimal pain control without compromising the patient's neurologic status, airway protection, or respiratory function. Titration of analgesics is not as straightforward as it might seem. While the patient is being aroused, pain may become a problem, and the patient may legitimately require additional analgesics. However, as soon as the patient is no longer stimulated, the same analgesics may contribute to respiratory failure, carbon dioxide retention, or hemodynamic compromise. The patient who has required large amounts of analgesics or sedatives in the early postoperative period must be carefully monitored to prevent respiratory deterioration and potential arrest, both in the PACU and after transfer to the hospital ward. Pulse oximetry is often used as the monitor of choice in these situations. *Although the pulse oximeter may provide information about oxygen saturation, it is not a monitor of ventilation.* For a patient who is receiving supplemental oxygen, oxygen saturation may be maintained in spite of dramatic increases in the partial carbon dioxide pressure. These patients require ongoing assessment of the respiratory rate and tidal volume as well as regular stimulation. Occasionally, capnography is required to document air movement and adequacy of ventilation because the obstructed patient will have chest wall movement for a short time even when there is no gas exchange—often misleading the clinician regarding airway patency.

A trend has emerged toward providing the patient with greater control over pain management in the postoperative period. The advantages of patient-controlled analgesia include better pain control, fewer analgesics, and improved patient satisfaction (11). Although patient-controlled analgesia administered through an intravenous line is now commonplace, alternative patient-controlled systems are also finding favor with patients and practitioners. For example, patient-controlled epidural analgesia and anesthesia have been found to be highly effective, and patient-controlled continuous infusions of anesthetic agents into catheters located near the brachial plexus and other locations are also being used with some success (12,13). These techniques have advantages, but they do not reduce the need for careful monitoring of the adequacy of the pain relief, appropriate placement of the catheters, and potential complications and side effects (Chapter 18).

Postoperative *nausea and vomiting* also require attention in the PACU. Although many newer anesthetic agents cause less nausea, problems remain. Nausea may occur more commonly in patients undergoing laparoscopic procedures. The incidence of postoperative nausea and vomiting is also higher in patients with preoperative hypovolemia and orthostatic dysfunction. Several agents are effective in treating nausea and vomiting, including droperidol, ondansetron, and dolasetron (14). Other therapies, including adequate fluid resuscitation in the operating room and use of dexamethasone, have been demonstrated to reduce the likelihood and duration of postoperative nausea (15).

CONCLUSIONS

The care of the patient undergoing surgery and anesthesia has improved significantly, allowing surgeons to perform procedures previously unavailable to many patients. The risks of anesthesia and surgery have also decreased. Patients with significant underlying disease are now able to undergo complex procedures with few complications. These advances are the result of improved technology and also (and probably more importantly) a better understanding of the risks and of ways to reduce them. At the same time, changes in the delivery of care are forcing physicians to reevaluate how they provide care, to whom, and where. To continue to provide these services to an aging and, in some cases, sicker patient population, anesthesiologists, surgeons, hospitalists, and other providers must coordinate their efforts to optimize the patient's preoperative status, tailor the intraoperative management to address these issues, and provide postoperative care based on an understanding of the likely risks and complications of the surgical procedure and their impact on the patient's underlying condition. This coordinated effort will allow physicians to minimize the complications of surgery and anesthesia for patients prior to, during, and after hospital discharge.

REFERENCES

1. Mallampati SR, Gatt SP, Gugino LD, et al. A clinical sign to predict difficult tracheal intubation: a prospective study. *Can J Anaesth* 1985;32:429–434.
2. Practice guidelines for management of the difficult airway. A report by the American Society of Anesthesiologists Task Force on Management of the Difficult Airway. *Anesthesiology* 1993;78:597–602.
3. Auerbach AD, Goldman L. Beta-blockers and reduction of cardiac events in noncardiac surgery: clinical applications. *JAMA* 2002;287:1445–1447.
4. Lazar HL, Chipkin SR, Fitzgerald CA, Bao Y, Cabral H, Apstein CS. Tight glycemic control in diabetic coronary artery bypass graft patients improves perioperative outcomes and decreases recurrent ischemic events. *Circulation* 2004;109:1497–1502.
5. Lobo SM, Salgado PF, Castillo VG, et al. Effects of maximizing oxygen delivery on morbidity and mortality in high-risk surgical patients. *Crit Care Med* 2000;28:3396–3404.
6. Rosenthal M. Intraoperative fluid management—what and how much? *Chest* 1999;115:106S.
7. Sibbald WJ, ed. *Fluid Management in the Acutely Ill: An Evidence-Based Educational Program.* Ontario, Canada: Core Health Services, 2001.
8. Frank SM, Fleisher LA, Breslow MJ, et al. Perioperative maintenance of normothermia reduces the incidence of morbid cardiac events: a randomized clinical trial. *JAMA* 1997;277:1127–1134.
9. Practice guidelines for acute pain management in the perioperative setting. A report by the American Society of Anesthesiologists Task Force on Pain Management, acute pain section. *Anesthesiology* 1995;82:1071–1081.
10. Ready LB. Acute perioperative pain. In: Miller RD, ed. *Anesthesia.* Philadelphia: Churchill Livingstone 2004;2323–2350.
11. Liu SS, Allen HW, Olsson GL. Patient-controlled epidural analgesia with bupivacaine and fentanyl on hospital wards: prospective experience with 1,030 surgical patients. *Anesthesiology* 1998;88:688–695.
12. Rawal N, Allvin R, Axelsson K, et al. Patient-controlled regional

analgesia (PCRA) at home: controlled comparison between bupivacaine and ropivacaine brachial plexus analgesia. *Anesthesiology* 2002;96:1290–1296.

13. Wheatley RG, Schug SA, Watson D. Safety and efficacy of postoperative epidural analgesia. *Br J Anaesth* 2001;87:47–61.

14. Domino KB, Anderson EA, Polissar NL, Posner KL. Comparative efficacy and safety of ondanstetron, droperidol, and metoclopramide for preventing postoperative nausea and vomiting: a meta-analysis. *Anesth Analg* 1999;88:1370–1379.

15. Coloma M, White PF, Markowitz SD, et al. Dexamethasone in combination with dolasetron for prophylaxis in the ambulatory setting: effect on outcome after laparoscopic cholecystectomy. *Anesthesiology* 2002;96:1346–1350.

ADDITIONAL READING

Kehlet H, Holte K. Effect of postoperative analgesia on surgical outcome. *Br J Anaesth* 2001;87:62–72.

Maurer WG, Borkowski RG, Parker BM. Quality and resource utilization in managing preoperative evaluation. *Anesthesiol Clin North America* 2004;22:155–175.

Rodgers A, Walker N, Schug S, et al. Reduction of postoperative mortality and morbidity with epidural or spinal anaesthesia: results from overview of randomised trials. *BMJ* 2000;321:1493.

Preoperative Evaluation

Joshua S. Adler

30

INTRODUCTION

Each year in the United States, millions of patients undergo surgical procedures using general, spinal, or epidural anesthesia. Most of these surgical procedures are completed without complications. Some 3%–10%, however, are associated with perioperative morbidity. Most perioperative morbidity and death occurs during the postoperative period and is of cardiac, pulmonary, neurologic, or infectious origin. Perioperative complications occur more frequently in older patients and in those with serious medical illnesses, particularly cardiovascular disease. The purpose of the preoperative evaluation is to assess perioperative risk and to guide interventions to reduce risk. The preoperative consultant must define clearly the patient's medical conditions, evaluate the stability and severity of each condition, determine the need for preoperative testing, and recommend therapy that may reduce the risk of complications. Close communication with the surgeon, anesthesiologist, and primary care physician is crucial to ensure that appropriate care is provided.

PREOPERATIVE EVALUATION IN THE INPATIENT SETTING

Over the past 10 years, surgeons have performed an increasing number of surgical procedures in the ambulatory setting. Furthermore, for many elective major surgical procedures, patients are admitted to the hospital on the morning of surgery. These patients generally are not seen by the inpatient preoperative consultant. Most patients seen by the inpatient preoperative consultant fall into one of three categories: patients undergoing urgent or emergent surgery, trauma victims, and patients with severe underlying medical illnesses who are undergoing major surgery. Compared with the ambulatory setting, the inpatient preoperative evaluation often must be done rapidly, and the urgency of the surgical condition may limit the consultant's ability to obtain desired diagnostic tests. Furthermore, any decision to delay surgery for further testing or to provide preoperative therapy must be weighed carefully against the potential risk of such delays. It is important for the preoperative consultant to understand the surgical procedures being considered as well as the common physiologic effects of anesthesia to facilitate discussions with the anesthesiologist and the surgical team, particularly if the surgical risk and the risk of delaying surgery are substantial. The inpatient preoperative consultant's most important role is to identify the most serious medical problems, provide an overall risk assessment, and recommend preoperative therapy to optimize organ function with little or no delay in surgical treatment.

The cornerstone of the preoperative evaluation is a history and physical examination. Emphasis is on assessing functional status, exercise tolerance, and cardiopulmonary signs and symptoms. In addition, the preoperative consultant must pay particular attention to any suggestion of previously unrecognized illness, particularly cardiac or pulmonary disease. Routine testing of patients whose history and physical examination do not reveal significant medical problems generally should include a 12-lead electrocardiogram in men over 40 years of age and women over 50 years of age to search for evidence of asymptomatic coronary artery disease. In multiple studies of patients undergoing major noncardiac surgery, the presence of minor abnormalities on the preoperative ECG, including axis deviation, ST segment changes, T-wave changes, and atrial or ventricular contractions are of prognostic importance only to the extent to which they are markers of the severity of underlying myocardial ischemia or heart failure; they are not independently associated with an increased risk of perioperative cardiac complications. Therefore, these findings do not, by themselves, justify detailed preoperative cardiac evaluation or perioperative interventions. Using routine laboratory tests and chest radiography in healthy patients has not been shown to add to the history and physical examination and is not recommended. Laboratory testing and chest radiography should be considered if a specific abnormality is suspected from the history or physical examination.

TYPE OF SURGERY

The perioperative risk for a patient undergoing a particular procedure depends on the characteristics of both the patient and the procedure. Using the technique of probabilistic decision making (Chapters 6 and 7), the risk assessment begins with a baseline risk that is modified by information obtained during the preoperative evaluation. The baseline risk for any patient is the average risk for a particular procedure at a particular institution. Although complication rates vary from institution to institution, certain generalizations can be made regarding the baseline risk of major cardiac complications (Table 30.1). The risk of other major complications likely follows a similar pattern. Note that procedures performed emergently are associated with more complications than those performed electively.

PREOPERATIVE MEDICATIONS

Most long-term medications should be continued during the perioperative period. This approach is particularly important for cardiac, pulmonary, and anticonvulsant medications. In

---

TABLE 30.1

RISK OF MYOCARDIAL INFARCTION OR CARDIAC DEATH FOR NONCARDIAC PROCEDURES

High risk (often >5%)

Aortic surgery and other major vascular surgery
Peripheral vascular surgery
Emergent major operations, particularly in the elderly
Anticipated prolonged surgical procedures associated with large
   fluid shifts or blood loss

Intermediate risk (1%–5%)

Intrathoracic and intraperitoneal surgery
Carotid endarterectomy
Head and neck surgery
Orthopedic surgery
Prostate surgery

Low risk (generally <1%)

Endoscopic procedures
Cataract surgery
Superficial procedures and biopsies
Breast surgery

Adapted with permission from ACC/AHA Guideline update for perioperative cardiovascular evaluation for noncardiac surgery—executive summary. *Anesth Analg* 2002;94:1052.

---

most situations, such medications can be administered up to and including the morning of surgery and then resumed postoperatively once the patient is eating. One important exception is *monoamine oxidase inhibitors,* which have been associated with intraoperative hemodynamic instability. Ideally, they should be discontinued at least two weeks prior to surgery. It is also generally recommended that metformin be discontinued prior to noncardiac surgery to reduce the risk of lactic acidosis. Metformin may be restarted once the patient is considered stable postoperatively.

CARDIAC EVALUATION

The cardiac complications of noncardiac surgery are the most well-studied area of perioperative risk assessment. The most important cardiac complications include nonfatal myocardial infarction, heart failure, and cardiac death. The principal predictors of cardiac complications are *advanced age,* the *presence and severity of coronary artery disease,* and *left-ventricular dysfunction.*

Multifactorial risk indices sum weights of a variety of cardiac and noncardiac conditions to predict an overall risk of cardiac complications after noncardiac surgery. The Revised Cardiac Risk Index was developed during the modern surgical era (1), has been validated on independent sets of patients, and represents the most useful of these tools currently available (Table 30.2). Preoperative consultants should use an index score to modify a baseline risk rather than as an absolute risk of cardiac complications. A low index score denotes a lower-than-baseline risk, a high score indicates a higher-than-baseline risk, and an intermediate score usually indicates an unchanged risk. This index is particularly useful if a preoperative evaluation must be done rapidly. Most of the data needed to use the index are available from a brief history and physical examination and basic laboratory studies. One important caution is that in patients at high risk for severe asymptomatic coronary-artery disease, this index may underestimate risk. This issue is particularly important in patients undergoing vascular surgery, where noncardiac functional limitations often prevent the occurrence of cardiac symptoms. In such patients, multifactorial indices are more useful if combined with a disease-specific assessment of cardiac risks.

CORONARY ARTERY DISEASE

Coronary artery disease accounts for the majority of severe perioperative cardiac complications, including myocardial infarction, unstable angina, and cardiac death. The magnitude of the increased risk associated with coronary artery disease depends on the severity and stability of ischemic symptoms. Patients with an unstable coronary syndrome (Table 30.3; see also Chapter 37) are at particularly high risk. In patients with stable anginal symptoms, consultants can estimate the perioperative risk by using a standardized scale

TABLE 30.2

REVISED CARDIAC RISK INDEX FOR ELECTIVE SURGERY

Factors—1 point each

High-risk surgery (intraperitoneal, intrathoracic, or suprainguinal vascular)

Ischemic heart disease (history of MI or positive exercise test; current angina or use of nitrates; or pathologic Q-waves on ECG)

Heart failure (history of heart failure, pulmonary edema, or paroxysmal nocturnal dyspnea; bilateral rales or S_3 gallop on physical examination; pulmonary vascular redistribution on chest radiograph)

Cerebrovascular disease (history of transient ischemia attack or stroke)

Insulin therapy for diabetes

Preoperative serum creatinine >2.0 mg/dL

Approximate risks of MI, cardiac arrest, or cardiac death with elective surgery[a]

0 factors	0.5%	Low risk
1 factor	1.0%	
2 factors	5%	Intermediate risk
≥ 3 factors	10%	High risk

[a] Based on 4,315 inpatients undergoing elective major surgery.
ECG, electrocardiogram; MI, myocardial infarction.
From Lee TH, Marcantonio ER, Mangione CM, et al. Derivation and prospective validation of a simple index for prediction of cardiac risk in major noncardiac surgery. *Circulation* 1999;100:1043–1049.

such as the Canadian Cardiovascular Society angina scale (Table 30.4). Patients with class I or II symptoms are at low risk for cardiac complications (4%–5% risk of myocardial infarction and roughly a 1% mortality rate). Those with class III or IV symptoms are at higher risk (>10% risk of my-

TABLE 30.3

UNSTABLE CORONARY SYNDROMES ASSOCIATED WITH A VERY HIGH RISK OF PERIOPERATIVE CARDIAC COMPLICATIONS

Myocardial infarction within 1 month with evidence of persistent ischemia
Unstable angina
Accelerated angina

ocardial infarction or death). In most patients for whom the stability and severity of anginal symptoms can be reliably determined from the history, further cardiac testing has not been shown to improve the accuracy of the risk assessment. Therefore, it is not recommended for routine use (2).

Noninvasive Ischemia Testing

Improvements in methods for clinical risk assessment and in interventions to reduce risk, particularly the use of perioperative β-adrenergic blocking agents, have combined to narrow the spectrum of patients who may benefit from preoperative noninvasive testing for inducible myocardial ischemia (3). For example, noninvasive ischemia testing does not improve the clinical risk assessment in patients with documented stable class I or II anginal symptoms, and it should not alter recommended perioperative management. In two types of patients, however, noninvasive cardiac testing may be useful (Chapter 36) because of difficulty in assessing the severity of anginal symptoms accurately: unreliable historians, and patients with severe orthopedic or

TABLE 30.4

CANADIAN CARDIOVASCULAR SOCIETY ANGINA SCALE

Class	Definition	Specific activity scale
I	Ordinary physical activity (e.g., walking and climbing stairs) does not cause angina; angina occurs with strenuous, rapid, or prolonged exertion at work or recreation.	Ability to ski, play basketball, light jog (5 mph), or shovel snow without angina
II	Slight limitation of ordinary activity; angina occurs on walking or climbing stairs rapidly; walking uphill; walking or stair climbing after meals, in cold, in wind, or under emotional stress, or only during the few hours after awakening; when walking >two blocks on level ground; or when climbing more than one flight of stairs at a normal pace and in normal conditions.	Ability to garden, rake, roller skate, walk at 4 mph on level ground, and have sexual intercourse without stopping
III	Marked limitation of ordinary physical activity; angina occurs on walking one to two blocks on level ground or climbing one flight of stairs at a normal pace in normal conditions.	Ability to shower or dress without stopping, walk at 2.5 mph, bowl, make a bed, and play golf
IV	Inability to perform any physical activity without discomfort; anginal symptoms may be present at rest.	Inability to perform activities requiring two or fewer metabolic equivalents (METs) without stopping

Adapted from Goldman L, Hashimoto B, Cook EF, Loscalzo A. Comparative reproducibility and validity of systems for assessing cardiovascular functional class: advantages of a new specific activity scale. *Circulation* 1981;64:1227–1234. Copyright 2002 The Cleveland Clinic Foundation, with permission.

vascular disease whose specific cardiac functional status is not known. Noninvasive testing may also be useful in clinically high-risk patients who may be candidates for preoperative coronary revascularization. Prior to testing, the physician should always ask whether the results are likely to change perioperative management.

Exercise electrocardiography can accurately stratify risk in patients who are able to exercise and who will undergo vascular or general surgery. Patients who achieve 85% of maximum predicted heart rate without ischemic electrocardiographic changes are at low risk for cardiac complications. Those who cannot achieve at least 75% of maximum predicted heart rate, with or without ischemic changes, are at substantially higher risk.

Dipyridamole-thallium scintigraphy can accurately predict cardiac complications in selected patients undergoing vascular surgery. In studies of consecutive unselected vascular surgery patients, however, thallium scintigraphy did not significantly alter the clinical risk assessment. This discrepancy likely is explained by a higher prevalence of severe coronary artery disease among the patients selected for testing by their physicians compared with unselected patients. In vascular surgery patients with an intermediate risk clinical assessment, a positive test, defined as an area of thallium redistribution after dipyridamole administration, is associated with a high cardiac complication rate, and a negative test is associated with a substantially lower rate. Although data are limited in nonvascular surgery patients, it is likely that thallium scintigraphy again is most useful diagnostically in patients at intermediate risk on clinical assessment.

In the largest study of preoperative dobutamine echocardiography in patients undergoing vascular surgery, a normal test, defined as the absence of any new regional wall motion abnormality with dobutamine administration, was associated with a very low risk of perioperative myocardial infarction or cardiac death (4). This finding was true for all patients in the study, regardless of whether they were at low, intermediate, or high risk by clinical assessment.

Noninvasive preoperative testing is worthwhile only when it will change perioperative management. In the era of β blockade, such testing is recommended primarily in patients with a history of angina or peripheral vascular disease and with poor or indeterminant functional status (Figure 30.1).

Preoperative Angiography and Revascularization

The role of preoperative coronary angiography and revascularization (with coronary artery bypass graft [CABG] surgery or percutaneous transluminal coronary angioplasty [PTCA], with or without stenting) is controversial. Data from the Coronary Artery Surgery Study trial registry indicate that patients who have undergone prior CABG surgery, particularly if within 5 years, are at lower risk for complications after subsequent noncardiac surgery compared with similar patients whose coronary artery disease was treated medically. In a recent trial (5), patients who underwent PTCA without intracoronary stent placement

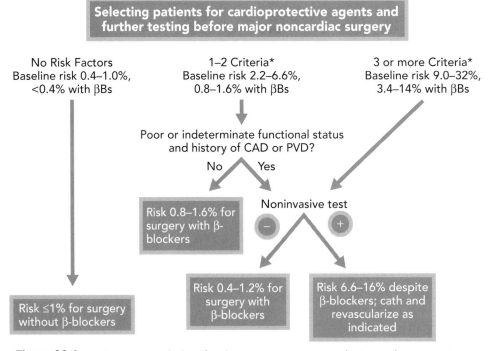

Figure 30.1 Perioperative β-Blockers for elective surgery: patient selection and preoperative risk stratification. *See Table 30.2 for criteria. βB, beta blocker.

had a 1.6% cardiac complication rate with subsequent noncardiac surgery. The rate was 0.8% when PTCA preceded noncardiac surgery by fewer than 4 years but 3.6% if the interval was greater than 4 years. On the other hand, patients who underwent noncardiac surgery within 2 weeks of intracoronary stent placement had a very high morbidity and mortality rate. The rate remained somewhat elevated for another 2–6 weeks and then became very low by about 9 weeks after stenting (5). The very high complication rate is attributable to in-stent restenosis when anticoagulant and antiplatelet therapies are discontinued prematurely. It is prudent, therefore, to delay nonemergent noncardiac surgery for at least 4 weeks, and preferably 9 weeks, after intracoronary stenting.

For low-risk patients, the risk of prophylactic revascularization with either CABG surgery or PTCA (1%–2% mortality in most studies) is likely to be at least as high as that associated with noncardiac surgery without revascularization. Prophylactic revascularization, therefore, is not recommended in low-risk patients. In a recent randomized trial of patients who were undergoing elective vascular surgery at 18 Veterans Affairs medical centers and who had significant, remediable coronary disease, the 258 patients assigned to coronary revascularization (either a percutaneous procedure or bypass surgery depending on the recommendations of their physicians) did no better than the 252 who were managed medically, immediately or over 2.7 years of follow-up (6). Based on these results, preoperative coronary revascularization should be reserved for patients who meet criteria for it independent of the planned surgery (Chapter 37).

Preoperative Medical Therapy

In very high-risk patients with an unstable coronary syndrome, noncardiac surgery should be delayed to allow for stabilization of ischemic symptoms. For high-risk patients undergoing elective surgery who are not candidates for angiography or revascularization, one approach to reduce risk is to delay surgery for several weeks to optimize medical therapy. Although this strategy may reduce risk, it has not been evaluated in clinical trials.

The most effective intervention to reduce risk is *the use of perioperative β-adrenergic blocking agents* (2,3). In the largest study of very high-risk patients (including positive stress echocardiogram results) undergoing vascular surgery, the perioperative cardiac morbidity rate was 3.4% among patients who received perioperative bisoprolol, compared with 34% in the placebo group. It appears that most of the benefit from perioperative β-blockers is mediated through heart rate control. The recommended goal is to achieve a heart rate less than 65 beats per minute throughout the perioperative period. Perioperative β-blockers are recommended for patients with known or suspected coronary artery disease undergoing intermediate-risk or high-risk surgery. Atenolol and bisoprolol have been the most

widely studied agents and are the preferred choices when initiating therapy (Table 30.5). However, patients already taking other β-blockers need not switch to one of these two agents prior to surgery (but they may need their dosage adjusted to achieve the desired heart rate).

In a meta-analysis, α-2 agonists have also been shown to reduce adverse perioperative cardiac complications (7). The largest experience is with mivazerol, which is not currently available for clinical use. Clonidine, an α-2 agonist similar to mivazerol, has been evaluated in a smaller number of patients but is a potential alternative in high-risk patients who cannot take β-blockers.

Intravenous nitroglycerin reduces perioperative ischemia but has not been shown to improve cardiac outcomes. Preliminary data suggest that patients on statins may have fewer postoperative ischemic cardiac events, but the therapy has not been subjected to randomized trials.

Invasive Intraoperative Monitoring

Two commonly used intraoperative monitoring techniques in patients with coronary artery disease are *pulmonary artery catheterization* and *transesophageal echocardiography*. Trials comparing routine versus selective use of intraoperative pulmonary artery catheterization showed no differences in outcomes (8). The limited data available on intraoperative transesophageal echocardiography have not demonstrated an improvement in cardiac outcomes. These monitoring techniques, therefore, should be considered only in high-risk patients, particularly those with unstable coronary syndromes undergoing high-risk procedures. In most situations, the anesthesiologist makes decisions regarding intraoperative monitoring.

The overall approach to patients with known or suspected coronary artery disease is summarized in Figure 30.1.

TABLE 30.5

DOSING SCHEDULE FOR THE ADMINISTRATION OF PROPHYLACTIC β-BLOCKERS

Bisoprolol	5–10 mg[a] given orally once daily, begun before surgery (ideally at least 7 days) and continued for 30 days postoperatively.[b]
Atenolol	5–10 mg[a] given intravenously every 12 hours beginning 1 hour before surgery and continued until the patient is eating; followed by 50–100 mg orally every 12 hours until postoperative day 7.

[a] The dose is titrated to achieve a heart rate <65 bpm.
[b] Intravenous atenolol or metoprolol may be used during the time when the patient is not eating.
Adapted from Mangano DT, Layug EL, Wallace AW, Tateo I. Effect of atenolol on mortality and cardiovascular morbidity after noncardiac surgery. *N Engl J Med* 1996;335:1713; and from Poldermans D, Boersma E, Bax JJ, et al. The effect of bisoprolol on perioperative mortality and myocardial infarction in high-risk patients undergoing vascular surgery. *N Engl J Med* 1999;341:1789, with permission.

HEART FAILURE

Patients with poorly controlled heart failure, defined as the presence of jugular venous distention, a third heart sound, or pulmonary edema seen on a chest radiograph, are at substantially increased risk for cardiac complications, including death. In these patients, heart failure should be controlled prior to surgery with diuretics and afterload-reducing agents. This approach probably reduces risk, although it has not been studied in controlled clinical trials. Patients with compensated left-ventricular systolic dysfunction, defined as an ejection fraction less than 50% on echocardiogram or radionuclide ventriculography without overt heart failure on preoperative evaluation, are at moderately increased risk for developing pulmonary edema after vascular surgery but are not at increased risk for other serious cardiac complications.

Any patient with heart failure who has not had an objective assessment of left ventricular function or in whom the cause of heart failure is unknown should undergo echocardiography prior to surgery. The cause and severity of ventricular dysfunction may affect intraoperative and early postoperative management. For example, fluid management will differ in patients with hypertrophic obstructive cardiomyopathy, who need to be well hydrated to avoid obstructive hypotension, and patients with dilated cardiomyopathy, who will need to be kept appropriately fluid restricted. If arranging for such testing requires a substantial delay in surgery, it is justified only in patients with worrisome signs or symptoms that cannot be controlled preoperatively.

VALVULAR HEART DISEASE

Patients with aortic stenosis and a gradient above 20–40 mm Hg have a small increase in perioperative cardiac risk, whereas patients with a gradient above 40 usually have a substantial increase in risk. Symptomatic patients appear to be at higher risk than asymptomatic patients with similar degrees of valvular stenosis. In patients with severe symptomatic aortic stenosis, elective noncardiac surgery should be delayed until valve surgery or balloon valvuloplasty can be performed. Preoperative balloon valvuloplasty may reduce perioperative cardiac complications, though this is an unproven strategy. If noncardiac surgery cannot be delayed, it is crucial that the anesthesiologist be aware of the severity of aortic valvular disease because it has significant implications for intraoperative and postoperative management.

The perioperative cardiac risks associated with other valvular lesions are not as well quantified. Patients with severe mitral stenosis appear to be at increased risk for atrial arrhythmias and heart failure. It is not known to what extent mitral or aortic regurgitation imparts any excess risk independent of that associated with heart failure. In any patient with valvular heart disease, preoperative optimization of cardiac function with medications is recommended (Chapter 41). If surgical correction of valvular heart disease is indicated, such surgery should precede elective noncardiac surgery. Echocardiography should be considered in patients with a previously undiagnosed heart murmur because it may reveal a lesion that requires antibiotic prophylaxis.

Several surgical procedures are known to produce transient bacteremia with organisms that commonly cause *endocarditis*. Nevertheless, the risk of developing endocarditis after a surgical procedure is low. Certain structural cardiac abnormalities are associated with an increased risk for the development of endocarditis and for increased morbidity once endocarditis develops. Controlled trials have not demonstrated that prophylactic antibiotics reduce the risk of developing postprocedure endocarditis. However, the morbidity associated with endocarditis is high (Chapter 71), and the risks associated with prophylactic antibiotics are low. As a result, if patients with high-risk or moderate-risk structural cardiac abnormalities are undergoing certain surgical procedures (Table 30.6), antibiotic prophylaxis is indicated (Table 30.7).

ARRHYTHMIAS

Most important cardiac arrhythmias are associated with underlying structural heart disease, particularly coronary artery disease and heart failure. It is likely that any association between rhythm disturbances and adverse cardiac outcomes results from the underlying structural heart disease. Cardiac rhythm disturbances in the absence of structural heart disease have not been associated with increased cardiac risk. The finding of an arrhythmia on a preoperative electrocardiogram should prompt an investigation for unsuspected structural heart disease. Preoperative treatment for arrhythmias should be guided by principles independent of surgery. Ventricular rate control should be ensured in patients who have atrial fibrillation. Symptomatic supraventricular (Chapter 42) and ventricular arrhythmias (Chapter 43) should be controlled prior to surgery. Asymptomatic arrhythmias do not require specific therapy. Patients who have an indication for a permanent pacemaker (Chapter 45) should have this placed prior to surgery. If noncardiac surgery is urgent, these patients require temporary transvenous pacing during and after surgery.

HYPERTENSION

Severe hypertension, defined as a systolic blood pressure greater than 200 mm Hg or a diastolic blood pressure greater than 120 mm Hg, during the immediate preoperative period is associated with an increased risk of postoperative myocardial infarction and heart failure. Lesser degrees of hypertension are associated with more frequent

TABLE 30.6

CARDIAC CONDITIONS AND SURGICAL PROCEDURES IN WHICH ENDOCARDITIS PROPHYLAXIS IS RECOMMENDED

Cardiac conditions	Surgical procedures[a]
High risk	Respiratory tract
Prosthetic heart valves	Tonsillectomy or adenoidectomy
Previous bacterial endocarditis	Rigid bronchoscopy
Complex cyanotic congenital heart disease	Surgical operations involving the respiratory mucosa
Surgically constructed pulmonary shunts or conduits	
Moderate risk	Gastrointestinal tract
Other congenital heart lesions	Sclerotherapy
Acquired valvular dysfunction	Esophageal stricture dilation
Hypertrophic cardiomyopathy	Endoscopic retrograde cholangiography with biliary obstruction
Mitral-valve prolapse with regurgitation or thickened leaflets	Surgical operations involving the intestinal mucosa
	Biliary-tract surgery
	Genitourinary tract
	Prostate surgery
	Cystoscopy
	Urethral dilation

[a] Dental procedures are not covered in this chapter.
Adapted from Dajani AS, Taubert KA, Wilson W, et al. Prevention of bacterial endocarditis, recommendations by the American Heart Association. *JAMA* 1997;277:1794, with permission.

TABLE 30.7

RECOMMENDED PROPHYLACTIC ANTIBIOTIC REGIMENS

Patient	Regimen
Oral, respiratory tract, or esophageal procedures	
Standard	Amoxicillin 2.0 g orally 1 hour before procedure or Ampicillin 2.0 g IM or IV within 30 minutes before procedure
Patients allergic to penicillin	Clindamycin 600 mg orally 1 hour before procedure or Cephalexin or cefadroxil 2.0 g orally 1 hour before procedure or Azithromycin or clarithromycin 500 mg orally 1 hour before procedure or Clindamycin 600 mg IV within 30 minutes before procedure or Cefazolin 1.0 g within 30 minutes before procedure
Gastrointestinal (excluding esophageal) and genitourinary procedures	
High-risk patients	Ampicillin 2.0 g IM or IV plus gentamicin 1.5 mg/kg IV or IM (not to exceed 120 mg) within 30 minutes of starting procedure and Ampicillin 1.0 g IM or IV or amoxicillin 1 g orally 6 hours later
High-risk patients allergic to penicillin	Vancomycin 1.0 g IV over 1–2 hours plus gentamicin 1.5 mg/kg (not to exceed 120 mg) IV or IM; complete injection/infusion within 30 minutes of starting procedure
Moderate-risk patients	Amoxicillin 2.0 g orally 1 hour before procedure or Ampicillin 2.0 g IM or IV within 30 minutes of starting procedure
Moderate-risk patients allergic to penicillin	Vancomycin 1.0 g IV over 1–2 hours; complete infusion within 30 minutes of starting procedure

IM, intramuscularly; *IV,* intravenously.
Adapted from Dajani AS, Taubert KA, Wilson W, et al. Prevention of bacterial endocarditis, recommendations by the American Heart Association. *JAMA* 1997;277:1794, with permission.

electrocardiographic occurrences of ischemia but not with adverse cardiac outcomes. Severe hypertension should be controlled prior to surgery with rapid-acting agents such as sodium nitroprusside or intravenous β-adrenergic blocking agents (Chapter 48). Moderate preoperative hypertension does not require specific preoperative therapy. Patients with moderate hypertension should be re-evaluated after surgery to determine whether chronic antihypertensive therapy is needed. Generally, a patient's chronic oral antihypertensive medications should be continued throughout the perioperative period.

PULMONARY DISEASE

Postoperative pulmonary complications are common following major surgery. Most of these complications, including atelectasis, bronchitis, and mild bronchospasm, are relatively minor in nature and do not lead to permanent morbidity or a prolongation of the hospital stay. They often require no specific therapy. The most serious postoperative pulmonary complications are pneumonia and prolonged mechanical ventilation, which may occur in up to 19% of patients undergoing cardiothoracic or upper-abdominal surgery. By comparison, serious pulmonary complications occur in less than 3% of patients after lower-abdominal, pelvic, or extremity surgery. Three patient characteristics have been associated with an increased risk of serious pulmonary complications: *obstructive lung disease, tobacco use,* and *morbid obesity.* Patients with chronic obstructive pulmonary disease (COPD) are at increased risk for both pneumonia and prolonged mechanical ventilation. In studies that have evaluated preoperative pulmonary-function testing in patients with COPD, results have been inconsistent. No single test or combination of tests can reliably predict the risk of pulmonary complications. One exception is that patients who have an FEV_1 <500mL appear to be at particularly high risk. Patients with asthma are at risk to develop severe bronchospasm during endotracheal intubation or extubation. If symptoms are well controlled prior to surgery, asthmatic patients do not appear to be at excessive risk for other pulmonary complications.

Patients who weigh more than 250 pounds are about twice as likely to develop postoperative pneumonia as nonobese patients. Current smokers have a twofold to threefold increased risk of developing pneumonia. Smoking cessation for at least 4 weeks prior to surgery reduces the risk of postoperative pulmonary complications, but one week of smoking cessation does not (9). Smoking cessation, nevertheless, should be recommended prior to any surgery as part of routine health care. In a large prospective cohort of U.S. veterans, additional risk factors for pulmonary complications included age over 60 years, dependent functional status, impaired sensorium, and prior stroke (10). A postoperative nasogastric tube is also associated with an increased risk of pneumonia.

Preoperative pulmonary function testing with spirometry or arterial blood-gas measurement is unlikely to change the management of most patients seen by the inpatient preoperative consultant and generally is not required. In patients with severe pulmonary compromise of unknown origin, preoperative testing may be useful to delineate the cause of lung dysfunction because intraoperative ventilator management may be affected by the results. In patients with known COPD who have more severe symptoms than usual at the time of surgery, spirometry may be a useful objective measure of pulmonary function to help identify the need for preoperative therapy.

Preoperative optimization of pulmonary function in patients with COPD or asthma (Chapters 55 and 56) may reduce the risk of postoperative complications. Therapy may include inhaled bronchodilators, theophylline (or aminophylline), or corticosteroids. Antibiotics may be helpful in patients with purulent sputum, especially if sputum can be cleared before surgery. Incentive spirometry and deep breathing exercises with pursed lips, continuous positive airway pressure (CPAP), and intermittent positive pressure breathing (IPPB) can reduce the risk of developing postoperative atelectasis and pneumonia and shorten the length of the hospital stay in patients after upper-abdominal surgery. In most studies, these interventions were equally effective. Incentive spirometry and deep breathing exercises are less expensive and easier to administer than CPAP and IPPB and are the preferred methods in most patients. Incentive spirometry should be used for at least 15 minutes four times daily, and deep breathing should be done hourly. These therapies should begin preoperatively and be continued for 1–2 days postoperatively. For patients undergoing esophageal or gastric resection, CPAP is significantly better than incentive spirometry or deep breathing exercises for reducing the risk of pulmonary complications and is, therefore, the preferred intervention (11).

NEUROLOGIC COMPLICATIONS

The most common serious perioperative neurologic complications are *stroke* and *delirium.* Perioperative stroke occurs in 1%–6% of patients undergoing cardiac, carotid, or peripheral vascular surgery but is rare (less than 1%) after most other surgical procedures. The risk factors for stroke following cardiac surgery include carotid stenosis greater than 50%, a calcified aorta, diabetes mellitus, prior stroke, age over 60 years, peripheral vascular disease, and cigarette smoking (12). In both the cardiac and noncardiac surgical settings, patients with symptomatic carotid stenoses of greater than 50% luminal narrowing are at a substantially increased risk for perioperative stroke. Patients with severe asymptomatic carotid stenoses undergoing noncardiac surgery may be at increased risk, but studies to date are not conclusive. An asymptomatic carotid bruit is not an independent predictor of perioperative stroke. It is not known whether patients who have undergone carotid endarterectomy are at lower risk for perioperative stroke with subsequent surgery than similar patients who have not undergone endarterectomy. As a result, prophylactic endarterectomy is not recommended prior to necessary noncarotid surgery. However, if carotid endarterectomy is indicated and the noncarotid surgery can be safely delayed, it is preferable to proceed with carotid surgery first.

Postoperative delirium is a common complication, occurring in nearly 10% of patients over the age of 50 after major surgery. Postoperative delirium is associated with significant morbidity, including the development of cardiac and pulmonary complications, prolonged hospital stays, and emotional distress for the patient and family. Several surgical and patient characteristics have been associated with the development of postoperative delirium (Table 30.8). If three or more of these characteristics are present, the risk of developing delirium approaches 50%.

Delirium may occur in 35%–65% of patients after hip fracture repair. In a randomized trial of hip fracture patients, a comprehensive intervention (maintenance of the hematrocrit above 30%; minimizing the use of benzodiazepine, anticholinergic, and antihistamine medications; maintenance of regular bowel function; early removal of urinary catheters; and daily visits by a geriatrician) reduced the incidence of postoperative delirium from 50%–32% (13).

Adverse neurologic outcomes are particularly common after CABG surgery. In a large prospective evaluation, the incidence of postoperative stroke was 2.7% and of encephalopathy was 6.9% (12). The risk factors for developing neurologic complications after CABG surgery include age over 70 years, proximal aortic atherosclerosis, or a history of neurologic or pulmonary disease.

Postoperative delirium in patients previously thought not to be demented is associated with a 3.5-fold higher rate of subsequently diagnosed dementia. This dementia is also associated with a significantly higher 5-year mortality rate (14).

HEMATOLOGIC EVALUATION

Several hematologic disorders may have an impact on surgical outcomes. Two common issues faced by the preoperative consultant are the *patient with anemia* and *assessing surgical bleeding risk.*

The most important issue in the anemic patient is to determine the need for preoperative transfusion. If time permits, it is preferable to determine the cause of anemia prior to surgery because certain disorders, particularly hemolytic anemias, may require specific perioperative therapy. Limited studies suggest that surgical outcomes are inversely related to the preoperative hemoglobin level, although these studies did not control for the underlying diseases. Hemoglobin levels below 8 g/dL are associated with the greatest risk. Preoperative transfusion in patients with a hemoglobin level below 8 g/dL may reduce perioperative complications. In patients with coronary artery disease, a preoperative hemoglobin level below 10g/dL has been associated with increased mortality. Thus, preoperative transfusion to a level of at least 10g/dL may be justified in these patients. In an individual patient, the presence of cardiopulmonary disease, the likelihood of surgical blood loss, and the hemoglobin level must be considered to determine the need for preoperative transfusion.

The most important component of the preoperative assessment for the risk of bleeding is a detailed history focused on factors suggestive of a bleeding disorder (see Table 30.9). Patients without evidence of abnormal bleeding on a directed history and physical examination are at extremely low risk for abnormal surgical bleeding (15). Laboratory tests of hemostasis, including the prothrombin time, activated partial thromboplastin time, platelet count, or bleeding time, are not needed. If the bleeding history is incomplete or unreliable, or if abnormal bleeding is suggested, then a formal evaluation of hemostasis is indicated (Chapter 98).

TABLE 30.8

RISK FACTORS FOR THE DEVELOPMENT OF POSTOPERATIVE DELIRIUM

Preoperative factors	Postoperative factors
Age >70 years	Use of meperidine or benzodiazepines
Alcohol abuse	
Poor cognitive status	
Poor physical function status	
Markedly abnormal serum sodium, potassium, or glucose level[a]	
Aortic aneurysm surgery	
Noncardiac thoracic surgery	

[a] Defined as follows: sodium <130 mEq/L or >150 mEq/L, potassium <3.0 mEq/L or >6.0 mEq/L, glucose <60 mg/dL or >300 mg/dL.
Adapted from Marcantonio ER, Goldman L, Mangione CM, et al. A clinical prediction rule for delirium after elective noncardiac surgery. *JAMA* 1994;271:134; and from Marcantonio ER, Juarez G, Goldman L, et al. The relationship of postoperative delirium with psychoactive medications. *JAMA* 1994;272:1518, with permission.

TABLE 30.9

FACTORS SUGGESTIVE OF A BLEEDING DISORDER

Unprovoked bruising on the trunk of >5 cm in diameter
Frequent, unprovoked epistaxis or gingival bleeding
Menorrhagia with iron deficiency
Hemarthrosis with mild trauma
Prior excessive surgical blood loss or reoperation for bleeding
Family history of abnormal bleeding
Presence of severe kidney or liver disease

Adapted from Baker R. Pre-operative hemostatic assessment and management. *Transfusion and Apher Sci* 2002;27:45, with permission.

ENDOCRINE DISORDERS

The perioperative management of patients with diabetes is discussed in Chapter 107.

GLUCOCORTICOID REPLACEMENT

Perioperative hypotension resulting from primary or secondary adrenocortical insufficiency is rare. The administration of high-dose glucocorticoid medications during the perioperative period to prevent complications is controversial. In the only clinical trial comparing high-dose with baseline-dose perioperative glucocorticoid administration in patients with proven secondary adrenocortical suppression, the perioperative complication rates were similar. However, the short-term use of high-dose glucocorticoids during the perioperative period also has not been associated with adverse outcomes. Physicians should consider high-dose glucocorticoid replacement in any patient who has received the equivalent of 20 mg of prednisone daily for 1 week or 7.5 mg of prednisone daily for 1 month within the past year. A commonly used regimen is 100 mg of hydrocortisone administered intravenously every 8 hours for 2 or 3 days. Patients on chronic glucocorticoid medications then should resume their usual dosage. The corticosteroids need not be tapered (also Chapter 109).

HYPOTHYROIDISM

Severe symptomatic hypothyroidism is associated with a variety of perioperative complications, including hypotension, heart failure, and death. If possible, surgery should be delayed in patients with hypothyroidism to allow for adequate thyroid hormone replacement (Chapter 108). For urgent or emergent surgery, it is not known whether one or two doses of thyroid hormone prior to surgery reduces the risk of complications; this strategy is not recommended and should be considered only after consultation with an endocrinologist. Mild or asymptomatic hypothyroidism may be associated with mild intraoperative hypotension but has not been shown to increase the risk of major perioperative complications. Surgery need not be delayed in such patients to allow for adequate hormone replacement.

KEY POINTS

- Delaying surgery is likely to be justified only if the perioperative risks are substantial, the risks of delaying needed surgery are not substantial, and a delay would lead to a significant reduction in perioperative risk.
- Coronary artery disease accounts for the majority of serious perioperative cardiac complications; patients with unstable coronary syndromes or severe stable angina are at the highest risk.
- Prophylactic β-blockers reduce morbidity and mortality in patients with coronary disease, especially those undergoing major surgery.
- Preoperative noninvasive ischemia testing using dipyridamole thallium scintigraphy or dobutamine stress echocardiography is most useful in patients whose cardiac functional status is unknown and cannot be determined by a standard exercise test.
- Decompensated heart failure is associated with substantial perioperative risk and should be controlled prior to surgery.
- The risk factors for postoperative pulmonary complications include cardiac, thoracic, or upper-abdominal surgery, COPD, morbid obesity, and current tobacco use.
- Maintenance of the hematocrit above 30%, early removal of urinary catheters, maintenance of regular bowel function, and avoidance of benzodiazepines, antihistamines, and anticholinergics may reduce the risk of postoperative delirium in hip fracture patients.
- The most important and reliable tool to assess the risk for abnormal surgical bleeding is a directed bleeding history.

REFERENCES

1. Lee TH, Marcantonio ER, Mangione CM, et al. Derivation and prospective validation of a simple index for prediction of cardiac risk in major noncardiac surgery. *Circulation* 1999;100:1043–1049.
2. Eagle KA, Berger PB, Calkins H, et al. ACC/AHA guideline update for perioperative cardiovascular evaluation for noncardiac surgery—executive summary. *Anesth Analg* 2002;94:1052–1064.
3. Auerbach AD, Goldman L. β-blockers and reduction of cardiac events in noncardiac surgery: scientific review. *JAMA* 2002;287:1435–1444.
4. Boersma E, Poldermans D, Bax JJ, et al. Predictors of cardiac events after major vascular surgery, role of clinical characteristics, dobutamine echocardiography, and β-blocker therapy. *JAMA* 2001;285:1865–1873.
5. Wilson SH, Fasseas P, Orford JL, et al. Clinical outcomes of patients undergoing non-cardiac surgery in the two months following coronary stenting. *J Am Coll Cardiol* 2003;42:234–240.
6. McFalls EO, Ward HB, Moritz TE, et al. Coronary-artery revascularization before elective major vascular surgery. *N Engl J Med* 2004;351:2795–2804.
7. Wijeysundera DN, Naik JS, Beattie WS. α-2 adrenergic agonists to prevent perioperative cardiovascular complications: a meta-analysis. *Am J Med* 2003;114:742–752.

8. Sandham JD, Hull RD, Brant RF, et al. A randomized controlled trial of the use of pulmonary artery catheters in high risk surgical patients. *N Engl J Med* 2003;348:5–14.
9. Nakagawa M, Tanaka H, Tsukuma H, Kishi Y. Relationship between the duration of the preoperative smoke-free period and the incidence of postoperative complications after pulmonary surgery. *Chest* 2001;120:705–710.
10. Arozullah AM, Khuri SF, Henderson WG, Daley J. Development and validation of a multifactorial risk index for predicting postoperative pneumonia after major noncardiac surgery. *Ann Intern Med* 2001;135:847–857.
11. Olsen MF, Wennberg E, Johnsson E, Josefson K, Lonroth H, Lundell L. Randomized clinical study of the prevention of pulmonary complications after thoracoabdominal resection by two different breathing techniques. *Br J Surg* 2002;89: 1228–1234.
12. McKhann GM, Grega MA, Borowicz LM, et al. Encephalopathy and stroke after coronary artery bypass grafting: incidence, consequences, and prediction. *Arch Neurol* 2002;59:1422–1428.
13. Marcantonio ER, Flacker JM, Wright RJ, Resnick NM. Reducing delirium after hip fracture: a randomized trial. *J Am Geriatr Soc* 2001;49:516–522.
14. Lundstrøm M, Edlund A, Bucht G, Karlsson S, Gustafson Y. Dementia after delirium in patients with femoral neck fractures. *J Am Geriatr Soc* 2003;51:1002–1006.
15. Baker R. Pre-operative hemostatic assessment and management. *Transfusion and Apher Sci* 2002;27:45–53.

ADDITIONAL READING

Armas-Loughran B, Kalra R, Carson JL. Evaluation and management of anemia and bleeding disorders in surgical patients. *Med Clin N Amer* 2003;87:229–242.

Blacker DJ, Flemming KD, Link MJ, Brown RD Jr. The preoperative cerebrovascular consultation: common cerebrovascular questions before general or cardiac surgery. *Mayo Clin Proc* 2004;79:223–230.

Glowniak JV, Loriauz DL. A double blind study of perioperative steroid requirements in secondary adrenal insufficiency. *Surgery* 1997;121:123–129.

Goldman L. Aortic stenosis in noncardiac surgery: underappreciated in more ways than one? *Am J Med* 2004;116:60–62.

McAlister FA, Khan NA, Straus SE, et al. Accuracy of the preoperative assessment in predicting pulmonary risk after nonthoracic surgery. *Am J Resp Crit Care Med* 2003;167:741–744.

Poldermans D, Boersma E, Bax JJ, et al. The effect of bisoprolol on perioperative mortality and myocardial infarction in high-risk patients undergoing vascular surgery. *N Engl J Med* 1999;341: 1789–1794.

Schiff RL, Welsh GA. Perioperative evaluation and management of the patient with endocrine dysfunction. *Med Clin N Amer* 2003;87:175–192.

Shammash JB, Ghali WB. Preoperative assessment and perioperative management of the patient with nonischemic heart disease. *Med Clin N Amer* 2003;87:137–152.

Postoperative Care

31

Richard H. Savel   Jeanine P. Wiener-Kronish
Michael A. Gropper

INTRODUCTION

Management of patients in the postoperative period has undergone substantial change in the past decade. Improvements in surgical and anesthetic techniques, such as those in laparoscopic surgery, allow sicker and more elderly patients to undergo major surgical procedures safely. An increasing percentage of surgical procedures is performed on an outpatient basis, so the remaining hospitalized patients tend to have more concurrent illnesses and to undergo more invasive surgical procedures. An essential component of caring for the postoperative patient is close communication with the surgeon and anesthesiologist, who can provide information that may have a significant impact on diagnosis and treatment of postoperative problems. Postoperative co-management by a hospitalist may reduce complication rates and, in some circumstances, be preferred by surgeons and nurses (1). This chapter focuses on problems commonly encountered in patients in the immediate postoperative period, both during and after their stay in the post-anesthesia care unit (PACU).

CARE OF THE HOSPITALIZED PATIENT

Initial Assessment

Initial assessment of the postoperative patient should focus on the respiratory and cardiovascular systems. Changes in these systems occur rapidly in the postoperative period and may require admission to the ICU. Patients with any respiratory difficulties (stridor, tachypnea, dyspnea, bradypnea, and hypoxemia) should be transferred to the ICU or kept in the PACU, where physicians skilled in airway management are immediately available. Respiratory status may be rapidly assessed by physical examination, pulse oximetry, and arterial blood gas (ABG) measurement. In general, all patients

should receive supplemental oxygen in the immediate postoperative period because of the high risk of hypoxemia. Patients who have had surgical procedures involving the chest, upper abdomen, neck, and axilla should have chest radiography to exclude pneumothoraces, as should all patients who have had successful or attempted central venous cannulation. Both hypertension and hypotension are common in the immediate postoperative period and require immediate attention. Hypotension and tachycardia may indicate hemorrhage that requires immediate volume resuscitation and surgical re-exploration; hemoglobin concentration should be determined without delay. Volume resuscitation, rather than vasopressors, should be used first in treatment of the hypotensive postoperative patient. Hypertension may indicate pain or significant myocardial ischemia. Mental status should be monitored and documented because changes in mental status may indicate major complications (e.g., carotid artery occlusion or hematoma, subarachnoid hemorrhage). Serum glucose should be assessed and treated as necessary based on recent evidence that tight glucose control and normoglycemia decrease mortality in the postoperative period (2).

Management of Acute Postoperative Pain

Pain associated with surgical procedures is a major determinant of postoperative morbidity and mortality. If pain is not controlled, patients are at increased risk of complications, especially myocardial ischemia and respiratory failure from atelectasis. In addition, fear of postoperative pain is often the single greatest cause of anxiety in surgical patients. The usual approach to postoperative pain has been to use opiates, delivered by intramuscular or intravenous injection and ordered on an "as needed" basis. This approach has been found to be inadequate; intramuscular injection of opiates leads to highly unpredictable levels, resulting in either undertreatment or accumulation of multiple doses, depending on the dosing frequency, site of injection, and tissue perfusion. *Instead, opiates should be administered on a regular schedule and should be given intravenously* (3). The advent of "patient-controlled analgesia" (PCA) (Figure 31.1) enables the patient to self-administer frequent, small doses of opiates instead of boluses that may result in overtreatment or undertreatment. The PCA's lockout mode prevents overdosing. Studies have shown that postoperative patients prefer PCA over other modes of pain management that produce equipotent analgesia, probably because patients can control their own medication.

As the majority of postsurgical pain is inflammatory in nature, *nonsteroidal anti-inflammatory drugs (NSAIDs)* should be administered in combination with opiates to treat this inflammatory component. When used in this manner, NSAIDs can decrease the total dose of opiates required. NSAIDs should not be used routinely in patients with renal insufficiency or a history of gastric ulceration. In addition, certain postsurgical patients at risk for bleeding, such as those following craniotomy or major vascular surgery, may not be candidates for NSAIDs for the first 24–36 postoperative hours.

Certain patients may benefit from *epidural analgesia,* which can deliver opiates and local anesthetics to the epidural space in small doses with minimal side effects. Although this technique requires placement of an epidural catheter, patients will receive superior analgesia and benefit from sympathectomy if local anesthetics are used.

Ambulation should be with assistance because patients may have partial motor blockade and diminished baroreflexes. A number of studies have demonstrated improved outcomes in patients who have undergone epidural anesthesia for surgery and who continue to receive epidural anesthesia for postoperative pain (4,5). Recent studies have also demonstrated earlier ambulation, earlier return of bowel function, and earlier discharge from the hospital if patients receive epidural anesthesia for postoperative pain after abdominal surgery. Common complications of epidural analgesia include urinary retention, pruritis, and, rarely, significant respiratory depression. Patients who receive epidural anesthesia, either with opiates or in combination with local anesthetics, should have specific postoperative orders to monitor for delayed respiratory depression and to limit the doses of additional opiates. One newer approach to epidural analgesia includes patient-controlled epidural analgesia (PCEA), which allows the patient to control the epidural infusion in much the same way as PCA for intravenous opioid doses.

Delirium

Postoperative delirium is commonly encountered, especially in elderly patients. General anesthesia results in imbalances of central cholinergic systems, which can cause delirium and confusion. The elderly are especially susceptible to this problem. Patients who develop delirium have

---

Patient Controlled Analgesia

Recommended initial settings:

1) **dose** of opiate (See below for equipotent dosing)

2) **lockout interval** = 6 minutes
   (this is the minimum interval between doses, regardless of the number of patient attempts)

2) **basal rate** = 0 (except for chronic pain patients)

3) **rescue dose** = usually twice the unit dose in #1 (administered by nurse at patient's request, once/hour)

Opiates: recommended initial unit dose
   morphine: 1 mg/injection
   meperidine*: 10 mg/injection
   hydromorphone: 0.2 mg/injection
   fentanyl: 10 mcg/injection

* Avoid in patients with renal insufficiency.

Figure 31.1 Patient-controlled analgesia. Recommended initial settings for PCA. Usual settings are dilaudid (hydromorphone) 0.2 mg/injection with 6-minute lockout, no basal rate, and a 0.4 mg/hour rescue dose that is administered on demand. Avoid meperidine in large doses and especially in patients with renal failure because of the possibility of seizures induced by the metabolite normeperidine.

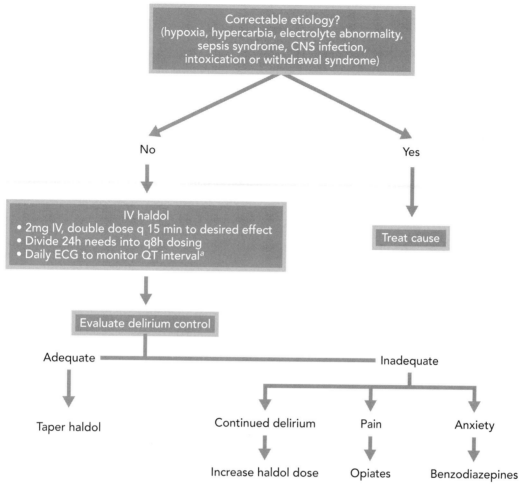

Figure 31.2 Flow Chart for Evaluation and Treatment of Delirium in Postoperative Patients. Correctable etiologies must be ruled out prior to initiation of pharmacologic therapy.[a] ECG monitoring must be done prior to therapy and at daily intervals to detect QT prolongation induced by haloperidol. CNS, central nervous system; ECG, electrocardiogram; IV, intravenous.

more complications, longer hospital stays, and an increased need for rehabilitative care. Attention to identifiable risk factors in elderly postoperative patients can reduce the risk of delirium (6) (see also Chapter 16 and Table 30.8).

It is important to identify hypoxemia, pain, and electrolyte disorders, all of which contribute to delirium even in the absence of neuroleptic drugs (Figure 31.2). Benzodiazepines should be used with caution in elderly patients because of the pharmacokinetic and pharmacodynamic changes that occur with aging. For example, the half-life of diazepam increases to nearly 60 hours in 70-year-old patients. In the evaluation and care of the delirious patient, it is often necessary to discontinue all psychoactive medications. In this setting, opiates such as fentanyl may be more predictable and reversible sedatives than are benzodiazepines and other drugs. If sedatives or opiates are used as a continuous infusion, the level of sedation should be assessed several times per day and titrated as needed, with a particular focus on minimizing the duration of mechanical ventilation (7).

Nausea and Vomiting

Postoperative nausea and vomiting are a significant source of preoperative anxiety, and they increase costs because of prolonged lengths of stay in the PACU and hospital. A number of agents used intraoperatively, especially opiates, have been associated with an increased incidence of nausea and vomiting. Laparoscopic, plastic, otolaryngologic, and neurologic surgeries have the highest incidence of postoperative nausea and vomiting. Patient risk factors include female sex, poorly controlled pain, hypotension, and history of motion sickness or previous nausea and vomiting.

A number of antiemetic agents have been evaluated for efficacy, but most studies have been in patients who are receiving cancer chemotherapy. Recently, 5HT$_3$ receptor antagonists, especially ondansetron and granisetron, have been used for both prophylaxis and treatment of postoperative nausea and vomiting. Other agents to consider include supplemental oxygen, dexamethasone, and lorazepam. Droperidol, which can cause QT prolongation and torsade de pointes, should be used only after other drug interventions have failed (8).

CARDIAC ISSUES

Prevention of Perioperative Ischemia

Perioperative ischemic events can be significantly decreased in patients at risk for cardiac events by the administration of a β-blocker immediately prior to the operation and throughout the hospitalization (up to 7 days) (Table 30.5, Chapter 30) (9,10). α-2 agonists such as clonidine are unproven but can be considered in patients who cannot tolerate β-blockers.

Perioperative Myocardial Infarction

The most common cause of morbidity and mortality after noncardiac surgery is myocardial infarction. The measurement of serum levels of cardiac troponin I is a sensitive and specific method for diagnosing perioperative infarction. Most postoperative myocardial infarctions occur in the first 5 days after surgery. Ischemic changes in the immediate postoperative electrocardiogram markedly increase the likelihood of a diagnosable myocardial infarction, and so an electrocardiogram is generally recommended soon after surgery. In contrast, serial electrocardiograms or troponin levels are not recommended except in patients with symptoms or new postoperative electrocardiographic changes (11). Remember, however, that *postoperative myocardial infarction may not present with typical pain* because of anesthesia, pain medications, and other postoperative pain. Therefore, nonspecific symptoms such as heart failure, tachycardia, unexplained dyspnea, or relative hypotension should also prompt an electrocardiogram. Elevations of cardiac troponin I or T carry a twofold to threefold increased risk of major myocardial ischemic events in the 6 months after surgery, even in patients without chest pain or diagnosed acute myocardial infarction.

Atrial Tachyarrhythmias

Atrial tachyarrhythmias, which are especially common after cardiac and thoracic surgery, can lead to serious consequences, including stroke, heart failure, myocardial ischemia, and prolonged stays in the intensive care unit and hospital. Atrial arrhythmias occur most frequently in the first 2–3 days after surgery, and they frequently recur. The risk of developing atrial tachyarrhythmias can be reduced by administering β-blockers and/or by not withdrawing β-blockers perioperatively. Atrial arrhythmias are typically precipitated by hypoxia, hyperthermia, electrolyte abnormalities, hypertension, infection, and medications.

Although pulmonary embolism and primary myocardial ischemia are uncommon causes, secondary myocardial ischemia is common. Treatment should focus on reversing the precipitating causes and on rate control (Chapter 42). After 24 hours of atrial fibrillation, anticoagulation therapy should be instituted if not otherwise contraindicated. Because conversion of atrial fibrillation to sinus rhythm does not appear to confer any added survival benefit over rate control alone, cardioversion need be undertaken in the hospital only in patients who cannot tolerate the arrhythmia or the anticoagulation needed for atrial fibrillation (Chapter 42) (12). In many patients, the arrhythmia will resolve as the clinical situation stabilizes, so no long-term therapy will be required.

Postoperative Hypertension

In patients who have postoperative hypertension, pain is the apparent cause in up to 35% of patients, with hypercarbia and sympathetic stimulation during emergence from anesthesia being the other common causes. Treatment should emphasize pain relief, sedation, oxygenation, and diuresis if necessary. When the blood pressure itself needs to be treated, the combined α/β-blocker labetalol is usually the preferred first-line agent. If a continuous infusion is required, options include labetalol, nitroglycerine, fenoldopam, and nitroprusside. Because of its toxicities, prolonged use of nitroprusside should be avoided (13).

INTERPLAY BETWEEN CARDIAC AND NONCARDIAC ISSUES

Patients who have postoperative cardiac complications are 6.4-fold more likely to have a variety of noncardiac complications, including wound infections, confusion, respiratory failure, deep venous thrombosis, and bacterial pneumonia (14). These complications also increase postoperative length of stay and increase 3-month mortality about threefold.

PULMONARY ISSUES

Postoperative Atelectasis and Pneumonia

The most common postoperative pulmonary complication is atelectasis, especially after surgery involving the upper abdomen. The consequences of atelectasis include hypoxemia, which can cause myocardial ischemia or stroke, infection, and delayed ambulation. Results are equivalent whether the atelectasis is treated with positive pressure treatment (intermittent positive pressure breathing) or negative pressure treatment (incentive spirometry), and incentive spirometry is much more cost-effective, so it should be instituted as soon as the patient is able to cooperate. Preoperative patient training in the use of incentive spirometry (Chapter 30) will improve performance.

Epidural opioid administration reduces atelectasis compared with systemic opioids. The incidence of pulmonary infections and overall pulmonary complications also appear to decrease.

Perioperative Anticoagulation

A variety of perioperative regimens have been advocated for patients taking preoperative anticoagulants (15). For patients whose chronic international normalized ratio (INR) is maintained between 2 and 3, the warfarin can be held 4 days in advance of surgery to reduce the INR to 1.5 on the day of surgery. For patients who have been on anticoagulants for more than 3 months since the last episode of venous thromboembolism, preoperative heparin is not needed. Although low-molecular-weight heparins are superior to unfractionated heparin in most clinical applications, they should be reserved for patients who are not likely to have significant postsurgical bleeding (such as patients undergoing routine surgery on an extremity) because of their longer half-life and inability to be reversed by protamine (Table 31.1; Chapter 98).

Careful attention should be paid to thromboembolism prophylaxis in the postoperative patient. A sample prophylaxis protocol is included (Figure 31.3).

GASTROINTESTINAL COMPLICATIONS

Postoperative Ileus

Residual effects of anesthetics, especially opioids, decrease motility and delay return of normal bowel function. Other causes of ileus include gut manipulation, denervation, pain, and sympathetic outflow. Ileus after abdominal surgery is usually pronounced for 24–48 hours and resolves over the next 2–3 days. Inability to feed orally due to ileus results in delayed hospital discharge, inadequate nutrition, and increased costs. Laparoscopic surgical techniques markedly decrease the incidence of postoperative ileus. In one randomized study of patients undergoing colorectal resections, patients who had laparoscopic procedures had persistalis first noticed 26 hours after the procedures, compared with 38 hours after the open resections. Furthermore, the first bowel movements occurred 70 hours after laparoscopic surgery versus 91 hours after conventional resection. Finally, oral feedings were tolerated 3.3 days after laparoscopic resections compared with 5 days after open resections (16).

Treatment of ileus should target its underlying cause. If peritonitis has occurred and is caused by a community-acquired infection (i.e., perforated appendix), single agents including ampicillin/sulbactam or ticarcillin/clavulanic acid can be used (17). Postoperative peritoneal infections tend to be caused by more resistant flora, including *Pseudomonas aeruginosa* and methicillin-resistant *Staphylococcus aureus* and *Candida* species. For these nosocomial infections, local nosocomial resistance patterns should dictate empiric treatment, and treatment will need

TABLE 31.1

RECOMMENDATIONS FOR PREOPERATIVE AND POSTOPERATIVE ANTICOAGULATION IN PATIENTS WHO ARE TAKING ORAL ANTICOAGULANTS[a]

Indication	Before surgery	After surgery
Acute venous thromboembolism	IV heparin	IV heparin
Month 1	No change	IV heparin
Months 2 and 3	No change	SC heparin[b]
Recurrent venous thromboembolism	IV heparin	SC heparin
Acute arterial embolism (Month 1)	IV heparin	IV heparin
Mechanical heart valve	No change	SC heparin
Nonvalvular atrial fibrillation	No change	SC heparin

[a] IV heparin denotes intravenous heparin at therapeutic doses; SC denotes subcutaneous.
[b] IV heparin should be used after surgery only if bleeding risk is low.
Consideration should also be given to insertion of an inferior vena caval filter if patient is at high risk for thromboembolism and cannot be anticoagulated. Patients should have daily platelet counts for the first 72 hours after initiation of unfractionated heparin therapy and then every 2–3 days to monitor for heparin-induced thrombocytopenia.
Adapted from Kearon C, Hirsh J. Management of anticoagulation before and after elective surgery. *N Engl J Med* 1997;336:1506–11, with permission.

UC~SF~ Medical Center

Adult Venous Thromboembolism Prophylaxis Order Form
These recommendations are for prophylaxis only, not treatment of acute thromboembolic disease. DO NOT USE THESE GUIDELINES IF THE PATIENT IS RECEIVING THERAPEUTIC ANTICOAGULATION

DATE		*TIME*		ALLERGIES	

1. ASSESSMENT   Check all pertinent risk factors (RFs)

RFs with value of 1 point		
q Age 41-60 years	q Pregnancy, or postpartum < 1 month	**RFs with value of 2 points**
q Prior history of postoperative DVT	q Obesity (>20% over IBW)	q Age 61-70 years
q Family history of DVT or PE	q Hyperviscosity syndromes	q Prior h/o unprovoked/idiopathic DVT
q Leg swelling, ulcers, stasis, varicose veins	q Estrogen therapy	q Major surgery
q MI/CHF		q Malignancy
q Stroke with paralysis		q Multiple trauma
q Inflammatory bowel disease		q Spinal cord injury with paralysis
q Central line		
q Bed confinement / immobilization >12 hours		**RFs with value of 3 points**
q General anesthesia time >2 hours		q Age over 70 years
		q Prior history of PE
		q Inherited thrombophilia
		q Acquired thrombophilia

TOTAL RISK FACTOR **SCORE** (RFS) = _____   (see reverse side for abbreviations and thrombophilia definitions)

2. CONTRAINDICATIONS TO PHARMACOLOGIC PROPHYLAXIS

Relative (check if applicable)	Absolute (check if applicable)
q History of cerebral hemorrhage	q Active hemorrhage
q Craniotomy within 2 weeks	q Heparin or warfarin use in active HIT
q GI, GU hemorrhage within the last 6 months	q Warfarin use in the first trimester of pregnancy
q Thrombocytopenia	q Severe trauma to head, spinal cord or extremities with
q Coagulopathy (PT >18 sec)	hemorrhage within the last 4 weeks
q Active intracranial lesions/neoplasms/monitoring devices	q Epidural/indwelling spinal catheter – placement or removal (see
q Proliferative retinopathy	reverse side)
q Vascular access/biopsy sites inaccessible to hemostatic control	

If contraindications exist to pharmacologic prophylaxis, consider sequential compression devices (SCDs).

3. REGIMENS FOR PROPHYLAXIS[a]

Low Risk (0 RFS)	Moderate Risk (1-2 RFS)	High Risk (3-4 RFS)	Very High Risk (>4 RFS)[b]
• Early ambulation	• LDUH (5000 U) q 8-12 h or	• LDUH (5,000 U) q 8h *or*	• LMWH *or*
	• LMWH *or*	• LMWH *or*	• Warfarin, INR 2-3 *or*
	• SCD	• SCD	• ADH

[a]See reverse side for dosing recommendations
[b]Consider consultation with the Comprehensive Hemostasis and Antithrombotic Service (CHAS) pager 719-4023
ADH = adjusted dose heparin, subcutaneous UFH to achieve aPTT at high range of normal (35 sec) six hours after dose.
ADDITIONAL CONSIDERATIONS
Renal impairment: Use low molecular weight heparins and fondaparinux with <u>caution</u> in patients with a Scr >2 or CrCL <30 mL/min.
Consider dose adjustments for pharmacologic prophylaxis in patients with a weight of < 50 kg. (Fondaparinux should not be used in patients < 50 kg.)
Obesity: Appropriate dosing for obese patients is not well established. Consider CHAS consult.

4. SELECTION OF THROMBOPROPHYLAXIS: (√ in box activates order)

A)   *NON-PHARMACOLOGIC*

q   **Early ambulation:** (Low Thromboembolic Risk)

q   **SCD (Knee High):** (High Bleed Risk) – Send order to Material Services

B)   *PHARMACOLOGIC* -- Send order to Pharmacy

q **Enoxaparin (LMWH)**	q **30 mg SQ Q12H**	q **40 mg SQ Q24H**
q **UFH** →	q **5000 U SQ Q12H**	q **5000 U SQ Q8H**

q   **Other** _____

(Follow CBC with platelets QOD if heparin or LMWH is used. Follow daily INR if warfarin is used.)

Signature _____ M.D.# _____ Time _____ Date _____ Pager _____

FLAG CHART Checked by _____ R.N. Time _____ Date_____

P&T Approved June 2002; Revised 1/17/2003

Figure 31.3   A sample Adult Venous Thromboembolism Prophylaxis order form.

Deep Venous Thrombosis Risk Factor Assessment

1.   Abbreviations:

VTE   venous thromboembolism   **LMWH** low molecular weight heparin
LDUH low dose unfractionated heparin **APLA** antiphospholipid antibody
ADH   adjusted dose heparin   **CHAS** Comprehensive Hemostasis & Antithrombotic Service
SCD   sequential compression device   (pager: 719-4023)
UFH   unfractionated heparin   **RFS**   risk factor score

2.   *Thrombophilia* includes:

Factor V Leiden	Prothrombin variant G20210A
APLA or lupus anticoagulant	Antithrombin III deficiency
Protein C or protein S deficiency	Hyperhomocysteinemia
Heparin induced thrombocytopenia (HIT)	Myeloproliferative disorders (polycythemia vera, essential thrombocytosis (ET))

3.   *Recommendations for the use of antithrombotic prophylaxis in patients with epidural catheters.*
      For patients receiving low-dose SC unfractionated heparin (5000units Q12H)
            Wait 4-6 hours after a prophylactic dose of UFH before placing or removing a catheter
            Initiate UFH thromboprophylaxis 1-2 hours after placing or removing a catheter
            Concurrent use of epidural or spinal catheter and SC low-dose unfractionated heparin is not
            contraindicated.
      For patients receiving prophylactic-dose LMWH
            Wait 24 hours after a prophylactic dose of LMWH before placing a catheter or performing a neuraxial
            block
            Wait 12-24 hours after a prophylactic dose of LMWH before removing a catheter
            Initiate LMWH thromboprophylaxis 2-4 hours after removal of the catheter
            Initiate LMWH thromboprophylaxis 24 hours after a "single shot" spinal procedure
            Concurrent use of an epidural catheter and LMWH thromboprophylaxis needs to be approved by the pain
            service
      For patients receiving fondaparinux
            Extreme caution is warranted given the sustained antithrombotic effect, early postoperative dosing, and
            "irreversibility".
            Until further clinical experience is available, an alternate method of prophylaxis should be utilized.

4.   Dosing recommendations for LMWH and fondaparinux (consider risk factors, caution in patients with renal
      insufficiency - CrCl < 30 mL/min):

Condition	*Recommended Dose
General Surgery	Enoxaparin 40 mg SQ q24h, 1st dose 2 h preop
Gynecologic Surgery	Enoxaparin 40 mg SQ q24h
Urologic Surgery	Enoxaparin 30 mg SQ q12h^c
Major Orthopedic Surgery	Enoxaparin 30 mg SQ q12h, Enoxaparin 40 mg SQ q24h, *or* Fondaparinux 2.5 mg SQ q 24 h start 6 h post-op
Neurosurgery	Enoxaparin 40 mg SQ q24h If pharmacologic prophylaxis is the chosen intervention.
Trauma and Acute Spinal Cord Injury	Enoxaparin 30 mg SQ q12h If pharmacologic prophylaxis is the chosen intervention.
Medical Conditions (e.g. MI, CHF, malignancy)	Enoxaparin 40 mg SQ q24h

For low-risk procedures, early postoperative mobilization may be the prophylactic approach of choice. ^{c}High-risk patients
include those undergoing more extensive, open procedures, including radical prostatectomy, cystectomy, or nephrectomy.

These recommendations are NOT intended to replace an individual clinician's judgment.

P&T Approved June 2002; Revised 1/17/2003

Figure 31.3 (*continued*)

to be altered on the basis of the results of a thorough microbiologic evaluation of infected fluid (18). Therapies for ileus *per se* are nasogastric intubation and decompression, correction of metabolic abnormalities, and intravenous hydration. Neuraxial blockade with epidural bupivacaine accelerates the return of postoperative gastrointestinal function in patients after colon surgery. Prophylactic nasogastric intubation does not appear to be effective and may result in electrolyte abnormalities and dehydration. Parasympathomimetic agents, such as bethanechol and neostigmine, do not appear to decrease the duration of postoperative ileus. These agents are not recommended because of their side effects. Metoclopramide acts as an antiemetic and prokinetic. Although it may decrease nausea and vomiting, it does not appear to decrease the duration of postoperative ileus.

Stress Ulceration

Routine stress ulcer prophylaxis is not recommended prior to surgical procedures. However, critically ill patients are at increased risk for the development of stress ulcers, and stress ulceration should be considered in patients with abdominal discomfort or distention. Prophylaxis is indicated for patients who have thrombocytopenia, increased serum creatinines, liver failure, respiratory failure, and multisystem organ failure (19).

POSTOPERATIVE RENAL FAILURE

In procedures involving the abdominal aorta, cross-clamping the aorta above the renal arteries results in renal ischemia and may lead to acute tubular necrosis. Other patients at risk for postoperative renal insufficiency include those with inadequate intraoperative or postoperative fluid resuscitation, those whose procedures involve large abdominal incisions (insensible fluid losses), or those with massive blood loss. Acute oliguria (urine output of less than 400 mL/day) may be caused by prerenal, renal, and postrenal causes (Table 31.2 and Chapter 100). Acute tubular necrosis from intraoperative renal ischemia may not manifest itself for 24–48 hours. Patients on high doses of opiates may require bladder catheterization to overcome urinary sphincter spasm.

KEY POINTS

- Physicians helping to manage patients postoperatively should maintain close communication with the surgeon and anesthesiologist during the intraoperative and postoperative periods.
- Hypertension and hypotension require immediate attention in postoperative patients because these patients may require urgent re-exploration.
- Aggressive pain management decreases morbidity, cost, and length of hospital stay.
- Patients at risk for perioperative myocardial infarction should be treated with β-blockers throughout the perioperative period.
- Postoperative myocardial infarction often presents without typical chest pain.

TABLE 31.2
ACUTE POSTOPERATIVE OLIGURIA

Prerenal

Decreased preload
  Inadequate fluid resuscitation
  Postoperative surgical/medical hemorrhage
Decreased perfusion pressure
  Myocardial ischemia or infarction
  Vasodilation—sepsis syndrome, pharmacologic, anaphylaxis
  Surgical—renal artery obstruction/thrombosis, emboli

Renal

Acute tubular necrosis—ischemia/reperfusion
Contrast induced nephropathy
Myoglobinuria—post-transfusion reaction
Rhabdomyolysis

Postrenal

Ureteral obstruction/injury
Urinary sphincter spasm—pain, inflammation, opiates

REFERENCES

1. Huddleston JM, Long KH, Naessens JM, et al. Medical and surgical comanagement after elective hip and knee arthroplasty: a randomized, controlled trial. *Ann Intern Med* 2004;141:28–38.
2. van den Berghe G, Wouters P, Weekers F, et al. Intensive insulin therapy in critically ill patients. *N Engl J Med* 2001;345: 1359–1367.
3. Liu LL, Gropper MA. Postoperative analgesia and sedation in the adult intensive care unit. *Drugs* 2003;63:755–767.
4. Wheatley RG, Schug SA, Watson D. Safety and efficacy of postoperative epidural analgesia. *Br J Anaesth* 2001;87:47–61.
5. Block BM, Liu SS, Rowlingson AJ, Cowan AR, Cowan JA Jr, Wu CL. Efficacy of postoperative epidural analgesia: a meta-analysis. *JAMA* 2003;290:2455–2463.
6. Inouye SK, Bogardus ST Jr, Charpentier PA, et al. A multicomponent intervention to prevent delirium in hospitalized older patients. *N Engl J Med* 1999;340:669–676.
7. Kress JP, Pohlman AS, Hall JB. Sedation and analgesia in the intensive care unit. *Am J Respir Crit Care Med* 2002;166:1024–1028.
8. Gan TJ. Postoperative nausea and vomiting—can it be eliminated? *JAMA* 2002;287:1233–1236.
9. Auerbach AD, Goldman L. β-blockers and reduction of cardiac events in noncardiac surgery: scientific review. *JAMA* 2002;287: 1435–1444.
10. Auerbach AD, Goldman L. β-blockers and reduction of cardiac events in noncardiac surgery: clinical applications. *JAMA* 2002; 287:1445–1447.
11. Garcia-Miguel FJ, Serrano-Aguilar PG, Lopez-Bastida J. Preoperative assessment. *Lancet* 2003;362:1749–1757.

12. Wyse DG, Waldo AL, DiMarco JP, et al. A comparison of rate control and rhythm control in patients with atrial fibrillation. *N Engl J Med* 2002;347:1825–1833.

13. Erstad BL, Barletta JF. Treatment of hypertension in the perioperative patient. *Ann Pharmacother* 2000;34:66–79.

14. Fleischmann KE, Goldman L, Young B, Lee TH. Association between cardiac and noncardiac complications in patients undergoing noncardiac surgery: outcomes and effects on length of stay. *Am J Med* 2003;115:515–520.

15. Dunn AS, Turpie AG. Perioperative management of patients receiving oral anticoagulants: a systematic review. *Arch Intern Med* 2003;163:901–908.

16. Schwenk W, Bohm B, Haase O, Junghans T, Muller JM. Laparoscopic versus conventional colorectal resection: A prospective randomised study of postoperative ileus and early postoperative feeding. *Langenbecks Arch Surg* 1998;383:49–55.

17. Solomkin JS, Mazuski JE, Baron EJ, et al. Guidelines for the selection of anti-infective agents for complicated intra-abdominal infections. *Clin Infect Dis* 2003;37:997–1005.

18. Mazuski JE. The Surgical Infection Society guidelines on antimicrobial therapy for intra-abdominal infections: evidence for the recommendations. *Surg Infections* 2002;3:175–233.

19. Cook D, Heyland D, Griffith L, Cook R, Marshall J, Pagliarello J for the Canadian Critical Care Trials Group. Risk factors for clinically important upper gastrointestinal bleeding in patients requiring mechanical ventilation. *Crit Care Med* 1999;27:2812–2817.

ADDITIONAL READING

Chassot PG, Delabays A, Spahn DR. Preoperative evaluation of patients with, or at risk of, coronary artery disease undergoing noncardiac surgery. *Br J Anaesth* 2002;89:747–759.

Manku K, Bacchetti P, Leung JM. Prognostic significance of postoperative in-hospital complications in elderly patients. Long-term survival. *Anesth Analg* 2003;96:583–589.

Mantilla CB, Horlocker TT, Schroeder DR, Berry DJ, Brown DL. Frequency of myocardial infarction, pulmonary embolism, deep venous thrombosis, and death following primary hip or knee arthroplasty, *Anesthesiology* 2002;96:1140–1146.

Pardo M, Gropper MA. Approach to the critically ill patient. In: Parsons P, Wiener-Kronish JP, eds. *Critical Care Secrets.* 2nd ed. Philadelphia: Hanley & Belfus, 2002.

Singri N, Ahya SN, Levin ML. Acute renal failure. *JAMA* 2003; 289:747–751.

Medical Complications of Pregnancy

32

Jeffrey Pickard   *Linda A. Barbour*   *Raymond O. Powrie*

INTRODUCTION

Pregnant women may be hospitalized for medical problems, during which time the hospital physician may be consulted. Before treating a pregnant woman, it is necessary to understand how pregnancy changes the relevant physiology and the way various diseases may present. Diagnosis may be difficult, and treatment may differ from that in the nonpregnant patient. Additionally, diseases specific to pregnancy may complicate evaluation and management.

CARDIAC DISORDERS

In pregnancy, important changes in cardiovascular physiology can alter the normal physical examination and may lead to significant maternal morbidity. By 24–28 weeks' gestation, cardiac output increases by 30%–50%; it then plateaus until delivery. Heart rate may increase slightly but should remain within the normal range. Stroke volume increases with a concomitant decrease in systemic vascular resistance. Blood volume increases by 40%–50%, and red blood cell mass increases by 30%; the result is the "physiologic anemia" of pregnancy. These changes cause the precordial pulse to become stronger and may cause a mild parasternal lift. Both heart sounds are louder and usually split. Up to three-quarters of pregnant women have a third heart sound during the second half of pregnancy. Benign pulmonic or tricuspid flow murmurs are often present, and a venous hum or mammary souffle may be heard occasionally (1).

Pregnancy may unmask or worsen underlying heart disease, especially late in the second trimester, during labor, and immediately postpartum—the three periods in which cardiac demand peaks. Regurgitant murmurs usually are well tolerated, whereas mitral and aortic stenosis may lead to pulmonary edema. Moderate to severe pulmonary hypertension of any cause is associated with a significant maternal mortality rate. Patients with Marfan syndrome who have a dilated aortic root are at risk for aortic dissection (1). Ischemic cardiac disease also is tolerated poorly during pregnancy and often leads to myocardial infarction. However, 30%–50% of myocardial infarctions during pregnancy are caused by coronary dissection and occur in women without underlying coronary disease. Virtually any relevant diagnostic or therapeutic procedure, including catheterization, angioplasty, and stenting, may be done during pregnancy.

Palpitations are common during pregnancy but sometimes represent significant tachyarrhythmias. Adenosine, calcium-channel blockers, β-blockers, and digoxin all may be used in the evaluation and treatment of these rhythm disturbances, as may cardioversion if the mother is hemodynamically unstable (2). Of the remaining antiarrhythmics, amiodarone may expose the fetus to unacceptably high iodine levels and therefore should be used only if all others have been ineffective. Cardiopulmonary resuscitation can be performed successfully during pregnancy and is likely to be more successful if the uterus is pulled to the left side to avoid compression of the inferior vena cava.

Pulmonary edema may present in a previously healthy pregnant woman because of marked volume shifts and decreased plasma oncotic pressure, especially in the setting of tocolytics (decreased filling time), preeclampsia (leaky capillaries), or large fluid boluses during epidural anesthesia. Pulmonary edema that does not reverse rapidly with diuretics may indicate that the patient has *peripartum cardiomyopathy*, which may present at any time between the third trimester and 6 months postpartum. Echocardiography reveals global myocardial hypokinesis. At least one third of patients with peripartum cardiomyopathy go on to suffer progressive heart failure.

RESPIRATORY DISORDERS

Pregnant women increase their minute ventilation because of a progesterone-stimulated increase in tidal volume. The increased minute ventilation lowers the normal arterial partial pressure of carbon dioxide to between 30–35 mm Hg, and a concomitant lowering of the serum bicarbonate results in a compensated respiratory alkalosis. Maternal arterial partial pressure of oxygen should be kept above 60 mm Hg at all times to avoid fetal distress.

Shortness of breath is a common complaint among pregnant women (Table 32.1). Dyspnea of pregnancy is a benign process. The pathophysiology is unclear but is thought to be related to progesterone, which stimulates the increase in tidal volume. It occurs in up to 70% of all pregnant women and resolves spontaneously after delivery if not before.

The treatment of asthma during pregnancy differs little from its treatment outside pregnancy (Chapter 56), and acute asthma exacerbations should be treated as if the woman were not pregnant (3,4). Inhaled β-agonists are used as first-line therapy for mild, intermittent asthma, whereas inhaled steroids are considered first-line therapy for all other types. In general, betamethasone and budesonide are preferred because of their safety record during pregnancy. Experience with fluticasone and flunisolide in pregnancy is limited, but they may be used, if necessary, to control maternal symptoms. Theophylline has an unparalleled safety profile during pregnancy and is an excellent choice as a second-line or third-line agent; serum levels should be kept between 8–12 mg/mL to minimize

TABLE 32.1

CAUSES OF SHORTNESS OF BREATH IN PREGNANCY

Pulmonary
  Pulmonary embolism
  Pneumonia
  Asthma
  Adult respiratory distress syndrome
  Pulmonary hypertension
  Pulmonary edema
Cardiac
  Valvular heart disease
  Peripartum cardiomyopathy
  Myocardial infarction
  Right-to-left intracardiac shunt
Other
  Dyspnea of pregnancy

effects on the fetus. Leukotriene inhibitors should be avoided at present because there are no safety data regarding their use during pregnancy. Intravenous methylprednisolone and oral prednisone do not cross the placenta to any significant degree and are considered safe for the fetus, although there may be an extremely small risk of cleft palates in infants exposed to prednisone during the first trimester.

HYPERTENSIVE DISORDERS

Hypertension, the most common medical problem seen in pregnancy, is the most important risk factor for the development of *preeclampsia.* Preeclampsia occurs in 5%–10% of all pregnancies and in 20% of women with chronic hypertension regardless of blood pressure control. Blood pressure usually decreases by 10–15 mm Hg during the first two trimesters but returns to prepregnancy levels near term. Pressures above 140/90 in the third trimester suggest either preeclampsia or previously unrecognized chronic hypertension (5).

The main symptoms of preeclampsia are visual disturbances (scintillations or scotomas), headaches, epigastric discomfort, edema (especially in the hands or face), and rapid weight gain. Signs of preeclampsia include hypertension, retinal vasospasm, hepatic tenderness, facial and hand edema, and hyperreflexia. Blood pressure greater than 140/90 or a rise of more than 30 mm Hg systolic or 15 mm Hg diastolic from baseline is considered abnormal and suggests the development of preeclampsia. Laboratory manifestations of preeclampsia include hemoconcentration, thrombocytopenia, proteinuria (>300 mg/dL over 24 hours), elevated creatinine level (>0.8 mg/dL in pregnancy), and hyperuricemia (>5 mg/dL in pregnancy). The *HELLP syndrome* is a severe form of preeclampsia in which *h*emolysis, *e*levated *l*iver-enzyme level, and *l*ow *p*latelet count occur; urgent delivery is indicated to protect mother and baby.

Women on antihypertensive medication at the time of conception generally can continue their medications during pregnancy (Table 32.2). However, *angiotensin-converting enzyme inhibitors and angiotensin receptor blockers are contraindicated* because they are associated with neonatal renal failure and death, as well as with pulmonary hypoplasia (5). Diuretic therapy may be continued during pregnancy but generally is not initiated once a woman becomes pregnant. Because β-blockers may cause intrauterine growth restriction if used throughout gestation, they are considered third-line or fourth-line agents. Treatment of mild hypertension first noted during pregnancy is controversial because there is no evidence that treatment benefits either the mother or the baby (6). Treatment should be initiated if the diastolic pressure exceeds 100 mm Hg or the systolic pressure exceeds 160 mm Hg. The goal of therapy is a diastolic pressure between 80–90 mm Hg.

TABLE 32.2

ANTIHYPERTENSIVE MEDICATIONS USED DURING PREGNANCY

Drug	Oral dose	Parenteral dose	Comments
Atenolol	50–100 mg/d	—	Intrauterine growth restriction a concern
Clonidine	0.1–0.3 mg b.i.d.	—	Used infrequently
Hydralazine	10–100 mg b.i.d.	5–10 mg intravenous/intramuscular q20–30 min; continuous infusion 0.5–10 mg/h	Safe; useful in hypertensive emergency; second line in chronic hypertension
Labetalol	100–300 mg b.i.d.	20 mg intravenous; then 20–80 mg q20 min; max 300 mg; continuous infusion 1–2 mg/min; at target blood pressure, stop or reduce to 0.5 mg/min	Gaining popularity in both chronic and urgent hypertension during pregnancy
Methyldopa	250–1,500 mg b.i.d. or t.i.d. (max 3,000 mg/d)	—	Safest antihypertensive in pregnancy
Metoprolol	50–200 mg b.i.d.	—	Intrauterine growth restriction a concern
Nifedipine	30–120 mg/d	—	Appears safe; no first-trimester data
Nitroprusside	—	0.5–10 mcg/kg/min continuous infusion	Risk of fetal cyanide toxicity if used longer than 24 h

Physicians other than obstetricians may become acutely involved in the care of a pregnant woman if preeclampsia becomes severe or eclampsia (seizure) supervenes. In contrast to nonpregnant patients, eclamptic seizures are best treated with intravenous magnesium sulfate given as a 6-gram load over 20–30 minutes in a 5% dextrose solution, followed by 2–4 grams per hour continuous infusion. Serum magnesium levels should be assessed (range 4.8–8.4 mg/dL), and calcium gluconate should be administered to reverse any magnesium toxicity (cardiac or respiratory depression) (7).

Blood pressure usually is elevated in severe preeclampsia/eclampsia. Target blood pressure should be around 150/100. However, treatment of the blood pressure has no effect on preeclampsia per se, so patients whose blood pressures are not elevated do not need antihypertensive medication. Aggressive blood-pressure reduction (systolic <140 mm Hg, diastolic <90 mm Hg) should be avoided because of the risk of uteroplacental hypoperfusion. Severe hypotension may occur if calcium-channel blockers are used concurrently with magnesium sulfate. Women with severe preeclampsia are at risk for pulmonary edema because of cardiomyopathy and pulmonary capillary leak. Intravenous fluids should be monitored carefully, and diuretics are required if pulmonary edema develops. Intracerebral hemorrhage may occur, as may oliguric renal failure, even in the absence of severe hypertension. Liver dysfunction of any severity also may complicate severe preeclampsia or eclampsia and should be differentiated from acute fatty liver of pregnancy. Other conditions in the differential diagnosis include systemic lupus erythematosus (Chapter 112) and hemolytic uremic syndrome/thrombotic thrombocytopenic purpura (Chapter 98). Preeclampsia may worsen or arise *de novo* within the first week postpartum despite the fact that delivery of the baby is the only definitive treatment of this potentially life-threatening disorder.

GASTROINTESTINAL DISORDERS

As pregnancy progresses, changes in gastrointestinal physiology presage the relevant problems seen in pregnant women. Lower esophageal sphincter tone and esophageal peristalsis diminish, increasing the likelihood of gastroesophageal reflux disease (8). Antacids, sucralfate, cimetidine, and ranitidine may be used as necessary during pregnancy. Experience with proton pump inhibitors, especially omeprazole, is growing, and they appear to be safe. Transit time through the gastrointestinal tract is prolonged, and nausea, vomiting, and constipation all are seen more frequently in women who are pregnant. Metoclopramide and prochlorperazine are safe to use. Occasionally nausea and vomiting become severe and prolonged (*hyperemesis gravidarum*) and require hospital admission. Hyperthyroidism, with depressed thyroid stimulating hormone (TSH) and elevated free thyroxine levels, often coexists with hyperemesis gravidarum due to the thyrotropic activity of human chorionic gonadotropin, but it usually is transient and rarely requires treatment.

During pregnancy, gallbladder volume increases, and emptying becomes sluggish; as a result, bile becomes more lithogenic. Biliary "sludge" occurs in up to 30% of pregnancies. Gallstones occur in 2%–4%, but intervention during gestation is required in less than 0.1% of all pregnancies. If intervention becomes necessary, it should be done during the second trimester, if possible, to minimize the likelihood of spontaneous abortion and fetal malformations (first trimester) and of premature labor and delivery (third trimester). Endoscopic retrograde cholangiopancreatography and cholecystectomy (open and laparoscopic) have been performed safely during pregnancy (Chapter 84).

The diagnosis of abdominal pain during pregnancy may be difficult because the expanding uterus may alter the location and presentation of common causes. In addition, diseases specific to pregnancy may present with abdominal pain (Table 32.3).

Acute fatty liver of pregnancy is an uncommon (1 in 13,000 deliveries) but serious disease characterized by fatty infiltration of the liver, hepatic failure, and encephalopathy developing in the third trimester. The mortality rate is approximately 20%. Acute fatty liver usually occurs after 34 weeks' gestation, and patients present with anorexia, nausea, vomiting, malaise, and right upper quadrant pain; it often is confused with HELLP. Abnormal laboratory values may include anemia with evidence of hemolysis, leukocytosis, increased uric acid, renal insufficiency, elevated liver aminotransferases (aspartate aminotransferase >alanine aminotransferase), prolonged prothrombin time, hyperbilirubinemia, and hypoglycemia (<60 mg/dL). There may be signs of fetal distress. Treatment includes supportive care for the mother (Chapter 82) and prompt delivery of the baby.

Inflammatory bowel disease (Chapter 81) is relatively common during childbearing years. If quiescent at conception, it usually remains so during gestation. Steroids, sulfasalazine, mesalamine, azathioprine, and mercaptopurine all have been used safely during pregnancy. Metronidazole also is considered safe, although some recommend delaying its use until after the first trimester.

Intrahepatic cholestasis of pregnancy (ICP) is a disease characterized by severe pruritis without a skin rash, generally starting in the palms and soles and progressing centripetally (9). It usually occurs during the third trimester.

TABLE 32.3

ABDOMINAL PAIN DURING PREGNANCY

Acute hepatitis from alcohol or toxins
Cholecystitis/cholelithiasis
Ureterolithiasis
Peptic ulcer disease (rare)
Pulmonary embolus
Pneumonia (especially right lower lobe)
Pancreatitis
Pyelonephritis
Appendicitis
Diabetic ketoacidosis
Acute fatty liver of pregnancy
Preeclampsia
HELLP syndrome

Aminotransferases and bilirubin are usually (60%) moderately elevated, but severe hyperbilirubinemia and jaundice are relatively uncommon (25%). Although the maternal course is usually benign, ICP may lead to preterm birth, fetal distress, and fetal demise. Delivery should occur as soon as fetal lungs are mature, usually by 37 weeks (9,10).

DIABETIC KETOACIDOSIS

Pregnant women with diabetes are at increased risk for ketoacidosis throughout gestation, but the risk increases significantly during the latter half of pregnancy. Because of the "accelerated starvation" that characterizes pregnancy and the decreased buffering capacity of maternal serum, diabetic ketoacidosis in a pregnant woman may occur with near-normal glucose levels (11). Therefore, a pregnant woman with diabetes admitted to the hospital because of intractable emesis should be evaluated for diabetic ketoacidosis regardless of her serum glucose. Pregnant women during the second and third trimesters require an additional 100–150 grams of glucose daily to meet the metabolic demands of the fetus and placenta (12). These women may require a 10% glucose infusion to provide adequate carbohydrates until oral intake can be resumed. Otherwise, fat will be burned for fuel, and ketosis will persist (13). Pregnant women with diabetes are also more susceptible to infections, especially of the urinary tract, which also can trigger diabetic ketoacidosis. Pregnancy does not change the recommended treatment of diabetic ketoacidosis (Chapter 107).

THYROTOXICOSIS IN PREGNANCY

Thyroid storm is a life-threatening condition to both mother and fetus. It usually develops in an inadequately treated woman with severe thyrotoxicosis who is subjected to additional physiologic stress such as severe infection, preeclampsia, induction of anesthesia, labor, or surgery (14). The incidence of thyroid storm during pregnancy is estimated at 1%–2% of women with preexisting hyperthyroidism and usually presents with severe symptoms of thyrotoxicosis, fever over 101° F, altered mental status, congestive heart failure, tachyarrhythmias, nausea and vomiting, diarrhea, or abdominal pain. Initial treatment is the same as in the nonpregnant patient. Cold iodide (e.g., Lugol solution, 10 drops every 8 hours, or saturated solution of potassium iodide, three drops every 8 hours) can be administered to the pregnant woman in thyroid storm to diminish the release of thyroid hormone but should be given 1–2 hours after propylthiouracil (15). Iodide can cause fetal goiter, but this is rare if the iodide is given for no more than 3 days. Esmolol (0.25 mg/kg intravenously over 1 minute, then 0.05–0.1 mg/kg/min infusion) and propranolol (20–60 mg orally every 6 hours) can be used to control maternal heart rate, but blood pressure must be carefully monitored. Hydrocortisone (100 mg every 8 hours) can help maintain maternal blood pressure. It diminishes the peripheral conversion of thyroxine to triiodothyronine (T_4 to T_3) and does not cross the placenta to any appreciable degree (Chapter 108).

THROMBOEMBOLISM

A pregnant woman is 5–10 times more likely to develop venous thromboembolism (VTE) than when she is not pregnant, and pulmonary embolism is a leading cause of maternal death (16,17). This hypercoagulable state exists throughout all three trimesters and persists until 4–6 weeks postpartum. Deep venous thrombosis is most common in the left lower extremity because of the vascular anatomy. It occurs antepartum and postpartum with equal frequency, and antepartum events are evenly distributed throughout gestation. Pulmonary embolism is more likely to occur postpartum, primarily because cesarean section increases the risk of pelvic-vein thrombosis. Other risk factors for thrombosis include previous thrombosis, obesity, venous insufficiency, prolonged bedrest, older age and higher parity, ovarian hyperstimulation, and underlying hypercoagulable states (17). Approximately 50% of pregnant women with thrombosis have a predisposing cause of thrombophilia, the most common being the factor V Leiden mutation or the prothrombin gene mutation (18) (Chapter 98).

It is critical to make the diagnosis of deep venous thrombosis or pulmonary embolism definitively because the diagnosis mandates the use of subcutaneous heparin throughout the remainder of the current and all future pregnancies and usually contraindicates the future use of oral contraceptives. The diagnostic approach should be similar to recommendations in the nonpregnant patient (Chapters 52 and 53); of note is that venography, if necessary, is safe during pregnancy (<0.05 rad) (19). D-dimers increase during pregnancy, and their predictive value for the diagnosis of VTE during pregnancy is unknown. The diagnosis of pulmonary embolism may be missed clinically during pregnancy, in part because the alveolar–arterial oxygen gradient is often normal, perhaps reflecting a younger population with greater pulmonary reserve. Ventilation–perfusion scanning is completely safe during pregnancy (<0.02 rad), but the interpretation is often not definitive. Helical computed tomography exposes the fetus to no more radiation than ventilation-perfusion scanning as long as the fetus can be kept out of the scanning field (20). Pulmonary angiography can be done without significant radiation to the fetus (<0.5 rad) and is recommended if there is any doubt regarding the diagnosis after computed tomography or ventilation-perfusion scanning (21). Magnetic resonance imaging may be used if pelvic vein thrombosis is suspected, but the utility and safety of other diagnostic modalities have not been adequately established.

The treatment of acute thromboembolism during pregnancy requires intravenous anticoagulation with heparin for 5 days. Subcutaneous heparin then should be given every 8–12 hours for 3–6 months after the acute event, keeping the partial thromboplastin time 1.5 times the control value throughout the dosing interval. After the patient receives at least 3 months of therapeutic anticoagulation, heparin doses of at least 10,000 units twice daily should be continued until term. Heparin requirements increase throughout pregnancy because of increased clearance, expanded plasma volume, increased protein binding, and degradation by the placenta. Upward dosage adjustments are often necessary in the second and third trimesters. Because of the increased levels of fibrinogen and factor VIII during pregnancy, some women will appear to be heparin resistant on the basis of monitoring with the activated partial thromboplastin time (aPTT). Anti-factor Xa levels (0.3–0.6 IU/ml throughout the dosing interval) may be used to guide therapy in these women (22). Heparin-induced thrombocytopenia (HIT) is rare during gestation (23), but women who develop HIT during pregnancy may be treated with danaproid sodium, which does not appear to cross the placenta (24). *Warfarin is relatively contraindicated during pregnancy because of the risk of both fetal bleeding and malformation.* Warfarin is safe to use during breastfeeding and may be used once the baby is delivered; it should be continued for at least 4–6 weeks postpartum because women remain hypercoagulable until then. Low-molecular-weight heparin does not cross the placenta, but dosing requirements during pregnancy have not been determined. If low-molecular-weight heparin is used to treat acute thromboembolism, anti-factor Xa levels should be monitored, and the dose should be adjusted to maintain peak anti-factor Xa levels between 0.5 and 1.2 IU/mL using twice-daily dosing (22). Thrombolytic therapy should be reserved for life-threatening situations because of the significant risk of maternal hemorrhage, preterm delivery, and fetal loss.

RENAL DISORDERS

During pregnancy, the increase in cardiac output and blood volume results in an increase in renal plasma flow; the glomerular filtration rate rises to 150–180 mL/min. Serum creatinine levels typically fall, so a serum creatinine of greater than 0.8 mg/dL is considered abnormal, as is a blood urea nitrogen level of greater than 14 mg/dL. Urinary protein excretion increases to 300 mg/d, and patients with underlying proteinuria may develop nephrotic range proteinuria (>3.5 gm/24 hours) during pregnancy. Renal compensation for the normal hyperventilation of pregnancy results in a serum bicarbonate fall of approximately 4 mEq/L. The influence of progesterone and the mechanical compression of the ureters and bladder by the gravid uterus result in a normal hydronephrosis of pregnancy, most notably on the right side. Both urinary stasis and reflux may increase as the ureters dilate, and they predispose the pregnant woman to pyelonephritis (mostly right-sided) and stone formation (Chapters 68 and 103) (25).

In addition to the usual nonobstetric causes of acute renal failure, severe preeclampsia, acute fatty liver of pregnancy, and postpartum hemorrhage are causes unique to pregnancy. Idiopathic postpartum renal failure may be pathophysiologically related to hemolytic uremic syndrome and thrombotic thrombocytopenic purpura (8). Renal biopsy should be performed, if necessary, prior to the third trimester. Hemodialysis and peritoneal dialysis can treat renal failure successfully during pregnancy. Dialysis should be performed earlier (blood urea nitrogen level > 60 mg/dL) and more often than in the nonpregnant patient because a blood urea nitrogen level greater than 80 mg/dL is toxic to the fetus. More frequent dialysis also reduces the need to remove large volumes of fluid and the resulting risk of hypotension and uteroplacental hypoperfusion.

Women who have had renal transplants (Chapter 102) usually maintain normal renal function during pregnancy and normally have no evidence of graft rejection. Prednisolone crosses the placenta to only a minimal degree and does not appear to adversely affect the fetus. Azathioprine crosses the placenta, but the fetal liver lacks the activating enzyme, so the fetus is protected from its effects. Cyclosporine does not appear to cause congenital anomalies but may be associated with fetuses that are small for gestational age. Experience with tacrolimus and mycophenolate mofetil is extremely limited during gestation, and these immunosuppressives are generally avoided during pregnancy (26,27).

CEREBROVASCULAR DISORDERS

Cerebrovascular disorders account for 8%–12% of all maternal deaths, and about 35% of all strokes that occur in women of childbearing age occur during pregnancy. Strokes may occur at any time from the second trimester through the first 4–6 weeks postpartum. *Cerebral venous thrombosis*, however, almost always occurs during the first 4 weeks postpartum in association with cesarean section, dehydration, hypercoagulable states, infection, or hyperviscosity.

Over 90% of headaches during pregnancy are migraine or "tension-type." Approximately two-thirds to three-quarters of women with chronic migraine report that their headaches improve or stay the same during gestation. Nevertheless, cerebral aneurysms and arteriovenous malformations (Chapter 117) may be more likely to bleed during pregnancy or postpartum. Women with new onset of severe headaches during pregnancy, especially with aura or mental-status changes, should be evaluated carefully (Table 32.4). Appropriate imaging studies such as computed tomography

TABLE 32.4

CAUSES OF "ABNORMAL" HEADACHES IN PREGNANCY

Hemorrhagic stroke
   Eclampsia
   Hypertensive encephalopathy
   Aneurysms
   Arteriovenous malformation
Nonhemorrhagic stroke
   Eclampsia
   Hypertensive encephalopathy
   Cardioembolism
   Thrombosis resulting from thrombophilia
   Illicit drugs
Cerebral venous thrombosis
   Dehydration
   Infection
   Hypercoagulable states
   Hyperviscosity
Other
   Pseudotumor cerebri
   Illicit drugs
   Tumor

with or without contrast or magnetic resonance imaging or angiography may be done safely during pregnancy and should be used to aid the diagnosis if necessary. Treatment of headaches during pregnancy should start with simple analgesics. Opiates may be used, if necessary, but should be limited to short-term use because they cross the placenta. Benzodiazepines and ergots generally are avoided during pregnancy, as is sumatriptan (although some believe that sumatriptan may be used in selected women [28]). β-blockers may be used if prophylaxis is indicated.

The treatment of epileptic seizures (Chapter 118) during pregnancy is generally the same as in the nonpregnant patient. Seizures that occur for the first time during the third trimester should be considered eclamptic until proven otherwise. If the seizures do not respond to magnesium sulfate, underlying stroke may be causing the epilepsy.

FEVER

Fever in a pregnant woman commonly indicates an infection, with a spectrum of infections similar to that in the nonpregnant woman. However, aspiration pneumonia and acute sinusitis are more common in the pregnant woman. Listeria infections can cause significant fetal injury and death unless treated promptly with penicillin or ampicillin (Chapter 70).

Pregnant women also are prone to urinary tract infections and pyelonephritis (Chapter 68), which must be treated aggressively to prevent sepsis. Most of the antibiotics used to treat these infections, including sulfa drugs and aminoglycosides, are safe during pregnancy. Quinolones have been used safely in a limited number of pregnant women despite initial reports that they impair cartilage formation in dogs. *Tetracyclines should be avoided after the first trimester* (29).

Endometritis and septic pelvic thrombophlebitis are important causes of postpartum fever. Endometritis is a polymicrobial infection with genitourinary pathogens such as *Streptococcus, Enterobacteriaceae,* and *Bacteroides* species, especially if the infection begins within the first 48 hours postpartum. Women who remain febrile despite what should be appropriate antibiotic therapy are often felt to have septic pelvic thrombophlebitis, even though blood clots usually are not found despite appropriate imaging studies. The recommended treatment for septic pelvic thrombophlebitis is empiric intravenous heparin, but there are no controlled studies to confirm its efficacy.

KEY POINTS

- Pregnancy causes significant cardiac stress that may unmask or worsen underlying heart disease.
- Severe preeclampsia or eclampsia causes significant injury and death and requires aggressive management. Eclamptic seizures are treated differently from epileptic seizures, so the diagnosis of seizures during pregnancy must be accurate.
- Diabetic ketoacidosis during pregnancy may present with glucose levels of less than 200 mg/dL.
- Thromboembolism is five times more common in pregnancy. All relevant imaging studies should be performed to ascertain the diagnosis because the amount of radiation to the fetus is well below that which is still considered safe.
- Most antibiotics, including penicillins, sulfa drugs, and aminoglycosides are safe during pregnancy. Tetracyclines should be avoided after the first trimester.

REFERENCES

1. Gei AF, Hankins GD. Cardiac disease and pregnancy. *Obstet Gynecol Clin North Am* 2001;28:465–512.
2. Pearson GD, Veille JC, Rahimtoola S, et al. Peripartum cardiomyopathy: National Heart, Lung, and Blood Institute and Office of Rare Diseases (National Institutes of Health) workshop recommendations and review. *JAMA* 2000;283:1183–1188.
3. Wendel PJ. Asthma in pregnancy. *Obstet Gynecol Clin North Am* 2001;28:537–551.
4. Luskin AT. An overview of the recommendations of the Working Group on Asthma and Pregnancy. National Asthma Education and Prevention Program. *J Allergy Clin Immunol* 1999;103(2 Pt 2):S350–S353.
5. Report of the National High Blood Pressure Education Program. Working group on high blood pressure in pregnancy. *Am J Obstet Gynecol* 2000;183:S1–S22.
6. Magee LA. Drugs in pregnancy. Antihypertensives. *Best Pract Res Clin Obstet Gynaecol* 2001;15:827–845.
7. Magpie Trial Collaboration Group. Do women with pre-eclampsia, and their babies, benefit from magnesium sulphate? The magpie trial: a randomised placebo-controlled trial. *Lancet* 2002; 359:1877–1890.
8. Winbery SL, Blaho KE. Dyspepsia in pregnancy. *Obstet Gyncol Clin North Am* 2001;28:333–350.
9. Mullally BA, Hansen WF. Intrahepatic cholestasis of pregnancy: review of the literature. *Obstet Gynecol Surv* 2002;57:47–52.
10. Milkiewicz P, Elias E, Williamson C, et al. Obstetric cholestasis: may have serious consequences for the fetus, and needs to be taken seriously. *BMJ* 2002;324:123–124.
11. Ramin KD. Diabetic ketoacidosis in pregnancy. *Obstet Gynecol Clin North Am* 1999;26:481–487.
12. Aldoretta PW, Hay WW. Metabolic substrates for fetal energy metabolism and growth. *Clin Perinatol* 1995;22:15–35.
13. Whiteman VE, Homdo CJ, Reece EA. Management of hypoglycemia and diabetic ketoacidosis in pregnancy. *Obstet Gynecol Clin North Am* 1996;23:87–107.
14. Masiukiewicz US, Burrow GN. Hyperthyroidism in pregnancy: diagnosis and treatment. *Thyroid* 1999;9:647–652.
15. Mestman J. Hyperthyroidism in pregnancy. *Clinical Obstet Gynecol* 1997;40:45–64.
16. Lindqvist P, Dahlback B, Marsal K. Thrombotic risk during pregnancy: a population study. *Obstet Gynecol* 1999;94:595–599.
17. Lockwood CJ. Inherited thrombophilias in pregnant patients: detection and treatment paradigm. *Obstet Gynecol* 2002;99:333–341.
18. Witlin AG, Mattar FM, Saade GR. Presentation of venous thromboembolism during pregnancy. *Am J Obstet Gynecol* 1999;181: 1118–1121.
19. Douketis JD, Ginsberg JS. Diagnostic problems with venous thromboembolic disease in pregnancy. *Haemostasis* 1995;25:58–71.
20. Winer-Muram HT, Boone HL, Jennings SG, et al. Pulmonary embolism in pregnant patients: fetal radiation dose with helical CT. *Radiology* 2002;224:487–492.
21. Spritzer CE, Evans AC, Kay HH. Magnetic resonance imaging of deep venous thrombosis in pregnant women with lower extremity edema. *Obstet Gynecol* 1995;85:603–607.
22. Bates SM, Greer IA, Hirsh J, et al. Use of antithrombotic agents during pregnancy: the seventh ACCP conference on antithrombotic and thrombolytic therapy. *Chest* 2004;126(3 suppl): 627s–644s.
23. Fausett MB, Vogtlander M, Lee RM. Heparin-induced thrombocytopenia is rare in pregnancy. *Am J Obstet Gynecol* 2001;185: 148–152.
24. Magnani HN. Heparin-induced thrombocytopenia (HIT): an overview of 230 patients treated with orgaran (Org10172). *Thromb Haemost* 1993;70:554–561.
25. Sanders CL, Lucas MJ. Medical complications of pregnancy. *Obstet Gyncol Clin* 2001;28:593–600.
26. Hou S. Pregnancy in chronic renal insufficiency and end-stage renal disease. *Am J Kidney Dis* 1999;33:235–252.
27. Davison JM. Renal disorders in pregnancy. *Curr Opin Obstet Gynecol* 2001;13:109–114.
28. Von Wald T, Walling AD. Headache during pregnancy. *Obstet Gynecol Surv* 2002;57:179–185.
29. Dashe JS, Gilstrap LC. Antibiotic use in pregnancy. *Obstet Gynecol Clin North Am* 1997;24:617–629.

ADDITIONAL READING

Barbour LA. ACOG Practice Bulletin. *Clinical Guidelines for Obstetricians and Gynecologists. Thromboembolism in Pregnancy,* Number 19, August 2000.

Barbour LA, Oja L, Schultz LK. A prospective trial that demonstrates that dalteparin requirements increase in pregnancy to maintain therapeutic levels of anticoagulation. *Am J Obstet Gynecol* 2004;191:1024–1029.

Gei AF, Hankins GD. Cardiac disease and pregnancy. *Obstet Gynecol Clin* 2001;28:465–512.

Holmes LB, Harvey EA, Coull BA, et al. The teratogenicity of anticonvulsant drugs. *N Engl J Med* 2001;344:1132–1138.

Koren G, Pastuszak A, Ito S. Drugs in pregnancy. *N Engl J Med* 1998;338:1128–1137.

Lee RV, Rosene-Montella K, Barbour LA, et al., eds. *Medical Care of the Pregnant Patient.* Philadelphia: American College of Physicians–American Society of Internal Medicine, 2000.

Watts DH. Management of human immunodeficiency virus infection in pregnancy. *N Engl J Med* 2002;346:1879–1891.

Care of Special Populations: Psychiatry

David F. Gitlin   Bernard Vaccaro

INTRODUCTION

Patients with primary or secondary psychiatric disorders commonly present to general hospitals for either psychiatric or medical care. Patients with previously known psychiatric conditions, such as schizophrenia or bipolar disorder, are often a challenge for the nonpsychiatrist with little previous exposure to these illnesses. In fact, these patients may be at greater risk of medical illness than the general population because of decreased self-care, limited access to medical care, and poor compliance with outpatient treatment. Hospital management of these patients should focus on the medical condition. However, additional attention to the comorbid psychiatric illness may be necessary if it complicates or interferes with medical management. Psychiatric medications may require adjustment in the setting of acute renal or hepatic insufficiency or because of potential drug interactions.

Patients without primary mental disorders may demonstrate acute neuropsychiatric symptoms in the hospital. An array of medical illnesses, such as myocardial infarction, stroke, or infections, may disrupt brain function and lead to delirium. Patients may develop acute anxiety or profound depressive mood because of uncertainty about their condition or concern about prognosis. Recognizing and addressing these psychiatric sequelae are essential for the optimal care of all patients.

Finally, some patients may have conditions bordering between medicine and psychiatry. Such patients may present with a variety of somatic complaints, but appropriate evaluation demonstrates no organic etiology. For many patients, a "psychosomatic" condition may exist. Hospital physicians must confront the challenge of understanding such a condition in patients whom they may never have seen before.

DEPRESSION

Depression is perhaps the most common psychiatric condition seen in the general hospital. Appropriate assessment and effective management are the hallmarks of care. Inadequate diagnosis or treatment occurs in over 50% of patients, however, and may result in serious results such as suicide. For a complete discussion of depression, see Chapter 119.

SUICIDE

Suicide, the most common and serious psychiatric emergency, is frequently seen in general hospital EDs and medical services. Suicide is the eighth leading cause of death in the United States, with a rate of 10–13 deaths/100,000 deaths each year. Suicide is the second leading cause of death in teens and young adults ages 15–24. Whites are twice as likely as nonwhites to commit suicide, men are more than four times as likely as women to kill themselves, and the highest suicide rate (41/100,000, or four times the general population) is seen in elderly men (1).

Over 90% of individuals who complete suicide have a psychiatric disorder, most commonly a depressive illness. Higher rates of suicide are also seen with schizophrenia, bipolar disorders, substance abuse disorders, and possibly anxiety and personality disorders. Approximately 20% of completed suicides are accompanied by medical illnesses, and the suicide rate increases with more severe or chronic conditions (1). Fifty percent of individuals who commit suicide saw a physician in the month before the event, but most did not identify their suicidal thoughts directly to the physician. Thus, assessment and management of suicidal risk are critical skills for the hospital physician.

Identification of suicidal potential and the acute management of suicidal behavior are the cornerstones of care for the hospital physician. Some patients will present with primary psychiatric derangements, including agitation, withdrawn behavior, poor self-care, psychosis, and overt suicidal intentions. Patients should be questioned about active suicidal behaviors, and appropriate medical interventions must be taken if overdose or self-inflicted injuries have occurred. The physician must assess suicidal risk and, if it is present, provide a safe and effective treatment environment, which should include the following:

1. *Location* in a secured setting, devoid of objects that the patient might use for self-harm.
2. *A search* of the individual for potentially dangerous objects, such as guns, knives, razor blades, and so on, and for medications that might be used in an overdose attempt. This search should be completed in a timely but, when possible, respectful manner.
3. *Constant observation* by staff.
4. *Physical and/or chemical restraint only as a last resort* in patients whose behavior cannot be adequately controlled with less-restrictive means.

For other patients, the risk of suicide may not be obvious. Patients with new illnesses or diagnoses or with further deterioration of a chronic medical condition may feel overwhelmed and hopeless. Physicians should be alert to signs and symptoms of depression, anxiety, and hopelessness, all of which increase the risk of suicidal ideation. Patients with organic brain disorders, such as delirium, dementia, and traumatic brain injury, may have increased impulsivity and behavioral dysregulation, which may lead to self-injurious behaviors. Asking patients about self-destructive thoughts and intents is the best way to identify patients at risk.

Once a potential risk is identified, it is important to request consultation from the hospital mental health staff, preferably an emergency or consultation-liaison psychiatrist. The psychiatrist will help in the assessment and acute management of underlying psychiatric disorders as well as provide expertise about the potential risk of suicide. The psychiatrist is typically the physician who will determine the appropriate level of care for the patient, including but not limited to psychiatric hospitalization, and help establish proper treatment and follow-up planning. Whenever possible, rapid access to a 24/7 hospital-based psychiatric consultation service is advantageous for effectively managing acutely suicidal individuals.

ANXIETY DISORDERS

Anxiety disorders are frequent in the acute hospital setting. The challenge is determining whether the anxiety is caused by the underlying medical condition, hypoxia, hypercapnea, delirium, alcohol/sedative withdrawal syndrome, a reaction to a new medication, or the stress of the medical hospitalization.

Patients with an underlying *panic disorder* may often present to an emergency department with chest pain or acute cardiac syndromes. Anxiety often accompanies cardiac or pulmonary disease as well, such as angina, heart failure, COPD, or asthma. For treatment of acute anxiety, low-dose benzodiazepines (e.g., lorazepam 0.5–2 mg b.i.d. or t.i.d.) are often effective. Longer-acting benzodiazepines such as diazepam or clonazepam are not usually recommended because of their long half-lives and their tendency to accumulate in the geriatric and the medically ill patient. For chronic anxiety, such as panic disorder or generalized anxiety disorder, the use of a selective serotonin reuptake inhibitor (SSRI) may be indicated (2). Serotonin reuptake inhibitors are best started at a low dose and then increased as tolerated (see Chapter 119 for information on selecting and starting SSRIs). Because they are known to suppress respiratory drive, benzodiazepines must be used cautiously in individuals with respiratory conditions such as COPD and sleep apnea.

PSYCHOSIS

Psychosis, by definition, is the presence of perceptual disturbances (hallucinations) and/or thought disturbances (delusions). The patient with psychotic symptoms is often misunderstood on a medical service. Chronic or recurrent psychotic symptoms, which can be present in a number of psychiatric disorders, are the hallmark of schizophrenia but also can occur in bipolar (manic depressive) disorder and major depressions. In the acute hospital setting, the key to assessing psychosis is to determine the course of symptoms. New and acute psychotic symptoms, especially in persons over 50 years of age, are almost always related to an organic brain syndrome, typically delirium or dementia, although occasionally they may represent the index episode of a primary psychiatric disorder. The presence of confusion or a disturbance in the level of consciousness can confirm the diagnosis of delirium. Psychosis associated with dementia typically occurs late in the course of the dementia, and a careful history will often elicit evidence of progressive cognitive impairment (Chapter 115).

When psychotic symptoms are mild and unobtrusive, they can often be managed with gentle reassurance and support. More often than not, however, psychosis is distressing to both patients and staff, and it requires antipsychotic (neuroleptic) medications. In patients with delirium, the psychosis is usually associated with agitation and behavioral disturbance and thus may require rapid response for control. *Haloperidol,* the most commonly used neuroleptic in general hospitals, may be administered intravenously, intramuscularly, or by mouth (Table 33.1). Parenteral haloperidol is often well tolerated, likely has fewer extrapyramidal side effects, and has a long history of use for behavioral dyscontrol caused by delirium (see the

TABLE 33.1
TYPICAL NEUROLEPTIC MEDICATIONS USED IN GENERAL HOSPITALS

Medication	Dosage range for acute psychosis/agitation	Maintenance dosage for psychosis	Available routes of administration
Haloperidol	0.5–5 mg q 30 min p.r.n.	0.5–10 mg	PO/IM/IV
Droperidol	2.5 mg. May repeat in 3 hrs	0.625-5 mg	IM/IV
Chlorpromazine	50–100 mg q 30–60 min p.r.n.	50–500 mg	PO/IM/IV
Risperidone	0.5–2 mg q 1–2 hrs p.r.n.	0.5–6 mg	PO
Olanzapine	2.5–5 mg q 1–2 hrs p.r.n.	2.5–20 mg	PO
Ziprasidone	20 mg q 1–2 hrs p.r.n.	20–160 mg	PO/IM
Quetiapine	25–50 mg q 1–2 hrs p.r.n.	25–400 mg	PO

section about management of delirium that follows). Patients with dementia often require a similar approach, but lower doses are typically used.

Although haloperidol and the other, older neuroleptics are generally safe and effective, the patient must be monitored for side effects that can limit their use (Table 33.2).

The new generation of *atypical antipsychotics* such as olanzapine, risperidone, and quetiapine are beginning to be used in treating acute psychosis and are becoming the mainstay of treatment for primary psychotic disorders (3). They carry a substantially lower risk of inducing of extrapyramidal side effects and other dopamine-blockade effects, such as tardive dyskinesia and the neuroleptic malignant syndrome. However, they carry higher risks of hyperglycemic complications, weight gain, and prolongation of the QT interval.

Patients with chronic psychiatric disorders also develop medical illnesses and are admitted to acute care hospitals. To prevent relapse or decompensation, it is important to maintain the patients on their antipsychotic medications unless otherwise contraindicated. Use of the hospital psychiatric consultant or close coordination with the patient's outpatient psychiatrist can often be helpful.

DELIRIUM

Delirium, or acute confusional states (Chapter 115), are common problems in hospitalized patients. As many as 15%–30% of patients on a general medical service suffer from delirium. The percentage can be as high as 50% in subspecialty populations (such as patients undergoing hip

TABLE 33.2
COMMON SIDE EFFECTS OF NEUROLEPTIC MEDICATIONS

Side effect	Characteristics	Management
Acute dystonic reaction	Sudden onset dystonia, typically of the mouth, jaw, neck, eyes; usually occurs in first few days	Diphenhydramine IM 50 mg b.i.d. or t.i.d.; benztropine 1–2 mg b.i.d., switch to low potency neuroleptic
Secondary Parkinsonism	Cogwheel rigidity, mask facies, pill-rolling tremor, and peri-oral movements; occur more commonly on the higher potency neuroleptics	Diphenhydramine 25–50 mg b.i.d.; benztropine 0.5–2 mg b.i.d., switch to low potency neuroleptic
Akathesia	Internal sensation of restlessness, inability to sit still	Propanolol 10–20 mg t.i.d.; Lorazepam 1–2 mg b.i.d.
Neuroleptic malignant syndrome	Rare but sometimes fatal complication; marked by confusion or mental status changes, lead-pipe rigidity in the limbs, elevated white blood count, elevated CK level, fever, and autonomic dysregulation	Immediately stop neuroleptic; IV hydration, antipyretics; bromocriptine or dantrolene if severe
Cardiac arrhythmias	Rare; QT prolongation leading to torsade de pointes; also seen with atypical neuroleptics	Avoid neuroleptic; close monitoring and correction of potassium, calcium, and magnesium levels; may be less common with olanzapine

Adapted from Norris ER, Cassem, NH. Cardiovascular and other side effects of psychotropic medications. In: Stern TA, Herman, JB, eds. *Massachusetts General Hospital Psychiatry Update & Board Preparation.* New York: McGraw-Hill, 2003;391–398, with permission.

replacement surgery or coronary bypass surgery patients ((4)) and up to 83% of ICU patients (5). A multicomponent intervention can help prevent delirium in older patients (6). The presumed underlying mechanism of delirium is an imbalance of dopamine and acetylcholine in the neural synapses. This mechanism may explain why dopamine blockers such as haloperidol have been helpful in controlling the agitation associated with delirium.

The primary management of delirium consists of recognizing the condition and thoroughly searching for underlying medical causes. The causes of delirium are extensive, including metabolic, neurologic, infectious, cardiac, pulmonary, and endocrinologic sources (Table 115.4, Chapter 115). Identifying potentially life-threatening causes is imperative: myocardial infarction, pulmonary embolus, Wernicke's encephalopathy, hypoglycemia, intracerebral bleeding, CNS infections, and stroke. One frequently unrecognized cause of delirium in the medically ill is withdrawal from alcohol or sedative-hypnotic drugs. Patients in withdrawal often develop sudden agitation and confusion 1–3 days into a hospitalization. Interviews with family members or other sources may reveal the drinking history or clarify prior doses of sedative-hypnotic medications. Clonidine can be used as prophylaxis against alcohol withdrawal symptoms (7).

Patients with *organic brain syndromes or psychiatric disorders caused by general medical illnesses* can also present with a myriad of symptoms, from acute confusion and delirium to odd or inappropriate behaviors. Common causes include cerebral hypoxia, stroke, and closed head injuries. Patients may have had falls or trauma in which a closed head injury may have occurred but other injuries were initially more prominent or urgent. Closed head injuries present as confusion, inattentiveness, forgetfulness, apathy, or socially inappropriate and disinhibited behavior. Computed tomography (CT) scans of the head may help identify underlying trauma such as a subdural hematoma or skull fracture, but the scans may be normal in many cases. A magnetic resonance image, which may identify diffuse axonal injury or hypoxic damage, may be diagnostic in cases in which the CT scan is unrevealing despite a strongly suggestive clinical history of head trauma.

Patients can be managed with nonpharmacologic or behavioral interventions as well as with pharmacotherapy. Often, patients who are quietly confused need little or no intervention. The presence of a family member or sitter may help calm the patient. Gentle reassurance and firm limits may be all that are required. If the patient does not respond to these interventions, neuroleptic medication is the treatment of choice. The application of mechanical restraints may also be required when all other appropriate interventions have been unsuccessful.

For mild delirium or delirium in a geriatric patient, initial therapy is haloperidol 0.5–2 mg intravenously, every 30 minutes, until the patient is calm. It is important to allow the 30 minutes for the medication to work before repeating the dose to avoid oversedation and other complications of neuroleptic use. For a moderately delirious patient, 2–3 mg is given, whereas 5–10 mg is recommended for a severely agitated patient. If the patient is not calmer after the initial dose, the dose may be repeated every 30 minutes until the desired affect is achieved. If a cumulative 10 mg dose of haldoperidol is inadequate, 1–2 mg of lorazepam every 30 minutes may act synergistically to help decrease the total amount of haloperidol required. The total required dose of medication needed to calm the patient is then calculated and given in divided doses b.i.d. or t.i.d. Once the patient's symptoms begin to decrease, the medication can be tapered as tolerated.

THE "DIFFICULT" PATIENT

Occasionally, managing a hospitalized patient is challenging because patients may refuse treatments or tests, undermine the staff's efforts to care for them, and react with mistrust and anger. These patients typically have personality traits or disorders that can be disruptive, and they often create strong emotional reactions in the staff who care for them.

A *personality disorder* is defined as a lifelong pattern of maladaptive behavior that does not serve to meet an individual's needs effectively. Signs of a personality disorder include overvaluation of some staff while devaluing others; rapid shifts in mood, especially when given unwanted news; and playing off some staff members against others, called *splitting*. Often these disruptive behaviors arise because the patient feels emotionally out of control, and it is the responsibility of hospital staff to help the patient feel self-contained.

The most important part of treating these patients is recognition of the personality problem itself. This recognition can help staff understand that splitting is occurring rather than personalize the difficult interactions with the patient. Psychiatric consultants can assist the team in understanding the patient's particular personality issues and help tailor the treatment plan to maximize success. Nursing and medical staff should come together to agree on a thoughtful and medically appropriate plan, especially around emotionally charged issues such as pain, anxiety medications, and discharge planning. Difficult patients often need acknowledgment of their suffering and the difficulty of their predicament as well as firm limits. The treatment plan should be communicated to the patient in the presence of the whole team (and documented accordingly) to minimize the opportunity for splitting.

FUNCTIONAL SOMATIC DISORDERS

Emotional distress can trigger physical symptoms, whether it is diaphoresis and tachycardia seen with anxiety or the insomnia, anorexia, and fatigue of depression. Most individuals who have somatic symptoms are able to differentiate whether they are physical or psychic in origin. However, some patients are unaware that their somatic symptoms have an emotional source. Subclinical somatic presentations are common and generally self-limiting.

Functional somatic disorders can present as atypical somatization disorder, hypochondriasis, or a conversion disorder. *Somatization disorder* is a chronic state of persistent and varied somatic symptoms for which there are no discernable organic causes. It typically occurs in young women, many of whom have had traumatic childhood histories. *Hypochondriasis* is manifest by a preoccupation with one's health to the exclusion of all else. Patients with hypochondriasis are convinced they have a serious medical disorder despite repeated evaluations, are difficult to persuade otherwise, and will often present multiple times to multiple health systems. *Conversion disorder* is a demonstrated loss of motor or sensory function not associated with any organic source, presumably as an expression of psychological distress. Common examples include psychogenic seizures, blindness, and paralysis.

Factitious disorders, including the rare variant known as *Munchausen's syndrome,* entail the conscious manufacturing of signs and symptoms by patients. Patients may produce false fevers by surreptitiously heating thermometers, alter laboratory tests with covertly ingested medications, or even inject urine and feces to create false infections. Despite conscious awareness of their behaviors, patients are likely unaware of the psychological process that underlies their actions (8).

Whether or not these patients are consciously aware of their symptom production, the signs and symptoms are caused by psychologic distress too unbearable for the patient to manage. Rather than deal with their psychic anguish, these patients experience their suffering somatically. They may have learned that physical illness can earn them love and attention from caregivers, whereas emotional illness leads to abandonment and criticism.

Hospital physicians may have intense reactions once they realize that a somatic syndrome is not likely caused by an organic etiology. A physician who has invested a great deal of time, concern, and resources may feel especially abused or manipulated or feel that he or she has been made to look foolish. The tendency is to respond angrily by confronting or even abandoning the patient, a response that will not rectify the situation because the patient will soon find another physician and/or health care system in an endless search for care.

Physicians must recognize their essential role in managing these patients. One requirement is to appreciate that the patient is quite ill with either a serious physical disorder or a serious mental disorder. By limiting unnecessary testing and invasive procedures, especially surgeries, the physician helps prevent iatrogenic complications. Although psychiatric consultation is important in understanding the patient's incentive toward illness, patients

with somatic disorders are generally averse to psychiatric intervention or treatment. The psychiatrist typically helps the hospital physician and primary care provider establish a treatment plan that can minimize patients' danger to themselves.

VIOLENT PATIENTS

Violent and aggressive behavior in hospitalized patients is predominantly a manifestation of derangement in brain function: delirium, dementia, head trauma, and drug intoxication/withdrawal states. Aggression can also be seen in patients with psychiatric conditions such as mania, psychosis, severe anxiety, borderline personality disorder, and agitated depression. Occasionally, violent behavior is volitional, representing sociopathy.

Violent behavior in an acute care hospital is relatively rare, but it can be devastating to staff and patients. Hospital physicians must recognize the risk for violence early in the assessment of patients and be sure all staff are warned about a particular patient's potential for aggressiveness. They should then assemble a multidisciplinary team, including nursing, social work, and psychiatry, to address the issue rapidly. Hospital security staff may also play an important role. When behavioral approaches fail, medications or physical restraints may be necessary (9).

INFORMED CONSENT, COMPETENCY, AND THE RIGHT TO REFUSE TREATMENT

A general tenet of good medical practice is to ensure that patients are adequately informed about their condition and understand the risks and benefits of the range of treatments available. Occasionally, patients do not agree with their physician's opinion and/or recommendation regarding evaluation and treatment. Although physicians typically defer to their patients' choices, the physician may at times question whether a patient has the decision-making capacity needed to refuse the treatment. When the risks of refusing treatment are substantial, the physician may request a psychiatric consultation to assess whether the patient is competent to refuse.

Over the past half-century, there has been a movement toward supporting a patient's autonomy for decision making rather than relying on the physician's beneficence (Chapter 17). The courts have adopted the concept of *informed consent,* whereby individual patients should expect their medical providers to inform them adequately but allow them to make the decision free of coercion. *Informed* means that patients are made aware of their condition and that the risks and benefits of treatment (plus all alternatives, including no treatment) are provided in a reasonable manner. The final aspect of the informed consent doctrine is that a patient's decision making is based upon a presumption of competency to make such a decision, including the following:

1. The ability to make a decision
2. The ability to understand information
3. The ability to appreciate the consequences of one's decision
4. The ability to think rationally (10)

If a physician believes that a patient does not have one or more of these abilities, he or she may conclude that the patient is not competent to make medical decisions. Although the physician may encourage the family (or hospital in lieu of family) to pursue some form of guardianship, the standard of care in most hospitals is to seek the opinion of a psychiatric consultant. The psychiatrist will not only assess the patient's decision-making ability, but also assist the patient, family, and medical team to collaborate effectively on decision making, thereby obviating the need for legal interventions. Occasionally the consultant may identify disruptions in the communications between medical team and patient and, as a result, catalyze increased consensus and agreement.

CIVIL COMMITMENT

Acutely decompensated, mentally ill patients frequently present to emergency departments of general hospitals with psychosis, depression, suicidal ideation or attempts, or potential violence. These patients may present on their own or be brought by police, family, or outside providers. Suicide attempts, including overdoses and self-inflicted injuries, may result in medical hospitalization despite ongoing suicidal risk. A hospitalist may need to decide rapidly whether involuntary psychiatric confinement is preferable to admission to a general hospital.

Most states have statutes that allow for the emergency involuntary hospitalization and confinement of mentally ill individuals who are considered to be an imminent danger to themselves or others. These commitment statutes are typically short-term, lasting anywhere from 2 days–3 weeks. In general, these statutes permit involuntary confinement but not involuntary treatment, which typically requires a separate hearing to assess whether the patient is competent to refuse the actual treatment.

Most jurisdictions permit licensed physicians to hold individuals in the hospital against their will if it is determined that they are a potential danger because of a mental illness. Some states require more than one physician's input, and others require evaluation by designated clinicians or psychiatrists. It is critical that every hospital physician know the local statutes regarding involuntary commitment. However, when the physician is uncertain about the state laws concerning commitment, it is prudent to protect the patient and community by holding the individual until the appropriate

psychiatric evaluation can occur. Hospital lawyers and psychiatrists are useful resources regarding local regulations.

TRANSFER/ADMISSION TO PSYCHIATRIC UNITS

Patients who present with acute psychiatric symptoms may benefit from psychiatric hospitalization. When patients are determined to be a potential danger to themselves or others, hospitalization is typically necessary, whether or not the patient agrees with this recommendation. Most states have two basic processes for psychiatric hospitalization: *voluntary* or *involuntary*.

Voluntary admission, as implied, is when a patient who might benefit from acute treatment in a psychiatric unit agrees to this treatment. For many of these patients, the inpatient treatment provides a more intensive, accelerated approach than can be provided in an outpatient setting. However, restrictions on insurance coverage for inpatient psychiatric care often preclude this option by covering only outpatient counseling or day treatment programs.

Patients who are considered a potential danger to themselves or others must be held in a safe environment until a formal psychiatric evaluation can be performed to determine whether the patient must be hospitalized. Patients who do not agree with this recommendation must be committed involuntarily to the psychiatric unit or hospital. In most states, this requires an evaluation by a qualified psychiatrist or mental health provider.

WHEN TO REQUEST PSYCHIATRIC CONSULTATION

Psychiatric consultation should be considered for patients with any of the following characteristics:

1. Suicidal ideation or behavior
2. Agitated or aggressive behavior
3. Unexplained somatic symptoms
4. Active primary psychiatric disorders
5. Significant emotional dysfunction associated with the primary medical condition
6. Personality traits and disorders that interfere with medical care

In addition, psychiatric consultation should be considered if the physician has serious questions regarding the patient's decision-making capacity.

KEY POINTS

- Patients with chronic psychiatric disorders also develop medical disorders, and careful evaluation is required to detect medical problems and distinguish them from psychiatric symptoms.

- Patients with medical disorders can develop acute psychiatric symptoms, which may represent a manifestation of the medical illness.
- Suicide is typically seen with depression or other mental disorders, and its frequency increases in patients with significant medical disorders.
- Early recognition and management of delirium can decrease morbidity and mortality.
- Antipsychotic medications are essential for the treatment of delirium and psychosis, but side effects of these medications can complicate medical illness.
- Consultation-liaison psychiatrists can assist in assessing and managing functional somatic disorders, difficult-to-manage patients with personality disorders, and potentially dangerous behavior.

REFERENCES

1. Mann JJ. A current perspective of suicide and attempted suicide. *Ann Intern Med* 2002;136:302–311.
2. Sheehan DV. The management of panic disorder. *J Clin Psychiatry* 2002;63(Suppl 14):17–21.
3. Lieberman JA, Tollefson G, Tohen M, et al. Comparative efficacy and safety of atypical and conventional antipsychotic drugs in first-episode psychosis: a randomized, double-blind trial of olanzapine versus haloperidol. *Am J Psychiatry* 2003;160: 1396–1404.
4. Pompei P, Foreman M, Rudberg MA, et al. Delirium in hospitalized older persons: outcomes and predictors. *J Am Geriatr Soc* 1994;42:809–815.
5. Ely EW, Inouye SW, Bernard GR, et al. Delirium in mechanically ventilated patients: validity and reliability of the confusion assessment method for the intensive care unit (CAM-ICU). *JAMA* 2001;286:2703–2710.
6. Inouye SK, Bogardus ST, Charpentier PA, et al. A multicomponent intervention to prevent delirium in hospitalized older patients. *N Engl J Med* 1999;340:669–676.
7. Dobrydnjov I, Axelsson K, Berggren I, et al. Intrathecal and oral clonidine as prophylaxis for postoperative alcohol withdrawal syndrome: a randomized double-blind study. *Anesth Analg* 2004;98:738–744.
8. Krahn LE, Li H, O'Connor MK. Patients who strive to be ill: factitious disorder with physical symptoms. *Am J Psychiatry* 2003; 160:1163–1168.
9. Buckley PF, Noffsinger SG, Smith DA, et al. Treatment of the psychotic patient who is violent. *Psychiatr Clin N Am* 2003;26: 231–272.
10. Appelbaum PS, Grisso T. Assessing patients' capacities to consent to treatment. *N Engl J Med* 1988;319:1635–1638.
11. Norris ER, Cassem NH. Cardiovascular and other side effects of psychotropic medications. In: Stern TA, Herman, JB, eds. *Psychiatry Update and Board Preparation*, 2nd ed. New York: McGraw-Hill, 2003;391–398.

ADDITIONAL READING

Allen MH, ed. *Emergency Psychiatry* (Review of Psychiatry Series, Volume 21, Number 3; Oldham JM, Riba MB, series editors). Washington, DC: American Psychiatric Publishing, 2002.

Bruce ML, Ten Have TR, Reynolds CF 3rd, et al. Reducing suicidal ideation and depressive symptoms in depressed older primary care patients: a randomized controlled trial. *JAMA* 2004;291:1081–1091.

Kane JM, Leuch TS, Carpenter D, et al. Expert consensus guideline series. Optimizing pharmacologic treatment of psychotic disorders. Introduction: methods, commentary, and summary. *J Clin Psychiatry* 2003;64(Suppl 12):5–19.

Phillips KA, ed. *Somatoform and Factitious Disorders* (Review of Psychiatry Series, Volume 20, Number 3; Oldham JM, Riba MB, series editors). Washington, DC: American Psychiatric Publishing, 2001.

Pomeroy C, Mitchell JE, Roerig J, et al. *Medical Complications of Psychiatric Illness.* Washington, DC: American Psychiatric Publishing, 2002.

Trauma

Deborah M. Stein   *Ronald Rabinowitz*   *Ellis Caplan*

34

INTRODUCTION

Victims of injury are not limited by age, race, gender, or socioeconomic class. Trauma is unbiased in who it afflicts, and it can occur at any time or place. All clinicians must be prepared to treat injured patients, who can present challenging diagnostic and management decisions.

Death from trauma can occur at three separate phases of injury. Those who die at the scene usually have unsalvageable major vascular disruption, high spinal cord injury, or massive head trauma. A second group of patients may lose their lives because of ongoing hemorrhage or evolving injuries. Trauma systems aim to treat these patients within minutes-to-hours following injury. A third group of patients succumb to infection and multiple organ system failure days-to-weeks following trauma.

EPIDEMIOLOGY

Accidents represent the fifth leading cause of death among all age groups, and the leading cause of death in people ages 1–34 (1). About 40,000 Americans are killed in motor vehicle collisions each year, and another 3.5 million suffer nonfatal injuries (2, 3). Another 30,000 deaths occur annually from firearm violence in the United States (4). Among the age groups 15–19, 20–24, and 25–34, accidents, homicides, and suicides cause more than 75%, 72%, and 51% of deaths, respectively (5).

Mechanisms

Injuries are divided into two broad classes. Penetrating trauma is caused by firearms, knives, and other sharp objects that can become impaled. Blunt trauma most commonly arises from motor vehicle or motorcycle collisions, pedestrians struck by vehicles, or falls. However, any significant force sustained by the human body can result in major injury. Sports injuries and industrial accidents are commonly seen. Some types of injuries can result in a combination of both blunt and penetrating damage.

Initial Evaluation

The basic philosophy in caring for a trauma patient is to assume that major injury exists until proven otherwise. The onus is on the health care team to rule out life-threatening injuries definitively and constantly to protect against destabilization of existing injuries. The American College of Surgeons Committee on Trauma has outlined a highly protocolized way of evaluating the trauma patient (6): The primary survey (composed of "A = airway, B = breathing, C = circulation, D = disability, E = exposure"); rapid diagnostic studies; and the secondary survey, which includes a complete history and physical examination of the patient and the performance of secondary diagnostic procedures.

Primary Survey

The primary survey consists of a sequence of systematic evaluations; each component must be addressed before proceeding. These steps must be constantly reevaluated throughout the workup of the injured patient.

- The first priority is the *evaluation and treatment of airway compromise*. The airway may be secured with simple positioning, insertion of oral or nasal airways, endotracheal or nasotracheal intubation, or surgical access (cricothyroidotomy). Care must always be taken to maintain cervical spine stability; this goal is accomplished with "in-line" traction techniques.
- The second priority is *adequate ventilation and oxygenation*. The physical examination should assess the presence of equal bilateral breath sounds and equal, symmetric rise of the chest. The chest wall should be palpated for crepitus or fractures. Adequate oxygenation can be confirmed with pulse-oximetry. All trauma patients should be administered supplemental oxygen.
- The third priority is *rapid evaluation of the circulation*. Vital signs are obtained, and large-bore IV access is secured. Control of hemorrhage is performed here, most commonly with direct pressure.
- The fourth priority is a *rapid assessment of the patient's neurologic status*. This task includes assessment of the Glascow Coma Scale (GCS) (Table 117.1) and presence (and level) of focal neurologic deficits.
- The next priority is to *expose the patient completely*, for a comprehensive external examination.

Rapid Diagnostic Studies

During the primary survey, a decision must be made as to the patient's overall stability. Patients who are unstable, as evidenced by shock or severe neurologic disability, should enter into a treatment algorithm that allows for rapid identification and treatment of life-threatening injuries. A chest and pelvic radiograph (at minimum) are required to make decisions about the next intervention. The FAST (*focused assessment with sonography for trauma*) exam is often used in hemodynamically unstable patients to determine whether the source of hemorrhagic shock is injured abdominal viscera that require immediate surgical intervention. In the case of an equivocal FAST, diagnostic peritoneal lavage can be utilized to identify the peritoneal cavity as the source of bleeding. In the technique, a catheter is inserted into the peritoneal cavity, and saline is instilled. Once the saline is removed, it can be examined for presence of blood or enteric contents to establish the diagnosis of visceral injury. It is crucial to conduct the secondary survey to identify all injuries soon after the patient is stabilized.

Secondary Survey

For patients deemed to be "stable," the secondary survey, which must be performed immediately, includes a history and physical examination to identify all injuries and prior-

itize treatment. An electrocardiogram (ECG), if needed, and blood samples should be obtained, and blood should be sent for type and crossmatch. The clinician must remember to reevaluate the ABCDEs and be prepared to change diagnostic and therapeutic priorities rapidly.

In the hemodynamically stable patient, the FAST is also performed as part of the secondary survey to identify free fluid in the pericardium and specific areas of the abdominal cavity. The test has a reported sensitivity and specificity as high as 90% and 99%, respectively, in the hands of experienced operators (7). The FAST examination can also identify fluid or air in the hemithoraces.

Diagnostic Studies

Most centers will perform chest, pelvic, and lateral cervical spine radiographs in the initial series. Additional views of the cervical spine may be obtained at this time to definitively exclude a cervical spine injury. Thoracic and lumbar spine radiographs are also obtained as clinically indicated.

Head CT scan should be performed in all patients with witnessed or suspected loss of consciousness or altered level of consciousness (GCS <15). If all 7 cervical vertebrae are not visualized on plain radiograph, a CT scan of the cervical spine with sagittal and coronal reconstructions should be performed. CT scans of the chest to evaluate the aorta are indicated for all patients with an abnormal mediastinum on chest radiograph (Figure 34.1). Abdominal and pelvic CT scans should be performed in any patient with an abnormal FAST, abdominal pain or tenderness, or injuries that suggest that a significant force was sustained. Clinical judgment must guide what CT scans or additional studies should be performed.

MANAGEMENT OF SPECIFIC INJURIES

Head Trauma

Blunt head injuries are generally divided initially into minor (GCS = 15–14), moderate (GCS = 13–9), and severe (GCS = 8–3). The CT scan and evolution of the clinical examination guide subsequent management. For patients with a normal CT scan and mild deficit, simple observation is all that is generally required. A patient with a normal CT scan and neurologic exam rarely deteriorates. Such patients can generally be sent home with a responsible observer, although they may still suffer from long-term memory or cognitive deficits. Patients who are intoxicated should be observed until their level of consciousness is normal.

Any patient with an abnormality on CT scan, GCS <12 (or motor component <5), or focal neurologic deficit should be evaluated by a neurosurgeon. Abnormal findings on CT scan include depressed skull fractures, epidu-

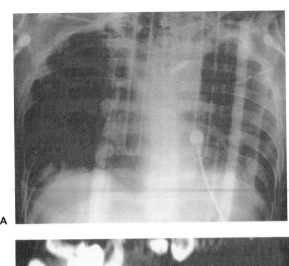

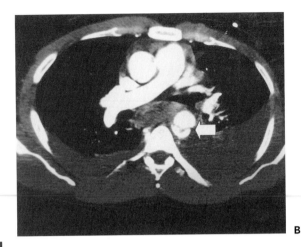

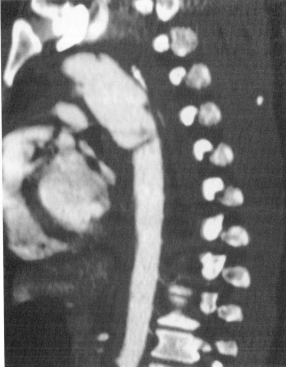

Figure 34.1 **A:** Chest radiograph demonstrating widened mediastinum suspicious for aortic injury. **B:** CT scan of the chest showing traumatic aortic injury (arrow). Also note mediastinal blood. **C:** Sagittal reconstructions of chest CT demonstrating aortic injury.

ral hematomas, subdural hematomas (Figure 34.2), subarachnoid blood, parenchymal contusions, and intraventricular blood. Patients with normal CT scans but an abnormal neurologic exam often have diffuse axonal injury. Immediate surgical intervention is indicated in patients who have extra-axial collections of blood with midline shift or worsening mental status. Seizure prophylaxis is often recommended (Table 34.1; see also Chapter 118) (8).

At the discretion of the neurosurgeon, intracranial pressure monitors may be placed. Strategies for management of elevated intracranial pressure include (9), but are not limited to, mild hyperventilation, sedation, paralytics, osmotic diuretics (generally mannitol, 1 gm/kg), hyperosmo-

lar therapy, placement of intraventricular drainage devices, barbiturates, and decompressive craniotomy. The aim of therapy is to maintain a low intracranial pressure while maintaining an adequate cerebral perfusion pressure (>60–70 mm/Hg) (cerebral perfusion pressure = mean arterial pressure–intracranial pressure). Intervention must prevent hypoxia and hypotension, both of which worsen long-term outcome (10). Patients with severe head injuries are at risk for coagulopathies and shock, even in the absence of other injuries. Transtentorial herniation, which is often heralded by the "blown" pupil and a Cushing reflex (bradycardia and hypertension), is treated with acute hyperventilation, osmotic diuretics, and immediate neurosurgical evaluation (see also Chapter 117).

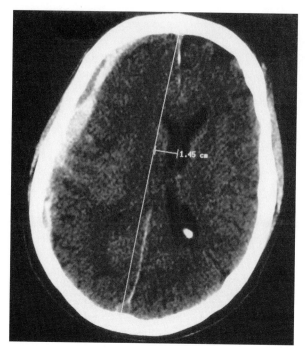

Figure 34.2 CT scan of brain with acute subdural hematoma with 1.45 cm midline shift.

Spinal Cord and Spine Fractures

Cervical, thoracic, and lumbar spine fractures are classified as stable vs. unstable injuries. Stable injuries do not pose risk to the spinal cord and are treated with methods ranging from simple pain control to immobilization with collars and braces. Unstable fractures, by definition, pose a risk to the spinal cord, and consultation with a spine surgeon is required for stabilization.

Spinal cord injuries, most of which occur in the cervical cord, are a major cause of short- and long-term morbidity in trauma patients. All patients with a significant mechanism of injury should be assumed to have a spinal cord injury or spine fracture until proven otherwise. Cervical collars and strict logroll precautions should be utilized. A

TABLE 34.1

INDICATIONS FOR SEIZURE PROPHYLAXIS

Glasgow Coma Score <10 (Table 117.1)
Intraparenchymal contusion
Depressed skull fracture
Subdural hematoma
Epidural hematoma
Intraparenchymal hematoma
Penetrating head injury
Evidence of seizure activity

careful neurologic examination for sensory and motor deficits is essential. All patients with spinal cord injury should be evaluated by a spine surgeon. In blunt spinal cord injury, the use of high dose methylprednisolone as a bolus (30 mg/kg), followed by a 23-hour infusion (5.4 mg/kg/hr), currently represents the standard of care, although it is not without controversy (11). It must be started within 8 hours of injury to be beneficial. Further intervention in these patients includes early operative decompression and the avoidance of hypotension, to prevent spinal cord ischemia. Mean arterial blood pressure should be maintained at 85–90 mm Hg for 7 days following injury (12), despite the hypotension that may accompany the loss of sympathetic innervation.

Neck

Blunt and penetrating trauma can result in life-threatening injuries in the neck. Penetrating injuries to the neck can cause exsanguinating hemorrhage, major neurologic morbidity, tracheal disruption, or esophageal/oropharyngeal disruption. Carotid injuries should be evaluated by angiography and treated in consultation with a trauma surgeon or neurosurgeon. All penetrating injuries that violate the platysma muscle also necessitate consultation with a surgeon.

Thoracic

Penetrating injuries to the chest can range from simple soft tissue injury to major vascular disruption. The diagnostic and therapeutic approach must be guided by the patient's stability and the assumed trajectory of the offending object. Simple pneumothorax or hemothorax is treated with tube thoracostomy. Massive hemothorax (initial drainage >1200 mL or >200 mL/hr for 2–3 hours) often requires surgical intervention. Precordial or transmediastinal injuries necessitate evaluation of mediastinal structures by a combination of echocardiography, pericardiocentesis, bronchoscopy, esophagoscopy, contrast studies, and CT scanning (Figure 34.1). All patients with penetrating injuries (other than simple hemothorax or pneumothorax) should be evaluated by a surgeon and all unstable patients require emergent surgical intervention.

Blunt thoracic trauma can also be a major source of morbidity and mortality. Simple rib fractures can lead to splinting and pneumonia if pain control is not adequate. Epidural analgesia by an experienced pain specialist can be extremely helpful. Simple pneumothoraces and hemothoraces are treated with tube thoracostomy. Pulmonary contusions, which can range from mild to severe, may require mechanical ventilation. All patients with potential myocardial injury, ranging from mild sinus tachycardia to major cardiac dysfunction, require an ECG. Hemodynamically stable patients should be treated supportively with telemetry monitoring (13). Major catastrophic injuries such as aortic rupture, severe disruptions of the tracheobronchial tree, esophageal injuries, and myocardial rupture mandate emergent evaluation by an experienced surgeon.

Abdominal

Penetrating abdominal and flank injuries must be evaluated to determine the risk of underlying injury. Any patient with hemodynamic instability, pneumoperitoneum, evisceration, or peritonitis on exam requires laparotomy. For patients without indications for surgical intervention, a variety of diagnostic modalities exist, including observation and serial physical examinations, peritoneal lavage, FAST, triple contrast CT scan (14), local wound exploration, diagnostic laparoscopy, and diagnostic laparotomy. As a general rule, peritoneal or retroperitoneal violation necessitates laparotomy.

The evaluation of blunt abdominal injuries is generally accomplished with a combination of abdominal exam, FAST, and CT scan. Any evidence of peritonitis, pneumoperitoneum, or hemodynamic instability attributable to abdominal injury should be evaluated by laparotomy. Although a detailed discussion of the management of these injuries is beyond the scope of this chapter, observation and angiography are cornerstones of the treatment of splenic and hepatic injuries (15) (Figure 34.3).

Pelvic Fractures

Pelvic fractures are a major source of morbidity and mortality in the trauma patient. Exsanguinating hemorrhage, from either arterial and/or venous disruption, can occur without outward signs of hemorrhage, particularly where there is major injury to the posterior elements of the pelvis. Patients with hemodynamic instability in the setting of a significant pelvic fracture are treated with a combination of fracture stabilization with abdominal binders, or external fixation and angiographic control of bleeding. MAST trousers can be used in the field or during initial presentation to control bleeding, but a simple bedsheet tied securely around the pelvis can be extremely effective in allowing temporary reduction of the pelvic elements. An exhaustive search for associated injuries, such as those of the rectum, vagina, bladder, and urethra, is mandatory. Long-term morbidity can also be caused by prolonged immobilization, which can lead to life-threatening deep venous thrombosis.

Extremity Trauma

Fractures should be stabilized and reduced by simple splinting. Early (within 48 hours) definitive stabilization and fixation is advocated for both isolated injuries and those occurring in the context of a polytrauma (16).

For open fractures or those associated with significant soft tissue trauma, operative irrigation and closure of the defect are necessary to avoid osteomyelitis. Tetanus and prophylactic antibiotics should be administered in all such cases. Major crush injuries may lead to rhabdomyolysis due

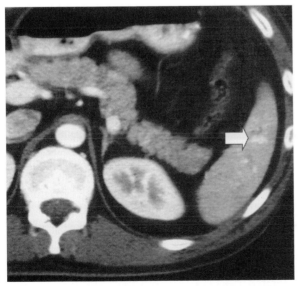
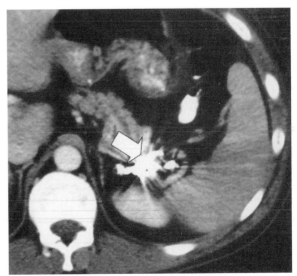

Figure 34.3 A. CT scan of abdomen demonstrating splenic "blush" consistent with active bleeding (arrow). B. CT scan of abdomen of the same patient after proximal coil embolization (arrow).

to muscle destruction, which should be treated aggressively to prevent renal failure (Chapter 100).

The fractured or injured extremity must always be evaluated for possible ischemia. Angiography may be required to determine the level and degree of injury and to plan vascular repair. The patient's clinical examination (changes in edema, warmth, and pulses) should be closely monitored for signs of compartment syndrome. This entity can be confirmed by exact pressure measurements done at appropriate intervals by an orthopedist.

SPECIAL CONSIDERATIONS AND COMPLICATIONS

The trauma patient is at unique risk for many complications.

Previous Medical Comorbidities

Information about past medical history is crucial to providing adequate treatment to the trauma patient. Significant cardiac, pulmonary, liver, and renal disease may impact the care of the trauma patient. A dialogue between the trauma team and the patient's primary or hospital physician can be of vital importance in assuring appropriate care.

Pregnancy

The pregnant trauma patient raises issues for the injured mother and the fetus. The general rule is that the mother's welfare takes priority. All diagnostic tests needed to identify the mother's injuries adequately should be performed in a timely fashion, minimizing radiation exposure when possible. Volume resuscitation should be liberal, due to the relative hypovolemia of pregnancy; the mothers of fetuses over 20 weeks of gestation should be placed on their left sides to decrease the pressure of the fetus on the vena cava. Early obstetrical consultation should be obtained and fetal monitoring performed for all patients more than 22 weeks and at the discretion of the obstetrician. The Kleihauer-Betke test can detect fetal blood in the maternal circulation. This test, performed in the lab, makes use of the relative resistance of fetal hemoglobin to acid denaturation. If the test is positive, Rhogam should be administered to all Rh– mothers.

Domestic Violence

Although domestic violence disproportionately affects women, all patients should be screened for it. Early in-volvement of social workers and specially trained clinicians is imperative. Because patients often deny the true cause of their injury, the index of suspicion must remain high to assure the safety of the patient in the hospital and after discharge.

Nutrition

Patients with major injuries are, by definition, catabolic, with extreme caloric and protein requirements. When possible, enteral nutrition should be provided by a nasogastric or naso-jejunal feeding tube (17). Post-pyloric tubes and promotility agents can aid the delivery of adequate nutrition. Parenteral nutrition is recommended only for patients who are unable to tolerate enteral feeds or where gastrointestinal trauma precludes enteral nutrition (see also Chapter 15).

Infectious Disease

Infections are a leading complication in the trauma patient. Prophylactic antibiotics are efficacious in limited circumstances related to trauma, especially penetrating abdominal wounds and open fractures. First generation cephalosporins are generally used in patients with open fractures for a duration of 48 hours (cefazolin 1 gm IV q8h). Patients with penetrating abdominal injury should receive 1 gram of cefotetan prior to surgery. If a hollow viscus is found to be violated, cefotetan (1 gm IV q 12 hrs) should be continued for 24–48 hours. Patients with open facial fractures should receive antibiotics targeting the anaerobes of the mouth, as well as *Staphylococcus aureus* (clindamycin or ampicillin/sulbactam) for 48 hours. Patients with other injuries are generally not given prophylactic antibiotics.

Prophylaxis for Deep Venous Thrombosis (DVT)

Prolonged immobilization, long bone fractures, pelvic fractures, closed head injuries, and, most importantly, spinal cord injuries put the trauma patient at extremely high risk for the development of DVT and subsequent pulmonary embolism (18). Some centers advocate placement of vena caval filters for all patients with spinal cord injuries. Surveillance duplex ultrasonography is recommended for patients with spinal cord injuries, closed head injuries, or prolonged immobilization (19). The approach to prophylactic anticoagulation is outlined in Chapter 52.

Prophylaxis for Gastrointestinal Stress Ulcers

Injured patients, particularly those with head trauma, are at risk for the development of stress ulcers, especially if they require long term (>48 hours) mechanical ventilation. All trauma patients should be treated with H_2 blockers or proton pump inhibitors. Early enteral feeding is also extremely effective at reducing the risk of stress ulcerations. Additional information on prophylaxis is found in Chapter 80.

Alcohol and Drug Abuse

Alcohol is often associated with motor vehicle collisions, and both drugs and alcohol are associated with crime and traumatic injury. Toxicology screening should be performed in suspected cases, and a positive toxicology screen should lead to an evaluation for substance abuse.

The management of hospitalized patients with drug or alcohol abuse or withdrawal is described in Chapters 121 and 122, respectively.

Multiple Organ Dysfunction Syndrome

Patients with multiple injuries and those who have significant shock states are at risk for the development of the systemic inflammatory response syndrome and subsequent organ dysfunction. Head trauma, multiple orthopedic injuries, massive blood transfusions, and pulmonary contusions place the trauma patient at an increased risk for the development of acute respiratory distress syndrome (ARDS) (Chapter 24). Cardiac dysfunction can result from direct myocardial injury or loss of sympathetic innervation to the heart. Renal failure may be precipitated by rhabdomyolysis from crush injuries or ischemia secondary to hypoperfusion (Chapter 100). Liver dysfunction and subsequent coagulaopathies can similarly result from direct injury or secondary hypoperfusion states (Chapter 82). Any organ can become profoundly dysfunctional from the direct effects of trauma or the subsequent inflammatory response. The treatment for organ dysfunction in this population is primarily supportive.

KEY POINTS

- The initial evaluation of the trauma patient must be performed in an orderly, step-wise fashion designed to identify and treat the most imminently life-threatening problems first. Always remember the ABCDEs: airway, breathing, circulation, disability, exposure.
- Hemodynamically unstable patients require aggressive resuscitation and identification of the cause of shock. Temporary stabilization and transfer to a definitive care center is indicated if specialized personnel are not available.
- The secondary survey identifies specific injuries and prioritizes treatment. Adjunctive studies are utilized as deemed necessary by the health care team.

- Neurologic injuries can be devastating. Maintaining adequate blood pressure and oxygenation is critical. The spinal cord must be stabilized until injury is definitively excluded.
- Penetrating injuries can range from mild to fatal. All hemodynamically unstable patients with possible penetrating injury should have emergent surgical consultation and likely will require operative intervention.
- Specific concerns in the hospitalized trauma patient include malnutrition, infectious complications, deep venous thrombosis, stress ulcers, and the sequelae of alcohol and substance abuse.
- The multiple injury or hypotensive patient may develop systemic inflammation and subsequent multiple organ system dysfunction. Prevention and rapid treatment of shock can reduce morbidity and mortality.

REFERENCES

1. CDC National Center for Health Statistics (NCHS). National Mortality Data, 2000. Hyattsville, MD: NCHS 2002 Available at: www.cdc.gov/nchs.html. Accessed March 5, 2005.
2. CDC National Center for Injury Prevention and Control. Available at: www.cdc.gov/ncipc. Accessed March 5, 2005.
3. Quinlan KP, Thompson MP, Annest JL, et al. Expanding the National Injury Surveillance System to monitor all nonfatal injuries treated in US hospital emergency departments. *Ann Emerg Med* 1999;34:637–645.
4. Nonfatal and fatal firearm-related injuries—United States, 1993–1997. *MMWR* 1999;48:1029–1034.
5. CDC National Center for Health Statistics (NCHS). National Mortality Data, 2000. Hyattsville, MD: NCHS 2002 Available at: www.cdc.gov/nchs.html. Accessed March 5, 2005.
6. American College of Surgeons Committee on Trauma. Advanced Trauma Life Support Course for Doctors, 1997. American College of Surgeons, Chicago, IL, USA.
7. Rozycki GS, Sisley A. The surgeon's use of ultrasonography in the trauma setting. *Prob Gen Surg* 1997;14:76–83.
8. Role of antiseizure prophylaxis following head injury. *J Neurotrauma* 2000;17:549–553.
9. Guidelines for the Management of Severe Head Injury. The Brain Trauma Foundation, 1995.
10. Management and Prognosis of Severe Traumatic Brain Injury. The Brain Trauma Foundation, 2000.
11. Pharmacological therapy after acute cervical spinal cord injury. *Neurosurgery* 2002;50:S63–S72.
12. Blood pressure management after acute spinal cord injury. *Neurosurgery* 2002;50:S53–S62.
13. Practice Management Guidelines for Screening of Blunt Myocardial Injury. EAST Practice Parameter Workgroup for Screening of Blunt Cardiac Injury. Eastern Association for the Surgery of Trauma, 1998. Available at: www.east.org/tpg.html. Accessed March 5, 2005.
14. Shanmuganathan K, Mirvis SE, Chiu WC, et al. Triple-contrast helical CT in penetrating torso trauma: a prospective study to determine peritoneal violation and the need for laparotomy. *Am J Roentgenol* 2001;177:1–10.
15. Practice Management Guidelines for the Nonoperative Management of Blunt Injury to the Liver and Spleen. EAST Practice Management Guidelines Work Group. Eastern Association for the Surgery of Trauma 2003. Available at: www.east.org/tpg.html. Accessed March 5, 2005.

16. Practice Management Guidelines for the Optimal Timing of Long Bone Stabilization in Polytrauma Patients. EAST Practice Management Guidelines Work Group. Eastern Association for the Surgery of Trauma 2000. Available at: www.east.org/tpg.html. Accessed March 5, 2005.

17. Practice Management Guidelines for Nutritional Support of the Trauma Patient. The EAST Practice Management Guidelines Work Group. Eastern Association for the Surgery of Trauma. Available at: www.east.org/tpg.html. Accessed March 5, 2005.

18. Practice Management Guidelines for the Management of Venous Thromboembolism in Trauma Patients. EAST Practice Parameter Work Group for DVT Prophylaxis. Eastern Association for the Surgery of Trauma. Available at: www.east.org/tpg.html. Accessed March 5, 2005.

19. Deep venous thrombosis and thromboembolism in patients with cervical spine injuries. *Neurosurgery* 2002;50:S63–S72.

ADDITIONAL READING

Rozycki GS. What's new in trauma and critical care. *J Am Coll Surg* 2004;198:798–805.

Cardiovascular
Medicine

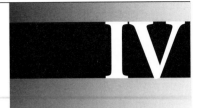

Signs, Symptoms, and Laboratory Abnormalities in Cardiovascular Diseases

35

Randall H. Vagelos   *Rachel Marcus*   *J. Edwin Atwood*

TOPICS COVERED IN CHAPTER
- Chest Pain 297
- Palpitations 303
- Lightheadedness 306
- Jugular Venous Pressure 306
- Arterial Pulses 307
- Heart Sounds 308
- Common Cardiac Murmurs 309
- Electrocardiogram 312
- Chest Radiograph 312
- Common Blood Tests 312

INTRODUCTION

The tempo of cardiovascular disease requires the clinician to diagnose rapidly and treat sometimes before the diagnosis is certain. This time pressure often creates a conflict between the need to be careful, conservative, and correct on the one hand, and the equally pressing need to institute effective interventions rapidly in the acutely ill patient on the other.

This chapter covers common symptoms, signs, and laboratory abnormalities elicited from cardiovascular patients at the time of their initial evaluation for hospitalization.

The evolution of these problems during the course of an inpatient stay is also considered. Symptoms to be reviewed include chest pain, palpitations, and lightheadedness, which all have causes that range from the extremely dangerous to the annoyingly benign; dyspnea (Chapter 54) and syncope (Chapter 44) are covered elsewhere. Common physical findings include the jugular venous pattern, pulse abnormalities, heart sounds, and cardiac murmurs; edema (Chapter 99) is discussed elsewhere. Finally, the electrocardiogram (ECG), chest radiograph, and common biochemical and hematologic test results are discussed.

CARDIAC SYMPTOMS

Chest Pain

History

Because most adults have experienced chest pain of some type in their past, the history of the current episode can be made more valuable by an assessment of its similarity to previous episodes. It is also extremely important to assess the clinical setting in which the chest pain presents itself: a 22-year-old athletic medical student who presents with substernal chest pain for the first time after hearing a lecture on cardiovascular pathology is much less likely to have active cardiovascular disease, no matter what the quality of the chest pain, than is a 63-year-old hypertensive, hypercholesterolemic man, all of whose progenitors died of coronary disease by age 55 (Chapter 6).

Chest pain can be associated with a number of cardiovascular, pulmonary, and gastrointestinal conditions (Table 35.1). In an individual patient, however, it may be frustratingly difficult to ascribe chest pain to a specific pathologic process. In general, the chest pain history is more useful than the physical examination. Important aspects of the history include the quality, location, radiation, frequency, and duration of the pain; precipitating or relieving factors; and associated symptoms (1–3).

The differential diagnosis of chest pain includes acute coronary syndrome (spectrum from unstable angina to ST elevation myocardial infarction [MI]), angina pectoris, myocardial ischemia resulting from valvular heart disease or cardiomyopathy, aortic dissection, pericarditis, pulmonary hypertension, pulmonary embolism, esophageal spasm/acid-peptic disease, gallbladder/pancreatic disease, pulmonary disease, and musculoskeletal pain. The critical importance of differentiating these entities (Table 35.2) revolves around both the need to intervene as early as possible in some clinical scenarios (i.e., acute MI, aortic dissection) and the fact that the beneficial therapy for a patient with one possible diagnosis (i.e., antiplatelet therapy, anticoagulation, and/or thrombolytic therapy for acute MI) might mean disaster for the patient with another (aortic dissection).

For both *acute MI* (Chapter 38) and *angina pectoris* (Chapter 37), the quality of chest discomfort is classically described as pressure, heaviness, squeezing, tightness, or constriction. However, some patients complain of burning, indigestion, fullness, or "gas". When a patient complains of sharp or stabbing chest discomfort that is reproduced by changes in position or palpation, it is much less likely to represent ischemic heart disease. The typical location of the chest discomfort of ischemic heart disease is substernal, but the discomfort may also be principally in the left precordial area. Common sites of radiation include the left shoulder, the base of the neck, and the left more often than the right arm. Less commonly, the pain may radiate to the jaw, teeth, or back. Pain that radiates to the abdomen or legs is unlikely to be related to ischemic heart disease.

Both MI and angina may be associated with shortness of breath and fatigue caused by ischemic myocardial dysfunction, ischemic mitral valve dysfunction, or both. MI is suggested if the pain lasts more than 20–30 minutes, especially if it occurred without obvious provocation. By contrast, anginal pain usually persists for less than 15 minutes and is more likely to be provoked by recognizable physiologic stress. Unstable angina is distinguished from stable angina by its occurrence at rest or with minimal exercise and by its change from any previous stable anginal pattern (Chapter 37). Complete response of chest pain to nitroglycerin within 5 minutes is most consistent with transient myocardial ischemia, although it can also be seen in esophageal spasm.

The presenting symptoms for acute MI may also be different for women and men. In women, shortness of breath is at least as common as acute chest pain, and prodromal symptoms of unusual fatigue are also more common in women, perhaps because their MIs tend to occur at a later age.

True myocardial ischemia may also be found in the absence of demonstrable coronary disease on angiography. For example, some patients may have angina related to episodic coronary artery spasm without underlying severe coronary stenoses, and some patients have true ischemia

TABLE 35.1
DIFFERENTIAL DIAGNOSIS OF CHEST DISCOMFORT

Cardiac disorders	Noncardiac disorders
Coronary artery disease	Gastrointestinal disorders
Stable angina	Esophageal disorders (spasm, reflux)
Unstable angina	Acid (peptic ulcer, gastritis)
Acute myocardial infarction	Cholecystitis/pancreatitis
Valvular disease	Pulmonary
Aortic valve disease (stenosis > insufficiency)	Pneumonia
Myocardial disease	Pleuritis
Hypertrophic cardiomyopathy	Pneumothorax
Other	Musculoskeletal
Aortic dissection	Chest wall pain
Pericarditis	Costochondritis (Tietze's syndrome)
Pulmonary hypertension (severe)	Thoracic outlet syndrome
Pulmonary embolism	Other
	Herpes zoster
	Psychogenic

TABLE 35.2

SOME HELPFUL FINDINGS IN THE INITIAL EVALUATION OF CHEST PAIN

	Physical examination	Electrocardiogram	Chest radiograph	Echocardiogram	Other tests
Coronary artery disease	■ Check CAD risks ■ Peripheral vascular disease ■ S_4, MR ■ Heart failure	■ ST depression or elevation ■ New Q waves ■ T-wave inversion ■ New conduction system disease	■ LV enlargement ■ Heart failure ■ Coronary calcification	■ LV segmental wall motion abnormality or ■ MR	■ Cardiac biomarkers
Aortic dissection	■ Hypertension ■ Cerebrovascular accident ■ Loss of carotid or peripheral pulses ■ Mesenteric or lower extremety ischemia ■ Marfanoid habitus ■ Aortic insufficiency ■ Pericarditis	■ Pericarditis (PR depression, J-point elevation) ■ Inferior ischemia or infarction	■ Widened mediastinum ■ Enlarged cardiac silhouette ■ Pleural effusion	*Transesophageal* ■ Aortic root dissection ■ Pericardial effusion ■ AR, MR	■ Hematocrit ■ CT scan ■ MRI
Pericarditis/ pericardial tamponade	■ Pericardial rub ■ Diminished heart sounds ■ Elevated JVP ■ Kussmaul's sign ■ Pulsatile liver ■ Ascites ■ Peripheral edema	■ PR depression (early) ■ Prominent or "peaked" T waves ■ J-point or ST elevation (diffusely) ■ Low voltage ■ Electrical alternans	■ Enlarged cardiac silhouette ■ Pericardial calcification ■ Pleural effusion without pulmonary congestion ■ Pericardial fat pad separation	■ Pericardial effusion ■ Pericardial thickening ■ Diastolic RA or RV collapse (c/w tamponade) ■ Doppler evidence of constriction	■ ESR, ANA ■ Hematocrit ■ BUN/ creatinine ■ Thyroid panel
Pulmonary embolus or infarction	■ Hypotension ■ Tachycardia ■ Tachypnea ■ RV heave ■ RV S_3 ■ Loud P_2 ■ Pleural rub	■ Sinus tachycardia ■ Right axis deviation ■ RVH or RV strain ■ S wave in lead I ■ Q wave in lead III ■ Inverted T wave in lead III	■ Hampton's hump (pleura-based wedge-shaped infarct) ■ Westermark's sign (focal oligemia) ■ Pleural effusion ■ Enlarged PAs ■ RV enlargement	■ RV dysfunction ■ Elevated PA systolic pressure ■ RA or RV thrombus ■ Proximal PA thrombus	■ Arterial blood gas ■ D-dimer ■ V/Q scan and/or spiral CT and/or lower-extremity Doppler exam
Gastrointestinal chest pain	■ RUQ or mid-epigastric pain on palpation ■ Peritonitis ■ Abnormal bowel sounds	■ Sinus tachycardia with pain or GI blood loss ■ Inverted septal T waves with esophageal spasm	■ Aspiration pneumonia ■ Hiatial hernia		■ Hematocrit, MCV ■ Amylase, liver enzymes ■ Stool for blood ■ Upper GI endoscopy and/or RUQ ultrasound
Musculoskeletal chest pain	■ Tenderness over ribs, spine, costochondral junction ■ Ecchymoses ■ Decreased range of motion	■ Sinus tachycardia with pain	■ Rib fractures ■ Vertebral fractures		

AR, aortic regurgitation; *CAD*, coronary artery disease; *GI*, gastrointestinal; *JVP*, jugular venous pressure; *LV*, left ventricle; *MR*, mitral regurgitation; *PA*, pulmonary artery; *RA*, right atrium; *RUQ*, right upper quadrant; *RV*, right ventricle; *RVH*, right ventricular hypertrophy; *V/Q*, ventilation–perfusion.

despite the absence of any demonstrable abnormalities in their epicardial coronary arteries (Syndrome X). A newly recognized syndrome has symptoms and ECG changes that clinically mimic acute infero-apical MI in the absence of obstructive coronary disease; it is generally seen in older women in the setting of hypertension and intense physical and/or psychological stress or somatic pain. Labeled the "Tako-Tsubo" syndrome (5) because the left ventricular apex balloons in a pattern likened to the Japanese pot used to catch octopus, it may be caused by microvascular spasm or regional myocarditis. Its transient ECG changes are similar to the acute cardiac findings in the setting of neurologic injuries. Myocardial ischemia can also be found in patients with aortic valvular disease, especially aortic stenosis, or hypertrophic cardiomyopathy because of an imbalance between myocardial oxygen demand and supply (Figure 38.1).

Anemia, thyrotoxicosis, fever, and other high-output states can exacerbate underlying causes of myocardial ischemia but do not usually cause myocardial ischemia themselves in the absence of other underlying abnormalities. The chest discomfort caused by myocardial ischemia resulting from these various conditions usually is clinically indistinguishable from that of angina pectoris.

Recent exposure to recreational drugs, pharmaceuticals, or diet supplements (e.g., cocaine, amphetamines, β-agonist inhalers, ephedrine) can cause coronary spasm or transient increases in myocardial oxygen demand secondary to sympathetic nervous system mediated increases in contractility or peripheral arterial tone. At least in the case of cocaine exposure, patients with significant ECG changes or elevations of cardiac biomarkers are at low risk of death or myocardial infarction (6).

Aortic dissection (Chapter 49) is a less common condition, usually associated with underlying hypertension or an abnormality such as Marfan syndrome that causes the aortic abnormalities. The pain is typically described as tearing or ripping, is excruciating in severity, and has a sudden onset (unlike that of acute MI, which tends to build in intensity over several minutes). The pain often indicates the location of the dissection, with ascending aortic dissections causing pain in the chest and upper back, and descending dissections causing pain in the upper back and mid to lower back and abdomen. The pain is not typically precipitated by exertion, although any stimulus that increases blood pressure or heart rate can exacerbate the dissection. An aortic dissection can compromise a coronary artery, primarily the right coronary artery, and cause acute inferior wall MI. Dissection retrograde into the pericardium can cause acute pericardial tamponade. If the dissection compresses the branch of any major artery, signs and symptoms of arterial insufficiency will be noted, with diminished or delayed pulses and end-organ dysfunction. When aortic dissection is clinically suspected, the physical examination should search carefully for evidence of delayed pulses or vascular insufficiency. The

chest radiograph may confirm an enlarged aorta. Transesophageal echocardiography is an excellent screening test, and computed tomography (CT) or magnetic resonance imaging (MRI) can confirm the diagnosis (7) (Chapter 36).

Pericarditis (Chapter 46) may present with dull or aching chest discomfort similar to that of an acute MI, or with pleuritic discomfort similar to that of pulmonary embolism, pneumonia, or other pleural disease. Pericarditis can also accompany acute MI, usually occurring a day or more after an acute Q-wave MI, and pericardial tamponade can occur with proximal aortic dissection back into the pericardium. The discomfort of pericarditis is often exacerbated by inspiration or coughing. Unless accompanied by acute MI or aortic dissection, the pain is unlikely to be associated with diaphoresis, nausea, or vomiting, and it seldom radiates to the arms. The pain is usually not related to exertion, and it tends to persist for hours or days. A key physical finding is a pericardial rub. In patients with evidence of tamponade or constriction, additional findings of hemodynamic compromise should be sought.

Although heart failure is not commonly associated with chest discomfort, a sense of pressure or fullness may be caused by pulmonary hypertension (Chapter 59) or the excessive stimulation or distention of the J-receptors in the lung parenchyma. Shortness of breath and orthopnea will almost always accompany any chest discomfort associated with heart failure, and the patient may also have jugular venous distention or peripheral edema consistent with secondary right-sided heart failure. Because heart failure may also be a manifestation of other serious causes of chest discomfort (e.g., acute MI, severe myocardial ischemia, aortic dissection, pericarditis, pulmonary embolism), these other possible precipitants of heart failure must be considered in the initial evaluation.

Cardiac arrhythmias commonly cause a sensation of palpitations (see below) rather than true chest discomfort. However, some arrhythmias may precipitate myocardial ischemia and its associated chest discomfort.

The chest discomfort of *pulmonary embolus* (8) or pulmonary infarction can be similar to that of coronary insufficiency when acute right ventricular (RV) strain and ischemia associated with the pulmonary hypertension are present. However, the pain of these conditions is more commonly described as pleuritic in nature and is usually peripheral rather than central in the chest.

The *gastrointestinal* causes of chest discomfort include esophageal motility disorders such as spasm and reflux, acid-peptic diseases such as ulcer and gastritis, and cholecystitis or pancreatitis. Esophageal spasm may mimic myocardial ischemia in terms of its quality and location; even more vexing, it may have a similar response to nitroglycerin. The diagnosis can often be made based on the relation of the pain to meals, exacerbation by recumbent position, and lack of relation to exercise. Esophageal reflux and spasm commonly respond to antacid therapy. However, a therapeutic trial of antacids in the emergency setting is notoriously inaccurate for making a diagnosis of esophageal or acid-peptic causes of chest discomfort because the resolution of pain caused by ischemic heart disease during the same time frame may be inappropriately attributed to this unrelated therapeutic trial. Gastrointestinal causes of chest discomfort are often associated with abnormalities on the abdominal examination, and, except for esophageal spasm, are unlikely to cause pain that radiates to the shoulder, neck, or arms. Gastrointestinal causes of pain also tend to have a reproducible relationship to eating, to be unrelated to exercise, and to persist for hours.

Pulmonary causes of chest discomfort include pneumonia, pleuritis, and pneumothorax, and tend to be exaggerated by breathing and sometimes by changes in position. The pain is commonly described as sharp and stabbing. The episodes range from fleeting pain associated with a particular precipitant to prolonged and constant discomfort; neither of these characteristics is typical of myocardial ischemia.

Musculoskeletal chest discomfort may be related to a variety of abnormalities of the muscles, bones, and nerves of the chest wall and shoulder. These causes of pain are commonly exacerbated by movement or local palpation, are not otherwise affected by exertion, and do not respond to nitroglycerin. It should be remembered that patients with substantial chest wall trauma may also have cardiac trauma, including myocardial contusion, valvular damage, or damage to the great vessels.

Although traditional cardiac risk factors, such as hypertension, hyperlipidemia, smoking, and diabetes mellitus, increase the likelihood that chest discomfort may be related to ischemic heart disease (and are present in up to 90% of patients with atherosclerotic coronary artery disease [9]), these long-term risk factors are not particularly helpful in the evaluation of the patient with acute chest pain. Rather, the evaluation must focus on attempts to establish a specific diagnosis; patients without a specific diagnosis will commonly require additional evaluation and observation until the most serious causes can be effectively excluded.

Physical Examination

For patients with chest discomfort, the focus of the physical examination should include evaluation of the pulse and blood pressure. If aortic dissection is seriously considered, blood pressure should be measured in both arms, and pulses should be checked in the legs to exclude pulse delay. Evaluation of jugular venous pressure is important to exclude right-sided heart failure or evidence of pericardial constriction and tamponade. The carotid pulse may be diminished in amplitude and its peak delayed in patients with aortic stenosis (Chapter 41), delayed or absent in

patients with aortic dissection, or associated with a bruit in patients with generalized atherosclerosis. Pulmonary evaluation may reveal a pleuritic rub suggestive of pleuritis, pulmonary infarction, or pneumonia; evidence of consolidation suggesting pneumonia; rales or wheezes of heart failure; or findings consistent with pneumothorax. Palpation of the chest wall and related areas may reveal a musculoskeletal cause of pain. On cardiac auscultation, a prominent second component of the second heart sound may suggest pulmonary hypertension, which may reflect pulmonary embolism. A pericardial rub or knock is found in acute pericarditis or pericardial constriction, respectively. Patients with ischemic heart disease may have transient third or fourth heart sounds or a murmur of mitral regurgitation caused by transient papillary muscle dysfunction. The murmur of aortic stenosis (Chapter 41) should be readily apparent, as should the murmur of hypertrophic obstructive cardiomyopathy (see later in this chapter). The murmur of aortic insufficiency may suggest a diagnosis of acute aortic dissection. A careful abdominal examination is critical to evaluate possible gastrointestinal diagnoses, such as cholecystitis or pancreatitis.

Electrocardiogram

The ECG is the most important single piece of information for the evaluation of the cause of acute chest pain. The ECG alone is probably as important as all other pieces of information combined. About 45% of patients with acute MI will have diagnostic findings (new ST-segment elevation or Q waves) on initial ECG. An additional 35% or so of patients will have ST-segment depression or T-wave inversions consistent with ischemia. In patients presenting to an emergency department with acute chest pain but who lack such ECG findings, the probability of acute MI is less than 10%; however, identification of these MI patients, who account for about 20% of all infarcts, is critical. It must be remembered that the ECG is relatively insensitive for detecting infarction of the posterior, lateral, and apical walls of the left ventricle (10), and its specificity is limited by individual variations in coronary anatomy and preexisting coronary disease.

In interpreting the ECG, several important points must be kept in mind. First, at the time the ECG is performed, notations should be made regarding whether the patient is having active chest pain. Changes with acute coronary insufficiency or arrhythmia can be dynamic and resolve completely when the symptom abates. Second, every effort must be made to obtain previous ECGs so that abnormalities can be compared with those on the old tracing. *Any ECG finding that cannot be proved to be old must be assumed to be new.* The physician must have a low threshold for repeating an ECG while the patient is under observation, especially if the symptoms change in quality, appear or disappear, or persist for more than 10–20 minutes.

Chest Radiograph

The chest radiograph will rarely be diagnostic for the cause of acute chest pain. However, it may establish a diagnosis of pneumonia or pneumothorax, reveal an increased cardiac silhouette consistent with pericardial effusion, indicate pulmonary hypertension, or demonstrate an abnormal aorta suggestive of aortic dissection. It may also show overt skeletal abnormalities or trauma consistent with musculoskeletal causes of pain. Once again, comparison with previous films is critical; in the absence of old films, any changes must be assumed to be new until proved otherwise.

Integrating Clinical Data

Based on the history, physical examination, and ECG, it is possible to arrive at an approximate probability that the patient is having an acute MI (3, 11) (Figure 35.1). These data, derived from patients presenting to emergency departments, may or may not be directly applicable to patients in whom chest pain develops while they are in the hospital.

Initial triage decisions for patients who present to emergency departments with acute chest pain are driven by the probability of acute MI in addition to the probability of complications requiring intensive care (Figure 37.2). The

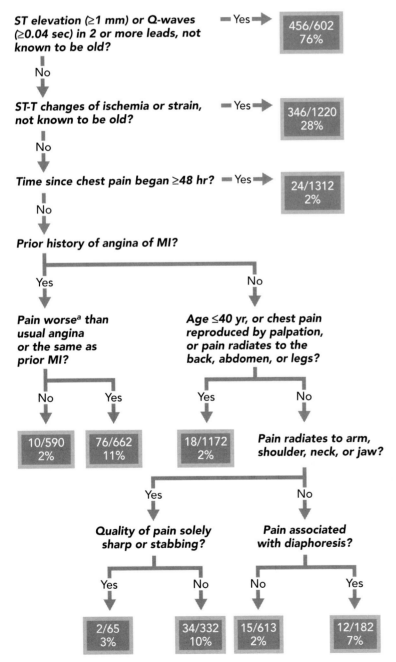

Figure 35.1 Flow diagram for estimating the risk for acute myocardial infarction in emergency department patients with acute chest pain. For each clinical subset, the numerator is the number of patients with the set of presenting characteristics in whom a myocardial infarction developed, whereas the denominator represents the total number of patients presenting with that characteristic or set of characteristics.[a] In frequency, severity, duration, or failure to respond to usual measures. (Adapted from Pearson SD, Goldman L, Garcia TB, et al. Physician response to a prediction rule for the triage of emergency department patients with chest pain. *J Gen Intern Med* 1994;9:241–247, with permission.)

hospital physician may participate in the initial triage decision and in the management of patients in the emergency department. Currently, many chest pain evaluation units (12, 13) are part of the emergency department itself, and hence the hospital physician may not directly participate in initial decision making. In some hospitals, however, the hospital physician may directly supervise the chest pain evaluation unit. In these situations, this physician will be involved in initial triage and management decisions. Patients should generally have telemetry monitoring, serial biomarker determinations and ECGs, and other tests as needed to exclude myocardial ischemia or other important causes of chest pain.

Chest pain evaluation units or observation units may be established in the emergency department itself or in other locations in the hospital. Such units provide continuous ECG telemetry monitoring with ward-level nursing intensity. These units usually have strict entry criteria and prohibit intravenous medications or major ECG changes; many insist that the patients have a low probability for MI by validated methods (Figure 35.1). These units also have strict transfer criteria, so that patients with recurrent angina, MI, or evidence of hemodynamic or arrhythmic instability must be transferred. Similarly, patients who have evidence of other important causes of chest pain, such as pulmonary embolism, aortic dissection, or pericarditis, must be moved to an appropriately intensive location. Chest pain units typically also have a maximum length of stay, usually no more than 12 hours (Chapters 37 and 38). These units may be established by admitting patients to observation status in otherwise empty beds in an ICU or step-down unit, by transforming an existing observation unit into a cardiac monitoring unit, or by using an area in the emergency department itself. Numerous studies have shown that when patients at low risk for MI are admitted to such units, they can receive appropriate care at markedly reduced expense compared with admission to traditional step-down units or ICUs. In most studies, only about 2% of patients admitted to these units are shown eventually to have MI, and only 10%–20% of such patients are admitted from such units (the others are sent home after appropriate observation and pre-discharge noninvasive testing).

Echocardiography can demonstrate wall motion abnormalities or other evidence of ischemia but is not generally recommended for establishing the diagnosis of acute coronary ischemia. Echocardiograms are critical for patients with suspected valvular abnormalities, cardiomyopathy, or pericarditis; transesophageal echocardiography is one of the most sensitive ways to diagnose aortic dissection. In patients with pulmonary embolism or other causes of pulmonary hypertension, the echocardiogram may reveal sufficient tricuspid or pulmonic regurgitation to allow estimation of pulmonary artery pressures, as well as assessment of right ventricular function, an important prognostic variable when deciding on the clinical utility of

thrombolytic therapy in the case of suspected pulmonary embolus.

Perfusion scintigraphy with sestamibi or thallium will commonly reveal abnormalities in patients with acute ischemia. However, it is not clear whether integrating such tests into routine practice will improve decision making in patients with acute chest discomfort (Chapter 36).

Coronary angiography remains the gold standard for diagnosing ischemic heart disease, despite the fact that some patients have ischemia with normal epicardial coronary arteries and other patients with coronary stenoses may have chest pain unrelated to the angiographic findings (Chapter 37). Catheterization may also be critical to diagnose pericardial tamponade or constriction (Chapter 46), localize the site of aortic dissection (Chapter 49), or perform pulmonary angiography to diagnose pulmonary embolism (Chapter 53).

A substantial number of patients with otherwise undiagnosed causes of chest pain may have underlying esophageal pathology. Strong consideration should be given to studies of esophageal motility and acid reflux in patients with recurrent chest pain of uncertain etiology.

When Chest Pain Presents after Admission

The evaluation of chest pain in the hospitalized patient is very similar to that in a patient who presents to the emergency department. The principal difference is that in-hospital chest pain is more likely to be precipitated by fever, anemia, hypoxia, pain, or the wide variety of stresses that are found in sick inpatients. In the hospitalized patient, attention to these precipitating causes may be critical to the evaluation and management of the chest pain itself. For example, the resolution of pain resulting from myocardial ischemia may depend critically on the control of postoperative fever and blood loss. Because patients who are already sick in the hospital typically have less physiologic reserve, attention to the underlying precipitating causes and prompt evaluation and treatment of the precise etiology of chest pain are of key importance.

Palpitations

Palpitations, like chest pain, can be a warning of severe underlying cardiac pathology but can also be completely benign (14). Patients complaining of palpitations may be experiencing bursts of ventricular tachycardia (VT) (Chapter 43), runs of supraventricular tachycardia (Chapter 42), or single premature atrial contractions (PACs), or they may just be keenly aware of a physiologic sinus tachycardia. The physician evaluating the patient must, through careful history and physical examination, select the appropriate diagnostic studies to ensure that the patient is not at risk for sudden death or any other significant adverse cardiovascular event (Table 35.3).

TABLE 35.3
EVALUATION OF PALPITATIONS

Basics
History
Physical examination
Electrocardiogram
Electrolytes/arterial blood gases as indicated

Document arrhythmia
Holter/event monitor
Exercise test (if exertional symptoms)
Electrophysiology study

Risk-stratify for malignant arrhythmia/cardiac morbidity/mortality
Echocardiogram (look for wall motion abnormality, abnormal ventricular function, valvular heart disease, hypertrophic obstructive cardiomyopathy)
Electrophysiology study

History

A careful history can be extremely helpful in determining the likely etiology of "palpitations" and the likelihood that they stem from serious underlying cardiac disease. The clinical context is crucial. A 65-year-old man with a recent history of MI and decreased left ventricular (LV) function is at higher risk for malignant arrhythmia than is a young person with no other evidence of structural or coronary heart disease.

One critical aspect of the history is the patient's precise definition of what is being experienced as palpitations. Asking patients to "tap out" what they feel, or tapping out some possibilities for them, can help distinguish a solitary premature contraction from atrial fibrillation or a sustained regular tachyarrhythmia.

Symptoms that accompany the palpitations can help diagnose the arrhythmia and define high- and low-risk patients. Palpitations accompanied by near-syncope (transient loss of consciousness) imply compromised cerebral blood flow. As a general rule, supraventricular tachycardias are less likely to cause presyncopal events than is VT. A notable exception is the case of a patient with reduced LV function, whose cardiac output may fall with any increase in heart rate. Chest pain associated with palpitations should raise concern for concomitant myocardial ischemia.

The next important aspect of the history is the description of precipitating factors. Certain arrhythmias are more likely to be encountered at times of high sympathetic tone, others at times of high vagal tone. Atrioventricular nodal reentrant tachycardia (AVNRT), an arrhythmia that is precipitated by a PAC, occurs more frequently at times of slow heart rates, especially at rest or in bed. Atrial fibrillation may occur at times of high vagal tone, during sleep, or immediately after exercise, but it can also occur in high catecholamine states, such as postoperatively or during exercise (this distinction can be helpful in the choice of therapy). Ventricular tachyarrhythmias are most commonly associated with high catecholamine states. The hereditary long-QT syndrome is characterized by polymorphic VT at times of emotional stress.

Some patients are keenly aware of the maneuvers they can perform to terminate palpitations. AVNRT is often easily terminated by vagal maneuvers, and some patients may note that their palpitations stop when they cough. Ventricular premature beats (VPBs) associated with low heart rates may cease with exercise.

Another important factor is the list of medications, both prescribed and over-the-counter. Patients on diuretics may experience VPBs or VT associated with hypokalemia or hypomagnesemia. Patients on antiarrhythmic medications, psychotropic medications, or some antihistamines are at risk for VPBs and polymorphous VT because of prolongation of the QT interval (Table 35.4). Theophylline derivatives can cause supraventricular tachycardia or VT. Substance abuse can also be an aggravating factor; cocaine, amphetamines, alcohol (e.g., "holiday heart"), and excess caffeine can precipitate palpitations and arrhythmia.

The period of time during which a patient has experienced symptoms is also helpful in determining their etiology. Bypass tract-mediated tachycardias often present in childhood, whereas atrial fibrillation and most VTs start in adulthood.

In the patient who is already in the hospital, the diagnosis of the arrhythmia is often evident (the patient is on monitor), and the physician should focus on the cause of the

TABLE 35.4
CAUSES OF LONG QT INTERVAL

Congenital
Electrolyte abnormalities
  Hypocalcemia
  Hypokalemia (long QT secondary to fusion of ST segment with "U" wave)
Ischemia
Medications
  Antiarrhythmic drugs
    Type IA: disopyramide, procainamide, quinidine
    Type IC: encainide, flecainide, propafenone
    Type III: amiodarone, sotalol
  Psychotropic medications
    Phenothiazines, butyrophenones (haloperidol), tricyclics
  Macrolide antibiotics: erythromycin, clarithromycin, troleandomycin
  Seldane
  Cisapride
  Pentamidine
  Ketoconazole
CNS disease: subarachnoid bleed
Hypothyroidism
Myocarditis
Hypothermia

arrhythmia. VPBs and VT are seen in critically ill patients with electrolyte disturbances, hypoxemia, sepsis, myocardial ischemia, and drug side effects. Atrial fibrillation is seen in similar situations; it is also seen with lung processes (e.g., pneumonia, chronic obstructive pulmonary disease), hyperthyroidism, valvular heart disease, and postoperatively.

Physical Examination

The physical examination is critical in the evaluation of a patient with palpitations. Unfortunately, most patients do not have symptoms at the time of examination, but evidence of any underlying heart disease can be helpful in determining the likelihood of a serious etiology of the palpitations.

The pulse can indicate evidence of VPBs or PACs or the irregularly irregular rhythm of atrial fibrillation. Pronounced bradycardia, although normal in the trained athlete, may be a marker of abnormal conduction or need for an "escape mechanism" (e.g., atrial fibrillation in the brady-tachy syndrome). Apical-to-peripheral pulse discrepancies can be found in many arrhythmias. Hypertensive heart disease is a prominent predisposing factor for atrial fibrillation.

Examination of the jugular venous pulse may give a clue to the etiology of the palpitations. For example, flutter or fibrillatory waves may be seen in the jugular venous pressure contour, and cannon *a* waves are often seen in AV dissociation.

The cardiac examination can also yield helpful clues. A laterally displaced point of maximal impulse, dyskinetic impulses or heaves, or palpable extra heart sounds denote the substrate for ventricular arrhythmias. A midsystolic click can diagnose the mitral valve prolapse syndrome, which is accompanied by both supraventricular and ventricular tachyarrhythmias. Significant murmurs may indicate underlying structural heart disease, especially aortic stenosis, mitral regurgitation, and hypertrophic obstructive cardiomyopathy, all of which predispose patients to arrhythmia.

Proptosis, lid lag, and tremors are markers for hyperthyroidism, which predisposes to atrial fibrillation. Tarnished nail enamel and knuckle scarring accompany bulimia nervosa, which leads to electrolyte imbalances that can cause ectopic beats.

Risk Stratification

After a careful history and physical examination, many patients can be stratified into high- or low-risk categories in terms of the likely morbidity associated with their palpitations. At low risk are young patients with isolated premature beats, no evidence of structural or ischemic heart disease on the basis of history and physical examination, no sustained arrhythmia, and no syncopal symptoms. Some patients will have evidence suggesting panic attacks. At high risk are older patients with known coronary artery disease, LV dysfunc-

tion, heart failure, evidence of structural or valvular heart disease on physical examination, or symptoms such as dizziness, syncope, chest discomfort, or dyspnea with the palpitations.

Diagnostic Tests

The easiest and least expensive diagnostic test for palpitations is the 12-lead ECG, which may show PACs, VPBs, a short PR interval, delta waves, Q waves, atrial abnormalities, a long QT interval, or LV or RV hypertrophy. PACs either may be the source of the sensation of palpitations or may trigger AVNRT (Chapter 42). VPBs may be the source of the palpitations or the marker of a more serious abnormality that might predispose to malignant arrhythmia. A short PR interval or a delta wave suggests a preexcitation syndrome such as Wolff-Parkinson-White syndrome. Q waves may indicate previous MI as the substrate for VT. LV hypertrophy may be a marker for hypertrophic cardiomyopathy in a young patient with a predisposition for atrial fibrillation and VT. Fascicular blocks, bundle branch blocks, and AV block are all markers for conduction system disease that may indicate bradyarrhythmia.

An echocardiogram is warranted if signs or symptoms suggestive of any structural heart disease are present (Chapter 44). The echocardiogram can reveal the substrate for malignant ventricular arrhythmias: wall motion abnormalities (suggestive of coronary artery disease or cardiomyopathy), hypertrophic cardiomyopathy, or valvular heart disease. Atrial enlargement, reduced LV function, or mitral annular calcification indicate a higher likelihood of atrial fibrillation. In a young patient with syncope, a cardiac MRI can occasionally be helpful to evaluate for RV dysplasia, an important cause of VT.

In a patient with very frequent symptoms, a 24-hour Holter monitor can diagnose the arrhythmia. For those patients whose arrhythmia is less frequent, an event monitor may be preferable in that the patient can keep the device for a month at a time and trigger it to record only when symptoms occur. Diaries are crucial to correlate arrhythmias with any symptoms.

Treadmill exercise testing can be helpful in a patient whose symptoms are precipitated by exercise. The exercise test can induce the arrhythmia and provide evidence of ischemic heart disease. A person with excellent functional capacity is less likely to have significant underlying pathology.

In a patient with alarming symptoms (e.g., syncope), symptoms refractory to medical management, or a documented substrate for malignant arrhythmia, an electrophysiology study may be warranted. These studies can document and treat bypass tract-mediated arrhythmias, AVNRT, atrial flutter, and ectopic atrial tachycardias (Chapter 42). Electrophysiologic studies can also diagnose and occasionally treat ventricular arrhythmias. These studies are the "gold standard" for the evaluation of palpitations, but they are invasive and should be reserved for those patients in whom they are necessary.

In the hospitalized patient, the approach to palpitations is similar with the exception that a variety of acute perturbations may precipitate arrhythmias. In hospitalized patients, fever, blood loss, hypotension, hypoxia, pain, and medications are common causes of arrhythmia. Attention to these precipitating causes may be at least as important as specific anti-arrhythmic treatment.

Lightheadedness

Like chest pain and palpitations, lightheadedness can also represent a spectrum of risk, from the completely benign to potentially catastrophic. It can be a difficult symptom for the patient to describe, and alternative terms include "dizzy," "woozy," "weak," "unsteady," and "faint".

Lightheadedness from a cardiovascular cause stems from decreased blood flow to the brain; if prolonged or more profound, syncope will occur (Chapter 44). However, cardiac symptoms must be distinguished from vertigo, decreased proprioception, and impaired visual acuity. Is the room spinning around? Is the sensation worse with poor lighting? Does the patient feel faint? An answer of "yes" to the first question implies vertigo; to the second, decreased proprioceptive or coordination abilities; and to the third, cardiovascular-related "lightheadedness."

The precipitants of the sensation of lightheadedness can also suggest its etiology. Does the patient feel lightheaded on rising from a sitting or lying position? If so, orthostasis is a likely mechanism. Does it occur when the patient is standing for some time? If so, orthostasis or a vasovagal cause is likely. Does it occur with exercise? If so, an arrhythmia, aortic stenosis, or hypetrophic obstructive cardiomyopathy are a possible etiologies. Does it occur when the patient is anxious? If so, hyperventilation should be suggested. Is it related to micturition, cough, or straining to defecate? If so, a vagally mediated response is likely.

Accompanying symptoms can also be helpful in determining the etiology of lightheadedness. Palpitations suggest an arrhythmia that decreases cardiac output. Chest pain suggests myocardial ischemia. Additional neurologic deficits suggest a primary central nervous system condition, such as a transient ischemic attack (Chapter 116) or intracranial mass (Chapter 117).

A thorough review of the patient's medication list is critical in determining both the cause and the severity of the condition. For example, with most antihypertensive medications and many psychotropic medications, lightheadedness can be caused by orthostasis.

The patient's problem list may also be very helpful in determining both the cause and the severity of the condition. Heart failure, coronary disease, and vascular disease all predispose to potentially serious causes of lightheadedness.

Anemia (if severe) or significant recent blood loss can be contributing or causative factors to the symptom. Parkinson's disease, as well as other primary neurologic disorders, may predispose to the Shy-Drager syndrome. Diabetes and alcohol abuse cause neuropathies that can lead to lightheadedness. Anxiety can lead to hyperventilation, which also causes this symptom.

Physical Examination

A slow pulse might indicate heart block or symptomatic bradycardia. A comparison of supine and standing blood pressures and heart rate, especially if it elicits symptoms, can be diagnostic.

Skin turgor, mucous membranes, and jugular venous pressure can be excellent indicators of volume status. Additionally, skin pallor can raise the question of anemia and blood loss.

The cardiac examination should be directed toward consideration of conditions that decrease cardiac output (e.g., aortic stenosis, hypertrophic obstructive cardiomyopathy, or enlarged and dysfunctional ventricles) or predispose to arrhythmias. A loud P_2 sound or right ventricular heave suggest pulmonary hypertension. Auscultatory evaluation for carotid bruits is critical in screening for cerebral vascular disease.

The neurologic examination may reveal evidence of previous central nervous system damage or diseases that would put the patient at increased risk for autonomic dysfunction (Shy-Drager syndrome). Abnormalities in visual acuity or evidence of inner ear pathology may provide noncardiovascular explanations for the lightheadedness.

Risk Stratification

Risk stratification and further evaluation of the patient with lightheadedness follow the same approach as the evaluation of palpitations, with all efforts focused on identifying underlying or occult structural or ischemic cardiac disease and electrophysiologic pathology.

CARDIOVASCULAR SIGNS

Jugular Venous Pressure

Before recent technologic advances became available (i.e., echocardiography and cardiac catheterization), correct assessments of abnormal jugular venous pressure were essential in certain diagnostic dilemmas, such as the differentiation of constrictive pericardial disease from cirrhosis and other noncardiac sources of peripheral edema and ascites. However, the subjectivity and difficulty of the examination have limited its current applicability. The key parameters are the height of jugular veins (easily assessed via the external jugular veins) and the jugular wave forms (best assessed in the internal jugular veins, which do not have valves to distort retrograde flow) (Table 35.5).

Perhaps the most reliable way of describing jugular venous distention is as elevated or not. Somewhat more precise estimates can be made by assuming that the "angle of Louis" at the clavicle is 5 cm above the center of the right atrium, and thus the jugular venous pressure is the number of centimeters above this angle added to 5 cm. Unfortunately, this assumption of 5 cm is quite variable, and the true value ranges between 2–8 cm. If the neck veins are obstructed from view, an alternative is to raise the hand and look for the height above the heart at which there is a loss of venous distention. The key wave forms are the *a* wave, which is retrograde flow during right atrial contraction, and the *v* wave, which corresponds to ventricular contraction and is exaggerated in the presence of tricuspid regurgitation.

The jugular veins are a very useful way of assessing a patient's intravascular volume status and right atrial pressure. Although not a direct measurement of left atrial or pulmonary capillary wedge pressure, the jugular venous pressure can indirectly reflect elevations in these pressures if there is no other cause of elevated right atrial pressure. In contrast, *Kussmaul's sign*, which is seen in constrictive pericarditis, is an exaggerated distention of the neck veins during inspiration, in contrast to the normal obliteration of venous distention during inspiration.

Hepatojugular reflux can be assessed with the patient at a 45-degree angle and approximately 30–40 mm Hg of pressure placed at the xiphosternal epigastric area and held for approximately 15–30 seconds. This sign is positive if jugular venous distention is sustained for that period of time and immediately falls on removal of pressure. In general,

hepatojugular reflux is an indicator of right-sided heart failure (15), which in most cases is a consequence of long-standing left atrial pressure elevation.

The *cannon a wave* is an indicator of AV dissociation or any second- or third-degree AV block in which the right atrium contracts against a closed tricuspid valve. Intermittent AV dissociation may lead to irregular cannon *a* waves, which are more easily recognized than the regular cannon *a* waves of a junctional rhythm or VT.

Giant v waves are often seen in patients with tricuspid insufficiency as a result of regurgitant blood being transmitted to the right atrium and subsequently to the jugular veins. Tricuspid insufficiency is often present in patients with right-sided heart failure resulting from either left-sided heart failure or pulmonary hypertension of any etiology, but can also represent primary tricuspid valve pathology as in the congenital Ebstein's anomaly or trauma caused by right ventricular endomyocardial biopsy. This latter procedure is a regular part of the surveillance of heart transplant recipients.

Arterial Pulses

Examination of the arterial pulses is an invaluable component of the cardiovascular examination (Table 35.6). It is the primary modality used to diagnose atherosclerotic peripheral vascular disease, and the presence of abnormalities in the peripheral pulses often suggest similar coronary pathology. Additionally, careful examination of the peripheral arteries facilitates the diagnosis of valvular heart lesions, pericardial tamponade, heart failure, and arrhythmias. However, the examination of peripheral arteries is complicated by its subjectivity and its ill-defined grading system.

Important qualities to note on the physical examination of the peripheral arteries include rhythm, contour, amplitude, and symmetry. Usually, the carotid artery is best suited for examination because of its close proximity to the heart. Examination of the carotid pulse requires a certain degree of caution, in that undue pressure on a carotid body may result in asystole or cerebral embolism. The amplitude of the carotid arterial pulse increases with age, owing to stiffening of the arterial wall. As the amplitude of the pulse is generally proportional to stroke volume, a low-amplitude pulse suggests reduced stroke volume, and increased amplitude suggests an increased stroke volume. Hypotension, aortic stenosis, and mitral regurgitation cause low-amplitude pulses. In contrast, hypertension, hyperthyroidism, high catecholamine states, and aortic insufficiency lead to high-amplitude pulses. In the peripheral vascular bed, low-amplitude pulses imply poor blood flow, either from reduced cardiac output or from peripheral vascular disease.

The contour of the arterial pulse represents the rise and fall of the arterial blood flow. The rise and fall of the pulse is a marker of the rapidity of the ejection of the stroke

TABLE 35.5
JUGULAR VENOUS PRESSURE FINDINGS

Normal
<7–10 cm H$_2$O (i.e., not elevated)

Elevated
Intracardiac causes of high RA pressures (e.g., RV failure/LV failure, RV infarct)

Other causes
Pericardial tamponade or constriction
Any cause of pulmonary hypertension
Superior vena caval obstruction

Key abnormalities to assess
Giant v wave—tricuspid regurgitation
Hepatojugular reflux (abdominojugular reflux)
RV dysfunction and elevated pulmonary capillary wedge pressure ≥15 mm Hg
Cannon a wave—AV dissociation
Kussmaul's sign—constrictive pericarditis

LV, left ventricular; RV, right ventricular; RA, right atrial; AV, atrioventricular.

TABLE 35.6

EXAMINATION OF ARTERIAL PULSE (PALPATION, AUSCULTATION)

Palpation
1. Amplitude (indirect measure of stroke volume)
   a. Weak, thready in hypotensive and/or hypovolemic states
   b. Reduced in aortic stenosis (parvus) and mitral regurgitation
   c. Increased in hyperdynamic states, aortic insufficiency, arteriovenous fistulae
   d. Pulsus paradoxus—inspiratory fall in systolic pressure >10 mm Hg seen in pericardial tamponade and exaggerated breathing in asthma or COPD
   e. Pulsus alternans—alternating weaker or stronger pulse in marked LV systolic dysfunction
2. Contour (rapidity of rise and fall of pulse)
   a. Delayed (tardus) in aortic stenosis
   b. Bisferiens pulse—double impulse classically seen with aortic insufficiency and often in hypertrophic obstructive cardiomyopathy
   c. Corrigan/Waterhammer (rapid, strong) pulse seen in aortic insufficiency
   d. Carotid shudder/thrill seen in aortic stenosis
3. Cadence
   a. Irregularly irregular—atrial fibrillation, frequent multifocal VPBs, PACs
   b. Regularly irregular—usually PACs, VPBs in a pattern
4. Symmetry
   a. Symmetric—normal
   b. Asymmetric—seen in aortic dissection or vascular obstruction

Auscultation
1. Bruits—sign of atherosclerotic vascular disease over that particular artery
2. Transmitted murmur—aortic stenosis (if palpable, called a thrill)
3. Systolic and diastolic bruits imply
   a. severe vascular obstruction
   b. aortic insufficiency
4. Arteriovenous fistula

Visual inspection
1. Subungual capillary pulsations (Quincke's pulsations)—seen in hyperdynamic states, aortic insufficiency, anemia
2. Retinal vessels—hypertensive and diabetic changes

COPD, chronic obstructive pulmonary disease; *LV,* left ventricular;

volume. In aortic insufficiency, for example, rapid high-volume/amplitude pulses are noted, whereas in mitral regurgitation, rapid low-volume pulses are palpated. In aortic stenosis, the slow ejection time translates to a *parvus et tardus* ("weak and delayed") pulse. Other special pulses include a bisferiens pulse (two impulses in each systole), found in aortic insufficiency and hypertrophic cardiomyopathy, and pulsus alternans, found in heart failure. The former represents the exaggerated dicrotic notch. Pulsus alternans is a manifestation of marked LV systolic dysfunction, in which one weak ejection is followed by a strong one. *Pulsus paradoxus,* which may be seen in cardiac tamponade (and also in severe obstructive lung disease with

exaggerated inspiratory effort), refers to a decline in blood pressure of more than 10 mm Hg during inspiration in comparison with expiration.

The arterial pulses may cue the examiner to the presence of an arrhythmia. Although normally the phrase "irregularly irregular" is used to describe the pulse of atrial fibrillation, frequent extrasystoles may also have this cadence. A "regularly irregular" cadence may correspond to extrasystoles in a fixed pattern with sinus beats.

The symmetry of peripheral pulses may be important in diagnosing vascular obstruction. In the setting of acute chest pain, asymmetric pulses may indicate aortic dissection. Sudden loss of pulses in one limb, accompanied by pain, can be a result of an embolic phenomenon or progressive vascular disease (Chapter 51).

Palpation of pulses is not limited to the periphery. Important information about the abdominal aorta can be gained by examination of its pulse. An enlarged pulsatile mass in the abdomen suggests aneurysmal dilatation (Chapter 50).

A comprehensive examination of the arterial tree includes auscultation in addition to palpation. Bruits are indicative of stenosis and can be heard in the carotid, femoral, renal, and abdominal aortic vessels. A to-and-fro bruit indicates severe obstruction or the presence of aortic insufficiency.

Direct inspection of the arterial tree is possible in a few locations in the body—namely, the eye grounds and the nail bed. Abnormalities of the retinal vessels are found in hypertension, and neovascularization is seen in diabetes mellitus. In the nail bed, dilated capillary loops may be seen with the ophthalmoscope in several collagen vascular diseases, and Quincke's pulses (subungual capillary pulsations) of aortic insufficiency may also be seen.

Heart Sounds

The stethoscope and the auscultatory skills necessary for its effective clinical use symbolize the diagnostic skill that has been lost in the more technologically oriented present-day practice of medicine. Combining clinical clues derived from the auscultatory examination with verification or reinterpretation by an imaging modality offers the best of both worlds. With the advent of high-quality echocardiographic and Doppler interrogation of the structure and function of the heart and valves, the role of the auscultatory examination is often to serve as a screening test to determine the need for further evaluation.

Abnormalities in heart sounds may reflect circulatory status, valvular abnormalities, or other cardiac abnormalities. The normal first heart sound, which represents closure of the mitral and tricuspid valves, is accentuated in rheumatic mitral or tricuspid valvular stenosis, provided that the valve is mobile enough to close completely. The first heart sound tends to be softer in patients with incomplete mitral or tricuspid valve closure (as in valvular insufficiency) or in patients in whom ventricular systolic pressures are insufficient to close these valves crisply before the beginning of systole. The second heart sound commonly includes discernible aortic closure followed by pulmonic closure. At expiration, the two valves close virtually simultaneously, but with inspiration and increased RV filling and ejection time, the pulmonic valve closes slightly later. The aortic second sound is generally increased in hypertension and decreased in calcific aortic stenosis. The pulmonic second sound is increased in intensity by any process that causes pulmonary hypertension, which delays RV outflow and may also widen the split of the second sound. With an atrial septal defect, the splitting of the second sound tends to be wide and fixed in both inspiration and expiration because increased RV filling and outflow occur regardless of the respiratory cycle.

An S_4 gallop (fourth heart sound) precedes the first heart sound and represents relatively poor distensibility of the ventricle during late diastole at the time of atrial contraction. A fourth heart sound is common in patients with hypertension, coronary disease, or any other condition that leads to ventricular stiffness and impaired compliance. A third heart sound (S_3 gallop) (16) corresponds to the phase of rapid ventricular filling in early diastole; although sometimes found in healthy young adults or pregnant women, it is often a sign of advanced ventricular failure. In patients with rapid rates, diastole may be sufficiently shortened that the third and fourth heart sounds become superimposed and form a summation gallop.

A pericardial knock, which is caused by impaired filling in early diastole in patients with constrictive pericarditis, occurs at about the same time as a third heart sound but is usually louder and more distinctive. The "tumor plop" associated with an atrial myxoma that is prolapsing into the ventricle also occurs at about the same time, but it is usually louder and distinctive from a third heart sound.

A pericardial rub, which is found with pericarditis, is a high-pitched, scratchy sound. It may have one, two, or three components corresponding to ventricular systole, rapid ventricular filling, and atrial contraction.

Common Cardiac Murmurs

The assessment of any cardiac murmur should include the following considerations: timing (systole, diastole), intensity (grades I through VI), frequency (high-diaphragm or low-bell), configuration (crescendo, decrescendo, plateau), quality (harsh, coarse, blowing, cooing, musical, rumble), duration (e.g., pansystolic), radiation (e.g., carotid, axilla, back), and dynamic changes [e.g., effect of ectopic beats or response to breathing, expiration against a closed glottis (Valsalva maneuver), handgrip, standing, or squatting].

Grading the intensity of the murmur is particularly important in ill patients, as alterations from previous baseline

evaluations or ongoing changes may explain the dynamic physiologic status of a patient. The standard grading for murmurs is as follows: I, faint, heard with concentration in a quiet setting; II, heard immediately on auscultation; III, moderate intensity; IV, loud murmur with palpable thrill; V, loud murmur heard with the stethoscope partly on the chest; VI, loud, heard with the stethoscope off the chest. All heart murmurs should also be classified as either systolic, diastolic, or continuous (Table 35.7).

The auscultatory examination can usually differentiate a nonpathologic or functional systolic murmur from a pathologic murmur and further differentiate among the various pathologic murmurs (17). The "flow," "functional," or "innocent" murmurs include the ejection murmur related to increased cardiac output (or increased volume or velocity of ejection) and the systolic murmur appreciated only because of the thinness of the chest wall or the unusually quiet surroundings of the examining room. The clinical settings most often responsible for nonpathologic systolic murmurs include fever, anemia, thyrotoxicosis, and vigorous exercise. Innocent murmurs tend to occur in early systole and be grade I to II; have a high frequency, a crescendo-decrescendo configuration, a vibratory or humming quality, and a short duration; and be most prominent at the left sternal border without radiation.

Unfortunately, the very conditions that create the "innocent" murmur (fever, sepsis, or anemia) are often present in sick patients in whom pathologic murmurs would have potentially serious implications. In these sick or unstable patients, there should be a very low threshold for obtaining an echocardiogram (Chapter 36) to evaluate the systolic murmur. Three specific clinical scenarios should also prompt a more aggressive evaluation of the possible "innocent" murmur: (a) the early (3–7 days) post-MI patient with evidence of new hemodynamic deterioration, in whom ischemic mitral regurgitation or a new ventricular septal defect should not be missed (Chapter 38); (b) the septic patient at risk for endocarditis (Chapter 71); and (c) the elderly patient with cardiac symptoms, in whom aortic stenosis must be considered (Chapter 41).

Pathologic murmurs commonly indicate valvular or congenital heart disease and often have characteristic auscultatory findings (Table 35.8). Once an organic murmur is appreciated or suspected, confidence in the auscultatory diagnosis can sometimes be increased with the addition of physiologic maneuvers (Table 35.9). These possible pathologic diagnoses should be confirmed by echocardiography.

Occasionally, neither the cardiac examination nor the echocardiographic evaluation can adequately confirm or exclude one of the previously described etiologies of an auscultatory cardiac abnormality. In some cases, such as the patient with severe chronic obstructive pulmonary disease, an excessively expanded lung parenchyma diminishes the quality of the transthoracic echocardiographic signal.

TABLE 35.7

CLASSIFICATION OF HEART MURMURS

A. Organic systolic murmurs
  1. Midsystolic (ejection)
    a. Aortic
      (1) Obstructive
        (a) Supravalvular—supraortic stenosis, coarctation of the aorta
        (b) Valvular—AS and sclerosis
        (c) Infravalvular—HOCM
      (2) Increased flow, hyperkinetic states, AR, complete heart block
      (3) Dilatation of ascending aorta, atheroma, aortitis, aneurysm of aorta
    b. Pulmonary
      (1) Obstructive
        (a) Supravalvular—pulmonary arterial stenosis
        (b) Valvular—pulmonic valve stenosis
        (c) Infravalvular—infundibular stenosis
      (2) Increased flow, hyperkinetic states, left-to-right shunt (e.g., ASD, VSD)
      (3) Dilatation of pulmonary artery
  2. Pansystolic (regurgitant)
    a. Atrioventricular valve regurgitation (MR, TR)
    b. Left-to-right shunt at ventricular level
B. Early diastolic murmurs
  1. AR
    a. Valvular: rheumatic deformity, perforation postendocarditis, posttraumatic, postvalvulotomy
    b. Dilatation of valve ring: aortic dissection, annuloectasia, cystic medial necrosis, hypertension
    c. Widening of commissures: syphilis
    d. Congenital: bicuspid valve, with VSD
  2. Pulmonic regurgitation
    a. Valvular: postvalvulotomy, endocarditis, rheumatic fever, carcinoid
    b. Dilatation of valve ring: pulmonary hypertension, Marfan syndrome
    c. Congenital: isolated or associated with tetralogy of Fallot, VSD, pulmonic stenosis
C. Mid-diastolic murmurs
  1. MS
  2. Carey-Coombs murmur (mid-diastolic apical murmur in acute rheumatic fever)
  3. Increased flow across nonstenotic mitral valve (e.g., MR, VSD, PDA, high-output states, and complete heart block)
  4. Tricuspid stenosis
  5. Increased flow across nonstenotic tricuspid valve (e.g., TR, ASD, and anomalous pulmonary venous return)
  6. Left and right atrial tumors
D. Continuous murmurs
  1. PDA
  2. Coronary AV fistula
  3. Ruptured aneurysm of sinus of Valsalva
  4. Aortic-pulmonary window
  5. Cervical venous hum
  6. Anomalous left coronary artery
  7. Proximal coronary artery stenosis
  8. Mammary soufflé
  9. Pulmonary artery branch stenosis
  10. Bronchial collateral circulation
  11. Small (restrictive) ASD with MS
  12. Intercostal AV fistula

AR, aortic regurgitation; AS, aortic stenosis; ASD, atrial septal defect; AV, arteriovenous; HOCM, hypertrophic obstructive cardiomyopathy; MR, mitral regurgitation; MS, mitral stenosis; PDA, patent ductus arteriosus; TR, tricuspid regurgitation; VSD, ventricular septal defect.
A and C modified from Oram S, ed. Clinical heart disease. London: Butterworth–Heineman, 1981. D modified from Fowler NO, ed. Reprinted from *Cardiac Diagnosis and Treatment*. Hagerstown, MD: Harper & Row, 1980, with permission.

TABLE 35.8

AUSCULATORY CHARACTERISTICS OF SOME COMMON CARDIAC MURMURS

Mitral valve prolapse
S_1 normal
S_2 normal splitting
Midsystolic click
  Earlier—standing, Valsalva
  Later—squatting, handgrip
Midsystolic to late systolic murmur
  Longer—standing, Valsalva
  Shorter—squatting, handgrip
Hypertrophic obstructive cardiomyopathy
A_2 normal
Paradoxical splitting S_2
S_4 usually present
Systolic ejection murmur
  ↑ Valsalva, standing, post-PVC
  ↓ handgrip, squatting
Bisferiens pulse
Mitral regurgitation
Diminished S_1
Wide splitting S_2
S_3 (with moderate to severe regurgitation)
High-frequency holosystolic murmur
Occasional diastolic filling rumble
Brisk and low-amplitude carotid pulse
Aortic stenosis
Ejection sound (noncalcified valve)
Diminished A_2 (immobile valve)
Paradoxical splitting S_2
S_3 and S_4 (if severe)
Late peaking systolic ejection murmur
Delayed and low-amplitude carotid pulse
Aortic regurgitation
S_1 diminished

Soft A_2 and narrow splitting S_2
S_3 common
Diastolic decrescendo murmur
Early peaking systolic ejection murmur common
  owing to increased systolic flow
Pulmonary stenosis
S_1 normal
S_2 wide splitting
Tricuspid regurgitation
S_1 normal
Holosytolic murmur
  ↑ with inspiration, squatting
  ↓with expiration, standing
Atrial septal defect
S_2 wide fixed splitting
Pulmonic systolic ejection murmur
Tricuspid mid-diastolic filling murmur if large flow
Mitral stenosis
Loud S_1
Narrow splitting S_2
Loud P_2
Opening snap
  Narrow A_2-OS interval (severe)
Diastolic rumble with presystolic accentuation
  (longer murmur with more severe stenosis)
Ventricular septal defect
S_1 normal
S_2 wide splitting
P_2 loud
S_3 often present
Holosystolic murmur
Mitral filling rumble if large flow

OS, opening snap; PVC, premature ventricular contraction.

TABLE 35.9

EFFECT OF PHYSIOLOGIC MANEUVERS ON SOME COMMON CARDIAC MURMURS

Maneuver	Physiologic change	Accentuates	Diminishes
Valsalva (phase II)	↓↓ VR ↓↓ AL ↓ CO	HOCM, MVP	MR, AS, AR
Inspiration	↑ VR	TR, TS, PS, PR	MR
Squat	↑ VR ↑ AL ↑↑ CO	MR, PS, TS, TR, AR	HOCM, MVP
Standing	↓ VR ↓↓ CO	HOCM, MVP	TR, PFM
Handgrip	↑↑ AL	MR, VSD, AR	HOCM, AS
Post-PVC (Long RR interval)	↑↑ C	HOCM, AS	No change in MR

AL, afterload (systemic vascular resistance); AR, aortic regurgitation; AS, aortic stenosis; C, contractility; CO, output; HOCM, hypertrophic obstructive cardiomyopathy; MR, mitral regurgitation; MVP, mitral valve prolapse; PFM, pulmonary flow murmur; PR, pulmonic regurgitation; PS, pulmonic stenosis; PVR, pulmonary venous return; TR, tricuspid regurgitation; TS, tricuspid stenosis; VR, systemic venous return: VSD, ventricular septal defect.

In other patients, mechanical prosthetic valves may cause enough acoustic artifact to hinder accurate diagnoses. In both of these examples, transesophageal echocardiography or magnetic resonance imaging may be necessary to make a correct diagnosis.

LABORATORY ABNORMALITIES

Key laboratory abnormalities that are found in patients with heart disease include abnormalities of the ECG, chest radiograph, and common blood tests. These abnormalities may be found in patients with known heart disease or may be the first suggestion of previously undiagnosed heart disease.

Electrocardiogram

In addition to being useful in diagnosing MI and abnormalities of heart rhythm or AV conduction, the ECG provides evidence regarding ventricular hypertrophy, interventricular conduction, ischemia, and electrolyte abnormalities. The normal QRS axis ranges from –30 degrees to +90 degrees. An axis more negative than 30 degrees (left axis deviation) indicates left anterior hemiblock, which is often associated with ischemic heart disease. An axis more positive than 90 degrees (right axis deviation) may be consistent with left posterior hemiblock, again suggestive of ischemic heart disease, or RV hypertrophy. Patients with right axis deviation should be carefully assessed for lung disease or other causes of pulmonary hypertension, such as pulmonary vascular disease or congenital heart disease. Evidence for RV hypertrophy is highly suggestive of pulmonary hypertension or pulmonic valve disease. Evidence of LV hypertrophy should raise questions regarding prior hypertension or left-sided valvular heart disease.

Bundle branch blocks may represent intrinsic conduction system disease or damage from prior MI. Bundle branch blocks may be constant or may be rate-related if the bundle branch is able to conduct normally at lower heart rates but not at more rapid rates. In the hospitalized patient, the new appearance of a bundle branch block, especially of the left bundle, should raise suspicion of acute myocardial ischemia.

ST-segment depression greater than 1 mm is highly suggestive of myocardial ischemia. T-wave inversion may also suggest myocardial ischemia. New ST-T–wave changes arising in the hospital will often require formal evaluation to exclude unstable angina (Chapter 37) or acute MI (Chapter 38). ST-T–wave changes can also be caused by medications (e.g., digoxin) or electrolyte abnormalities (especially hypokalemia).

Chest Radiograph

The finding of previously unsuspected cardiomegaly on a chest radiograph should raise the question of ventricular dilatation (and heart failure) or pericardial fluid. Echocardiography is indicated to clarify otherwise unexplained cardiomegaly.

An enlarged or tortuous aorta often signifies atherosclerotic disease. However, in a patient with chest discomfort, the possibility of aortic dissection must be considered and appropriate tests obtained (Chapter 49).

The chest radiograph may provide the first evidence of heart failure by showing unsuspected increases in pulmonary vasculature. Heart failure typically leads to increased pulmonary vascular markings in the upper lung fields, whereas a left-to-right shunt typically increases vascular markings in the lower lung fields. A previously unsuspected unilateral right pleural effusion or bilateral pleural effusions may indicate heart failure.

Common Blood Tests

Elevation of the blood urea nitrogen (BUN) may indicate intrinsic renal disease but, especially if out of proportion to the serum creatinine level, often indicates decreased renal perfusion resulting from heart failure. In patients with right-sided heart failure, aminotransferase, alkaline phosphatase, and bilirubin levels may be minimally or even markedly elevated. Some patients will have evidence of poor synthetic function resulting from marked hepatic congestion, with elevated prothrombin time and reduced albumin levels. Patients with right-to-left shunts and hypoxia typically have compensatory erythrocytosis with abnormally elevated hemoglobin and hematocrit levels, while anemia is now recognized as a common finding in late stage heart failure.

KEY POINTS

- In the differential diagnosis of chest pain, the evaluation must focus on the most serious possible causes (e.g., acute myocardial infarction, unstable angina, aortic dissection, pulmonary embolism, and pericarditis).
- The electrocardiogram is the single best predictor of acute ischemic heart disease in patients with chest pain.
- In patients in whom the cause of chest pain is uncertain, a chest pain evaluation unit may provide a rapid and efficient approach to diagnosis.
- Palpitations are very common, and their evaluation is guided in large part by whether there is evidence of concomitant symptoms or underlying structural heart disease.
- Lightheadedness has many cardiovascular and noncardiovascular causes; as with palpitations, further evaluation is guided by the history and physical examination.
- Abnormal jugular venous pressure may be indicative of heart failure, pericardial disease, tricuspid regurgitation, or arrhythmias.

- Arterial pulse examination is critical for diagnosing peripheral vascular disease and aortic dissection. It is also useful in the assessment of valvular heart disease.
- Careful cardiac auscultation of heart sounds and heart murmurs is critical for the cardiovascular assessment; auscultation serves as the key screen to determine whether noninvasive diagnostic testing is appropriate.
- Electrocardiographic changes may point to previously unsuspected ventricular hypertrophy, myocardial ischemia, or electrolyte abnormalities.
- In hospitalized patients, abnormalities on the chest radiograph (e.g., cardiomegaly, pulmonary vascular congestion) may be the first clues of underlying heart disease.
- Abnormalities of renal function, hepatic function, or the hematocrit may be clues to previously unsuspected heart disease.

REFERENCES

1. Braunwald E, Jones RH, Mark DB, et al. Diagnosing and managing unstable angina. *Circulation* 1994;90:613–615.
2. Goldman L. Approach to the patient with chest pain. In: Goldman L, Braunwald E, eds. *Primary Cardiology*, 2nd ed. Philadelphia: WB Saunders, 2003.
3. Panju AA, Hemmelgarn BR, Guyatt GH, et al. Is this patient having a myocardial infarction? *JAMA* 1998;280:1256–1263.
4. McSweeney JC, Cody M, O'Sullivan P, et al. Women's early warning symptoms of acute myocardial infarction. *Circulation* 2003;108:2619–2623.
5. Girod P, Messerli AW, Zidar F, et al. Tako-tsubo-like transient left ventricular dysfunction. *Circulation* 2003;107:e120–e121.
6. Weber JE, Shofer FS, Larkin GL, et al. Validation of a brief observation period for patients with cocaine-associated chest pain. *N Engl J Med* 2003;348:510–517.
7. Nienaber CA, von Kodolitsch Y, Nicolas V, et al. The diagnosis of thoracic aortic dissection by noninvasive imaging procedures. *N Engl J Med* 1993;328:1–9.
8. Wells PS, Ginsburg JS, Anderson DR, et al. Use of a clinical model for safe management of patients with suspected pulmonary embolism. *Ann Intern Med* 1998;129:997–1005.
9. Khot UN, Khot MB, Bajzer CT, et al. Prevalence of conventional risk factors in patients with coronary artery disease. *JAMA* 2003;290:898–904.
10. Zimetbaum PJ, Josephson MJ. Use of the electrocardiogram in acute myocardial infarction. *N Engl J Med* 2003;348:933–940.
11. Goldman L, Cook EF, Brand DA, et al. A computer protocol to predict myocardial infarction in emergency department patients with chest pain. *N Engl J Med* 1988;318:797–803.
12. Reilly BM, Evans AT, Schaider JJ, et al. Impact of a clinical decision rule on hospital triage of patients with suspected acute cardiac ischemia in the emergency department. *JAMA* 2002;288:342–350.
13. Farkouh ME, Smars PA, Reeder GS, et al. A clinical trial of a chest pain observation unit for patients with unstable angina. *N Engl J Med* 1998;339:1882–1888.
14. Zimetbaum P, Josephson ME. Evaluation of patients with palpitations. *N Engl J Med* 1998;338:1369–1373.
15. Ewy GA. The abdominojugular test: technique and hemodynamic correlates. *Ann Intern Med* 1988;109:456–460.
16. Westman EC, Matchar DB, Samsa GP, et al. Accuracy and reliability of apical S_3 gallop detection. *J Gen Intern Med* 1995;10:455–457.
17. Etchells E, Bell C, Robb K. Does this patient have an abnormal systolic murmur? *JAMA* 1997;277:564–571.

ADDITIONAL READING

Cho S, Atwood JE. Peripheral edema. *Am J Med* 2002;113:580–586.
Ganz LI. Approach to the patient with asymptomatic electrocardiographic abnormalities. In: Braunwald E, Goldman L, eds. *Primary Cardiology*, 2nd ed., Philadelphia: WB Saunders 2003.
Lee TH, Goldman L. Evaluation of the patient with acute chest pain. *N Engl J Med* 2000;342:1187–1195.

Diagnostic Tests in Cardiology

36

Karen P. Alexander   Eric D. Peterson

INTRODUCTION

The past two decades have witnessed a phenomenal expansion in diagnostic technologies for patients with cardiovascular disease. New stress imaging protocols have improved the detection of coronary artery disease (CAD), and the widespread availability of echocardiography and cardiac catheterization have enabled the accurate measurement of ventricular and valvular function. Although these diagnostic innovations have enhanced patient care, their associated costs have substantially added to health care expenditures. This chapter outlines the general issues regarding test selection and interpretation. It also reviews the major cardiovascular tests for the diagnosis of ischemia (stress electrocardiography, nuclear perfusion imaging, and stress echocardiography) and the assessment of heart structure and function (transthoracic and transesophageal echocardiography, nuclear ventriculography, cardiac magnetic resonance imaging [MRI] and cardiac catheterization). The arrival of several newer diagnostic modalities and electron-beam computerized tomography (CT) are also discussed. The basic electrocardiogram (ECG) and tests for syncope (Chapter 44) and arrhythmias (Chapters 42 and 43) are covered elsewhere.

TEST SELECTION

In the hospital setting, cardiovascular tests are typically ordered for one of four indications. First, they can assist the clinician in identifying a cardiac cause for presenting symptoms such as chest tightness, dyspnea, or syncope. Second, they may be ordered to evaluate physical examination or laboratory findings suggestive of cardiac pathology, such as a new murmur or an enlarged cardiac silhouette on the chest radiograph. Third, cardiac studies can define changes in the severity of known cardiac conditions (e.g., progression of ventricular or valvular dysfunction). Finally, cardiovascular tests can identify patients who are at high risk for subsequent cardiac events (e.g., preoperatively or following infarction).

To select the most appropriate diagnostic test from the available technologies, the clinician should begin by reviewing what is already known about the patient. The likelihood of coronary disease, and the prognosis, can be estimated based on the patient's presenting symptoms, clinical risk factors, and ECG. *The potential incremental value of the diagnostic study is determined by this "pretest" clinical assessment in addition to the intrinsic sensitivity and specificity of the proposed test* (see discussion of Bayes' theorem, Chapter 6). In general, a diagnostic test provides the most new information in a patient whose pretest likelihood is in the intermediate range. For example, a positive stress study result in a patient with a high pretest probability of disease (such as a 60-year-old male patient with typical angina) merely confirms the diagnosis, whereas a negative study result leaves a posttest likelihood of disease of greater than 20%.

In addition, clinicians should strive to use all the information provided by a given test. For example, exercise ECG testing provides important information concerning hemodynamic responses to exercise and overall cardiovascular fitness in addition to demonstrating ECG signs of ischemia.

Local clinical expertise can also affect test accuracy. Therefore, the diagnostic accuracy of technologies at leading centers described in published reports may differ from that found in local practice. A final consideration is that tests should be reserved for situations in which these results are likely to influence subsequent treatment decisions.

TESTS FOR ISCHEMIA

Stress Induction

Stress testing measures the response of the cardiovascular system to graded increases in workload and oxygen demand. Whereas treadmill and bicycle protocols result in similar maximal heart rates, treadmill testing induces a 6% to 25% higher maximal oxygen uptake and is a more familiar form of exercise for most patients in the United States. However, it is estimated that up to 50% of patients presenting for stress testing are either unable to exercise at all or exercise submaximally because of musculoskeletal, neurologic, or other limitations. In these patients, pharmacologic stress with inotropes (e.g., dobutamine or arbutamine) or vasodilators (e.g., dipyridamole or adenosine) are alternative methods for inducing stress.

Detection of Patterns of Ischemia and Perfusion

Regardless of how the stress is induced, the goal of stress testing is to diagnose obstructive coronary disease, either by inducing functional ischemia or by altering myocardial perfusion patterns. Some patients may experience symptoms such as angina or dyspnea. Ischemia alters normal ventricular repolarization and causes ST-segment depression during ECG stress testing. The ischemia can also cause systolic dysfunction that can be detected as wall motion abnormalities on stress echocardiography. Scintigraphic defects in perfusion with agents such as thallium or technetium (Tc) 99m sestamibi represent areas of myocardium that receive relatively less blood flow than neighboring tissue transiently during stress only (*"reversible" deficits*) or both at rest and during stress (*"fixed" deficits*).

Safety

When performed in a monitored setting, stress ECG testing is remarkably safe, with fewer than 1 death and 5 myocardial infarctions (MIs) occurring per 10,000 tests, and the complication rate may even be as low as 0.8/10,000 tests (1) in patients without contraindications (Table 36.1). Dipyridamole and adenosine pharmacologic stress testing is relatively contraindicated in patients with reactive airway disease because of the potential for bronchoconstriction, and adenosine may induce transient heart block in patients with underlying conduction system disease. Theophylline-containing drugs and caffeine interfere with the action of dipyridamole and adenosine and should be discontinued 24 hours before testing with these agents. Dobutamine is relatively contraindicated in patients with hypertrophic cardiomyopathy, severe hypertension, aortic aneurysms, or a history of serious ventricular arrhythmia.

TABLE 36.1

CONTRAINDICATIONS TO EXERCISE STRESS TESTING

Absolute contraindications
Acute MI (within 2 days)
High-risk unstable angina pectoris
Uncompensated heart failure
Uncontrolled cardiac dysrhythmia
Acute endocarditis, pericarditis, or myocarditis
Symptomatic severe aortic stenosis
Acute pulmonary embolus
Acute aortic dissection

Relative contraindications
Left main coronary artery stenosis
Symptomatic heart failure
Severe arterial hypertension
Significant pulmonary hypertension
Hypertrophic cardiomyopathy
Moderate valvular or myocardial heart disease
Fixed-rate artificial pacemaker
Psychiatric disorder causing an inability to cooperate with testing
Advanced atrioventricular block (may use stress imaging)
Drug- or electrolyte-induced ECG abnormalities (may use stress imaging)

MI, myocardial infarction; *ECG,* electrocardiogram.

Stress Electrocardiogram

Stress ECG testing is the most widely used and least expensive coronary disease screening modality. It is continued until the patient becomes fatigued or achieves 85% of the maximum predicted heart rate (approximately 220 minus the patient's age). Tests may be terminated earlier if signs or symptoms of severe ischemia (angina, ST-segment elevation, ST-segment depression >0.3 mV, or a fall in blood pressure of 10 mm Hg), arrhythmias, or heart block develop (2).

Test Information

ST-segment depression is considered "significant" if 1 mV or more of flat or downsloping depression is measured 60 msec past the J-point in three consecutive complexes (Figure 36.1A). If ST-segment depression is present on the baseline ECG, twice the resting ST-segment depression is usually required for a positive result (e.g., patients having a baseline depression of 1 mV would require an additional 2mV of ST-segment depression with exercise). In general, the likelihood of multivessel disease is proportional to the degree, distribution, and duration of ST-segment depression. ST-segment depression that is upsloping, however, is normally seen with rapid heart rates during exercise and does not constitute a positive test result (Figure 36.1B).

Lead II   **Lead V5**

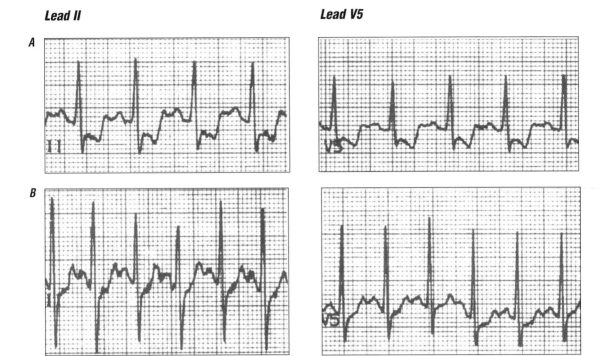

Figure 36.1 Exercise electrocardiographic (*ECG*) tracings at peak exertion on standard Bruce protocol. **A.** Downsloping ST-segment depression of 3 mm at peak exercise in ECG leads II and V5 in a patient who stopped exercising at 5 minutes (stage 2) because of severe chest pain at a heart rate of 115 beats/min (a "significant" test for ischemia). **B.** Upsloping ST-segment depression at peak exercise in ECG leads II and V5 in a different patient, who exercised for more than 10 minutes (stage 4) without chest pain and achieved a heart rate of 165 beats/min. This does not constitute a positive test result.

Exercise-induced ST-segment elevation in leads with diagnostic Q waves usually indicates preexisting regional wall motion abnormalities. However, ST-segment elevation seen in leads without existing Q waves can represent coronary artery spasm or even exercise-induced acute myocardial injury.

Exercise-induced premature ventricular contractions and nonsustained ventricular tachycardia occur in up to one-third of patients and are more common in those with CAD. Frequent ventricular ectopy in the recovery phase of testing correlates with an increased risk of death during 5-year follow-up (3), but other arrhythmias are not specific markers for coronary disease unless accompanied by other evidence of ischemia. Finally, exercise-induced supraventricular tachycardias occur rarely and are not generally related to underlying coronary disease.

Patients who can exercise longer than 9 minutes on a standard Bruce protocol or achieve 13 times the metabolic equivalents required at rest (METS) have a very good prognosis regardless of ischemic ECG changes. Chronotropic incompetence (failure to reach age-appropriate heart rate response), abnormal heart rate recovery (a decline in the heart rate of <10 beats per minute in first minute of recovery), and abnormal blood pressure responses (decline in systolic blood pressure with exercise) are important signs of severe coronary disease and poor prognosis (Table 36.2).

Scoring systems such as the Duke Treadmill Score and the VA Treadmill Score have been developed to integrate information provided by the exercise test.

Patient Selection and Indications

The clinical uses for stress ECG testing are broad (Table 36.3). It is most commonly used for the diagnosis of chest

---

TABLE 36.2

STRESS ELECTROCARDIOGRAPHIC INDICATORS OF SEVERE CORONARY DISEASE*a* OR POOR PROGNOSIS

Downsloping ST-segment depression ≥3 mV
Involvement of five or more leads with ST-segment depression
Early ST-segment depression (<5 METS)
Prolonged ST-segment depression late into recovery
Failure to complete stage II of Bruce protocol
Failure to obtain HR >120/min (off negative chronotropic drugs)
Exertional hypotension

---

a Severe coronary disease is >75% stenosis of three vessels or >50% stenosis of the left main coronary artery.
HR, heart rate; *METS*, metabolic equivalents.

TABLE 36.3
INDICATIONS FOR EXERCISE TESTING

Diagnosis
- Patients with interpretable electrocardiogram and an intermediate pretest probability of CAD, based on gender, age, and symptoms
- Before and after revascularization
  - Demonstration of ischemia before revascularization
  - Evaluation of patients with recurrent symptoms suggesting ischemia after revascularization

Risk assessment/prognosis
- Patients undergoing initial evaluation with suspected or known CAD
- Patients with suspected or known CAD with significant change in clinical status
- Post-myocardial infarction
  - Before discharge for prognostic assessment, activity prescription, or evaluation of medical therapy (submaximal at about 2 to 7 days)
  - Early after discharge for prognostic assessment, activity prescription, evaluation of medical therapy, and cardiac rehabilitation if the pre-discharge exercise test was not done (symptom-limited at about 14 to 21 days)
  - Late after discharge for prognostic assessment, activity prescription, evaluation of medical therapy, and cardiac rehabilitation if the early exercise test was submaximal (symptom-limited at about 3 to 6 weeks)

Other
- Selection of appropriate settings in patients with rate-adaptive pacemakers
- Evaluation of exercise capacity and response to therapy in patients with heart failure who are being considered for heart transplantation
- Assistance in differentiating cardiac from pulmonary limitations as a cause of exercise-induced dyspnea or impaired exercise capacity when the cause is uncertain.

CAD, coronary artery disease.
Reprinted with permission from Gibbons RJ, Balady GJ, Beasley JW, et al. ACC/AHA guidelines for exercise testing: a report of the American College of Cardiology/American Heart Association Task Force on Practice Guidelines, Committee on Exercise Testing. *J Am Coll Cardiol* 1997;30:260–315.

pain in patients who are able to exercise and who have an interpretable baseline ECG (Figure 36.2).

Test Interpretation and Accuracy

A meta-analysis of 58 consecutive published studies of stress ECG reported a sensitivity and specificity of 67% and 72%, respectively, for the diagnosis of coronary disease, although these figures varied considerably across studies depending on the population examined and the study design. For detecting multivessel disease, the sensitivity of stress ECG increases to 81% (1). Estimates of diagnostic accuracy are affected by "workup bias," which occurs when disease status is not known on all patients tested. When workup bias is minimized, the sensitivity of ECG changes declines to about 45%, but specificity rises to near 90% (4). Diagnostic accuracy of stress ECG is lower in patients who have abnormal baseline ECGs (hypertrophy and repolarization changes) or who are taking medications (digoxin) that alter the ECG or heart rate. Diagnostic accuracy is also lower in the elderly, who are less likely to reach maximal heart rate targets, and in women, who are more likely to have false-positive ST-segment depression.

Treadmill testing provides important prognostic information. Patients with a normal ECG tracing at stage 3 of a Bruce protocol have an excellent short-term prognosis (1-year mortality <1%). Stress ECG testing following MI effectively identifies a low-risk population (negative predictive value of 90%), although its positive predictive value is more limited (16% to 20%) (5).

Nuclear Perfusion Imaging

Stress myocardial perfusion imaging can be performed with exercise or pharmacologic stress. A radioactive tracer agent is injected approximately 60 seconds before maximal stress or exertion; on completion of the stress, either planar or tomographic (single-photon emission computed tomography, or SPECT) images are obtained. For comparison, resting images are obtained either immediately before or several hours after stress imaging.

Nuclear perfusion imaging commonly uses either thallium (Tl) 201 or ^{99m}Tc-sestamibi. Dual-isotope scanning techniques (e.g., resting ^{201}Tl and stress ^{99m}Tc-sestamibi) can decrease the overall rest-stress imaging time to just 90 minutes.

Test Information

Stress perfusion imaging can demonstrate both "reversible defects" and "fixed defects," which have been equated with territories of ischemia and prior infarction, respectively (Figure 36.3). The size, severity, and distribution of these defects carry important diagnostic and prognostic significance, and their location can be correlated with areas of coronary circulation. Nuclear perfusion imaging can also be used to determine myocardial viability; for example, perfusion deficits that redistribute on delayed repeated imaging (6 to 24 hours following stress) or following administration of a second tracer bolus correlate with areas of *"hibernating" myocardium*, which is myocardium that does not contract normally because of chronic ischemia but will recover function if and when perfusion is restored. Tracer uptake by the lungs indicates exercise-induced increases in pulmonary pressures suggestive of left ventricular (LV) dysfunction and multivessel coronary disease. Nuclear studies also can provide information on ventricular function with stress (first-pass studies or radionuclide angiography). Typically, LV function is

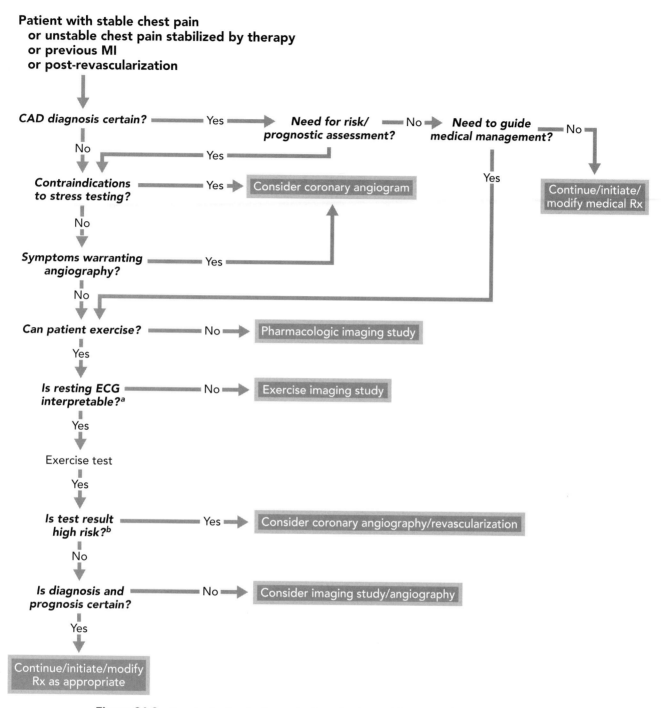

Figure 36.2 Exercise testing for the evaluation of patients with suspected ischemic heart disease.

[a]Electrocardiogram is interpretable unless preexcitation, electronically paced rhythm, left bundle branch block, or resting ST-segment depression >1 mm is present.

[b]For example, high-risk if Duke treadmill score predicts average annual cardiovascular mortality >3%. *MI*, myocardial infarction; *CAD*, coronary artery disease; *ECG*, electrocardiogram.

Reprinted with permission from Gibbons RJ, Balady GJ, Beasley JW, et al. ACC/AHA guidelines for exercise testing: a report of the American College of Cardiology/American Heart Association Task Force on Practice Guidelines (Committee on Exercise Testing). *J Am Coll Cardiol* 1997;30:260–315.

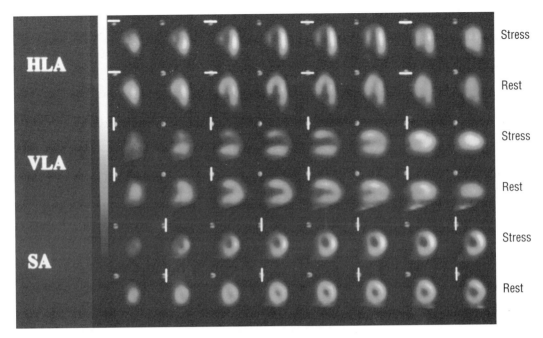

Figure 36.3 Single-photon emission computed tomography (*SPECT*) nuclear perfusion imaging with ^{99m}Tc-sestamibi. SPECT cardiac images displayed at stress (*rows 1, 3, 5*) and rest (*rows 2, 4, 6*) in the horizontal long axis (*HLA*) from anterior to inferior (*left to right*), vertical long axis (*VLA*) septal to lateral (*left to right*), and short axis (*SA*) from apex to base (*left to right*). Normal perfusion is seen in rest images, but decreased perfusion to the anteroseptal and antero-apical walls occurs at peak stress. Courtesy of Dr. Salvadore Borges-Neto, Department of Radiology, Duke University Medical Center, Durham, NC.

augmented by 5% to 15% with exercise; a blunted increase (<5%) can signal the presence of multivessel disease and poor prognosis, particulary in men.

Patient Selection and Indications

Given its higher cost, perfusion imaging should be reserved for the diagnosis of coronary disease in patients for whom stress ECG is not indicated or when localization of ischemia is important for management decisions (6) (Figure 36.2).

Test Interpretation and Accuracy

Nuclear perfusion imaging is significantly more accurate for the diagnosis of coronary disease than is stress ECG. The reported overall sensitivity and specificity for stress myocardial perfusion imaging range from 80% to 90% in most clinical series and in two meta-analyses (6). SPECT imaging appears to have slightly superior diagnostic accuracy relative to planar imaging, although overall diagnostic accuracy does not seem to vary significantly by type of stress, radioisotope, or type of analysis (quantitative vs. qualitative). False-negative nuclear perfusion studies can occur when collateral circulation masks single-vessel disease or "balanced" hypoperfusion disguises multivessel disease. False-positive studies, in contrast, occur because of tissue attenuation (diaphragmatic attenuation of the inferior wall, breast attenuation of the anterior wall) or left bundle branch block (septal perfusion defects).

Myocardial perfusion imaging can also provide important prognostic information. In a recent large series of patients with suspected or known CAD, the annual rate of cardiac death or MI was 0.8% for patients with a normal test result but 3.9% in those with severely abnormal test findings (7). High-risk test results include large areas of ischemia, multiple territory involvement, LV dilatation, and increased lung uptake. Following MI, the positive predictive value of an abnormal study result for death or recurrent MI was 17%, and the negative predictive value was 95% (5).

Stress Echocardiography

Stress echocardiography is a sensitive way to examine exercise-induced changes in LV wall function. For exercise stress, bicycle protocols have the advantage over treadmill protocols because they allow imaging during exertion. Dobutamine echocardiography and dipyridamole echocardiography are alternatives for those unable to exercise.

Test Information

The contractile force of each segment of the LV is quantitatively assessed at rest and after stress. New or worsening wall motion abnormalities indicate ischemia (Figure 36.4). Flow must be decreased by at least 50% in 5% of the myocardium to cause ischemia sufficient to induce wall motion abnormalities under stress. Conversely, resting wall

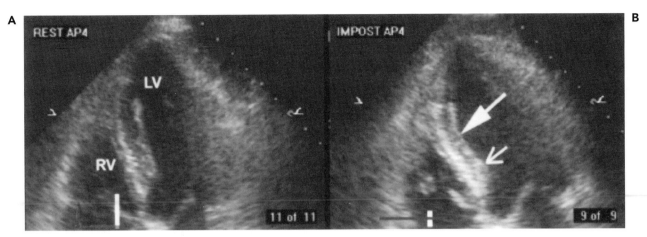

Figure 36.4 Stress echocardiography with stress induced regional wall motion abnormality. **A:** Apical four chamber 2-D image of left ventricle at rest. **B:** Anteroseptal wall becomes dyskinetic with peak stress. Solid arrowhead shows the anteroseptal wall bulging away from the left ventricular cavity with systole, and the open arrowhead shows the hinge point between normal and abnormal myocardial contraction.

motion abnormalities do not always indicate prior infarction. Improvement of abnormal resting wall motion with low doses of dobutamine (5 mcg/kg per minute) suggests hibernating but viable myocardium.

Patient Selection and Indications

For the diagnosis of coronary disease, stress echocardiography is particularly advantageous in situations in which ECG tracings are less accurate (women, patients with LV hypertrophy or resting ECG abnormalities) (8). Choice between stress echocardiography and nuclear imaging modalities may be determined by patient factors (e.g., tissue attenuation, imaging windows) or by local experience, availability, and cost. Stress echocardiography may be less helpful in patients with chronic lung disease, because of poor image quality, and in those with baseline wall motion abnormalities.

Test Interpretation and Accuracy

Inducible wall motion abnormalities under stress have a sensitivity of 80% to 90% and a specificity of 85% for detecting CAD (8). The level of stress at onset and the degree of induced wall motion abnormality are predictive of the extent of disease. Failure to achieve maximal stress, delayed post-stress imaging, or poor image quality may all adversely affect test accuracy. Although roughly equivalent to exercise SPECT nuclear perfusion imaging, exercise stress echocardiography generally has a lower sensitivity and higher specificity for detecting CAD. Stress echocardiography is less sensitive for single-vessel disease but more sensitive for multivessel disease because "balanced ischemia" may be unappreciated during nuclear testing.

Dobutamine stress echocardiography has the ability to predict functional improvement in viable myocardium after revascularization, with a sensitivity of 80% and specificity

of 90% (8). After MI, stress echocardiography has a positive predictive value of 48% and a negative predictive value of 86% for subsequent MI and death (5).

ASSESSMENT OF CARDIAC STRUCTURE AND FUNCTION

The assessment of cardiac structure and function has assumed a central role in the evaluation of cardiac patients. Echocardiography, radionuclear angiography, and cardiac catheterization can each provide aspects of this important diagnostic and prognostic information.

Echocardiography

Test Information

The major advantage of transthoracic echocardiography is the ease and speed with which a study can be performed. Its major limitation is obtaining adequate images through the patient's chest wall. *Transesophageal echocardiography* (TEE) is not limited by imaging through air or rib spaces and is particularly suited for the assessment of cardiac valves, atria, and aortic arch because of their posterior location and proximity to the probe. Major clinical applications of TEE include evaluation of valves for endocarditis, prosthetic valve function, intracardiac masses (including thrombi in the left atrial appendage), and aortic arch pathology (dissection, coarctation).

Although TEE is generally quite safe, it carries minor risks of conscious sedation, hypoxia, aspiration, or damage to the hypopharynx, esophagus, or laryngeal nerves. Relative contraindications to TEE include esophageal pathology, active upper gastrointestinal bleeding, and severe cervical arthritis.

Patient Selection and Indications

Major indications for the use of echocardiography include the evaluation of murmurs found during cardiac auscultation and the evaluation of symptoms such as dyspnea, fatigue, and edema (8) (Table 36.4). In addition, echocardiography can assess ejection fraction and resting wall motion abnormalities in patients with chest pain or with known CAD, especially after MI. Echocardiograms are also indicated to evaluate valvular heart disease, LV hypertrophy, suspected aortic dissection, pericardial disease, as well as cardiac sources of emboli in stroke patients, and for serial assessments of ventricular size and function in patients with known heart failure or valvular disease, especially in the setting of worsening symptoms.

Test Interpretation and Accuracy

Systolic function can be qualitatively estimated as an overall ejection fraction and by the contractile function of each regional wall. Wall motion is described as either normal, hyperkinetic, hypokinetic, akinetic, or dyskinetic (aneurysmal). Left atrial (LA) and LV chamber dimensions and ventricular hypertrophy are measured in standard views.

Intraatrial cavitary defects (as in atrial myxoma or atrial thrombus) may be visualized particularly well with TEE. Intraventricular masses (tumor or LV thrombus) can also be diagnosed. Finally, amyloid cardiomyopathy can be suspected on the basis of thickening and a "ground glass" appearance of the myocardium.

Valvular Regurgitation

The structure, motion, and morphology of the cardiac valves can be clearly seen with two-dimensional (2-D) imaging. Prolapse of mitral leaflets, chordal rupture, widening of the annular ring with decreased coaptation, and valvular degeneration give clues to the presence of regurgitation. Color Doppler is very sensitive in detecting turbulence and regurgitation of flow through valves (Figure 36.5). The width of the origin and the volume of the regurgitant jet on color flow images provide a semiquantitative estimate of the severity of mitral and aortic regurgitation.

Spectral Doppler can be used to measure the velocity of the regurgitant jet directly. These measurements have several clinical applications, as the velocity (V) of flow through the valve is related to the pressure gradient (DP) across the valve by the modified Bernoulli equation ($DP = 4V^2$). For example, when tricuspid valve regurgitation is present, this relationship between velocity and pressure gradients is useful in estimating pressures in the right side of the heart. Specifically, right ventricular (RV) systolic pressure can be estimated by adding the assumed RA pressure (5 to 10 mm Hg in normal patients) to the tricuspid regurgitation pressure gradient (DP).

Valvular Stenosis

Stenosis is suggested by diminished valve mobility, thickening, or calcifications on 2-D echocardiographic images, and by turbulent flow through the valve on color Doppler images (Figure 36.6). The diagnosis is confirmed by using spectral Doppler to detect elevated velocities as blood travels through the narrowed valve orifice. Velocities can be converted to peak and mean pressure gradients across the aortic valve by using the modified Bernoulli equation ($DP = 4V^2$).

The severity of mitral stenosis is typically assessed from the pressure gradient half-time equation (the time required for the peak pressure gradient between the LA and LV to decline to half of its value). Planimetry, which is direct measurement of the mitral valve orifice on a freeze-frame image, can also be used to assess mitral valve area.

Pericardial Disease

Two-dimensional images enable the identification and assessment of pericardial effusions. An effusion is seen as an "echo-free space" surrounding the heart and can be focal or circumferential. The effusions are visually estimated to be small (<100 cc), moderate (100 to 500 cc), or large (>500 cc). Findings that suggest compromise to RV filling and impending tamponade include early diastolic collapse of the RV, invagination of the right atrial (RA) wall, and respiratory variation in Doppler flow across the mitral and tricuspid valves (Chapter 46).

Septal Defects

Atrial or ventricular septal defects are often associated with abnormal motion of the septum on 2-D images. Color Doppler can occasionally detect septal defects if the direction of flow is parallel to the Doppler signal; otherwise, the diagnosis must be made by observing the flow of agitated saline contrast. The appearance of agitated saline contrast injected through a peripheral intravenous line into the LV establishes the existence of an abnormal connection between structures in the right and left sides of the heart, such as an atrial or ventricular septal defect or a patent foramen ovale.

Radionuclide Angiography

Radionuclide angiography techniques provide the most reproducible and accurate studies for assessing ventricular function under most conditions. These studies are most useful for serial evaluation of ejection fraction in patients with heart failure or those receiving cardiotoxic agents (e.g., doxorubicin). Although they provide highly accurate assessments of ventricular ejection fraction, radionuclide angiography studies are nearly as expensive as Doppler echocardiography and do not provide detailed information regarding cardiac structure or valves.

TABLE 36.4

MAJOR AHA/ACC CLASS I INDICATIONS FOR ECHOCARDIOGRAPHY[a]

Evaluation of valvular disease
- Murmur in a patient with cardiorespiratory symptoms
- Changing symptoms in patient with known valvular disease or with a prosthetic valve
- Asymptomatic patients with severe valvular disease
- Assessment of severity and leaflet morphology in mitral valve prolapse
- Bacteremia without known source
- Documentation of severity in valvular stenosis or regurgitation (e.g., left ventricular and right ventricular size, function, and hemodynamics)
- Timing of surgical valvular repair or selection of alternative therapies
- Identification of valvular lesions and associated abnormalities (e.g., abscesses) in infective endocarditis

Diagnosis and prognosis in myocardial ischemic syndromes
- Identification of cardiac disease in patients with chest pain or severe hemodynamic instability
- Assessment of baseline LV function and infarct size
- Assessment for possible RV infarction or mechanical complications in patients with hemodynamic instability

Patients with dyspnea, edema, or cardiomyopathy
- Assessment of LV size and function in patients with cardiomyopathy or heart failure
- Dyspnea, unexplained hypotension, or edema with clinical signs of elevated central venous pressure or other signs of heart disease
- Changing symptoms in patients with cardiomyopathy

Pericardial disease
- Suspected pericardial disease (e.g., effusion, constriction, or effusive-constrictive process)
- Pericardial friction rub developing in acute myocardial infarction
- Suspected bleeding in the pericardial space (e.g., trauma, perforation)

Cardiac masses and tumors
- Evaluation of patients with clinical syndromes suggesting an underlying cardiac mass
- Surveillance studies after removal of masses known to have a high likelihood of recurrence (e.g., myxoma)
- Surveillance for cardiac involvement and staging in patients with known primary malignancies

Diseases of the great vessels
- Evaluation for aortic dissection, aneurysm, or rupture
- Degenerative or traumatic aortic disease with clinical atheroembolism
- Evaluation for aortic root dilatation in patients or their first-degree relatives with Marfan syndrome or connective tissue diseases

Pulmonary disease
- Suspected or known pulmonary hypertension (e.g., pulmonary artery pressures)
- Pulmonary emboli and suspected clots in the right atrium or ventricle or main pulmonary artery branches
- Lung disease with clinical suspicion of cardiac involvement (suspected cor pulmonale)

Hypertension
- Detection and assessment of functional significance of concomitant coronary artery disease and resting LV function, hypertrophy, or concentric remodeling
- Follow-up assessment of LV size and function in patients with LV dysfunction when there has been a documented change in clinical status or to guide medical therapy

Suspected cardioembolic events
- Patients of any age with abrupt occlusion of a major peripheral or visceral artery
- Younger patients (age <45 y) with cerebrovascular events
- Older patients (age >45 y) with neurologic events but no evidence of cerebrovascular disease or other obvious cause

Arrhythmias, palpitations, and syncope
- Arrhythmias with clinical suspicion of structural heart disease or a family history of a genetically transmitted cardiac lesion associated with arrhythmia
- Before cardioversion in patients in whom extended anticoagulation before cardioversion is not desirable
- Peri-exertional syncope or any syncope in a patient with clinically suspected heart disease

[a] Transesophageal echocardiography (TEE) is preferred over transthoracic echocardiography (TTE) for the evaluation of the great vessels (e.g., possible aortic dissection), intracardiac masses (e.g., tumors, clots, vegetations), and prosthetic valves.
LV, left ventricle; RV, right ventricle.
Reprinted with permission from Cheitlin MD, Alpert JS, Armstrong WF, et al. ACC/AHA guidelines for the clinical application of echocardiography: a report of the American College of Cardiology/American Heart Association, Task Force on Practice Guidelines. *Circulation* 2003;42:954–970.

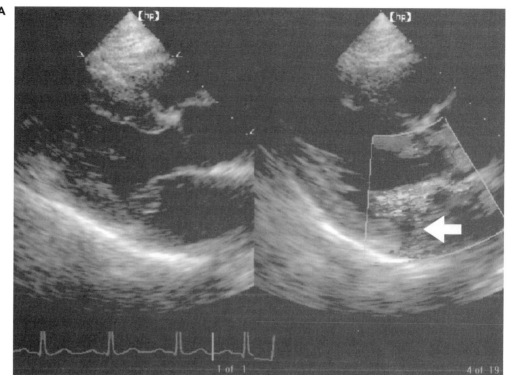

Figure 36.5 Parasternal long-axis echocardiographic images showing mitral regurgitation. The panel on the left **(A)** is a two-dimensional image in the parasternal long axis without mitral regurgitation. The panel on the right **(B)** is the same view showing regurgitant flow by Doppler (see arrow), which would be depicted in a color Doppler image as a mosaic of colors, through the mitral valve into the left atrium during peak systole. Color Doppler provides information on the direction of flow by coding signals as moving toward (red/yellow) or away from (blue) the transducer. Turbulent flow is depicted as a mosaic of colors.

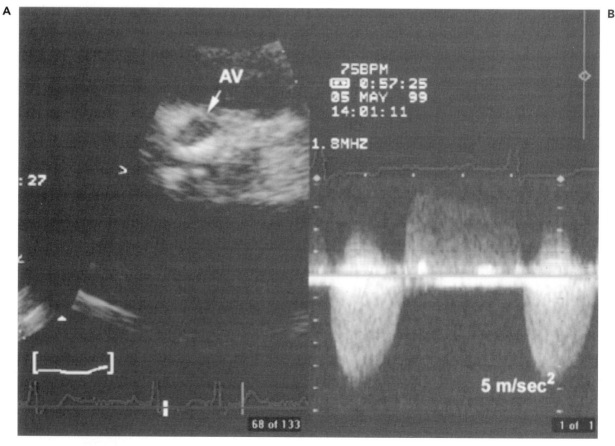

Figure 36.6 2-D and Doppler images of severe aortic valve stenosis. **A.** Parasternal short axis view of a calcified aortic valve (AV). **B.** Doppler gradient through the aortic valve. Peak velocity of blood through the valve is 4.8 m/sec, corresponding to a peak transvalvular gradient of 92 mm Hg.

Cardiac Catheterization

Cardiac catheterization generally describes a number of percutaneous catheter-based procedures (e.g., coronary and bypass graft angiography, ventriculography, and aortic angiography) for imaging the heart and its major vessels. In addition, catheterization of the left and right sides of the heart is used to record intracardiac pressures.

Percutaneous peripheral vascular access is obtained in the femoral (Judkins technique), brachial (Sones technique), or radial arteries for catheterization of the left side of the heart, and the femoral or jugular veins for catheterization of the right side. Patients on full systemic anticoagulation or intravenous anti-platelet agents can undergo diagnostic catheterization without difficulty, but for outpatient procedures, low-dose heparin is all that is required (9).

Coronary Angiography

Coronary angiography is the standard for defining coronary anatomy and assessing coronary artery obstructive disease. Coronary arteries are assessed for extent of distribution, flow pattern, collaterals, and luminal irregularities. Stenoses are characterized as concentric or eccentric, discrete or tubular; the presence of luminal filling defects, calcium, or dissections is also noted. Coronary bypass grafts are injected at their site of origin from the aorta or, in the case of the internal mammary arteries, at their origin from the subclavian artery.

Visual interpretation of the degree of stenosis can vary significantly between interpreters and is subject to several types of error. Stenoses may be overestimated or underestimated if the lesion is not concentric or if the reference segment of the vessel is also diseased. In general, qualitative (visual) estimates of stenoses tend to overestimate severity in comparison with quantitative measurements (in which calipers or computer algorithms are used). These limitations of coronary angiography can be improved by the use of *intravascular ultrasound*, which can display a 3-D ultrasonic view of the plaque mass.

Ventriculography

Ventriculography provides information on regional wall motion and overall ventricular function (qualitatively, or quantitatively measured as the ejection fraction or end-systolic LV volume divided by end-diastolic LV volume). Pressure tracings are also obtained in the aorta and LV (which can be used to diagnose aortic stenosis or subvalvular outflow tract obstruction). The mean LV end-diastolic pressure is useful for assessing LV function, and the contour of the waveform is helpful in diagnosing abnormal filling and relaxation patterns.

Aortic Angiography

The aortic root is imaged by injecting a volume of contrast above the level of the aortic valve (aortic arch angiography) or into the abdominal aorta (usually at the level of the diaphragm). Aortic arch angiography opacifies the coronary arteries sufficiently to locate their origins if these are anomalous and demonstrates the size and contour of the ascending aorta. It also can be used to assess the severity of aortic regurgitation. Abdominal aortic angiography opacifies the descending aorta and its branch vessels in the leg and is helpful in identifying aortic aneurysms, renal artery stenosis, or peripheral vascular disease.

Catheterization of the Right Side of the Heart

Catheterization of the right side of the heart provides hemodynamic measurements and waveform recordings from the RA, RV, pulmonary artery, and pulmonary capillary wedge position, in addition to measuring cardiac output. Although it is not a routine part of cardiac catheterization for patients with CAD, it is often performed in those with associated LV dysfunction, cardiomyopathy, shunts, or valvular disease. Characteristic waveforms are present in valvular regurgitation (large *c-v* waves on RA pressure tracing for tricuspid regurgitation, or on pulmonary wedge tracing for mitral regurgitation), and abnormal filling patterns can provide clues to constrictive or restrictive physiology. In mitral valvular stenosis, the gradient between the pulmonary capillary wedge pressure and LV end-diastolic pressure can be used to calculate peak and mean gradients.

Cardiac output is usually determined by the Fick method, which calculates oxygen consumption. Combining cardiac output with pressure gradients across vascular beds can determine the pulmonary and systemic resistance. If intracardiac shunts are suspected, blood gases are drawn from various sites in the right side of the heart to look for an unexpected step-up in oxygenation. For example, if oxygenation increases by more than 5% between the RA and pulmonary artery, a left-to-right intracardiac shunt between these sites probably exists.

Patient Selection and Indications

The most frequent indication for cardiac catheterization is the evaluation of patients with suspected obstructive coronary artery disease (9). For patients with an acute coronary syndrome, early cardiac catheterization followed by any indicated revascularization procedure is of proven benefit (10). Catheterization is indicated for stable angina when it is unresponsive to medical therapy or associated with evidence of LV dysfunction, or with high-risk features on stress testing. Patients with high-risk occupations (e.g., airline pilot) may proceed directly to catheterization for definitive evaluation of any symptoms consistent with potential my-ocardial ischemia.

When performed safely, cardiac catheterization has a very low rate of complications, but it can result in serious vascular injury, MI, bleeding, neurologic events (transient ischemic attack, stroke), contrast reaction, and mortality (9) (Table 36.5). Other complications include vasovagal events, worsening renal insufficiency, and hematomas at the puncture site. Overall, the risk to life should be less than 0.2%, and the risk for other serious adverse events should be less than 0.5%. Relative contraindications include recent stroke (within 1 month), progressive renal insufficiency, fever or active infection, severe anemia, thrombocytopenia, electrolyte imbalance, uncontrolled hypertension, or allergy to angiographic contrast media. Patients at highest risk for mortality include the very old and those with New York Heart Association class III or IV symptoms, severe LV or valvular dysfunction, acute or unstable ischemic syndromes, and high-risk noninvasive test results. Patients at highest risk for vascular complications include women, those who are very old or obese, and those with a history of peripheral vascular disease. Hydration and administration of N-acetylcysteine (Mucomyst) prior to cardiac catheterization may reduce the nephrotoxicity associated with the contrast agents.

The indications for and risks of pulmonary artery (right side of the heart) catheterization in severely ill patients are described in Chapter 25.

NEW AND EMERGING DIAGNOSTIC TESTS

Cardiac Magnetic Resonance Imaging (MRI)

MRI is a rapidly evolving technology that produces high-resolution images of cardiac structure and function without interference from surrounding bone or air, biological hazards, or the need for nephrotoxic contrast agents. MRI is useful when evaluating patients for pericardial abnormalities (e.g., constrictive pericarditis or pericardial hematoma) or certain myocardial diseases (e.g., cardiac amyloid or RV dysplasia). Intracardiac masses (e.g., myxoma or thrombus) can also be imaged in detail. MRI can be combined with pharmacologic stress testing to determine both viability and perfusion of ischemia myocardium. Proximal coronary arteries can often be visualized, but MRI is not currently a substitute for coronary arteriography (11).

Electron-beam Computed Tomography (EBCT)

EBCT uses a single focused electron beam and one stationary detector to measure the calcium content of coronary arteries rapidly. The magnitude of coronary artery calcification (coronary calcium score) predicts the presence of coronary stenoses and the future occurrence of cardiac events with a sensitivity above 90%, but a specificity of only 20% to 50%. Despite this good sensitivity, some plaques lack calcium yet can become unstable and produce symptoms and cardiac events. EBCT may add incremental information for high-risk primary patients who have no symptoms or have atypical chest pain, but a randomized trial showed no benefit from EBCT in terms of the effectiveness of subsequent interventions to improve cardiac risk factors (12). As a result, its routine use as a screening test cannot be recommended.

COST AND RESOURCE USE

Clearly, it is important for physicians to have information about the economic aspects of cardiovascular diagnostic testing (Table 36.6). The full economic implications of a diagnostic test also go well beyond its initial cost and include indirect costs associated with each testing strategy. For example, if a screening study provides a false-positive result, it may prompt further evaluation and increased resource use. Alternatively, a false-negative test result may lead to the high costs (both financial and clinical) associated with a delayed or missed diagnosis. In addition to cost, the efficiency of a testing strategy must be considered. For example, to assess ventricular function and diagnose coronary disease, the physician may order an echocardiogram and stress myocardial perfusion imaging, a rest and exercise echocardiogram or radionuclide ventriculogram, or a cardiac catheterization.

TABLE 36.5
RISK OF COMPLICATIONS DURING DIAGNOSTIC CATHETERIZATION [a]

Mortality	0.11%
Myocardial infarction	0.05%
Cerebrovascular accident	0.07%
Arrhythmia	0.38%
Vascular complications	0.43%
Contrast reaction	0.37%
Hemodynamic complications	0.26%
Perforation of heart chamber	0.03%
Other complications	0.28%
Total complications	1.7%

[a] Scanlon PJ, Faxon DP, Audet A, et al. ACC/AHA Guidelines for coronary angiography: executive summary and recommendations. *Circulation* 1999;99:2345–2357.

KEY POINTS

■ Clinicians should consider a patient's diagnostic and prognostic estimates based on clinical factors before ordering additional diagnostic studies. Diagnostic testing

TABLE 36.6

MEDICARE CHARGES FOR VARIOUS TESTING MODALITIES (2003, IN U.S. DOLLARS)

Tests for ischemia	Medicare allowable charges ($)		
	Facility	**Professional**	**Total**
Exercise electrocardiogram	56	50	106
Exercise perfusion imaging[a]	463	122	585
Exercise ventriculography	289	72	361
Exercise echocardiography	118	123	241
Tests for left ventricular function			
Radionuclide ventriculography	183	44	227
Echocardiography (2-D/Doppler)	302	65	367
Left-sided heart catheterization	1,869	337	2,206
Cardiac MRI	393	86	479

[a] Excluding cost of isotope. All charges are for participating Medicare providers. Electron beam computed tomography (cost, about $600) is not approved for Medicare reimbursement.

usually provides the most new information in patients with intermediate pretest estimates.

- Most tests provide multiple forms of information, and all information should be considered.
- Stress electrocardiographic testing is an inexpensive strategy for the diagnosis of coronary disease in symptomatic ambulatory patients with interpretable baseline electrocardiograms.
- Exercise stress enables a correlation between symptoms and physical workload and provides information on exercise capacity in addition to ischemia. Pharmacologic stress is an alternative for those unable to exercise.
- Nuclear perfusion imaging and stress echocardiography similarly improve the sensitivity and specificity of stress electrocardiographic testing in the diagnosis of coronary disease.
- Compared with stress echocardiography, nuclear perfusion imaging has slightly superior sensitivity for detecting single-vessel disease but slightly lower specificity and higher costs.
- Decisions regarding which stress test to order should be individualized according to the patient's clinical characteristics and local availability, expertise, and cost.
- Echocardiography has become the standard means for noninvasive assessment of cardiac structure and function.
- For patients with a high clinical likelihood of coronary disease before testing, cardiac catheterization may be the best initial diagnostic test.
- EBCT provides information about coronary calcification (calcium score) and is being evaluated to assess its proper role as an adjunct to risk factor assessment in primary prevention strategies. It is not recommended as a routine screening test or as a diagnostic test in patients with known coronary disease.

- Cardiac MRI provides detailed structural images of the heart and pericardium, but accurate noninvasive coronary artery imaging is not yet a reality.

REFERENCES

1. Gibbons RJ, Balady GJ, Bricker JT, et al. ACC/AHA 2002 guideline update for exercise testing: A report of the American College of Cardiology/American Heart Association Task Force on Practice Guidelines, Committee on Exercise Testing, 2002. American College of Cardiology Web site. Available at: www.acc.org/clinical/guidelines/exercise/dirIndex.htm.
2. Gibbons RJ, Balady GJ, Bricker JT, et al. ACC/AHA 2002 guideline update for exercise testing: summary article. A report of the American College of Cardiology/American Heart Association Task Force on Practical Guidelines (Committee to Update the 1997 Exercise Testing Guidelines). *J Am Coll Cardiol* 2002;40:1531–1540.
3. Frolkis JP, Pothier CE, Blackstone EH, et al. Frequent ventricular ectopy after exercise as a predictor of death. *N Engl J Med* 2003;348:781–790.
4. Froelicher VF, Lehmann KG, Thomas R, et al. The electrocardiographic exercise test in a population with reduced workup bias: Diagnostic performance, computerized interpretation, and multivariable prediction. VA Cooperative Study in Health Services (QUEXTA) Study Group. *Ann Intern Med* 1998;128:965–974.
5. Peterson ED, Shaw LJ, Califf RM. Risk stratification after myocardial infarction. *Ann Intern Med* 1997;126: 561–582.
6. Klocke FJ, Baird MG, Bateman TM, et al. ACC/AHA/ASNC guidelines for the clinical use of cardiac radionuclide imaging: A report of the American College of Cardiology/American Heart Association Task Force on Practice Guidelines (ACC/AHA/ASNC Committee to Revise the 1995 Guidelines for the Clinical Use of Radionuclide Imaging (2003) American College of Cardiology Web Site. Available at: http://www.acc.org/clinical/guidelines/radio/index.pdf.
7. Berman DS, Kang X, Hayes SW, et al. Adenosine myocardial perfusion single-photon emission computed tomography in women compared with men: Impact of diabetes mellitus on incremental prognostic value and effect on patient management. *J Am Coll Cardiol* 2003;41:1125–1133.
8. Cheitlin MD, Armstrong WF, Aurigemma CP, et al. ACC/AHA/ASE 2003 guideline update for the clinical application of

echocardiography—summary article: A report of the American College of Cardiology/American Heart Association Task Force on Practice Guidelines. *Circulation* 2003;108:1146–1162.

9. Scanlon PJ, Faxon DP, Audet A, et al. ACC/AHA Guidelines for coronary angiography: Executive summary and recommendations. *Circulation* 1999;99:2345–2357.

10. Boden WE. Interpreting new treatment guidelines for non-ST segment elevation acute coronary syndrome. *Am J Cardiol* 2001; 88:19K–24K.

11. Dearls, JP, Ho VB, Foo TK, et al. Cardiac MRI: Recent progress and continued challenges. *J Mag Res Imag* 2002;16:111–127.

12. O'Malley PG, Feuerstein IM, Taylor AJ. Impact of electron beam tomography, with or without case management, or motivation, behavior change, and cardiovascular risk profile: a randomized controlled trial. *JAMA* 2003;289:2215–2223.

ADDITIONAL READING

Feigenbaum H, Armstrong WF, Ryan T. Echocardiography. 6th ed. Malvern, PA: Lippincott Williams & Wilkins, 2004.

U.S. Preventive Services Task Force. Screening for coronary heart disease: recommendation statement. *Ann Intern Med* 2004;140: 569–572.

Angina and Unstable Angina

37

Daniel B. Mark

INTRODUCTION

Although clinicians commonly refer interchangeably to angina pectoris, myocardial ischemia, and coronary artery disease, these three terms are not equivalent. *Angina pectoris*, first described in detail by William Heberden in 1772, is a syndrome of characteristic symptoms centering on reproducible exercise or stress-induced precordial chest discomfort that is promptly relieved by rest or nitroglycerin. There is no gold standard for this clinical diagnosis. *Unstable angina* is a progression of the symptom pattern, often with prolonged episodes of angina at rest. Unstable angina portends an increased risk for adverse cardiac events.

Myocardial ischemia is a pathophysiologic disorder caused by reduced perfusion of myocytes. Myocardial ischemia results from an imbalance between myocardial oxygen supply (perfusion) and demand (cellular consumption). Disordered myocyte metabolism results in impaired contraction of the affected heart muscle. Severe, prolonged ischemia may produce irreversible cellular damage and myocardial infarction (MI). Although many clinical tests are thought to assess myocardial ischemia, no diagnostic gold standard exists. Of the diagnostic technologies currently available, positron emission tomography (PET) comes the closest to allowing repeated assessment of the metabolic state of the myocardium.

Coronary artery disease (CAD) typically refers to an anatomic disorder of the epicardial segments of the coronary arteries. It is most commonly caused by focal accumulations of atherosclerotic material in the intima of these arteries. Pathologic examination is the best way to diagnose CAD. The coronary angiogram serves as a more convenient, if imperfect, surrogate standard.

Although these distinctions may appear semantic, confusing these concepts leads to errors in diagnosis and management. The presence of classic anginal symptoms is not pathognomonic for either myocardial ischemia or CAD, and the diagnosis of angina pectoris is not disproved by the absence of CAD on diagnostic testing. Furthermore, myocardial ischemia frequently occurs silently, without angina, and the pathway from myocardial ischemia to anginal symptoms is much more complex than has been previously appreciated. It is possible for anginal symptoms to be produced experimentally without myocardial ischemia, and vice versa. Finally, many people have coronary atherosclerotic disease but have neither angina nor myocardial ischemia. Unfortunately, such preclinical atherosclerotic disease is not always benign; it may progress without warning to either acute MI or sudden cardiac death. Thus, when evaluating these patients, the clinician must be aware of the imperfect relationships among symptoms (angina), the metabolic state of the myocardium (ischemia), and anatomic CAD.

This chapter briefly reviews the relevant epidemiology and pathophysiology of angina and unstable angina and then focuses on the identification and hospital management of symptomatic angina patients. In the current era of cost containment and managed care, it is uncommon for a patient with stable angina to require admission for evaluation or therapy. Clinicians admit patients with anginal symptoms to the hospital because they deem it either unsafe or of uncertain safety to continue outpatient evaluation and management. Most of these inpatients will have either unstable angina pectoris or acute MI. The patient's presenting symptoms need to be integrated with early test data to formulate an initial assessment of prognosis and an initial management strategy (see Issues at the Time of

Admission). As the patient progresses through the hospital course, the clinician must reevaluate the diagnosis and management strategy and make appropriate modifications (see Issues During the Course of Hospitalization). Finally, the clinician must decide when it is safe to discharge the patient from the hospital (see Issues at the Time of Hospital Discharge).

EPIDEMIOLOGY

CAD is the leading cause of death in the United States (about 500,000 deaths each year). The prevalence of angina pectoris approximates 7 million cases, with an annual incidence of 350,000. Unstable angina is the principal diagnosis in about 700,000 hospitalizations annually. Almost 60% of unstable angina patients are over age 65 and nearly half are women. Another 1.5 million Americans have an acute MI each year. Thus, the acute coronary syndromes (acute MI, unstable angina) collectively comprise the most frequent cause of hospitalization for adults in the United States. Hospitalization for unstable angina has increased during the last decade, whereas hospitalization for MI has declined. Whether these trends are a consequence of risk factor reduction, improvements in pharmacotherapy, or changes in discharge coding practices remains unsettled. However, the routine measurement of troponin during the last 4 years has resulted in many patients who would have been diagnosed with unstable angina now being classified as non-ST elevation myocardial infarction, so these trends will likely reverse after 2000 (1).

PATHOPHYSIOLOGY

Determinants of Myocardial Ischemia

In normal subjects, it is nearly impossible to create ischemia by voluntarily increasing myocardial demand (Figure 37.1). Thus, for ischemia to develop, there must be an abnormal reduction in coronary blood flow, an abnormal increase in myocardial oxygen demand, or both.

The heart differs from most other organs in that maximal oxygen extraction already occurs in the resting state. When myocardial oxygen demand increases, the heart muscle is obligated to increase coronary blood flow. Coronary blood flow occurs predominantly during diastole and has three principal determinants: aortic diastolic perfusion pressure, coronary vascular resistance, and the length of the diastolic phase of the cardiac cycle. Factors that reduce coronary blood flow include lower aortic diastolic pressure, obstructive coronary lesions, and tachycardia. In some patients in whom severe obstructive CAD develops, coronary collaterals may mitigate the effects of reduced antegrade coronary flow.

Myocardial oxygen demand is primarily determined by how much work the heart is doing. Higher heart rates (as occur with exercise or tachyarrhythmias) and increased contractility (from increased circulating catecholamines) will increase myocardial oxygen demand. Factors that increase left ventricular (LV) wall tension, including higher systolic blood pressure, ventricular chamber enlargement, and LV hypertrophy, also increase oxygen demand.

Atherosclerotic Plaque Events

Atherosclerosis is a progressive disorder that often begins in childhood, with significant lesions evident at autopsy by the third decade of life. This pathophysiologic process is characterized by the formation of atherosclerotic plaques comprised of smooth-muscle cells, inflammatory cells, cellular debris, lipid, and other material within the intima of medium-size and large arteries. Complex recurrent cycles of endothelial injury, inflammation, and healing produce these lesions. Endothelial injury, believed to be the initiating event, has been linked to hypercholesterolemia, hypertension, cigarette smoking, diabetes, viruses, chlamydia infection, and homocysteine.

Atherosclerotic plaques vary in their composition, consistency, and vulnerability to rupture. Mature plaques contain a soft, lipid-rich, atheromatous gruel center supported by outer, collagen-rich, sclerotic components. Plaques may contain varying amounts of hard and soft components. A

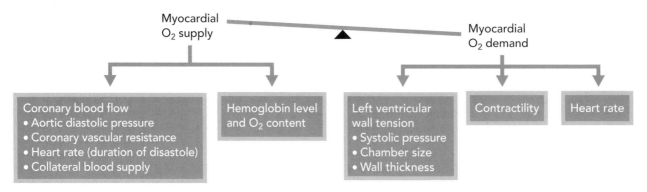

Figure 37.1 Major determinants of myocardial oxygen supply and demand.

plaque that is made up of only collagenous tissue is sometimes referred to as a *"nonvulnerable" plaque*, because it is not believed to pose a risk for rupture. In contrast, a *"vulnerable" plaque* has a core of soft, extracellular, highly thrombogenic, lipid-rich gruel (usually >40% of the plaque volume) and a fibrous cap that varies in composition, strength, and thickness. Most plaque ruptures start at the plaque shoulder, where the cap is often thinnest and most heavily infiltrated with inflammatory cells. It is unclear whether plaque rupture is caused by an inflammatory process at the shoulder of the plaque cap or by external triggers that physically disrupt the cap at its weakest point. The circadian patterns of major cardiac events suggest that sympathetic nervous system activity (which would increase blood pressure, heart rate, myocardial contractility, and coronary flow rates) can provide sufficient stress to disrupt a vulnerable plaque. Some plaque events appear to be caused by erosion of the plaque surface with subsequent thrombus formation. The relative importance of plaque erosion versus plaque rupture in unstable angina has been difficult to define because few unstable angina patients undergo autopsy examination. *Plaque "events" (rupture or erosion) underlie most episodes of acute coronary disease*, which range from a worsening of effort angina at the lower-risk end of the spectrum to acute MI and sudden cardiac death at the other.

Importantly, many of the plaques that are most predisposed to rupture appear angiographically as "insignificant" stenoses (i.e., stenoses that narrow the diameter of the arterial lumen by 50% or less). Lesions causing severe, subtotal stenosis of the arterial lumen tend more often to be bulky fibrous plaques and have a much lower propensity to rupture. Revascularization therapies directed at obstructive coronary disease can relieve symptoms and (indirectly) reduce the risk of death from a major plaque event, but they do not reduce the risk of a clinical plaque event. To achieve this latter goal, additional therapies must be directed at the pathophysiologic process of atheroma formation, the development of vulnerable plaques, and the thrombotic response to plaque rupture.

ISSUES AT THE TIME OF ADMISSION

The two major components involved in the initial assessment of the patient with suspected angina are assessment of the diagnosis and assessment of the short-term prognosis. Patients who require hospital admission either have a history of known CAD with recurrent or worsening symptoms or present with symptoms that are at least suggestive of possible CAD. In both of these scenarios (i.e., new presentation and patient with preestablished CAD), the clinician must assess the likelihood that the patient's symptoms represent ischemic atherosclerotic disease (see Initial Assessment of Diagnosis). Concurrently, the clinician must decide whether the patient needs immediate therapy or can be

treated once the results of initial testing have been obtained (see Initial Assessment of Prognosis).

Initial Assessment of Diagnosis

Diagnostic Features of the History

When the patient gives a history that conforms closely to the template of characteristics initially described by Heberden and other early cardiologists, the terms *"typical" angina* or *"definite" angina* are often used. *"Atypical" angina* describes symptoms that are not classic in one or more key features. *"Probable" angina* and *"possible" angina* are alternative terms that define greater shades of uncertainty. "Non-anginal" symptoms clearly favor another diagnosis (e.g., gall bladder disease or peptic ulcer disease) or are completely inconsistent with typical angina. These terms summarize the likelihood that a patient's symptoms are being caused by underlying obstructive CAD. Seven features of the history should be considered in this assessment: quality, location, duration, and severity of the discomfort; precipitants; factors providing relief; and associated symptoms.

Quality of Discomfort

Because the myocardium and the other thoraco-abdominal viscera are not well equipped with sensory nerves, ischemia in these organs produces sensations that are difficult for patients to describe. Some angina patients deny that they have "chest pain" because they do not consider the symptoms painful. Consequently, the patient should be asked about any *discomfort* and allowed to supply the descriptive terms that are most appropriate. Frequently, the patient with typical angina will use words such as *tightness, pressure, squeezing, aching, fullness, constriction,* or *heaviness*; terms such as *burning, indigestion, cramping,* and *gas* are also commonly used by patients with angina, but these sensations often occur in patients without angina and hence are less typically associated with the diagnosis. Descriptions that point to a diagnosis of non-anginal pain include knifelike, sharp, stabbing, and throbbing, or any discomfort that is clearly altered by a change in posture or respiratory movements.

Location

Myocardial ischemic discomfort can be perceived anywhere between the jaw and the diaphragm. The most typical location is substernal (retrosternal). Because of the visceral origin of these symptoms, patients may not only have trouble describing but also localizing them. Occasionally, a patient with typical angina will spontaneously clench a fist over the sternum while describing symptoms (*Levine's sign*). In contrast, the patient who can point with one finger to the location of the discomfort does not have typical angina. Similarly, isolated right-sided chest discomfort is almost never anginal (unless the patient has dextrocardia), and discomfort limited to the region below or lateral to the left breast is also unlikely to represent myocardial ischemia. Typical angina commonly radiates down one or both arms (the left more frequently than the right), to the neck, or to the left shoulder; some typical angina patients may have symptoms confined to these locations. However, symptoms of exertional tightness or less commonly an ache in more unusual locations—the lower jaw, teeth, or ear region—are also consistent with a diagnosis of angina. In the unstable angina patient who presents only with symptoms in these unusual locations at rest, the clinician must maintain a high index of suspicion to arrive at the correct diagnosis. Radiation of the discomfort to the lower abdomen or lower extremities, in contrast, is inconsistent with a diagnosis of typical or definite angina.

Duration

Typical stable anginal episodes usually last for ≤5 minutes unless the precipitating factors have not been removed. The discomfort characteristically resolves completely between episodes. A duration of discomfort of ≥20 minutes, particularly if the discomfort is severe, should prompt consideration of acute CAD (which is discussed further below). Symptoms that last only for seconds (sometimes described as "lightning-like") are very unlikely to be caused by myocardial ischemia and are inconsistent with a diagnosis of typical angina. Symptoms that last for >20 minutes but do not present the features of acute coronary disease are not characteristic of typical angina.

Severity

Anginal symptoms occur on a continuum ranging from mild effort-related angina at one end to acute MI with severe, unrelenting discomfort at the other. The most widely used classification of anginal symptom severity is the Canadian Cardiovascular Society Classification (Table 37.1). Although such information is useful in making treatment decisions, symptom severity does not help in making an assessment of the likelihood of underlying CAD.

Precipitants

Typical angina is characteristically precipitated by factors that increase the cardiac workload, such as exercise or psychological stress. However, not all patients with angina caused by myocardial ischemia can provide information about precipitants, especially if their symptoms are recent in origin or present with an unstable pattern.

Reproducibility of symptoms is a cardinal feature of typical angina. The patient who relates that certain exertional or stress-related activities predictably elicit the discomfort and that this discomfort is relieved promptly by rest or sublingual nitroglycerin has described the core features of typical angina. If the quality and location of the discomfort are consistent with typical angina but the episodes occur sporadically without any obvious precipitants, the diagnosis of atypical angina is more appropriate. The major exception is unstable angina, which may have all the features of typical angina except that symptoms occur at rest. Under these circumstances, a diagnosis of typical or definite angina would still be appropriate.

Factors Providing Relief

Stable exertional angina is characteristically relieved by rest in 3–5 minutes and by sublingual nitroglycerin within 1–3 minutes. If >10 minutes is consistently required to obtain relief with nitroglycerin, acute coronary disease may be present; or, if this pattern is chronic and stable, a diagnosis of atypical angina may be more appropriate. Patients often say that relief of symptoms is obtained by belching or taking antacids or other over-the-counter medications. Although these features may sway the clinician away from a diagnosis of typical angina, it should be remembered that even patients with acute MI may occasionally make such associations. Thus, in patients with suspected acute coronary disease, these historical elements alone should not be used as reasons for rejecting a diagnosis of typical angina if other features are consistent with the diagnosis.

TABLE 37.1

CANADIAN CARDIOVASCULAR SOCIETY CLASSIFICATION OF ANGINAL SYMPTOM SEVERITY

Class	Description
I	No symptoms with ordinary activity (e.g., walking, climbing stairs). Symptoms may occur with strenuous, rapid, or prolonged exertion.
II	Slight limitation of ordinary activity. Discomfort induced by walking or climbing stairs rapidly, walking uphill, walking more than 2 blocks on level ground, or climbing more than 1 flight of stairs at a normal pace.
III	Marked limitation of ordinary activity. Symptoms may occur after walking 1 or 2 blocks on level ground or climbing 1 flight of stairs at a normal pace.
IV	Severe limitation. Inability to carry on any level of exertion without inducing discomfort. Discomfort may also be present at rest.

From Campeau L. Grading of angina pectoris. *Circulation* 1976;54:522–523, with permission.

Associated Symptoms

During an anginal episode, a variety of associated symptoms may occur, including dyspnea, nausea, sweating, weakness, and palpitations. These symptoms by themselves are of little use in deciding whether a patient's symptoms represent typical angina. Dyspnea resulting from myocardial ischemia is common with anginal discomfort and may also occur in isolation as an "anginal equivalent". In the latter situation, it should have the other features of typical angina (e.g., reproducibly provoked by exertion or stress and relieved by rest or nitroglycerin).

Diagnostic Features of the Physical Examination

The physical examination contributes relatively little to the diagnosis of typical angina with underlying coronary disease. The physician should be very wary of rejecting the diagnosis of angina just because the patient agrees that a particular type of palpation of the chest wall or a certain movement causes chest pain. For this sign to be reliable, the pain must be *completely reproduced* by palpation.

Occasionally, the clinician has the opportunity to examine the patient during an episode of angina. Although the results of such an examination may be unremarkable, if the patient is noted to have a transient systolic murmur of mitral regurgitation, an S_3, or a paradoxically split S_2, and if these findings resolve after the anginal episode has been relieved, the diagnosis of typical angina with underlying ischemia is greatly strengthened. The presence of vascular bruits or pulse deficits suggesting extracardiac vascular disease (carotid, peripheral, aortic, renal) is associated with a higher likelihood of significant CAD. Physical examination can also provide useful information on alternative diagnoses, such as hypertrophic cardiomyopathy or aortic valve disease.

Diagnostic Features of Initial Laboratory Tests

At the initial evaluation of the patient with suspected angina caused by CAD, a resting 12-lead electrocardiogram (ECG) (Table 37.2) and a chest radiograph should be obtained. The chest radiograph is not useful for the diagnosis of CAD but may be helpful in the differential diagnosis and assessment of prognosis. Laboratory markers of myocardial necrosis are indicated for patients with a presumptive diagnosis of unstable angina to exclude acute MI (see Initial Assessment of Prognosis).

Assessment of the Likelihood of Coronary Artery Disease

The likelihood (i.e., probability) that a patient has significant CAD (defined as stenosis ≥75% of the vessel diameter on a coronary angiogram) can be estimated with moderate accuracy from five features of the initial clinical examination and ECG (in order of importance): the

TABLE 37.2

ELECTROCARDIOGRAPHIC FINDINGS USEFUL FOR ESTABLISHING THE LIKELIHOOD OF CORONARY ARTERY DISEASE

Finding	Most likely cause	Alternate causes
ST-segment elevation ≥1 mm in 2 or more contiguous leads	Acute MI	Acute pericarditis Early repolarization Left ventricular aneurysm Coronary spasm
ST-segment depression ≥0.5 mm	Ischemia or acute MI	Normal heart Hyperventilation LV hypertrophy with strain Digitalis Hypokalemia Hypomagnesemia
Inverted T waves in 2 or more contiguous leads (≥2 mm in leads with dominant R waves, or marked symmetric precordial T-wave inversion)	Ischemia or acute MI	Normal heart Central nervous system disease Hypertrophic cardiomyopathy
Pathologic Q waves in 2 or more contiguous leads	Recent or old MI	Myocarditis Hypertrophic cardiomyopathy Chronic obstructive lung disease Pulmonary embolism Left ventricular hypertrophy Idiopathic cardiomyopathy

LV, left ventricular; *MI*, myocardial infarction.
From Braunwald E, Mark DB, Jones RH, et al. Unstable angina: diagnosis and management. Agency for Health Care Policy and Research. Publication 94-0602, Rockville, MD.

physician's assessment of the patient's symptoms (as typical angina, atypical angina, or non-anginal pain); evidence of a prior MI (by history and pathologic Q waves on the ECG); gender; age; and number of major risk factors (diabetes, hypercholesterolemia, smoking, hypertension). A summary estimate of the patient's likelihood of significant CAD can be generated either informally by the clinician or by using one of several quantitative tools developed to assist in that process (Table 37.3).

If the patient has known CAD (e.g., a history of prior revascularization or CAD established by coronary angiography), then the diagnostic question of interest is whether the patient's symptoms are caused by CAD. This judgment is best based on the elements of the angina history described earlier.

Definition of Unstable Angina

Unstable angina is conceptually defined as the clinical syndrome that falls between stable angina (lower risk) and acute MI (higher risk). Operationally, it is often not possible (nor is it necessary) to separate patients with unstable angina from those with non-ST-elevation acute MI during the initial assessment process. What is important is to recognize that the patient has an *acute coronary syndrome* (ACS) and to decide quickly about the proper pace of evaluation and treatment.

The 1994 Agency for Health Care Policy and Research (AHCPR) guideline for unstable angina proposed three principal presentations of unstable angina (2). Prolonged (≥20 minutes) episodes of rest angina are what most clinicians think of as unstable angina. However, the unstable angina guideline proposed two other circumstances in which a patient's short-term risk of cardiac events may be increased. All patients with new-onset angina are considered by some to be "unstable" because they have changed from a state of no symptoms to at least one symptom. However, this increased risk does not relate to the onset of symptoms *per se* but rather to the tempo, severity, and frequency of symptoms. Thus, new-onset or preexisting effort angina that progresses to the point where the patient cannot perform less-than-ordinary activity (Class III, Table 37.1) without provoking angina would be considered unstable angina.

The 2000 American College of Cardiology (ACC)/American Heart Association (AHA) Guideline used the term *unstable angina/non-ST elevation myocardial infarction* (NSTEMI) to emphasize the continuum between these manifestations of acute coronary disease (3). The term *acute coronary syndrome* (ACS) serves a similar purpose. The distinction of greatest initial therapeutic importance is between the patient with acute ST-elevation MI, who is eligible for reperfusion therapy, and other types of ACS.

Initial Assessment of Prognosis

Predicting the presence of a vulnerable but unruptured atherosclerotic plaque is not yet possible with available technology. Thus, assessment of prognosis focuses on

TABLE 37.3

LIKELIHOOD OF SIGNIFICANT CORONARY ARTERY DISEASE IN PATIENTS WITH SYMPTOMS SUGGESTING UNSTABLE ANGINA

High likelihood (e.g., 0.85–0.99)	Intermediate likelihood (e.g., 0.15–0.84)	Low likelihood (e.g., 0.01–0.14)
Any of the following features: History of prior MI, sudden death, or other known history of CAD Definite angina: men ≥60 or women ≥70 years old Transient hemodynamic or ECG changes during pain Variant angina (pain with reversible ST-segment elevation) ST-segment elevation or depression ≥1 mm Marked symmetrical T-wave inversion in multiple precordial leads	*No high-likelihood features and any of the following:* Definite angina: men <60 or women <70 years old Probable angina: men ≥60 or women ≥70 years old Chest pain probably not angina in patients with diabetes Chest pain probably not angina and 2 or 3 risk factors other than diabetes[a] Extracardiac vascular disease ST depression 0.05–1 mm T wave inversion ≥2 mm in leads with dominant R waves	*No high- or intermediate-likelihood features but may have the following:* Chest pain classified as probably not angina One risk factor other than diabetes[a] T-wave flattening or inversion <2 mm in leads with dominant R waves Normal ECG

[a] Coronary artery disease risk factors include diabetes, smoking, hypertension, and elevated cholesterol. *CAD*, coronary artery disease; *ECG*, electrocardiogram; *MI*, myocardial infarction.
NOTE: Likelihood of significant coronary artery disease is a complex, multivariable problem that cannot be fully specified in a table such as this. Therefore, the table is meant to illustrate major relationships rather than offer rigid algorithms.
Adapted with permission from Braunwald E, Mark DB, Jones RH, et al. Unstable angina: diagnosis and management. Rockville, Maryland: U.S. Department of Health and Human Services; 1994.

TABLE 37.4

SHORT-TERM RISK OF DEATH OR NONFATAL MYOCARDIAL INFARCTION IN PATIENTS WITH SYMPTOMS SUGGESTING UNSTABLE ANGINA

High risk	Intermediate risk	Low risk
At least one of the following features must be present:	*No high-risk feature, but must have any of the following:*	*No high- or intermediate-risk feature, but may have any of the following features:*
Prolonged ongoing (>20 min) rest pain	Prolonged (>20 min) rest angina, now resolved, with moderate or high likelihood of CAD	Increased anginal frequency, severity, or duration
Pulmonary edema, most likely related to ischemia	Nocturnal angina	Angina provoked at a lower threshold
Angina at rest with dynamic ST-segment changes ≥0.5 mm	Angina with dynamic T-wave changes (>0.2 mV)	New onset angina with onset 2 weeks to 2 months before presentation
Angina with new or worsening mitral regurgitation murmur, S_3, new or worsening rales, or hypotension	New onset CCSC III or IV angina in the past 2 weeks with moderate or high likelihood of CAD	Normal or unchanged ECG
Age >75 years	Pathological Q waves, or resting ST-segment depression ≥0.5 mm	
Troponin T or I level >0.1 ng/mL	Age >65 years	

CCSC, Canadian Cardiovascular Society classification (see Table 37.1); other abbreviations as in Table 37.3.
NOTE: Estimation of the short-term risks of death and nonfatal MI in unstable angina is a complex multivariable problem that cannot be fully specified in a table such as this. Therefore, the table is meant to offer general guidance and illustration rather than rigid algorithms.
Adapted with permission from Braunwald E, Mark DB, Jones RH, et al. Unstable angina: diagnosis and management. Rockville, Maryland: U.S. Department of Health and Human Services; 1994.

two main concepts: identifying the CAD patient with a plaque event early enough in the course to prevent progression to a catastrophic complication, and identifying those CAD patients who lack sufficient cardiac reserve to survive should a major plaque event occur.

Clinical and Electrocardiographic Factors Related to Short-term Prognosis

The tempo of a patient's anginal syndrome is assessed from the cardiac history, the 12-lead ECG, and examination of the patient during a symptomatic episode (when possible). Important adverse prognostic elements of the history include: a higher current frequency of episodes, an increase in the frequency of episodes during the last 4–6 weeks (and particularly during the last week), an increase in the duration or severity of symptoms (with emphasis on any symptom episodes lasting ≥20 minutes), progression from effort- or stress-related symptoms to symptoms at rest, new onset of symptoms that awaken the patient from sleep, and a significant decrease in the amount of effort needed to provoke symptoms. By using these features, the clinician can separate patients into high-, moderate- and low-risk subgroups (Table 37.4).

Factors Related to Both Short-term and Long-term Prognosis

The four factors most strongly predictive of survival should an acute plaque event occur are LV function, extent of obstructive CAD, age, and comorbid conditions. *LV function is the single most important predictor;* the worse the LV function, the more likely that a major plaque event will be fatal. A fatal outcome is also more likely when all three coronary arteries have significant stenosis in comparison with lesser degrees of CAD. Among comorbidities, diabetes and chronic renal insufficiency are particularly important for identifying high-risk patients (4, 5).

Integrated Clinical Risk Stratification

Two generations of risk stratification models have been developed for use in ACS patients. Earlier models, such as that by Goldman and colleagues in the Multicenter Chest Pain Study, were designed to improve decision making and triage in the emergency department (Figure 37.2). These models use history and ECG data but not cardiac biomarker data. More recent models focus on management decisions for patients admitted with ACS. These are typified by the TIMI (Thrombolysis in Myocardial Infarction) risk score for unstable angina/non-ST elevation MI (6) (Table 37.5).

Laboratory Markers of Myocardial Necrosis

Traditional risk stratification for acute coronary syndrome patients has rested on the clinician's initial history and physical examination and on the interpretation of the 12-lead ECG. During the last several years, new approaches have been developed based on markers of myocardial necrosis (Table 37.6).

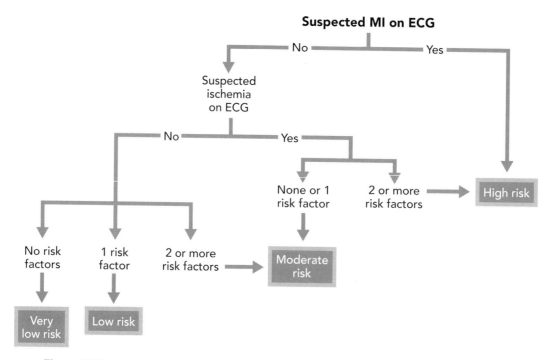

Figure 37.2 Stratification of patients with acute chest pain into 4 risk groups based on the initial electrocardiogram and the presence of clinical risk factors. Criteria for suspected myocardial infarction on the electrocardiogram were ST-segment elevation ≥1 mm or pathologic Q waves in 2 or more leads, with these findings not known to be old. Criteria for suspected ischemia were ST-segment depression ≥1 mm or T-wave inversion in 2 or more leads, with these findings not known to be old. Risk factors included systolic blood pressure <110 mm Hg, rales above the lung bases bilaterally, and worsening symptoms of known ischemic heart disease. The recommended triage is generally admission to an intensive care unit for high- and moderate-risk patients. If appropriate, low- and very low-risk patients should generally be admitted to an intermediate care unit and a chest pain evaluation unit (if available), respectively. (Redrawn from Goldman L, Cook EF, Johnson PA, et al. Prediction of the need for intensive care in patients who come to emergency departments with acute chest pain. *N Engl J Med* 1996;334:1498–1504, with permission.)

Troponins have replaced creatine kinase (CK)-MB as the gold standard for detection of myocardial necrosis (7). The troponins are structural proteins that comprise part of the myocardial contractile apparatus. *Troponin T* (cTnT) exists in the myocyte, with about 95% bound to other structural proteins and 5% free in the cytosol. After damage to myocytes, elevated cTnT is detectable in the serum as early as 4–6 hours, and elevated levels remain detectable for 10–14 days. About 98% of *troponin I* (cTnI)

is bound to other myocyte proteins, and 2% is free in the cytosol. After myocardial damage, cTnI rises slightly later than cTnT, at about 6 hours, and remains elevated for 7–10 days. Both cTnT and cTnI are cleared more slowly in the presence of renal insufficiency. Thus, interpretation of elevated levels in this setting remains more difficult. Because cardiac troponins are immunologically distinct from troponins in non-cardiac muscle, they are extremely specific for the diagnosis of myocardial necrosis. Because of their prolonged period of elevation, they have also supplanted the use of lactate dehydrogenase (LDH) and LDH isoenzymes in the diagnosis of MI in patients who present late (i.e., >24–36 hours) after the onset of symptoms.

Studies of serial troponin testing have suggested that optimal risk stratification is obtained by measuring a troponin level at presentation and at 8 hours after presentation. Patients with negative troponin levels at 0 and 8 hours have a low mortality rate, and no further prognostic information is learned by obtaining a level at 16 hours. However, a negative finding before 8 hours does not provide the same level of reassurance and should not be used for purposes of triage.

TABLE 37.5

TIMI RISK SCORE FOR UNSTABLE ANGINA

1 point each for:

- Age ≥65
- ≥3 risk factors for CAD
- Known CAD ≥50% stenosis
- ST deviation on presenting ECG
- ≥2 anginal events in past 24 hours
- Use of aspirin in prior 7 days
- Elevated cardiac biomarkers

0–2 = low risk
3–4 = intermediate risk
5–7 = high risk

TABLE 37.6

LABORATORY MARKERS OF MYOCARDIAL NECROSIS

	Myoglobin	Total CK	CK-MB (mass assay)	cTnT	cTnI
Cardiac-specific	No	No	Very	Extremely	Extremely
Affected by renal function	Yes	No	Yes	Yes	Yes
Initial detection	1–3 h	4–8 h	3–4 h	4–6 h	4–6 h
Duration of elevation	18–24 h	12–24 h	24–36 h	10–14 d	7–10 d
Rapid laboratory assay	Yes	Yes	Yes	Yes	Yes
Bedside assay	Yes	Yes	Yes	Yes	Yes

CK-MB, myocardial-specific isoenzyme of creatine kinase; cTnT, troponin T; cTnI, troponin I.
Reprinted with permission from Newby LK, Ohman EM, Christenson RH. The role of troponin and other markers for myocardial necrosis in risk stratification. In: Topol EJ, ed. *Acute Coronary Syndromes*. New York: Marcel Dekker, 1998:405–435.

With the advent of these more heart-specific and sensitive troponin assays, some patients in whom unstable angina would have been diagnosed have been redefined as having small, non-ST-elevation MIs. Whether these patients should be labeled as "MIs" remains controversial and is actually less important than recognizing their positive troponin result as a marker of elevated risk. For example, in a meta-analysis of 16 studies involving around 4,500 non-ST elevation ACS patients, a positive troponin indicated a 5-fold increased risk (8). Mortality also increased linearly with increasing troponin levels. Troponin T and I had similar prognostic importance.

CK-MB, the myocardium-specific isoenzyme of creatine kinase, indicates myocardial necrosis but is not as specific as troponin (about 5% of skeletal muscle CK is of the CK-MB form). Non-heart-related elevations of CK-MB may be seen after surgery on or trauma to the small intestine, uterus, prostate, tongue, or diaphragm. Levels of CK-MB may also be elevated in chronic renal failure; in this situation, the absence of a characteristic rise and fall during several days should confirm the noncardiac etiology.

Initial Management

General Measures

When the patient is first seen, the clinician must decide if immediate stabilization measures need to be instituted during the initial diagnostic assessment. One of the most important initial questions the clinician must address is whether the patient is having an ST-elevation acute MI and has indications for emergency reperfusion therapy.

Patients with stable angina can usually be managed on an outpatient basis unless they have evidence of substantially increased risk, such as a high-risk result on a noninvasive stress test. Thus, most angina patients admitted to the hospital will have ACS.

As soon as the clinician has established a working diagnosis of unstable angina/acute coronary syndrome, therapy should be directed toward two goals: stabilizing the patient to prevent further disease progression and relieving symptoms (Table 37.7). Therapy should not be delayed until a decision has been made to admit the patient from the office or emergency department to the inpatient unit but rather should be guided by the prognostic risk assessment. For low-risk patients, further evaluation and therapy may be conducted on an outpatient basis. Generally, patients with intermediate- and high-risk features will require hospital admission. For some intermediate-risk patients, further evaluation and therapy can be performed in a chest pain unit or a short-stay unit, whereas others may be admitted to a step-down unit or an ICU. High-risk patients will typically start out in an ICU.

For all hospitalized ACS patients, initial therapy includes such general measures as bed rest until stabilization occurs, continuous ECG monitoring, and supplemental oxygen for those with respiratory distress or documented hypoxemia. As part of the early evaluation process, secondary causes for the development of a progressive or unstable course should be sought. These include tachyarrhythmias and bradyarrhythmias, high fever, hypotension or severe hypertension, and severe anemia. The initial evaluation may also suggest other responsible or contributory cardiac disorders (e.g., aortic valve disease, hypertrophic cardiomyopathy), hyperthyroidism, medical noncompliance (e.g., failure to refill prescriptions), or a recent increase in physical activity or emotional stress.

Antithrombin and Antiplatelet Therapy

In addition to these general measures, clinicians should generally use antithrombin and antiplatelet therapy in intermediate- and high-risk patients. All patients should promptly receive aspirin (an initial dose of 160, followed

TABLE 37.7

ACUTE MANAGEMENT OF ACS IN RELATION TO RISK FOR MYOCARDIAL INFARCTION OR DEATH

	High risk	Intermediate risk	Low risk
General			
Treatment setting	ED → CCU	ED → CCU, step-down, or ward	ED → home
ECG monitoring	≥48 h	24 to 48 h	ED only
IV	Yes	Yes	No
Analgesic	IV opiate	Usually none unless recurrent chest discomfort	None
Anti-ischemic therapy			
Nitrates	Sublingual stat, IV infusion	Sublingual stat, or PRN oral or topical	Sublingual PRN, oral or topical
β-blocker	IV or oral	Oral	Oral
β-blocker failure or contraindicated	Diltiazem or verapamil substituted	Diltiazem or verapamil substituted	Diltiazem or verapamil substituted
Antiplatelet therapy			
Daily ASA	Yes	Yes	Yes
ASA intolerance or allergy	Clopidogrel	Clopidogrel	Clopidogrel
Platelet GP IIb/IIIa receptor inhibitors	Bolus → IV ≥48 h	Patients with planned cath/PCI	No
Anticoagulant therapy			
Heparin or enoxaparin	Routine	Routine	No
Angiography and revascularization	For most patients	Early invasive or early conservative strategies	Reserve for failure of optimal medical therapy

ACS, acute coronary syndrome; *ASA*, aspirin; *ED*, emergency department; *GP*, glycoprotein; *PCI*, percutaneous coronary intervention
Adapted with permission from Cairns J, Theroux P, Armstrong P, et al. Unstable angina—report from a Canadian expert roundtable. *Can J Cardiol* 1996;12:1279–1292.

by 80 to 160 mg per day) unless it is contraindicated. For patients who are truly aspirin-allergic, clopidogrel (loading dose of 300 mg, followed by 75 mg/d) is a reasonable alternative. Based on the CURE trial, the ACC/AHA Guidelines recommend clopidogrel be administered in addition to aspirin in all non-ST elevation ACS patients who will not be referred for early intervention (i.e., first 24–36 hours) (9). In patients who are referred for early catheterization, clopidogrel should be held until the need for urgent coronary bypass surgery is assessed.

Intravenous heparin or subcutaneous enoxaparin (a low-molecular-weight heparin) should be started in most intermediate- and all high-risk patients who lack contraindications. Two randomized trials (ESSENCE and TIMI 11B) have demonstrated that enoxaparin reduced death or MI by 23% relative to unfractionated heparin in this population and has an equivalent risk of bleeding (10). In addition, it is more convenient to administer and does not require laboratory monitoring to assess the level of anticoagulation, as is necessary with unfractionated heparin (see Chapter 98).

Two intravenous glycoprotein IIb/IIIa (GP 2b/3a) receptor antagonists, eptifibatide and tirofiban, have been approved for use in acute coronary syndrome patients in the United States, and abciximab is approved for use in percu-

taneous coronary interventions (PCI). A GP IIb/IIIa antagonist should be administered in all ACS patients for whom catheterization and PCI are planned (11). Eptifibatide or tirofiban should also be given in high-risk patients (e.g., continuing ischemia, elevated troponin) who are not planned for PCI.

Symptomatic Therapy

Control of anginal symptoms is based on the use of nitrates, β-blockers, and opiates (Table 37.7). For patients with ongoing or recent prolonged or severe symptoms, parenteral therapy should be initiated. For others, nonparenteral (oral, topical) therapy may be sufficient. The use of calcium channel blockers in acute coronary syndromes remains controversial, but there is general agreement that these drugs should be reserved for symptom relief in patients in whom β-blocker therapy has failed or is contraindicated.

Response to Therapy

The vast majority of acute coronary syndrome patients respond within 30 minutes to the medical management described above with a clear improvement in symptoms and other evidence of stabilization. Failure of patients to respond within this time frame should prompt the clinician to (re)consider other causes of severe chest discomfort (e.g., acute MI, aortic dissection, pulmonary embolus, or pneumothorax). If acute coronary disease still appears to be the correct diagnosis, consideration should be given to early referral for diagnostic cardiac catheterization and revascularization, placement of an intra-aortic balloon pump, or both. While arrangements are being made for these therapies, aggressive pharmacologic therapy should be continued in a carefully monitored setting.

Risk Stratification in a Chest Pain Unit

Approximately one-fourth of U.S. hospitals now have a chest pain unit in the emergency department. Patients admitted to a chest pain unit are typically those for whom the diagnosis of acute coronary syndrome or the risk level is uncertain after evaluation of initial clinical and ECG data (12).

Testing in the chest pain unit typically includes serial cardiac biomarkers: every 3 to 4 hours for CK-MB or at 0 and 8 hours for cTnT. Patients with positive biomarkers by 8–9 hours are admitted for further evaluation. In some centers, patients with nondiagnostic ECGs may also undergo acute imaging with echocardiography or a nuclear perfusion agent to detect evidence of severe ischemia or infarction. Patients with negative biomarkers may then undergo an exercise or pharmacologic stress test in the chest pain unit before the final triage decision is made. Numerous test combinations are possible to provide adequate risk stratification for clinical management and triage purposes (Chapter 36). In the experience of several large centers, only about 15% of chest pain unit patients will require hospital admission.

ISSUES DURING THE COURSE OF HOSPITALIZATION

The hospital course of patients with acute coronary disease can be conceptually divided into three major phases: completion of stabilization, risk stratification, and selection of definitive therapy.

Completion of Stabilization

It is desirable for patients initially requiring ICU or step-down care to experience a 24-hour period of freedom from recurrent ischemic episodes, hemodynamic abnormalities, decompensated heart failure, or other complications before being transferred to a less intensive environment. Patients who have been symptom-free for ≥24 hours before admission and do not have evidence of heart failure or other complications may proceed directly to the risk-stratification phase.

Aspirin should be continued at a daily dose of 80–160 mg. In general, patients who are at sufficiently high risk to require therapy with either unfractionated or low-molecular-weight heparin should continue this therapy for 2–5 days or until a revascularization procedure is performed. In large clinical trials of acute coronary syndrome patients, U.S. physicians typically use antithrombin therapy for 2.5–3 days, whereas physicians in Canada and Western Europe tend to use such therapy for 4–5 days or more. These trials do not show any difference in event rates associated with the duration of therapy. Because the shorter duration of U.S. therapy is coupled with a substantially higher rate of revascularization procedures, it is unclear whether the U.S. pattern of care also defines the minimum duration of antithrombin therapy needed when a less invasive management style is practiced.

The duration of glycoprotein IIb/IIIa inhibitor therapy in clinical trials has generally been for 72 hours or until the time of revascularization. For patients undergoing percutaneous revascularization, eptifibatide and tirofiban are usually continued for another 24 hours after the procedure.

Risk Stratification

Management of the patient with ACS requires ongoing risk stratification with appropriate modification of therapy. Initial risk stratification is based on the admission evaluation and the clinical course during the early hospital stay. Once the patient's condition has stabilized, the clinician needs to assess the longer-term prognosis, especially for the next 3–6 months, and decide what additional tests and modifications of therapy are required to protect the patient from (further) cardiac complications, to reassure the patient, and to return the patient to as full and unimpaired a lifestyle as possible. Three main options are available: (1) proceed directly to diagnostic cardiac catheterization; (2) perform a noninvasive exercise or pharmacologic stress test; or (3) neither. For almost all patients hospitalized with ACS, some form of risk stratification testing should be performed once they have been stable without angina or heart failure for 48 hours. Patients with extensive comorbidity who would not be candidates for revascularization are a potential exception.

Two approaches to the use of cardiac catheterization in this setting have been studied: early invasive and early conservative (11). In the *early invasive strategy*, diagnostic catheterization is performed routinely in all hospitalized unstable angina patients who do not have contraindications, usually within 48 hours of admission. In the *early conservative strategy*, diagnostic catheterization is performed routinely in patients with one or more of the following high-risk indicators: persistent or recurrent angina/ischemia despite intensive medical therapy, elevated troponin, prior revascularization (coronary artery bypass graft, percutaneous coronary intervention), associated heart failure or depressed LV function (ejection fraction <0.40) by noninvasive study, malignant ventricular arrhythmias, and a high-risk noninvasive stress test result.

If the early conservative strategy is chosen, choice of the stress testing modality for the non-high-risk patients should be based on a consideration of 3 factors: the patient's resting 12-lead ECG, the ability of the patient to walk on a treadmill or pedal a bicycle, and the local expertise and testing modes available. Although imaging stress tests have better sensitivity and specificity for the diagnosis of significant CAD than does an exercise ECG test, there is no convincing evidence that their improved accuracy translates into improved patient management among patients with a normal baseline ECG who are not taking digoxin. Hence, the exercise treadmill test is the standard choice for these patients. Patients with significant resting ST-segment depression ($\geq$1 mm), ST changes associated with digoxin, left bundle branch block, intraventricular conduction delay, or LV hypertrophy should have an exercise imaging test (e.g., a sestamibi or thallium perfusion scan or an echocardiogram). Patients unable to exercise should have a pharmacologic stress imaging study. At centers where multiple testing options are available, choice of testing mode should be based primarily on local expertise (see also Chapter 36).

The results of stress testing can be partitioned into low-risk, intermediate-risk, and high-risk categories. Patients with low-risk test results generally have an annual cardiac mortality rate below 1% and can be safely managed medically. High-risk test results typically predict an annual cardiac mortality rate of 4% or more and should usually prompt referral for cardiac catheterization. Patients with intermediate-risk test results typically require either an additional stress test or cardiac catheterization to clarify their prognosis. Alternatively, a rest echocardiogram may be performed. If depressed resting LV function is found in a patient with an intermediate-risk stress test result, referral to catheterization should strongly be considered. If the resting LV function is normal, medical therapy or a second stress test are reasonable options.

Selection of Definitive Therapy

The available evidence supports three general conclusions: First, a patient who cannot be adequately stabilized with appropriate medical therapy or who has clear indication of high risk based on clinical or stress test criteria, as discussed in the previous section, should usually be referred promptly for coronary angiography. Second, with current medical therapy, there does not appear to be any excess risk if angiography is deferred for the remaining patients. For example, in patients in the conservative arm in TACTICS-TIMI 18 who did not undergo angiography (49%), the death and nonfatal MI rate at 30 days was 2.4% (13). Patients over age 65, however, may benefit from a routine aggressive strategy (14). Third, controlling the atherosclerotic disease process provides the key to reducing the risk for a future cardiac event. Hence, *all patients should have a careful evaluation of their modifiable cardiac risk factors*, particularly lipids, smoking, blood pressure, and diabetes. Patients

with a low-density lipoprotein (LDL) cholesterol level above 100 mg/dL should begin statin therapy, with an LDKL goal of about 60 mg/dL (15). Blood pressure and blood glucose control should be reviewed in patients in whom these parameters are elevated. Smoking cessation resources in the local environment should be identified and offered to patients who smoke.

ISSUES AT THE TIME OF HOSPITAL DISCHARGE

The achievements of the hospitalization should be compared at least daily with the management goals established by the clinician in conjunction with the patient. These goals typically include stabilization of the clinical course, effective relief of symptoms, completion of the most important diagnostic tests, and design of a longer-term management strategy. The need for continued hospitalization is then based on whether these goals have been achieved. In the modern era, with its tremendous financial pressures on hospitals and providers, the clinician must decide which goals need to be achieved in the hospital and which can be shifted to the post-discharge outpatient phase. In general, effective stabilization of the clinical course, relief of symptoms, and risk stratification should be achieved in the hospital. Lower-risk patients who have responded well to therapy can then be targeted for accelerated discharge.

Patients who have undergone successful revascularization will usually have their post-procedure length of stay defined by the evolving standard practice for the given procedure. Patients who are treated medically include both a low-risk group that can be discharged virtually immediately after their primary risk stratification test (e.g., stress test or cardiac catheterization) and a higher-risk group. These latter patients, who are typically either unwilling to have or unsuitable for revascularization, may require additional time to stabilize their disease.

Unless the diagnosis of CAD has been effectively excluded during the hospitalization, all patients should be discharged on aspirin therapy at a daily dose of 80–160 mg. Recent data have suggested an increased risk of bleeding with chronic aspirin doses above 160 mg (16). There are also data indicating less complete platelet inhibition with lower doses of aspirin, so the optimal dose for the ACS patient remains controversial. Patients with a true aspirin allergy should be given 75 mg/day of clopidogrel as an alternative antiplatelet agent. Continued anti-anginal therapy is required after discharge except in patients who have undergone successful revascularization earlier in the hospitalization. β-blockers are the cornerstone of anti-anginal therapy and should be strongly considered for secondary prevention in all CAD patients without contraindications. Long-acting nitrates often provide incremental anti-anginal benefit. Calcium channel blockers should be reserved for patients who require triple anti-anginal drug therapy or who truly cannot tolerate (or have contraindications to) β-blockers; current recommendations are to avoid short-acting dihydropyridine calcium channel blockers (e.g., nifedipine) in patients with CAD. Patients who are not revascularized and who required medical therapy to achieve stabilization should be continued on the regimen found to be effective (e.g., nitrates, β-blockers). In general, long-acting agents are preferred to maximize compliance. However, efforts should also be made to determine whether there are financial barriers for the patient to continue the prescribed regimen. It is better to have the patient take a few effective, affordable medications than to not take an elegant but expensive multidrug regimen. In addition to the longer-acting agents, all patients likely to experience recurrent angina should be given sublingual nitroglycerin and instructed in its use.

A well-defined risk factor modification plan should be in place at the time of hospital discharge. Because of the current brevity of many hospital stays, some of the objectives of the plan will necessarily have to be achieved on an outpatient basis. Specific issues to consider include the following:

- No patient who smokes at the time of admission should be allowed to leave the hospital without being strongly advised to quit smoking permanently. If the patient lives in a household where others smoke (e.g., spouse, children), these household members should also be strongly advised to quit.
- Pharmacologic assistance and smoking cessation counseling programs should be strongly considered.
- Blood pressure and blood glucose control are critical.
- A lipid panel (total, LDL, and HDL cholesterol; triglycerides) should ideally be checked within 24 hours of hospital admission and appropriate therapy started or adjusted. Otherwise, lipids should be checked 8 weeks after admission by the patient's outpatient physician.

An elevated level of *plasma homocysteine* has recently been added to the list of potentially modifiable risk factors for CAD (17). One recent clinical trial demonstrated that dietary folate supplementation significantly decreases plasma homocysteine levels, and epidemiologic studies have associated supplemental intake of folate and vitamin B_{12} with reduced risk for coronary heart disease. Increasing numbers of clinicians are advising their CAD patients to take supplemental B vitamins on empiric grounds. Clinical trials of vitamin E have not shown overall benefit.

Whenever possible, the initial follow-up visit should be set at the time of discharge. Low-risk patients and those with successful uncomplicated revascularization should generally be seen for an outpatient visit 2–6 weeks after discharge. Higher-risk patients should usually be seen sooner (e.g., 1–2 weeks).

In the pre-discharge encounter, the patient should be given instructions about appropriate activities (e.g., resumption of sexual activity, driving), returning to work, daily exercise, and diet. There is very little evidence to guide such recommendations, so they tend to be based on clinical judgment and experience. Referral to an outpatient cardiac rehabilitation program can help the patient achieve the dietary, behavioral, and exercise goals necessary to maximize recovery potential.

COST CONSIDERATIONS AND RESOURCE USE

In the admission phase, use of a chest pain unit with appropriate evaluation and triage protocols can reduce the cost and improve the efficiency of evaluation for patients about whom the clinician remains uncertain after initial evaluation (12). Appropriate risk stratification can also improve care efficiency and reduce costs by ensuring that only the highest-risk patients are admitted to the the ICU, most expensive hospital unit.

As soon as the patient has been been stabilized for 24 hours, the clinician can begin planning the approach to risk stratification, either early aggressive or early conservative. Although the early aggressive strategy is initially more expensive, in TACTICS-TIMI 18 the early conservative strategy lost some of its initial cost advantage because of an increased rate of follow-up rehospitalizations.

KEY POINTS

- Initial diagnostic and prognostic assessment in the emergency department or clinic is based on the history, physical examination findings, and 12-lead ECG data and determines the need for immediate therapy and the next set of diagnostic tests.
- A troponin level measurement at 0 and 8 hours provides powerful additional prognostic information.
- All ACS patients should receive daily aspirin therapy unless contraindicated. Addition of clopidogrel to aspirin for the first 9 months is supported by the CURE trial.
- Intermediate- and high-risk patients should also have parenteral antithrombin (heparin or enoxaparin) and parenteral antiplatelet (eptifibatide or tirofiban) therapy for 2–5 days.
- Patients who fail to stabilize or who have high-risk features should be considered for early coronary angiography.
- Non-high-risk patients with a 24-hour symptom- and complication-free period can be managed with either routine coronary angiography or noninvasive stress testing (angiography reserved for those with high-risk test results).
- All patients should have careful assessment of lipid levels, smoking status, blood pressure, and diabetes status.

REFERENCES

1. Newby LK, Alpert JS, Ohman EM, et al. Changing the diagnosis of acute myocardial infarction: Implications for practice and clinical investigations. *Am Heart J* 2002;144:957–980.
2. Braunwald E, Mark DB, Jones RH, et al. Unstable angina: diagnosis and management. Agency for Healthcare Policy and Research 1994;94–0682.
3. Braunwald E. ACC/AHA guidelines for the management of patients with unstable angina and non-ST-segment elevation myocardial infarction. *J Am Coll Cardiol* 2000;36:970–1062.
4. Roffi M, Chew DP, Mukherjee D, et al. Platelet glycoprotein IIb/IIIa inhibitors reduce mortality in diabetic patients with non-ST-segment-elevation acute coronary syndromes. *Circulation* 2001;104:2767–2771.
5. Al Suwaidi J, Reddan DN, Williams K, et al. Prognostic implications of abnormalities in renal function in patients with acute coronary syndromes. *Circulation* 2002;106:974–980.
6. Antman EM, Cohen M, Bernink PJ, et al. The TIMI risk score for unstable angina/non-ST elevation MI: A method for prognostication and therapeutic decision making. *JAMA* 2000;284:835–842.
7. Antman EM. Decision making with cardiac troponin tests. *N Engl J Med* 2002;346:2079–2082.
8. Ottani F, Galvani M, Nicolini FA, et al. Elevated cardiac troponin levels predict the risk of adverse outcome in patients with acute coronary syndromes. *Am Heart J* 2000;140:917–927.
9. Yusuf S, Zhao F, Mehta SR, et al. Effects of clopidogrel in addition to aspirin in patients with acute coronary syndromes without ST-segment elevation. *N Engl J Med* 2001;345:494–502.
10. Antman EM, Cohen M, Radley D, et al. Assessment of the treatment effect of enoxaparin for unstable angina/non-Q-wave myocardial infarction. TIMI 11B-ESSENCE meta-analysis. *Circulation* 1999;100:1602–1608.
11. Braunwald E, Antman EM, Beasley JW, et al. ACC/AHA 2002 guideline update for the management of patients with unstable angina and non-ST-segment elevation myocardial infarction-summary article: a report of the American College of Cardiology/American Heart Association task force on practice guidelines (Committee on the Management of Patients With Unstable Angina). *J Am Coll Cardiol* 2002;40:1366–1374.
12. Farkouh ME, Smars PA, Reeder GS, et al. A clinical trial of a chest pain unit observation for patients with unstable angina. Chest Pain Evaluation in the Emergency Room (CHEER) Investigators. *N Engl J Med* 1998;339:1882–1888.
13. Cannon CP, Weintraub WS, Demopoulos LA, et al. Comparison of early invasive and conservative strategies in patients with unstable coronary syndromes treated with the glycoprotein IIb/IIIa inhibitor tirofiban. *N Engl J Med* 2001;344:1879–1887.
14. Bach RG, Cannon CP, Weintraub WS, et al. The effect of routine, early invasive management on outcome for elderly patients with non-ST-segment elevation acute coronary syndromes. *Ann Intern Med* 2004;141:186–195.
15. Cannon CP, Braunwald E, McCabe CH, et al. Intensive versus moderate lipid lowering with statins after acute coronary syndromes. *N Engl J Med* 2004;350:1495–1504.
16. Topol EJ, Easton D, Harrington RA, et al. Randomized, double-blind, placebo-controlled, international trial of the oral IIb/IIIa antagonist lotrafiban in coronary and cerebrovascular disease. *Circulation* 2003;108:399–406.
17. Hackam DG, Anand SS. Emerging risk factors for atherosclerotic vascular disease: a critical review of the evidence. *JAMA* 2003;290:932–940.

ADDITIONAL READING

Alpert JS, Thygesen K, Antman E, et al. Myocardial infarction redefined—a consensus document of The Joint European Society of Cardiology/American College of Cardiology Committee for the redefinition of myocardial infarction. *J Am Coll Cardiol* 2000;36:959–969.

Boersma E, Harrington RA, Moliterno DJ, et al. Platelet glycoprotein IIb/IIIa inhibitors in acute coronary syndromes: a meta-analysis of all major randomised clinical trials. *Lancet* 2002;359:189–198.

Kaul P, Newby LK, Fu Y, et al. Troponin T and quantitative ST-segment depression offer complementary prognostic information in the risk stratification of acute coronary syndrome patients. *J Am Coll Cardiol* 2003;41:371–380.

Sabatine MS, Morrow DA, de Lemos JA, et al. Multimarker approach to risk stratification in non-ST elevation acute coronary syndromes: simultaneous assessment of troponin I, C-reactive protein, and B-type natriuretic peptide. *Circulation* 2002;105:1760–1763.

Wiviott SD, Cannon CP, Morrow DA, et al. Differential expression of cardiac biomarkers by gender in patients with unstable angina/non-ST-elevation myocardial infarction: a TACTICS-TIMI 18 (Treat Angina with Aggrastat and determine Cost of Therapy with an Invasive or Conservative Strategy-Thrombolysis In Myocardial Infarction 18) substudy. *Circulation* 2004;109:580–586.

Acute Myocardial Infarction

38

Daniel I. Simon   **James C. Fang**   **Naomi Kenmotsu Rounds**

INTRODUCTION

The contemporary management of acute myocardial infarction (MI) exemplifies the notion that evidence-based medical therapies save lives. Guided by prospective, randomized clinical trials in well over 250,000 patients worldwide and further refined by meta-analyses, current MI therapy has contributed significantly to the marked reduction of average in-hospital MI mortality. Rates dropped from approximately 30% in the 1960s to less than 10% in the present era of reperfusion (i.e., fibrinolysis and primary percutaneous coronary intervention [PCI]). An expedient approach to the assessment and treatment of patients with acute MI focuses on diagnosis, risk stratification, and evidence-based pharmacologic and mechanical interventions aimed at maximizing survival in the context of streamlined critical pathways.

MI commonly occurs secondary to atherosclerotic plaque rupture and thrombosis that results in acute coronary artery occlusion. Less commonly (<10% of cases), MI results from coronary artery embolism, spasm, spontaneous dissection, vasculitis, or a variety of congenital abnormalities (e.g., anomalous coronary artery origin, myocardial bridge). Clinical, pathologic, and experimental data have reshaped the current pathophysiologic understanding of acute ischemic syndromes. Angiography performed in the acute MI setting has demonstrated that mild or moderate (<50% of vessel diameter) rather than severe stenosis is responsible for plaque rupture in most infarct-related arteries. In vulnerable plaques populated by a variety of inflammatory cells, including macrophages and T lymphocytes, a thin, fibrous cap separates the thrombogenic lipid core from the lumen. Inflammation secondary to metabolic, environmental, physical, and possibly infectious injury is an important mechanism of vulnerable plaque development. Clinical cardiologists and vascular biologists now focus on the fine structure of the plaque and the integrity of extracellular matrix proteins in the vessel wall, such as collagen and elastin, as determinants of the clinical manifestations and complications of atherosclerosis.

ISSUES AT THE TIME OF ADMISSION

Clinical Presentation

The alerting symptom of MI is chest pain, which is typically described as severe and prolonged pressure, crushing, burning, or constricting discomfort. However, many patients use different descriptors, such as aching, burning, fullness, or even indigestion or gas. Ischemic chest pain is classically located in the retrosternal, left thoracic, or epigastric regions and may radiate to the neck and shoulders, jaw, back, or arms. Accompanying symptoms may include nausea, vomiting, diaphoresis, dyspnea, and lightheadedness. Not all patients present with typical symptoms of MI. Up to 25% of nonfatal MIs occur silently or with vague, atypical symptoms. Atypical presentations, which occur more commonly in women, the elderly, and in patients with diabetes mellitus, are characterized by severe weakness, heart failure, neurologic manifestations resulting from cerebral hypoperfusion (syncope and mental status changes), and evidence of peripheral embolization.

DIFFERENTIAL DIAGNOSIS AND INITIAL EVALUATION

The differential diagnosis for patients who present with chest pain (Chapter 35) includes pericarditis, aortic dissection, pleuritis, pulmonary embolism, gastrointestinal disease, and musculoskeletal pain. *Pericarditis* (Chapter 46) is characterized by retrosternal pain with positional change (improvement with sitting up and leaning forward). Its pain may be described in the same way as that of classic myocardial ischemia or may be pleuritic in nature. The pain of *aortic dissection* (Chapter 49) is described as sudden, severe, or "ripping" retrosternal discomfort that radiates to the back or legs, worst at its onset, and often associated with pulse deficits. *Pleuritis*, frequently associated with pneumonia, consists of a sharp, knifelike pain that is exacerbated with inspiration. *Pulmonary embolism* (Chapter 53) presents with pleuritic pain accompanied by dyspnea and occasionally hemoptysis. The pain of *costochondritis* is localized and often aggravated by palpation of costochondral joints. *Gastrointestinal causes of chest discomfort* include reflux esophagitis, esophageal spasm, peptic ulcer disease, and cholecystitis.

MI is a medical emergency. The rapid diagnosis of MI is prerequisite for early, life-saving treatment. The diagnosis of MI is based on the presence of at least two of three criteria: a clinical history of ischemic chest discomfort (Chapter 35), changes in serial electrocardiograms (ECGs), and a pattern of rise and fall in serum cardiac markers (Table 37.6). Within 10 minutes of a patient's arrival at the emergency department, a 12-lead ECG should be obtained. ST-segment elevation of 1 mm or more in at least two contiguous leads or a new left bundle branch block is highly suggestive of ST-elevation MI (STEMI). These patients should be screened immediately for reperfusion therapy with fibrinolysis or primary PCI (see later in this chapter).

Patients with ST-segment depressions or new T-wave inversions may be experiencing a non-ST-segment elevation MI (NSTEMI) or unstable angina and should also be treated as if they are having an MI. Differentiating patients presenting with ST-segment elevation from those without ST-segment elevation is useful clinically, for both prognostic and treatment purposes. In general, STEMIs are larger (as assessed by peak biomarker levels) and are associated with higher rates of in-hospital mortality. In contrast, NSTEMIs are smaller and associated with lower in-hospital mortality, but they are notable for at least equivalent rates of recurrent ischemia and MI in the subsequent year. Importantly, from a management standpoint, certain interventions that have resulted in significant mortality reductions in STEMI, such as fibrinolysis, are not beneficial in patients who present with only ST-segment depression or T-wave inversion (i.e., NSTEMI).

Indications for Hospitalization

All patients with MI or suspected MI should be admitted to the hospital. The clinical presentation and outcomes of patients with MI are heterogeneous. Therefore, rapid risk stratification of MI patients is crucial for appropriate therapies and management. Mortality from MI ranges from 1.5% in low-risk groups to more than 80% in high-risk groups. The Killip and Forrester classifications were developed in the era before fibrinolysis and are based on simple physical examination findings or hemodynamic variables, respectively (Table 38.1). The more current Thrombolysis in Myocardial Infarction (TIMI) risk classification is based on nine risk factors easily obtained from clinical history, physical examination, and ECG (Table 38.2). Age is a particularly powerful independent predictor of both in-hospital and 6-month mortality rates. The GISSI (Gruppo Italiano per lo Studio della Sopravvivenza nell'Infarto Miocardico) investigators reported that in patients who presented with a first MI and received thrombolytic therapy, overall in-hospital mortality was 1.9% among patients less than 40 years old but nearly 32% among those more than 80 years old. Multivariate analysis showed that relative risk increased by about 6% annually.

Indications for Initial Coronary Care Admission

Patients with STEMI who present within 24 hours of symptom onset should be admitted to the cardiac care unit

---

TABLE 38.1

RISK STRATIFICATION OF PATIENTS WITH ACUTE MYOCARDIAL INFARCTION

A. Based on clinical examination			B. Based on invasive monitoring		
Class	Definition	Mortality	Subset	Definition	Mortality
I	Rales and S$_3$ absent	6%	I	Normal hemodynamics, PCWP <18, CI >2.2	3%
II	Rales or S$_3$	30%	II	Pulmonary congestion, PCWP >18, CI >2.2	9%
III	Rales over >50% of lung fields (pulmonary edema)	38%	III	Peripheral hypoperfusion, PCWP <18, CI <2.2	23%
IV	Shock	81%	IV	Pulmonary congestion and peripheral hypoperfusion, PCWP >18, CI <2.2	51%

CI, cardiac index; *PCWP*, pulmonary capillary wedge pressure.
A modified from Killip T, Kimball J. Treatment of myocardial infarction in a coronary care unit. A two-year experience with 250 patients. *Am J Cardiol* 1967;20:457. *B* modified from Forrester JS, Diamond GA, Juan HJC. Correlative classification of clinical and hemodynamic function after acute myocardial infarction. *Am J Cardiol* 1997;39:137–145, with permission.

TABLE 38.2

RISK STRATIFICATION: TIMI CLASSIFICATION

Risk factors (No.)[a]	Patients (%)	Mortality (%)
0	26	1.5
1	42	2.3
2	21	7.0
3	7	13.0
≥4	3	17.2

[a] Risk factors: anterior myocardial infarction, prior myocardial infarction, age >70 y, female sex, diabetes, atrial fibrillation, rales >1/3 of lung fields, hypotension (systolic blood pressure <100 mm Hg), and sinus tachycardia (heart rate >100 beats/min).
Reprinted with permission from Hillis LD, Forman S, Braunwald E, and the Thrombolysis in Myocardial Infarction (TIMI) Investigators. Risk stratification before thrombolytic therapy in patients with acute myocardial infarction. *J Am Coll Cardiol* 1990;16:313–315.

(CCU). In addition, all high-risk MI patients (large MI, Killip class II through IV, history of previous MI, age >70 years), patients with persistent ischemic chest pain, early sustained ventricular arrhythmias, or heart block, and patients requiring devices such as an intraaortic balloon pump or temporary pacemaker require CCU level of care. In some hospitals, low-risk MI patients (age <70 years, small MI, no previous MI, Killip class I) may be admitted directly to an intermediate care telemetry unit with ECG monitoring and defibrillation equipment.

Initial Therapy

The goal of MI therapy is to prolong survival by limiting infarct size, repeated infarction, and mechanical complications that lead to pump failure and by preventing sudden death secondary to arrhythmias. It is useful to categorize interventions into those that increase coronary blood flow—recanalization therapy (thrombolytic agents, primary PCI, antithrombotic agents), decrease myocardial oxygen consumption (β-blockers, nitrates, calcium channel blockers), or prevent sudden arrhythmic death (lidocaine, β-blockers) (Table 38.3). Some treatments such as magnesium and angiotensin-converting enzyme (ACE) inhibitors, have multiple effects that may together have a positive impact on MI therapy. Management of MI patients should focus on the pharmacologic and mechanical interventions that unequivocally save lives as determined by prospective, randomized trials: thrombolytic therapy, primary PCI, aspirin, β-blockers, and ACE inhibitors (Table 38.3).

ST Elevation MI

All patients with STEMI should be rapidly assessed for treatment with fibrinolysis or primary PCI with balloon angioplasty and/or stenting. The goal of early recanalization

therapy is to salvage ischemic but viable myocardium, thereby preserving left ventricular (LV) function. Because the wavefront of irreversible ischemic injury progresses over time from subendocardium toward the subepicardium, with nearly transmural necrosis occurring by 6 hours of coronary occlusion in animal models, the degree of myocardial salvage with reperfusion is highly time-dependent.

Although fibrinolysis remains the standard in many institutions, substantial data suggest the superiority of prompt primary PCI. Primary PCI at experienced centers is a superior method of canalization; its routine use in clinical practice is limited (presently about 20% of patients with STEMI in the United States) by lack of availability or unavoidable delays in mobilizing the cardiac catheterization laboratory. Rapid triage of patients to fibrinolysis or to the cardiac catheterization laboratory for PCI requires an algorithmic approach (Figure 38.1).

Recanalization Fibrinolysis

During the past decade, several intravenous (IV) fibrinolysis trials have demonstrated an unequivocal reduction in mortality. Meta-analysis of all trials of fibrinolytic therapy (versus control) that randomized more than 1,000 patients indicates that thrombolytic therapy reduces 35-day mortality on average by 18%, with significant benefits observed with treatment from 0 to 12 hours after the onset of symptoms. Thrombolytic therapy has been estimated to save 39 lives per 1,000 patients treated in the first hour, compared with fewer than 7 lives saved per 1,000 patients treated 13

TABLE 38.3

THERAPIES FOR MYOCARDIAL INFARCTION

Increased myocardial oxygen supply
  Reperfusion therapy: Thrombolytic agents,[a] PTCA[a]
  Antithrombin agents: Unfractionated heparin, low-molecular-weight heparin
  Direct antithrombins: Hirudin, hirulog, argatroban
  Antiplatelet agents: Aspirin,[a] glycoprotein IIb/IIIa inhibitors
Decrease myocardial oxygen consumption
  β-Blockers[a]
  ACE inhibitors[a]
  Nitrates
  Calcium channel blockers
Anti-arrhythmics
  β-Blockers[a]
  Lidocaine
  Magnesium
Multifactorial
  β-Blockers[a]
  ACE inhibitors[a]
  HMG CoA reductase inhibitors (statins)[a]
  Magnesium

[a] Large randomized trials have demonstrated a mortality benefit.
ACE, angiotensin-converting enzyme; *HMG CoA,* hydroxymethylglutaryl coenzyme A; *PTCA,* percutaneous transluminal coronary angioplasty.

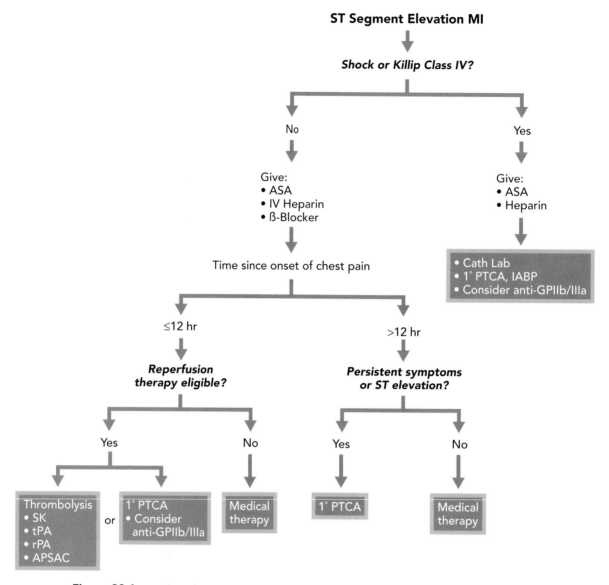

Figure 38.1 An algorithmic approach to the management of the patient with acute myocardial infarction with ST-segment elevation. *APSAC,* anisoylated plasminogen streptokinase activator complex; *ASA,* aspirin; *IABP,* intraaortic balloon pump; *PTCA,* percutaneous transluminal coronary angioplasty; *rPA,* recombinant plasminogen activator; *SK,* streptokinase; *t-PA,* tissue plasminogen activator.

to 24 hours after the onset of chest pain. Fibrinolysis may also be considered in certain patients who present late (>12 hours), but clinical benefit may be marginal, as suggested by the preponderance of trial experience (Table 38.4).

The comparative efficacy of different thrombolytic regimens (Table 38.5) is a controversial topic. Three large trials have directly compared these agents. GISSI-2 compared streptokinase (SK) and non-accelerated tissue plasminogen activator (t-PA), with or without subcutaneous heparin, and found no mortality difference (8.9% vs. 8.5%). ISIS-3 (Third International Study of Infarct Survival) examined SK, t-PA, and anisoylated plasminogen streptokinase activator complex (APSAC) and found all three were associated with sim-

ilar mortality rates (10.5%, 10.3%, and 10.6%, respectively). Because both trials were criticized for inadequate IV heparin therapy, especially with t-PA, GUSTO-1 investigated four thrombolytic strategies utilizing accelerated t-PA, SK, and IV or subcutaneous (SC) heparin (1). A 14% relative mortality reduction was seen with the accelerated t-PA regimen (6.3% t-PA vs. 7.3% SK), resulting in 9 net lives saved per 1,000 patients treated with t-PA in comparison with SK.

Several variants of t-PA have also been approved as fibrinolytic agents, including rPA (reteplase) and single bolus TNK-tPA (tenecteplase). Double bolus rPA does not offer any advantage over accelerated t-PA except for its ease of administration, which facilitates more rapid treatment and may reduce medication errors. Single-bolus

TABLE 38.4
REPERFUSION THERAPY

Recommendations	Class I	IIa	IIb	III	Level of Evidence
Reperfusion therapy is indicated in all patients with history of chest pain/discomfort of <12 h and associated with ST-segment elevation or (presumed) new bundle-branch block on the ECG	X				A
Primary PCI					
• preferred treatment if performed by experienced team <90 min after first medical contact	X				A
• indicated for patients in shock and those with contraindications to fibrinolytic therapy	X				C
• GP IIb/IIIa antagonists and primary PCI					
no stenting	X				A
with stenting		X			A
Rescue PCI					
• after failed fibrinolysis in patients with large infarcts		X			B
Fibrinolytic treatment					
In the absence of contraindications (see Table 38.5) and if primary PCI cannot be performed within 90 min after first medical contact by an experienced team, pharmacological reperfusion should be initiated as soon as possible	X				A
• choice of fibrinolytic agent depends on individual assessment of benefit, risk, availability, and cost					
In patients presenting late (>4 h after symptom onset), a more fibrin-specific agent such as tenecteplase or alteplase is preferred		X			B
For dosages of fibrinolytic and antithrombin agents, see Tables 39.5 and text					
• pre-hospital initiation of fibrinolytic therapy if appropriate facilities exist	X				B
• readministration of a non-immunogenic lytic agent if evidence of reocclusion and if mechanical reperfusion is not available		X			B
• if not already on aspirin, 150–325 mg chewable aspirin (no enteric-coated tablets)	X				A
• with alteplase and reteplase, a weight-adjusted dose of heparin should be given with early and frequent adjustments according to the aPTT	X				B
• with streptokinase, heparin is optional		X			B

Class I, eividence and/or general agreement that treatment is effective; Class II, conflicting evidence on efficacy (A-weight of evidence favors treatment; B-effectiveness less well established); Class III, evidence and/or general agreement that treatment is not effective and may be harmful. Adapted from Task Force on the Management of Acute Myocardial Infarction of the European Society of Cardiology. Management of Acute Myocardial Infarction in Patients presenting with ST-Segment Elevation *EurHeart J* 2003;24:28–66.

weight-adjusted TNK-tPA is equivalent to accelerated t-PA in terms of 30-day mortality and is associated with significantly lower rates of non-cerebral bleeding and need for transfusion.

Regardless of the choice of thrombolytic agents, the important goal appears to be early coronary artery patency. The angiographic substudy of GUSTO-1 demonstrated the lowest mortality (4.4%) in patients with normal coronary blood flow (TIMI grade 3) 90 minutes after fibrinolysis, in comparison with those having no or minimal flow (TIMI grade 0 or 1, 8.9% mortality) or delayed flow (TIMI grade 2, 7.4% mortality) (1). The most common complications of thrombolytic therapy involve bleeding. Although most bleeding is minor, vascular interventions after fibrinolysis may lead to more serious hemorrhagic complications at the groin site. The incidence of intracranial hemorrhage ranges from 0.26% to 2.2%; a higher risk is associated with older age (>65 years), hypertension, and use of t-PA rather than SK. Another potential complication of SK or APSAC involves allergic reactions, which may occur in 1.7% of patients; the risk is greater in those with previous exposure to streptococcal infection or SK products. Recent data suggest

TABLE 38.5

THROMBOLYTIC REGIMENS AND CRITERIA FOR FIBRINOLYSIS IN ACUTE MYOCARDIAL INFARCTION

Indications	Contraindications
Indications	**Contraindications**

Indications

- Chest pain consistent with acute MI
- Electrocardiographic changes
  ST-segment elevation >0.1 mV in at least two contiguous leads
  New or presumably new left bundle branch block
- Time from onset of symptoms <12 h

Regimens

- APSAC 30-U IV bolus over 2–5 min
- Reteplace (r-PA): 10-U IV bolus over 2–5 min, followed 30 min later by an additional 10-U IV bolus
- Streptokinase (SK): 1.5 million IU IV over 60 min
- Alteplace (t-PA):
  >67 kg: 15-mg IV bolus, followed by 50 mg infused over the next 30 min, and then 35 mg infused over the next 60 min
  <67 kg: 15-mg IV bolus, followed by 0.75 mg/kg infused over the next 30 min not to exceed 50 mg, and then 0.5 mg/kg over the next 60 min not to exceed 35 mg
- Tenecteplace (TNK-tPA)
  single IV bolus
  30 mg if <60 kg
  35 mg if 60 to <70 kg
  40 mg if 70 to <80 kg
  45 mg if 80 to <90 kg
  50 mg if ≥90 kg

Contraindications

Absolute
- Active internal bleeding (excluding menses)
- Suspected aortic dissection
- Recent head trauma or known intracranial neoplasm
- History of cerebrovascular accident known to be hemorrhagic
- Major surgery or trauma <2 wk previously

Relative[a]
- Blood pressure >180/110 mm Hg on at least two readings
- History of chronic, severe hypertension with or without drug therapy
- Active peptic ulcer
- History of cerebrovascular accident
- Known bleeding diathesis or current use of oral anticoagulants regardless of INR
- Prolonged or traumatic cardiopulmonary resuscitation
- Diabetic hemorrhagic retinopathy or other hemorrhagic ophthalmic condition
- Pregnancy

[a] These should be considered on a case-by-case analysis of risk versus benefit. In instances in which these contraindications (particularly 1 through 5) have paramount importance, such as active peptic ulcer with history of bleeding, they become absolute contraindications when weighed against a less than life-threatening, evolving acute MI.

MI, myocardial infarction; APSAC, anisoylated plasminogen steptokinase activator complex; r-PA, recombinant plasminogen activator; t-PA, tissue plasminogen activator; SK, streptokinase; INR, international normalized ratio.

Adapted from AHA Medical/Scientific Statement Special Report. ACC/AHA guidelines for the early management of patients with acute myocardial infarction. *Circulation* 1990;82:707, and from Anderson HV, Willerson JT. Thrombolysis in acute myocardial infarction. *N Engl J Med* 1993;329:703, with permission.

that routine post-thrombolysis coronary angiography and appropriate subsequent interventions improve 1-year outcomes compared iwth a conservative strategy.

Recanalization by Primary PCI

Canalization with primary revascularization by PCI or by-pass grafting offers an alternative way to salvage ischemic but viable myocardium. Primary balloon angioplasty results in early and rapid patency recanalization of the infarct-related artery, with a technical success rate above 90% and in-hospital mortality rates <7–8%. The landmark Primary Angioplasty in Myocardial Infarction (PAMI) trial demonstrated significantly decreased death or nonfatal re-infarction at 6 months with immediate balloon angioplasty (9%), compared to fibrinolysis with t-PA (17%). In addition, angioplasty was accompanied by a 0% stroke rate and shorter mean time to resolution of chest pain (290 versus 354 minutes).

More than 20 head-to-head randomized trials have randomly assigned nearly 8,000 thrombolytic-eligible patients with STEMI to primary PCI (balloon angioplasty or stenting) or thrombolytic therapy. Recent meta-analysis of these trials

showed that primary PCI was better than thrombolytic therapy at reducing short-term death (7% vs. 9%, $P = 0.0002$), non-fatal reinfarction (3% vs. 7%, $P < 0.0001$), stroke (1% vs. 2%, $P = 0.0004$), and the combined endpoint of death, non-fatal reinfarction, and stroke (8% vs. 14%, $P < 0.0001$) (2). The results seen with primary PCI remained better than those with thrombolytic therapy during long-term follow-up, and were independent of the type of thrombolytic agent used and whether or not the patient was transferred for primary PCI. This meta-analysis suggests that for every 1,000 patients treated with primary angioplasty rather than thrombolytic therapy, an additional 20 lives are saved, 43 reinfarctions are prevented, 10 fewer strokes occur, and 13 intracranial hemorrhages are prevented. Myocardial salvage is greater with PCI, and primary PCI gives better results than thrombolytic therapy even in community hospitals without on-site surgical back-up (3). Most importantly, primary PCI reduces death, recurrent MI, or stroke compared with front-loaded t-PA (8.5% versus 14.2%, $P < 0.002$) even when patients need to be transferred by ambulance (taking up to 3 hours) to reach an interventional center (4).

Unfortunately, the current average door-to-balloon times in the United States exceed the 2-hour goal, and transfer patients average more than 3 hours (4). Efforts to improve clinical outcome when timely angioplasty is unavailable have focused on "facilitated angioplasty," which is the combination of pharmacologic reperfusion with mechanical revascularization (5). However, randomized trials have found that facilitated angioplasties are either inferior to or no better than primary PCI alone (6).

Treatments that may be Common to STEMI and NSTEMI

Treatment of patients with NSTEMI/unstable angina is covered extensively in Chapter 37. Differentiating patients with STEMI and NSTEMI is critical from a management standpoint, since certain interventions that have resulted in significant mortality reductions in STEMI are not beneficial in patients who present with NSTEMI. In general, all patients presenting with acute coronary syndromes should be treated with aspirin, heparin, and clopidogrel. In higher risk patients, such as those presenting with STEMI or NSTEMI/unstable angina with refractory ischemia, positive cardiac biomarkers, ST-segment depression, hemodynamic instability, signs of left ventricular dysfunction, or history of revascularization within 6 months, intravenous glycoprotein (GP) IIb/IIIa receptor antagonists are usually added. Planning for timely reperfusion with fibrinolysis (door-to-needle <30 min) or PCI (door-to-balloon <120 min) is mandatory for STEMI, but may be delayed in patients presenting with NSTEMI/unstable angina unless refractory ischemia develops. Based on clinical trial evidence, all patients with NSTEMI should proceed to the cardiac catheterization laboratory (after a period of medical stabilization) for delineation of coronary anatomy and revascularization by PCI or CABG. Although guidelines have recommended cardiac catheterization with 48 hours of presentation, a recent study found significant clinical benefit of an early (<6 hours) invasive strategy, compared to delayed cardiac catheterization (72–120 hours) after medical stabilization (7). There is no role for fibrinolysis in patients presenting with NSTEMI/unstable angina.

Antiplatelet Therapy

Aspirin

Platelet activation and aggregation play an important role in thrombus formation at the site of plaque rupture in acute MI. Aspirin functions as an antiplatelet agent by irreversibly acetylating cyclo-oxygenase and inhibiting thromboxane A_2. In patients with acute MI, aspirin alone reduces mortality by 23% at 35 days and reduces nonfatal MI and stroke by 49% and 46%, respectively, in comparison with placebo (8,9). When aspirin is given with SK in STEMI, mortality is reduced by 42%. A daily dose of 81 to 325 mg of aspirin should be administered to all patients with an MI and continued indefinitely.

Clopidogrel

Clopidogrel blocks the platelet P2Y12 ADP-receptor and provides potent platelet inhibition when added to aspirin therapy. Clopidogrel is an irreversible inhibitor of platelet function that is not correctable by platelet transfusion. Approximately 5 days are required for significant attenuation of clopidogrel's anti-platelet effect. The combination of aspirin (325 mg daily) and clopidogrel (300 mg bolus dose followed by 75 mg daily) is now the standard antithrombotic regimen following PCI with stenting, based on the results of clinical trials demonstrating 3-5-fold reductions in subacute stent thrombosis compared with treatment with aspirin plus warfarin or aspirin alone. There is growing clinical evidence that pre-treatment with clopidogrel improves clinical outcomes in patients undergoing PCI. However, since clopidogrel is a pro-drug that requires hepatic cytochrome P450-dependent activation, pre-treatment with a 300 mg bolus dose requires approximately 6 hours to achieve clinically beneficial effects. This time lag may be reduced to 2 hours when a 600 mg bolus dose is utilized. The potential beneficial effect of pre-treatment must be balanced against the potential increased risk of bleeding in the event that emergency CABG is required because of unfavorable anatomy or PCI-induced complications.

Patients undergoing primary PCI for STEMI should be treated with aspirin and clopidogrel for a minimum of 30 days. Patients receiving a drug-eluting stent require more prolonged treatment (90 days for sirolimus- and 180 days for paclitaxel-eluting stent). Evidence guiding the use of clopidogrel after thrombolytic therapy for STEMI is lacking. Based on clinical trial results, patients with unstable angina/NSTEMI should receive clopidogrel for 9–12 months.

Glycoprotein IIb/IIIa Inhibitors

Newer, more potent antiplatelet agents block platelet GP IIb/IIIa fibrinogen binding, the final common molecular pathway of platelet aggregation. Two pharmacologic strategies have been employed in designing inhibitors of GP IIb/IIIa: blockade with a humanized monoclonal antibody Fab fragment (e.g., abciximab or ReoPro) or inhibition with agents that mimic the physiologic arginine-glycine-aspartic acid (RGD) ligand-binding sequence of fibrinogen (e.g., eptifibatide and tirofiban). Meta-analysis of three clinical trials in patients undergoing PCI for unstable angina or non-STEMI shows that GP IIb/IIIa inhibitors reduce death and MI by 33% in the 48–72 hours prior to PCI and by 45% peri- and post-PCI. Guidelines now recommend GP IIb/IIIa inhibitors in conjunction with aspirin and heparin in all high risk patients (refractory ischemia, ST-segment depression, troponin-positive, hemodynamic instability, prior PCI or CABG within 6 months) prior to diagnostic angiography and PCI, which is generally performed with 24–48 hours after admission.

Most interventionalists use GP IIb/IIIa blockers for patients undergoing primary PCI for STEMI based on a series of randomized trials. Potent platelet inhibition with abciximab is associated with substantial reductions in death, reinfarction, and the need for urgent revascularization. Early use of eptifibatide, tirofiban, or abciximab in addition to aspirin plus heparin in the emergency department is strongly encouraged since angiographic studies have shown that each of these agents improves patency of the infarct-related artery as well as microvascular flow.

Antithrombin Therapy

Heparin

Trials document that low-molecular-weight heparin (enoxaparin or nadroparin) significantly reduces major adverse cardiac outcomes, including death, MI, and recurrent angina, compared with unfractionated heparin, in patients with non-STEMI. Studies also suggest perhaps a slight benefit for low-molecular-weight heparin in combination with fibrinolytic agents in STEMI (10), but data are conflicting (11). The current recommendation is heparin for patients who do not receive reperfusion therapy, those undergoing PCI or surgical revascularization, patients receiving t-PA, and patients who are at high risk for systemic emboli. The recommended dosing regimen for low-molecular-weight heparin is enoxaparin 1 mg/kg sc BID (requires dose adjustment for renal insufficiency and obesity). If unfractionated heparin is used, the recommendation is an IV bolus of 60 units/kg (maximum 4000 U) followed by an infusion of 12 units/kg per hour (maximum 1000 units/h) with subsequent adjustment (3, 6, 12, 24 h after start of treatment) to achieve an activated partial thromboplastin time (a PTT) of 50 to 70 seconds.

Direct Antithrombin Agents

Direct antithrombin agents such as hirudin, hirulog, and argatroban inhibit thrombin directly and do not require antithrombin III as a cofactor. Direct antithrombins offer the theoretical advantage of inhibiting clot-bound thrombin more effectively than unfractionated heparin or low-molecular-weight heparin. Two large trials evaluating the use of hirudin versus unfractionated heparin as adjunctive therapy to fibrinolysis in STEMI revealed no significant difference in mortality in the two groups. Bivalirudin with streptokinase compared to unfractionated heparin with streptokinase significantly reduced reinfarction for 48 hours with no effect on 30 day mortality, at the cost of a modest and non-significant increase in non-cerebral bleeding complications. Therefore, to date the direct antithrombin agents do not seem to provide additional benefits over heparin in STEMI. The use of bivalirudin in patients undergoing primary PCI for STEMI is under active investigation.

Warfarin

Trials of anticoagulants following MI demonstrate favorable reductions in late mortality, stroke, and recurrent MI

when compared to placebo (12). Some studies have also suggested that warfarin is superior to aspirin alone or that the addition of warfarin to low-dose aspirin may also be beneficial. However, the impact of other antiplatelet agents, such as clopidogrel, on the role of warfarin is unknown. Current guidelines suggest the use of warfarin anticoagulation when aspirin cannot be taken or when other indications for anticoagulation exist (atrial fibrillation, thromboembolic events, LV thrombus). If warfarin is added to aspirin, the aspirin dose should be lowered to 81 mg qd and the target INR should be 2.0–2.5.

Treatments to Decrease Myocardial Oxygen Consumption

β-blockers

β-blockers effectively reduce myocardial oxygen consumption by decreasing heart rate, contractility, and wall stress. Their anti-adrenergic properties also confer protection from significant ventricular arrhythmias. The use of immediate IV β-blockers followed by oral therapy reduces in-hospital mortality by 13%, repeated infarction by 19%, and cardiac arrest and ventricular fibrillation (VF) by 16%. Long-term β-blockade also plays an essential role in secondary prevention, with 22% and 27% reductions in mortality and repeated infarction, respectively, at 1 year. Data also support the use of early β-blockade, even in patients with moderate heart failure and significant left ventricular dysfunction. In one trial, carvedilol 25 mg PO bid reduced all cause mortality by 23% in patients who had a recent MI (day 3–21) and an ejection fraction of less than 40%, but who did not have uncontrolled heart failure or required ongoing diuretic or inotropic therapy, and who were taking a stable dose of an ACE inhibitor (13). The current recommendations are to initiate β-blockade as soon as possible in all patients without contraindications, especially in those with persistent or recurrent ischemic chest discomfort and those with atrial or ventricular tachyarrhythmias. Relative contraindications include bradycardia, systolic blood pressure below 100 mm Hg, presence of heart failure, history of chronic obstructive pulmonary disease or asthma, or signs of advancing atrioventricular (AV) block (PR interval >0.22, type I or II second-degree AV block, complete heart block). β-blocker regimens include the following: (a) metoprolol, 5 mg IV every 15 minutes three times, followed by 25 to 50 mg PO every 6 hours; (b) propranolol, 0.033 mg/kg IV three times, followed by 20 to 80 mg every 6 hours; and (c) atenolol, 5 mg IV every 10 minutes two times, followed by 50 mg PO every 12 hours. If concerns about toxicity are substantial, a trial of the ultra-short-acting agent esmolol (500 mcg/kg per minute, then 50 to 250 mcg/kg per minute), which has a half-life of 9 minutes, may be warranted. In general, β-blockers should be titrated to the target doses used in the clinical trials (metoprolol 100 mg PO bid, atenolol 100 mg PO qd, and propranolol 60–80 mg PO tid) unless heart rate, blood pressure, or other symptoms prohibit these doses.

Angiotensin-Converting Enzyme Inhibitors

Three trials have demonstrated that ACE inhibitors may be safely started in the early hours of MI (0 to 36 hours), with a statistically significant mortality benefit in all patients after acute MI at 4–6 weeks, irrespective of LV function (14). The average 7% reduction in mortality compared with placebo therapy translates into approximately 5 lives saved per 1,000 patients treated with ACE inhibitors. Sub-group analysis of these trials suggests that patients with anterior MI benefit to a much greater extent than those with inferior MI (11 lives saved per 1,000 patients treated vs. 1 life saved per 1,000 patients treated with inferior MI). Clinical trial data support a broad recommendation that ACE inhibitors should be considered in all patients with a systolic blood pressure above 100 mm Hg and no contraindications to ACE inhibitors and commenced within 1–2 days of acute MI. Acute ACE inhibitor regimens include (a) lisinopril, 5 mg PO on the first day, 5 mg PO at 24 hours, then 10 mg daily thereafter; (b) captopril, 6.25 mg PO on the first day, titrated up to 50 mg twice daily thereafter; and (c) zofenopril, 7.5 mg twice daily on the first day, titrated up to 30 mg twice daily thereafter. The mechanism of action of ACE inhibitors is multifactorial, and the clinical benefits observed may be secondary to a reduction in angiotensin II–mediated vasoconstriction and sodium retention; an increase in bradykinin and prostaglandins, which improves hemodynamics and ventricular remodeling; and a decrease in plasma levels of plasminogen activator inhibitor-1, which promotes endogenous fibrinolysis.

Like β-blockers, ACE inhibitors play an important role in secondary prevention by preventing recurrent ischemic events, heart failure and sudden death, thereby providing a 20% reduction in long-term mortality in patients with a previous MI and symptomatic LV dysfunction (14).

More complete blockade of the renin-angiotensin-aldosterone system with selective aldosterone blockade lowers mortality further. For example, the selective aldosterone blocker, eplerenone reduced total mortality by 15% in patients with acute myocardial infarction complicated by left ventricular dysfunction and heart failure (15), but the rate of serious hyperkalemia was 5.5% compared with 3.9% in the placebo group. Selective aldosterone blockade (eplerenone 25–50 mg PO qd) should be considered when heart failure complicates STEMI after ACE inhibitors and β-blockers have been maximized, but only if renal function is preserved (creatinine <2.5 mg/dL) and hyperkalemia (potassium level ≥5.0 mmol/l) is not present.

Nitrates

Nitrates are venous and arterial vasodilators that reduce preload and afterload, thereby decreasing wall stress and myocardial oxygen consumption. In addition, these agents improve coronary blood flow. However, recent randomized trials failed to demonstrate a reduction in mortality when nitrates were added to current standard therapy. Furthermore, they may cause excessive bradycardia and hypotension, especially when right ventricular infarction is present. IV or topical nitrate preparations followed by oral therapy reduce episodes of angina after infarction. Therefore, nitrates should be considered in patients with ongoing ischemic chest pain or uncontrolled heart failure if the systolic blood pressure is greater than 90 mm Hg, the heart rate is greater than 50 beats per minute, and right ventricular infarction is not present.

Calcium Channel Blockers

There is no survival benefit with use of calcium channel antagonists in the initial treatment or secondary prevention of MI. In fact, the use of nifedipine in acute myocardial infarction is contraindicated.

Prevention of Sudden Death

Sudden death, the most feared complication of MI, is usually caused by ventricular tachycardia or fibrillation and less frequently by complete heart block, asystole, or mechanical catastrophes such as free wall rupture or massive pulmonary embolism. Empowering trained nurses in the coronary care unit to recognize and defibrillate sustained ventricular arrhythmias without direct physician supervision has had the greatest impact on sudden death from MI. Other strategies include the use of medication and implantable cardiac defibrillators (ICDs) for patients at highest risk for sudden death.

Antiarrhythmic Medications

Lidocaine, a Vaughan-Williams class Ib (sodium channel blocker) antiarrhythmic agent, is indicated for treatment of VF or ventricular tachycardia (VT) in acute MI. Although the prophylactic use of lidocaine may decrease the overall incidence of VF, this potential clinical benefit is offset by an increased number of deaths associated with severe bradycardia, asystole, or pulseless electrical activity. The drug should therefore be reserved for the treatment of sustained or symptomatic VT. Its neurologic toxicity may produce confusion, tremor, and seizures, especially in the elderly and those with heart failure or impaired hepatic function.

Amiodarone blocks adrenergic β-receptors and various membrane channels including potassium (Vaughan-Williams Class III effect), calcium, and sodium. It is effective and is used for the treatment of recurrent ventricular fibrillation and hemodynamically significant ventricular tachycardia, especially in lidocaine-resistant patients. In two long-term post-MI studies in high-risk patients, amiodarone appeared to lower arrhythmic death and cardiac arrest but not total mortality. Unfortunately, 40% of patients stopped the drug. When given intravenously, amiodarone may cause phlebitis (especially when given through a peripheral IV), heart block, hypotension, and heart failure.

Magnesium is not recommended in acute MI because its use has been associated with a nonsignificant increase in mortality and heart failure.

Implantable Cardiac Defibrillators (ICDs) are small devices (50–70 ccs) that implanted in the left pectoral region, continuously monitor the heart rhythm, and can be combined with pacing and hemodynamic monitoring. In two randomized trials of patients with previous myocardial infarction and reduced ejection fraction (less than 30–35% at 3–4 weeks post-infarction), prophylactic ICDs reduced mortality by 54% in patients with nonsustained ventricular tachycardia and by 31% when nonsustained VT was not an entry criteria, compared with standard medical therapy (16).

Indications for Early Consultation

Complicated MI patients with hemodynamic instability, recurrent ischemia, heart failure, or arrhythmias, and those requiring PCI, an intraaortic balloon pump, or temporary pacing should be evaluated and managed by a cardiologist. Consultation with an electrophysiologist should be considered in all post-infarct patients with severe left ventricular dysfunction (ejection fraction < 0.30), especially if they have nonsustained ventricular tachycardia.

ISSUES DURING THE COURSE OF HOSPITALIZATION

The early hospital management of acute MI focuses on pharmacologic and mechanical interventions that save lives (careful monitoring and treatment of arrhythmias, recurrent ischemia, and heart failure), assessment of risk factors, and patient and family education (Table 38.6; Figures 38.2, and 38.3). After initial assessment in the emergency department and institution of treatment with aspirin, β-blockers, heparin, nitrates, and fibrinolysis or PCI (for ST-segment elevation MI), the patient is admitted to the CCU. Following successful PCI of the infarct-related artery, low-risk patients (age <70 years, small MI, Killip class I, no previous MI) may be admitted directly to an intermediate care unit. Streamlined critical pathways for patients with MI treated either with fibrinolysis or PCI are outlined in Figures 38.2 and 38.3.

Activity should be restricted to bed rest for the first 12 hours. Hemodynamically stable patients may have bedside commode privileges. During hospital days 0 and 1, serial determinations of troponin levels or, less commonly, CK-MB (myocardium-specific isoenzyme of creatine kinase) are performed (every 8 hours three times), serial ECGs are obtained, and an ACE inhibitor is added to the above medical regimen if hemodynamically tolerated. If ischemia is detected at any time during the hospitaliza-

tion, the patient should undergo cardiac catheterization to guide revascularization. During the first 24 to 48 hours of an acute MI, the lipid profile remains near baseline levels (total, low-density lipoprotein [LDL], and high-density lipoprotein [HDL] cholesterol; triglycerides), and it should be checked on admission or soon thereafter. All patients should be started on a "heart-healthy" diet with subsequent nutritional education.

During day 1, low-risk patients (age <70, small MI, Killip class I, no previous MI) may be transferred to a step-down floor with continued ECG monitoring. These patients should increase activity, with frequent bed-to-chair transfers and ambulation in the room. Moderate- to high-risk patients should remain in the CCU; if hemodynamically stable, they should undergo active range-of-motion exercises to all extremities, with bed-to-chair transfers for 1 to 2 hours a day. All patients should be considered candidates for HMG CoA reductase inhibitors (statins), independent of lipid values, with an LDL goal of 60 mg/dL (17). Ezetimibe can be added if a statin cannot achieve this goal. Niacin or fibric acids can be used when triglyceride levels are greater than 200 mg/dl and/or the HDL is less than 35 mg/dl despite statins.

During day 2, low-risk patients should increase ambulation around the step-down floor. In the absence of ischemia, heart failure, or ventricular arrhythmia, non-low-risk pa-

---

TABLE 38.6

RISK STRATIFICATION FOLLOWING ACUTE MYOCARDIAL INFARCTION

Ischemia
Assessment: stress test (exercise or pharmacologic) with electrocardiography, perfusion scintigraphy, or echocardiography
Low risk: absence of spontaneous or provokable ischemia
High risk: presence of spontaneous or provokable ischemia
If high risk, catheterization and revascularization

Left ventricular dysfunction
Assessment: echocardiography
Low risk: absence of heart failure symptoms, normal LVEF
High risk: heart failure symptoms, LVEF <40%
If high risk, heart failure symptoms: ACE inhibitors, diuretics, digoxin
LVEF <40%: strongly consider catheterization to rule out three-vessel CAD given survival benefit with revascularization
LVEF <35%: strongly consider prophylactic AICD

Electrical instability
Assessment: routine clinical information; Holter monitor not routinely indicated
Low risk: none or non-sustained VT or VF <48 h post-MI
High risk: sustained VT or VF >48 h post-MI
If high risk, rule out ischemia, catheterization/revascularization if indicated; AICD indicated

---

ACE, angiotensin-converting enzyme; *AICD*, automated implantable cardioverter̄defibrillator; *CAD*, coronary artery disease; *EPS*, electrophysiologic study; *LVEF*, left ventricular ejection fraction; *VF*, ventricular fibrillation; *VT*, ventricular tachycardia.

	Day 0: Emerg. Dept.	Day 0: CCU	Day 1: Stepdown Unit/CCU	Day 2: Stepdown Unit	Day 3: Stepdown Unit	Day 4: Stepdown Unit	Day 5: Stepdown Unit	Post-Discharge
Goals	• Door-to-needle <30 minutes	• Admit CCU	**Low Risk** (Age <70, small MI, no prev. MI, Killip I): • Transfer to stepdown • Get ETT/cath slots	**Low Risk** • Ambulate **Not Low Risk** In absence of ischemia/CHF/VT • Transfer to stepdown	**Low Risk** • am ETT - If Neg: D/C home - If Pos: Cath	• ETT • Consider D/C home	• D/C home in am	
Assessment	• Vitals • Hx: Contra-indication?	• Vitals q 1-2 h • Cont. ECG monitor	• Vitals q 4h • Continuous ECG	• Vitals q 8h **Low Risk** • D/C cont. ECG monitor	• Vitals q 8h **Not Low Risk** • Cont. ECG	• Vitals q 8h • D/C cont. ECG		
Tests	• Admit labs: CBC, Chem 20, CK-MB, Troponin, Lipid Profile, PT/PTT, Clot • ECG	• Troponin q8 x2 • PTT 6, 12 h • ECG on CCU arrival • Follow STs on monitor	• ECG in am • CBC, Chem 7 • PTT in am, 6 h post change in heparin	• Chem 7 • PTT, CBC if on heparin • Echo (if ant / large MI, CHF, prior MI, Q waves)	**Not Low Risk** • Chem 7			
Medications	• Thrombolysis • ASA 325 chewed • Heparin IV (as necessary) • Metoprolol IV • SL/IV nitro prn • Morphine prn	• Ensure ASA given • IV heparin • Metoprolol PO • IV nitro - wean • ACEI (if SBP>100)	• ASA • IV heparin • Metoprolol PO • IV nitro - D/C • Lipid lower-ing prn • ACE inhibitor	• ASA • IV heparin • Metoprolol PO • Lipid lower-ing prn • ACE inhibitor	• ASA • D/C heparin • Warfarin prn • ß-Blocker • Lipid lower-ing prn • ACE inhibitor	• ASA • Warfarin prn • ß-Blocker • Lipid lower-ing prn • ACE inhibitor	• ASA • Warfarin prn • ß-Blocker • Lipid lower-ing prn • Cont. ACEI if EF <40, CHF, Ant. or prior MI	
Treatments	• Cont. ECG monitor • 20 gauge IV • O₂ as needed	• If ischemia, shock, or failed throm-bolysis → Cath • O₂	• If ischemia → Cath • D/C Foley • O₂	• If ischemia → Cath • D/C O₂	• If ischemia → Cath	• If ischemia → Cath		
Activity/ Rehab	• Bedrest	• Bedrest	• Bedrest	**Low Risk** • Ambulate **Not Low Risk** • Bedrest	• Routine activity	• Routine activity	• Routine activity	
Diet	• NPO	• Heart Healthy Diet	• Dietary consult	• Heart Healthy	• Heart Healthy	• Heart Healthy	• Heart Healthy	
Education/ Pt/Family	• Family to CCU • Explain Dx to pt/family	• Explain Dx to pt/family	• Discuss with family readi-ness for D/C	• Discuss meds/Risk factors with pt/family	• Discharge instructions	• Discuss meds/Risk factors	• Discharge instructions	
Discharge Planning	• Book bed in CCU with charge nurse	• Notify primary MD • Notify case manager	• Soc. Serv. consult prn	• Arrange VNA prn • Lipid manag. plan • Exercise plan/ Rehab prn • Appt to 1° MD	**Low Risk** • If ETT-neg: Discharge in am • Call 1° MD • D/C letter	• Recheck D/C arrangements	• D/C in am • Call 1° MD • D/C letter	• F/U call in 24-48 h

Figure 38.2 Critical pathway for the patient receiving fibrinolysis. *ACEI*, angiotensin converting enzyme inhibitor; *ASA*, aspirin; *CATH*, cardiac catheterization; *CBC*, complete blood count; *CCU*, coronary care unit; *CHF*, congestive heart failure; *D/C*, discharge or discontinue; *Dx*, diagnosis, *ECG*, electrocardiogram; *EF*, ejection fraction; *ETT*, exercise treadmill testing; *Hx*, history; *IV*, intravenous; *MI*, myocardial infarction; *SL*, sublingual; *VT*, ventricular tachycardia.

tients can be transferred to a step-down unit; their activity level should include increased bed-to-chair transfers with gradual ambulation. During the remaining hospitalization, β-blocker and ACE inhibitor doses should be titrated to achieve optimal heart rate and blood pressure response. Se-lective aldosterone blockers should be considered in patients with heart failure and significant LV dysfunction.

Risk Stratification After Myocardial Infarction

Risk stratification after MI should assess the presence of spontaneous or provokable ischemia, the status of the LV, and the risk for ventricular arrhythmias. An echocardiogram generally should be obtained in virtually all patients.

	Day 0: Emerg. Dept.	Day 0: Cath Lab	Day 0 Low Risk: Stepdown / NOT Low Risk: CCU	Day 1 Low Risk: Stepdown / NOT Low Risk: CCU	Day 2 NOT Low Risk: Stepdown	Day 3 NOT Low Risk: Stepdown	Day 2 Low Risk: Floor bed / Day 4 NOT Low Risk: Stepdown	Day 3 Low Risk / Day 5 NOT Low Risk: Stepdown	Post-Discharge / Post-Discharge
Goals	• Call Cath Lab in <15 min • Leave ED in <30 min	• Room ready <15 min • P<I <30 min from cath lab arrival • Door-to-balloon <60 min	*Low Risk* (<70, small MI, No prev. MI, EF>45, <3VD, succ. P<I, no complic.) • Admit to Stepdown • Remove sheath *Not Low Risk* • Admit CCU	*Low Risk* • Ambulate in room *Not Low Risk* • Transfer to Stepdown • Remove sheaths			• Ambulate	• D/C home in am	
Assessment	• Hx:prior CABG, allergies • PE:vitals, rales, shock, PVD	• Vitals • Cont. ECG monitoring • O₂ sats	• Vitals q 1-2h • Cont. ECG monitor • Fem sheath monitor • Monitor groin q2h	• Vitals q 4h • Cont. ECG • Monitor groin site	• Vitals q 8h	• Vitals q 8h	• Vitals q shift • D/C Cont. ECG monitor	• Vitals q shift	
Tests	• CBC, Chem 20, CK-MB, Troponin, PT/PTT, Lipid Profile, Clot • ECG	• ACT >350 (ACT 200-250 if IIb/IIIa antagonist)	• Troponin q8x2 • PTT 6h post PTCA • ECG	• CK total in am • ECG in am • CBC, Chem 7 • PTT if on heparin	• Chem 7 • PTT	• Chem 7 • PTT	• Echo (if no LVGram, Ant/large/Q wave, prior MI, or CHF)		
Medications	• ASA 325 chew • Heparin IV • Metoprolol IV • SL, IV nitro prn • Morphine prn	• IV Heparin • IV IIb/IIIa antagonist • Metoprolol IV • IV nitro prn • MS/Fentanyl prn	• IV Heparin • Metoprolol PO • IV nitro-wean • ACE inhibitor • Pain meds prn	• ASA *Low Risk* • D/C heparin in am for sheath removal *Not Low Risk* • Restart heparin • Metoprolol • Lipid lowering prn • ACE inhibitor	• ASA • β-Blocker • Lipid low. prn • ACE inhibitor • IV heparin	• ASA • D/C Heparin • Warfarin prn • β-Blocker • Lipid low. prn • ACE inhibitor	• ASA • Warfarin prn • β-Blocker • Lipid low. prn • ACE inhibitor	• ASA • Warfarin prn • β-Blocker • Lipid low. prn • Continue ACE inhibitor if: EF <40, CHF, Ant. or prior MI	
Treatments	• 20 gauge IV • O₂ prn	• PTCA *Not Low Risk* • IABP prn	• O₂ • Foley prn	• D/C O₂ • D/C Foley					
Activity/ Rehab	• Bedrest • Cath Lab MD to transport pt	• Bedrest • MD Transport to CCU/Step-down	• Bedrest, leg straight • If anti-IIb/IIIa: sheath removal when ACT <180	• Bedrest 6h p sheath removal • Ambulate in room	• Ambulate in room	• Routine activity	• Ambulate	• Routine activity	
Diet	• NPO	• NPO	• Heart Healthy Diet	• Dietary consult	• Heart Healthy	• Heart Healthy	• Heart Healthy	• Heart Healthy	
Education/ Pt/Family	• Explain procedure • Cath Consent	• Explain diagnosis to patient and family	• Explain procedure, results	• Discuss readiness for D/C			• Discuss risk factors/ meds	• D/C instructions	
Discharge Plan	• Book bed with CCU charge RN	• Cath report in chart • Notify Team/ 1° MD • Notify Case Manager		• Soc. Serv. consult prn			• Call VNA prn • Lipid manag. plan prn • Exercise plan (Card Rehab prn)	• D/C in am • Appt 1° MD • Call 1° MD • D/C letter	• F/U call 24-48h p D/C

Figure 38.3 Critical pathway for the patient treated with percutaneous coronary intervention (PCI). *ACEI*, angiotensin converting enzyme inhibitor; *ACT* activated clotting time; *ASA*, aspirin; *CATH*, cardiac catheterization; *CBC*, complete blood count; *CCU*, coronary care unit; *CHF*, congestive heart failure; *D/C*, discharge or discontinue; *Dx*, diagnosis, *ECG*, electrocardiogram; *EF*, ejection fraction; *ETT*, exercise treadmill testing; *Hx*, history; *IV*, intravenous; *MI*, myocardial infarction; *SL*, sublingual; *VT*, ventricular tachycardia (Adapted from cardiovascular critical pathways developed at Brigham and Women's Hospital by Drs. Elliott Antman, John Bittl, Christopher Cannon, James K. Kirshenbaum, Patrick O'Gara, and Peter Stone, Reprinted with permission.)

On day 3, low-risk patients should undergo a submaximal exercise test, during which they exercise until anginal symptoms occur, ECG ischemia is seen, or the exercise protocol is completed (approximately 5 METS [metabolic equivalents]). In patients with baseline ECG abnormalities that preclude interpretation of a stress ECG, an exercise perfusion scintigram or exercise echocardiogram should be performed. If patients are unable to exercise, stress perfusion scintigraphy or echocardiography with dipyridamole or dobutamine can mimic the stress of exercise and allow risk stratification (Chapter 36). The goals of post-MI stress testing are to (a) assess exercise capacity and the patient's ability to perform daily home and work activities; (b) evaluate the efficacy of the current medical regimen; and (c) assess the risk for a subsequent cardiac event. If the stress test result is strongly positive ($\geq$2 mm ST-segment depression; large or multiple stress-induced perfusion abnormalities; stress-induced echocardiographic changes), the patient should undergo cardiac catheterization with a view toward revascularization. If the test result is negative, the patient can be discharged on a medical regimen consisting of aspirin, a β-blocker, a statin, and, if indicated, an ACE inhibitor. A symptom-limited exercise test should be obtained at 3 to 6 weeks after discharge.

Moderate- to high-risk patients should be continually monitored through day 3, with an increased level of ambulation; IV heparin can then be discontinued. These patients should undergo a submaximal exercise test on day 4 or 5. If the test result is negative, the patient can be discharged on a medical regimen consisting of aspirin, a β-blocker, a statin, and, if indicated, an ACE inhibitor.

Cardiac catheterization and revascularization should be strongly considered in patients with LV dysfunction, given the established survival benefits of coronary artery bypass grafting in patients with two- or three-vessel coronary artery disease and a reduced LV ejection fraction. For patients with nonsustained ventricular arrhythmias 24–48 hours after infarction, consultation with an electrophysiologist should assess the advisability of further testing to refine the risk of sudden death and/or placement of a prophylactic ICD before discharge.

COMPLICATIONS OF MYOCARDIAL INFARCTION

Heart failure, hypotension, and shock often require invasive hemodynamic monitoring with a pulmonary artery catheter and an arterial line. Measurement of filling pressures and cardiac output guide further management with regard to volume status, need for inotropic agents, and therapeutic response to afterload reduction. LV failure should be treated with diuretics, afterload reduction with easily titratable agents such as IV nitroprusside or IV nitroglycerin, and possibly inotropic agents, such as dopamine and dobutamine (Chapter 39). Right ventricular (RV) failure in the setting of RV MI requires aggressive volume repletion to raise right-sided filling pressures and right ventricular inotropic support until the RV recovers. Saline should be used to keep the central venous pressure 10–15 mm Hg and inotropic agents, such as dobutamine 1–5 mcg/kg/min, can be used to keep the systolic blood pressure > 90 mm Hg. Patients in cardiogenic shock or with persistent ischemia require intra-aortic balloon pumping, which functions to augment coronary perfusion pressure and reduce LV afterload; these patients should also be taken immediately to cardiac catheterization. Timely revascularization of patients with cardiogenic shock has been associated with significant reductions in in-hospital mortality.

Mechanical Complications

Mechanical complications such as *free wall rupture, ventricular septal defect*, and *papillary muscle rupture* most commonly occur 3 to 5 days after the MI. They occur dramatically and are associated with a high mortality rate (up to 90%) with medical management alone. Free wall rupture usually involves the anterior or lateral wall of the LV in a large Q-wave MI, resulting in hemopericardium. The clinical presentations range from sudden death to hypotension and pericardial chest pain. The diagnosis can be made by urgent pericardiocentesis or, if the patient is stable, by urgent echocardiography. Survival rate is low and depends on patient stability and prompt surgical intervention.

Ventricular septal defects occur in approximately 2% of patients with an acute MI. Defects in anterior MI are often apical, whereas those in inferior MI tend to be in the basal septum and are associated with a worse prognosis. The clinical presentation usually involves the new appearance of a harsh, loud holosystolic murmur at the left lower sternal border. Within a few hours or days, biventricular failure ensues. Diagnosis is made by echocardiographic visualization or shunt detection via pulmonary artery catheter sampling of oxygen saturation. Survival depends on early detection, RV and LV function, and size of the defect. Treatment consists of surgery or catheter-based clamshell device closure. Surgical mortality approaches 50%.

Papillary muscle rupture is a rare, dramatic, and often fatal complication of MI. Rupture of the posteromedial papillary muscle, which is associated with inferior MI, occurs more frequently than does anterolateral papillary muscle rupture (associated with anterolateral MI). Patients present with acute, severe mitral regurgitation, hypotension, and heart failure. The apical murmur is often subtle and may become inaudible as arterial hypotension occurs. The diagnosis is made by echocardiography or ventriculography. A pulmonary artery catheter will reveal large *c-v* waves in the pulmonary capillary wedge pressure tracings. Surgical treatment involves repair or replacement of the mitral valve and is associated with a mortality rate of 40% to 90%.

Arrhythmias

Arrhythmias in MI occur as a result of ischemia, increased adrenergic state, and electrolyte abnormalities. Frequent ventricular premature beats (VPBs) are commonly observed in patients with acute MI and do not predict the likelihood of progression to VF. Antiarrhythmic agents are not indicated in this setting and may increase the risk for adverse bradycardic events. Non-sustained VT (more than three consecutive ventricular beats at a rate >100 beats/min lasting <30 seconds) in the first 24–48 hours after acute myocardial infarction is not associated with an increased acute or long-term mortality rate after MI. In contrast, sustained VT (lasting longer than 30 seconds or causing hemodynamic compromise requiring intervention) is associated with a 20% in-hospital mortality. Hemodynamically compromised patients with sustained VT should be treated with synchronized cardioversion. Stable patients should be treated with an intravenous antiarrhythmic agent such as: (a) lidocaine, initial bolus of 1 to 1.5 mg/kg to a maximum of 3 mg/kg, and infusion of 1 to 4 mg/min; (b) procainamide, initial dose of 12 to 17 mg/kg over 30 minutes, followed by maintenance infusion of 1 to 4 mg/min; (c) amiodarone, initial dose of 150 mg over 10 minutes, followed by infusion of 1 mg/min for 6 hours and then maintenance rate of 0.5 mg/min. Primary VF during acute MI increases in-hospital mortality but is not a predictor for long-term risk. Secondary VF in the setting of significant LV dysfunction and cardiogenic shock is associated with in-hospital mortality rates of 40% to 60%. VF should be promptly treated with defibrillation. Pharmacologic prevention of recurrent episodes includes the use of β-blockers, lidocaine, amiodarone, or bretylium (5 to 10 mg/kg).

In acute MI, the incidence of atrial fibrillation (AF) is 10% to 16%. Atrial flutter and supraventricular tachycardia occur less frequently. In the hemodynamically compromised patient with AF, atrial flutter, or supraventricular tachycardia, immediate synchronized cardioversion is indicated. In the stable patient, IV intravenous β-blockers or digoxin should be administered. Although not considered first-line agents, calcium channel blockers may also be used in patients with preserved LV function. Because electrolyte abnormalities may exacerbate or precipitate both ventricular and atrial arrhythmias, all patients should have a potassium level above 4.0 mEq/L and a magnesium level above 2.0 mEq/L.

Bradyarrhythmias also occur in the acute MI setting. Inferoposterior MI is more often associated with sinus bradycardia resulting from vagal stimulation of the heart, first-degree AV block, and Mobitz type I second-degree AV block. These bradyarrhythmias are usually transient and do not require therapy unless associated symptoms are present. Treatment includes a reduction in β-blocker or calcium channel blocker dose, the use of atropine, or temporary pacing. Anteroseptal MI is associated with more advanced AV block, including Mobitz type II second-degree AV block and complete AV block. These patients should be treated with temporary transvenous pacing. Temporary pacing should also be strongly considered in patients with new bifascicular bundle branch block or alternating right and left bundle branch block. Specific arrhythmias are covered in more detail in Chapters 42, 43, and 45.

Thromboembolism

Patients in the post-MI setting are at risk for venous thrombosis, pulmonary embolic, and arterial thromboembolic events. IV heparin during the first 48 to 72 hours of hospitalization and early ambulation reduces the risk for deep venous thrombosis and pulmonary embolism. Large anterior MI and LV dysfunction are risk factors for thrombus formation and systemic embolization; in such patients, an echocardiogram should be performed, and heparin anticoagulation should be instituted if a thrombus is found. Although the risk of ventricular mural thrombus in association with large infarctions has not been defined in the modern reperfusion and ACE inhibitor era, strong consideration should be given to the prophylactic use of antithrombotic agents such as coumadin when LV function is very poor or extensive wall motion abnormalities are present.

DISCHARGE ISSUES

Patients who have undergone recanalization therapy and have no heart failure, recurrent ischemia, or significant ventricular arrhythmias may be discharged after a submaximal exercise test at 3 to 5 days. Patients who have experienced any complications require a more prolonged hospitalization, with discharge dependent on clinical stability after appropriate medical and surgical interventions.

Before discharge, all patients and families should receive education regarding medications, secondary prevention, and risk factor modification. All patients should be discharged on aspirin, a β-blocker, a statin, and, if indicated, an ACE inhibitor. Patients should be instructed on how to use sublingual nitroglycerin. Patients with significant LV dysfunction and heart failure may also require a diuretic, a selective aldosterone antagonist, an ICD, and/or digitalis. Risk factor changes include dietary modification, lipid lowering medications, smoking cessation, blood pressure and diabetic management, weight loss, and exercise, if indicated. Nicotine patches or gum or bupropion are recommended (along with counseling) to aid in smoking cessation. Patients should receive instructions regarding physical activity in the immediate post-MI period. Low-level ambulation and aerobic activity should be encouraged, but isometric exercises such as heavy lifting should be avoided. Most patients should enroll in a cardiac rehabilitation program that includes both supervised physical exercise and education.

Patients should undergo a symptom-limited exercise test at 3 to 6 weeks, with subsequent follow-up by a cardiologist. Because significant improvement in LV function has been observed in serial echocardiographic studies obtained in the peri- and post-infarction setting, many cardiologists obtain a follow-up assessment of ventricular function at 6 weeks post-MI.

ASSESSMENT AND MANAGEMENT OF THE PATIENT PRESENTING WITH MYOCARDIAL INFARCTION DURING A HOSPITALIZATION

MI in patients hospitalized for other illnesses or surgery can present with atypical signs and symptoms, including hypoxia, nausea and vomiting, hypotension, mental status changes, and heart failure on examination or chest radiography. In the setting of postoperative anesthesia/analgesia and ICU sedation, symptoms may be difficult to elucidate. Therefore, careful interpretation of the ECG and measurement of cardiac enzymes, especially troponin T or I, after surgery may be useful. In addition, echocardiography to assess regional wall motion abnormalities may aid in the diagnosis. All patients should receive β-blockers, in addition to aspirin and heparin, if not contraindicated. Reperfusion therapy with thrombolytic agents or primary PCI (especially in a patient who has undergone noncardiac surgery) should be considered for patients in whom the MI began within the last 24 hours or in whom symptoms persist. Because diagnostic uncertainty is common, cardiac catheterization is often required in patients presenting with an MI during hospitalization. In hemodynamically unstable patients, invasive monitoring with a pulmonary artery catheter may be used to assess filling pressures and cardiac output before and during pharmacologic management.

COST CONSIDERATIONS AND RESOURCE USE

For the treatment of MI, issues regarding cost and resource use are complex. Clinical investigators have applied cost-effectiveness analysis to a number of randomized clinical trials to help guide physician practice. Compared with t-PA treatment, reperfusion by primary PCI improves clinical outcome with similar or reduced costs; total hospital charges, including the cost of cardiac catheterization and physician charges for PCI, were not significantly different from those of patients treated with t-PA ($27,653 ± $13,709 vs. $30,227 ± $18,903; $p = .21$) (18). The choice of thrombolytic agent also has significant cost implications. Patients who received t-PA had higher costs ($2,845) but also a higher survival rate (9 to 10 lives saved per 1,000 patients treated) than did SK-treated patients; the cost of t-PA was $32,678 per year of life saved, a dollar amount that compares favorably with that of other therapies whose added medical benefit for dollars spent has been judged by society to be worthwhile (19). In the GUSTO trial, Canadian

patients underwent fewer invasive cardiac procedures and had fewer visits to specialists, but Canadian patients also had more cardiac symptoms and worse functional status 1 year after acute MI than the U.S. patients did. Cost issues will remain paramount as newer therapies, such as glycoprotein IIb/IIIa inhibitors and drug-eluting coronary stents, add significant charges (approximately $500–1,000 and $3,200, respectively). However, by significantly reducing ischemic events and the need for repeated revascularization, these technologic innovations may be cost-effective.

In treating an individual patient, the treating physician has a significant impact on cost considerations with respect to length of stay. Critical pathways (Figures 38.2 and 38.3) provide a safe, streamlined approach to shortening hospital stays.

KEY POINTS

- The ECG and a focused history and physical examination are critical for early triage and treatment decisions.
- Recanalization therapy with primary PCI or fibrinolysis is indicated in all patients with ST-elevation myocardial infarction seen within 12 hours of the onset of symptoms.
- Routine coronary angiography with revascularization as indicated (an early aggressive strategy) improves outcomes in NSTEMI.
- Aspirin, β-blockers, and intravenous heparin are recommended in all patients who lack contraindications.
- Angiotensin-converting enzyme inhibitor therapy is often beneficial.
- Patients should be monitored for arrhythmia, heart failure, recurrent chest pain, and mechanical complications.
- Risk stratification should be performed before discharge.
- Risk factor management (especially aggressive lipid-lowering therapy, smoking cessation, and blood pressure control) is routinely indicated.
- Cardiac rehabilitation is usually beneficial.
- To assess the process of care, the following data should be collected: monitor door-to-needle time (goal: <30 minutes); monitor door-to-balloon time (goal: <120 minutes); maximize β-blocker, aspirin, angiotensin-converting enzyme inhibitor, and statin use; assess percentage of patients who undergo exercise testing for risk stratification; monitor cardiac catheterization and revascularization rates; tabulate length of stay for low- and high-risk patients.

REFERENCES

1. The GUSTO Investigators. An international randomized trial comparing four thrombolytic strategies for acute myocardial infarction. *N Engl J Med* 1993;329:673–682.
2. Keeley EC, Boura JA, and Grines CL. Primary angioplasty versus intravenous thrombolytic therapy for acute myocardial infarction: a quantitative review of 23 randomized trials. *Lancet* 2003; 361:13–20.

3. Aversano T, Aversano LT, Passamani GL, et al. Thrombolytic therapy versus primary percutaneous coronary intervention for myocardial infarction in patients presenting to hospitals without on-site cardiac surgery: a randomized controlled trial. *JAMA* 2002;287:1942–1951.

4. Van de Werf F, Ardissino D, Betriu A, et al. Management of acute myocardial infarction in patients presenting with ST-segment elevation. *Eur Heart J* 2003;24:28–66.

5. Stone GW. Primary angioplasty versus "earlier" thrombolysis—time for a wake-up call. *Lancet* 2002;360:814–816.

6. Kastrati A, Mehilli J, Schlotterbeck K, et al. Early administration of reteplase plus abciximab vs abciximab alone in patients with acute myocardial infarction referred for percutaneous coronary intervention: a randomized controlled trial. *JAMA* 2004;291:947–954.

7. Cho L, Bhatt DL, Marso SP, et al. An invasive strategy is associated with decreased mortality in patients with unstable angina and non-ST-elevation myocardial infarction: GUSTO IIb trial. *Am J Med* 2003;114:106–11.

8. Task Force on the management of acute myocardial infarction of the European Society of Cardiology. Management of acute myocardial infarction in patients presenting with ST-segment elevation. *Eur Heart J* 2003;24:28–66.

9. Antman EM, Anbe DT, Armstrong PW, et al. ACC/AHA guidelines for the management of patients with ST-elevation myocardial infarction—executive summary: a report of the American College of Cardiology/American Heart Association Task Force on Practice Guidelines (Writing Committee to Revise the 1999 Guideliness for the Management of Patients With Acute Myocardial Infarction). *Circulation* 2004;110:588–636.

10. Blazing MA, de Lemos JA, White HD, et al. Safety and efficacy of enoxaparin vs unfractionated heparin in patients with non-ST-segment elevation acute coronary syndromes who receive tirofiban and aspirin: a randomized controlled trial. *JAMA* 2004;292:55–64. Erratum in: *JAMA* 2004;292:1178.

11. Ferguson JJ, Califf RM, Antman EM, et al. Enoxaparin vs unfractionated heparin in high-risk patients with non-ST-segment elevation acute coronary syndromes managed with an intented early invasive strategy: primary results of the SYNERGY randomized trial. *JAMA* 2004;292:45–54.

12. Hurlen M, Abdelnoor M, Smith P, et al. Warfarin, aspirin, or both after myocardial infarction. *N Engl J Med* 2002;347:969–974.

13. Dargie HJ. Effect of carvedilol on outcome after myocardial infarction in patients with left-ventricular dysfunction: the CAPRICORN randomised trial. *Lancet* 2001;357:1385–1390.

14. Group AIMIC. Indications for ACE inhibitors in the early treatment of acute myocardial infarction: systematic overview of individual data from 100,000 patients in randomized trials. ACE Inhibitor Myocardial Infarction Collaborative Group. *Circulation* 1998;97:2202–2212.

15. Pitt B, Remme W, Zannad F, et al. Eplerenone, a selective aldosterone blocker, in patients with left ventricular dysfunction after myocardial infarction. *N Engl J Med* 2003;348:1309–1321.

16. Moss AJ, Zareba W, Hall WJ, et al. Prophylactic implantation of a defibrillator in patients with myocardial infarction and reduced ejection fraction. *N Engl J Med* 2002;346:877–883.

17. Cannon CP, Braunwald E, McCabe CH, et al. Intensive versus moderate lipid lowering with statins after acute coronary syndromes. *N Engl J Med* 2004;350:1495–504.

18. Stone GW, Grines CL, Rothbaum D, et al. Analysis of the relative costs and effectiveness of primary angioplasty versus tissue-type plasminogen activator: the Primary Angioplasty in Myocardial Infarction (PAMI) trial. The PAMI Trial Investigators. *J Am Coll Cardiol* 1997;29:901–7.

19. Mark DB, Hlatky MA, Califf RM, et al. Cost effectiveness of thrombolytic therapy with tissue plasminogen activator as compared with streptokinase for acute myocardial infarction. *N Engl J Med* 1995;332:1418–24.

ADDITIONAL READING

Fernandez-Aviles F, Alonso JJ, Castro-Beiras A, et al. Routine invasive strategy within 24 hours of thrombolysis versus ischaemia-guided conservative approach for acute myocardial infarction with ST-segment elevation (GRACIA-1): a randomised controlled trial. *Lancet* 2004;364:1045–1053.

Popma JJ, Berger P, Ohman EM, Harrington RA, Grines C, Weitz JI. Antithrombotic therapy during percutaneous coronary intervention: the Seventh ACCP Conference on Antithrombotic and Thrombolytic Therapy. *Chest* 2004;126(3 Suppl):576S–599S.

Zhu MM, Feit A, Chadow H, et al. Primary stent implantation compared with primary balloon angioplasty for acute myocardial infarction: a meta-analysis of randomized clinical trials. *Am J Cardiol* 2001;88:297–301.

Heart Failure

39

Carey D. Kimmelstiel   **David DeNofrio**
Marvin A. Konstam

INTRODUCTION

In addition to being a disabling and life-threatening condition, heart failure represents an ever-increasing financial burden to society. More than 5 million Americans carry the diagnosis of heart failure, and 400,000 new cases are discovered annually (1). The prevalence has steadily increased during recent years, and heart failure now represents the single most frequent diagnosis leading to hospitalization in patients older than age 65 (2).

Guidelines on the evaluation and management of patients with heart failure have been published by several entities, most notably the American College of Cardiology (ACC) and the American Heart Association (AHA). The ACC/AHA guideline categorizes patients into clinical subgroups of acute decompensation of chronic left ventricular (LV) failure, acute cardiogenic pulmonary edema, and cardiogenic shock (3). Although the groupings are useful, there is a fair amount of overlap in the pathophysiologic processes and therapeutic principles used in evaluating and treating these patients.

ISSUES AT THE TIME OF ADMISSION

The most common cause of LV systolic dysfunction in the United States is ischemic cardiomyopathy. Other causes include hypertension, valvular disease, and primary cardiomyopathies. Regardless of etiology, impairment of LV systolic function eventuates in a predictable sequence of hemodynamic and neurohormonal events. Although the precise triggers that activate these neurohormonal systems remain obscure, they are presumably linked to altered hemodynamics and altered responses of the cardiopulmonary barorecep-

tors. Activation of the sympathetic nervous system can lead to vasoconstriction, with consequent augmentation of afterload, which serves to maintain blood pressure at the expense of further reductions in cardiac output. Increased circulating levels of antidiuretic hormone lead to augmented preload by means of salt and water retention; these adaptations aid in maintaining cardiac output via the Frank-Starling mechanism but often lead to increases in LV filling pressure, which can cause alveolar edema and resulting dyspnea. Reduction in cardiac output is associated with reduced renal perfusion pressure, leading to enhanced formation of angiotensin II and aldosterone, which lead to further retention of salt and water in addition to vasoconstriction.

Indications for Hospitalization and Intensive Care Unit Admission

Published guidelines have delineated the patients with heart failure who typically benefit from hospitalization (Table 39.1). Patients with cardiogenic shock or with pulmonary edema that requires intubation require ICU admission. Other subsets of patients routinely admitted to an ICU are those in whom heart failure coexists with acute ischemia, and those with hypoxia or hypotension. Any patient in whom a pulmonary artery catheter is judged to be necessary (see later in this chapter) requires hospitalization in an ICU.

Initial Evaluation

General Principles

The initial evaluation and therapy of patients with acute heart failure proceed in tandem. It is important to clarify the precipitating cause and underlying disease in order to

TABLE 39.1

INDICATIONS FOR HOSPITAL ADMISSION FOR HEART FAILURE

- Evidence for acute myocardial ischemia[a]
- Pulmonary edema or severe respiratory distress[a]
- Hypoxia[a]
- Associated acute illness
- Hypotension/cardiogenic shock[a]
- Syncope
- Anasarca
- Heart failure refractory to oral medications
- Need for pulmonary artery catheterization (Table 39.4)[a]

[a] These are also indications for intensive care unit admission.

define the severity of the syndrome, to estimate prognosis, and to create a therapeutic protocol for all patients admitted with this syndrome. If an acute intervening problem has caused or led to acute heart failure, therapy must be targeted to the underlying disorder. Examples of such underlying causes include acute myocardial ischemia (MI), rapid atrial fibrillation, uncontrolled hypertension, valvular heart disease such as mitral or aortic stenosis, pulmonary embolism, pericardial constriction, sepsis, severe anemia, hyperthyroidism, and hypothyroidism (Table 39.2).

CLINICAL PRESENTATIONS

Acute Decompensation of Chronic Heart Failure

In this patient population, a directed history most frequently reveals a prior history of LV dysfunction. More than half of the patients have a prior MI as a cause of LV dys-

TABLE 39.2

SOME COMMON PRECIPITATING CAUSES OF HEART FAILURE

- Myocardial ischemia or infarction
- Atrial fibrillation or other supraventricular tachycardias
- Uncontrolled hypertension
- Valvular disease
- Ventricular tachycardia
- Pulmonary embolism
- Pericardial disease
- Sepsis
- Anemia
- Nutritional and medical noncompliance
- Adverse drug effects
- Hyperthyroidism or hypothyroidism

function. The clinical evaluation most frequently reveals signs and symptoms of pulmonary or systemic vascular congestion and low cardiac output. Patients often report increasing dyspnea on exertion and sometimes even at rest, fatigue, orthopnea, increasing edema, or paroxysmal nocturnal dyspnea, with most patients having symptoms for days to weeks before hospitalization (Figure 39.1). Physical examination frequently reveals elevated jugular venous pressure, pitting edema, and hepatomegaly. Chest auscultation commonly reveals pulmonary crackles. Cardiac examination frequently finds an inferolaterally displaced and sustained apical impulse, tachycardia, gallop rhythms, and systolic murmurs of mitral or tricuspid regurgitation.

In the initial evaluation of the patient with decompensation of chronic heart failure, it is critical to look for a precipitating cause. In addition to previously noted disorders, poor compliance with medications or diet contributes to half or more of admissions. Adverse drug effects (e.g., nonsteroidal anti-inflammatory agents or medications, such as antibiotics, that contain a high concentration of sodium) are another common precipitant. In a substantial percentage of patients, however, no specific precipitant can be found because the decompensation relates to the progressive natural history of the underlying disease process.

In the patient with decompensated chronic heart failure, the most useful diagnostic information comes from a directed history and physical examination. In some patients, the history and physical examination may be inconclusive in assessing the cause of acute dyspnea. Rapid measurement of *B-type natriuretic peptide* (BNP) can help distinguish heart failure from other causes of dyspnea because a value ≤100 pg/mL makes heart failure very unlikely (4). Therefore, the use of BNP measurements in this setting can reduce unnecessary hospitalization and the costs of care (5). Conversely, an initial BNP level ≥200 pg/mL in the emergency department predicts a worse 90-day outcome (6). Routine blood work should exclude anemia, renal insufficiency, electrolyte disorders, and liver dysfunction. Electrocardiography should be performed, and there should be a low threshold for measuring cardiac biomarkers if there is any possibility that acute MI may have precipitated clinical deterioration. All patients should undergo noninvasive testing, usually with echocardiography or alternatively with radionuclide ventriculography, to assess LV function (Chapter 36), unless this measurement is already known. If the ejection fraction has already been demonstrated to be low, repeated testing is of less value unless there is a need to document possible further deterioration.

Some patients with heart failure have normal systolic function but abnormal diastolic function that causes high filling pressure and a clinical picture that is often undistinguishable from heart failure caused by reduced systolic functions (7). Patients hospitalized with diastolic heart failure are more likely to be older women than those with systolic heart failure (8). The entity of diastolic heart failure remains mostly a clinical diagnosis, often supported by

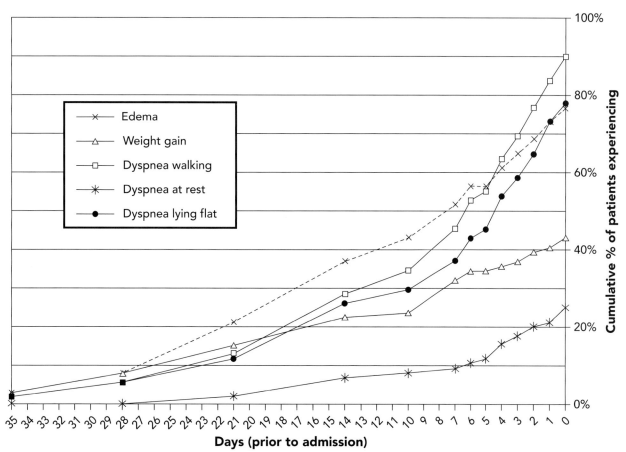

Figure 39.1.   Number of days from onset of selected heart failure symptoms to hospital admission: cumulative percentage of patients.
Reprinted with permission from Schiff GD, Fung S, Speroff T, et al. Decompensated heart failure: symptoms, patterns of onset, and contributing factors. *Am J Med* 2003;114:625–630.

BNP levels but without reliable, universally accepted echocardiographic criteria (9).

In patients hospitalized with heart failure, anemia is a risk factor for adverse outcomes, and limited data suggest that treatment is beneficial (10). Both renal function and the hematocrit should be routinely measured and followed during the hospitalization.

Myocardial ischemia in the absence of a frank MI may precipitate acute heart failure. In such patients, especially those with rest angina or exercise-limiting symptoms, coronary angiography should be performed, followed when possible by revascularization. Several studies have demonstrated the value of documenting myocardial viability as a guide for selecting patients for revascularization and for predicting subsequent outcomes. These studies have generally indicated lower rates of adverse events after revascularization in selected patients with heart failure.

Pulmonary Edema

Acute pulmonary edema represents a medical emergency, and its diagnosis is usually clear from the history and physical examination, although a chest radiograph may sometimes be required for diagnosis. In patients with cardiogenic pulmonary edema, a relatively acute elevation in LV filling pressure (pulmonary capillary wedge pressure) secondary to LV dysfunction leads to transudation of fluid from pulmonary capillaries into the lung interstitium. As a consequence of this process, pulmonary compliance declines, and subjective breathlessness, frank hypoxia, or both, ensue. Physical examination usually reveals diffuse pulmonary rales. Cardiac examination is frequently difficult because of the patient's clinical status and labored breathing, but it often shows tachycardia with a third or fourth heart sound or a summation gallop. The extremities are often cool and diaphoretic, reflecting the low cardiac output with shunting of blood away from the periphery.

Occasionally, patients with pulmonary edema are mistakenly thought to have a pulmonary infectious process such as pneumonia (Chapters 65 and 66). Although patients with pulmonary edema are at risk for pulmonary sepsis, purulent cough and hyperpyrexia are typical in pneumonia. Exacerbations of chronic obstructive pulmonary disease (COPD) (Chapter 55) are usually not difficult to distinguish from pulmonary edema. Prominent use of accessory muscles of respiration, marked diminution of breath sounds, hyperresonance to percussion, subxiphoid location of the apical impulse, and a flattened diaphragm are all common in decompensated emphysema and unusual in pulmonary edema. Similarly, hypercarbia and cyanosis in the setting of a history of productive cough are commonly seen in decompensated chronic bronchitis but are not usually seen in patients with pulmonary edema. Cardiogenic pulmonary edema must be distinguished from *noncardiogenic pulmonary edema* (also known as acute respiratory distress syndrome, or ARDS), which is not secondary to poor LV performance with deranged hemodynamics but rather occurs as a consequence of altered capillary permeability, usually in the setting of trauma, sepsis, or aspiration (Chapter 24).

Cardiogenic Shock

Cardiogenic shock, which is defined as cardiogenic hypotension accompanied by fluid overload and pulmonary edema, represents a medical emergency that most commonly is caused by an acute MI. Cardiogenic shock develops when approximately 40% of the LV is affected by current or repetitive ischemic insult and occurs in about 10% to 15% of patients with acute MI (Chapter 38). Clinically, the diagnosis is usually not difficult to recognize. Patients present most frequently with hypotension, tachycardia, tachypnea, rales, and a reduced pulse pressure. When hypotension is not associated with pulmonary congestion, the diagnosis of cardiogenic shock cannot be made unless and until the low blood pressure fails to respond to the documented achievement of adequate left ventricular filling pressures. Signs of diminished cardiac output include diaphoresis, cool extremities, and confusion. Tissue hypoperfusion and pulmonary congestion usually cause hypoxia and a metabolic acidosis.

Indications for Early Consultation

Prompt specialty consultation (Table 39.3) is especially important in patients who are thought to have ongoing ischemia or a mechanical complication of a myocardial infarction (MI) as a precipitant of decompensation. In these patients, early catheterization can aid in the choice of appropriate and often life-saving therapies, such as revascularization or valve repair.

Pulmonary Artery Catheterization

Although not routinely indicated, a pulmonary artery catheter can help diagnostically and therapeutically when there is uncertainty regarding a cardiogenic etiology, when there is concomitant pulmonary congestion and low or

TABLE 39.3

INDICATIONS FOR EARLY CONSULTATION

- Failure to improve clinically
- Myocardial ischemia
- New murmur
- Abnormal renal function
- Uncontrolled hypertension
- Heart failure with normal left ventricular function
- Heart failure complicated by shock

borderline blood pressure or hypoperfusion, or when the patient has acute ischemia or MI that is thought to be complicated by acute mitral regurgitation or ventricular septal rupture (Table 39.4). Hemodynamic data derived from pulmonary artery catheters are also useful in patients whose clinical courses deteriorate despite application of appropriate therapies, and such data can help to guide therapy in patients in whom volume status cannot be reliably ascertained because of coexisting conditions such as morbid obesity or obstructive lung disease. It must be remembered, however, that a pulmonary artery catheter provides diagnostic information and is not in itself therapeutic (Chapter 25). The duration of catheterization should be minimized to avoid complications.

MEDICAL TREATMENT

General Principles

The goals of therapy in acute heart failure are to correct the hemodynamic derangement leading to decompensation while simultaneously improving symptoms. In all cases, the diagnosis of heart failure implies that pulmonary or

TABLE 39.4

SITUATIONS IN WHICH PULMONARY ARTERY CATHETERIZATION MAY BE BENEFICIAL IN PATIENTS WITH HEART FAILURE

- Uncertain etiology of pulmonary edema
- Pulmonary congestion with any of the following:
   hypotension
   acute ischemia or infarction
   acute mitral regurgitation
   ventricular septal rupture
- Clinical deterioration despite application of usual therapy
- Uncertain volume status
- Oliguria

systemic venous pressure is elevated, with or without reduction in cardiac output and blood pressure. Therapy, therefore, is directed at reducing venous pressure by the use of diuretics, venodilators, or both.

Whenever filling pressures are elevated or a significant amount of extravascular fluid (pulmonary or peripheral edema, or ascites) is present, diuresis should be attempted. In the presence of renal dysfunction or hypoperfusion, intravenous (IV) inotropic agents and vasodilators and/or diuretics should be used concomitantly. The response to therapy in these patients often suggests that their ventricles had been on the descending limb of the Starling curve; that is, a reduction in filling pressures *improves* cardiac performance through reductions in tricuspid and mitral regurgitation and relief of ventricular-interdependent constraints on LV filling. Diuresis-induced reduction in right-sided pressures may improve effective LV compliance, thereby improving cardiac output and renal perfusion. Agents with inotropic and arteriolar dilating action may also be used if a low-output state exists and diuretics are found to be ineffective or exacerbate renal dysfunction.

The hospitalization is also a crucial time to initiate or titrate chronic pharmacologic therapies that will have long-term benefit, including an angiotensin-converting enzyme (ACE) inhibitor (or other vasodilator if ACE inhibitors cannot be used), a β-blocker, and often an aldosterone antagonist. Device therapies also should be considered.

Although there is a great deal of individual variability, the hemodynamic goals of therapy are generally to maintain blood pressure above 90 mm Hg (preferably >100 mm Hg), pulmonary capillary wedge pressure below 20 mm Hg, and right atrial pressure below 10 mm Hg. In patients with chronic heart failure and systolic dysfunction, the pulmonary capillary wedge pressure may be persistently elevated, and "normal" filling pressures may not be achievable without inducing or aggravating shock.

Acute Decompensation of Chronic Heart Failure

Diuretics

Patients who require hospitalization are often unresponsive to oral diuretics, possibly because of malabsorption resulting from bowel edema. The recommended initial approach is therefore to use IV loop diuretics, such as furosemide. These agents usually begin to reduce right ventricular (RV) and LV filling pressures within 5 minutes because of rapid venodilation. Diuresis follows shortly thereafter and continues for up to 3 hours following IV administration.

Therapy typically begins with an IV furosemide dose equal to the usual oral dose, followed by upward titration; doses are increased as required to effect diuresis and lower filling pressures. In patients not previously receiving diuretics, low-dose therapy (e.g., 20 to 40 mg of furosemide) is initially recommended. In patients on chronic high-dose oral diuretic therapy, even IV agents may not yield a rapid diuresis. This refractoriness may be a consequence of diminished renal perfusion or renal tubular dysfunction induced by the nephrotoxic effects of medications such as aspirin and nonsteroidal anti-inflammatory drugs, antihypertensive agents, cimetidine, and occasionally ACE inhibitors. When there is no response within 1 hour after IV administration of a diuretic, the dose is increased by 50% to 100% and readministered. When patients exhibit resistance to initial therapy with intermittent parenteral doses of loop diuretics, alternatives include a continuous infusion (often 5 to 10 mg/h) of a loop diuretic, such as furosemide, or the combination of a loop diuretic with a thiazide diuretic (e.g., metolazone) that acts synergistically at a different segment of the nephron. If these alternatives fail or if diuresis is accompanied by increasing renal dysfunction, attempts should focus on increasing cardiac output with inotropic agents or reducing resistance to renal perfusion with dopaminergic doses of dopamine (≤ 2 g/kg per minute). In truly refractory cases with escalating renal failure, dialysis is the only alternative.

As long as filling pressures are elevated and a significant amount of extravascular fluid (edema, ascites, pulmonary fluid) is present, diuresis should be continued. Diuresis-induced reduction in right-sided pressures may improve effective LV compliance, thereby improving cardiac output and renal perfusion. Reductions in ventricular filling pressures will also improve cardiac performance if tricuspid or mitral regurgitation is reduced.

Angiotensin-Converting Enzyme (ACE) Inhibitors

ACE inhibitors should be considered a distinct class of drugs with vasodilator effects, instead of simply a subgroup of vasodilators. The long-term effectiveness of these agents in reducing morbidity and mortality in patients with heart failure and a reduced LV ejection fraction has been documented more clearly than that of any other class of agents (3). They have unequivocally been demonstrated to improve survival, reduce the frequency of hospitalization, prevent disease progression, and improve quality of life in both symptomatic and asymptomatic patients with ventricular systolic dysfunction and heart failure. At least some of these benefits are likely to be mediated by myocardial and vascular effects, including prevention or regression of myocardial and possibly vascular remodeling, independent of afterload reduction.

In the setting of an acute exacerbation of heart failure, vasodilation is most practically achieved with direct, short-acting vasodilators, such as nitrates, rather than with ACE inhibitors, which have relatively long half-lives and tend to reduce the glomerular filtration rate by means of renal efferent arteriolar dilation. However, *given the clear long-term benefit of ACE inhibitors, one of the goals of hospitalization should be to initiate and titrate ACE inhibitors toward the target doses that have been identified in large-scale clinical trials and in clinical practice guidelines* (Table 39.5). ACE inhibitors should be introduced and titrated carefully in patients with marginal renal function and blood pressure. Other adverse effects include cough, which is seen in about 5% more patients treated with these agents than with placebo in randomized trials, and, rarely, angioedema. Treatment is often initiated with a shorter-acting agent, such as captopril, before or after hospital discharge; however, most patients can be switched to a longer-acting agent, such as enalapril, lisinopril, quinapril, or ramipril, to maximize long-term compliance.

Angiotensin Receptor Blockers

Angiotensin receptor blockers (ARBs) directly inhibit the angiotensin II (AT$_1$ type) receptor and do not induce cough as a side effect. These agents reduce mortality in patients who cannot tolerate an ACE inhibitor by about the same 25% seen for ACE inhibitors compared with placebo (11, 12), and in head-to-head studies, ARBS are at least equivalent to ACE inhibitors (13, 14). Although data are not conclusive, recent studies also suggest that ARBs can further reduce adverse outcomes by about 15% when added to an ACE inhibitor (15).

Based on aggregate data, it is reasonable to conclude first that the benefit on cardiovascular morbidity and mortality of primary ARB therapy is extremely close to that of ACE inhibitors. Although some believe that ACE inhibitors should remain the first-line therapy in patients with heart failure, and cost is a factor, ARBs are better tolerated, and some contend that these agents are an acceptable alternative first-line therapy. Second, ARBs should routinely be prescribed in patients who are intolerant of ACE inhibitors because of cough or angioedema. Third, the combination of ACE inhibitors and ARBs remains controversial. For patients in whom addition of an aldosterone blocker is indicated (see below), there are insufficient supportive data (and reason for safety concern) regarding the combination of an ACE inhibitor, an ARB, and an aldosterone blocker. At present, many would contend that addition of either an aldosterone blocker or an ARB (but not both) should be tried in patients already receiving an ACE inhibitor and a β-blocker and whose potassium levels are not elevated and can be closely followed.

Other Combinations

The combination of hydralazine and isosorbide dinitrate diminishes mortality and improves LV performance in heart failure when compared with placebo, but this combination did not achieve the same level of survival benefit as an ACE inhibitor in the largest study. In African American patients, however, the combination of hydralazine and nitrates may be substantially more effective than in whites, with a benefit that appears to be at least of the magnitude found with ACE inhibitors (16). Whether this combination will become first-line therapy in African Americans will depend on clinical experience and side effects. In whites, the combination of hydralazine and isosorbide dinitrate should be considered a reasonable alternative only in patients who cannot tolerate either an ACE inhibitor or angiotensin receptor blocker therapy.

β-blockers, Aldosterone Receptor Blockers, and Digoxin

In patients with heart failure and reduced LV systolic function, augmented adrenergic tone may be helpful in the short term but cause long-term complications. Results with carvedilol (3.125 mg twice daily titrated up to 25 mg twice daily based on the patient's clinical condition, blood pressure, and heart rate), bisoprolol (1.25 mg daily titrated to 5 to 10 mg daily), and long-acting metoprolol (Table 39.5) document long-term benefit in reducing morbidity and mortality. Carvedilol appears to be the preferred β-blocker (17). These agents should be considered when patients are otherwise euvolemic and well compensated, usually a day or two before (18) or in the first week or so after hospital discharge. β-blockers have no documented short-term benefit, can be deleterious during an acute exacerbation, must be used cautiously in patients with bradyarrhythmias, but have been shown to be beneficial in patients with mild, moderate, and severe symptoms (i.e., including class IV) of heart failure (19).

Spironolactone 25 mg per day reduces morbidity and mortality when added to standard care for class III or IV heart failure (20). Gynecomastia will develop in about 10% of men. Hyperkalemia is uncommon even with concomitant ACE inhibitors. More recently, in patients with post-infarction heart failure, the addition of the selective aldosterone receptor antagonist eplerenone to standard therapy, on top of treatment with an ACE inhibitor and β-blocker, has been documented to reduce mortality (21). It is essential that serum potassium and renal function be carefully monitoring following initiation of treatment and during titration of aldosterone receptor blockers because a substantial minority of patients will develop sufficient hyperkalemia to mandate discontinuation of the aldosterone receptor antagonist.

Clinical trials have confirmed the long-term benefit of digoxin in preventing recurrent hospitalization and improving symptoms and functional capacity in patients with heart failure (22); it does not, however, reduce mortality. Although there is no evidence for a benefit of digoxin in the setting of an acute exacerbation, it is reasonable to initiate treatment during hospitalization, in the absence of abnormal atrioventricular conduction (first-, second-, or third-degree heart block or slow ventricular response to atrial

TABLE 39.5

MEDICATIONS USED IN THE TREATMENT OF HEART FAILURE

Agent	Usual initial dose	Target dose[a]	Comments
Diuretics			
Furosemide	20–200 mg IV intermittent therapy 5–10 mg/h continuous infusion 20 mg qd–240 mg bid PO	Titrate to clinical response	May cause metabolic alkalosis. When used with ACE inhibitors, may cause deterioration in renal function.
Bumetanide	0.5–3.0 mg IV 0.5 mg qd–10 mg qd PO	Titrate to clinical response	Same as furosemide.
Ethacrynic acid	5–100 mg IV (0.5–1.0 mg/kg) 50 mg qd–200 mg bid PO	Titrate to clinical response	Beware of ototoxicity.
Metolazone	2.5–10 mg qd PO	Titrate to clinical response	Enhanced sodium excretion when combined with loop diuretics.
Inotropic/vasopressor agents			
Dobutamine	2.5–20 mcg/kg per minute IV	Titrate to clinical response	Increases in contractility and stroke volume do not lead to increased myocardial oxygen consumption because of reduction in afterload and filling pressures. Major concerns relate to tachycardia and arrhythmogenesis.
Milrinone	Initial 50-mcg/kg bolus over continuous infusion at 10 min, followed by 0.25–1.0 mcg/kg per minute	Titrate to clinical response	Dose reduction necessary in presence of renal dysfunction. Greater vasodilatory potency than dobutamine, which may cause more profound reductions in filling pressures and BP. Major concerns related to tachycardia and arrhythmogenesis.
Dopamine	1–20 mcg/kg per minute	Titrate to clinical response	Dopaminergic doses (<2 mcg/kg per minute) promote renal and splanchnic vasodilation. Doses of 2–10 mcg/kg per minute are primarily inotropic. At 10–20 mcg/kg per minute, vasoconstriction predominates.
Norepinephrine	2–12 mcg per minute	Titrate to clinical response	May reduce cardiac output because of increased afterload.
Digoxin	0.125–0.375 mg	Titrate to clinical response	Narrow therapeutic-toxic ratio. Serum level increased by many medications. Dose adjustment necessary in renal dysfunction.
Vasodilators			
Nitroglycerin	0.3–0.6 mg SL 0.2–10 mcg/kg per minute IV	Titrate to clinical response	Continuous therapy for ≥24 h leads to tolerance.
Nitroprusside	0.2–10 mcg/kg per minute	Titrate to clinical response	Is light-sensitive. Must be carefully titrated to BP.
Hydralazine	10–75 mg qid PO	Titrate to clinical response	Used in combination with oral nitrates in African-American patients and other patients intolerant to ACE inhibitors and angiotensin receptor blockers. Can cause tachycardia and lupus-like syndrome.
Nesiritide	2 mcg/kg bolus 0.01–0.03 mcg/kg/min	Titrate to clinical response	May cause hypotension. Prolonged infusions of >48 hour have been poorly studied.
ACE inhibitors			
Enalapril	2.5–10 mg bid	10–20 mg bid	Reduction in dose or increase in dosing interval may be necessary in renal failure. Cough relatively frequent (about 5%) side effect.
Captopril	6.25–50 mg bid	50 mg tid	
Lisinopril	5–20 mg qd	20–35 mg bid	
Quinapril	5–20 mg bid	Not established	
Ramipril	1.25–5 mg bid	5 mg bid	

(continued)

TABLE 39.5

MEDICATIONS USED IN THE TREATMENT OF HEART FAILURE *(continued)*

Agent	Usual initial dose	Target dose[a]	Comments
Angiotensin II (AT$_1$ type) receptor antagonists			
Losartan	25–50 mg qd PO	Not established	Used in patients intolerant to ACE inhibitors or sometimes
Valsartan	80–160 mg qd PO	Not established	in those who need it added to an ACE inhibitor.
β-Blocking agents			
Carvedilol	3.125–25 mg bid	25–50 mg bid	Not for use in acute heart failure; indicated in patients with
Metoprolol	12.5–25 mg qd	200 mg qd	NYHA class II–IV heart failure resulting from systolic
Bisoprolol	1.25–5 mg qd	10 mg qd	dysfunction.
Aldosterone antagonists			
Spironolactone	12.5–25 mg qd	25 mg qd	Data indicate incremental benefit.
Eplerenone	25–50 mg qd	50 mg qd	Data indicate benefit in post-infarction LV dysfunction.

[a] Dose shown to be beneficial in randomized trials. This dose often is not achievable acutely in the hospital, but it should be the goal in patients with chronic heart failure unless they cannot tolerate it.

fibrillation). A loading dose is not necessary. Treatment can begin with a dose of 0.25 mg/d; lower doses should be used in the setting of reduced renal function or concern regarding atrioventricular conduction. No data support the use of serum levels to guide the digoxin dose. In addition, it is not clear that higher doses are more efficacious than lower ones in the clinical management of heart failure.

Limited data suggest that the acute use of a vasopressin antagonist may be useful in hospitalized patients whose heart failure does not respond to standard measures (23). However, the therapy remains experimental at the current time.

Pulmonary Edema

In the presence of acute pulmonary edema, *nitrate therapy* may be begun with sublingual nitroglycerin, which, in the absence of hypotension, can be repeated at 5- to 10-minute intervals (Table 39.6). Nitroglycerin is especially useful in patients with known or possible myocardial ischemia. Ongoing treatment may then be initiated with IV nitroglycerin. More effective afterload reduction may be achieved with IV nitroprusside. This agent should particularly be considered when blood pressure is normal ($\geq$110 mm Hg systolic) or elevated.

In patients who have pulmonary edema and who are experiencing ongoing dyspnea at rest, *morphine sulfate* given in doses of 2–6 mg IV can alleviate symptoms by reducing preload and relieving anxiety while more definitive therapy is being prepared. Care should be taken to avoid hypotension. Morphine should be used with great caution in patients with obstructive lung disease, especially those with respiratory acidosis.

Arteriolar dilation with ACE inhibitors, nitroglycerin, nitroprusside, nesiritide, or low-dose (<2 mcg/kg per minute) dopamine reduces afterload, augments cardiac output, increases renal perfusion, and improves responsiveness to diuretics. Nitrates also act as systemic and pulmonary arteriolar dilators, thereby reducing ventricular afterload. Nitrates may reduce myocardial oxygen demand via a decrease in wall stress. In addition, nitroglycerin acts as a coronary arterial dilator, increasing coronary blood flow in the presence of coronary artery disease. Nitroglycerin (1–50 mcg/kg/min) is suggested in patients with underlying ischemic heart disease. Nesiritide (2 mcg/kg bolus, followed by 0.01–0.03 mcg/kg/min) can also be used, although experience with it remains more limited. Inotropic agents, including dobutamine, dopamine, epinephrine, norepinephrine, and milrinone, increase cardiac output and peripheral perfusion and are indicated instead of or in addition to vasodilators in patients with marginal blood pressure.

TABLE 39.6

TREATMENT APPROACH TO PULMONARY EDEMA

- Supplemental oxygen.
- Nitrate therapy: initially sublingual, then IV—induces venodilation, which reduces filling pressures and relieves myocardial ischemia. If hypertension is present, use nitroprusside.
- Morphine sulfate—initial therapy for preload reduction and anxiety reduction.
- IV diuresis—reduces alveolar edema.
- Inotropic therapy (e.g., dopamine, dobutamine) in presence of hypotension, low cardiac output.
- Actively investigate possibility of myocardial ischemia and treat if present.

Cardiogenic Shock

For additional discussion of cardiogenic shock, the reader is referred to Chapter 25.

Pharmacologic management of heart failure in the presence of both hypotension and elevated filling pressures includes diuresis to relieve pulmonary and systemic venous congestion as well as inotropic therapy to increase cardiac output and systemic perfusion (Table 39.7). One approach is to use *furosemide with dopamine*, the latter at a dose of 5.0 mcg/kg per minute with upward titration as necessary (Table 39.5). Although the target systolic blood pressure is generally ≥90 mm Hg, this target must be tailored to the individual patient. Some patients manifest clinical hypoperfusion at a systolic blood pressure of 90 to 95 mm Hg, whereas others may be well compensated at a systolic pressure of 85 mm Hg or even slightly lower. Dopamine doses in excess of those required to maintain adequate blood pressures should be avoided because the progressive α-adrenergic agonism at increasing doses will reduce cardiac output through excessive afterload. Dopamine is dosed based on lean rather than actual weight. If increased doses of dopamine do not improve blood pressure, addition of a more selective α-adrenergic agonist, such as *norepinephrine*, should be considered. However, high-dose dopamine, norepinephrine, and other vasoconstrictors should be used judiciously so as to maintain adequate systemic and myocardial perfusion because progressive increases in afterload raise myocardial oxygen demand and diminish renal blood flow. Norepinephrine is usually initiated at a dose of 2 mcg/min and titrated to blood pressure, with the dose usually increased every 15–20 minutes to a maximum of approximately 12 mcg/min.

Agents with both inotropic and vasodilator actions, such as *dobutamine* and *milrinone*, are valuable adjunctive agents. They reduce left- and right-sided filling pressures while augmenting cardiac output without reducing systolic blood pressure to the extent that pure vasodilators do. These agents may be combined with vasodilators when clinical or hemodynamic improvement is not otherwise achieved, particularly in diuretic-resistant patients. Long-term dobutamine infusion can be considered in refractory patients (24).

In patients in whom medical therapy is not successful in improving clinical status, *intraaortic balloon counterpulsation* should be considered, principally in patients with an identifiable, reversible precipitant of cardiogenic shock, especially if emergent percutaneous PCI coronary intervention (PCI) is not feasible. This technique improves tissue and coronary perfusion through augmentation of diastolic pressure, and it decreases ventricular afterload. The result is improved cardiac output and reduced myocardial oxygen consumption. Intraaortic balloon counterpulsation is specifically indicated in the setting of severe acute mitral regurgitation or ventricular septal rupture, situations in which considerable benefit may be derived from reduction in aortic impedance. It is contraindicated in the presence of significant aortic regurgitation because of the adverse effect of increases in aortic diastolic pressure.

TABLE 39.7

TREATMENT APPROACH TO CARDIOGENIC SHOCK

- Pulmonary artery catheterization to guide hemodynamic management.
- Supplemental oxygen/mechanical ventilation in patients with hypoxia/respiratory embarrassment.
- Blood pressure support (e.g., dopamine) increases cardiac output and systemic perfusion.
- Inotropic vasodilators (e.g., dobutamine, milrinone) reduce filling pressures while increasing cardiac output.
- Diuretics (e.g., IV furosemide) relieve pulmonary and systemic venous congestion.
- IV fluid administration in patients with depleted intravascular volume.
- Mechanical therapy (e.g., intra-aortic balloon counterpulsation), which unloads the ventricle while augmenting coronary perfusion, is recommended when pharmacotherapy is ineffective in patients with a reversible cause of shock (e.g., ischemia). It also can be used as a bridge to definitive therapy (e.g., PCI in patients with suitable anatomy).

PCI, percutaneous coronary intervention.

DEVICE THERAPY FOR HEART FAILURE

Cardiac Resynchronization Therapy

Pacing modalities that use left ventricular stimulation to optimize cardiac pump function through synchronization of right and left ventricular contraction are referred to as cardiac resynchronization therapy. In contrast to dual-chamber pacemakers, this therapy uses a third lead placed through the coronary sinus and into a left ventricular free wall vein to allow simultaneous pacing of the ventricles. An estimated 30% to 50% of patients with chronic heart failure have significant intraventricular conduction delay, which is most often exhibited as a left bundle branch block pattern. This conduction delay leads to loss of coordination between right and left ventricular (LV) contraction.

Several recent studies have demonstrated that cardiac resynchronization therapy improves patient quality of life, increases exercise capacity, and lowers NYHA heart failure classification (25, 26). Based on these data, cardiac resynchronization therapy should be considered in Class III–IV patients who remain symptomatic despite optimal medical therapy for heart failure.

Implantable Cardioverter Defibrillators

For patients with heart failure, as much as half the mortality resulting from LV systolic dysfunction can be attributable to sudden cardiac death. In contrast to antiarrhythmic agents, which have been either harmful or neutral when used in the treatment of patients with a prior myocardial infarction and impaired LV function, implantable cardioverter defibrillators (ICDs) have been of clear benefit for primary and secondary prevention of sudden death. Data from large, randomized clinical trials have demonstrated reduced mortality in patients with both ischemic and non-ischemic cardiomyopathy who undergo ICD implantation (27, 28). Based on available data, most symptomatic heart failure patients with marked reduction in LV systolic function should be viewed as candidates for ICD implantation. Furthermore, the combination of cardiac resynchronization therapy with an ICD significantly improves survival in patients with advanced heart failure and a prolonged QRS interval (26).

Ventricular Assist Devices

Ventricular assist device (VAD) therapy is an option for patients with end-stage heart failure whose symptoms fail to improve with medical therapy. However, given the risk of short- and long-term device-related complications following implantation, VAD therapy should be considered only after all meaningful medical therapeutic options have been exhausted (but before progression to irreversible end-organ failure has occurred). These devices have been successful as both a bridge-to-cardiac transplantation and permanent therapy for patients with end-stage heart failure (29). Two intracorporeal VADs approved by the U.S. Food and Drug Administration as a bridge-to-transplantation are the HeartMate VE (Thoratec, Pleasanton, CA) and the Novacor LVAS (Novacor World Heart Corporation, Oakland, CA). Both are pulsatile devices with external controllers and batteries that are connected to the pump by transcutaneous leads and have a flow rate of approximately 10 liters/min. These two devices have been very successful when utilized as a bridge-to-transplantation, with a success rate for survival to transplant of approximately 70%.

Limitations to existing treatment options for patients with end-stage heart failure, including the severe shortage of donor organs, have prompted the use of VADs not only as a bridge-to-transplantation, but also as an alternative to transplantation in patients who are ineligible for cardiac transplantation. One randomized trial showed a 48% reduction in the risk of death from any cause with an LVAD (30), but the frequency of serious adverse events in the device group was more than double that in the medical therapy group. Based on the results of the REMATCH trial, Medicare has approved payment for LVAD use as destination therapy in patients with chronic end-stage heart disease who are not eligible for cardiac transplantation (Chapter 40).

PATIENT SUBSETS

Patients with Predominant Right Ventricular (RV) Failure

Patients who present with signs and symptoms of RV dysfunction most frequently do so as a consequence of LV failure. Other causes include direct RV myocardial dysfunction, RV pressure or volume overload, or impediments to RV inflow. Examples of RV myocardial dysfunction include RV MI and dilated cardiomyopathy. RV pressure overload may be related to chronic LV failure, chronic mitral valve disease (e.g., mitral regurgitation), or cor pulmonale (e.g., COPD, pulmonary emboli). RV volume overload may be secondary to pulmonic or tricuspid regurgitation, a left-to-right intracardiac shunt, or other causes.

Clinical findings in RV failure are influenced by the elevated systemic venous pressure and the depressed cardiac output, and vary depending on the chronicity of these abnormalities. Patients with acute RV failure, as may be found in RV MI and acute pulmonary embolism, may exhibit signs of low cardiac output and elevated jugular venous pressure with prominent v waves. Other findings may include the murmur of tricuspid regurgitation, right-sided S_3 gallop, and Kussmaul's sign. In patients with chronic RV pressure overload, signs of pulmonary hypertension and RV hypertrophy are often present, including RV S_4 gallop, RV heave, and a loud pulmonic component to the second heart sound.

Regardless of the cause, patients with chronic RV failure most often present with edema and ascites. In addition, visceral edema may cause signs and symptoms of hepatic, renal, and gastrointestinal dysfunction. Impaired parietal pleural drainage may lead to pleural effusions.

In patients with chronic RV failure, IV diuretics are useful in decreasing sodium and water retention, central venous pressure, and edema. Diuretics can improve forward output by decreasing the degree of tricuspid regurgitation and by decreasing RV distention, thus reducing a ventricular-interdependent restraint on LV filling. In addition to loop diuretics, spironolactone can be effective in reducing edema resulting from RV failure because activation of the renin–angiotensin–aldosterone system is involved in sodium retention in these patients.

Systemic arteriolar dilators useful in LV failure (e.g., ACE inhibitors, nitrates, nitroprusside) also act as pulmonary vasodilators and thus improve RV output by reducing RV afterload. Because RV afterload may be augmented by hypoxia in patients with COPD, supplemental oxygen may decrease pulmonary hypertension and should be used acutely and perhaps on a long-term basis in decompensated COPD patients with RV failure. In addition, bronchodilators may improve symptoms and RV function in patients with decompensated COPD through a combination of bronchodilation, pulmonary vasodilation, and inotropy.

Concomitant Myocardial Ischemia

Myocardial ischemia or MI can precipitate heart failure by acutely diminishing systolic and diastolic performance and by causing mitral regurgitation. It is essential to maintain a low threshold for considering ischemia as a precipitant of heart failure because ischemia is reversible by medical therapy or coronary revascularization and because uncorrected ischemia is associated with a poor prognosis.

Heart failure and active ischemia may present together in a pathophysiologic vicious cycle. Heart failure is frequently characterized by LV dilation and tachycardia, which increase myocardial oxygen consumption and can precipitate ischemia in patients with coronary artery disease and diminished coronary reserve. Abnormal systolic and diastolic function lead to elevation in LV diastolic pressure; the resulting reduction in the transcoronary pressure gradient predisposes to subendocardial ischemia. Conversely, acute myocardial ischemia compromises both diastolic and systolic LV performance, which leads to a rise in filling pressures and to symptoms secondary to pulmonary congestion and low output.

Patients with regional asynergy and global LV dysfunction may have significant recovery of contractile function following revascularization with coronary artery bypass surgery or PCI. Such patients may have severe coronary stenosis with reduced myocardial blood flow that is adequate to maintain regional myocardial viability but not to provide normal function at rest or with minimal stress. The resulting *"hibernating myocardium"* can regain normal function following the restoration of myocardial blood flow after coronary revascularization.

Although there have been no randomized trials of revascularization among patients presenting with heart failure, revascularization in the setting of LV dysfunction appears to be associated with lower rates of morbidity and mortality than medical treatment. In addition, most studies of patients with angina and LV dysfunction suggest a survival benefit for those patients who undergo coronary revascularization.

It is currently recommended that *heart failure patients with exercise-limiting angina or recurrent pulmonary edema undergo coronary arteriography and subsequent revascularization when feasible.* Heart failure patients without significant angina but with a history of MI should undergo a physiologic test for myocardial viability (Chapter 36) and, when appropriate, angiography followed by revascularization.

When acute MI leads to cardiogenic shock, emergent cardiac catheterization is indicated (Chapter 38). Acute primary PCI is likely to result in improved survival in comparison with thrombolysis (31).

Heart Failure Caused by Valvular Heart Disease

For additional discussion of this topic, please see Chapter 41.

Several valvular lesions, when severe enough, can lead to symptoms of heart failure. Symptomatic patients with physical or imaging findings suggestive of *critical aortic stenosis* have improved survival following aortic valve replacement, which also usually improves LV performance. Medical management can provide short-term benefit but is not a substitute for prompt valve surgery. Patients with either heart failure symptoms or evidence of LV dysfunction and dilation secondary to *chronic aortic regurgitation* are best treated with aortic valve replacement. Therapy with vasodilators such as ACE inhibitors, hydralazine, and nifedipine can improve hemodynamics and symptoms of aortic regurgitation before surgery.

Patients with *mitral stenosis* should undergo correction (balloon valvuloplasty, open commissurotomy, or mitral valve replacement) whenever symptoms become difficult to manage with a combination of diuretics and heart rate control. Mitral valve repair or replacement is recommended as soon as it is feasible in *acute symptomatic mitral regurgitation*. Patients with *chronic mitral regurgitation* should, in general, undergo mitral valve repair or replacement when heart failure symptoms are present or when diagnostic testing documents abnormal LV function or LV dilatation (end-systolic dimension >45–50 mm).

Heart Failure with Normal Ejection Fraction

A majority of patients hospitalized for heart failure have a low resting LV ejection fraction. A significant minority, however, have a normal LV ejection fraction. In some patients, ejection fraction may be normal when measured but was abnormal when the symptoms developed; these patients may have transient ischemia, arrhythmias, toxic exposure (e.g., alcohol), or severe hypertension. Other patients may have a normal ejection fraction but heart failure related to mitral regurgitation. In some patients, the diagnosis of heart failure may be incorrect, and the symptoms may have other causes, such as pulmonary disease.

In other patients, a variety of different disorders can lead to abnormal ventricular relaxation and compliance, increased vascular stiffness, and/or reduced renal sodium clearance, with consequent elevation in ventricular filling pressures leading to pulmonary venous and capillary hypertension. Such patients cannot increase cardiac output in response to stress without inordinate increases in LV filling pressure and associated pulmonary congestion. The single most common etiology is hypertension. *Restrictive cardiomyopathies* are caused by conditions such as sarcoidosis, amyloidosis, hemochromatosis, and radiation injury. Other causes include hypertrophic cardiomyopathy and pericardial constriction. Echocardiography may suggest abnormal diastolic function in a patient with a thickened myocardium, a predisposing condition, or pericardial disease.

The ARB candesartan showed a trend toward reducing the primary endpoint of cardiovascular mortality or heart failure hospitalization in these patients, but this finding did not reach statistical significance (32). A number of additional studies are under way. Based on physiologic considerations, as well as findings in patients with hypertension and LVH (33), the general consensus is to recommend an ACE inhibitor or ARB in patients with heart failure, preserved ejection fraction, and a history of hypertension. In patients with heart failure with normal ejection fraction, diuretics are often needed to normalize fluid balance. Doses should be titrated carefully because these patients are often volume-sensitive and many have marginal renal function. Hypertension should be aggressively managed (monitoring renal function carefully) (Chapter 48). In patients who continue to be hypertensive despite ACE inhibitors and diuretics, a β-blocker or calcium blocker should be considered. β-blockers are particularly useful in patients with tachycardia, including those with atrial fibrillation, in whom rate control represents a major therapeutic goal. Myocardial ischemia should be treated with medications and, when appropriate, revascularization (Chapters 37 and 38).

ISSUES DURING HOSPITALIZATION

Patients with acute decompensation of chronic heart failure usually manifest rapid clinical improvement in response to IV diuretics, especially if coexisting illnesses are properly treated. Patients usually note marked symptomatic improvement, with resolution of rest dyspnea, by the end of the first hospital day. As the patient approaches his or her dry body weight, IV therapy is withdrawn and oral agents are reinstituted.

For patients with pulmonary edema, the hospital course is influenced by whether or not a precipitant for decompensation is identified. If IV diuresis is effective and any concomitant ischemia is successfully treated, the patient may be asymptomatic on the first hospital day; attention should then be focused on definition of the coronary anatomy and potential revascularization. Similarly, if valvular disease (such as mitral regurgitation) is responsible for decompensation, valvular repair or replacement preceded by coronary angiography should be strongly considered (Chapter 41).

Patients with cardiogenic shock have a high mortality regardless of etiology. Emergent PCI is indicated for cardiogenic shock in the presence of acute MI. For patients with papillary muscle rupture or an acute ventricular septal defect, emergency repair is recommended (Chapter 38). In patients who are not eligible for these therapies, consideration should be given to intra-aortic balloon counter pulsation or ventricular assist devices if a definable acute and potentially recoverable event is responsible for the abrupt deterioration or if cardiac transplantation (Chapter 40) is being considered.

DISCHARGE ISSUES

In general, patients admitted to the hospital for heart failure may be discharged when symptoms have been controlled and reversible precipitants have been treated. Noncompliance with medication and dietary recommendations is the most common identifiable causes of readmission. Thus, care should be taken before discharge to initiate and reinforce education regarding a diet restricted to approximately 2 g of sodium per day, self-monitoring through daily weights, and the importance of compliance with medications. Unusual patients who have not recovered to the point of unassisted ambulation may benefit from a short stay in a skilled nursing facility for rehabilitation.

All patients should be on an ACE inhibitor or angiotensin receptor blocker unless it is absolutely not tolerated. β-blockers also reduce mortality in patients with class II–IV heart failure. Although initiation of these agents requires a degree of clinical stability, there is increasing evidence that they can be initiated safely in low doses and titrated slowly in patients hospitalized with heart failure (18). Aldosterone receptor blockade has been shown to be beneficial, in addition to ACE inhibitors, in patients with class IV, or recent class IV, symptoms, and in patients following myocardial infarction, reduced ejection fraction, and signs or symptoms of heart failure. These agents may ultimately prove to be useful in broader populations of patients with heart failure. Digoxin is beneficial for symptoms but not longevity.

A mechanism for achieving careful follow-up must be established before discharge. Such follow-up generally includes an office visit within 2 weeks of discharge. Programs in *heart failure disease management* may reduce the frequency of readmission and maintain or improve the quality of life (34, 35). These programs, which serve as an extension of care beyond hospitalization and the office visit, focus on optimizing patient compliance and providing a rapid medical response to subtle changes in the patient's condition. They are generally delivered by nurses linked to primary care physicians and utilize a mixture of home visits and telephone monitoring. Such programs have the potential to reduce length of stay by providing patients and hospital physicians with a sense of security regarding post-acute care. Effective programs may also reduce readmission rates and emergency department visits. Exercise training can improve functional capacity but its impact on reducing mortality is less certain (36).

The response to inpatient treatment typically results in reductions in BNP levels. High predischarge levels predict readmission and death, even among patients who have responded clinically during hospitalization (37, 38).

Loss of weight unrelated to diuresis portends a poor outcome in patients with heart failure (39), as does progressive renal dysfunction (40); the only known treatment is better control of the heart failure. For anemia, transfusion or erythropoietin to raise the hemoglobin level should be considered, but the target level remains uncertain (10).

WHEN HEART FAILURE PRESENTS DURING HOSPITALIZATION

The physiologic stresses associated with any of a variety of illnesses can cause decompensation in patients with known or unsuspected LV dysfunction. In addition, previously undiagnosed valvular disease may become clinically manifested during the tachycardia and fluid administration attendant to surgery. One example is the diagnosis of heart failure in a previously healthy young woman in whom pulmonary congestion develops after administration of fluid or blood products after parturition (Chapter 32). These patients are usually easily managed with diuresis.

In patients with known and previously undiagnosed LV dysfunction in whom heart failure becomes manifest during hospitalization for another illness, it is of primary importance to correct the underlying disorder that prompted hospitalization; heart failure should be managed according to symptoms and the clinical examination as detailed above. When heart failure occurs in the setting of acute MI, medications with inotropic and especially chronotropic action (e.g., dobutamine) should be avoided if possible because they may increase myocardial oxygen consumption and thereby potentially worsen ischemia and increase infarct size. Like patients admitted primarily for heart failure, patients with previously unrecognized LV dysfunction should have standard long-term therapy instituted before hospital discharge.

COST CONSIDERATIONS AND RESOURCE USE

Heart failure is the single most common cause for hospitalization among patients old enough to receive Medicare benefits. Care for patients with heart failure has been estimated to cost about $20 billion annually, with approximately 75% of that cost expended within the hospital setting (1, 2). Importantly, there has been a focus on reducing the readmission rate, which has been reported to be as high as 40% during 6 months. Although it would also be valuable to reduce length of stay, hospitalization should not be shortened at the expense of a markedly increased readmission rate; it is essential that patients not be discharged before stability is achieved, needed medications are instituted, and adequate follow-up is arranged.

KEY POINTS

- Patients hospitalized with heart failure require simultaneous emergent evaluation of possible causes of decompensation and individualized therapy focusing on the principal hemodynamic perturbation.
- Once filling pressures have been reduced and depressed cardiac output and blood pressure treated, plans for long-term management should be addressed. Management should include administration of pharmacologic agents with proven survival benefits: angiotensin-converting enzyme inhibitors, angiotensin receptor blockers, and β-blockers; aldosterone receptor blockers, at least in patients with class IV or recent class IV symptoms; and cardiac resynchronization therapy, implantable cardioventral defibrillators, and coronary revascularization in appropriately selected patients. Renal function, electrolytes, hematocrit, and clinical status should be carefully monitored during up-titration of drug therapy.
- Plans for focused follow-up are crucial to ensure successful ongoing management. They include careful evaluation of dietary and medication compliance, optimization of medical treatment, constant re-evaluation, and early response to changes in volume status.

REFERENCES

1. American Heart Association. 2004 Heart and Stroke Statistical Update. American Heart Association, Dallas, TX; 2003.
2. Graves EJ, Owings MF, National Center for Health Statistics summary. National hospital discharge survey. Advance data from vital and health statistics. No. 301. Hyattsville, MD: Public Health Service [DHHS publication No. (PHS)98-1250], 1998:1–12.
3. Hunt SA, Baker DW, Chin MH, et al. ACC/AHA guidelines for the evaluation and management of chronic heart failure in the adult: A report of the American College of Cardiology/American Heart Association Task Force on Practice Guideline (Committee to revise the 1995 guidelines for the evaluation and management of heart failure), 2001 American College of Cardiology. Available at: http://www.acc.org/clinical/guidelines/failure/hf_index.htm
4. Maisel AS, Krishnaswamy P, Nowak RM, et al. Rapid measurement of B-type natriueretic peptide in the emergency diagnosis of heart failure. *N Engl J Med* 2002;347:161–167.
5. Mueller C, Scholer A, Laule-Kilian K, et al. Use of B-type natriuretic peptide in the evaluation and management of acute dyspnea. *N Eng J Med* 2004;350:647–654.
6. Maisel A, Hollander JE, Guss D, et al. Primary results of the rapid emergency department heart failure outpatient trial (REDHOT): A multicenter study of B-type natriuretic peptide levels, emergency department decision making, and outcomes in patients presenting with shortness of breath. *J Am Coll Cardiol* 2004;44:1328–33.
7. Aurigemma GP, Gaasch WH. Diastolic heart failure. *N Engl J Med* 2004;351:1097–1105.
8. Klapholz M, Maurer M, Lowe AM, et al. Hospitalization for heart failure in the presence of a normal left ventricular ejection fraction: Results of the New York Heart Failure Registry. *J Am Coll Cardiol* 2004;43:1432–1438.
9. Maurer MS, Burkhoff D, Kronzon I, et al. Diastolic dysfunction: Can it be diagnosed by Doppler echocardiography? *J Am Coll Cardiol* 2004;44:1453–1459.
10. Felker GM, Adams KF, Gattis WA, et al. Anemia as a risk factor and therapeutic target in heart failure. *J Am Coll Cardiol* 2004;44:959–966.
11. Cohn JN, Tognoni G, et al. A randomized trial of the angiotensin-receptor blocker valsartan in chronic heart failure. *N Engl J Med* 2001;345:1667–1675.
12. Granger CB, McMurray JJV, Yusuf S, et al. Effects of candesartan in patients with chronic heart failure and reduced left-ventricular systolic function intolerant to angiotensin-converting enzyme inhibitors: the CHARM-alternative trial. *Lancet* 2003; 362:772–776.
13. Pitt B, Poole-Wilson PA, Segal R, et al. Effect of losartan compared with captopril on mortality in patients with symptomatic heart failure: Randomised trial-the losartan heart failure survival study (ELITE II). *Lancet* 2000;355:1582–1587.

14. Pfeffer MA, McMurray JJ, Velazquez EF, et al. Valsartan is an effective as captopril in patients with heart failure or left ventricular dysfunction after MI. *N Engl J Med* 2003;349:1893–1906.

15. McMurray JJV, Ostergren J, Swedberg K, et al. Effects of candesartan in patients with chronic heart failure and reduced left-ventricular systolic function taking angiotensin-converting enzyme inhibitors: the CHARM-added trial. *Lancet* 2003;362:767–771.

16. Taylor AL, Ziesche S, Yancy C, et al. Combination of isosorbide dinitrate and hydralazine in blacks with heart failure. *N Engl J Med* 2004;351:2049–2057.

17. Poole-Wilson PA, Swedberg K, Cleland JG, et al. Comparison of carvedilol and metoprolol on clinical outcomes in patients with chronic heart failure in the Carvedilol OR Metoprolol European Trial (COMET): randomised controlled trial. *Lancet* 2003;362:7–13.

18. Gattis WA, O'Connor CM, Gallup DS, et al. Predischarge initiation of carvedilol in patients hospitalized for decompensated heart failure: results of the Initiation Management Predischarge: Process for Assessment of Carvedilol Therapy in Heart Failure (IMPACT-HF) trial. *J Am Coll Cardiol* 2004;43:1534–1541.

19. Packer M, Coats AJS, Fowler MB, et al. Effect of carvedilol on survival in severe chronic heart failure. *N Engl J Med* 2001;344:1651–1658.

20. Pitt B, Zannad F, Remme WJ, et al. The effect of spironolactone on morbidity and mortality in patients with severe heart failure. *N Engl J Med* 1999;341:708–717.

21. Pitt B, Remme W, Zannad F, et al. Eplerenone, a selective aldosterone blocker, in patients with left ventricular dysfunction after myocardial infarction. *N Engl J Med* 2003;348:1309–1321.

22. The Digitalis Investigation Group. The effect of digoxin on mortality and morbidity in patients with heart failure. *N Engl J Med* 1997;336:525–533.

23. Gheorghiade M, Gattis WA, O'Connor CM, et al. Effects of tolvaptan, a vasopressin antagonist, in patients hospitalized with worsening heart failure: a randomized controlled trial. *JAMA* 2004;291:1963–1671.

24. Nanas JN, Tsagalou EP, Kanakakis J, et al. Long-term intermittent dobutamine infusion, combined with oral amiodarone for end-stage heart failure: A randomized double-blind study. *Chest* 2004;125:1198–204.

25. Cazeau S, Leclercq C, Lavergne T, et al. Effects of multisite biventricular pacing in patients with heart failure and intraventricular conduction delay. *N Engl. J Med* 2001; 344:873–880.

26. Bristow MR, Saxon LA, Boehmer J, et al. Cardiac-resynchronization therapy with or without an implantable defibrillator in advanced chronic heart failure. *N Engl J Med* 2004; 350:2140–2150.

27. Brady GH, Lee KL, Mark DB, et al. Amiodarone or implantable cardioverter defibrillator for congestive heart failure. *N Engl J Med* 2005; 352:225–237.

28. Kadish A, Dyer A, Daubert JP, et al. Prophylactic defibrillator implantation in patients with non-ischemic dilated cardiomyopathy. *N Engl J Med* 2004; 350:2151–2158.

29. Goldstein DJ, Oz MC, Rose EA. Implantable left ventricular assist devices. *N Engl J Med* 1998; 339:1522–1533.

30. Rose EA, Gelijns AC, Moskowitz AJ, et al. Long-term use of a left ventricular assist device for end-stage heart failure. REMATCH Study Group. *N Engl J Med* 345:1435–1443.

31. Hochman JS, Sleeper LA, Webb JG, et al. Early revascularization in acute myocardial infarction complicated by cardiogenic shock. SHOCK Investigators. Should We Emergently Revascularize Occluded Coronaries for Cardiogenic Shock. *N Engl J Med* 1999;341:625–634.

32. Pfeffer MA, Swedberg K, Granger CB, et al. Effects of candesartan on mortality and morbidity in patients with chronic heart failure: the CHARM-overall programme. *Lancet* 2003;362:759–766.

33. Dahlöf B, Devereux RB, Kjeldsen SE, et al. Cardiovascular morbidity and mortality in the Losartan Intervention For Endpoint reduction in hypertension study (LIFE): a randomised trial against atenolol. *Lancet* 2002;359:995–1003.

34. Kimmelstiel C, Levine D, Perry K, et al. Randomized, controlled evaluation of short- and long-term benefits of heart failure disease management within a diverse provider network: The SPAN-CHF trial. *Circulation* 2004;110:1450–1455.

35. McAlister FA, Stewart S, Ferrua S, et al. Multidisciplinary strategies for the management of heart failure patients at high risk for admission: A systematic review of randomized trials. *J Am Coll Cardiol* 2004;44:810–819.

36. Smart N, Marwick TH. Exercise training for patients with heart failure: a systematic review of factors that improve mortality and morbidity. *Am J Med* 2004;116:693–706.

37. Logeart D, Thabut G, Jourdain P, et al. Predischarge B-type natriuretic peptide assay for identifying patients at high risk of readmission after decompensated heart failure. *J Am Coll Cardiol* 2004;43:635–641.

38. Bettencourt P, Azevedo A, Pimenta J, et al. N-terminal-pro-brain natriuretic peptide predicts outcome after hospital discharge in heart failure patients. *Circulation* 2004;110:2168–2174.

39. Anker SD, Negassa A, Coats AJ, et al. Prognostic importance of weight loss in chronic heart failure and the effect of treatment with angiotensin-converting enzyme inhibitors: an observational study. *Lancet* 2003;361:1077–1083.

40. Forman DE, Butler J, Wang Y, et al. Incidence, predictors at admission, and impact of worsening renal function among patients hospitalized with heart failure. *J Am Coll Cardiol* 2004;43:61–67.

ADDITIONAL READING

Doust JA, Glasziou PP, Pietrzak E, et al. A systematic review of the diagnostic accuracy of natriuretic peptides for heart failure. *Arch Intern Med* 2004;164:1978–1984.

Hogg K, Swedberg K, McMurray J. Heart failure with preserved left ventricular systolic function: epidemiology, clinical characteristics, and prognosis. *J Am Coll Cardiol* 2004;43:317–327.

McAlister FA, Ezekowitz JA, Wiebe N, et al. Systematic review: cardiac resynchronization in patients with symptomatic heart failure. *Ann Intern Med* 2004;141:381–90.

Schiff GD, Fund S, Speroff T, et al. Decompensated heart failure: symptoms, patterns of onset, and contributing factors. *Am J Med* 2003;114:625–630.

Heart Transplantation

40

Maria Ansari   Teresa DeMarco

INTRODUCTION

Despite advances in pharmacologic therapy and mechanical assist devices, the mortality for end-stage heart failure remains 50% at 1 year. With improved surgical techniques and the availability of cyclosporine, the overall 1-year actuarial survival after heart transplantation is 85%, and the 5-year actuarial survival is 71% (1, 2). More than 40,000 transplants have been performed worldwide since 1982. In the United States, approximately 2,200 donor hearts are available per year, but nearly 10,000 patients are referred annually for cardiac transplantation.

EVALUATING A PATIENT FOR CARDIAC TRANSPLANTATION

Selection Criteria

Cardiac transplantation is indicated in patients with terminal heart failure in whom all other conventional therapies have failed or are inappropriate (Table 40.1). Cardiomyopathy, coronary heart disease, and valvular heart disease are the three most common indications for adult cardiac transplantation (2). Candidates are usually New York Heart Association class III or IV, with an unacceptable quality of life and a 1-year predicted survival less than could be achieved with transplantation. Patients with peak oxygen consumption (VO_2 max) during exercise of less than 14 mL/kg per minute have a 1-year survival of about 32% and should therefore be referred immediately for transplantation (3). By comparison, patients with a VO_2 max above 14 mL/kg per minute have a 1-year survival close to 90% with medical therapy and are not candidates for immediate transplant. It is important that patients undergo repeated testing if the clinical condition changes.

Exclusion Criteria

Contraindications for transplantation (Table 40.2) include comorbid conditions with a poor prognosis, ongoing unresolved medical diseases or neoplasms, and important psychosocial issues that may lead to life-threatening noncompliance. A physiologic age over 65 years is a controversial relative contraindication based on data showing a significant decrease in posttransplant survival for each decade of age and a clinically significant decrease in survival after the age of 65.

Short- and long-term survival postcardiac transplant is closely linked to the preoperative pulmonary vascular resistance (PVR). Patients with a PVR below 2.5 Wood units, pulmonary artery pressure below 50 to 60 mm Hg systolic, and a mean transpulmonary gradient (mean pulmonary artery pressure minus pulmonary capillary wedge pressure) of 15 mm Hg or less have a better prognosis than do patients with higher values (4). Patients with a high PVR who respond to intravenous (IV) nitroprusside (PVR <2.5 Wood units with adequate systemic pressure) also have a favorable prognosis.

Listing a Patient for Transplant

After patients have been selected as appropriate candidates for cardiac transplantation, they are placed on the United Network for Organ Sharing (UNOS) waiting list in one of two categories. Status I patients require IV vasoactive drugs or mechanical support in an ICU to maintain adequate hemodynamics. All other patients are Status II. Status I patients generally wait weeks-to-months for an available organ. Status II patients often wait 6 months to several years, and 20–40% of Status II patients die while awaiting a donor heart.

TABLE 40.1

INDICATIONS FOR CARDIAC TRANSPLANTATION

- Refractory class III or IV heart failure despite optimal contemporary therapy
- Recurrent and refractory symptomatic ventricular arrhythmias with unacceptable quality of life
- Recurrent and refractory unstable ischemic heart disease with major functional limitations
- Maximum oxygen consumption ($\dot{V}O_2max$) <14 mg/kg per minute

BRIDGE TO CARDIAC TRANSPLANTATION

The cardiac organ donor supply is inadequate to meet demands. When intense interventions (Chapter 39) fail to stabilize a patient with unstable refractory heart failure, mechanical support is required. Among patients who are at high risk for dying of irreversible myocardial failure despite maximum inotropic support with or without an intraaortic balloon pump but who do not have irreversible end-organ damage, *left ventricular assist devices* (LVADs) can provide a successful bridge to transplantation in about 75% of cases. Complications of LVADs include thromboembolism, infection, and right ventricular (RV) failure from increased PVR. Use of a LVAD is usually part of a two-step process: first the insertion of the device and correction of vital organ hypoperfusion; second, orthotopic heart transplantation as soon as a donor is available, usually within weeks to months. However, the LVAD is also being evaluated as a bridge to recovery in patients with reversible causes of heart failure, and even as a permanent ventricular support device. In selected patients with end-stage heart failure, these devices have been used for 3 years or longer with improved quality of life and an acceptable mortality rate (5), thereby serving as a reasonable alternative in patients who are not candidates for transplantion (Chapter 39).

CARDIAC TRANSPLANTATION SURGERY

Donor Organ Selection

Donor hearts must be ABO-compatible with the recipient, but HLA matching is neither necessary nor feasible. All transplant recipient candidates are screened for allo-antibodies by means of a panel-reactive antibody (PRA) test of recipient serum against a panel of allogeneic lymphocytes with known HLA antigens. For potential recipients who react to 15% or more of the panel, prospective lymphocyte cross-matching is performed by mixing recipient serum with potential heart donor lymphocytes; a positive cross-

TABLE 40.2

EXCLUSION CRITERIA FOR CARDIAC TRANSPLANTATION

- Physiologic age >65 y
- Active infection
- Active peptic ulcer disease
- Severe diabetes mellitus
- Severe peripheral vascular disease
- Severe chronic obstructive pulmonary disease
- Renal failure (creatinine >2 mg/dL and or creatinine clearance <50 mL/min, unless caused by low cardiac output)
- Liver disease with serum bilirubin >2.5 mg/dL, aminotransferases more than twice the upper limit of normal, prothrombin time >14 sec
- Pulmonary artery systolic pressure >60 mm Hg
- Pulmonary vascular resistance >3.0 Wood units despite vasodilator trial
- Mean transpulmonary gradient >15 mm Hg
- Active substance abuse
- Psychosocial impairment limiting medical compliance

Adapted from Stevenson LW. Candidates for heart transplantation: selection and management. In Poole-Wilson PA, Colucci WS, Massie BM, et al., eds. *Heart Failure: Scientific Principles and Clinical Practice.* New York: Churchill Livingstone, 1997:807–826.

match excludes that donor heart for the recipient. Potential donor hearts must also be free of significant infectious agents (i.e., viral hepatitis, HIV). Donor heart function is examined by echocardiography; coronary angiography should be performed if the donor is at high risk for coronary artery disease (CAD). Potential organ donor weight must be within 20% of the recipient weight to match cardiac size. Finally, the donor heart must be within a 1,000-mile radius of the recipient to ensure an ischemic time of less than 6 hours to minimize damage to the donor heart during transport.

Operative Methods

Orthotopic heart transplantation involves the partial removal of recipient atria and the entire removal of the ventricles. In the *bicaval technique*, which is now the standard of care, the recipient's right atrium is excised with a cuff left intact around both the superior and the inferior vena cava (6). Most of the recipient's left atrium and all of the interatrial septum are removed.

CARE OF THE HOSPITALIZED PATIENT

Early Post-transplant Care

Unique Physiologic Properties

Because of preservation injury, the newly transplanted heart is a model of *stunned ischemic myocardium*, characterized by transient systolic and diastolic dysfunction, bradycardia, and RV dysfunction. It is also devoid of autonomic innervation. Inotropic and chronotropic support, usually with a combination of isoproterenol and dopamine, is generally needed for the first 3 to 5 postoperative days. The target heart rate for the early postoperative period is between 110 and 130 beats/min to maximize cardiac output (cardiac index >2.5 L/min per square meter.) When the above combination is inadequate to attain optimal hemodynamics, milrinone, epinephrine, or both may be required. RA filling pressures are maintained at 8 to 15 mm Hg to attain adequate cardiac output. Diuretics are usually initiated after the first day to achieve normal RA pressures. In cases of pulmonary hypertension, pulmonary vasodilators such as nitroprusside, prostacycline, or inhaled nitric oxide can be employed (Chapter 59).

Bradycardia and Tachycardia

In the early posttransplant period, bradycardia (sinus or junctional bradycardia, or AV block) is common as a consequence of preservation injury, sinus node edema from ischemia during surgery, conduction system injury inflicted at the time of harvest, electrolyte disturbances, preoperative administration of amiodarone, or allograft rejection (Table 40.3).

Treatment for bradycardia early after transplant includes isoproterenol or nonglycoside inotropes. Atropine, whose chronotropic action is based on a vagolytic mechanism, will not be effective in increasing donor sinus rate in a denervated heart but may reverse vagally-mediated peripheral vasodilation. Bradycardia generally resolves within several days after transplant. However, a small percentage of patients (3–15%) require permanent pacemakers.

Several weeks after transplantation, the denervated heart exhibits a resting sinus tachycardia because of the loss of parasympathetic tone. The heart rate rises more slowly with exercise and is attenuated at peak exercise. Compared with the normal heart, the denervated heart depends more on an augmented stroke volume than on an increased heart rate to increase cardiac output.

Ventricular and Supraventricular Dysrhythmias

Ventricular or supraventricular tachycardias (Table 40.4) after transplant may be signs of preservation injury (early posttransplant), allograft rejection, ischemia, or electrolyte disturbance. The most common cause of early posttransplant tachyarrhythmias is preservation injury, which tends to resolve in several days. Myocardial ischemia from transplant CAD is a cause of late dysrhythmias.

Drugs that primarily act through the autonomic nervous system will have no effect on the transplanted heart. For example, digoxin, a vagotonic agent, will not be effective in managing supraventricular arrhythmias in the usual clinical doses. Type Ia anti-arrhythmics (e.g., quinidine, procainamide) exert not only vagotonic properties (which will not be observed in the transplanted heart) but also direct effects (which will be observed); these agents slow both the sinus rate and AV conduction, which makes them effective agents for tachyarrhythmias. Calcium channel blockers and β-blockers directly slow the sinus rate and AV conduction in the transplanted heart; because of their negative inotropic and chronotropic effects, they must be used cautiously in the early transplant period, when allograft function is marginal.

TABLE 40.3
ELECTRICAL DISTURBANCES AFTER CARDIAC TRANSPLANT

Bradycardia

Cause	Onset	Treatment
Sinus node preservation injury	Early	Time/temporary pacer
Conduction system injury at harvest	Early	Time/temporary and/or permanent pacer
Amiodarone	Early	Time/temporary pacer
Electrolyte derangement	Early or late	Electrolyte normalization
Allograft rejection	Early or late	Increased immunosuppression

Ventricular or supraventricular tachycardia

Cause	Onset	Treatment
Preservation injury	Early	Time, antiarrhythmics
Hypomagnesemia, hypokalemia	Early or late	Electrolyte normalization
Allograft rejection	Early or late	Increased immunosuppression
Myocardial ischemia (transplant coronary artery disease)	Late	Nitrates, β-blockers, aspirin, lipid-lowering agents, revascularization, re-transplantation

TABLE 40.4

SIGNS AND SYMPTOMS OF ACUTE ALLOGRAFT REJECTION

Signs and symptoms	Pathophysiology
Fever	Cytokine release from injured myocardium and activation of inflammatory pathways
Fatigue, decreased exercise tolerance	Cytokine release, decreased cardiac function
Cough	Increased pulmonary vascular pressures from systolic or diastolic dysfunction
Syncope, near-syncope	Bradycardia/VT/SVT
Palpitations	VT/SVT
Dyspnea	Increased pulmonary venous pressures
Sudden death	Terminal arrhythmia
Decreased urine output	Decreased cardiac output and decreased renal perfusion
Pulmonary crackles	Increased pulmonary venous pressures
Loud pulmonic heart sound	Increased pulmonary arterial pressures
S_3 gallop	High left ventricular end-diastolic pressures from low cardiac output
New regurgitant murmur (tricuspid or mitral	Dilation of right and/or left ventricle
Jugular venous distention	Right or left ventricular failure

SVT, supraventricular tachycardia; *VT*, ventricular tachycardia.

Right Ventricular Failure

Heart transplant recipients with preexisting pulmonary hypertension are at high risk for the development of RV failure soon after transplant surgery. RV failure is initially treated with pulmonary vasodilators such as nitroprusside, prostacycline, or inhaled nitric oxide. Isoproterenol, milrinone, or both are often required to support the compromised RV. For RV failure refractory to pharmacologic intervention or in cases of concomitant systemic hypotension, an RVAD should be placed until intrinsic pulmonary hypertension reverses and RV function improves.

Biventricular Failure

Biventricular failure after transplantation should always prompt the suspicion of allograft rejection, although there are other causes (Table 40.4). Immediately after transplant, the cause is usually hyperacute allograft rejection from preformed allo-antibodies. In the early posttransplant period, biventricular pump failure can be a manifestation of organ preservation injury, tamponade, or acute allograft rejection. Posttransplant tamponade tends to occur in a posterolateral closed space and is almost always a consequence of postoperative bleeding; surgical decompression is necessary. Biventricular failure for 2–10 days postoperatively can be a manifestation of preservation injury; this is a diagnosis of exclusion and is treated with hemodynamic support.

Allgraft Rejection

Allograft rejection occurs at a rate of 0.5 to 2.5 episodes per patient during the first posttransplant year. *Hyperacute allograft rejection* presents in the operating room or immediately postoperatively and results in primary nonfunctioning of the graft. *Acute cellular allograft rejection* usually occurs within the first 6 months after cardiac transplantation but can occur later; it is the most common form of allograft rejection. *Chronic rejection* presents with slowly developing symptoms of fatigue and dyspnea suggestive of transplant CAD.

Prophylaxis

Prophylactic immunosuppression regimens are transplant center-specific. (For a general discussion of available immunosuppressive regimens, see Chapter 102, particularly Table 102.4.) Maintenance prophylaxis involves triple therapy: prednisone, azathioprine (or mycophenolate mofetil), and cyclosporine (or tacrolimus).

Indications for Hospital and Intensive Care Unit Admission

Because allograft rejection can be clinically silent, surveillance endomyocardial biopsies are performed to exclude occult allograft rejection (every week for the first four weeks, then every other week for two more weeks, then quarterly twice, semi-annually twice, and then yearly thereafter). Additional endomyocardial biopsies are performed whenever allograft rejection is suspected.

Any patient with hemodynamic instability, signs of heart failure, or symptomatic dysrhythmias should be admitted to the ICU for cardiac rhythm monitoring, invasive hemodynamic monitoring, inotropic support, and intensified nursing care (Table 40.5). By comparison, moderate acute cellular rejection without hemodynamic compromise or dysrhythmias is usually treated in the outpatient setting, as supervised by a transplant center.

Treatment of Allograft Rejection

The treatment of acute cellular rejection includes optimization of immunosuppression (Table 40.5). Acute humoral rejection must be treated aggressively with immunosuppression and plasmapheresis to remove circulating immunoglobulin and reduce anti-allograft immunoglobulin titers.

Indications for Early Consultation

Every cardiac transplant patient admitted for possible allograft rejection to any hospital requires an urgent consultation with a transplant cardiologist. The cardiologist will assist in the evaluation of suspected allograft rejection, which includes an endomyocardial biopsy. Once the diagnosis is established, treatment should begin under the direction of the cardiologist.

DISCHARGE ISSUES

Patients admitted with cardiac allograft rejection often have hospital stays ranging from several days to several weeks, depending on the clinical manifestations of the rejection

TABLE 40.5
TREATMENT OF ALLOGRAFT REJECTION

Endomyocardial biopsy grade	Clinical status	Treatment
Acute cellular rejection		
1A, 1B, 2	Subclinical	No augmentation of immunosuppression
2	Overt[a]	Optimize immunosuppression[b] Prednisone pulse[c]
3A	Subclinical	Optimize immunosuppression Prednisone pulse
3A	Overt	Optimize immunosuppression Methylprednisolone pulse[d]
3B	Subclinical, ≤3 mo from transplant	Optimize immunosuppression Methylprednisolone pulse
3B	Overt, >3 mo from transplant	Optimize immunosuppression Methylprednisolone pulse
3B, 4	Overt, ≤3 mo from transplant, subclinical or overt >3 mo from transplant	Optimize immunosuppression ATG or OKT3[e]
Acute humoral rejection		
Not applicable	Subclinical/overt	Plasmapheresis (60 mL/kg qod) Methylprednisolone pulse Cyclophosphamide 1 mg/kg per day PO Optimize immunosuppression IV immunoglobulin
Hyperacute rejection		
Not applicable	Overt	Mechanical ventricular assist devices Total artificial heart Urgent re-transplantation

[a]Overt: Hemodynamic compromise, allograft dysfunction clinically or on echocardiogram, arrhythmias.
[b]Optimize immunosuppression: Increased doses within conventional range as toxicity permits; consider changing azathioprine to mycophenolate mofetil (1–1.5 g PO bid); consider changing cyclosporine to tacrolimus (0.1 mg/kg PO bid); consider the addition of methotrexate 5–7.5 mg PO qd for 3–5 days for refractory rejection.
[c]Prednisone pulse: 1.5 mg/kg PO qd (or divided doses) for 5 days, then rapid taper.
[d]Methylprednisolone pulse: 1 g IV qd × 3, then subsequent prednisone taper.
[e]ATG (anti-thymocyte globulin): 10 mg/kg per day IV × 7–10 doses or OKT3 5 mg/d IV × 10 doses.

episode and the therapeutic response. A patient is ready for discharge when a clinical response to augmented immunosuppression leads to improved symptoms and acceptable hemodynamics on a stable oral medication regimen. Discharge planning is a coordinated effort between the inpatient hospital team, the transplant cardiology consult team, and the patient's primary care provider in the community. Patients often live far away from a center that provides transplant cardiology care, so outpatient follow-up with the patient's primary physician is extremely important.

Some immunosuppressive medications (e.g., cyclosporine, tacrolimus, mycophenolate-mofetil) may not be readily available at community pharmacies. It is critical to anticipate discharge and to have medications available when the patient leaves the hospital. The patient generally returns in 1 to 2 weeks for an endomyocardial biopsy to assess response to therapy. The scheduling of subsequent endomyocardial biopsies is adjusted based on the frequency of rejection episodes and the presence or absence of persistent rejection.

Late Posttransplant Care

Long-term immunosuppressive therapy in the cardiac transplant patient has many potential sequelae, including infection, malignancy, and other organ-specific complications (Table 40.6).

Infections

For additional discussion of infection in immunocompromised hosts, see Chapter 63.

The blood and lungs are the most common sites of infection after heart transplantation. Cardiac transplant patients are particularly prone to pancreaticobiliary disease and especially acalculous cholecystitis, in which the usual signs and symptoms of cholecystitis may be blunted or absent. There should be a low threshold to image the gallbladder and biliary system when gastrointestinal complaints are present (Chapter 84).

Renal Insufficiency

Patients presenting with decreased urine output, lower-extremity edema, or easy bruisability should be evaluated for renal insufficiency, which may be caused by cyclosporine or tacrolimus. Cyclosporine and tacrolimus cause prerenal azotemia by constricting afferent renal arterioles; this effect can be modified by reducing doses when permitted. Cyclosporine and tacrolimus also produce a

TABLE 40.6

COMMON LONG-TERM COMPLICATIONS OF CARDIAC TRANSPLANTATION

Complications	Etiology
Opportunistic Infections	Immunosuppression
Renal failure	Cyclosporine alone or in combination with other drugs
	Renal hypoperfusion (e.g., because of sudden death, arrhythmias, or sepsis)
	Hemolytic uremic syndrome
Musculoskeletal	
Myopathy, rhabdomyolysis, gout	Drug-induced (lipid-lowering agents with cyclosporine)
Central nervous system	
Seizures, depression, psychosis, headache, tremor, focal deficits	Drug-induced (cyclosporine, steroids)
	Hemolytic uremic syndrome
	Infections (*Nocardia*, *Aspergillus*)
	Malignant hypertension
Metabolic	
Hyperglycemia, electrolyte abnormalities, adrenal crisis, hyperlipidemia	Drug-induced (cyclosporine, steroids)
Vasculopathy	
Transplant coronary artery disease	Endothelial injury and repair
Malignancy	
Lymphoproliferative disorders, skin, lips, solid organs	Immunosuppression

generally reversible renal tubular dysfunction characterized by potassium retention, magnesium wasting, and diminished uric acid secretion.

Cyclosporine/tacrolimus renal failure can be exacerbated by other nephrotoxic agents (nonsteroidal antiinflammatory agents, amphotericin B, aminoglycosides, angiotensin-converting enzyme inhibitors, or angiotensin II receptor blockers) or drugs that alter the metabolism of cyclosporine/tacrolimus (Chapter 102). Other causes of renal insufficiency include heart failure and hypotension. A rare complication of cyclosporine/tacrolimus is the hemolytic uremic syndrome (Chapter 98).

Musculoskeletal System

There is a small risk of rhabdomyolysis with the use of antihyperlipidemic agents (statins and fibrates) in combination with cyclosporine. Statins should be started at doses lower than usual, and creatine kinase levels should be checked, especially if there are any symptoms of myalgias or muscle weakness. Because pravastatin is not extensively metabolized by the cytochrome P450 system, it is less likely than other statins to cause myopathy in patients taking cyclosporine.

Central Nervous System

Cyclosporine/tacrolimus can lead to drug-induced central nervous system changes, such as alterations in cognition and personality, seizures, headaches, tremors, and cortical blindness. These changes are dose-related and generally resolve with a reduction (or discontinuation) of cyclosporine/tacrolimus doses.

Transplant patients are also subject to opportunistic central nervous system infections, such as nocardiosis and aspergillosis. Malignant (cyclosporine-induced) hypertension may also present with mental status changes and headaches.

Affective disorders are common after heart transplantation. Many patients will require antidepressants and long-term follow-up with a psychiatrist or psychologist; these interventions may enhance compliance with immunosuppressive therapy, as well as quality of life.

Metabolic Disturbances

Heart transplant patients are at risk for all the usual complications of high-dose steroids. Stress-dose corticosteroids (usually 100 mg of hydrocortisone three times a day for the first day) are required to avert adrenal crisis at times of increased stress (Chapter 109).

Transplant Coronary Artery Disease

Transplant CAD, which develops at a rate of about 10% annually, results in diffuse and concentric narrowing of distal intramural coronary arteries and veins in addition to typical focal stenoses of epicardial arteries; it is the primary determinant of long-term survival following cardiac transplantation. Because of cardiac denervation following transplant surgery, the classic signs of myocardial ischemia (angina pectoris) are usually absent. This primary presenting features of transplant CAD are heart failure, ventricular dysrhythmia, and sudden death. An elevated C-reactive protein level is a strong predictor of vasculopathy (7).

As a consequence of the absence of angina pectoris, cardiac transplant patients must be routinely screened for CAD. The combination of denervation and diffuse, distal CAD makes traditional noninvasive screening tests both insensitive and nonspecific; the current recommendation is annual coronary angiography.

Primary prevention of transplant CAD includes risk factor modification, such as smoking abstinence and control of hyperlipidemia with diet and aggressive use of statins (8). Diltiazem, verapamil, and nicardipine, which alter the metabolism of cyclosporine and tacrolimus, must be used carefully. Everolimus is better than azothioprine for the prevention of cardiac-allograft vasculopathy (9).

Because of the diffuse and concentric nature of transplant CAD, coronary interventions and coronary artery bypass surgery are not as successful as in non-transplant CAD. Repeated cardiac transplantation is the only reasonable alternative for many patients with severe, uncorrectable transplant CAD, but survival after a second cardiac transplant is not as good as after a primary transplant, mainly as a consequence of increased surgical mortality and an increased probability of malignancy.

Malignancy

All organ transplant recipients are at increased risk for the development of malignancy because of immunosuppressive therapy. *Posttransplant lymphoproliferative disorders*, particularly non-Hodgkin's lymphoma, are the most common malignancies and occur in 2% of the cardiac transplant population. The peak occurrence is 1 year after transplant, but they can develop as early as 1 week after transplant. The Epstein-Barr virus genome is found in these polyclonal/monoclonal B cells. Sometimes the presentation can mimic allograft rejection because of constitutional symptoms and involvement of the myocardium (20% of cases). Although not all posttransplant lymphoproliferative disorders are "malignant" (i.e., not all are monoclonal), they behave biologically like aggressive proliferative lymphomas. Once a diagnosis is made by biopsy of the affected organ, the usual practice is to lower immunosuppression and initiate full-dose IV ganciclovir. Lymphoma chemotherapy may also be given (Chapter 94) but the prognosis of patients requiring such therapy is poor.

Malignant solid tumors also occur at a rate greater than in the general population. Cancers of sun-exposed areas (lips and skin) are common, as are cancers of the gastrointestinal tract and lung.

KEY POINTS

■ Cardiac transplantation is a viable treatment option to improve survival and quality of life in selected patients with terminal heart failure.

■ Early postoperative complications include electrical and mechanical disturbances, often caused by allograft rejection, preservation injury, tamponade, immunosuppressive drugs, electrolyte disturbances, or sinus node dysfunction.

■ Allograft rejection may present as an emergency or as a nonspecific complaint; a high degree of clinical suspicion is often required for the diagnosis to be made.

■ Treatment of allograft rejection should be guided by a transplant cardiologist. Clinical responses are demonstrated by improvement in cardiac function, abatement of dysrhythmias, and resolution of cellular infiltrate on follow-up endomyocardial biopsies.

■ Immunosuppression and rejection can lead to infection, malignancy, and transplant coronary artery disease, which is difficult to treat.

REFERENCES

1. 2003 Heart and stroke statistical update. Dallas: American Heart Association. 2003.
2. Hertz MI, Taylor DO, Trulock EP et al. The registry of the International Society for Heart and Lung Transplantation: nineteenth official report–2002. *J Heart Lung Transplant* 2002;21:950–970.
3. Mancini DM, Eisen H, Kussmaul W. Value of peak oxygen consumption for optimal timing of cardiac transplantation in ambulatory patients with heart failure. *Circulation* 1991;83:778–783.
4. Costard-Jackle A, Fowler MB. Influence of preoperative pulmonary artery pressure on mortality after heart transplantation: testing of potential reversibility of pulmonary hypertension with nitroprusside is useful in defining a high-risk group. *J Am Coll Cardiol* 1992;19:48–54.
5. Rose EA, Gelijns AC, Moskowtiz AJ, et al. Long-term use of a left ventricular assist device for end-stage heart failure. *New Engl J Med* 2001; 345:1435–1443.
6. Trento A, Czer LS, Blanche C. Surgical techniques for cardiac transplantation. *Semin Thorac Cardiovasc Surg* 1996;8:126–132.
7. Hognestad A, Endresen K, Wergeland R, et al. Plasma C-reactive protein as a marker of cardiac allograft vasculopathy in heart transplant recipients. *J Am Coll Cardiol* 2003;42:477:482.
8. Wenke K, Meiser B, Thiery J, et al. Simvastatin reduces graft vessel disease and mortality after heart transplantation: a four-year randomized trial. *Circulation* 1997;9:1398–1402.
9. Eisen HJ, Tuzcu EM, Dorent R, et al. Everolimus for the prevention of allograft rejection and vasculopathy in cardiac-transplant recipients. *N Engl J Med* 2003;349:847–858.

ADDITIONAL READING

Copeland JG, Smith RG, Arabia FA, et al. Cardiac replacement with a total artificial heart as a bridge to transplantation. *N Engl J Med* 2004;351:859–867.
Fishman JA, Rubin RH. Infection in organ-transplant recipients. *N Engl J Med* 1998;338:1741–1751.
Gammie JS, Edwards LB, Griffith BP, Pierson RN 3rd, Tsao L. Optimal timing of cardiac transplantation after ventricular assist device implantation. *J Thorac Cardiovasc Surg* 2004;127:1789–1799.
Velanovich V, Ezzat W, Horn C, Bernabei A. Surgery in heart and lung transplant patients. *Am J Surg* 2004;187:501–504.
Weis M, Von Scheidt W. Cardiac allograft vasculopathy. A review. *Circulation* 1997;96:2069–2077.

Valvular Heart Disease

41

Richard A. Lange   L. David Hillis

INTRODUCTION

Valvular heart disease affects tens of thousands of people annually in the United States and leads to more than 50,000 valve surgeries per year. It contributes to the development of heart failure, and in some subjects is responsible for sudden cardiac death. The pathophysiology and hemodynamic consequences of valvular disease are determined by the valvular abnormality and, to a lesser degree, by its underlying etiology and associated cardiac abnormalities. Of central importance in the management of the patient with valvular heart disease is a determination of the timing of surgical intervention.

AORTIC STENOSIS

Issues at the Time of Admission

Valvular aortic stenosis (AS) is most often caused by degeneration and calcification of (a) a congenitally bicuspid valve (in subjects who become symptomatic before 70 years of age) or (b) a tricuspid valve (in those who develop symptoms after age 70 years). Rheumatic disease usually causes a mixture of AS and aortic regurgitation and is almost always accompanied by mitral valve involvement. Regardless of the etiology of AS, the gradual increase in obstruction to left ventricular (LV) outflow causes compensatory LV hypertrophy, which serves to normalize LV wall stress and maintain forward output despite a stenotic valve orifice.

Clinical Presentation

The subject with AS usually is encountered initially in the ambulatory setting, often having been referred for the evaluation of a systolic murmur. The asymptomatic patient with AS (irrespective of its severity) can be followed expectantly until the appearance of symptoms (1). The cardinal symptoms of AS are angina pectoris, syncope, and heart failure. Angina pectoris is the initial symptom in about one-third of patients with AS, many of whom do not have significant atherosclerotic coronary artery disease (CAD). In these subjects, angina pectoris results from a relatively fixed myocardial oxygen supply in the setting of increased oxygen demand (caused by an increased LV wall tension). Syncope or near-syncope, usually exertional, is the initial symptom in about 15% of patients with AS. The remaining 50% of subjects with AS first note symptoms of heart failure (dyspnea, orthopnea, or fatigue). Any patient with one of these cardinal symptoms and a systolic murmur consistent with AS requires further evaluation.

Differential Diagnosis and Initial Evaluation

A severely stenotic aortic valve delays LV emptying and results in the characteristic findings on physical examination. The carotid arterial pulse is diminished in amplitude, and its upstroke is delayed (*pulsus parvus et tardus*). The precordial impulse is usually normal. Auscultation reveals the typical systolic ejection (crescendo–decrescendo) murmur at the aortic area, with radiation to the carotid arteries. Because of slow LV emptying, the murmur peaks in mid to late systole. The electrocardiogram (ECG) usually shows LV hypertrophy. On the chest radiograph, the cardiac silhouette is usually normal in shape and size. In the symptomatic patient, the findings upon physical examination should be corroborated by noninvasive testing. Two-dimensional echocardiography typically reveals concentric LV hypertrophy and a calcified aortic valve with reduced leaflet mobility. Doppler examination permits estimation of the transvalvular pressure gradient and calculation of the valve area (Table 41.1). Although invasive assessment (by catheterization) remains the gold standard for determining valve area, the echocardiographically measured valve area

TABLE 41.1

RELATIONSHIP BETWEEN AORTIC VALVE AREA AND THE SEVERITY OF AORTIC STENOSIS

Normal AVA	3 to 4 cm^2
Trivial AS	>1.3 cm^{2a}
Mild AS	1.1–1.3 cm^2
Moderate AS	0.7–1.0 cm^2
Severe AS	<0.7 cm^2
"Critical" AS	<0.5 cm^2

^{a}With a pressure gradient.
AS, aortic stenosis; AVA, aortic valve area.

correlates well with that determined at catheterization. Catheterization should be reserved for the symptomatic patient who is being considered for valve replacement. Coronary angiography is indicated in subjects over 40 years old to assess the presence or absence of CAD that may require concomitant bypass graft surgery at the time of valve replacement. At the time of catheterization, pressures on either side of the stenotic valve are recorded simultaneously (Figure 41.1), and the flow across the valve is quantified. From these data, the valve area is calculated with the Gorlin equation:

$$\text{Valve Orifice Area (cm}^2\text{)}$$
$$= \text{Flow across the Valve/Constant}$$
$$\times \text{(Mean Pressure Gradient)}^{1/2}$$

The mean pressure gradient is the average gradient during systole (for aortic or pulmonic valves) or diastole (for mitral or tricuspid valves).

The systolic ejection murmur of *hypertrophic obstructive cardiomyopathy* may be confused with that of AS. However, careful examination reveals the dynamic nature of obstruction in the patient with hypertrophic obstructive cardiomyopathy. The murmur of hypertrophic obstructive cardiomyopathy diminishes in intensity with squatting, handgrip,

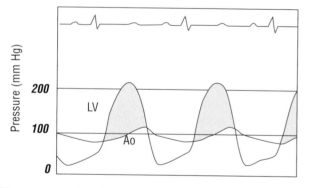

Figure 41.1. Simultaneous pressure recordings from the left ventricle (*LV*) and aorta (*Ao*) demonstrating a systolic gradient in a patient with aortic stenosis. The pressure gradient is shaded. (Redrawn from Lange RA, Hillis LD. Diagnostic and therapeutic catheterization. In Humes DG, ed. *Textbook of Internal Medicine*, 4th ed. Philadelphia: Lippincott Williams & Wilkins, 2002, p. 628, with permission.)

and other maneuvers that increase LV filling and reduce the outflow tract pressure gradient. It increases in intensity with standing and the Valsalva maneuver, since these maneuvers reduce LV filling. The murmur of AS does not change with these maneuvers, since LV outflow tract obstruction is fixed. Other infrequently encountered forms of LV outflow obstruction include congenital abnormalities, such as subvalvular membranes or supravalvular stenosis, which often resemble *valvular* AS symptomatically and on physical examination.

Indications for Hospitalization

The patient with severe AS and symptoms of unstable angina, syncope, or heart failure should be hospitalized. During hospitalization, the diagnostic evaluation should be completed and a decision reached regarding surgery.

Indications for Initial Intensive Care Unit Admission

Any patient with AS and decompensated heart failure is appropriate for admission to the ICU. Moreover, any patient whose hospitalization is complicated by a major comorbid condition (i.e., systemic infection, atrial fibrillation with a rapid ventricular response, uncontrolled diabetes mellitus, renal or hepatic failure, altered mental status) should be admitted to an ICU or step-down unit because of the risk of acute decompensation.

Initial Therapy

Occasionally, a discrete, identifiable event (i.e., a febrile illness or the onset of atrial fibrillation) precipitates symptoms of AS in a previously asymptomatic patient. The noncompliant, hypertrophied LV depends on a forceful atrial "kick" to maintain adequate filling and hence cardiac output. Because atrial tachyarrhythmias may cause hemodynamic deterioration, they should be treated promptly with pharmacologic rate control, direct current cardioversion, or both (Chapter 42). Other therapy often includes the judicious use of diuretics in the patient with AS and concomitant pulmonary congestion. Afterload-reducing agents generally are contraindicated in the patient with known AS. Similarly, exercise testing should be avoided.

Indications for Consultation

Consultation with a cardiologist is appropriate for the symptomatic patient with AS. The specialist can (a) assist with ongoing medical care, (b) suggest further studies (echocardiography, cardiac catheterization) when indicated, and (c) determine the appropriate timing for surgical intervention.

TABLE 41.2
INDICATIONS FOR VALVE SURGERY

Aortic stenosis (AS)	Onset of symptoms (angina, syncope, or heart failure) in the presence of moderate or severe AS
Aortic regurgitation (AR)	Onset of symptoms in the presence of moderate or severe AR -or- Asymptomatic LV systolic dysfunction (LV ESD^a ≥5.5 cm or LV EF^b ≤0.55)
Mitral stenosis (MS)	Symptoms refractory to medical therapy (heart failure, fatigue, systemic thromboembolism) in the presence of moderate or severe MS
Mitral regurgitation (MR)	Onset of symptoms in the presence of moderate or severe MR -or- Asymptomatic LV systolic dysfunction (LV ESD^a ≥4.5 cm or LV EF^b ≤0.65)

^{a}Left ventricular end-systolic dimension determined by transthoracic echocardiogram.
^{b}Left ventricular ejection fraction determined by radionuclide or contrast ventriculograhy.

Issues During the Course of Hospitalization

The symptomatic patient with severe AS treated *medically* has a poor prognosis, with a median survival of 5 years in those whose initial symptom is angina, 3 years in those whose symptom is syncope, and 2 years in those with heart failure. Therefore, *once symptoms develop in the patient with moderate or severe AS, valve replacement is imperative* (Table 41.2). Since balloon aortic valvuloplasty yields only temporary modest improvement in adults with AS, it is rarely indicated.

Discharge Issues

The asymptomatic patient with AS should be seen regularly and should receive antibiotic prophylaxis at the time of dental or genitourinary procedures (Table 30.10). Outpatient visits should focus on the appearance of the cardinal symptoms of AS (angina, syncope, heart failure), which, if they occur in the patient with moderate or severe AS, mandate surgery. On average, the aortic valve area decreases by about 0.1 cm^2 annually in patients with AS (2). Recent studies suggest that this rate of progression is slowed by the administration of a statin (e.g., HMG CoA reductase inhibitor) medication (3).

AORTIC REGURGITATION

Issues at the Time of Admission

Aortic regurgitation (AR) may be congenital or acquired and could be acute or chronic. The clinical presentation and management depend on the severity and chronicity of regurgitation. *Acute AR* is usually caused by (a) valve leaflet damage from infective endocarditis, (b) aortic dissection, or (c) trauma; and it usually requires urgent valve replacement.

Chronic AR may result from disease of the valve leaflets or dilatation of the ascending aorta, which distorts the leaflets and prevents their coaptation during LV diastole. Rheumatic involvement of the aortic valve frequently leads to AR, which may occur in subjects with certain systemic illnesses, including systemic lupus erythematosus, rheumatoid arthritis, ankylosing spondylitis, Whipple's disease, and Crohn's disease. Disorders that may lead to aortic dilatation and resultant AR include systemic arterial hypertension, coarctation of the aorta, bicuspid aortic valve, syphilitic aortitis, and diseases of connective tissue (i.e., Marfan syndrome, cystic medial necrosis, osteogenesis imperfecta, and idiopathic annulo-aortic ectasia).

In the patient with chronic AR, the LV is exposed to diastolic volume overload, which results in the development of LV hypertrophy and chamber dilatation. Early in the process, LV end-systolic volume is normal; therefore, LV stroke volume and ejection fraction are greatly increased. Myocardial function remains normal until relatively late in the disease process, at which time the LV begins to fail. With acute AR, the ventricle does not have time to dilate; therefore, the individual with acute AR has a markedly elevated left ventricular diastolic pressure, which usually leads to severe pulmonary vascular congestion. Severe, acute AR may cause premature closure of the mitral valve during diastole, because LV and LA pressures equalize before the end of diastole; in this situation, net forward cardiac output is markedly reduced. As a result, urgent valve replacement usually is indicated in the patient with severe, acute AR.

Clinical Presentation

Similar to the patient with AS, the patient with AR may be asymptomatic and come to medical attention for the evaluation of a murmur. In the asymptomatic individual with normal LV systolic function, endocarditis prophylaxis

(Table 30.10), and careful clinical follow-up are sufficient (4). Often, early symptoms of AR are attributable to the increased LV stroke volume and consist of an awareness of a forceful heartbeat and prominent carotid arterial pulsations. Eventually, the patient with AR notes symptoms of heart failure (dyspnea, orthopnea, and fatigue). Angina, syncope, and sudden death are less common in patients with AR than in those with AS.

Differential Diagnosis and Initial Evaluation

In the subject with chronic AR, the characteristic findings on physical examination include bounding peripheral arterial pulses with a rapid upstroke (from the increased LV stroke volume) and rapid runoff (from regurgitation into the LV). The precordial impulse is hyperdynamic and displaced inferiorly and laterally. Auscultation reveals a high-pitched, decrescendo murmur commencing immediately after S_2 and extending through part or all of diastole. A systolic ejection murmur in the absence of valvular stenosis is caused by the markedly increased LV stroke volume. An apical diastolic rumble (the Austin Flint murmur) represents turbulent flow across the mitral valve with its anterior leaflet held partially closed by aortic regurgitant flow.

The ECG typically shows LV hypertrophy. The chest radiograph reveals an enlarged cardiac silhouette and a dilated ascending aorta. Echocardiography permits a determination of LV dimensions during diastole and systole, an assessment of LV systolic function, and measurement of ascending aortic width. Doppler echocardiography, which can measure the regurgitant jet width at the valve orifice and the regurgitant jet volume (into the LV), permits an estimate of the severity of AR. Invasive evaluation by catheterization includes aortography (to assess the severity of AR) and left ventriculography (to determine LV volumes and function). The presence and severity of AR may be evaluated qualitatively by aortography, with which the amount of radiographic contrast material that regurgitates into the LV during diastole can be observed (Table 41.3). To obtain a quantitative assessment of the severity of AR, the regurgitant fraction (RF) can be calculated. The RF is the percentage of total angiographic LV output that regurgitates into the LV:

$$RF = (\text{Angiographic Cardiac Output} - \text{Forward Cardiac Output})/\text{Angiographic Cardiac Output}$$

Typically, valvular regurgitation with an RF of 0.6 or more is considered to be severe; 0.40–0.59, moderate; 0.20–0.39, mild; and below 0.2, trivial.

Indications for Hospitalization

Although heart failure often can be treated in the outpatient setting, hospitalization is required for the subject with refractory heart failure. Heart failure caused by moderate-to-severe AR is an indication for prompt evaluation for valve replacement.

Indications for Initial Intensive Care Unit Admission

Heart failure resistant to standard medical therapy (diuretics and vasodilators) is often seen in severe acute AR and may require invasive hemodynamic monitoring and intravenous sodium nitroprusside (for afterload reduction) as temporizing measures before valve replacement. These measures are rarely necessary in the patient with chronic AR, whose LV has adapted gradually to the altered loading conditions.

Initial Therapy

Initial therapy of the patient with chronic AR should include diuretics and afterload reduction (with hydralazine,

TABLE 41.3

RELATIONSHIP BETWEEN APPEARANCE OF REGURGITANT CONTRAST AFTER AORTOGRAPHY AND SEVERITY OF AORTIC REGURGITATION

Angiographic grade	Definition[a]	Descriptor
1+	Regurgitant contrast clears LV with each systole	Trivial
2+	Regurgitant contrast does not clear from LV; LV density < aortic	Mild
3+	Regurgitant contrast does not clear from LV; LV density = aortic	Moderate
4+	Regurgitant contrast does not clear from LV; LV density > aortic or LV fills (from aorta) in one diastole	Severe

[a] Contrast is injected into ascending aorta (aortogram) immediately above the aortic valve. Incompetent aortic valve permits regurgitation of contrast into left ventricle (LV).

an angiotensin-converting enzyme inhibitor, or a dihydropyridine-class calcium channel antagonist). Chronic afterload reduction has been shown to improve symptoms, reduce the need for hospitalization, and delay the need for valve replacement in patients with chronic AR.

Although the etiology of chronic AR is not usually important for guiding therapy, it is critical that the patient with acute AR be evaluated for possible infective endocarditis. Symptomatic acute AR is generally an indication for urgent surgery. In patients with endocarditis, however, the indications for surgery must be balanced against the benefits of administering antibiotics before surgery (Chapter 71).

Issues for Early Consultation

The cardiologist can assist with the choice of initial medical therapy, further evaluation (i.e., echocardiography, cardiac catheterization), and the decision to operate or to continue medical therapy. Early consultation may reduce hospitalization and procedural costs and improve outcome.

Issues During the Course of Hospitalization

The key issue during hospitalization is the determination of the need for and timing of surgical intervention. Unlike valvular stenosis, valvular regurgitation may progress insidiously and may cause LV compromise before symptoms develop. In general, the symptomatic patient with moderate-to-severe AR should be considered for valve surgery. In addition, the asymptomatic patient with moderate-to-severe AR and evidence of LV systolic dysfunction should be referred for evaluation and probable valve replacement (Table 41.2) (4).

Discharge Issues

The asymptomatic patient with AR and normal LV systolic function can be followed expectantly, with periodic echocardiographic assessments of LV function and chamber dimensions. The onset of symptoms or a deterioration in LV systolic function (manifested as an increased LV end-systolic dimension or a decreased LV ejection fraction) should prompt cardiac consultation with an eye toward valve replacement. Surgical intervention before the development of severe LV systolic dysfunction is imperative.

MITRAL STENOSIS

Issues at the Time of Admission

Mitral stenosis (MS) is almost always the result of previous rheumatic carditis. The mitral valve leaflets thicken and become scarred and fused at the commissures, and the chordae tendineae shorten and become fused. Eventually, the valve leaflets become calcified and immobile. Symptoms attributable to MS usually do not develop until 15–20 years after the initial rheumatic injury.

Clinical Presentation

The patient with MS usually first notes dyspnea or fatigue. Dyspnea results from an elevated left atrial (LA) pressure, with resultant pulmonary congestion. Fatigue is caused by failure to augment cardiac output appropriately during exertion. When MS is mild, the patient may experience dyspnea only in association with a tachycardia (i.e., during physical exertion, pregnancy, infection, or the appearance of atrial fibrillation). Tachycardia shortens the LV diastolic filling period (when flow across the mitral valve occurs), thereby increasing LA pressure. As the stenosis becomes more severe, dyspnea occurs with less exertion and eventually at rest. Other, less common symptoms of MS include chest pain, hemoptysis, sequelae of systemic arterial thromboembolism, and hoarseness resulting from compression of the recurrent laryngeal nerve by an enlarged LA (Ortner's syndrome).

Differential Diagnosis Initial Evaluation

In the patient with MS, the carotid arterial pulsation usually is normal and the precordial impulse is normal. A right ventricular (RV) lift may be palpated if concomitant pulmonary hypertension is present. Auscultation reveals an opening snap (OS) usually between 0.08 and 0.12 seconds after S_2, followed by a diastolic murmur. The opening snap is caused by sudden tensing of the mitral valve leaflets after the cusps have completed their opening excursion. A short A_2–OS interval suggests severe MS. The diastolic murmur of MS is low-pitched, rumbling, and heard best with the bell of the stethoscope at the cardiac apex with the patient in the left lateral decubitus position. S_1 is typically loud, though it softens if the valve becomes progressively fixed and regurgitant. S_2 is normal initially, but P_2 becomes louder (and may be louder than A_2) as pulmonary hypertension develops. In the subject with pulmonary hypertension, a Graham Steell murmur of pulmonic regurgitation may be present.

In the patient with MS, the ECG frequently shows atrial fibrillation. LA enlargement is noted in most subjects with severe MS who are in sinus rhythm, RV hypertrophy may be seen in the setting of pulmonary hypertension, and the chest radiograph usually reveals LA enlargement. With pulmonary hypertension, the pulmonary arteries, RV, and right atrium (RA) may be enlarged. Echocardiography reveals LA enlargement and a thickened and usually calcified mitral valve with decreased leaflet mobility. LV systolic function is usually normal but may be mildly depressed in some patients. The severity of MS (Table 41.4) can be

TABLE 41.4

RELATIONSHIP BETWEEN MITRAL VALVE AREA AND SEVERITY OF MITRAL STENOSIS

Normal MVA	4 to 6 cm
Trivial MS	>2.0 cm^{2a}
Mild MS	1.5–2.0 cm^2
Moderate MS	1.0–1.5 cm^2
Severe MS	<1.0 cm^2

^{a} With a pressure gradient.
MS, mitral stenosis; MVA, mitral valve area.

determined by (a) planimetry of the valve orifice by transthoracic echocardiography or (b) measurement of the decay of the transvalvular pressure gradient (pressure half-time method) by Doppler echocardiography. In addition, echocardiography allows one to assess the suitability of the valve for *percutaneous mitral balloon valvuloplasty* (PMBV), in that certain echocardiographic features of the mitral valve and its subvalvular apparatus (i.e., leaflet thickening, leaflet mobility and calcification, and subvalvular thickening) influence the results of PMBV (5). Catheterization permits the simultaneous measurement of LA (often measured as pulmonary capillary wedge) and LV pressures (pressure gradient across the valve) (Figure 41.2), a determination of cardiac output, and, therefore, calculation of the valve area by the Gorlin equation (see Aortic Stenosis). In addition, the presence and severity of concomitant mitral regurgitation (MR), aortic valvular disease, and CAD can be assessed.

Indications for Hospitalization

The patient with symptomatic MS requires hospitalization only if outpatient therapy is inadequate to control

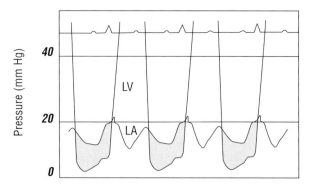

Figure 41.2. Simultaneous pressure recordings from the left atrium (*LA*) and left ventricle (*LV*) demonstrating a diastolic gradient in a patient with mitral stenosis. The gradient is shaded. (Redrawn from Lange RA, Hillis LD. Diagnostic and therapeutic catheterization. In: Humes DG, ed. *Textbook of Internal Medicine*, 4th ed. Philadelphia: Lippincott Williams & Wilkins, 2002, p. 628, with permission.)

pulmonary congestion or if complications such as atrial fibrillation with a rapid ventricular response develop. Most subjects with dyspnea (from pulmonary congestion) and fatigue (from a low cardiac output) can be evaluated and treated as outpatients.

Indications for Initial Intensive Care Unit Admission

The patient with MS rarely has such severe pulmonary congestion that ICU admission is required. However, intensive care may be required for pulmonary edema or markedly diminished cardiac output, either of which may be caused by atrial arrhythmias.

Initial Therapy

Pulmonary congestion is treated with diuretics. Maintenance of sinus rhythm is important in patients with MS, in whom a normal atrial "kick" may account for 20%–25% of cardiac output. In subjects with atrial fibrillation, the ventricular response rate should be controlled (Chapter 42). Electrical cardioversion to sinus rhythm can be attempted after the patient has received anticoagulant therapy for at least 3–4 weeks or if a transesophageal echocardiogram shows no evidence of a left atrial thrombus. The restoration of sinus rhythm often improves symptoms and reduces the risk of systemic thromboembolisim. Following successful cardioversion, the patient with MS and an enlarged left atrium should remain on chronic anticoagulant therapy indefinitely.

Issues for Early Consultation

Consultation with a cardiologist is appropriate as part of the care of any patient with symptomatic MS. As with patients with other valvular abnormalities, the cardiologist can help to determine initial medical therapy, appropriate diagnostic studies, and the need for nonmedical intervention (surgery or PMBV).

Issues During the Course of Hospitalization

The subject with MS often first seeks medical attention with pulmonary congestion associated with an inciting event, such as the onset of atrial fibrillation, pregnancy, or an infection. Unlike patients with the valvular abnormalities discussed previously, *the patient with MS should be managed medically until symptoms are limiting* (Table 41.2). In these "medically refractory" subjects, the choice of surgery or percutaneous valvuloplasty should be discussed with the consulting cardiologist. In general, PMBV is most efficacious in younger patients with minimal valvular calcification. It should be avoided in the patient with LA thrombus, heavy valvular calcification, subvalvular thickening, or moderate or severe MR. If PMBV is not available or is contraindicated, mitral valve surgery (commissurotomy or valve replacement) should be performed.

Discharge Issues

Outpatient therapy includes endocarditis prophylaxis at the time of dental and genitourinary procedures (Table 30.10) and treatment of pulmonary congestion, when present. In addition, because the subject with MS and atrial fibrillation or an enlarged LA is particularly prone to LA thrombus formation, prophylactic warfarin anticoagulation to an International Normalized Ratio (INR) of 2.5–3.5 is indicated. The patient with atrial fibrillation may benefit from receiving a β-adrenergic or calcium channel blocking agent to slow the ventricular response and increase the LV diastolic filling time, thereby decreasing LA pressure and diminishing pulmonary congestion. Symptoms that persist despite therapy should prompt referral to a cardiologist for consideration of balloon valvuloplasty or surgery.

MITRAL REGURGITATION

Issues at the Time of Admission

Mitral regurgitation (MR) may be caused by any disorder that affects one or more of the components of the mitral valve apparatus, including the annulus, leaflets, chordae tendineae, and papillary muscles. In the United States, the most common cause of isolated, chronic MR is myxomatous valvular degeneration. Chronic MR also may result from rheumatic injury, rupture of the chordae tendineae, and papillary muscle dysfunction or rupture. LV enlargement of any cause results in annular dilatation, which may lead to incomplete leaflet coaptation and resultant MR. In addition, chronic MR may occur as a result of certain congenital or heritable diseases (i.e., Marfan syndrome, Ehlers-Danlos syndrome, endocardial cushion defects). *Acute MR* most often results from (a) ruptured chordae tendineae (due to myxomatous degeneration, infective endocarditis, trauma, or rheumatic disease), (b) papillary muscle dysfunction or rupture (caused by myocardial ischemia or infarction), or (c) leaflet damage caused by infective endocarditis.

When MR is present, total LV output consists of forward output (from the LV to the systemic arterial circulation) and regurgitant flow (from the LV to the LA). Forward output is maintained by compensatory LV dilatation and hypertrophy. The patient with *chronic MR* is often asymptomatic for years. Eventually, the chronic diastolic LV volume overload causes symptoms of pulmonary congestion or asymptomatic LV systolic dysfunction, which is signaled by an increased LV end-systolic dimension or a decreased LV ejection fraction.

Clinical Presentation

The patient with chronic MR may be asymptomatic for months or even years. The initial symptom is usually dyspnea (caused by pulmonary congestion) or fatigue (caused by a decreased forward output). As the disease progresses, the patient notes dyspnea with less exertion, orthopnea, and paroxysmal nocturnal dyspnea. In some patients with chronic MR, pulmonary hypertension develops, which may lead to right-sided heart failure, with peripheral edema, ascites, and hepatic congestion.

Differential Diagnosis and Initial Evaluation

On physical examination, the patient with MR has a normal carotid arterial upstroke. The precordial impulse is hyperdynamic (because of an increased LV stroke volume) and displaced inferolaterally. The typical MR murmur is holosystolic, blowing in quality, and heard best at the apex, with radiation to the axilla. There is no correlation between the intensity of the murmur and the severity of MR. Even a relatively soft murmur deserves further evaluation (with echocardiography) if the patient has pulmonary congestion, systemic arterial hypotension, or evidence of a diminished cardiac output. The murmur of MR may be confused with that of (a) a ventricular septal defect, which is heard best along the left sternal border and is often accompanied by a palpable thrill; (b) tricuspid regurgitation, which is heard best at the left lower sternal border and increases in intensity with inspiration; and (c) AS, especially in the elderly or in patients whose MR is due to dysfunction of the posterior mitral valve leaflet.

The ECG reveals LA enlargement in most patients with chronic MR and LV hypertrophy in about a third. Frequently, the patient is in atrial fibrillation. The chest radiograph demonstrates LA and LV dilatation. Two-dimensional echocardiography (a) reveals LA enlargement, (b) documents LV chamber dimensions and function, and (c) helps to define the underlying pathophysiology of MR (i.e., ruptured chordae tendineae or papillary muscle, mitral valve prolapse, vegetation of infective endocarditis). Doppler echo permits quantification of the MR. Invasive evaluation by catheterization allows an assessment of the severity of MR by left ventriculography (Table 41.5) and determination of a regurgitant fraction (see Aortic Regurgitation). Moreover, left ventriculographic volumes permit an assessment of LV systolic function. Finally, coronary angiography can be performed; in general, it should be reserved for patients being considered for valve surgery.

Indications for Hospitalization

Most patients with chronic MR can be managed in the ambulatory setting. As noted, the most common initial symptom is dyspnea (caused by pulmonary congestion), which

TABLE 41.5

RELATIONSHIP BETWEEN APPEARANCE OF REGURGITANT CONTRAST AFTER VENTRICULOGRAPHY AND SEVERITY OF MITRAL REGURGITATION

Angiographic grade	Definition[a]	Descriptor
1+	Regurgitant contrast clears LA with each beat	Trivial
2+	Regurgitant contrast does not clear LA; LA density <LV	Mild
3+	Regurgitant contrast does not clear LA; LA density = LV	Moderate
4+	Regurgitant contrast does not clear from LA; LA density > LV or LA fills (from LV) in one systole or contrast refluxes into pulmonary veins	Severe

[a] Contrast is injected into left ventricle (LV) (ventriculogram). Incompetent mitral valve permits regurgitation of contrast into left atrium (LA).

is treated with diuretics, digitalis, and afterload reduction. Once the patient with MR is symptomatic, evaluation of the severity of MR and its effect on LV systolic function is imperative (6). Referral for possible surgical intervention is indicated in patients with (a) persistent symptoms and normal LV systolic function or (b) evidence of mild or moderate LV systolic dysfunction even without symptoms (Table 41.2).

Indications for Initial Intensive Care Unit Admission

The patient with MR due to rupture of chordae tendineae (caused most commonly by trauma or infective endocarditis), papillary muscle dysfunction or rupture (from myocardial ischemia or infarction), or leaflet injury (from infective endocarditis) often has severe pulmonary congestion and, therefore, may require urgent intervention. On physical examination, the patient is tachypneic and often prefers the upright to the supine position. The acute process does not permit the development of LA enlargement and alterations in the pulmonary vasculature; as a result, LA pressure is markedly elevated. Acute MR usually requires prompt surgical intervention.

Initial Therapy

The patient with acute MR may be supported temporarily with inotropic agents and afterload reduction (vasodilators, intraaortic balloon counterpulsation, or both). Echocardiography should be performed preoperatively in an attempt to define the valvular pathology, assess reparability, determine LV function, and document other cardiac abnormalities. Coronary angiography should be performed in patients over 40 years of age or in those with previous myocardial infarction or risk factors for atherosclerosis. Subjects with severe MR and pulmonary edema require

diuretic therapy and afterload reduction (with sodium nitroprusside or intraaortic balloon counterpulsation) to alleviate pulmonary congestion. In the patient with only mildly decompensated heart failure, the combination of digitalis, diuretics, and angiotensin-converting enzyme inhibitors may render him or her asymptomatic. Importantly, no large, long-term studies demonstrating the efficacy of angiotensin-converting enzyme inhibitors or other vasodilators in patients with chronic MR have been performed. Therefore, once symptoms appear or LV systolic dysfunction is noted, surgery is the most appropriate therapy (Table 41.2) (7).

Issues for Early Consultation

For the patient with MR, the cardiologist can assist with the selection of appropriate initial medical therapy, further evaluation, and the decision regarding referral for valve surgery.

Issues During the Course of Hospitalization

Perioperative morbidity and mortality are influenced by the patient's clinical and hemodynamic condition, LV systolic function, the presence of concomitant CAD, and other comorbidities (renal, hepatic, or pulmonary disease). In addition, the ability to repair—rather than to replace—the valve has prognostic import (8). Until Carpentier and Duran popularized mitral valve repair, valve replacement with chordal transection was the only surgical option for the patient with MR. Nowadays, mitral valve repair (with or without an annuloplasty ring) or valve replacement with chordal preservation have improved short- and long-term outcomes in patients requiring mitral valve surgery. Patients who undergo valve repair do not require long-term anticoagulation if they remain in sinus rhythm, and they avoid possible late prosthetic valve dysfunction. In addition, chordal and papillary muscle-sparing procedures help to maintain normal LV geometry and systolic function postoperatively.

Discharge Issues

Similar to patients with AR, the asymptomatic patient with MR should be seen and evaluated periodically for the development of symptoms or evidence of LV systolic dysfunction. Endocarditis prophylaxis should be administered for dental and other procedures (Table 30.10).

TRICUSPID REGURGITATION

Issues at the Time of Admission

Tricuspid regurgitation (TR) most often results from dilatation of the RV and, hence, the tricuspid annulus. Annular dilatation prevents normal leaflet coaptation and results in functional or "secondary" TR. RV enlargement usually is secondary to pulmonary hypertension from MS, LV failure, cor pulmonale, or pulmonary embolic disease. Other etiologies of TR include rheumatic valvular disease, endocarditis, tricuspid valve prolapse, Ebstein's anomaly, phentermine–fenfluramine toxicity, and carcinoid heart disease (9).

Clinical Presentation

In the absence of pulmonary hypertension, TR is generally well tolerated. However, when pulmonary hypertension and TR coexist, cardiac output declines, and right-sided venous congestion ensues.

Differential Diagnosis and Initial Evaluation

Physical examination reveals jugular venous distention with prominent *v* waves and a prominent *y* descent. The RV is hyperdynamic, as reflected by an RV lift. The liver is often enlarged and tender; it may even be pulsatile. Ascites and peripheral edema may be present. Auscultation reveals a high-pitched, pansystolic murmur heard best at the left lower sternal border. The murmur increases in intensity with inspiration (Carvallo sign). A right-sided S_3 may be heard, and P_2 is prominent in the setting of pulmonary hypertension. If tricuspid valve prolapse is present, a midsystolic click may be audible. Holosystolic murmurs that may be mistaken for TR include those of MR (see Mitral Regurgitation) and ventricular septal defect. With TR, the ECG may show an incomplete right bundle branch block, and the patient frequently is in atrial fibrillation. Chest radiography reveals distention of the caval and azygous venous systems. Echocardiography permits (a) detection and assessment of the severity of TR, (b) estimation of pulmonary

arterial systolic pressure, (c) assessment of RV function, and (d) assessment of RV and RA size. In addition, echocardiography may identify the etiology of TR (i.e., valvular prolapse, vegetation in the case of endocarditis, valvular thickening with carcinoid). At catheterization, RA pressure is elevated, increases with inspiration, and may even qualitatively resemble RV pressure if the TR is severe.

Issues During the Course of Hospitalization

In the absence of pulmonary hypertension, TR usually does not require surgery. The patient is often given diuretics to relieve peripheral venous congestion. Effective treatment of the underlying pulmonary hypertension (Chapter 59) usually leads to an improvement in secondary tricuspid regurgitation. When surgery is required, valve repair can be performed with or without an annuloplasty ring. When valve replacement is required, a bioprosthesis (rather than a mechanical valve) is preferred, as the relatively low velocity of flow in the right heart chambers increases the likelihood of thrombus formation on a mechanical valve. Because of the relatively low right-sided pressures, tricuspid valve bioprostheses have excellent longevity (10).

PROSTHETIC HEART VALVES

When a patient with a prosthetic heart valve develops fever or heart failure, a thorough evaluation of the prosthesis is mandatory. Prosthetic heart valves may be bioprosthetic or mechanical; the latter, in turn, may be composed of a tilting disc (single or bileaflet) or ball-in-cage. Central to the assessment of prosthetic valve function is an understanding of the normal auscultatory findings for each valve type in the mitral or aortic position (10). In patients in whom prosthetic valve dysfunction is suspected, several imaging modalities may be used to assess valve function. In subjects with mechanical valves, cinefluoroscopy is a simple, inexpensive technique for assessing prosthetic structural integrity. Diminished motion of the disk or ball suggests obstruction by thrombus or tissue ingrowth, whereas excessive tilt ("rocking") of the base ring is consistent with partial dehiscence of the valve's sewing ring. Cinefluoroscopy cannot be used to visualize the leaflets of bioprosthetic valves. Two-dimensional transthoracic echocardiography can be used to assess sewing-ring stability and leaflet motion of bioprosthetic valves, but mechanical valves are often difficult to visualize because of intense echo reverberations from the metal. Transesophageal echocardiography may better visualize the mitral valve, but assessment of a prosthesis in the aortic position may be limited (because of echo reverberations), especially when another prosthesis is present in the mitral position.

New-onset heart failure is an important complication following implantation of a prosthetic valve. Of the various causes of heart failure, *prosthetic valve thrombosis* is potentially catastrophic; it is usually manifested as acute hemodynamic deterioration, pulmonary congestion, poor peripheral perfusion, or systemic thromboembolism. Valve thrombosis most often results from inadequate anticoagulant therapy; it affects mechanical valves more often than bioprostheses and involves those placed in the mitral position more commonly than the aortic. Once the diagnosis of valve thrombosis has been established, intravenous heparin therapy should be instituted promptly. More aggressive therapy (valve replacement or thrombolysis) is indicated when the thrombus burden is large (more than 5 mm in diameter) or when the patient does not improve with systemic heparinization alone.

In the subject with a prosthetic heart valve, other causes of heart failure include (a) perivalvular leakage (caused by spontaneous dehiscence of the suture line or endocarditis), (b) structural failure of the prosthetic valve (caused, for example, by disc dislodgement or ball fracture of mechanical valves or leaflet avulsion of a bioprosthesis), and (c) bioprosthesis leaflet damage (from thickening and retraction or endocarditis). Structural failure of a mechanical prosthesis is rare. One exception, the Bjork-Shiley single tilting disc valve, was withdrawn from use after reports of fracture of the valve ring structure, resulting in displacement and embolization of the disk. Structural failure of bioprosthetic valves necessitates replacement of 20%–30% over the ensuing 10–15 years. Most patients whose valves fail have severe regurgitation caused by a tear or rupture of one or more of the valve cusps, which have become calcified and rigid; only an occasional subject develops severe bioprosthetic valve stenosis. The incidence of bioprosthetic valve failure is particularly high in patients under 40 years old and in those with mitral prostheses. The magnitude of valve dysfunction can be assessed by echocardiography or catheterization.

Prosthetic valve infection occurs at some time in 3%–6% of patients. *"Early"* endocarditis (occurring less than 60 days after valve replacement) usually results from perioperative bacteremia that develops from skin or wound infections or contaminated intravascular devices. The most common offending organisms, therefore, are *Staphylococcus epidermidis*, *S. aureus*, gram-negative bacteria, diphtheroids, and fungi. *"Late"* prosthetic valve endocarditis (occurring more than 60 days postoperatively) is usually caused by the organisms responsible for native valve endocarditis, most often streptococci. The risk of endocarditis is similar in patients with mechanical and bioprosthetic valves.

Long Term Follow-up of Prosthetic Valves

The patient with a prosthetic valve should be seen and evaluated regularly to assess the presence of new symptoms or murmurs. The presence of either warrants a complete and thorough evaluation, including an echocardiogram. All patients with prosthetic valves should receive endocarditis prophylaxis for dental or other procedures. The possibility of prosthetic valve endocarditis should be entertained in the patient with an unexplained or persistent fever and should prompt the acquisition of several blood samples for culture prior to the administration of antibiotic therapy (Chapter 71). The causative organism can be identified by routine blood culture in over 90% of patients who have not recently received antibiotics. In addition to fever, other findings of prosthetic valve endocarditis include a new or changing murmur, systemic embolization, and heart failure. All patients with a mechanical valve should receive chronic anticoagulant therapy, with the precise target INR determined by the type of valve and its position (10).

COST CONSIDERATIONS AND RESOURCE USE

The asymptomatic patient with valvular heart disease can be followed in the outpatient setting until the onset of symptoms or the appearance of early, often asymptomatic, LV systolic dysfunction. At such time, the decision to continue medical therapy or to pursue surgical intervention should be made. Consultation with a cardiologist is the appropriate next step. The cardiologist can (a) provide guidance concerning medical therapy that may reduce the need for hospitalization and delay valve surgery; (b) help to determine which diagnostic studies are indicated, thereby avoiding costly and unwarranted testing; and (c) assist in the decision of when to operate by weighing the risks and potential benefits of surgery.

KEY POINTS

- The asymptomatic patient with *aortic stenosis* may be followed expectantly until symptoms develop. Once angina, syncope, near-syncope, or heart failure develops in the patient with moderate-to-severe aortic stenosis, valve replacement should be performed promptly.
- Symptomatic patients with *aortic regurgitation* should undergo valve replacement. Asymptomatic patients should be treated with afterload-reducing agents to slow disease progression. In addition, the patient should be monitored for evidence of LV systolic dysfunction, and surgical correction should be pursued if this develops.
- Patients with *mitral stenosis* should be managed medically until symptoms persist despite such therapy. Anticoagulation should be maintained to reduce the risk of systemic embolization.
- Similar to patients with aortic regurgitation, those with *mitral regurgitation* should undergo mitral valve surgery for the relief of symptoms or deterioration of left ventricular systolic function (even without symptoms).

Advances in mitral valve surgery, including valve repair and valve replacement with chordal preservation, have improved perioperative and long-term outcomes in patients with mitral regurgitation.

■ *Tricuspid regurgitation* is usually caused by right ventricular dilatation (functional or "secondary" tricuspid regurgitation) resulting from pulmonary hypertension associated with mitral stenosis, left ventricular failure, cor pulmonale, or pulmonary embolic disease. In the absence of pulmonary hypertension, tricuspid regurgitation usually does not require surgical therapy.

REFERENCES

1. Rosenhek R, Binder T, Porenta G, et al. Predictors of outcome in severe, asymptomatic aortic stenosis. *N Engl J Med* 2000;343: 611–617.
2. Bahler RC, Desser DR, Finkelhor RS, et al. Factors leading to progression of valvular aortic stenosis. *Am J Cardiol* 1999;84: 1044–1048.
3. Novaro GM, Tiong IY, Pearce GL, et al. Effect of hydroxymethylglutaryl coenzyme A reductase inhibitors on the progression of calcific aortic stenosis. *Circulation* 2001;104:2205–2209.
4. Dujardin KS, Enriquez-Sarano M, Schaff HV, et al. Mortality and morbidity of aortic regurgitation in clinical practice: a long-term follow-up study. *Circulation* 1999;99:1851–1857.
5. Palacios IF, Sanchez PL, Harrell LC, et al. Which patients benefit from percutaneous mitral balloon valvuloplasty? Prevalvuloplasty and postvalvuloplasty variables that predict long-term outcome. *Circulation* 2002;105:1465–1471.
6. Otto, CM. Evaluation and management of chronic mitral regurgitation. *N Engl J Med* 2001;345:740–746.
7. Bonow RO, Carabello B, deLeon AC Jr, et al. ACC/AHA guidelines for the management of patients with valvular heart disease: a report of the American College of Cardiology/American Heart Association Task Force on Practice Guidelines (Committee on Management of Patients with Valvular Heart Disease). *J Am Coll Cardiol* 1998;32:1486–1588.
8. Yau TM, El-Ghoneimi YA, Armstrong S, et al. Mitral valve repair and replacement for rheumatic disease. *J Thorac Cardiovasc Surg* 2000;119:53–60.
9. Westberg G, Wangberg B, Ahlman H, et al. Prediction of prognosis by echocardiography in patients with midgut carcinoid syndrome. *Br J Surg* 2001;88:865–872.
10. Vongpatanasin W, Hillis LD, Lange RA. Prosthetic heart valves. *N Engl J Med* 1996;335:407–416.

ADDITIONAL READING

Carabello BA. Aortic stenosis. *N Engl J Med* 2002;346:677–682.

Enriquez-Sarano M, Tajik AJ. Aortic regurgitation. *N Engl J Med* 2004;351:1539–1546.

Rahimtoola SH. The year in valvular heart disease. *J Am Coll Cardiol* 2004;43:491–504.

Rahimtoola SH. Choice of prosthetic heart valve for adult patients. *J Am Coll Cardiol* 2003;41:893–904.

Rahimtoola SH, Durairaj A, Mehra A, et al. Current evaluation and management of patients with mitral stenosis. *Circulation* 2002; 106:1183–1188.

Atrial Fibrillation, Atrial Flutter, and Other Supraventricular Tachyarrhythmias

42

Leonard I. Ganz

INTRODUCTION

Supraventricular tachyarrhythmias (SVTs) frequently cause emergency department visits and hospital admissions, and they also occur commonly in patients hospitalized for other reasons. SVTs require atrial or atrioventricular (AV) junctional tissue for their initiation and maintenance, whereas ventricular tachyarrhythmias require only ventricular tissue for their initiation and maintenance (Chapter 43). SVTs may be classified according to whether AV junctional or only atrial tissue is critical to the tachycardia (Table 42.1).

TACHYCARDIAS ARISING IN ATRIAL TISSUE

In *atrial fibrillation* (AF), the most common SVT, the orderly sequence of sinus rhythm (SR) is replaced by rapidly firing foci and/or multiple reentry circuits in the atria that bombard the AV node, resulting in a rapid and irregular ventricular rate. In some patients, the AF has a "focal" origin, typically in the pulmonary veins near where they enter the left atrium. In *atrial flutter*, a single macroreentry circuit in the right atrium inscribes regular, sawtooth flutter waves.

AF and atrial flutter may be *paroxysmal*, with episodes that revert spontaneously, or *persistent*, with episodes that persist unless the patient is cardioverted to sinus rhythm. If efforts at cardioversion are unsuccessful, AF is considered *permanent*. *Atrial tachycardia* (AT), also called ectopic or unifocal AT, occurs if an isolated atrial focus fires at a rate substantially higher than that of the sinus node. In *multifocal AT* (MAT), patients have at least three different P-wave morphologies with irregular ventricular rates greater than 100 beats/min.

TACHYCARDIAS ARISING IN THE AV JUNCTION

Most regular SVTs require the participation of the AV node. Two mechanisms, *AV nodal reentrant tachycardia* (AVNRT) and *AV reentrant tachycardia* (AVRT), constitute the majority of what are called paroxysmal supraventricular tachycardias (PSVT) (1, 2). In AVNRT, dual AV nodal pathway physiology provides the substrate for a reentry circuit involving the AV node (Figure 42.1). In AVRT, an accessory pathway, which connects an atrium and corresponding ventricle, can serve as a limb in a reentry circuit (Figure 42.2). Some patients with this arrhythmia manifest

TABLE 42.1

CLASSIFICATION OF SUPRAVENTRICULAR TACHYARRHYTHMIAS

Atrial	A-V Junctional
Sinus tachycardia	A-V nodal reentrant tachycardia
Atrial fibrillation	A-V reentrant tachycardia
Atrial flutter	Junctional ectopic tachycardia
Atrial tachycardia	Nonparoxysmal junctional tachycardia
Multifocal atrial tachycardia	

A-V, atrioventricular.

ventricular preexcitation, known as the *Wolff-Parkinson-White* (WPW) *syndrome.* In other patients, the accessory connection is concealed during sinus rhythm and becomes evident only during an SVT. AVRT has two forms, orthodromic and antidromic. In orthodromic AVRT, antegrade conduction is over the AV node, resulting in a narrow QRS complex, and retrograde conduction goes up the accessory pathway. These accessory pathways can be manifest or concealed accessory pathways. Much less common is an-

tidromic AVRT, in which the circuit is reversed, resulting in a wide and bizarre QRS complex. This phenomenon occurs only in WPW syndrome. Patients with WPW syndrome merit special attention because of the possibility of extremely rapid ventricular rates during AF or atrial flutter and the risk that these rhythms will deteriorate into ventricular fibrillation.

PREVALENCE AND ASSOCIATED CONDITIONS

Associated cardiovascular disease, including hypertension, is encountered frequently in patients with AF. The prevalence of AF increases with age as approximately 2%–5% of patients in their seventies and 4%–10% in their eighties have AF. Fewer epidemiologic data exist regarding other forms of supraventricular arrhythmia. PSVT may be seen in patients of all ages, both in the absence and presence of structural heart disease. Overall, the prevalence of PSVT is on the order of several per thousand; the prevalence of the WPW pattern on an electrocardiogram (ECG) is similar.

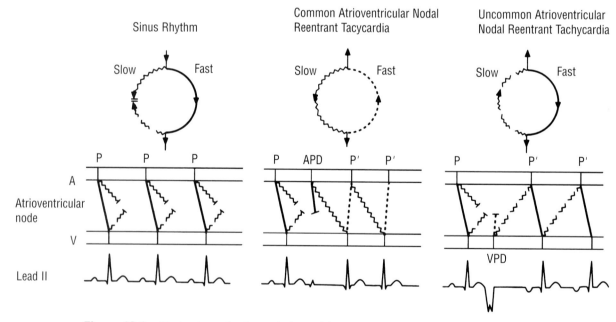

Figure 42.1. Mechanisms of atrioventricular nodal reentrant tachycardias. Each panel shows the AV node (*top*), a ladder diagram (*middle*), and surface ECG lead II (*bottom*). *Solid lines* indicate anterograde conduction and *broken lines* retrograde conduction; *straight lines* represent fast pathway conduction and *wavy lines* slow pathway. During sinus rhythm, the slow pathway is not apparent, as the impulse travels down the fast pathway, turns around, and retrogradely penetrates into the slow pathway. An atrial premature depolarization (*APD*) blocks in the fast pathway, conducts down the slow pathway, and then can conduct retrograde up the fast pathway, initiating atrioventricular nodal reentrant tachycardia. Less commonly, a ventricular premature depolarization (*VPD*) conducts up the slow pathway, initiating the uncommon form of atrioventricular nodal reentrant tachycardia. *A,* atrium; *P,* sinus P waves; *P′,* atrial echoes from atrioventricular nodal reentry; *V,* ventricle. (Reprinted from Ganz LI, Friedman PL. Supraventricular tachycardia. *N Engl J Med* 1995;332:162–173, with permission.)

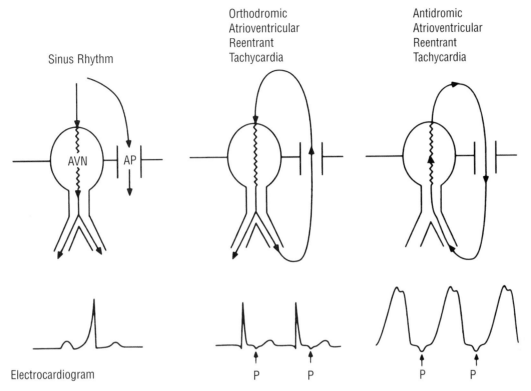

Figure 42.2. Mechanisms of atrioventricular reentrant tachycardias. During sinus rhythm the initial part of the *QRS*, the delta wave, results from ventricular preexcitation over the accessory pathway. During orthodromic atrioventricular reentrant tachycardia, antegrade conduction is over the normal His–Purkinje system, inscribing a normal *QRS*. Rarely, antidromic atrioventricular reentrant tachycardia causes a wide, bizarre *QRS*, because the entire ventricle is depolarized over the accessory pathway, with retrograde conduction over the normal His–Purkinje system and atrio-ventricular node. (Reprinted from Ganz LI, Friedman PL. Supraventricular tachycardia. *N Engl J Med* 1995;332:162–173, with permission.)

Wide-complex Tachycardia

SVTs usually present with a narrow QRS complex. Wide-complex tachycardias may be due to ventricular tachycardia (VT) or SVT with aberrant conduction into the ventricles. Aberrancy may be fixed (i.e., bundle branch block occurring at any heart rate), rate-related (i.e., narrow QRS at normal sinus rates but bundle branch block at rapid rates), or caused by antidromic conduction over an accessory pathway (i.e., only in patients with WPW syndrome). Whereas VT occurs primarily in patients with structural heart disease (e.g., coronary artery disease or cardiomyopathy) and can cause cardiac arrest, SVT is rarely life-threatening (except for WPW syndrome with AF or atrial flutter).

Algorithms can aid in determining whether a wide-complex tachycardia is VT or SVT (Figure 42.3) (3). Several issues warrant emphasis, however. First, among wide complex tachycardias, VT occurs much more frequently than SVT with aberrancy. Second, in patients with structural heart disease, particularly coronary artery disease or cardiomyopathy, wide-complex tachycardia is almost always caused by VT. Finally, misdiagnosis of SVT as VT rarely causes untoward consequences, but misdiagnosis of VT as

SVT and treatment with an intravenous (IV) AV nodal blocking agent can precipitate cardiac arrest. Thus, *unless a wide-complex tachyarrhythmia is known to be supraventricular in origin, it should be presumed to be VT and treated as such until proven otherwise.* Therapy should be direct current (DC) cardioversion in unstable patients and IV drug therapy in hemodynamically stable patients.

In hemodynamically stable patients, intravenous amiodarone is increasingly used because it is effective for both VT and SVT and is safe, even in patients with left ventricular dysfunction (4). Lidocaine may be most effective for VT caused by acute ischemia or myocardial infarction (MI). Procainamide may be more effective in other settings and is the agent of choice in patients with WPW and AF, or atrial flutter. IV adenosine has been proposed as a diagnostic or therapeutic challenge in patients with hemodynamically tolerated wide-complex tachycardia, because it terminates most PSVT and unmasks atrial flutter by transiently blocking AV conduction. However, in rare cases adenosine can cause hemodynamically-tolerated VT to deteriorate into cardiac arrest. Thus, if adenosine is to be administered to patients with wide-complex tachycardia, a defibrillator should be immediately available.

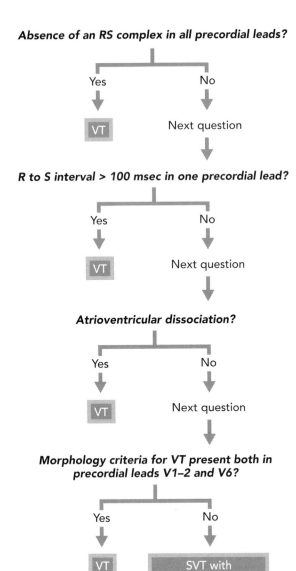

Absence of an RS complex in all precordial leads?

Yes → VT

No → Next question

R to S interval > 100 msec in one precordial lead?

Yes → VT

No → Next question

Atrioventricular dissociation?

Yes → VT

No → Next question

Morphology criteria for VT present both in precordial leads V1–2 and V6?

Yes → VT

No → SVT with aberrant conduction

Figure 42.3. Algorithm for diagnosis of wide-complex tachycardia proposed by Brugada and colleagues. If there is no RS complex in any precordial lead, ventricular tachycardia (VT) is diagnosed. If an RS complex exists in any precordial lead, the longest RS interval (from onset of QRS to nadir of S wave) is measured in the precordium; if the longest RS interval is greater than 100 msec, VT is diagnosed. If not, atrioventricular dissociation is sought; if present, VT is diagnosed. If absent, morphologic criteria are applied to leads V_1 and V_6 to differentiate VT from a supraventricular tachyarrhythmia (SVT) with aberrancy. (From Brugada P, Brugada J, Mont L, et al. A new approach to the differential diagnosis of a regular tachycardia with a wide QRS complex. Reprinted with permission from *Circulation* 1991;83:1649–1659.)

ARRHYTHMIAS PRESENTING AT THE TIME OF ADMISSION

Clinical Presentation

Symptoms referable to AF and other supraventricular arrhythmias span a wide range (Table 42.2). Some AF

TABLE 42.2	
SYMPTOMS ASSOCIATED WITH SUPRAVENTICULAR TACHYARRHYTHMIAS	
Mild	**Moderate–Severe**
Asymptomatic	Chest pain
Fatigue/malaise	Heart failure
Poor exercise capacity	Near syncope
Dyspnea	Syncope
Lightheadedness	Sudden death
Palpitations	

patients are truly asymptomatic, and severe symptoms most commonly are seen in patients with significant structural heart disease. Many patients with structurally normal hearts have fairly mild symptoms. However, patients with WPW syndrome and AF, or with atrial flutter, can develop hemodynamic instability or even ventricular fibrillation.

Differential Diagnosis and Initial Evaluation

A 12-lead electrocardiogram (ECG) should be obtained in all stable patients. Tachyarrhythmias should be classified as wide- or narrow-complex, and regular or irregular (Figure 42.4). Irregularly irregular rhythms without organized P-wave activity are AF; MAT is distinguished by multiple discrete P-wave morphologies. A normal dominant P-wave morphology distinguishes sinus tachycardia with premature atrial complexes. AF with conduction over an accessory pathway in patients with WPW syndrome presents as an irregular tachycardia with wide as well as variable-width QRS complexes; ventricular rates may be extremely rapid. Atrial flutter in these patients may be conducted 1:1 into the ventricle with uniformly wide QRS complexes.

Narrow-complex regular tachycardias are frequently atrial flutter with 2:1 AV conduction, AVNRT, AVRT, or, less commonly, AT with 1:1 AV conduction. Atrial flutter typically presents with an atrial rate of approximately 300 beats/min, 2:1 AV conduction, and a ventricular rate of about 150 beats/min. The underlying atrial rate may be slower in elderly patients or those on antiarrhythmic drugs. The typical sawtooth pattern usually is visible on an ECG, particularly in the inferior leads (II, III, aVF). If there are retrograde P waves, or if no P waves are visible at all, the diagnosis is usually AVNRT or AVRT. Tachycardias with an abnormal P-wave morphology that precedes the QRS complex may be AT or atypical forms of AVNRT or AVRT. ATs may present with 1:1, 2:1, or variable AV conduction. The distinction between AT and atrial flutter is based on the atrial rate and P-wave morphology: the atrial rate in atrial flutter tends to be more rapid than in ATs, and, in AT, discrete P waves are separated by an isoelectric segment in

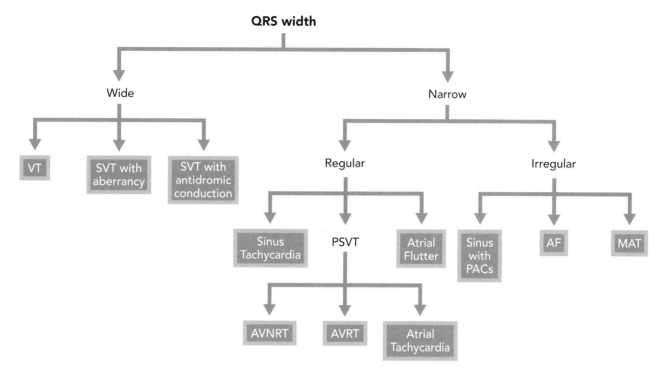

Figure 42.4. Decision algorithm for ECG diagnosis of supraventricular tachyarrhythmia (*SVT*). *AVNRT*, atrioventricular nodal reentrant tachycardia; *AVRT*, atrioventricular reentrant tachycardia; *MAT*, multifocal atrial tachycardia; *PAC*, premature atrial contraction; *PSVT*, paroxysmal supraventricular tachycardia; *VT*, ventricular tachycardia.

contrast with the sawtooth pattern of continuous atrial activity in atrial flutter.

The induction of transient block at the AV node is very useful diagnostically and therapeutically in patients with regular SVT (Figure 42.5). A rhythm strip, preferably in several simultaneous leads, should be recorded continuously during such maneuvers. Vagal maneuvers such as the Valsalva maneuver or carotid sinus massage should be tried first; if unsuccessful, IV AV nodal blocking agents may be administered. Induced block at the AV node with adenosine or verapamil (Table 42.3) terminates AVNRT and AVRT; tachycardias that persist in the atrium despite transient AV block must be AT or atrial flutter. Some ATs are adenosine-sensitive, so the ECG recording must be scrutinized to determine the mechanism of termination.

It is also important to identify conditions that may accompany or even may have triggered the SVT. AF may be associated with acute MI, pulmonary embolus, stroke, and thyrotoxicosis. MAT is seen almost exclusively in the setting of acute pulmonary disease. Digitalis toxicity may cause AT.

Indications for Hospitalization

If the tachyarrhythmia is secondary to an acute condition such as acute MI or pulmonary embolus, admission is obviously necessary. Absent such associated conditions, many patients with AF or atrial flutter can be safely started on medical therapy without hospital admission. In particular, patients with minimal symptoms, a ventricular rate that is not too rapid, and no signs of ischemia, heart failure, or hemodynamic instability can be started on an AV nodal blocking agent and warfarin if careful outpatient follow-up is available. Patients with ischemia, heart failure, or hemodynamic instability caused by AF should be admitted. Frequently these patients have rapid ventricular rates as well as structural heart disease. Patients with AF of unknown duration but no acute symptoms do not necessarily require admission solely for the initiation of anticoagulation with IV heparin. For patients with AF of less than 24–36 hours' duration, cardioversion should be considered to avert the need for prolonged anticoagulation (see the section on "Issues During the Course of Hospitalization" later in this chapter).

If PSVT can be terminated in the emergency department, admission frequently is not required. Exceptions include patients with severe symptoms of angina, heart failure, syncope, or near-syncope resulting from SVT. These patients often have structural heart disease, and admission is frequently useful to expedite initiation of medical therapy or consideration of electrophysiologic studies and radiofrequency (RF) catheter ablation. Patients with WPW syndrome who have AF or atrial flutter or symptoms of syncope

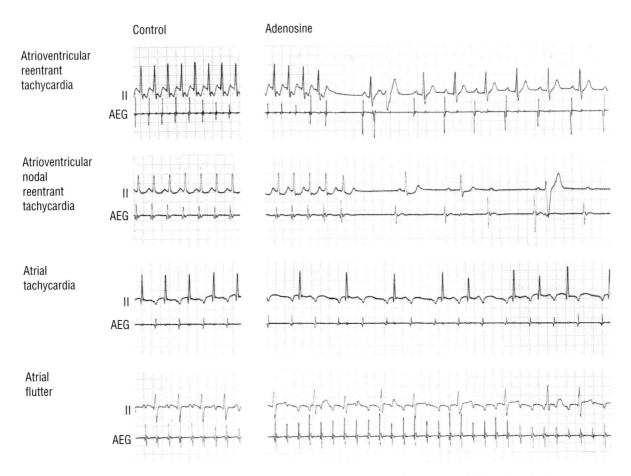

Figure 42.5. Use of adenosine to diagnose patients with a regular supraventricular tachyarrhythmia. Each panel shows surface electrocardiogram lead II and an intracardiac atrial electrogram (*AEG*) to show the timing of atrial depolarization, both at baseline and after adenosine administration. Adenosine induces transient atrioventricular block, terminating atrioventricular reentrant tachycardia and atrioventricular nodal reentrant tachycardia. With atrial tachycardia and atrial flutter, tachycardia continues in the atrium despite transient atrioventricular block, revealing the correct diagnosis. (Reprinted from Ganz LI, Friedman PL. Supraventricular tachycardia. *N Engl J Med* 1995;332: 162–173, with permission.)

or near-syncope should be admitted for electrophysiologic studies and RF catheter ablation.

In general, patients admitted for SVT should have continuous cardiac monitoring. Exceptions include those with chronic AF admitted for noncardiac reasons.

Indications for Initial ICU Admission

Admission to an ICU is infrequent, unless the arrhythmia is a complication of a condition such as MI or pulmonary embolus that itself requires ICU admission. ICU admission is also reasonable in patients with symptoms of significant ischemia, heart failure, or hemodynamic instability caused by arrhythmia. Patients with the WPW syndrome and pre-excited AF or atrial flutter also might benefit from initial ICU admission.

Initial Management

The initial management strategy depends on the stability of the patient. Synchronized DC cardioversion should be considered for unstable patients. For stable AF and atrial flutter, initial efforts are directed at controlling the ventricular rate with AV nodal blocking agents (Table 42.3). *Intravenous calcium channel blockers and β-blockers are far more effective than digoxin for acutely slowing a rapid ventricular response.* Careful monitoring for complications, such as bronchospasm, hypotension, heart failure, or an excessively slow ventricular rate, is necessary.

For unstable patients with the WPW syndrome and AF, or with atrial flutter, cardioversion is appropriate. Hemodynamically stable patients should not initially receive AV nodal blocking agents (calcium channel

TABLE 42.3

DRUGS USED IN MANAGING SUPRAVENTRICULAR TACHYARRHYTHMIAS

Arrhythmia	Goal	Drug	Dosage
Atrial fibrillation and atrial flutter	Anticoagulation	Heparin (IV)	Varies; target aPTT 2 times control
		Warfarin (po)	Varies; target INR 2.0–3.0
	Acute termination	Ibutilide (IV)	Patient 60 kg or more: 1 mg[a]
			Patient less than 60 kg: 0.01 mg/kg[a]
	Acute rate control	Diltiazem (IV)	0.25 mg/kg, then 5–15 mg/h
		Verapamil (IV)	2.5–10 mg q4h prn
		Propranalol (IV)	1–3 mg q4h prn
		Metoprolol (IV)	5–10 mg q4h prn
		Esmolol (IV)	0.5 mg/kg, then 0.05–0.2 mg/kg/min
	Chronic rate control	Diltiazem ER (po)	120–300 mg qd
		Verapamil ER (po)	120–240 mg qd
		Metoprolol (po)	25–100 mg bid
		Atenolol (po)	25–200 mg qd
		Propranalol ER (po)	80–240 mg qd
		Digoxin (po)	0.125–0.25 mg qd
	Sinus rhythm maintenance (suppression of recurrences of fibrillation/flutter)	Quinidine Gluconate (po)	324 mg tid
		Procainamide ER (po)	500–100 mg qid
		Disopyramide ER (po)	150–300 mg bid
		Propafenone (po)[b]	150–300 mg tid
		Propafenone SR (po)[b]	225–425 mg bid
		Flecainide (po)[b]	50–100 mg bid
		Sotalol (po)	80–160 mg bid
		Dofetilide (po)	125–500 mcg bid
		Amiodarone (po)	100–200 mg qd (after load)
Paroxysmal supraventricular tachycardia	Acute termination	Adenosine (IV)	6–12 mg push
		Verapamil (IV)	2.5–10.0 mg
	Chronic Suppression	Diltiazem ER (po)	120–300 mg qd
		Verapamil ER (po)	120–240 mg qd
		Metoprolol (po)	25–100 mg bid
		Atenolol (po)	25–200 mg qd
		Propranalol ER (po)	80–240 mg qd
		Digoxin (po)	0.125–0.25 mg qd

[a] Initial dose over 10 minutes, can be repeated one time.
[b] Use in associaton with AV nodal blocker (β-blocker, diltiazem, verapamil, digoxin).
aPTT, activated partial thromboplastin time; *ER*, extended release formulation that permits once-daily dosing; *INR*, international normalized ratio; *IV*, intravenous; *po*, oral.

blockers, β-blockers, digoxin, or adenosine) because these agents can shunt conduction over the accessory pathway, thereby increasing the ventricular rate and the risk of degeneration to ventricular fibrillation. Intravenous procainamide, which slows conduction throughout the heart, is the agent of choice.

Induction of transient AV block with vagal or pharmacologic maneuvers is the initial approach for PSVT. AV block terminates AVNRT and AVRT, and it unmasks most ATs and atrial flutter. Following termination of the SVT, another ECG should be obtained; to diagnose WPW syndrome, an ECG must be obtained with the patient in sinus rhythm. Patients with WPW syndrome typically should not be treated empirically with digoxin or calcium channel blocking agents even if they present with PSVT, because of the risk of more rapid ventricular rates should AF or atrial flutter occur. Rather, patients with symptomatic WPW syndrome (i.e.,

SVT, AF, or atrial flutter) generally should be advised to undergo electrophysiologic studies and RF catheter ablation (1, 2). Symptomatic patients with WPW syndrome who refuse this approach typically require treatment with a membrane-active drug (i.e., class IA, IC, or III; Table 42.4), often in combination with an AV nodal blocking agent; chronic monotherapy with a β-blocker may be an alternative, though few data are available regarding safety and efficacy. In the past, most asymptomatic patients with ventricular preexcitation have been observed. Recent data suggest, however, that if atrial fibrillation or AVRT is inducible at diagnostic electrophysiologic studies, then prophylactic catheter ablation may be preferable, particularly in younger patients (5).

Most patients with PSVT without the WPW syndrome have either AVNRT or AVRT resulting from a concealed accessory pathway. In either case, the risk of sudden death is

TABLE 42.4

CLASSIFICATION OF ANTIARRHYTHMIC DRUGS

Class I Sodium channel blockers			Class II β-blockers	Class III Prolong refractoriness (K channel blockers)	Class IV Calcium channel blockers (Nondihydropyridine)
Class IA	Class IB	Class IC			
Procainamide	Lidocaine	Flecainide	Propranalol	DL Sotalol[c]	Diltiazem
Quinidine	Mexilitene	Propafenone	Metoprolol	Ibutilide[d]	Verapamil
Disopyramide	Moricizine		Atenolol	Dofetilide	
			Nadolol	Amiodarone[e]	
			Carvedilol[a]		
			Labetalol[a]		
			Betaxalol		
			Bucindolol[b]		
			Pindolol		
			Acebutalol[b]		

[a] combined β- and α-blocker; carvedilol has additional antioxidant properties
[b] partial β agonist effects; may be preferred in tachy-brady syndrome
[c] combined β-blocker/Class III agent
[d] Sodium channel enhancer, rather than potassium channel blocker
[e] Amiodarone has Class I, I, III, and IV electrophysiologic effects

extremely low. It is reasonable to follow the patient without chronic oral therapy after an initial episode of PSVT if symptoms were mild. For recurrent episodes or extremely symptomatic first episodes, choices for initial therapy include chronic therapy with an AV nodal blocking agent (e.g., β-blocker, diltiazem, verapamil, or digoxin) or electrophysiologic study and RF catheter ablation (1, 2).

Unless the clinical situation dictates otherwise, few tests are indicated in the routine evaluation of new AF or other SVTs. A careful history and physical examination, ECG, transthoracic echocardiogram, and a serum thyroid stimulating hormone (TSH) measurement should be adequate in most patients. Screening laboratory studies (e.g., complete blood count, electrolytes, and renal function) and a chest radiograph are reasonable, though supporting data are limited. Cardiac biomarker measurements to exclude MI, exercise stress testing to exclude ischemia, arterial blood gas measurement, and ventilation–perfusion or CT scanning to exclude pulmonary embolus are not routinely necessary.

Indications for Early Consultation

Cardiology consultation is reasonable if cardiac catheterization is being considered, especially in patients with MI, significant ischemia, or heart failure. Similarly, early cardiology consultation may be appropriate if transesophageal echocardiography (TEE; see the section on "Issues During the Course of Hospitalization" that follows) or DC cardioversion is contemplated. Consultation with a cardiac electrophysiologist is recommended in all patients with WPW syndrome and in other patients in whom the option of RF catheter ablation is being weighed. In patients with

tachycardia-bradycardia (tachy-brady) syndrome, consultation regarding permanent pacemaker implantation (Chapter 45) is often useful.

ISSUES DURING THE COURSE OF HOSPITALIZATION

Atrial Fibrillation

Management of AF has three components: anticoagulation, control of the ventricular rate, and restoration and maintenance of SR. Each must be considered in developing a treatment strategy (Figure 42.6) (5–8).

The risk of stroke resulting from thromboembolism is markedly increased by AF (8); anticoagulation with warfarin significantly attenuates this risk (8–10). Although young patients with idiopathic AF are at low risk, most other patients with AF (Table 42.5) should be anticoagulated (target international normalized ratio [INR] 2.0–3.0) unless contraindications exist. The recently proposed CHADS$_2$ index (Figure 42.7) allows calculation of a given patient's risk of stroke without anticoagulation (11). The thromboembolic risk of atrial flutter probably approximates that of AF, and guidelines for anticoagulation are the same. Patients with contraindications to anticoagulation should receive aspirin, which attenuates the risk of stroke somewhat. Newer antithrombotic agents are under development. One promising oral agent, ximelagatran (12), was denied FDA approval in late 2004 because of reports of serious liver toxicity.

AF of very short duration frequently terminates spontaneously. If it does not, it is reasonable to have the patient fast

Atrial Fibrillation / Flutter

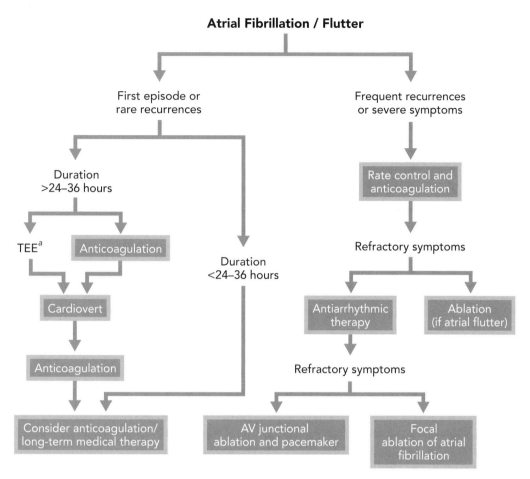

Figure 42.6. Management algorithm for atrial fibrillation or flutter. *TEE,* transesophageal echocardiogram. ªWith appropriate anticoagulation.

overnight and cardiovert the next morning (see later in this chapter) to obviate the need for anticoagulation. If the duration of AF is not known to be extremely short, warfarin should be initiated immediately. For patients with new-onset AF that does not convert spontaneously, two alternative approaches with similar efficacy and outcomes may be

---

TABLE 42.5

ANTICOAGULATION IN ATRIAL FIBRILLATION

Age	Risk factors	Recommendation
<65	Present	Warfarin (INR 2.0–3.0)
	Absent	ASA
65–75	Present	Warfarin (INR 2.0–3.0)
	Absent	Warfarin or ASA
>75		Warfarin (INR 2.0–3.0)

Risk factors for embolism—Clinical: prior TIA/stroke, hypertension, congestive heart failure, diabetes mellitus, coronary artery disease, mitral stenosis, prosthetic heart valves (more intense anticoagulation indicated), thyrotoxicosis; Echocardiographic: left-atrial enlargement, left-ventricular dysfunction.
Adapted from Albers G, Dalen J, Laupacis A, et al. Antithrombotic therapy in atrial fibrillation. *Chest* 2001;119(1 Suppl): 194S–206S, with permission.

considered (13). In one approach, patients with AF of more than 24–36 hours' duration are anticoagulated for at least 3 weeks prior to any attempt at cardioversion, whether electric or pharmacologic. Because restoration of atrial mechanical function can lag behind establishment of sinus rhythm, anticoagulation should be continued for at least 4 weeks after successful cardioversion. An alternative to prolonged anticoagulation prior to cardioversion is an expedited approach using transesophageal echocardiography. Once anticoagulation is initiated, transesophageal echocardiography is performed. If the atria are free of thrombus, cardioversion is performed. Anticoagulation must continue for at least 4 weeks following restoration of sinus rhythm. It is reasonable to administer heparin during hospitalization. Target activated partial thromboplastin times (aPTTs) are typically two times control. In patients who have tachy-brady syndrome and in whom permanent pacemaker implantation may be required, initiation of warfarin may be delayed.

Direct current cardioversion can be performed in the presence or absence of antiarrhythmic drug therapy. It carries a low risk of systemic embolism if patients have been in AF for less than 24–36 hours, have no evidence of clot on transesophageal echocardiography, or are on chronic

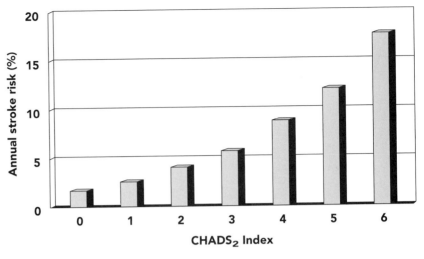

Clinical Risk Factor	Points
C Recent **C**HF	1
H **H**ypertension	1
A **A**ge ≥75 years	1
D **D**iabetes mellitus	1
S$_2$ Prior **S**troke or TIA	2

Figure 42.7. CHADS$_2$ index for calculating risk of stroke in patients with AF. For each point, the annual risk of stroke increases by 50%. Left: CHADS$_2$ index. Right: Annual risk of stroke. Adapted with permission from Gage BF, et al. Validation of clinical classification schemes for predicting stroke-results from the national registry of atrial fibrillation. *JAMA* 2001;285:2864–2870.

therapeutic anticoagulation. If cardioversion is contemplated, the patient should receive nothing orally after midnight. Biphasic external defibrillators are far more effective at restoring sinus rhythm than the older monophasic devices. Because of the efficacy of biphasic external cardioversion, pharmacologic cardioversion is used less frequently. If pharmacologic cardioversion is preferred, *ibutilide*, a novel type III agent, is approved for the acute conversion of AF and flutter of relatively short duration. Administered as an IV bolus, ibutilide is more effective for atrial flutter than for AF. As with other type III agents, there is a risk of *torsades de pointes*; ibutilide should not be used in patients receiving other antiarrhythmic drugs. If ibutilide fails to restore SR, DC cardioversion can then be performed.

Four weeks following cardioversion should be the absolute minimum period of anticoagulation. Contemporary practice generally recommends anticoagulation for much longer periods, often indefinitely, even if efforts at maintaining sinus rhythm appear to be successful. Exceptions are situations in which the AF had a well-defined trigger (e.g., hyperthyroidism, cardiac surgery, etc.) and the risk of AF recurrence therefore seems extremely low.

Reduction of the ventricular rate with AV nodal blocking agents often markedly improves symptoms of AF. Few data exist comparing the available agents, which include β-blockers, the nondihydropyridine calcium channel blockers diltiazem and verapamil, and digoxin. Digoxin has a delayed onset compared with other agents and is the least effective agent if catecholamine tone is high, as in postoperative patients or with physical exertion. Frequently, a combination of digoxin with a β-blocker or calcium channel blocker is necessary to achieve adequate rate control. In patients with extremely poor ventricular function or acute congestive heart failure, though, digoxin may be the only agent that is tolerated.

Intravenous agents frequently are used initially to manage the ventricular rate (Table 42.3). Diltiazem and esmolol are given as a continuous infusion; verapamil, metoprolol, and propranalol can be given as IV boluses. The target heart rate depends on the clinical scenario; rates of 60–80 at rest and 90–110 with mild-to-moderate exertion are reasonable. Oral agents should be started as soon as rate control is achieved with the IV agent.

The use of antiarrhythmic drugs to suppress recurrences of AF and maintain sinus rhythm is being reassessed, given their limited efficacy and adverse effects, including life-threatening proarrhythmia (14). With a first episode of AF, it is reasonable to cardiovert without maintenance antiarrhythmic therapy. For recurrent episodes, either rate control with long-term anticoagulation or rhythm control with antiarrhythmic therapy can be chosen (Table 42.6). In several trials (15–17), the strategy of rate control and anticoagulation provided very similar functional and clinical outcomes to a strategy of aggressive attempts to maintain sinus rhythm. Antiarrhythmic drug therapy should therefore be reserved for patients who remain symptomatic despite attempts at rate control. If antiarrhythmic therapy is selected, the particular agent should fit the clinical scenario (Table 42.4). DL-sotalol, dofetilide, and amiodarone are reasonable in patients with coronary artery disease. For younger patients with paroxysmal AF and structurally normal hearts, flecainide and propafenone are often well tolerated and effective. With flecainide and propafenone, an AV nodal blocking agent (Table 42.4) should be used as well. Procainamide, quinidine, and disopyramide, though used frequently in the past, are neither safer nor more effective than newer agents, and they are less well tolerated. Amiodarone may be the most effective agent and likely poses the smallest risk of ventricular proarrhythmia, but its noncardiac adverse effects must be carefully considered. Amiodarone is

TABLE 42.6

RHYTHM CONTROL VERSUS RATE CONTROL IN ATRIAL FIBRILLATION

Rhythm control	Rate control
Theoretic advantages	
Symptomatic improvement	Safe
Hemodynamic improvement	Medications well tolerated
Reduced risk of thromboembolism	Medications fairly inexpensive
Possible discontinuation of anticoagulation	
Theoretic disadvantages	
Adverse extracardiac effects	Bradycardia
Proarrhythmia	Life-long anticoagulation
Frequently ineffective	Cardiomyopathy if rate poorly controlled chronically
Expensive	Incomplete resolution of symptoms

Adapted from Ganz LI, Antman EM. Long-term pharmacologic management of atrial fibrillation for control of rate and rhythm. *Cardiac Electrophysiology Review* 1997;1/12:40–43, with permission.

the most frequently used antiarrhythmic agent in patients with cardiomyopathy or significant left-ventricular dysfunction; dofetilide may also be reasonable in these patients. Prescription of dofetilide is limited to physicians who have completed a training program regarding its use.

For selected patients with symptomatic and refractory AF, catheter ablation of triggering foci typically in and around the pulmonary venous ostia may be curative. These procedures are currently being performed at tertiary care centers. Patients with idiopathic paroxysmal AF are the best candidates for curative ablation; recently, many centers have extended the indications for curative ablation to include patients with mild structural heart disease and persistent AF (18). Success rates vary by center and type of patients treated, and truly long-term follow-up is not yet available. With improvements in techniques, procedural complications such as pulmonary vein stenosis, stroke, and tamponade have decreased in frequency.

Patients whose AF is extremely refractory to pharmacologic therapy may benefit from RF catheter ablation of the AV junction and implantation of a permanent pacemaker (Chapter 45). Although this approach generally markedly improves symptoms, potential downsides include pacemaker dependence and the adverse effects related to chronic right ventricular pacing. Biventricular pacing (known as cardiac resynchronization therapy [CRT]) is preferable to standard right ventricular pacing in many patients who undergo catheter ablation of the AV junction.

Atrial Flutter

For patients with recurrent atrial flutter in the absence of AF, RF catheter ablation of the tricuspid annulus–inferior vena cava isthmus is effective in preventing recurrent flutter, though AF may recur. Atrial flutter may occur in association with or independent of AF. Pharmacologic rate control is typically much more difficult to achieve with atrial flutter than with AF. Recommendations for anticoagulation of atrial flutter mirror those for AF.

With a first episode of atrial flutter, direct current cardioversion after appropriate anticoagulation is reasonable. If atrial flutter is recurrent, or if a first episode is accompanied by 1:1 A:V conduction or severe symptoms, radiofrequency catheter ablation should be strongly considered. Catheter ablation in the tricuspid valve-inferior vena cava isthmus offers approximately 90% likelihood of freedom from recurrent atrial flutter. AF may occur after atrial flutter ablation (even in patients who have not previously manifested it), but this is generally easier to manage pharmacologically than atrial flutter.

Multifocal Atrial Tachycardia (MAT)

In MAT, efforts should be focused on correcting the underlying metabolic or pulmonary abnormalities. Digoxin or theophylline excess rarely plays a role, while repletion of potassium and magnesium may be helpful. Verapamil lowers the ventricular rate (Table 42.3); β-blockers have similar effects but may be contraindicated by obstructive lung disease. Unlike most SVTs, MAT is nonreentrant, and cardioversion is unlikely to be beneficial.

PSVT (AVNRT, AVRT, and AT)

For patients admitted with AVNRT, AVRT, or AT, attention should immediately be turned to long-term therapy (Figure 42.8). For patients with symptomatic WPW syndrome, electrophysiologic testing and catheter ablation generally are recommended as initial therapy. In the absence of WPW syndrome, either medical therapy or catheter ablation can be used initially for other PSVTs (AVNRT, AVRT utilizing a concealed accessory pathway, and AT). If catheter ablation is to be performed during the same admission, no long-acting agent should be given, as this therapy might render the patient noninducible at electrophysiologic testing. In the absence of WPW syndrome, the initial choice for chronic drug therapy should be an AV nodal blocker; digoxin, a calcium channel blocker, or a β-blocker (Table 42.3). Combinations of agents also can be used. Given the risks of proarrhythmia, catheter ablation should be recommended in these patients rather than the use of type I or III antiarrhythmic agents (Figure 42.8).

DISCHARGE ISSUES

In patients with AF or atrial flutter, careful follow-up is required to monitor the INR and the dose of warfarin. If AF is chronic or of unknown duration, discharge need not always be delayed until the INR is therapeutic. Rather,

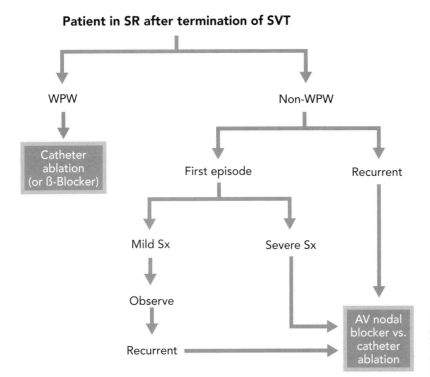

Patient in SR after termination of SVT

WPW

Non-WPW

Catheter ablation (or ß-Blocker)

First episode

Recurrent

Mild Sx

Severe Sx

Observe

AV nodal blocker vs. catheter ablation

Recurrent

Figure 42.8. Management algorithm for paroxysmal supraventricular tachycardia. *SR*, sinus rhythm; *SVT*, supraventricular tachycardia; *Sx*, symptoms; *WPW*, Wolff-Parkinson-White syndrome.

warfarin may be started and the patient discharged with a plan in place quickly to realize a therapeutic INR (2.0–3.0). If a patient undergoes TEE-expedited cardioversion, IV heparin should be administered until the INR is therapeutic. Subcutaneous low-molecular-weight heparin is equivalent to unfractionated heparin as a "bridge" to a therapeutic INR in this setting (19). Because confusion ensues if several physicians modulate warfarin dosing, a single physician or office should be designated for this task. Dedicated anticoagulation clinics or services have been shown to improve outcomes compared with less organized approaches. Weekly INR checks are reasonable until a steady maintenance dose is established (Chapter 98).

Despite the high prevalence of AF and atrial flutter, optimal long-term treatment strategies remain uncertain. Clinical trials (15–17) document that long-term anticoagulation and rate-control is a more attractive strategy than vigorous antiarrhthmic use in many patients, particularly those with few or mild symptoms (Table 42.6). In high-risk patients, the combination of moderate intensity warfarin anticoagulation plus an antiplatelet agent may be better than warfarin alone (20).

Patients who are receiving rate-control agents should be followed carefully to assess adequacy of therapy, symptomatic status, and potential side effects. *Patients on antiarrhythmic drugs require meticulous follow-up because of the risk of adverse effects* (14). The QT_c interval and heart rate must be monitored in patients on procainamide, quinidine, disopyramide, amiodarone, dofetilide, and DL-sotalol. Ventricular proarrhythmia in these patients is torsade de pointes, typically precipitated by bradycardia or pauses; this compli-

cation appears much more rare in patients treated with amiodarone compared with other QT-prolonging drugs. For patients started on flecainide or propafenone, exercise stress testing on a steady state of drug is useful to screen for exercise-induced proarrhythmia. Patients on amiodarone must be followed for pulmonary, thyroid, and hepatic dysfunction; annual or biannual pulmonary function testing or chest radiographs and biannual or quarterly blood testing is recommended. Finally, an annual ophthalmologic evaluation is also recommended, as rare cases of optic neuritis have been reported in patients taking amiodarone.

Patients who are considering RF catheter ablation may desire a visit with a cardiac electrophysiologist to discuss the procedure. After successful RF catheter ablation for PSVT, patients are frequently treated with antithrombotic agents (e.g., aspirin) for 4–6 weeks to reduce the risk of procedure-related thromboembolism. After catheter ablation of AF or atrial flutter, patients are anticoagulated with warfarin; the optimal duration of anticoagulation following successful ablation has not yet been established. A follow-up visit in several weeks to confirm healing of the femoral catheterization sites and assess procedural success is reasonable.

SUPRAVENTRICULAR ARRHYTHMIAS DEVELOPING IN THE HOSPITAL

SVTs, primarily AF and to a lesser extent atrial flutter, are frequent complications in both medical and surgical patients. Because PSVT requires a conducive electrophysiologic substrate (i.e., dual AV nodal pathways or an accessory pathway), these arrhythmias occur de novo much less frequently in patients admitted for other reasons. AF and atrial flutter are particularly difficult to control in acutely ill patients with problems such as sepsis, pain, and hemodynamic instability. SVTs that develop in hospitalized patients are commonly precipitated by conditions such as infection, hypoxia, drugs, electrolyte abnormalities, or other causes of hypo- or hypervolemia. Although attention must be paid to acute hemodynamic stability, ischemia secondary to the SVT, and rate control, treatment of the underlying condition is also necessary and often sufficient to control the arrhythmias. Some important precipitants are reviewed here.

Acute Myocardial Infarction

AF is an occasional complication of MI (Chapter 38). β-blockers are the agents of choice for ventricular rate control, given their other beneficial effects in acute MI. If AF persists for more than 24 hours, cardioversion should be considered, particularly if no other indication for long-term anticoagulation is present. No data exist regarding the use of low-molecular-weight heparins, clopidogrel, glycoprotein IIa-IIIb inhibitors, or thrombolytic agents in the management of AF; data are few with respect to antiarrhythmic drug use for AF in acute MI. Nonparoxysmal junctional tachycardia also has been reported infrequently during MI.

Acute Pulmonary Embolus

Initial treatment of AF due to acute pulmonary embolus (Chapter 53) should be directed at controlling the ventricular rate using IV calcium channel blockers or β-blockers. As patients with pulmonary emboli routinely are anticoagulated, AF does not pose an additional burden in this regard. Antiarrhythmic drug data are scarce in this setting.

Thyrotoxicosis

SVTs resulting from thyrotoxicosis are extremely refractory, in terms of both ventricular rate control and maintenance of sinus rhythm. Amiodarone is a common cause of hyperthyroidism (as well as hypothyroidism) and complicates its management; since amiodarone loads the thyroid gland with iodine, radioactive iodine ablation is generally ineffective. β-blockers are most effective, given the hyperadrenergic state, in combination with antithyroid therapy (Chapter 108). Anticoagulation should be undertaken as well. If AF persists after a euthyroid state is reached, cardioversion should be performed.

Pulmonary Disease

MAT, AT, AF, and atrial flutter all may accompany acute or chronic lung disease. In chronic pulmonary conditions, these atrial arrhythmias recur frequently. Other than the fact that β-blockers are frequently contraindicated in these patients, management is just as in other patients with these arrhythmias. Atrial arrhythmias may be refractory in patients with elevated right heart pressures and right atrial enlargement. Amiodarone must be used cautiously in patients with advanced pulmonary disease.

Postoperative Atrial Fibrillation

AF is a common postoperative complication (Chapter 31), particularly after cardiac, thoracic, and vascular surgery. AF also may occur following other major operations such as hip replacement or abdominal surgery. Potential causes of AF after any operation include atrial stretch from volume overload, high catecholamine levels, and β-blocker withdrawal in patients on these agents preoperatively. Pericarditis likely plays an important role in the high incidence of AF and atrial flutter after cardiac and thoracic surgery. Other contributory factors after cardiac surgery may include atrial ischemia and inadequate atrial protection during cardiopulmonary bypass. If left-ventricular function is unknown, a transthoracic echocardiogram may help guide drug selection. In patients who are otherwise doing well, serial cardiac biomarker studies need not be obtained to exclude perioperative MI just because AF has developed. Patients should be transferred, however, to a cardiac telemetry unit.

Noncardiothoracic Operations

Postoperative AF typically occurs with very rapid ventricular rates; unstable patients should be cardioverted. Stable patients should be treated with IV β-blockers or calcium channel blockers. Frequently, AF in this setting terminates spontaneously. If not, it is reasonable to cardiovert if AF persists more than 24–36 hours to avoid the need for anticoagulation. Oral β- or calcium channel blockers may be continued for several weeks to attenuate the ventricular rate if AF recurs. If AF is recurrent or persists for more than 24–36 hours, anticoagulaton is recommended, and antiarrhythmic drug therapy may be considered.

Thoracic Surgery

Ventricular rates are frequently extremely rapid in AF after thoracic surgery. Aggressive use of IV β-blockers or calcium channel blockers is necessary to reduce the ventricular response. Though commonly used in this setting, procainamide is of uncertain efficacy in effecting conversion to sinus rhythm and preventing recurrent AF. A 4- to 6-week course of oral β-blockers or calcium channel blockers is reasonable, as pericarditis may provoke recurrent AF after hospital discharge. It is reasonable to consider cardioversion if AF persists for 24–36 hours to obviate the need for anticoagulation. If AF is recurrent or persists for more than 24–36 hours, then careful anticoagulation is recommended and antiarrhythmic therapy may be considered.

Cardiac Surgery

AF, and to a lesser extent atrial flutter, are the most common complications after cardiac surgery (21). The prevalence is 20%–40% after coronary artery bypass grafting, and significantly higher after valvular procedures. β-blockers should be initiated prophylactically as early as possible postoperatively in all patients without contraindications to reduce the likelihood of postoperative AF (Chapter 31). Digoxin and verapamil are less effective prophylactically than β-blockers; few data exist for diltiazem. Prophylactic amiodarone also reduces the incidence of AF after cardiac surgery.

Despite the importance of this problem, the optimal treatment strategy for AF in this setting is unknown. Though frequently used, procainamide is neither particularly effective nor well tolerated. Initial efforts should be directed at control of the ventricular rate with IV β-blockers or calcium channel blockers; digoxin should be used initially only if ventricular function is poor. If AF does not convert spontaneously, cardioversion after 24–36 hours is reasonable. Patients who remain in sinus rhythm after a single brief episode of AF are typically discharged on aspirin and oral β-blockers or calcium channel blockers. If AF is recurrent or persists for more than 24–36 hours, careful anticoagulation is recommended, and AF suppression with antiarrhythmic drugs may be considered.

Discharge Issues

Most patients who develop AF in the postoperative setting need not be discharged on medications if the AF was transient and clearly related to serious noncardiac problems that are not expected to recur. If recurrence is a major concern, discharge on an oral AV nodal blocking agent is reasonable. Patients who have AF of more than 24–36 hours' duration or have paroxysmal AF, and certainly those discharged in AF, require anticoagulation with warfarin. Postoperative patients are at very high risk of developing a supratherapeutic INR and having bleeding complications, perhaps because of poor oral intake and/or the use of broad-spectrum antibiotics. Cardioversion should be considered following appropriate anticoagulation if AF persists for more than a few weeks postoperatively, particularly in patients who have not had AF previously. Patients treated with antiarrhythmic agents require the careful follow-up care described previously.

COST CONSIDERATIONS

Few data exist regarding the cost effectiveness of various therapeutic approaches to AF and other SVTs. By preventing strokes, chronic anticoagulation for AF is not only cost-effective but also likely cost-saving. Cost-effectiveness data generally support TEE-expedited cardioversion compared with the traditional approach, and rate control compared with the rhythm control strategy. In PSVT, RF catheter ablation is clearly cost-effective for medically refractory patients, but data are unavailable for less refractory patients. Similarly, data are not yet available regarding the cost effectiveness of catheter ablation for atrial flutter. In refractory AF, AV junctional ablation with permanent pacemaker implantation improves quality of life and reduces health care resource utilization; biventricular pacing (CRT) will likely prove to be preferable to standard right ventricular pacing. Subcutaneous low-molecular-weight heparins may have the potential to shorten hospital stays by replacing prolonged courses of IV unfractionated heparin anticoagulation until the INR is therapeutic on warfarin; clinical trials are ongoing. Clinical trials are also currently evaluating newer antithrombotic compounds that may provide clinical efficacy similar to warfarin for preventing strokes, but without the need for INR monitoring and dose adjustments, and perhaps with a lower risk of bleeding (12). AF after cardiac surgery increases length of stay and costs significantly, highlighting the importance of defining an optimal treatment strategy.

KEY POINTS

- Wide-complex tachycardia should be presumed to be VT until proven otherwise and treated as such.
- Long-term anticoagulation is indicated in the majority of patients with AF or atrial flutter to reduce the risk of thromboembolic complications such as stroke.
- Aggressive use of AV nodal blocking drugs to attenuate the ventricular rate is frequently very effective in improving symptoms due to AF.
- The potential risks and benefits should be weighed carefully prior to starting antiarrhythmic drug therapy in any patient with AF or other SVT.
- In the absence of WPW syndrome, PSVT is rarely life-threatening, and hospital admission is not routinely necessary.
- Symptomatic WPW syndrome patients should generally undergo diagnostic electrophysiologic studies and RF catheter ablation; diagnostic electrophysiologic testing and catheter ablation should be considered in selected asymptomatic patients as well.
- Electrophysiologic studies and RF catheter ablation should be considered early in the management of patients with recurrent or refractory PSVT or atrial flutter.
- Routine exercise stress testing, ventilation–perfusion scanning, and assays of cardiac biomarkers are unnecessary in patients with SVTs, unless the clinical scenario is suggestive of ischemia, pulmonary embolus, or MI, respectively. Transthoracic echocardiography and serum TSH screening are reasonable in the diagnostic workup of new SVTs.

■ Patients treated with amiodarone and other antiarrhythmic drugs require extremely careful follow-up, because of the potential for both cardiac and extracardiac toxicity.

REFERENCES

1. Blomström-Lunqvist CB, Scheinman MM, Aliot EM, et al. ACC/AHA/ESC guidelines for the management of patients with supraventricular arrythmias—executive summary. *J Am Coll Cardiol* 2003;42:1493–1531.
2. Ferguson JD, DiMarco JP. Contemporary mangement of paroxysmal supraventricular tachycardia. *Circulation* 2003;107:1096–1099.
3. Brugada P, Brugada J, Mont L, et al. A new approach to the differential diagnosis of a regular tachycardia with a wide QRS complex. *Circulation* 1991;83:1649–1659.
4. Guidelines 2000 for advanced cardiovascular life support. *Circulation* 2000;102 (suppl 8):I112–I128.
5. Pappone C, Santinelli V, Manguso F, et al. A randomized study of prophylactic catheter ablation in asymptomatic patients with the Wolff-Parkinson-White Syndrome. *N Engl J Med* 2003;349:1803–1811.
6. Fuster V, Ryden LE, Asinger RW, et al. ACC/AHA/ESC guidelines for the management of patients with atrial fibrillation. *J Am Coll Cardiol* 2001;38:1852–1923.
7. Falk RH. Atrial fibrillation. *N Engl J Med* 2001;344:1067–1078.
8. Atrial Fibrillation Investigators. Risk factors for stroke and efficacy of antithrombotic therapy in atrial fibrillation. *Arch Intern Med* 1994;154:1449–1457.
9. Singer DE, Albers GW, Dalen JE, et al. Antithrombotic therapy in atrial fibrillation. *Chest* 2004;126 (3 Suppl.):429S–456S.
10. Lip GYH, Hart RG, Conway DSG. Antithrombotic therapy for atrial fibrillation. *Br Med J* 2002;325:1022–1025.
11. Gage BF, Waterman AD, Shannon W, Boechler M, Rich MW, Radford MJ. Validation of clinical classification schemes for predicting stroke—results from the national registry of atrial fibrillation. *JAMA* 2001;285:2864–2870.
12. Halperin JL. Ximelagatran: oral direct thrombin inhibition as anticoagulant therapy in atrial fibrillation. *J Am Coll Cardiol* 2005;45:1–9.
13. Klein AL, Grimm RA, Murray RD, et al. Use of transesophageal echocardiography to guide cardioversion in patients with atrial fibrillation. *N Engl J Med* 2001;344:1411–1420.
14. Ganz LI, Antman EM. Antiarrhythmic drug therapy in the management of atrial fibrillation. *J Cardiovasc Electrophys* 1997;8:1175–1189.
15. AFFIRM Investigators. A comparison of rate control with rhythm control in patients with atrial fibrillation. *N Engl J Med* 2002;347:1825–1833.
16. Van Gelder IC, Hagens VE, Bosker HA, et al. A comparison of rate control and rhythm control in patients with recurrent persisten atrial fibrillation. *N Engl J Med* 2002;347:1834–1840.
17. Opolski G, Torbicki A, Kosior DA, et al. Rate control vs. rhythm control in patients with nonvalvular persistent atrial fibrillation: the results of the Polish How to Treat Chronic Atrial Fibrillation (HOT CAFE) Study. *Chest* 2004;126:476–486.
18. Oral H, Scharf C, Chugh A, et al. Catheter ablation for paroxysmal atrial fibrillation: Segmental pulmonary vein ostial ablation versus left atrial ablation. *Circulation* 2003;108:2355–2360.
19. Stellbrink C, Nixdorff U, Hofmann T, et al. Safety and efficacy of enoxaparin compared with unfractionated heparin and oral anticoagulants for prevention of thromboembolic complications in cardioversion of nonvalvular atrial fibrillation: the Anticoagulation in Cardioversion using Enoxaparin (ACE) trial. *Circulation* 2004;109:997–1003.
20. Perez-Gomez F, Alegria E, Berjon J, et al. Comparative effects of antiplatelet, anticoagulant, or combined therapy in patients with valvular and nonvalvular atrial fibrillation: a randomized multicenter study. *J Am Coll Cardiol* 2004;44:1557–1566.
21. Crystal E, Connolly SJ, Slek K, et al. Interventions on prevention of postoperative atrial fibrillation in patients undergoing heart surgery. A meta-analysis. *Circulation* 2002;106:75–80.

ADDITIONAL READING

Halligan SC, Gersh BJ, Brown RD, et al. The natural history of lone atrial flutter. *Ann Intern Med* 2004;140:265–268.
Karamanoukian HL, Chang AH. Post operative atrial fibrillation. Key References. *Heart Surgery Forum.* Available at www.hsforum.com/vol6/issue1/2002-34343.html.
Koster RW, Dorian P, Chapman FW, Schmitt PW, O'Grady SG, Walker RG. A randomized trial comparing monophasic and biphasic waveform shocks for external cardioversion of atrial fibrillation. *Am Heart J* 2004;147:e20.
Pappone C, Rosanio S, Augello G, et al. Mortality, morbidity, and quality of life after circumferential pulmonary vein ablation for atrial fibrillation: outcomes from a controlled nonrandomized long-term study. *J Am Coll Cardiol* 2003;42:185–197.
Rockson SG, Albers GW. Comparing the guidelines: anticoagulation therapy to optimize stroke prevention in patients with atrial fibrillation. *J Am Coll Cardiol* 2004;43:929–935.
Tsai CF, Tai CT, Chen SA. Pulmonary vein ablation: role in preventing atrial fibrillation. *Curr Opin Cardiol* 2003;18:39–46.

Ventricular Arrhythmias and Cardiac Arrest

43

Graham Gardner   H. Leon Greene   Peter Zimetbaum

INTRODUCTION

Epidemiology

Sudden cardiac death is the most common cause of mortality in the United States. Approximately 250,000 people each year die within one hour of the onset of cardiovascular symptoms. The most common mechanism for sudden cardiac death is an arrhythmia, usually ventricular fibrillation (VF). Though the overall mortality rate from cardiovascular diseases has been decreasing in the past few years, sudden arrhythmic cardiac death remains a major problem.

Epidemiologic studies clearly show an association between the number of cardiac risk factors and the occurrence of sudden cardiac death. Nearly three-quarters of all patients who experience a cardiac arrest resulting from ventricular arrhythmias have previously recognized cardiac disease, either angina pectoris, prior myocardial infarction (MI), hypertension, or heart failure. Many patients are completely asymptomatic until collapse (or have no change in their chronic symptoms), although others, in whom MI precipitates the ventricular arrhythmias, may have chest pain prior to the collapse. Nevertheless, prospective identification of the patient who will develop serious ventricular arrhythmias, so that appropriate therapy can be instituted, remains an elusive goal.

Several cardiac rhythms can produce cardiac arrest. The initial rhythm identified on the monitor depends on how quickly monitoring is begun. Most patients who suffer cardiac arrest in the community are believed to have VF as the mechanism of arrest (1). The incidence of VF in the community may be declining, such that VF is now thought to be responsible for a minority of in-hospital and fully monitored cardiac arrests (2, 3). This trend may be related to improvements in treating underlying coronary artery disease as a result of better revascularization and more aggressive pharmacologic management. In addition, patients with symptoms of acute coronary syndrome may be presenting to medical attention earlier—leading to a shift in the occurrence of cardiac arrest from the outpatient to the inpatient setting. To date, however, no evidence supports such a trend (2). Still, telemetry monitoring for hospitalized patients could lead to the earlier identification of aberrant rhythms. Often VF is preceded by a short run of ventricular tachycardia (VT), but sustained VT without subsequent VF rarely causes clinical cardiac arrest. Patients seen late after their cardiac arrest commonly have asystole recorded as the initial rhythm, although the rhythm actually responsible for collapse is more likely to have been VT/VF (4). Pulseless electrical activity or electromechanical dissociation is less common but may be increasing in relative frequency.

The success of resuscitation depends on many factors, which may be different for the patient resuscitated in the hospital as opposed to the patient resuscitated out of the hospital. Reported resuscitation success varies. It is less than 1% in some inner-city areas in which medic response time is prolonged, but the success rate is over 40% in Seattle, in patients who have VF as the initially recorded rhythm and who receive early defibrillation followed by the administration of amiodarone en route to the hospital (5). Under the best circumstances, approximately two-thirds of patients who have VF on the arrival of medics are resuscitated and survive to hospital admission. Approximately half these cardiac arrest patients who are admitted to the hospital (one-third of the total VF population) ultimately are discharged from the hospital alive and well. However, in settings in which the medic response time is longer, resuscitation efforts are less successful. If patients have electromechanical dissociation or asystole as the first recorded rhythm, their prognosis is poor, with a long-term survival of only about 6% with electromechanical dissociation and 1% with asystole.

The most important factor determining survival in VF is rapid defibrillation (6). Provision of early cardiopulmonary resuscitation (CPR), although useful, is a temporizing measure. Even excellent CPR provides only about 15% of normal cerebral blood flow and 5% of normal cardiac perfusion.

Recurrent risk of cardiac arrest is high in survivors of VF, and aggressive risk factor modification is necessary to help prevent subsequent episodes. In addition, antiarrhythmic medications and implantable cardioverter defibrillators (ICDs) have been shown to improve survival in this group (7). However, survivors of VF represent only a small percentage of the total cardiac arrest population. For this reason, identifying high-risk patients and initiating primary prevention have taken on increasing urgency.

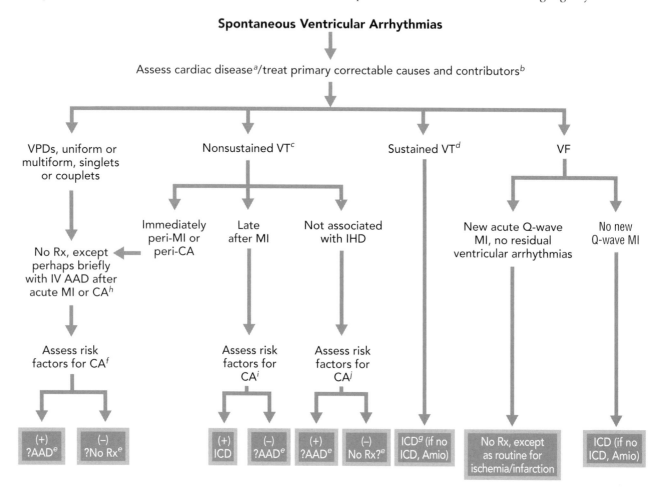

^{a} History; physical examination; serial ECGs and cardiac biomarkers; echocardiogram; cardiac catheterization; chest radiograph; ?exercise test; ?cardiac MRI or CT

^{b} Electrolytes; blood gases; ischemia/infarction; drug toxicity; CHF; as appropriate, use aspirin, β-blockers, ACE inhibitors

^{c} ≥3 complexes, ≥100 beats per minute

^{d} ≥30 seconds, ≥100 beats per minute; if CAD, remote (>48 hours) after MI without recurrent ischemia

^{e} Indications uncertain (for AAD, Amio is usually the drug of choice)

^{f} Clinical factors, ejection fraction, Holter, EPS, heart rate variability, baroreflex sensitivity, QT alternans, QT disperson, T-wave alternans, signal-averaged ECG, ECG MI score, vulnerability index, complexity index, activation recovery interval

^{g} Or consider guided arrhythmia surgery or catheter ablation for sustained monomorphic VT

^{h} Lidocaine, procainamide, amiodarone, or bretylium

^{i} Ejection fraction, Holter, EPS

^{j} Ejection fraction, Holter, ?others

Figure 43.1   Spontaneous ventricular arrhythmias. *AAD*, antiarrhythmic drug; *ACE*, angiotensin-converting enzyme; *Amio*, amiodarone; *CA*, cardiac arrest; *CAD*, coronary artery disease; *CHF*, congestive heart failure; *CT*, computed tomography; *ECG*, electrocardiogram; *EPS*, electrophysiologic study; *ICD*, implantable cardioverter defibrillator; *IHD*, ischemic heart disease; *IV*, intravenous; *MI*, myocardial infarction; *MRI*, magnetic resonance imaging; *Rx*, treatment; *VF*, ventricular fibrillation; *VPD*, ventricular premature depolarization; *VT*, ventricular tachycardia.

CATEGORIZATION OF VENTRICULAR ARRHYTHMIAS

Ventricular arrhythmias can be classified as sustained or nonsustained, symptomatic or asymptomatic, and tolerated or nontolerated. *Sustained VT* is defined as 30 seconds or more of a ventricular rhythm at greater than 100 beats per minute. Sustained VT that is one uniform morphology is called monomorphic. If sustained VT is multiform in morphology, it is called polymorphic VT. *Nonsustained VT* is characterized by three or more ventricular beats at a rate of greater than 100 beats per minute that last less than 30 seconds. *Symptomatic VT* refers to VT with the sensation of palpitations, chest pain, shortness of breath, dizziness, presyncope, or syncope. *Tolerated VT* suggests an absence of associated significant hypotension or cardiac ischemia. Isolated ventricular premature beats (VPBs) or couplets can also be symptomatic or asymptomatic (Figure 43.1). They may represent an independent risk for recurrent ventricular arrhythmia in patients with coronary artery disease or other cardiac pathology—particularly when they are frequent (greater than 6–10 beats per hour).

GENERAL PRINCIPLES OF THERAPY

Though ventricular arrhythmias identify patients at higher risk of sudden arrhythmic cardiac death, specific treatment of these ventricular arrhythmias is not always indicated. Treatment strategy should first focus on the primary disease process and then on assessing the risk of further symptomatic ventricular arrhythmias. No single test adequately predicts serious ventricular arrhythmias, which means that evaluating the risk of sudden death often involves several testing modalities. These include echocardiogram, Holter monitoring, stress testing, cardiac catheterization, and electrophysiologic study. The role for some of these tests remains controversial, and the extent of workup may depend on the goals of the patient and the patient's family, as well as the experience of the cardiologist.

WHEN VENTRICULAR ARRHYTHMIAS PRESENT ON ADMISSION

Clinical Presentations and Indications for Admission

Symptomatic ventricular arrhythmias requiring hospital admission include resuscitated VF (cardiac arrest) as well as sustained and nonsustained VT with symptoms of syncope, near-syncope, dizziness, or lightheadedness. Patients with any of these symptoms should be admitted to the ICU, coronary care unit, or (for patients with tolerated VT who have not suffered loss of consciousness) a telemetry unit. If a patient is asymptomatic and (a) it has been previously demonstrated that the ventricular arrhythmia is chronic, (b) the arrhythmia has been completely evaluated, and (c) the arrhythmia has not been associated with serious hemodynamic compromise or symptoms (e.g., idiopathic VT), hospital admission may not be necessary. Patients with ICDs who present with recurrent ventricular arrhythmias that have been appropriately treated by their ICD (e.g., defibrillation or pacing) also do not require hospitalization.

Etiology

A wide range of diseases and conditions is associated with ventricular arrhythmias and may produce sudden cardiac death (Table 43.1). These conditions must be distinguished from nonarrhythmic conditions that can also cause sudden collapse, such as cardiac tamponade, aortic dissection, sudden blood loss, stroke, tension pneumothorax, sepsis, and pulmonary embolus.

On the initial evaluation, it is useful to distinguish the more typical monomorphic sustained VT (Figure 43.2 A) from polymorphic VT (Figure 43.2 B and C). *Polymorphic VT* is characterized by beat-to-beat alterations in the morphology of the QRS complex. If the polymorphic VT has a pattern that appears to be rotating around a baseline and is associated with QT prolongation (Figure 43.2 C), it is called *torsade de pointes*. Torsade de pointes may be caused by congenital prolongation of the QT interval, either at rest or with

TABLE 43.1

DISEASES ASSOCIATED WITH SUDDEN ARRHYTHMIC CARDIAC DEATH

Coronary artery disease	Congenital heart disease
Acute ischemia/infarction	Coronary artery anomalies
Chronic coronary disease with prior myocardial infarction	Valvular heart disease
	Tetralogy of Fallot
	Left ventricular diverticulum
Ruptured myocardium	Right ventricular dysplasia
Coronary arteritis	Wolff-Parkinson-White syndrome
Coronary spasm	
Cardiomyopathy	Long QT syndromes
Dilated	Congenital
Hypertrophic	Acquired
Symmetric	Drug toxicity
Asymmetric	Electrolyte abnormalities
Myocarditis	Toxins (e.g., cocaine)
Infiltrative myocardial disease	Proarrhythmic effects of antiarrhythmic drugs
Tumor	
Infection	Electrolyte abnormalities
Sarcoid	Mitral valve prolapse
Other	Cardiac tumors
Valvular heart disease	Pulmonary hypertension
	Cardiac trauma
	Electrocution
	Primary electrical disease (e.g., Brugada syndrome, idiopathic VF)

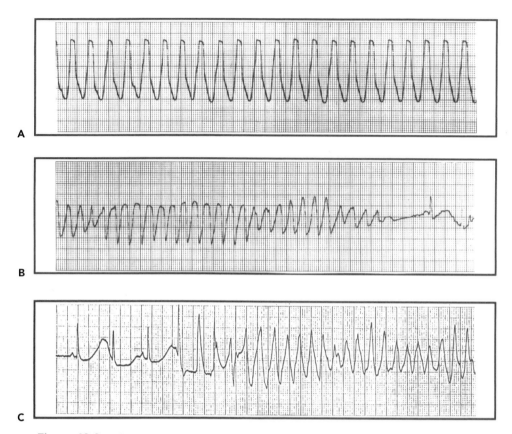

Figure 43.2. Electrocardiographic monitor strips from three different patients. **A.** Monomorphic sustained ventricular tachycardia *(VT)* in a patient with a previous myocardial scar. The QRS morphology is identical from beat to beat. **B.** Polymorphic VT in a patient with ongoing ischemia. The QRS changes from beat to beat, and the VT terminates spontaneously. Though it is difficult to measure on this single lead, the QT interval was normal on a 12-lead electrocardiogram. **C.** Torsade de pointes VT in a patient taking quinidine. The QT is prolonged. The QRS changes dramatically from beat to beat, twisting around an imaginary baseline. This VT also ultimately terminated spontaneously, as is common for torsade de pointes VT.

exercise. More commonly, however, polymorphic torsade de pointes is acquired and is caused by antiarrhythmic drugs (especially quinidine, procainamide, disopyramide, dofetilide, sotalol, or rarely amiodarone), tricyclic antidepressants, phenothiazines, some antibiotics (especially erythromycin and pentamidine), some antihistamines (terfenadine and astemizole), and other drugs (probucol and cisapride). It also may be precipitated by electrolyte disorders such as hypokalemia, hypocalcemia, and hypomagnesemia. Polymorphic VT in the absence of a prolonged QT may occur after MI or with myocardial ischemia. By comparison, *monomorphic sustained VT* (Figure 43.2A) has a constant appearance from beat to beat and is commonly seen in patients with underlying coronary artery disease (especially with left-ventricular scar) or other myocardial disease. Only rarely do patients with monomorphic sustained VT lack underlying heart disease (when they do, this is termed idiopathic VT, and it is rarely life threatening).

Sudden death in the young person or athlete carries its own differential diagnosis (8). The most common causes are hypertrophic obstructive cardiomyopathy (HOCM)

and anomalous coronary arteries. Direct trauma to the heart (commotio cordis) is also an important cause. Other etiologies include arrhythmogenic right ventricular dysplasia (ARVD), long QT syndrome, Brugada syndrome, and idiopathic VF (VF without underlying structural heart disease).

Wolff-Parkinson-White syndrome (WPW) is a special circumstance in which atrial fibrillation conducted over an accessory pathway can precipitate VF. Administration of drugs that directly or indirectly accelerate conduction of atrial fibrillation over the accessory pathway (e.g., digoxin, verapamil) can facilitate the development of VF in patients with WPW. Definitive therapy is radiofrequency ablation (Chapter 42).

Differential Diagnosis

Ventricular arrhythmias can usually be distinguished from wide-complex supraventricular arrhythmias (Chapter 42) by the presence of atrioventricular dissociation, the axis of the QRS vector, the width of the QRS complex, and several morphological criteria. *In patients with pre-existing heart disease or risk factors for sudden cardiac death, any arrhythmia about which there is a question should be evaluated and treated as ventricular in origin until proven otherwise.*

Initial Evaluation and Treatment

Evaluation

The evaluation for the etiology of the cardiac arrest should begin immediately after the resuscitation because the treatment of any provoking factors will help stabilize the patient and prevent an immediate recurrence of the arrhythmia (Figure 43.3). An electrocardiogram (ECG) and cardiac biomarker levels should be obtained to identify patients with active ischemia or infarction who may benefit from early revascularization. Evaluation of telemetry and any rhythm strips provided by the paramedics is also critical. Unfortunately, complications from the arrest, such as acidemia, electrolyte abnormalities, and myocardial stunning, can sometimes make the interpretation of noninvasive tests more difficult. Similarly, because arrests are frequently unwitnessed and patients may not be responsive, the history is often unhelpful in determining whether cardiac ischemia preceded the arrest. In these circumstances, physicians may choose to proceed with cardiac catheterization to exclude the possibility of coronary artery disease. Cardiac catheterization with catheter-based revascularization, if available, is preferred to thrombolysis in the patient with active ischemia who has received CPR (9).

For patients with polymorphic VT, attention must be paid to possible precipitating causes, including illicit drugs, prescribed medications, and electrolyte abnormalities. Electrolyte abnormalities should be corrected aggressively, although it is important to remember that certain abnormalities, such as hypokalemia, may be the consequence of the high catecholamine state associated with cardiac arrest and not necessarily the precipitating factor. For this reason, a full cardiac workup should be simultaneously pursued in these patients. Potentially offending medications must be discontinued immediately.

Approximately 20% of patients develop new Q waves, and 50% develop biomarker abnormalities consistent with MI. Cardiac troponin assays are more specific and more sensitive than creatine kinase MB levels for myocardial damage, especially after CPR. Patients who have an acute Q-wave MI at the time of VF have only about a 2% risk of recurrent VF and do not warrant aggressive long-term antiarrhythmic drug or device therapy, particularly if they have been revascularized. By comparison, *patients who have neither new Q waves nor biomarker elevations are at the highest risk for recurrent VT/VF*, and patients without new Q waves but with biomarker elevations have an intermediate risk. Other risk factors for the recurrence of VT or VF include male sex, advanced age, history of prior MI, low ejection fraction, and a history of heart failure.

Early attention should also be directed toward the patient's underlying neurologic status. Although diffuse anoxic encephalopathy is the most common cause of stupor or coma after cardiac arrest, persistent abnormal mental states after admission or any suggestion of localizing central nervous system signs should prompt computed tomography or magnetic resonance imaging of the head to evaluate for treatable intracranial pathology. It is important to realize, and to help the family understand, that dramatic recovery can occur, particularly within the first 72 hours. Families often insist upon withdrawal of support immediately, based on the patient's previously expressed wishes to avoid "being hooked to machines," without realizing that nearly full recovery may be possible following a brief period of mechanical support. Supportive efforts should not be withdrawn based upon lack of return of neurologic function if the patient has been exposed to drugs that might depress central nervous system function or if seizures are uncontrolled (e.g., barbiturate overdose).

Finally, the initial workup of a cardiac arrest should focus on conditions that can accompany an arrest (Figure 43.3). This workup includes a chest radiograph to evaluate for pulmonary edema or aspiration pneumonia. A nasogastric tube must be placed to prevent gastric distention and to evaluate for gastrointestinal bleeding. Urinary output should be monitored by Foley catheter. Laboratory data to monitor the patient's renal function and acid-base status will also help identify complications such as acute renal failure, rhabdomyolysis, and lactic acidosis. Frequently, an initial lactic acidosis may be caused by poor peripheral tissue perfusion; however, persistent lactic acidosis should be a clue to additional damage, such as bowel ischemia.

Management

Management of recurrent VF or pulseless VT begins with early defibrillation, along with administration of intravenous antiarrhythmic medication (Table 43.2). Patients who undergo a primary arrest in the hospital or who develop recurrent VF after presentation should be defibrillated with 200–360 joules of energy applied to the chest wall. Defibrillation should be performed as quickly as possible because the chance of success in terminating the arrhythmia decreases with time (6).

Antiarrhythmic medications may also have a role in the acute setting. In the ARREST trial, early administration of intravenous amiodarone, given as a 300 mg intravenous push, led to a significant improvement in survival to hospitalization among patients who experienced a cardiac arrest from VF or VT that was initially unresponsive to defibrillation (5). Although the study failed to detect a difference in long-term survival between the groups that received amiodarone versus placebo, *amiodarone is now considered first-line therapy for the management of VF or*

	In field or ER (OOH arrest) or on general hospital ward (IH arrest)	Day 1[a]: First 4 hours and continuing, as needed	Day 1: Remainder and continuing, as needed	Day 2	Day 3	Day 4–7[b]	Day ≥8

Evaluation/ Tests/ Procedures	• BCLS/ACLS
	• Defibrillation
	• Intubation
	• Central IV line
	• Rhythm monitoring[?]
		• Detailed Hx/PE
		  - from Pt (rarely)
		  - from relatives/ friends/bystanders
		  - from primary MD
		• Arterial line
		• ± Swan Ganz catheter
		• Foley catheter
		• NG tube
		• Lytes/CBC/UA/PT/ PTT
		• CXR
		• ECG
		• Cardiac biomarkers
		• Toxicology screen
		• Pulse oximetry
		• ABGs
		• ± Head CT/MRI
		• ± Chest CT/MRI
		• ± Echocardiogram
			• Cardiac biomarkers
			• ABGs
			• Social work consult prn
				• CXR
				• Lytes/CBC
				• ECG
				• Cardiac biomarkers
				• ABGs
				• Echocardio-gram[d]
				• Neurology consult[d]
				• Pulse oximetry
					• CSF CK-BB
					• ± CXR
					• Lytes/CBC
					• ECG
					• EP consult
					• Nutrition screen/consult
					• Physical/occu-pational thera-py consult prn
						• D/C Swan-Ganz
						• D/C arterial line
						• CXR prn
						• ECG prn
						• Cardiac cath/other diagnostic tests prn
						• ± PTCA/CABG
						• Cardiac surgery consult
							• ICD[c]
							• If severe brain anoxia, ethics consult prn
							• Nursing home placement ± DNAR
							• ± Feeding tube, gastrostomy, or TPN

Medications and Theraputics	• ± Lidocaine or other AAD	• ± Cath/PTCA
		• ± Thrombolysis
		• ± ASA
		• Ventilate to correct
		  - pCO$_2$
		  - pO2 (maintain saturation ≥92%)
		  - pH
		• ± K$^+$, Mg^{++}
		• Heparin (DVT prophylaxis)
		• ± Inotropes
		• ± Vasodilators
		• ± Vasopressors
		• ± Diuretics
		• ± ACE inhibitors
		• H$_2$ blockers/ antacids
		• Pain meds/ sedation prn
				• Abx if aspira-tion pneumo-nia	• D/C lidocaine
					• Ventilator weaning parameters
					• ± Extubation
						• D/C IV as appropriate
						• Heparin lock IV[e]
							• D/C IV as appropriate

Nursing Assessment	• VS q15 min until stable	• VS q4h (mini-mum) • Weight • I + O • Hemodynamics • Neuro exam q shift • Pulse/circulatory exam q shift • Bedrest • Eye/Skin care • Restraints prn	• VS q4h (minimum) • I + O	• VS/weight • I + O	• VS/weight • I + O	• VS/weight • I + O • Sit in chair, ambu-late as tolerated • D/C I + O • Transfer to telemetry unit	

Figure 43.3 Critical pathway: cardiac arrest. *AAD*, antiarrhythmic drug; *ABG*, arterial blood gas; *Abx*, antibiotics; *ACE*, angiotensin-converting enzyme; *ACLS*, advanced cardiac life support; *ASA*, aspirin; *BCLS*, basic cardiac life support; *CABG*, coronary artery bypass graft; *CBC*, complete blood count; *CK*, creatine kinase; *CSF*, cerebrospinal fluid; *CT*, computed tomography; *CXR*, chest radiograph; *D/C*, discontinue; *DNAR*, do not attempt resuscitation; *DVT*, deep venous thrombosis; *ECG*, electrocardiogram; *EP*, electrophysiologic; *ER*, emergency room; *Hx*, history; *H$_2$*, histamine; *ICD*, implantable cardioverter defibrillator; *IH*, in-hospital; *I+O*, intake and output; *IV*, intravenous; *MD*, physician; *MRI*, magnetic resonance imaging; *NG*, nasogastric; *NHP*, nursing home placement; *NPO*, nothing by mouth; *OOH*, out-of-hospital; *PE*, physical examination; *Pt*, patient; *PT*, prothrombin time; *PTCA*, percutaneous transluminal coronary angioplasty; *PTT*, partial thromboplastin time; *TPN*, total parenteral nutrition; *UA*, urinalysis; *VS*, vital signs; *VT*, ventricular tachycardia.

	In field or ER (OOH arrest) or on general hospital ward (IH arrest)	Day1[1]: First 4 hours and continuing, as needed	Day 1: Remainder and continuing, as needed	Day 2	Day 3	Day 4–7[2]	Day ≥8
Nutrition		• NPO • IV fluids/glucose				• Clear liquids, advance diet as tolerated, or feeding per feeding tube, or parenteral nutrition	
Patient/Family Education		• Orient to procedures/tests • Introduce therapeutic options • Begin education re: prognosis (cardiac and neurological)				• Teaching regarding tests, therapeutics • Frequent orientation to surroundings, tests, procedures (near-term memory loss)	• Discharge teaching
Discharge Planning		• Discuss projected timetable with family				• Assess discharge needs (NHP, rehabilitation facility, home) • Notify primary MD of progress/plans	• Review with patient and family • Return appointments • Return signs and symptoms • Notify primary MD

[a] *Under care of cardiologist/internist*
[b] *For sustained VT without anoxic brain damage, the algorithm starts approximately at day 4*
[c] *After all infectious sources cleared*
[d] *If not already performed*
[e] *Continue until definitive therapy is achieved, usually day 8 or after*

Figure 43.3   (*continued*)

TABLE 43.2
ACUTE INTRAVENOUS ANTIARRHYTHMIC DRUGS FOR VT/VF

	Loading dose	Maintenance dose	Therapeutic levels
Lidocaine	1–2 mg/kg bolus	1–4 mg/min	2–5 mg/mL
Procainamide	15–20 mg/kg over 30–60 min	1–4 mg/min	4–10 mg/mL
Amiodarone	150 mg over 10 min, 360 mg over 6h, 540 mg over 18h	0.5–1.0 mg/min	Not useful
β-blockers			
Esmolol	500 mcg/kg over 1 min (additional 500 mcg/kg over 1 min q5 min)	50 mcg/kg/min for 4 min; adjust up or down q5 min to maximum of 200 mcg/kg/min	Not useful
Metoprolol	5 mg bolus × 3, separated by 2 min	5–10 mg/h	Not useful
Propranolol	0.1 mg/kg at 1 mg/min; may repeat after 5 min (maximum 0.2 mg/kg)	3–15 mg/h	Not useful

VT-mediated cardiac arrest. Lidocaine may have a role in the acute management of ischemia-mediated VF or VT, although the ALIVE trial indicated that amiodarone was more effective than lidocaine in improving survival to hospitalization (10). Magnesium sulfate is recommended for the treatment of torsade de pointes and hypomagnesemic states.

The induction of mild-to-moderate hypothermia (target core body temperature of 32–34°C for 24 hours) has been shown to improve neurologic recovery in patients who are successfully resuscitated after cardiac arrest (11–13). At this time, the logistics involved in cooling patients quickly and effectively has limited its broad application. However, newer technologies designed to achieve efficient and isolated CNS cooling may prove useful in helping patients retain their functional status after suffering an arrest.

Prognosis

Even in the acute phase, long-term prognosis can be estimated with simple prognostic indices such as the Glasgow Coma Scale (Table 117.1), the APACHE classification system (Chapter 22), or other simple algorithms (Table 43.3) (14). The time elapsed in the coma itself is also predictive of subsequent awakening. For example, the patient who has not awakened by the end of day 2 has only a 27% probability of ever awakening; the probability remains about 20% even at three weeks (14). The probability of awakening without gross motor and cognitive deficits, however, is much lower. Fully one-third of even those patients who are awake on admission have some neurologic impairment in the long term, and after four days of coma, essentially 100% of patients have both motor and cognitive deficits in the long term. Seizures and myoclonus are also bad prognostic signs. Patients may be observed for a variety of post-resuscitation complications (Table 43.4).

Measurement of *cerebrospinal fluid creatine kinase BB* at 48 to 72 hours following cardiac arrest is predictive of the patient's awakening (15). If the level of cerebrospinal fluid creatine kinase BB is less than 50 units/L, substantial neurologic recovery is likely; values of more than 204 units/L are associated with nearly zero chance of awakening.

ISSUES DURING THE COURSE OF HOSPITALIZATION

Acute Cardiac Issues

In patients surviving cardiac arrest, the rhythm usually stabilizes within the first 24 hours, and acute antiarrhythmic drugs can often be discontinued 48–72 hours after admission. Frequent recurrent arrhythmias, particularly during the first 24 hours after admission, may indicate an ongoing ischemic process. However, other causes should be sought, such as drug intoxication and electrolyte abnormalities, especially in patients with prolonged QT intervals and polymorphic VT. Likewise, cardiac output and blood pressure usually stabilize by 48 hours, although dramatic fluctuations in blood pressure may continue, requiring variable doses of vasodilating and vasopressor drugs.

Definitive Cardiac Evaluation

Definitive cardiac evaluation should begin as soon as possible after hospital admission (Chapter 36). Echocardiography is useful to measure left ventricular ejection fraction, to assess valve function, and to exclude pulmonary hypertension and the presence of dilated or hypertrophic cardiomyopathies. Remember, however, that transient myocardial stunning may follow cardiac arrest from any cause. Thus, an accurate measurement of left ventricular function may need to be delayed 48–72 hours. If it is suspected that transient myocardial ischemia triggered the ventricular arrhythmia, an invasive or noninvasive

TABLE 43.3A

PREDICTION OF AWAKENING: DETERMINATION OF SCORE

Motor response	+ 3 × pupillary light response	+ Spontaneous eye movements	+ First blood-glucose level
0, Absent	0, Absent	0, Absent	0, ≥300 mg/dL
1, Extensor posturing	1, Present	1, Present	1, <300 mg/dL
2, Flexor posturing			
3, Nonposturing			
4, Withdrawal or localizing			

Note: Sum of subscores gives score on admission.

TABLE 43.3B

PREDICTION OF AWAKENING: CORRELATION OF SCORE WITH PROBABILITY

Score on admission	Probability of awakening (%)
0, 1, 2	5
3, 4	24
5, 6, 7	74
8, 9	95

assessment of coronary perfusion should be performed. Holter monitoring and electrophysiologic testing may be critical for diagnosis, but studies have suggested that expedited progression to placement of an ICD is often appropriate in patients who have suffered a near-fatal cardiac arrest (7).

Risk factors for recurrence of sustained VT or VF include male sex, advanced age, lack of development of a new Q-wave MI with the episode of VF, history of prior MI, low ejection fraction, and history of heart failure. The only reliable single indicator of low risk of recurrent VT/VF is the development of a new Q-wave MI at the time of VF.

WHEN THE DISEASE PRESENTS DURING HOSPITALIZATION

Cardiac Arrest

Frequently, cardiac arrest resulting from VT or VF occurs in a patient already hospitalized for another condition. Patients with in-hospital arrests may have the same spectrum of diseases as patients who present with arrests that occurred out of the hospital, but inpatients are more likely to have had an arrest because of an MI, pulmonary embolus, or blood loss related to their coexisting diseases. Nevertheless, the evaluation and treatment of these patients should be as extensive as it is in the patient with an out-of-hospital presentation. Often the patient is unconscious or in the operating room at the time of the arrhythmia and cannot provide the history of chest pain that might otherwise have been noted as an ischemic precipitant. These patients often are sicker because of the combination of the cardiac disease and other coexisting pathology, and the success of the initial resuscitation in fact may be lower than that for out-of-hospital arrest, even though the response time is faster. However, under certain circumstances, such as in the cardiac catheterization laboratory, resuscitation rates can approach 100% because of nearly immediate defibrillation of VT or VF.

A VT/VF arrest that occurs in an already critically ill patient often portends irreversibility of the underlying disease process. If such an arrest occurs in a patient with a preterminal condition, such as an advanced malignancy, aggressive resuscitation may be inappropriate (Chapter 17). It is critical that the physician quickly understand the patient's overall situation to guide in-hospital CPR attempts. It is tempting to blame a low potassium level, catecholamines, drugs, or hypoxia for the arrhythmia, but hospitalized patients commonly also have an underlying propensity to ventricular arrhythmias unrelated to any transient condition. They may well need even more extensive testing than out-of-hospital patients to be certain that the VT/VF has a reversible cause. Furthermore, they ultimately have worse long-term outcomes than patients with out-of-hospital VT/VF.

TABLE 43.4

COMPLICATIONS OF CARDIAC ARREST AND RESUSCITATION

Early	Late
Rib fractures/flail chest	Acute respiratory distress syndrome
Pneumothorax/hemothorax	
Stomach/esophageal rupture	Sepsis
Liver laceration	Gastrointestinal bleeding
Rhabdomyolysis	Anoxic encephalopathy
Limb ischemia	
Bowel ischemia	
Aspiration pneumonia	
Renal failure	
Coma	
Trauma (especially head trauma) related to fall, automobile accident, etc., secondary to cardiac arrest	
Pericardial effusion	
Complications related to central line placement	
Laceration of subclavian artery or vein	
Hematoma	
Arteriovenous fistula	
Complications related to endotracheal intubation	
Selective intubation of right or left mainstream bronchus	
Vocal-cord damage	
Cardiac laceration or rupture	
Splenic laceration	
Skin burns from repeated defibrillation	

Because hospitalized patients usually have other comorbid diseases that precipitate the arrhythmia, the first step is to identify these causes and correct them if possible. It is critical to distinguish polymorphic VT from monomorphic VT because of the often differing underlying causes and their therapeutic implications.

For the patient with *drug-induced polymorphic VT with a long QT interval*, electrolyte abnormalities must be corrected, and potentially causative medications must be discontinued. A bolus of magnesium (1–2 g over 10 minutes, followed by a continuous infusion) followed by emergent insertion of a temporary transvenous pacemaker or administration of intravenous isoproterenol to increase the cardiac rate is indicated. In a patient with unstable ischemic heart disease and polymorphic VT, aggressive treatment with β-blockers, nitrates, and possibly intravenous amiodarone may be effective; prompt revascularization is the ideal treatment. For patients with congenital or idiopathic long QT syndrome, cardiologic consultation is required to plan therapy.

For the patient with *monomorphic VT*, direct-current cardioversion is the treatment of choice. Lidocaine, procainamide, or amiodarone (Table 43.2) can be used as adjunctive therapy after successful cardioversion or for loading doses prior to repeat cardioversion in patients in whom initial cardioversion has been unsuccessful. In some instances, tolerated sustained monomorphic VT can be ablated in the electrophysiology laboratory. In most cases of tolerated VT associated with structural heart disease, or in cases of untolerated VT, an ICD is indicated.

OTHER PRESENTATIONS OF VENTRICULAR ARRHYTHMIAS

Patients may present not with VF and cardiac arrest, but rather with more well-tolerated arrhythmias such as hemodynamically stable sustained VT (30 seconds or more of VT), nonsustained VT, or frequent VPBs. Many patients with VPBs or nonsustained VT require no specific antiarrhythmic therapy. These arrhythmias are commonly seen in hospitalized patients (especially those who are critically ill) and often are related to marked sympathetic stimulation from hypotension, fluid overload, sepsis, respiratory failure, or other critical illnesses. If the VPB or nonsustained VT is a manifestation of an exacerbation of ischemic heart disease, aggressive therapy should target the ischemic heart disease itself (Chapter 37). If the nonsustained VT or frequent VPBs themselves cause hemodynamic complications, suppression with intravenous antiarrhythmic drugs (Table 43.2) may be helpful and generally is indicated. However, the patient's ultimate prognosis is depends more on the outcome of treatment of the underlying severe illness than on the treatment of the ventricular arrhythmias themselves. In some critically ill patients, VPBs may be precipitated by a right heart catheter; withdrawal of the catheter back into the central venous system is curative. Remember that *VPBs in patients without structural heart disease do not carry an increased risk for cardiac events.*

Nonsustained VT may herald more serious arrhythmias, however. For that reason, basic evaluation is essential, though it need not necessarily be performed completely in the hospital, nor need it always result in long-term treatment. On occasion, a patient may have recurrent episodes of nonsustained VT documented for a considerable length of time without symptoms. In such cases, in-hospital evaluation is not required. Nonsustained VT or even torsade de pointes VT usually can be managed in either the critical care unit or a monitored telemetry unit. Patients with coronary artery disease or with heart failure or low left ventricular ejection fraction who have nonsustained VT are at higher risk of cardiac arrest than similar patients without these arrhythmias. Higher-risk patients should be managed in consultation with a cardiac electrophysiologist as they often require specialized electrophysiologic testing, ICD implantation, or antiarrhythmic drugs.

With the proliferation of ICDs, more patients are presenting to hospitals with a history of a shock or shocks from the ICD. These shocks may be either single, isolated events or repeated shocks over a short period of time. Single, isolated ICD shocks require an evaluation for acute factors such as electrolyte abnormality, drug intoxication, ischemia, or device malfunction. However, most patients with ICD shocks can be discharged from the physician's office or the emergency department without hospitalization. Frequent, closely spaced shocks or symptomatic episodes may require hospitalization for evaluation for primary causes, the initiation of antiarrhythmic drugs, or electrophysiologic study with VT ablation.

Another common issue is the question of whether to replace an ICD at the time of battery depletion if no shocks or antitachycardia pacing therapies have been delivered since the original implantation. In general, it is appropriate to replace these devices because patients have a continued moderate risk for recurrence of ventricular arrhythmias.

DISCHARGE ISSUES

Long-Term Therapy

It is important to address the primary cause of the arrhythmia, usually coronary artery disease. Evidence of reversible ischemia will usually lead to a percutaneous coronary intervention or to coronary artery bypass graft (CABG) surgery. However, unless transient ischemia was responsible for the arrhythmia, revascularization alone may not be sufficient to prevent further arrhythmic episodes. Aortic or mitral valve disease should be corrected if appropriate, but patients with valve disease probably remain at risk for further VT/VF even after correction of their valvular abnormality.

In patients with polymorphic VT, avoidance of precipitating medications may be the only treatment needed. However, many patients with polymorphic VT have myocardial ischemia or an ongoing tendency to develop precipitating electrolyte abnormalities and may require more definitive therapy.

Based on the results of multiple clinical trials (7, 16–20), *it is now widely accepted that the ICD is the most efficacious therapy for patients with a history of VF or sustained VT with syncope or serious hemodynamic compromise*, except in situations in which there are contraindications (7) (Tables 43.5 and 43.6). In fact, in patients with heart failure that remains symptomatic, an ICD can be combined with cardiac resynchronization therapy to improve outcome (16). Multiple trials suggest that high-risk patients, even those without a previously documented history of VT or VF arrest, also benefit from implantation of an ICD for the primary prevention of sudden cardiac death (17–21).

In addition to ICD implantation, other therapies can be considered in consultation with a cardiac electrophysiolo-

TABLE 43.5

WHEN AN IMPLANTABLE CARDIOVERTER DEFIBRILLATOR IS *NOT* INDICATED FOR THE PATIENT WITH SUSTAINED VENTRICULAR TACHYCARDIA/FIBRILLATION

Temporarily
  Patient has ongoing infection
  Patient has a poor neurologic recovery, soon after arrest
Permanently
  VF associated with new Q-wave myocardial infarction
  Patient fails to improve neurologically over time
  Patient refusal
  Coexisting disease that will seriously limit chance of survival
  ? Class IV CHF, unless the patient is a transplant candidate
  VT/VF occurred early (≤48h) after myocardial infarction, percutaneous coronary angioplasty, or coronary artery bypass graft

CHF, congestive heart failure; *VF*, ventricular fibrillation; *VT*, ventricular tachycardia.

TABLE 43.7

CLASSIFICATION OF ANTIARRHYTHMIC DRUGS FOR VT/VF

Class I	IA	Quinidine
		Procainamide
		Disopyramide
	IB	Tocainide
		Lidocaine (intravenous only)
		Mexiletine
	IC	Flecainide
		Propafenone
Class II		β-blocking agents
Class III		Amiodarone
		Sotalol
		Bretylium

gist. Radiofrequency ablation in patients with monomorphic VT may reduce symptoms and decrease device firing. Antiarrhythmic medications (Table 43.7) may also help to suppress recurrent arrhythmias, although medications should not replace the implantation of an ICD in appropriate candidates. Concomitant use of antiarrhythmic medications with an ICD is common practice (in as high as 70% of patients). Amiodarone is generally considered first-line therapy (particularly for patients with heart failure), although it has a number of potential toxicities. Because of this, amiodarone should be loaded in the hospital in patients with VT who do not have an ICD. In general, decisions about the use of amiodarone or alternative antiarrhythmic medications should be made in consultation with a cardiologist.

Other Long-Term Issues

Patients who do not survive the hospitalization after initial resuscitation from their ventricular arrhythmias usually die of either cardiogenic shock or devastating neurologic impairment. Lack of neurologic function itself may limit the ability to perform diagnostic tests or even to obtain

TABLE 43.6

CONDITIONS FOR WHICH TREATMENT OF CHOICE IS UNCERTAIN

Nonsustained VT, especially if asymptomatic and/or noninducible at electrophysiology study
VT/VF associated with transient, supposedly reversible cause
Sustained VT that is minimally symptomatic with minimal hemodynamic consequences
Unexplained syncope

VF, ventricular fibrillation; *VT*, ventricular tachycardia.

consent for procedures. It is common for a patient to be discharged to a nursing home or a rehabilitative facility without definitive cardiac evaluation or treatment for ventricular arrhythmias, with subsequent cardiac evaluation deferred for weeks or even months until the patient's neurologic status renders evaluation appropriate.

Return of neurologic function is commonly slow and progressive. Patients often retain excellent long-term memory but virtually no short-term memory. In fact, patients who have had a VF arrest almost always have total amnesia for the event, including the minutes or hours preceding the arrest, whereas patients with only sustained VT (and therefore maintenance of at least some cardiac output) usually have preserved memories.

Activities that could put the patient or others at risk should an arrhythmia recur should be addressed. Guidelines for driving are variable from state to state and often ill defined (22). Most physicians restrict driving for approximately six months after the most recent cardiac arrhythmia that caused loss or near loss of consciousness. Restriction is not directly related to subsequent therapy, such as the ICD, but it reflects the hazards that may occur should the patient become temporarily incapacitated and lose control of a vehicle because of an arrhythmia.

Other potentially risky activities, such as traveling to remote areas, swimming, climbing ladders, working in exposed areas (e.g., on the roof of a house), and piloting an airplane must also be restricted. Recommendations should be individualized, based upon the characteristics of the patient's myocardial function and symptoms with arrhythmias. In considering these recommendations, the physician should also take account of risks to other parties.

OUTPATIENT FOLLOW-UP

The patient can be discharged after complete cardiac evaluation and definitive therapy for both the primary and secondary conditions. Except for some specific situations, an ICD is now the recommended therapy for survivors of sustained VT/VF; hospital discharge is appropriate soon after recovery from anesthesia for implantation. Patients can usually be discharged home, although they sometimes must be discharged to a nursing home or rehabilitation facility for further neurologic and cardiac recovery.

A return outpatient visit with the primary care physician and cardiologist should be scheduled for one to four weeks after hospital discharge. In addition, close follow-up with a device clinic is required for patients who have undergone ICD implantation. Patients usually are seen at two- to four-month intervals thereafter.

COST CONSIDERATIONS AND RESOURCE USE

Two weeks is the average length of hospital stay for the patient who survives a cardiac arrest from out-of-hospital sustained VT/VF and who has an ICD implanted. Patients who have severe myocardial dysfunction often die soon after hospital admission; other patients with severe neurologic impairment may require prolonged hospital stays, including time in a rehabilitation facility or nursing home. Therefore, the treatment of cardiac arrest is expensive.

The development of the ICD has raised major issues regarding the cost and quality of care for patients with VT and VF. In the Multicenter Automatic Defibrillator Implantation Trial (MADIT) (17), the average hospitalization cost for patients treated with antiarrhythmic drugs was about $19,000, compared with $45,000 for patients treated with an ICD (23). Nevertheless, compared with antiarrhythmic drugs, the cost per year of life saved by an ICD was only about $23,000, well within the range of other commonly offered therapies in the United States. However, in another trial, the cost was considerably higher (7). Clearly, careful selection of patients is essential to avoid implantation of ICDs in patients who are unlikely to have a recurrence of VT/VF.

KEY POINTS

- In patients presenting with ventricular arrhythmias, investigation for the cause of the arrhythmia should begin immediately after successful resuscitation.
- Clinicians should search vigorously for treatable other conditions that may accompany cardiac arrest.
- Neurologic recovery may be slow, and one needs to allow adequate time for recovery before estimating prognosis with certainty.

- Randomized trials have concluded definitively that patients with a history of VF or symptomatic VT benefit from implantation of an ICD and that this intervention is relatively cost effective.
- Polymorphic VT must be differentiated from monomorphic VT because the former has different causes and treatments.
- Do not overtreat otherwise asymptomatic patients with nonsustained VT or VPBs in the absence of structural heart disease.

REFERENCES

1. Demirovic J, Myerburg RJ. Epidemiology of sudden cardiac death: an overview. *Prog Cardiovasc Dis* 1994;37:39.
2. Cobb LA, Fahrenbruch CE, Olsufka M, Copass MK. Changing incidence of out-of-hospital ventricular fibrillation, 1980–2000. *JAMA* 2002;288:3008–3013.
3. Pederdy MA, Kaye W, Ornato JP, et al. Cardiopulmonary resuscitation of adults in the hospital: a report of 14,720 cardiac arrests from the National Registry of Cardiopulmonary Resuscitation. *Resuscitation* 2003;58:297–308.
4. Greene HL. Sudden arrhythmic cardiac death-mechanisms, resuscitation and classification: the Seattle perspective. *Am J Cardiol* 1990;65:4B–12B.
5. Kudenchuk PJ, Cobb LA, Copass MK, et al. Amiodarone for resuscitation after out-of-hospital cardiac arrest due to ventricular fibrillation. *N Engl J Med* 1999;341:871–878.
6. Thompson RJ, McCullough PA, Kahn JK, O'Neill WW. Prediction of death and neurologic outcome in the emergency department in out-of-hospital cardiac arrest survivors. *Am J Cardiol* 1998;81:17–21.
7. The Antiarrhythmics Versus Implantable Defibrillators (AVID) Investigators. A comparison of antiarrhythmic drug therapy with implantable defibrillators in patients resuscitated from near-fatal ventricular arrhythmias. *N Engl J Med* 1997;337:1576–1583.
8. Maron BJ. Sudden death in young athletes. *N Engl J Med* 2003; 349:1064–1075.
9. Spaulding CM, Joly L-M, Rosenberg A, et al. Immediate coronary angiography in survivors of out-of-hospital cardiac arrest. *N Engl J Med* 1997;336:1629–1633.
10. Dorian P, Cass D, Schwartz B, Cooper R, Gelaznikas R, Barr A. Amiodarone as compared with lidocaine for shock resistant ventricular fibrillation. *N Engl J Med* 2002;346:884–890.
11. Felberg RA, Krieger DW, Chuang R, et al. Hypothermia after cardiac arrest: feasibility and safety of an external cooling protocol. *Circulation* 2001;104:1799–1804.
12. The Hypothermia after Cardiac Arrest Study Group. Mild therapeutic hypothermia to improve neurologic outcome after cardiac arrest. *N Engl J Med* 2002;346:549–556.
13. Bernard SA, Gray TW, Buist MD, et al. Treatment of comatose survivors of out-of-hospital cardiac arrest with induced hypothermia. *N Engl J Med* 2002;346:557–563.
14. Longstreth WT. The neurologic sequelae of cardiac arrest. *West J Med* 1987;147:175–180.
15. Tirschwell DL, Longstreth WT Jr, Rauch-Matthews RE, et al. Cerebrospinal fluid creatine kinase BB isoenzyme activity and neurologic prognosis after cardiac arrest. *Neurology* 1997;48: 352–357.
16. Higgins SL, Hummel JD, Niazi IK, et al. Cardiac resynchronization therapy for the treatment of heart failure in patients with intraventricular conduction delay and malignant ventricular tachyarrhythmias. *J Am Coll Cardiol* 2003;42:1454–1459.
17. Moss AJ, Hall WJ, Cannom DS, et al. Improved survival with an implanted defibrillator in patients with coronary disease at high risk for ventricular arrhythmia. *N Engl J Med* 1996;335: 1933–1940.

18. Moss AJ, Zareba W, Hall WJ, et al. Prophylactic implantation of a defibrillator in patients with myocardial infarction and reduced ejection fraction. *N Engl J Med* 2002;346:877–883.
19. Buxton AE, Lee KL, Fisher JD, Josephson ME, Prystwosky EN, Hafley G. A randomized study of the prevention of sudden death in patients with coronary artery disease. *N Engl J Med* 1999; 341:1882–1890.
20. Kadish A, Dyer A, Daubert JP, et al. Prophylactic defibrillator implantation in patients with nonischemic dilated cardiomyopathy. *N Engl J Med* 2004;350:2151–2158.
21. Bardy GH, Lee KL, Mark DB, et al. Amiodarone or an implantable cardioverter-defibrillator for congestive heart failure. *N Engl J Med* 2005;352:225–237.
22. Epstein AE, Miles WM, Benditt DG, et al. Personal and public safety issues related to arrhythmias that may affect consciousness: implications for regulation and physician recommendations. A medical/scientific statement from the American Heart Association and the North American Society of Pacing and Electrophysiology. *Circulation* 1996;94:1147–1166.
23. Mushlin AI, Hall WJ, Zwanziger J, et al. The cost-effectiveness of automatic implantable cardiac defibrillators: results from MADIT. Multicenter Automatic Defibrillator Implantation Trial. *Circulation* 1998;97:2129–2135.

ADDITIONAL READING

Crawford MH, Bernstein SJ, Deedwania PC, et al. ACC/AHA guidelines for ambulatory electrocardiography. A report of the American College of Cardiology/American Heart Association Task Force on Practice Guidelines (Committee to Revise the Guidelines for Ambulatory Electrocardiography). Developed in collaboration with the North American Society for Pacing and Electrophysiology. *J Am Coll Cardiol* 1999;34:912–948.

Gregoratos G, Abrams J, Epstein AE, et al. ACC/AHA Guidelines for implantation of cardiac pacemakers and antiarrhythmia devices: a report of the American College of Cardiology/American Heart Association Task Force on Practice Guidelines (Committee on Pacemaker Implantation). *J Am Coll Cardiol* 2002;40:1703–1719.

Zipes DP, DiMarco JP, Gillette PC, et al. Guidelines for clinical intracardiac electrophysiological and catheter ablation procedures: a report of the American College of Cardiology/American Heart Association Task Force on Practice Guidelines (Committee on Clinical Intracardiac Electrophysiologic and Catheter Ablation Procedures), developed in collaboration with the North American Society of Pacing and Electrophysiology. *J Am Coll Cardiol* 1995; 26:555–573.

Syncope

Wishwa N. Kapoor   David J. McAdams

44

INTRODUCTION

Syncope is a common problem that accounts for 1%–6% of hospital admissions and 3% of visits to emergency departments. The incidence is about six first episodes of syncope per 1,000 person-years among adults (1). The differential diagnosis of syncope is broad, and assigning a cause of syncope can be challenging. Furthermore, subgroups of patients, especially those with cardiac disease, have a high risk of sudden death. Because of these issues, patients with syncope are often admitted and subjected to a large number of tests that have low yield (1–3).

ISSUES AT THE TIME OF ADMISSION

Clinical Presentation

Syncope is defined as a sudden transient loss of consciousness associated with a loss of postural tone, with spontaneous recovery. Usually, the first issue to determine is whether a given patient had syncope or another state of altered consciousness that resembles syncope. Patients requiring chemical or electrical cardioversion are defined as having survived sudden death rather than as having experienced syncope. The absence of loss of consciousness defines dizziness and presyncope, as well as "drop attacks." Vertigo has an associated sense of motion.

Seizure and syncope can be difficult to separate clinically for several reasons. First, hypotension leading to cerebral ischemia may cause convulsions; experimental cerebral ischemia lasting 15 seconds or more has been associated with seizure-like activity. Second, akinetic seizures have been described despite a negative interictal electroencephalogram (EEG). Finally, many patients with syncope may have myoclonic jerks or urinary incontinence, which may mistakenly be attributed to seizures. The patient may not recall convulsive symptoms during an unwitnessed spell. In differentiating seizures from syncope, disorientation after the loss of consciousness is the best distinguishing feature suggesting seizure rather than syncope. Patients whose loss of consciousness lasts more than five minutes are also more likely to have had a seizure than an episode of syncope. Features suggesting syncope rather than seizure include pallor during the episode, sweating, nausea, and vomiting.

Differential Diagnosis and Initial Evaluation

The causes of syncope can be divided into four broad categories (Table 44.1). A brief general description of these disorders is provided here, and greater details are found elsewhere.

1. *Neurally mediated syncope.* This category encompasses the most common causes of syncope and includes vasovagal, situational (micturition, cough, defecation, swallow), and carotid sinus syncope, as well as many other types of syncope such as neuralgia, panic and generalized anxiety disorders, and spells associated with exercise in athletes without heart disease. Neurally mediated syncope is also termed neurocardiogenic or vasovagal syncope.

   In these disorders, syncope results from sudden reflex-mediated hypotension and/or bradycardia. Although the exact mechanism is poorly understood, these disorders may be triggered by stimulation of receptors that respond to stretch (mechanoreceptors). These receptors are located diffusely throughout the body (such as in the bladder, esophagus, respiratory tract, and carotid sinus). In susceptible individuals, the stimulation of these receptors results in transmission of impulses to the medulla. Efferent discharges from the medullary centers lead to hypotension and/or bradycardia.

2. *Orthostatic hypotension.* Orthostatic hypotension is defined as a decline of 20 mm Hg or more in systolic pressure or 10 mm Hg or more in diastolic pressure after the patient assumes an upright position. The clinical diag-

TABLE 44.1

CAUSES OF SYNCOPE ACCORDING TO SEX AND THE PRESENCE OR ABSENCE OF CARDIOVASCULAR DISEASE AT BASELINE

Cause	Cardiovascular disease absent (N = 599)		Cardiovascular disease present (N = 223)		Total sample (N = 822)
	Men	Women	Men	Women	
	Percentage of subjects				
Cardiac	6.5	3.8	26.7	16.8	9.5
Unknown[a]	31.0	41.7	31.0	37.4	36.6
Stroke or transient ischemic attack	1.7	2.5	9.5	9.4	4.1
Seizure	7.3	3.3	6.9	2.8	4.9
Vasovagal	24.1	24.5	11.2	14.0	21.2
Orthostatic	9.5	10.9	6.9	6.5	9.4
Medication	7.3	6.5	4.3	9.4	6.8
Other[b]	13.0	6.8	3.5	3.7	7.5

[a] When a participant did not seek medical attention for syncope and the history, physical examination, and electrocardiographic findings were not consistent with any of the specific causes, the cause was considered to be unknown.
[b] Cough syncope, micturition syncope, and situational syncope were included in the category of other causes.
From Soteriades ES, Evans JC, Larson MG, et al. Incidence and prognosis of syncope. *N Engl J Med* 2002;347:881, with permission.

nosis of orthostatic hypotension requires the presence of symptoms in association with a decrease in blood pressure. Symptoms of orthostatic hypotension include dizziness or light-headedness, blurring or loss of vision, weakness, and syncope. Loss of consciousness is usually brief. These symptoms are often worse when a person arises in the morning and may be especially prominent after meals or exercise.

Orthostatic hypotension has many causes. Decreased intravascular volume and adverse effects of drugs are the most common causes of symptomatic orthostatic hypotension. Elderly patients are especially vulnerable to symptoms from drugs and volume depletion because of decreased baroreceptor sensitivity, decreased cerebral blood flow, excessive renal sodium wasting, and a reduced thirst response with aging. Any condition that impairs peripheral sympathetic tone, such as the use of many antihypertensive medications and the neuropathy of diabetes mellitus, also predisposes patients to orthostatic hypotension and syncope.

3. *Neurologic diseases.* Syncope is a rare manifestation of cerebrovascular disease. Only about 15% of patients with vertebrobasilar transient ischemic attacks (TIAs) have drop attacks, and syncope is even less common. Loss of consciousness is almost always accompanied by other neurologic symptoms of brain stem ischemia. Syncope is generally not a manifestation of carotid artery ischemia unless accompanied by disease of the vertebrobasilar arteries. Subclavian steal syndrome due to subclavian stenosis and reversal of blood in the ipsilateral vertebral artery may also lead to brain stem is-

chemia. A difference in blood pressure (usually >20mm Hg) and pulse intensity between arms is a helpful clue to this diagnosis. A "faint sensation" is reported in 12%–18% of patients with migraine and may often be a vasovagal reaction to pain. Basilar artery migraine, a rare disorder that affects adolescents, may cause syncope because of spasm of the basilar arterial tree. The clinical presentation includes syncope and headaches in association with symptoms of brain stem ischemia. Seizures can also mimic syncope and are important to recognize, as discussed earlier.

4. *Cardiac diseases.* Cardiac etiologies include those diseases associated with severe obstruction to cardiac output (4), various other cardiac diseases associated with sudden decrease in cardiac output, and rhythm disturbances. Although cardiac disease is sometimes first discovered after a patient presents with syncope, it is more typical for patients with known, preexisting cardiac disease to present cardiogenic syncope (see Table 44.1).

Outflow obstruction can critically reduce cerebral blood flow and may be caused by structural lesions of the left or right side of the heart. All types of heart disease may produce exertional syncope when the cardiac output is fixed and does not rise (or even falls) with exercise. Examples include severe aortic stenosis, hypertrophic cardiomyopathy, pulmonary hypertension, pulmonic stenosis, and pulmonary emboli. All can result in both exertional or nonexertional syncope.

Other organic cardiac diseases that cause syncope include myocardial infarction, unstable angina, coronary artery spasm, aortic dissection, and other conditions where cardiac output suddenly decreases.

Arrhythmias may cause syncope by reducing cardiac output. Excessive vagal tone, decreased sympathetic tone, or sinus node disease may cause sinus bradycardia. Many parasympathomimetic agents, sympatholytic agents, and β-blocking agents can cause bradycardia (Chapter 45). Syncope occurs in 25%–70% of patients with sick sinus syndrome. Electrocardiographic manifestations of this disorder include sinus bradycardia, pauses, arrest, or exit block. Supraventricular tachycardia or atrial fibrillation may also occur in association with bradycardia or atrial fibrillation with slow ventricular response (tachycardia-bradycardia syndrome).

Ventricular tachyarrhythmias almost always occur in the setting of known organic heart disease (Chapter 43). Torsade de pointes (or polymorphic ventricular tachycardia) occurs in patients with congenital prolongation of the QT interval (with or without associated deafness) as well as acquired long QT syndromes caused by drugs (such as quinidine, procainamide, amiodarone, and sotalol), electrolyte abnormalities, and central nervous system disorders. Other tachyarrhythmias that may cause syncope include atrial fibrillation or flutter with rapid ventricular response, AV nodal re-entrant tachycardia, and supraventricular tachycardia in patients with Wolff-Parkinson-White syndrome (Chapter 42). About 18% of patients have multiple causes of syncope (5). Such patients have a significantly worse prognosis than patients with a single cause.

Diagnostic Evaluation

Figure 44.1 shows a flow diagram for approach to patients with syncope. Initial history, physical examination, and electrocardiography (ECG) form the cornerstone of the evaluation of syncope. This initial assessment may be diagnostic of a cause (such as orthostatic hypotension), in which case treatment can be initiated without the need for additional workup for the etiology of syncope. Alternatively, history, physical examination, and ECG may suggest a cause (such as symptoms consistent with pulmonary emboli). In these instances, specific tests can be done, and if diagnostic, treatment can be started. The remainder of the patients have unexplained syncope after history, physical examination, and ECG. These patients can be considered under three categories: those with organic heart disease, the elderly, and those without heart disease. The evaluation of patients with structural heart disease revolves around assessment of the extent and severity of underlying heart disease and detection of arrhythmias. In patients without heart disease or when arrhythmias are not likely, the evaluation centers on neurally mediated syncope, psychiatric illnesses, or, rarely, bradyarrhythmias.

Some specific observations and recommendations follow:

1. The history and physical examination identify a cause in 45% of cases. Examples of such diagnoses include orthostatic hypotension, situational syncope, and drug-induced syncope. Baseline laboratory tests rarely point to a cause of syncope but may be needed for evaluation and management of comorbid conditions and effect of drugs.

2. The ECG directly identifies the cause of syncope in less than 5% of patients, but ECG abnormalities are found in up to 50% of patients and can be important clues to possible causes. Examples include bundle-branch block and long QT interval.

3. Electroencephalography provides diagnostic information in less than 2% of patients, almost all of whom have symptoms suggestive of seizure or a history of a convulsive disorder. Computed tomographic (CT) scans of the head provide new diagnostic information in about 4% of patients, almost all of whom have focal neurologic findings or history consistent with a seizure.

4. Testing for arrhythmias: Arrhythmias are found mainly in patients with structural heart disease or an abnormal ECG. Predictors of arrhythmic syncope or cardiac death at one year include: age greater than 45 years, history of congestive heart failure, abnormal ECG other than nonspecific ST changes, and history of ventricular arrhythmias (frequent or repetitive premature ventricular contractions [PVCs]). Arrhythmia testing is recommended in patients who have at least one predictor of arrhythmic syncope or cardiac death and whose symptoms are suggestive of cardiac syncope (sudden brief loss of consciousness without prodrome). In patients with structural heart disease, a cardiovascular evaluation (such as stress testing and echocardiogram) is often needed in addition to tests for arrhythmias, because management of underlying heart disease is closely linked to treatment plans for arrhythmias. The tests for arrhythmias include the following:

   ■ *Ambulatory monitoring.* In studies of ambulatory Holter monitoring performed for 12–24 hours, symptoms with concurrent arrhythmias are found in 5% (leading to diagnosis of arrhythmic syncope) and symptoms without arrhythmias, in 17% (potentially excluding arrhythmic syncope) (6). In 79%, brief arrhythmias or no arrhythmias are found, and there is no clear link to symptoms. Arrhythmic syncope cannot be excluded in these patients.

   ■ *External loop event monitoring.* External loop recorders can be used for monitoring patients for weeks to months, making it possible to capture a rhythm strip during symptoms in patients with infrequent events. Arrhythmias during syncope are found in 8%–20%, and normal rhythm during symptoms in 12%–27% of patients by the use of external event monitoring. Overall, event monitors are significantly more likely to establish or exclude arrhythmias as a cause of

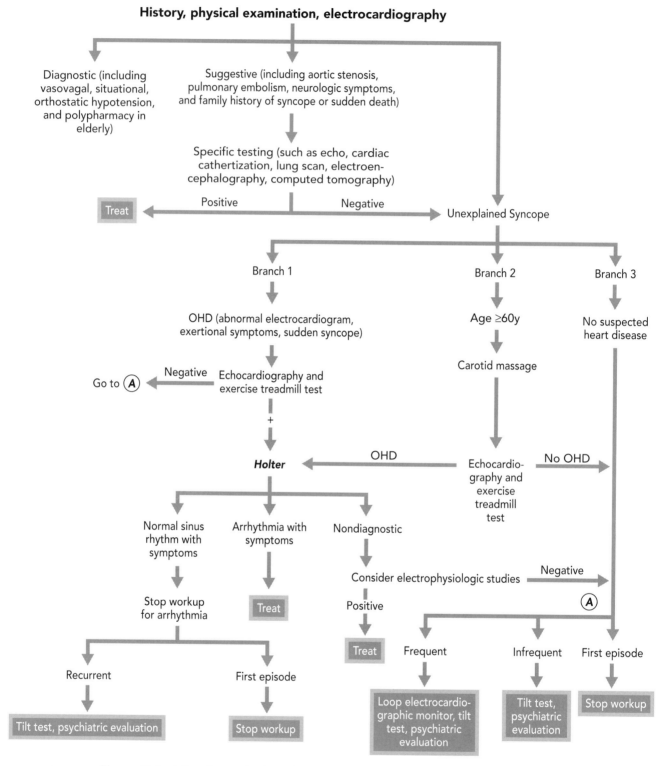

Figure 44.1 A flow diagram for the evaluation of syncope. *OHD,* organic heart disease. (Adapted from Linzer M, Yang EH, Estes NA 3rd, Wang P, Vorperian VR, Kapoor WN. Diagnosing syncope. Part 1: Value of history, physical examination, and electrocardiography. *Ann Intern Med* 1997;126: 989–996, with permission.)

syncope than is Holter monitoring. Major limitations of external event monitoring include lack of an event during monitoring and failure of the patient to activate the device during symptoms, sometimes because symptoms are so severe. Implantable loop recorders, which are inserted surgically and can provide continuous monitoring for 12–18 months, can diagnose arrhythmias in approximately 25% of patients who have previously undiagnosed syncope despite prior monitoring (8). In a randomized trial, a diagnosis of the cause of syncope was made significantly more often in patients who were evaluated with prolonged implanted loop recorders (55%) than in patients who had "conventional" evaluation with tilt-table testing, external loop monitors, and electrophysiologic studies (19%). The most frequent arrhythmia found was bradycardia (9).

- *Electrophysiologic studies.* In syncope patients, electrophysiologic tests are abnormal mainly in those with structural heart disease or an abnormal ECG. In patients with heart disease, approximately 21% have inducible ventricular tachycardia and 34%, bradycardia (14% have multiple diagnoses). In patients with ECG abnormalities, 3% have inducible ventricular tachycardia and 19%, bradycardia. In patients without heart disease, 1% have ventricular tachycardia and 10%, bradycardia. Several studies have suggested that the sensitivity and specificity of electrophysiologic tests for bradyarrhythmias is poor.
- *Signal-averaged ECG (SAGE).* The presence of late potentials demonstrated by SAGE has a high sensitivity and specificity (approximately 70%–90%) for inducible ventricular tachycardia by electrophysiologic testing. A normal SAGE may help avoid electrophysiologic studies if ventricular tachycardia is the only concern (9). However, electrophysiologic tests in patients with syncope often are done for other arrhythmias in addition to ventricular tachycardias. Thus, SAGE testing rarely obviates the use of electrophysiologic testing.

5. Upright tilt testing: Upright tilt testing is used for evaluation of the autonomic nervous system. In patients presenting with syncope, it is generally used to evaluate the predisposition to neurally mediated or vasovagal syncope, although dysautonomic responses and postural tachycardia syndrome are also rarely diagnosed by tilt testing. To test for predisposition to vasovagal syncope, methodologies include passive tilt testing (without the use of chemical stimulation) or the use of various drugs (most commonly isoproterenol in the United States and nitroglycerin in Europe) during testing. In patients with unexplained syncope, positive responses occur in approximately 50% with passive testing and in approximately 66% with isoproterenol protocols. The results with nitroglycerin appear similar to those with isoproterenol. The specificity of tilt testing without chemical stimulation is approximately 90%, and approximately

75% with isoproterenol. Specificity with isoproterenol appears to be higher when a high-dose (5 mcg/min) infusion is not used. This test is often (15%–35%) not reproducible when repeated on the same day or later.

Indications for tilt testing include recurrent unexplained syncope when arrhythmias are either unlikely (such as in patients without structural heart disease or abnormal ECG) or have been excluded by appropriate testing in patients with structural heart disease. Rarely, tilt testing is suggested for the evaluation of a single episode of unexplained syncope associated with trauma or in certain high-risk occupations (e.g., pilots), but these indications are controversial.

6. Unsuspected abnormalities by echocardiogram are found in 5%–10% of patients but only rarely lead to the determination of the cause of syncope. Examples include aortic stenosis or hypertrophic cardiomyopathy, but these disorders are usually suspected from the history and physical examination. Echocardiography is indicated whenever valvular diseases are suspected clinically, and it is often needed for the evaluation of cardiac function in patients suspected of having arrhythmic syncope. The yield of stress testing for the diagnosis of syncope is less than 1%, although the test is widely used for this purpose.

Indications for Hospitalization

Table 44.2 shows common indications for admission for syncope. Hospitalization is considered if there is a concern

---

TABLE 44.2
INDICATIONS FOR HOSPITAL ADMISSION IN PATIENTS WITH SYNCOPE

Indicated:

History of coronary-artery disease, heart failure, or ventricular arrhythmia
Accompanying symptoms of chest pain
Physical signs of significant aortic stenosis, hypertrophic cardiomyopathy, heart failure, stroke, or focal neurologic disorder
Electrocardiogenic findings of ischemia, arrhythmia (serious bradycardia or tachycardia), prolonged QT interval, or bundle-branch block

Often indicated:

Sudden loss of consciousness with injury, rapid heart beat, or exertional syncope
Frequent spells, suspicion of coronary disease or arrhythmia (for example, use of medications associated with torsade de pointes)
Moderate-to-severe orthostatic hypotension
Age over 70 years

Adapted from Linzer M, Yang E, Estes NA 3rd, Wang P, Vorperian VR, Kapoor WN. Diagnosing syncope. Part 1: Value of history, physical examination, and electrocardiography. *Ann Intern Med* 1997;126:989–996, with permission.

for arrhythmic syncope and sudden cardiac death or if immediate treatments need to be initiated. The predictors of arrhythmic syncope or cardiac death (at one year) include history of congestive heart failure, history of ventricular arrhythmia, abnormal ECG (other than nonspecific ST changes), and age over 45 years. The presence of two or more of these factors is associated with 10% or greater incidence of syncope or cardiac death. These predictors, along with symptoms suggestive of cardiac syncope in patients with underlying structural heart disease, can be used to guide admission decisions.

Indications for Initial ICU Admission

Telemetry or monitoring in a cardiac unit (see Tables 44.3 and 44.4) is indicated for patients with structural heart disease or abnormal ECG when arrhythmias are clinically suspected.

Initial Therapy

Initial therapy depends on the etiologies of syncope under consideration. Many of the etiologies of syncope have specific known treatment approaches; a full discussion is beyond the scope of this chapter. The following issues are important in initial therapeutic approaches:

1. If a cause of syncope can be identified based on initial evaluation (history, physical examination, and ECG), treatment of those disorders can be initiated without the need for further diagnostic evaluation for other causes of syncope. Examples include orthostatic hypotension, drug-induced syncope, and symptomatic supraventricular tachycardia.

2. When a disease has been identified as suggestive of causes of syncope, further testing is done in a directed fashion. If specific entities are confirmed, treatment is

TABLE 44.3

INDICATIONS FOR INITIAL ICU ADMISSION

Acute cardiovascular conditions
Aortic dissection
Acute myocardial infarction or unstable angina
Pulmonary edema
Circulatory collapse (cardiogenic shock or other types of shock)
Long QT with ventricular arrhythmias
Massive pulmonary embolism
Acute noncardiac problems
Multiple seizures or status epilepticus
Drug overdoses
Gastrointestinal bleeding
Acute stroke or intracranial bleed

Adapted from Linzer M, Yang E, Estes NA 3rd, Wang P, Vorperian VR, Kapoor WN. Diagnosing syncope. Part 1: Value of history, physical examination, and electrocardiography. *Ann Intern Med* 1997;126:989–996, with permission.

TABLE 44.4

INDICATIONS FOR CONSULTATION

Recommended at the time of admission

Structural heart disease
History of ventricular arrhythmias
Diagnosis of bradyarrhythmias
Acute cardiovascular disease
Bundle-branch block and unexplained syncope
Suspected seizure or other neurologic events

Evaluation and management of findings during hospitalization

Severe aortic stenosis
Aortic dissection
Treatment of arrhythmias found on monitoring
Tilt testing for recurrent syncope
Evidence of possible seizure or other neurologic events

initiated. An example would be a patient with syncope and findings consistent with severe aortic stenosis. Further assessment with echocardiogram, possible cardiac catheterization, and consultation with cardiology and cardiothoracic surgery are needed for management.

3. When syncope occurs in an elderly patient, it is important to recognize that such patients often have multiple comorbid illnesses and take medications that may result in alterations of vascular tone or in volume depletion. Additionally, elderly patients may have physiologic impairments that predispose them to syncope (decreased baroreceptor sensitivity, renal sodium wasting, decreased cerebral blood flow, and impaired thirst). The initial approach is to search for a single cause of syncope. If a specific cause cannot be identified, treatment of multiple abnormalities should be initiated prior to considering invasive or extensive diagnostic testing. Medications should always be reviewed in detail, and unnecessary ones should be discontinued.

4. For patients with neurally mediated syncope, initial therapy should focus on avoiding situations that trigger symptoms, increasing fluid and salt intake, avoiding alcohol, and reducing or discontinuing diuretics and vasodilators (10). These measures alone will effectively treat many patients, especially those with a single or rare episodes. Uncontrolled studies suggest that tilt training (repeatedly subjecting the cardiovascular system to orthostatic stress as a means of fatiguing the symptomatic response) may decrease recurrences of syncope. Drinking 500 ml of water acutely can significantly reduce orthostatic hypotension (11). Patients can also be taught to use isometric handgrip exercise to increase systemic blood pressure and thereby abort impending neurally mediated syncope (12).

The effectiveness of most drugs currently used in the treatment of neurally mediated syncope is unclear.

Despite a lack of controlled studies, fludrocortisone and increased salt intake are widely utilized. One short-term (one-month) randomized trial of β-blockers showed a lower rate of recurrent syncope, but several controlled trials have not confirmed their effectiveness (13). Midodrine has been effective in reducing recurrences in small studies (14). A small randomized trial of paroxetine showed a reduction of recurrent episodes at two years (15). The effectiveness of permanent pacemakers in highly symptomatic patients with positive tilt tests (consisting of hypotension and bradycardia) has been assessed in four randomized trials; of these, the three unblinded studies showed decreased recurrences, but the one blinded study did not (16–18).

ISSUES DURING THE COURSE OF HOSPITALIZATION

The issues during the course of hospitalization fall into the following categories:

1. *Establishing a cause of syncope.* Figure 44.1 shows an approach to the evaluation of a patient with syncope. The sequence of testing is the major issue in the course of hospitalization. In patients with structural heart disease or when arrhythmias are considered likely based on clinical presentation and risk stratification, cardiac testing (e.g., stress testing and echocardiogram) should be done prior to considering electrophysiologic studies. In patients with moderately severe coronary disease, revascularization or medical therapy should be considered prior to electrophysiologic testing or tilt testing because of the risk from possible provocation of hypotension during these tests. Once arrhythmias are excluded, further evaluation can generally be planned on an outpatient basis. Most laboratories perform tilt testing immediately after electrophysiologic testing; this approach is recommended in patients with recurrent syncope. To use resources efficiently, hospitalization should be limited to that required to confirm or exclude serious causes of syncope and to treat disorders that need inpatient care. The remainder of the workup can be done in the outpatient setting. Coordination and communication with the referring physician or patient's primary care physician is vitally important.
2. *Treatment of disorders found in the hospital.* Many of the diseases and disorders found during the hospital course have specific treatments. Once these diagnoses are made, treatments can be initiated. Examples include severe aortic stenosis (for which aortic valve replacement is indicated) or a seizure disorder (for which anticonvulsants can be started).
3. *Recurrent unexplained syncope.* In patients followed over the past two decades, no cause of syncope was found in approximately 36% of patients (Table 44.1) (1). However, most observers believe that the wider use of tilt

testing, event monitoring, attention to psychiatric illnesses, and recognition that syncope in the elderly may be multifactorial has decreased the size of the "syncope of unknown origin" (SUO) group to less than 10% in the modern era. Currently, it is estimated that approximately 50% of the SUO group has neurally mediated syncope that is not diagnosed clinically but can be provoked by upright tilt testing. An additional 10%–20% have psychiatric disorders (panic, anxiety, somatization, major depression, alcohol and substance abuse). Other etiologies are found in follow-up in less than 5% of the SUO group (e.g. supraventricular tachycardia, seizure). A small fraction is elderly patients in whom comorbid illnesses and medications may interact to cause syncope.

In patients with recurrent syncope and without heart disease or an abnormal ECG, the diagnoses to focus on are neurally mediated syncope, psychiatric disorders, and, rarely, bradyarrhythmias (11). A consultation with cardiology (particularly for tilt testing) and with psychiatry may be needed to arrive at a cause. Prior to considering psychiatric causes, screening psychiatric instruments (such as PRIME-MD) or a focused psychiatric interview is recommended. Loop event monitoring is recommended if symptoms are recurrent and suggestive of cardiac syncope.

DISCHARGE ISSUES

Patients should be instructed in the following areas:

1. *Preventing loss of consciousness.* Examples of patient instructions are shown in Table 44.5.
2. *Driving.* The risk of syncope during driving depends on frequency of syncope and length and duration of driving. Injury (to the patient or bystanders) during driving is estimated to be quite unusual (up to 0.33% per driver per year), but there are few data on this issue. Restrictions on driving vary from state to state and may change over time. Physicians caring for syncope patients should consult their state's motor vehicle departments and follow their state's regulations.

TABLE 44.5
PATIENT INSTRUCTIONS

Preventing syncope or vasovagal spells

Avoid alcohol, lack of sleep, hot environment
Maintain adequate hydration and food intake
Avoid drugs that lead to hypotension (e.g., vasodilators, diuretics)
Avoid activities that precipitate syncope (e.g., exercise for exertional syncope)

Preventing loss of consciousness or injury

Assume supine position upon onset of prodrome
Avoid driving and other activities that could lead to injury

3. *Preventing injury from recurrent syncope.* Patients should be instructed to assume a supine or at least sitting position at the first hint of prodromal symptoms. A patient with recurrent spells should swim with a companion who knows that patient has had recurrent syncope. Patients can play team and contact sports unless they have had post-exercise syncope, in which case exercise should be avoided until symptoms are controlled with therapy. Climbing ladders, taking hot showers, standing by fires, and using power tools pose risks and should be avoided until the patient has been symptom-free for several months. Alcohol should be avoided. Patients should also not be employed as police officers, airline pilots, drivers, or heavy machinery operators.

4. *Follow-up.* The recurrence rate of syncope is approximately 30% at three years. Unfortunately, the patient whose initial episode of syncope eluded diagnosis will only rarely be diagnosed after a recurrence (19). Therefore, patients with recurrent, undiagnosed syncope should be followed closely to determine whether therapy was effective.

KEY POINTS

- A cause of syncope is currently identified in more than 90% of patients.
- Initial clinical assessment (history, physical examination, and ECG) leads to a diagnosis in approximately 50% of patients.
- EEG and CT scan of the head provide diagnostic information in 2%–4%; almost all these patients have a history of a seizure disorder or focal neurologic signs and symptoms.
- Arrhythmias are mainly of concern in patients with structural heart disease, a history of ventricular arrhythmias, or an abnormal ECG (other than nonspecific ST changes).
- In diagnosing arrhythmias as a cause, attempts should be made to correlate arrhythmias with symptoms by using Holter, external, or implantable loop recorder monitoring. Implantable loop recorders are preferred when the diagnosis is elusive and the need to establish a diagnosis is high.
- Sensitivity and specificity of electrophysiologic studies is poor for the diagnosis of bradyarrhythmias.
- Upright tilt testing provokes vasovagal syncope in the laboratory and shows positive responses in 50%–66% of patients with unexplained syncope. Tilt testing is recommended in patients with recurrent unexplained syncope because treatments are available (although not widely tested by randomized controlled trials).
- Treatment should be directed toward the cause of syncope. Patients with rare or single episodes of neurally mediated syncope can be treated without medications. Neurally mediated syncope may respond to volume loading (fludrocortisone plus salt), but β-blockers, paroxetene (a selective serotonin reuptake inhibitor), or permanent pacing may be required.

REFERENCES

1. Soteriades ES, Evans JC, Larson MG, et al. Incidence and prognosis of syncope. *N Engl J Med* 2002;347:878–885.
2. Benditt D, Ferguson D, Grubb B, et al. Tilt table testing for assessing syncope. *JACC* 1996;28:263–275.
3. Sarasin FP, Louis-Simonet M, Carballo D, et al. Prospective evaluation of patients with syncope: a population-based study. *Am J Med* 2001;111:177–184.
4. Alboni P, Brignole M, Menozzi C, et al. Diagnostic value of history in patients with syncope with or without heart disease. *J Am Coll Cardiol* 2001;37:1921–1928.
5. Chen LY, Gersh BJ, Hodge DO, Wieling W, Hammill SC, Shen WK. Prevalence and clinical outcomes of patients with multiple potential causes of syncope. *Mayo Clin Proc* 2003;78:414–420.
6. Sheldon R, Rose S, Ritchie D, et al. Historical criteria that distinguish syncope from seizures. *J Am Coll Cardiol* 2002;40:142–148.
7. Sivakumaran S. A prospective randomized comparison of loop recorders versus Holter monitors in patients with syncope or presyncope. *Am J Med* 2003;115:1–5.
8. Krahn AD, Klein GJ, Yee R, Takle-Newhouse T, Norris C. Use of an extended monitoring strategy in patients with problematic syncope. *Circulation* 1999;99:406–410.
9. Krahn A, Klein G, Yee R, Skanes AC. Randomized assessment of syncope trial: conventional testing versus a prolonged monitoring strategy. *Circulation* 2001;104:46–51.
10. Bloomfield D. Strategy for the management of vasovagal syncope. *Drugs Aging* 2002;19:179–202.
11. Schroeder C, Bush VE, Norcliffe LJ, et al. Water drinking acutely improves orthostatic tolerance in healthy subjects. *Circulation* 2002;106:2806–2811.
12. Brignole M, Croci F, Menozzi C, et al. Isometric arm counter-pressure maneuvers to abort impending vasovagal syncope. *J Am Coll Cardiol* 2002;40:2053–2059.
13. Ventura R, Maas R, Zeidlev D, et al. A randomized and controlled pilot trial of β-blockers for the treatment of recurrent syncope in patients with positive or negative response to head-up tilt test. *Pacing Clin Electrophysiol* 2002;25:816–821.
14. Perez-Lugones A, Schweikert R, Pavia S, et al. Usefulness of midodrine in patients with severely symptomatic neurocardiogenic syncope: a randomized control study. *J Cardiovasc Electrophysiol* 2001;12:935–938.
15. Di Girolamo E, Di Iorio C, Sabatini P, Leonzio L, Barbone C, Barsotti A. Effects of paroxetine hydrochloride, a selective serotonin reuptake inhibitor, on refractory vasovagal syncope: a randomized, double-blind, placebo-controlled study. *J Am Coll Cardiol* 1999;33:1227–1230.
16. Ammirati F, Colivicchi F, Santini M, Syncope Diagnosis and Treatment Study Investigators. Permanent cardiac pacing versus medical treatment for the prevention of recurrent vasovagal syncope: a multicenter, randomized, controlled trial. *Circulation* 2001;104:52–57.
17. Connolly SF, Sheldon R, Thorpe KE, et al. Pacemaker therapy for prevention of syncope in patients with recurrent severe vasovagal syncope: Second Vasovagal Pacemaker Study (VPS II): a randomized trial. *JAMA* 2003;289:2224–2229.
18. Kapoor WN. Is there an effective treatment for neurally mediated syncope? *JAMA* 2003;289:2272–2275.
19. Mathias CJ. Observations on recurrent syncope and presyncope in 641 patients. *Lancet* 2001;357:348–353.

ADDITIONAL READING

Brignole M, Alboni P, Benditt D, et al. Guidelines on management (diagnosis and treatment) of syncope. *Eur Heart J* 2001;22:1256–1306.

Kapoor WN. Current evaluation and management of syncope. *N Engl J Med* 2002;106:1606–1609.

Schnipper JL, Kapoor WN. Diagnostic evaluation and management of patients with syncope. *Med Clin North Am* 2001;85:423–456.

Bradycardia and Pacemakers

45

Richard H. Hongo   *Nora F. Goldschlager*

INTRODUCTION

This chapter outlines an approach to the two most common indications for hospitalization because of bradycardia and for permanent pacemaker implantation: sinus node dysfunction and acquired atrioventricular (AV) block. Conditions occurring during hospitalization that may warrant temporary cardiac pacing are also addressed. In addition, the chapter contains a review of the basic features of permanent pacemakers and discusses potential problems encountered with pacing systems.

ISSUES AT THE TIME OF ADMISSION

Sinus Node Dysfunction

Sinus node dysfunction, a degenerative process involving the sinus node and sinoatrial area, includes a variety of disorders such as sinus bradycardia, sinus node exit block, sinus pause, and sinus arrest. The AV node and intraventricular conduction system are also involved in up to 25%–30% of patients who have sinus node dysfunction (1).

Sinus bradycardia is generally defined as a sinus rate of less than 50 beats per minute (bpm). This rate is not necessarily pathologic but is a marker of sinus node dysfunction in specific clinical contexts. In sinus node exit block, impulses are formed within the sinus node but encounter varying degrees of blockage in the surrounding sinoatrial tissue as they try to exit to the atrial conduction system. Sinus pauses are caused by disorders of impulse formation within the sinus node. Sinus arrest, which is total failure of sinus impulse generation, cannot be distinguished from complete sinoatrial exit block on the surface electrocardiogram.

Clinical Presentation

If an inadequate heart rate causes cerebral hypoperfusion, clinical symptoms result, including presyncope, syncope, confusion, memory loss, and, rarely, seizure activity. Inability of the heart rate to increase in response to increased physiologic demand results in effort intolerance, fatigue, weakness, and breathlessness. Sudden death from ventricular asystole or bradycardia-dependent polymorphic ventricular tachycardia can also occur. Occasionally, patients with AV block complain of no symptoms; many of these patients, however, feel significantly better after pacemaker implantation. Patients with a variant of sinus node dysfunction, the *tachycardia-bradycardia syndrome*, can present with palpitations. These patients have concomitant supraventricular tachycardias (Chapter 42) that may include atrial tachycardia, atrial flutter, atrial fibrillation, or AV nodal reentrant tachycardia. Symptoms are related to either the rapid heart rate or the pauses in atrial rate, caused in part by overdrive suppression of the sinus node. It is often necessary to treat the tachycardia with medications that further slow the sinus rate (e.g., β-blockers or class I or III antiarrhythmic agents) (Table 42.4). As a result, a permanent pacemaker commonly is required for rate support.

Differential Diagnosis and Initial Management

Sinus node dysfunction can result from medications, vagally mediated states, and, rarely, acute myocardial infarction. Medication profiles should be examined, and potassium and drug levels should be obtained. In patients who present with the tachycardia-bradycardia syndrome, thyroid disease must be considered, although it is a rare cause. Initial management of patients with bradycardia should be directed at identifying and treating reversible causes and at providing rate support. Oral theophylline has been used with some success in the treatment of bradycardia caused by sinus node dysfunction. Symptomatic patients without reversible causes are candidates for permanent pacemaker implantation.

Indication for Hospitalization

Patients who require permanent pacemaker therapy according to the American College of Cardiology/American Heart Association Task Force guidelines should be hospitalized for pacemaker implantation (Table 45.1). All patients should be admitted to a monitored setting to ensure prompt diagnosis and treatment of any severe bradycardia.

TABLE 45.1
INDICATIONS FOR PERMANENT PACING IN SINUS NODE DYSFUNCTION

Class I (conditions for which there is evidence and/or general agreement that a given procedure or treatment is useful and effective)

1. Sinus node dysfunction with documented symptomatic bradycardia, including frequent sinus pauses that produce symptoms; in some patients, bradycardia is iatrogenic and occurs as a consequence of essential long-term drug therapy of a type and dose for which there are no acceptable alternatives
2. Symptomatic chronotropic incompetence

Class II (conditions for which there is conflicting evidence and/or divergence of opinion about the usefulness/efficacy of a procedure or treatment)

Class IIa (weight of evidence/opinion is in favor of usefulness/efficacy)

1. Sinus node dysfunction, occurring spontaneously or as a result of necessary drug therapy, with heart rate <40 bpm, when a clear association between significant symptoms consistent with bradycardia and the actual presence of bradycardia has not been documented
2. Syncope of unexplained origin when major abnormalities of sinus node function are discovered or provoked in electrophysiological studies

Class IIb (usefulness/efficacy is less well established by evidence/opinion)

1. In minimally symptomatic patients, chronic heart rate <40 bpm while awake

Class III (conditions for which there is evidence and/or general agreement that a procedure/treatment is not useful/effective and in some cases may be harmful)

1. Sinus node dysfunction in asymptomatic patients, including those in whom substantial sinus bradycardia (heart rate <40 bpm) is a consequence of long-term drug treatment
2. Sinus node dysfunction in patients with symptoms suggestive of bradycardia and clearly documented as not associated with a slow heart rate
3. Sinus node dysfunction with symptomatic bradycardia due to nonessential drug therapy

Adapted from Gregoratos G, Abrams J, Epstein AE, et al. ACC/AHA/NASPE 2002 guideline update for implantation of cardiac pacemakers and antiarrhythmia devices—summary article. *J Am Coll Cardiol* 2002;40:1703–1719. Copyright 2002 by the American College of Cardiology and American Heart Association, Inc., with permission.

TABLE 45.2
COMMON INDICATIONS FOR TEMPORARY CARDIAC PACING

1. Therapeutically, for symptomatic bradycardia
   a. Persistent bradycardia, until permanent pacemaker implantation can be accomplished
   b. Transient bradycardia (e.g., acute myocardial infarction or Lyme myocarditis)
2. Therapeutically, to maintain or restore AV synchrony
   a. In acute myocardial infarction (especially inferior-wall and right-ventricular)
   b. In congestive heart failure
   c. In ventricular hypertrophy states (e.g., hypertrophic obstructive cardiomyopathy)
3. Prophylactically, for potential bradycardia that may produce symptoms or hemodynamic embarrassment in acute myocardial infarction
   a. New bundle-branch block
   b. New bi- or trifascicular block with 1st-degree AV block
   c. Type I 2nd-degree AV block with wide QRS complexes at slow rate
   d. Type II 2nd-degree AV block or higher degrees of AV block
4. Prophylactically, to prevent pause-dependent ventricular tachyarrhythmias

AV, atrioventricular.

Indications for Initial Coronary Care Unit Admission

Patients should be admitted to the coronary care unit (CCU) if the cause of the sinus node dysfunction itself necessitates a CCU admission (e.g., myocardial infarction) or if temporary rate support by pacing is needed while awaiting definitive therapy (Table 45.2).

Acquired Atrioventricular Block

In AV block, the delay in conduction can be at the level of the AV node or can be infranodal (at or below the His bundle). In first-degree AV block, the PR interval exceeds 200 ms. Second-degree AV block indicates that not all supraventricular impulses are conducted. Second-degree AV block can take the form of progressive delay in conduction followed by failure of conduction (Wenckebach, or type I second-degree block) or abrupt failure of conduction (type II second-degree block). In third-degree (complete) AV block, no impulses are conducted. Accurate differentiation between type I (Wenckebach) and type II second-degree AV block is difficult if there is 2:1 conduction, because a single PR interval prior to a nonconducted P wave does not allow evaluation of successive PR intervals. However, certain features may be helpful in distinguishing the two. If the PR interval of the conducted P wave is prolonged and the QRS complexes are narrow and appear normal, type I second-degree AV block is probably present. If the PR interval of the conducted P wave is normal and the

QRS complexes have a bundle-branch block pattern, type II second-degree AV block is probably present. The two can be more definitively differentiated either by recording a long rhythm strip that might document changing AV conduction ratios or by using various maneuvers. Intravenous atropine and exercise improve AV conduction at the AV nodal level but often worsen AV block at the infranodal level. Conversely, carotid sinus massage can worsen AV block at the AV nodal level and improve AV conduction at the infranodal level because a slower sinus rate permits conduction to occur. *High-grade AV block* is defined by the presence of more nonconducted P waves than conducted ones (e.g., 3:1 AV conduction). High-grade AV block should be considered a precursor to complete AV block and, as such, should be managed aggressively.

Clinical Presentation

Symptoms depend on the severity and site of AV block. In the absence of an adequate escape rate, symptoms of AV block are similar to those of sinus-node dysfunction, and the two conditions often coexist. If there is complete AV block or prolongation of the PR interval to more than 300 ms, asynchronous atrial and ventricular depolarization-contraction sequences can result in elevated atrial pressures, pulmonary congestion, and, at times, peripheral edema and refractory hypotension.

Differential Diagnosis and Initial Management

The most common causes of AV block are idiopathic sclerodegeneration of the conduction system, acute myocardial infarction, medications, and vagal stimulation. Rarer causes of block include inflammation (e.g., myocarditis), infection (e.g., infective endocarditis, especially involving the aortic valve ring), infiltrative disease (e.g., amyloidosis), and trauma (e.g., following aortic valve surgery).

AV block associated with anterior-wall myocardial infarction often indicates extensive myocardial necrosis and disruption of the infranodal conduction system. This combination results in a wide QRS complex escape rhythm with a slow rate and in variable constancy that is unresponsive to autonomic nervous system input. AV block associated with inferior-wall myocardial infarction generally indicates AV nodal ischemia that is often transient and, in part, vagally mediated; a narrow, relatively normal-appearing QRS

complex escape rhythm arises from the AV junction and is variably responsive to autonomic input. Medications that precipitate AV block include β-blockers (oral and ophthalmic), some calcium channel blockers (e.g., verapamil, diltiazem), digoxin, and some antiarrhythmic drugs. Serum digoxin levels should be obtained, although a normal level does not exclude digoxin toxicity. Vagally mediated AV block is suggested by the transient nature of the episode, concomitant slowing of the sinus rate, inconstant PR intervals, and reversal with atropine or enhanced sympathetic tone (Figure 45.1). Vagally mediated AV block is common in hospitalized patients (e.g., during suctioning, vomiting, coughing, and endoscopic procedures) and generally does not require specific treatment. Hyperkalemia can exacerbate AV nodal block.

Pharmacologic rate support is often achievable with atropine; however, infranodal block may worsen or be unresponsive to vagolytic agents. Intravenous infusion of isoproterenol generally is not recommended because of the risk of precipitating myocardial ischemia and producing or aggravating ventricular arrhythmias.

Indication for Hospitalization

Reversible causes of AV block should always be excluded. Patients with a Class I indication for permanent pacemaker therapy according to the American College of Cardiology/American Heart Association Task Force guidelines (see Tables 45.3 and 45.4) should be admitted to the hospital for pacemaker implantation (2). This heterogeneous group includes all patients with symptomatic AV block, regardless of severity. The management of asymptomatic patients is less straightforward, and identifying high-risk patients who would not tolerate bradycardia because of an inadequate escape mechanism is important. These asymptomatic high-risk patients include those with the following: third-degree AV block and asystole lasting longer than 3 seconds or an escape rate less than 40 bpm; third-degree AV block that precipitates bradycardia-dependent ventricular arrhythmias; third-degree AV block caused by drugs that are needed for coexisting medical conditions; and bifascicular block associated with type II second-degree or higher degrees of AV block (2). Patients with Class II indications for pacing therapy (see Table 45.1) are less well defined; a decision not to implant a pacemaker requires close outpatient follow-up.

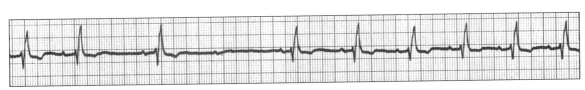

Figure 45.1 Vagally mediated atrioventricular block. The MCL1 rhythm strip illustrates slowing of the sinus rate prior to the nonconducted P wave; the PR intervals also vary. These findings are commonly seen in states of high vagal input and during sleep, when sympathetic tone is low. Vagally mediated rhythms are almost always benign and do not require treatment.

TABLE 45.3

INDICATIONS FOR PERMANENT PACING IN ACQUIRED ATRIOVENTRICULAR BLOCK

Class I

1. 3rd-degree and advanced 2nd-degree AV block at any anatomic level, associated with any one of the following conditions:
   a. Bradycardia with symptoms (including heart failure) presumed to be due to AV block
   b. Arrhythmias and other medical conditions that require drugs that result in symptomatic bradycardia
   c. Documented periods of asystole $\geq$3.0 s or any escape rate <40 bpm in awake, symptom-free patients
   d. After catheter ablation of the AV junction
   e. Postoperative AV block that is not expected to resolve after cardiac surgery
   f. Neuromuscular diseases with AV block (e.g., myotonic muscular dystrophy, Kearns-Sayre syndrome, Erb's limb-girdle dystrophy, and peroneal muscular atrophy) with or without symptoms, because there may be unpredictable progression of AV conduction disease
2. 2nd-degree AV block with associated symptomatic bradycardia, regardless of the type or site of block

Class IIa

1. Asymptomatic 3rd-degree AV block at any anatomic site with average awake ventricular rates of $\geq$40 bpm, especially if cardiomegaly or left ventricular dysfunction is present
2. Asymptomatic type II 2nd-degree AV block with narrow QRS; when type II 2nd-degree AV block occurs with a wide QRS, pacing becomes a Class I recommendation
3. Asymptomatic type I 2nd-degree AV block at intra- or infra-His levels found at electrophysiologic study performed for other indications
4. 1st- or 2nd-degree AV block with symptoms similar to those of *pacemaker syndrome*[a]

Class IIb

1. Marked 1st-degree AV block (>0.30 s) in patients with left ventricular dysfunction and symptoms of congestive heart failure in whom a shorter AV interval results in hemodynamic improvement
2. Neuromuscular disease (e.g., myotonic muscular dystrophy, Kearns-Sayre syndrome, Erb's limb-girdle dystrophy, and peroneal muscular atrophy) with any degree of AV block (including 1st-degree AV block) with or without symptoms, because there may be unpredictable progression of AV conduction disease

Class III

1. Asymptomatic 1st-degree AV block
2. Asymptomatic type I 2nd-degree AV block at the supra-His (AV node) level or not known to be intra- or infra-Hisian
3. AV block expected to resolve and/or unlikely to recur (e.g., drug toxicity, Lyme disease, or during hypoxia in sleep apnea syndrome in absence of symptoms)

See Table 45.1 for definitions of classes.
[a] A symptom complex of fatigue, weakness, dizziness, hypotension, effort intolerance, and pulmonary and central venous hypertension caused by inappropriate relationships between atrial and ventricular depolarization-contraction sequences.
AV, atrioventricular.
Adapted from Gregoratos G, Abrams J, Epstein AE, et al. ACC/AHA/NASPE 2002 guideline update for implantation of cardiac pacemakers and antiarrhythmia devices—summary article. *J Am Coll Cardiol* 2002;40:1703–1719. Copyright 2002 by the American College of Cardiology and American Heart Association, Inc., with permission.

Indications for Initial Coronary Care Unit Admission

Patients should be admitted to the CCU if the cause of the AV block necessitates admission (e.g., acute myocardial infarction) or if temporary pacemaker support is needed while awaiting definitive therapy. Temporary pacing may be needed for both transient and persistent AV block. Patients not requiring a CCU admission should be observed in a telemetry setting. Atropine should be readily available. Transcutaneous pacing allows rate support in emergent situations.

Pacemakers

The basic pacing system includes the pulse generator, lead(s), and electrodes. The permanently implanted pulse generator is a hermetically sealed titanium "can" contain-

TABLE 45.4

INDICATIONS FOR PERMANENT PACING AFTER THE ACUTE PHASE OF A MYOCARDIAL INFARCTION

Class I

1. Persistent 2nd-degree AV block in the His-Purkinje system with bilateral bundle-branch block or 3rd-degree AV block within or below the His-Purkinje system
2. Transient advanced (2nd- or 3rd-degree) infranodal AV block and associated bundle-branch block; if the block site is uncertain, an electrophysiologic study may be necessary
3. Persistent and symptomatic 2nd- or 3rd-degree AV block

Class IIa

None

Class IIb

1. Persistent 2nd- or 3rd-degree AV block at the AV node level

Class III

1. Transient AV block in the absence of intraventricular conduction defects
2. Transient AV block in the presence of isolated left anterior fascicular block
3. Acquired left anterior fascicular block in the absence of AV block
4. Persistent 1st-degree AV block in the presence of bundle-branch block that is old or age-indeterminate

See Table 45.1 for definitions of classes.
AV, atrioventricular.
Adapted from Gregoratos G, Abrams J, Epstein AE, et al. ACC/AHA/NASPE 2002 guideline update for implantation of cardiac pacemakers and antiarrhythmia devices—summary article. *J Am Coll Cardiol* 2002;40:1703–1719. Copyright 2002 by the American College of Cardiology and American Heart Association, Inc., with permission.

ing a lithium power source and circuitry for sensing cardiac electrical activity. The pacing lead contains a metal wire (or wires) insulated by either polyurethane or silastic rubber. The lead can be either bipolar or unipolar. Bipolar leads contain two electrodes: a proximal (ring) electrode and a distal (tip) electrode. The interelectrode distance is small, usually 1–3 cm. Unipolar leads contain only a tip electrode (cathode); the pulse generator serves as the anode. The interelectrode distance is, therefore, much greater in a unipolar system than in a bipolar one, which results in both larger stimulus artifacts on the surface electrocardiogram and a larger "antenna" that senses electrical activity.

A "demand" pacing system provides a stimulus output when no electrical activity is sensed. Conversely, it inhibits its output when electrical activity is sensed. The magnitude of the stimulus output can be described in terms of voltage or current (usually the former), and the duration of the stimulus output is the pulse width. The capture threshold is the minimum stimulus output required to initiate a depolarization. The sensing threshold is the smallest intracardiac signal that can be detected by the sensing amplifier. Appro-

priate sensing is important in preventing unwanted inhibition of output or competitive output from the pacemaker.

The North American Society of Pacing and Electrophysiology—Heart Rhythm Society has adopted a five-letter code to describe the function of pacing systems. The first letter describes the chamber or chambers in which pacing occurs (*V*, ventricle; *A*, atrium; *D*, dual [atrium and ventricle]). The second letter describes the chamber or chambers in which sensing occurs (and has the same codes as for pacing). The third letter describes the response to a sensed event (*T*, triggered output in response to a sensed event; *I*, inhibited output in response to a sensed event; *D*, dual [triggered and inhibited, e.g., an atrial sensed event inhibits atrial output and triggers a ventricular output after a preset AV interval]). In today's pulse generators, the fourth letter, *R*, indicates rate modulation. The fifth letter describes antitachycardia functions (Table 45.5). More recent codes incorporate designations for multisite pacing and special lead features such as steroid elution.

The mode of function that is programmed depends upon the underlying atrial rhythm, the status of AV conduction, the need for AV synchrony (appropriate relationships between atrial and ventricular depolarization-contraction sequences), and the presence or absence of chronotropic competence (ability of the sinus rate to increase in response to increases in metabolic need). Although intact AV conduction theoretically can reduce or eliminate

TABLE 45.5

COMMONLY USED PACING MODES AND FUNCTIONS

Mode	Definition
AAI	Atrial pacing on demand; output inhibited by sensed atrial signals
AAIR	Atrial pacing on demand; output inhibited by sensed atrial signals; atrial pacing rates can increase and decrease in response to sensor input, up to the programmed sensor-based upper rate limit
VVI	Ventricular pacing on demand; output inhibited by sensed ventricular signals
VVIR	Ventricular pacing on demand; output inhibited by sensed ventricular signals; ventricular pacing rates can increase and decrease in response to sensor input, up to the programmed sensor-based upper rate limit
DDD	Paces and senses in both the atrium and the ventricle; paces the ventricle in response to sensed atrial activity, up to the programmed upper rate limit
DDDR	Paces and senses in both the atrium and the ventricle; atrial and ventricular pacing rates increase and decrease in response to sensor input, up to the programmed sensor-based upper rate limit

Asynchronous pacing (sensing function eliminated) is the usual mode of function in response to magnet application to the pulse generator.

TABLE 45.6
PACEMAKER EMERGENCIES

Postimplantation complications
    Immediate
        Pneumothorax, hemothorax
        Cardiac tamponade
        Myocardial perforation
    Late
        Subclavian vein thrombosis
        Superior vena cava syndrome
        Lead thrombus
        Pulmonary emboli
        Infection of pacing system
        Pericarditis
Undersensing ("failure" to sense)
Failure to output (no pacing stimulus delivered)
Failure to capture (pacing stimulus delivered, but no myocardial
    depolarization)
Inappropriate changes in pacemaker rate
    Inappropriately slow rate (most often because of oversensing; can
        indicate end of life of pulse generator)
    Inappropriately fast rate (most often because of normal tracking of
        atrial arrhythmias or inappropriately programmed rate-adaptive
        settings)

the need for a ventricular lead, up to 30% of patients with sinus node dysfunction also have AV block or bundle-branch block. AV dyssynchrony that results in loss of atrial contribution to ventricular filling is tolerated poorly in patients with noncompliant ventricles, including patients with acute ischemia and infarction. Chronotropic incom-

petence can result in exercise intolerance; sensors for rate adaptation lead to increases and decreases in pacing rate in response to parameters such as body motion, minute ventilation, and QT interval. Programmed modes of function and rates may not be appropriate in specific patients or circumstances, and changes in programmed parameters often become necessary in hospitalized patients to adapt to specific clinical situations.

Pacemaker Emergencies

Pacemaker emergencies (Table 45.6) include complications of the implant procedure itself, "failure" to sense (undersensing) (Table 45.7 and Figure 45.2), failure to output, failure to capture (Table 45.8 and Figure 45.3), and inappropriate or unwanted changes in pacemaker rate. Undersensing is manifested on the surface electrocardiogram by delivered pacing stimuli when inhibition of output is expected. Absence of output, which results in pauses in paced rhythm, can be caused by normal inhibition, oversensing (unwanted sensing of noncardiac electrical signals) (Figure 45.4), or end of life of the pulse generator. Unanticipated end of generator life, which is rare today because most patients are followed in specialized pacemaker clinics, is a medical emergency. Failure to capture is manifested by pacemaker stimuli that do not initiate a depolarization, provided that there is temporal opportunity to do so; "functional" noncapture exists if the pacemaker stimulus falls in the atrial or ventricular refractory period and thus cannot initiate depolarization. For a patient with potential pacemaker dysfunction or a pacemaker emergency, urgent

TABLE 45.7
DIFFERENTIAL DIAGNOSIS OF UNDERSENSING ("FAILURE" TO SENSE)

Normal pacing system function	Comment/management
Inappropriately low programmed sensitivity	Reprogram sensitivity
Poor intracardiac signal	Most common cause of undersensing; reprogram sensitivity
"Functional" undersensing	Sensing amplifier is transiently refractory to incoming electrical signals as part of its normal operation; causes confusion in electrocardiogram interpretation; program new parameters of function where appropriate

Abnormal pacing system function	
End of battery life	Requires generator replacement
Open circuit	
Poor connection between lead and pulse generator	Requires revision
Lead fracture	Chest radiograph may reveal subclavian crush; interrogation documents high lead impedance; revision required
Insulation failure	Chest radiograph can help detect; interrogation documents low lead impedance; revision required

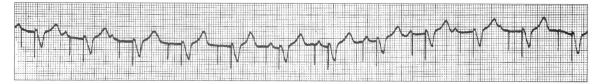

Figure 45.2 Atrial undersensing ("failure" to sense) in a DDD pacing system. Spontaneous P waves do not inhibit the atrial output from the pulse generator, resulting in atrial stimulus outputs at the programmed base rate. This rhythm strip also illustrates "functional noncapture" of atrial stimulus outputs due to myocardial tissue refractoriness rather than to a true noncapture problem.

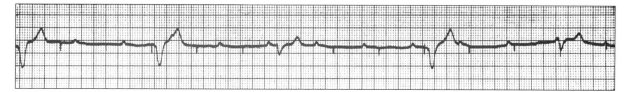

Figure 45.3 Intermittent failure to capture with a ventricular pacing system in a patient with hyperkalemia resulting from renal failure. The first, second, and fourth QRS complexes are paced. Most pacing stimuli do not stimulate myocardial tissue despite the temporal opportunity to do so. This problem should be managed by correcting the electrolyte abnormality. On occasion, programming a higher pacemaker output can be a successful temporary measure to restore pacing function.

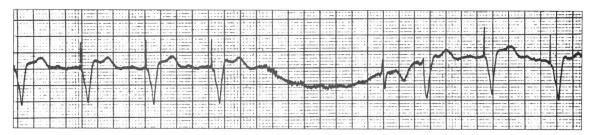

Figure 45.4 Pause in paced rhythm resulting from myopotential oversensing. The ventricular lead senses the myopotentials (which can reach amplitudes of 3–5 mV), with resulting inhibition of output. The asystolic period is terminated by a narrow QRS complex escape beat. The problem is best managed by lowering the sensitivity (increasing the signal amplitude that the pacemaker will sense); take care to avoid undersensing ("failure" to sense) spontaneous QRS complexes. Reprogramming the lead from a unipolar to bipolar mode of function may also solve this problem. In this example, myopotentials are readily visible in the rhythm strip; in most instances, however, the oversensed signal is not appreciable from the surface electrocardiogram and must be inferred. The presence of oversensing can be confirmed by visualizing the signal from the intracardiac lead using the pacemaker analyzer.

cardiologic consultation is mandatory. Physicians unfamiliar with the intricacies of pacemakers should not attempt to reprogram the pacemaker.

Temporary Cardiac Pacing

Temporary (Table 45.2) pacing provides effective rate support for transient bradycardias and can serve as a bridge to permanent pacing. Temporary pacing can be accomplished using transcutaneous, transesophageal, and transvenous routes. *Transcutaneous pacing* involves application of two large surface patch electrodes (70 to 120 cm²) on the torso (negative cathodal electrode positioned anteriorly; positive anodal electrode positioned posteriorly). Programmable parameters of the transcutaneous pacemaker include rate, output, and sensitivity. Stimulus output ranges from 0 to 200 mA. The capture threshold usually ranges between 35 and 80 mA; the stimulus output should be set at 5 to 10 mA above the capture threshold. Successful temporary pacing can be achieved in up to 70% of patients. Complications of transcutaneous pacing include uncomfortable, often painful, cutaneous nerve stimulation at stimulus outputs greater than 30 mA. Ease of application has made transcutaneous pacing a valuable tool in the emergent treatment of bradycardias as a bridge to permanent therapy. However, transcutaneous pacing is much less reliable than transvenous pacing, and, in patients who are pacemaker-dependent (spontaneous QRS rate of less than 30 bpm or symptoms at slow rates), transcutaneous pacing should serve only as a temporary measure until a transvenous lead is inserted.

Transesophageal pacing, which is a relatively simple form of pacing, involves swallowing an electrode. The proximity of the esophagus to the left atrium allows access to atrial pacing. The ideal atrial pacing site is indicated by the atrial

TABLE 45.8
DIFFERENTIAL DIAGNOSIS OF FAILURE TO CAPTURE

Cause	Chest radiograph	Capture threshold	Lead impedance	Comment/management
Inappropriately low programmed output	Normal or unchanged	Normal	Normal	Interrogation confirms the programmed output; determine capture thresholds and reprogram output
High pacing thresholds	Normal or unchanged	High	Normal	Hyperkalemia, flecainide, acidosis are usual causes
Battery failure	Normal or unchanged	High	Normal	Interrogation confirms end of life
Open circuit				
Lead fracture	Often abnormal	High	High	Lead fracture may not be visible on chest radiograph
Lead dislodgment	May be abnormal	High	High	May be able to program increased output; pacing system revision may be required
Insulation failure	Often abnormal	High	Low	Insulation break may not be visible on chest radiograph
"Functional" noncapture	Normal	Normal	Normal	Stimulus falls in refractory period of myocardial tissue; assess electrocardiogram; identify cause; reprogram if warranted

electrogram that has the largest magnitude (about 35–40 cm from the teeth). Ventricular pacing can be performed through the esophagus but with less reliability than atrial pacing because of the greater distance between the esophagus and the ventricles. Thus, esophageal pacing should not be used in patients with AV block. Complications are minimal and include epigastric discomfort and phrenic-nerve stimulation with high stimulation outputs.

Transvenous pacing is the most reliable method of temporary pacing. The left subclavian vein should be avoided, if possible, so that it can be used for a permanent pacing lead if required. The temporary pacing lead is positioned under fluoroscopic guidance in the right-atrial appendage for atrial pacing and right-ventricular apex for ventricular pacing. Stimulus outputs range between 0.1 mA and 20 mA and should be set two to three times above the capture threshold. The ideal atrial and ventricular capture thresholds are no more than 1.0 mA. Sensitivity is usually set at 25%–50% of the sensing threshold.

Indication for Early Consultation

Cardiology consultation is recommended if the patient has a life-threatening cardiac disorder associated with bradycardia, if the patient is pacemaker-dependent and is admitted to the CCU for rate support, or if the patient has (or is suspected of having) a malfunctioning pacemaker. Implantation and follow-up of permanent pacing systems are usually performed by a cardiologist with expertise in the field. Interrogation of the pulse generator is the only method by which programmed values, battery status, and lead impedances can be determined. Optimal programming, sensing, and capture threshold evaluations require familiarity with pacemaker technology and appropriate equipment. These determinations are best performed by an experienced cardiologist, whether the pacing system is a temporary or a permanent one.

ISSUES DURING THE COURSE OF HOSPITALIZATION

The major issues accompanying hospitalization of the patient with bradycardia include identifying and treating the cause of bradycardia, deciding whether or not permanent pacemaker implantation is necessary, arranging for implantation of a permanent pacemaker if appropriate, and subsequent postimplant evaluation. The initial goals are to stabilize the patient and evaluate the cause and severity of the bradycardia. After the exclusion of or failure to rectify potentially reversible causes of bradycardia, a permanent pacemaker should be implanted on day 2 unless there is active infection. Rhythm monitoring in a telemetry facility is recommended until hospital discharge, usually on the day after implant.

Following pacing-system implantation and prior to discharge, a 12-lead electrocardiogram should be obtained to document the patient's spontaneous rhythm and rate, if possible, and the morphology and axis of paced P waves and QRS complexes. Normal sensing and pacing function must be established prior to discharge. After permanent or temporary pacemaker placement, a chest radiograph should be obtained to exclude pneumothorax and to assess lead position as well as connector block (lead connections to pulse generator) integrity.

Pacemakers can have unexpected and unwanted decreases or increases in rate. A decrease in pacemaker rate can be caused by sensor-driven rate reduction, by magnet application with a device-specific rate reduction, by phantom programming (with the pacemaker unknowingly reprogrammed by either someone else or electromagnetic noise), or by end of battery life. Increases in paced rates can result from sensor-driven rate increases, tracking of atrial tachyarrhythmias, and pacemaker-mediated tachycardias in which the pacemaker lead itself participates in a reentry pathway; pacemaker-mediated tachycardias rarely occur with newer pacemaker systems.

Rate-adaptive pacing is designed to increase and decrease the heart rate to meet the physiologic demands of the patient. Depending on the sensor and the programmed parameters, however, increases in paced rate can be inappropriate for a given clinical circumstance (e.g., body motion sensor input in a shivering patient or minute ventilation sensor in a hyperventilating patient).

Pacemaker Malfunction

Medical sources of electromagnetic interference can have adverse effects on pacemakers. Direct-current cardioversion and defibrillation deliver a large current of energy and can adversely affect pacemaker function. These effects can be minimized by maintaining a cardioversion/defibrillation vector perpendicular to the vector of the pacing system and by keeping the cardioversion/defibrillation electrodes more than 5 cm from the pacing system.

Magnetic resonance imaging should not be performed in patients with pacemakers because of potential complications, including reports of postimaging death (3). Surgeons must be careful to use electrocautery according to established recommendations (4) to avoid pacemaker oversensing and output inhibition.

Patients with pacemakers who require therapeutic radiation should avoid high-energy neutron radiation. Direct exposure of the pulse generator to the radiation beam should be prevented by shielding. Complete pacing system replacement should be anticipated if the pulse generator is within the radiation field. Lithotripsy can damage the pacemaker. Transcutaneous electrical nerve stimulation therapy can result in oversensing and output inhibition (particularly in unipolar pacemakers), as well as in atrial oversensing and triggered rapid ventricular pacing.

DISCHARGE ISSUES

In the absence of medical conditions necessitating continued hospitalization, the patient can be discharged as early as on the day of implant. The patient should be instructed not to perform vigorous upper-extremity activities for at least a week to prevent lead dislodgment. Fever or any abnormality over the pocket site (pain, warmth, swelling, redness, discharge, or bleeding) should be reported immediately, as should palpitations, syncope, presyncope, and shortness of breath. These symptoms should prompt immediate outpatient evaluation.

Pacemakers can interact with nonmedical sources of electromagnetic interference. The most common sources are cellular phones, which can result in oversensing, output inhibition, and noise-reversion pacing (temporary asynchronous pacing in response to electrical signals sensed as "noise"), particularly if the phone is used ipsilaterally in proximity (<10 cm) to the pulse generator and if the phone is digital (5). Cellular phone users with pacemakers should use the ear contralateral to the pulse generator and should avoid placing the telephone directly over the pacemaker. Airport-security metal detectors and antitheft surveillance systems generally do not cause a problem if patients do not linger in the vicinity of the detectors (6). Sporadic cases of transient output inhibition or noise-reversion pacing have been reported with the use of some household appliances (microwaves, electric shavers, electrical blankets, and ham radios) and also with acupuncture. Scuba diving can cause deformation of the titanium pulse generator at depths greater than 132 feet.

At discharge, the patient should be given a card identifying the manufacturer of the pulse generator and lead(s), including model and serial numbers. Copies of the interrogated data should be given to the patient and placed in the patient's medical record. The patient should have a follow-up pacemaker check within one week and again at one month and then be enrolled in a telephone pacemaker-surveillance program. Careful medical follow-up is also important because more than 50% of patients will die of noncardiac causes (7).

Postimplantation pocket infections occur in 1% to 6% of patients. Clinical manifestations include warmth, erythema, and discharge from the pocket site, as well as fever. Although some studies report successful outcomes using intravenous antibiotics alone, the preferred therapy is removal of the entire pacemaker system accompanied by use of antibiotics (8). Blood cultures should be obtained prior to administration of antibiotics. Initial antibiotic therapy should be intravenous and cover the two most common offending organisms, *Staphylococcus aureus* and *Staphylococcus epidermidis*. The latter is more often associated with late infections (occurring later than one month after implantation).

COST CONSIDERATIONS AND RESOURCE USE

The most effective strategy for the efficient use of resources is early identification and implantation of a permanent pacing system in patients who require lifelong rate support. Early implantation avoids the use and associated cost of temporary pacing and, in the absence of medical conditions necessitating continued hospitalization, reduces length of hospital stay. Data from randomized trials suggest that dual-chamber pacing (atrial-based pacing) does not significantly reduce stroke or death compared with single-chamber ventricular pacing in patients with sinus node dysfunction (9,10). However, dual-chamber pacing does appear to reduce the frequency of atrial fibrillation and the development of chronic atrial fibrillation. Its use also results in fewer hospitalizations for heart failure and improved quality of life (9, 11–13). As a result, it is cost effective compared with single chamber ventricular pacing (14).

Evidence suggests that ventricular dyssynchrony caused by right ventricular apical pacing can be detrimental in patients with depressed left ventricular function (ejection fraction of 40% or less), evidenced by the development of heart failure and a higher mortality rate (15). Although biventricular pacing has been found to be effective in improving heart failure symptoms and signs in patients with ventricular dyssynchrony (Chapter 39), the benefit of biventricular pacing in patients with bradycardia who do not have heart failure (for the sole purpose of correcting right ventricular pacing-induced dyssynchrony) has yet to be established.

KEY POINTS

- All patients with symptomatic bradycardia should be treated with permanent cardiac pacing unless the cause of bradycardia is clearly reversible.
- Permanent cardiac pacing is indicated in patients with bradycardia caused by necessary drug therapy.
- Vagally mediated bradycardia is common in hospitalized patients and usually does not require temporary or permanent cardiac pacing.
- Transcutaneous pacing should not be used in patients for prolonged periods because it is both uncomfortable and unreliable.
- In patients with chronotropic incompetence, always attempt to implant a permanent pacing system that allows the heart rate to adapt to changing metabolic needs.
- Data from randomized controlled trials show that in patients with sinus node dysfunction, dual-chamber pacing does not significantly reduce stroke or death compared with ventricular pacing; however, dual-chamber pacing does appear to reduce the frequency of atrial fibrillation and the progression to chronic atrial fibrillation, prevent hospitalizations for heart failure, and improve quality of life.
- Magnetic resonance imaging is contraindicated in patients with pacemakers; special precautions may be required during electrocautery, ionizing radiation, lithotripsy, transcutaneous nerve stimulation, and cellular-phone use.
- When patients present with pacemaker pocket infections, explantation of the entire pacing system is recommended.

REFERENCES

1. Rosen KM, Loeb HS, Sinno MZ, Rahimtoola SH, Gunnar RM. Cardiac conduction in patients with symptomatic sinus node disease. *Circulation* 1971;43:836–844.
2. Gregoratos G, Abrams J, Epstein AE, et al. ACC/AHA/NASPE 2002 guideline update for implantation of cardiac pacemakers and antiarrhythmia devices. *J Am Coll Cardiol* 2002;40:1703–1719.
3. Sommer T, Vahlhaus C, Lauck G, et al. MR imaging and cardiac pacemakers: in-vitro evaluation and in-vivo studies in 51 patients at 0.5 T. *Radiology* 2000;215:869–879.
4. Levine PA, Balady GJ, Lazar HL, Belott PH, Roberts AJ. Electrocautery and pacemakers: management of the paced patient subject to electrocautery. *Ann Thorac Surg* 1986;41:313–317.
5. Hayes DL, Wang PJ, Reynolds DW, et al. Interference with cardiac pacemakers by cellular telephones. *N Engl J Med* 1997;336:1473–1479.
6. Mugica J, Henry L, Podeur H. Study of interactions between permanent pacemakers and electronic antitheft surveillance systems. *PACE* 2000;23:333–337.
7. Flaker G, Greenspan A, Tardiff B, et al. Mode Selection Trial (MOST) Investigators. Death in patients with permanent pacemakers for sick sinus syndrome. *Am Heart J* 2003;146:887–893.
8. Chua JD, Wilkoff BL, Lee I, Juratli N, Longworth DL, Gordon SM. Diagnosis and management of infections involving implantable electrophysiologic cardiac devices. *Ann Intern Med* 2000;133:604–608.
9. Lamas GA, Lee KL, Sweeney MO, et al. Ventricular pacing or dual-chamber pacing for sinus-node dysfunction. *N Engl J Med* 2002;346:1854–1862.
10. Connolly SJ, Kerr CR, Gent M, et al. Effects of physiologic pacing versus ventricular pacing on the risk of stroke and death due to cardiovascular causes. *N Engl J Med* 2000;342:1385–1391.
11. Lamas GA, Orav EJ, Stambler BS, et al. Quality of life and clinical outcomes in elderly patients treated with ventricular pacing as compared with dual-chamber pacing. *N Engl J Med* 1998;338:1097–1104.
12. Tang AS, Roberts RS, Kerr C, et al. Relationship between pacemaker dependency and the effect of pacing mode on cardiovascular outcomes. *Circulation* 2001;103:3081–3085.
13. Skanes AC, Krahn AD, Yee R, et al. Progression to chronic atrial fibrillation after pacing: the Canadian Trial of Physiologic Pacing (CTOPP). *J Am Coll Cardiol* 2001;38:167–172.
14. Rinfret S, Cohen DL, Lamas GA, et al. Cost effectiveness of dual-chamber pacing as compared with ventricular pacing for sinus node dysfunction. *Circulation* 2005;111:165–172.
15. Wilkoff BL, Cook JR, Epstein AE, et al. Dual-chamber pacing or ventricular backup pacing in patients with an implantable defibrillator: the Dual Chamber and VVI Implantable Defibrillator (DAVID) Trial. *JAMA* 2002;288:3115–3123.

ADDITIONAL READING

Hayes DL, Strathmore NF. Electromagnetic interference with implantable devices. In: Ellenbogen KA, Kay GN, Wilkoff BL, eds. *Clinical Cardiac Pacing and Defibrillation.* 2nd ed. Philadelphia: W. B. Saunders, 2000:939–943.
Kusumoto FM, Goldschlager NF, eds. *Cardiac Pacing for the Clinician.* Philadelphia: Lippincott Williams & Wilkins, 2001:284–307.
Mangrum JM, DiMarco JP. The evaluation and management of bradycardia. *N Engl J Med* 2000;342:703–709.

Pericardial Disease

46

Fady Malik   Elyse Foster

INTRODUCTION

Although pericardial disease is a rare cause of hospital admission, it can be life threatening, and it may be the first manifestation of other systemic illnesses. After diagnostic testing, pericardial disease usually still is considered idiopathic, and the disease is often self-limited without specific therapy. Thus, the challenges for the clinician are to decide when to hospitalize, when to proceed with further testing, and when to prescribe empiric treatment. In the case of a pericardial effusion, the physician also must decide when to perform pericardiocentesis, either diagnostic or therapeutic.

PERICARDIAL ANATOMY AND PHYSIOLOGY

Hippocrates (c. 460–370 BC) described a normal pericardium as "a smooth mantle surrounding the heart and containing a small amount of fluid resembling urine" (1). In truth, the pericardium comprises two distinct layers in continuity with each other. The visceral pericardium is a single cellular layer that covers the surface of the heart. At the origins of the great vessels, this layer reflects back on itself and acquires an outer fibrous layer to form a sac around the heart. The pericardial sac is tethered in place by ligamentous attachments to the sternum, spine, and diaphragm. Normally, the potential space enclosed by the inner and outer layers of the pericardium is filled with about 50 ml of clear fluid. The function of the pericardium is unclear, and its congenital absence may have little consequence (1). The intact pericardium does serve as a barrier to the spread of infection from the pleural space. Because the parietal layer is stiff, the pericardium may provide support to the more compliant walls of the right atrium and right ventricle, limiting their distension under pressure loads. The hemodynamic consequences of pericardial disease can arise from changes in the elastic properties of the pericar-

dial layers or from inflammation and fluid accumulation within the pericardial sac.

CLINICAL SYNDROMES

Acute pericarditis (2) is an inflammation of the pericardium from any of a variety of causes (Table 46.1). The syndrome may be self-limited, or it may be associated with an enlarging pericardial effusion that can lead to pericardial tamponade or that requires drainage because of suspected purulent bacterial pericarditis. In some patients, chronic or recurrent pericarditis leads to *constrictive pericarditis*. It is critical to differentiate among these various syndromes to guide decisions regarding need for admission as well as subsequent diagnostic and therapeutic interventions.

The physical examination remains the single most important test in evaluating the type and severity of pericardial disease. Careful evaluation of the jugular venous pulse and pressure is essential. In uncomplicated pericarditis and in the absence of other complicating heart disease, the jugular venous pressure (JVP) is normal. Pericardial effusion leads to an increase in JVP, with a blunting of the *y* descent if there is an increase in intrapericardial pressure. Patients with cardiac tamponade will nearly always have elevated neck veins, along with hypotension and tachycardia. The two exceptions to this general rule are seen in patients who have had recent open chest surgery (which can lead to localized hematoma behind the left atrium, leaving the JVP normal) and in patients who are frankly hypovolemic (who may also have normal JVP). In constrictive pericarditis, the JVP is elevated with prominent *x* and *y* descents. Paradoxical inspiratory increase of the JVP (*Kussmaul's sign*) is seen in constrictive pericarditis but usually not in cardiac tamponade. *Pulsus paradoxus*, present in cardiac tamponade, is a lowering of systolic blood pressure more than 10 mm Hg during inspiration. The cause is an increase in filling of the right cardiac chambers during inspiration, resulting in compression

TABLE 46.1

CAUSES OF ACUTE PERICARDITIS

Idiopathic
Infectious
  Viral
  Bacterial
  Mycobacterial
  Fungal
  Protozoal
Neoplastic
  Primary (mesothelioma: rare)
  Secondary (especially breast, lung, melanoma, lymphoma,
    leukemia)
Immune/inflammatory
  Connective tissue diseases, sarcoidosis, familial Mediterranean
    fever
  Myocardial infarction
  Dressler's (after MI) syndrome
  Postcardiotomy
Metabolic
  Uremia
  Dialysis-associated
  Myxedema
  Amyloidosis
Iatrogenic
  Radiation injury
  Cardiac perforation (catheters or automatic implantable
    cardioverter defibrillator placement)
  Drugs (hydralazine, procainamide, isoniazid, anticoagulants,
    minoxidil, methysergide)
Other
  Aortic dissection
  Blunt or penetrating trauma
  Chylopericardium
Congenital
  Pericardial cysts
  Congenital absence of pericardium
  Mulibrey nanism

of the left cardiac chambers and subsequent decrease in left-ventricular stroke volume.

Auscultation of the heart may reveal a pericardial friction rub in cases of acute pericarditis. The sound has been likened to the crunch of walking on dry snow. The rub may occur only during ventricular systole; the presence of additional distinct components during atrial systole and ventricular diastole leads to the classic (but often not heard) three-component rub. In constrictive pericarditis, a pericardial knock, representing the end of rapid diastolic filling, sometimes is heard. The timing is similar to an S3 gallop, but the sound's character is distinctly different. Distant, muffled heart tones may imply the presence of a pericardial effusion. Cardiac gallops usually are not seen in tamponade and imply the coexistence of heart failure.

If a pericardial effusion is present, the echocardiogram may provide corroborative evidence of tamponade, including diastolic collapse of the right ventricle and right atrium. Nevertheless, tamponade remains a clinical diagnosis, suggested by *a triad of hypotension, elevated JVP, and tachycardia*

in the presence of a pericardial effusion. Echocardiographic signs may be less reliable in the presence of severe heart failure or in ventilated patients. Occasionally, a therapeutic pericardiocentesis with subsequent improvement of vital signs may be the only way to confirm the diagnosis of tamponade.

In constrictive pericarditis, transthoracic echocardiography has a low sensitivity for detecting pericardial thickening. However, the absence of normal "sliding" between the pericardial layers suggests adhesion. Transesophageal echocardiography has been shown to be accurate in measuring pericardial thickness (3). Doppler echocardiography can assess the velocity of blood flow across tricuspid and mitral valves, which in constriction (as in tamponade) shows excessive respiratory variation. As in tamponade, the inferior vena cava is dilated because of high right-atrial pressures. Other echocardiographic signs are not diagnostic of constriction. On chest radiograph, the pericardium may appear as a calcified shell surrounding the heart. Computed tomography and magnetic resonance imaging can help assess pericardial thickening, but normal pericardial thickness does not exclude constrictive pericarditis. Invasive hemodynamic measurements in the cardiac catheterization laboratory are usually necessary to support the diagnosis of constrictive pericarditis and differentiate it from restrictive cardiomyopathy.

ACUTE PERICARDITIS

Issues at the Time of Admission

Clinical Presentation

Classic pericarditis presents as a sharp retrosternal discomfort that improves on sitting up and worsens on lying down. The pain can be quite severe, burning in nature, radiating to the shoulder or back, and sudden in onset. It is frequently pleuritic and worsens with inspiration. The pain is variable in nature and location and may mimic cardiac ischemia, an acute abdomen, or aortic dissection. Dyspnea may be present in the absence of pulmonary edema on the chest radiograph. Often pericardial pain follows a prodrome of fever, malaise, and myalgia. A pericardial friction rub is commonly present. The usual electrocardiographic manifestation early in the course of acute pericarditis is widespread ST elevation (concave upward and usually less than 5 mm) with depression of the PR segment below baseline (the T-P segment) (Figure 46.1). These changes (stage I) are diagnostic of acute pericarditis. Occasionally, ST-segment elevation can be confined to the inferior or anterior electrocardiogram (ECG) leads in pericarditis, simulating myocardial infarction. The clinician must take care not to confuse stage I changes of pericarditis with those of acute myocardial infarction (leading to inappropriate thrombolysis) or to mistake a large antero-

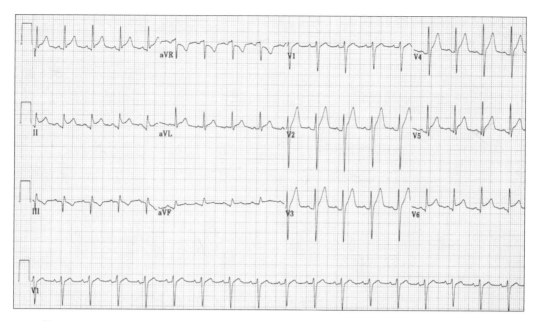

Figure 46.1 Electrocardiogram (stage I) from a patient with acute pericarditis. Widespread ST elevations are present with PR-segment depression in lead II. In stage II, the ST segments return to baseline with flattening of the T waves. In stage III, the T waves become inverted, and in stage IV, the electrocardiogram returns to normal. The evolution typically occurs over two weeks, although the T-wave inversions may persist.

lateral infarction for pericarditis. In stage II, the ST segments return to baseline with flattening of the T waves. In stage III, the T waves invert, and in stage IV, the electrocardiogram returns to normal. The evolution typically occurs over two weeks, although T-wave inversions may persist. If pericarditis presents as a manifestation of a systemic illness, it can be asymptomatic and found incidentally on the ECG or echocardiogram.

Differential Diagnosis and Initial Evaluation

Because the hallmark of acute pericarditis is chest pain, the clinician must rapidly consider and exclude other more life-threatening illnesses, including aortic dissection, pulmonary embolism, esophageal rupture, and either acute or recent myocardial infarction. Thus, the initial evaluation must include (a) rapid assessment of hemodynamic status, noting the presence of tachycardia, hypotension, jugular venous distension, and pulsus paradoxus; (b) cardiac auscultation; (c) ECG; and (d) chest radiograph. Initial laboratory evaluation should include electrolytes, blood urea nitrogen, creatinine, complete blood count, activated partial thromboplastin time, and prothrombin time. Cardiac biomarkers (e.g., troponins or creatine kinase MB levels) should be obtained to exclude myocardial infarction or coexisting myocarditis. However, it is important to recognize that cardiac biomarkers are frequently elevated in acute pericarditis because of coincident subepicardial myocarditis (2,4). When these biomarkers are abnormal, acute myocardial infarction must be excluded definitively before concluding that the diagnosis is acute pericarditis.

Early in the evaluation, echocardiography reveals a pericardial effusion in about 60% of cases of acute pericarditis (5,6) and can help distinguish between myocardial infarction and pericarditis if the ECG changes are nondiagnostic. Occasionally, coronary angiography is required to exclude an acute coronary syndrome definitively, especially if wall motion abnormalities are present on echocardiography. If mediastinal widening appears on chest radiography or aortic root dilation on echocardiography, a transesophageal echocardiogram should be obtained to exclude aortic dissection.

Once the diagnosis of pericarditis is clear, the clinician must consider the available history, physical examination, and initial laboratory results to look for clues to a cause (see Table 46.1). For example, a patient with a fever and an elevated, left-shifted neutrophil count may have purulent pericarditis or endocarditis. A history of breast cancer or the presence of a breast mass might suggest neoplastic invasion and a malignant pericardial effusion. Possible causes should be pursued further by prompt and appropriate additional testing. Pericardiocentesis should be performed if infection or neoplasm is suspected, but it is not required for an asymptomatic effusion discovered incidentally. As most cases of pericarditis remain idiopathic, extensive testing early in the course is discouraged.

In the initial evaluation and triage of patients with acute pericarditis, the sensitivities of low frontal-plane voltage and electrical alternans for cardiac tamponade are only 25% and 8%, respectively (7), rendering the ECG a poor tool for this diagnosis. The presence of an enlarged cardiac silhouette on the chest radiograph suggests a large pericardial effusion, for which echocardiographic assessment and pericardiocentesis are indicated, given the correlation of large effusions with poor outcomes (8).

Emergent echocardiography is not required in patients with normal blood pressure, no tachycardia, normal JVP, normal cardiac biomarkers, and normal cardiac silhouette (Figure 46.2), but such patients should have an echocardiogram at the earliest convenience. Echocardiography may show a large pericardial effusion or evidence of right-atrial or right-ventricular collapse, greatly raising the level of concern regarding the risk for, or presence of, tamponade.

Indications for Hospitalization

The main reasons for hospital admission include pain control and observation for the development of tamponade. In two large Spanish series of consecutive admissions for acute pericarditis, the development of cardiac tamponade in acute idiopathic pericarditis was as high as 15% (5,6). Some high-risk indicators generally are acknowledged (Table 46.2), but no prospectively validated criteria exist by which to risk-stratify patients for development of cardiac tamponade.

Young patients (age under 40 years) with normal vital signs, normal jugular venous pressure, negative cardiac biomarkers, and pain that is easily controlled in the emergency department might be considered candidates for outpatient management if family or friends can carry out adequate observation. Echocardiography before discharge from the emergency department is indicated to exclude a very large pericardial effusion, because effusion size correlates with outcome (8). Patients over age 40 or with other significant coronary risk factors should be routinely evaluated in a coronary observation or chest-pain evaluation unit for 8–12 hours or admitted to a telemetry unit, given the risk of missing an atypical presentation of acute myocardial infarction.

Indications for Initial ICU Admission

Without question, the most important diagnostic test in the triage of patients with primary acute pericarditis is a careful examination of the JVP. Presence or absence of pulsus paradoxus should be ascertained. Elevated JVP in the presence of tachycardia or a positive pulsus paradoxus forewarns early tamponade. Such patients should have emergent echocardiography. If a large effusion is present, then these patients should be monitored in an ICU and receive early cardiology consultation, with the anticipation of urgent pericardiocentesis. Patients with suspected pericarditis secondary to another condition warranting ICU admission, such as myocardial infarction, should be triaged appropriately.

In pericardial tamponade, stroke volume falls and heart rate increases in an attempt to maintain cardiac output; therefore, tachycardia is an early clinical sign of impending tamponade. Pulsus paradoxus may be difficult to diagnose

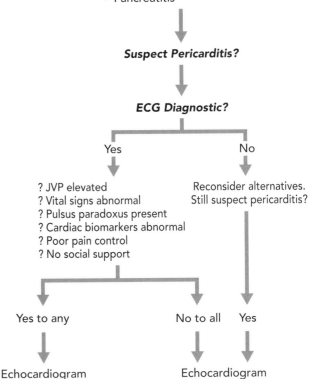

Figure 46.2 Emergency evaluation of possible acute pericarditis. *CBC,* complete blood count; *CXR,* chest radiograph; *D/C,* discharge; *ECG,* electrocardiogram; *F/U,* follow-up; *JVP,* jugular venous pressure; *NSAIDs,* nonsteroidal anti-inflammatory drugs.

TABLE 46.2

INDICATORS OF HIGH RISK FOR COMPLICATIONS OF PERICARDITIS

Study	Indicator
Physical examination	Tachycardia
	Pulsus paradoxus
	Elevated jugular venous pressure
Laboratory examination	Leukocytosis
	Uremia
	Elevated cardiac biomarkers
Chest radiograph	Enlarged cardiac silhouette
Echocardiogram[a]	Large pericardial effusion
	Right-atrium or -ventricle collapse
	Respiratory variation of mitral and tricuspid inflow

[a] Echocardiogram should be obtained immediately if other high-risk indicators are present.

in patients with severe hypotension or atrial fibrillation. However, in patients with pulsus paradoxus, a systolic arterial pressure less than 120 mm Hg, tachycardia, dyspnea, or any evidence of systemic hypoperfusion, pericardial tamponade must be suspected seriously. Echocardiography should be performed unless the patient is so ill that there is no time for it. Echocardiography usually shows exaggerated leftward motion of the interventricular septum and exaggerated increase in right-ventricular filling during inspiration. Right-atrial or right-ventricular collapse during diastole indicates equilibration of intrapericardial pressures with right-ventricular diastolic pressures and also indicates cardiac tamponade (Figures 46.3 and 46.4). These findings often are seen even before the patient has decompensated.

Once pericardial tamponade has been diagnosed clinically, the patient should be moved to a cardiac catheteriza-tion laboratory emergently to undergo catheterization and pericardiocentesis in a controlled setting. In hospitals without catheterization laboratories or in situations that are too emergent to permit catheter guidance, pericardiocentesis can be performed at the bedside (Figure 46.5). Echocardiography can identify the location on the chest wall where the fluid is closest to the transducer. Care is taken to avoid the intercostal and internal mammary arteries, and the transducer angle is used to determine the optimal trajectory of the needle (9). After pericardiocentesis, an intrapericardial catheter generally is left in place as part of a closed drainage system for about 24 hours to be sure that tamponade does not recur. Subsequently, the catheter may be removed. If fluid recurs, percutaneous balloon pericardiotomy or a limited subxiphoid pericardiotomy may be required.

Initial Therapy

If cardiac tamponade is absent and no specific cause is readily apparent, the early management of acute primary pericarditis is focused on relief of symptoms. Treatment is initiated with high-dose nonsteroidal anti-inflammatory drugs, such as 650 mg of aspirin every three to four hours or 800 mg of ibuprofen every eight hours. In patients with severe pain in need of more immediate relief, 60 mg of parenteral ketorolac may promote the more the rapid resolution of symptoms (10). *Anticoagulants generally should be avoided* because of the risk of intrapericardial hemorrhage; for patients requiring anticoagulant therapy, levels should be maintained in the lower end of the indicated therapeutic range.

In some patients, pericarditis may be caused by infectious conditions, uremia, tumor, radiation, or autoimmune diseases. *Tuberculous pericarditis* is not usually associated with evidence of pulmonary tuberculosis. It should be suspected in patients with persistent fever and otherwise unexplained pericardial effusion, especially in

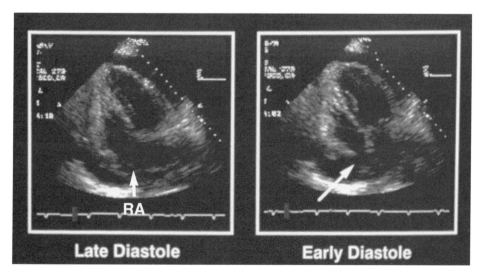

Late Diastole   **Early Diastole**

Figure 46.3   Right-atrial (*RA*) collapse (*arrow*) in a patient with pericardial tamponade.

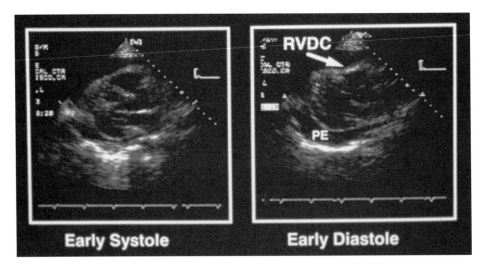

Figure 46.4 Right-ventricular diastolic collapse (*RVDC*) in a patient with pericardial tamponade. *PE*, pericardial effusion.

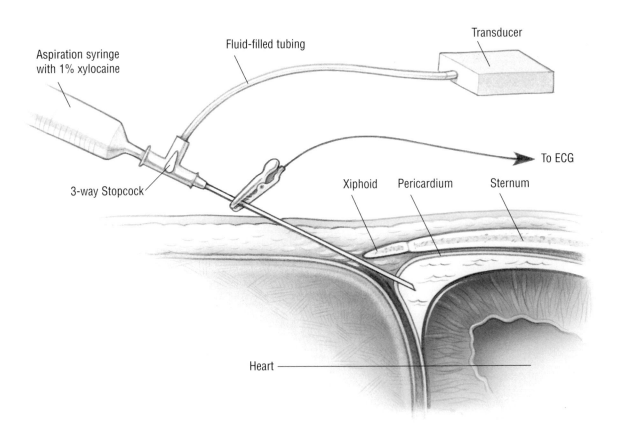

Figure 46.5 Pericardiocentesis using the subxiphoid approach, which avoids the major epicardial vessels. A hollow needle, which is attached via a stopcock to an aspiration syringe and to a short length of connecting tubing leading to a transducer, is used to enter the pericardial space. If fluid is aspirated initially, the pressure waveform at the needle tip should be examined briefly to confirm that the needle tip is in the pericardial space. A floppy-tipped guide wire then is passed through the hollow needle, and the needle is exchanged for a soft flexible catheter with end and side holes to facilitate safe and thorough drainage of the pericardial sac. *ECG*, electrocardiogram. (Adapted from Lorell BH, Grossman W. Profiles in constrictive pericarditis, restrictive cardiomyopathy, and cardiac tamponade. In Grossman W, Baim DS, eds. *Cardiac Catheterization, Angiography, and Intervention.* Philadelphia: Lea and Febiger, 1991:643, with permission.)

patients who are otherwise at high risk for tuberculosis. Both pericardial fluid and tissue often are required to make the diagnosis. In many patients, the effusion may resolve spontaneously and progress insidiously to constrictive pericarditis. Multidrug antituberculosis therapy is required and usually is supervised by an infectious-disease specialist.

Bacterial pericarditis (often referred to as purulent pericarditis) is usually a complication of an adjacent pneumonia with *Staphylococcus, Pneumococcus,* or *Streptococcus* organisms or is associated with thoracic surgery or bacterial endocarditis. It is usually an aggressive, acute illness with fevers, chills, and evidence of sepsis. Cardiac tamponade may develop rapidly. Treatment requires early surgical drainage, often including pericardiectomy, and appropriate intravenous antibiotics.

Fungal pericarditis is unusual. Most cases are caused by histoplasmosis, which can cause massive pericardial effusions. The diagnosis of fungal pericarditis is made based on known exposure to histoplasmosis or coccidioidomycosis, positive titers, and often confirmatory biopsy material.

Uremic pericarditis may occur prior to or during dialysis. Treatment is usually intensification of dialysis and use of nonsteroidal anti-inflammatory drugs.

Malignant pericarditis is usually caused by lung cancer, breast cancer, leukemia, or lymphoma. Patients often have other evidence of tumor in the chest, liver, or lymphatic system. Pericardiocentesis is diagnostic in about 85% of cases. The preferred treatment is catheter drainage of the pericardial space or subxiphoid pericardiectomy. It is critical to realize that some patients with malignancies may have idiopathic pericarditis or radiation pericarditis. For example, radiation pericarditis develops in about 0.5%–5% of patients after radiation for Hodgkin's disease or breast cancer. Pericardiocentesis should be performed only in patients with possible pericardial tamponade.

Autoimmune pericarditis occurs in 20% or more of patients with systemic lupus erythematosus or rheumatoid arthritis. It is more likely to occur if the underlying disease is active. Patients commonly have chest pain and a pericardial rub. Pericarditis usually responds to aggressive treatment of the underlying disease.

Indications for Early Consultation

Prompt cardiology consultation is indicated if there is clinical suspicion of cardiac tamponade, such as the presence of pulsus paradoxus, hypotension, tachycardia, or elevated JVP. Patients with these symptoms are more likely to require pericardiocentesis, which is most safely performed in a cardiac catheterization laboratory with echocardiographic or fluoroscopic guidance. Other indications for cardiology consultation include the failure to improve in the first 24 hours, more than mild elevations of cardiac biomarkers, unexplained electrocardiographic changes, and new arrhythmias.

Issues During the Course of Hospitalization

The purpose of hospitalization in acute pericarditis is the relief of pain and monitoring for the development of cardiac tamponade. As most cases of pericarditis are idiopathic, early conservative therapy is justified. The prognosis is favorable in patients who do not have tamponade and who have early relief of symptoms. Such patients do not require further testing, as the likelihood of discovering significant underlying disease is reported to be less than 3% (5). Failure to improve over 24 hours or the development of tamponade warrant a more aggressive approach to establishing an etiologic cause (Figure 46.6).

In the first 24 hours, patients who do not present with cardiac tamponade should be treated aggressively with nonsteroidal anti-inflammatory drugs. The patients' vital signs and JVP should be evaluated three to four times a day. Patients with deteriorating vital signs or increasing JVP should receive immediate echocardiography and cardiology consultation. In stable patients, repeat cardiac biomarker studies and an ECG should be obtained at 24 hours.

Although pericardial chest pain and fever in acute idiopathic pericarditis may persist for up to a week, patients who fail to show improvement after 24 hours should have further evaluation, including an echocardiogram to assess the presence and size of the pericardial effusion. Additional laboratory testing should be considered to screen for common underlying etiologies of acute pericarditis: occult infection, rheumatoid arthritis, hypothyroidism, HIV disease, malignancy, or tuberculosis. Patients should remain hospitalized until it is clear that they do not have enlarging pericardial effusions (on serial echocardiograms) or life-threatening causes of pericarditis, such as bacterial infection. If pain is refractory to nonsteroidal anti-inflammatory drugs, a one-week course of prednisone 60 mg/d, followed by a one-week taper, usually provides relief. Tuberculosis and bacterial infection should be excluded before beginning corticosteroids. Table 46.3 briefly outlines the management of specific causes of pericarditis; for further discussion, see the "Additional Reading" list at the end of the chapter.

Patients with acute pericarditis frequently have pericardial effusions regardless of the underlying cause. Routine diagnostic pericardiocentesis is generally not useful; the appearance of the fluid (e.g., serous compared with sanguinous) does not reliably distinguish between idiopathic and nonidiopathic causes (11). In one series, only 7% of patients presenting with pericarditis had specific diagnoses (which included tuberculosis, purulent pericarditis, and neoplasm) established by examination of pericardial fluid (5). Pericardial biopsy was not useful. The findings of a large pericardial effusion, impending cardiac tamponade, or failure to resolve fever and illness after five to seven days of conservative treatment predict poorer outcome and a higher diagnostic yield of pericardiocentesis (5,8). In patients with AIDS, the presence of a pericardial effusion portends a dire prognosis (12). Patients with any

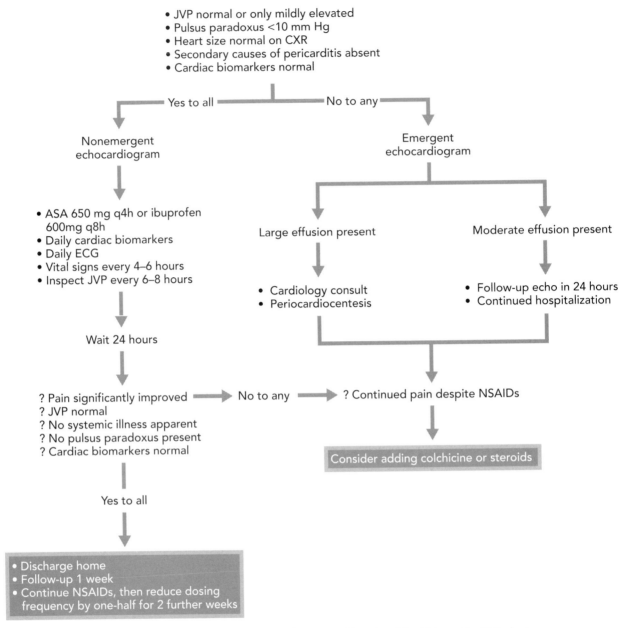

- JVP normal or only mildly elevated
- Pulsus paradoxus <10 mm Hg
- Heart size normal on CXR
- Secondary causes of pericarditis absent
- Cardiac biomarkers normal

Yes to all — No to any

Nonemergent echocardiogram

Emergent echocardiogram

- ASA 650 mg q4h or ibuprofen 600mg q8h
- Daily cardiac biomarkers
- Daily ECG
- Vital signs every 4–6 hours
- Inspect JVP every 6–8 hours

Large effusion present

Moderate effusion present

- Cardiology consult
- Periocardiocentesis

- Follow-up echo in 24 hours
- Continued hospitalization

Wait 24 hours

? Pain significantly improved
? JVP normal
? No systemic illness apparent
? No pulsus paradoxus present
? Cardiac biomarkers normal

No to any — ? Continued pain despite NSAIDs

Consider adding colchicine or steroids

Yes to all

- Discharge home
- Follow-up 1 week
- Continue NSAIDs, then reduce dosing frequency by one-half for 2 further weeks

Figure 46.6 Initial hospital management of patients with pericarditis. *ASA*, aspirin; *CXR*, chest radiograph; *ECG*, electrocardiogram; *JVP*, jugular venous pressure; *NSAIDs*, nonsteroidal anti-inflammatory drugs.

of these characteristics merit cardiology consultation for consideration of diagnostic or therapeutic pericardiocentesis. Patients with moderate-size effusions and no other evidence of underlying disease may continue conservative management with nonsteroidal anti-inflammatory drugs and undergo a second echocardiogram in 24 hours to document stable effusion size. Small effusions may be followed clinically.

Elective pericardiocentesis should be done in a cardiac catheterization laboratory by a physician experienced in the procedure. Rare emergency situations may require bed-

side pericardiocentesis with only electrocardiographic monitoring. As large a volume as possible should be removed and sent for cell count, bacterial culture, mycobacterial culture, and cytology. If tuberculous pericarditis is suspected, elevated levels of adenosine deaminase activity (>40 units/L) support the diagnosis, but culture or biopsy are the standards of diagnosis (2,13). Other laboratory tests generally have low specificity. A follow-up echocardiogram should be performed the next day. If the effusion reaccumulates rapidly, it may be necessary to repeat the pericardiocentesis to avoid the development of cardiac tampon-

TABLE 46.3

PRESENTATION AND TREATMENT OF THE MOST COMMON SPECIFIC CAUSES OF PERICARDITIS

Type of cause	Pathogenesis/ etiology	Diagnosis	Treatment	Complications	Comments
Viral	Coxsackie B Echovirus type 8 Epstein–Barr	Leukocytosis Elevated erythrocyte sedimentation rate Mild cardiac biomarker elevation	Symptomatic relief NSAIDs	Tamponade Relapsing pericarditis	Peaks in spring and fall
Tuberculosis	Mycobacterium tuberculosis	1. Isolation of organism from fluid or biopsy 2. Granulomas not specific	1. Triple drug antituberculosis regimen 2. Pericardial drainage followed by early (4–6 wk) pericardiectomy if signs of tamponade or constriction develop	Tamponade Constrictive pericarditis	1%–8% of patients with tuberculosis pneumonia; R/O HIV infection
Bacterial	Group A Streptococcus Staphylococcus aureus S. pneumoniae	1. Leukocytosis with marked left shift 2. Pericardial fluid purulent	1. Pericardial drainage by catheter or surgery 2. Systemic antibiotics 3. Pericardiectomy if constrictive physiology develops	Tamponade in one-third of patients	Very high mortality rate if not recognized early
Post-myocardial infarction	12 h–10 d post-infarction	1. Fever 2. Pericardial friction rub 3. Echo: effusion	1. ASA 2. Prednisone	Tamponade rare	More frequent in large Q-wave infarctions Anterior > inferior
Uremic	Untreated renal failure: 50% Chronic dialysis: 20%	Pericardial rub: 90%	1. Intensive dialysis 2. Indomethacin: probably ineffective 3. Steroids: high complication rate 4. Catheter drainage 5. Surgical drainage	1. Tamponade 2. Hemodynamic instability on dialysis	Avoid NSAIDs About 50% respond to intensive dialysis
Neoplastic	In order of frequency: Lung cancer Breast cancer Leukemia/ lymphoma Others	1. Chest pain, dyspnea 2. Echo: effusion 3. CT, MRI: tumor metastases to pericardium 4. Cytologic examination of fluid positive in 85%	1. Catheter drainage 2. Subxiphoid pericardiectomy 3. Chemotherapy directed at underlying malignancy	Tamponade Constriction	

ASA, aspirin; *CT,* computed tomography; *MRI,* magnetic resonance imaging; *NSAIDs,* nonsteroidal anti-inflammatory drugs; *R/O,* rule-out.

ade. In refractory cases with recurrent effusions, surgical creation of a pericardial "window" (with samples sent for pathological examination and culture) may be necessary. However, note that these pericardial "windows" may not remain patent, so recurrent tamponade may occur.

Following complete drainage of the pericardial fluid either percutaneously or surgically, a small percentage of patients develop constrictive physiology because of coexistent pericardial thickening. This entity, *"effusive–constrictive" pericarditis,* is most common with neoplastic invasion of the pericardium. Further treatment depends on the prognosis of the patient.

Pericarditis Developing in the Hospital

Patients hospitalized with other illnesses may develop a pericardial effusion or symptoms of acute pericarditis. Frequently, the cause is related to the underlying illness; however, evaluation still requires consideration of other unrelated causes (Table 46.1). Silent myocardial infarction with resulting pericarditis is an example. Intrapericardial bleeding also should be considered in hospitalized patients, especially those on anticoagulants or who have had intracardiac procedures. Echocardiography is warranted as initial evaluation to assess for presence and size of effusion as well as to evaluate ventricular wall motion. Evaluation, therapy, and indications for pericardiocentesis are otherwise similar to primary acute pericarditis.

Discharge Issues

After 24 hours, patients with improving clinical status, defined by marked improvement of chest pain, normal vital signs, lack of elevated JVP and pulsus paradoxus, normal cardiac biomarkers, and no evidence of myocardial ischemia on ECG, may be considered ready for discharge to home. In the absence of a large cardiac silhouette on the chest radiograph or evidence of cardiac tamponade, echocardiography is not necessary prior to discharge. If high-dosage nonsteroidal anti-inflammatory treatment was begun in the hospital, it should be continued for one to two weeks. The dose may then be halved, and treatment should continue for a total duration of four weeks. Patients should be instructed on discharge to return for evaluation if their symptoms worsen or if they develop shortness of breath, palpitations, or light-headedness.

Follow-up may consist of outpatient visits to the primary care physician or consulting cardiologist at one- to two-week intervals until complete resolution is documented. Development of mild cardiac constrictive disease may occur in the first month (9% of cases) but usually resolves spontaneously (14). Persistently elevated neck veins and new peripheral edema should prompt further investigation. The most common complication of acute pericarditis is recurrent pericarditis, which develops in one-quarter of cases (14) and occasionally becomes refractory. Patients with such complications may require courses of colchicine, steroids, or immunosuppressive agents under the care of a cardiologist.

Patients who improve more slowly require longer hospitalizations. Patients with stable moderate-size or small effusions documented during hospitalization but otherwise negative evaluations generally may be discharged home after 2–3 days of hospitalization. These patients should be followed at 2- to 3-day intervals initially as outpatients and undergo repeat echocardiography to ensure stable effusion size. Continuing fever, pain, or growing effusion size should prompt referral for pericardiocentesis as discussed earlier.

CONSTRICTIVE PERICARDITIS

Issues at the Time of Admission

Clinical Presentation

Constrictive pericarditis usually has a slow, insidious onset resembling heart failure or chronic liver disease. Patients complain of fatigue and dyspnea and often note growing abdominal girth and increasing lower-extremity edema. Careful history might reveal a predisposing condition such as mediastinal irradiation, cardiac surgery, tuberculosis, neoplasm, connective tissue disease, renal disease, or previous history of pericarditis; however, most cases are idiopathic. Physical examination reveals elevated neck veins. The classic finding on physical examination is *Kussmaul's sign*, which is an increase in jugular venous pressure during deep inspiration because of the inability of the right ventricle to accommodate the increase in venous return caused by the negative intrathoracic pressure. Pulsus paradoxus is not seen in constrictive pericarditis unless the patient has effusive–constrictive pericarditis, which is a clinical syndrome with some characteristics of both pericardial tamponade and constrictive pericarditis. A pericardial knock may be heard. The chest radiograph may show pericardial calcification, although this finding occurs in fewer than half of the cases. The ECG is nonspecific; atrial fibrillation occurs in about one-third of cases (1).

Differential Diagnosis and Initial Evaluation

Although constrictive pericarditis may resemble chronic liver disease with ascites and abnormalities of the liver function tests, the presence of elevated neck veins points to a cardiac cause. Primary pulmonary hypertension, pulmonic or tricuspid stenosis, or right-heart failure resulting from mitral stenosis or chronic left-to-right shunting may give the same clinical picture as constrictive pericarditis. Restrictive cardiomyopathies also may have a similar clinical presentation. Distinguishing constrictive pericarditis from a restrictive cardiomyopathy can be difficult, even after careful hemodynamic assessment on cardiac catheterization (Figure 46.7). Moreover, these two entities can coexist.

Initial evaluation of the patient with possible constriction consists of careful history and physical, ECG, chest radiograph, and laboratory tests as outlined for acute pericarditis. There are no pathognomonic electrocardiographic changes in constrictive pericarditis, although atrial fibrillation and nonspecific repolarization changes are common. Given evidence of elevated JVP and edema, the patient should also have an echocardiogram to evaluate ventricular and valvular function. Because the diagnosis of constrictive pericarditis includes documentation of pericardial thickening or adhesion and confirmatory hemodynamics, early magnetic resonance imaging or computed tomography, as

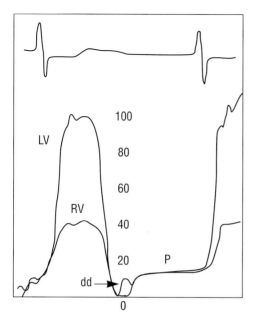

Figure 46.7 Intracardiac pressures in a patient with constrictive pericarditis. Simultaneous pressures obtained in left (*LV*) and right ventricles (*RV*) show equalization of the diastolic pressures. In both ventricles, there is an early diastolic dip (*dd*) that rises rapidly to a plateau (*P*). The patient is in atrial fibrillation. (Adapted from Spodick DH. *The Pericardium: A Comprehensive Textbook.* New York: Marcel Dekker, 1997:243, with permission.)

well as cardiac catheterization, should be part of the initial evaluation. Additional evaluation for specific causes should be guided by the history and index of clinical suspicion.

Indications for Hospitalization

Constrictive pericarditis is slowly progressive, so hospitalization is usually not necessary. However, severe heart failure occasionally may require admission. Patients with anasarca, hypotension, excessive tachycardia, abnormal renal function, or failure to oxygenate adequately should be admitted.

Indications for Initial Intensive Care Unit Admission

Patients with hypotension requiring intravenous vasopressors or patients in a low cardiac output state manifested by renal failure and poor urine output should be admitted to a cardiac care unit. Patients with hypoxia and excessive oxygen requirements or respiratory rate also should be triaged to a cardiac care unit.

Initial Therapy

Patients with evidence of volume overload (elevated JVP, ascites, and edema) should be sodium restricted and receive an intravenous diuretic such as furosemide. The desired rate of diuresis is for output to exceed intake by

500–1,000 mL per day. Patients should have careful assessment of fluid intake and output, vital signs, and daily weights. Patients in atrial fibrillation should be treated with digoxin alone to achieve a target heart rate of 90–100 beats/min. β-blockers and calcium channel blockers are poorly tolerated because of their negative inotropic effects and excessive slowing of heart rate. Medical therapy is usually only palliative for constrictive pericarditis. Patient care is facilitated by rapidly confirming the diagnosis and proceeding with definitive surgical management.

Indications for Early Consultation

Patients with suspected constriction who are admitted to cardiac care units or who have deteriorating renal function should have initial cardiology consultation. Consultation is also indicated in any patient in whom the diagnosis of constrictive pericarditis is established. Cardiac catheterization is required to confirm the hemodynamics of constriction and to exclude coronary artery disease. Myocardial biopsy may be indicated to exclude infiltrative myocardial disease (such as amyloid) if other clinical data do not clearly differentiate restrictive compared with constrictive physiology.

Issues During the Course of Hospitalization

The goal of hospitalization is to relieve the congested state, to establish the diagnosis of constrictive pericarditis, and to proceed to pericardial stripping if appropriate. Diuresis should proceed as described previously while renal function and electrolytes are monitored daily. Once the diagnosis is confirmed, cardiothoracic surgery consultation should be obtained. The decision to recommend surgery should not be made lightly, especially in the severely debilitated elderly patient. The surgical mortality rate ranges from 6%–19% in optimally selected patients and is as high as 40% in the most severely affected individuals (15). The coexistence of restrictive cardiomyopathy and radiation-induced constriction may be associated with poorer surgical outcome, as may the coexistence (with constriction) of coronary artery disease, valvular disease, and renal or hepatic insufficiency. Involvement of the visceral pericardium also negatively impacts surgical outcome.

Patients in atrial fibrillation should be anticoagulated. Cardioversion to normal sinus rhythm may improve cardiac function, but it is unlikely that this sinus rhythm will be sustained. Medications that control the ventricular response rate should be employed judiciously because excessive slowing of the heart rate may lead to clinical deterioration.

Discharge Issues

In postsurgical patients, time to discharge depends on the postsurgical course. If the patient is not considered to be a surgical candidate, discharge depends on the relief of congestion. In general, patients should be able to ambulate and perform their activities of daily living. Elderly or debilitated patients are candidates for referral to a short-term rehabilitation facility. If surgery is delayed, patients may proceed to discharge if their vital signs normalize and effective diuresis is maintained using oral diuretics.

Even after pericardial stripping, it may take several weeks or months for the filling pattern of the heart to return to normal. Patients should continue oral diuretics and have follow-up every 2–4 weeks to be observed for fluid retention. After several weeks, the patient may attempt to taper and eventually discontinue diuretics under supervision. Failure to improve may be a result of inadequate pericardiectomy or any of the other factors discussed previously.

COST CONSIDERATIONS AND RESOURCE USE

Limited diagnostic testing in low-risk patients with acute pericarditis is the primary means of reducing hospitalization costs. Clinical criteria and simple diagnostic tests remain the most effective tools for risk stratification of patients. Selective discharge from the emergency department using echocardiography as a risk-stratification tool may be a cost-effective strategy that does not compromise patient safety. Cost-effectiveness studies are not available and are unlikely to be forthcoming owing to the relative infrequency of acute pericarditis.

KEY POINTS

Acute Pericarditis

- The chest pain of pericarditis is usually pleuritic but can mimic the pain of myocardial infarction, aortic dissection, and pulmonary embolus.
- Patients at high risk for complications include those with fever, tachycardia, pulsus paradoxus, or elevated jugular venous pressure.
- Other indicators of high risk include uremia, history of neoplasm, enlarged cardiac silhouette on chest radiograph, and a large effusion on echocardiography.
- Initial treatment is with nonsteroidal anti-inflammatory drugs for pain relief, except in uremic pericarditis, in which dialysis is indicated.
- Pericardiocentesis is always indicated if there is clinical evidence of tamponade and usually indicated if patients fail to improve with conservative management.

Constrictive Pericarditis

- The onset is usually insidious with symptoms and signs of venous congestion.

- Hospitalization is recommended to relieve symptoms of severe congestion and for low cardiac output.
- Definitive diagnosis requires demonstration of both pericardial thickening and adhesions, as well as hemodynamics consistent with constriction.
- Pericardial stripping carries a 5%–10% or higher mortality rate and should not be recommended lightly.

REFERENCES

1. Hoit BD. Pericardial heart disease. *Current Prob Cardiol* 1997;22: 355–400.
2. Lange RA, Hillis, LD. Acute pericarditis. *N Engl J Med* 2004; 351:2195–2202.
3. Ling LH, Oh JK, Tei C, et al. Pericardial thickness measured with transesophageal echocardiography: feasibility and potential clinical usefulness. *J Am Coll Cardiol* 1997;29:1317–1323.
4. Bonnefoy E, Godon P, Kirkorian G, Fatemi M, Chevalier P, Touboul P. Serum cardiac troponin I and ST-segment elevation in patients with acute pericarditis. *Eur Heart J* 2000;21:832–836.
5. Levy PY, Corey R, Berger P, et al. Etiologic diagnosis of 204 pericardial effusions. *Medicine* (Baltimore) 2003;82:385–391.
6. Troughton RW, Asher CR, Klein AL. Pericarditis. *Lancet* 2004; 363:717–727.
7. Eisenberg MJ, Munoz de Romeral L, Heidenreich PA. The diagnosis of pericardial effusion and cardiac tamponade by 12-lead ECG. *Chest* 1996;110:318–324.
8. Eisenberg MJ, Oken K, Guerrero S, Saniei MA, Schiller NB. Prognostic value of echocardiography in hospitalized patients with pericardial effusion. *Am J Cardiol* 1992;70:934–939.
9. Tsang TS, Freeman WK, Barnes ME, Reeder GS, Packer DL, Seward JB. Rescue echocardiographically guided pericardiocentesis for cardiac perforation complicating catheter-based procedures. The Mayo Clinic experience. *J Am Coll Cardiol* 1998;32:1345–1350.
10. Arunasalam S, Siegel RJ. Rapid resolution of symptomatic acute pericarditis with ketorolac tromethamine: a parenteral nonsteroidal anti-inflammatory agent. *Am Heart J* 1993;125:1455–1458.
11. Chui J, Atar S, Siegel RJ. Comparison of serous and bloody pericardial effusion as an ominous prognostic sign. *Am J Cardiol* 2001;87:924–926.
12. Heidenreich PA, Eisenberg MJ, Kee LL, et al. Pericardial effusion in AIDS: incidence and survival. *Circulation* 1995;92:3229–3234.
13. Koh KK, Kim EJ, Cho CH, et al. Adenosine deaminase and carcinoembryonic antigen in pericardial effusion diagnosis, especially in suspected tuberculous pericarditis. *Circulation* 1994;89:2728–2735.
14. Haley JH, Tajik AJ, Danielson GK, et al. Transient constrictive pericarditis: causes and natural history. *J Am Coll Cardiol* 2004;43:271–275.
15. Houghtaling PL, Lytle BW, Blackstone EH, Lauer MS, Klein AL. Constrictive pericarditis: etiology and cause-specific survival after pericardiectomy. *J Am Coll Cardiol* 2004;43:1445–1452.

ADDITIONAL READING

Hoit BD. Management of effusive and constrictive pericardial heart disease. *Circulation* 2002;105:2939–2942.
Maisch B, Seferovic, Ristic AD, et al. Guidelines on the diagnosis and management of pericardial diseases: executive summary. *Eur Heart J* 2004;25:587–610.
Spodick DH. Acute pericarditis: current concepts and practice. *JAMA* 2003;289:1150–1153.
Spodick DH. Acute cardiac tamponade. *N Engl J Med* 2003;349: 684–690.

Vascular Medicine

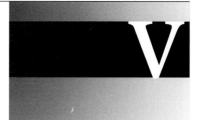

Signs, Symptoms, and Laboratory Abnormalities in Peripheral Arterial Disease

47

Stanley G. Rockson

TOPICS COVERED IN CHAPTER

- Claudication 456
- Symptoms of Critical Leg Ischemia 457
- Pulse Examination 457
- Pallor and Rubor 458
- Cyanosis 458
- Ankle-Brachial Index 458
- Blood tests 459
- Exercise Testing 459
- Segmental Pressure Analysis 460
- Pulse Volume Recording 460
- Imaging Studies 460

INTRODUCTION

Peripheral arterial disease (PAD) is the term most commonly applied to the clinical syndrome that accompanies chronic obstruction of the arterial blood flow to one or more extremities. Most commonly, but not exclusively, this disease is encountered in the legs and represents a manifes- tation of atherosclerosis. As such, PAD often coexists with identifiable occlusive disease in other major arterial con- duits, most notably in the heart and the extracranial cere- bral vasculature. Approximately 40% of patients with PAD have concurrent coronary artery or cerebrovascular disease, and 8.6% of patients have disease in all three vascular beds.

Although there has been a substantial increase in the awareness of PAD within the medical community, this dis- ease remains under-diagnosed in usual medical practice. This under-diagnosis poses a barrier to effective secondary prevention of the substantial ischemic cardiovascular and cerebrovascular risk associated with PAD.

SYMPTOMS

A detailed medical history is mandatory for proper evalua- tion and management of the patient with suspected lower extremity arterial insufficiency. The initial history should include questions designed to define the walking distance, velocity, and incline that are required to elicit the patient's symptoms. These variables constitute a baseline measure of disability and assist in the future monitoring of the efficacy of therapeutic intervention.

Claudication

Intermittent claudication is the hallmark symptom of peripheral arterial insufficiency. Claudication is classically described as a sensation of fatigue or cramping that is elicited during muscular activity (e.g., walking) of the involved extremity. The symptom usually arises after a consistent, reproducible level of exertion and resolves promptly within minutes of cessation of effort, either by sitting or standing still. The location of pain within the extremity is useful in the identification of the likely vascular site of hemodynamically significant arterial stenosis. Disease of the superficial femoral or popliteal arteries typically elicits claudication in the calf muscles, whereas disease of the iliofemoral arteries or obstruction of the aorta leads to claudication in the buttocks, hips, or thighs. Ankle or foot claudication more often arises with stenosis of the tibial and peroneal arteries.

The symptom of claudication is primarily caused by an inadequate blood supply to the extremity caused by a flow-limiting lesion of a conduit artery. If a pressure gradient is present, its magnitude increases in a non-linear manner, thereby magnifying the symptomatic importance of an arterial stenosis as the arterial flow rates increase. A stenosis that does not provoke a gradient at rest may very well cause a gradient during exercise, as a consequence of the augmented cardiac output and reduced vascular resistance. Thus, as the stenosis increases, the distal perfusion pressure is not maintained. The increase in the intramuscular pressure during exercise, if it exceeds the arterial pressure distal to the stenosis, can further compromise blood flow.

When the impaired blood supply is insufficient to meet the increased metabolic demands of the exercising muscle, anaerobic metabolism supervenes in the recipient muscular bed. Accumulation of lactate and other metabolites, such as acylcarnitines, adenosine diphosphates, and hydrogen ions, ensues. Increasing local concentrations of these metabolites activates local sensory receptors: the patient perceives limb discomfort, which, in peripheral arterial disease, is called claudication.

Several standard questionnaires have been developed to identify the patient with claudication and to help assess its severity. The Rose, San Diego, and Edinburgh Questionnaires have been developed for the epidemiologic assessment of the prevalence of angina and claudication. The Medical Outcomes Short Form 36 (SF-36) Questionnaire is intended to evaluate the functional status and well-being of patients with chronic conditions. The Walking Impairment Questionnaire, the most recently developed of these instruments, evaluates the symptoms and assigns a point score to the elicited responses. Although these instruments were developed to facilitate prospective studies of PAD,

they can be utilized as the source for a series of questions for the patient. The questions can be particularly helpful in assessing the patient's functional impairment as a consequence of the suspected vascular insufficiency (Table 47.1). By comparison, clinicians who rely on a classic history of claudication to detect PAD are likely to miss the diagnosis in 85%–90% of patients.

Dynamic leg discomfort is the hallmark of PAD, but nonvascular causes of exertional leg pain should be considered in the differential diagnosis of true claudication (Table 47.2). Alternate, nonvascular diagnoses include lumbosacral radiculopathy and spinal stenosis, arthritis of the hips and knees, and various musculoskeletal diseases.

Venous claudication (defined as exertional lower extremity aching in the absence of peripheral arterial insufficiency) can be observed in patients with venous regurgitation and produces discomfort that occurs during exertion and that might mimic the calf claudication of arterial insufficiency. Various clinical characteristics, including peripheral edema, stasis, pigmentation, and varicosities, help to identify the patient with chronic venous insufficiency. A symptomatic Baker's cyst or a chronic compartment syndrome can similarly cause discomfort at the level of the calf, although the nature and location of the pain, which is characteristically associated with a particular position, should help distinguish these patients from those with PAD.

TABLE 47.1

SUBJECTIVE ASSESSMENT OF THE PATIENT WITH POSSIBLE PERIPHERAL ARTERIAL DISEASE

These questions are derived from the Walking Impairment Questionnaire (WIQ)

Walking distance

How much difficulty do you experience in walking
- Around your home?
- 50 feet?
- 1/2 block?
- 1 block?
- 2 blocks?
- 3 blocks?
- 5 blocks?

Walking speed

How difficult is it for you to
- Walk 1 block slowly?
- Walk 1 block at an average speed?
- Walk 1 block quickly?
- Run or jog 1 block?

Stair climbing

How difficult is it for you to climb
- 1 flight of stairs?
- 2 flights of stairs?
- 3 flights of stairs?

TABLE 47.2

DIFFERENTIAL DIAGNOSIS OF INTERMITTENT CLAUDICATION

Calf	Hip/thigh buttock	Foot
Venous claudication	Arthritis	Arthritis
Chronic compartment syndrome	Spinal cord compression	Inflammation
Nerve root compression		
Baker's cyst		

Arthritis of the hips and knees clearly can be responsible for leg discomfort and pain with ambulation. However, the resulting pain is characteristically a persistent ache, typically localized to the affected joints, and, unlike the pain of PAD, is commonly precipitated by exercise of variable intensity. The clinician should attempt to elicit complaints of arthralgia using range-of-motion examinations.

Lumbosacral radiculopathy typically presents as a consequence of degenerative disc disease or spinal stenosis. In this condition, walking short distances may evoke pain with a quality very similar to claudication, but relief is obtained not with rest alone, but rather by sitting or leaning against a support. This symptom complex, which is called neurogenic claudication or pseudoclaudication, is common in the elderly and often coexists with PAD.

Symptoms of Critical Leg Ischemia

Pain at Rest

Patients with critical limb ischemia present with relentless lower extremity pain (Table 47.3). The classic description is a burning discomfort in the ball of the foot and in the toes, typically exacerbated at night, in the supine position. The latter manifestation can be explained by the loss of gravity-assisted blood flow to the lower extremities. The patient may try to minimize discomfort by suspending the legs over the side of the bed or sleeping in an upright or semi-sitting position. The protracted dependency of the lower extremities produces considerable peripheral edema, which

TABLE 47.3

DIFFERENTIATING CRITICAL LIMB ISCHEMIA FROM CLAUDICATION

Critical limb ischemia	Claudication
Rest pain with legs horizontal	Ischemic symptoms are present only during exercise
ABI <0.5	ABI typically >0.5
Ischemic ulcers or lesions on foot	No loss of skin integrity

might not otherwise be characteristic of arterial insufficiency in the absence of venous disease.

Non-healing Wounds

In critical leg ischemia, non-healing wounds of the lower extremity and/or foot are common. Failure to heal is typically defined after a 4–12 week trial of therapy. Such wounds often result from trauma caused by an injury or improperly fitted shoe. When the blood supply falls to extremely low levels, gangrene, usually of the toes, may develop.

Differential Diagnosis

Other clinical entities, such as night cramps, arthritis, or diabetic sensory neuropathy, must be considered in the differential diagnosis of critical leg ischemia. Patients with night cramps usually have relief after muscle massage, walking, or the administration of an antispasmodic drug. Arthritis typically produces intermittent pain at defined intervals, in contrast to the constant pain that is characteristic of critical limb ischemia. The pain of diabetic sensory neuropathy is not necessarily associated with recumbency.

The differential diagnosis of critical limb and digital ischemia should also include the connective tissue disorders, such as systemic lupus erythematosus and scleroderma (Table 51.1). Other entities to be considered include vasculitis (in particular, thromboangiitis obliterans), atheroembolism, diabetic sensory neuropathy, reflex sympathetic dystrophy, and acute gouty arthritis.

General Symptomatic Evaluation for Atherosclerosis

Because PAD may represent only one of several manifestations of systemic atherosclerosis, a detailed interrogation for the symptoms of coronary and cerebrovascular insufficiency should be undertaken. Hospitalized patients with coronary artery disease are particularly likely to harbor the undetected diagnosis of PAD (1). Hypertension is a major risk factor for the development of PAD (2), and poorly controlled hypertension predisposes patients to a higher incidence of coronary and cerebrovascular events.

SIGNS

Pulse Examination

A careful pulse examination must be performed in all extremities. It is most practical to grade pulses according to whether they are absent (0), diminished (1), or normal (2). Unusually prominent pulses should also be noted. Auscultation for bruits is an integral part of the circulatory examination and includes the neck, abdomen, flank, and groin.

Patients with aortoiliac disease will often have attenuated femoral pulse amplitudes, at times accompanied by audible femoral bruits. In the presence of hemodynamically significant disease in the superficial femoral artery, the femoral pulse will be palpable, but popliteal and tibial pulses will be diminished or absent. A history of calf claudication with absent pedal pulses and preserved pulse amplitude in the femoral and popliteal vessels is likely to represent tibioperoneal disease, seen commonly in diabetics.

The general examination may reveal hypertension, arrhythmias, abnormal heart sounds, or findings suggestive of the presence of anemia. Blood pressure should be measured in both upper extremities, and any observed pressure gradients should be noted. The abdomen must be palpated to exclude the presence of a pulsatile mass.

Pallor and Rubor

Pallor on elevation and dependent rubor represent reciprocal, physical changes of ischemia. The rapidity with which the pallor occurs can be used as a semiquantitative bedside assessment of the severity of ischemia. The leg of a supine patient is passively elevated by the examiner to a 60-degree angle. Pallor will be observed within 25 seconds with severe disease, within 30 seconds with moderate insufficiency, and within 60 seconds in the presence of mild obstructive disease. With dependency after elevation (i.e., the patient resumes the sitting position, with the legs descending passively from the edge of the exam table), a venous filling time of 20–45 seconds denotes more severe disease; in a normal patient, the venous filling time is nearly instantaneous. In severe disease, capillary refill (the return of color to the skin after blanching) will be comparably delayed: whereas capillary refill is nearly instantaneous in the normal patient, delays of 20 seconds or more are commonly seen in severe arterial insufficiency. Rubor on dependency (the reddish-purple hue assumed by the skin with sitting or standing) can similarly be elicited in such patients.

Dependent rubor is characteristic of poor arterial inflow, but can only be qualitatively defined as present or absent. Cutaneous changes in the affected extremity indicate the presence of significant longstanding arterial disease. It is only over many months that cutaneous and subcutaneous atrophy, along with hair loss and poor nail plate growth, become evident.

Cyanosis

Livedo reticularis or cyanosis of the digits suggest a recent atheroembolic event. Additional manifestations of acute arterial occlusion can include painful cyanosis of one or more of the digits. Acute occlusion can occur de novo in patients at risk for thromboemboli, or can punctuate the natural history of patients with pre-existing PAD; such events are highly characteristic after thrombotic occlusion of a pre-existent bypass graft.

Prompt assessment of limb viability is mandatory. Signs of irreversible ischemia include major tissue loss, absent capillary return (marbling), profound muscle weakness or paralysis, profound sensory loss, and inaudible arterial and venous Doppler signals (see Ankle-Brachial Index). Critical limb ischemia is characterized by severe ischemic pain at rest, often accompanied by skin breakdown, gangrene, and ineradicable tissue infection.

LABORATORY TESTS AND IMAGING STUDIES

Ankle-Brachial Index

Bedside quantification of lower extremity arterial insufficiency is eminently feasible and should be considered an element of the standard physical examination of patients with suspected PAD. The results of this diagnostic maneuver, performed with a hand-held Doppler probe and a sphygmomanometer, is commonly called the *Ankle-Brachial Index* (ABI). The ABI is expressed, for each leg, as a ratio of the greater of the 2 ankle systolic pressures, measured at the malleolar level, and the greater of the 2 brachial systolic pressures. Systolic blood pressure is measured by Doppler ultrasonography in each arm and in the dorsalis pedis (DP) and posterior tibial (PT) arteries at each ankle (Figure 47.1). An ABI of ≥1.0 is considered normal, recognizing that systolic blood pressure is normally higher in the legs than in the arms. Patients with PAD typically have Ankle-Brachial Index values between 0.41 and 0.90. Critical leg ischemia, to be discussed later, is typified by an ABI <0.4. However, the predictive accuracy of the ABI relies upon normal compressibility of the infrapopliteal arterial vasculature. In older patients, and especially in patients with diabetes, vascular calcification reduces the elasticity of the arterial wall. As a result, the higher external pressures that are required to compress these inelastic vessels will produce an overestimation of the true, intraluminal arterial pressure. An ABI >1.30 suggests the presence of noncompressible, calcified vessels. In such patients, pulse volume recordings (see later) may be required to validate the presence of an attenuated pulse volume characteristic of arterial insufficiency.

The ABI is particularly useful to identify and evaluate asymptomatic patients with risk factors or other symptoms suggestive of atherosclerosis (3, 4). In one study, about 7% of persons ages 45–74 years had an ABI of ≤0.95, but only 22% of these patients had symptoms (3). An ABI <0.5 is the most important measure of the severity of disease and predictor of the subsequent need for surgery or amputation (5). Skin perfusion pressure on the foot may be an even better predictor of the likelihood of leg amputation or the need for revascularization in patients with critical leg ischemia (6).

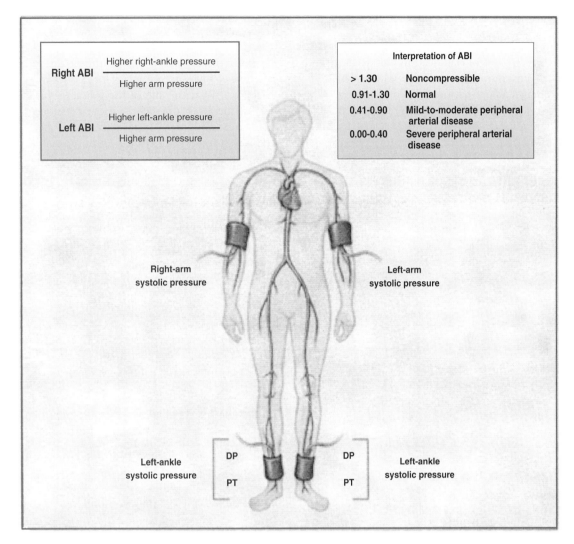

Figure 47.1 Measurement and calculation of the Ankle-Brachial Index (ABI). For details, please see text. (Reproduced from Hiatt WR. Medical treatment of peripheral arterial disease and claudication. *N Engl J Med* 2001;344:1608–1621, with permission.)

Blood Tests

Routine laboratory testing of the suspected claudicant should include a complete blood count (CBC), fasting glucose level and/or hemoglobin A_{1C} level, a fasting lipid profile, a creatinine level, and levels of lipoprotein (a) and serum homocysteine. In patients with premature atherosclerosis or very aggressive, rapidly progressive vascular disease, additional investigations may include plasma fibrinogen levels, an antiphospholipid antibody screen, assay for antithrombin III antibodies, and coagulation studies designed to detect deficiencies in protein C and S, Factor V Leiden, and others. Identification of such so-called "novel" risk factors for PAD, such as hyperhomocysteinemia, may help to explain the racial disproportions in disease prevalence that have been observed in population studies. Laboratory confirmation of limb-threatening arterial occlusion can be sought in the form of elevated serum levels of muscle enzymes and myoglobinuria.

Exercise Testing

Treadmill exercise testing can evaluate the severity of the peripheral arterial stenosis and provide objective evidence of the patient's walking capacity. Two accepted treadmill protocols are: the constant-workload protocol, which uses a constant speed and grade (typically 2 mph and 12% grade), and the graded test, which provides constant speed but varies the grade from an initial horizontal position in predefined steps (e.g., 2%) at predefined intervals (e.g., 2 minutes). The reproducibility of the two testing methods is comparable except when claudication distances are very short, in which case the graded test is superior (7).

The initial claudication distance is defined as the workload at which symptoms of claudication first develop, and the absolute claudication distance is the point at which the patient is no longer able to continue walking because of severe leg discomfort. Together, these two measures provide a useful, quantitative assessment of the patient's disability and can be monitored after therapeutic interventions (8).

Segmental Pressure Analysis

Segmental pressure analysis, which quantifies systolic blood pressure at selected sites along the length of each extremity, is one of the most useful ways to evaluate PAD. Blood pressure cuffs are applied at the thigh, above and below the knee, and above the ankle. A hemodynamically significant stenosis should be suspected if a segmental pressure decrement of ≥15% is observed. Segmental pressure analysis is often supplemented by color flow Doppler ultrasound of the major conduit vessels. The Doppler probe is placed over an artery distal to the cuff to assess the velocity of blood flow. In the lower extremities, the probe is usually placed over the posterior tibial artery behind and below the medial malleolus. The dorsalis pedis artery can also be interrogated on the dorsum of the metatarsal arch. In the upper extremity, the brachial, radial, and ulnar arteries are suitable imaging targets.

Pulse Volume Recording

Pulse volume recordings are obtained along the axis of the limb with specifically placed transducers. The goal is to record segmental pulse volumes at the thigh, calf, ankle, and toes. The morphology of the arterial waveform can be analyzed when the changes in volume are displayed with a graphic recorder. In the presence of a hemodynamically significant stenosis, the amplitude of the pulse volume is reduced, and the normal dicrotic notch is lost, with conversion from the normal biphasic waveform to an abnormal monophasic pattern.

Imaging Studies

Duplex Ultrasound Imaging

Duplex imaging provides a direct noninvasive means of assessing both the anatomic characteristics of peripheral arteries and the functional significance of stenoses that are detected. The acoustic properties of the vascular wall can be discriminated from those of the surrounding tissues, thereby enabling them to be imaged readily. Normal arteries have laminar flow, with the highest velocity of flow detected at the center of the artery. The representative image is usually homogeneous, with a nearly constant hue and intensity. With a stenosis, blood flow velocity through the narrowed lumen increases; proportional desaturation of the color display and flow disturbance distal to the lesion provoke changes in hue and color. A doubling of peak systolic velocity at the site of the lesion serves to identify a 50% reduction in diameter. If the artery is occluded, no signal can be obtained. The sensitivity and specificity of this technique for the identification of arterial stenosis have been reported to be 85% and 95%, respectively.

Magnetic Resonance Angiography

Magnetic resonance angiography provides a noninvasive technique to visualize the peripheral arterial vasculature and the aorta. The technique has been reported to be highly sensitive and specific. Resolution of the vascular anatomy with gadolinium-enhanced magnetic resonance imaging approaches that of conventional contrast digital subtraction angiography. Its greatest current utility may be in patients who require anatomic definition of disease for therapeutic decision making but who are at high risk for renal, allergic, or other complications of conventional angiography.

Contrast Angiography

Conventional angiography is performed when the arterial anatomy must be defined prior to a revascularization procedure. Occasionally, a diagnostic procedure is performed when the diagnosis is in doubt, but revascularization would be warranted if the symptoms and/or signs could be linked to PAD.

EVALUATION AND TREATMENT

The evaluation and management of patients with peripheral arterial disease is covered in Chapter 51. For most patients with critical leg ischemia, early consideration will be given to an attempt at revascularization of the ischemic limb, using a variety of thrombolytic, catheter-based, and surgical approaches. In all such cases, angiographic documentation of the relevant anatomy is mandatory. In patients who are not amenable to surgery or endovascular intervention, the primary, urgent management issues include control of pain, treatment of non-healing wounds and/or infection, improvement of tissue perfusion, and prevention of tissue loss.

When critical limb ischemia occurs, patients require palliation of pain, aggressive wound care, antibiotic therapy of supervening infections, and interventions to prevent the loss of limb. Other long-term management goals include control or elimination of modifiable risk factors such as smoking, diabetes, hypertension, and dyslipidemias.

KEY POINTS

- The medical history is crucial to the diagnosis of PAD and to avoiding substantial underdiagnosis.
- Physical findings usually occur late in PAD.
- The ABI is the key diagnostic test for PAD.

REFERENCES

1. Dieter RS, Tomasson J, Gudjonsson T, et al. Lower extremity peripheral arterial disease in hospitalized patients with coronary artery disease. *Vasc Med* 2003;8:233–126.
2. Murabito JM, D'Agostino RB, Silbershatz H, et al. Intermittent claudication: a risk profile from The Framingham Heart Study. *Circulation* 1997;96:44–49.
3. Hirsch AT, Criqui MH, Treat-Jacobson D, et al. Peripheral arterial disease detection, awareness, and treatment in primary care. *JAMA* 2001;286:1317–1324.
4. Ouriel K. Peripheral arterial disease. *Lancet* 2001;358:1257–1264.
5. Hafner J, Schaad I, Schneider E, et al. Leg ulcers in peripheral arterial disease (arterial leg ulcers): impaired wound healing above the threshold of chronic critical limb ischemia. *J Am Acad Dermatol* 2000;43:1001–1008.
6. Castronuovo JJ, Jr., Adera HM, Smiell JM, et al. Skin perfusion pressure measurement is valuable in the diagnosis of critical limb ischemia. *J Vasc Surg* 1997;26:629–637.
7. Labs KH, Nehler MR, Roessner M, et al. Reliability of treadmill testing in peripheral arterial disease: a comparison of a constant load with a graded load treadmill protocol. *Vasc Med* 1999;4:239–246.
8. Labs KH, Dormandy JA, Jaeger KA, et al. Transatlantic Conference on Clinical Trial Guidelines in Peripheral Arterial Disease: Clinical trial methodology. Basel PAD Clinical Trial Methodology Group. *Circulation* 1999;100:e75–e81.

ADDITIONAL READING

Hiatt WR. Medical treatment of peripheral arterial disease and claudication. *N Engl J Med* 2001;344:1608–1621.
Schmieder FA, Comerota AJ. Intermittent claudication: magnitude of the problem, patient evaluation, and therapeutic strategies. *Am J Cardiol* 2001;87:3D–13D.

Urgent and Emergent Hypertension

48

William B. White

INTRODUCTION

Hypertensive emergencies are defined not by the absolute value of blood pressure (BP) but by the presence of acute end organ damage secondary to a rapidly increasing blood pressure with attendant vascular injury (Table 48.1). Hypertensive patients with longstanding blood pressure elevations tolerate much higher pressures prior to manifesting rapid decompensation of vital organ function compared with previously normotensive patients, who may present with clinical signs of accelerated disease at lower pressures that have developed more acutely (e.g., pregnancy and acute glomerulonephritis). Hypertensive emergencies dictate immediate hospitalization with management in a critical care unit setting and reduction of blood pressure within minutes to hours. In contrast, severe, uncontrolled hypertension without acute or ongoing end-organ damage is typically defined as a *hypertensive urgency.* This type of patient can be managed vigilantly on an outpatient basis with the aim to reduce blood pressure within 1 to several days.

The incidence of uncontrolled and severe hypertension has been significantly reduced in the United States over the past few decades, driven by increased awareness regarding the importance of managing high blood pressure as an outpatient. In fact, the seventh report of the Joint National Committee (1) demonstrated this improvement in control rates for hypertension (systolic BP <140 mm Hg and diastolic BP <90 mm Hg). Because of this progress, hypertensive emergencies now occur in less than 1% of the hypertensive population (2). Despite these successes, however, many Americans remain unaware of their hypertension, and hypertensive urgencies continue to be relatively common.

ISSUES AT THE TIME OF ADMISSION

Clinical Presentation

Patients presenting with severe hypertension (>180/110 mm Hg) are usually asymptomatic. On the rare occasion at which the patient becomes symptomatic or has evidence of acute target-organ injury, it becomes an "emergent" syndrome. There is no "typical" presentation; emergent hypertension can present with symptoms ranging from headaches, visual disturbances, confusion, weakness, and seizures to chest pain and shortness of breath.

Initial Evaluation

The history is an important first step in determining the level of urgency. The focus should be on eliciting cerebrovascular or cardiac symptoms. Questions that should be priorities are those regarding cardiovascular decompensation (myocardial ischemia, acute pulmonary edema, or aortic dissection), central nervous system compromise (encephalopathy, cerebral hemorrhage, or ischemic stroke), and acute renal failure. Other important details include a previous history of hypertension, current medications including oral contraceptives, drug abuse (e.g., cocaine), alcohol intake, smoking, peripheral vascular disease, and pregnancy. If the history is unrevealing, pain or anxiety can also elevate blood pressure and need to be excluded.

The physical examination first should establish that the elevated blood pressure reading is accurate. Inaccurate measurement is a simple but common issue in severe hypertension. A large sphygmomanometer bladder should be used if the arm circumference exceeds 32 cm; during the measurement, the arm should be at heart level. Second, the physical

TABLE 48.1

TYPES OF HYPERTENSIVE EMERGENCIES

Central nervous system

Hypertensive encephalopathy
Hypertension with intracranial hemorrhage
Hypertension with ischemic stroke
Hypertension with acute subarachnoid hemorrhage
Head trauma with or without subdural hematoma

Cardiovascular system

Hypertension with myocardial infarction
Hypertension with unstable angina
Dissecting aortic aneurysm
Hypertension with congestive heart failure
Hypertension after coronary artery bypass graft surgery

Retina

Grade III Keith-Wagner retinopathy—exudates or flame
    hemorrhages
Grade IV Keith-Wagner retinopathy—papilledema

Miscellaneous

Eclampsia
Dissecting renal artery
Adrenergic crisis (pheochromocytoma, cocaine, monoamine-
    oxidase inhibitors with tyramine interactions, hyperthyroidism)

examination should focus on signs of acute end organ damage. Examinations that should be expedited are funduscopic (flame hemorrhages, exudates, and papilledema; Figure 48.1 A, B), cardiovascular (S3 gallop, rales, or new regurgitant murmur), renal (abdominal or flank tenderness associated with a dissecting artery), and neurologic (focal signs).

Laboratory investigations should include an electrocardiogram (ECG). This will alert the physician to underlying ischemia/infarction, conduction abnormalities, and electrolyte disturbances (e.g., hyperkalemia) and guide the optimal form of therapy, which should begin immediately. Serum electrolytes, blood urea nitrogen, creatinine, and hematocrit should be ordered at the time of presentation. A urinalysis should assess for proteinuria, red blood cells, and red cell casts. A chest radiograph should be performed to assess for pulmonary vascular congestion (which should first be established clinically) as well as for a widened mediastinum that may be due to aortic dissection. It should be emphasized, however, that therapy should be instituted immediately after obtaining the focused history, physical examination, and electrocardiogram without waiting for the results of these other tests.

Other radiographic or biochemical evaluations should be performed, depending on the emergency at hand. For example a computed tomographic scan of the chest or a transesophageal echocardiogram may be necessary to exclude an aortic dissection (Chapter 49). Computed tomography would be warranted if neurologic symptoms are present and especially to differentiate between hemorrhage and ischemia (Chapters 116 and 117). A urine toxicology screen to exclude cocaine or amphetamine overdose is pertinent in a patient who appears clinically to have excessive sympathetic nervous system activity.

Diagnostic investigations for secondary hypertension should also be considered at the time of presentation. Urine collection of catecholamines, metanephrines, and VMAs also can be initiated if the suspicion of a pheochromocytoma exists. Persistent tachycardia and widened pulse pressure may alert a physician to send thyroid function tests. Captopril renography and measurement of plasma renin activity may be useful in a patient who has an abdominal

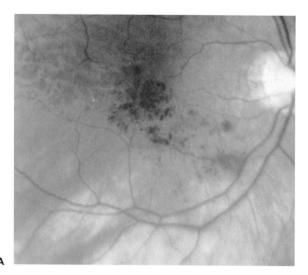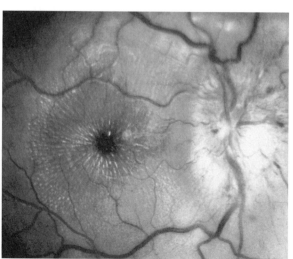

Figure 48.1 Effects of malignant or accelerated hypertension on the retina. **A.** The fundus shows marked hemorrhage and infarction. **B.** The fundus shows loss of integrity of the optic disc with papilledema. These findings on physical examination indicate acute target injury regardless of the level of blood pressure.

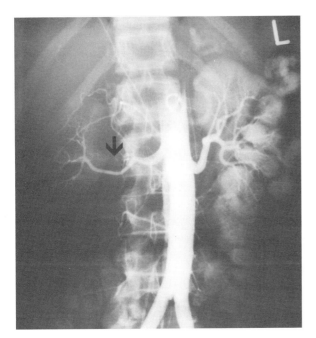

Figure 48.2 Aortogram in a young man who presented with malignant hypertension, seizures, and hematuria. The right renal artery shows an acute and spontaneous dissection that led to right renal ischemia/infarction and renin-dependent hypertension. Initially, blood pressure was controlled with intravenous enalaprilat and labetalol. This patient later underwent right nephrectomy and has been normotensive for 6 years postoperatively.

bruit, significant peripheral vascular disease, worsening renal function on an angiotensin-converting enzyme inhibitor, or severe flank pain, all of which may be signs of renovascular hypertension, including renal artery dissection (Figure 48.2). Unprovoked hypokalemia during the course of hospitalization should be evaluated by obtaining paired serum aldosterone and plasma renin activity measurements, though hyperaldosteronism only rarely presents with severe, accelerated hypertension.

Indications for Hospitalization

A spectrum of clinical manifestations warrants emergent treatment and hospitalization (Figure 48.3). Patients who present with severe elevations in blood pressure but who have no evidence of acute target organ damage and appear to be reliable usually do not require hospitalization; they can be managed as outpatients with careful and early follow-up (within 10 days after the initial presentation).

Initial Therapy

Hypertensive emergencies should be treated in an intensively monitored environment. In a patient with suspected hypertensive encephalopathy, therapy should be instituted immediately prior to any diagnostic testing other than an electrocardiogram. Placement of an arterial line is appropriate in individuals for whom continuous readings are

necessary. However, most patients can be managed with noninvasive blood pressure recorders or traditional sphygmomanometry. Ideal drug therapies are medications that have a rapid onset of action, are short-acting and easy to titrate, have a predictable dose-response curve with minimal side effects (in particular, they do not alter the patient's mental status), and do not induce significant reductions in cerebral, renal, or coronary blood flow.

Blood pressure reduction should be performed quickly but with caution so as not to alter cerebral blood flow too rapidly and cause deterioration of neurologic symptoms. *Normalization of blood pressure need not be achieved and should not be the aim of therapy for hypertensive urgency or emergency.* Cerebral autoregulation of blood flow in normotensive patients occurs between mean arterial pressures (MAPs) of 50–150 mm Hg (MAP = diastolic blood pressure + 1/3 [systolic blood pressure − diastolic blood pressure]). If blood pressure falls below the lower limit of autoregulation (typically 25% below the pretreatment MAP), the brain extracts more oxygen from the circulation to compensate for the reduction in blood flow until a point may be reached at which ischemic damage ensues. The dangers of precipitously lowering the blood pressure include serious complications such as blindness, stroke, coma, or even death.

In elderly hypertensive patients and patients with cerebrovascular disease, adaptive changes in cerebral blood flow cause higher MAPs to become the lower limit of autoregulation (Figure 48.4). Hence, care should be taken to avoid marked reductions that dangerously reduce blood pressure below that lower-limit set point for autoregulation. Intravenous medication is recommended initially either by constant infusion or by repeated small injections to give a rapid pharmacologic onset and a controlled duration of action (Table 48.2). The general consensus is that *the blood pressure reduction for the first several hours should not be by more than 20% of the resting MAP that is observed on admission.* During this time, neurologic status should be closely monitored; if it deteriorates, the rate of administration of the antihypertensive drug should be reduced to allow the MAP to recover. Although certain conditions of ongoing end-organ damage may demand a more rapid reduction in blood pressure (e.g., cardiac ischemia, aortic dissection, pulmonary edema, and hypertensive encephalopathy), the physician should be cognizant of the patient's neurologic status at all times.

Specific Drug Therapies

Sodium nitroprusside, a potent vasodilator and venodilator, is the time-tested drug for management of hypertensive emergencies, because of its high (80%) rate of efficacy. However, hypotension, reflex tachycardia, and thiocyanate toxicity are clinically significant adverse effects of this drug. Thiocyanate toxicity is more likely to occur in patients with renal insufficiency, prolonged use (>48 hours) of the

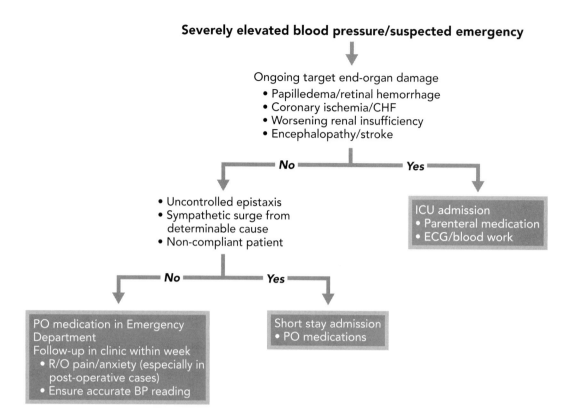

Figure 48.3 Triage of the severely hypertensive patient. The presence of severe and acute target organ injury requires admission to a critical care unit, laboratory evaluation, and immediate or nearly immediate blood pressure lowering with parenteral therapy. Severely hypertensive patients with symptoms who lack overt target organ injury should be placed in observation units until stable. Most other patients with severe hypertension can be managed with close follow-up in the ambulatory setting. *BP*, blood pressure; *CHF*, congestive heart failure; *ECG*, electrocardiogram; *ICU*, intensive care unit; *PO*, oral.

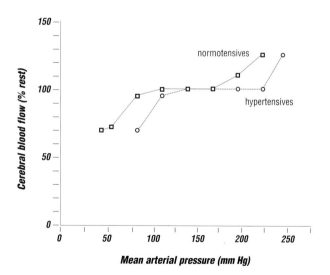

Figure 48.4 Autoregulation of cerebral blood flow. Cerebral blood flow is autoregulated as a protective mechanism. However, if systemic arterial pressure is accelerated to extremely high values, this autoregulatory process is lost and cerebral edema may occur. Loss of autoregulation in normotensive individuals occurs at lower levels of systemic mean arterial pressure than in hypertensive patients.

medication, and plasma thiocyanate levels exceeding 1.7 mmol/L (3). Manifestations of the toxicity include nausea, vomiting, headache, delirium, and psychosis. Infusion rates of sodium nitroprusside need to be started at 0.1–0.2 mcg/kg/min and meticulously monitored; maximal rates of infusion are 2.0 mcg/kg/min.

Fenoldopam is a newer intravenous dopaminergic agonist that dilates most vascular beds but has its greatest effects in the splanchnic and renal vessels. Thus, it is a potent renal and systemic vasodilator that lowers the MAP promptly and smoothly, comparable to the effects of sodium nitroprusside (4). Unlike sodium nitroprusside, fenoldopam does not cause as large an increase in heart rate, because of its limited action on α- and β-agonist receptors. In addition, fenoldopam is associated with a natriuresis that makes it useful for patients with heart failure or renal failure and that may obviate the need for a loop diuretic in some patients (5). Despite these small advantages, sodium nitroprusside remains the first line agent in most settings, in large part because it is substantially less expensive.

TABLE 48.2
PARENTERAL ANTIHYPERTENSIVE MEDICATIONS RECOMMENDED FOR HYPERTENSIVE EMERGENCIES

Medication	Dosage	Mechanism of action	Onset-duration of action	Special indications	Cautions and contraindications
For general use					
Sodium nitroprusside (Nipride)	0.2–10 mcg/kg/min; increase at rate of 0.05 mcg/kg/min q15 min to meet BP goal	Arterial and venous vasodilator	1–2 min/10 min	Encephalopathy, stroke/bleed MI/heart failure/aortic dissection (with β-blockers)	Pregnancy; caution in renal failure due to thiocyanate toxicity; methemoglobinemia, muscle twitching, hypotension; delivery system must be light-resistant
Fenoldapam mesylate (Corlopam)	0.1–1.7 mcg/kg/min; increase at rate of 0.1 mcg/kg/min q20 min to meet BP goal	Dopamine (D1) receptor agonist—systemic and renal vasodilator	1–5 min/10 min	Renal insufficiency; postoperative and all other hypertensive emergencies	May increase intraocular pressure and should be used with caution in glaucoma; flushing
Labetalol hydrochloride IV (Normodyne, Trandate)	5–10 mg IV bolus q10 min or 0.5–2.0 mg/min; total dose: 300 mg/d	α- and β-receptor blocker; IV ratio: 7:1; oral ratio: 3:1	5–10 min/1.8–6 h	Hyperadrenergic syndromes: cardiac and cerebral events, eclampsia, MAO inhibitor–tyramine interaction	2nd-degree or greater heart block, bronchoconstriction, orthostatic hypotension; sick-sinus syndrome
For special situations					
Diltiazem (Cardizem)	0.25 mg/kg over 2 min as a bolus; repeat in 15 min or 5–15 mg/h infusion	Calcium-channel blocker	2–5 min/12 h	Atrial fibrillation and supraventricular tachycardia	2nd-degree or greater heart block
Nitroglycerin IV	5–200 mcg/min	Venodilator: coronary arteries and veins	2–5 min/3–5 min	Unstable angina, MI	Methemoglobinemia headache; tachycardia; special delivery system due to drug binding to tubing; BP effects are variable
Furosemide (Lasix)	20–120 mg q6 hourly not to exceed 600 mg/d	Loop diuretic	15 min/6 h	Congestive heart failure/volume-overload states	Ototoxicity; prerenal azotemia
Enalaprilat (Vasotec)	0.625–1.25 mg q6–8 h	Angiotensin-converting enzyme inhibitor	30 min/4–6 h	Most useful in high renin states, e.g., renal artery stenosis	Bilateral renal-artery stenosis; hyperkalemia; contraindicated in pregnancy
Hydralazine hydrochloride (Apresoline)	IV: 5–20 mg slowly at 1 mg/min; IM: 10–50 mg	Vasodilator: Arterial > venous	IV: 10–15 min, IM: 20–30 min/IV: >1 h, IM: 4–6 h	Eclampsia, severe hypertension during pregnancy	Tachycardia, increase in dp/dt, increase in intracranial pressure; avoid in aortic dissection, central nervous system, or cardiovascular complications
Phentolamine (Regitine)	1–5 mg IV q5–15 minutes	Nonselective α-receptor blocker	2–5 min/30–120 min	Drug of choice in pheochromocytoma; MAO inhibitor—tyramine interaction	Tachycardia and increase in dp/dt; orthostatic hypotension
Nicardipine IV (Cardene)	Infusion at 2–4 mg/h and increase by 1–2.5 mg/h to maximum of 15 mg/h	Dihydropyridine calcium-channel blocker	10–15 min/short until 12 h or infusion, then >4 h	Cyclosporine-induced hypertension, similar spectrum to sodium nitroprusside	Increases intracranial pressure

BP, blood pressure; dp/dt, change in pressure per change in time; IM, intramuscular; IV, intravenous; MAO, monoamine oxidase; MI, myocardial infarction.

TABLE 48.3
ORGAN-SPECIFIC DISEASE AND THERAPY

End-organ damage	Incidence (%) (6)	Recommended treatment	Medications to be avoided
Cerebral infarction	24.5	No treatment (7), SNP, fenoldopam, labetalol	Clonidine and α-methyldopa (because of central nervous system depression)
Encephalopathy	16.3	SNP, fenoldopam, labetalol	Clonidine and α-methyldopa
Intracerebral/ subarachnoid hemorrhage	4.5	No treatment (6), SNP, fenoldopam, labetalol	Clonidine and α-methyldopa
Myocardial ischemia/ infarction	12.0	NTG, labetalol, SNP, fenoldopam	Hydralazine, diazoxide, minoxidil
Acute pulmonary edema	14.3	Fenoldopam, SNP with loop diuretic, NTG with loop diuretic	Hydralazine, diazoxide, minoxidil
Aortic dissection aortic valve and arch beyond aortic arch	2.0	Surgery SNP with β-blocker, labetalol	Hydralazine, diazoxide, minoxidil
Eclampsia	4.5	Labetalol, hydralazine, calcium channel blockers, diazoxide	Diuretics, β-blockers, trimethaphan, angiotensin-converting enzyme inhibitor
Acute renal failure	NA	Fenoldopam, labetalol, and SNP (with caution)	β-blocker (reduce glomerular filtration rate), trimethaphan
Keith–Wagner III/IV changes (Figure 48.1)	NA	Fenoldopam, SNP, labetalol, calcium-channel blockers	Clonidine, α-methyldopa, β-blockers
Microangiopathic hemolytic anemia	NA	Fenoldopam, SNP, labetalol, calcium-channel blockers	β-blockers

NA, not available; *NTG*, nitroglycerin; *SNP*, sodium nitroprusside.

Patients who present with specific causes of hypertensive urgencies and emergencies may benefit from specific types of medications (Table 48.3) (6, 7). *Labetalol*, an α- and β-blocker, is especially useful in patients with ischemic heart disease. Labetalol or pure β-blockers are also indicated to control or reverse the reflex tachycardia often induced by nitroprusside. Although *nitroglycerin* is not generally as effective as nitroprusside, it may be preferable in patients with unstable angina or myocardial infarction because it better maintains blood flow to ischemic myocardium.

Diuretics should be administered only if fluid overload is evident on examination. If diuretics are administered to hypertensive patients who are volume-depleted, they cause more harm (such as a precipitous drop in blood pressure) than benefit.

Nifedipine has an unreliable dose-response curve and is *not* recommended for urgent or emergent hypertension. The once-popular use of sublingual nifedipine, in particular, is dangerous and should be abandoned.

Indications for Early Consultation

A consultant is not always necessary unless there is failure to respond to initial therapy or an issue regarding the appropriate diagnostic evaluation. In some cases, cardiology, nephrology, or neurology consultation may be appropriate depending on the primary manifestations of target organ injury.

ISSUES DURING HOSPITALIZATION

As with many other medical emergencies, the initial therapy is of great importance. The patient should be kept fasting in view of possible pending procedures or because of suboptimal or wavering mental status. The patient should remain in the ICU for approximately 24–48 hours before transfer to a regular medical floor. The critical care pathway for each patient must be individualized according to the type of end-organ damage involved. For example, a patient

TABLE 48.4
WHAT TO THINK ABOUT IF THE PATIENT FAILS TO IMPROVE AS EXPECTED

Causes	Indicators	Tests	Treatment
Secondary HTN Pheochromocytoma	Flushing, palpitations, persistant tachycardia, episodic/severe elevations in blood pressure, worsening on β-blockers alone, significant improvement on α-blockers	24-h urine for catecholamines, magnetic resonance imaging of adrenal gland with "light bulb" effect on T2-weighted images	α-blockers, β-blockers if tachycardic, surgery
Renal-artery stenosis/dissection (Figure 48.2)	Abdominal bruit, flank pain; premorbid indicators: AODM, PVD, smoking Hypercholesterolemia	Plasma renin activity, captopril renal scan, renal arteriogram	Angiotensin-converting enzyme inhibitor, angioplasty, surgery
Hyperaldosteronism	Persistent/unprovoked hypokalemia	Plasma renin activity Serum and urine aldosterone	Medication: spironolactone, eplerenone, amiloride Surgery (if adenoma)
Use of drugs (e.g., cocaine)	Hyperthermia, mydriasis, agitation, chest pain, nasal mucosal injury/lesions	Urine toxicology screen	α- and β-blockers in combination
Problems with the delivery system	Ensure adequate dosing—errors commonly made with IV infusions Light-resistant system for sodium nitroprusside Special tubing for IV nitroglycerin	Check infusion concentrations and rates	Improve delivery system (Chapter 21)

AODM, adult-onset diabetes mellitus; *BP,* blood pressure; *dp/dt,* change in pressure per change in time; *IM,* intramuscular; *IV,* intravenous; *MAO,* monoamine oxide; *MI,* myocardial infarction; *PVD,* peripheral vascular disease.

with myocardial ischemia or infarction follows a specific pathway that addresses blood pressure reduction in the face of ischemia and potential left-ventricular dysfunction. Failure to respond to common therapies should always alert the physician to the possibility of secondary forms of hypertension (Table 48.4).

Although blood pressure need not be normalized prior to discharge, there should be substantial improvement in blood pressure and reversal or stabilization of target organ damage. Inpatient education is essential, as most patients are either newly diagnosed or noncompliant. Emphasis should be placed on the fact that medications are likely to be required for the rest of the patient's life, with grave danger of repeated cardiovascular or cerebrovascular insults if the patient is noncompliant. Detailed written instructions regarding discharge medications should be reviewed with the patient and family. Long-acting drugs with once- or twice-a-day dosing promote compliance.

Patient-directed home blood pressure monitoring using automated devices should be strongly considered. These devices facilitate the management of the hypertension and require the patient to take more responsibility for his or her care. If home monitoring is not an option (i.e., because of lack of patient motivation or resources), other mechanisms may be established to assist in blood pressure monitoring. Early follow-up (within 2–10 days) is recommended after discharge.

ASSESSMENT AND MANAGEMENT OF A PATIENT WITH "URGENT" HYPERTENSION DURING A HOSPITALIZATION

The initial evaluation of an urgently hypertensive patient already admitted to the hospital is similar to the evaluation for an outpatient. The most common in-hospital scenario is the postoperative patient. Severe hypertension can occur as the patient awakens and as the discontinuation of positive pressure ventilation permits a sudden increase in venous return. Preferred medications in the postoperative period include intravenous labetalol or enalaprilat in repeated scheduled bolus injections. Transdermal clonidine is also a practical option but takes 1–2 days before blood pressure is effectively lowered. Nifedipine capsules and hydralazine are not recommended. Analgesia should be a priority because excessive sympathetic nervous system activity associated with pain often increases blood pressure and heart rate.

Another type of urgent hypertension encountered in the hospital is seen in post-transplant patients receiving immunotherapy (high-dosage corticosteroids or cyclosporine) who develop elevations in the blood pressure secondary to their disease processes or treatment. Elevations in blood pressure may demand urgent attention, because of severe accompanying thrombocytopenia. Volume status should be evaluated, as fluid overload is common in these patients and responds well to loop diuretics. Cyclosporine produces widespread vasoconstriction and severe hypertension that responds best to dihydropyridine calcium channel blockers (e.g., nifedipine, amlodipine, nicardipine). By comparison, verapamil and diltiazem increase cyclosporine levels and may precipitate hepatotoxicity and nephrotoxicity; they should not be used in this setting. If the patient is unable to take medication orally, intravenous nicardipine is preferred. Angiotensin-converting enzyme inhibitors typically produce a limited response because the renin-angiotensin system is already suppressed (9). Labetalol may be used alone or in combination with the dihydropyridines.

COST CONSIDERATIONS

A patient with a hypertensive emergency can incur a significant cost, primarily because of the ICU stay in the initial 24–48 hours. Of note, fenoldopam is 25–50 times more expensive than sodium nitroprusside or labetalol. Of course, the most cost-effective maneuver is prevention, which is best assured by patient education and adherence to chronic antihypertensive therapy.

KEY POINTS

- Hypertensive emergencies are diagnosed not on the absolute blood pressure value but by clinical evidence for acute target-organ damage.
- Hypertensive urgencies can be managed as an outpatient with vigilant follow-up.
- Treatment should be immediate and not be delayed while awaiting laboratory results.
- The goal of initial therapy is to reduce blood pressure by 20% of the original MAP and not necessarily to achieve a normal (<140/90 mm Hg) blood pressure rapidly.
- Fenoldopam, a parenteral dopamine-1 agonist, is as effective as sodium nitroprusside and induces less reduction in renal blood flow; however, it is much more costly.
- Short-acting nifedipine is not indicated or approved by the U.S. Food and Drug Administration for hypertensive

urgencies or emergencies and may cause excessive hypotension.
- Patient education regarding lifelong therapy and compliance should be started in the hospital, because of the significant morbidity and mortality rates associated with the disease.

REFERENCES

1. Chobanian AV, Bakris GL, Black HR, et al. National Heart, Lung, and Blood Institute Joint National Committee on Prevention, Detection, Evaluation, and Treatment of High Blood Pressure; National High Blood Pressure Education Program Coordinating Committee. The seventh report of the Joint National Committee on Prevention, Detection, Evaluation, and Treatment of High Blood Pressure: the JNC 7 report. *JAMA* 2003;289:2560–2572.
2. Tuncel M, Ram VC. Hypertensive emergencies: etiology and management. *Am J Cardiovasc Drugs* 2003;3:21–31.
3. Cherney D, Straus S. Management of patients with hypertensive urgencies and emergencies: a systematic review of the literature. *J Gen Intern Med* 2002;17:937–945.
4. White WB, Halley SE. Comparative renal effects of intravenous administration of fenoldopam mesylate and sodium nitroprusside in patients with severe hypertension. *Arch Intern Med* 1989;149:870–874.
5. White WB, Radford MJ, Gonzalez FM, et al. Selective dopamine-1 agonist therapy in severe hypertension: effects of intravenous fenoldopam. *J Am Coll Cardiol* 1988;11:1118–1123.
6. Elliott WJ. Management of hypertension emergencies. *Curr Hypertens Rep* 2003;5:486–492.
7. Semplicini A, Maresca A, Boscolo G, et al. Hypertension in acute ischemic stroke: a compensatory mechanism or an additional damaging factor? *Arch Intern Med* 2003;163:211–216.
8. Rehman F, Mansoor GA, White WB. "Inappropriate" physician habits in prescribing oral nifedipine capsules in hospitalized patients. *Am J Hypertens* 1996;9:1035–1039.
9. Rodicio JL. Calcium antagonists and renal protection from cyclosporine nephrotoxicity: long-term trial in renal transplantation patients. *J Cardiovasc Pharmacol* 2000;35(Suppl 1):S7–S11.

ADDITIONAL READING

Haas CE, LeBlanc JM. Acute postoperative hypertension: a review of therapeutic options. *Am J Health Syst Pharm* 2004;61:1661–1673.
Phillips RA, Greenblatt J, Krakoff LR. Hypertensive emergencies: diagnosis and management. *Prog Cardiovasc Dis* 2002;45:33–48.
Varon J, Marik PE. Clinical review: the management of hypertensive crises. *Crit Care* 2003;7:374–384.

Aortic Intramural Hematoma and Dissection

49

Lee Goldman

INTRODUCTION

Diseases of the aorta include intramural hematoma, aortic dissection, and aneurysms of the thoracic and abdominal aorta. Hematoma or dissection can involve the ascending aorta, aortic arch, or descending aorta. Because not all aortic hematomas or dissections result in aneurysmal dilatation of the aorta, the terms *aortic intramural hematoma and dissection* are preferred to "dissecting aneurysm". Aneurysms of the thoracic and especially the abdominal aorta commonly occur in the absence of dissection; such aneurysms are discussed in Chapter 50. The key clinical challenges are to suspect aortic hematomas and dissection from the patient's symptoms, to diagnose them expeditiously, and to treat the patient rapidly and appropriately.

AORTIC DISSECTION AND INTRAMURAL HEMATOMA

In *dissection of the aorta*, there is a sudden tearing of the intima of the aorta, with communication between the false and the true aortic lumens (Figure 49.1). The phasic aortic pressure waves then are delivered directly into the false lumen, tearing the media down the aorta, compromising arterial branches that arise from it, and creating ischemia of organs and tissues that these vessels supply. With external rupture of the adventitia, there is hemorrhage and, frequently, rapid death. *Intramural hematoma* is also a potentially lethal condition because of the possibility of additional hemorrhage within the arterial wall, which is thought to be most commonly caused by rupture of the vasa vasorum. Although no intimal tear is initially present, the hematoma can extend to compromise distal vessels and the organs they supply. It can also rupture either into the lumen, hence becoming a more typical aortic dissection, or externally. In 10% of patients who die, only an intramural hematoma is found. These patients, who are increasingly diagnosed by noninvasive imaging, would be missed by angiography because they lack an intimal tear. The increasing recognition of intramural hematomas suggests that, in many patients with aortic dissection, formation of the hematoma is the initial event (i.e., it precedes tearing of the abnormal media and later rupture into the aortic lumen). In some patients, however, it is still possible that the initial event is an intimal tear.

The clinical picture is determined by the organs made ischemic by compromised blood vessels and by the place at which an aortic rupture occurs. *Proximal hematomas and dissections* involve the ascending aorta with or without distal dissection; *distal hematomas or dissections* are defined as those that do not involve the ascending aorta.

Because the driving force for dissection is the left-ventricular systolic pressure, the rate of rise of the aortic pressure (dP/dt) and the aortic systolic pressure itself are the two major determinants of progression. It is common for dissection to proceed and suddenly stop, only to begin again.

Issues at the Time of Admission

Clinical Presentation

Hematomas and dissection of the aorta are seen most commonly in the fifth through the seventh decades of life. They occur twice as often in men as in women, and most patients have a history of hypertension or are hypertensive. In younger patients, dissection usually is seen either with a connective tissue disorder, commonly Marfan's syndrome or Turner's syndrome, or in women in association with a pregnancy. Other disorders that predispose to aortic dissection include bicuspid aortic valve, coarctation of the aorta, and, to a much lesser degree, aortic stenosis.

The most common presenting symptom for intramural hematoma and dissection is *pain*, which occurs in about 90% of cases (1–3) (Table 49.1). The pain, which usually is described as sudden in onset and extremely severe, often is described as "tearing" or "ripping". It usually occurs in or radiates into the regions in which the aorta is involved. The pain is frequently in the anterior precordium or substernal area and, less frequently, in the interscapular area, the epigastrium, and the lumbar region.

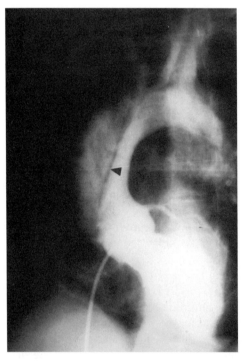

Figure 49.1 Angiogram in the left anterior oblique view, injection into the left ventricle. The catheter is passed through a patent foramen ovale into the left atrium and then into the left ventricle. The patient is a 62-year-old nurse with severe anterior chest pain. The angiogram shows a proximal dissection with the false lumen less opacified than the true lumen. Notice the radiolucent flap of the dissected aorta with contrast on both sides (*black arrowhead*); this finding is pathognomonic of aortic dissection. The total aortic diameter is normal, not aneurysmal, and the true lumen is compressed.

Frequently the pain mimics that of an acute myocardial infarction. Features that help to distinguish an aortic dissection are that the pain frequently begins abruptly at its maximum degree without the gradual build-up in severity seen with an acute myocardial infarction, and that the pain can start in one or more locations and move from one area to another as the aortic dissection progresses (Chapters 35 and 38). At times, the prominent symptom of dissection is that of a myocardial infarction (caused by occlusion of an arterial branch), abdominal or back pain (caused by splenic or renal artery occlusion), or arm or leg pain (caused by subclavian artery or femoral artery occlusion).

In the minority of patients in whom pain is not a prominent feature, *neurologic involvement* is common and may explain the absence of pain. A classic stroke can occur. Alternatively, the patient may present with syncope, which can be neurologic or can signify acute cardiac tamponade resulting from rupture of the ascending aorta into the pericardial sac (Chapters 44 and 46).

The final event is the *external rupture*. Because the proximal two-thirds of the ascending aorta is intrapericardial, there is no external compression on the adventitia; cardiac tamponade occurs rapidly and is usually fatal. The next most frequent site of rupture, the descending thoracic aorta, results in mediastinal hematoma or bleeding into the left pleural cavity causing a left pleural effusion. Rupture also can occur retroperitoneally or into the abdominal cavity.

On physical examination, the classic description is the patient with chest pain or back pain who is pale and sweaty, appears to be in shock, and sometimes has elevated blood pressure. In proximal dissection, aortic regurgitation occurs about half the time. Because the dissection spirals around the aorta and because some of the vessels are supplied from the false lumen, about 30% of patients have arterial pulse deficits. As the intramural hematoma progresses, the pressure in the false lumen can change abruptly, decreasing compression of the true lumen as the false lumen collapses; as a result, arterial pulses may be present at one time and absent at the next examination.

Younger patients with dissection are more likely to have Marfan's syndrome, a bicuspid aortic valve, or prior aortic surgery, and less likely to be hypertensive (4). Older patients are more likely to have hypertension, known atherosclerosis, and a prior aortic aneurysm (5).

Differential Diagnosis and Initial Evaluation

If aortic dissection is suspected clinically, immediate evaluation is required. In about 65% of patients, the chest radiograph is abnormal, with dilatation of the ascending aorta, dilatation of the aortic knob, or lateral bowing of the descending aorta (Figure 49.2). However, all these findings are relatively common in elderly patients without dissection because they can result from atherosclerosis with lengthening and uncoiling of the aorta. Overall, the finding of an enlarged aorta on the chest radiograph increases the

TABLE 49.1
PREVALENCE OF PRESENTING FINDINGS IN AORTIC DISSECTION

	Reference 1	Reference 2	Pooled series (reference 3)
History			
Hypertension	72%		64%
Marfan syndrome	5%		5%
Prior cardiac surgery	19%		
Caused by angioplasty or coronary bypass surgery	4%		
Pain			
Any	96%		90%
Abrupt onset	85%	79%	84%
Severe or worst ever	91%	86%	90%
Tearing or ripping	51%	62%	39%
Anterior chest	61%	76%	57%
Posterior chest	36%	50%	32%
Back	53%		32%
Physical Exam			
Hypertensive	49%	41%	49%
Aortic insufficiency	32%	40%	20%
Pulse deficit	15%	38%	31%
Chest Radiograph			
Widened mediastinum	62%		64%
• in ascending dissection	63%		
• in descending dissection	56%		

likelihood of dissection two-fold, but the absence of enlargement does not exclude dissection.

With transesophageal echocardiography, it is possible to visualize the entire ascending aorta, part of the arch, and the entire descending thoracic aorta (Figure 49.3). CT with contrast, especially spiral CT, can picture the entire aorta from the origin to the iliac bifurcation. Magnetic resonance imaging (MRI) provides an excellent view of the entire aorta without the use of contrast (Figure 49.4). Whereas in classic dissection the key finding is the intimal flap, in intramural hematoma, the characteristic appearance is that of high signal intensity in the aortic wall (Figure 49.5). With MRI, however, the imaging time is longer and the patient is relatively inaccessible to treatment during imaging.

Because each of these techniques has about the same sensitivity and specificity (both about 95%) for dissection, if one study is negative and there is still strong suspicion that the patient has aortic dissection, a second imaging technique should be used. If, however, suspicion is low–to moderate for aortic dissection, then a negative study is sufficient to exclude the diagnosis (Chapter 6). *Angiography is*

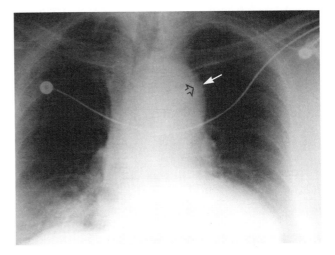

Figure 49.2 Chest radiograph, posteroanterior view. A 70-year-old man entered the hospital with tearing anterior chest pain. Notice the large aortic knob. The *open black arrow* indicates intimal calcification. The *small white arrow* indicates the outside wall of the aorta. The 6-mm thickness of the aortic wall between the arrows is consistent with blood in the false lumen of an aortic dissection.

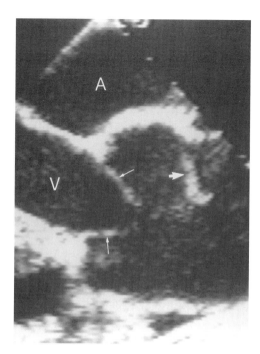

Figure 49.3 Transesophageal echocardiogram, long axis view. *Small arrows* indicate aortic leaflets, the *large arrow* indicates intimal flap in the ascending aorta just above the sinus of valsalva. *A*, left atrium; *V*, left ventricle.

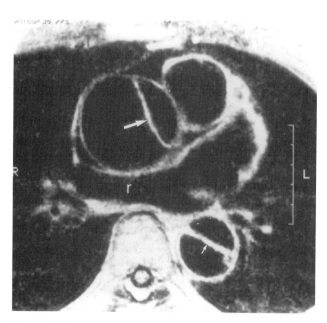

Figure 49.4 Magnetic resonance imaging; horizontal section at the level of the ascending aorta and the right pulmonary artery as it passes posterior to the ascending aorta. The *large arrow* indicates dissected intimal flap in the ascending aorta; the *small arrow* indicates dissected intimal flap in the descending aorta. This patient had a proximal aortic dissection. *r*, right pulmonary artery.

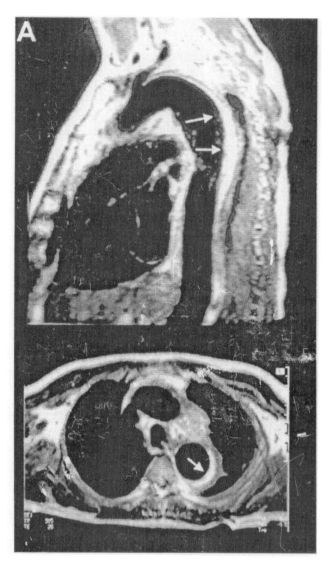

Figure 49.5 An aortic intramural aortic hematoma. In the acute phase, MRI shows a high signal intensity suggestive of intramural hematoma. Top, sagittal view demonstrates the hematoma in the upper and middle third of the descending thoracic aorta; bottom, the intramural hematoma is seen as a crescent in the axial view. This particular hematoma, which was observed without surgical treatment, later progressed (over 4 years of follow-up) to localized dissection and formation of a pseudoaneurysm.

(Reprinted with permission from Evangelista A, Dominguez R, Sebastia C, et al. Long-term follow-up of aortic intramural hematoma: predictors of outcome. *Circulation* 2003;108:583–589).

not the gold standard because its sensitivity is too low for dissection and it is not good at detecting intramural hematoma.

Indications for Hospitalization

All patients with suspected acute or chronic aortic dissections, either proximal or distal, should be admitted to the hospital unless the diagnosis can be excluded effectively by an evaluation in the emergency department. It is critical that blood pressure be lowered aggressively and that the patient be placed on β-blockers to eliminate reflex sympathetic stimulation while the diagnosis is being actively considered and until it has been excluded.

Indications for Initial Intensive Care Unit Admission

An ICU admission is indicated in patients with proximal aortic intramural hematomas or dissections if they cannot be taken immediately to the operating room from the emergency department. In patients with distal hematomas or dissections, ICU admission is required if there is ongoing pain, ischemia of vital organs, or other complications. In most hospitals, ICU care is indicated to monitor the intravenous medications or intra-arterial catheters required to achieve strict blood pressure control; in some hospitals, however, a step-down unit may suffice if blood pressure control has been achieved rapidly and if nursing capabilities are sufficient to monitor intravenous medications and blood pressure.

Treatment

While the diagnosis is being established, *all patients should be started on β-blockers and, if needed, vasodilators,* unless there is an absolute contraindication. Intravenous morphine should be given for pain relief. Labetolol, a combined alpha- and β-blocker, is an excellent first choice as an IV bolus of 5–10 mg followed by 0.5–2 mg/min. Alternatively, propanolol is administered intravenously in 0.5-mg increments at 1- to 5-minute intervals until target blood pressure of 100–110 mm Hg is reached or a total dose of 0.15 mg/kg of body weight has been given. Alternatively, metoprolol can be given intravenously as 5 mg every 5 minutes for 3 doses, then 25–50 mg 3 times per day orally. Intravenous esmolol has a rapid onset and offset of action; it must be diluted to a concentration of no more than 10 mg/mL because of venous irritation. An initial inravenous loading dose of 0.5 mg/kg is given over 1 min, followed by an infusion of 0.05 mg/kg/min. The infusion rate can be increased every 4 minutes by 0.05 mg/kg/min, up to 0.3 mg/kg/min. If β-blockers alone do not reduce systolic blood pressure to 100–110 mm Hg, intravenous nitroprusside should be added to reduce blood pressure promptly, starting at 0.5 mcg/kg/min and increasing gradually up to 10 mcg/kg/min until the target blood pressure is achieved.

Patients with *proximal* aortic dissections have a high risk of early life-threatening complications (Table 49.2) and should undergo immediate operative repair unless there are absolute contraindications. Risk factors for death include age over 70 years, abrupt onset of pain, renal failure, abnormal electrocardiogram, a pulse deficit, or the presence of hypotension, pericardial tamponade, or shock (6). For *proximal intramural hematomas,* resorption without progression to clinical complications may occur in half to two-thirds of patients (7, 8). Although the likelihood of progressive dissection or other complications is lower than in patients with hematoma than in those who initially present with a frank dissection (particularly in patients with smaller hematomas and normal aortic dimensions) (9, 10), the 25%–50% risk of progression has led many experts to recommend early surgery. However, a strategy of serial follow-up imaging studies, with surgery reserved for those who progress, may be a reasonable alternative, especially in patients who are elderly or have comorbid conditions that increase the risk of surgery (11, 12). For *distal* hematomas or dissections, medical management is reasonable if there are no secondary complications and the aorta stabilizes without marked dilatation, especially if the patient has severe coronary artery disease; otherwise, surgical repair is indicated.

The goal of surgery for dissection is to eliminate the proximal intimal tear, at which most of the external

---

TABLE 49.2
IN-HOSPITAL COMPLICATIONS AND MORTALITY RATES IN PROXIMAL AORTIC DISSECTION

In-hospital complications	Pulse deficit(s) present	Pulse deficit(s) absent	P
Mortality	41.1	24.7	<0.0001
Any neurologic deficits	35.1	11.2	<0.0001
Coma/altered consciousness	26.8	9.1	<0.0001
Myocardial ischemia/infarction	8.9	11.1	0.47
Mesenteric ischemia/infarction	4.8	3.0	0.34
Acute renal failure	10.3	4.6	0.009
Hypotension	34.5	22.4	0.006
Cardiac tamponade	20.1	15.5	0.21
Limb ischemia	28.8	2.1	<0.0001

Values are given as percentages.
From Nienaber CA and Eagle KA. Aortic dissection diagnosis and management: Part I. From etiology to diagnostic strategies. *Circulation* 2003;108:628–35.

ruptures occur, and to close the false channel at this site. For ascending aortic dissections, surgery usually involves transection of the aorta at the proximal level of the dissection while on cardiopulmonary bypass, obliteration of the false lumen by suturing its inner and outer walls, and placement of a graft beyond the dissected aorta to the takeoff of the innominate artery (13, 14). If the aortic valve is prolapsed, it can be successfully resuspended by sewing the commissures to the proximal graft. Other patients may require a prosthetic valve or, if the dissection extends into the sinuses of Valsalva, a composite tube graft with an aortic valve and reimplantation of the coronary arteries. The likelihood of being alive without further events with medical management can be as high as 70% at 8 years for distal dissections (15), but is less than 50% at 5 years and only about 20% at 10 years for proximal dissection (16).

In the open surgical option for distal dissections, the aorta is transected proximal to the intimal tear, the false lumen is obliterated by suturing, and an interposed tube graft is placed. If the aortic dissection is chronic, then the interposed graft is sewed to the outer wall to allow the false lumen to be perfused in case important arteries might arise totally from the false lumen. Alternatively, endovascular exclusion and/or closure of the entry tear has been reported to have excellent results at 2–3 years for distal dissections in experienced centers (17, 18).

The surgical mortality rate in nonruptured aortic dissection is between 10% and 15%. By comparison, the in-hospital mortality rate after endovascular repair of distal dissections is reported to be about 4%.

Indications for Early Consultation

All patients with suspected or proven aortic intramural hematoma or dissection should have early consultation with a cardiologist to aid in diagnosis. As soon as there is strong supportive evidence from any testing modality, consultation with a cardiothoracic surgeon is mandatory. In hospitals without cardiothoracic surgery capabilities, arrangements should be made urgently to transfer the patient to a hospital with such capabilities as soon as the diagnosis is established.

Issues During the Course of Hospitalization

For aortic intramural hematomas or dissections that do not involve the ascending aorta or the aortic arch and are classified as distal dissections, outcomes are generally comparable for medical and surgical therapy. Surgical therapy can be reserved for patients with continued expansion of the aneurysm, uncontrolled pain, ongoing ischemia of organs supplied by compromised vessels, or saccular aneurysm formation. If observation is chosen for proximal intramural hematoma, observation and treatment in the hospital is similar as for distal dissections. Surgery is also recommended for patients with dissections resulting from Marfan syndrome, regardless of the location.

Some patients may be diagnosed as having "chronic" dissection of either the proximal or distal aorta. These patients, who are generally defined by being diagnosed more than 2 weeks after the presumed acute event, are usually reasonably stable at the time of diagnosis. For chronic proximal dissections, surgery is generally recommended if the patient has severe aortic regurgitation, a localized aneurysm, or symptoms related to compression of surrounding structures. For chronic distal dissections, symptoms or aneurysmal enlargement to >6.0 cm are indications for surgery.

During the hospital phase, *blood pressure control is critical.* The long-term goal should be to maintain ambulatory blood pressure at no more than 110 mm Hg, with an emphasis on β-blockers to reduce myocardial contractility. If β-blockers alone are insufficient, calcium channel blockers, which also decrease contractility, are recommended. Other medications utilized in patients with hypertension can be added as needed, with the exception that α-blockers should be avoided.

The reemergence of pain generally indicates ongoing dissection and the failure of medical therapy. In such situations, aggressive therapy similar to what is recommended at the time of admission must be instituted. Urgent surgery commonly is required.

Discharge Issues

Patients generally are ready for discharge after several days without pain and at least 1 day of desired blood pressure with oral medications. Plans must be made for careful outpatient follow-up to ensure strict blood pressure control. Usually a patient is followed by a cardiovascular specialist. Follow-up should include a chest radiograph every 3 months for the first year and a contrast CT scan or MRI every 6 months for the first 2 years and then annually thereafter. For distal dissections, progressive asymptomatic growth, especially with persistent blood flow in the false lumen, may be an indication for elective surgery (19). Blood pressure control should generally continue to emphasize β-blockers and calcium channel blockers, both of which have negative inotropic properties.

Of patients who survive hospitalization, about 80% survive for the next 5 years. Long-term complications include aortic regurgitation (in patients with proximal dissections), recurrent dissection, or formation of true or false aneurysms.

KEY POINTS

- Aortic dissection must be considered in any patient with acute chest pain, especially if it radiates to the back. Rapid evaluation includes assessment of any pulse or blood pressure deficits, a chest radiograph, and a sensitive diagnostic test (transesophageal echocardiography, CT, or MRI).

- Aortic dissection requires emergent blood pressure control and β-adrenergic blockade followed by emergent surgery for proximal dissections or complicated distal dissections and most proximal intramural hematomas; uncomplicated distal dissections and most chronic dissections and perhaps some proximal intramural hematomas can be managed medically.

REFERENCES

1. Hagan PG, Nienaber CA, Isselbacher EM, et al. The International Registry of Acute Aortic Dissection (IRAD): new insights into an old disease. *JAMA* 2000;283:897–904.
2. Von Kodolitsch Y, Schwartz AG, Nienaber CA. Clinical prediction of acute aortic dissection. *Arch Intern Med* 2000;160;2977–2982.
3. Klompas M. Does this patient have an acute thoracic aortic dissection? *JAMA* 2002;287:2262–2272.
4. Januzzi JL, Isselbacher EM, Fattori R, et al. Characterizing the young patient with aortic dissection: results from the International Registry of Aortic Dissection (IRAD). *J Am Coll Cardiol* 2004;43:665–669.
5. Mehta RH, Bossone E, Evangelista A, et al. International Registry of Acute Aortic Dissection Investigators. Acute type B aortic dissection in elderly patients: clinical features, outcomes, and simple risk stratification rule. *Ann Thorac Surg* 2004;77:1622–1628.
6. Mehta RH, Suzuki T, Hagan P, et al. Predicting death in patients with acute type A aortic dissection. *Circulation* 2002;105:200–206.
7. Nishigami K, Tsuchiya T, Shono H, et al. Disappearance of aortic intramural hematoma and its significance to the prognosis. *Circulation* 2000;102 (Suppl):243–247.
8. Song JK, Kim HS, Song JM, et al. Outcomes of medically treated patients with aortic intramural hematoma. *Am J Med* 2002;113: 181–187.
9. Evangelista A, Dominguez R, Sebastia C, et al. Long-term follow-up of aortic intramural hematoma: predictors of outcome. *Circulation* 2003;108:583–589.
10. Song JM, Kim HS, Song JK, et al. Usefulness of the initial noninvasive imaging study to predict the adverse outcomes in the medical treatment of acute type A aortic intramural hematoma. *Circulation* 2003;108 (Suppl):324–328.
11. Motoyoshi N, Moizumi Y, Komatsu T, et al. Intramural hematoma and dissection involving ascending aorta: the clinical features and prognosis. *Eur J Cardiothorac Surg* 2003;24:237–242.
12. Von Kodolitsch Y, Csösz SK, Koschyk DH, et al. Intramural hematoma of the aorta: predictors of progression to dissection and rupture. *Circulation* 2003;107:1158–1563.
13. Kallenbach K, Oelze T, Salcher R, et al. Evolving strategies for treatment of acute aortic dissection type A. *Circulation* 2004;110 (Suppl):243–249.
14. Tan ME, Dossche KM, Morshuis WF, et al. Operative risk factors of type A aortic dissection: analysis of 252 consecutive patients. *Cardiovasc Surg* 2003;11:277–285.
15. Hata M, Shiono M, Inoue T, et al. Optimal treatment of type B acute aortic dissection: long-term medical follow-up results. *Ann Thorac Surg* 2003;75:1781–1784.
16. Yu HY, Chen YS, Huang SC, et al. Late outcome of patients with aortic dissection: study of a national database. *Eur J Cardiothorac Surg* 2004;25:683–690.
17. Lambrechts D, Casselman F, Schroeyers P, et al. Endovascular treatment of the descending thoracic aorta. *Eur J Vasc Endovasc Surg* 2003;26:437–444.
18. Bortone AS, De Cillis E, D'Agostino D, et al. Endovascular treatment of thoracic aortic disease: four years of experience. *Circulation* 2004;110 (Suppl):262–267.
19. Sueyoshi E, Sakamoto I, Hayashi K, et al. Growth rate of aortic diameter in patients with type B aortic dissection during the chronic phase. *Circulation* 2004;110 (Suppl):256–261.

ADDITIONAL READING

Blanchard DG, Sawhney NS. Aortic intramural hematoma: current diagnostic and therapeutic recommendations. *Curr Treat Options Cardiovasc Med* 2004;6:99–104.

Nienaber CA, Eagle KA. Aortic dissection diagnosis and management: Part I. from etiology to diagnostic strategies. *Circulation* 2003;108: 628–635.

O'Gara PT. Recognition and management of patients with diseases of the aorta: aneurysms and dissection. In: Braunwald E, Goldman L, eds. *Primary Cardiology*, 2nd ed. Philadelphia: W.B. Saunders, 2003:643–658.

Aortic Aneurysm

50

Frank A. Lederle

INTRODUCTION

Aortic aneurysm can develop anywhere along the course of the aorta, from the ascending aorta to the iliac bifurcation. The diameter of the aorta gradually decreases so that the descending thoracic aorta is only about two-thirds the size of the ascending aorta. The ascending and thoracic aorta have vessels called vasa vasora to nourish the aortic wall. As the thoracic aorta becomes the abdominal aorta, the vasa vasora diminish; nourishment of the abdominal aortic wall is mainly from the lumenal blood. Because of the additive effect of transmitted pressure waves and waves reflected from the aortic bifurcation, systolic aortic pressure and thus the distending pressure of the aorta are higher in the abdominal aorta than more proximally. Aortic aneurysms are caused by the distending pressure on the aortic wall as well as the failure of material components of the wall.

Aortic aneurysms can be classified by their geometric shapes (fusiform [cylindrical] or saccular) and their extent (focal or diffuse). Aortic aneurysms can also be classified as false or true aneurysms. True aneurysms involve all three layers of the aortic wall; false aneurysms are contained aortic ruptures in which the wall of the aneurysm is formed by the aortic adventitia as well as adherent adjacent tissues (e.g., pleural and mediastinal).

Most aortic aneurysms result from an idiopathic degenerative process involving the elastin and collagen of the arterial media, probably related to matrix metalloproteinases released by macrophages (Table 50.1) (1). Aneurysms of the thoracic aorta also may be caused by connective tissue diseases, such as Marfan syndrome, or idiopathic aortitis, such as granulomatous aortitis and Takayasu's disease. Prior trauma also can cause a false aneurysm that usually occurs in the thoracic aorta just beyond the takeoff of the left subclavian artery. Syphilitic aortitis is now uncommon.

Ninety percent of abdominal aneurysms involve the infrarenal abdominal aorta, where an aortic diameter greater than 3.0 cm, as determined by ultrasound or computed tomography (CT), is abnormal. In the United States, aortic aneurysm result in 15,000 deaths per year, including those resulting from treatment, making it the 15th leading cause of death. Although thoracic and abdominal aortic aneurysms are indistinguishable on gross or microscopic pathology, thoracic aneurysms occur equally in men and women, whereas abdominal aortic aneurysms are four times more frequent in men than women. There are also genetic influences, as demonstrated by the six-fold increase in abdominal aortic aneurysms in first-degree relatives of patients with such aneurysms.

AORTIC ANEURYSM AND RUPTURE

Most aneurysms of the thoracic aorta, thoracoabdominal aorta, and abdominal aorta are totally asymptomatic until they rupture suddenly, at which time they are usually rapidly fatal. For aortic aneurysms at each of these locations, patients may present moribund, with refractory hypotension resulting from exsanguinating hemorrhage. Other patients may have pain and an incipient leak, which permits emergent surgery in a relatively stable patient. Still others are somewhere on a continuum between these two extremes. All patients with rupture require emergent evaluation, to confirm the diagnosis and determine the site of the leak, and emergent surgical repair. Surgery after rupture carries a 50% or greater mortality rate, whereas operation in the asymptomatic patient carries a low mortality rate.

By comparison, other patients may be diagnosed as having asymptomatic aortic aneurysms that either require serial follow-up evaluations or are large enough to mandate semi-elective surgery. These patients normally do not re-

TABLE 50.1
ETIOLOGY OF AORTIC ANEURYSMS

Smoking
Aortitis
Specific etiology; e.g., syphilis
Unknown etiology
Takayasu's disease
Granulomatous aortitis
Connective-tissue disease; e.g., Marfan syndrome, Ehlers-Danlos
    syndrome
Cystic medial necrosis
Postsurgical
Mycotic aneurysm
Aneurysm associated with coarctation of the aorta
Traumatic aneurysm
Dissection of the aorta

quire hospitalization or prolongation of an existing hospitalization, because most of the preoperative evaluation can be performed on an outpatient basis.

Non-traumatic aortic rupture is nearly always because of aneurysm. Dissection nearly always occurs in the thoracic aorta (Chapter 49). Thus, abdominal aortic aneurysms rupture, whereas thoracic aneurysms can either dissect or rupture with approximately equal frequency (2). The risk of dissection is increased by the presence of a thoracic aneurysm, but *about 80% of dissections occur in non-aneurysmal aortas.* Finally, about one-fourth of aortic dissections result in aneurysm, and chronic aortic dissection is the cause of about one-fifth of all thoracic aneurysms.

THORACIC AORTIC ANEURYSM

Thoracic aortic aneurysms can involve the aortic root (annuloaortic ectasia), the ascending aorta, the aortic arch, the descending aorta, and the thoracoabdominal aorta. The larger the aneurysm is, the higher the risk of leaking or rupture. Thoracic aneurysms are often detected in patients with a previously diagnosed abdominal aortic aneurysm.

Issues at the Time of Admission

Clinical Presentation

Although most thoracic aortic aneurysms are asymptomatic, ascending aortic aneurysms can cause signs or symptoms by their pressure on adjacent structures, such as the superior vena cava. Deep chest pain, described as throbbing or aching, is seen if there is erosion of ribs or vertebrae. Aneurysms of the aortic arch can involve the great vessels and cause ischemia of the organs they supply. Aneurysms of the aortic arch also can compress mediastinal structures, the thoracic spine, or tracheobronchial structures and cause cough, dyspnea, or tracheal deviation. Pressure on the esophagus may cause dysphagia; stretch of the left recurrent laryngeal nerve may cause hoarseness. Aneurysms of descending aorta or thoracoabdominal aorta rarely compress any structures or cause symptoms until they rupture.

With rupture of a thoracic aneurysm, there may be massive cardiac tamponade (ascending aorta) or exsanguinating hemorrhage, usually into the left pleural cavity, depending on the site. Hemoptysis, sometimes intermittent over days or weeks, may occur if a descending aortic aneurysm is adherent to the lung and ruptures into it.

The physical examination is of little help in detecting thoracic aortic aneurysms unless they are very large or involve the aortic valve (causing aortic regurgitation). By the time a hemorrhagic pleural effusion can be detected by physical examination, the patient is usually *in extremis.*

Differential Diagnosis and Initial Evaluation

The differential diagnosis includes other causes of chest pain, hypertension, or thoracic mass. Aneurysms usually are suspected after examination of the chest radiograph: spherical aneurysms can deform the aortic silhouette, and cylindrical aneurysms can increase the mediastinal shadow and simulate a progressive uncoiling of the aorta.

With intimal calcification, which is very common in the elderly, it is possible to identify the lateral borders of the aorta and sometimes even the medial border. A calcified aortic aneurysm can be detected on the plain chest radiograph. The diagnosis of a thoracic aneurysm is usually confirmed by a spiral CT scan, MRI, transesophageal echocardiography, or aortogram.

Initial Therapy

Aneurysms that produce symptoms or are associated with bleeding should be treated emergently as impending rupture. The correct management of asymptomatic thoracic aneurysms is less clear. No randomized trials have compared early elective repair with surveillance, and data on natural history are limited. Nationwide, elective surgical treatment of thoracic aortic aneurysms carries a perioperative mortality rate of 20%–25% (3, 4), though centers that choose to publish their results tend to report much lower rates. The risks of dissection and rupture increase with the diameter of the aneurysm. A population-based study from Olmsted County, Minnesota, found a 5-year rupture risk of 0% for thoracic aneurysms smaller than 4.0 cm in diameter, 16% for those 4.0–6.0 cm, and 31% for those larger than 6.0 cm (5). The Yale prospective database of 721 patients with thoracic aortic aneurysm reported an annual rupture or dissection rate of 6.9% (2). Based on these natural history data, the Yale group has recommended elective repair of asymptomatic aneurysms larger than

6.5 cm in the descending thoracic aorta or 5.5 cm in the ascending aorta. However, these recommendations were based on a 9% operative mortality in their own series, or less than half the national average. The authors of the nationwide studies have recommended that these recommendations be re-evaluated (4). Others have recommended that elective repair be undertaken when the 1-year rupture risk exceeds the operative mortality (6). Using this criterion, there are insufficient data to recommend elective repair of thoracic aneurysms of any diameter. Better data, ideally from randomized trials, will be needed to resolve this issue.

Elective repair of thoracic aneurysms 5.5–6.5 cm may be justifiable for patients with *Marfan syndrome*. Marfan patients appear to have significantly higher rates of dissection or rupture, and significantly lower operative mortality rates (2). In one study of 675 Marfan patients who had aortic root replacement at a mean age of 34, one-year survival was 93% (7).

In Marfan patients with smaller aneurysms, close observation is indicated. β-blockers are now widely used in Marfan patients, though their benefit has not been proven (8).

Surgical Issues

Annuloaortic ectasia requires replacement of the ascending aorta with a graft that includes a prosthetic aortic valve and implantation of the coronary ostia into a site in the graft above the valve. Ascending aortic aneurysms require replacement of the aorta from just above the coronary ostia to just below the takeoff of the innominate artery. Operation for aneurysm of the transverse arch is the most difficult and hazardous because the brain must be perfused while the aorta is cross-clamped.

One serious potential surgical complication is spinal-cord injury and paralysis. Thoracoabdominal aneurysms are more difficult to treat, because both the thoracic and the abdominal cavities must be entered. The celiac, superior mesenteric, and renal arteries must be reimplanted in the graft.

Indications for Hospitalization and Early Consultation

Patients with leaking or ruptured thoracic aortic aneurysms usually go directly from the emergency department to the operating room. An asymptomatic thoracic aortic aneurysm may require further evaluation, but this evaluation usually does not need to occur emergently and does not require hospitalization. For patients with asymptomatic aneurysms, consultation with a cardiologist and often a vascular surgeon is indicated to guide evaluation and follow-up.

Issues During the Course of Hospitalization

Adequate blood pressure control may slow progression of the aneurysm in patients who are not initially managed surgically. β-blockers and vasodilators are commonly used for this purpose.

Discharge Issues

For patients with asymptomatic thoracic aortic aneurysms, the aneurysm itself should not affect discharge decisions other than by creating a need for appropriate follow-up. For smaller aneurysms, suitable follow-up should be arranged, usually at 6-month intervals for 1–2 years and annually thereafter, usually with a CT scan or MRI study.

ABDOMINAL AORTIC ANEURYSM

Issues at the Time of Admission

Clinical Presentation

Any patient who has abdominal or back pain and evidence of an abdominal aortic aneurysm by imaging study or abdominal paplation could be leaking or rupturing; such patients must be evaluated and treated emergently. Ruptured abdominal aortic aneurysms can be surprisingly difficult to diagnose. Most ruptures occur in previously undiagnosed abdominal aortic aneurysm, and delays and errors are common. Physicians can be misled by symptoms of dysfunction of the gastrointestinal or genitourinary tracts (due to mass effect and compromised circulation), leukocytosis, and preservation of blood pressure and hematocrit, all of which are characteristic of rupture of an abdominal aortic aneurysm. If retroperitoneal bleeding has been extensive, ecchymoses may appear in the skin of the flanks and the lateral abdominal wall. Abdominal aortic aneurysms sometimes can attach to viscera and rupture into the lumen of the gastrointestinal tract, especially the small intestine, resulting in an *aortoenteric fistula* and causing massive gastrointestinal bleeding. Occasionally, the bleeding can be intermittent and gradual, simulating a chronic lower gastrointestinal bleed. After initially successful abdominal aortic aneurysm surgery, a similar syndrome also is seen in patients who leak adjacent to the graft months or years later, often in association with a focal site of bacterial endarteritis.

In some patients, abdominal aortic aneurysms develop layers of mural thrombus that can result in distal embolization of either thrombus or atheromatous debris, especially after trauma from a catheter (Chapter 51). Patients can present with sudden pain or numbness in the foot or lower leg caused by peripheral ischemia or with hypertension, hematuria, or renal failure resulting from atheromatous embolization to the kidney. Livedo reticularis is often present. As with thoracic aneurysms, patients with frank rupture can present with severe or refractory hypotension resulting from exsanguinating hemorrhage.

Differential Diagnosis and Initial Evaluation

Asymptomatic abdominal aortic aneurysms are often palpable, most commonly in men over age 50 who have smoked. In nonobese patients, it is usually possible to feel pulsation of the normal abdominal aorta. If the physician places both hands flat against the abdominal wall on either side of the palpable aorta and gently compresses the abdominal wall, the width of the abdominal aorta can be estimated.

Unfortunately, the ability to feel an abdominal aortic aneurysm is limited by the size of the abdomen. In one study of 200 patients ages 51–88, half of whom had abdominal aortic aneurysms, sensitivity of abdominal palpation by examiners unaware of the diagnosis was 91% when abdominal girth was less than 100 cm but only 53% when girth was 100 cm or greater (9). No abdominal aortic aneurysm of 5.0 cm or larger was missed when abdominal girth was less than 100 cm.

Aneurysms smaller than 4.0 cm in diameter rarely rupture. Aneurysms expand by an average of about 0.3 cm/y, but expansion is variable from year to year, even in an individual patient. For aneurysms of 4.0–5.5 cm in diameter that are followed by ultrasound surveillance, the annual rupture rate is about 1% per year; it is substantially higher for larger aneurysms.

A lateral abdominal radiograph may show intimal calcification, but abdominal ultrasound is the preferred test, with a specificity and positive predictive value approaching 100% (Figure 50.1). CT with or without contrast and MRI provide additional detail for preoperative evaluation.

Indications for Hospitalization

Any patient with a suspected leaking abdominal aortic aneurysm must be admitted emergently for evaluation. Commonly, such patients go directly from the emergency department to the surgical ICU or to the operating room. Patients with asymptomatic abdominal aortic aneurysms do not require hospitalization unless the aneurysm is sufficiently large to require surgery.

Initial Therapy

Patients with symptomatic abdominal aneurysms require immediate hospitalization, emergent diagnostic imaging, and immediate consultation with a vascular surgeon. Even as resuscitative efforts begin, patients with ruptured aortic aneurysms must be taken immediately to the operating room to control hemorrhage, exclude the aneurysm, and place a bypass graft. Currently, fluid resuscitation prior to repair of a ruptured abdominal aortic aneurysm is an area of controversy. Although fluids may reduce the adverse sequellae of shock, they may also cause clot disruption,

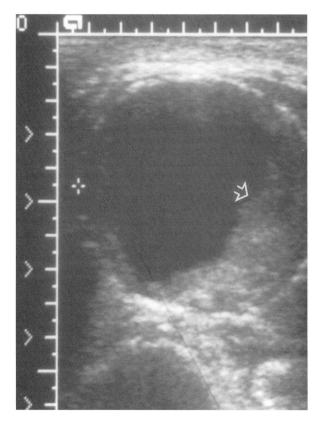

Figure 50.1 Abdominal aortic ultrasound showing a large abdominal aortic aneurysm 7.5 cm in diameter just distal to the takeoff of the renal arteries. The *open arrow* indicates mural thrombus. Small scale markers are 0.5 cm.

hemodilution, and coagulopathy. Although there are no studies that address this question directly, one large randomized trial of patients with stab wounds and shock found that preoperative fluid resuscitation significantly increased mortality (10). For preoperative management of patients with ruptured abdominal aortic aneurysm, resuscitation to a systolic pressure of 90 mm Hg is sometimes recommended as a compromise.

The mortality rate once the aneurysm has ruptured is very high. More than 50% of patients die before reaching the operating room, and operative mortality for open repair remains about 50%, resulting in an 80% overall mortality for ruptured abdominal aortic aneurysm (11). Endovascular repair is emerging as a potentially important therapy for ruptured abdominal aortic aneurysm, sometimes accompanied by drainage of the retroperitoneal hematoma. In two randomized trials, endovascular repair had a lower operative mortality and complication rate (12, 13), but long-term follow-up is not yet available.

Although repair of some type is usually attempted for ruptured abdominal aortic aneurysm because the alternative is certain death, the indications for elective repair of an unruptured abdominal aortic aneurysm must be carefully weighed against peri-operative risk, especially cardiac risk (Chapter 30). In the absence of any clinical or electrocardiographic evidence of coronary artery disease in an active patient with good exercise capacity, surgery for abdominal aortic aneurysm is relatively safe, with low rates of morbidity and mortality from cardiac events. If there is evidence of coronary artery disease and the patient is stable and has good exercise tolerance (i.e., can climb two flights of stairs without difficulty), it is probably safe to proceed to surgery. If the patient is at high risk (i.e., has decreased left-ventricular systolic function, signs of heart failure, or myocardial ischemia at low levels of exercise), preoperative testing (Chapter 30) is indicated. Coronary revascularization is not recommended before abdominal aortic surgery unless the patient has severe coronary disease and would be a candidate for coronary revascularization independent of the need for the abdominal aortic surgery (14).

Various surgical and endovascular approaches to elective repair are associated with operative mortality rates of about 2%–5%. Surgery does not remove the aneurysm but rather involves the placement of a prosthesis to connect normal proximal and distal aortic lumens, either within the aneurysmal sac itself or adjacent to a ligated and excluded aneurysmal sac. Alternatively, a stent graft can be placed into the aneurysmal aorta via the femoral artery. Currently, these various approaches have reasonably similar success rates. The endovascular approach may ultimately be preferred in patients with severe cardiac or pulmonary disease, although experience with this technique varies from hospital to hospital, success rates are highly dependent on individual operators, and long-term outcomes are unknown.

Indications for Early Consultation

Any patient with suspected leaking from an abdominal aortic aneurysm requires emergent surgical consultation because of the need for emergent surgery. For patients with asymptomatic abdominal aortic aneurysms 5.5 cm or larger, surgical consultation should be obtained to consider elective surgery.

Issues During the Course of Hospitalization

If a leaking abdominal aortic aneurysm is suspected during the course of hospitalization, the approach is similar to the recommendations for a patient who is admitted with abdominal aortic aneurysm rupture. For patients with asymptomatic abdominal aortic aneurysms discovered during hospitalization, noninvasive testing with ultrasound, or rarely CT or MRI, should be obtained to determine the maximum diameter of the aneurysm.

Discharge Issues

For patients who do not undergo surgery, an asymptomatic aortic aneurysm usually does not prolong hospitalization unless it is large enough to warrant surgery. Two large randomized trials have evaluated immediate open surgical repair compared with imaging surveillance every 6 months in good operative candidates with abdominal aortic aneurysms of 4.0–5.5 cm in diameter (15, 16). Both studies reported no survival benefit from immediate repair, thereby indicating that repair can be deferred until the AAA enlarges to ≥5.5 cm. In the Department of Veterans Affairs trial, the survival trend favored surveillance (versus immediate repair) regardless of age or the diameter of the aneurysm, despite a low 30-day operative mortality of 2%. These studies suggest that the surveillance strategy can reduce the number of elective abdominal aortic aneurysm repairs in this population by about 20%. The most likely reason that early repair was not beneficial in these trials was that the rate of rupture of abdominal aortic aneurysm in patients randomized to surveillance was less than 1% per year. In patients who are at high operative risk, elective repair may be further deferred until the abdominal aortic aneurysm enlarges to the point at which the risk of rupture is thought to warrant the risk of repair. However, patients at high operative risk may also be at especially high risk for rupture; in a series of 199 such patients in whom repair was not undertaken because of high operative risk or because they refused surgery, risk of rupture was 10% at one year for abdominal aortic aneurysms 5.5–6.9 cm and more than 30% at one year for abdominal aortic aneurysms ≥7.0 cm (17). β-blocker therapy does not slow the rate of growth of abdominal aortic aneurysms and should not be prescribed for this purpose (18).

KEY POINTS

- Most thoracic aortic aneurysms are asymptomatic unless they dissect, rupture, or compress adjacent structures; elective surgery (at centers of excellence) may be indicated for large thoracic aneurysms.
- A symptomatic abdominal aortic aneurysm requires emergent evaluation because such symptoms commonly indicate leaking and impending rupture.
- Elective surgical repair is indicated for abdominal aortic aneurysms at least 5.5 cm in diameter. For aneurysms smaller than 5.5 cm, surveillance ultrasonography is recommended, every 6 months for abdominal aortic aneurysms ≥4.0 cm, and every 1–2 years for smaller abdominal aortic aneurysms.
- Careful evaluation is required to assess operative risk prior to elective aortic aneurysm surgery.
- The choice of surgical technique depends on local expertise; endovascular stenting is a new and promising alternative to the open surgical approach, especially in patients with rupture or substantial comorbid cardiac or pulmonary disease.

REFERENCES

1. Curci JA, Liao S, Huffman MD, et al. Expression and localization of macrophage elastase (matrix metalloproteinase-12) in abdominal aortic aneurysms. *J Clin Invest* 1998;102:1900–1910.

2. Davies RR, Goldstein LJ, Coady MA, et al. Yearly rupture or dissection rates for thoracic aortic aneurysms: simple prediction based on size. *Ann Thorac Surg* 2002;73:17–28.

3. Lawrence PF, Gazak C, Bhirangi L, et al. The epidemiology of surgically repaired aneurysms in the United States. *J Vasc Surg* 1999;30:632–640.

4. Derrow AE, Seeger JM, Dame DA, et al. The outcome in the United States after thoracoabdominal aortic aneurysm repair, renal artery bypass, and mesenteric revascularization. *J Vasc Surg* 2001;34:54–61.

5. Clouse WD, Hallett JW Jr, Schaff HV, et al. Improved prognosis of thoracic aortic aneurysms. *JAMA* 1998;280:1926–1929.

6. Juvonen T, Ergin MA, Galla JD, et al. Prospective study of the natural history of thoracic aortic aneurysms. *Ann Thorac Surg* 1997;63:1533–1545.

7. Gott VL, Greene PS, Alejo DE, et al. Replacement of the aortic root in patients with Marfan's syndrome. *N Engl J Med* 1999;340:1307–1313.

8. Shores J, Berger KR, Murphy EA, Pyeritz RE. Progression of aortic dilatation and the benefit of long-term beta-adrenergic blockade in Marfan's syndrome. *N Engl J Med* 1994;330:1335–1341.

9. Fink HA, Lederle FA, Roth CS, et al. The accuracy of physical examination to detect abdominal aortic aneurysm. *Arch Intern Med* 2000;160:833–836.

10. Bickell, WH, Wall MJ, Pepe PE, et al. Immediate versus delayed fluid resuscitation for hypotensive patients with penetrating torso injuries. *New Engl J Med* 1994;331:1105–1109.

11. Adam DJ, Mohan IV, Stuart WP, et al. Community and hospital outcome from ruptured abdominal aortic aneurysm within the catchment area of a regional vascular surgical service. *J Vasc Surg* 1999;30:922–928.

12. Greenhalgh RM, Brown LC, Kwong GP, et al., EVAR trial participants. Comparison of endovascular aneurysm repair with open repair in patients with abdominal aortic aneurysm (EVAR trial 1), 30-day operative mortality results: randomized controlled trial. *Lancet* 2004;364:843–848.

13. Prinssen M, Verhoeven EL, Buth J, et al.; Dutch Randomized Endovascular Aneurysm Management (DREAM) Trial Group. A randomized trial comparing conventional and endovascular repair of abdominal aortic aneurysms. *N Engl J Med* 2004;351:1607–1618.

14. McFalls EO, Ward HB, Moritz TE, et al. Coronary-artery revascularization before elective major vascular surgery. *N Engl J Med* 2004;351:2795–2804.

15. The UK Small Aneurysm Trial Participants. Long-term outcomes of immediate repair compared with surveillance of small abdominal aortic aneurysms. *N Engl J Med* 2002;346:1445–1452.

16. Lederle FA, Wilson SE, Johnson GR, et al. Aneurysm Detection and Management (ADAM) Veterans Affairs Cooperative Study Group. Immediate repair compared with surveillance of small abdominal aortic aneurysms. *N Engl J Med* 2002;346:1437–1444.

17. Lederle FA, Johnson GR, Wilson SE, et al. Veterans Affairs Cooperative Study #417 Investigators. Rupture rate of large abdominal aortic aneurysms in patients refusing or unfit for elective repair. *JAMA* 2002;287:2968–2972.

18. The Propranolol Aneurysm Trial Investigators. Propranolol for small abdominal aortic aneurysms. Results of a randomized trial. *J Vasc Surg* 2002;35:72–78.

ADDITIONAL READING

Fleming C. Whitlock EP, Beil TL, Lederle FA. Screening for abdominal aortic aneurysm: a best-evidence systematic review for the U.S. Preventive Services Task Force. *Ann Intern Med* 2005;142:203–211.

Peripheral Arterial Disease

51

Eric P. Brass   **William R. Hiatt**   **Mark R. Nehler**

INTRODUCTION

Peripheral arterial disease (PAD) is an atherosclerotic disease associated with cardiovascular risk factors (particularly diabetes and smoking) and aging. Because the Western population is rapidly aging, an increase in hospitalized patients with PAD can be anticipated. PAD includes two overlapping but distinct pathophysiologic processes. Patients may present with clinical problems related to *chronic, atherosclerotic PAD,* including critical leg ischemia or ischemic ulcerations. Alternatively, patients may present with *acute arterial occlusion* or *insufficiency* as a result of embolic or thrombotic events in the arteries supplying the lower extremities. The majority of hospitalized patients with acute peripheral arterial problems are suffering sequelae of chronic PAD.

The major symptom of PAD is *intermittent claudication.* Claudication means to limp, but more specifically it refers to exercise-induced discomfort in the calf, thigh, or buttocks that is reliably brought on by a given level of exercise and relieved within 10 minutes of rest (Chapter 47). The pain should not begin at rest or with change in position. The pathophysiology of claudication is primarily a supply-demand mismatch, with inadequate oxygen delivery to meet the metabolic demand of exercising skeletal muscle.

The prevalence of PAD from a variety of population studies ranges from 7%–20% in individuals older than 55 years, although two-thirds of these patients may be asymptomatic and their disease unrecognized (1). In addition to involving the vessels in the lower extremity, atherosclerosis is a systemic disease. By clinical history, about 40%–60% of patients with PAD have had events indicating the presence of concomitant coronary disease; however, by angiographic studies, 90% have concomitant, significant coronary disease and as many as 80% have significant carotid artery disease. Given these associations, an ankle-brachial index below 0.90 at rest (ABI) (see Chapter 47) has been shown to be a strong, independent predictor of cardiovascular death. A number of epidemiologic studies have shown an approximate 4%–5% rate of myocardial infarction, stroke, or vascular mortality per year in patients with claudication. Moreover patients with critical leg ischemia have an annual mortality of 20%, with 80% of these deaths due to vascular causes. Thus, inpatient treatment goals for this disorder are primarily to relieve symptoms and preserve the lower extremity, as well as to ensure that the greatly increased risk of cardio- and nuerovascular injury and death in these patients is subsequently addressed.

The prevalence of intermittent claudication is lower than that of PAD, as defined by ABI measurements. Based on a variety of trials, the prevalence of claudication is ≤1% in individuals younger than 50 years, 3%–5% in 50- to 59-year-olds, 5%–10% in 60- to 69-year-olds, and ≥10% in those older than 70 years. Males are overrepresented in the claudication population, with a male:female ratio between 1.5:1 and 2.5:1. However, the gender ratio is approximately 1:1 when PAD is defined as the presence of an abnormal ABI. Natural-history studies of patients with claudication reveal that 75% of individuals have –stable symptoms if followed over 5 years, and only 25% –clinically worsen; only 5% require revascularization, and about 2%–4% will have amputations over the same 5-year period. Thus, most patients with claudication have a stable natural history and can be managed as outpatients with medical therapies. Progression of disease is more likely in patients who continue to smoke or who have diabetes; for example, PAD patients with diabetes are

2–10 times more likely to progress to amputation than are PAD patients without diabetes.

Critical leg ischemia is the most severe manifestation of PAD. Patients with critical leg ischemia by definition have one or more hemodynamically significant occlusive lesions that reduce blood flow to the extremity at rest. This severe compromise of limb blood flow results in the clinical manifestations of either ischemic rest pain, ischemic ulceration, or gangrene principally affecting the distal ankle and foot. The pathophysiology of critical leg ischemia is severe blood-oxygen supply-demand mismatch manifest in the resting state, principally involving the skin of the distal lower extremity. Ischemic rest pain typically occurs at night with the patient supine. The pain progressively becomes more severe and is relieved upon dangling the foot to augment distal blood flow. Ischemic ulcerations, which principally affect the toes and distal forefoot or heel, are usually the result of minor trauma in a limb with a compromised circulation. Ischemic ulcers have dark necrotic centers and are painful, similar to the ischemic pain experienced in the remainder of the foot. As ischemic ulceration progresses, it leads to gangrene, and ultimately loss of the extremity. Several studies have reported an incidence of critical leg ischemia of approximately 500–1,000 new cases per million adults per year, with an estimated prevalence between 500,000 and 1,000,000 in the United States. Seventy-five percent of those affected with critical leg ischemia are older than 60 years. Patients with critical leg ischemia have a poor natural history regarding both limb and life. Without revascularization, the amputation rate at 3-month follow-up is about 12%, and it may be as high as 35% at 6 months. The annual mortality rate is approximately 20% per year (2).

Importantly, some patients with acute arterial insufficiency are experiencing an embolic or thrombotic occlusion in an otherwise normal arterial circulation (Table 51.1) rather than as a complication of chronic, occlusive PAD. These patients without chronic arterial insufficiency have fewer collateral vessels, are less able to tolerate acute severe ischemia, and are more likely to require amputation than patients with chronic, occlusive PAD in whom collateral formation is better established. Several studies have demonstrated that among patients with acute onset of critical leg ischemia symptoms and no history of PAD, more than 50% require amputation.

Patients with acute arterial insufficiency or severe, symptomatic chronic PAD should be admitted to the hospital for possible revascularization procedures in an attempt to relieve claudication or ischemic rest pain, to promote wound healing, and to prevent amputation. These interventions also are designed to prevent limb loss and to improve the functional status of the patient. Since these patients are at high risk for cardiovascular events in the perioperative period, physicians must consider the appropriate cardiac evaluation and therapy needed during the perioperative course (Chapters 30 and 31).

TABLE 51.1

CAUSES OF PERIPHERAL ARTERIAL INSUFFICIENCY

Chronic arterial occlusive disease

Atherosclerosis
Buerger's disease (thromboangiitis obliterans)
Arteritis
   Giant-cell arteritis
   Takayasu's arteritis
   Fibromuscular dysplasia

Embolic

Cardiac origin
   Left-ventricular thrombus (from underlying myocardial infarction or cardiomyopathy)
   Left-atrial thrombus
   Mitral or aortic-valve thrombus (from infectious endocarditis [vegetation] or marantic endocarditis)
   Prosthetic-valve thrombus or vegetation
Paradoxic embolism of venous clot via a right-to-left shunt, principally an atrial septal defect or patent foramen ovale
Noncardiac atheroembolism from proximal aneurysm or atherosclerosis

In situ arterial thrombosis

Postprocedure/pseudoaneurysm
Hypercoagulable states
Heparin-induced thrombocytopenia

Other

Trauma
Aneurysm
Cyst
Vasoconstrictor drugs
   Cocaine
   Ergots
   Cyclosporine
Radiation

ACUTE LIMB ISCHEMIA

Issues at the Time of Presentation

Clinical Presentation

The pain in acute limb ischemia is usually of sudden onset, but occasionally it may develop gradually over several hours, depending on the location and extent of the arterial occlusion. This pain is unrelenting, diffuse foot pain, often extending above the ankle, and is not affected by dependent position of the limb. Alert patients are in extreme discomfort, so the diagnosis is usually not subtle. The patient complains of paresthesias, numbness, and, as symptoms progress, weakness and paralysis in the affected limb. A history of prior revascularization procedures, antecedent claudication, diabetes, tobacco use, cardiac disease, arrhythmias, or chronic anticoagulation therapy may be helpful in defining the etiology.

Acute arterial insufficiency not related to PAD is frequently the result of *cardiac emboli, atheroembolism,* or *in situ arterial thrombosis,* with rare additional causes (Table 51.1). The most common presentation of acute ischemia in patients with known PAD is *occlusion of an existing bypass graft.* These patients present with either rest pain or increasing claudication, depending on the degree of the resulting ischemia.

Cardiac embolism most commonly is encountered in patients who have mural thrombus of the ventricle as a complication of prior myocardial infarction or cardiomyopathy, atrial thrombosis as a complication of mitral valve disease or atrial fibrillation or flutter, or valvular thrombus or vegetation. The most frequent sites of hemodynamically significant lower extremity embolization involve the aortic and femoral bifurcations. Patients may suffer severe ischemia caused by a lack of existing collateral circulation at the time of occlusion.

Arterial-arterial embolization (atheroembolism) usually is observed as one of two types, spontaneous or iatrogenic. Patients with spontaneous atheroembolism present with painful, cyanotic digits of acute onset. Occasionally, the majority of the forefoot is involved. Bilateral findings indicate an aortic source; unilateral findings suggest an iliac or femoral source. Aneurysms of the aorta, femoral, or popliteal arteries are also potential causes of distal emboli. Unless the entire foot is involved, the patient typically has a palpable pedal pulse and a normal or only slightly diminished ABI because the circulation from the digital arteries to the embolic source remains relatively uninterrupted.

Iatrogenic atheroembolism may complicate aortic catheterization procedures. The clinical picture of limb atheroembolism in this setting can vary from mild livedo reticularis that slowly resolves, to severe limb pain and cyanosis and eventual tissue loss, with concurrent elevated plasma muscle enzyme levels and myoglobinuria. Peripheral pulses are usually unaffected, as the atheroemboli lodge distal to the dorsalis pedis or posterior tibial arteries. Atheroembolism frequently includes cholesterol emboli, which can be confirmed by skin biopsy of peripheral lesions demonstrating cholesterol crystals in the capillaries. Rising creatinine, oliguria, and urine eosinophils are often present in patients with emboli involving the renal circulation. The diagnosis is usually not difficult if the lower extremities are also involved. Severe abdominal pain (indicating intestinal ischemia) following arteriography is a recognized indication for laparotomy. Direct surgical treatment of arteries occluded by atheroembolic material is usually not possible, given the small particle and vessel size. Because of the nonthrombotic nature of the embolus, anticoagulation and thrombolytic therapy are also relatively ineffective and may even be deleterious, and are thus not recommended for the management of the ischemic limb. Statins, by causing plaque stabilization, may reduce the risk of recurrent atheroemboli in affected patients who recover from an acute embolic event. Most patients with catheter-induced atheroembolism have diffuse aortic disease not amenable to surgical treatment. An exception occurs if catheter-induced atheroembolism calls attention to an arterial aneurysm as the suspected source of the embolic material.

In situ arterial thrombosis occurs in two common scenarios. First, patients with a hypercoagulable state (Chapter 98), often previously unrecognized, may have an acutely occluded native artery (frequently with previous subclinical thromboses of small arteries). Second, patients with severe aortoiliac occlusive disease may develop iliac artery thrombosis secondary to catheter trauma from coronary angiography (resulting either from dissection of the iliac artery from the catheter or overzealous compression and occlusion of the groin postcatheterization).

In acute ischemia, the extremity is often pale and cool to palpation; pulses are often absent. It is particularly important to palpate the femoral as well as pedal pulses because a reduced femoral pulse indicates obstruction of the inflow vessels (aorto-iliac) that may be amenable to angioplasty. In contrast, a relatively normal femoral pulse with absent pedal pulses indicates occlusive disease distal to the inguinal ligament; in these patients, relief of limb ischemia typically requires a bypass operation to the distal vessels (popliteal or tibial). Doppler studies are critical and can be used to calculate an ABI. Determination of limb viability is made primarily based on physical examination and the judgment of the surgeon; thus, early vascular surgery consultation is required for all patients with suspected limb ischemia.

Differential Diagnosis and Initial Evaluation

The initial evaluation of the patient with suspected acute limb ischemia is directed toward confirming the ischemia and assessing limb viability. Paralyzed, insensate extremities with fixed skin mottling, and especially extremities with hard calf musculature, are not salvageable and require primary amputation as soon as the patient is medically prepared for the procedure and the margin of viability is clearly determined. However, the majority of acutely ischemic limbs are salvageable, because skeletal muscle generally can tolerate warm ischemia for 6 hours, or even longer in patients with chronic arterial occlusive disease, prior to irreversible loss. The decision about whether to proceed with limb salvage in marginal cases usually relies on the judgment of the vascular surgeon.

Acute limb ischemia rarely is confused with other processes. Infections (particularly necrotizing fasciitis), trauma, or conditions such as Raynaud's disease occasionally may cause initial diagnostic confusion. Once the diagnosis of acute arterial insufficiency is made, the differential diagnosis principally involves distinguishing embolic from thrombotic occlusion. Patients with emboli in normal arteries typically present with sudden onset of clinical symptoms, without a preceding history of claudication, and may have a known embolic source; the unaffected extremity has normal pulses and Doppler signals. Patients with arterial emboli to the limb also should be carefully evaluated for emboli in other arterial beds. In contrast, patients with thrombotic occlusions typically have an antecedent history of claudication or rest pain, prior vascular grafts, and clinical and laboratory evidence of occlusive disease in both lower extremities.

Differential diagnosis of acute ischemia includes emboli from a cardiac source or atheroemboli from large vessel atherosclerosis or aneurysm (Table 51.1). *In situ* thrombosis of native vessels or in bypass grafts also are recognized causes of acute arterial ischemia. Cardiac emboli associated with acute limb ischemia typically affect proximal vessels and lead to the sudden loss of a femoral pulse and a pale, cool extremity. In contrast, atheroemboli typically affect the most distal vessels and result in blue, intensely painful toes (*blue toe syndrome*).

Atrial fibrillation as a potential cause of cardiac emboli may be diagnosed from the electrocardiogram. Identification of mitral stenosis, left-atrial enlargement, or mural thrombus by echocardiography also may indicate a proximal source for the emboli. In addition, ultrasound or computed tomographic imaging of the aorta and femoral or popliteal vessels may identify aneurysms as a source of atheroemboli. However, although these options are useful in individual clinical situations, angiography provides more definitive diagnosis; an acute embolic source typically is identified by a "meniscus sign," and *in situ* thrombosis usually is accompanied by extensive atherosclerosis. Additionally, angiography provides vascular access for either angioplasty or thrombolysis, if indicated.

Additional laboratory evaluation is typically not necessary, except as required for pre-operative evaluation (Chapter 30). A sedimentation rate or ultra-sensitive C-reactive protein may be obtained if the clinical presentation is consistent with arteritis (Chapter 111), and an evaluation for hypercoagulable states (Chapter 98) is indicated in selective cases of unusual *in situ* thrombosis in otherwise healthy individuals.

Indications for Hospitalization or Intensive Care Unit Admission

The majority of patients presenting with acute limb ischemia need hospital admission. Occasionally patients with mild ischemia may be managed with oral analgesia and elective admission or nonoperative outpatient management. Most patients require hospital admission for pain control, rapid anticoagulation with heparin, and evaluation directed at either revascularization or amputation.

Most patients can be managed in a non-ICU setting. Considerations for ICU admission include requirements for management of comorbid conditions, level and severity of

ischemic pain, and rapidity of planned interventions. For example, if high-dose analgesia, rapid central venous access, or urgent heparinization or fluid resuscitation are needed prior to surgery or angiography, the ICU is often a more practical place to perform these interventions quickly. Postprocedural monitoring usually is performed in the ICU, as these patients have a high risk of needing other interventions and of developing hemorrhage at the operative site because of the frequent concomitant anticoagulation. In addition, the incidence of postintervention myocardial infarction is high in this group of vascular patients. Complications of myoglobinuria and limb reperfusion require careful acid-base monitoring and hydration and are also best managed in the ICU (Chapters 100 and 105).

Initial Therapy and Issues During Hospitalization

Initial therapy for all patients with acute limb ischemia (Figure 51.1) includes prompt heparinization (unless contraindicated) and administration of oxygen. Heparin therapy may be associated with rapid improvement of symptoms and helps stabilize the patient prior to more definitive management. Other systemic factors that may contribute to poor limb perfusion and oxygenation need to be optimized as indicated in individual patients. For example, patients with hypotension or heart failure should be stabilized hemodynamically to maximize limb perfusion. Patients with evidence of secondary bacterial infection should receive appropriate antibiotic therapy (Chapter 69). Most patients need diagnostic or therapeutic arteriography and thus should have an urgent evaluation of their renal function and receive hydration in preparation for this procedure. In patients with diabetes and renal insufficiency, use of N-acetylcysteine may reduce the risk of contrast-induced renal failure. Definitive therapy of the patient with acute limb ischemia requires re-establishment of arterial perfusion. Thus, all patients with acute peripheral ischemic syndromes should receive emergent consultation from a vascular surgeon.

The priorities in early management of the patient with graft occlusion include assessment of limb viability and current circulatory status, determination of the nature of previous operations (patients frequently have undergone multiple procedures at different institutions, and operative reports are often critical), and achievement of rapid, therapeutic heparin anticoagulation to prevent propagation of thrombus. Also important are decisions concerning timing of arteriography (emergent or next day), timing of exploration and graft thrombectomy (unusually emergent), and management of comorbid diseases or risks (hydration to prepare for arteriography, evaluation and therapy of associated cardiac arrhythmias or ischemia). Another practical issue is obtaining central venous access. These patients frequently need repeat vascular reconstructions, often using arm veins for the conduit (because the leg veins have

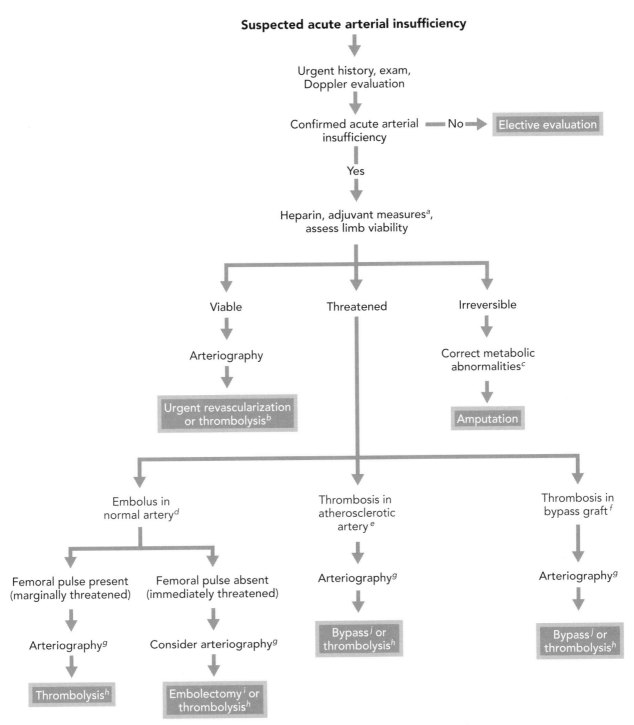

Figure 51.1 Algorithm for management of acute arterial insufficiency. [a]Adjuvant measures include antibiotics for infection and wound care if appropriate. [b]In a viable limb, there is usually time to attempt a course of thrombolysis. [c]Potential metabolic abnormalities include acidosis, hyperkalemia, and creatinine kinase elevations with myoglobinuria. [d]The acute occlusion of a primarily normal artery is usually caused by an embolus. In this situation, collateral vessels are usually not well developed, so there is a high risk for rapid progression to irreversible ischemia. [e]The acute occlusion of a previously atherosclerotic artery is usually because of a thrombosis. Typically these vessels have extensive collaterals that partially protect the leg from progression to irreversible ischemia. [f]Most graft occlusions are caused by thrombosis. [g]The decision to perform arteriography is based, in part, on time constraints in obtaining the procedure before irreversible changes occur. Duplex imaging of the leg may provide anatomic information more rapidly than arteriography. However, an arteriogram is always required for catheter-directed thrombolysis. [h]Thrombolysis is most useful for (a) embolic occlusion of a marginally threatened leg (these patients usually have a palpable femoral pulse); (b) lack of angiographically defined outflow (in this situation, there is no target for a bypass graft); (c) thrombosis of a new inflow graft; (d) lack of definitive surgical options; and (e) hypercoagulable states. [i]Embolectomy is usually performed for (a) proximal embolus (absent femoral pulse) in a leg that is immediately threatened; and (b) failure of lysis or contraindications for lysis. [j]Bypass grafting is performed for (a) outflow (leg) graft occlusion and (b) old inflow graft occlusion.

frequently been used for previous bypass operations); central venous access allows these veins to be preserved.

Patients with mild ischemia may undergo elective arteriography to plan the most suitable procedure. Patients presenting with fixed nonviable extremities ultimately come to amputation. Therefore, these patients are evaluated and managed primarily to determine the timing and the level of amputation. All other patients need urgent evaluation and therapy to restore perfusion rapidly to a potentially viable limb. In patients with acute peripheral arterial emboli, the decision of whether to proceed directly to operation for embolectomy (almost always involving a groin and popliteal approach) or to proceed with angiography and regional catheter-directed thrombolysis depends on the severity of the ischemia. Thrombolysis relieves the occlusion more slowly but offers the advantages of more complete resolution of the thrombus and avoiding catheter-induced endothelial trauma, which often leads to later fibrointimal hyperplasia and branch stenosis or occlusion of the involved arteries. If the limb is moderately threatened but time is available, angiography can be performed, followed by catheter-directed thrombolysis of the emboli. In contrast, if profound limb ischemia is present (often the case if the femoral pulse is absent and an embolus is present at or above the inguinal ligament), patients are best treated with operative embolectomy.

In patients with suspected *in situ* arterial thrombosis, arteriography is usually critical in decision making. The physical examination helps to localize the problem but offers insufficient anatomic information to plan needed surgery.

In patients with acute occlusion of an arterial graft, the location of the graft is important to subsequent management. If the graft is an inflow conduit (aortofemoral, axillofemoral, iliofemoral, or femorofemoral), then often the surgeon can proceed directly to graft thrombectomy and revision of the graft. The vast majority of inflow graft stenoses are located at the distal anastomosis, and a simple groin approach allows access to the graft. The primary problem with this approach is exposure of the prosthetic bypass material to potential infections. If the inflow graft cannot be opened with thrombolysis or surgery, an alternative option is an extra-anatomic bypass. Some surgeons believe occluded infrainguinal bypass grafts should be replaced with a new graft. Additional studies are required to define the necessity of this approach.

Several randomized trials have evaluated the efficacy of approaches for managing acute ischemia. In one study, 114 patients with acute arterial occlusions (thrombotic/embolic) or graft occlusions were randomized to either surgery or thrombolysis followed by angioplasty or surgery if needed (3). At 1 year, the limb salvage rate was equal (82%) in both groups. However, patient survival at 1 year was 84% in the thrombolytic group compared with 58% in the surgical group. Thus, this series would suggest that thrombolytic therapy may be associated with a lower 1-year mortality rate (the mechanism of this observed benefit remains unexplained). Two larger randomized trials, Surgery versus Thrombolysis for Ischemia of the Lower Extremity (STILE)

and Thrombolysis or Peripheral Artery Surgery (TOPAS), did not show any differences in 1-year mortality rates between thrombolytic and surgical management (4, 5). The amputation rate was greater in the thrombolytic group compared with the surgical group at one year in STILE (6), but there was no difference in TOPAS. Importantly, catheter-directed thrombolysis, which is superior to systemic administration of thrombolytic agents, is required. Currently, the question of optimal management using thrombolytic therapy or operation in acute limb ischemia remains unsettled (7, 8).

CHRONIC LIMB ISCHEMIA

Issues at the Time of Presentation

Clinical Presentation

Patients presenting with chronic limb ischemia as defined here typically do not present emergently for revascularization. Rather, the typical history is that of a patient with longstanding severe claudication who develops rest pain, a traumatic injury to the foot or digit, or an ischemic ulcer. The rest pain commonly occurs at night and is relieved with dependency or short ambulation.

Ischemic ulcers usually are found at the toes and distal points of the foot and are usually painful. However, chronic diabetic malperforans ulcers (sole of the foot at metatarsal heads) and venous ulcers (medial malleolus area) can be seen in patients with concomitant arterial ischemia. These conditions must be excluded in patients with refractory lesions. In general, any patient with an open foot wound needs to have adequate arterial circulation confirmed by careful hemodynamic assessment or Duplex ultrasound imaging (including ABI measurement) of the affected limb. Failure to do so is a common error that occasionally leads to delays in appropriate therapy and to unnecessary limb loss.

Differential Diagnosis and Initial Evaluation

Confirmation of the diagnosis of arterial insufficiency requires hemodynamic assessment of the critical components of the arterial tree. In the absence of previously documented atherosclerotic PAD, hemodynamics can be assessed noninvasively by measuring the ABI, the toe:brachial index, or segmental pressures in the affected limb. Initial evaluation also must exclude other causes of acute deterioration, such as hypotension. Patients with arteritis present with a typical clinical syndrome including systemic manifestations of their disease, an elevated sedimentation rate, and loss of pulses in the upper or lower extremity. Patients with Buerger's disease (*thromboangiitis obliterans*) have histories of substantial tobacco use; the arteriogram often shows corkscrew collaterals around an occluded medium-sized vessel. Biopsy is rarely necessary to confirm this diagnosis. Viability of the tissue should be addressed as discussed previously.

The differential diagnosis in these patients includes several entities in addition to atherosclerotic disease. Patients with diabetic neuropathy may present with symptoms consistent with ischemic pain and with nonhealing neuropathic ulcers, but their pedal pulses are normal, unless there is coexistent PAD. Reflex sympathetic dystrophy, which may develop after surgical or other forms of trauma, leads to a painful, discolored, swollen extremity; although this disorder typically is an autonomic neuropathy, arterial perfusion may be maintained. Patients with arteritis, particularly those with Buerger's disease and a strong smoking history, may present with ischemic limbs (Chapter 111). Acute limb ischemia, discussed above, must also be considered.

Indications for Hospitalization or Intensive Care Unit Admission

Admission to the hospital is guided primarily by the associated analgesic requirements to control pain, the need for intravenous antibiotics for associated infection, or the presence of comorbid conditions. In the absence of these considerations, revascularization usually can be planned in an elective manner.

Initial Therapy and Issues During Hospitalization

Initial management of these patients involves pain relief (Chapter 18). Although nonsteroidal anti-inflammatory drugs may work initially, most patients with ischemic rest pain require opiates for relief.

Patients with more severe disease including ischemic ulceration or gangrene also need wound care and prevention of further trauma to the extremity. Heel protection is critical to prevent pressure necrosis to the Achilles area. Hospitalized patients should not be allowed to bear weight on the affected limb. Patients with an infected ulcer must be treated with antibiotics. The empiric antibiotic selected should have broad Gram-positive and Gram-negative coverage, and the specific antibiotic regimen selected should be based on local microbial resistance patterns, the presence of comorbid conditions such as diabetes, and local formulary considerations.

Numerous trials of drugs of the prostaglandin class (including analogs of prostacyclin and PGE) in critical leg ischemia have shown only marginal success. Antiplatelet therapy may be necessary not only to attempt to preserve graft patency but also to reduce the systemic risk of myocardial infarction and stroke. Aspirin (325 mg/day) promotes the patency of peripheral bypass grafts and angioplasty procedures. Clopidogrel (75 mg/day) has been shown to reduce the risk of cardiovascular events in patients with PAD.

Anticoagulation is often used in the perioperative period to maintain graft patency after peripheral bypass procedures. The use of unfractionated or low-molecular-weight heparin in the immediate postoperative period may improve the patency of infrainguinal bypass grafts, but with the tradeoff of an increased risk of bleeding. In contrast, there is less evidence to support long-term anticoagulation to prevent graft occlusion. The largest experience suggests that anticoagulation (with warfarin to an INR of 2–3) may improve patency of vein grafts. Finally, several ongoing clinical trials are evaluating the use of growth factors to promote revascularization in chronic severe leg ischemia.

Definitive evaluation and management requires arterial imaging to localize the lesions, followed by revascularization or primary amputation (Figure 51.2). The choice between angioplasty and bypass surgery is complex and is based on the specific vascular anatomy, availability of appropriate conduit, previous revascularizations, and local expertise. Currently, the patient's own veins (greater saphenous, lesser saphenous, and arm veins) provide the optimal bypass vessels. Current 5-year patency rates for tibial bypass grafts are 60%–70% (9–12), with limb salvage rates of 80% or more. Operative mortality is less than 5% in most series, but may reach 10% in patients older than 80 years (13). The decision to amputate, and at what level to perform the amputation, remains largely one of clinical judgment.

Despite successful revascularization, post-operative recovery may be problematic (14, 15). Leg incisions or ischemic ulcers heal poorly, with mean healing times of 2 and 4 months, respectively. During this time, the wounds should be kept clean and inspected for infection and breakdown. Use of topical agents or growth factors applied directly to the wound have not been shown to offer any clinical benefit over usual local wound care. About 20%–30% of bypasses require operative revision, usually within the first year, to repair a stenotic lesion in the vein graft (15). Up to 20% of patients require at least one readmission for wound care issues, usually associated with an operative incision. The majority of patients develop significant ipsilateral lymphedema, which, if left uncontrolled, retards incisional wound healing.

The vast majority of patients with salvaged limbs walk on them, in contrast to the poor postamputation mobility in the elderly (16). Early consultation with a vascular surgeon helps prevent progression to a necrotic forefoot lesion too advanced to heal despite revascularization and aggressive debridement. Such unfortunate delays are a common cause of limb loss.

Discharge Issues

Patients who survive an episode of acute limb ischemia are almost always suffering from a systemic, chronic disease. Patients with PAD are at high risk for cardiac and cerebrovascular events; they require aggressive cardiovascular risk factor modification programs and long-term antiplatelet therapy as for patients who have angina or who have survived a myocardial infarction (Chapters 37 and 38). In patients with

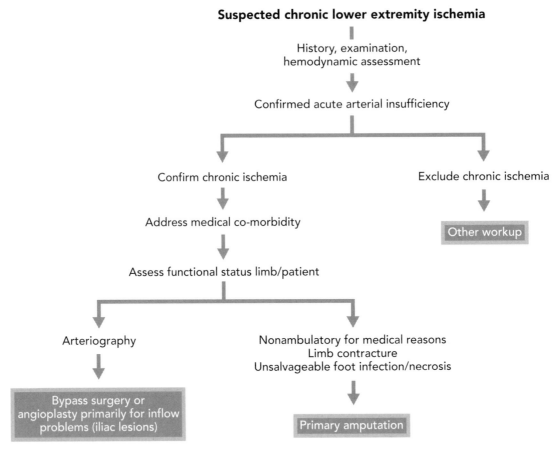

Suspected chronic lower extremity ischemia

History, examination,
hemodynamic assessment

Confirmed acute arterial insufficiency

Confirm chronic ischemia   Exclude chronic ischemia

Address medical co-morbidity   Other workup

Assess functional status limb/patient

Arteriography   Nonambulatory for medical reasons
                                Limb contracture
                                Unsalvageable foot infection/necrosis

Bypass surgery or
angioplasty primarily for inflow
problems (iliac lesions)   Primary amputation

Figure 51.2.   Algorithm for management of ischemic complications of peripheral arterial disease.

PAD who also have a history of myocardial infarction, acute coronary syndrome, or stroke, either aspirin or clopidogrel would be appropriate antiplatelet therapy. However, in patients with PAD who do not have other clinically evident cardiovascular disease, evidence supports clopidogrel as first-line therapy. Aggressive therapy of hyperlipidemia with statins is mandatory and can improve walking distance (17). Participation in a supervised exercise rehabilitation program is effective in improving claudication-limited exercise capacity. Management of any residual wounds, including amputation sites, is an important factor in long-term outcome. Referral to specialized wound care clinics may assist in management. Despite optimal care, however, the long-term prognosis for this population remains poor (2).

KEY POINTS

■ PAD presenting as critical leg ischemia may be the result of acute arterial ischemia or progression of chronic atherosclerotic PAD.

■ Initial management is focused on emergent vascular surgery consultation, identifying the level and type of arterial obstruction, assessing limb viability, and optimization of other comorbid disease processes (i.e., infection, congestive heart failure).

■ The goal of therapy is to preserve the affected limb and the patient's functional status.

■ Definitive therapy currently is guided primarily by the vascular surgeon's judgment and assessment because of the limited evidence from clinical trials.

■ Discharge planning must recognize the chronic nature of the underlying disease processes, and their impact on long-term morbidity and mortality rates.

■ Long-term outcome is critically dependent on treatment of the underlying systemic arterial pathophysiology, because most patients with PAD die from cardiac or cerebral events.

REFERENCES

1. Hirsch AT, Criqui MH, Treat-Jacobson D, et al. Peripheral arterial disease detection, awareness, and treatment in primary care. *JAMA* 2001;286:1317–1324.
2. Dormandy J, Heeck L, Vig S. The fate of patients with critical leg ischemia. *Sem Vasc Surg* 1999;12:142–147.
3. Ouriel K, Shortell CK, DeWeese JA, et al. A comparison of thrombolytic therapy with operative revascularization in the initial treatment of acute peripheral arterial ischemia. *J Vasc Surg* 1994; 19:1021–1030.
4. Ouriel K, Veith FJ, Sasahara AA. Thrombolysis or peripheral artery surgery: phase 1 results. TOPAS investigators. *J Vasc Surg* 1996; 23:64–75.

5. STILE investigators. Results of a prospective randomized trial evaluating surgery versus thrombolysis for ischemia of the lower extremity: the STILE trial. *Ann Surg* 1994;220:251–268.

6. Weaver FA, Comerota AJ, Youngblood M, et al. Surgical revascularization versus thrombolysis for nonembolic lower extremity native artery occlusions: results of a prospective randomized trial. The STILE Investigators. Surgery versus Thrombolysis for Ischemia of the Lower Extremity. *J Vasc Surg* 1996;24:513–523.

7. Ouriel K. Current status of thrombolysis for peripheral arterial occlusive disease. *Ann Vasc Surg* 2002;36:1104–1111.

8. Berridge DC, Kessel D, Robertson I. Surgery versus thrombolysis for acute limb ischemia: intial management. *Cochrane Database Syst Rev* 2002;CD002784.

9. Taylor LM, Edwards JM, Porter JM, et al. Present status of reversed vein bypass: five year results of a modern series. *J Vasc Surg* 1990; 11:193–205.

10. Gentile AT, Lee RW, Moneta GL, et al. Results of bypass to the popliteal and tibial arteries with alternative sources of autogenous vein. *J Vasc Surg* 1996;23:272–280.

11. Shah DM, Leather RP, Darling RC III, et al. Long-term results of using the in situ saphenous vein bypass. *Adv Surg* 1996;30: 123–140.

12. Harris RW, Andros G, Salles-Cunha SX, et al. Alternative autogenous vein grafts to the inadequate saphenous vein. *Surgery* 1986; 100:822–827.

13. Nehler MR, Moneta GL, Edwards JM, et al. Surgery for chronic lower extremity ischemia in patients eighty or more years of age:

operative results and assessment of postoperative independence. *J Vasc Surg* 1993;18:618–626.

14. Nicoloff AD, Taylor LM Jr, McLafferty RB, et al. Patient recovery after infrainguinal bypass grafting for limb salvage. *J Vasc Surg* 1998; 27:256–266.

15. Tretinyak AS, Lee ES, Kuskowski MN, et al. Revascularization and quality of life for patients with limb-threatening ischemia. *Ann Vasc Surg* 2001;15:84–88.

16. Harris KA, van Scie L, Carroll SE, et al. Rehabilitation potential of elderly patients with major amputations. *J Cardiovasc Surg* 1991; 32:463–467.

17. Mohler ER 3rd, Hiatt WR, Creager MA. Cholesterol reduction with atorvastatin improves walking distance in patients with peripheral arterial disease. *Circulation* 2003;108:1481–1486.

ADDITIONAL READING

Bittl JA, Hirsch AT. Concomitant peripheral arterial disease and coronary artery disease: therapeutic opportunities. *Circulation* 2004; 109:3136–3144.

McDermott MM, Liu K, Greenland P, et al. Functional decline in peripheral arterial disease: associations with the ankle brachial index and leg symptoms. *JAMA* 2004;292:453–461.

TASC Working Group. Management of peripheral arterial disease (PAD): TransAtlantic Inter-Society Consensus (TASC). *Eur J Vasc Endovasc Surg* 2000: 19(Suppl A): S1–S244.

Deep Venous Thrombosis

52

David A. Garcia   Mark A. Crowther

INTRODUCTION

Recent advances in the management of acute deep venous thrombosis (DVT) and pulmonary embolism (PE) have revolutionized the treatment of these common clinical problems. Two such advances are the demonstration that more than 90% of patients with acute venous thrombosis can be managed safely and effectively as outpatients (1) and the development and validation of diagnostic algorithms, which reduce practice variations and eliminate unnecessary diagnostic testing.

Traditionally, patients with acute venous thrombosis (including DVT and PE) have been admitted to the hospital for treatment with intravenous unfractionated heparin (UFH) for two reasons. First, it was felt that these patients required careful clinical monitoring to allow immediate treatment of PE, which could be fatal. Second, intravenous UFH requires laboratory monitoring. Outpatient treatment of DVT was made possible by the realization that most patients with acute DVT do not require in-hospital clinical monitoring and by the introduction of the low-molecular-weight heparins, which do not require laboratory monitoring of their anticoagulant effect.

The primary concerns of the physician treating patients with proven, acute proximal DVT are to triage those patients who require hospital admission and to arrange outpatient treatment for those who do not. DVT should no longer be the sole reason for admission to the hospital, except in selected circumstances (Table 52.1).

Although there is considerable overlap between the syndromes of DVT and PE, this chapter focuses on the diagnosis and treatment of patients with proximal DVT. PE is covered in Chapter 53.

WHEN THE DISEASE PRESENTS ON ADMISSION

Issues at the Time of Admission

In all cases, the diagnosis of acute DVT should be verified by an objective test. Although the gold standard for diagnosis remains contrast venography, this test is rarely needed. Rather, the diagnosis can usually be made with ultrasonography. In many symptomatic patients, compression ultrasound of the proximal venous system of the leg (or arm) reveals noncompressibility of a venous segment. This finding, in the setting of typical clinical signs and symptoms, has a specificity of 97% for acute DVT. A variety of other noninvasive testing methods, such as impedance plethysmography (IPG), thermography, and hand-held Doppler flow meters, lack sufficient sensitivity to reliably diagnose acute DVT. The use of contrast CT scanning to examine the legs for DVT ("CT venography") is generally confined to situations in which a spiral CT of the chest is being performed for suspected PE. It is further described in Chapter 53.

Recently, the use of both whole-blood and plasma D-dimer assays has been studied as an aid to the diagnosis of acute DVT (2, 3). D-dimer, which is a byproduct of fibrinolysis, is elevated in patients with active thrombosis. However, D-dimer levels also are elevated in the postoperative period, and in patients with malignancy, pregnancy, or septicemia. D-dimer levels can be assayed using a variety of techniques: plasma-based latex or enzyme-linked immunosorbent assays (ELISA), which quantify D-dimer levels, and whole-blood (bedside) assays, which are semiquantitative. Large prospective clinical evaluations have shown that a whole-blood D-dimer assay (the

TABLE 52.1

FACTORS THAT MAY PRECLUDE (OR COMPLICATE) OUTPATIENT DVT TREATMENT

The patient has
- renal insufficiency (calculated creatinine clearance <30 ml/min)
- hemodynamically apparent pulmonary embolism
- severe pain requiring parenteral opiates
- increased risk of bleeding

A system to monitor INR every 2–3 days is not available.

SimpliRED D-dimer) has a sensitivity of about 93% and a negative predictive value of 98% for proximal DVT. The specificity of the test, however, is only about 77%, because disorders other than acute DVT and PE can cause elevated D-dimer levels. Quantifying D-dimer levels using ELISA-based assays increases the sensitivity of the test but, in most cases, decreases its specificity (4). Clinicians must become familiar with the characteristics of the particular assay available at their institution, since reliance on an insensitive D-dimer could result in the inappropriate exclusion of deep vein thrombosis, placing patients at risk for pulmonary embolism (see also Chapter 53).

When evaluating a patient with possible acute DVT, the use of a clinical decision model can help determine which diagnostic tests to perform. Based on the history and clinical examination, the pretest probability of DVT can be reliably determined (Table 52.2). In a study by Wells et al., patients presenting with suspected DVT were evaluated using a validated pretest probability model. Subsequently, DVT was objectively confirmed in 5% of patients with a low pretest probability, 33% of patients with an intermediate probability, and 85% of those with a high pretest probability.

Translation of the study results into clinical practice will simplify the approach to patients with suspected DVT (Figure 52.1). Patients with a *low pretest probability* can be screened with a clinically tested D-dimer assay. A negative result rules out the diagnosis of proximal DVT (negative predictive value >99%) (5). Patients with an *intermediate* or *high pretest probability* should undergo an objective test, either a compression ultrasound or, if that is unavailable, a venogram. If the patient has a moderate or high pretest probability of DVT and negative compression ultrasound, a validated D-dimer assay should then be performed to rule out the possibility of extending calf vein thrombosis not detected by the ultrasound. If the D-dimer test is also negative, DVT can be excluded and anticoagulaton safely withheld. If the D-dimer is positive, further testing with either serial compression ultrasonography or venography must be performed.

Once the diagnosis of acute DVT has been confirmed objectively, a decision regarding hospital admission should be made. Patients with evidence of a hemodynamically significant PE should be admitted to the hospital. All patients

should be assessed for bleeding risk. Initial laboratory investigations should include a hemoglobin and platelet count. Although routinely performed, an activated partial thromboplastin time (aPTT) or international normalized ratio (INR) value is not required in otherwise well patients without a history of clinically significant bleeding. Patients who are admitted with acute DVT should be treated with

TABLE 52.2

ASSESSING THE PROBABILITY OF DEEP VENOUS THROMBOSIS BASED ON THE CLINICAL PRESENTATION

Major points

Active cancer
Paralysis, paresis, or recent plaster cast immobilization of the lower limb
Recently bed-ridden >3 d or major surgery within 4 wk
Localized tenderness along the distribution of the deep venous system
Thigh and calf swollen
Calf swelling 3 cm >symptomless side
More than two 1st-degree relatives with history of objectively documented deep venous thrombosis

Minor points

History of trauma (within 60 d) to the affected leg
Pitting edema in the symptomatic leg only
Dilated superficial veins in the symptomatic leg only
Hospitalization within the previous 6 mo
Erythema

Clinical probability

High

≥3 major points and no alternative diagnosis
≥2 major points and ≥2 minor points and no alternative diagnosis

Low

1 major point + 2 minor points + alternative diagnosis
1 major point + 1 minor point + no alternative diagnosis
0 major points + 3 minor points + alternative diagnosis
0 major points + 2 minor points + no alternative diagnosis

Moderate

All other combinations

Clinical pretest probability	Number of patients evaluated	Number of patients with deep venous thrombosis (%)	95% confidence interval
High	85	72 (85)	75%–92%
Moderate	143	47 (33)	25%–41%
Low	301	16 (5)	3–8.5%

Modified from Wells PS, Hirsh J, Anderson DR, et al. Accuracy of clinical assessment of deep-vein thrombosis. *Lancet* 1995;345:1326–1330, with permission.

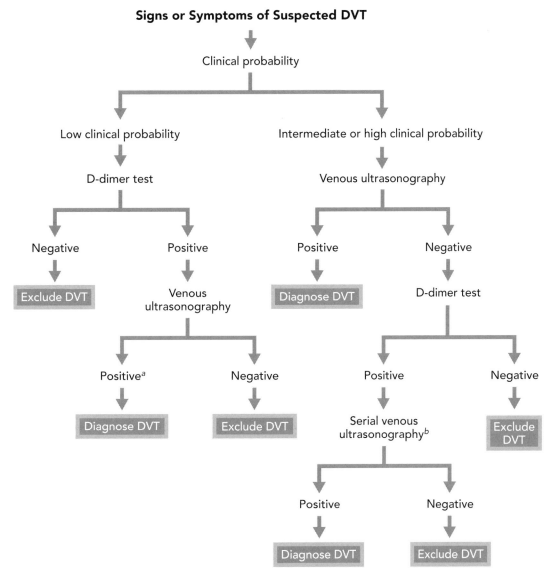

Figure 52.1 Algorithm for patient with suspected deep venous thrombosis. *DVT,* deep venous thrombosis. Clinical probabilities are drawn from Table 52.2. [a]Re-evaluate history and review ultrasound for features suggestive of old rather than new thrombosis. If ultrasound findings are inconclusive, venography should be considered. [b]In patients with a high clinical probability or those who cannot return for serial ultrasonography, venography is recommended. Venography can also be considered in patients with cardiorespiratory compromise. (Reproduced from Hirsh J, Lee AY. How we diagnose and treat deep vein thrombosis. *Blood* 2002; 99:3102–3110, with permission.)

either unmonitored, weight-adjusted subcutaneous low-molecular-weight heparin or intravenous UFH monitored using the aPTT. Intravenous UFH is preferred in patients with acute DVT or PE at high risk for bleeding because once the infusion of UFH is discontinued, the majority of its anticoagulant effect is lost within 2 hours, whereas the anticoagulant effect of subcutaneous low-molecular-weight heparin persists for up to 24 hours. Furthermore, the anticoagulant effect of unfractionated heparin can be rapidly reversed with protamine sulfate; protamine sulfate cannot neutralize all of the anticoagulant effect of low-molecular-weight heparin.

If the patient is younger than 65 and does not have a risk factor for DVT (e.g., recent surgery, immobilization, or malignancy), screening for a hypercoagulable state should be considered (see Table 98.6 for a standard laboratory workup). This can be done either before anticoagulation is initiated or after it is completed. Testing for a hypercoagulable state while the patient is receiving therapy is problematic: heparin lowers antithrombin levels and may interfere with testing for both activated protein C resistance and the lupus anticoagulant; warfarin lowers the plasma levels of proteins C and S and may interfere with testing for both activated protein C resistance and the lupus anticoagulant.

Appropriate screening tests are discussed subsequently, and a more extensive discussion of hypercoagulable states is found in Chapter 98.

Issues During the Course of Hospitalization

All patients who are proven to have acute DVT and who do not have a contraindication to anticoagulation should be treated with therapeutic unfractionated or low-molecular-weight heparin beginning at diagnosis. Hospitalized patients should receive an initial bolus of UFH followed by a continuous infusion of UFH adjusted to maintain the anti-Xa heparin level in a range of 0.35–0.70 units/mL. Because heparin levels are not widely available, most laboratories have published aPTT values that correspond to this anti-Xa range. Studies have demonstrated that the use of a weight-based heparin nomogram improves outcomes and decreases complications (Table 53.2). Outpatients or inpatients at low risk for bleeding may be treated with one of the commercially available low-molecular-weight heparins. Monitoring of the anticoagulant effect of low-molecular-weight heparins is unnecessary in the majority of patients with acute DVT or PE. Dose adjustment or monitoring of anti-Xa levels may be advisable in patients with renal failure, those with significant obesity (>150 kg), and pregnant patients. The published experience using low-molecular-weight heparins for such patients is limited because they have been excluded from most clinical trials evaluating low-molecular-weight heparins (6).

Warfarin should be initiated on the day of diagnosis, after heparin has been started. Warfarin "loading doses" (e.g., 10 mg on the first 2 days of treatment) can be associated with early overanticoagulation. For most patients (including the elderly or those with significant co-morbidities), warfarin is best initiated at a dose likely to be required for maintenance (usually around 5 mg/d) (7). (Chapter 53 for a warfarin nomogram [Table 53.3] and a list of warfarin drug interactions [Table 53.5].) A higher initial warfarin dose may be appropriate for otherwise healthy, young outpatients (8). The heparin should not be discontinued until the INR has stabilized between 2.0 and 3.0 on 2 consecutive days, and heparin has been administered for a minimum of 4–5 days.

Patients may present with, or develop, unusual manifestations of thromboembolism. Patients with DVT of the renal veins, inferior vena cava, cerebral veins, portal vein, or in the upper venous circulation should be treated similarly to those with proximal DVT in the leg. Patients with mesenteric vein thrombosis often have associated ischemic bowel, which may require surgical removal. Hepatic vein thrombosis (Budd–Chiari syndrome) is a potentially life-threatening condition for which optimal therapy is unknown. All patients with these unusual thrombi should be screened for a hypercoagulable state (Chapter 98). Occasionally, pa-

TABLE 52.3

OPTIMAL DURATION OF WARFARIN ANTICOAGULATION IN PATIENTS WITH DEEP VENOUS THROMBOSIS

	Target INR	Duration
Calf DVT (i.e. does not involve veins proximal to the popliteal fossa)	2.0–3.0	Minimum: 6 wk; maximum: 12wk[a]
Transient risk factor that now is resolved, e.g., thrombosis after arthroscopy	2.0–3.0	Minimum: 6 wk; maximum: 12wk
Transient risk factor that is persistent, e.g., thrombosis with current plaster-cast immobilization, pregnancy	2.0–3.0	Continue for 6 wk after risk factor resolved
Thrombosis with malignancy	2.0–3.0	Indefinite anticoagulation[b]
Idiopathic thrombosis, i.e. thrombosis with no identified precipitant	2.0–3.0	≥6months anticoagulation Discuss risks and benefits of extended anticoagulation with patient
Recurrent idiopathic thrombosis occurring off anticoagulants, e.g., thrombosis in patient with previous episode of DVT/PE	2.0–3.0	Life-long anticoagulation
Recurrent thrombosis occurring while on anticoagulants, e.g. new DVT or PE in patient therapeutically anticoagulated with warfarin	LMWH, or warfarin with target INR >3.0	Life-long anticoagulation; consider placement of IVC filter

[a] If anticoagulation withheld, serial noninvasive studies should be performed over 7–14 days to ensure thrombus has not extended to involve proximal veins.
[b] Consider prolonged monotherapy with LMWH instead of warfarin (9).
DVT, deep venous thrombosis; INR, international normalized ratio; IVC, inferior vena cava; LMWH, low-molecular-weight heparin; PE, pulmonary embolism.

tients present with venous gangrene caused by a large proximal DVT. In such cases, thrombolytic therapy or catheter-directed therapy may be used to acutely reduce the venous outflow obstruction. There is no high quality evidence, however, that thrombolytics or cathether-directed techniques provide long-term benefit beyond those obtained with heparin (either low-molecular-weight or unfractionated) and warfarin.

The management of patients with a contraindication to anticoagulant therapy is more difficult. Patients with acute DVT of the leg and such a contraindication should have an inferior vena cava (IVC) filter placed, because IVC filters substantially reduce the short-term risk of PE. However, a randomized controlled trial found that IVC filters do not improve long-term survival, and that permanent IVC filters increase the risk of recurrent thrombosis nearly twofold in the 2 years following their placement (10). Patients with IVC filters frequently experience worsening of their leg symptoms, secondary to proximal extension of their thrombus. Therefore, if the contraindication to anticoagulation is transient (such as temporary thrombocytopenia secondary to chemotherapy or gastrointestinal bleeding from a reversible lesion), patients with filters should be anticoagulated as soon as possible to reduce the severity of their leg symptoms. "Temporary" removeable IVC filter devices may offer short-term protection from pulmonary embolism without increasing the long-term risk of recurrent DVT. Although not well studied, such devices are now available in many centers.

It is controversial whether *upper-circulation deep vein thrombi* can cause clinically important PE; traditional teaching is that they cannot. It is clear, however, that children with upper-extremity thrombosis do suffer PE and other complications such as post-phlebitic syndrome (Figure 52.2). The rate of these complications in adults is unknown but sufficiently high that patients should be treated as for lower-extremity DVT. In our opinion, extended duration therapeutic anticoagulation should be given to patients with involvement of deep, proximal (e.g. axillary, subclavian, internal jugular) veins. The optimal management of patients with upper-circulation DVT and a contraindication to anticoagulation (a scenario found frequently in oncology patients with indwelling central venous catheters) is unclear. Our practice is to either simply observe the patient closely without treatment or treat with prophylactic doses of low-molecular-weight heparin after discussing the risks of thromboembolism and hemorrhage with the patient.

During the course of hospitalization, the patient should be monitored for bleeding and for the development of *heparin-induced thrombocytopenia* (HIT). HIT is a potentially devastating complication and should be considered if the platelet count drops below normal (or by more than 50% from baseline), or if the patient develops recurrent thrombosis (arterial or venous) despite heparin therapy. The management of HIT is discussed in Chapter 98.

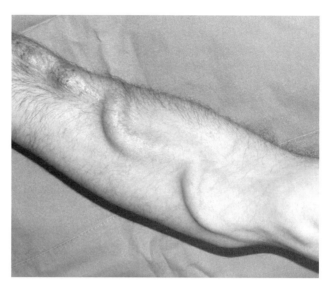

Figure 52.2 This upper-extremity thrombosis was associated with an AV fistula used for hemodialysis. While hospitalized and receiving IV unfractionated heparin, this patient died suddenly, seconds after reporting that his fistula had started working again. Autopsy showed the cause of death to be pulmonary embolism.

Bleeding is a common complication of anticoagulant therapy, occuring in 2%–5% of patients who are therapeutically anticoagulated. The risk of bleeding is highest during the initial days of heparin therapy. Bleeding can be managed by withdrawing heparin and, if acute neutralization is required, by the use of protamine sulfate. Bleeding in patients receiving warfarin usually can be controlled by mechanical means (such as pressure). If rapid reversal of warfarin's anticoagulant effect is required, intravenous vitamin K (1 or 2 mg) is effective. If immediate reversal is required, frozen human plasma or coagulation factor concentrates should be administered in concert with intravenous vitamin K. Recombinant factor VIIa may stop bleeding in patients receiving warfarin who present with major or life-threatening hemorrhage. However, this therapy is expensive and has not been well studied (11).

Discharge Issues

At the time of discharge, the patient should be advised to avoid situations that might precipitate bleeding. In addition, arrangements should be made for outpatient monitoring of the INR. Initially this should be performed frequently (i.e., every 2–4 days). The interval can be increased to as little as once per month once the patient has stable INR values. The target INR value for all patients with acute DVT or PE should be 2.0–3.0. The optimal duration of anticoagulant therapy varies as a function of the suspected cause of the DVT; common scenarios are shown in Table 52.3.

For patients who present with DVT without an identified precipitant, the ideal duration of anticoagulant therapy is controversial. These patients have a high risk of recurrent thrombosis (15%–30% 2-year risk of recurrence) if their warfarin is stopped after 3 months of treatment. Although warfarin is very effective at preventing a DVT while patients are taking the drug, prolonged warfarin therapy does not appear to confer any long-term protection against recurrent DVT after anticoagulation is discontinued (12). It has been proposed that patients with an unprovoked DVT will benefit from lowering the target INR range (to 1.5–2.0) after 3–6 months of "full-dose" anticoagulation. There are now two randomized, controlled studies confirming that "low-intensity" warfarin provides substantial protection against recurrent venous thromboembolism (13, 14). Surprisingly, there is no evidence from these trials to support the hypothesis that reducing the target INR will decrease the risk of major hemorrhage among chronically anticoagulated patients. For now, it is our recommendation that all patients who have a DVT without an identified precipitant should be maintained on warfarin (target INR range 2.0–3.0) for at least 6 months. Patients who have had more than one DVT without an identified precipitant should likely receive indefinite conventional-intensity (target INR 2.0– 3.0) anticoagulation. In many cases, a discussion with the patient about the risks and benefits of anticoagulation is invaluable.

The most common acquired conditions that predispose to DVT are antiphospholipid antibodies (lupus anticoagulant or anticardiolipin antibody) and malignancy. Current evidence suggests that patients with DVT and convincing evidence of antiphospholipid antibodies are best treated with indefinite duration warfarin administered to achieve an INR of 2.0–3.0 (15). One in 10 patients presenting with idiopathic DVT is found to have a malignancy within 12–18 months of follow-up. Although some authors have recommended aggressive investigation for malignancy in patients presenting with a single, acute idiopathic DVT or PE, there is no evidence that such investigations improve the outcome of these patients. For patients who present with recurrent thrombosis, particularly in the face of therapeutic anticoagulation, the clinician should perform a thorough review of systems and physical exam, with special attention to signs and symptoms that could be attributed to malignancy. Classically, carcinoma of the pancreas, breast, prostate, or bowel are associated with DVT, although DVT (and unusual complications such as migratory superficial thrombophlebitis) can accompany any type of malignancy.

The decision to screen a patient for an inherited or acquired hypercoagulable state (Table 98.5) should be made only if it is clear that the results of the testing will influence clinical management. Because the presence of a hypercoagulable state might influence the duration of anticoagulant therapy and subsequent decisions about medication use, screening of patients with idiopathic DVT is often indicated, although screening of asymptomatic populations and patients with known risk factors is not. Evidence-based strategies for screening and counseling are currently being developed.

The major long-term complication of DVT is the *postphlebitic syndrome*. This syndrome, which is caused by ele-vated venous pressure in the deep veins of the leg as a result of destruction of the venous valves by the thrombus, is associated with leg pain and swelling (particularly after prolonged standing) and, occasionally, venous stasis ulceration. Graduated compression stockings improve patient symptoms and may reduce the risk of ulcers (16). Physical activity improves symptoms in many patients, presumably by increasing venous outflow from the leg. Although the risk of post-phlebitic syndrome was once thought to be as high as 30%–50%, evidence now suggests the risk of severe post-phlebitic syndrome is less than 10%.

WHEN THE DISEASE PRESENTS DURING HOSPITALIZATION

Acute DVT is frequently found in already-hospitalized patients. Typically, inpatients with new DVTs present with leg (or arm) swelling that cannot be explained by their clinical conditions. Risk factors include immobilization, recent surgery (particularly orthopedic surgery), the presence of malignancy, major trauma, chemotherapy, or overwhelming infections. The incidence of DVT among hospitalized patients may be reduced if clinicians employ one of a variety of effective prevention strategies (17) (Table 52.4). For patients undergoing major orthopedic surgery, an indirect factor Xa inhibitor, fondaparinux, has been recently added to the options for thromboprophylaxis (18).

Certain groups of hospital patients are at such high risk of DVT that routine surveillance for DVT has been recommended; for example, in some centers patients who undergo orthopedic surgery on the legs are screened routinely at discharge for DVT. These patients do not require predischarge screening if they receive adequate antithrombotic prophylaxis (Table 52.4). Recent studies suggest that 28–35 days of thromboprophylaxis (with either low-molecular-weight heparin, fondaparinux, or therapeutic dose warfarin) is more effective in reducing the risk of VTE than 7–10 days of prophylaxis in patients with high risk of DVT, such as those who have had total joint arthroplasty or repair of a fractured hip (19–22).

Diagnostic testing options in symptomatic inpatients are similar to those available for outpatients. Compression ultrasound is the diagnostic test of choice. If the clinical suspicion is high and the ultrasound is normal, either serial ultrasonography or venography should be performed. The D-dimer (previously discussed) has not been well studied in inpatients. This test is likely to be less useful in this population because many inpatients have conditions that elevate plasma D-dimer levels (e.g., recent surgery, malignancy, infection).

Issues During the Course of Hospitalization

The clinical course of patients who have acute DVT that develops during hospitalization is primarily dependent upon their underlying conditions. Treatment with unfractionated or low-molecular-weight heparin should be initi-

TABLE 52.4

EVIDENCE-BASED STRATEGIES TO PREVENT DEEP VENOUS THROMBOSIS AND PULMONARY EMBOLISM IN HOSPITALIZED PATIENTS

Group	Subgroup	Level of risk	Effective strategies[a]
Surgical patients	General surgery[b]	Low risk (<40 y of age, minor operations, no clinical risk factors)	No prophylaxis other than early ambulation and possibly compression stockings
	General surgery	Moderate (>40 y of age, major surgery, but no additional clinical risk factors for DVT/PE)	LDUH, LMWH, IPC, or ES
	General surgery	Higher risk (>40 y of age, major surgery, and with additional clinical risk factors for DVT/PE)	LDUH or higher-dose LMWH; if prone to wound complications (e.g., hematoma or infection), IPC is a good alternative
	General surgery	Very high risk[c] (multiple risk factors for DVT/PE)	LDUH or LMWH and IPC; in selected patients postoperative warfarin (target INR of 2–3)
	Elective hip replacement[c]		Fondaparinux (started 8–10 h after surgery), LMWH (started 12–24 h after surgery) or warfarin (INR 2–3; started preoperatively or immediately after surgery)[d], or adjusted-dose heparin started preoperatively; adjuvant prophylaxis with ES or IPC may provide additional efficacy
	Elective knee replacement		Fondaparinux (started 8–10 hours after surgery), LMWH or warfarin or IPC
	Hip-fracture surgery[c]		Fondaparinux (started 8–10 hours after surgery), preoperative LMWH, or warfarin (INR 2–3, started perioperatively or immediately after surgery)
	Intracranial neurosurgery		IPC with or without ES; LMWH or LDUH may be acceptable alternatives; in high-risk patients, combining a physical modality (IPC or ES) and pharmacologic modality (LMWH or LDUH) may be more effective
	Acute spinal-cord injury		LMWH; ES and IPC may be added to LMWH; note that LDUH, ES, and IPC are ineffective if used alone
	Trauma	With risk factors for DVT/PE	LMWH if no contraindication; consider IPC if LMWH delayed or contraindicated; consider IVC filter if patient at high risk for DVT/PE and unable to receive optimal prophylaxis
Medical conditions	Myocardial infarction		LDUH (full anticoagulation is also effective); IPC and possibly ES may be useful if heparin contraindicated
	Ischemic stroke and lower-extremity paralysis		LDUH or LMWH are effective; IPC and ES are probably effective
	General medical patients	With risk factors for DVT/PE (especially congestive heart failure or pulmonary infection)	LDUH or LMWH (Fondaparinux may be effective but has not been approved for this indication by regulatory bodies)

[a] In patients having a spinal puncture or an epidural catheter placed, LMWH should be used with caution.
[b] Aspirin is not recommended for prophylaxis in general surgery patients because other methods (shown in table) are more effective.
[c] Consider extended anticoagulation (29- to 35-d) based on studies demonstrating a reduced risk of thrombosis.
[d] Optimal duration of LMWH or warfarin prophylaxis is uncertain. At least 7–10 d is mandatory; emerging data suggest that a 29- to 35-d duration of LMWH offers additional protection.
adjusted-dose heparin, 3,500 U unfractionated heparin given subcutaneously q8 h, with postoperative dose adjustments by ±500 U to maintain aPTT at high-normal values; *aPTT,* activated partial thromboplastin time; *ES,* elastic stockings; *higher-dose LMWH,* enoxaparin 4,000 U qd or 3,000 U bid, or its equivalent; *INR,* international normalized ratio; *IPC,* intermittent pneumatic compression; *IVC,* inferior vena cava; *LDUH,* low-dose unfractionated heparin (5,000 U q8–12 h); *LMWH,* low-molecular-weight heparin at standard doses (e.g., enoxaparin 2,000 U qd or its equivalent.)

ated, and the patient should be started on warfarin the same day. Heparin (or low-molecular-weight heparin) then should be discontinued 48 hours after the INR has risen to a level between 2.0 and 3.0, provided the patient has received heparin for a minimum of 4 days. Patients

usually begin to notice reduced pain and swelling in their leg within 48 hours of starting the intravenous heparin. Some patients, however, have prolonged symptoms that may persist for months after the diagnosis of DVT. Occasionally patients (particularly those with malignancy or those who develop heparin-induced thrombocytopenia) develop severely impaired venous outflow from the leg with associated venous gangrene. A variety of different interventional techniques have been employed in these patients, including venous angioplasty and catheter-directed clot lysis. However, none of these interventions has been studied in a methodologically rigorous manner. Some patients, particularly those with malignancy and those with disseminated intravascular coagulation, may develop DVT in the setting of thrombocytopenia. In such cases, it generally is safe to anticoagulate the patient if his or her platelet count is more than 50,000/mL. Patients with DVT and platelet counts less than 30,000/mL should have a removeable IVC filter placed if possible. Occasionally patients are found to have an asymptomatic DVT discovered during an ultrasound performed for other reasons. In general, all deep vein thrombi proximal to the knee or involving the deep circulation of the arm should be treated, irrespective of whether they produce symptoms. The incidentally discovered calf vein thrombosis is more problematic; either serial evaluation for proximal extension using ultrasonography or treatment with heparin and an abbreviated course of warfarin is probably adequate. Patients who develop DVT or PE as inpatients, but who are otherwise eligible for discharge, can be discharged on outpatient low-molecular-weight heparin and treated as described previously.

Superficial phlebitis is a commonly encountered clinical problem. Although it can occur in any superficial vein, it is most commonly encountered in the long saphenous vein of the leg. Superficial phlebitis is usually a self-limiting disease responding to conservative treatment with anti-inflammatory medications. Up to 15% of patients with extensive superficial phlebitis have a DVT on objective testing. Such patients should be treated for their DVTs, as discussed previously. Patients who have less extensive superficial phlebitis, or those with extensive phlebitis who do not have DVT on objective testing, often benefit from a short course (5–7 days) of low-dose subcutaneous UFH (5,000–12,500 units subcutaneously twice daily), which the patient can self-administer at home. Subsequently, patients can be managed in most cases with anti-inflammatory medications. Recalcitrant or recurrent superficial phlebitis (particularly superficial phlebitis that recurs in patients who are therapeutically anticoagulated) can be a manifestation of underlying malignancy.

Catheter-related thrombosis is encountered with increasing frequency. Most commonly encountered in the upper extremity, catheter-related thrombosis presents with either arm or neck swelling, signs of impaired venous outflow, or catheter occlusion. Treatment is controversial; in particular, it is unknown whether a functioning catheter should be removed. Treatment with UFH or low-molecular-weight heparin and warfarin is usually administered to prevent proximal extension of the clot, superior vena cava syndrome, PE, and worsening of clinical symptoms. If the thrombus is not causing clinical symptoms but is associ-

ated with dysfunction of the catheter, it can be cleared in some cases with the local installation of thrombolytic medication. If the catheter cannot be removed, treatment with therapeutic doses of UFH or low-molecular-weight heparin and warfarin may reduce symptoms. Although systemic thrombolytic therapy has been employed in such patients (Chapter 98), its use cannot be recommended, because there are no rigorous studies demonstrating its utility. At least one systematic review suggests the risk of catheter-associated thrombosis can be reduced by either prophylactic dose low-molecular-weight heparin or warfarin. However, the quality of available evidence is "fair" at best.

Septic thrombophlebitis is an uncommon clinical problem, and there is no consensus regarding its management. When deep veins are involved, treatment with therapeutic doses of low-molecular-weight heparin or UFH followed by warfarin is appropriate. Antibiotics should be administered, and the patient followed for evidence of septic embolization. Although both surgical removal of thrombus and thrombolytic therapy have been used in selected patients, their use as initial therapy in uncomplicated cases cannot be endorsed in the absence of appropriate studies demonstrating benefit.

Discharge Issues

All patients with symptomatic DVT should be discharged on warfarin unless they have completed a full treatment course in the hospital. The INR value should be maintained between 2.0 and 3.0, and arrangements should be made for monitoring as often as every 2–3 days for a short time after hospital discharge. Patients should be educated at the time of discharge (or soon thereafter) about precautions relevant to warfarin therapy and signs of bleeding or recurrent thrombosis. The optimal duration of anticoagulation is described in Table 52.3.

COST CONSIDERATIONS AND RESOURCE USE

Outpatient treatment of acute DVT substantially reduces the cost of treating this disorder. The vast majority of patients (more than 90% in our experience) can be successfully treated as outpatients. Further cost savings, without compromised patient care, could be realized by judicious use of a diagnostic strategy employing clinically tested D-dimer assays in patients who have a low pretest probability of DVT.

The treatment course of heparin should not be shortened to less than 4 days. However, patients frequently require heparin therapy for more than 5 days because of difficulties achieving adequate initial anticoagulation with warfarin. The proportion of patients who achieve a therapeutic aPTT within 2 days and a therapeutic INR value within 5 days can be increased with the use of validated heparin and warfarin initiation nomograms, respectively (Chapter 53).

KEY POINTS

- Patients presenting with suspected acute DVT should have the diagnosis confirmed by objective testing.
- Once the diagnosis of DVT has been confirmed, the majority of patients can be treated as outpatients with low molecular weight heparin, although patients with comorbid conditions or those with symptomatic PE should be admitted to the hospital.
- Inpatients should be treated with intravenous UFH with frequent monitoring of the aPTT, or with unmonitored, weight-adjusted subcutaneous low molecular weight heparin.
- The duration of anticoagulant therapy should be individualized based on the cause of the patient's DVT.
- The anticoagulant effect of warfarin should be monitored closely throughout the treatment course (see Chapter 53 for drug interactions).
- Patients who have had a previous DVT or PE have a lifelong increased risk of having a second event and should thus monitor themselves closely for symptoms suggesting recurrence.
- Hospitalized patients, particularly those with hip fractures or who have undergone orthopedic surgery, are at high risk for acute DVT and PE. Patients at risk should receive prophylaxis with one of several effective pharamacologic or nonpharmacologic modalities (Table 52.4).
- Extending prophylaxis for 3–6 weeks after surgery should be considered in all patients who have undergone major orthopedic surgery on their legs.

REFERENCES

1. Hyers TM, Agnelli G, Hull RD, et al. Antithrombotic therapy for venous thromboembolic disease. *Chest* 2001;119:176S–193S.
2. Kearon C, Ginsberg JS, Douketis J, et al. Management of suspected deep venous thrombosis in outpatients by using clinical assessment and D-dimer testing. *Ann Intern Med* 2001;135: 108–111.
3. Tamariz LJ, Eng J, Segal JB , et al. Usefulness of clinical prediction rules for the diagnosis of venous thromboembolism: a systematic review. *Am J Med* 2004;117:676–684.
4. Van der Graaf F, van den Borne H, van der Kolk M, et al. Exclusion of deep venous thrombosis with D-dimer testing—comparison of 13 D-dimer methods in 99 outpatients suspected of deep venous thrombosis using venography as reference standard. *Thrombosis & Haemostasis* 2000;83:191–198.
5. Wells PS, Anderson DR, Rodger M, et al. Evaluation of D-dimer in the diagnosis of suspected deep-vein thrombosis. *N Engl J Med* 2003;349:1227–1235.
6. Hirsh J, Warkentin TE, Shaughnessy SG, et al. Heparin and low-molecular-weight heparin: mechanisms of action, pharmacokinetics, dosing, monitoring, efficacy, and safety. *Chest* 2001; 119:64S–94S.
7. Crowther MA, Ginsberg JB, Kearon C, et al. A randomized trial comparing 5-mg and 10-mg warfarin loading doses. *Arch Intern Med* 1999;159:46–48.
8. Kovacs MJ, Rodger M, Anderson DR, et al. Comparison of 10-mg and 5-mg warfarin initiation nomograms together with low-molecular-weight heparin for outpatient treatment of acute

venous thromboembolism. A randomized, double-blind, controlled trial. *Ann Intern Med* 2003; 138:714–719.
9. Lee AY, Levine MN, Baker RI, et al. Randomized comparison of low-molecular-weight heparin versus a coumarin for the prevention of recurrent venous thromboembolism in patients with cancer. *N Engl J Med* 2003;349:146–153.
10. Decousus H, Leizorovicz A, Parent F, et al. A clinical trial of vena caval filters in the prevention of pulmonary embolism in patients with proximal deep-vein thrombosis. Prevention du risque d'embolie pulmonaire par interruption cave study group. *N Engl J Med* 1998;338:409–415.
11. Deveras RA, Kessler CM. Reversal of warfarin-induced excessive anticoagulation with recombinant human factor VIIa concentrate. *Ann Intern Med* 2002;137:884–888.
12. Agnelli G, Prandoni P, Santamaria MG, et al. Three months versus one year of oral anticoagulant therapy for idiopathic deep venous thrombosis. Warfarin Optimal Duration Italian Trial Investigators. *N Engl J Med* 2001;345:165–169.
13. Kearon C, Ginsberg JS, Kovacs MJ, et al. Comparison of low-intensity warfarin therapy with conventional-intensity warfarin therapy for long-term prevention of recurrent venous thromboembolism. *N Engl J Med* 2003;349:631–639.
14. Ridker PM, Goldhaber SZ, Danielson E, et al. Long-term, low-intensity warfarin therapy for the prevention of recurrent venous thromboembolism. *N Engl J Med* 2003;348:1425–1434.
15. Crowther MA, Ginsberg JS, Julian J, et al. A comparison of two intensities of warfarin for the prevention of recurrent thrombosis in patients with the antiphospholipid antibody syndrome. *N Engl J Med* 2003;349:1133–1138.
16. Kahn SR, Ginsberg JS. Relationship between deep venous thrombosis and the postthrombotic syndrome. *Arch Intern Med* 2004; 164:17–26.
17. Geerts WH, Heit JA, Clagett GP, et al. Prevention of venous thromboembolism. *Chest* 2001;119:132S–175S.
18. Turpie AG, Bauer KA, Eriksson BI, et al. Fondaparinux vs enoxaparin for the prevention of venous thromboembolism in major orthopedic surgery: a meta-analysis of 4 randomized double-blind studies. *Arch Intern Med* 2002;162:1833–1840.
19. Prandoni P, Bruchi O, Sabbion P, et al. Prolonged thromboprophylaxis with oral anticoagulants after total hip arthroplasty: a prospective controlled randomized study. *Arch Intern Med* 2002;162:1966–1971.
20. Hull RD, Pineo GF, Stein PD, et al. Extended out-of-hospital low-molecular-weight heparin prophylaxis against deep venous thrombosis in patients after elective hip arthroplasty: a systematic review. *Ann Intern Med* 2001;135:858–869.
21. Bergqvist D, Agnelli G, Cohen AT, et al. Duration of prophylaxis against venous thromboembolism with enoxaparin after surgery for cancer. *N Engl J Med* 2002;346:975–980.
22. Eriksson BI, Lassen MR. Duration of prophylaxis against venous thromboembolism with fondaparinux after hip fracture surgery: a multicenter, randomized, placebo-controlled, double-blind study. *Arch Intern Med* 2003;163:1337–1342.
23. Klerk CP, Smorenburg SM, Buller HR. Thrombosis prophylaxis in patient populations with a central venous catheter: a systematic review. *Arch Intern Med* 2003;163:1913–1921.

ADDITIONAL READING

Hirsh J, Lee AY. How we diagnose and treat deep vein thrombosis. *Blood* 2002;99:3102–3110.
Hutten BA, Prins MH. Duration of treatment with vitamin K antagonists in symptomatic venous thromboembolism (Cochrane Review). In: *The Cochrane Library,* Issue 1, 2003. Oxford: Update Software.
Seventh ACCP Conference on Antithrombotic and Thrombolytic Therapy. *Chest* 2004;126(Suppl).
Van den Belt AGM, Prins MH, Lensing AWA, et al. Fixed dose subcutaneous low-molecular-weight heparins versus adjusted dose unfractionated heparin for venous thromboembolism (Cochrane Review). In: *The Cochrane Library,* Issue 1, 2003. Oxford: Update Software.

Pulmonary Embolism

53

Thomas M. Hyers

INTRODUCTION

Pulmonary embolism is a common disease, with an incidence of 205 per 100,000 person-years. It accounts for as many as 250,000 hospitalizations and 50,000 deaths annually in the United States. Diagnosing pulmonary embolism remains one of the most challenging problems in hospital medicine. Clinical signs and symptoms are nonspecific, and treatment involves significant risk for bleeding. Even when pulmonary embolism is diagnosed and treated, the 1-year mortality rate approaches 25% (1). It is essential that every physician caring for hospitalized adult patients be proficient in diagnosing and treating this disorder. This chapter focuses specifically on the diagnosis and management of pulmonary embolism. The prevention, diagnosis, and treatment of deep venous thrombosis are covered in Chapter 52.

ISSUES AT THE TIME OF ADMISSION

Clinical Presentation

The symptoms and signs of pulmonary embolism are nonspecific and are present in similar proportions of patients with and without pulmonary embolism. However, 97% of patients with pulmonary embolism have at least one symptom of the following: dyspnea, pleuritic chest pain, or tachypnea (2). Hemoptysis is uncommon. Chest wall tenderness suggests a musculoskeletal etiology for chest pain. Unilateral leg tenderness or edema may be signs of deep venous thrombosis. In severely ill or postoperative patients, signs and symptoms may be particularly subtle.

Given the lack of specificity of signs and symptoms, one's index of suspicion for pulmonary embolism often depends on whether a patient has predisposing factors for the disease. Patients at greatest risk for pulmonary embolism are those with a history of venous thromboembolism and those with cancer, congestive heart failure, recent surgery, or immobilization. Other risk factors include use of oral contraceptives or postmenopausal estrogen, pregnancy, and inherited or acquired hypercoagulable disorders (Table 98.5).

INITIAL EVALUATION AND DIFFERENTIAL DIAGNOSIS

The goal of the initial laboratory evaluation is to exclude other diseases in the differential diagnosis and to refine the clinical probability of disease. The initial laboratory evaluation includes an arterial blood gas determination, chest radiograph, and electrocardiogram. Eighty-one percent of patients with pulmonary embolism have an arterial oxygen tension (PaO_2)<80 mm Hg and 89% have an alveolar–arterial gradient >20 mm Hg. However, hypoxia is common in patients with illnesses that mimic pulmonary embolism. The main value of the arterial blood gas is, therefore, to recognize and treat hypoxia rather than to rule in or rule out pulmonary embolism.

A chest radiograph is essential for excluding conditions such as pneumonia, pneumothorax, aortic dissection, and cancer, and for aiding in interpretation of the lung scan. The most common radiographic findings in pulmonary embolism (atelectasis, parenchymal infiltrates, and pleural effusions) are commonly seen with other diseases. Normal chest radiographic findings occur in only 12% of patients with pulmonary embolism.

The electrocardiographic findings are also frequently unhelpful. The "classic" finding of S_1–Q_3–T_3 is both rare and nonspecific. The primary value of the electrocardiogram is, then, to exclude the diagnoses of myocardial infarction and pericarditis.

After completing the history, physical examination, and simple laboratory tests, the clinician should estimate the probability of pulmonary embolism. Although research has not identified precisely how to estimate this probability, studies indicate that experienced clinicians can do so reproducibly. The probability of pulmonary embolism is low in the absence of a predisposing factor, when the history or physical findings suggest another disease, or when the arterial blood gas values are normal. When patients have a predisposing factor or when their history or physical examination findings are consistent with pulmonary embolism without an alternative diagnosis, the probability of pulmonary embolism is high. Other patients (the majority) fall into the intermediate clinical probability group.

DIAGNOSTIC STUDIES

A New Diagnostic Strategy Using Spiral Computed Tomography (CT) Scanning

Although the literature has traditionally used the ventilation-perfusion scan as the lynchpin of the diagnostic algorithm, a number of recent prospective studies using spiral contrast chest CT scanning as the principal or only screening study for pulmonary embolism (PE) have shown that a negative spiral CT identifies a population at very low risk (<2%) for subsequent venous thromboembolism (VTE) (3–5). In a few studies, the venous phase of the contrast has also been used to produce an image of the deep veins of the legs following imaging of the pulmonary vasculature. The venous CT of the legs appears to have similar sensitivity and specificity to that of duplex ultrasound of the legs (6) (see Chapter 52). Moreover, the test is readily available and

can also identify other pathology that may mimic PE. Because of these virtues, in many centers spiral contrast chest CT has replaced ventilation-perfusion lung scanning as the initial screening test for PE. The major drawback of the study is the risk of contrast-induced renal injury in patients with borderline renal function, especially in diabetics. In this setting, the ventilation-perfusion lung scanning continues to be the initial test of choice.

If spiral CT scanning is used as the initial diagnostic test, an effective algorithm should incorporate both a clinical probability estimate and the use of leg ultrasound or leg venous CT. The rationale behind leg testing is the relatively low sensitivity of the chest spiral CT when pulmonary emboli involve subsegmental or smaller pulmonary arteries. As advanced multidetector CT scanners come into use, the current sensitivity of spiral CT (around 80%) for PE will likely improve, which may influence the algorithm. For now, the combination of chest spiral CT scan and a leg study improves the overall sensitivity for detecting VTE to greater than 90%. A positive result for either the chest CT scan or leg study mandates anticoagulation. If both chest and leg studies are negative and the clinical probability estimate is low or intermediate, anticoagulation can reasonably be withheld. If both tests are negative but the clinical probability estimate is high, the physician should perform pulmonary angiography. Figure 53.1 shows an algorithm for utilizing spiral contrast chest CT in diagnosing PE. This approach has recently been reviewed in greater detail (7).

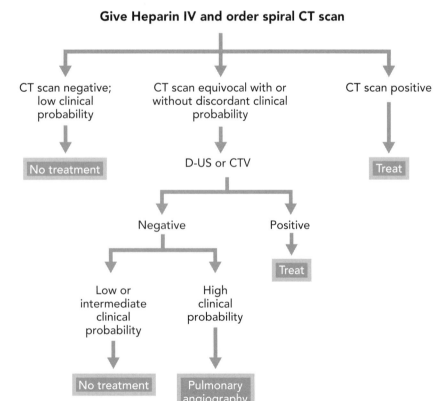

Figure 53.1 Diagnostic strategy for suspected pulmonary embolism using spiral contrast chest CT scanning. *CTV,* venous phase imaging of legs—following contrast bolus injection for chest CT scan; *D-US,* duplex ultrasound of the lower extremities.

TABLE 53.1

PROBABILITY OF PULMONARY EMBOLISM BASED ON COMBINATIONS OF CLINICAL PROBABILITY AND LUNG SCAN RESULTS

Clinical probability	High-probability lung scan	Low-probability lung scan
>80%	96%	40%
20%–79%	88%	16%
<20%	56%	2%

From Value of the ventilation/perfusion scan in acute pulmonary embolism: results of the Prospective Investigation of PE Diagnosis (PIOPED). The PIOPED Investigators. *JAMA* 1990;263:2753–2759, with permission.

Other Tests for Pulmonary Embolism

Ventilation-Perfusion Lung Scanning

The ventilation-perfusion lung scan result is classified as normal, low probability, intermediate probability, or high probability. A normal perfusion lung scan excludes pulmonary embolism. Pulmonary embolism is present in 86%–87% of patients with a high-probability scan and in 30%–34% of patients with an intermediate-probability scan. In two prospective series, patients with a low-probability scan had a 14%–31% incidence of pulmonary embolism (8). Looking at it another way, only 41% of patients with angiographically proven pulmonary embolism have a high-probability scan; an intermediate-probability scan is present in 42%, and a low-probability scan in 16%.

As in CT-scan based algorithms, an estimate of the clinical probability of pulmonary embolism should be combined with the lung scan interpretation to further refine the diagnostic probabilities (see Table 53.1). In patients for whom the lung scan and clinical probability agree (high-probability lung scan and high clinical probability, or low-probability lung scan and low clinical probability), the lung scan is highly accurate, and clinicians will generally assume (high-probability scan) or exclude (low-probability scan) the diagnosis of pulmonary embolus without further testing. When the lung scan probability and clinical probability are discordant, the probability of disease is about 40%–56%, which suggests that additional studies are needed. Additional studies are also needed when the scan is read as intermediate probability because *an intermediate-probability scan has a likelihood ratio of 1* (meaning that the posttest probability is the same as the pretest probability of pulmonary embolism; see Chapter 6).

Venous Studies

Pulmonary embolism and deep venous thrombosis are two manifestations of one illness, VTE. Because patients with pulmonary embolism frequently have deep venous thrombosis, a commonly used adjunct to the ventilation-perfusion diagnostic algorithm is evaluation of the legs for deep venous thrombosis. In this strategy, duplex ultrasonography is performed in patients with low- or intermediate-probability lung scans. Patients with high-probability lung scans or positive findings on venous studies are treated with anticoagulation therapy. Patients with low- or intermediate-probability lung scans ("nondiagnostic") and negative initial results on leg ultrasonography undergo a second venous study 4–7 days later. The purpose of this follow-up is to detect the proximal migration of a distal deep venous thrombosis, which may not have been evident on the initial duplex ultrasonogram. If the venous study does not show deep venous thrombosis, the patients are followed. In large studies of patients with normal or nondiagnostic lung scans and negative results on venous studies, the incidence of deep venous thrombosis or pulmonary embolism at 3-month follow-up was approximately 2% (9). Patients with poor cardiovascular reserve were excluded from these studies because of fear that they might not tolerate emboli missed by this diagnostic strategy.

Conventional Pulmonary Angiogram

The demonstration of an intraluminal filling defect by pulmonary angiogram is the "gold standard" diagnostic test for pulmonary embolism. A negative result on pulmonary angiography excludes acute pulmonary embolism in 99.4% of patients. Pulmonary angiography is indicated when (a) the diagnosis is uncertain after CT or lung scanning *and* leg studies, (b) the patient has a high-probability lung scan but is at high risk for bleeding from anticoagulation, and (c) thrombolytic therapy is anticipated.

Complications of pulmonary angiography are uncommon. Death attributable to the procedure occurs in 0.5% of patients. Major complications occur in 1% and include renal failure, bleeding at the puncture site that requires transfusion, and respiratory distress leading to intubation or cardiopulmonary resuscitation. Complications appear to be more common in patients with pulmonary hypertension. Minor complications occur in 5% of patients and include urticaria, pruritus, and mild renal insufficiency.

New Diagnostic Tests

Several new tests are being used to diagnose pulmonary embolism. *Magnetic resonance angiography* appears to be a promising new test for pulmonary embolism. In comparison with standard angiography, its sensitivity ranges from 75%–100% and its specificity from 95%–100% (10). Additional studies in larger numbers of patients from different centers are needed to fully assess the performance of this test. Studies using a whole blood-based assay or a rapid enzyme-linked immunosorbent assay

(ELISA) for D-dimer demonstrate a high negative predictive value of a low or normal D-dimer level. D-dimer assays are most useful in low- to moderate-risk outpatients (11). D-dimer assays are not particularly useful for excluding venous thromboembolism in higher-risk hospital inpatients because the great majority of these patients will have elevated D-dimer levels for nonspecific reasons. In general, a negative D-dimer assay in an outpatient with a low clinical probability of PE is as useful as a normal lung scan (12). The test is further described in Chapter 52.

Diagnostic Strategy Using Ventilation-Perfusion Lung Scanning

Figure 53.2 outlines a widely recommended, more traditional diagnostic strategy based on ventilation-perfusion lung scanning. It begins with a careful history to identify predisposing factors, a physical examination, and initial laboratory tests to determine the pretest probability of disease. A ventilation-perfusion scan is performed next and interpreted in the context of the clinical suspicion of disease. Patients with a high clinical pretest probability and a high-probability ventilation-perfusion scan have a 96% likelihood of disease, and should be treated without further tests. Patients with a high-probability lung scan and a low clinical probability of disease have a 56% likelihood of disease. Patients with a high-probability lung scan and a prior

history of pulmonary embolism have a 75% likelihood of disease (3). These latter two groups of patients should undergo either duplex ultrasonography, CT scanning, or pulmonary angiography to confirm the presence of thromboembolism. If ultrasonography is chosen first and the result is negative, CT scanning or angiography should be performed.

Low- or intermediate-probability scans are best thought of as nondiagnostic. The exception is in those patients with low-probability scans and a low clinical probability of disease, in whom the probability of pulmonary embolism is sufficiently low (2%) that other diagnoses can be pursued. In all other cases of nondiagnostic scans, duplex ultrasonography, CT scanning, or pulmonary angiography should be performed. Because the research evaluating the use of serial negative venous studies excluded patients with significant cardiopulmonary disease, such patients should either go directly to pulmonary angiography or undergo duplex ultrasonography first and then pulmonary angiography if the results of ultrasonography are negative. In patients without cardiopulmonary disease, strategies employing serial duplex ultrasonography or pulmonary angiography are both reasonable. Finally, the diagnostic strategy should be modified in patients who are at high risk for bleeding from anticoagulation or in whom thrombolytic therapy will be used. Pulmonary angiography should be performed on these patients.

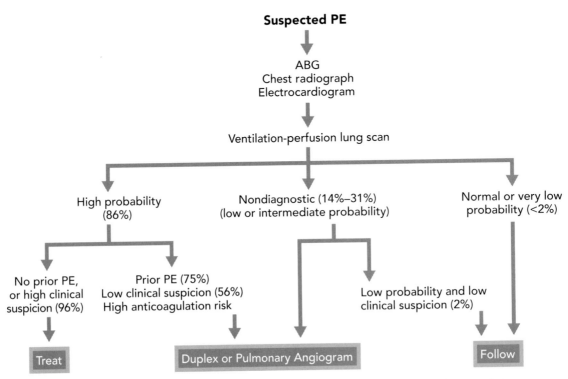

Figure 53.2 Diagnostic strategy for suspected pulmonary embolism using ventilation-perfusion lung scanning. Numbers in parentheses represent probability of pulmonary embolism for the subset of patients. *ABG*, arterial blood gas; *PE*, pulmonary embolism.

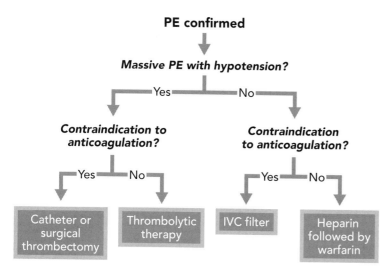

Figure 53.3 Treatment algorithm for pulmonary embolism.

INDICATIONS FOR INTENSIVE CARE UNIT ADMISSION AND CONSULTATION

Patients with hemodynamic instability or severe hypoxia, particularly in the presence of comorbid conditions, should be monitored in the ICU. A pulmonary consultation may be helpful, particularly if ventilatory or vasopressor support is anticipated.

INITIAL THERAPY

Intravenous (IV) heparin should be started immediately, even before a definitive diagnosis is made, if there is no contraindication to anticoagulation. The goal of heparin therapy is to prevent the recurrence or continued growth of thrombi. Heparin does not prevent embolism or promote thrombus resolution. Thrombolytic therapy is reserved for patients with hemodynamic compromise resulting from massive pulmonary emboli. A vena cava filter is indicated when anticoagulation is contraindicated or unsuccessful (Figure 53.3).

Unfractionated heparin is administered by continuous IV infusion after an initial bolus of 80 units/kg. The activated partial thromboplastin time (aPTT) is measured 6 hours later, and the heparin dose is adjusted to maintain the aPTT at 1.5 to 2 times normal. A weight-based nomogram (Table 53.2) should be used to choose the dose because studies demonstrate that using the old standard dose of 1,000 units/h usually results in subtherapeutic aPTT values (13). Moreover, because aPTT values vary from site to site, every laboratory should establish target aPTT values that correspond to therapeutic anti-Xa heparin levels (Chapter 98). If the aPTT is subtherapeutic after the initial heparin bolus and infusion, the infusion is increased after a repeated bolus. *Heparin-induced thrombocytopenia* occurs in approximately 3% of patients who receive heparin for at least 7 days and can lead to arterial and venous thrombosis. The

TABLE 53.2

WEIGHT-BASED NOMOGRAM FOR UNFRACTIONATED HEPARIN ADMINISTRATION

	Dose change (U/kg per hour)	Additional action
Initial dose	18 U/kg per hour	Bolus 80 U/kg
aPTT results after 4–6 hours:		
<35 (<1.2 × control)	Increase 4 U/kg	Repeat bolus 80 U/kg
35–45 (1.2–1.5 × control)	Increase 2 U/kg	Repeat bolus 40 U/kg
46–70 (1.5–2.3 × control)	No change	None
71–90 (2.3–3.0 × control)	Decrease 2 U/kg	None
>90 (>3 × control)	Decrease 3 U/kg	Hold infusion for 1 hour

aPTT, activated partial thromboplastin time.
From Raschke RA, Reilly BM, Guidry JR, Fontana JR, Srinivas S. The weight-based heparin dosing nomogram compared with a "standard care" nomogram. *Ann Intern Med* 1993;119:874–881, with permission.

thrombocytopenia usually appears between days 5 and 9 of therapy, but a delayed-onset variant can appear after heparin has been discontinued (14). Heparin is associated with mild liver enzyme elevations after 5–10 days of treatment. Long-term use of heparin can lead to osteoporosis and can rarely cause hyperkalemia from hypoaldosteronism.

Warfarin should be started on the day of diagnosis. Warfarin reduces protein C levels (an inhibitor of coagulation) more quickly than it reduces factors II, IX, and X and may create a relative hypercoagulable state for the first 4 days. For this reason, warfarin should not be started until after heparin has been administered (although it is not necessary to wait for a therapeutic aPTT), and heparin is continued at least for 5 days, even if the prothrombin time is within the therapeutic range sooner. A 5-mg loading dose of warfarin should generally be used instead of 10 mg because 5 mg produces less excess anticoagulation (15). Heparin is discontinued when the prothrombin time has been in the therapeutic range (international normalized ratio [INR] of 2 to 3) for 2 days. Table 53.3 provides a warfarin dosing protocol.

Recent evidence suggests that *low-molecular-weight heparin* is an effective and safe alternative to unfractionated IV heparin in the treatment of pulmonary embolism (16,17).

TABLE 53.3

ORAL ANTICOAGULATION WITH WARFARIN

Day	INR	Warfarin dose
1		5.0 mg
2	<1.5	5.0 mg
	1.5–1.9	2.5 mg
	2.0–2.5	1.0–2.5 mg
	>2.5	0.0
3	<1.5	5.0–10.0 mg
	1.5–1.9	2.5–5.0 mg
	2.0–3.0	0.0–2.5 mg
	>3.0	0.0
4	<1.5	10.0 mg
	1.5–1.9	5.0–7.5 mg
	2.0–3.0	0.0–5.0 mg
	>3.0	0.0
5	<1.5	10.0 mg
	1.5–1.9	7.5–10.0 mg
	2.0–3.0	0.0–5.0 mg
	>3.0	0.0
6	<1.5	7.5–12.5 mg
	1.5–1.9	5.0–10.0 mg
	2.0–3.0	0.0–7.5 mg
	>3.0	0.0

Initial dose is 5 mg (7.5 mg for patients >85 kg).
For inpatients, INR should be monitored daily; any increase >0.3–0.4 U/d should result in warfarin dose reduction.
INR, international normalized ratio.
From Harrison L, Johnston M, Massicotte MP, Crowther M, Moffat K, Hirsh J. Comparison of 5 mg and 10 mg loading doses in initiation of warfarin therapy. *Ann Intern Med* 1997;126:133–136; and Crowther MA, Harrison L, Hirsh J. Warfarin: less may be better. *Ann Intern Med* 1997;127:332–333, with permission.

This class of drugs has the advantages of not requiring aPTT monitoring and of being administered by subcutaneous injection once or twice per day. However, it costs more and has a longer half-life, and its effects cannot be completely reversed by protamine, features which make it less attractive than unfractionated heparin for routine use in hospitalized patients with complicated disease. Whether stable patients with pulmonary embolism can be managed as outpatients on low-molecular-weight heparin has not yet been clearly demonstrated, and at this time patients with pulmonary embolism are nearly always hospitalized. However, an outpatient treatment strategy (if proved safe and effective) would save considerable resources and is used in low-risk patients in some settings (18). The risks for bleeding, recurrent disease, and death are comparable to those of unfractionated heparin. Thrombocytopenia occurs less frequently with low-molecular-weight than with unfractionated heparin, but low-molecular-weight heparin is contraindicated in patients with thrombocytopenia caused by unfractionated heparin because of cross-reactivity between the two types of heparin. There are limited data contrasting the various low-molecular-weight heparin preparations (Chapter 98).

Thrombolytic therapy should be considered (in the absence of contraindications) for patients with massive pulmonary embolism complicated by hypotension. Efforts to enlarge the indications for thrombolytic therapy in pulmonary embolism have been hampered by the higher incidence of major bleeding associated with lytic therapy and the lack of a proven survival benefit. A recent study that proposed wider indications for thrombolytic therapy in PE reported a very low bleeding rate that has not generally been matched in the clinical use of alteplase (19). If possible, patients should first undergo pulmonary angiography to document the presence of disease even though bleeding often occurs at the puncture site. Thrombolytics reduce pulmonary artery pressure and improve pulmonary artery perfusion within 2 hours. Within 5 days of treatment, however, the perfusion of patients receiving heparin (as measured by lung scan) is equal to the perfusion of patients receiving thrombolytic treatment. The studies evaluating thrombolytics have been too small to demonstrate reduced mortality, and there are limited data comparing different drugs and doses (Table 53.4).

Absolute contraindications to thrombolytics include active internal bleeding, stroke or other active intracranial process within 2 months, and surgery within 10 days. Although a number of other relative contraindications exist, thrombolytic therapy is a potentially life-saving measure in the context of a massive pulmonary embolism and hypotension. In this setting, if thrombolytics are contraindicated, transvenous catheter embolectomy should be tried (20). Surgical embolectomy is indicated only as a last resort, and even then only if the clot is located in a surgically accessible site.

TABLE 53.4

ANTICOAGULANTS USED TO TREAT PULMONARY EMBOLISM

Drug	Dose	Cost[a]
Unfractionated heparin	Weight-based (Table 53.2)	$5–$7 daily
Low-molecular-weight heparin		
Dalteparin (Fragmin)	100 U/kg twice daily	$51 daily
Enoxaparin (Lovenox)	1 mg/kg twice daily	$55 daily
Nadroparin (Fraxiparin)	90 U/kg twice daily	NA
Tinzaparin (Logiparin)	175 U/kg once daily	$41 daily
Thrombolytic agents		
Streptokinase (Streptase)	250,000 IU loading dose 100,000 IU/h for 24 h	$904–$1,228 per course
Urokinase (Abbokinase)	4,400 IU/kg loading dose 4,400 IU/kg/h for 12 h	$5,460 per course
Alteplase/tissue plasminogen activator (Activase)	100 mg over 2 h or 40 mg over 2 min	$2,750 per course $1,100 per course
Warfarin sodium (Coumadin)	5 mg loading dose (Table 53.3) Maintenance dose varies	$0.57 daily

[a] Cost based on average wholesale price, May 1998.
NA, not approved in the United States.

Inferior vena cava filters are indicated for patients with (a) deep venous thrombosis or pulmonary embolism when anticoagulation is contraindicated, (b) recurrent thromboembolism despite adequate anticoagulant therapy, and (c) deep venous thrombosis or pulmonary embolism and such severe concomitant cardiopulmonary disease that a subsequent embolus might be fatal.

Several types of inferior vena cava filters are available; the best known are the Greenfield and the Bird's Nest. Both are placed IV into the inferior vena cava to prevent a clot from passing from the lower-extremity venous system into the pulmonary circulation. Mortality from filter insertion is rare. Complications are unusual; they include misplacement, air embolism, hematoma, infection, pneumothorax, filter migration, and deep venous thrombosis. In one clinical trial, prophylactic insertion of filters in patients with proximal deep venous thrombosis reduced the risk for pulmonary embolism but nearly doubled the risk for recurrent deep vein thrombosis (21). Therefore, in the absence of a contraindication, anticoagulation therapy should be initiated after insertion of the filter.

ISSUES DURING THE COURSE OF HOSPITALIZATION

The first few hours after presentation are the most critical. Diagnostic tests should be promptly conducted and anticoagulation initiated without delay. Patients with massive pulmonary embolism may die within hours of the onset of symptoms; the overall in-hospital mortality rate is about 10% (1). Pulmonary embolism recurs in about 8% of patients within 1 year of diagnosis and is associated with a 45% mortality rate. Only 2.5% of patients with pulmonary embolism die of the embolism itself; most deaths occur in patients with recurrent disease and are caused by underlying diseases such as cancer and infection (1).

Although they vary a great deal depending on size and location, pulmonary emboli begin to resolve within 24 hours on average, and by 2 weeks 50% of perfusion has returned. Clinical improvement should parallel the perfusion changes, with significant improvement seen by day 2 or 3. The symptoms and signs in a patient not improving include continued or worsening dyspnea, new chest pain, fever, tachycardia, and hypoxia. Failure to improve after 2 to 3 days of therapy suggests the possibility of recurrent pulmonary embolism, worsening of the underlying disorder (i.e., congestive heart failure), bleeding, or development of a new problem, such as pneumonia or myocardial infarction. Arterial blood gases, hemoglobin level, and aPTT should be determined, and a chest radiograph and electrocardiogram should be obtained. The diagnosis of recurrent pulmonary embolism is demonstrated by the finding of a new perfusion defect on lung scan or a new intraluminal filling defect on pulmonary angiogram or chest CT scan. It is important to diagnose recurrent pulmonary embolism promptly because the insertion of an inferior vena cava filter is indicated in patients who have failed anticoagulation. Even in the absence of a recurrence, the condition of a patient who was initially hemodynamically stable may deteriorate so that the patient becomes a candidate for thrombolytic therapy.

There is an increased incidence of cancer in the first 6 months after the diagnosis of VTE (with 40% of cancers having distant metastases) (22). Such cancers can usually be identified by a thorough history, physical examination, and routine laboratory studies. See Chapter 98 for a fuller discussion of hypercoagulable states.

DEVELOPMENT OF PULMONARY EMBOLISM IN THE HOSPITAL

The presentation of pulmonary embolism may be quite subtle in the postoperative or hospitalized patient; as a result, the diagnosis will be missed unless consciously considered. The majority of patients in whom an embolism develops during their hospital stay are not receiving adequate thromboembolic prophylaxis. A typical patient presents several days after orthopedic, oncologic, or neurologic surgery or after admission for congestive heart failure, stroke, or pneumonia. The diagnostic workup and treatment are identical to those for patients presenting to the hospital. However, thrombolytic therapy is contraindicated in patients who have recently undergone surgery.

General issues regarding prophylaxis for deep venous thrombosis and pulmonary embolism are covered in Chapter 52.

DISCHARGE ISSUES

Stable patients can be discharged from the hospital on warfarin therapy once the INR is 2 to 3, or 48 hours after an inferior vena cava filter has been placed. The patient should be seen in the office within 2 weeks to evaluate clinical status, review current medications, emphasize the need for regular measurement of the INR, and reinforce that new medications must not be taken without speaking to the doctor. Patients and physicians should be aware of the many medications that can interact with warfarin (Table 53.5). The duration of warfarin therapy varies, depending on the presence of ongoing predisposing factors and whether the thromboembolic event was the first or recurrent; however, recent research supports longer treatment courses for many patients (23) (Chapter 52).

Two strategies designed to shorten hospital stay can be considered in stable patients who are otherwise healthy. First, a patient might be transferred to a subacute facility to continue IV unfractionated heparin therapy until the prothrombin time is therapeutic. Alternatively, some patients can be discharged home after a switch from IV unfractionated heparin to low-molecular-weight heparin a few days into the hospitalization, or even treated completely on an outpatient basis. In either case, low-molecular-weight heparin is discontinued once the prothrombin time is therapeutic on warfarin. Preliminary evidence suggests that some patients with both deep venous thrombosis and pulmonary embolism can be safely treated at home with low-molecular-weight heparin (24), but more research is needed before outpatient therapy can be recommended as standard treatment for pulmonary embolism (18).

TABLE 53.5

DRUGS THAT ALTER ANTICOAGULANT RESPONSE TO WARFARIN[a]

Prothrombin time increased by

Antimicrobials
- Ciprofloxacin
- Erythromycin
- Isoniazid
- Metronidazole
- Fluconazole
- Itraconazole
- Ketoconazole

Analgesics
- Piroxicam

HMG CoA reductase inhibitors
- Any "statin" (e.g., lovastatin or simvastatin)

Antiarrhythmics
- Amiodarone
- Propafenone

Sulfa agents
- Disulfiram
- TMP/SMX

Miscellaneous
- Omeprazole
- Cimetidine
- Clofibrate

Prothrombin time decreased by

Agents that induce cytochrome P-450
- Barbiturates
- Carbamazepine
- Rifampin

Vitamin K
- Polyvitamin preparations

Miscellaneous
- Griseofulvin
- Nafcillin
- Bile resins (e.g., cholestyramine)
- Sucralfate
- Dicloxacillin

Warfarin interacts with coagulation factors that are dependent on vitamin K. Any disease state or drug therapy that affects vitamin K will also affect warfarin response.

Drugs that affect platelet function (e.g., aspirin, ticlopidine, NSAIDs, and the anti-GP IIb/IIIa inhibitors) may increase the risk for bleeding when used in conjunction with warfarin.

Warfarin should not be administered during pregnancy.

[a] This list is not all-inclusive. It is recommended that the INR be checked after any drug therapy is initiated or modified.

GP, glycoprotein; INR, international normalized ratio; TMP/SMX, trimethoprim/sulfamethoxazole.

Table courtesy of Steve Kayser, Pharm.D., and Julie Hambleton, M.D., with permission.

The long-term prognosis depends on the patient's underlying medical problems. The 1-year mortality rate is about 24% (1). The conditions associated with increased 1-year mortality in patients with pulmonary embolism are malignancy, left-sided congestive heart failure, and chronic lung disease.

COST CONSIDERATIONS

The drug costs of low-molecular-weight heparin are 10 times those of unfractionated heparin. The early-discharge strategies previously described (to a subacute facility for continued IV heparin or to home for low-molecular-weight heparin) are relatively untested but have the potential to reduce both hospital length of stay and cost. It is important to determine whether the patient's insurance plan will pay for outpatient treatment with low-molecular-weight heparin or for subacute rehabilitation.

KEY POINTS

- The signs and symptoms of pulmonary embolism are nonspecific. However, 97% of patients with pulmonary embolism have one or more of the following symptoms: dyspnea, pleuritic chest pain, or tachypnea.
- Normal findings on a perfusion lung scan effectively exclude important pulmonary embolism. Pulmonary embolism is present in 86%–87% of patients with a high-probability scan and in 14%–31% of patients with a low-probability scan.
- Only 41% of patients with pulmonary embolism have a high-probability ventilation-perfusion lung scan. An intermediate-probability scan is present in 42%, and a low-probability scan in 16%.
- A negative spiral CT scan coupled with a negative leg study (either duplex ultrasound or "CT venogram") identifies a patient at low risk for venous thromboembolism. It appears that anticoagulation can be withheld in these patients.
- Pulmonary embolism and deep venous thrombosis are two manifestations of one illness, venous thromboembolism, and a commonly used diagnostic strategy includes evaluation of the legs for deep venous thrombosis.
- A weight-based algorithm should be used to choose the dose of intravenous heparin because studies demonstrate that using a fixed dose of 1,000 U/h usually results in a subtherapeutic activated partial thromboplastin time. The role of low-molecular-weight heparin in the treatment of pulmonary embolism is still being defined.
- A 5–10 mg loading dose of warfarin should be used instead of higher doses because the 5–10 mg dose produces less excess anticoagulation.

REFERENCES

1. Carson JL, Kelley MA, Duff A, et al. The clinical course of pulmonary embolism. *N Engl J Med* 1992;326:1240–1245.
2. Stein PD, Saltzman HA, Weg JG. Clinical characteristics of patients with acute pulmonary embolism. *Am J Cardiol* 1991;68:1723–1724.
3. van Strijen MJ, de Monye W, Schiereck J, et al. Single-detector helical computed tomography as the primary diagnostic test in suspected pulmonary embolism: a multicenter clinical management study of 510 patients. *Ann Intern Med* 2003;138:307–314.
4. Swensen SJ, Sheedy PF 2nd, Ryu JH, et al. Outcomes after withholding anticoagulation from patients with suspected acute pulmonary embolism and negative computed tomographic findings: a cohort study. *Mayo Clin Proc* 2002;77:130–138.
5. Perrier A, Howarth N, Didier D, et al. Performance of helical computed tomography in unselected patients with suspected pulmonary embolism. *Ann Intern Med* 2001;135:99–97.
6. Loud PA, Katz DS, Bruce DA, Klippenstein DL, Grossman ZD. Deep venous thrombosis with suspected pulmonary embolism: detection with combined CT venography and pulmonary angiography. *Radiology* 2001;219:498–502.
7. Fedullo PF, Tapson VF. The evaluation of suspected pulmonary embolism. *N Engl J Med* 2003;349:1247–1256.
8. Value of the ventilation/perfusion scan in acute pulmonary embolism: results of the Prospective Investigation of PE Diagnosis (PIOPED). The PIOPED Investigators. *JAMA* 1990;263:2753–2759.
9. Hull RD, Raskob GE, Ginsberg JS, et al. A noninvasive strategy for the treatment of patients with suspected pulmonary embolism. *Arch Intern Med* 1994;154:289–297.
10. Meaney JF, Weg JG, Chenevert TL, Stafford-Johnson D, Hamilton BH, Prince MR. Diagnosis of pulmonary embolism with magnetic resonance angiography. *N Engl J Med* 1997;336:1422–1427.
11. Wells PS, Anderson DR, Rodger M, et al. Evaluation of D-dimer in the diagnosis of suspected deep-vein thrombosis. *N Engl J Med* 2003;349:1227–1235.
12. Stein PD, Hull RD, Patel KC, et al. D-dimer for the exclusion of acute venous thrombosis and pulmonary embolism: a systematic review. *Ann Intern Med* 2004;140:589–602.
13. Raschke RA, Reilly BM, Guidry JR, Fontana JR, Srinivas S. The weight-based heparin dosing nomogram compared with a "standard care" nomogram. *Ann Intern Med* 1993;119:874–881.
14. Warkentin TE, Kelton JG. Delayed-onset heparin-induced thrombocytopenia and thrombosis. *Ann Intern Med* 2001;135:502–506.
15. Harrison L, Johnston M, Massicotte MP, Crowther M, Moffat K, Hirsh J. Comparison of 5-mg and 10-mg loading doses in initiation of warfarin therapy. *Ann Intern Med* 1997;126:133–136.
16. The Columbus Investigators. Low-molecular-weight heparin in the treatment of patients with venous thromboembolism. *N Engl J Med* 1997;337:657–662.
17. Simonneau G, Sors H, Charbonnier B, et al. A comparison of low-molecular-weight heparin with unfractionated heparin for acute pulmonary embolism. The THESEE Study Group (tinzaparine ou héparine standard: évaluations dans l'embolie pulmonaire). *N Engl J Med* 1997;337:663–669.
18. Wells PS, Buller HB. Outpatient treatment of patients with pulmonary embolism. *Semin Vasc Med* 2001;1:229–234.
19. Konstantinides S, Geibel A, Heusel G, et al. Heparin plus alteplase compared with heparin alone in patients with submassive pulmonary embolism. *N Engl J Med* 2002;347:1143–1150.
20. Koning R, Cribier A, Gerber L, et al. A new treatment for severe pulmonary embolism: percutaneous rheolytic thrombectomy. *Circulation* 1997;96:2498–2500.
21. Decousus H, Leizorovicz A, Parent F, et al. A clinical trial of vena caval filters in the prevention of pulmonary embolism in patients with proximal deep-vein thrombosis. *N Engl J Med* 1998;338:463–464.
22. Sorensen HT, Mellemkjaer L, Blot WJ, et al. The risk of a diagnosis of cancer after primary deep venous thrombosis or pulmonary embolism. *N Engl J Med* 1998;338:1169–1173.

23. Ridker PM, Goldhaber SZ, Danielson E, et al. Long-term, low-intensity warfarin therapy for the prevention of recurrent venous thromboembolism. *N Engl J Med* 2003;348:1225–1234.

24. Wells PS, Kovacs MJ, Bormanis J, et al. Expanding eligibility for outpatient treatment of deep venous thrombosis and pulmonary embolism with low-molecular-weight heparin: a comparison of patient self-injection with homecare injection. *Arch Intern Med* 1998;158:1809–1812.

ADDITIONAL READING

Hyers TM. Venous thromboembolism. *Am J Respir Crit Care Med* 1999;159:1–14.

Hyers TM. Management of venous thromboembolism: past, present and future. *Arch Intern Med* 2003;163:759–768.

Seventh ACCP Conference on Antithrombotic and Thrombolytic Therapy. *Chest* 2004;126(Suppl).

Pulmonary Medicine

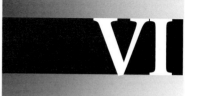

Signs, Symptoms, and Laboratory Abnormalities in Pulmonary Medicine

54

Meshell D. Johnson   *Paul G. Brunetta*

TOPICS COVERED IN CHAPTER

■ Crackles 518
■ Wheezes 518
■ Dullness 519
■ Tactile Fremitus 520
■ Cyanosis 520
■ Cough 521
■ Dyspnea 522
■ Hemoptysis 523
■ Pulmonary Function Testing 525
■ Arterial Blood Gases 527
■ Chest Radiograph 527

INTRODUCTION

Technology has drastically transformed the evaluation and diagnosis of pulmonary disease. During the past 20 years, bronchoscopy, computed tomography (CT), and nuclear medicine studies have greatly advanced our ability to see within the chest. More recently, spiral CT has become an important tool in the diagnosis of pulmonary embolism (Chapter 53), and high-resolution CT has enhanced our ability to assess interstitial lung disease (Chapter 57). Positron emission tomography (PET) is becoming an important noninvasive method of staging mediastinal lymph nodes in lung cancer and is having an impact on the evaluation of solitary pulmonary nodules (Chapter 61).

Despite these advances, excellence in history taking and physical examination remains extremely important in pulmonary medicine. Like the skin and gastrointestinal tract, the lungs function mainly to interface with the environment. This fact makes the occupational, substance abuse, and travel history vital parts of the initial patient assessment. The control of respiration during sleep has a great effect on daily life and activity, and disorders of sleep and obstructive apnea are extremely common and increasingly recognized. This chapter describes several basic signs, symptoms, and laboratory abnormalities in pulmonary disease and provides a general framework for their evaluation.

SIGNS

The physical examination of the chest is an important element in diagnosing respiratory disease. Signs elicited on examination, such as crackles or dullness to percussion, when combined with other findings, can be invaluable in assessing a patient with respiratory symptoms. Given the nonspecific nature of the signs discussed in this chapter, the approach to most signs is the same whether they are present on admission or emerge during a hospitalization. Therefore, we focus on differential diagnosis rather than on the timing of presentation. Various disease entities present with a pattern of individual signs (see Table 54.1).

Crackles

When Crackles Are Present at the Time of Admission

Description and Differential Diagnosis

The American Thoracic Society has adopted the term *crackles* to describe what was previously referred to as *rales* or *crepitations* (1). Crackles are adventitial lung sounds that are discontinuous in nature. They are often described as short, explosive sounds that are nonmusical in quality. When fluid is present inside an airway and there is distal collapse of the alveoli, a crackle can be generated from the sudden opening of many small airways with the equalization of pressure that occurs during normal breathing (2). Crackles can be fine or coarse, early or late, and inspiratory or expiratory. Coarse crackles are produced from larger airways and finer crackles from smaller ones. Crackles are present in a variety of disorders, including bronchitis, pneumonia, pulmonary edema, atelectasis, and fibrosis. Pulmonary edema resulting from congestive heart failure (CHF) often yields early, fine crackles, whereas pulmonary fibrosis produces late, fine crackles. Late, coarse crackles are a common feature of pneumonia.

Evaluation

A thorough history and physical examination, in addition to a chest radiograph, can be helpful in determining the etiology of crackles heard on auscultation. Fevers, productive cough, dyspnea, and leukocytosis in conjunction with a chest radiograph demonstrating parenchymal consolidation are consistent with pneumonia. Orthopnea, elevated jugular venous pressures, a third heart sound (S_3), and pedal edema in the face of a chest radiograph revealing perihilar interstitial infiltrates suggest pulmonary edema. When the diagnosis is not clear, further evaluation may be required to establish the etiology of crackles. For example, pulmonary function tests and high-resolution CT may be needed to diagnose pulmonary fibrosis (Chapter 57).

Management

Management depends on the etiology of the process generating the abnormality.

When Crackles Appear During Hospitalization

The differential diagnosis for crackles appearing during the course of hospitalization is identical to that for crackles present on admission. Nosocomial or aspiration pneumonia and fluid overload resulting in pulmonary edema are common complications during hospitalization that can give rise to crackles. The evaluation of the patient with crackles that develop during hospitalization is also similar to the admission evaluation. Attention should be paid to possible iatrogenic causes of crackles (e.g., fluid overload, inadequate diuresis, or oversedation leading to aspiration). Depending on the diagnosis, therapy may entail diuresis or antibiotics (the latter directed toward gram-negative organisms for nosocomial pneumonias or mixed aerobic and anaerobic organisms for aspiration pneumonias).

Wheezes

When Wheezes Are Present at the Time of Admission

Description and Differential Diagnosis

Wheezes are produced when airways are narrowed to the point of closure and the opposing walls begin to vibrate (3). The pitch of the sound depends on rate of flow of air and is independent of the length or caliber of the airway.

TABLE 54.1

PHYSICAL SIGNS OF COMMON PULMONARY DISEASES

Disease	Tracheal deviation	Percussion	Tactile fremitus	Crackles
Pneumothorax	Away or none	Hyperresonant	Decreased	None
Asthma	None	Normal (or hyperresonant if severe air trapping)	Normal or decreased	None
Atelectasis	Toward or none	Dull	Increased	None or few
Pneumonia	None	Dull	Increased	Present
Pleural effusion	Away or none	Dull	Decreased	None

Wheezing is indicative of bronchospasm. Although asthma is the most common cause of wheezing, *"all that wheezes is not asthma."* Generalized wheezing on examination can indicate exacerbation of chronic obstructive pulmonary disease (COPD), aspiration, pulmonary edema, pulmonary embolism (transient bronchospasm caused by release of local mediators of inflammation), or anaphylaxis. Upper airway wheezing, or stridor, can be caused by laryngospasm, a laryngeal or tracheal tumor, epiglottitis, foreign body aspiration, or vocal cord dysfunction. Localized wheezing can result from airway tumors, mucous plugging, or foreign body aspiration.

Evaluation

The degree of respiratory distress accompanying the wheezing guides the pace of the evaluation. If the patient presents with respiratory failure, it is necessary to proceed urgently with intubation (Chapter 24). Establishing adequate oxygenation and ventilation is paramount. A chest radiograph can help determine the cause of generalized wheezing if it shows consolidation or pulmonary edema. The presence of an aspirated foreign body may explain a unilateral wheeze. A patient with localized wheezing and negative chest radiographic findings may benefit from a chest CT, which can better visualize the area in question. Bronchoscopy may be necessary to rule out an airway lesion. If stridor is present, an ear, nose, and throat (ENT) consultation is recommended to evaluate the upper airway; if the patient is clinically stable, pulmonary function tests with flow-volume loops can be obtained to determine the presence of intrathoracic or extrathoracic obstruction, which may be the cause of upper airway wheezing.

Management

Again, the management of wheezing depends on the etiology of the wheeze. If stridor is present and the patient shows signs of respiratory compromise, immediate treatment with intravenous (IV) methylprednisolone, nebulized racemic epinephrine, and possible intubation is vital. ENT consultation should be obtained. If the wheezing is caused by an exacerbation of obstructive lung diseases such as asthma or emphysema, β_2-agonist nebulizers and steroids, if necessary, can be administered (Chapters 55 and 56). Pulmonary edema can be treated with diuretics and afterload reduction (Chapter 39). If foreign body aspiration is the suspected etiology of the wheeze, the method of retrieval depends on where the object is lodged. A pulmonary consultant can assist with extraction.

When Wheezes Appear During Hospitalization

Exacerbations of COPD can develop in patients who are hospitalized for other reasons. Anaphylaxis is important to consider, and foreign body aspiration may occur, especially after oral instrumentation (e.g., endoscopy or bronchoscopy). Pulmonary embolism should always be included in the differential diagnosis. Evaluation of wheezing is similar whether it presents during hospitalization or at the time of admission; therefore, the etiology of the wheeze should guide the management.

Dullness

When Dullness Is Present at the Time of Admission

Description and Differential Diagnosis

Percussion over normal lung should produce a resonant, high-amplitude, low-pitched sound. Dullness may normally be elicited between the third and fifth intercostal spaces to the left of the sternum, an area that correlates with the position of the heart anteriorly. Dullness to percussion elsewhere indicates a barrier of the lung's ability to transmit sound from the alveoli, either because the alveoli are filled with something other than air or the alveolar units are compressed. Dullness usually indicates pneumonia, pleural effusion, atelectasis, a large intrathoracic mass, or an elevated hemidiaphragm.

Evaluation

A chest radiograph is the most helpful way to evaluate dullness uncovered on physical examination, as it can reveal consolidation, elevation of the hemidiaphragm, or pleural effusion. A chest CT is standard in the evaluation of an intrathoracic mass. Diaphragm movement can be elicited by checking for dullness during a respiratory cycle. During inspiration, the diaphragm moves downward, allowing for resonance on percussion in the lower lung fields. On expiration, the diaphragm and liver move upward, resulting in dullness to percussion in the previously resonant areas. Normal diaphragmatic movement is approximately 4 cm. Failure of hemidiaphragm movement can be confirmed with a *"sniff"* test. Patients are asked to sniff deeply while their diaphragmatic movement is visualized under fluoroscopy. Absence of movement indicates diaphragmatic paralysis, which is most often a consequence of phrenic nerve palsy. Causes of unilateral diaphragmatic paralysis include direct trauma, postoperative complications, mechanical compression (substernal thyroid, vascular aneurysm), sequelae of mediastinal infection (bacterial, viral, syphilitic, or tuberculous), malignancy, or neuropathy. Quite often, the cause is idiopathic.

Management

The management of dullness to percussion elicited on physical examination depends on the underlying cause. If a pleural effusion is present, bilateral decubitus films should be obtained to determine whether the effusion is free flowing and to evaluate the parenchyma that is obscured by the effusion. Thoracentesis should be performed if there are no relative contraindications (such as if the effusion is very small or an underlying bleeding disorder is present) (Chapter 60). If unilateral diaphragmatic paralysis is present and malignancy is not the etiology, the patient may be referred for plication of the hemidiaphragm. If bilateral diaphragmatic paralysis is present, therapy depends on the underlying cause. If an injury has occurred in the cervical region, diaphragmatic pacing may be an option. Nocturnal ventilation may be considered in those with neuromuscular disease.

When Dullness Appears During Hospitalization

The diagnoses to be considered for dullness noted on physical examination during hospitalization are the same as for dullness present on admission. Evaluation and management should be the same as described earlier.

Tactile Fremitus

When Abnormal Tactile Fremitus Is Present at the Time of Admission

Description and Differential Diagnosis

Sound from the larynx creates vibrations that are conducted through the bronchi to the lung parenchyma and chest wall. These palpable vibrations are known as tactile fremitus (3). Tactile fremitus is elicited by placing the ulnar side of the hand against the chest wall and having the patient say "ninety-nine" as the entire chest wall is examined. Conditions such as pneumonia or atelectasis increase lung density and increase the transmission of sound waves, thereby increasing tactile fremitus. Pneumothorax, pleural effusion, bronchial obstruction, or chest wall thickening (from muscle or fat) decrease sound wave transmission, thus reducing tactile fremitus.

Evaluation

The finding of increased or decreased tactile fremitus can help distinguish consolidation from pneumothorax or pleural effusion (see Table 54.1). The signs can be misleading, however, so examination findings should be confirmed with a chest radiograph. Although decreased tactile fremitus can represent pleural effusion, there may be a small area of increased tactile fremitus at the top limit of the effusion that represents atelectatic lung. Tactile fremitus, along with dullness to percussion, can therefore allow approximation of the level of the effusion.

Management

If a pneumothorax is small (<15% of the hemithorax) and the patient is not short of breath, then a chest tube is not indicated. Further management is described in Chapter 60. Often, if a pleural effusion is present and free flowing (as demonstrated by decubitus films), both tactile

fremitus and dullness to percussion can establish the fluid level so that a thoracentesis can be performed. If there is any evidence of loculation or a question regarding the size of the effusion, either ultrasonography or CT of the chest should be obtained before any invasive procedure is performed.

Cyanosis

When Cyanosis Is Present at the Time of Admission

Description and Differential Diagnosis

Cyanosis can occur when blood is inadequately oxygenated or when it becomes deoxygenated in areas of venous stasis. The blue-gray discoloration of cyanosis in the lips, buccal mucosa, nail beds, ears, malar regions, and skin is *central cyanosis*. This finding indicates insufficient oxygenation from any of various causes: transbronchial obstruction, alveolar barriers (asthma, atelectasis, pulmonary edema), defective alveoli (emphysema, pulmonary fibrosis, pneumonia), inefficient circulation (pulmonic stenosis, right-to-left shunts, arteriovenous malformations), nonoxygenated hemoglobin (methemoglobinemia, hemoglobinopathies), and hypoventilation resulting from conditions such as the obesity-hypoventilation syndrome. *Peripheral cyanosis*, in which cyanosis is found in an extremity, is predominantly caused by an increased circulatory time of deoxygenated blood secondary to low cardiac output or vasoconstriction. In central cyanosis, the skin is warm and oxygen corrects the cyanosis. In peripheral cyanosis, the skin is cool and supplemental oxygen may only marginally improve cyanosis. If the patient appears to have central cyanosis and supplemental oxygen does not correct the cyanosis, methemoglobinemia should be considered.

Evaluation

Because cyanosis is not a reliable indicator of hypoxemia, arterial blood gases should be measured, and oxygen should be administered. Cyanosis can be seen when the arterial oxygen pressure (PaO_2) drops below 60 mm Hg, but it may be nearly impossible to detect in dark-skinned patients. Evaluation should be directed toward uncovering the cause of the hypoxemia. The history and constellation of other findings noted on examination can help distinguish inadequate oxygenation from pneumonia, atelectasis, or pulmonary fibrosis from nonpulmonary causes. An echocardiogram can detect valvular abnormalities or the presence of right-to-left shunts (Chapter 36). A history of daytime somnolence, lethargy, and apnea during sleep with polycythemia or CHF suggests a hypoventilation syndrome. Polysomnography is indicated to make the diagnosis. Patients with methemoglobinemia typically have pulse oximetry readings of about 85%. Arterial blood gas testing can detect the percentage of methemoglobinemia.

Management

Oxygen therapy should be the first step in managing the cyanotic patient. However, if the patient has *obstructive sleep apnea,* oxygen should be supplied with caution because it can aggravate the degree of nocturnal hypoventilation and further elevate carbon dioxide levels by removing hypoxic ventilatory drive. If a patient becomes more somnolent after supplemental oxygen therapy, blood gases should be measured to assess the level of hypercapnia. Patients may have compensated for hypoxemia during the course of months and may suddenly decompensate on oxygen therapy. In these cases, the target oxygen saturation may be only 90%. The use of continuous positive airway pressure, most often nocturnally, can help decrease carbon dioxide levels, daytime somnolence, morning headache, and polycythemia and pulmonary hypertension.

If *methemoglobinemia* is present, offending drugs should be eliminated. These include nitrates, nitroprusside, chlorates, sulfonamides, antimalarials, and dapsone. High levels of oxygen therapy should be instituted. In addition, 1 to 2 mg of methylene blue per kilogram should be given IV over 5 minutes if hypoxia is present or if the level of methemoglobinemia is above 30%. The dose can be repeated in 1 hour and then every 4 hours for a total dose of 7 mg/kg.

When Cyanosis Appears During Hospitalization

Cyanosis arising during hospitalization is often a consequence of inadequate gas transfer secondary to a pulmonary process that develops or worsens, such as pneumonia. It also is caused by conditions that can decrease cardiac output and increase vasoconstriction, such as cardiogenic shock. A blood gas determination, chest radiograph, and echocardiogram can be used to evaluate pulmonary and cardiac disease. Again, oxygen administration is key if cyanosis is detected.

SYMPTOMS

Cough

When Cough Is Present at the Time of Admission

Description and Differential Diagnosis

Cough is a common complaint. It is caused by activation of a series of reflexes mediated between receptors in the larynx and tracheobronchial tree and the medullary cough center (4). This reflex complex, transmitted by the vagus nerve, is designed to expel foreign bodies or excessive secretions and occurs after inspiration with a sudden contraction of the respiratory musculature and opening of a closed glottis. Cough can signify allergic, pulmonary, laryngeal, or cardiac

processes. Although the differential diagnosis is broad, multiple studies have shown that approximately 95% of chronic cough cases are caused by postnasal drip syndromes, asthma, gastroesophageal reflux disease, chronic bronchitis, bronchiectasis, eosinophilic bronchitis, or angiotensin-converting enzyme inhibitor use. The remaining 5% of cases are caused by other diseases such as bronchogenic cancer, sarcoidosis, left-ventricular failure, and aspiration secondary to pharyngeal dysfunction. Causes for chronic cough can be established in 88%–100% of cases, and specific therapies are successful in 84%–98% of these cases (5).

The character of the cough may help elucidate its etiology. A dry, nonproductive cough may suggest an alveolar process without central mucous production and is typical of hypersensitivity pneumonitis, connective tissue disease with pulmonary involvement, or interstitial lung disease. Pink, frothy sputum classically suggests decompensated CHF. Thick, green sputum can signify infection, inflammation, or both. Cough in the setting of wheezing suggests obstructive disease, but the combination of cough and wheeze is not specific for COPD; cardiac asthma and pulmonary embolus should be considered. Rarely, tympanic membrane irritation can trigger cough.

Chronic cough *per se* will rarely be a reason for hospital admission. However, cough can have several side effects, some of which may necessitate admission (e.g., syncope or hemoptysis). Recurrent paroxysms can occasionally fracture ribs in debilitated patients or in those with metastatic cancer. Prolonged paroxysms interrupt normal ventilation and can lead to desaturation in patients with poor pulmonary reserve.

Evaluation

Abnormal vital signs, such as fever with hypoxia, point to the diagnosis of pneumonia, and tachypnea suggests compensation for a primary pulmonary process. Physical examination of the ears, nose, and throat should be performed to assess for any abnormalities to suggest sinus disease or tympanic membrane irritation as a cause of cough. Absence of a gag reflex may suggest increased susceptibility to aspiration. Examination of the neck to determine jugular venous distention, tracheal shift, or thyroid enlargement is important. Full cardiac and pulmonary examinations should be performed on all patients to look for consolidation (egophony, fremitus), obstruction, or effusion. A chest radiograph should be obtained in most patients with persistent cough, and determination of oxygen saturation is routine. Evidence of bronchospasm should be followed with peak flow measurements and bedside spirometry, with serial repetitions of peak flow measurement performed to chart a trend if the findings are initially abnormal.

Patient demographics are important in the evaluation of a cough. Patients with risk factors for and associated symptoms of tuberculosis (weight loss, hemoptysis, night sweats, fatigue) should be identified; such patients should be isolated pending the return of three sputum smears for acid-fast bacilli (Chapter 67). If patients are producing sputum, it is important to acquire an adequate sample before antibiotics are administered, as the yield for detecting a dominant organism drops dramatically afterward. Standard criteria for an adequate specimen (>25 polymorphonuclear leukocytes, <10 epithelial cells per low-power field) should be followed before sending a specimen for bacterial culture. A suspicion of *Pneumocystis jirovecii* pneumonia (HIV risk factors, dyspnea, interstitial process on chest radiograph, hypoxia) should prompt sputum induction and a search for organisms. Other special tests in the evaluation of cough may include esophageal pH monitoring (to look for reflux, which can induce bronchospasm and cough), chest CT to rule out bronchiectasis, or sinus CT to rule out sinusitis. The decision to perform these tests is based on clinical suspicion, which rises when a diagnosis is not determined through initial studies.

Management

Cough should be aggressively treated because it is extremely uncomfortable for hospitalized patients and can interfere with eating and sleeping. Cough after abdominal or thoracic surgery is particularly painful and, if excessive, can threaten suture lines. Nocturnal cough may signal postnasal drip, and decongestants can provide relief if sinus disease is the culprit. Similarly, esophageal reflux disease can be relieved by elevating the head of the bed and administering antacids, histamine$_2$ blockers, or proton pump inhibitors (Chapter 79). Suspicion of cough induced by angiotensin-converting enzyme inhibitors should prompt discontinuation or replacement. Cardiogenic cough is frequently relieved quickly with diuresis, oxygen, and low-dose morphine. For other coughs, the standard combination of dextromethorphan and guaifenesin is adequate for mild symptoms. All opiates are effective antitussives, but sedation, constipation, or nausea may ensue. Many patients, even those without a history of asthma, have temporary bronchoconstriction during an acute infection, and bronchodilators will often provide relief from cough. Suspicion of bronchospasm should be confirmed with peak flow measurement. Smoking cessation should be discussed and may decrease cough from tobacco-related diseases.

When Cough Appears During Hospitalization

Description and Differential Diagnosis

Cough as a new symptom in the inpatient setting is cause for concern. Nosocomial pneumonia is a constant threat (Chapter 66). Drug reactions, aspiration after administration of sedatives, and precipitation of CHF by volume overload are all common scenarios. Nasal cannulae for administration of oxygen and nasoenteric or nasogastric tubes can be irritating to the sinuses and precipitate nasotracheal secretions and cough.

Of particular concern is cough that develops or worsens after procedures such as central line placement, chest tube placement or withdrawal, bronchoscopy, and extubation. In all these situations, one must be concerned about and exclude an iatrogenic complication.

Evaluation

Pneumothorax or new infiltrates should be ruled out with a chest radiograph, and a history of associated pleuritic chest pain, dyspnea, or fever should be noted. Postextubation stridor and cough warrant evaluation for tracheal stenosis, an uncommon side effect of endotracheal tube placement. As in the patient presenting with cough, a complete examination with determination of oxygen saturation and performance of chest radiography are warranted.

Management

Management is the same as for cough at admission, with therapy directed at the primary etiology. Treating cough without understanding the primary etiology may mask an important precipitant, such as pulmonary embolism or volume overload.

Dyspnea

When Dyspnea Is Present at the Time of Admission

Description and Differential Diagnosis

Dyspnea is a general sense of breathlessness, inadequate ventilation, or "discomfort" during breathing. The neurologic pathways that are activated to produce dyspnea are poorly understood, but they link the cortex and brainstem respiratory complex and chemoreceptors (peripheral and medullary) with lung and cardiovascular receptors (6). Dyspnea may be caused by acute or chronic obstructive pulmonary disease, pneumonia, pleural effusion, atelectasis, cardiac dysfunction (CHF, valvular anomalies, intracardiac shunts), pulmonary embolism, or restrictive defects—in short, any abnormality of pulmonary or cardiac function. Acidosis is a metabolic cause of dyspnea, as in diabetic ketoacidosis, aspirin overdose, sepsis, or renal tubular acidosis. The resultant compensatory respiratory alkalosis with increased minute ventilation often causes patients to notice deep breathing at rest or to feel that they are unable to catch their breath. Orthopnea classically suggests left-ventricular failure, but it may also be caused by diaphragmatic paralysis or abdominal masses. Platypnea (increased dyspnea in the upright position) may be a consequence of orthodeoxia (decreased oxygenation associated with positional change) resulting from basilar arteriovenous malformations, hepatopulmonary syndrome, or atrial septal defects. Nocturnal dyspnea may be caused by asthma, CHF, gastroesophageal reflux, or nasal congestion. Dyspnea is frequently associated with anxiety, but it should not be considered psychogenic until medical etiologies have been excluded.

Evaluation

A history of the precipitants of dyspnea, aggravating or relieving factors, orthopnea, infectious symptoms (fever, purulent sputum), recurrent dyspnea, and renal or hepatic dysfunction are all important. Examination findings of tachypnea or desaturation are also important. Cyanosis suggests an emergently low oxygen level and should prompt immediate oxygen use and a blood gas determination. A chest radiograph should be obtained, and negative findings in the setting of hypoxia should immediately suggest pulmonary vascular abnormalities, such as pulmonary embolism or pulmonary hypertension. Given the potential metabolic causes, an arterial blood gas determination should be obtained. A patient with dyspnea and any degree of respiratory acidosis or unexpected hypercarbia must be observed carefully because of the possibility of muscle fatigue and respiratory arrest. Pulmonary embolism is a life-threatening diagnosis that is frequently missed, and clinical suspicion (hypoxia, tachypnea, tachycardia, respiratory alkalosis) should prompt a workup (Chapter 53). A complete blood cell count, chemistry panel, and blood urea nitrogen and creatinine determinations should be obtained, and an electrocardiogram should be performed if the patient is over the age of 40. Patients who show any evidence of alveolar hypoventilation or muscle weakness should be evaluated for neurogenic disorders, such as Guillain-Barré syndrome or myasthenia gravis. Parameters of pulmonary mechanics, such as the maximum inspiratory force and vital capacity, should be measured in this setting, and if uncertainty remains, electromyographic and nerve conduction studies should be performed. Other special tests may include exercise testing, methacholine challenge, and echocardiography.

Management

Hypoxia should be corrected to maintain adequate saturation (>92%), and, if it is difficult to correct or is associated with hypercarbia, the patient should be monitored in the ICU. If pulmonary embolism is a possibility, patients without contraindications should immediately be started on anticoagulation with IV heparin while arrangements are made for nuclear medicine studies or spiral CT. Bronchodilators and generally corticosteroids should be used if obstructive disease is present in the hospitalized patient.

When Dyspnea Appears During Hospitalization

Dyspnea may be caused by iatrogenic volume overload or problems with oxygen delivery. Dyspnea is frequently seen in patients who become deconditioned after a critical illness. Such patients have a high dead space fraction (normal <30%) and are prone to development of atelectasis. Incentive spirometry should be encouraged, and patients should sit up in bed or transfer to chairs as soon as possible to unload the diaphragm, which performs 70%–90% of the work of breathing. The classic critical care scenario for pulmonary embolism is a sudden increase in minute ventilation with associated tachycardia. Patients in the postoperative period are especially vulnerable to volume overload, new infections, and embolic disease. Evaluation is the same as at admission, as is management, although tests can be performed more rapidly and empiric therapy started more quickly in the inpatient setting. Such speed is particularly important when embolic disease is suspected.

Hemoptysis

When Hemoptysis Is Present at the Time of Admission

Description and Differential Diagnosis

Hemoptysis is an important initial complaint and is very alarming to patients. The differential diagnosis for this symptom covers a range of inflammatory, infectious, and malignant etiologies (Table 54.2). *Pseudohemoptysis* is important to recognize early; the patient coughs up blood that does not originate in the tracheobronchial system. Hemoptysis is often characterized as "ordinary" (<200 mL/24 h) or "massive" (>600mL/24 h). The precise volume history is difficult to obtain in many cases, as patients often describe hemoptysis in terms of tablespoons of a mixture of blood and sputum. Certainly any bleeding that

---

TABLE 54.2

CAUSES OF HEMOPTYSIS

Pseudohemoptysis

Upper gastrointestinal bleeding
Epistaxis
Gingival or oral bleeding
Oropharyngeal or laryngeal cancer
Hereditary hemorrhagic telangiectasia

Hemoptysis

Bronchitis
Bronchiectasis
Lung cancer or metastases
Foreign body
Cystic fibrosis
Pneumonia
Pulmonary embolism
Lung abscess
Trauma
Fungal infection (especially aspergilloma)
Catamenial hemoptysis
Pulmonary-renal syndromes
Pulmonary edema
Mitral stenosis
Collagen vascular diseases
Coagulopathy
Thrombocytopenia
Idiopathic (5%–15%)

compromises oxygenation or is increasing in volume should be considered life threatening, even if it fails to meet the arbitrary volume cutoff (7).

Physicians are taught that the most common cause of hemoptysis is bronchitis, and although true, this catechism may falsely lead them to discount its importance. The vast majority of patients hospitalized for hemoptysis should undergo bronchoscopy, which may rapidly identify the location and cause of bleeding, provide diagnostic and prognostic information, and correctly determine the best approach to further testing or intervention.

Evaluation

Initial tests should include a chest radiograph, determination of oxygen saturation, complete blood cell count, electrolytes and renal function, and a coagulation panel. The chest radiograph may localize the source of bleeding, but it can be misleading. For example, a patient may have a tracheal source yet present with a right lower lobe infiltrate from dependent flow of blood into this region. Both tracheal and main bronchial bleeding can be rapidly fatal because blood can be distributed to both lungs quickly, but this is true of any source that bleeds rapidly. Hypoxia in the setting of hemoptysis is an ominous sign and suggests significant compromise of a large surface area of the lung. A purified protein derivative of tuberculin (PPD) should be placed and respiratory precautions observed if tuberculosis is suspected. Hemoptysis with anemia may also provide clues about the chronicity or severity of the symptom. An elevated white cell count might suggest a primary cavitary pneumonia, eosinophilia might suggest a fungal etiology (aspergillosis), and lymphocytosis or monocytosis could suggest a more indolent bronchiectasis associated with tuberculosis. Renal function should be checked to determine whether the patient has a pulmonary–renal syndrome, such as Wegener granulomatosis or Goodpasture syndrome, both of which can present with hemoptysis. Abnormal renal function is a separate risk factor for diffuse alveolar hemorrhage, as are advanced age and a compromised immune system. In addition, a low platelet count or abnormal prothrombin time or partial thromboplastin time suggests a bleeding diathesis, which should be rapidly corrected.

The initial examination must include a complete survey of the entire body for clues to extrapulmonary causes. The conjunctivae should be checked for pallor and the sclerae for icterus or signs of liver disease and coagulopathy. The nose and throat must be inspected for evidence of bleeding or inflammation, and a history of epistaxis should be pursued. Poor dentition might suggest a lung abscess. Cervical or other adenopathy might suggest tuberculosis or malignancy. A recent history of tracheostomy might suggest that cuff- or suture-related inflammation has eroded into a blood vessel—a condition that can be rapidly fatal. The presence of a rash may suggest an underlying collagen vascular disorder such as Wegener granulomatosis or lupus. Careful observation of the extremities may reveal clubbing

or cyanosis resulting from hypoxia, or edema resulting from renal or cardiac dysfunction. The pulmonary and cardiac examinations may localize sources of risk. Isolated crackles may suggest alveolar blood, whereas wheezing may be stimulating cough, which can be relieved with bronchodilators. An apical diastolic murmur may suggest the diagnosis of mitral stenosis, most commonly seen in patients with a history of rheumatic heart disease. Fever can be caused by pulmonary hemorrhage alone; the fever is typically low grade. Tachypnea, in the setting of even mild hypoxia, should immediately prompt consideration of intubation with a relatively large (outer diameter >7.5 mm) endotracheal tube for rapid bronchoscopy and immediate suctioning if hemoptysis suddenly worsens.

Management

If the airway is compromised or threatened, immediate pulmonary and thoracic surgical consultations are mandatory. Any doubt about a patient's airway should trigger transfer to the ICU for careful monitoring while definitive therapy is planned. Patients intubated in the emergency department for hemoptysis may be best served by being sent directly to the operating room for *rigid bronchoscopy*, which allows for superior suctioning. In these cases of very rapid bleeding, flexible bronchoscopy may not only be futile (because all that is visualized is blood) but also actually delay surgical intervention. *Embolization* of the involved bronchial arteries can be accomplished in the interventional radiology suite and is effective in up to 90% of cases. If this approach fails to control bleeding, *surgical resection* of the involved lobe may be the only recourse. Temporizing measures before embolization or surgery can include intubation with a double-lumen tube, placement of a bronchial blocker (Fogarty catheter), or even temporary intubation of the main bronchus of the uninvolved lung (8).

For the awake patient with brisk hemoptysis and no evidence of airway compromise, several specific rules are worth following. First, always have suction set up and immediately available at the bedside. Second, continuous or frequent pulse oximetry should be used to highlight any trends that should hasten intervention. Third, it is important to try to identify the location of bleeding and, if it is unilateral, to place the *"bad side" down* to deter aspiration of blood into the unaffected lung. Fourth, cough suppressants are useful because cough can stimulate further bleeding. Finally, because the status of patients with hemoptysis can change rapidly, consultants should be called quickly and updated frequently.

When Hemoptysis Appears During Hospitalization

Description and Differential Diagnosis

Hemoptysis during hospitalization is common and usually mild in nature. Bloody secretions may be caused by frequent endotracheal suctioning in the ICU. Patients who have been hospitalized for thoracic or ENT surgery may have hemoptysis in the immediate postoperative period, but this is typically very short lived. In patients who have received chemotherapy with resultant neutropenia, several etiologies for hemoptysis might be possible: thrombocytopenia, nosocomial pneumonia, recrudescence of a prior fungal disease, or diffuse alveolar hemorrhage.

Evaluation

As on admission, a full examination, determination of oxygen saturation, chest radiograph, and history (looking for recent nasal, oral, or tracheal instrumentation) should be obtained. If the patient is immunocompromised and the chest radiographic findings are abnormal, bronchoscopy should be considered early to diagnose immediately treatable diseases and narrow antibiotic coverage. Bronchoalveolar lavage findings of increasingly bloody lavage return or hemosiderin-laden alveolar macrophages support the diagnosis of diffuse alveolar hemorrhage (Chapter 57).

Management

There are few differences between the management of hemoptysis present at admission and hemoptysis developing during hospitalization. The inpatient setting may allow for more immediate bedside consultation with other services (i.e., thoracic surgery, ENT, interventional radiology). Correction of abnormal coagulation parameters is important, and this intervention, along with cough suppression and removal of inciting trauma, may be adequate to control the bleeding. Hemoptysis in any setting can be life threatening, and careful attention must be paid to changes in oxygen saturation, examination findings, and the extent of bleeding.

LABORATORY STUDIES

Oxygen Saturation

Oxygen saturation has become the fifth vital sign (9), and, because of the noninvasive way in which it is measured and its relatively close correlation with PaO_2, it is a highly useful parameter. The pulse oximeter emits two frequencies of light that are differentially absorbed by oxygenated hemoglobin (HbO_2) and reduced hemoglobin (Hb). The oxygen saturation is then determined by the ratio of HbO_2 to Hb (10). Soft tissue, bone, skin, and venous and arterial blood absorb most of the light. At each arterial pulse, the amounts of absorption are calculated to produce an oxygen saturation (SaO_2). To ensure an accurate reading of the SaO_2, it is important that the pulse oximeter is simultaneously able to capture an adequate waveform. Readings are confounded by nail polish, intravascular dyes or pigments (bilirubin, methylene blue), motion artifact, severe anemia, external light sources, and poor distal perfusion.

Normal SaO_2 is 95%–99% on room air. The SaO_2 and PaO_2 are related by the oxygen dissociation curve. When the SaO_2 is between 50% and 90%, the relationship is linear, with the estimated PaO_2 equal to the SaO_2 minus 30. The accuracy of most oximeters is ± 4% and drops significantly when the SaO_2 is less than 70% (11). The oximeter will overestimate saturations in the presence of elevated levels of carbon monoxide (smoke inhalation, smoking) because the absorption wavelengths of HbO_2 and HbCO are very similar.

If difficulty is encountered in obtaining a saturation level, decreasing patient movement, warming the extremity, applying a vasodilator such as nitropaste, or using an ear oximeter may prove beneficial. In any case, an arterial blood gas determination is indicated if questions of accuracy remain.

Pulmonary Function Testing

Pulmonary function testing allows for the evaluation of the mechanics of airway function and gas exchange. By measuring lung volumes, the rates of airflow, and the diffusing capacity, various lung diseases can be diagnosed. Pulmonary function testing can also be employed as a tool to estimate the severity of disease, monitor disease progression, and assess response to therapy. Other indications for pulmonary function testing include monitoring of patients treated with pulmonary toxins (amiodarone, bleomycin, radiation therapy), assessment of disability, and preoperative testing. Contraindications include active airborne infection, recent massive hemoptysis, and pneumothorax. Although pulmonary function may not return to baseline for a few months after an insult, interval measures of lung function can be a helpful adjunct to observation of symptoms in assessing the speed and course of recovery.

Spirometry

Spirometry is used to differentiate between *obstructive* and *restrictive* lung disease. Maximum expiratory flow rates and certain lung volumes can be measured with simple spirometry. The forced vital capacity (FVC) is the maximal volume of air that can be exhaled after a maximal inhalation. The FEV_1 is the volume of air forcibly exhaled after 1 second. The values obtained are generally reported as a percentage of those predicted; "normal" values have been obtained from healthy, nonsmoking adults and adjusted for age, height, and race. Degrees of impairment can be assigned according to the guidelines put forth by the American Thoracic Society (see Table 54.3).

Obstructive lung disease is defined as a decrease in the FEV_1 to below 80%, a reduced or normal FVC, and a ratio of FEV_1 to FVC below 70% of that predicted. *Restrictive* lung disease is defined as a decrease in the FVC to below 80% of that predicted but with a ratio of FEV_1 to FVC that is normal or higher than predicted. Although spirometry can suggest

TABLE 54.3

TYPICAL PULMONARY FUNCTION TEST FINDINGS

	FVC[a]	FEV$_1$[a]	FEV$_1$/FVC[b]	FEF$_{25\%-75\%}$[a]	TLC[a]
Normal	>80	>80	>70	>65	>80
Mild obstruction[c]	66–80	66–80	60–70	50–65	66–80
Severe obstruction	<50	<50	<45	<35	<50
Mild restriction[c]	Varies with process	Varies with process	Generally normal or elevated	Varies with process	66–80
Severe restriction	Generally decreased	Varies with process	Generally normal or elevated	Varies with process	<50

[a] Percentage of predicted value.
[b] Ratio, expressed as a percentage of absolute values.
[c] Patients with moderate obstruction/restriction have values between those of mild and severe states.
FEV$_1$, forced expiratory volume in 1 second; FEF$_{25\%-75\%}$, forced expiratory flow, mid-expiratory phase; FVC, forced vital capacity; TLC, total lung capacity.

restrictive disease, a reduced total lung capacity (TLC) is definitive for a restrictive process. Restriction cannot be diagnosed by spirometry if moderate to severe airflow obstruction is present. The FEF$_{25\%-75\%}$ is the volume expired between 25% and 75% of the FVC. This measurement is more sensitive to small-airway function than is the FEV$_1$, which is more dependent on the resistance of the larger central airways. A reduction in this value suggests small-airway disease. Increases in the FEV$_1$ or FVC of more than 12% along with a 200-mL increase in volumes after two inhalations of a bronchodilator are indicative of a positive bronchodilator response. A negative bronchodilator response during formal testing does not exclude the possibility of clinical benefit from bronchodilators.

Flow–volume loops are often included in spirometric measurements. Based on their shape, obstructive or restrictive disease can be inferred. More importantly, patient effort and the presence of airflow limitation secondary to upper airway obstruction can be assessed (12) (Figure 54.1). A plateau on the expiratory limb in conjunction with a reduced peak flow and a normal inspiratory limb suggests a nonfixed intrathoracic airway obstruction (intratracheal neoplasm). A plateau present on the inspiratory limb in conjunction with reduced flow suggests a nonfixed extrathoracic obstruction (vocal cord neoplasm or tracheomalacia of the extrathoracic trachea). A plateau of both the inspiratory and expiratory limbs of the flow–volume loop suggests fixed upper airway obstruction (tracheal stenosis).

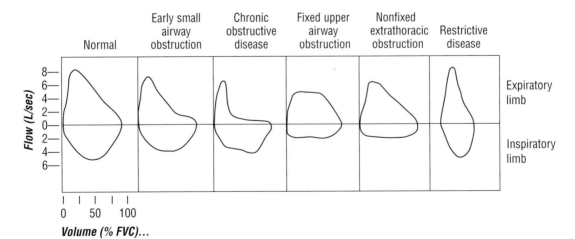

Figure 54.1 Flow–volume curves. (From Kiss GT. Pulmonary disease. In: Ferri FF, ed. *Practical Guide to the Care of the Medical Patient.* 2nd Ed. St. Louis: Mosby, 1991, with permission.)

Lung Volumes

Measurement of lung volumes can verify the presence of obstructive or restrictive lung disease. There are three ways to measure lung volumes: helium dilution, nitrogen washout, and body plethysmography. The latter is the most accurate measurement, as it measures the total volume of compressible air in the chest and is not significantly altered by air trapping.

In restrictive diseases, the TLC is reduced. In obstructive diseases, the FVC is usually normal or reduced, and the residual volume (RV) and the ratio of RV to TLC are increased. This represents air trapping caused by increased airway resistance. In some disease states, obstruction and restriction are combined (e.g., sarcoidosis, lymphangiomatosis, cystic fibrosis, hypersensitivity pneumonitis, eosinophilic granuloma).

Diffusing Capacity

The diffusing capacity (DLCO) is a measure of the ability of gases to diffuse from the alveoli into the pulmonary capillary bed. Thus, qualitative as well as quantitative differences in the status of the alveolar–capillary membrane affect the diffusing capacity. The diffusing capacity depends on age, body size, lung volume, hemoglobin concentration, the presence of carboxyhemoglobin, and changes in body position. The diffusing capacity is reduced in diseases that affect the interstitium of the lung, which can either decrease the total area of alveolar–capillary membrane available for gas diffusion or thicken the membrane, which makes diffusion more difficult. Examples of disease processes causing reduced diffusing capacity are emphysema, pulmonary vascular disease, pneumocystis pneumonia, and fibrosis. The diffusing capacity can be increased with erythrocytosis, severe liver disease, obesity, increased pulmonary blood volume (CHF, atrial septal defect), and alveolar hemorrhage.

Arterial Blood Gases

Whereas spirometry enables assessment of the mechanics of the respiratory system, determination of arterial blood gases enables assessment of the adequacy of oxygen uptake and carbon dioxide elimination. In a blood gas determination, the pH, PO_2, and PCO_2 are measured, and the bicarbonate concentration (HCO_3) is calculated.

Hypoxemia is defined as a PO_2 below 80 mm Hg on room air at sea level. Causes of hypoxemia are low inspired oxygen tension (high altitude), hypoventilation (central sleep apnea and obesity hypoventilation syndrome), ventilation–perfusion (V/Q) mismatch (pneumonia, asthma, pulmonary embolus, CHF), shunt (atrial septal defect, pulmonary arteriovenous malformation), and diffusion abnormality (interstitial pulmonary fibrosis, sarcoidosis, emphysema, pneumocystis pneumonia).

The alveolar–arterial oxygen gradient $[(A-a)DO_2]$ is normally between 10 and 15 mm Hg because everyone has a right-to-left shunt approximating 3%–5% of the right ventricular cardiac output. The $(A-a)DO_2$ increases with age. If the $(A-a)DO_2$ is greater than 15 mm Hg or greater than what is expected for a person of a particular age who is breathing room air, pulmonary disease is present and is interfering with gas exchange. If the $(A-a)DO_2$ fails to correct when breathing 100% oxygen, a shunt is present.

The acid–base status of the body is determined by the pH. Acidosis is present if the pH is below 7.35. Alkalosis is present if the pH is above 7.45. Determining the etiology of the acid–base abnormality first requires deciding whether the primary disturbance is metabolic or respiratory.

- Acidosis is metabolic if the serum $[HCO_3^-]$ is low and the PCO_2 is low.
- Acidosis is respiratory if the serum $[HCO_3^-]$ is high and the PCO_2 is high.
- Alkalosis is metabolic if the serum $[HCO_3^-]$ is high and the PCO_2 is low.
- Alkalosis is respiratory if the serum $[HCO_3^-]$ is normal to low and the PCO_2 is low.

Next, the duration of the primary disturbance is determined. Various rules exist to determine whether the acidosis or alkalosis is acute or chronic and whether it is compensated. In general, respiratory compensation occurs rapidly, whereas complete renal compensation takes on the order of 3–5 days. Maximum respiratory compensation reduces the PCO_2 to 12–15 mm Hg unless significant respiratory disease is present. If it is, the pH will remain low.

In acute respiratory acidosis, for each increase in the PCO_2 of 1 mm Hg, there is a fall of 0.008 in the pH. In chronic respiratory acidosis, for each elevation of 10 mm Hg in the PCO_2, the $[HCO_3^-]$ increases by 4 mEq/L.

In acute respiratory alkalosis, for each decrease in the PCO_2 of 1 mm Hg, there is an increase of 0.008 in the pH. In chronic respiratory acidosis, for each decline of 10 mm Hg in the PCO_2, the $[HCO_3^-]$ decreases by 5 mEq/L.

Many patients with COPD will have an elevated PCO_2 and respiratory acidosis, and a metabolic alkalosis will develop when they are placed on steroids or diuretics. It is important to remember that maintaining adequate oxygenation should override any concerns of hypercarbia. A low pH and lower-than-expected PCO_2 are suggestive of the combination of metabolic acidosis and respiratory alkalosis, as is seen with salicylate overdose and sepsis. Further discussion of acid–base abnormalities is found in Chapter 105.

Chest Radiograph

The chest radiograph is central to the evaluation and diagnosis of pulmonary diseases and is extremely useful for generating an overview of clinical signs and symptoms (13). As a general rule, patients with new pulmonary symptoms should routinely undergo chest radiography. A few limited exceptions include patients with recent bronchitis outside the hospital who have normal pulmonary examination findings and patients with hemoptysis clearly determined to be of nasal origin who have a normal oxygen saturation. All patients presenting with pulmonary symptoms requiring hospitalization should have a chest radiograph, as should any patient experiencing a significant change in pulmonary status after the initial chest radiograph. Daily chest radiographs are not mandatory for stable ICU patients, but they are often performed in this rapidly changing population. It is traditional teaching that patients with endotracheal tubes, central lines, or feeding tubes warrant serial radiographs to ensure appropriate placement, although a recent study found no advantage of daily chest radiographs over performing these radiographs only when clinically indicated in mechanically ventilated ICU patients (14).

Pneumothorax

In most cases, pneumothorax (Chapter 60) is readily apparent on anteroposterior views of the chest and is predominantly apical in distribution. This finding is usually quantified as a percentage, to allow for comparison with the anticipated repeated chest radiograph taken within 6 to 8 hours after chest tube placement. Patients experiencing an iatrogenic pneumothorax after a procedure (thoracentesis, transbronchial biopsy, subclavian line placement) may not necessarily need tube thoracostomy if the chest radiographic findings remain stable. A pneumothorax in the supine ICU patient may not be readily apparent. The *sulcus sign* is noted when trapped air causes the costophrenic angle to appear lower and more radiotranslucent than expected. *Subcutaneous emphysema* should always prompt concern for undiagnosed pneumothorax or pneumomediastinum. Critically ill patients on positive pressure ventilation are susceptible to this condition, and CT is more sensitive than chest radiography for definitive diagnosis. Severe bullous disease may greatly resemble pneumothorax, and emphysematous patients frequently present with pulmonary symptoms. If the patient is clinically stable, a chest CT can prevent the inadvertent placement of a chest tube into a bullous air collection.

Interstitial Pattern

Any entity that causes fluid collection in the draining interlobular septa will cause linear densities on the chest radiograph. This fluid can be lymphatic drainage, as in CHF or Kaposi's sarcoma lesions; in these cases, Kerley B lines form at the perimeter. Lines may be inflammatory, as in fibrotic conditions, or infectious, as in pneumocystis pneumonia. Unilateral reticular changes can be seen in carcinomatosis from lung primary tumors or metastases. Reticular (linear) changes are extremely nonspecific, and the chest radio-

graph often underestimates their severity and distribution in comparison with high-resolution chest CT, the next study of choice. High-resolution CT will also help designate a site for lavage and transbronchial biopsy if indicated, and the findings can be nearly pathognomonic in some conditions (bronchiectasis, "tree and bud" pattern of inflammatory disease, nodules along bronchovascular bundles as in sarcoidosis) (Chapter 57).

Air Space (Alveolar) Disease

Infiltrates seen on chest radiographs in patients with air space disease have an indistinct edge and are "fluffy" and often confluent. Miliary disease falls within this category and can represent mycobacterial or fungal infection. Air space disease is typically caused by fluid overload, infection, inflammation, or hemorrhage. Many pulmonary processes show a combination of alveolar and interstitial changes.

Pleural Fluid

Extrapulmonary fluid is suggested by a meniscus sign, blunting of a costophrenic angle, or homogenous haziness of the lower or dependent aspects of the lungs. Pleural fluid may be free-flowing or loculated, and this important distinction is usually determined by lateral decubitus films. Tactile fremitus and chest percussion (see "Signs," earlier in this chapter) will frequently correlate accurately with the amount of fluid seen on chest radiographs. Supine films may miss a small effusion. Large effusions on supine chest radiographs, especially if unilateral, can be mistaken for infiltrates. CT is the best alternative if any confusion persists. Pleural effusions are discussed in Chapter 60.

Consolidation

Any density confined to the lobar anatomy is considered a consolidation and should be suspected of being infectious if accompanied by specific symptoms (Chapters 65 and 66). It is difficult to distinguish atelectasis from pneumonia on chest radiographs—this is a clinical and not a radiographic distinction. A greater number of involved lobes bodes a worse prognosis, particularly in community-acquired pneumonia. Upper-lobe infiltrates are more typical of recurrent tuberculosis, and middle- or lower-lobe infiltrates are more common in primary tuberculous pneumonia. Lower-lobe disease is common in aspiration pneumonia, given its dependent location. The bulging fissure sign is considered classic for *Klebsiella* pneumonia, a diagnosis more commonly seen in alcoholics and those with poor dentition. Lung cancer can mimic pneumonia or cause a postobstructive pneumonitis. For this reason, patients at risk for lung cancer (smoking history, emphysema, family history) should routinely have a repeat chest radiograph 6 weeks after discharge for pneumonia. Persistent findings after this interval are more suggestive of cancer and may need to be evaluated. Air bronchograms are commonly seen in consolidated lung and suggest that the proximal airways are open. Lobar collapse may mimic consolidation and has the same features on physical examination. An elevated hemidiaphragm and shift of the mediastinum toward the collapse is common.

Normal Chest Radiographic Findings

Persistent symptoms and normal chest radiographic findings do not guarantee that the patient is free of a pulmonary illness; they often demonstrate that radiography is not a very sensitive test. Diffuse abnormalities can be missed on the chest radiograph but picked up on pulmonary function tests or high-resolution CT. Cough, pleurisy, hemoptysis, and hypoxia are all classic signs of pulmonary embolism, which usually presents with normal chest radiographic findings (Chapter 53). Persistent cough may be caused by a mediastinal mass that is not well localized on a chest radiograph and can be visualized only on CT.

KEY POINTS

- Hemoptysis that impairs oxygenation is considered life threatening and should be evaluated by specialists in the ICU.
- Determination of arterial blood gases is an accurate, informative test and should be performed if there is any doubt about oxygenation or acid–base status.
- Chest radiography is a valuable test but insensitive for detecting diseases confined to the airways or pulmonary vasculature.
- Oxygen saturation does not detect alveolar hypoventilation and hypercarbia.
- All that wheezes is not asthma. Consider other causes of wheezing if initial therapy for asthma is unsuccessful.
- Pulmonary function tests can be helpful in the initial evaluation of respiratory symptoms such as cough and dyspnea.

- High-resolution computed tomography is a useful imaging test for symptoms of dyspnea and cough.

REFERENCES

1. Murray JF. History and physical. In: Murray JF, Nadel JA, Mason RJ, Boushey HA, eds. *Textbook of Respiratory Medicine.* 3rd ed. Philadelphia: W. B. Saunders, 2000:594.
2. Piirila P, Sovijarvi A. Crackles: recording, analysis and clinical significance. *Eur Respir J* 1995;8:2139–2148.
3. Murray JF. History and physical. In: Murray JF, Nadel JA, Mason RJ, Boushey HA, eds. *Textbook of Respiratory Medicine.* 3rd ed. Philadelphia: W. B. Saunders, 2000:595.
4. Irwin R, Widdicombe J. Cough. In: Murray JF, Nadel JA, Mason RJ, Boushey HA, eds. *Textbook of Respiratory Medicine.* 3rd ed. Philadelphia: W. B. Saunders, 2000:553–556.
5. Irwin RS, Madison JM. The diagnosis and treatment of cough. *New Engl J Med* 2000;343:1715–1721.
6. American Thoracic Society. Dyspnea. Mechanisms, assessment, and management: a consensus statement. *Am J Respir Crit Care Med* 1999;159:321–340.
7. Jean-Baptiste E. Clinical assessment and management of massive hemoptysis. *Crit Care Med* 2000;28:1642–47.
8. Lordan JL, Gascoigne A, Corris PA. The pulmonary physician in critical care—illustrative case 7: assessment and management of massive haemoptysis. *Thorax* 2003;58:814–819.
9. Tierney LM Jr, Whooley MA, Saint S. Oxygen saturation: a fifth vital sign? *West J Med* 1997;166:285–286.
10. Schnapp LM, Cohen NH. Pulse oximetry. *Chest* 1990;98: 1244–1250.
11. Epstein SK. Oxygen therapy. In: Goldstein RH, O'Connell JJ, Karlinsky JB, eds. *A Practical Approach to Pulmonary Medicine.* Philadelphia: Lippincott-Raven, 1997:543–560.
12. Kiss GT. Pulmonary disease. In: Ferri FF, ed. *Practical Guide to the Care of the Medical Patient.* 2nd ed. St. Louis: Mosby, 1991.
13. Novelline RA. *Squire's Fundamentals of Radiology.* 6th ed. Cambridge, MA: Harvard University Press, 2004.
14. Krivopal M, Shlobin DA, Schwartzstein RM. Utility of daily routine portable chest radiographs in mechanically ventilated patients in the medical ICU. *Chest* 2003;123:1607–1614.

ADDITIONAL READING

Crapo RO. Pulmonary function testing. *N Engl J Med* 1994;331: 25–30.
McGee S. *Evidence-Based Physical Diagnosis.* Philadelphia: W. B. Saunders, 2001:311–365.

Chronic Obstructive Pulmonary Disease

55

Matthew B. Stanbrook   Kenneth R. Chapman

INTRODUCTION

Chronic obstructive pulmonary disease (COPD) is the fourth most common cause of death in the United States and Canada and is a leading cause of disability. The annual U.S. health care expenditure for this condition has been estimated at $6.6 billion in direct medical costs (1). Acute exacerbations of COPD are responsible for 9–13 hospital admissions per 1,000 population each year, with the average COPD patient experiencing 1–4 such exacerbations per year. The average length of stay for a typical COPD exacerbation is approximately twice that required for an acute exacerbation of asthma.

In the Americas and Europe, most COPD is the consequence of decades of cigarette smoking; occupational exposures to various respiratory irritants such as grain dust are thought to be cofactors of lesser importance. In large parts of Africa and Asia, COPD is more likely to result from years of exposure to cooking and heating with biomass fuels, and it affects women more commonly than men. Regardless of the source of the airway or parenchymal injury, genetic predisposition to COPD probably also has a role; clinically important disease develops in only 1 in 6 regular smokers. The only genetic predisposition to COPD that has been identified clearly is α-1-antitrypsin deficiency, which should be considered in nonsmokers or younger patients with minimally reversible airflow obstruction. Damage to the lung parenchyma in COPD is irreversible, but the rate of decline in lung function can be slowed if smoking is discontinued. In addition, some COPD patients have a component of reversible airway obstruction; this can be clinically indistinguishable from asthma and may respond to effective anti-asthma therapy, such as inhaled steroids (Chapter 56). COPD symptoms usually begin after at least 20 pack-years of tobacco exposure. For this reason, COPD usually presents in the fifth decade of life or later, so that the prevalence of COPD in a population reflects the prevalence of tobacco consumption a few decades earlier. Thus, the frequency of hospital admissions for COPD will continue to increase significantly in the near future despite recent decreases in smoking rates. In fact, current data show that women now suffer from COPD as commonly as men and tend to develop their disease at an earlier age.

ISSUES AT THE TIME OF ADMISSION

Clinical Presentation

An exacerbation of COPD can best be defined as an acute and persistent worsening of the patient's respiratory symptoms, beyond that which can be attributed to normal day-to-day variations, and requiring a change in medications (2). Common symptoms include, but are not limited to, increased dyspnea, increased sputum purulence, or increased sputum volume (3). Although the COPD exacerbation is commonly viewed and treated as a respiratory tract infection that causes a worsening of airflow, an exacerbation may have many etiologies.

For the newly hospitalized patient with an apparent exacerbation of previously undiagnosed COPD, it is necessary to verify the presence of obstructive lung disease and distinguish COPD from asthma. It is also important to determine whether the precipitant of the exacerbation is primarily respiratory or nonrespiratory. Common precipitating factors are listed in Table 55.1. A typical history is that of an upper respiratory tract "infection" in the preceding days to weeks, followed by increasing dyspnea. Cough

TABLE 55.1

COMMON PRECIPITANTS OF EXACERBATIONS OF CHRONIC OBSTRUCTIVE PULMONARY DISEASE

Infections (Viral, Bacterial)
Environmental irritants
Gastroesophageal reflux or aspiration
Cardiac arrhythmias
Congestive heart failure
Myocardial infarction
Pulmonary embolism
Pneumothorax
Lung cancer
Postoperative status
Medications
End-stage respiratory disease

typically becomes productive of larger volumes of yellow-green and viscous sputum, but in some breathless patients sputum production is paradoxically decreased. Chest tightness or wheezing may be present. Less commonly, fever will occur. Physical examination reveals tachypnea, suprasternal and intercostal retractions, and the use of accessory muscles of respiration. Pursed-lip breathing may be seen. Breath sounds are usually decreased, accompanied by diffuse expiratory wheezes. A "silent" chest may indicate severe obstruction. A forced expiratory maneuver that is prolonged beyond 6 seconds has moderate predictive value for obstructive lung disease but does not obviate the need to measure lung function objectively.

Differential Diagnosis

Chronic obstructive pulmonary disease must be distinguished from other acute respiratory and nonrespiratory syndromes. The presence of fever, chills, or bronchial breath sounds should alert the clinician to a possible underlying pneumonia. Pleuritic chest pain suggests pulmonary embolism, pneumothorax, or a pleural complication of pneumonia. Congestive heart failure can generally be distinguished by a history of cardiac disease, signs of volume overload, and characteristic chest radiographic features. This differentiation can be more difficult in patients with severe underlying lung disease, some of whom will ultimately develop cor pulmonale.

Initial Evaluation

The initial evaluation should be directed toward rapid assessment of the severity of respiratory compromise. Measurement of oxygen saturation via pulse oximetry is a widely available and cost-effective means of determining

the adequacy of oxygenation. In addition, arterial blood gas measurement is indicated in all patients with a COPD exacerbation to assess exacerbation severity, to identify the presence of hypercapnia, and to determine the potential need for mechanical ventilation (invasive or noninvasive).

During COPD exacerbations, chest radiographs commonly show findings not identified on physical examination but which subsequently alter management, such as new infiltrates or pulmonary edema. The chest radiograph may also be helpful in distinguishing COPD from other conditions; this is particularly true for patients not previously identified as having COPD in whom typical findings (e.g., hyperinflation, flattened diaphragm, and decreased parenchymal markings) suggest the diagnosis.

An early measurement of bedside spirometry may be useful in some circumstances. For patients without an established diagnosis of COPD, a simple flow-volume loop can distinguish other conditions with similar acute presentations (such as congestive heart failure) from obstructive lung disease and thus avoid inappropriate empiric therapy. Establishing the baseline FEV_1 at the time of admission may also be helpful subsequently for comparison in monitoring response to therapy and facilitating discharge planning. However, patients in exacerbation are often too ill initially to generate valid spirometric results. Also, unlike in asthma, spirometry and peak flow measurements have been found to correlate poorly with the severity of a COPD exacerbation. Therefore, in patients with *well-documented* COPD, such measurements may be omitted.

Electrocardiographic (ECG) features such as tall P waves and right-sided changes, although nonspecific, support the diagnosis of COPD; an ECG may be more useful in patients with previously undiagnosed disease than in those with known COPD. However, in patients with an irregular pulse, careful ECG interpretation is important to separate those with multifocal atrial tachycardia from those with atrial fibrillation; multifocal atrial tachycardia is associated with COPD and responds well only to treatment of the underlying condition (Chapter 42).

In addition to the blood gas determination, diagnostically useful blood work includes a complete blood cell count, which may reveal polycythemia resulting from chronic hypoxemia. A theophylline level should be checked in patients taking this medication.

Indications for Hospitalization

The need for management in the hospital rather than as an outpatient depends on the severity of the exacerbation and of the patient's underlying lung disease, as well as the availability of resources for support and surveillance of a community-based treatment attempt. The likelihood of outpatient treatment failure increases in proportion to the frequency of previous exacerbations and is also higher for patients using home oxygen (4). Hospital admission is clearly indicated for patients with a decreased level of consciousness, hypercapnia or hypoxemia representing a significant change from baseline, or severe symptoms. Hospitalization is also appropriate for patients with persistent or progressive symptoms despite an attempt at outpatient management and for those who cannot provide adequate self-care in their current environment.

Indications for Initial Intensive Care Unit Admission

The usual reason for ICU admission with a COPD exacerbation is respiratory failure currently requiring or likely to require intubation and mechanical ventilation (Chapter 24). Signs on physical examination such as cyanosis, asterixis, paradoxical abdominal movement (or other evidence of respiratory muscle fatigue), decreased level of consciousness, or hemodynamic instability should alert the clinician to this situation. Patients with persistent hypoxemia refractory to oxygen supplementation (which may suggest a secondary cause for the exacerbation, such as pneumonia or pulmonary embolism) or with severe hypercapnia also require ICU admission.

Patients with tachypnea and respiratory acidosis or severe hypoxemia are candidates for noninvasive ventilation, an intervention best monitored in an ICU or "step-down" setting. Some centers with appropriate numbers of trained personnel may be equipped to employ this modality in the medical wards.

Chronic obstructive pulmonary disease is a chronic and largely irreversible disease in which respiratory exacerbations recur frequently and baseline disability may be significant. Such patients may have issued advance directives indicating their wishes regarding mechanical ventilation or other life-sustaining therapies. It is prudent to address these issues with patients or their appropriate surrogates at the time of hospital admission in all cases, whether they appear likely to require ICU management or not (Chapter 17). Mortality after a COPD exacerbation that requires ICU admission is high. However, contrary to popular belief, mortality rates and duration of mechanical ventilation are no greater in patients with COPD than in patients suffering respiratory failure from other causes.

Initial Therapy

Hypoxemia must be corrected with an appropriate amount of *supplemental oxygen*. In patients who chronically retain carbon dioxide, a frequently expressed concern is that excessive oxygenation will lead to increased hypercapnia. Although traditionally this was attributed to depression of central respiratory drive, most of the increase in carbon dioxide pressure following oxygen administration is the consequence of altered ventilation-perfusion matching and simple biochemistry (oxygen competitively reduces the capacity of hemoglobin to carry carbon dioxide, a phenomenon known as the Haldane effect). *Oxygen therapy must not be withheld from a hypoxemic patient because of concerns that hypercapnia may result.* Instead, it should be administered carefully and levels reassessed frequently. A target range of 88%–92% for oxygen saturation is both safe and adequate.

Noninvasive ventilation via facial or nasal mask has been demonstrated in multiple randomized trials to decrease mortality, hasten improvement of hypercapnia and acidosis, reduce respiratory rate, avoid complications associated with intubation, and decrease hospital length of stay (5). Suitable candidates are patients with moderate respiratory acidosis (pH <7.35) and hypercapnia despite an increased respiratory rate. Conversely, noninvasive ventilation is unlikely to be beneficial in those with milder (pH ≥7.35) exacerbations and is contraindicated in patients with decreased respiratory drive, decreased level of consciousness, hemodynamic instability, or very severe (pH <7.20) exacerbations, who instead require intubation. Noninvasive ventilation is best delivered by experienced personnel able to monitor patient respiratory status, titrate pressures, and allay patient anxiety. The technique is well described in Chapter 23. Improvement should be seen within the first 4 hours; if not, intubation should be considered.

Inhaled bronchodilators are the safest, most rapid, and most effective means of improving airway caliber to the degree possible. Both β_2–adrenergic agonists and inhaled anticholinergic agents (e.g., ipratropium bromide) improve spirometric parameters and relieve symptoms in acute COPD exacerbations. In this setting, the optimal dose of β-agonist based on dose-response studies in COPD patients, is the equivalent of 800–1,000 mg of albuterol via metered-dose inhaler (MDI) (approximately six to eight puffs), or 2.5 mg via nebulizer. Higher doses may increase bronchodilation but also cause more adverse effects, such as tachyarrhythmias and tremor. Similarly, optimal benefit from ipratropium bromide has been demonstrated at a dose of 80–120 mg (4–6 puffs) via MDI, or 0.5 mg via nebulizer. It is common practice to treat with both classes of bronchodilator together, although studies to date have been too limited to establish whether combined therapy is superior to single-agent therapy early in the acute exacerbation (6). However, in the setting of stable disease, the combination produces greater spirometric benefit than does monotherapy, making it plausible that the acutely ill COPD patient will benefit from the combination approach sometime during the recovery. In general, administration of bronchodilators via MDI with a spacer device achieves bronchodilation equal to that achieved via nebulizer but at lower cost. An added advantage of this approach is the in-hospital opportunity to assess and teach inhaler technique. Moreover, current concerns about the spread of highly contagious respiratory infections such as SARS in the hospital setting will discourage the use of nebulizers that are likely to aerosolize infectious droplets. Patients unable to hold their breath for 3 seconds may require initial nebulizer therapy with appropriate infection control procedures in place.

Systemic corticosteroids have been shown in multiple randomized trials to be effective in reducing treatment failure, hastening the recovery of lung function, and decreasing length of stay (7). Studies comparing different doses are lacking, but a dose of 0.5 mg/kg of prednisone or equivalent, given once daily either orally or intravenously, appears to be sufficient. Inhaled steroids have not been well evaluated in the management of exacerbations. The only exception is nebulized budesonide, which appears to improve lung function, but tends to be less effective overall than systemic steroids and is more expensive (8).

Antibiotics can be beneficial in COPD exacerbations, primarily in patients with productive cough and purulent-appearing sputum. For patients with mucoid sputum or no sputum, antibiotics do not appear to alter recovery (9). Acquisition of a new strain of *Haemophilus influenzae, Streptococcus pneumoniae*, and *Moraxella catarrhalis* (but not of *Pseudomonas aeruginosa* or *Staphylococcus aureus*) has been found to be associated with exacerbations (10), so the antibiotic chosen should cover these three pathogens, taking into account local resistance patterns. Reasonable choices include a second-generation cephalosporin, a second-generation macrolide, a tetracycline, a second-generation fluoroquinolone, or amoxicillin clavulanate.

Intravenous aminophylline appears to add little benefit, produces troublesome side effects, and interacts with multiple other medications. Its use in the setting of acute COPD exacerbation *must be considered hazardous*, and we do not recommend it. Although some argue that theophylline may be a ventilatory stimulant or may relieve fatigued respiratory muscles, these attributes are of questionable benefit in acute COPD, a disease in which most patients already have an increased drive to breathe. The best treatment for fatigued respiratory muscles is rest with supportive ventilation. Oral theophylline may be continued in patients who have been taking it before their acute illness; indeed, abrupt discontinuation during an exacerbation may be detrimental (11). The theophylline level should be checked.

Mucolytic agents such as *N*-acetylcysteine have not been shown to be useful. Long-acting bronchodilators (e.g., formoterol) and heliox have been the subject of preliminary investigations, but do not currently have a defined role in acute exacerbations.

Medications that depress the respiratory system, such as opiates and sedative/hypnotics, should be avoided or minimized. However, if patients are "end-stage" and the goal of care is comfort, their use is permissible and sometimes essential (Chapter 19).

Indications for Early Consultation

Most COPD exacerbations can be managed by the generalist without difficulty. Consultation by a specialist in pulmonary medicine should be considered in patients with severe disease, complicated disease, or atypical features. This last category might include COPD occurring before age 50 or in the absence of a significant smoking history. Those whose FEV$_1$ value is better (>1 L or approximately >35% of the predicted value) than one would guess from the degree of symptoms or arterial blood gas abnormalities should receive subspecialty assessment. The markedly breathless patient with an FEV$_1$ value greater than 1 L may have concomitant congestive heart failure or some other condition to explain the disproportionate symptoms. The use of the B-type natriuretic peptide (BNP) can aid in the diagnosis of CHF in patients with asthma or COPD (12) (Chapter 39). The patient with hypercapnic respiratory failure despite only moderate obstruction may have a previously undiagnosed sleep apnea syndrome and should undergo formal evaluation.

ISSUES DURING THE COURSE OF HOSPITALIZATION

A critical pathway for acute exacerbations of COPD is shown in Figure 55.1.

In the period immediately following admission, bronchodilators must be given aggressively to provide symptomatic relief, and oxygen needs must be met. The respiratory therapist plays a key role at this time. β_2-agonists may be given as often as every 20 minutes; the severity and persistence of symptoms should guide the frequency of administration. Ipratropium is commonly given initially and administration repeated every 2–4 hours, although there is little research to guide optimal dosing frequency in this setting. In patients whose clinical or blood gas findings indicate impending respiratory failure, supportive ventilation must be initiated by invasive or noninvasive means. The management of mechanical ventilation in patients with airway obstruction is reviewed in Chapter 23.

For the majority of patients who stabilize with treatment, the subsequent goal is gradual improvement in respiratory function toward baseline within the next few days. Use of oxygen and bronchodilators is guided by the same principles as before, but the patient's less precarious status allows for less frequent administration of bronchodilators and fewer assessments of blood gases. As improvement is seen, bronchodilator dose and frequency of administration can be decreased to typical maintenance regimens. Steroids and antibiotics are continued and should be given orally whenever possible unless there is concern that absorption may be impaired by a coexisting condition such as congestive heart failure. The optimal duration of steroid therapy is 5 days to 2 weeks (13); longer steroid use should be discouraged because it can lead to muscle wasting (including respiratory muscles), metabolic alkalosis, hyperglycemia, and increased risk of infections. Tapering of the steroid dose is not necessary, since adrenal suppression is not an issue with short courses of steroids in the acute setting. Patients should be encouraged to increase their activities as tolerated. Physiotherapy may be helpful

	Day 1 *Initial management*	*Subsequent* *days*	*Discharge day* *(average day 5–9)*
Tests	• O$_2$ sat • ABG. Repeat in 30–60 minutes to assess trend if initial PaCO$_2 \geq 45$ or if level of consciousness changes • Chest radiograph • CBC/diff • Theophylline level • ECG • Bedside spirometry (where appropriate)	• Repeat bedside spirometry on day 3 (if baseline done) ***If not improving:*** • Consider repeat chest radiograph, ABG • ? exacerbating factors • ? other disease contributing • ? pulmonary consult • See Table 55.2	• PFTs before discharge as baseline for follow-up

Medications and therapeutics	• O$_2$ to keep sats 88%–92% or pO$_2$ >55
	• ***Bronchodilators:***
	  - Ipratropium + β-2 agonist q2 to 4h via MDI if possible or via nebulizer
	  - β-2 agonist up to q20 min prn
	• Prednisone 0.5 mg/kg po daily
	• Antibiotics (if purulent sputum)
	Consider:
	• Noninvasive ventilation if resp rate >23, pH <7.35, pCO$_2$ >45
	• SQ heparin if non-ambulatory
		• Continue bronchodilators; reduce to qid
		• Continue po steroids for 5–14 day course
		• Continue po antibiotics for 5–10 day course
		• Wean O$_2$ if possible
			• Choose maintenance bronchodilator regimen (e.g., ipratropium 2 puffs qid + β-agonist prn)
			• Consider influenza or pneumococcal vaccine before discharge

Nursing/ assessment	• Vitals • Reassess O$_2$ sat • Reassess for prn β-agonist • Admission weight • RT to evaluate and follow	• Vitals • Reassess O$_2$ sat • Reassess need for prn β-agonist • Assist with ADLs	• Vitals • Reassess O$_2$ sat
Activity	• Bed rest with bathroom privileges	• Encourage activity as tolerated • RT to perform exercise oximetry	• Ambulation + ADLs back to baseline
Nutrition	• Diet as tolerated	• Diet as tolerated	
Communications/ discharge planning	• Notify primary MD • Assess home situation • Involve SW if indicated	• MD/RN/SW communication re: patient status and discharge • Assess need for home O$_2$ therapy	• Discharge needs met (home O$_2$, meds, transportation) • Follow-up appointment made • Instruction sheet given
Patient education	• Assess MDI technique • Orient to unit	• Discharge teaching (meds, MDIs) • Smoking cessation counseling	Review with patient and family: • Meds/MDIs/O$_2$ • Return signs and symptoms

Figure 55.1 A critical pathway for the hospitalized patient with chronic obstructive pulmonary disease. *ABG*, arterial blood gas; *ADLs*, activities of daily living; *CBC*, complete blood count; *MDI*, metered dose inhaler; *PFTs*, pulmonary function tests; *RT*, respiratory therapist; *SW*, social worker.

to prevent deconditioning; however, traditional chest physiotherapy by means of percussion and postural drainage (which is useful in other obstructive lung diseases such as bronchiectasis) has not been shown to be of benefit in COPD and may even be detrimental.

Duration of illness varies among patients; an average hospitalization generally ranges from 5–15 days, with the median length of stay being 9 days. In some managed care markets in the United States, an average length of stay of 3 to 5 days is now seen without obvious untoward effects. In the stable patient, some of the final days can potentially be spent in a post-acute setting.

A successful treatment outcome is usually heralded by an improvement in FEV$_1$ within the first 2 days after admission (11). If patients fail to improve, one must search for underlying diseases or factors impeding recovery. Possi-

bilities and suitable approaches in this circumstance are outlined in Table 55.2.

The hospital admission provides a major opportunity for patient education. *Smoking cessation* is the most important intervention in COPD and has been proved to reduce the decline in lung function; a hospitalization thus represents a particularly appropriate time for counseling. *Teaching optimal inhaler technique* is a simple but often overlooked factor that can improve symptom control and reduce readmission rates.

DISCHARGE ISSUES

The patient is ready for discharge when the presenting symptoms have been substantially reduced or abolished,

TABLE 55.2

CONSIDERATIONS IN PATIENTS FAILING TO IMPROVE AFTER EMPIRIC THERAPY FOR ACUTE EXACERBATION OF CHRONIC OBSTRUCTIVE PULMONARY DISEASE

Reason for failure to improve	Recommended approach
Respiratory muscle fatigue	Look for physical signs. Consider mechanical ventilation.
Respiratory depression	Repeat arterial blood gases. Review medications carefully. Assess for other causes of decreased level of consciousness (delirium, sepsis). Consider mechanical ventilation (noninvasive or invasive).
Underlying precipitant not reversed	Repeat history and physical, review medications, repeat chest radiograph and basic bloodwork. Consider sputum culture for atypical mycobacteria. Consider pulmonary consult if cause remains unclear.
Pneumothorax	Repeat chest examination and chest radiograph. Suspect particularly in patients with known bullous disease or if positive pressure ventilation has been used.
Poor inhaler technique	Reassess technique and reinforce teaching as appropriate. Encourage use of spacer device.
Psychological misperception of dyspnea	Repeat objective measurements of pulmonary function. Refer for pulmonary rehabilitation incorporating breathing retraining, coping, and self-management techniques.
Lung disease at end-stage	Repeat history with focus on patient's level of function during recent months. Obtain past pulmonary function results for comparison. Consider pulmonary consultation. Consider palliative management.

requirements for oxygen and other medications have stabilized, and any precipitating causes have been reversed. Although resolution of symptoms is typically seen by day 7 on average, recovery to pre-exacerbation levels of physical function may take up to 3 months (3). In the interval between discharge and full recovery to usual self-care, patients may need assistance at home on a temporary basis.

Patients who have not previously required long-term oxygen therapy may exhibit mild persistent hypoxemia in the recovery period. Nevertheless, if they are otherwise stable, they may safely be discharged with home oxygen therapy. The criteria for home oxygen are listed in Table 55.3. Appropriate arrangements should be made before discharge. Because only about 20% of such patients will require the oxygen supplementation indefinitely, follow-up blood gas studies should be scheduled.

TABLE 55.3

CRITERIA FOR LONG-TERM OXYGEN

Room air P_{O_2} ≤55 mm Hg or O_2 saturation ≤88%
Room air P_{O_2} 56–60 mm Hg or O_2 saturation 89–90% and any of the following:
  cor pulmonale
  pulmonary hypertension
  persistent erythrocytosis

Maintenance bronchodilator therapy should be prescribed and a plan for discontinuation of oral steroids established. Several studies have reported that stable but exacerbation-prone patients with severe airflow obstruction are less likely to suffer exacerbations if inhaled corticosteroids are used regularly as maintenance therapy; these findings are reflected by current international and national COPD management guidelines. Whether such therapy should be initiated after the first COPD exacerbation or whether it is more appropriate to await a pattern of exacerbations is a matter of current debate. Some experts would currently regard a severe exacerbation requiring hospitalization to be reasonable grounds for long-term inhaled anti-inflammatory therapy. The use of long-acting bronchodilators seems to reduce the exacerbation risk, as has been reported for both tiotropium (14) and salmeterol (15). Studies are currently underway to define the role of combination therapy with inhaled long-acting bronchodilators and inhaled corticosteroids in COPD.

Advice should also be given regarding what to do if symptoms recur. For some patients, a self-management plan with instructions to start antibiotics or steroids in the face of an exacerbation may prevent a visit to the emergency department or hospitalization. Factors associated with an increased risk of readmission include the degree of baseline lung function impairment, the frequency of previous admissions for COPD, a limited capacity for self-care, and polypharmacy (16).

Follow-up should be arranged with the patient's primary care physician or pulmonary specialist. Pneumococcal and influenza vaccines are indicated in all COPD patients and may be given before discharge when appropriate. It may also be useful to repeat spirometry before discharge to provide a baseline for the outpatient return visit. Patients observed to have a sudden decrease in FEV_1, the appearance of bullae on radiographic tests, or severe respiratory disease but who otherwise have a good medical status may be appropriate candidates for surgical interventions, such as lung volume reduction surgery or bullectomy (Chapter 58). The follow-up visit also represents an appropriate opportunity for the primary physician to discuss advance directives, if these have not already been addressed.

EXACERBATIONS OF CHRONIC OBSTRUCTIVE PULMONARY DISEASE PRESENTING DURING HOSPITALIZATION

Exacerbations of COPD frequently commence after patients are hospitalized for other reasons. As such, symptoms often go unrecognized initially or are attributed to other processes. A typical example is the postoperative patient who fails extubation or has difficulty being weaned from supplemental oxygen; commonly, underlying COPD has been previously unsuspected. In some instances, the COPD exacerbation will be triggered by the primary event responsible for the hospitalization. When a patient with COPD experiences respiratory difficulties after a cholecystectomy, for example, it is not difficult to understand how postoperative sedation, atelectasis, and an upper abdominal incision would impair gas exchange and respiratory muscle function.

Some hospital interventions may contribute more subtly to worsening COPD. A frequently overlooked culprit is β-blocker eyedrops, which may be absorbed in sufficient amounts to produce systemic effects. In exacerbations arising in the hospital, identification and treatment of the underlying precipitant is of primary importance. Management is otherwise similar to that for community-acquired cases, although empiric antibiotic treatment may not be useful. In-hospital presentations more frequently represent *de novo* diagnoses of COPD, and so more attention may need to be paid to investigation and follow-up.

COST CONSIDERATIONS AND RESOURCE USE

Although previous estimates have been higher, a population-based study found the average cost of a COPD admission in the United States to be $2,700, using data from the early 1990s (1). A simple but often neglected way to minimize costs is to administer medications by less expensive but equally efficacious routes. Two examples are administration of bronchodilators by MDI with spacer instead of by nebulizer, and oral (in place of IV) administration of antibiotics and steroids at the earliest appropriate juncture. Patient education can also be a simple way to decrease resource utilization: establishing self-management plans for patients to initiate during exacerbations has been shown to reduce hospitalizations and emergency room visits (17).

KEY POINTS

- Chronic obstructive pulmonary disease is a major cause of morbidity, mortality, and hospitalization, and its prevalence continues to increase.
- The initial approach to an exacerbation of chronic obstructive pulmonary disease consists of identifying obstructive lung disease, distinguishing chronic obstructive pulmonary disease from asthma and other causes of acute respiratory symptoms, and determining the precipitating factor(s).
- The severity of respiratory compromise is determined from the physical examination findings and arterial blood gas measurement.
- Hypoxemia must be corrected with appropriate and carefully monitored oxygen therapy.
- Treatment of acute exacerbations generally involves inhaled bronchodilators, systemic corticosteroids, and antibiotics.
- Noninvasive ventilation can reduce morbidity and mortality significantly in selected patients.
- Exacerbations of chronic obstructive pulmonary disease in patients hospitalized for other reasons are common, but recognition is often delayed.

REFERENCES

1. Ward MM, Javitz HS, Smith WM, et al. Direct medical cost of chronic obstructive pulmonary disease in the U.S.A. *Respir Med* 2000;94:1123–1129.
2. Rodriguez-Roisin R. Toward a consensus definition for COPD exacerbations. *Chest* 2000;117:398S–401S.
3. Seemungal TAR, Donaldson GC, Bhowmik A, et al. Time course and recovery of exacerbations in patients with chronic obstructive pulmonary disease. *Am J Respir Crit Care Med* 2000;161:1608–1613.
4. Dewan NA, Rafique S, Kanwar B, et al. Acute exacerbation of COPD: factors associated with poor treatment outcome. *Chest* 2000;117:662–671.
5. Lightowler JV, Wedzicha JA, Elliott MW, et al. Noninvasive positive pressure ventilation to treat respiratory failure resulting from exacerbations of chronic obstructive pulmonary disease: Cochrane systematic review and meta-analysis. *BMJ* 2003;326:185.
6. McCrory DC, Brown CD. Anti-cholinergic bronchodilators versus β2-sympathomimetic agents for acute exacerbations of chronic obstructive pulmonary disease (Cochrane Review). In: *The cochrane Library*, Issue 2, 2003. Oxford: Update Software.
7. Singh JM, Palda VA, Stanbrook MB, et al. Corticosteroid therapy for patients with acute exacerbations of chronic obstructive pulmonary disease: a systematic review. *Arch Intern Med* 2002;162:2527–2536.

8. Maltais F, Ostinelli J, Bourbeau J, et al. Comparison of nebulized budesonide and oral prednisolone with placebo in the treatment of acute exacerbations of chronic obstructive pulmonary disease: a randomized controlled trial. *Am J Respir Crit Care Med* 2002; 165:698–703.

9. Stockley RA, O'Brien C, Pye A, et al. Relationship of sputum color to nature and outpatient management of acute exacerbations of COPD. *Chest* 2000;117:1628–1645.

10. Sethi S, Evans N, Grant BJB, et al. New strains of bacteria and exacerbations of chronic obstructive pulmonary disease. *N Engl J Med* 2002;347:465–471.

11. Niewoehner DE, Collins D, Erbland ML for the Department of Veterans Affairs Cooperative Study Group. Relation of FEV_1 to clinical outcomes during exacerbations of chronic obstructive pulmonary disease. *Am J Respir Crit Care Med* 2000;161:1201–1205.

12. McCullough PA, Hollander JE, Nowak RM, et al. Uncovering heart failure in patients with a history of pulmonary disease: rationale for the early use of B-type natriuretic peptide in the emergency department. *Acad Emerg Med* 2003;10:198–204.

13. Stanbrook MB, Goldstein RS. Steroids for acute exacerbations of COPD: how long is enough? *Chest* 2001;119:675–676.

14. Brusasco V, Hodder R, Miravitlles M, et al. Health outcomes following treatment for six months with once daily tiotropium compared with twice daily salmeterol in patients with COPD. *Thorax* 2003;58:399–404.

15. Calverley P, Pauwels R, Vestbo J, et al. for the TRISTAN (TRial of Inhaled STeroids ANd long-acting β2-agonists) study group. Combined salmeterol and fluticasone in the treatment of chronic obstructive pulmonary disease: a randomised controlled trial. *Lancet* 2003;361:449–456.

16. Roberts CM, Lowe D, Bucknall CE, et al., on behalf of the British Thoracic Society Audit Subcommittee of the Standards of Care Committee and the Royal College of Physicians of London. Clinical audit indicators of outcome following admission to hospital with acute exacerbation of chronic obstructive pulmonary disease. *Thorax* 2002;57:137–141.

17. Bourbeau J, Julien M, Maltais F, et al., for the Chronic Obstructive Pulmonary Disease axis of the Respiratory Network, Fonds de la Recherche en Santé du Québec. Reduction of hospital utilization in patients with chronic obstructive pulmonary disease: a disease-specific self-management intervention. *Arch Intern Med* 2003; 163:585–591.

ADDITIONAL READING

Bach PB, Brown C, Gelfand SE, et al. Management of acute exacerbations of chronic obstructive pulmonary disease: a summary and appraisal of published evidence. *Ann Intern Med* 2001;134: 600–620.

Johnson MK, Stevenson RD. Management of an acute exacerbation of COPD: Are we ignoring the evidence? *Thorax* 2002;57(Suppl II):ii15–ii23.

Kim S, Emerman CL, Cydulka RK, et al. Prospective multicenter study of relapse following emergency department treatment of COPD exacerbation. *Chest* 2004;125:473–481.

Man SF, McAlister FA, Anthonisen NR, et al. Contemporary management of chronic obstructive pulmonary disease: clinical applications. *JAMA* 2003;290:2313–2316.

O'Donnell DE, Aaron S, Bourbeau J, et al. Canadian Thoracic Society recommendations for management of chronic obstructive pulmonary disease. *Can Respir J* 2004;11(Suppl B):7B–59B.

Pauwels RA, Buist SA, Calverley PMA, et al. Global strategy for the diagnosis, management, and prevention of chronic obstructive pulmonary disease. NHLBI/WHO Global Initiative for Chronic Obstructive Lung Disease (GOLD) Workshop Summary. *Am J Respir Crit Care Med* 2001;163:1256–1276.

Exacerbations of Asthma

Homer A. Boushey

INTRODUCTION

The causes, pathophysiology, clinical presentation, and treatment of asthma exacerbations share many features with those of exacerbations of Chronic obstructive pulmonary disease (COPD), discussed in the previous chapter. There are, however, important differences in the presentations and treatments of the two disorders that must be understood to avoid potentially serious errors in management.

EXACERBATIONS OF ASTHMA

Asthma is the most common respiratory emergency encountered in clinical practice. About 7% of the U.S. population suffers from asthma. In 1998, asthma accounted for 13.9 million visits for outpatient care, 2 million visits for urgent care, and 423,000 hospitalizations (1). The costs for hospitalization account for over half of the more than $6 billion in direct medical costs of asthma (2).

The incidence of asthma peaks in childhood, but new asthma may present at any age. The condition is now recognized as a chronic disorder of the airways, so the risk for attacks extends over the lifetime of most patients, especially for those with asthma in adulthood. National and international guidelines have classified asthma as "mild intermittent," "mild persistent," "moderate," or "severe," based on the frequency and severity of symptoms, the disturbance in pulmonary function, and the requirement for medications (3) (see Table 56.1). Although this classification has proved useful in providing general guidelines for therapy, it does not recognize all forms of asthma, such as "sudden asphyxic asthma" or "brittle asthma" (4). In general, the frequency of attacks requiring urgent treatment varies with severity, but severe and even fatal attacks can occur in patients with mild forms of asthma. The risks for severe morbidity or death from attacks increase with age, probably because of the development of complicating coexistent diseases, especially of the cardiovascular system.

Acute asthma exacerbations in patients presenting to the emergency department are a common and potentially serious complication of asthma. Between 20%–30% of asthmatic patients presenting for emergency care require hospitalization (5). The most common precipitating factor—accounting for as much as 80% of exacerbations in children—is infection with one of the viruses responsible for the common cold, especially rhinovirus (6). However, infections with other respiratory pathogens, including influenza, parainfluenza, and respiratory syncytial viruses, adenoviruses, and the bacteria *Mycoplasma pneumoniae* and *Chlamydia pulmonis*, can also trigger severe attacks. Other precipitants are exposure to allergens or irritants (e.g., sulfur dioxide, particulate pollutants), use of medications (especially nonsteroidal anti-inflammatory agents or oral or topical β-blocking drugs), and medication noncompliance. Asthmatic patients with anaphylactic sensitivity to an allergen such as peanuts or insect venom have especially severe sudden attacks on encountering the allergen.

Knowing the cause of an attack can be useful for predicting the duration of treatment likely to be necessary and for educating patients about measures they should take to avoid severe attacks in the future, but it has no effect on initial management. Regardless of the cause of the attack, the first steps are to assess the severity of airflow obstruction and begin treatment. It is also necessary to identify risk factors for a poor outcome, including death, to determine

TABLE 56.1

CLASSIFICATION OF ASTHMA SEVERITY: CLINICAL FEATURES BEFORE TREATMENT

	Days with symptoms	Nights with symptoms	PEF or FEV$_1$	PEF variability
Severe persistent	Continual	Frequent	≤60%	>30%
Moderate persistent	Daily	≥5/mo	61–79%	>30%
Mild persistent	3–6/wk	3–4/mo	≥80%	20–30%
Mild intermittent	≤2/wk	≤2/mo	≥80%	<20%

Patients should be assigned to the most severe group in which any feature occurs. Clinical features for individual patients may overlap across groups. A patient's classification may change over time. Patients with chronic asthma at any level of severity can have mild, moderate, or severe exacerbations of asthma. Some patients with intermittent asthma experience severe and life-threatening exacerbations separated by long periods of normal lung function and no symptoms. Patients with two or more asthma exacerbations per week (i.e., progressively worsening symptoms that may last hours or days) tend to have moderate to severe asthma.
FEV_1, forced expiratory volume in 1 second; *PEF*, peak expiratory flow.
From National Asthma Education and Prevention Program, Expert Panel Report 2. *Guidelines for the diagnosis and management of asthma.* NIH publication No. 97-4051, April 1997, with permission.

whether admission to intensive care or to a hospital ward will likely be necessary, and to identify comorbid diseases that may complicate management, such as pneumothorax, pneumonia, and bacterial sinusitis.

ISSUES AT THE TIME OF ADMISSION

Clinical Presentation

The cardinal symptoms of asthma are wheeze, chest tightness, and shortness of breath, often associated with cough. When a patient with a prior history of asthma presents with dyspnea and diffuse wheezes throughout the lung fields, the diagnosis is not difficult. The fundamental abnormality accounting for these features is diffuse, inhomogeneous narrowing of the airways throughout the lungs, but the signs and symptoms of asthma correlate poorly with the severity of airflow obstruction. Except for patients with an obviously severe attack, the initial assessment should therefore include some objective assessment of airflow. Simple measurements of lung function, such as forced expiratory volume in 1 second (FEV_1) or peak expiratory flow (PEF), provide quantitative, reproducible information, and serial measurements help the clinician to assess the response to therapy and avoid both unnecessary admission and premature discharge. Performing a maximal inspiratory-expiratory maneuver can itself provoke bronchoconstriction, especially in the absence of bronchodilator treatment. Therefore, in the patient suffering an obviously severe acute attack, it is prudent to wait until an hour or two after treatment has started before the first measurement of FEV_1 or peak flow.

Differential Diagnosis and Initial Evaluation

Cough, shortness of breath, and wheeze are nonspecific symptoms, and other diagnoses need to be considered, especially in patients without a prior diagnosis of asthma. In children under the age of 3 years, the most common cause of these symptoms is acute viral bronchitis/bronchiolitis, often resulting from infection with respiratory syncytial virus. Pneumonia is a cause of dyspnea, cough, and sputum production, but it is associated with localized wheezing at most. In elderly patients or in those with risk factors for cardiac disease, pulmonary edema must be considered, as acute elevations in left atrial pressure can cause airway narrowing and wheezing ("cardiac asthma"). The frequency with which acute pulmonary embolism presents with wheezing is probably overestimated, but the association is authentic. The disorder most commonly confused with an asthma exacerbation is probably acute bronchitis. Strictly speaking, the label of "acute bronchitis" may be correctly applied to the condition of asthmatic patients presenting with dyspnea and cough productive of purulent sputum, for they do indeed have an acute inflammation of the bronchial mucosa. The problem is that the diagnosis is insufficient, and the treatment prescribed, generally a broad-spectrum antibiotic, is inappropriate and ineffective. In fact, the correct diagnosis is often delayed by this error, and many patients are not given a diagnosis of asthma until they have taken multiple courses of antibiotics over several years to treat "bronchitis."

The most important mimic of asthma is *mechanical obstruction of the upper airway.* Unusual cases include laryngeal edema, an aspirated foreign body, benign or malignant tumors of the larynx or trachea, or mediastinal masses compressing the central airways. The most common cause of upper airway obstruction is *vocal cord dysfunction,* a frequently overlooked psychophysiologic disorder in which contraction of intrinsic muscles of the larynx causes adduction of the vocal cords (7). Patients may be diagnosed with this disorder only after multiple emergency department visits and hospitalizations for asthma; many are treated (inappropriately) with high daily doses of an oral corticosteroid. Patients with vocal cord dysfunction are heterogeneous, but a substantial subgroup consists of overweight females with a history of sexual or emotional abuse. Another risk factor appears to be gastroesophageal reflux with repeated microaspiration of gastric acid. Regardless of an individual patient's demographics, upper airway obstruction should be considered when auscultation reveals monophonic wheezing over the lung fields that is loudest over the neck. Other clues include dysphonia and inspiratory stridor. The consequences can be dramatic; vocal cord dysfunction can even result in hypoventilation and carbon dioxide retention. The diagnosis may be confirmed by a flow–volume curve indicating fixed limitation of inspiratory flow (Chapter 54), but it usually requires laryngoscopy showing paradoxical adduction of the vocal cords during inspiration. The distinction of vocal cord dysfunction from asthma is important because β_2-agonists and systemic corticosteroids are ineffective in the former, and the emergency treatment for severe attacks of vocal cord dysfunction—intravenous administration of a short-acting sedative such as midazolam—is contraindicated for asthma. Long-term management of vocal cord dysfunction often requires psychological counseling and consultation with a speech therapist.

The low mortality of asthmatics who present for emergency care is partly attributable to improved recognition of the features of potentially fatal attacks so that early transfer to an ICU is facilitated. It is sometimes easy to recognize an attack as life threatening. Obvious clues are an altered sensorium, an upright posture, diaphoresis, telegraphic speech, cyanosis, and fatigue. When any of these signs is present, objective assessment of the severity of airflow obstruction is not necessary before treatment is started (and, as noted earlier, may actually be risky). However, the absence of these signs does not exclude an attack from being potentially life threatening. Other clues are an inspiratory fall in systolic blood pressure (pulsus paradoxus) of more than 15 mm Hg, intercostal retractions, poor air movement ("silent chest"), a PEF or FEV_1 value that is below 25% of the predicted value, PEF below 100 L/min, and FEV_1 below 1.0 L. Pneumothorax is a life-threatening complication of asthma; wide swings in pleural pressure can rapidly cause progression to lung collapse and tension pneumothorax (Chapter 60).

Although a portable chest radiograph should be obtained whenever pneumothorax is suspected, chest radiography is not necessary for routine assessment of a patient with an asthma exacerbation. Bacterial pneumonia rarely causes exacerbations, and the purulent sputum sometimes produced by asthmatic patients usually reflects inflammation of the bronchial airways caused by viral infections or allergen inhalation rather than bacterial bronchitis or pneumonia. Chest radiographs are thus reserved for the assessment of patients with fever in addition to purulent sputum, those with localized wheezing, and those in whom pneumothorax is suspected. Similarly, measurement of the white blood cell count and Gram stain of the sputum need not be performed in assessing acute attacks of asthma unless pneumonia is suspected.

Measurement of arterial blood gases is rarely necessary in the initial assessment. Patients having mild attacks usually have mild hypoxemia with normal oxygen saturation (PaO_2 66 to 69 mm Hg), hypocapnia ($PaCO_2$ 33–36 mm Hg), and respiratory alkalosis. Hypoxemia can be detected by simple percutaneous oximetry and can be corrected by administering supplemental oxygen. *The practical purpose of measuring arterial blood gases is detection of carbon dioxide retention.* Respiratory drive is invariably increased in asthma exacerbations, and a normal value for PCO_2 may indicate extremely severe airflow obstruction (FEV_1 <15%–20% of predicted value) and fatigue of the muscles of respiration. However, even patients with carbon dioxide retention often respond quickly to therapy, so the important goal of initial assessment is to recognize that an attack is severe and to administer effective treatment. The information obtained from arterial blood gas measurement becomes particularly important when an attack does not respond to initial therapy, as it can help with the decision regarding the need for intubation and mechanical ventilation. In severe attacks, arterial blood gas values may also indicate the presence of acidosis, variably from metabolic and respiratory causes (lactic acidosis and alveolar hypoventilation, respectively); this rarely requires any treatment beyond effective oxygenation and relief of airflow obstruction.

Initial Treatment

Treatment should be started as soon as an asthma exacerbation is recognized and its severity assessed (Figure 56.1). While treatment is being administered, a focused history and physical examination pertinent to the exacerbation should be obtained. Lung function should be measured periodically, usually 2 hours after initial treatment and prior to hospital admission or discharge. The following are the key treatment modalities:

1. *Supplemental oxygen* (by nasal cannulae or mask) should be administered to maintain an oxygen saturation above 90% (>93% in children and pregnant women). Oxygen saturation should be monitored until a clear response to bronchodilator therapy occurs.

2. An inhaled short-acting β_2-agonist should be administered promptly. In the emergency department, it is

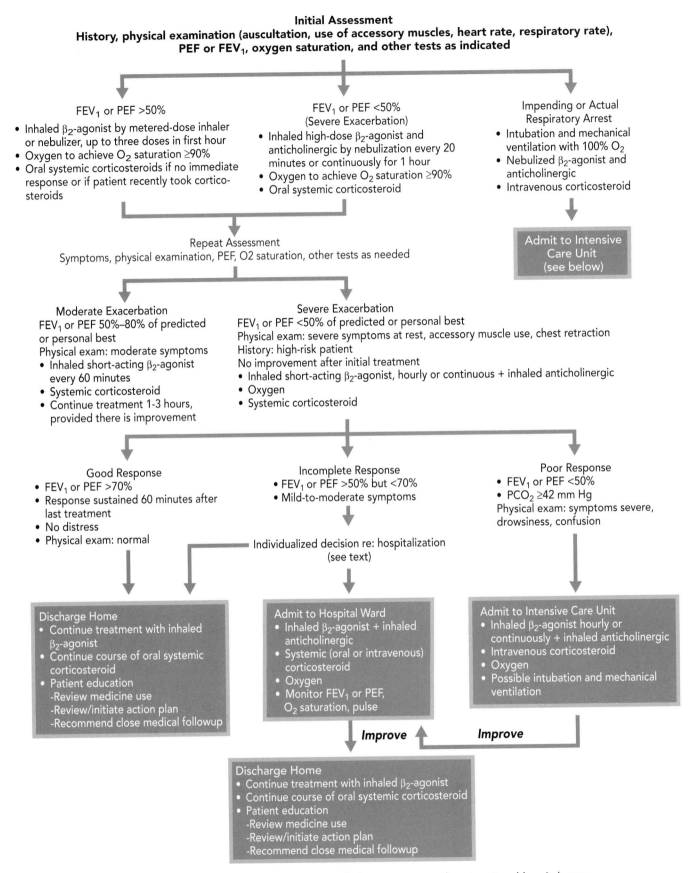

Figure 56.1 Management of asthma exacerbations: emergency department and hospital care. Adapted from the NIH guidelines for the diagnosis and management of asthma. Expert panel report 2. United States Department of Health and Human Services publication no. 97-4051.

usually given via a nebulizer (albuterol 2.5–5.0 mg in 1.5–2.0 mL isotonic saline) powered by a compressed oxygen–air mixture every 20 minutes for the first hour and hourly thereafter, or until clear improvement occurs. An alternative, but no more effective, strategy is to give the same total dose by continuous nebulization over 4–6 hours (8). Another equally effective approach for patients who can coordinate the use of a metered dose inhaler is to give albuterol by metered-dose inhaler (MDI) with a spacer, four to six puffs (90 mg per puff) every 20–30 minutes for the first hour and hourly thereafter. After this initial period of intense treatment, the frequency of administration varies according to the improvement in airflow obstruction and associated symptoms.

3. For severe exacerbations, an *anticholinergic agent* should be added to the nebulized β_2-agonist. The addition of a high dose of ipratropium bromide (0.5 mg in adults) to an aerosolized solution of albuterol has been shown to enhance bronchodilation and reduce the rate of hospitalization in asthmatic patients with severe airflow obstruction (9).

4. For moderate to severe exacerbations, and for exacerbations incompletely responsive to initial β_2-agonist therapy, begin an *oral corticosteroid "burst" regimen* (e.g., 40–60 mg of prednisone per day or 1–2 mg/kg per day), given in a single or divided doses for 3–7 days. Also provide supplemental doses of oral corticosteroids to patients who take them regularly, even if the exacerbation is mild. Prednisone and methylprednisolone are well absorbed when taken orally, so intravenous administration is not necessary. Systemic corticosteroids do not act immediately (the earliest demonstrable improvement is noted at 6 hours), but they have been proven to reduce the rates of hospitalization and relapse (10). In the past, treatment of patients hospitalized for severe asthma with an inhaled corticosteroid was thought to be contraindicated, for fear that the inhaled particles would irritate the airways and provoke bronchoconstriction. The opposite has been found to be the case, and some exploratory studies have suggested that early treatment with high doses of a potent inhaled corticosteroid may reduce or eliminate the need for systemic corticosteroid therapy after the third hospital day (11,12). At the least, starting patients on an inhaled corticosteroid before discharge provides an opportunity to instruct patients in their use and may reduce the risk of relapse even if oral corticosteroids are continued for 10–14 days after the attack (13,14).

5. *Methylxanthines are no longer recommended* because they appear to add no benefit to optimal inhaled β_2-agonist therapy and may increase adverse effects. In patients currently taking a theophylline preparation, the serum level should be measured to rule out theophylline toxicity.

6. The place of antibiotics in treatment is not established. Only two prospective, blinded clinical trials have examined the question, and neither showed beneficial effect (15). Antibiotic treatment may be necessary for comorbid conditions (e.g., pneumonia, bacterial sinusitis), and it should be considered for patients with fever and purulent sputum or pulmonary infiltrates on chest radiography. The use of macrolide antibiotics has some theoretical attractiveness because they are active against the atypical bacteria *Mycoplasma pneumoniae* and *Chlamydia pneumoniae,* which are identified in around 5% of asthma exacerbations. There is even a possibility that some asthmatic patients have a chronic, low-grade bronchial epithelial infection with these organisms (16) that flares with viral respiratory infection. This unproven hypothesis may account for the frequency with which macrolide antibiotics, especially azithromycin, are prescribed for asthma exacerbations.

7. If the response to treatment is favorable (no shortness of breath or wheezing, PEF or FEV_1 greater than 70% of predicted or "personal best" value), the patient can be discharged from the emergency department or short-stay unit with instructions to take a continued, tapering burst of oral corticosteroids and an inhaled β_2-agonist as needed. Inhaled corticosteroid therapy should be initiated or continued, and arrangements should be made for appropriate follow-up.

8. If the response is incomplete or poor (persistence of symptoms, PEF less than 70% of baseline), an inhaled, short-acting β_2-agonist should be given hourly and systemic corticosteroids begun. Treatment and monitoring can be continued for 1–3 hours provided improvement is noted. If the response is still incomplete (the patient remains symptomatic, PEF <70% of baseline), consider hospitalization for more intensive therapy and monitoring.

In summary, in the emergency department or hospital, the primary therapies—oxygen, inhaled β_2-agonist, and systemic corticosteroids—are constant, but the dose and frequency of administration and the frequency of assessing the patient's response may vary.

Indications for Hospitalization

The decision to hospitalize a patient is based on several considerations: duration and severity of symptoms, severity of airflow obstruction (measurements of FEV_1 or PEF), course and severity of prior exacerbations, medication use at the time of the exacerbation, access to medical care and medications, adequacy of support and home conditions, and presence of comorbidities, especially psychiatric illness.

In general, patients with an incomplete response to therapy in the emergency department (FEV_1 or PEF >50% but <70% of predicted value or "personal best") and persistence of mild to moderate symptoms require an individualized decision regarding hospitalization. Patients with an FEV_1 below 50% after 2 or 3 hours of initial treatment will generally require hospitalization; those who still appear fatigued or severely distressed or who still have severe airflow obstruction (FEV_1 or PEF <30% of predicted value) should be admitted to an ICU.

Identifying Patients at High Risk

Patients at high risk for asthma-related death require special monitoring and intensive education and care. The elements to consider in defining asthma severity and identifying those at risk for death are shown in Table 56.2.

It is not yet entirely resolved whether excessive use of an inhaled β-agonist is simply a marker of life-threatening asthma or in itself leads to an increased risk for death, but it is clear that the use of more than two canisters of an inhaled β-agonist per month is associated with a significant increase in the risk for death or near-death from asthma (17).

Indications for Intensive Care Unit Admission

A small subset of patients will require admission to an ICU for monitoring or for intubation and mechanical ventilation. These are patients with asthma that is unresponsive to

TABLE 56.2
RISK FACTORS FOR DEATH FROM ASTHMA

Past history of sudden severe exacerbations
Prior intubation for asthma
Prior admission for asthma to an ICU
Two or more hospitalizations for asthma in the past year
Three or more emergency care visits for asthma in the past year
Use of >2 canisters per month of inhaled short-acting $β_2$ agonist
Current use of systemic corticosteroids or recent withdrawal from systemic corticosteroids
Difficulty perceiving airflow obstruction or its severity
Comorbidity, such as cardiovascular diseases or chronic obstructive pulmonary disease
Serious psychiatric disease or psychosocial problems
Low socioeconomic status and urban residence
Illicit drug use
Sensitivity to *Alternaria*

From Kallenbach JM, Frankel AH, Lapinsky SE, et al. Determinants of near fatality in acute severe asthma. *Am J Med* 1993;95:265–272; Rodrigo C, Rodrigo G. Assessment of the patient with acute asthma in the emergency department: a factor analytic study. *Chest* 1993;104: 1325–1328; Suissa S, Ernst P, Boivin JF, et al. A cohort analysis of excess mortality in asthma and the use of inhaled β-agonists. *Am J Respir Crit Care Med* 1994;149:604–610; Greenberger PA, Miller TP, Lifschultz B. Circumstances surrounding deaths from asthma in Cook County (Chicago), Illinois. *Allergy Proc* 1993;14:321–326; O'Hollaren MT, Yunginger JW, Offord KP, et al. Exposure to an aeroallergen as a possible precipitating factor in respiratory arrest in young patients with asthma. *N Engl J Med* 1991;324:359–363, with permission.

the usual methods of treatment (*status asthmaticus*) or who manifest severe airway obstruction and impending respiratory arrest. Clinical features include an altered level of consciousness, obvious physical exhaustion, cyanosis or severe hypoxia (PaO_2 <60 mm Hg), pulsus paradoxus of more than 15 mm Hg, diminished breath sounds on auscultation ("silent chest"), tachycardia (>130 beats/min), and low arterial pH with a high $PaCO_2$. An FEV_1 value below 0.6 L or a PEF rate below 60 L/min that is unresponsive to bronchodilator therapy also heralds impending respiratory failure.

Such patients require the aggressive treatment and close monitoring that are possible only in an ICU setting. Arterial blood gases should be reassessed periodically until improvement occurs. Because of the dangers of intubation in severe asthma, additional treatments are sometimes attempted. One study found that the addition of intravenous montelukast improved FEV_1 and lessened the need for β agonist treatments but did not reduce the need for hospitalization (18). Slow (over 20–30 minutes) intravenous administration of magnesium sulfate (1–2 grams in adults) has not been proven effective but is safe, and it may be beneficial for some patients with severe acute asthma unresponsive to bronchodilators, oxygen, and corticosteroids (19). The same may be said of substitution of a mixture of helium and oxygen ("heliox") for oxygen-enriched air. Resistance to flow is a function of gas density, and use of a 70% helium, 30% oxygen mixture does lead to transient improvements in airflow and in clinical status, but the benefits wane after about an hour, so the treatment can be regarded only as temporizing, given in the hopes that other therapy becomes effective before intubation is necessary (20). A more promising approach to forestalling the need for intubation may be to apply noninvasive mechanical ventilation (21).

The addition of these unproven therapies may prevent the need for some intubations, but *intubation should not be delayed once it is deemed clinically necessary*. The intubation and ventilation of asthmatic patients is fraught with hazard and should be performed in a controlled setting by a physician with extensive experience in intubation and airway management (Chapters 23 and 24). Because respiratory failure can develop rapidly once a patient becomes fatigued, it may be necessary to intubate the patient in the emergency department or inpatient ward and subsequently transfer the patient to an ICU.

Once intubation has been performed, mechanical ventilation is complicated by a dramatic shift in intrathoracic pressures, with wide swings from inspiration to expiration in response to a continuously positive pressure. Venous return falls sharply, and the consequent fall in arterial pressure requires aggressive IV administration of crystalloid. The general strategy in mechanically ventilating a patient with respiratory failure from asthma is to avoid dynamic hyperinflation and high airway pressures and the associated risks of barotrauma (22) (Chapter 23). Expiratory time is thus made as long as possible to allow complete exhalation, and if the ventilation necessary to maintain a normal PCO_2 cannot be achieved without excessive airway pressure, "permissive hypercapnia" is accepted. Adequate tissue oxygenation is ensured by administration of high inspired oxygen tensions. Hypercapnia is intensely uncomfortable to the patient, so profound sedation and paralysis are necessary for this strategy.

ISSUES DURING THE COURSE OF HOSPITALIZATION

Treatment with inhaled β-agonists and oral or intravenous prednisone or methylprednisolone is almost invariably effective, but not always promptly. The rate of response roughly parallels the rate of deterioration, and the most rapid improvements occur in patients with sudden, severe attacks (e.g., after ingestion of sulfites or nonsteroidal anti-inflammatory medication, or after a food-provoking anaphylaxis). Slower responses to treatment are typically seen in attacks provoked by viral respiratory infections, especially if the attack has developed during several days and is associated with mucous hypersecretion. Clear improvement is sometimes not apparent until the third or fourth hospital day. In such cases, it is important to continue to monitor the patient closely because *improvement is not always smoothly progressive, and asthma sometimes worsens after initial improvement.* Nocturnal deterioration seems particularly common, and most respiratory arrests in hospitalized patients occur in the early hours of the morning. Monitoring FEV_1 or peak flow each morning and evening can provide useful information; wide diurnal swings suggest extreme bronchial lability and a heightened risk for respiratory arrest. Impatience with the slowness of response sometimes provokes the use of injudicious or unproven therapies, such as chest physical therapy or aerosolized mucolytic agents. Both can cause distress or fatigue, and an aerosolized mucolytic agent (e.g., acetylcysteine) can irritate the airway, thereby worsening cough and airflow obstruction.

DISCHARGE ISSUES

The criteria for discharge from the hospital resemble those for discharge from the emergency department. Discharge is appropriate when symptoms and physical findings are minimal and the PEF or FEV_1 remains above 70% of the predicted or "personal best" value for 3 or 4 hours after administration of a standard dose of an inhaled β-agonist from an MDI.

The requirement for hospitalization is a signal event, indicating an increased risk for asthma mortality during the subsequent year and probably also an inadequate understanding of triggers to be avoided or the actions that should be taken to abort attacks once they start. Before patients are discharged from the emergency department or hospital, they should be educated (or re-educated) regarding the need for maintenance "long-term controller" therapy (e.g., with an inhaled corticosteroid), avoidance of triggers (e.g., removing allergens and irritants from the home environment), and development of self-assessment skills (e.g., monitoring symptoms and peak flow). A peak flow meter should be given to the patient, along with instructions on how to measure and record peak flow values in a diary (see Table 56.3).

Before discharge, the provider and patient should review the nature and purposes of prescribed medications, with an emphasis on the importance of correct inhaler technique. Patients given systemic corticosteroids should continue them for 7–10 days. Inhaled corticosteroids, or the combination of an inhaled corticosteroid and a long-acting β-agonist should also be started before discharge. A follow-up appointment should be scheduled at about the time the course of oral corticosteroid therapy is to be completed.

Finally, the patient should be given at least a simple plan for actions to be taken if symptoms, signs, and PEF values suggest recurrent airflow obstruction (see Figure 56.2). The plan can be based on symptoms or peak flow, but it should follow the principle that therapy must be intensified (e.g., by increasing the dose of inhaled corticosteroid fourfold) as soon as asthma begins to worsen, with even more aggressive treatment undertaken (e.g., initiating a short course of prednisone) if the attack progresses. Action plans should be coupled with instructions for early contact with a provider to prevent recurrences of severe or life-threatening episodes.

COST CONSIDERATIONS AND RESOURCE USE

The high cost of asthma is largely attributable to the costs of hospitalization, emergency department visits, and unscheduled office visits. The risks for these events increase with increasing severity of disease and can be reduced by the regular use of "long-term controller" therapies, such as an inhaled corticosteroid and a long-acting inhaled β-agonist. The logical approach to reducing costs is thus improving the care of those patients most likely to require emergency care or hospitalization—patients with moderate or severe persistent asthma. One marker of severity is the need for hospitalization, and attention to the exacerbation itself should not distract providers from the opportunity hospitalization presents for intense patient education about the principles of self-assessment and care.

The measure that most powerfully reduces the costs of treatment of individual attacks is reducing the duration of

TABLE 56.3
HOSPITAL DISCHARGE CHECKLIST FOR PATIENTS WITH ASTHMA EXACERBATIONS

Intervention	Dose/timing	Education/advice (with M.D./R.N. initials)
Inhaled medications (MDI + spacer/ holding chamber)	Select agent, dose, and frequency (e.g., albuterol)	Teach purpose Teach technique
β_2-agonist	2–6 puffs q3–4h p.r.n.	Emphasize need for spacer/ holding chamber
Corticosteroids	Medium dose	Check patient technique
Oral medications	Select agent, dose, and frequency (e.g., prednisone 20 mg b.i.d. for 3–10 days)	Teach purpose Teach side effects
Peak flow meter	Measure a.m. and p.m. PEF and record best of three tries each time	Teach purpose Teach technique Distribute peak flow diary
Follow-up visit	Make appointment for follow-up care with primary clinician or asthma specialist	Advise patient (or caregiver) of date, time, and location of appointment (should be within 7 days of hospital discharge)
Action plan	Before or at discharge	Instruct patient (or caregiver) on simple plan for actions to be taken when symptoms, signs, and PEF values suggest recurrent airflow obstruction

MDI, metered dose inhaler; *PEF*, peak expiratory flow.
From: National Asthma Education and Prevention Program, Expert Panel Report 2. *Guidelines for the diagnosis and management of asthma.* NIH publication No. 97-4051, April 1997.

hospitalization. Prompt initiation of patient education in self-monitoring and treatment appears to increase the comfort of the inpatient medical and nursing staff with the idea of allowing the patient to go home so that a hospital stay is shortened by about a day. Additional savings can be achieved by avoiding unnecessary laboratory tests (especially arterial blood gas determinations, chest radiographs, and blood and sputum cultures) and avoiding inappropriate administration of antibiotics. Even severe airflow obstruction responds well to β-agonist administration by MDI with a spacer device. The costs for the personnel, equipment, and medication needed to deliver nebulized therapy are much greater, so savings can be achieved by reserving nebulized therapy for patients with severe attacks and switching to treatment by MDI as soon as possible. Institution of all these measures is enhanced by institution of a "clinical pathway" for inpatient asthma (23).

KEY POINTS

- Management of patients with asthma, particularly those with acute exacerbations, should begin with a risk assessment that considers the clinical presentation, the history, and objective measures of the severity of the attack.
- Respiratory drive is invariably increased in acute attacks of asthma, so detection of an elevated or even normal carbon dioxide tension (PCO_2) on arterial blood gas measurement indicates an attack of life-threatening severity.
- Hospital management of acute attack consists principally of oxygen supplementation, the frequent use of bronchodilators (especially inhaled β-adrenergic agonists), and systemic administration of corticosteroids.
- The place of antibiotics in the treatment of exacerbations of asthma is not established. Because viral respiratory infections are the most common precipitant of exacerbations, antibiotics should not be given routinely. There is some theoretical basis for the use of a macrolide antibiotic, but its clinical value has not been established.
- Hospitalization for asthma is a predictor of increased risk for readmission for subsequent attacks and for death from asthma. Full advantage must be taken of the opportunity presented by hospitalization to evaluate and improve the patient's knowledge of the disease and skills for self-monitoring and treatment.

Date_____

When to Monitor Peak Flow Numbers

☐ In the morning soon after waking up
☐ Before supper
☐ Before bed
☐ Before and 5-15 minutes after inhaled treatments
☐ With increased respiratory symptoms
☐ _____

Important Peak Flow Numbers

Baseline _____

_____ % baseline =_____
_____ % baseline =_____

If your peak flow number drops below _____ or you notice:

• Increased use of inhaled treatments to manage asthma
• Increased asthma symptoms upon awakening
• Awakening at night with asthma symptoms

Follow these treatment steps:

☐ Increase inhaled steroids.
   Take _____ puffs of _____ _____ times a day.

☐ Begin/increase treatment with oral steroids.
   Take _____ mg of _____
   in the ☐ morning and/or ☐ before supper.
☐ Other_____

If your peak flow number drops below _____ or you continue to get worse after increasing treatment according to the directions above, follow these treatment steps:

☐ Begin/increase treatment with oral steroids.
   Take _____ mg of _____
   in the ☐ morning and/or ☐ before supper.
☐ Contact your health care provider.
☐ Other_____

Contact your health care provider if:

☐ Asthma symptoms worsen while you are taking oral steroids, or
☐ Inhaled bronchodilator treatments are not lasting 4 hours, or
☐ Your peak flow number falls below _____.
☐ If you cannot contact your health care provider go directly to the Emergency Room.

Directions for Resuming Normal Treatment:

☐ Continue increased treatment until symptoms and peak flow number have returned to normal; then continue increased inhaled steroids or _____ mg of oral steroids for the same number of days it took to return to normal. If your peak flow number has not returned to normal in 5 days, contact your health care provider.

☐ Call your health care provider for specific instructions.

If you have questions please call:

_____ After hours_____
Name   Phone   Name   Phone

Physician Signature _____Date_____

Patient/Family Signature _____ Staff Signature_____

Figure 56.2   Adult self-management instructions for asthma action plan.
Adapted from the NIH guidelines for the diagnosis and management of asthma. Expert panel report 2. United States Department of Health and Human Services publication No. 97-4051.

REFERENCES

1. Mannino DM, Homa DM, Akinbami LJ, Moorman JE, Gwynn C, Redd SC. Surveillance for Asthma—United States, 1980–1999. *MMWR* 2002;51:1–13.
2. Smith DH, Malone DC, Lawson KA, Okamoto LJ, Battista C, Saunders WB. A national estimate of the economic costs of asthma. *Am J Respir Crit Care Med* 1997;156:787–793.
3. Practical guide for the diagnosis and management of asthma. Bethesda, MD: National Institutes of Health/National Heart, Lung, and Blood Institute/National Asthma Education and Prevention Program, 1997.
4. Ayres JG. Classification and management of brittle asthma. *Brit J Hospital Med* 1997;57:387–389.
5. McFadden ER Jr. Acute severe asthma. *Am J Respir Crit Care Med* 2003;168:740–759.
6. Message SD, Johnston SL. Viruses in asthma. *Br Med Bull* 2002; 61:29–43.
7. Bahrainwala AH, Simon MR. Wheezing and vocal cord dysfunction mimicking asthma. *Curr Opin Pulm Med* 2001;7:8–13.
8. Besbes-Ouanes L, Nouira S, Elatrous S, Knani J, Boussarsar M, Abroug F. Continuous versus intermittent nebulization of salbutamol in acute severe asthma: a randomized, controlled trial. *Ann Emerg Med* 2000;36:198–203.
9. Plotnick LH, Ducharme FM. Combined inhaled anticholinergics and β2-agonists for initial treatment of acute asthma in children. *Cochrane Database Syst Rev* 2000;CD000060.
10. Rowe BH, Spooner CH, Ducharme FM, Bretzlaff JA, Bota GW. Corticosteroids for preventing relapse following acute exacerbations of asthma. *Cochrane Database Syst Rev* 2000; CD000195.
11. Lee-Wong M, Dayrit FM, Kohli AR, Acquah S, Mayo PH. Comparison of high-dose inhaled flunisolide to systemic corticosteroids in severe adult asthma. *Chest* 2002;122:1208–1213.
12. Leuppi JD, SR Downie, CM Salome, Jenkins CR, Woolcock AJ. A single high dose of inhaled corticosteroids: a possible treatment of asthma exacerbations. *Swiss Med Wkly* 2002;132:7–11.
13. Rowe BH, Bota GW, Fabris L, Therrien SA, Milner RA, Jacono J. Inhaled budesonide in addition to oral corticosteroids to prevent asthma relapse following discharge from the emergency department: a randomized controlled trial. *JAMA* 1999;281: 2119–2126.
14. Edmonds ML, Camargo CA Jr, Brenner BE, Rowe BH. Replacement of oral corticosteroids with inhaled corticosteroids in the treatment of acute asthma following emergency department discharge: a meta-analysis. *Chest* 2002;121:1798–1805.
15. Expert panel report: guidelines for the diagnosis and management of asthma. Bethesda, MD: National Institutes of Health/National Heart, Lung, and Blood Institute/National Asthma Education and Prevention Program,2002;5074.
16. Kraft M, Cassell GH, Pak J, Martin RJ. Mycoplasma pneumoniae and Chlamydia pneumoniae in asthma: effect of clarithromycin. *Chest* 2002;121:1782–1788.
17. Spitzer WO, Suissa S, Ernst P, et al. The use of β-agonists and the risk of death and near-death from asthma. *N Engl J Med* 1992; 326:501–506.
18. Camargo CA Jr., Smithline HA, Malice MP, Green SA, Reiss TF. A randomized controlled trial of intravenous montelukast in acute asthma. *Am J Respir Crit Care Med* 2003;167:528–533.
19. Rowe BH, Bretzlaff JA, Bourdon C, Bota GW, Camargo CA Jr. Magnesium sulfate for treating exacerbations of acute asthma in the emergency department. *Cochrane Database Syst Rev* 2000; CD001490.
20. Ho AM, Lee A, Karmakar MK, Dion PW, Chung DC, Contardi LH. Heliox vs air-oxygen mixtures for the treatment of patients with acute asthma: a systematic overview. *Chest* 2003;123: 882–890.
21. Fernandez MM, Villagra A, Blanch L, Fernandez R. Non-invasive mechanical ventilation in status asthmaticus. *Intensive Care Med* 2001;27:486–492.
22. Shapiro JM. Management of respiratory failure in status asthmaticus. *Am J Respir Med* 2002;1:409–416.
23. Johnson KB, Blaisdell CJ, Walker A, Eggleston P. Effectiveness of a clinical pathway for inpatient asthma management. *Pediatrics* 2000;106:1006–1012.

ADDITIONAL READING

Kalltrom TJ. Evidence-based asthma management. *Respir Care* 2004; 49:783–792.

McFadden E Jr. Acute severe asthma. *Am J Respir Crit Care Med* 2003;168:740–759.

Roy SR, Milgrom H. Management of the acute exacerbation of asthma. *J Asthma* 2003;40:593–604.

Interstitial Lung Disease

57

Talmadge E. King, Jr.

INTRODUCTION

The interstitial lung diseases (ILDs) are a heterogeneous group of parenchymal lung disorders that are classified together because of similar clinical, roentgenographic, physiologic, or pathologic manifestations. Environmental or occupational exposures, especially to inorganic or organic dusts, are the most common known causes of ILD. Sarcoidosis, idiopathic pulmonary fibrosis (IPF), and pulmonary fibrosis associated with connective tissue diseases (CTD) are the most common ILDs of unknown etiology.

The incidence and prevalence of ILDs are unknown. Studies suggest a prevalence of 80.9 per 100,000 for men and 67.2 per 100,000 for women, with both incidence and prevalence rising with age. In 1988, an estimated 30,000 hospitalizations (compared with 665,000 hospitalizations for chronic obstructive pulmonary disease and asthma) and 4,851 deaths in the United States were attributed to pulmonary fibrosis. The death rate for pulmonary fibrosis appears to have increased during the past 20 years, but vital statistics are sparse and unreliable.

Table 57.1 outlines the major causes of ILD. In the vast majority of ILDs, the symptoms and signs unfold over months or years (e.g., IPF, sarcoidosis, and pulmonary histiocytosis X). In other ILDs, the onset may be acute (days to weeks) or subacute (weeks to months). These latter processes may be confused with community-acquired pneumonias because they often present with diffuse radiographic opacities, fever, or recurrent episodes of disease activity. Examples of acute or subacute processes include acute idiopathic interstitial pneumonia (AIP), diffuse alveolar hemorrhage syndromes (DAH), bronchiolitis obliterans with organizing pneumonia (BOOP), some drug-induced ILDs, eosinophilic pneumonias, hypersensitivity pneumonitis (HSP), and the acute immunologic pneumonia that complicates CTDs (especially systemic lupus erythematosus or polymyositis). Because these acute and subacute groups most frequently lead to hospitalization, this chapter focuses on these processes.

ISSUES AT THE TIME OF ADMISSION

Clinical Presentation

Patients with ILD most commonly come to clinical attention because of the insidious onset of progressive breathlessness on exertion (dyspnea), a persistent nonproductive cough, or an incidental finding associated with another disease, such as a CTD. Acute presentations are usually associated with the development of spontaneous pneumothorax, hemoptysis, wheezing, or chest pain.

Differential Diagnosis

Acute Interstitial Pneumonia (Hamman-Rich Syndrome)

Acute interstitial pneumonia is a rare fulminant form of lung injury that presents acutely (days), usually in a previously healthy person over the age of 40 (1). Fever, cough, and dyspnea are the most common clinical signs and symptoms. There is no sexual predilection. Results of routine laboratory studies are nonspecific and generally not helpful. Diffuse, bilateral opacification is seen on chest radiographs. Computed tomography (CT) shows bilateral, patchy, symmetric areas of "ground glass" attenuation. Most patients have moderate to severe hypoxemia, and in

TABLE 57.1
CLINICAL CLASSIFICATION OF INTERSTITIAL LUNG DISEASE

Environmental and occupational exposures

I. Inorganic dust
  A. Silica
  B. Silicates (i.e., asbestos, talc, and kaolin or "china clay")
  C. Hard-metal dusts (i.e., cadmium and titanium oxide)
  D. Beryllium
II. Organic dusts (hypersensitivity pneumonitis or extrinsic allergic alveolitis)
  A. Thermophilic bacteria (i.e., *Micropolyspora faeni*, *Thermoactinomyces vulgaris*, and *T. sacchari*)
    1. Farmer's lung
    2. Grain handler's lung
    3. Humidifier or air conditioner lung
  B. Other bacteria (i.e., *Bacillus subtilis* and *B. cereus*)
    1. Humidifier lung
  C. True fungi (i.e., *Aspergillus*, *Cryptostroma corticale*, *Aureobasidium pullulans*, and penicillin species)
III. Animal proteins (e.g., bird fancier's disease)
IV. Bacterial products (byssinosis)
V. Chemical sources, gases, fumes, vapors, aerosols, paraquat, and radiation

Drug-induced lung disease (partial list)

I. Acute onset
  A. Diffuse alveolar damage (DAD): "crack" cocaine, amiodarone, nitrofurantoin, and any cytotoxic agent (e.g., bleomycin, carmustine, busulfan, mitomycin, procarbazine, methotrexate, gefitinib, and trastuzumab)
  B. Noncardiogenic pulmonary edema (probably DAD): cytosine arabinoside, aspirin and related compound, and opiates
  C. Diffuse alveolar hemorrhage (DAH): "crack" cocaine, penicillamine, phenytoin, anticoagulants, thrombolytic agents, and cytotoxic drugs that cause diffuse alveolar damage
II. Acute or subacute onset
  A. Eosinophilic pneumonia: nonsteroidal anti-inflammatory agents and antibiotics (ampicillin, minocycline, sulfonamides, nitrofurantoin, and sulfasalazine)
  B. Bronchiolitis obliterans organizing pneumonia (BOOP): amiodarone, methotrexate, and bleomycin
  C. Desquamative interstitial pneumonia (DIP): nitrofurantoin and sulfasalazine

Fibrotic disorders of unknown etiology

I. Acute interstitial pneumonia (AIP)
II. Idiopathic pulmonary fibrosis (IPF)
III. Lymphocytic interstitial pneumonia (LIP)
IV. Idiopathic bronchiolitis obliterans organizing pneumonia (cryptogenic organizing pneumonia)
V. Respiratory bronchiolitis-associated interstitial lung disease (RB-ILD)/DIP

Connective tissue disease-associated interstitial lung disease

Primary or unclassified

I. Sarcoidosis
II. Pulmonary Langerhans' Cell Histiocytosis
III. Lymphangioleiomyomatosis
IV. Lymphangitic carcinomatosis
V. Vasculitides (Wegener's granulomatosis, Churg-Strauss syndrome)
VI. Chronic gastric aspiration
VII. Alveolar proteinosis
VIII. Eosinophilic pneumonia (acute and chronic)
IX. Chronic pulmonary edema
X. Diffuse alveolar hemorrhage (vasculitides, collagen vascular diseases, other autoimmune diseases, and drugs)
XI. Chronic uremia
XII. Hemorrhagic syndromes (Goodpasture syndrome and idiopathic pulmonary hemosiderosis)

many patients, respiratory failure requiring mechanical ventilation develops.

The diagnosis of AIP requires the demonstration of organizing *diffuse alveolar damage* (DAD) on lung tissue examination. Consequently, a lung biopsy (now generally performed thoracoscopically) is required to confirm the diagnosis. DAD is a nonspecific reaction to lung injury and is therefore the underlying lesion seen in many insults, including in the acute respiratory distress syndrome and cytotoxic drug injury. The characteristic histology of DAD includes the presence of interstitial and intra-alveolar edema, capillary congestion and microthrombi, and intra-alveolar hyaline membranes.

The mortality associated with AIP is high (>60%), with the majority of patients dying within 6 months of presentation. However, those who recover usually do not have a recurrence of the disease, and many have a substantial or complete recovery of lung function. The main treatment is supportive care; corticosteroids have not been demonstrated to be beneficial.

Diffuse Alveolar Hemorrhage

Diffuse alveolar hemorrhage (DAH) is a syndrome of diffuse intra-alveolar bleeding originating from the alveolar capillaries and occasionally the precapillary arterioles and postcapillary venules (2). The most frequent underlying associated histology is *pulmonary capillaritis*, which is an infiltration of neutrophils into the interstitium of the lung. Pulmonary capillaritis has been reported with variable frequency and severity among the vasculitides (Chapter 111). A bland form of pulmonary hemorrhage *without* capillaritis can be found as a complication of anticoagulation or thrombolytic therapies, various coagulopathies, and mitral stenosis.

Patients with DAH have several days of cough, dyspnea, and (most importantly) hemoptysis. Patients presenting to the hospital with DAH may be having a first episode, a recurrent episode, or the initial manifestation of an underlying disease. DAH should be suspected if there is an acute pneumonic presentation, a chest radiograph demonstrating diffuse alveolar opacities, or an unexplained anemia. It is important to note that one can have significant alveolar bleeding without hemoptysis. The demonstration of sequential hemorrhagic bronchoalveolar lavage specimens can verify the presence of DAH if hemoptysis is absent. Although the diagnosis of pulmonary capillaritis can be made by fiberoptic bronchoscopy with transbronchial biopsy, thoracoscopic biopsy is often required to be certain of the diagnosis. In addition, certain ancillary laboratory tests, such as antineutrophil cytoplasmic antibodies, antinuclear antibodies, and antiglomerular basement membrane antibodies, may help diagnose an underlying disease (Chapters 111 and 112). Therapy depends on the underlying process that gave rise to the pulmonary capillaritis and usually includes corticosteroids and cyclophosphamide or

azathioprine. Thus, it is crucial that infection be excluded as a cause of the acute illness. In more than 50% of DAH cases, regardless of cause, mechanical ventilation is required. Furthermore, many of the causes of DAH are associated with recurrent episodes.

Cryptogenic Organizing Pneumonia

Cryptogenic organizing pneumonia (COP), or *idiopathic bronchiolitis obliterans with organizing pneumonia* (idiopathic BOOP), is a clinicopathologic syndrome of unknown etiology that is often confused with community-acquired pneumonia. The disease usually presents in the fifth and sixth decade and affects men and women equally. Almost three-fourths of the patients have their symptoms for less than 2 months, and few have symptoms for more than 6 months before diagnosis. A flulike illness, characterized by cough, fever, malaise, fatigue, and weight loss, heralds the onset of COP in two-fifths of the patients. Inspiratory crackles are found on chest examination. Results of routine laboratory studies are nonspecific. Pulmonary function is usually impaired; a restrictive defect is the most common finding. Resting or exercise arterial hypoxemia is also common. The roentgenographic manifestations are quite distinctive and include bilateral, diffuse alveolar opacities (often recurrent and migratory) in the presence of normal lung volumes. Chest CT may reveal much more extensive disease than is expected from the plain radiographic findings. Corticosteroid therapy is the most commonly used treatment and results in clinical recovery in two-thirds of these patients.

Lung biopsy (usually via thoracoscopy) is required to confirm the diagnosis. The histopathologic process is characterized by an excessive proliferation of granulation tissue within small airways (*proliferative bronchiolitis*) and alveolar ducts associated with chronic inflammation in the surrounding alveoli. This organizing pneumonia ("BOOP pattern") is a nonspecific reaction to lung injury that can occur as a secondary finding adjacent to many pathologic processes (e.g., malignancy) or as a component of other primary pulmonary disorders (e.g., cryptococcosis, Wegener's granulomatosis, lymphoma, HSP, and eosinophilic pneumonia) (3). In cases of COP, however, the "BOOP pattern" is the only lesion found.

Drug-Induced Interstitial Lung Disease

Many drugs are capable of causing interstitial lung reactions, usually during the therapeutic period or immediately thereafter (4). Pulmonary reactions can occur acutely after a single dose of a drug such as nitrofurantoin or after inhalation of "crack" cocaine. Factors that increase the likelihood of a drug-induced ILD include older age of the patient, higher initial dosing, higher cumulative dose, and the use of several cytotoxic drugs in combination. Patients who receive cytotoxic chemotherapy for underlying malignancy with either bleomycin, busulfan, or carmustine are also at risk for the development of DAD after radiation therapy or treatment with high concentrations of oxygen. Patients being treated with amiodarone who undergo a surgical procedure in which high concentrations of oxygen are administered may also develop DAD. The diagnosis of drug toxicity is confirmed when withdrawal of the drug is followed by improvement and eventual resolution of the ILD. Further proof of a drug-related ILD is the return of the pneumonitis with reinstatement of the drug (not a recommended strategy).

Connective Tissue Diseases

Because of the systemic nature of CTDs, all components of the respiratory system can be involved. Although the pulmonary complication may occur simultaneously with the onset of the systemic disorder, it is more common for the pulmonary disorder to complicate a previously established CTD. An acute presentation, often mimicking that of community-acquired pneumonia, is most likely to occur in systemic lupus erythematosus but has also been noted in other CTDs (polymyositis–dermatomyositis, scleroderma, and mixed CTD). The possible underlying histologies for this acute pneumonitis include BOOP (usually seen with rheumatoid arthritis or polymyositis–dermatomyositis) (Figure 57.1), DAD, DAH (usually in patients with systemic lupus erythematosus and nephritis), nonspecific interstitial pneumonia, and lymphocytic interstitial pneumonia (often in patients with Sjögren syndrome, either primary or associated with rheumatoid arthritis). Pul-

monary hypertension (Chapter 59) and vasculitis (Chapter 111) can complicate the clinical course of patients with CTD. Although pulmonary complications of CTDs are not uncommon, the clinician must carefully consider infection or side effects of drug treatment as the cause of acute worsening in any patient with a CTD.

Idiopathic Pulmonary Fibrosis

The clinical manifestations of IPF are dyspnea on exertion, nonproductive cough, and "Velcro-type" inspiratory crackles on chest examination. In advanced disease, signs of cor pulmonale, digital clubbing, and cyanosis may be noted on physical examination. The chest roentgenogram and high-resolution CT typically reveal reduced lung volumes with patchy reticular opacities in the lower lung zones in a predominantly peripheral distribution. Honeycombing (small cystic lesions), traction bronchiectasis, subpleural fibrosis, and signs of pulmonary hypertension also may be present, depending on the stage of the disease. Pulmonary function studies often reveal restrictive impairment, reduced diffusing capacity for carbon monoxide, and hypoxemia.

Clinical deterioration in patients with IPF is expected. Most patients experience progressive breathlessness and decreased exercise tolerance during months to years. End-stage IPF frequently leads to incapacitating respiratory insufficiency, with patients unable to carry out activities of daily living without extreme distress. The goals of hospitalization are usually to search for a treatable cause of worsening symptoms or to provide comfort (oxygen, sedation)

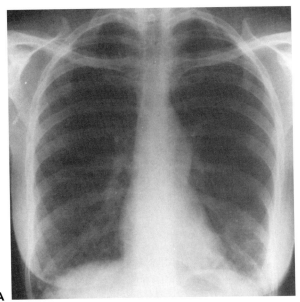
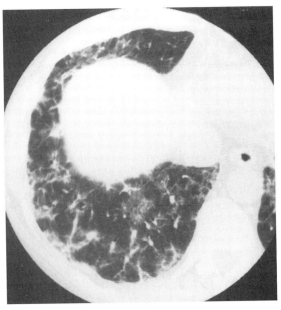

A

B

Figure 57.1 Dermatomyositis. **A.** This 51-year-old woman with long-standing dermatomyositis presented with cough, fever, and dyspnea of 2 weeks duration. The chest roentgenogram shows diffuse bilateral alveolar opacities, most prominent at the left lung base. **B.** High-resolution, thin-section computed tomogram shows predominantly patchy, "ground glass" opacities and consolidation, especially in the lower lobes. Thoracoscopic lung biopsy showed the pattern of bronchiolitis obliterans with organizing pneumonia (BOOP).

to the patient at the end of life (Chapter 19). Weaning patients with IPF from mechanical ventilation is extremely difficult; therefore, a decision to start mechanical ventilation should be made with extreme caution. Death usually ensues as a result of intractable hypoxemia and respiratory failure.

Some patients have acute or rapidly progressive disease ("acute exacerbation" or "accelerated stage" of IPF). This presentation is generally characterized by severe worsening dyspnea or cough and systemic symptoms, such as fever, fatigue, and weight loss. Usually, the illness duration prior to presentation is 2–4 weeks (5). The episodes often represent the superimposition of another process, such as DAD, DAH, or BOOP. In the evaluation of subacute or acute clinical deterioration in patients with IPF, disease progression may be difficult to distinguish from disease-associated complications and adverse effects of therapy (6). The incidence of pulmonary infections is slightly increased in IPF and is a major factor in the death of 2%–4% of patients. Therapeutic interventions, especially corticosteroids and cytotoxic agents, may further increase the risk for infection and reactivation of latent infections by suppression of cell-mediated immunity. Heart failure and ischemic heart disease are common problems in patients with IPF, accounting for nearly one-third of deaths. Right ventricular failure may develop as a result of pulmonary hypertension (present in approximately 70% of patients) (5). Pneumothorax is uncommon and may be extremely difficult to treat because the lung is stiff and difficult to re-expand. Prolonged chest tube drainage, with high levels of negative pressure (20–40 mm Hg), may be necessary. Some patients may require thoracotomy, bleb resection, and pleurectomy to close the air leak. Acute pulmonary embolism may cause a sudden worsening of dyspnea, with unexplained deterioration in arterial blood gas levels. Pulmonary embolism causes 3%–7% of deaths in IPF.

Interstitial Lung Disease Associated with Respiratory Bronchiolitis

Interstitial lung disease associated with respiratory bronchiolitis is a distinct and unusual clinical syndrome found in current or former cigarette smokers in their fourth or fifth decades of life. ILD associated with respiratory bronchiolitis and desquamative interstitial pneumonia are now thought to be different stages of the same process. Most patients present with a subacute (weeks to months) illness characterized by dyspnea and cough. Diffuse, fine, reticular or nodular interstitial opacities are found on chest radiographs; lung volumes are usually normal. Other features include bronchial wall thickening, prominence of peribronchovascular interstitium, small regular and irregular opacities, and small peripheral ring shadows. High-resolution CT shows similar features with hazy opacities. A mixed obstructive–restrictive pattern is common on lung function testing. Arterial blood gas levels show mild hy-

poxemia. The clinical recognition of ILD associated with respiratory bronchiolitis and of desquamative interstitial pneumonia is important because the process is associated with a good prognosis. Smoking cessation is the main treatment. Hospitalization is generally unnecessary (when it occurs, it is usually to facilitate initial evaluation and lung biopsy). The estimated mortality rate is 5% within 5 years, and overall survival is about 70% after 10 years.

Pulmonary Langerhans' Cell Histiocytosis

Pulmonary Langerhans' Cell Histiocytosis (previously called Pulmonary Histiocytosis X) is a rare, smoking-related diffuse lung disease that primarily afflicts young adults (usually men) between the ages of 20 and 40. The clinical presentation is variable, ranging from an asymptomatic state to a rapidly progressive condition. The most common clinical findings at presentation are cough, dyspnea, chest pain, weight loss, and fever. Pneumothorax occurs in about 25% of patients and is the most common reason for hospitalization. It is occasionally the first manifestation of the illness. Hemoptysis and diabetes insipidus are other, rare manifestations. The physical examination findings are usually normal. The radiographic changes include a combination of ill-defined or stellate nodules (2 mm–10 mm in size), reticular or nodular opacities, upper zone cysts or honeycombing, preservation of lung volume, and costophrenic angle sparing. The most frequent pulmonary function abnormality is a markedly reduced diffusing capacity for carbon monoxide, although varying degrees of restrictive disease, airflow limitation, and diminished exercise capacity have been described. Discontinuance of smoking is the key treatment; it results in clinical improvement in one-third of patients. Most patients with Pulmonary Langerhans' Cell Histiocytosis suffer persistent or progressive disease, and about 10% die of respiratory failure.

Sarcoidosis

Sarcoidosis is a systemic disorder of unknown origin characterized by granulomatous inflammation in a variety of organs, most commonly the lung. This disease is usually seen in younger persons between the ages of 20 and 40. The clinical presentation is quite variable; some patients are asymptomatic, some have generalized constitutional symptoms, and others have symptoms associated with specific organ involvement. Dyspnea, cough, and chest pain are common thoracic manifestations. The lungs often seem normal on auscultation even when parenchymal abnormalities are present on the chest roentgenogram. Hypercalcemia, hypergammaglobulinemia, and abnormal serum liver chemistries are frequently found. Symmetric, bilateral hilar adenopathy is the most common chest radiographic finding, but parenchymal opacities occur in roughly half of subjects (Figure 57.2). Pulmonary function testing may show a normal, restrictive, or mixed obstructive–restrictive

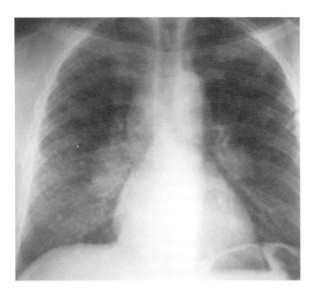

Figure 57.2 Sarcoidosis. This 38-year-old man was hospitalized because of worsening cough and breathlessness of 3–4 weeks duration. Previous chest radiographic findings were normal. This film shows bilateral hilar lymphadenopathy and diffuse nodular opacities (stage II sarcoidosis).

pattern. Hypoxemia or exercise-induced desaturation and a reduced diffusing capacity for carbon monoxide may also be seen. The diagnosis is occasionally made on clinical grounds, but in most cases, examination of lung tissue obtained by transbronchial biopsy is useful in confirming a suspected diagnosis of sarcoidosis.

Life-threatening situations that require hospitalization are very uncommon. These include progressive fibrosis with development of respiratory failure; cardiac disease (which often has a relatively rapid onset and high mortality because of ventricular arrhythmias, supraventricular arrhythmias, or heart block); renal failure secondary to granulomatous interstitial nephritis and hypercalcemia with hypercalciuria; hepatic disease with development of hepatic vein occlusion or bleeding esophageal varices; and neurosarcoidosis (meningitis, space-occupying lesions, cranial nerve involvement, diabetes insipidus, seizure disorders, peripheral neuropathies). Treatment with corticosteroids is indicated for symptomatic patients and those with involvement of vital organs, such as the eyes, central nervous system, and heart. Although sarcoidosis is generally very responsive to steroids, it is unclear whether the natural history of this disease is altered by therapy.

Eosinophilic Pneumonia

Acute eosinophilic pneumonia presents as a community-acquired pneumonia causing several days of dyspnea, nonproductive cough, and low-grade fever (7). It tends to appear in young persons. A recent history of the onset of cigarette smoking is present in some patients. The chest radiograph shows diffuse bilateral alveolar opacities. Most cases are idiopathic, but drug toxicity (particularly to non-steroidal anti-inflammatory agents and tetracycline and its related compounds) can also be responsible. Peripheral and bronchoalveolar lavage eosinophilia is often found.

Chronic eosinophilic pneumonia is a recurrent disease, appearing intermittently during several years and, in some patients, leading to extensive lung fibrosis. Most patients are between the fifth and eighth decades, and the onset is subacute, with cough and dyspnea present for weeks to months. More than half the patients with chronic eosinophilic pneumonia have a prominent background of asthma or allergies, and wheezing with evidence of airflow obstruction on lung function studies may therefore be present. Another important finding is an increased serum level of immunoglobulin E, seen in approximately two-thirds of the patients. The chest radiograph often shows alveolar opacities that are peripherally distributed ("photographic negative of pulmonary edema") (Figure 57.3). With recurrent disease, pulmonary fibrosis can develop, most prominently in the upper lung zones.

When patients are hospitalized with eosinophilic pneumonia, it is usually because of impending respiratory failure and the need to make a definite diagnosis. Intensive care is rarely needed if the diagnosis is made promptly and treatment initiated with corticosteroids. Both acute and chronic cases of eosinophilic pneumonia have an excellent response to corticosteroid treatment. Unfortunately, in

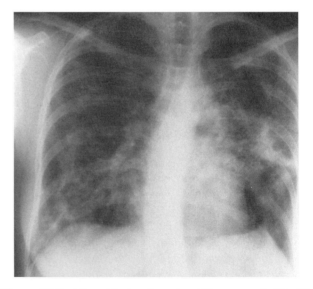

Figure 57.3 Idiopathic chronic eosinophilic pneumonia. This 35-year-old woman was hospitalized because of a progressive nonproductive cough, fever, malaise, and a 10-pound weight loss of 4 weeks duration. She had noted progressive breathlessness and night sweats during the week before admission. The chest roentgenogram shows bilateral diffuse peripheral opacities. There was a dramatic response to corticosteroid therapy, with complete resolution of the chest radiographic abnormalities within 1 month following discharge. She unfortunately has had multiple recurrences after withdrawal or lowering of her corticosteroids.

chronic eosinophilic pneumonia relapse frequently results when the steroids are tapered. Maintenance therapy with low doses of prednisone (5 mg–20 mg) is often required to prevent recurrence.

Inhalation Injury Secondary to Toxic Fumes, Gases, Chemicals, Aerosols, or Mists

Exposure to noxious and toxic fumes and gases is a significant industrial and environmental hazard (8). Oxides of nitrogen are the most common and best-described agents that cause acute and chronic lung injury, particularly nitrogen dioxide (NO_2). Silo filler's disease is a well-studied example, with an annual incidence of 5.0 cases per 100,000 silo-associated farm workers. Several outcomes are possible after an exposure, based on the setting, degree, and type of exposure: (a) Sudden death may occur in persons exposed to high concentrations of these substances. Death is caused by bronchiolar spasm, laryngospasm, reflex respiratory arrest, or simple asphyxiation. (b) In persons with mild exposures, symptoms may be limited to upper airway and visual disturbances. Some patients will experience cough, dyspnea, fatigue, cyanosis, vomiting, hemoptysis, arterial hypoxemia, vertigo, somnolence, headache, emotional difficulties, and loss of consciousness. These symptoms usually resolve in hours but may persist for several weeks before complete recovery occurs. (c) Pulmonary edema is a common complication at higher concentrations. Frequently, these patients have deceptively mild symptoms initially, but severe, acute DAD develops within several (3 to 30) hours. Most patients recover with no significant sequelae, but death may occur at this stage from progressive respiratory insufficiency. (d) In patients who have recovered or who suffered no acute illness after exposure, cough and dyspnea may recur or develop 2–6 weeks later.

In patients with acute lung injury, rales are usually present on auscultation of the lungs. The chest roentgenogram often demonstrates pulmonary edema. In survivors, these changes often clear rapidly. The roentgenographic pattern in the late stage can be variable, either normal or hyperinflated. Arterial hypoxemia, which is common, is caused by ventilation–perfusion mismatching resulting from altered airway dynamics and interstitial and alveolar edema. Methemoglobinemia may contribute to the arterial hypoxemia. Severe metabolic acidosis occurs when nitrogen dioxide dissolves in body fluids to form nitrous and nitric acid and tissue hypoxia leads to lactic acidosis. Decreased diffusing capacity is also common. These abnormalities gradually resolve in most patients.

Histopathologically, there may be severe pulmonary edema and evidence of DAD. Autopsy studies reveal marked intra-alveolar edema and exudation, in addition to thickening of the alveolar walls with lymphocytic cellular infiltrates. An organizing DAD with a component of proliferative bronchiolitis obliterans is seen in some patients who survive but have persistent lung injury. Widespread

constrictive bronchiolitis, obliterans or not, is found in patients in whom progressive obstructive lung disease develops.

Hospitalization for 24–48 hours is required after acute exposure, and the patient should be followed weekly or biweekly for 6–8 weeks. If arterial blood gas or pulmonary function test values are abnormal, treatment with corticosteroids should be started immediately. Corticosteroid therapy has been demonstrated to be useful in the management of both nitrogen dioxide-induced pulmonary edema and bronchiolitis obliterans. Treatment should be continued for a minimum of 8 weeks to avoid relapses. Bronchodilators are occasionally helpful. Antibiotics should be used only when clinically indicated and directed at a specific pathogen. The prognosis for survivors is generally good, although about one-third of persons exposed to nitrogen dioxide die acutely.

Hypersensitivity Pneumonitis

Hypersensitivity pneumonitis (HSP) denotes a group of diseases produced by repeated inhalation of finely dispersed organic dusts or simple chemicals in susceptible persons. Respiratory symptoms, fever, chills, and abnormal chest roentgenographic findings are often temporally related to working (*farmer's lung*) or engaging in a hobby (*pigeon breeder's disease*). Granulomatous inflammatory responses in these people produce diffuse or patchy patterns of interstitial and alveolar disease in the lungs. The list of antigens and sources or reservoirs of antigens potentially related to HSP continues to grow. Bacterial and fungal overgrowth in air conditioners, humidifiers, and evaporative coolers, in addition to bird droppings and proteins, are important causes of disease in urban settings.

The disease may present acutely, presumably after heavy or new antigen exposure, with the patient complaining of fever, chills, dyspnea, and cough. Inspiratory rales and mild hypoxemia are common. Chest radiographic findings may be normal or show fleeting reticular, nodular, or alveolar opacities, predominantly in the middle to lower lung zones (Figure 57.4). Leukocytosis is common, but eosinophilia is generally absent. Restrictive pulmonary function is seen early in the disease course, but lung function frequently is normal between exposures.

Hospitalization is rarely necessary, as the symptoms and signs usually resolve several hours after exposure has ended; symptoms often reappear on repeated exposure. In most patients who are hospitalized, the diagnosis is not suspected. Often, the patient is thought to have a community-acquired pneumonia and improves rapidly on treatment with antibiotics. After discharge, the patient commonly suffers a rapid and sometimes severe relapse when exposed again to the antigen.

HSP may present in a much less dramatic fashion. Low-level, persistent antigen exposure may cause a progressive deterioration in function associated with irreversible

Section VI: Pulmonary Medicine

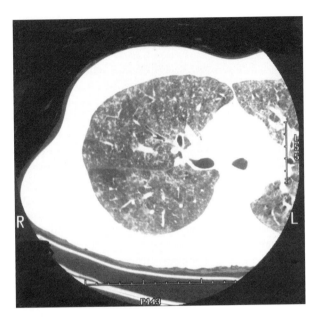

Figure 57.4 Hypersensitivity pneumonitis. This 39-year-old woman was hospitalized because of severe cough, dyspnea, and hypoxemia (oxygen saturation of 83% while breathing room air). She gave a history of a recurrent illness characterized by cough, breathlessness, and low-grade fever 4–6 hours after using her hot tub. Her admission chest examination revealed bilateral basilar crackles. Her chest radiographic findings were normal. High-resolution, thin-section computed tomography (Figure) showed a diffuse increase in lung attenuation with profuse, small, poorly defined centrilobular nodules. Thoracoscopic lung biopsy showed diffuse inflammation and numerous ill-formed granulomas.

pulmonary fibrosis. Mixed obstructive and restrictive pulmonary function is present, and predominantly upper lobe fibrosis with volume loss on chest radiography is typical of late-stage disease. Lung biopsy is often required for diagnosis and commonly shows bronchiolitis obliterans, fibrosis, and honeycombing in addition to areas of persistent interstitial pneumonitis with ill-formed granulomas. The diagnosis is often made on clinical grounds, especially in the early form of the disease. Precipitating antibodies to antigens commonly associated with HSP (e.g., thermophilic actinomycetes, *Micropolyspora faeni*, avian proteins) are often not present, and when present, they are not diagnostic. Avoidance of antigen exposure is the only established therapy for HSP. Steroids are often used to treat all forms of this disorder, but there are few data to confirm that they alter the natural history.

Initial Evaluation

History

The initial evaluation of patients with ILD should include a complete history and physical examination. Key areas of focus in the past history include occupational and environmental exposures and the smoking, medication, and family history. A strict chronologic listing of the patient's lifelong modes of employment must be sought, including specific duties and known exposures to dusts, gases, and chemicals. The degree, duration, and latency of exposure and the use of protective devices should be elicited. A review of the environment (at home and at work, and including the environments of spouse and children) is also valuable. Exposures to pets (especially any birds), air conditioners, humidifiers, hot tubs, and evaporative cooling systems (e.g., swamp coolers) and the presence of any water damage in the home or work environment is important to determine. The history of tobacco use is important because some diseases occur largely among never-smokers and former smokers (sarcoidosis and HSP) or among current and former smokers (desquamative interstitial pneumonitis, respiratory bronchiolitis, pulmonary histiocytosis X, and IPF). A detailed history of the medications taken by the patient is needed to exclude the possibility of drug-induced disease, including over-the-counter medications, oily nose drops, and amino acid supplements. Importantly, lung disease may occur weeks to years after the drug has been discontinued. The family history is occasionally helpful because familial associations have been identified in cases of IPF, sarcoidosis, tuberous sclerosis, and other rare conditions.

Physical Examination

The physical examination findings are commonly not specific but can be useful by revealing tachypnea, reduced chest expansion, and bilateral basilar end-inspiratory dry crackles. The cardiac examination findings are usually normal except in the middle or late stages of the disease, when findings of pulmonary hypertension (i.e., augmented P_2, right-sided lift, and S_3 gallop) and cor pulmonale may become evident (Chapter 59). Signs of pulmonary hypertension and cor pulmonale are generally secondary manifestations of advanced ILD, although they may be primary manifestations of a connective tissue disorder (e.g., progressive systemic sclerosis). Clubbing of the digits is common in some disorders (IPF, asbestosis) and rare in others (sarcoidosis, HSP, histiocytosis X). In most patients, clubbing is a late manifestation suggesting advanced derangement of the lung.

Laboratory Evaluation

The routine laboratory evaluation is often not helpful. Serologic studies should be obtained if clinically indicated by features suggestive of a CTD or vasculitis: sedimentation rate, antinuclear antibodies, rheumatoid factor, antineutrophil cytoplasmic antibodies, and antibasement membrane antibody (Chapters 111 and 112). A recent chest roentgenogram should be obtained, and it also is important to review all old chest roentgenograms to assess the tempo of change in disease activity. Complete lung function testing (spirometry, lung volumes, diffusing capacity) and a determination of resting arterial blood gases in room air should be obtained. Common diseases, such as chronic obstructive pulmonary disease, anemia, heart failure, and mycobacterial or fungal disease, can mimic ILD, so they must be ruled out. Most causes of ILD will be identified by the history, physical examination, and laboratory studies.

Chest Imaging Studies

The most common radiographic abnormality is a reticular or nodular pattern; however, mixed patterns of alveolar filling and increased interstitial markings are not unusual. Most ILDs have a predilection for the lower lung zones. As the disease progresses, widespread opacities are associated with reductions in lung volume and the appearance of pulmonary hypertension. A subgroup of ILDs has a predilection for the upper lung zones, and these ILDs often produce nodular opacities that cause an upward contraction of the pulmonary hilus. With progression of the disease, small cystic structures, which represent fibrous replacement of the normal alveolar architecture, and radiographic honeycombing appear. Although the chest roentgenogram is useful in suggesting the presence of ILD, the correlation between the roentgenographic pattern and the stage of disease (clinical or histopathologic) is generally poor. Only the radiographic finding of *honeycombing* (small cystic spaces) correlates with the pathologic findings; when present, it portends a poor prognosis. High-resolution CT is well suited for the evaluation of diffuse pulmonary parenchymal disease and often reveals disease patterns that aid in the diagnosis.

Lung Function Testing

Measurement of lung volumes and spirometry are important tests in assessing the severity of lung involvement in patients with ILD. Also, the finding of an obstructive or restrictive pattern is useful in narrowing the number of possible diagnoses. Most of the interstitial disorders have a *restrictive defect*, associated with a reduced total lung capacity (TLC), functional residual capacity (FRC), and residual volume (RV). Flow rates are decreased (forced expiratory volume in 1 second—FEV_1—and forced vital capacity—FVC), but these decreases are related to the decreased lung volumes. The ratio of FEV_1 to FVC is usually normal or increased. The smoking history must be considered when the functional studies are interpreted. A few disorders are associated with interstitial opacities on the chest roentgenogram and obstructive airflow limitation on lung function testing (e.g., sarcoidosis, lymphangioleiomyomatosis, HSP, tuberous sclerosis, and chronic obstructive pulmonary disease with superimposed ILD).

A reduction in the diffusing capacity for carbon monoxide is very commonly found but is not specific for any particular type of ILD. The decrease partly represents the degree of effacement of the alveolar capillary units, but more importantly the extent of ventilation–perfusion mismatching in the alveoli.

The resting arterial blood gas values may be normal or reveal hypoxemia (secondary to ventilation–perfusion mismatching) and respiratory alkalosis. Carbon dioxide retention is rare and usually a manifestation of far-advanced, end-stage disease. A normal resting value for arterial oxygen tension (or oxygen saturation by oximetry) does not rule out significant hypoxemia during exercise or sleep. Because resting hypoxemia is not always evident and because severe exercise-induced hypoxemia may go undetected, it is important to perform exercise testing with serial measurement of arterial blood gases. There is evidence that serial assessment of gas exchange at rest and during exercise is the best method to identify disease activity and responsiveness to treatment. Lung function testing is also discussed in Chapter 54.

Lung Biopsy

Occasionally, the bronchoalveolar lavage cellular distribution (not a recommended test; see below), chest radiographic or high-resolution CT appearance, or specific laboratory results in conjunction with the clinical story may be sufficient to establish a specific diagnosis. However, in most cases, histologic examination of lung tissue is required to make the diagnosis. In some disorders, transbronchial biopsy may yield a specific diagnosis; examples include alveolar proteinosis, sarcoidosis, and lymphangitic carcinomatosis. However, a transbronchial biopsy that shows only nonspecific inflammation or fibrosis is not acceptable. In these cases, *video-assisted thoracoscopic lung biopsy* by an experienced chest surgeon is recommended to establish a specific diagnosis.

Indications for Hospitalization

Hospitalization of patients with ILD usually occurs as a result of sudden worsening of dyspnea or cough, often associated with hypoxemia. Hospitalization is usually required to determine the diagnosis (especially to rule out or treat acute pneumonia) or to manage and monitor the severe hypoxemia that complicates the course of many of these patients. When associated with pleural pain, such hypoxemia may indicate a spontaneous pneumothorax or pulmonary embolism. *Spontaneous pneumothorax* is a characteristic finding in pulmonary histiocytosis X, tuberous sclerosis, lymphangioleiomyomatosis, and neurofibromatosis.

Indications for Initial Intensive Care Unit Admission

Few patients with ILD will require admission to an ICU during the initial phase of hospitalization. Those who do require intensive care have respiratory failure that is often associated with hemodynamic instability (hypovolemia or sepsis), significant concomitant medical disease (usually cardiovascular disease or renal failure), or severe hypoxemia requiring frequent monitoring of arterial blood gases or mechanical ventilation. The presence of hypercapnia is rare and portends a grave prognosis. Intubation and mechanical ventilation should be undertaken only after the patient's long-term prognosis has been carefully assessed. Patients with end-stage lung fibrosis of any cause are difficult to ventilate and are rarely successfully weaned from mechanical ventilation. ILD patients are rarely candidates for or tolerant of noninvasive ventilation.

Initial Therapy

The management of most ILDs is difficult, and the approach depends on the specific entity (Table 57.2) (6). Regardless of etiology, end-stage fibrosis is irreversible and untreatable. Thus, patients at this stage of illness should be spared the potential toxicity of agents such as corticosteroids. Pursuing a diagnosis and instituting appropriate therapy early in the disease course, before the development of extensive fibrosis, is likely to improve responsiveness to therapy and, it is hoped, delay or prevent the functional limitation and disability that commonly occur in these patients.

The major therapies for ILD involve the administration of corticosteroids, either alone or with a cytotoxic agent (cyclophosphamide or azathioprine). Many patients with ILD are elderly; consequently, the decision to treat them with immunosuppressive drugs should not be taken lightly, as the toxicity and side effects of these medications can be substantial. Among patients who present acutely and require hospitalization, those with underlying DAD have the worst prognosis. Conversely, patients with hypersensitivity pneumonitis, BOOP, or nonspecific interstitial pneumonia often demonstrate an excellent response to corticosteroid treatment (Table 57.2).

TABLE 57.2

LIKELIHOOD OF TREATMENT RESPONSE BASED ON HISTOLOGIC PATTERNS OF INTERSTITIAL LUNG DISEASE

Probability of response	Histologic entity
High	Bronchiolitis obliterans organizing pneumonia (BOOP)
	Cellular interstitial pneumonia
	Lymphocytic interstitial pneumonia (LIP)
	Eosinophilic pneumonia
	Pulmonary capillaritis
	Granulomatous pneumonitis
Medium	Diffuse alveolar damage (DAD)
	Desquamative interstitial pneumonia (DIP)
	Alveolar proteinosis
Low	Usual interstitial pneumonia (UIP)
	Honeycomb (end-stage) lung

Treatment of drug-induced ILD is based on recognition of the potential etiology and withdrawal of the suspected offending agent. In some cases, severe gas exchange abnormalities develop after the initiation of mechanical ventilation with high-flow oxygen. In this situation, corticosteroid medications are effective. This is especially true of drug-induced eosinophilic pneumonia, BOOP, and some cellular (nonspecific) interstitial pneumonias. In some patients with DAD secondary to cytotoxic drugs, corticosteroids can have a beneficial effect. Unfortunately, some patients with drug-induced DAD may progress to pulmonary fibrosis despite corticosteroid therapy. There is no rationale for the use of other immunosuppressive medication in cases that do not respond to corticosteroids. However, the failure to respond to both discontinuation of the drug and the addition of corticosteroid medication should raise the possibility of another cause for the interstitial pulmonary reaction.

Corticosteroid Therapy

The optimal dose of corticosteroids in the treatment of most ILDs is not known. Because most of the ILDs are chronic processes, patients who are hospitalized usually are on maintenance corticosteroid or cytotoxic therapy. It is the author's practice to treat acute exacerbations of established cases of AIP or new-onset AIPs with intravenous methylprednisolone (250–500 mg every 6 hours for up to 5 days). The patient is then placed on 40–60 mg of oral prednisone daily for 10–12 weeks, after which the dose is tapered to 20 mg and maintained for an additional 6–12 months. Intermittent, high-dose parenteral corticosteroid treatment ("pulse therapy") has also been used in patients with aggressive and severe disease. Treatment with 2 g of intravenous methylprednisolone once a week plus 0.25 mg of oral prednisone per kilogram daily suppresses the alveolitis present in many ILDs, but this treatment has not been clearly shown to improve the long-term outcome of patients with the lung disease.

The proper length of therapy in patients who respond to treatment is not known. The usual aim for a duration of therapy is at least 1 year. Rapid tapering or a shortened course of corticosteroid treatment can result in disease recurrence. Unfortunately, most patients experience declining lung function and worsening exercise tolerance despite corticosteroid therapy. If the patient's condition continues to decline on corticosteroids, a second agent is often added, and the prednisone dose is lowered to or maintained at 0.25 mg/kg/day. However, the addition of azathioprine or cyclophosphamide, particularly in patients with DAD, is of questionable benefit.

Cytotoxic Therapy

There is little experience with the use of intermittent ("pulse") intravenous cyclophosphamide therapy in patients with rapidly progressive disease. The author has used a dose of 2 mg/kg of ideal body weight administered over 30–60 minutes once daily for 3–5 days. Following this, daily oral therapy is initiated.

Although side effects are frequently encountered when corticosteroid or cytotoxic therapy is used, they usually do not necessitate discontinuation of therapy. Patients should be carefully monitored for the development of side effects from both corticosteroids and cytotoxics (see Figure 111.2).

Indications for Early Consultation

The initial presentation of patients with ILD frequently suggests that of acute community-acquired pneumonia. Consequently, the initial evaluation should follow the critical pathway outlined for the management of this problem (Figure 65.3). If there is concern that the illness is of non-infectious etiology, then pulmonary medicine consultation is recommended. Other indications for specialized testing and referral to a pulmonologist include the following: no specific cause of dyspnea or cough can be found; symptoms exceed the physiologic or radiographic abnormalities identified; empiric management (antibiotics, bronchodilators, diuretics, smoking cessation) results in an atypical or unsatisfactory clinical outcome; specialized testing is needed for diagnostic purposes (e.g., fiberoptic bronchoscopy with bronchoalveolar lavage; transbronchial, video-assisted thoracoscopic, or open lung biopsy); and therapy with immunosuppressive or cytotoxic drug is contemplated.

ISSUES DURING THE COURSE OF HOSPITALIZATION

Correction of the hypoxemia with appropriate levels of supplemental oxygen is the most important first step. The levels of oxygen required to maintain saturations above 90% can be much higher than those usually employed in other lung diseases. Wheezing should be managed with inhaled bronchodilators. Often, these are best delivered by nebulizer because the patient is too breathless to use a metered-dose inhaler properly (Chapter 56). Parenteral antibiotics are often given empirically because the presentation of acute exacerbations in patients with ILD is similar to that of a community-acquired pneumonia (fever with cough productive of purulent sputum). The critical pathway for community-acquired pneumonia (Figure 65.3) should be followed during the initial phases of hospitalization. The failure to improve after empiric therapy (usually by day 3 of hospitalization; Table 65.3) or the presence of other complications (pneumothorax, hemoptysis, worsening pulmonary status) prompts further pulmonary workup. Despite their often extreme breathlessness, patients should be encouraged to increase or maintain their level of activity, as tolerated, to prevent further deconditioning. Counseling regarding smoking cessation may be particularly effective during the hospital stay.

When appropriate, pneumococcal and influenza vaccination should be given before discharge.

DISCHARGE ISSUES

Patients with ILD, especially IPF, should be enrolled in a pulmonary rehabilitation program at discharge. Typically, patients are sufficiently dyspneic with exertion that they have stopped regular exercise and in fact might be frightened even to carry out normal daily activities that require physical exertion. These patients need encouragement to develop a routine conditioning program to improve muscle strength and cardiovascular efficiency. Education in energy management techniques may enable patients to perform more of their daily activities and hence improve their quality of life. For example, using labor-saving devices to simplify work, planning daily priorities, pacing physical activity, and improving breathing and body mechanics can significantly contribute to energy conservation.

Severe hypoxemia (PaO_2 <55 mm Hg) at rest or during exercise should be managed with supplemental oxygen. Usually, this can be accomplished by prescribing low-flow oxygen therapy via nasal cannula at home. Often, patients with ILD need higher oxygen flow rates (4–6 L/min, especially when walking) than are commonly employed in other chronic lung disorders. This must be taken into consideration when the oxygen prescription is written.

The patient and family should receive information and education about the medications used in treatment, especially because side effects are frequently encountered during corticosteroid or cytotoxic therapy (see Figure 111.2 for sample discharge instructions). Routine follow-up with the primary care physician should be scheduled within 2–3 weeks of discharge or sooner if significant comorbidities are present.

Many cases of ILD are chronic and irreversible. Consequently, these patients should be encouraged to issue advance directives indicating their wishes regarding life-sustaining therapies (Chapter 17). This issue should be discussed with the patient and family at the time of admission or at discharge.

COST CONSIDERATIONS AND RESOURCE USE

No studies have examined resource utilization in patients with ILD. Recent data show that surgical lung biopsy substantially changes the level of diagnostic certainty and is required in the patient with ILD whose clinical evaluation fails to establish a "certain" diagnosis. Also, studies have demonstrated that some tests previously touted in the assessment of ILD are not helpful, so reducing their use will result in lower costs. One such test is bronchoalveolar lavage, which may be valuable in ruling out certain acute processes (hemorrhage or infection) but has not proved to be clinically useful in the routine evaluation of the state of the pulmonary inflammatory response. In addition, the cellular analysis is time consuming and improperly performed by most clinical laboratories, so the data obtained can be invalid. The role and value of serial bronchoalveolar lavage in assessing the clinical progress of patients with IPF have also not been defined. Other frequently unhelpful tests include measurement of the sedimentation rate, angiotensin-converting enzyme levels, and circulating immune complex levels (none is helpful in diagnosis or follow-up) and gallium lung scanning (which is nonspecific and difficult to interpret).

Most ILD patients have progressive lung disease and cannot return to full employment after hospital discharge. The hospital or primary physician often needs to document the patient's level of impairment on an application for disability coverage. Lung transplantation may be offered to young patients with end-stage ILD but without significant comorbidities and to those with progressive, severe disease that is unresponsive to other forms of treatment. Lung transplantation is a costly procedure, and the guidelines for the selection of ILD patients are discussed elsewhere (Chapter 58).

KEY POINTS

- The interstitial lung diseases are a heterogeneous group of disorders with typical manifestations of cough, dyspnea, crackles on chest examination, diffuse interstitial opacities on chest radiograph, and a restrictive ventilatory defect.
- The vast majority of interstitial lung diseases are chronic; however, in some cases, the onset may be acute (days to weeks), subacute (weeks to months), or progressive, with the patient requiring hospitalization. These latter processes are often confused with community-acquired pneumonia.
- Important disorders to consider in hospitalized patients include acute idiopathic interstitial pneumonia, diffuse alveolar hemorrhage syndromes, bronchiolitis obliterans with organizing pneumonia, some drug-induced interstitial lung diseases, eosinophilic pneumonias, hypersensitivity pneumonitis, and the acute immunologic pneumonia that complicates connective tissue disease (especially systemic lupus erythematosus or polymyositis).

- In most cases, a specific diagnosis requires histologic examination of lung tissue. Therefore, lung biopsy (usually a video-assisted thoracoscopic lung biopsy) should be performed early in the clinical course.
- Treatment responses vary among these processes, and the likelihood of response is based mostly on the histologic patterns of the interstitial lung disease.

REFERENCES

1. Vourlekis JS, Brown KK, Cool CD, et al. Acute interstitial pneumonitis: case series and review of the literature. *Medicine* 2000;79:369–378.
2. Specks U. Diffuse alveolar hemorrhage syndromes. *Curr Opin Rheumatol* 2001;13:12–17.
3. Lohr RH, Boland BJ, Douglas WW, et al. Organizing pneumonia. Features and prognosis of cryptogenic, secondary, and focal variants. *Arch Intern Med* 1997;157:1323–1329.
4. Camus P. Drug-induced infiltrative lung disease. In: Schwarz MI, King TE Jr, eds. *Interstitial Lung Diseases.* 4th ed. Hamilton, Ontario, Canada: B. C. Decker, 2003:485–534.
5. Collard HR, King TE Jr. Demystifying idiopathic interstitial pneumonias. *Arch Intern Med* 2003;163:17–29.
6. Panos RJ, Mortenson R, Niccoli SA, King TE Jr. Clinical deterioration in patients with idiopathic pulmonary fibrosis. causes and assessment. *Am J Med* 1990;88:396–404.
7. Shorr AF, Scoville SL, Cersovsky SB, et al. Acute eosinophilic pneumonia among US military personnel deployed in or near Iraq. *JAMA* 2004;292:2997–3005.
8. King TE Jr. Bronchiolitis. In: Schwarz MI, King TE Jr., eds. *Interstitial Lung Diseases.* 4th ed. Hamilton, Ontario, Canada: B. C. Decker, 2003:787–824.

ADDITIONAL READING

Allen JN, Davis WB. Eosinophilic lung diseases. *Am J Respir Crit Care Med* 1994;150:1423–1438.
American Thoracic Society/European Respiratory Society. International multidisciplinary consensus classification of the idiopathic interstitial pneumonias. *Am J Respir Crit Care Med* 2002;165:277–304.
Hunninghake GW, Costabel U, Ando M, et al. Statement on sarcoidosis. *Am J Respir Crit Care Med* 1999;160:736–755.
King TE Jr. Idiopathic interstitial pneumonias. In: Schwarz MI, King TE Jr., eds. *Interstitial Lung Diseases.* 4th ed. Hamilton, Ontario, Canada: B. C. Decker, 2003:701–786.
Lynch JP III, McCune WJ. Immunosuppressive and cytotoxic pharmacotherapy for pulmonary disorders. *Am J Respir Crit Care Med* 1997;155:395–420.
Raghu G, Brown KK. Interstitial lung disease: clinical evaluation and keys to an accurate diagnosis. *Clin Chest Med* 2004;25:409–419.
Schwarz MI. The acute (noninfectious) interstitial lung disease. *Compr Ther* 1996;22:622–630.

Lung Transplantation and Lung Volume Reduction Surgery

58

Steven G. Peters   David E. Midthun

INTRODUCTION

Over the past decade, surgical options have emerged for patients with end-stage lung diseases that have been unresponsive to medical therapy. Lung transplantation is an established option for a subset of patients with obstructive lung diseases, restrictive diseases, and pulmonary hypertension, whereas lung volume reduction surgery has been evaluated for patients with emphysema. This chapter focuses on the evolving status of these procedures.

Patients with chronic obstructive pulmonary disease comprise the largest pool of candidates for transplantation. Chronic obstructive pulmonary disease is the fourth leading cause of death in the United States, accounting for more than 8 million physician visits, 726,000 hospitalizations, and approximately 119,000 deaths in 2000 (1). The majority of outpatient visits are for exacerbations of chronic bronchitis, and the majority of deaths are related to emphysema.

The pathophysiology of emphysema is characterized by irreversible destruction of distal air spaces with loss of alveolar walls and development of bullae. The combined effects of loss of elastic recoil and increased airway resistance lead to hyperinflation and decreased airflow. Ventilation–perfusion (V/Q) mismatching occurs, with regions of abnormally high V/Q acting as physiologic dead space, with impairment of CO_2 elimination, and areas of low V/Q contributing to venous admixture and shunting, resulting in hypoxemia. Surgical approaches may be directed toward replacement or toward removal of diseased areas to improve physiologic function.

LUNG TRANSPLANTATION

History

The first human *single-lung transplant* (SLT) was reported by Hardy and colleagues in 1963. The patient died of renal failure after 18 days. During the next 20 years, approximately 38 SLT procedures were performed, with poor results (2). The majority of patients died within 2 weeks of surgery of primary graft failure, rejection, or infection. Of 12 survivors beyond 2 weeks, seven died of dehiscence of the bronchial anastomosis. Enthusiasm for this procedure increased greatly in 1986 after the report by the Toronto Lung Transplant Group of successful SLT in patients with pulmonary fibrosis in a closely supervised program of perioperative pulmonary rehabilitation, limited use of preoperative corticosteroids, use of omentum to wrap the bronchial anastomosis, and immunosuppression with cyclosporine (3).

The beginning of *double-lung transplantation* (DLT) has been attributed to Yacoub and colleagues (2). Use of a single tracheal anastomosis was complicated by a high frequency of airway ischemia and dehiscence. Subsequent success has been achieved with bilateral bronchial anastomoses. Vascular anastomoses for SLT and DLT include the pulmonary artery and venous return via a cuff of donor left atrium. The indications for single versus double lung transplantation continue to evolve and are discussed below.

Heart–lung transplantation emerged in the early 1980s as an option for patients with pulmonary vascular diseases, especially congenital cardiac disease with Eisenmenger's syndrome, and primary pulmonary hypertension. Early postoperative complications included graft failure, acute rejection, and infection. As experience with heart–lung transplantation grew, the late complication of obliterative bronchiolitis (OB) emerged as the major contributor to morbidity and mortality. Although it was hoped that OB would not be as prevalent a complication of SLT and DLT, current experience indicates that this life-threatening complication may occur in more than half of lung transplant recipients who survive beyond 2–3 years.

Indications and Selection Criteria

Current indications for lung transplantation are shown in Table 58.1. Contraindications include active infection, malignancy, current cigarette smoking, drug abuse, and unstable psychological status, especially if the patient is unable to understand and comply with a complicated postoperative medical program. Additional relative contraindications include diabetes, osteoporosis, obesity, prior long-term use of corticosteroids, or a current requirement of more than 5–10 mg of prednisone daily. Systemic diseases that would be expected to affect outcome or survival following transplantation are considered contraindications. The presence of a connective tissue disease such as scleroderma resulting in pulmonary fibrosis or pulmonary hypertension is a contraindication in many but not all transplant programs. Prior thoracic surgery including open lung biopsy complicates possible removal of the lung and increases the risk for serious bleeding, but usually does not represent a contraindication to transplantation. Negative serologic status for Epstein-Barr virus (EBV) greatly increases the risk for posttransplantation lymphoproliferative disorder, which is discussed further

below. Whether negative EBV serology should preclude consideration of transplantation is controversial.

Preoperative Evaluation

Patients with emphysema, pulmonary fibrosis, cystic fibrosis, or pulmonary hypertension are referred most frequently for consideration of transplantation (4). Although SLT may be adequate for many of these patients, bilateral transplantation or heart–lung transplantation has often been performed, depending on surgical recommendation, donor availability, and underlying cardiac function. Patients with suppurative lung diseases, including bronchiectasis and cystic fibrosis, are considered for bilateral lung transplantation.

Data from the 2002 Registry of the International Society for Heart and Lung Transplantation show that SLT is currently carried out for emphysema (excluding α_1-antitrypsin deficiency) in approximately 54% of cases, α_1-antitrypsin deficiency emphysema in 9%, idiopathic pulmonary fibrosis in 24%, and primary pulmonary hypertension in only 1% (5). DLT or bilateral transplantation is performed for cystic fibrosis in 34%, emphysema in 22%, α_1-antitrypsin deficiency emphysema in an additional 10%, primary pulmonary hypertension in 8%, pulmonary fibrosis in 9%, and a variety of conditions in the remainder of cases.

Potential candidates are evaluated with a complete history and physical examination and by pulmonary function testing, arterial blood gas determination, and exercise testing, including 6-minute walking distance. Cardiac catheterization is carried out for assessment of right-sided pressures, and coronary angiography is performed for older adults and previous cigarette smokers. Laboratory studies include blood typing and serologic studies for cytomegalovirus (CMV), EBV, herpes viruses, *Toxoplasma*, and fungal organisms. Renal function is assessed in anticipation of impairment induced by cyclosporine, tacrolimus, or other immunosuppressive and anti-infective agents. Bone mineral density frequently is abnormal in transplant candidates because of corticosteroid therapy and prolonged inactivity. Although newer anti-resorptive agents have improved the outlook for patients with osteoporosis, measurements below the fracture threshold may represent a relative barrier to successful transplantation and rehabilitation. All candidates participate in an ongoing program of pulmonary rehabilitation, with goals of maintaining cardiorespiratory conditioning and functional status to the greatest extent possible. Because waiting periods currently exceed 2 years in most centers, management during the waiting time may have an important impact on outcome.

Outcomes

Currently, overall survival following lung transplantation is approximately 75% at 1 year, 65% at 2 years, and 50% at 4–5

TABLE 58.1

SELECTION CRITERIA FOR LUNG TRANSPLANTATION

Age <65y
End-stage pulmonary disease despite maximal medical therapy
Limited life expectancy without transplantation
Satisfactory rehabilitation potential
Ability to comply with medical program
Satisfactory psychosocial status
No active systemic disease expected to worsen outcome
No other major organ system dysfunction

years (5). Survival for patients with emphysema is approximately 10% greater at any time after transplant than for patients with idiopathic fibrosis or pulmonary hypertension. For patients with emphysema, bilateral lung transplantation is associated with statistically improved 3- to 5-year survival compared to SLT. However, criteria for patient selection have varied, and organ supply remains limited, so that the choice of transplant procedure remains controversial. For the individual patient, survival figures must be considered in light of the existing quality of life and expected survival without further intervention. Physiologic improvement following successful lung transplantation is characterized by increased vital capacity and expiratory flows and by improved gas exchange. Maximal oxygen consumption and 6-minute walking distance typically double by 3 months after transplantation. Functional status may improve proportionally, with approximately 80% of patients performing daily activities without restriction at 1 year after surgery. Approximately 20% of patients are reported to be working full-time and 10% part-time at 1 year. The major causes of morbidity and mortality following transplantation, including infection, rejection, OB, and malignancy, are discussed below.

CARE OF THE HOSPITALIZED PATIENT FOLLOWING LUNG TRANSPLANTATION

Postoperative Care and Immunosuppression

Complications following organ transplantation usually reflect the conflict between the need to administer immunosuppressive drugs to prevent rejection and the side effects of these agents. Most current protocols for immune suppression are based on the use of a combination of *cyclosporine or tacrolimus (FK-506), azathioprine or mycophenolate mofetil, corticosteroids, and antilymphocyte antibodies* (antilymphocyte globulin, antithymocyte globulin, or OKT3) (6).

In lung-transplant patients receiving regimens containing cyclosporine, close monitoring is necessary. The most common adverse effects of cyclosporine are renal insufficiency and hypertension. At maintenance dosing levels, renal clearance typically falls and serum creatinine rises to average values of 1.5–2.0 mg/dL. Within 1 year following lung transplantation, the serum creatinine level is greater than 2.5 mg/dL in approximately 8% of patients. Hypertension requiring additional treatment is present in the majority of patients at 1 year. Early studies, including both retrospective data and prospective comparisons, suggest that tacrolimus may be superior to cyclosporine for maintenance immunosuppression and for treatment of rejection episodes (7). Although no improvement in overall survival has been demonstrated, the frequency of acute rejection episodes and of late development of OB is reported to be less with tacrolimus regimens. Recent registry data indicate that approximately 40% of lung transplant recipients are receiving tacrolimus for maintenance immunosuppression (5).

Similarly, early data support a potential role for mycophenolate mofetil as an alternative to azathioprine in anti-rejection therapy for solid organ transplants. Preliminary data in lung transplant recipients suggest that this agent may also be useful in the treatment of chronic rejection and bronchiolitis obliterans. In an effort to reduce the long-term adverse effects of corticosteroids (including obesity, osteoporosis, and myopathy), many solid organ transplant programs attempt to wean from steroids stable patients who have not had recurrent rejection episodes. However, experience with steroid withdrawal in lung transplant recipients is limited, and concern remains regarding the risks for chronic rejection or OB. Finally, monoclonal OKT3 has been used in cardiothoracic transplantation for induction immunosuppression and for acute rejection.

Complications Requiring Hospitalization

In the first year following lung transplantation, approximately 55% of patients are readmitted, most frequently for infection and rejection. Common complications are listed in Table 58.2.

Early graft dysfunction may result from a variety of insults, including acute lung injury after implantation, airway ischemia, dehiscence or stenosis, and pulmonary vascular complications. Acute rejection may present with any combination of dyspnea, cough, and fever; as an asymptomatic decline in pulmonary function test values; or as radiographic pulmonary infiltrates. In addition to these complications, infections constitute the main differential diagnostic considerations in the early weeks following transplantation.

As indicated in Table 58.2, a relatively small number of organisms account for most infections following lung transplantation. Bacterial infection with gram-negative or

---

TABLE 58.2

COMMON COMPLICATIONS FOLLOWING LUNG TRANSPLANTATION

Early graft failure
Implantation lung injury
Airway anastomotic complications
Pulmonary vascular complications
Acute rejection
Infection
Bacterial
  Viral, especially CMV, herpes, EBV
  Fungal, especially *Aspergillus, Cryptococcus*
  Pneumocystis jirovecii, Nocardia, Toxoplasma
  Mycobacteria: tuberculosis, atypical
Obliterative bronchiolitis
Posttransplant lymphoproliferative disorder (PTLD)
Other malignancies
Other complications (e.g., renal failure, hypertension, diabetes)

CMV, cytomegalovirus; *EBV*, Epstein-Barr virus.

-positive organisms is common, and, although these infections are usually treated successfully, they contribute significantly to early postoperative mortality. CMV infection is a common cause of morbidity and mortality, especially if the recipient is CMV antibody-negative and receives an organ from a CMV-positive donor. Early manifestations may range from asymptomatic viral shedding identified in blood or urine to pneumonitis or extrapulmonary involvement of gastrointestinal, hepatic, neurologic, or hematologic systems. Prophylaxis for CMV-mismatched patients is commonly administered in the form of ganciclovir or valganciclovir. Prophylactic therapy also is given for fungal organisms. Although *Candida* isolates rarely result in organ injury, *Aspergillus* species can cause significant morbidity and mortality in lung transplant patients. Disease may be localized to the native or transplanted lung, and dissemination is usually a fatal late complication. Prophylaxis with itraconazole has probably decreased these complications, but controlled data are not available. *Pneumocystis jirovecii* pneumonia is generally prevented by prophylactic trimethoprim-sulfamethoxazole, but pneumonitis remains a life-threatening complication in patients who discontinue or cannot tolerate these medications.

Bronchoscopy plays an early and important role in differentiating rejection and infection. Bronchoalveolar lavage should have a yield of at least 80% for most of the pathogens listed in Table 58.2, especially CMV and pneumocystis. Transbronchoscopic lung biopsy increases the yield of infectious agents only slightly but may identify or confirm an inflammatory response (e.g., granulomas or CMV inclusions). However, the chief purpose of transbronchoscopic lung biopsy is to establish and quantify the presence of rejection. Acute rejection is characterized by perivascular lymphocytic infiltrates and is classified according to a standardized scale (grade 0, none; grade 4, severe). Acute rejection is treated by augmentation of immunosuppression, most commonly with high-dose methylprednisolone. Bronchoscopic biopsies are usually repeated after treatment to confirm resolution. Persistent rejection is often treated with further corticosteroids, antilymphocyte antibodies, or cytotoxic agents.

Obliterative bronchiolitis has been identified as the most common cause of late morbidity and mortality following lung transplantation. The prevalence of OB approaches 50% at 1 year, and the entity accounts for the majority of posttransplant deaths at 5 years. The onset is characterized by a gradually progressive decline in pulmonary function, most often defined as a decrease in the forced expiratory volume in 1 second (FEV_1) of more than 10% of the baseline postoperative value. Radiographic changes can include hyperinflation and loss of peripheral vascular markings, but these can be subtle on plain films. Computed tomography may show a mosaic pattern of increased lucency representing focal air trapping, especially evident on expiratory views. Histologic changes are characterized by patchy fibroproliferative occlusion of bronchioles. Al-

though the specific causes of these chronic and progressive inflammatory changes are unknown, the major risk factors appear to be recurrent acute rejection episodes and possibly prior CMV pneumonitis. Although the specific diagnosis of OB requires histologic confirmation, the yield with transbronchoscopic lung biopsy is low, and open lung biopsy is performed infrequently because other diagnoses are unlikely in the appropriate clinical setting and therapeutic options are limited. The OB syndrome can be diagnosed in the setting of a decline in FEV_1 in the absence of infection, acute rejection, or other apparent etiology. Treatment with augmented immunosuppression has been disappointing. A definition of the potential role of tacrolimus and mycophenolate mofetil in the possible prevention and treatment of OB awaits further experience, although many programs use these agents as primary immune suppression, or switch from cyclosporine and azathioprine if acute or chronic rejection is detected.

Following solid organ transplantation, malignancies develop in 5%–10% of patients, at an average interval of 4–5 years after surgery. Squamous cell carcinomas of the skin and lips are most common, accounting for nearly half of all neoplasms. *Posttransplantation lymphoproliferative disorders* (PTLD) account for 15%–20% of malignancies. The overall frequency of PTLD following solid organ transplants is approximately 3%, but the risk is higher for lung transplant recipients. Histologically, PTLD usually are identified as B-cell neoplasms of recipient origin and may be monoclonal or polyclonal. Extranodal disease is common, including lung, liver, and central nervous system nodular lesions. EBV infection following transplantation has been implicated as the major risk factor for PTLD. In a Mayo Clinic series of solid organ transplant patients, PTLD developed in 3 of 367 (0.8%) patients who were EBV-seropositive before transplant, and in 11 of 22 (50%) who were EBV-negative (8). Additional risk factors include CMV mismatch (seronegative recipient) and OKT3 immune suppression. Because the relative risk for PTLD is high in EBV-negative patients, EBV seronegative status is considered a relative contraindication for potential lung recipients at some centers. Some cases of PTLD have been observed to resolve after immunosuppression is decreased, so the current empiric approach to therapy usually includes a period of several weeks of observation after cyclosporine is reduced by approximately 50%, azathioprine is decreased or discontinued, and prednisone is reduced to approximately 5–10 mg. Combination chemotherapy protocols for lymphoma (Chapter 94) are considered if disease persists or progresses.

The hospital physician may encounter a variety of other complications of immunosuppression or of the underlying disease. These include diabetes, hypertension, complications of osteoporosis, renal failure, neurologic disease, and gastrointestinal bleeding, ulceration, or perforation. These conditions are relatively uncommon causes of late death following transplantation but are frequent contributors to major morbidity.

LUNG VOLUME REDUCTION SURGERY

History

Pulmonary resection for emphysema has been performed for more than 40 years, most commonly for localized large bullae that compress adjacent lung tissue. Physiologic improvement results from recruitment of functioning alveoli, increased elastic recoil of the lungs, and improvement in chest wall and diaphragm mechanics. The origin of lung resection for diffuse emphysema (in the absence of giant bullae) is attributed to Brantigan in 1957. Initially, high morbidity and mortality prevented widespread acceptance of the procedure. In recent years, a variety of approaches have been taken to remove or obliterate peripheral bullous disease, including wedge resections using midline sternotomy, thoracotomy or thoracoscopic techniques, and laser treatment of the lung surface. Cooper and colleagues (9) are credited with developing the current approach to lung volume reduction surgery (LVRS), in which approximately 20%–30% of each lung (usually tissue from upper zones where the severity of the emphysema is the greatest) is excised by means of a linear stapling device buttressed with strips of bovine pericardium intended to prevent air leaks. This procedure has shown better short-term outcomes than has laser bullectomy. Following bilateral LVRS, FEV_1 improves by an average of approximately 50%, residual volume falls by 28%, and symptoms of dyspnea improve. Physiologic improvement has been attributed to increased lung elastic recoil, decreased chest wall compliance, improvement in respiratory muscle function, and increased airway conductance.

The reported success of LVRS led to the widespread application of surgical procedures for emphysema, with varying results from a large number of centers and practitioners, most of which have not been reported. The value of the intervention, considerations of cost versus benefit, and the potential role of randomized, controlled trials in the assessment of surgical procedures have been debated publicly. In a new paradigm for clinical research, the Health Care Financing Administration (now called the Center for Medicare and Medicaid Services) and the National Heart, Lung, and Blood Institute jointly sponsored the National Emphysema Treatment Trial (NETT). This study was designed to compare medical therapy, including pulmonary rehabilitation, with similar therapy plus LVRS. The hospital physician might encounter patients who are candidates for LVRS, or who have undergone this type of surgery. Less invasive methods than surgery for achieving volume reduction in emphysema are emerging. The bronchoscopic placement of one-way valves has shown the ability to reduce volume in applied segments in animals (10). Human studies in patient with emphysema are underway.

Results

Results from three small-randomized control trials of LVRS versus medical therapy showed that bilateral LVRS improved static lung function, gas exchange and quality of life compared to medical therapy and pulmonary rehabilitation alone (11–13). However, not every patient showed improvement and mortality with surgery was higher. Results of the NETT study are summarized in Table 58.3. A total of 1,218 participants with severe emphysema completed pulmonary rehabilitation and were then randomized to continued medical therapy or LVRS (14). After a mean follow-up of 29.2 months, overall mortality was the same in both arms. However, LVRS showed a significantly greater improvement at 24 months in exercise capacity, FEV_1, quality of life and dyspnea. These improvements were greatest at 6 months, but waned in follow-up at 12 and 24 months.

The NETT study found a survival benefit with surgery only in a subset of patients with predominantly upper-lobe emphysema and low exercise capacity after rehabilitation (14). A higher risk of death was demonstrated with surgery compared to medical treatment in participants with non-upper lobe disease and high exercise capacity.

Selection Criteria for Lung Volume Reduction Surgery

General criteria for LVRS have evolved with clinical experience in patients with diffuse emphysema. These include severe and disabling disease, thoracic hyperinflation, and

TABLE 58.3

NATIONAL EMPHYSEMA TREATMENT TRIAL (NETT) RESULTS

Therapy	# patients	Mortality		% with improvement in FEV_1			% with improvement in exercise capacity	% with improvement in QOL
		90-day	overall	6 mos.	12 mons.	24 mos.	24 months	24 months
Medical	610	1.3%	26.2%	27	26	19	3	9
Surgical	608	7.9%	25.8%	65	56	43	15	33

QOL, quality of life.
From Fishman A, Martinez F, Naunheim K, et al. A randomized trial comparing lung-volume-reduction surgery with medical therapy for severe emphysema. *N Engl J Med* 2003;348:2059–2073.

TABLE 58.4

SELECTION CRITERIA FOR LUNG VOLUME REDUCTION SURGERY

Severe emphysema with hyperinflation
Maximal medical therapy, including pulmonary rehabilitation
Age <80 years
FEV_1 ≤45% predicted, TLC ≥100% predicted, RV ≥150% predicted
Bronchodilator response <30% improvement
pCO_2 ≤55 mm Hg, pO_2 ≥45 mm Hg on room air
High resolution chest CT showing emphysema
Mean pulmonary artery pressure ≤35 mm Hg (peak ≤45 mm Hg)
No smoking
No recurrent infections, chronic bronchitis, or bronchiectasis
No severe cachexia

CT, computed tomography; *FEV_1*, forced expiratory volume in 1 second; *RV*, residual volume; *TLC*, total lung capacity.

nonhomogeneous "target areas" for resection. Commonly accepted indications are listed in Table 58.4 (15).

The intent of these selection criteria is to identify candidates whose disease is severe enough to warrant this intervention and who are most likely to benefit, given the data available. Prior to consideration of LVRS, patients requiring steroids are weaned to the lowest possible level, typically a dose of prednisone of less than 10–20 mg daily. Patients are also expected to complete at least a 6-week pulmonary rehabilitation program. Respiratory failure requiring mechanical ventilation has been considered a contraindication, although successful outcomes of LVRS have been reported in this setting. Although malignancy has also been an exclusion criterion, volume reduction has been carried out at the time of lung cancer resection in patients who otherwise might have been considered inoperable because of poor lung function. Using relatively strict criteria, Cooper and colleagues (9) excluded approximately 80% of patients referred for LVRS, most commonly for homogeneous disease, insufficient lung hyperinflation, or other medical conditions. The NETT identified a subgroup who were at high risk of death from LVRS. Patients who had a FEV_1 that was no more that 20% of their predicted value and either a homogeneous distribution of emphysema on CT or a carbon monoxide diffusing capacity (DLCO) of no more that 20% of predicted, had a 30-day mortality of 16% (16). There were no deaths in patients with these criteria in the nonsurgical treatment arm (P <0.001). Therefore, *LVRS should not be offered to patients meeting these criteria.*

Preoperative evaluation with CT and stress echo appear to be appropriate. A number of studies have assessed the quantification and distribution of emphysema with high resolution CT, spiral CT, CT morphometry, or V/Q scanning. In general, heterogeneous distribution of emphysema is the best predictor of post-operative increase in static function but not of exercise tolerance or dyspnea. Bossone et al, showed that, despite the difficulty of performing echocardiograms in patients with marked hyperinflation, a negative dobutatmine stress echo was a perfect predictor of an absence of major cardiac events following LVRS (17).

Care of the Hospitalized Patient Following Lung Volume Reduction Surgery

The average length of hospital stay following volume reduction surgery has been approximately 10–15 days, including shortening of stay with experience. Overall operative mortality has been approximately 4%–6%, with 1-year mortality in the range of 10%. Common complications are listed in Table 58.5.

Many patients have persistent *air leaks* following surgery. In the series of Cooper et al. (9), 46% of 150 patients had an air leak beyond 7 days. One randomized study showed that buttressing the staple line with bovine pericardium reduced air leaks and drainage time but did not change length of hospital stay compared to patients with nonbuttressed staples (18). Unless a large pneumothorax is present, chest tubes are frequently left attached to a water seal because suction is felt to perpetuate surface leaks. Approximately 5%–10% of patients require postoperative mechanical ventilation beyond 24–48 hours. Respiratory failure may reflect the severity of the underlying emphysema or be related to any of the complications listed above. In addition to air leaks, *postoperative pneumonia* has been a common and serious complication. Fewer than 5% of patients in reported series have required tracheostomy for prolonged ventilator support. Myocardial infarction and cardiac arrest have been observed rarely following LVRS, a finding that reflects the careful selection process and the quality of surgical and anesthetic management in reported series. Gastrointestinal complications, including ileus, bleeding, and bowel perforation, have occurred infrequently.

TABLE 58.5

COMPLICATIONS FOLLOWING LUNG VOLUME REDUCTION SURGERY

Prolonged air leaks, pneumothorax
Intrathoracic bleeding
Respiratory insufficiency requiring prolonged mechanical ventilation
Pneumonia
Cardiovascular complications (e.g., myocardial infarction, cardiac arrest, atrial arrhythmia)
Gastrointestinal complications (e.g., ileus, bleeding, bowel perforation)

Lung Volume Reduction Surgery vs. Lung Transplantation

Some patients hospitalized with exacerbations of severe chronic obstructive pulmonary disease may have exhausted medical therapy and ask the hospital physician about surgical options. Consideration of either LVRS or transplant requires that the patient be in generally good health aside from severe lung disease. Most patients with emphysema and severe airway obstruction will not be candidates for transplantation (but may be candidates for LVRS) based on age above 65 years. However, younger patients may require a decision between the two procedures. At this point, the best option for any given 50-year-old patient with severe emphysema is unclear. The 5-year survival rate for lung transplant is approximately 30%–40% and the only 5-year data for LVRS suggest that survival is similar (19). Attractive features of LVRS include the lack of immunosuppression, lesser expense, and the opportunity to fall back on transplant if surgery is not successful in alleviating symptoms or if improvement wanes. Senbaklavaci et al. reported that successful LVRS (resulting in improvement in FEV_1 by $\geq 20\%$ over baseline) delayed the subsequent need for transplantation, improved nutritional state and reduced perioperative mortality following subsequent lung transplant (20). Those patients who had unsuccessful LVRS ($<20\%$ improvement in FEV_1 over baseline) required transplant 11 months sooner and had a higher perioperative mortality than those with successful LVRS. Further study will need to clarify which procedure is the best option for the young patient with emphysema.

CONCLUSIONS

Lung transplantation and LVRS have emerged as surgical options for the treatment of severe emphysema. Evaluation of potential candidates requires thorough examination, laboratory and pulmonary function testing, and assessment of other medical conditions and risk factors for adverse outcomes. Even with careful patient selection, postoperative complications requiring prolonged hospitalization or readmission are frequent. Because of limited donor availability, lung transplantation remains an option for relatively few patients each year. The National Emphysema Treatment Trial showed improvement in exercise capacity and pulmonary function with LVRS. However, the surgery confered no survival advantage over medical therapy.

KEY POINTS

- Lung transplantation is an option for a subset of patients with end-stage lung diseases unresponsive to maximal medical therapy and with satisfactory rehabilitation potential. Currently, transplantation is carried out most often for emphysema, cystic fibrosis, pulmonary fibrosis, and pulmonary hypertension.
- The most common complications of lung transplantation are infection, rejection, adverse drug effects, obliterative bronchiolitis, and posttransplant lymphoproliferative disorders.
- Bronchoscopy with bronchoalveolar lavage and transbronchoscopic biopsy is an early and important step in the evaluation of new symptoms or pulmonary infiltrates in the transplant recipient.
- Obliterative bronchiolitis occurs in the majority of lung transplant patients beyond 2–3 years after surgery and is a major cause of late mortality and morbidity.
- The risk for posttransplant lymphoproliferative disorder is greatly increased in patients who are seronegative for Epstein-Barr virus at the time of transplantation. Additional risk factors include cytomegalovirus mismatch and OKT3 immune suppression.
- Lung volume reduction surgery has emerged as a promising therapy for highly selected patients with heterogeneous involvement by severe emphysema.
- Major complications of lung volume reduction surgery include prolonged air leaks, bleeding, pneumonia, respiratory insufficiency requiring mechanical ventilation, and death.
- The National Emphysema Treatment Trial showed no overall difference in mortality at 2-years between medical therapy and LVRS. Patients at high risk and not considered candidates include those with an FEV_1 of $<20\%$ predicted and either homogeneous distribution of emphysema on CT or a diffusing capacity of $<20\%$ predicted.
- The NETT study showed the LVRS improved pulmonary function, exercise capacity, dyspnea, and quality of life when compared with medical therapy. A survival advantage was seen with LVRS in those patients with upper-lobe predominant emphysema and low-exercise capacity after rehabilitation.

REFERENCES

1. Mannino DM, Homa DM, Akinbami LJ, et al. Chronic obstructive pulmonary disease surveillance—United States, 1971–2000. *Morbidity and Mortality Weekly Report* 2002;51:1–16.
2. Daly RC, McGregor CGA. Surgical issues in lung transplantation: options, donor selection, graft preservation, and airway healing. *Mayo Clin Proc* 1997;72:79–84.
3. Toronto Lung Transplant Group. Unilateral lung transplantation for pulmonary fibrosis. *N Engl J Med* 1986;314:1140–1145.
4. Peters SG, McDougall JC, Scott JP, et al. Lung transplantation: selection of patients and analysis of outcome. *Mayo Clin Proc* 1997;72:85–88.
5. Hertz, MI, Taylor DO, Trulock EP, et al. The registry of the International Society for Heart and Lung Transplantation: nineteenth official report—2002. *J Heart Lung Transplant* 2002;21:950–970.
6. Midthun DE, McDougall JC, Peters SG, et al. Medical management and complications in the lung transplant recipient. *Mayo Clin Proc* 1997;72:175–184.

7. Griffith BP, Bando K, Hardesty RL, et al. A prospective randomized trial of FK506 versus cyclosporine after human pulmonary transplantation. *Transplantation* 1994;57:848–851.

8. Walker RC, Paya CV, Marshall WF, et al. Pretransplantation seronegative Epstein-Barr virus status is the primary risk factor for posttransplantation lymphoproliferative disorder in adult heart, lung, and other solid organ transplantations. *J Heart Lung Transplant* 1995;14:214–221.

9. Cooper JD, Patterson GA, Sundaresan RS, et al. Results of 150 consecutive bilateral lung volume reduction procedures in patients with severe emphysema. *J Thorac Cardiovasc Surg* 1996;112:1319–1330.

10. Maxfield RA. New and emerging minimally invasive techniques for lung volume reduction. *Chest* 2004;125:777–783.

11. Criner GJ, Cordova FC, Furukawa S, et al. Prospective randomized trial comparing bilateral lung volume reduction surgery to pulmonary rehabilitation in severe chronic obstructive pulmonary disease. *Am J Respir Crit Care Med* 1999;160:2018–2027.

12. Geddes D, Davies M, Koyama H, et al. Effect of lung–volume reduction surgery in patients with severe emphysema. *N Engl J Med* 2000;343:239–245.

13. Pompeo E, Marino M, Nofroni I, et al. Reduction pneumoplasty versus respiratory rehabilitation in severe emphysema: a randomized study. Pulmonary Emphysema Research Group. *Ann Thorac Surg* 2000;70:948–953.

14. Fishman A, Martinez F, Naunheim K, et al. A randomized trial comparing lung-volume-reduction surgery with medical therapy for severe emphysema. *N Engl J Med* 2003;348:2059–2073.

15. Rationale and design of the National Emphysema Treatment Trial (NETT): a prospective randomized trial of lung volume reduction surgery. *J Thorac Cardiovasc Surg* 1999;118:518–528.

16. National Emphysema Treatment Trial Research Group. Patients at high risk of death after lung volume reduction surgery. *N Engl J Med* 2001;345:1075–1083.

17. Bossone E, Martinez FJ, Whyte RI, et al. Dobutamine stress echocardiography for the preoperative evaluation of patients undergoing lung volume reduction surgery. *J Thorac CV Surg* 1999;118:542–546.

18. Stammberger U, Klepetko W, Stamatis G, et al. Buttressing the staple line in lung volume reduction surgery: a randomized three-center study. *Ann Thorac Surg* 2000;70:1820–1825.

19. Gelb AF, McKenna RJ, Brenner M, et al. Lung function 5 years after lung volume reduction surgery for emphysema. *Am J Respir Crit Care Med* 2001;163:1562–1566.

20. Senbaklavaci O, Wisser W, Ozpeker C, et al. Successful lung volume reduction surgery brings patients into better condition for later lung transplantation. *Eur J Cardio-Thorac Surg* 2002; 22:363–367.

ADDITIONAL READING

Burns KE, Keenan RJ, Grgurich WF, et al. Outcomes of lung volume reduction surgery followed by lung transplantation: a matched cohort study. *Ann Thoracic Surg* 2002;73:1587–1593.

Cassivi SD, Meyers BF, Battafarano RJ, et al. Thirteen year experience in lung transplantation for emphysema. *Ann Thoracic Surg* 2002;74(5):1663–1669.

Cordova FC, Criner GJ. Surgery for chronic obstructive pulmonary disease: the place for lung volume reduction and transplantation. *Curr Opin Pulm Med* 2001;7:93–104.

Flaherty KR, Martinez FJ. Lung volume reduction surgery for emphysema. *Clin Chest Med* 2000;21:819–848.

Meyers BF, Yusen RD, Guthrie TJ, et al. Results of lung volume reduction surgery in patients meeting a national treatment trial high-risk criterion. *J Thorac Cardiovasc Surg* 2004;127:829–835.

Pulmonary Hypertension

59

Lewis J. Rubin

INTRODUCTION

The normal pulmonary circulation is a high-flow, low-pressure circuit that is capable of accepting the entire right ventricular (RV) output at a pressure one-fifth of that in the systemic circulation. When pulmonary artery pressure is increased, either as a result of intrinsic diseases affecting the pulmonary vessels, disturbances in ventilation or intrapulmonary gas exchange, or downstream cardiac disease, RV afterload increases. Ultimately, the increased ventricular work imposed by the elevations in pulmonary vascular resistance results in RV dysfunction, right-sided heart failure, and death. Pulmonary hypertension is considered to be present when the mean pulmonary artery pressure exceeds 25 mm Hg at rest or 30 mm Hg during exercise (1). This chapter reviews the causes of pulmonary hypertension, their presenting signs and symptoms, and the initial approach to diagnosis and management.

ISSUES AT THE TIME OF ADMISSION

Clinical Presentation

The most common presenting symptom of patients with pulmonary vascular disease is dyspnea, which results from the inability of the right side of the heart to increase cardiac output and systemic oxygen delivery to meet the demands of physical activity. Dyspnea typically develops with exertion, but as pulmonary hypertension and RV dysfunction progress, it occurs with lesser degrees of activity. Exertional chest pain, similar to angina pectoris, may occur in severe pulmonary hypertension. It is thought to be a consequence of RV ischemia. Dizziness or syncope, particularly during

or immediately after exertion, is an ominous prognostic sign, indicating an inability to maintain cerebral perfusion because of marked limitations in RV output. Less common presenting symptoms of chronic pulmonary hypertension include a nonproductive cough, hoarseness (resulting from compression of the recurrent laryngeal nerve by enlarged main pulmonary arteries), and hemoptysis. The reader is referred to Chapter 53 regarding the presentation of patients with acute pulmonary hypertension associated with acute pulmonary embolism.

Although the findings of pulmonary hypertension on physical examination are often subtle, particularly in the early stages, important clues to the etiology may be evident. Examination of the jugular venous pulse may disclose a prominent *a* wave indicative of a poorly compliant RV, prominent *c-v* waves indicating the presence of tricuspid insufficiency, or venous distention suggesting an elevated right atrial pressure. Examination of the chest may reveal signs of severe airway obstruction, parenchymal lung disease, or hypoventilation as a consequence of body habitus or thoracic cage deformities. Patients with chronic thromboembolic pulmonary hypertension (CTEPH) may have bruits audible in the chest, which represent flow through partially obstructed vessels (2). An accentuated pulmonic component to the second heart sound (P_2), an S_3 or S_4 gallop, and murmurs of tricuspid or pulmonic insufficiency may be appreciated on cardiac examination. Fixed splitting of S_2, with or without a soft diastolic murmur audible at the base of the heart, is suggestive of an atrial septal defect with Eisenmenger's syndrome. The presence of ascites or hepatomegaly may be clues to either right-sided heart failure or significant intrinsic liver disease with associated pulmonary hypertension (portal–pulmonary hypertension syndrome). Examination of the extremities may demonstrate clubbing, which is suggestive of chronic pulmonary disease, congenital heart disease, or chronic liver disease. Central cyanosis suggests severe hypoxemia, caused either by disturbances in ventilatory function or right-to-left shunting with congenital heart disease. Peripheral cyanosis and edema are the result of a severely reduced cardiac output and right-sided heart failure, respectively. Examination of the skin and joints may show signs of a connective tissue disease, such as systemic sclerosis, systemic lupus erythematosis, or rheumatoid arthritis. Patients with portal–pulmonary hypertension caused by cirrhosis may have numerous truncal spider angiomas.

Differential Diagnosis and Initial Evaluation

Once the suspicion of pulmonary vascular disease has been raised by the patient's symptoms or signs, the approach should be directed toward establishing the presence of pulmonary hypertension and clarifying its etiology. A classification of conditions causing pulmonary hypertension is shown in Table 59.1. A meticulous history may provide important clues regarding causes. Prior or recent use of cocaine, anorexigenics (3), or intravenous (IV) drugs, in addition to risk factors for exposure to HIV, should be explored because all have been implicated in the development of pulmonary hypertension. A family history of pulmonary hypertension or death at a relatively young age from "heart disease" may suggest familial primary pulmonary hypertension (PPH), which accounts for approximately 7%–10% of all cases of that disease, or a familial prothrombotic state predisposing to chronic thromboembolic disease. A prior history of deep venous thrombosis or pulmonary embolism should raise the suspicion of CTEPH. A history of Raynaud's phenomenon suggests the presence of a connective tissue disease, although approximately 20% of patients with PPH may also experience this condition. Heavy alcohol use or infection with viral hepatitis raises the possibility of cirrhosis as the underlying etiology. Daytime somnolence, nightmares, and snoring suggest the presence of disordered breathing during sleep, with nocturnal hypoxemia and hypercapnia.

The initial diagnostic approach is outlined in Figure 59.1. Routine tests, including the chest radiograph and electrocardiogram, may disclose evidence of pulmonary hypertension, although the sensitivity of these studies is low for early disease. Echocardiography is often the first study that demonstrates findings of pulmonary hypertension, including right-sided chamber enlargement, flattening or displacement of the interventricular septum (which suggests RV pressure overload), and tricuspid regurgitation. The pulmonary artery systolic pressure can be estimated noninvasively by Doppler techniques based on the magnitude of the tricuspid regurgitant jet. Additionally, valvular disease, congenital heart disease, and conditions affecting left ventricular function can be excluded by transthoracic or transesophageal echocardiography. Contrast echocardiog-

TABLE 59.1

CLASSIFICATION OF PULMONARY HYPERTENSION

Intrinsic pulmonary vascular disease

Primary pulmonary hypertension
Connective tissue diseases (systemic sclerosis, systemic lupus erythematosis)
Pulmonary vasculitis
Eisenmenger's syndrome
Portal–pulmonary hypertension syndrome
HIV-associated pulmonary hypertension
Exogenous substances (anorexigens, cocaine, L-tryptophan, contaminated rapeseed oil)
Chronic thromboembolic pulmonary hypertension

Pulmonary vascular disease resulting from chronic respiratory disease

Parenchymal lung disease (interstitial lung disease, obstructive airways disease, mixed disorders)
Disorders of ventilation (sleep apnea and obesity hypoventilation syndromes, restrictive chest wall disease)
Chronic hypoxic exposure (altitude)

Pulmonary vascular disease resulting from disorders of left-sided heart filling

Left ventricular systolic or diastolic dysfunction
Mitral valve disease

Pulmonary vascular disease resulting from mechanical obstruction

Mediastinal fibrosis
Foreign bodies (talc, fibers)
Tumor
Parasites
Granulomatous vascular disease

raphy may also disclose the presence of a patent foramen ovale, which occurs frequently in the setting of right atrial pressure overload.

A number of additional studies should be obtained to assist in establishing the etiology of pulmonary hypertension. Serologic studies (e.g., antinuclear antibody, rheumatoid factor, HIV antibody) can exclude connective tissue diseases and HIV infection. Of note, antinuclear antibodies are frequently present in patients with PPH, although usually in a low titer and nonspecific pattern. More detailed serologic testing may be necessary if a specific connective tissue disorder is suspected. Standardized tests of lung function should be performed to exclude significant lung disease. Mild reductions in lung volumes or the diffusing capacity are nonspecific and may be seen in PPH in addition to most other forms of pulmonary vascular disease. Measurement of arterial blood gases while the patient is breathing ambient air and 100% oxygen is important, not

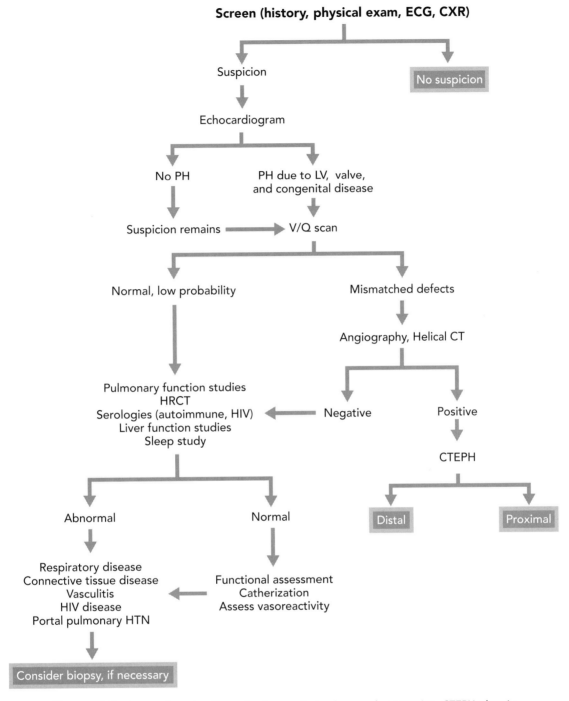

Figure 59.1 Approach to the diagnosis of suspected pulmonary hypertension. *CTEPH*, chronic thromboembolic pulmonary hypertension, *CXR*, chest X-ray; *ECG*, electrocardiogram; *HRCT*, high-resolution CT scan; *HTN*, hypertension; *LV*, left ventricular; *PH*, pulmonary hypertension.

only to clarify the need for supplemental oxygen therapy but also to determine whether a shunt exists. Similarly, measurement of oxygen saturation during activity, either by direct analysis of an arterial blood sample or by noninvasive measurement (pulse oximetry), may disclose desaturation, which can be effectively avoided through the use of ambulatory supplemental oxygen. Polysomnography is indicated when sleep apnea is suspected.

Imaging studies play a key role in differentiating between causes of pulmonary hypertension. Of these, the ventilation–perfusion lung scan is the most important because it may provide the sentinel clue to the presence of occult chronic thromboembolic disease. Because the ventilation–perfusion scan underestimates the extent of vascular involvement with chronic thrombosis, pulmonary angiography should be performed if the scan shows any

572 Section VI: Pulmonary Medicine

mismatched perfusion defects. Pulmonary angiography not only confirms the presence of thromboembolic disease but also delineates the sites and extent of involvement, information that is necessary to assess candidacy for pulmonary thromboendarterectomy. The lung scan in PPH is typically normal, whereas a patchy, nonsegmental perfusion pattern may be observed in pulmonary veno-occlusive disease. Other studies that can be helpful include spiral and high-resolution computed tomography, which can detect proximal thrombotic disease and occult interstitial lung disease, respectively.

Cardiac catheterization is usually the final diagnostic procedure performed in the evaluation of a patient with suspected pulmonary hypertension. A comprehensive study should include the measurement of right- and left-sided intracardiac and vascular pressures and cardiac output, and a search for the presence of intracardiac shunts or valvular disease. In the appropriate circumstances, testing for the presence of pulmonary vasoreactivity by means of short-acting vasodilators may also be performed during initial hemodynamic study.

Examination of lung tissue is rarely needed to establish an etiology for pulmonary hypertension. Furthermore, lung biopsy is often poorly tolerated by patients with pulmonary vascular disease, owing to their fragile cardiopulmonary status. When a definitive diagnosis cannot be made on clinical grounds, or when the management depends on the histopathologic findings (as in pulmonary vasculitis or other inflammatory conditions), thoracoscopically-guided biopsy is less invasive and carries a lower risk for adverse events than does open lung biopsy. The transbronchial biopsy specimens obtained via fiberoptic bronchoscopy are inadequate for establishing a diagnosis in most cases of pulmonary hypertension. Furthermore, the risk for uncontrollable hemorrhage is significant.

Indications for Hospitalization

The main indications for hospitalization are shown in Table 59.2. In general, much of the initial evaluation can be performed in the outpatient setting in most cases. However, patients with a rapid onset of symptoms, those with signs of progressive deterioration of right-sided heart function or severe hypoxemia, and patients who will be undergoing cardiac catheterization with acute vasodilator testing should be admitted.

Indications for Intensive Care Unit Admission

Patients who are hemodynamically unstable, defined as having systemic hypotension or severe hypoxemia requiring high concentrations of supplemental oxygen to maintain an adequate oxygen saturation, or those with evidence of severe right-sided heart failure (ascites, marked pedal edema) should be admitted to the ICU for management. This approach facilitates close monitoring of the patient's status as diagnostic and therapeutic approaches are initiated.

Initial Therapy

The initial therapy of pulmonary hypertension depends on the etiology. Patients with pulmonary vascular disease resulting from severe respiratory disease should be treated with modalities that will improve lung function and gas exchange (4). For example, sleep apnea should be managed with nocturnal use of noninvasive positive pressure ventilation, chronic airflow obstruction should be aggressively treated with bronchodilators and anti-inflammatory agents (Chapter 55), and interstitial lung disease should be treated with corticosteroids or other immunosuppressant or anti-inflammatory agents (Chapter 57), as appropriate. Supplemental oxygen therapy should be used in patients with hypoxemia at rest or during physical activity, both to optimize oxygen delivery to the peripheral tissues and to reduce the contribution of hypoxic pulmonary vasoconstriction to the altered pulmonary hemodynamic state. Patients with CTEPH should undergo placement of an inferior vena cava filter device, initiation of anticoagulation, and evaluation for pulmonary thromboendarterectomy (2) (Chapter 53). Patients with a connective tissue disease should receive the appropriate therapies for their systemic condition (Chapters 111 and 112).

Acute testing of pulmonary vasoreactivity is mandatory before a patient with PPH or connective tissue disease is given a course of vasodilator therapy, because less than 50% of patients respond to vasodilators. Vasodilators can cause significant deterioration in unresponsive patients by producing systemic hypotension, worsening hypoxemia, and diminishing cardiac output (5). Acute testing should be performed during careful hemodynamic study by physicians who have experience with vasodilators and the responses to these drugs in the setting of pulmonary hypertension. Short-acting agents are preferred because they can be discontinued rapidly if adverse effects are noted. The drugs of choice for acute testing are *inhaled nitric oxide, IV prostacyclin (epoprostenol), and adenosine.* A

TABLE 59.2

INDICATIONS FOR HOSPITALIZATION

Initial invasive evaluation (including cardiac catheterization and evaluation of responses to vasodilator testing)
Initiation of oral or intravenous vasodilator therapy
Symptoms consistent with New York Heart Association functional class IV (syncope, bed-bound, anasarca)
Hypoxemia refractory to supplemental oxygen
Worsening renal function
Symptomatic systemic hypotension
Hemorrhagic complications of anticoagulant therapy

TABLE 59.3

DOSE RANGES AND ROUTES OF ADMINISTRATION OF COMMONLY USED VASODILATOR AGENTS

Drug	Route	Dose range
Nitric oxide (NO)	Inhalation	5–40 ppm
Prostacyclin (epoprostenol, PGI$_2$)	Intravenous	1–12 ng/kg per minute acutely (Doses vary for long-term use.)
Adenosine	Intravenous	50–300 mcg/kg per minute
Nifedipine[a]	Oral	30–240 mg/d
Diltiazem[a]	Oral	120–900 mg/d
Amlodipine[a]	Oral	5–20 mg/d
Bosentan	Oral	62.5 mg twice daily, increase to 125 mg twice daily after 4 weeks

[a] Not recommended for acute testing of vasoreactivity. Doses listed are for long-term therapy only.

positive response is defined as a reduction in mean pulmonary artery pressure and pulmonary vascular resistance to normal or near-normal levels (e.g., <30–35 mm Hg and <5 units, respectively), without significant changes in systemic blood pressure or oxygen saturation or substantial side effects. The response to these agents administered acutely has been shown to predict responsiveness to long-term oral vasodilator therapy. Table 59.3 lists the most useful agents for acute testing and long-term therapy.

Long-term therapy in responders can be initiated with oral calcium channel blockers, which produce sustained hemodynamic and symptomatic improvement and are well tolerated by most patients (5). In general, the doses required to achieve an optimal effect are larger than those used to treat systemic vascular disease, although dose requirements and tolerance are variable. Therapy should be initiated with low doses and increased slowly during several days as vital signs, symptoms, and physical examination findings allow.

Until recently, there were no pharmacologic options for patients who failed to respond to acute testing. However, recent studies have demonstrated that several medications can be useful in the management of pulmonary hypertension that is unresponsive to oral vasodilators. Continuous IV infusion of epoprostenol improves hemodynamics, exercise tolerance, and survival in patients with PPH who fall into New York Heart Association functional classes III and IV (6, 7). Interestingly, continuous epoprostenol infusion produces improvement even in those patients who fail to respond to it acutely, which suggests that the long-term ef-

fects of this drug are a consequence of properties other than vasodilation. Epoprostenol is currently approved by the U.S. Food and Drug Administration for the treatment of PPH and PAH due to connective tissue disease refractory to conventional therapy. Experience with epoprostenol for other forms of severe pulmonary hypertension (connective tissue disease, congenital heart disease) has been limited, but beneficial results have been observed in this population also. Bosentan, a dual endothelin receptor antagonist that is administered orally, has recently been approved for symptomatic PAH (8).

Indications for Early Consultation

The management of patients with pulmonary vascular disease is highly complex and evolving rapidly. Consultation or referral to a center specializing in this area is recommended for those patients with PPH, CTEPH, and pulmonary hypertension associated with connective tissue disease or congenital heart disease because these patients may require complex medical or surgical interventions. Additionally, referral to specialized centers affords these patients access to investigational therapies. Patients with underlying pulmonary disease and persistence of pulmonary hypertension despite maximal medical therapy, and those in whom the etiology remains obscure, may also be candidates for referral or consultation.

ISSUES DURING THE COURSE OF HOSPITALIZATION

General Issues

The physician and patient should discuss the impact of pulmonary hypertension on survival, the avoidance of medications or illicit substances that can aggravate the underlying condition, and the options for management. For women of childbearing age, the issue of pregnancy must be discussed in detail. Pregnancy imposes significant cardiovascular stresses on the patient with pulmonary hypertension, particularly in the later stages, is poorly tolerated, and the mortality is high. Additionally, oral contraceptive agents may aggravate pulmonary hypertension, so alternative methods of contraception are advised. Exposure to high altitude is also not recommended because symptoms may be accentuated by even modest hypoxia.

General Medical Management

As stated previously, *supplemental oxygen therapy* is indicated when arterial oxygen saturation falls below approximately 90%, either at rest or during ambulation. Ambulatory systems allow the patient a greater degree of mobility, and the use of oxygen-conserving devices that deliver gas during inspiration enables patients to remain out of the home for longer periods of time. Patients with severe hypoxemia requiring high flow rates of oxygen may benefit from the placement of a transtracheal catheter for oxygen delivery, as this approach is more comfortable and may accomplish the goal of achieving a satisfactory oxygen saturation level with lower flow rates. Oxygen should be used for at least 18 hours daily by patients with resting hypoxemia, although continuous use is strongly advised.

Diuretics are useful when there is evidence of right-sided heart failure, including edema or ascites. However, caution should be exercised with their administration because the RV is highly preload-dependent and excessive diuresis can result in clinical deterioration. Loop diuretics such as furosemide are generally effective as first-line therapy. In patients with severe right-sided heart failure, these drugs should initially be given IV, as absorption through the gut may be impaired. Patients with ascites may benefit from the addition of aldosterone antagonists, such as spironolactone. Refractory heart failure may necessitate the administration of more potent diuretics, such as metolazone. Diuresis may also relieve severe hypoxemia resulting from shunting through a patent foramen ovale by reducing the transatrial pressure gradient.

The role of *cardiac glycosides* for isolated right-sided heart dysfunction resulting from pulmonary hypertension is controversial. Some investigators have advocated the use of digoxin when calcium channel blockers are given to counteract the negative inotropic effects of the latter. Digoxin therapy is associated with a decrease in neurohumoral activation, but convincing evidence of improvement in right-sided heart function is lacking. Additionally, the risk for digitalis toxicity may be increased when hypoxemia and diuretic-induced hypokalemia are present.

Anticoagulation

The management of acute pulmonary embolism is discussed in Chapter 53. Patients with CTEPH should be treated with warfarin for life unless absolute contraindications exist. The dose should be adjusted to achieve an international normalized ratio (INR) of approximately 2.5. Persons who are at increased risk for recurrence or who may be resistant to anticoagulation at these levels, such as those with a "lupus anticoagulant" or with the anticardiolipin antibody syndrome, should be treated with doses of warfarin adjusted to achieve an INR of 3–4 (Chapter 98). Anticoagulation has been demonstrated to improve survival in PPH (9), but no data are available for other pulmonary hypertensive conditions. Most experts recommend anticoagulation for patients with severe pulmonary hypertension regardless of the etiology, as these patients are at risk for thromboembolism and have little, if any, pulmonary vascular reserve to draw on if the pulmonary circulation is compromised further.

Vasodilator Therapy

Patients who respond to acute vasodilator testing may be candidates for long-term oral vasodilator therapy. The calcium channel blockers are the drugs of choice, with the most experience to date with nifedipine, diltiazem, and amlodipine (5). Verapamil is not recommended because it is a less potent pulmonary vasodilator and is more likely to produce negative inotropic effects. Although the beneficial effects of angiotensin-converting enzyme inhibitors in systemic hypertension and left-sided heart failure have been well documented, these agents do not appear to be effective in pulmonary hypertension.

Oral vasodilator therapy should be initiated under close monitoring, with gradual adjustment of doses as tolerated. Side effects include headache, dizziness, worsening hypoxemia, and edema. There are no clear advantages of one calcium blocker over another (with the exception of verapamil's lack of efficacy), and intolerance of one drug does not preclude tolerance of another. Edema during calcium channel blocker therapy may be a consequence of the salt and water retention properties of this class of drugs or of worsening cardiac function. If the former is the cause, administration of low doses of diuretics usually results in resolution.

Continuous Intravenous Epoprostenol

Continuous IV epoprostenol is indicated for patients with PPH who fall into New York Heart Association class III or IV. Epoprostenol is administered by continuous IV infusion by means of a portable infusion pump attached to a permanent indwelling central venous catheter. Patients must be trained in the preparation of medication, troubleshooting the delivery system, and sterile technique. Although dosing should generally begin slowly and be increased as tolerated, a more aggressive approach is needed in patients who are severely ill. Side effects of therapy are common but manageable, and include headache, jaw or foot pain, skin rash, and diarrhea. Interruption of the infusion, either through pump malfunction or loss of venous access, is poorly tolerated and can be life-threatening. Dose requirements increase with time, which necessitates close follow-up in the outpatient setting. Continuous IV epoprostenol has been used either as a primary mode of therapy or as a bridge to transplantation, depending on the patient's response to and tolerance of long-term therapy, candidacy for transplantation, and personal preference (6, 7).

Oral Bosentan

Bosentan, a dual endothelin receptor antagonist, may be considered for patients with PAH who fall into New York Heart Association Class III or IV. The target therapeutic dose is 125 mg twice daily (8). Because the main adverse effect of bosentan is altered liver function, monthly liver function testing is required. Mild increases in aminotransferases (<3 times normal) are common and do not require changes in dosing, while more severe increases (>5 times normal) require discontinuation of the drug.

Pulmonary Thromboendarterectomy

Pulmonary thromboendarterectomy has been demonstrated to produce substantial and sustained hemodynamic improvement in patients with proximal, unresolved pulmonary thromboembolic disease in major vessels. Patients who appear to have this condition should be referred to a center specializing in its diagnosis and treatment to assess their candidacy for thromboendarterectomy.

Transplantation

Single-lung, double-lung, and combined heart–lung transplantation have all been performed for pulmonary hypertension (10). Most centers reserve heart–lung transplantation for patients who have pulmonary vascular disease with irreversible cardiac disease, such as complex congenital heart disease, severe left-sided valvular disease, or left ventricular dysfunction. The median waiting time for single-lung or double-lung transplantation in the United States is currently approaching 2 years, which underscores the importance of early referral for evaluation. The 3-year survival after lung transplantation is approximately 60% (compared with a 20%–30% 3-year survival for untreated patients in New York Heart Association classes III and IV), with most deaths attributable to bronchiolitis obliterans, chronic rejection, or opportunistic infection.

The timing of lung transplantation poses a considerable challenge. Patients must be sufficiently ill to warrant transplantation, yet not so ill that surviving the surgery is unlikely. Close coordination of care between the physician overseeing medical management and the transplant center is crucial. A complete discussion of lung transplantation is presented in Chapter 58.

DISCHARGE ISSUES

Medications should be reviewed at discharge, with special emphasis on the risks associated with warfarin, drug interactions, and the importance of taking vasodilator medications as prescribed without interruptions. Patients discharged on continuous epoprostenol should have a list of emergency phone numbers and a letter to be kept on file in their local emergency department describing the nature of their treatment and emergency procedures to be followed in the event of interruption of the infusion. Dietary instructions, particularly salt and fluid restrictions or supplemental nutrition, should be reviewed. Patients should be encouraged to undertake physical activity to their level of tolerance but to avoid those activities that produce

sustained or serious adverse effects, such as chest pain, extreme dyspnea, dizziness, and syncope. A bracelet or medallion on which the diagnosis, medications, and emergency contact information are inscribed is recommended. A schedule should be developed for routine blood work, as necessary. Follow-up appointments should also be arranged, usually for 2–4 weeks after discharge. Finally, patients should be instructed to call immediately if changes in their condition develop, particularly syncope, hemoptysis, severe dizziness, or worsening edema.

COST CONSIDERATIONS AND RESOURCE USE

Most of the components of medical care for patients with pulmonary hypertension are costly and beyond the means of most people. Accordingly, patients should be encouraged to maintain adequate levels of medical insurance or to apply for government-supported coverage if eligibility can be established. Unfortunately, many patients with severe disease are unable to resume full-time employment after hospital discharge; their applications for disability often require substantial support and documentation by their physician. The unstable nature of this condition (11) necessitates the timely completion of disability applications to ensure that medical coverage does not lapse, even briefly.

Although diuretics and warfarin are relatively inexpensive, drugs such as calcium channel blockers can cost up to $100 a month. Supplemental oxygen is usually covered by third-party payers as long as hypoxemia is documented. Epoprostenol therapy costs between $50,000 and $150,000 a year depending on dose, but it is covered by insurance when prescribed for its approved indication. Bosentan therapy costs approximately $25,000 per year. The average cost for lung transplantation is $125,000–$150,000. Annual costs after transplantation vary, depending on the need for rehospitalization, but are estimated at $25,000–$50,000 a year, including the costs of medications. Complex treatments, such as epoprostenol and transplantation, are most efficiently and successfully performed at referral centers that have allocated resources to and gained experience with these approaches. In these centers, training for home epoprostenol therapy can usually be accomplished with short (5–7 days) inpatient stays. Some centers combine even briefer inpatient stays with outpatient training to minimize cost.

KEY POINTS

- Pulmonary hypertension is not a disease *per se*, but rather a hemodynamic abnormality that is common to a large number of divergent conditions. Determining the etiology of pulmonary hypertension is crucial to developing an individualized therapeutic approach.

- The presenting signs and symptoms of pulmonary hypertension are often subtle and nonspecific, particularly early in its course. Dyspnea out of proportion to evidence of heart or lung disease is an important clue.

- Several conditions are associated with pulmonary hypertension and should be explored during the initial assessment, including use of anorexigenics and illicit drugs, HIV infection, portal hypertension, and hereditary conditions.

- A systematic noninvasive approach to diagnosis will usually provide sufficient information to establish an etiology without the need for histologic confirmation.

- Complete cardiac catheterization, which is mandatory in patients with pulmonary hypertension, is used to confirm the severity and source of the hemodynamic abnormalities, help in estimating prognosis, and assess pulmonary vasoreactivity in response to potent, short-acting, titratable vasodilator agents.

- Patients with severe pulmonary hypertension who require complex treatments, such as pulmonary thromboendarterectomy, continuous epoprostenol therapy, or transplantation, should be referred to centers with expertise in these approaches.

REFERENCES

1. Rubin LJ. Primary pulmonary hypertension. *N Engl J Med* 1997;336:111–117.
2. Fedullo PF, Auger WR, Kerr KM, Rubin LJ. Chronic thromboembolic pulmonary hypertension. *N. Eng J Med* 2001;345:1465–1472.
3. Abenhaim L, Moride Y, Brenot F, et al. Appetite-suppressant drugs and the risk of primary pulmonary hypertension. *N Engl J Med* 1996;335:609–616.
4. Salvaterra CG, Rubin LJ. Investigation and management of pulmonary hypertension in chronic obstructive pulmonary disease. *Am Rev Respir Dis* 1993;148:1414–1417.
5. Rich S, Kaufmann E, Levy PS. The effect of high doses of calcium channel blockers on survival in primary pulmonary hypertension. *N Engl J Med* 1992;327:76–81.
6. Sitbon O, Humbert M, Nunes H, et al. Long-term intravenous epoprostenol infusion in primary pulmonary hypertension: prognostic factors and survival. *J Am Coll Cardiol* 2002;40:780–788.
7. Barst RJ, Rubin LJ, Long WA, et al. A comparison of continuous intravenous epoprostenol (prostacyclin) with conventional therapy for primary pulmonary hypertension. *N Engl J Med* 1996;334:296–301.
8. Rubin LJ, Badesch DB, Barst RJ, et al. Bosentan therapy for pulmonary arterial hypertension. *N Eng J Med* 2002;346:896–903.
9. Fuster V, Steele PM, Edwards WD, et al. Primary pulmonary hypertension: natural history and the importance of thrombosis. *Circulation* 1984;70:580–587.
10. Pasque MK, Trulock EP, Kaiser LR, et al. Single-lung transplantation for pulmonary hypertension. *Circulation* 1991;84:2275–2279.
11. D'Alonzo GE, Barst RJ, Ayres SM, et al. Survival in patients with primary pulmonary hypertension: results from a national prospective registry. *Ann Intern Med* 1991;115:343–349.

ADDITIONAL READING

Chin K, Channick R. Bosentan. *Expert Rev Cardiovasc Ther* 2004;2:175–182.

Farber HW, Loscalzo J. Pulmonary arterial hypertension. *N Engl J Med* 2004;351:1655–1665.

Mehta S. Drug therapy for pulmonary arterial hypertension. What's on the menu today? *Chest* 2003;124:2045–2049.

Rubin LJ, Rich S, eds. *Primary Pulmonary Hypertension.* New York: Marcel Dekker Inc, 1997.

Rubin LJ, American College of Physicians. Diagnosis and management of pulmonary arterial hypertension. ACCP evidence-based clinical practice guidelines. *Chest* 2004;126(1 suppl):7S–10S.

Stupi AM, Steen VD, Owens GR, et al. Pulmonary hypertension in the CREST syndrome variant of systemic sclerosis. *Arthritis Rheum* 1986;29:515–524.

Pleural Effusion and Pneumothorax

60

Steven A. Sahn   John E. Heffner

INTRODUCTION

The accumulation of fluid or air within the pleural space represents the most common clinical expression of pleural disease. Radiographic evidence of a pleural effusion may develop from a primary disorder of pleural membranes, a complication of intrathoracic pathology, or a manifestation of an underlying systemic disease. A pneumothorax may occur as a consequence of underlying lung disease or traumatic injury to the lung or chest wall. The occurrence of a pleural effusion or pneumothorax commonly represents the initial clinical manifestation of an underlying thoracic or extrathoracic disorder. A well-organized diagnostic approach to patients with pleural abnormalities provides a specific etiologic diagnosis for the majority of patients who present with these conditions.

Pleural effusions occur when (a) an increased inflow of fluid into the pleural space outstrips the resorptive capacity of pleural lymphatics, or (b) the pleural fluid resorptive mechanisms become impaired. *Transudative effusions* have low protein content and occur in patients with normal pleural membranes. They result from increased pulmonary capillary hydrostatic pressure (e.g., congestive heart failure), decreased oncotic pressure (e.g., nephrosis), translocation of infradiaphragmatic fluid into the pleural space (e.g., ascites), decreased intrapleural pressure (e.g., atelectasis), or erosion of central lines through intrathoracic venous structures. Less common causes of transudative effusions include constrictive pericarditis, trapped lung, and superior vena cava syndrome. *Exudative effusions* result from increased permeability of pleural capillaries to protein (e.g., pneumonia), introduction of chyle into the pleural space (chylothorax), impairment of lymphatic drainage (mediastinal lymph node tumors), or obstruction of

lymphatic stomas on the parietal pleura (e.g., pleural malignancy).

Pneumothoraces are categorized as spontaneous, traumatic, or iatrogenic (e.g., after barotrauma or invasive procedures). Spontaneous pneumothoraces are further categorized as primary (occurring in patients without clinically apparent lung disease) or secondary (occurring in patients with underlying lung disease, such as chronic obstructive pulmonary disease).

This chapter outlines a clinical approach to the diagnosis and management of patients who present with a pleural effusion or pneumothorax. Emphasis is placed on discriminating between patients who require extensive diagnostic evaluations and those who can be managed with observation or empiric therapy alone.

PLEURAL EFFUSIONS

Clinical Presentation

The cardinal symptom of pleural effusions is dyspnea, which may first present as exertion-related shortness of breath in patients with slowly developing effusions (malignant effusions) or severe resting dyspnea in patients with sudden-onset, rapidly progressing effusions (traumatic hemothorax). Coexisting lung disease with chronic respiratory impairment allows smaller fluid collections to produce earlier and more severe symptoms. Inflammatory conditions of the pleural space cause pleuritic chest pain, which may remit as enlarging fluid collections separate the visceral and parietal pleural surfaces. Pleural mesotheliomas cause a constant, nonpleuritic pain of the chest wall. Patients are often asymptomatic and present with radiographic evidence of a small pleural effusion as an incidental finding. Symptoms related to pleural effusions may be obscured by underlying cardiopulmonary conditions, such as congestive heart failure or pneumonia. Additional symptoms include cough, positional dyspnea, and a "feeling of fullness or heaviness" in the chest.

Physical findings include dullness to percussion, egophony, and tubular breath sounds over atelectatic lung regions just above the level of the effusion (Chapter 54). Pleural rubs can occur in patients with pleural inflammation. Rubs are heard best over the posterolateral chest.

Differential Diagnosis and Initial Evaluation

In most patients, radiographic detection of a pleural effusion warrants a diagnostic evaluation that utilizes imaging studies and pleural fluid analysis. A decubitus chest radiograph that detects free-flowing fluid with 1 cm or more of fluid layering indicates that thoracentesis can be performed with minimal risk for complications. Failure of the decubitus radiograph to detect free-flowing fluid does not exclude a pleural effusion and indicates a need for ultrasonographic or computed tomographic (CT) studies to detect loculated fluid. Ultrasonography can confirm the presence of fluid, demonstrate the thickness of pleural membranes, identify the presence of loculations, and localize fluid collections for thoracentesis. A contrast-enhanced chest CT can distinguish pleural fluid from pleural masses and underlying parenchymal consolidation and abscesses. CT imaging may also provide evidence of pleural inflammation, such as pleural enhancement, thickened extrapleural subcostal tissues, and increased attenuation of extrapleural fat. The resolution of CT imaging localizes loculations along the chest wall and in the mediastinum. Conditions associated with pleural effusions, such as mediastinal lymphadenopathy, central line erosions through venous structures with mediastinal hygromas, and pleural calcifications, can be identified by CT.

The finding of a previously undiagnosed pleural effusion mandates thoracentesis for pleural fluid analysis in the majority of patients. Exceptions include patients with typical congestive heart failure and clinically stable patients with asymptomatic pleural effusions in the early postpartum or postoperative period. These patients should be monitored for resolution of pleural fluid.

Pleural fluid obtained by thoracentesis is analyzed for gross appearance, which may be diagnostic or highly suggestive of an underlying diagnosis in some clinical settings (1, 2) (Table 60.1). Chemical analysis determines the exudative or transudative nature of effusions, which narrows the differential diagnosis. Exudates have been traditionally defined by the presence of any one of the following findings (Light's criteria): (a) pleural fluid-to-serum protein ratio above 0.5; (b) pleural fluid-to-serum lactate dehydrogenase (LDH) ratio above 0.6; or (c) pleural fluid LDH concentration above 67% of the laboratory's upper limit of

TABLE 60.1

GROSS APPEARANCE AND BIOCHEMICAL ANALYSIS OF PLEURAL FLUID

Gross appearance

White, opaque	Chylous or pseudochylous (cholesterol) effusion
Purulent	Empyema
Malodiferous	Anaerobic empyema
Brown, red-brown, "anchovy"	Empyema caused by *Entamoeba histolytica*
Yellow-green	Rheumatoid pleurisy
Black	Empyema caused by *Aspergillus niger*
Ammonia odor	Urinothorax

Biochemical analysis

Exudative criteria	1. PF LDH >67% upper limits of normal serum or PF/S protein >0.5, *and* 2. PF LDH >67% upper limits of normal serum LDH, *or* PF protein >2.9 g/dL *or* PF cholesterol >45 mg/dL.
Glucose <40 mg/dL	Empyema, complicated parapneumonic effusion, rheumatoid pleurisy, malignant pleural effusion, tuberculous pleurisy, lupus pleuritis.
Amylase-rich effusion	Ruptured esophagus with or without empyema (salivary amylase), acute pancreatitis and pancreatic pseudocyst (>100,000 IU/L) (both pancreatic amylase). Malignant pleural effusion (salivary)
PF/S creatinine >1	Urinothorax.
Triglyceride >110 mg/dL	Chylothorax
pH <7.30	Complicated parapneumonic effusion/empyema, rheumatoid pleurisy, lupus pleuritis, tuberculous pleurisy, malignant effusion, esophageal rupture

LDH, lactate dehydrogenase; *PF*, pleural fluid; *S*, serum.

normal for serum LDH. Pleural fluid LDH and pleural fluid-to-serum LDH ratio are highly correlated, however, because they both contain test results for the pleural fluid LDH. Some experts, therefore, recommend using an "abbreviated Light's criteria" that incorporates pleural fluid-to-serum protein ratio and pleural fluid LDH (3).

Other studies have proposed a higher cut off point for the pleural fluid LDH (>80% of the upper limits of the laboratory normal value) to diagnose exudative effusions (4). A meta-analysis determined that pleural fluid cholesterol, pleural fluid-to-serum cholesterol ratio, and pleural fluid-to-serum albumin gradient are about as accurate as each of the three tests within Light's criteria in identifying exudates (3). Light's criteria and other dichotomous test strategies with single cut off points frequently misdiagnose exudates in those patients with congestive heart failure who

TABLE 60.2

MULTILEVEL LIKELIHOOD RATIOS FOR LIGHT'S CRITERIA IN DETERMINING THE POSTTEST PROBABILITY OF AN EXUDATIVE EFFUSION

Protein ratio	MLR	LDH PF	MLR	LDH ratio	MLR
>0.70	168.65	>1.00	44.33	>1.10	38.92
0.66–0.70	53.26	0.91–1.00	10.09	1.01–1.10	16.71
0.61–0.65	6.92	0.81–0.90	2.17	0.91–1.00	5.92
0.56–0.60	3.02	0.71–0.80	3.60	0.81–0.90	1.99
0.51–0.55	1.78	0.61–0.70	2.12	0.71–0.80	1.34
0.46–0.50	0.49	0.51–0.60	0.64	0.61–0.70	0.99
0.41–0.45	0.28	0.41–0.50	0.43	0.51–0.60	0.46
0.36–0.40	0.12	0.31–0.40	0.26	0.41–0.50	0.18
0.31–0.35	0.06	0.21–0.30	0.07	0.31–0.40	0.08
≤0.30	0.04	≤0.20	0.04	≤0.30	0.05

Protein ratio denotes pleural fluid-to-serum protein ratio; LDH denotes lactate dehydrogenase; LDH PF denotes pleural fluid LDH; LDH ratio denotes pleural fluid-to-serum LDH; MLR denotes multilikelihood ratio. To use the table in practice, let's work through a hypothetical example:

A patient with congestive heart failure presents with a pleural effusion. After diuresis, the effusion persists and thoracentesis is performed. Results for Light's criteria are shown below:

- Pleural fluid-to-serum protein ratio = 0.45
- Pleural fluid LDH (fraction of upper limit laboratory normal) = 0.65
- Pleural fluid-to-serum LDH ratio = 0.75

By Light's criteria, the pleural fluid is an exudate because the pleural fluid-to-serum LDH ratio is greater than 0.6. The physician, however, has a low suspicion of an exudate and suspects that the patient has a transudate due to heart failure. The physician estimates the pretest probability of an exudate as only 20% and uses serial multilevel likelihood ratios to calculate the posttest probability of an exudate.

The physician first calculates the pretest odds of an exudate using the formula, pretest odds = pretest probability/(1 − pretest probability) = 0.20/(1 − 0.20) = 0.25.

The physician then refers to Table 60.2 to find the multilevel likelihood ratio related to each of the patient's pleural fluid test results:

- Pleural fluid-to-serum protein ratio of 0.45 = multilevel likelihood ratio of 0.28
- Pleural fluid LDH of 0.65 = multilevel likelihood ratio of 2.12
- Pleural fluid-to-serum LDH ratio of 0.75 = multilevel likelihood ratio of 1.34

The physician can now calculate a posttest odds by multiplying the pre-test odds by each of the multilevel likelihood ratios:

$$0.25 \times 0.28 \times 2.12 \times 1.34 = 0.20$$

The physician now calculates the posttest probability of an exudate from the posttest odds with the equation, posttest probability = posttest odds/(1 + posttest odds) = 0.17 or 17%. (See Chapter 6 for more on Bayesian reasoning.)

With the use of serial multilevel likelihood ratios, the patient's pleural fluid test results decreased the physician's pretest estimate of the probability that the patient has an exudate (from 20% to 17%).

have clinical evidence of transudative effusions (5). Multilevel likelihood ratios used in a Bayesian strategy more accurately discriminate between exudative and transudative effusions (6) (Table 60.2). This strategy allows the features of the patient's clinical presentation to be integrated with the pleural fluid test results.

Confirmation of a transudative effusion usually allows the effusion to be attributed to a clinically apparent process, such as congestive heart failure. In most patients, no additional diagnostic evaluation is required. Exudative pleural effusions require exclusion of parapneumonic effusions related to an underlying pneumonia, pleural malignancies, pleural tuberculosis, and pulmonary embolism. Less common causes of pleural effusions, categorized by their transudative or exudative nature, are listed in Table 60.3. Thoracentesis can definitively diagnose the cause of

pleural effusions in 25% of patients and help narrow the differential diagnosis in an additional 50% (1).

Lymphocyte-predominant exudative pleural effusions that remain undiagnosed after thoracentesis may require closed pleural needle biopsy, especially if tuberculosis is considered; closed pleural biopsy is less often positive when the etiology is malignancy. The sensitivity of pleural fluid cytology for the diagnosis of malignancy ranges from 60%–90%. Pleural fluid culture and pleural tissue culture and histology has a sensitivity of up to 85% for tuberculosis. Thoracoscopy can be performed in patients whose condition remains undiagnosed, provided that a specific diagnosis would provide clinically meaningful prognostic or therapeutic information. Thoracoscopy by skilled operators has a sensitivity that approaches 100% for both pleural malignancy and tuberculosis.

TABLE 60.3

CAUSES OF TRANSUDATIVE AND EXUDATIVE PLEURAL EFFUSIONS

Transudative
Congestive heart failure
Hepatic hydrothorax
Nephrotic syndrome
Urinothorax
Pulmonary embolism (up to 23% of patients with pulmonary emboli)
Central venous catheter eroded through vascular structures (saline infusion)
Atelectasis
Trapped lung
Constrictive pericarditis
Duro-pleural fistula (cerebrospinal fluid leak)

Exudative
Parapneumonic effusions and empyemas
Malignancy
Tuberculosis
Chylothorax
Pulmonary infarction
Hemothorax
Collagen vascular disease (rheumatoid arthritis, systemic lupus erythematosus)
Yellow-nail syndrome
Drug-induced effusions
Pancreatitis and pancreatic pseudocyst
After cardiac injury syndrome
After coronary artery bypass surgery

Parapneumonic effusions, which are effusions that occur in association with pneumonia, may respond to antibiotics alone (*uncomplicated parapneumonic effusions*) or require drainage (*complicated parapneumonic effusions*) to prevent progression to an *empyema* (frank intrapleural pus). A Bayesian approach (Chapter 6) to determining the need for drainage on the basis of pleural fluid biochemical results and the patient's clinical features is shown in Figure 60.1 (2).

Indications for Hospitalization

Most patients with pleural effusions who require hospitalization are admitted because of the underlying condition that caused the effusion rather than because of the effusion itself. Patients with symptoms caused by a large, slowly progressive effusion who do not otherwise require hospitalization usually can be stabilized with a therapeutic thoracentesis in the emergency department or office. Massive pleural effusions, rapidly progressing effusions, hemothoraces, cardiopulmonary symptoms that do not improve after thoracentesis, a trapped lung associated with moderate-to-severe respiratory symptoms, and parapneumonic effusions or empyemas represent indications for hospitalization.

Indications for Intensive Care Unit Admission

Pleural effusions by themselves rarely merit admission to an ICU. However, large, bilateral effusions can cause respiratory failure, especially in patients with underlying pulmonary dysfunction. Spontaneous hemothoraces complicating anticoagulation therapy or pleural malignancies require close hemodynamic monitoring and observation for the need for emergency thoracotomy. Patients in whom pulmonary edema develops after large-volume thoracentesis ("reexpansion" pulmonary edema) may benefit from short-term observation in a subacute care unit or ICU.

Initial Therapy

The therapy for pleural effusions depends on the underlying etiology of the pleural fluid collection. Patients with transudative pleural effusions require management of the underlying condition. With vasodilator and diuretic therapy for congestive heart failure (Chapter 39), for instance, pulmonary edema will generally resolve in a few days, and any associated pleural effusion will resolve a few days later. Patients with translocation of ascitic fluid into the pleural space may improve after paracentesis. Rare patients with chronic, symptomatic transudative pleural effusions unresponsive to therapy may benefit from either chemical pleurodesis to obliterate the pleural space or the placement of long-term, indwelling pleural drainage catheters.

Parapneumonic and malignant pleural effusions commonly require therapeutic interventions directed at the pleural space. For patients with parapneumonic effusions, urgent drainage must be considered. Delayed drainage in patients with complicated parapneumonic effusions prolongs hospitalization and worsens clinical outcome (7). Free-flowing, complicated parapneumonic effusions of low viscosity respond to *chest tube drainage* in 60%–90% of patients. When the effusion is not free-flowing, percutaneous catheters can be inserted into loculi under ultrasonographic or CT guidance and are highly effective in properly selected patients. Patients with parapneumonic effusions who fail to respond to chest tube drainage because of viscous effusions or intrapleural loculations may improve with the *intrapleural instillation of fibrinolytic agents*, such as streptokinase and urokinase (8). Although the use of these agents is not supported by large prospective, randomized, placebo-controlled trials, uncontrolled case series suggest that loculated, viscous pleural fluid can be drained and surgical interventions avoided in some patients. Measurable systemic fibrinolysis does not occur with the intrapleural instillation of these agents.

Patients with parapneumonic effusions who fail chest tube drainage may be candidates for *video-assisted thoracoscopic surgery* (VATS) if extensive pleural fibrosis and progression to a frank empyema have not occurred. More extensive, "organized" empyema (>6 weeks in duration) requires a standard thoracotomy with decortication. Open drainage

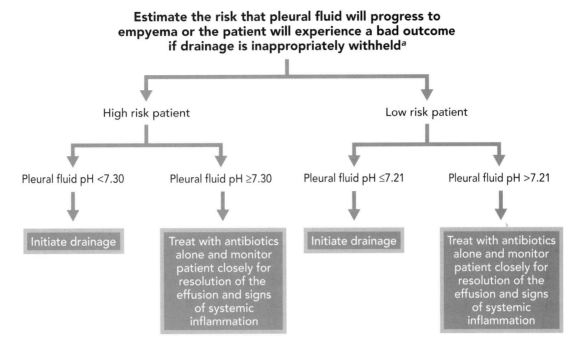

Estimate the risk that pleural fluid will progress to empyema or the patient will experience a bad outcome if drainage is inappropriately withheld[a]

High risk patient

Low risk patient

Pleural fluid pH <7.30

Pleural fluid pH ≥7.30

Pleural fluid pH ≤7.21

Pleural fluid pH >7.21

Initiate drainage

Treat with antibiotics alone and monitor patient closely for resolution of the effusion and signs of systemic inflammation

Initiate drainage

Treat with antibiotics alone and monitor patient closely for resolution of the effusion and signs of systemic inflammation

[a] Risk Factors for Empyema or Bad Outcome in Parapneumonic Effusion:
- Large effusion (>40% of hemithorax)
- Positive pleural fluid Gram stain or culture
- Multiple pleural loculations
- Toxic/unstable patient with limited cardiopulmonary reserve
- Presence of a virulent pathogen (e.g., *Staphyloccus aureus*, *Klebsiella pneumoniae*, or *Pseudomonas aeruginosa*)

Figure 60.1 Algorithm for selecting patients for drainage of a parapneumonic effusion according to pleural fluid chemical analysis results.

with rib resection is an alternative surgical procedure for extremely ill patients who are not candidates for decortication and have localized collections of pleural pus. The key to successful management is early and effective drainage of the pleural space that results in the complete removal of intrapleural pus and apposition of the lung to the chest wall.

Hospitalized patients with malignant exudative pleural effusions may require therapeutic thoracentesis if symptoms of dyspnea or decreased exercise tolerance are attributable to pleural fluid. Removal of a large volume (>500 cc) of fluid during a single thoracentesis may result in *reexpansion pulmonary edema*, especially in patients with ipsilateral mediastinal shift, which suggests the presence of an obstructing endobronchial lesion or trapped lung. This complication is uncommon if the thoracentesis is interrupted as soon as patients experience chest discomfort, mild dyspnea, or cough. Patients with recurrent malignant pleural effusions may be candidates for *pleurodesis*, a procedure in which the effusion is first drained and then a chemical agent is instilled through the chest tube to cause pleural inflammation and fibrosis. Available compounds include talc slurry, bleomycin, and doxycycline (9). Talc (5 g) has the lowest cost ($6–$12 per treatment) and the highest efficacy (90%–95%), as demonstrated in uncontrolled stud-

ies. It is usually well tolerated, although a small number of patients (<1%) experience life-threatening respiratory failure with its use. Doxycycline has a success rate of 75%–90% and is not associated with serious adverse reactions. Bleomycin is the least effective of these three agents and has a drug acquisition cost of $800–$1,000 per treatment. Most experts recommend the use of talc slurry or doxycycline for chemical pleurodesis by chest tube. Pleurodesis can also be performed by thoracoscopy with talc poudrage (the insufflation of dry talc). Thoracoscopic pleurodesis has the advantage over chest tube pleurodesis of allowing the lysis of pleural adhesions that interfere with lung reexpansion. A chronic indwelling catheter, which allows the pleural space to drain to relieve dyspnea, results in spontaneous pleurodesis (over a median time period of about 1 month) in 40%–50% of patients (10).

PNEUMOTHORAX

Primary Spontaneous Pneumothorax

Primary spontaneous pneumothorax (PSP) has an estimated incidence of 2.5–18 cases per 100,000 persons. PSP most commonly occurs in tall, thin men between the ages of 10 and 30 years. Smoking increases the risk for pneumothorax approximately 20-fold in males.

PSP occurs most commonly when an apical pleural bleb ruptures. The blebs are usually acquired as a result of bronchial inflammation but may be congenital. Abrupt changes in barometric pressure have been associated with an increased incidence of spontaneous pneumothorax. About 10% of patients with PSP have an associated small hemorrhagic pleural effusion that may be related to pleural injury from rupture of the bleb or traction on adhesions.

Clinical Presentation

About 90% of cases of PSP occur at rest. The most common symptoms are ipsilateral pleuritic chest pain (96%) and acute dyspnea (80%). The severity of the pain varies from mild to severe and has been described initially as sharp and later as a steady ache. Cough occurs in 10% of patients. Despite the persistence of the pneumothorax, symptoms frequently abate spontaneously by 24 hours. A regular tachycardia is the most common physical finding. There may be reduced chest wall excursion ipsilaterally, a hyper-resonant percussion note, absent fremitus, and reduced breath sounds. With a small pneumothorax, chest examination findings may be normal (Chapter 54).

The diagnosis is usually confirmed by visualization of the visceral pleural line removed from the chest wall on an upright posteroanterior chest radiograph; however, an end-expiratory radiograph or a lateral decubitus radiograph with the affected side in the superior position may be necessary to identify the pneumothorax. An arterial blood gas determination typically shows mild-to-moderate hypoxemia and a respiratory alkalosis. In PSP, there is a reduction in forced vital capacity, impaired ventilation–perfusion matching, and some shunting, depending on the size of the pneumothorax.

The risk for recurrence following the initial PSP has been reported to be 32%–52%, and the recurrent PSP is usually ipsilateral. The recurrence rate increases with each subsequent pneumothorax and does not appear to be affected by standard chest tube drainage.

Secondary Spontaneous Pneumothorax

A number of pulmonary disorders are associated with SSP (Table 60.4). Secondary spontaneous pneumothorax is most commonly associated with chronic obstructive pulmonary disease. The incidence of SSP is similar to that of PSP; however, the peak incidence occurs in the seventh decade of life.

Secondary spontaneous pneumothorax can be caused by hyperexpansion of the distal air spaces from obstruction or inflammation in the airways. This leads to alveolar rupture and retrograde movement of air along the bronchovascular sheath to the mediastinum, with eventual rupture through the mediastinal parietal pleura. A second mechanism is rupture of the visceral pleura from an inflammatory parenchymal process.

TABLE 60.4

CAUSES OF SECONDARY SPONTANEOUS PNEUMOTHORAX

Diseases of the airways
Chronic obstructive pulmonary disease
Cystic fibrosis
Status asthmaticus

Interstitial lung disease
Langerhans cell granulomatosis
Sarcoidosis
Lymphangioleiomyomatosis
Tuberous sclerosis
Rheumatoid disease
Idiopathic pulmonary fibrosis
Radiation fibrosis

Infectious diseases
Necrotizing gram-negative pneumonia
Anaerobic pneumonia
Staphylococcal pneumonia
AIDS with pneumocystis pneumonia
Mycobacterium tuberculosis infection

Malignancy
Sarcoma
Lung cancer

Other
Catamenial
Pulmonary infarction
Wegener's granulomatosis
Marfan syndrome
Ehlers-Danlos syndrome

Clinical Presentation

Dyspnea is more severe in SSP than in PSP because of the impaired pulmonary reserve. Chest pain appears to be both less common and less severe. Life-threatening hypoxemia or hypotension occurs in about 15% of patients. In contrast to the symptoms of PSP, those of SSP typically do not resolve spontaneously.

The underlying lung disease may result in subtle physical findings. Clinical suspicion of pneumothorax should remain heightened in patients with chronic obstructive pulmonary disease in whom dyspnea and unilateral chest pain develop. However, the presence of underlying lung disease often makes radiographic identification of the visceral pleural line more problematic. Pleural adhesions may result in loculated pneumothoraces, and the edge of a large bulla may simulate the visceral pleural line. In critically ill patients, the supine radiograph will show the pneumothorax gas in a juxtacardiac position or in the costophrenic sulcus, where it may produce a "deep sulcus" sign. CT may be necessary to diagnose pneumothorax in these patients (Chapter 54).

Arterial blood gas measurements in the patient with SSP generally show significant hypoxemia and hypercapnia. The recurrence rate is similar to that for PSP.

Iatrogenic Pneumothorax

Iatrogenic pneumothoraces are complications of diagnostic and therapeutic procedures and are caused by transthoracic needle biopsies, subclavian venous catheter insertions, thoracentesis, pleural biopsy, transbronchial lung biopsy, and mechanical ventilation (Chapter 23).

Tension Pneumothorax

Tension develops in a pneumothorax when the pleural pressure exceeds atmospheric pressure during the entire respiratory cycle because of an unidirectional flow of air from the lung into the pleural space. Tension pneumothorax can be fatal if not treated promptly. Air continues to accumulate in the pleural space from a "check-valve" mechanism. Experimental studies suggest that the circulatory collapse in tension pneumothorax is related to decreased oxygen delivery to tissues as a result of hypoxemia rather than impaired venous return. Tension pneumothorax occurs in about 1%–2% of cases of spontaneous pneumothorax and more commonly in traumatic pneumothorax and pneumothorax occurring with positive pressure ventilation.

Clinical Presentation

The patient with a pneumothorax under tension presents with severe respiratory distress, cyanosis, marked tachycardia, and hypotension. The ipsilateral hemithorax may be noticeably larger. It can be problematic to differentiate between the involved and uninvolved hemithorax, and the predominant symptoms may be related to hemodynamic instability rather than respiratory distress.

The characteristic triad of tension pneumothorax on chest radiograph includes contralateral mediastinal shift, depression of the ipsilateral diaphragm, and lung collapse.

Management of Tension Pneumothorax

Immediate decompression of the involved hemithorax is mandatory to save the patient's life. With decompression, there is an immediate fall in heart rate and respiratory rate and restoration of the blood pressure. Valuable time should not be wasted awaiting results of radiologic studies, as the clinical presentation is usually highly suggestive of the diagnosis. A large-bore catheter should be inserted into the pleural space of the suspected hemithorax through the second anterior intercostal space. A rush of air seen or heard bubbling through a fluid-filled syringe confirms the diagnosis; symptoms should improve rapidly. A large-bore chest tube should then be inserted without delay.

Management of Spontaneous Pneumothorax

The initial goal in the management of pneumothorax is to remove air from the pleural space and to reexpand the lung, with a secondary goal of preventing recurrence. After the pneumothorax gas equilibrates with tissue gases, a small nitrogen gradient for absorption exists and the pneumothorax gas is absorbed from the pleural space at a rate of 1.25% of the volume of the hemithorax daily. Figures 60.2 and 60.3 are algorithms for the initial management of patients with PSP and SSP, respectively.

Observation

Patients with a small PSP (<15%) usually do not require pleural space drainage if they are asymptomatic, have normal vital signs, are under age 40, and have no other abnormalities on chest radiograph. In addition, the pneumothorax must have occurred within the previous 24 hours, and there should be no radiographic progression during 6 hours of observation in the emergency department. These patients may be discharged from the emergency department and reevaluated with a chest radiograph in 24–48 hours.

All patients with SSP should be admitted to the hospital, and *virtually all will require chest tube drainage.* Rare patients with small SSPs can be initially observed without tube thoracostomy if they are asymptomatic with normal vital signs, if no progression is shown on a repeat chest radiograph 6 hours later, and if the patient is not a candidate for pleurodesis. However, most patients with SSP have significant symptoms, and therefore observation alone is usually not an option.

Supplemental Oxygen

Administration of supplemental oxygen results in a fourfold increase in pleural gas absorption. Oxygen causes a washout of nitrogen from the blood and reduces total pleural capillary gas pressure, which significantly increases the nitrogen gradient across the pleura.

Simple Manual Aspiration

Simple manual aspiration has a success rate similar to that of intercostal tube drainage for patients with their first PSP (10). Catheter aspiration is simple, causes less morbidity than chest tube insertion, and when successful does not require hospitalization.

A catheter is placed in the pleural space by either a catheter-over-needle device or the modified Seldinger technique (Chapter 27). With a 50-mL syringe attached to a three-way stopcock, air is removed until resistance occurs or 4 L of air has been aspirated, the latter defining a persistent leak necessitating chest tube drainage. An aspiration is successful when the pneumothorax resolves symptomatically and radiographically without evidence of a persistent air leak.

Catheter aspiration is most likely to be successful in PSP when the pneumothorax is several days old, which increases the likelihood that the air leak has stopped. Simple aspiration should not be used for SSP because of the higher

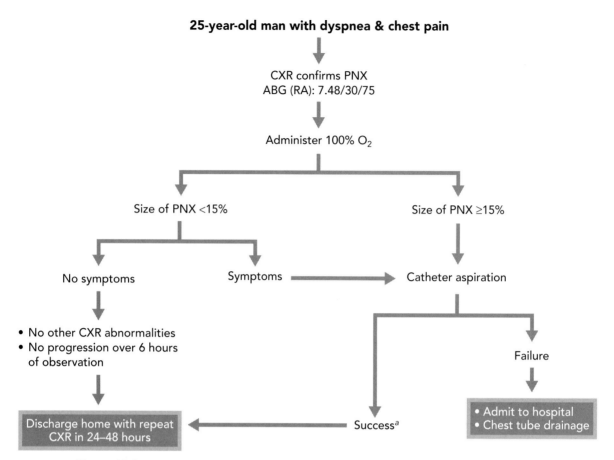

Figure 60.2 Initial management of a hypothetical patient with primary spontaneous pneumothorax. *ªSuccessful catheter aspiration: Air is withdrawn from the pleural space until no more can be aspirated and CXR reveals complete lung expansion. ABG*, arterial blood gas; *CXR*, chest X-ray; *PNX*, pneumothorax; *RA*, room air.

likelihood of persistent air leak and the more precarious state of the patient.

Chest Tube Drainage

Tube thoracostomy is the treatment of choice for virtually all patients with SSP, with the exception of stable, asymptomatic patients with small (<15%) pneumothoraces who would not be candidates for pleurodesis.

The majority of patients with a spontaneous pneumothorax can be treated with small thoracostomy tubes (8F to 16F). Drainage of the pleural space can be accomplished with either a Heimlich valve or a water seal. Some physicians apply suction to the system immediately, whereas others reserve this option for cases in which complete expansion is not attained by 24 hours. When the lung is completely expanded on chest radiograph, the air leak has ceased, and the drainage system is deemed functional, the tube can be removed within the next 24–48 hours. Some clinicians prefer to clamp the tube for a period of time; others simply observe with continued suction. Randomized trials are not available to help inform this decision.

Chemical Pleurodesis Through a Chest Tube

When standard chest tube or small-bore catheter placement has resulted in complete lung expansion, a chemical agent can be instilled into the pleural space in an attempt to create pleurodesis. Chemical pleurodesis was commonly performed for spontaneous pneumothorax in the past, but it has now been largely supplanted by video-assisted thoracoscopic surgery (VATS) with pleurodesis.

Thoracoscopy

VATS has become the preferred alternative to standard thoracotomy to identify and repair the visceral pleural lesion in patients with SSP and patients with recurrent PSP (11). Wedge resection of the blebs can be accomplished with an endoscopic stapler, or ablation of the blebs with an Nd:YAG (neodymium:yttrium-aluminum garnet) laser. When the bleb is identified and repaired, followed by pleural abrasion or talc poudrage, the recurrence rate approaches zero. VATS also requires only a short hospital stay, is associated with low morbidity, and has a high rate of patient acceptance. Axillary thoracotomy has similar

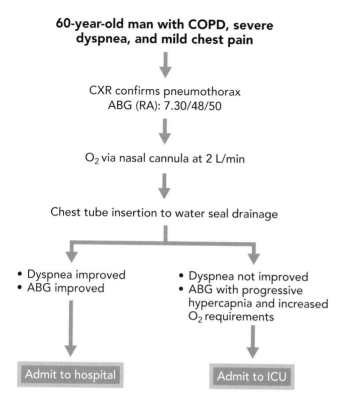

60-year-old man with COPD, severe dyspnea, and mild chest pain

↓

CXR confirms pneumothorax
ABG (RA): 7.30/48/50

↓

O₂ via nasal cannula at 2 L/min

↓

Chest tube insertion to water seal drainage

- Dyspnea improved
- ABG improved

- Dyspnea not improved
- ABG with progressive hypercapnia and increased O₂ requirements

Admit to hospital

Admit to ICU

Figure 60.3 Initial management of a hypothetical patient with secondary spontaneous pneumothorax.

efficacy and safety to VATS and is preferred where VATS is not available (12).

For patients with their first PSP treated with chest tubes, spontaneous resolution of air leaks tends to occur by 48 hours. There is little to be gained in PSP, therefore, by conservative treatment of air leaks that persist for longer than 72 hours. In contrast, the relatively high surgical risk for patients with SSP and severe underlying lung dysfunction may prompt a longer trial (7–10 days) of chest tube drainage before proceeding to VATS or limited thoracotomy.

Surgical intervention (VATS) is indicated in patients with recurrent pneumothoraces, persistent air leak, bilateral pneumothoraces, and a single episode of pneumothorax when a recurrence is thought to put the patient at great risk. Because spontaneous pneumothorax is usually poorly tolerated in patients with underlying lung disease, most patients with SSP qualify for pleurodesis after their first episode. A recent decision-analysis indicated that VATS could be optimal therapy for the first episode of PSP in men who fail simple manual aspiration (13). Patient preferences should determine whether VATS is performed after the first or second PSP.

COST CONSIDERATIONS AND RESOURCE USE

The treatment of patients with recurrent spontaneous pneumothorax should be individualized and guided by expert opinion, as few randomized, controlled trials have been performed. Simple aspiration in the Emergency Department allows many patients with PSP to avoid hospitalization.

KEY POINTS

- Discriminating between pleural fluid exudates and transudates is the first step in evaluating pleural effusions.
- The "abbreviated Light's criteria" using pleural fluid-to-serum protein and pleural fluid LDH has similar diagnostic performance to the traditional 3-component Light's criteria.
- Confirming a transudate generally narrows the differential diagnosis to a clinically apparent process.
- Factors that indicate a need for drainage of a nonpurulent parapneumonic effusion include a large effusion (>40% of hemithorax), a positive pleural fluid Gram's stain or culture, multiple loculations, a low pleural fluid pH or glucose level, and a high pleural fluid level of lactate dehydrogenase.
- Therapeutic thoracentesis should be performed cautiously in the patient with a large pleural effusion and ipsilateral mediastinal shift, as there is a high risk of unilateral plumonary edema.
- Primary spontaneous pneumothoraces occur most commonly in tall, thin male smokers in the second and third decades of life; they recur in 30%–50% of patients.
- Simple aspiration can be successful in primary spontaneous pneumothorax (and hospitalization avoided) if clinical evaluation suggests that the air leak has stopped.
- Tube thoracostomy is the treatment of choice for virtually all patients with secondary spontaneous pneumothorax.
- Video-assisted thoracoscopic surgery (VATS) is the preferred surgical procedure for recurrent spontaneous pneumothorax; the recurrence rate approaches zero if the bleb is identified and treated. Most patients with SSP should undergo pleurodesis after their first pneumothorax.

REFERENCES

1. Collins TR, Sahn SA. Thoracentesis: clinical value, complications, technical problems, and patient experience. *Chest* 1987;91: 817–822.
2. Heffner JE, Brown LK, Barbieri C, et al. Pleural fluid chemical analysis in parapneumonic effusions. A meta-analysis. *Am J Respir Crit Care Med* 1995;151:1700–1708.
3. Heffner JE, Brown LK, Barbieri C. Diagnostic value of tests that discriminate between exudative and transudative pleural effusions. *Chest* 1997;111:970–979.
4. Joseph J, Badrinath P, Basran GS, et al. Is the pleural fluid transudate or exudate? A revisit of the diagnostic criteria. *Thorax* 2001;56:867–870.
5. Romero-Candeira S, Hernandez L, Romero-Brufao S, et al. Is it meaningful to use biochemical parameters to discriminate between transudative and exudative pleural effusions? *Chest* 2002;122:1524–1529.

6. Heffner JE, Sahn SA, Brown LK. Multilevel likelihood ratios for identifying exudative pleural effusions. *Chest* 2002;121: 1916–1920.
7. Heffner JE, McDonald J, Barbieri C, et al. Management of parapneumonic effusions. An analysis of physician practice patterns. *Arch Surg* 1995;130:433–438.
8. Bouros D, Schiza S, Patsourakis G, et al. Intrapleural streptokinase versus urokinase in the treatment of complicated parapneumonic effusions: a prospective, double-blind study. *Am J Respir Crit Care Med* 1997;155:291–295.
9. Shaw P, Agarwal R. Pleurodesis for malignant pleural effusions. *Cochrane Database Syst Rev* 2004;1:CD002916.
10. Noppen M, Alexander P, Driesen P, et al. Manual aspiration versus chest tube drainage in first episodes of primary spontaneous pneumothorax: a multicenter, prospective, randomized pilot study. *Am J Respir Crit Care Med* 2002;165:1202–1203.
11. Ayed AK, Al-Din HJ. The results of thoracoscopic surgery for primary spontaneous pneumothorax. *Chest* 2001;118:235–238.
12. Miller JD, Simone C, Kahnamoui K, et al. Comparison of videothoracoscopy and axillary thoracotomy for the treatment of spontaneous pneumothorax. *Am Surg* 2000;66:1014–1015.
13. Morimoto T, Fukui T, Koyama H, et al. Optimal strategy for the first episode of primary spontaneous pneumothorax in young men. A decision analysis. *J Gen Intern Med* 2002;17:193–202.

ADDITIONAL READING

Antony VB, Loddenkemper R, Astoul P, et al. Management of malignant pleural effusions. *Eur Respir J* 2001;18:402–419.

Baumann MH, Noppen M. Pneumothorax. *Respirology* 2004;9: 157–164.

Colice GL, Curtis A, Deslauriers J, et al. Medical and surgical management of parapneumonic effusions: an evidence-based guideline. *Chest* 2000;118:1158–1171 (published erratum in *Chest* 2001;119:319).

Light RW, Lee YC. *Textbook of Pleural Diseases.* London: Arnold Publishers, 2003.

Sahn SA. Diagnostic value of pleural fluid analysis. *Semin Respir Crit Care Med* 1995;16:269–278.

Sahn SA. The pleura. *Am Rev Respir Dis* 1988;138:184–234.

Pulmonary Nodules and Mass Lesions

61

Michael K. Gould   Glen A. Lillington

INTRODUCTION

In this chapter, we discuss three categories of spherical intrapulmonary lesions, with a particular focus on the hospitalized patient: (a) the *solitary pulmonary nodule* (SPN), a spherical and fairly well-circumscribed radiographic opacity with a diameter of 3 cm or less; (b) the *pulmonary mass lesion*, which is roughly spherical and fairly well circumscribed but greater than 3 cm in diameter; and (c) *multiple nodules*, which are spherical and may be of different sizes. As the management of patients in the three categories differs considerably, we discuss each separately.

SOLITARY PULMONARY NODULES

The SPN is a spherical radiographic opacity that measures up to 30 mm in diameter. Use of the term "solitary" indicates that there is only one nodule and that there is no associated atelectasis, post-obstructive pneumonia, mediastinal widening or pleural effusion. We further distinguish nodules that measure less than 8–10 mm in diameter because they are difficult to biopsy or characterize by imaging tests. Most of these "sub-centimeter" nodules are detected incidentally on chest computed tomography (CT) and should be managed by repeating the CT scan every 3–6 months to check for growth, although the optimal interval for follow-up has not been determined.

About 20%–40% of SPNs that measure between 8 and 30 mm in diameter are malignant, mostly bronchogenic carcinomas (Table 61.1). Benign nodules are usually healed granulomas or benign tumors, but a variety of uncommon types include noninfectious granulomas, parasitic lesions, healed infarcts, and pulmonary arteriovenous malformations (1).

The primary management goal is to resect malignant nodules promptly while avoiding thoracotomies for benign nodules. Some nonmalignant SPNs require prompt investigation and treatment, however, particularly when they occur in immunocompromised patients.

Diagnostic Techniques

Most SPNs are incidentally found by *chest radiography*, which can detect most nodules that measure at least 1 cm in diameter. Ideally, nodules located within the chest should be visible in more than one radiographic projection, but nodules are sometimes difficult to visualize in the lateral view. Occasionally, nipple shadows, skin tumors or articular surfaces of ribs can be mistaken for pulmonary nodules. In these circumstances, repeated films in which nipple markers or apical lordotic projections are used will typically help differentiate normal anatomic structures from nodular parenchymal abnormalities.

In general, plain radiography provides few clues regarding etiology. Larger nodules and those with irregular, spiculated margins are more likely to be malignant. Although the sensitivity of chest radiography for detecting intranodular calcification is only 50% (2), certain patterns of calcification (central, laminated, diffuse and "popcorn") strongly point to a benign diagnosis. These nodule characteristics are often better evaluated by computed tomography (CT). Rarely, a (non-solitary) nodule is associated with an ipsilateral pleural effusion, mediastinal fullness, or atelectasis from bronchial obstruction, in which case bronchogenic carcinoma is likely.

Prior chest radiographs provide crucial information about nodule growth or stability over time. Thus, a critically important first step in SPN diagnosis is to locate any old films for radiographic comparison.

TABLE 61.1

ETIOLOGY OF SOLITARY PULMONARY NODULES

Malignant

Bronchogenic carcinoma 30%
Carcinoid tumors 5%
Solitary metastases 5%

Benign

Healed granulomas 35%
Granulomatous infection or inflammation, active 15%
Benign tumors (e.g., hamartoma) 5%
Miscellaneous causes 5%

Computed tomography of the thorax is usually advisable. This provides accurate information about the diameter of a nodule, the pattern of any calcification present, the characteristics of the nodule edge, and the presence or absence of hilar/mediastinal adenopathy. The latter has important implications for staging in patients with malignant nodules, although CT is neither sensitive nor specific for identifying mediastinal metastases (3). Selected high-resolution sections will show attenuation patterns within the nodule, which in some cases (e.g., hamartoma) may be diagnostic. Although the technique is not widely used in current clinical practice, a multicenter study of CT with dynamic contrast enhancement showed that absence of contrast enhancement (<15 Hounsfield units) strongly predicted a benign diagnosis (4).

Positron emission tomography (PET) is a newer and potentially useful functional imaging test for pulmonary nodule diagnosis. The sensitivity and specificity of PET for detecting malignancy are approximately 94% and 83%, respectively (5). The technique is also useful for detecting tumor involvement in the hilar/mediastinal lymph nodes and in distant organs (6).

Non-thoracotomy biopsy of the SPN often differentiates malignancy from benignity. Bronchoscopic biopsy is relatively insensitive unless the nodule is central in location and large. Transthoracic needle aspiration biopsy (TTNAB) under CT guidance is very helpful when it reveals a specific benign or malignant diagnosis, but nondiagnostic results and pneumothorax requiring chest tube placement can be expected in approximately 20% and 5% of cases, respectively (7). With the use of appropriate techniques and needles, it is possible to establish a specific diagnosis by TTNAB in about 50% of patients with benign nodules. The diagnostic yield for malignancy is over 90%, although the yield depends on several factors, including the size and location of the nodule.

Thoracotomy is required in some cases to establish the diagnosis, and it is particularly useful if the probability of cancer is high. In recent years, video-assisted thoracoscopic surgery (VATS) has become increasingly favored over classic thoracotomy for biopsy and resection of peripheral nodules. Most thoracic surgeons convert the VATS procedure to a classic thoracotomy when malignancy is identified on frozen section (8).

Issues at the Time of Admission

By definition, patients with solitary pulmonary nodules are asymptomatic, and therefore the presence of an SPN is not in itself an indication for admission to the hospital. In most cases, the symptoms and signs that have resulted in a hospital admission are caused by an unrelated disease process that will dominate investigation and management. Investigation of the coexistent ("incidental") SPN, although important, is usually deferred, at least temporarily.

Occasionally, the pulmonary nodule and the clinical syndrome that prompted hospital admission will appear to be related and must be investigated concurrently. Several clinical patterns may be encountered in which such a relationship appears likely.

Remote Metastases Pattern

Metastatic deposits from a malignant nodule may be regional or distant. Regional metastases may result in superior vena cava obstruction or upper airway obstruction due to tracheal compression. The diagnostic clue is the detection on chest CT of extensive mediastinal adenopathy. Distant (remote) tumor deposits may result in a variety of neurologic, hepatic, skeletal, and adrenal syndromes. For patients with non-small cell lung cancer, appropriate imaging studies should be ordered when one of these syndromes is suggested by a thorough history and physical examination. Although biopsy of metastatic lesions usually confirms the diagnosis, TTNAB of the SPN itself may occasionally be necessary.

Paraneoplastic Syndrome Pattern

Paraneoplastic syndromes secondary to bronchogenic carcinoma may be the impetus for hospital admission. These syndromes may include symptomatic hypercalcemia, inappropriate secretion of antidiuretic hormone (SIADH), Cushing's syndrome, cerebrocerebellar dysfunction, gynecomastia, and pseudomyasthenia. The clinical characteristics usually suggest the diagnosis, and biopsy evidence of malignancy is confirmatory.

Immunosuppression Pattern

An SPN may be a manifestation of an opportunistic infection, particularly in AIDS patients (9) and organ transplant recipients (10, 11). Other lung lesions are often present. Tests include sputum cultures, blood cultures, bronchoscopy with collection of bronchoalveolar lavage fluid, transbronchial needle aspiration, and TTNAB. The sensitivities of all these tests are low, and in some instances, a thoracotomy may be needed to determine the etiology. Empiric antibiotic therapy is often advisable if there is evidence of infection.

Incidental Nodule Pattern

In most hospitalized patients with an SPN, the clinical circumstances indicate that the nodule is incidental to the illness that precipitated hospital admission. If it seems likely that the two problems are unrelated, the prudent course is to diagnose and treat the acute illness and defer investigation of the nodule until the acute illness is resolving.

An incidental SPN may be detected in patients admitted to the hospital for acute coronary syndrome. If coronary bypass surgery seems necessary, the usual practice has been to defer consideration of the nodule until the patient has recovered from the cardiac surgery. However, if the probability that the nodule is malignant is high, resection of the nodule at the time of the cardiac procedure may be a reasonable alternative in selected cases (12).

Similarly, patients admitted to the hospital for lung volume reduction surgery (Chapter 58) have a concomitant SPN in up to 10% of cases. The nodule can be resected during the volume reduction procedure in selected instances (13).

Issues During the Course of Hospitalization

Once the illness for which the patient was hospitalized is being resolved, attention may be turned to the SPN. If it is still present and unchanged after therapy for the acute illness, further investigation is warranted. This can be initiated in the hospital and completed on an outpatient basis.

Two features that indicate a very high probability of benignity are (a) radiologic detection of *intranodular calcification in a benign pattern*, and (b) *stability* (no increase in size during a period of at least 2 years, as determined by serial chest roentgenograms). In either of these cases, exploratory thoracotomy can usually be deferred, but obtaining serial chest roentgenograms or CT scans every 6 months for another year or two is usually prudent, especially in patients with small nodules (14).

Management strategies for the *uncalcified nodule of unknown stability* include (a) prompt thoracotomy, (b) nonsurgical biopsy of the nodule, and (c) observation ("wait and watch"), a prospective determination of stability through serial chest roentgenograms. If the choice is to pursue nonsurgical biopsy of a solitary nodule, many studies have shown that TTNAB has a much greater sensitivity for malignancy than bronchoscopy since most solitary nodules are located peripherally.

While most clinicians use intuition to estimate the clinical likelihood (or pretest probability) of malignancy in a given patient, more precise estimates can be obtained by using one of several quantitative models that have been developed (15–17). Although the calculated probabilities of cancer do not permit an exact separation of malignant from benign nodules, they are useful for guiding management. For example, a decision analysis showed that watchful waiting was preferred when pretest probability of cancer was less than 3%; surgery was preferred when pretest probability was greater than 68%; and needle biopsy was preferred at intermediate probabilities, although the choice of strategy was a "close call" (18). A more recent cost-effectiveness analysis (19) concluded that PET imaging is now preferred over needle biopsy when the probability of malignancy falls in the range between 20% and 68% (Figure 61.1).

SPHERICAL MASS LESIONS

For purposes of this presentation, a mass lesion is defined as a roughly spherical and well-circumscribed opacity of the lung that is greater than 3 cm in diameter. Mass lesions have somewhat different etiologies than SPNs (Table 61.2), are more likely to be malignant, and require different management approaches. Although pulmonary masses are usually solitary, we include in this discussion the uncommon instances in which a patient has multiple mass lesions.

Issues at the Time of Admission

Unlike SPNs, the major types of mass lesions are often accompanied by symptoms and signs that can warrant hospitalization. The clinical picture provides clues to the diagnosis and will guide the choice of management strategies. Several presenting patterns are described.

Pneumonia Pattern

This includes acute onset, fever, cough, purulent sputum, leukocytosis, and dyspnea. The mass lesion is likely to be an example of *spherical pneumonia*, which is more common in children than in adults and is usually bacterial (20). Air bronchograms are often detectable within the mass. A trial of empirical antibiotic therapy is warranted in patients who are mildly symptomatic or asymptomatic. When the presentation is severe and fulminant, prompt attention to ascertaining the specific organisms involved is critical. The diagnostic approach may include blood cultures, sputum cultures, analysis of bronchial secretions collected by bronchoalveolar lavage or a plugged cascading catheter, and cultures of pleural effusions, if present. TTNAB is sometimes advisable. Occasionally, spherical pneumonia is caused by fungal infections.

Immunosuppression Pattern

The clinical picture suggests infection, and the presence and the specific cause (AIDS, organ transplants, drugs) of

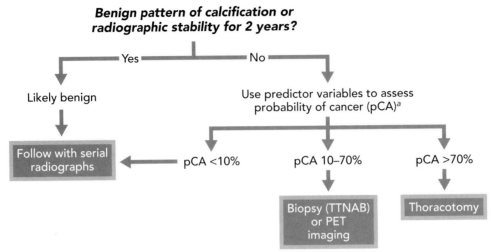

^aPredictor variables:

Age (years)
Smoking status (current or former = 1, never = 0)
Extrathoracic cancer diagnosed >5 years ago (yes = 1, no = 0)
Nodule diameter (mm)
Nodule Spiculation (yes = 1, no = 0)
Upper lobe location (yes = 1, no = 0)

$pCA = e^x/(1 + e^x)$,
Where $x = -6.8272 + (0.0391 \times$ Age$) + (0.7917 \times$ smoking status$) +$
$(1.3388 \times$ extrathoracic cancer$) + (0.1274 \times$ diameter$) +$
$(1.0407 \times$ spiculation$) + (0.7838 \times$ upper lobe location$)$

Figure 61.1 Proposed algorithm for management of solitary pulmonary nodules. A benign diagnosis is suggested by radiographic stability for at least 2 years, or by a benign pattern of calcification (central, laminated, diffuse, or popcorn pattern). In the absence of these characteristics, the probability of cancer (*pCA*) may be calculated by using a prediction equation that incorporates age, smoking status, history of previous extrathoracic malignancy, nodule diameter, nodule spiculation, and nodule location. When the pCA is less than 10%, follow-up with serial radiographs is recommended. When the pCA is more than 70%, immediate thoracotomy is usually warranted, unless surgery is contraindicated. For intermediate values of the pCA, initial biopsy is often prudent, although use of PET imaging may be preferable in centers where it is available. In these situations, it is especially important to consider patient preferences because the choice of strategy is a close call. *SPN*, solitary pulmonary nodule; *TTNAB*, transthoracic needle aspiration biopsy. (From Swensen SJ, Silverstein MD, Ilstrup DM, et al. *Arch Intern Med* 1997;157:849–855, with permission.)

TABLE 61.2

ETIOLOGY OF PULMONARY MASS LESIONS

Malignant

Bronchogenic carcinoma (including alveolar cell tumors)
Lymphoma, malignant teratoma
Plasmacytoma, others

Benign

Benign tumors and pseudotumors
Granulomas, infectious and noninfectious
Spherical pneumonia
Arteriovenous aneurysm, pulmonary infarct
Cysts (hydatid, bronchogenic, sequestration)
Conglomerate pneumoconiosis
Rounded atelectasis
Mucoid impaction
Pulmonary hematoma

the immunosuppressed state will usually be apparent. A mass lesion in these circumstances is usually fungal or bacterial. The development of cavitation in the mass is common. Other lung lesions are often visible. Vigorous diagnostic efforts are indicated. TTNAB is often helpful, but an open thoracotomy with biopsy may be required occasionally.

Diffuse Metastases Pattern

Lung masses are often malignant, and extensive regional and distant metastases can produce a clinical pattern with one or more of the following: neurologic deficits, convulsions, superior vena caval obstruction, bone pain or pathologic fractures, hypercalcemia, hepatic abnormalities, and Addison's disease. Mediastinal adenopathy is often prominent. The diagnosis may be established by imaging studies of multiple organs plus biopsy of the lung lesion, the mediastinal nodes, or another accessible lesion. In general, the clinician should select a biopsy site that establishes the most advanced stage of disease, while minimizing the risk of serious complications.

Endocrine Pattern

Clinical patterns of hypercalcemia, hypercortisolism, gynecomastia, inappropriate secretion of antidiuretic hormone (SIADH), and pseudomyasthenia suggest ectopic hormone secretion by a chest mass associated with bronchogenic carcinoma. Biopsy of the mass or enlarged mediastinal nodes will usually establish the diagnosis.

Systemic Vasculitis Pattern

The patient with Wegener's granulomatosis may present with the clinical picture of persistent fever, malaise, weight loss, rhinitis and sinusitis, uveitis, anemia, hematuria, renal insufficiency, and single or multiple pulmonary nodules or masses. The pulmonary lesions are often basilar in location and may be poorly circumscribed. The diagnosis is supported by the presence of elevated cytoplasmic antineutrophil cytoplasmic antibody (c-ANCA) titers, but open or thoracoscopic lung biopsy is often necessary (Chapter 111).

Pleural Pattern

Mass lesions can appear in conjunction with radiologic evidence of pleural disease in several situations:

1. A juxtapleural mass with an ipsilateral effusion suggests a bronchogenic carcinoma with direct intrapleural extension. TTNAB and/or thoracentesis are usually diagnostic.
2. In a patient with a chronic effusion that waxes and wanes with therapy, intrafissural loculation of the fluid may present as one or more sharply circumscribed large opacities. Comparison of roentgenograms in two projections often reveals loculated fluid, but chest CT is sometimes necessary to establish the diagnosis.
3. A pleural fibroma or a benign mesothelioma may present as an intrathoracic mass that may be quite large. Thoracotomy is often required for diagnosis.
4. In a patient with a history of significant asbestos exposure, a basilar mass can be a manifestation of rounded atelectasis. Several findings must be present to establish the diagnosis by CT criteria, including juxtapleural location, associated pleural thickening, evidence of ipsilateral volume loss and the presence of a "comet tail" that points toward the hilum. This condition is usually asymptomatic.

Issues During the Course of Hospitalization

While the evaluation of a solitary pulmonary nodule in a hospitalized patient can frequently be deferred, it is often prudent to initiate the work-up of a patient with a lung mass prior to discharge. In most cases, bronchoscopy, TTNAB, or both are indicated, and the mass will often prove to be neoplastic. Benign asymptomatic masses include hamartoma, teratoma, postinflammatory pseudotumor (i.e., plasma cell granuloma), fungal granuloma, intrapulmonary sequestration, hydatid cyst, and posttraumatic pulmonary hematoma. The investigation of such lesions is beyond the scope of this presentation (21).

MULTIPLE PULMONARY NODULES

For the purposes of discussion, this category includes multiple nodules that are 5 mm or more in diameter. It excludes miliary (micronodular, fine nodular) patterns. The number of visible nodules may vary from two to dozens.

Issues at the Time of Admission

Multiple lung nodules may have a number of causes (Table 61.3), but hematogenous metastatic spread from an extrapulmonary primary tumor is the most common. Metastatic deposits in the lung may be asymptomatic or associated with cough and dyspnea. Multiple pulmonary nodules are occasionally found incidentally during hospitalization for another disorder. A wide variety of clinical patterns can be present.

Immunosuppression Pattern

The presence of an immunosuppressed state may be known or suspected from the clinical history. Multiple pulmonary nodules in the AIDS patient can represent Kaposi's sarcoma, lymphoma, or opportunistic infections. Multiple pulmonary nodules in organ transplant recipients can be infectious or neoplastic. The diagnostic approach is similar to that in immunosuppressed patients with a solitary nodule.

TABLE 61.3

ETIOLOGY OF MULTIPLE PULMONARY NODULES

Malignant

Metastatic carcinoma or sarcoma
Kaposi's sarcoma
Lymphoma
Multicentric alveolar cell carcinoma

Benign

Benign tumors
Granulomas, infectious and noninfectious
Septic emboli, hematogenous pneumonias
Opportunistic infections
Miscellaneous

Diffuse Metastatic Pattern

The lung lesions may represent diffuse metastases from an extrapulmonary primary malignancy, and the clinical consequences of the deposits on other organs may have caused the illness requiring hospitalization. Common primary sites include breast, colon, kidney, pancreas, bone, and liver. If the primary tumor has been recognized and diagnosed, the cause of the diffuse pulmonary or multisystem involvement can be inferred, although biopsy confirmation is advisable in most instances.

Systemic Vasculitis Pattern

These patients have evidence of multisystem disease, including fever, arthritis, skin rashes, renal dysfunction, and elevated sedimentation rate. The nodular pulmonary lesions can be rheumatoid nodules, Wegener's granulomatosis, or lymphomatoid granulomatosis. The nodules tend to be large and limited in number. The diagnosis can often be established from the extrapulmonary manifestations (both serologic and histologic), but open or thoracoscopic biopsy of the pulmonary lesions is occasionally required (Chapters 111 and 112).

Asthma Pattern

Multiple nodules in an asthmatic patient can represent areas of mucoid impaction in a patient with allergic bronchopulmonary aspergillosis. The nodules may be single or multiple, large or small, and are primarily perihilar in location. Some of the lesions are elongated, serpentine or branching rather than spherical. Fever, increased dyspnea, marked eosinophilia, and expectoration of semisolid or rubbery "plugs" are common clinical manifestations. Diagnosis is most specifically established with measurement of high serum levels of *Aspergillus*-specific immunoglobulin E (IgE) antibodies. The response to systemic adrenocortical steroid therapy is usually excellent. A 16-week trial of adjunctive therapy with itraconazole demonstrated a clinical response in 46% of participants in the treatment group compared with 19% in the control group (22), so combined therapy with steroids and antifungal therapy should now be considered in all patients. In its early stages, Churg-Strauss syndrome mimics asthma and occasionally presents with multiple lung nodules. Marked eosinophilia, multiorgan involvement, and a positive perinuclear ANCA (p-ANCA) test results provide clues, and biopsy is confirmatory.

Hypoxemic Pattern

Multiple nodules may be a manifestation of pulmonary arteriovenous aneurysms, with right-to-left shunting and hypoxemia. The diagnostic clues are the presence on chest roentgenography or CT of enlarged vessels entering and leaving the nodules, the family history, and the presence of skin or mucosal lesions of hereditary hemorrhagic telangiectasia.

Acute Sepsis Pattern

Multiple nodules can be a manifestation of hematogenous bacterial pneumonia, most commonly resulting from staphylococcal infection and often associated with right-sided bacterial endocarditis (Chapter 71). Intravenous drug abuse is the usual cause. Some cases are a consequence of pelvic infection, pyelonephritis, or osteomyelitis, and organisms can include anaerobes and gram-negative aerobes. The lung lesions are typically "shaggy" in appearance and cavitation is common when staphylococcus is the causitive organism. The diagnosis can be suspected by the identification of a potential source for the infection and confirmed with sputum and blood cultures. Transthoracic or transesophageal echocardiography is helpful in establishing the diagnosis of endocarditis.

Issues During the Course of Hospitalization

If the cause of the illness requiring hospital admission is recognized and treated, it may then become apparent that the multiple lung lesions are *incidental*. The most common cause in such cases is metastatic malignancy. Less common causes include "alveolar" sarcoidosis, benign metastasizing leiomyomas, pulmonary chondromas in Carney's syndrome, healed infectious granulomas, rheumatoid nodules (including Caplan's syndrome), hamartomata, and asbestos-derived pleural plaques. Lung biopsy of one form or another is usually required.

Discharge Issues

In most patients with multiple lung nodules, the diagnosis will be established during the course of hospitalization. Patients with lung nodules undiagnosed at the time of hospital discharge require follow-up to exclude infection, vasculitis, or malignancy. In unusual cases, this will entail clinical observation for recurrent symptoms; more often, it will require outpatient biopsy or follow-up radiographic studies to demonstrate resolution or stability.

Cost Effectiveness and Resource Use

Little is known about cost effectiveness in the management of focal pulmonary lesions. Sputum cytology appears to be cost-effective under some circumstances, especially for centrally located lung masses. Recent studies indicate that selective use of PET imaging is likely to be highly cost-effective, especially when the diagnosis is particularly uncertain (i.e., when the pretest probability of malignancy and the CT results disagree—for example, when the clinical pretest probability is low but CT does not suggest a benign cause) (19, 23, 24).

In many cases, the time, expense, and risk for morbidity associated with aggressive diagnostic workups can be avoided by examining old films and confirming radiographic stability over time. The small investment in time required to locate old films for comparison is well worth the effort.

KEY POINTS

■ The prevalence of cancer in non-calcified solitary pulmonary nodules is high. Tissue diagnosis is often necessary.

■ Solitary pulmonary nodules are usually benign when intranodular calcification is present in a central, laminated, diffuse or "popcorn" pattern, or when the nodules have been radiographically stable for at least 2 years.

■ Solitary lung masses are larger than solitary pulmonary nodules and are even more likely to be malignant.

■ Multiple pulmonary nodules can represent hematogenous metastases but also infection or vasculitis.

■ For all pulmonary nodules, initial efforts should be directed at obtaining prior films, categorizing the clinical pattern, and treating acute illnesses. Cancer is highly probable in persistent nodules, and tissue diagnosis is generally required.

REFERENCES

1. Ost D, Fein AM, Feinsilver SH. The solitary pulmonary nodule. *N Engl J Med* 2003;348:2535–2542.
2. Berger WG, Erly WK, Krupinski EA, et al. The solitary pulmonary nodule on chest radiography: can we really tell if the nodule is calcified? *Am J Roentg* 2001;176:201–204.
3. Dwamena BA, Sonnad SS, Angobaldo JO, Wahl RL. Metastases from non-small cell lung cancer: mediastinal staging in the 1990s-meta-analytic comparison of PET and CT. *Radiology* 1999;213:530–536.
4. Swensen SJ, Viggiano RW, Midthum DE, et al. Lung nodule enhancement at CT: multicenter study. *Radiology* 2000;214:73–80.
5. Gould MK, Maclean CC, Kuschner WG, et al. Accuracy of positron emission tomography for diagnosis of pulmonary nodules and mass lesions: a meta-analysis. *JAMA* 2001;285:914–924.
6. Pieterman RM, van Putten JW, Meuzelaar JJ, et al. Preoperative staging of non-small-cell lung cancer with positron-emission tomography. *N Engl J Med* 2000;343:254–261.
7. Lacasse Y, Wong E, Guyatt GH, Cook DJ. Transthoracic needle aspiration biopsy for the diagnosis of localized pulmonary lesions: a meta-analysis. *Thorax* 1999;54:884–893.
8. Jimenez MF. The Spanish Video-Assisted Thoracic Surgery Study Group. Prospective study on video-assisted thoracoscopic surgery in the resection of pulmonary nodules: 209 cases from the Spanish Video-Assisted Thoracic Surgery Study Group. *Euro J Cardio-Thorac Surg* 2001;19:562–565.
9. Martinez-Marcos FJ, Viciana P, Canas E, et al. Etiology of solitary pulmonary nodules in patients with human immunodeficiency virus infection. *Clin Infect Dis* 1997;24:908–913.
10. End A, Helbich T, Wisser W, et al. The pulmonary nodule after lung transplantation. Cause and outcome. *Chest* 1995;107:1317–1322.
11. Haramati LB, Schulman LL, Austin JH. Lung nodules and masses after cardiac transplantation. *Radiology* 1993;188:491–497.
12. Mariani MA, van Boven WJ, Duurkens VA, et al. Combined off-pump coronary surgery and right lung resections through midline sternotomy. *Ann Thorac Surg* 2001;71:1343–1344.
13. Mentzer SJ, Swanson SJ. Treatment of patients with lung cancer and severe emphysema. *Chest* 1999;116:477S–479S.
14. Yankelevitz DF, Henschke CI. Does 2-year stability imply that pulmonary nodules are benign? *Am J Radiol* 1997;168:325–328.
15. Cummings SR, Lillington GA, Richard RJ. Estimating the probability of malignancy in solitary pulmonary nodules. A Bayesian approach. *Am Rev Resp Dis* 1986;134:449–452.
16. Gurney JW, Lyddon DM, McKay JA. Determining the likelihood of malignancy in solitary pulmonary nodules with Bayesian analysis. Part II. Application. *Radiology* 1993;186:415–422.
17. Swensen SJ, Silverstein MD, Ilstrup DM, et al. The probability of malignancy in solitary pulmonary nodules. Application to small radiologically indeterminate nodules. *Arch Intern Med* 1997;157:849–855.
18. Cummings SR, Lillington GA, Richard RJ. Managing solitary pulmonary nodules. The choice of strategy is a "close call." *Am Rev Resp Dis* 1986;134:453–460.
19. Gould MK, Sanders GD, Barnett PG, et al. Cost-effectiveness of alternative management strategies for patients with solitary pulmonary nodules. *Ann Intern Med* 2003;138:724–735.
20. Wagner AL, Szabunio M, Hazlett KS, Wagner SG. Radiologic manifestations of round pneumonia in adults.[comment]. *Am J Roentg* 1998;170:723–726.
21. Lillington GA. Multiple nodular lesions. In *A Diagnostic Approach to Chest Diseases: Differential Diagnosis Based on Roentgenographic Patterns.* 3rd ed. Lillington GA, ed. Baltimore: Williams & Wilkins; 1987:158–172.
22. Stevens DA, Schwartz HJ, Lee JY, et al. A randomized trial of itraconazole in allergic bronchopulmonary aspergillosis. *N Engl J Med* 2000;342:756–762.
23. Gambhir SS, Shepherd JE, Shah BD, et al. Analytical decision model for the cost-effective management of solitary pulmonary nodules. *J Clin Oncol* 1998;16:2113–2125.
24. Dietlein M, Weber K, Gandjour A, et al. Cost-effectiveness of FDG-PET for the management of solitary pulmonary nodules: a decision analysis based on cost reimbursement in Germany. *Eur J Nucl Med* 2000;27:1441–1456.

ADDITIONAL READING

Blank N. *Nodules and Neoplasms. Chest Radiographic Analysis.* New York: Churchill Livingstone, 1989.
Webb WR, Muller NL, Nadich DP. *High-Resolution CT of the Lung,* 3rd ed. Philadelphia: Lippincott Williams & Wilkins, 2000.

Infectious Diseases

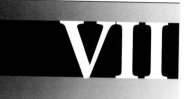

Signs, Symptoms, and Laboratory Abnormalities in Infectious Diseases

62

Richard A. Jacobs   Karen C. Bloch

TOPICS COVERED IN CHAPTER

- Fever 597
- Fever and Rash 600
- Fever in the Returning Traveler 602
- Fever of Unknown Origin 604
- Hypothermia 607
- Relative Bradycardia 607
- Atypical Lymphocytosis 608
- Interpreting Culture Results and Microbiologic Serologies 609

INTRODUCTION

Many of the signs, symptoms, and laboratory abnormalities associated with infections are nonspecific. They are seen in clinical entities as varied as adverse drug reactions, malignancy, and vasculitis. The challenge in evaluating a patient with potential infection is to determine whether historical information and objective findings detected by physical examination and laboratory evaluation are most compatible with infection or other disease states. If infection is suspected, the organ system involved must be identified. Once there is localization of infection, relatively accurate predictions about bacteriology can be made, and rational choices about appropriate antibiotic therapy can be made. The microbiology laboratory can be a "friend" or a "foe" in the diagnostic and therapeutic process. It can be invaluable in assisting the clinician in making a specific microbiologic diagnosis and defining appropriate therapy by sensitivity testing. However, the usefulness of information is dependent upon the reliability of the specimen submitted and the ability of the clinician to interpret the results. Submission of inappropriate material and misinterpretation of data can result in misdiagnosis and unneeded or even harmful therapy.

In this chapter, common signs, symptoms, and laboratory abnormalities frequently seen in hospitalized patients with infection are reviewed, with an emphasis on differential diagnosis. In addition, appropriate use of the microbiology laboratory and accurate interpretation of results are discussed.

SIGNS

Fever

Fever at Time of Admission

Hyperpyrexia, occurring in 30% of patients admitted to the medicine service, is a common but nonspecific sign and symptom. Classically, fever has been defined as an oral temperature higher than 38°C (100.4°F). A more precise definition of fever that accounts for normal circadian rhythms is an oral temperature higher than 37.2°C (99°F) in the morning or 37.8°C (100°F) irrespective of time of day. Rectal temperatures may be extrapolated by adding 0.6°C (1°F) to the oral reading.

Fever at the time of admission is attributable to community-acquired infections in more than 50% of cases. The exact frequencies of various community-acquired infections vary based on factors such as season, geography, and population demographics. In general, the most common community-acquired infections requiring hospitalization are pneumonia, pyelonephritis, cellulitis, and bacteremia (1). Noninfectious causes, accounting for approximately one-quarter of febrile admissions, include a diverse array of diseases involving multiple organ systems (Table 62.1). In the remainder of febrile admissions, no definitive underlying cause is identified.

Although much has been written about the use of fever patterns to aid in diagnosis, the low sensitivity and specificity of a given pattern greatly limits clinical usefulness.

Furthermore, fever may be blunted in the elderly or by the use of systemic corticosteroids. As a general rule, a fever higher than 102°F is unusual in the majority of inflammatory conditions (Table 62.1), and a temperature exceeding this level supports an alternative diagnosis. Extreme pyrexia, defined as a temperature higher than 41°C (106°F), may be seen with a limited number of conditions. Infection, most commonly Gram-negative bacteremia, is the leading cause of extreme hyperpyrexia, followed by a variety of conditions causing impaired thermoregulation (Table 62.2).

The protean causes of fever require a thorough history and physical examination to direct further testing and therapy. History of recent and remote travel, occupation, vaccinations, sexual encounters, and exposure to sick contacts, arthropods, or animals should be elicited, as these may provide important clues to diagnosis. Lymphadenopathy, splenomegaly, the presence of rash, or evidence of embolic phenomena may direct the clinician toward a specific diagnosis.

Appropriate laboratory studies include a complete blood count with differential, electrolytes, tests of renal

TABLE 62.1

NONINFECTIOUS CAUSES OF FEVER AT THE TIME OF ADMISSION

Disorders	T ≤102°F[a]	Characteristics	Disorders	T ≤102°F[a]	Characteristics
Neurologic			Endocrinologic		
Spinal cord injury		Restricted to lesions at T8 or higher	Pheochromocytoma		Associated with large, necrotic tumors
Hypothalamic injury		Trauma, tumor, vasculitis, hemorrhage	Thyrotoxicosis		Associated hypermetabolic state
Intracranial hemorrhage			Adrenal insufficiency		May mimic sepsis with hypotension
Seizures		89% of fevers last <48 h	Miscellaneous		
Subdural hematoma	X		Dissecting aortic aneurysm	X	Prolonged course of fever (5–11 weeks)
Malignancies		Prolonged fevers without systemic toxicity	Hematoma	X	
			Pancreatitis	X	Poor prognostic factor
Rheumatologic/ autoimmune					
Connective tissue disorders	X	Systemic lupus erythematosus, mixed connective tissue disease, etc.	Dehydration/ gastrointestinal bleeding	X	Caused by vasoconstriction/ decreased sweating
Vasculitides		Polyarteritis nodosa, Giant cell arteritis, polymyalgia rheumatica, etc.	Sarcoid	X	
			Deep venous thrombosis	X	
			Pulmonary embolus	X	
Rheumatoid arthritis	X	Still's disease: high fever, rash, leukocytosis	Myocardial infarction	X	89% febrile, duration of fever ≤1 week
Eosinophilia-myalgia syndrome		Associated with use of tryptophan pills	Narcotic abuse		Cocaine and phencyclidine
Crystal arthropathies		Fever seen only with active joint disease	Drug fever		Median delay in onset of 8 d

[a] Typically cause fever ≤102°F.

TABLE 62.2

NONINFECTIOUS CONDITIONS THAT MAY CAUSE EXTREME HYPERPYREXIA (TEMPERATURE >41°C)

Condition	On admission	During hospitalization
Hypothalamic injury		
Central nervous system malignancy	X	
Trauma	X	
Intracranial hemorrhage	X	X
Illicit drug use		
Cocaine	X	
Phencyclidine	X	
Miscellaneous		
Thyrotoxic crisis	X	
Drug fever	X	X
Heat stroke	X	
Exertional hyperthermia	X	
Neuroleptic malignant syndrome	X	X
Malignant hyperthermia		X

and liver function, and a urinalysis. If the clinical presentation supports a rheumatic or autoimmune process, specific confirmatory blood tests should be obtained. A chest radiograph is generally appropriate if there are signs or symptoms of respiratory involvement or concern for an intrathoracic process. Further radiologic studies should be directed by suggestive findings on the history and physical examination. Admission blood cultures from febrile patients have a yield of only 10%. However, the usefulness of a positive result in establishing a diagnosis, directing therapy, and defining length of treatment mandates that two sets be obtained ideally before antibiotics are administered.

Fever is a physiologic response to an underlying medical condition, and therapy should be directed against the cause rather than overzealous suppression of the sign. If the initial evaluation is suggestive of an infectious cause, antimicrobial therapy should be promptly initiated (Chapter 64). Fever may serve an adaptive function by inhibiting bacterial replication, promoting immune function, and increasing antimicrobial bactericidal activity. Antipyretics should be reserved for situations in which there is extreme patient discomfort, cardiopulmonary disease that may be exacerbated by fever-induced tachycardia, or temperature in excess of 40°C, as prolonged episodes of extreme hyperpyrexia may lead to permanent central nervous system damage or cause cardiac arrhythmias.

Two primary methods exist for ameliorating fever: *antipyretics* and *external cooling*. The latter, reserved for patients with extreme pyrexia, utilizes ice baths, alcohol sponges, cooling blankets, and, in emergency situations, intra-venous or intraperitoneal administration of cool fluids. Antipyretic options are limited to salicylates, nonsteroidal anti-inflammatory agents, and acetaminophen. Salicylates have been associated with Reye's syndrome in children with varicella or influenza and should not be used in this population. Naproxen (375 mg orally every 12 hours) is the preferred choice for patients with neoplastic fever. Persistent temperature elevation after more than three doses of naproxen essentially excludes the diagnosis of neoplastic fever.

Fever During the Course of Hospitalization

Causes of fever in the second or third hospital day are similar to those at admission, with one-third to one-half of cases attributable to community-acquired infection, and 30% of cases attributable to noninfectious causes (Table 62.1). Fever occurring more than 3 days into the hospital course should prompt investigation for a *nosocomial infection* or *drug fever*. Common hospital-acquired infections include urinary tract infections (particularly in patients with Foley catheters; see Chapter 68), nosocomial pneumonia (Chapter 66), vascular catheter-related infections (either localized or with bacteremia; see Chapter 72), wound infections, and antibiotic-associated colitis (2). Less common infections include infected decubitus ulcers, acalculous cholecystitis, and nosocomial sinusitis.

Not all nosocomial fevers require intervention. Postoperative patients frequently develop fever within the first several days of surgery, but this is rarely infectious, and is generally self-limited. True postoperative infections typically occur 1–2 weeks after surgery (exceptions include wound infections with group A *Streptococcus* or *Clostridium perfringens*, which may occur within several days of surgery) and are associated with local signs of infection. Patients undergoing esophageal (transesophageal echocardiograhy or upper endoscopy) or bronchial (bronchoscopy) instrumentation may develop transient fevers due to micro-aspiration of acidic gastrointestinal contents causing a chemical pneumonitis (Mendelson's syndrome).

While most causes of nosomial fevers can be identified by careful history and physical exam, occult causes of fever exist. This is particularly true in the ICU, where patients often are sedated or intubated, and abnormal laboratory findings such as leukocytosis and elevated liver-function tests are typically multifactorial. Particular attention should be paid to intravenous catheters and postoperative wounds for tenderness, purulence, or erythema. Decubitus ulcers can be a source of fever and bacteremia and should be diligently sought. Decubiti covered with an eschar should be unroofed, because significant deep-tissue involvement requiring debridement and antibiotics may be underlying the eschar. Acalculous cholecystitis, typically seen in postoperative or posttrauma patients receiving hyperalimentation, classically presents with fever, leukocytosis, right upper quadrant pain, and abnormal liver-function tests.

Nosocomial sinusitis has been reported to cause up to 5% of febrile episodes in the ICU, especially in patients with nasal packing, nasogastric tubes, and nasotracheal intubation. Diagnosis is suggested by the presence of more copious secretions from the oropharynx than from the endotracheal tube.

Febrile drug reactions have been reported to occur in 10% of hospitalized patients. Almost every pharmacologic agent has been anecdotally associated with drug fever. The median delay from the start of a new pharmacologic agent to the onset of fever is 8 days; however, there is substantial variation, with the median delay in fevers attributable to antineoplastic agents being shorter than 1 day. Careful review of pharmacy records may reveal a temporal relationship between starting a new agent and the onset of fever, although idiopathic reactions to medication have been reported to occur months to years after starting therapy. Clues to the diagnosis of drug fever include the presence of relative bradycardia (see subsequent section) and the lack of subjective discomfort during febrile episodes. Although cutaneous eruptions occur in only about 20% of febrile drug reactions, the presence of rash strongly supports an allergic etiology (3). Other noninfectious causes of fever in hospitalized persons include thromboembolic disease, myocardial infarction, Dressler's syndrome, adrenal insufficiency, gout or calcium pyrophosphate disease, and ischemic bowel disease.

Laboratory studies may not be particularly helpful in pinpointing a cause for fever. Total white blood cell count may be normal, high, or low even in the presence of serious infection. Leukocytosis or eosinophilia is present in only 22% of cases of drug fever, and both findings are associated with a number of other conditions included in the differential diagnosis of fever (3). Focality in the history or physical examination should prompt directed cultures. Patients with a new productive cough should have sputum sent for Gram's stain and culture. Those with an indwelling Foley catheter should have urine cultured, but results must be interpreted with caution. Colonization of the urine with Gram-negative organisms is common, but true infection as a cause of fever is unusual unless there is inflammation, as evidenced by the presence of significant pyuria. Similarly, *Candida* species frequently colonize the urine but are not associated with invasive disease unless there are preexisting abnormalities (stones, malignancy, or obstruction). Therapy is not routinely indicated for candiduria in the absence of pyuria.

Patients with new onset of diarrhea should have stool assayed for the presence of *Clostridium difficile* toxin. Testing for the presence of fecal leukocytes is neither a sensitive nor specific surrogate marker for the presence of *C. difficile* toxin and should not be done. Similarly, culturing stools and examining stools for ova and parasites in patients who develop diarrhea in the hospital is not cost-effective and is not recommended. Although meningitis frequently is considered as a cause of fever (usually in the ICU patient who is sedated and in whom mental status cannot be assessed), meningitis rarely develops in inpatients in the absence of head trauma, manipulation of the spinal cord (i.e., epidural catheterization), or recent neurosurgery. Thus, in the absence of meningeal signs or one of the above predisposing conditions, a lumbar puncture is generally not indicated. The yield of blood cultures in febrile inpatients is only 20%; however, as there are no reliable surrogate markers for bloodstream infection, all febrile patients should have two sets of blood cultures sent.

Chest radiographs may be helpful, as abnormalities suggest infection, aspiration, or pulmonary embolism. The role of sinus computed tomography (CT) scans in diagnosing sinusitis has not been rigorously studied. Most recumbent ICU patients with nasal tubes in place have fluid in their sinuses, and mucosal thickening is a common and nonspecific finding. To make a definitive diagnosis of acute sinusitus, a sinus aspirate with culture is needed. If there are abdominal findings or if there is a suspicion of acalculous cholecystitis or ischemic bowel disease, an abdominal ultrasound or CT scan is indicated.

The management of fever in hospitalized patients is identical to that for fever in a newly admitted patient. Elevated temperature should be viewed as a sign of an underlying disease, and therapy should be directed at the likely source. (Refer to Chapter 64 and chapters discussing specific nosocomial infections for discussion of potential antibiotic regimens). Most drugs causing fevers have short half-lives, and drug fever usually resolves within 48–72 hours of discontinuing the offending drug. Fever resulting from drugs with long half-lives may take substantially longer to resolve. The indications for antipyretic therapy are identical to those discussed in the previous section.

Fever and Rash

Fever and Rash at Time of Admission

The febrile patient with a cutaneous eruption requires urgent evaluation. Although many of the underlying conditions presenting with rash are relatively benign, a few are life threatening, and the rapid institution of appropriate antibiotics may prevent a fatal outcome. Furthermore, a number of these infections are highly contagious, and require prompt isolation of the index patient and identification of potential contacts to avoid secondary cases. Infectious disease emergencies associated with cutaneous manifestations include *meningococcemia*, *Rocky Mountain spotted fever*, *toxic shock syndrome*, and *bacterial sepsis*. *Smallpox* and *anthrax* have gained widespread attention as possible markers of a bioterrorist attack. Identification of the specific pathogen causing fever and a rash hinges on the characteristics of the skin eruption (Table 62.3, and see also Chapter 73).

TABLE 62.3

INFECTIONS ENDEMIC TO THE UNITED STATES CAUSING FEVER WITH PROMINENT CUTANEOUS MANIFESTATIONS

Infection	Petechial, Purpuric	Maculopapular	Vesicular	Other	Comments
Viral infections:					
Acute HIV		X			Adenopathy, pharyngitis, malaise
Enterovirus	X	X	X		Typically summer and early fall
Rubeola (measles)		X			Unvaccinated populations
Adenovirus	X	X			Keratopharyngitis variably seen
Lymphocytic choriomeningitis		X			Rodent exposure, more common in fall
Rubella (German Measles)	X	X			Unvaccinated populations
Varicella (zoster or chickenpox)			X		Acute varicella in unvaccinated. Zoster typically dermatomal
Herpes simplex			X		Predominately genital and perioral
Cytomegalovirus (CMV)		X			Associated with infectious mono sydrome
Epstein-Barr virus (EBV)	X	X			Associated with infectious mono syndrome; often appears after amoxicillin ingestion
Parvovirus B-19		X			Erythema infectiosum
Human herpesvirus 6		X			Roseola infantum
Smallpox			X		First lesions on face, palate, or forearms. Bioterror agent.
Bacterial infections:					
Chlamydia psittaci		X			Associated with bird exposure, pneumonia
Mycoplasma pneumoniae		X	X		Bullous myringitis in ~5%
Rickettsia spp.	X	X	X		Spotted-fever group typically petechial, typhoidal group maculopapular with eschar; rickettsial pox with vesicles
Ehrlichia spp.	X	X			Tick-borne pathogens, associated with leukopenia, thrombocytopenia
Bartonella spp.		X		Vascular cutaneous lesions	Bacillary angiomatosis in HIV infected
Franciscella tularensis		X			Ulceroglandular type, typhoidal type
Rat-bite fever agents	X	X			
Secondary syphilis		X	X		Lesions on palms and soles
Neisseria spp.	X	X			Purpura, petechial lesions on palms and soles
Leptospira spp.	X	X	X		Associated with aseptic meningitis, renal failure, hepatitis
Borrelia spp.	X	X			Erythema migrans in Lyme disease
P. aeruginosa		X			Ecthyma gangrenosum
S. aureus	X	X			Impetigo with localized infection, petechia with endocarditis
Group A streptococci		X			Scarlet fever, impetigo
Capnocytophaga canimorsus	X	X			Dog exposure, sepsis in asplenic host
Bacillus anthrasis (Anthrax)		X	X	Necrotic eschar late in course	Potential bioterrorism agent
Vibrio vulnificus			X		Exposure to salt water, particularly in patients with liver disease

Adapted from Weber DJ, Cohen MS, Fine JD. The acutely ill patient with fever and rash. In Mandell GL, Bennett JE, Dolin R, eds. *Principles and Practice of Infectious Diseases*, 5th ed. New York: Churchill Livingstone, 2000: 633–650.

The history and physical examination are the mainstays of the initial evaluation. Many of the syndromes in the differential diagnosis can be excluded if there has been no foreign travel (see subsequent section), no outdoor activities suggestive of arthropod exposure, no sexual activity, and no animal exposures. Menstrual history may support a diagnosis of tampon-associated toxic shock syndrome or disseminated gonorrhea. History regarding the initial site, appearance, and rapidity of spread of the rash may aid diagnosis. The physical examination should focus on the distribution of the cutaneous eruption and include a thorough search for associated findings such as pharyngitis, adenopathy, arthritis, nuchal rigidity or altered mental status, genital lesions, or cervical discharge. Gram stain and culture of selected cutaneous lesions may yield a rapid diagnosis. Gram-negative diplococci aspirated from petechiae are consistent with either disseminated meningococcemia or gonorrhea; Gram-positive cocci suggest *Staphylococcus aureus* sepsis. Culture of scrapings from the base of ecthyma gangrenosum ulcers may facilitate diagnosis of *Pseudomonas aeruginosa* sepsis. Bullous lesions should be unroofed under sterile conditions and the fluid sent for viral and bacterial diagnostic tests. A skin biopsy is often necessary to diagnose a vasculitic process, infection with *Bartonella* organisms (bacillary angiomatosis), or disseminated fungal infection. Therapy should be directed at the underlying cause of the syndrome and should include aggressive supportive measures as needed (see Chapter 26 for discussion of the sepsis syndrome).

Fever and Rash During Hospitalization

The most common cause of this syndrome is a cutaneous drug reaction, which develops in approximately 3% of hospitalized patients. These reactions are typically maculopapular and are pruritic in only one-half of cases. Infectious causes of rashes in hospitalized patients include bacterial sepsis (with or without disseminated intravascular coagulation), postoperative toxic shock syndrome (particularly among patients with indwelling nasal packings), and disseminated fungal disease (among immunosuppressed patients, those receiving total parenteral nutrition, or those on long term, broad-spectrum antibiotics). Exposure to a sick visitor or health care worker may provide an important clue in the patient with an exanthem and symptoms suggestive of a viral syndrome.

Infectious and noninfectious syndromes causing fever in hospitalized patients are best differentiated by the general appearance of the patient. Drug reactions typically cause minimal prostration, even during periods of extreme hyperpyrexia. Patients with sepsis, toxic shock syndrome, or fungemia often are critically ill or hypotensive and may have alterations in level of consciousness. Cultures of blood, wound discharge, urine, cutaneous lesions, and sputum should be obtained as clinically indicated. Skin biopsy may be necessary if cultures remain negative or if there is rapid progression of skin lesions. Therapy should be directed at the underlying cause of the syndrome, as elucidated by the initial evaluation.

Fever in the Returning Traveler

At Time of Admission

The differential diagnosis of fever in the returning traveler is broad, ranging from self-limited viral illness to fulminant, life-threatening infection. For the purposes of this chapter, the discussion will be limited to infections that typically require hospitalization for supportive care and treatment. The evaluation of the febrile traveler is best performed by identifying a syndrome (Table 62.4), and refining the differential based on the travel history and specific exposures. The travel history should include directed questions regarding geography (rural versus urban), animal or arthropod contact, unprotected sexual intercourse, ingestion of untreated water or raw foods, and history of pretravel immunizations and adherence to malaria prophylaxis. Routine laboratory studies usually include complete blood count with differential, electrolytes, liver function tests, urine analysis, and blood cultures. Thick and thin smears for malaria should be done if there has been any travel to endemic areas. If the initial smear is negative but the suspicion remains high, thick and thin smears should be repeated in the next 12–24 hours. Other studies are directed by the results of history, physical examination, and intial laboratory tests. They may include stools for ova and parasites, chest x-ray, HIV test, and specific serologies (dengue, leptospirosis, rickettsial illness, schistosomiasis, etc.).

Several general principles are helpful in evaluating the returning traveler with fever:

- Up to 50% of patients have either a self-limited illness that goes undiagnosed or have a "cosmopolitan" fever—one that is neither infectious in etiology nor travel-related. Thus, it is helpful to construct two differentials, one that includes the travel history and one that ignores it.
- People who visit family and friends while abroad or who are adventure travelers (hiking and camping in remote areas with less control of their food and water sources) are more likely to develop travel-related illnesses than are short-term visitors who frequent more standard tourist destinations.
- The goal of the initial evaluation is to identify those patients with acute, potentially life-threatening diseases that are treatable, or those with transmissible diseases that require isolation.
- The incubation period can be helpful in excluding certain diseases. Dengue, leptospirosis, yellow fever, rickettsial diseases, and Q fever usually present clinically within the first 3 weeks after exposure. In contrast, typhoid fever, malaria, tuberculosis, and hepatitis can

TABLE 62.4

INFECTIOUS SYNDROMES IN THE RETURNED TRAVELER

Syndrome	Initial evaluation	Specific pathogens	Syndrome	Initial evaluation	Specific pathogens
Fever & rash	Blood cultures Serologies (guided by history)	Dengue Viral hemorrhagic fever Leptospirosis Meningococcemia Yellow fever Typhus *Salmonella typhi* (Rose spot) HIV (acute)	Diarrhea	Blood cultures Fecal leukocytes Stool bacterial cultures Stool for O & P	Bacterial dysentery *E. histolytica* Cyclospora Disseminated strongyloidiasis
			Jaundice	Liver function tests Evaluation for hemolysis Thick/thin smear Serologies (guided by history)	Hepatitis A Yellow fever Hemorrhagic fever Leptospirosis Malaria
Pulmonary infiltrate	PPD Sputum for AFB Sputum for O & P	Tuberculosis Ascaris Paragonimus Strongyloides	Fever without localizing signs or symptoms	Blood cultures Thick/thin smears Serologies (guided by history) Bone marrow (typhoid fever)	Malaria Acute HIV Rickettsial illness *Salmonella typhi* Visceral leishmania Trypanosomiasis Dengue
Meningo-encephalitis	Blood cultures Thick/thin smears Lumbar puncture Serologies (guided by history) Nape biopsy (if rabies a concern)	*N. meningitidis* Leptospirosis Arboviruses Rabies Malaria (cerebral)			

present acutely, but may have longer incubation periods of greater than 6 weeks.

The most common infectious etiologies of fever in the returning traveler are malaria, respiratory infections, diarrhea, dengue, leptospirosis, typhoid fever, and rickettsial infections. Numerous other infections have been described and have been reviewed (4).

Malaria

Malaria presents with nonspecific symptoms of fever, chills, drenching sweats and headache. The typical pattern of fever every 48–72 hours occurs uncommonly, but when present strongly suggests infection with *Plasmodium vivax*, *P.ovale* (48 hours) or *P. malariae* (72 hours). Fevers with *P. falciparum* are more hectic and rarely synchronized. Splenomegaly and thrombocytopenia are frequent findings, but rash and lymphadenopathy are unusual. *P. falciparum*, the most severe form of disease, is more likely to be seen in patients traveling to Africa, whereas the other forms of malaria are more likely to occur after travel to Asia and Latin America. *P. falciparum* has a relatively short incubation, with 90% of patients presenting within 1month of return. In contrast, other forms of malaria are more indolent; only 50% develop symptoms within 1 month of return. Because clinical manifestations are nonspecific, any febrile traveler who has been in an endemic area should have thick and thin smears performed.

Respiratory Infections

Respiratory infections are usually "cosmopolitan" and due to viruses (including influenza), *S. pneumoniae*, my-

coplasma and legionella species. It is important to remember that tuberculosis is common in many less developed areas of the world and can present months after return. Other respiratory pathogens that should be considered depending on area of travel include histoplasmosis and coccidioidomycosis (Mexico). Q fever can also cause resiratory symptoms, and helminths that may migrate through the lung (ascariasis, strongyloidiasis).

Diarrhea

Travel-related diarrhea usually presents within the first month after return. Viruses and bacteria (enteroinvasive and enterohemorrhagic *E. coli*, *Salmonella*, *Shigella*, *Campylobacter*) commonly occur shortly after return and are usually self-limited. In patients with diarrhea that persists for several weeks, *Giardia lamblia*, *Entamoeba histolytica*, cryptosporidia and microsporidia should be considered. In patients with prolonged diarrhea and malabsorption, giardiasis and other small bowel parasites are likely. The diagnosis is usually made by stool culture or examination for ova and parasites. If an etiologic agent is not identified after stool examination and symptoms persist, many would treat empirically with a fluoroquinolone if symptoms suggestive of invasive disease of the large bowel are present (fevers, frequent small volume bloody stools), or metronidazole if bloating and watery diarrhea are present (giardia is the most common cause of these symptoms).

Dengue

Dengue is a mosquito-transmitted disease that has a short incubation period (almost always less than 10 days). It is common in tropical and subtropical areas (Asia, Central and South America, the Carribean), but some cases occur in travelers returning from Africa. Dengue presents with nonspecific symptoms of fever, chills, myalgia, artharalgias, and headache. Severe retroorbital pain exacerbated by eye movement is characteristic, and helps distinguish dengue from other travel-related febrile illnesses. Up to 50% of patients will have a maculopapular, diffuse erythematous rash that may be petechial in nature. Leukopenia and thrombocytopenia are common laboratory abnormalities. The diagnosis is usually made clinically and confirmed serologically. Therapy is supportive. Severe complications of dengue (dengue hemorrhagic fever and dengue shock syndrome) are not seen in first-time travelers. These complications are thought to be immunologically mediated and are seen in those sustaining a repeat infection with a different serotype of the virus.

Leptospirosis

Leptospirosis occurs worldwide, whenever humans come into contact with water that has been contaminated by urine from animal reservoirs. Spirochetes enter through abrasions in the skin, mucous membranes or conjunctiva. Following an incubation period of 1–3 weeks, nonspecific symptoms of fever, chills, and headache develop. Severe myalgias (sometimes mimicking an acute abdomen) and conjunctival suffusion may be present and should suggest the diagnosis. Recent outbreaks have been associated with hemorrhagic pneumonitis. The disease is often biphasic. After 3–7 days of illness there is a brief period of well-being followed by onset of fever, meningitis (immune mediated), uveitis and rash. Severe complications include renal failure, hepatitis, and shock. Although organisms can be isolated from blood, CSF, and urine in the first phase of the disease, the diagnosis is usually made clinically and confirmed serologically. Treatment within the first 3 days of illness improves outcome. Penicillin is the treatment of choice in severe disease. Doxycycline is used in mild to moderate disease, or in patients with IgE-mediated reactions to penicillin. Following treatment, the Jarisch-Herxheimer reaction can occur.

Typhoid Fever and Enteric Fever

Typhoid fever (caused by *Salmonella enterica* serotype *typhi*) and enteric fever (caused by other serotypes of salmonella) present with fever, headache, and gastrointestinal symptoms (abdominal pain and constipation are common, whereas diarrhea is rare). An evanescent rash (rose spots) is occasionally present, but the physical examination is usually not helpful in making a diagnosis. Most cases occur in travelers returning from India, Latin America, and the South Pacific. Blood cultures are positive in the majority of cases; salmonella can also be isolated from stool for several weeks after infection. Although multi-drug resistant organisms have been isolated, including a few strains resistant to fluoroquinolones, empirical therapy with either

ciprofloxacin or a third generation cephalosporin is indicated if the diagnosis is suspected.

Rickettsial Infections

Rickettsial infections are transmitted by mites and ticks, have a short incubation period (less than 3 weeks), and present with nonspecific influenza-like symptoms. Helpful clues to the diagnosis include a history of exposure (travel in grassy or wooded areas), a maculopapular rash, and the presence of a painless eschar at the inoculation site. The diagnosis is made clinically and confirmed serologically. Therapy with a tetracycline is indicated if the diagnosis is suspected.

Fever of Unknown Origin

At the Time of Admission

The "classic" 1961 definition of fever of unknown origin (FUO) included patients who had been ill for 3 weeks, had a fever over 38.3°C (101°F) on several occasions, and who remained undiagnosed after 1 week of study in the hospital. The time intervals in this definition are arbitrary and were chosen to exclude individuals with protracted but self-limited viral illnesses and to allow time for standard radiographic, serologic, and cultural data to be collected. With changes in health care delivery, these intervals have been modified to include patients who are undiagnosed after three outpatient visits or 3 days in the hospital. Over the ensuing decades, several new categories of FUO have been included (5):

1. *Nosocomial FUO:* hospitalized patients with fever of 38.3°C or higher on several occasions, caused by a process not present or incubating from admission, in whom the diagnosis remains uncertain after at least 3 days of investigation and in whom microbiologic cultures have been incubating at least 2 days (see pp 609–610)
2. *Neutropenic FUO:* fever of 38.3°C or higher on several occasions in patients with less than 500 neutrophils per cubic millimeter or expected to fall below that level within 2 days, in which the diagnosis remains unknown after at least 3 days of investigation with at least 2 days for cultures to incubate (Chapter 63)
3. *HIV-associated FUO:* a fever of 38.3°C or higher in an HIV-seropositive patient who has been febrile more than 4 weeks as an outpatient or 3 days as an inpatient, in whom the diagnosis remains uncertain after 3 days of investigation with at least 2 days for cultures to incubate (Chapter 74)

Although not formally considered a separate category, FUO in recipients of solid organ transplants is a common scenario with a unique differential diagnosis (Chapter 63).

The differential diagnosis of FUO is extensive (Table 62.5) and includes infection in 25%–40%, neoplasms in 20%–35%, and rheumatologic diseases in 10%–20% of

TABLE 62.5

CAUSES OF FEVER OF UNKNOWN ORIGIN IN THE ADULT

Type	Comment
Infections	
Localized	
Abscesses: liver, subphrenic, abdominal, pelvic	Previous surgery or gastrointestinal procedure are risk factors
Biliary system: cholecystitis, cholangitis	Preexisting cholelithiasis or pancreatitis
Urinary tract: perinephric abscess, intrarenal abscess, prostatic abscess, chronic prostatitis	Negative or intermittently positive urine cultures; obstruction may be present
Infective endocarditis	Culture negative (previous antibiotics for another suspected infection) or fastidious organism (HACEK[a] group)
Osteomyelitis	
Generalized: tuberculosis	Usually extrapulmonary (renal, peritoneal, miliary, meningeal)
Other (less common): Whipple's disease, cat-scratch disease and other *Bartonella* infections, toxoplasmosis, malaria, disseminated histoplasmosis or coccidioidomycosis, Q fever, brucellosis, leptospirosis, borreliosis, cytomegalovirus, Epstein-Barr virus, splenic, pulmonary and dental abscesses	
Malignancy	Many malignancies cause fever in association with liver metastases or obstruction with associated infection
Hodgkin's disease	
Lymphoma	
Renal cell carcinoma	
Hepatoma	
Other solid tumors	
Rheumatologic diseases	
Still's disease (adult juvenile rheumatoid arthritis)	Usually presents without joint manifestations or classic serologic abnormalities
Systemic lupus erythematosus	
Polyarteritis nodosa	
Rheumatoid arthritis	
Vasculitis	
Polymyalgia rheumatica	
Cryoglobulinemia	
Granulomatous disease	
Granulomatous hepatitis	Need to rule out treatable causes of granulomatous hepatitis
Sarcoidosis	
Inflammatory bowel disease	Without prominent gastrointestinal symptoms
Temporal arteritis	
Other disorders	
Factitious fever	
Familial mediterranean fever	
Wegener's granulomatosis	
Alcoholic hepatitis	
Metabolic disorders: hyperthyroidism, thyroiditis, pheochromocytoma	
Addison's disease	
Recurrent pulmonary emboli	

[a] *Haemophilus aphrophilus, Actinobacillus actinomycetocomitans, Cardiobacterium hominis, Eikenella corrodens, Kingella kingii.*

cases (5). Several general principles are helpful in approaching patients with classic FUO:

- Most cases of FUO represent unusual manifestations of common diseases, not rare or exotic diseases. About 50% of patients with FUO have one of the following diseases as a cause: tuberculosis, endocarditis, lymphoma, solid tumor, adult Still's disease, vasculitis, or a common rheumatologic disease (systemic lupus erythematosus, Sjögren's syndrome).

- Even after extensive evaluation, the diagnosis remains elusive in 10%–15% of patients. In the majority of these patients (about 75%) fever abates spontaneously, the patient improves, and a diagnosis is never made. In the remainder, classic manifestations of the underlying disease emerge, making the diagnosis obvious.

- Patients with prolonged fever (6 months or longer) have infection, malignancy, or rheumatologic disease as the cause in only 20% of cases. Instead, other diagnoses such as granulomatous diseases, factitious fever, and exaggeration of the normal circadian rhythm become much more likely.

■ Patients with episodic or recurrent fevers (i.e., classic definition of FUO with periods of 2 weeks or longer without fever), like patients with prolonged fever, usually do not have infection, malignancy, or rheumatologic disorder but instead have a number of miscellaneous causes such as Crohn's disease, allergic alveolitis, and Familial mediterranean fever. Approximately 50% of this group remains undiagnosed, but symptoms resolve.

These points are important in determining how aggressive to be in the evaluation. By the time most patients have been admitted to the hospital, noninvasive tests have been performed, and decisions must be made about more aggressive tests that may be associated with adverse effects. It is important to remember that, with time, the cause is likely to become obvious and, provided the patient is stable (not toxic, with stable weight, and able to carry on daily functions), continued observation or only limited additional evaluation is a reasonable option.

FUO is such a heterogeneous disease state that a routine cost-effective approach to diagnosis has not been established. Potential diagnostic clues should be elicited by careful history taking and physical examination, and further workup should pursue any abnormalities that are revealed. Careful attention to family history, social history (sexual practice, use of intravenous drugs), travel, vocational or recreational exposures, animal exposures, and dietary habits (unpasteurized milk products, raw meats) may provide clues to diagnosis. Careful and repeated physical examinations are important to detect evanescent rashes or subtle physical findings such as conjunctivitis, uveitis, and isolated lymph nodes.

Infection remains a leading cause of FUO, and blood cultures (two or three sets over 24 hours) off antibiotic therapy for at least 48–72 hours are routine in the evaluation. The laboratory should be asked to hold cultures for 2 weeks if bacteremia or endocarditis with fastidious organisms is suspected (e.g., HACEK group, *Brucella* spp.). Cultures on special media should be requested if *Legionella* or *Bartonella* organisms or nutritionally deficient streptococci are considered. If exposure suggests endocarditis caused by *Chlamydia psittaci* or *Coxiella burnetii*, serologic tests are required. "Screening" tests with immunologic or microbiologic serologies have a low yield and should not be done. Specific tests for rheumatologic diseases are indicated if history or physical examination suggest a specific diagnosis. Serologic tests for infections ("febrile agglutinins") are almost never helpful, with the exception of tests for syphilis.

Certain radiographic studies are considered routine. These include chest radiograph, upper gastrointestinal series with small bowel follow-through, and barium enema. The value of gastrointestinal radiography and endoscopy in patients without localizing symptoms is probably low,

but these tests should be considered in patients with prolonged fever in whom gastrointestinal pathology is more common. Radionuclide scanning (i.e., indium-labeled leukocyte scan or gallium 67–citrate) is theoretically attractive for detecting infection and malignancy, but in reality these studies are of little use as screening tests because of the high rates of false positive and negative results. PET scans may be useful in diagnosing infection and malignancy, but large-scale formal studies are lacking. Abdominal and pelvic CT scans are done in most patients with FUO and are powerful tools for detecting intra-abdominal pathology, but an invasive procedure almost always is needed to make a tissue diagnosis. It is also important to remember that a negative CT scan does not obviate the possible need for more aggressive studies. CT scanning is valuable in detecting anatomic abnormalities, but certain diseases such as vasculitis, peritoneal tuberculosis, or peritoneal carcinomatosis may not be detected by CT and may require invasive procedures for diagnosis. Thus, in patients for whom the diagnosis remains elusive despite a negative noninvasive evaluation, laparotomy or laparoscopy should be considered if they have abdominal pain and clinically are incapacitated or deteriorating. Ultrasonography and echocardiography as screening tests are of little value. If a specific diagnosis of endocarditis is suggested, a transesophageal echocardiogram is indicated. Even if this is negative, it does not exclude the diagnosis of endocarditis, and if suspicion is high, a repeat study should be done in 1–2 weeks (especially if a prosthetic value is present).

Biopsy of potentially pathologic tissue, if suggested by physical examination or abnormal laboratory value, is always indicated, as is aspiration of abnormal fluid collections. Even though the yield of a bone-marrow biopsy is low in FUO (about 5%), the risk is small and this test is usually done. Liver biopsy is more controversial. Abnormal liver function tests are common in FUO, and liver biopsy is associated with potentially serious complications. Nonetheless, a specific diagnosis by liver biopsy is made in about 15% of patients, and if less invasive tests have not yielded the diagnosis and liver function tests are abnormal, a biopsy should be considered. Although not formally studied, a temporal artery biopsy is reasonable in elderly patients with elevated sedimentation rates and no alternative diagnosis.

Whenever an invasive procedure is performed, as much tissue as possible should be obtained so that routine, mycobacterial, and fungal stains and cultures can be done. Newer investigational diagnostic tests such as polymerase chain reaction (PCR) may be helpful if specific diagnoses such as Whipple's disease, herpes simplex infection, or bartonellosis are considered.

If a specific diagnosis accounting for FUO is made, therapy is directed at the underlying cause. Difficulties arise if, despite extensive evaluation, the diagnosis remains elusive. A therapeutic trial is reasonable if a specific diagnosis is strongly suspected (e.g., antituberculous therapy if pulmonary or disseminated tuberculosis is suspected, intravenous antibiotics if endocarditis is suggested, or tetracycline for brucellosis). In the seriously ill or rapidly deteriorating patient, empiric therapy should be considered. Antituberculous medications (particularly in the elderly or foreign-born patient) and broad-spectrum antibiotics are reasonable in this setting. Two important caveats apply. First, before starting therapy, be sure that all relevant cultures have been obtained. Second, therapeutic end-points must be set. If there is no clinical response after several weeks of therapy, therapy should be discontinued and the situation carefully reevaluated.

There is often a temptation to suppress fever by using corticosteroids. This practice should be discouraged, because infection remains a leading cause of FUO, and many infections can become more invasive and disseminate in the presence of steroid therapy. Suppression of fever by low doses of naproxen (375 mg orally every 12 hours) is said to be relatively specific for fever associated with neoplasm.

FUO During Hospitalization

For information on FUO during hospitalization, see the section on "Fever During the Course of Hospitalization" on page 599.

Hypothermia

Hypothermia at Time of Admission

Hypothermia, defined as a core temperature of 35°C or less, is most often the consequence of accidental exposure to cold and is seen in individuals who are unable to move to a warm environment (e.g., the homeless, alcoholics, the elderly, those who overdose on drugs resulting in unconsciousness, and those who are immobile). Concomitant illnesses frequently are present in those with accidental exposure. These include bacteremia, hypothyroidism, pancreatitis, cirrhosis, diabetes with ketoacidosis, stroke, hypopituitarism, adrenal insufficiency, and hypoglycemia. Drugs such as alcohol, barbiturates and phenothiazines may worsen hypothermia by producing vasodilation, inhibiting shivering, or affecting central thermoregulation. Certain acute illnesses, including bacteremia, uremia, diabetes, congestive heart failure, and hypoglycemia, have been associated with hypothermia in the absence of exposure.

Clinical thermometers often do not read temperatures below 35°C. Therefore, if hypothermia is suspected, an incubator thermometer should be used. In addition to ordering routine laboratory tests, thyroid function studies, amylase, arterial blood gases, chest radiograph, head CT scan (if there is associated mental status change or focal neurologic findings), and blood, urine, and cerebrospinal fluid (if clinically indicated) cultures should be obtained. Thirty to forty percent of patients admitted with hypothermia have a concomitant serious infection (usually bacteremia, pneumonia, cellulitis, peritonitis, or meningitis), and classic

signs and symptoms may be delayed in appearance up to 72 hours (6). Although hemodynamic monitoring may be helpful in distinguishing those with bacteremia, other parameters such as blood pressure, arterial pH, oxygenation, azotemia, and degree of leukocytosis are not reliable predictors (7).

Supportive care including fluids, treatment of acidosis and arrhythmias, and rewarming (either active external or active core rewarming depending on the degree of hypothermia) are indicated. Because of the difficulty in distinguishing the infected from the noninfected patient, and because the mortality rate is higher if infection is present, *all hypothermic patients should be given empiric broad-spectrum antibiotics* to cover both Gram-positive and enteric Gram-negative organisms while awaiting culture results. If there is any suspicion of adrenal insufficiency, stress-dosage glucocorticoids should be administered after a cosyntropin stimulation test is performed (Chapter 109).

Hypothermia During the Course of Hospitalization

Hypothermia developing in the hospital may result from cardiac bypass surgery or continuous arteriovenous hemofiltration. In the absence of these factors, hypothermia is strongly suggestive of sepsis. Hypoglycemia also should be considered, particularly in patients with diabetes or liver disease. Hospitalized patients should be evaluated for potential sites of infection as outlined in the discussion of fever. After cultures are obtained, broad-spectrum antibiotics should be started while awaiting culture results.

Relative Bradycardia

Relative Bradycardia at Time of Admission

Heart rate is directly proportional to temperature, with an expected increase of between 2.4 and 10 beats/min for each 1°F rise in temperature. An inappropriately low heart rate, commonly termed relative bradycardia or Faget's sign, has been associated with a number of conditions (Table 62.6), particularly infection with an intracellular pathogen. Unfortunately, the lack of a standardized definition for relative bradycardia coupled with the low sensitivity and specificity of this finding limit its clinical utility (8). Furthermore, relative bradycardia is of limited significance in patients who are prescribed negative chronotropic agents (such as β-blockers or verapamil) or who have intrinsic cardiac conduction abnormalities.

With these caveats, if this finding is present, particular emphasis should be placed on obtaining a thorough travel history, because many of the infectious agents in Table 62.4 are found solely in developing countries or are endemic to restricted regions of the United States. *C. burnetii* may be acquired from domesticated animals (particularly parturient cats) and raw milk, and these exposures should be

TABLE 62.6

CONDITIONS THAT MAY BE ASSOCIATED WITH RELATIVE BRADYCARDIA

Infectious
Flaviviruses
　Dengue fever
　Yellow fever
Bacteria
　Salmonella typhi
　Salmonella paratyphi
　Leptospira spp.
　Brucella spp.
　Chlamydia psittaci
　Chlamydia pneumoniae

Rickettsia prowazekii (epidemic typhus)
Coxiella burnetti (Q fever)
Ehrlichia chaffeensis
Legionella spp.
Parasites: malaria
Noninfectious
　Drug fever
　Lymphoma
　Central fever

sought. An erythematous, blanching, maculopapular skin eruption resembling the rose spots of typhoid fever in a patient without a history of foreign travel suggests Horder's spots, associated with *C. psittaci*, or the rash commonly seen with epidemic typhus.

The low positive predictive value of relative bradycardia does not allow restriction of the laboratory evaluation to the entities listed in Table 62.6. Routine cultures must be performed, in addition to studies directed at diagnosing the organisms classically associated with relative bradycardia. Relative bradycardia in a patient with respiratory complaints suggests an atypical pneumonia, prompting supplementary evaluation for *Legionella* organisms, *C. burnetii*, and *Chlamydia pneumoniae*. Clinical suspicion of infection with *Ehrlichia*, *Chlamydia*, or *Legionella* organisms, *C. burnetii*, leptospirosis, or epidemic typhus may be confirmed by acute and convalescent serum titers. *Legionella* urinary antigen may provide a more rapid diagnosis than serology, but will only detect *L. pneumophila* serogroup 1.

Relative Bradycardia During Hospitalization

A new finding of relative bradycardia in a hospitalized patient suggests either nosocomially acquired *Legionella* pneumonia or a drug fever. Nosocomial legionellosis primarily occurs among patients with a history of heavy alcohol use or smoking, advanced age, or immunosuppression. Although relative bradycardia may be seen with drug fever, it is uncommon, occurring in 10% of cases (3). The evaluation of the patient with nosocomial-onset relative bradycardia is identical to that undertaken in any febrile hospitalized patient.

LABORATORY ABNORMALITIES

Several laboratory abnormalities frequently are associated with infection. Leukocytosis is discussed in Chapter 89 and eosinophilia in Chapter 120.

Atypical Lymphocytosis

Atypical Lymphocytosis at Time of Admission

Atypical lymphocytes, sometimes referred to as Downey cells or reactive lymphocytes, are large cells characterized by morphologic abnormalities such as vacuolated cytoplasm, lobulated nuclei, and prominent nucleoli. A peripheral smear with more than 10% atypical lymphocytes is highly suggestive of the infectious mononucleosis syndrome (9). A number of infectious and noninfectious causes have been associated with atypical lymphocytosis (Table 62.7). However, this may be an incidental finding in otherwise healthy children.

Ascertainment of exposures such as sick contacts, sexual history [cytomegalovirus (CMV), HIV, human T-cell lymphotropic virus (HTLV)], cat exposure (toxoplasmosis), travel (hepatitis A), tick exposures (ehrlichiosis), injection drug use (HIV, hepatitis B and C, HTLV), vaccination history (rubella), and blood transfusion (HIV, HTLV, and CMV) are important in pinpointing an infectious etiology. Common but nonspecific physical abnormalities associated with the infectious mononucleosis syndrome include exudative pharyngitis and cervical lymphadonopathy (9). Rash that develops after the administration of ampicillin is classic for Epstein-Barr virus infection. Jaundice and, rarely, autoimmune hemolytic anemia may be present with the

TABLE 62.7

SYNDROMES ASSOCIATED WITH ATYPICAL LYMPHOCYTOSIS

Syndrome	Description
Heterophile-positive mononucleosis	
Epstein-Barr virus	Triad of pharyngitis, fever, lymphadenopathy
Heterophile-negative mononucleosis	
Epstein-Barr virus	See text
Cytomegalovirus	Approximately 25% of heterophile-negative cases; minimal pharyngitis and lymphadenopathy
Viral hepatitis	Not associated with pharyngitis
Toxoplasmosis	Choreoretinitis variably present
Rubella	Maculopapular exanthem
Adenovirus	Pharyngoconjunctival fever
Human herpesvirus 6	Acute infection
HIV	Acute infection, often with rash
Human T-cell lymphotrophic virus	Primarily in immigrants and their sex partners from endemic areas
Other	
Ehrlichia chaffeensis	Usually with leukopenia
Large granular lymphoma	Clonal lymphocytes

infectious mononucleosis syndrome. A positive heterophile antibody test suggests Epstein-Barr virus but is insensitive; approximately 20% of heterophile-negative cases of mononucleosis are attributable to Epstein-Barr virus and represent false negative test results. Further diagnostic testing for cases of heterophile-negative infectious mononucleosis should be guided by findings on the history and physical examination and limited to diseases such as hepatitis or HIV in which a diagnosis would lead to a therapeutic or public health intervention. Epstein-Barr virus and CMV-related infectious mononucleosis syndromes are generally self-limited and require only supportive care.

Atypical Lymphocytosis During Hospitalization

The development of atypical lymphocytosis after hospital admission is distinctly unusual, with the exception of post-transfusion CMV infections. The risk of primary CMV infection in a previously seronegative patient is approximately 2% per unit of transfused whole blood and is highest in neonates and transplant patients. Nosocomial infections caused by CMV have declined because of the use of concentrated blood products and filters that decrease the number of leukocytes per unit, cold storage of blood products, and screening of donated blood prior to transfusion for high-risk, CMV-negative recipients. Treatment of post-transfusion CMV-related mononucleosis is restricted to supportive therapy.

Interpreting Culture Results and Microbiologic Serologies

The usefulness of the information provided by the microbiology laboratory is directly dependent upon the reliability of the specimen submitted and the ability of the clinician to interpret the results accurately. Specimens submitted for culture should be representative of the suspected infection and should be obtained in such a way as to avoid contamination. For example, cultures from draining sinuses misrepresent the true microbiology of the deeper infection. Sinus tract cultures obtained in association with chronic osteomyelitis are only 50% sensitive and specific for organisms isolated directly from bone at the time of surgery. Similarly, positive cultures from surgical drains that have been in place for days or weeks likely represent colonization of the drainage tube and do not reflect the underlying infection. During the acquisition of cultures, one should try to avoid contamination by indigenous flora and submit an adequate amount. Swabs often are abused. Cultures of swabs of skin or mucous membranes are often uninterpretable or give misleading data because of contamination by normal flora. In addition, swabs contain minimal material and can give false-negative results. Whenever possible, fluid and tissue specimens should be obtained rather than swabs of evacuated abscess or tissue. Specimens should reach the laboratory in a timely manner,

and ideally should be obtained prior to the administration of antibiotics. The clinician should communicate directly with the interventional radiologist or surgeon to emphasize the importance of obtaining adequate specimens. By providing the laboratory with clinical data, specific pathogens can be sought by a variety of culturing techniques.

Upon reaching the laboratory, many specimens undergo direct microscopic examination for bacteria, mycobacteria, and fungi. Because microscopy is much less sensitive than culture, a negative stain does not exclude the presence of infection. The sensitivity of direct stains depends upon microbial load. For example, cerebrospinal fluid is positive in 60%–80% of patients with meningitis; peritoneal fluid is positive in 30%–50% with bacterial peritonitis, sputum for acid-fast bacilli positive in up to 50% of patients with pulmonary tuberculosis, and joint fluid specimens positive in about 50%–70% of cases of septic arthritis. A positive stain indicates the presence of a significant number of organisms and should never be ignored. A negative culture in the presence of a positive Gram's stain suggests prior antibiotic therapy or infection with a fastidious organism.

Most specimens are cultured in a way that allows the amount of growth to be semi-quantitated, and this information can be extremely helpful. Specimens usually are inoculated on growth plates by making three separate streaks on the plates and then are placed in a liquid broth. Growth in liquid medium only is reported by the microbiology laboratory as growth in "broth only" or as "very few" organisms being present. Such results must be interpreted cautiously because they frequently represent contamination, especially when organisms of low virulence (e.g., *Staphylococcus epidermidis* or *Corynebacterium* spp.) are isolated. If the culture report is broth only, submission of another specimen is often helpful in resolving the issue of contamination versus infection. The presence of moderate or numerous organisms is almost always indicative of infection, provided the specimen is appropriate. In some circumstances, the organism isolated and the immune status of the patient are more important than the quantity of organism isolated. For example, isolation of *Nocardia* species, *Cryptococcus neoformans*, or *Coccidioides immitis* from sputum, regardless of quantity, is likely to be indicative of infection. These organisms are not part of the normal flora and when present, they almost always correlate with disease. Similarly, although *Aspergillus* organisms may colonize patients who have received prolonged antibiotic therapy, isolation of even a single colony from an immunosuppressed patient may be significant and requires further evaluation.

A number of nonculture technologies have been applied in the microbiology laboratory to improve diagnostic yield. Common examples include direct fluorescent antibody testing for *Legionella* in sputum, herpesviruses in vesicular fluid, antigen detection for CMV in blood, group A streptococci on throat swabs, *C. neoformans* in blood and CSF, *Legionella* and *Histoplasma capsulatum* in the urine, and giardia and rotavirus in stool. Polymerase chain reaction (PCR)-based genomic tests are available for parvovirus B19 and herpesviruses in the CSF. In general, these tests are very specific (over 90%), but sensitivity is variable (although better than culture). A negative test does not always exclude the diagnosis. Sensitivity is in excess of 90% for antigen detection of *C. neoformans* in cerebrospinal fluid, PCR for herpes in cerebrospinal fluid, PCR for parvovirus B19 in aplastic anemia and detection of CMV antigenemia in immunocompromised patients with CMV end-organ disease.

Interpretation of culture results ultimately depends upon the clinical response to antimicrobial therapy. Often the clinician can localize the source of the infection, predict bacteriology based upon the organ system involved, and choose empiric therapy based on predicted bacteriology and historic sensitivity patterns. If culture results confirm the initial impression, therapy can be continued with confidence. Laboratory data that contradict initial impressions about bacteriology must be reexamined carefully. If the specimen was obtained from a normally sterile site and organisms are isolated that do not support the original predictions of etiology, a change in therapy may be needed. On the other hand, isolation of an organism from a nonsterile site may represent colonization; if the patient is improving, a change in therapy may not be required. Cultures obtained after starting antimicrobial therapy must be interpreted carefully. Significant infections may take several days to respond even to appropriate therapy, and prolonged fever and leukocytosis may be part of the natural history of the infection. Before changing antibiotics, consultation with an infectious-diseases subspecialist might be helpful to assess whether the clinical course is consistent with an appropriate but delayed response. If a patient is truly not responding to therapy, additional considerations include appropriateness of drug dosage, penetration of the antibiotic into the site of infection, presence of undrained pus, presence of a foreign body, superinfection, emergence of a resistant organism, or the possibility of polymicrobial infection in which not all of the causative organisms are being treated.

Optimally, the diagnosis of an infection is based on isolation of the specific pathogen, but in many circumstances this is not possible. In these situations, confirmation of diagnosis may be sought by using serologic techniques. Making a specific diagnosis by serologic techniques is fraught with difficulty and rarely helps with the acute management of patients. The major pitfalls in serologic interpretation are the assumptions that a negative titer excludes disease and a positive titer indicates that a given organism is causative. Neither of these statements is entirely true.

Many different serologic tests are in existence, and these vary in sensitivity and specificity. Furthermore, the immunologic response to infection is variable. In general, IgM antibodies appear at 1–2 weeks after infection, peak at 3–4 weeks, and persist for several months before becoming undetectable. IgG antibodies appear later (2–3 weeks), peak later, and can persist for months or years. Thus, depending on which test is performed, when disease samples are tested, and which antibody class is tested, initial results may be negative. Prior antibiotic therapy may delay or abort the development of specific antibodies, and immunosuppressed patients may not develop antibodies even if significant infection is present.

Conversely, a positive titer is not necessarily indicative of active infection. Because IgG antibodies may persist for life, previous exposure to an organism can result in positive serologic tests. To make a definite serologic diagnosis of an infectious disease, one must demonstrate seroconversion or a fourfold rise or fall in antibody titers in paired sera drawn several weeks apart. A single very high titer may be suggestive of disease, but this must be interpreted with caution, because previous infection may result in persistently elevated high titers.

KEY POINTS

- Serious underlying infection may be present in the absence of localizing symptoms or signs.
- Careful attention to historical aspects of illness, as well as meticulous and repeated physical examinations, may reveal subtle clues that allow diagnoses to be made.
- Although often nonspecific, laboratory abnormalities interpreted in a clinical context frequently allow a presumptive diagnosis of infection to be made and empiric antimicrobial therapy to be instituted.
- The microbiology laboratory is invaluable in diagnosis and treatment but requires submission of reliable specimens for culture and accurate interpretation of results.
- Direct communication with the laboratory is critical in examining microbiolic information that can directly impact patient care and outcome.

REFERENCES

1. McGowan JE Jr., Rose RC, Jacobs NF, et al. Fever in hospitalized patients: with special reference to the medical service. *Am J Med* 1987;82:580–586.
2. O'Grady NP, Barie PS, Bartlett JG, et al. Practice guidelines for evaluating new fever in critically ill adult patients. *Clin Infect Dis* 1998;26:1042–1059.
3. Mackowiak PA, LeMaistre CF. Drug fever: a critical appraisal of conventional concepts. An analysis of 51 episodes in two Dallas hospitals and 97 episodes reported in the English literature. *Ann Intern Med* 1987;106:728–733.
4. Ryan ET, Wilson ME, Kain KC. Current concepts: illness after international travel. *N Engl J Med* 2002;347:505
5. Durack DT, Street AC. Fever of unknown origin: reexamined and redefined. In Remington JS, Swartz MN, eds. *Current Clinical Topics in Infectious Diseases*. Boston: Blackwell Scientific Publications, 1991:35–51.

6. Lewin S, Brettman LR, Holzman RS. Infections in hypothermic patients. *Arch Intern Med* 1981;141:920–925.
7. Morris DL, Chambers HF, Morris MG, et al. Hemodynamic characteristics of patients with hypothermia due to occult infection and other causes. *Ann Intern Med* 1985;102:153–157.
8. Ostergaard L, Huniche B, Andersen PL. Relative bradycardia in infectious diseases. *J Infect* 1996;33:185–191.
9. Cheeseman SH. Infectious mononucleosis. *Semin Hematol* 1998; 24:261–268.

ADDITIONAL READING

de Kleijn EMHA, Vandenbroucke JP, van der Meer JWM, and the Netherlands FUO Study Group. Fever of unknown origin (FUO): I. a perspective multicenter study of 167 patients with FUO, using fixed epidemiologic entry criteria. *Medicine* 1997;76:392–400.

de Kleijn EMHA, van Lier HJJ, van der Meer JWM, and the Netherlands FUO Study Group. Fever of unknown origin (FUO): II. diagnostic procedures in a prospective multicenter study of 167 patients. *Medicine* 1997;76:401–414.

Hirschmann JV. Fever of unknown origin in adults. *Clin Infect Dis* 1997;24:291–302.

Mackowiak PA, Bartlett JG, Borden EC, et al. Concepts of fever: recent advances and lingering dogma. *Clin Infect Dis* 1997; 25:119–138.

Mackowiak PA. Physiological rationale for suppression of fever. *Clin Infect Dis* 2000;31:S185–189.

Mourad O, Palda V, Detsky AS. A comprehensive evidence-based approach to fever of unknown origin. *Arch Intern Med* 2003; 163:545–551.

Schlossberg D. Fever and rash. *Infect Dis Clin North Am* 1996; 10: 101–110.

Spira AM. Assessment of travellers who return home ill. *Lancet* 2003;361:1459–1469.

Infections in Immunocompromised Hosts

63

Nesli Basgoz

INTRODUCTION

Features of the Compromised Host

A compromised host is an individual who has one or more alterations or defects in the body's defenses, defects that render the individual more susceptible to severe infections. There are several important principles that should guide the approach to these patients:

- The inflammatory response to infection is attenuated, thereby abolishing or diminishing the typical signs and symptoms of inflammation and making early diagnosis difficult. This is particularly dangerous in a patient population in which morbidity and mortality rates from infection are high.
- Therefore, the clinician's approach to even subtle signs and symptoms needs to be rapid and aggressive. Because the range of possible infections is vast, therapy should be tailored to the specific clinical presentation if possible and not be purely "algorithmic."
- However, localizing signs, symptoms, or cultures are not always present. Therefore, empiric broad-spectrum treatment of suspected infection is mandatory in high-risk patients whether or not they have localizing findings of infection.

Host defects can be divided into two major categories, nonspecific defects and specific immune defects. *Nonspecific defects* predisposing patients to invasion or infection are present in many hospitalized patients. They include alterations in the anatomy and function of major organ systems and alterations of indigenous microbial flora. Chief among anatomic alterations is disruption of skin and mucous membranes. This may occur through chemotherapy-induced mucositis, intravenous catheters, or infections such as herpes simplex and *Clostridium difficile*. Perturbation in organ function also may occur. Treatment of pain syndromes with opiates may result in central nervous system dysfunction and predispose to stasis, obstruction, and infection in the respiratory, gastrointestinal, or genitourinary tracts. Measures to protect mucocutaneous barriers include oral and dental evaluation and treatment before elective procedures such as transplantation, and ongoing hygiene including topical antibacterial and antifungal agents such as Peridex and clotrimazole or nystatin; prevention or treatment of constipation; tailoring of pain regimens to avoid unnecessary sedation; and paying careful attention to vascular access. If signs or symptoms of infection occur in patients who have a disrupted mucocutaneous barrier, empiric therapy targeting flora indigenous to that site should be started.

Microbial flora are altered by many factors. Chronic disease, debilitation, hospitalization, and stasis are associated with a shift in oropharyngeal and respiratory tract flora toward Gram-negative aerobes and with migration of colonic flora into the small bowel. However, antimicrobial therapy has the most dramatic effect on indigenous flora. Broad-spectrum antibiotics with anaerobic activity eliminate "colonization resistance," the ability of avirulent anaerobes to prevent colonization by potentially more virulent aerobes or yeast. Results may be particularly disastrous if colonizing nosocomial flora are highly resistant, such as vancomycin-resistant enterococci (Chapter 64). Alteration in microbial flora can be avoided by providing care in an outpatient rather than an inpatient setting; appropriate hand hygiene; preventing stasis or obstruction in the gastrointestinal, genitourinary, and respiratory tracts; and using antimicrobials prudently.

PATTERNS OF IMMUNOCOMPROMISE

Specific defects in immune function are associated with typical infectious disease syndromes; knowledge of these defects and syndromes can direct diagnostic testing and early therapy. The major categories of immune dysfunction are humoral immune dysfunction, granulocytopenia (neutropenia), and cellular immune dysfunction (Table 63.1). Patients develop both granulocytopenia and cellular immune dysfunction after bone marrow transplantation. This chapter describes a general approach to adult patients with the major categories of immune defects, a task made more difficult by the heterogenous nature of the patient population, and the lack of systematic study of many areas.

SPECIFIC IMMUNOCOMPROMISED STATES

Humoral Immune Dysfunction

Patients with hypogammaglobulinemia lack opsonizing antibodies to encapsulated bacteria, leading to severe infections with *Streptococcus pneumoniae, Haemophilus influenzae, Neisseria meningitidis* and, less commonly, *Escherichia coli* and other encapsulated pathogens. Patients with multiple myeloma, chronic lymphocytic leukemia, and splenectomy may have hypogammaglobulinemia. Asplenic patients also lack the filtering function of this reticuloendothelial organ. Asplenia may be anatomic or functional (e.g., resulting from sickle-cell disease).

Systematic studies of therapeutic strategies in these patients are lacking. However, because infection may be fulminant, any hypogammaglobulinemic or asplenic patient who develops a fever should attempt to access medical care within 1 hour, at which time blood cultures and other appropriate evaluation should be performed with antibiotic treatment started immediately. In adult patients who appear nontoxic, outpatient therapy with oral ampicillin, 500 mg four times a day, or amoxicillin 500 mg three times per day, is likely sufficient, as this covers most pneumococci, unencapsulated *H. influenzae* (which predominates in adults), and *N. meningitidis*.

TABLE 63.1

SPECIFIC DEFECTS IN IMMUNE FUNCTION AND COMMON ASSOCIATED PATHOGENS

Humoral immune dysfunction: encapsulated bacteria
  Streptococcus pneumoniae
  Haemophilus influenzae
  Neisseria meningitidis
  Escherichia coli
Granulocytopenia or neutropenia
  Bacteria
    Gram-positive
      Coagulase-negative staphylococci
      Staphylococcus aureus
      Viridans streptococci, pneumococci, other streptococci
      Corynebacterium spp., especially group JK
      Bacillus spp.
    Gram-negative
      Escherichia coli
      Klebsiella pneumoniae
      Pseudomonas aeruginosa
  Fungi
    Candida albicans and other *Candida* spp.
    Aspergillus spp.

Cellular immune dysfunction
  Bacteria
    Salmonella spp.
    Listeria monocytogenes
    Legionella pneumophila
    Nocardia spp.
    Mycobacterium tuberculosis and atypical mycobacteria
  Fungi
    Cryptococcus neoformans
    Histoplasma capsulatum
    Coccidioides immitis
    Aspergillus spp.
  Protozoa
    Pneumocystis jirovecii
    Toxoplasma gondii
    Cryptosporidium spp.
  Viruses
    Herpes simplex
    Varicella zoster
    Cytomegalovirus
    Epstein-Barr virus
  Helminth: *Strongyloides stercoralis*

In adult patients who appear ill, admission and intravenous therapy are required. For pneumococcal coverage, antibiotic selection should depend on the local prevalence of penicillin-resistant *Pneumococcus*, particularly if central nervous system infection is suspected. If the likelihood of penicillin resistance is low, penicillin at a dose of 12–24 million units per day (depending on whether central nervous system infection is suspected) or ampicillin (12 g/d) may be sufficient. If there is a significant risk of penicillin resistance, vancomycin or ceftriaxone should be added until cultures and results of susceptibility testing are available (Chapter 64). In pediatric patients, especially those who did not receive *H. influenzae* vaccination before splenectomy, an agent that treats β-lactamase–producing strains of *H. influenzae* should be used. Possible choices include a second- or third-generation cephalosporin such as cefuroxime or ceftriaxone (in maximal meningeal doses if needed). These agents have the added benefit of treating strains of Gram-negative bacilli that may not be susceptible to ampicillin or amoxicillin.

Hospitalized patients who have a microbiologically-documented infection should be treated with the most effective and cost-effective regimen for that organism in that site. In febrile patients who lack a microbiologically-documented infection, those with no demonstrable source of bacterial infection, no initial toxicity, and rapid defervescence are at low risk for complications. In such patients, it is reasonable to stop antibiotics after 3 or more days of therapy (particularly if a source of fever other than bacterial infection has become apparent) or to complete a 7- to 14-day course of an antibiotic. Depending on the organism suspected and its local epidemiology, oral agents such as ampicillin, amoxicillin, or second- or third-generation cephalosporins may be used to complete the course.

Finally, all asplenic patients should have available and take an oral antibiotic if they have a fever and cannot access care in 1 hour. Traditionally, this antibiotic has been amoxicillin or ampicillin. However, if encapsulated *H. influenzae* or ampicillin-resistant Gram-negative organisms are of concern, other potential options include ampicillin–clavulanate, oral second-generation cephalosporins, and levofloxacin (1).

Neutropenia

Clinical Features of the Febrile, Neutropenic Host

The differential diagnosis of neutropenia is reviewed in Chapter 89. Patients at high risk of developing infections during granulocytopenia include those with leukemia, those receiving chemotherapy for leukemia or lymphoma, and those receiving chemotherapy for other cancers, including small-cell lung carcinoma, testicular cancer, and sarcomas. Patients with aplastic anemia, cyclic neutropenia, HIV infection, and other chronic conditions in which neutropenia may be a feature appear to be at lower risk of neutropenic infection.

Many factors influence the risk of infection and the mortality rate in patients with neutropenia. These include the depth of the absolute neutrophil count (ANC) (with the highest risk at <100 cells per mL and a demonstrably increased risk at 500–1,000 cells per mL), a rapid rate of decline of ANC, and longer durations of neutropenia. Modern bone-marrow transplantation usually results in 3–4 weeks of neutropenia; the neutropenia from induction therapy of nonlymphocytic leukemia is shorter. The neutropenia resulting from chemotherapy of solid tumors usually lasts less than 1 week.

Evaluation

Patients who are febrile and neutropenic should have a meticulous history taken, focusing on even minor changes in symptoms and on any recent exposures. There is no strict definition of fever in this population; any temperature above normal may be significant. Many studies consider a single oral temperature >38.3°C or a sustained temperature (over 1 hour) >38.0°C to define the febrile state. Whatever the definition, all fever in the setting of neutropenia should be presumed initially to be infectious. Noninfectious causes of fever, including drug fever, transfusion reactions, thromboembolic disease, or fever caused by persistence or recrudescence of the underlying disease also should be considered. Fever may not always be present even with established infection, so other signs of clinical deterioration (e.g., relative hypothermia or hypotension, tachypnea, altered mental status) also should prompt evaluation and possibly treatment in neutropenic patients, especially in those at high risk (ANC <500 cells per milliliter).

At least two sets of peripheral blood cultures, plus one set from each port of any indwelling catheters, should be obtained prior to antibiotics. A urinalysis and a urine culture also should be done. In the patient who has recently received antibiotics or who has any gastrointestinal symptoms, a stool for *C. difficile* toxin should be obtained. The yield of stool examination for bacteria, ova and parasites, and viruses in patients hospitalized for more than 3 days is low, and it is reasonable to do these tests only if symptoms persist and *C. difficile* toxin is not present. Examination of spinal fluid is not recommended unless signs or symptoms of central nervous system involvement appear. A chest radiograph should be performed; in patients with gastrointestinal symptoms, upright and supine radiographs should also be considered. In patients who have localizing symptoms or signs, and have negative plain x-rays, chest or abdominal CT scan should be obtained. Skin lesions other than simple cellulitis should be aspirated or biopsied for appropriate pathologic examination, stains, and cultures.

The majority of infections in patients with neutropenia occur at a few sites. These include peridontium and oropharynx, lung, gastrointestinal tract (including the esophagus, small bowel, colon, and rectal and perirectal areas), vascular catheter access sites, other skin sites, and urinary tract, particularly if a catheter is in place. A thorough examination should include evaluation of all of these sites and of the optic fundus.

Decision to Admit

Although admission has been the standard for febrile neutropenic patients because of the high overall risk of medical complications, it is increasingly apparent that low-risk patients can be identified and safely partially or fully treated at home, as discussed in the Infectious Disease Society of America (IDSA) guidelines for the use of antibiotics in febrile, neutropenic patients (2). Low-risk patients lack co-morbid illnesses, systemic toxicity, or uncontrolled cancer; have no evidence of significant localized infection; can be adequately observed at home; and have telephone contact with the providers and rapid access to the hospital. The degree of the neutropenia also has influenced the risk in some studies. Both intravenous antibiotics and oral antibiotics have been studied in the ambulatory setting. Oral therapy improves convenience, avoids catheter use and decreases cost of treatment. Options include newer quinolones such as levofloxacin, oral first-, second- or third-generation cephalosporins, and the combination of ciprofloxacin plus amoxicillin-clavulanate. This latter combination regimen was equivalent to parenteral therapy in a placebo-controlled trial of low risk patients, and is specifically endorsed by the guidelines.

Initial Inpatient Antibiotic Therapy

Initial therapy should take into account the severity of illness, the site suggested by the patient's presentation, allergies, risks for toxicities or drug interactions, and the local and national epidemiology of infection in neutropenic patients. Historically, in patients presenting with presumed infection, a clinical diagnosis of infection is made in 40%–60% of febrile episodes. The infection is confirmed microbiologically in only about one-half of these clinically diagnosed cases. In the past decade, documented infections have shifted from aerobic Gram-negative bacilli (i.e., *E. coli* and *Klebsiella, Proteus,* and *Pseudomonas* organisms) toward Gram-positive bacteria (*Staphylococcus epidermidis,* streptococci including vancomycin-resistant enterococci, and corynebacteria). Although cultures of the nares, oropharynx, and stool may aid in infection control and demonstrate the colonizing flora in neutropenic patients, these cultures are not specific for infection, and their routine use is not recommended. Respiratory-tract cultures for *Aspergillus* organisms may be an exception to this rule.

Several different initial empiric antibiotic regimens have been proposed for the febrile neutropenic patient; many are equivalently efficacious. Figure 63.1 summarizes a set of recommendations adapted from the IDSA guidelines.

Subsequent Management of Antibiotics

Guidelines for management of antibiotics after initial therapy are summarized in Figures 63.2 and 63.3.

Early Defervescence on Therapy

The median time to defervescence on antibiotics in neutropenic patients is 5 days. Patients who defervesce within this period can be divided into those in whom a likely site or pathogen is identified and those in whom it is not. If a likely infection is identified, therapy should be altered to provide optimal treatment with minimal toxicity and lowest cost, but broad-spectrum coverage still should be continued. Antibiotic treatment should continue for at least as long as a similar infection in a normal host would be treated. A longer duration should be considered if the initial presentation was particularly severe, if the organism is virulent, if clinical or microbiologic response was slow, or if potential sites of invasion are still present. If patients improve and the ANC is >1,000 cells per mL therapy usually can proceed in the outpatient setting with intravenous or oral antibiotics. Ideally, the ANC should be >500 cells per mL before stopping. However, if all clinical signs and symptoms of infection have resolved and a reasonable duration of therapy has been given, discontinuation of antibiotics with careful observation appears safe.

If no cause is identified, patients can be stratified into low- and high-risk groups. Low-risk patients, whose features are summarized in Figure 63.2, are unlikely to require broadening of their initial regimen, are likely to do well on oral antibiotics in the outpatient setting, and are unlikely to develop relapse or other complications after discontinuation of antibiotics. They can be managed with brief courses of mostly oral therapy, completed in the outpatient setting. Approaches to higher-risk patients who respond to empiric antimicrobials are also outlined in the figure.

Persistent Fever During the First Five Days of Therapy

Persistent fever may represent a slower than average response to treatment, an infection with bacteria resistant to the antibiotics used, a loculated infection, a nonbacterial infection, or a noninfectious cause of fever (Figure 63.3). Patients who are well and have ANCs >500 cells per mL may not require alteration or even continuation of therapy in this setting. However, patients who have an ANC <500 cells per mL and who have had no response in fever or clinical status should have therapy altered as follows:

- If an indwelling line is present or there is significant epidemiologic risk for penicillin-resistant pneumococci or viridans streptococci, add vancomycin. If the initial regimen did not include coverage of a resistant Gram-negative pathogen known to be present in the patient or the hospital environment, consider a switch to a β-lactam with better activity or addition of an aminoglycoside. If the ini-

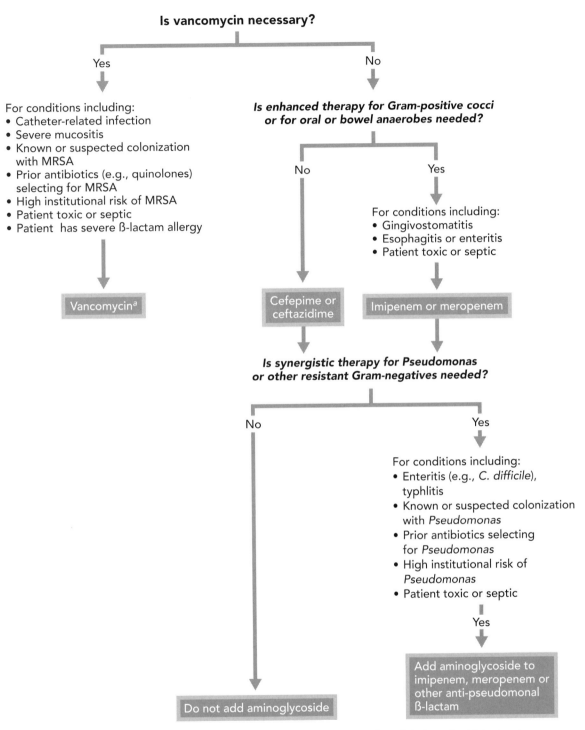

Figure 63.1 Initial inpatient therapy of fever and neutropenia. [a]If no clinical or microbiologic evidence suggests MRSA, MRSE, or other infection requiring vanomycin by 3–4 days, stop therapy. *MRSA*, methicillin-resistant *Staphylococcus aureus*; *MRSE*, methicillin-resistant *Staphylococcus epidermidis*.

tial regimen did not include good anaerobic activity, consider its addition. Also consider unusual infections.

■ If loculated infection is suspected, appropriate imaging and local drainage should be performed. Indwelling catheters that have tunnel infections and clinically unre-

sponsive exit-site infections may require line removal for cure. In addition, patients with persistently positive cultures for any organism or infections with Bacillus or Candida spp. also should have indwelling lines removed.

■ Evaluate and exclude noninfectious sources of fever.

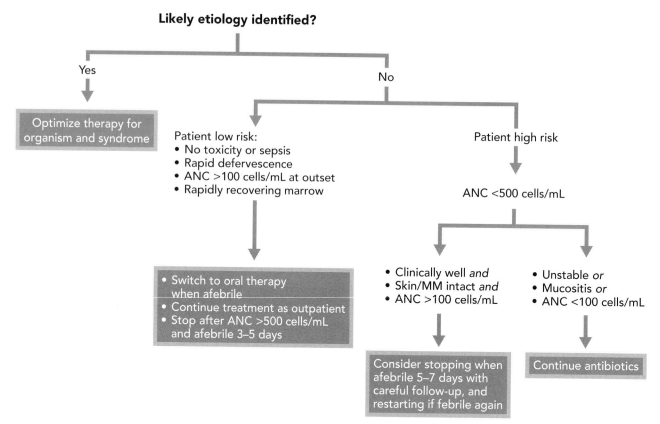

Figure 63.2 Inpatient management of neutropenia with early defervescence on therapy. *ANC*, absolute neutrophil count; *MM*, mucous membranes.

Patients who remain neutropenic for extended periods are at risk for invasive mycoses. Antemortem diagnosis is difficult because of the poor sensitivity of diagnostic techniques. Given the morbidity and mortality rates of late or disseminated infection, empiric therapy is required. Presumptive or early treatment of aspergillus has been hampered by the lack of a sensitive diagnostic test. This creates a tension: empiric therapy of aspergillus is expensive and may be toxic, yet by the time clinical and chest CT findings of the disease emerge, mortality is un-

acceptably high. A recently licensed blood test, the *Platelia Aspergillus galactomannan assay*, has been evaluated for early diagnosis in immunocompromised hosts. Depending on patient population, sensitivity is in the 80% range, with even higher specificity. While much needs to be learned about the optimal use of this assay, it already provides a useful adjunct for the early diagnosis of invasive aspergillus (3).

In general, empiric antifungal therapy is indicated for patients who remain neutropenic and febrile (or who

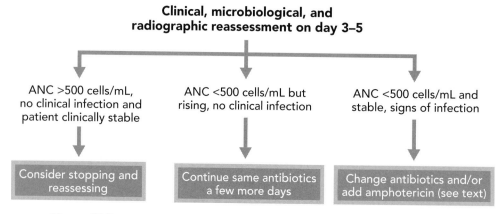

Figure 63.3 Inpatient management of neutropenia with persistent fever on therapy.

redevelop a fever) despite approximately 5–7 days of broad-spectrum antibacterial therapy (4). Amphotericin B is a broad spectrum agent with potent fungicidal activity against most yeasts and molds. There is extensive experience with this drug and most guidelines still favor its use for empiric therapy in febrile neutropenic patients. Voriconazole is an alternative for empiric antifungal therapy. In patients in whom *Candida* organisms appear most likely, doses of 0.5–0.6 mg/kg of amphotericin B per day may be used. This includes patients during the recovery phase of neutropenia, in whom hepatosplenic candidiasis is more common, and patients with any clinical, laboratory, or radiographic signs of this syndrome. Patients with mucous membrane lesions such as mucositis or colitis are also at risk for invasion of colonizing *Candida* organisms. Patients in whom *Aspergillus* organisms are suspected should be started on 1.0–1.5 mg/kg of amphotericin per day. This may include patients who have prolonged neutropenia, respiratory-tract colonization with *Aspergillus* organisms; concurrent defects in cellular immunity; or cutaneous, pulmonary, or central nervous system signs or symptoms suggesting aspergillosis. Liposomal amphotericin preparations are up to 10 or 20 times more expensive, and should be reserved for patients who cannot tolerate the conventional drug or have significant preexisting renal insufficiency. Caspofungin is not recommended for empiric therapy (5).

Patients should be rapidly assessed for deep fungal infection as empiric therapy is being started, with chest radiograph (and computed tomography scan if there are any upper or lower respiratory tract signs or symptoms, or if the respiratory tract is colonized with *Aspergillus* organisms) and abdominal computed tomography or magnetic resonance imaging if hepatosplenic candidiasis is suspected. If a causative agent and clinical syndrome are documented, this should determine the dose and course of antifungal therapy. Treatment of documented candidemia can be completed with fluconazole or amphotericin preparations, depending on speciation and fluconazole susceptibility of the *Candida* species. Intravenous caspofungin is an alternative for patients with species of *Candida* likely to be susceptible, especially those intolerant of the traditional regimens. In *Aspergillus* infection limited to the lung, monotherapy with voriconazole (oral favored over intravenous administration) or amphotericin is reasonable. Though data are limited, in CNS infection or suspected disseminated infection, many experts would favor combination therapy with voriconazole plus caspofungin, with or without high doses of an amphotericin preparation. However, if no fungal infection is found, duration of therapy should be individualized according to the degree of persistent neutropenia and the risk for deep fungal infection.

Prevention of Infection in Neutropenic Patients

Hand cleansing is highly effective. A "neutropenic diet" avoiding fresh fruits and vegetables containing high titers

of bacteria is simple and inexpensive. Although studies show some efficacy for systemic bacterial prophylaxis with oral trimethoprim–sulfamethoxazole (TMP-SMX) or quinolones, their use cannot be recommended routinely. This is because they have no demonstrable effect on mortality rate (since most infection can be successfully addressed by early empiric therapy) and because of the enormous concern over emergence of resistant organisms (Chapter 64). However, they may be appropriate for short periods in patients who have periods of particularly high risk for bacterial infection, such as those undergoing instrumentation. Systemic antifungal prophylaxis is associated with emergence of resistant fungi and is also not routinely recommended. There is no role for active or passive immunization in febrile neutropenic patients. Hematopoietic growth factors should not be employed routinely. Their use is discussed further in Chapter 90.

CELLULAR IMMUNE DYSFUNCTION

Clinical Features of the Host with Cellular Immune Dysfunction

Cell-mediated immunity refers to those aspects of the immune response that are mediated by T lymphocytes, natural killer cells, and mononuclear phagocytes. Although cell-mediated immunity is critical in the control of infection caused by intracellular pathogens such as viruses, fungi, and mycobacteria, it is also important in the control of many extracellular pathogens such as *Pneumocystis jirovecii* and in regulation of the global immune response. Table 63.2 lists some of the conditions causing defective cell-mediated immunity (see Table 63.1 for commonly associated infections). The most commonly encountered condition in adult medicine is iatrogenic immunosuppression. The drugs referred to in Table 63.2 and reviewed in Table 102.4 are used in the treatment of many conditions, including lymphoreticular and other malignancies, connective tissue diseases and other autoimmune diseases. However, solid-organ transplant recipients are the prototypical patients with prolonged and profound depression in cell-mediated immunity. This section focuses on principles of infection in this patient population, though these principles are applicable to other patients listed in Table 63.2. Because infection results in excessive deaths and injuries as well as hospitalization and cost, the most important principle is effective prevention of infection.

Principles of Antimicrobial Prophylaxis in Solid-Organ Transplant Recipients

Prevention must be stressed for two reasons: first, the previously mentioned attenuation in typical inflammatory responses; and second, the interactions and additive toxicities

TABLE 63.2

CONDITIONS ASSOCIATED WITH IMPAIRED CELL-MEDIATED IMMUNITY

Primary immunodeficiencies
Physiologically decreased CMI in the fetus, the neonate, and the aged
Immunodeficiency secondary to malignancies
   Hodgkin's disease and other lymphoid malignancies
   Hairy cell leukemia
   Thymoma
Immunodeficiency resulting from metabolic factors
   Malnutrition
   Uremia
Immunodeficiency resulting from coexisting infections
   HIV infection
   Other viral infections, e.g., CMV, EBV, VZV, hepatitis B and C
   Disseminated mycobacterial, fungal, parasitic infections
Iatrogenic immunodeficiency
   Total lymphoid irradiation
   Immunosuppressive drugs

CMI, cellular mediated immunity; *CMV,* cytomegalovirus; *EBV,* Epstein-Barr virus; *VZV,* varicella zoster virus

of antimicrobial agents with immunosuppressive agents (Table 102.4) (6). Three types of interactions may be seen between cyclosporine, tacrolimus and antimicrobial agents. Several drugs, most notably rifampin, upregulate the metabolism of cyclosporine and tacrolimus by the hepatic cytochrome P450 system, thus decreasing levels of immunosuppression and potentially leading to allograft rejection. Other drugs, such as macrolides and imidazoles, downregulate the metabolism of cyclosporine and tacrolimus, leading to higher levels, potentially with increased toxicity and overimmunosuppression. Finally, additive toxicities include renal toxicity of agents such as amphotericin, aminoglycosides, and high-dosage TMP-SMX with cyclosporine and tacrolimus, and bone marrow toxicity of agents such as high-dosage TMP-SMX with azathioprine or mycophenolate. Careful monitoring for antimicrobial toxicity and for changes in cyclosporine and tacrolimus levels is required in this setting.

The risk of infection is determined by epidemiologic exposures along with the patient's state of immunosuppression. Potential epidemiologic exposures in the hospital include recognized nosocomial pathogens such as *Aspergillus* and *Legionella* organisms, *C. difficile,* and resistant Gram-negative rods. Epidemiologic surveillance and measures to prevent transmission are critical. The net state of immunosuppression is primarily determined by the dose, duration, and temporal sequence of immunosuppressive drugs. Kidney transplants generally require the least immunosuppression, with increasing doses required for hepatic, cardiac, and pulmonary allografts. Prophylactic regimens are continued longer in transplant patients requiring more prolonged immunosuppression. In addition to both nonspecific and specific immune defects that contribute to immunosuppression, many transplant patients have other factors listed in Table 63.2, most notably infection with the chronic, immunomodulating viruses.

Prevention can be accomplished by using antimicrobial drugs in two different modes. The first is the *prophylactic mode,* in which the antimicrobial is given to every patient. This requires an infection that is common enough and antimicrobials that are safe enough to make prophylaxis worthwhile. The second is the *preemptive mode,* in which antimicrobials are given to a subgroup of patients before they develop symptomatic disease. The preemptive mode requires the use of a clinical or laboratory characteristic to identify a subgroup of patients at high risk, who would be expected to derive maximal benefit from the treatment. Given the current, standard immunosuppressive regimens, there is an expected temporal sequence in which infections occur posttransplant, although patients sometimes deviate from it. A discussion of the evaluation and management of the great variety of syndromes and infections that occur despite prophylaxis is beyond the scope of this chapter. Expert consultation should be sought early to facilitate rapid diagnostic and therapeutic decisions.

First Month Posttransplant

Rare causes of infection in this time period include untreated infection in the recipient and infection conveyed by the allograft. Before the transplant, meticulous evaluation of the donor as well as control of any infection present in the recipient should occur. However, most infections occurring in this time period are the same bacterial or candidal infections of the wound, lungs, urinary tract, or vascular access catheters that occur in nonimmunosuppressed surgical patients. The most important factor in prevention is technically faultless surgery to prevent bleeding and other fluid collections, devitalized tissues, anastamotic leaks, and so forth. Decreasing duration of intubation, of indwelling devices, and of immobilization are also critical. Well-established indications for prophylaxis during this time period include perioperative prophylaxis, prophylaxis of urinary tract infection, and prevention of intraabdominal infection in liver transplantation.

Perioperative antibiotics targeted to the skin and urinary tract, such as cefazolin begun intraoperatively and continued for less than 24 hours postoperatively, are effective in preventing infection in renal transplant patients and have been applied to liver and heart transplantation. In the case of lung transplantation, studies are lacking, but practice has been to use antibiotics targeted to the respiratory flora of the donor and recipient.

Without prophylaxis, the incidence of urinary tract infection in renal transplant recipients is 30%–60%. Urinary tract infection in this setting frequently is associated with signs of upper tract infection, bacteremia, and a high rate of relapse with standard short-course therapy. Prophylaxis with TMP-SMX, one single-strength tablet daily, or (if sulfa allergic) ciprofloxacin 250 mg at bedtime, decreases the incidence to 5%, is highly cost-effective, and typically is continued for 6–12 months. TMP-SMX has the added advantage of providing prophylaxis against *Pneumocystis jirovecii*, *Nocardia asteroides*, *Listeria monocytogenes*, and *Salmonella* spp. For patients in whom urinary-tract infections recur after this period, long-term UTI prophylaxis may be appropriate after anatomic factors have been evaluated and corrected.

Factors that increase the risk of infection after liver transplantation include intraperitoneal hemorrhage, need for reexploration, and the use of a choledochojejunostomy (rather than a choledochocholedochostomy) as an anastamosis. A decrease in postoperative infection has been reported with prophylactic regimens including quinolones alone, oral gentamicin, polymyxin and nystatin or amphotericin B, and cefazolin followed by TMP/SMX plus clotrimazole or nystatin. It is common for the biliary tree to be colonized postoperatively. If biliary drainage tubes are used, cultures may reveal enterobacteriaceae, enterococci, and coagulase-negative staphylococci, or more resistant flora if there has been prior hospitalization and antibiotics. In one center, a dose of preemptive therapy with antibiotics targeted to known or suspected biliary flora, given before biliary tract manipulation or liver biopsy, has decreased the rate of cholangitis or intrahepatic abscess.

Although additional prophylaxis may delay the onset of these infections and may be appropriate for short periods while technical or anatomic problems are being addressed, its routine use selects for resistance and should be avoided. Occurrence of typical opportunistic pathogens during this time suggests either excessive nosocomial exposure or significant immunosuppression preceding the transplant.

One to Six Months Posttransplant

Bacterial or candidal infections established in the immediate postoperative period may persist. However, this is the time period during which the typical opportunistic pathogens listed in Table 63.1 appear. Several infections are common enough to warrant routine prophylaxis. Incidence of *P. jirovecii* pneumonia (PCP) in solid-organ transplantation ranges from 10%–15%. This is effectively eliminated by one TMP-SMX single-strength tablet daily given for the first 6–12 months of transplantation or, in the case of lung transplantation, for the patient's lifetime. Alternatives in allergic patients include atovaquone, dapsone, or aerosolized pentamidine. The incidence of deep fungal infection is not high enough to warrant routine prophylaxis. However, mucocutaneous fungal infections are common, and the incidence is decreased by clotrimazole 10 mg twice per day or nystatin swish and swallow 3 mL twice per day. Cytomegalovirus (CMV) causes very significant direct and indirect morbidity and mortality in this population (as summarized in Table 63.3) (7). In seronegative recipients,

TABLE 63.3
EFFECTS OF CYTOMEGALOVIRUS IN TRANSPLANT RECIPIENTS

Direct effects
    Acute viral syndrome, may include:
        Fever, myalgias, arthralgias, headache
        Leukopenia, thrombocytopenia, hepatitis
    End organ disease
        Allograft
            Other tissues
            Gastrointestinal tract including bowel, liver, pancreas
            Pneumonitis
            Encephalitis or retinitis
            Myocarditis
Indirect effects
    Allograft rejection and injury
    Superinfection
    Increased risk of post-transplant lymphoproliferative disease associated with Epstein-Barr virus
Possible associations
    Bronchiolitis obliterans in lung transplants
    Accelerated coronary artery disease in heart transplants
    Vanishing bile duct syndrome in liver transplants
    Glomerulopathy in kidney transplants

prevention of primary infection using CMV-negative blood products is critical. With the availability of an orally bioavailable formulation of ganciclovir (valganciclovir), some higher risk patients now warrant routine CMV prophylaxis (8). These include patients who are donor seropositive and recipient seronegative for CMV, patients receiving antilymphocyte globulins or other significantly augmented immunosuppression for rejection, and patients early after lung transplantation. Preemptive therapy of viral replication (without symptomatic disease) may be appropriate in many other transplant patients. Treatment of documented viral replication or clinical disease should be done in conjunction with an infectious disease specialist. These same patients at high risk for disease are also at risk for drug resistance, particularly if they receive inadequate doses or durations of antiviral treatment.

More than Six-Months Posttransplant

Patients with a functioning allograft fall into two groups. The first includes those with good allograft function, on decreasing doses of immunosuppression, and free of chronic viral infection. These patients increasingly develop infections observed in the community (e.g., influenza, bacterial pneumonia, urinary tract infection), although opportunistic infections still are seen. The second group is characterized by poor allograft function, one or more episodes of acute or chronic rejection requiring increased immunosuppression, and infection with the chronic viruses. These patients remain at high risk for opportunistic infections, and it may be appropriate to employ prophylaxis for mucocutaneous fungal and viral infections and for PCP for much longer.

BONE-MARROW TRANSPLANTATION

General principles of bone-marrow transplantation and unique infectious disease considerations are discussed in Chapter 96. Principles of therapy of febrile neutropenia in these patients are similar to those already described.

KEY POINTS

- Compromised hosts may have specific or nonspecific defects in immune function, and these defects are associated with typical infectious disease syndromes. Because the inflammatory response to infection in these patients is attenuated and the morbidity from infection is high, early diagnosis and empiric therapy are critical.

- In patients with impaired humoral immunity, early treatment directed at encapsulated pathogens is essential.

- In the case of febrile neutropenic patients, in whom both bacterial pathogens and fungi are important, guidelines exist for rational empiric antibacterial and antifungal therapy. Although this therapy previously was provided entirely in the inpatient setting, it is increasingly possible to identify patients who can be either managed in the outpatient setting or discharged home early.

- In patients with solid-organ or bone marrow transplants and long-term immunosuppression, knowledge of the likely pathogens and the usual timing of their occurrence is increasingly allowing design of effective and cost-effective strategies to prevent infection.

REFERENCES

1. Davidson RN, Wall RA. Prevention and management of infections in patients without a spleen. *Clin Microbiol Infect* 2001;7:657–660.
2. Hughes WT, Armstrong D, Bodey GP, et al. 2002 guidelines for the use of antimicrobial agents in neutropenic patients with cancer. *Clin Infectious Dis* 2002;34:730–751.
3. Wheat LJ. Rapid diagnosis of invasive aspergillus by antigen detection. *Transpl Infect Dis* 2003;5:157.
4. Wingard JR. Empirical antifungal therapy in treating febrile neutropenic patients. *Clin Infect Dis* 2004;39(Suppl 1):S38–S43.
5. Rapp RP. Changing strategies for the management of invasive fungal infections. *Pharmacotherapy* 2004;24:4S–28S.
6. Fishman JA, Rubin RH. Infection in organ transplant recipients. *N Engl J Med* 1998;338:1741–1751.
7. Gandhi MK, Khanna R. Human cytomegalovirus: clinical aspects, immune regulation, and emerging treatments. *Lancet Infect Dis* 2004;4:725–738.
8. Egan JJ, Carroll KB, Yonan N, Woodcock A, Crisp A. Valacyclovir prevention of cytomegalovirus reactivation after heart transplantation: a randomized trial. *J Heart Lung Transpl* 2002;21:460–464.

ADDITIONAL READING

Picazo JJ. Management of the febrile neutropenic patient: a consensus conference. *Clin Infect Dis* 2004;39(Suppl 1):S1–S6.
Playford EG, Webster AC, Sorell TC, Craig JC. Antifungal agents for preventing fungal infections in solid organ transplant recipients. *Cochrane Database Syst Rev* 2004;3:CD004291.
Rubin RH, Young LS, eds. *Clinical Approach to Infection in the Compromised Host*, 4th ed. New York: Kluwer Academic Publishing, 2002.

Parenteral Antibiotics and Antibiotic Resistance

64

Lisa G. Winston   Henry F. Chambers III

INTRODUCTION

Antimicrobial Resistance

Bacterial resistance to antimicrobial therapy has emerged as a significant problem over the past 20 years, with concerns escalating in the 1990s. Local patterns of resistance vary widely, but the percentage of bacterial pathogens with resistance to a single or multiple antibiotics increases yearly. Risk factors for infection with resistant organisms include direct exposure to people carrying them (e.g., the spread of penicillin-resistant *Streptococcus pneumoniae* in day-care centers) or environmental contamination (e.g., colonization with vancomycin-resistant enterococci in hospital wards and intensive care units). However, the true driving force behind the emergence of antibiotic resistance is the use of antibiotics themselves. Indiscriminate prescription of antibiotics, for example for symptoms that are almost always caused by viral infections (1), is part of the problem. In addition, the availability of antimicrobial agents without a prescription in many parts of the world adds to the overuse. In recent years, patterns of prescribing physicians have begun to change in response to growing concerns about bacterial antimicrobial resistance. For example, some practitioners no longer prescribe antibiotics for routine acute otitis media in children because research has shown that most cases resolve without specific treatment.

This paradox of increasing antimicrobial resistance fueling increased use of broad-spectrum antibiotics often leaves the clinician with the dilemma of how best to care for individual patients. Familiarity with local bacterial resistance patterns, the usual pathogens in common infections, and specific therapy for a few resistant organisms helps clinicians make rational decisions regarding empiric and pathogen-specific selection of antibiotics.

Mechanisms of Resistance

A basic knowledge of the mechanisms that underlie bacterial resistance is important in understanding the potential for clinical failures and for the selection of appropriate antibiotics if resistant pathogens have been isolated or are suspected (Figure 64.1). There are three general mechanisms of bacterial resistance: inability of the antibiotic to reach its target; inactivation of the antibiotic before it reaches its target; or alteration of the antibiotic target itself. These mechanisms may operate independently but often work in concert.

Impaired penetration may result from either the failure of the drug to cross a membrane barrier (e.g., the outer membrane of Gram-negative bacteria) or the presence of a transmembrane efflux pump that transports drug out of the cell. Antibiotics penetrate the outer membrane of Gram-negative organisms via outer-membrane protein channels. Absence of the proper channel, or down-regulation of its production, can prevent or greatly reduce drug entry into the cell.

Antibiotic inactivation is the principle mechanism of resistance to β-lactam antibiotics and aminoglycosides.

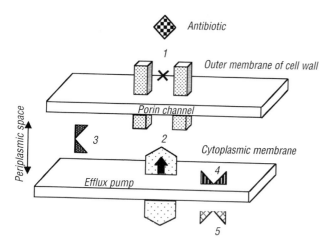

Figure 64.1 Schematic of the envelope of a Gram-negative bacterium illustrating mechanisms of antibiotic resistance. 1. The antibiotic may fail to reach its target secondary to absence or down-regulation of the outer membrane protein channel. 2. The antibiotic may be transported out of the cell by a transmembrane efflux pump. 3. The antibiotic may be inactivated before it reaches its target (e.g., by a β-lactamase in the periplasmic space). 4. A membrane-associated target (e.g., a penicillin-binding protein) may be altered. 5. An intracellular target (e.g., DNA gyrase or topoisomerase) may be altered.

β-lactamases are enzymes that hydrolyze the β-lactam ring. β-lactamases produced by commonly encountered organisms such as *Staphylococcus aureus*, *Haemophilus species*, *Bacteroides fragilis*, and *Escherichia coli* are predominantly penicillinases with relatively weak activity against cephalosporins. β-lactamases produced by more resistant species (e.g., *Pseudomonas*, *Enterobacter*, and *Serratia* spp.) are primarily cephalosporinases, although these enzymes also have penicillinase activity. β-lactamases of gram-negative species are located in the periplasmic space between the cytoplasmic and outer membranes, which effectively produces an enzymatic barrier to antibiotic penetration.

Target alteration is the basis of penicillin resistance in pneumococci, methicillin resistance in staphylococci, vancomycin resistance in enterococci, and fluoroquinolone resistance in both Gram-negative and Gram-positive organisms. In the cases of penicillin and methicillin resistance, the penicillin binding protein targets have been modified in such a way that they bind β-lactams poorly, so usual drug concentrations are ineffective. Vancomycin resistance in enterococci is caused by alteration of the drug's target in the nascent cell wall. Resistance to fluoroquinolones is caused by one or more point mutations in the primary target of the drug (DNA gyrase in *E. coli* and topoisomerase IV in staphylococci).

Resistance may be acquired vertically by selecting subpopulations with advantageous mutations or horizontally by transfer of genetic material encoding resistance determinants. Horizontal transmission has several potential advantages from the standpoint of bacterial survival. The trait can be widely and rapidly disseminated to other strains with high-level resistance achieved in a single step, and the problem of lethal mutation is avoided. Horizontally acquired resistance genes often are plasmid-encoded, and plasmids can harbor many resistance factors simultaneously.

Goals of Antibiotic Therapy

The general goals of antibiotic therapy are to eradicate infection as quickly as possible and to minimize toxicity. Choosing safe antibiotics with rapidly bactericidal activity is always desirable. Using an antibiotic with the narrowest possible spectrum of action likely helps prevent the emergence and spread of resistant organisms. In addition, broad-spectrum antibiotics dramatically alter normal host flora, which leaves patients vulnerable to organisms of intrinsically low virulence, such as enterococci and yeast. Finally, traditional antibiotics with more focused bacterial coverage frequently are less costly. Thus, in hospitalized patients for whom broad-spectrum or long-term antibiotic therapy is being considered, it is essential that appropriate cultures be taken before antibiotics are started so that therapy can be narrowed once specific pathogens are isolated. It is also important to recognize that many signs, symptoms, and laboratory abnormalities in the hospitalized patient that appear to be infectious in nature (such as fever or opacities on a chest radiograph) in fact may not be (Chapter 62). Therefore, their presence should not automatically lead the clinician to broaden antimicrobial coverage.

Combination Therapy

The use of antibiotic combinations to treat serious bacterial infections is common in hospitalized patients. There are four circumstances in which a clinician should select combination therapy: (1) if synergy between two agents has been shown to result in faster killing of organisms and potentially better outcomes for patients; (2) if combination therapy has been demonstrated to prevent the emergence of resistance; (3) if the agents chosen have distinct anatomic sites of action; or (4) if the infection is polymicrobial, mixed aerobic-anaerobic, or caused potentially by one of several organisms so that no single drug is likely to cover all pathogens. Enterococcal endocarditis is one example of an infection that requires the use of a synergistic combination (e.g., ampicillin plus gentamicin) to produce the bactericidal activity that is required to cure this infection (Chapter 71). Tuberculosis is, perhaps, the best example of a disease in which combination therapy is known to prevent the emergence of resistance (Chapter 67). Although synergism and prevention of resistance have been invoked as reasons for combination therapy for invasive infections caused by certain Gram-negative bacilli, this practice is quite controversial. *Pseudomonas aeruginosa* has been most extensively studied, and evidence supporting the use of combination therapy for *P. aeruginosa* infection is most compelling (see pages 627–628). Use of rifampin-containing regimens for the treatment of staphylococcal prosthetic valve endocarditis is an example of combination therapy to target different bacterial populations. Rifampin penetrates into and sterilizes valve ring and suture-associated abscesses, whereas vancomycin, β-lactams, and aminoglycosides—the other antibiotics used to treat this infection—do not. Rifampin cannot be used alone in such cases because resistance emerges rapidly. Finally, combination therapy often is used in the treatment of intra-abdominal infections, which frequently are polymicrobial (Chapter 87).

CARE OF THE HOSPITALIZED PATIENT

This section describes the features of the most commonly used antibiotics and the treatment of particularly challenging pathogens. It does not discuss the initial, empiric selection of antibiotics for common infections in hospitalized patients; this is specifically addressed in other chapters. However, it should be emphasized that *an attempt to cover all possible organisms is almost never indicated.* Instead, one should focus on the most common organisms that cause particular clinical syndromes and select an antibiotic regimen that covers these pathogens well, taking local resistance patterns into account. In general, patients who are more severely ill merit broader initial coverage, because one cannot afford to leave an unusual pathogen uncovered.

Overview of the Major Classes of Antibiotics

Aminoglycosides include streptomycin, neomycin, kanamycin, amikacin, gentamicin, tobramycin, sisomicin, and netilmicin. Aminoglycosides inhibit bacterial protein synthesis and are most active against Gram-negative enteric bacteria. They have no activity against anaerobes. Aminoglycosides often are used in combination with another antibiotic, usually a β-lactam. Resistance may be caused by production of an inactivating enzyme, impaired entry into the cell, or target alteration. Aminoglycosides are absorbed very poorly if administered orally, and systemic levels can be achieved only by intramuscular or intravenous administration. Aminoglycosides are highly polar compounds that do not enter cells or penetrate infected tissue and abscesses readily. Clearance is directly proportional to creatinine clearance. They are ototoxic and nephrotoxic. Toxicity is more likely to occur if aminoglycosides are administered for more than 5 days at high dosages in the elderly in the setting of renal insufficiency, or with diuretics or other potentially nephrotoxic agents (e.g., vancomycin or amphotericin-B). In most cases, once-daily dosing of aminoglycosides is the preferred mode of administration. Daily dosing appears to have less toxicity and is as efficacious as more frequent administration. However, daily dosing should not be used in cases of endocarditis and still requires dose adjustment in patients with renal failure.

β-*lactam antibiotics* include penicillins, cephalosporins, carbapenems, and monobactams. They all are similar chemically, mechanistically, pharmacologically, immunologically, and clinically. β-lactams are the most widely prescribed antibiotics, and their extensive use has exerted enormous selective pressure favoring resistant organisms. Broad-spectrum β-lactams eradicate normal flora, predisposing patients to colonization and superinfection with opportunistic, drug-resistant species. β-lactam antibiotics inhibit bacterial growth by inhibiting bacterial cell-wall synthesis. These compounds are structural analogues of the natural cell-wall substrate D-alanyl–D-alanine, and they covalently bind to penicillin-binding proteins at the active site of cell-wall synthesis. β-lactams are bactericidal only if cells are actively dividing. Resistance to β-lactams results from β-lactamase inactivation of the drug, alteration in target penicillin-binding proteins, or impaired antibiotic entry into Gram-negative bacteria. β-lactams are remarkably nontoxic; most of the serious adverse effects are caused by hypersensitivity. Allergic reactions include anaphylactic shock (0.05% of recipients), serum sickness, and skin rashes.

Penicillins can be divided into three groups: *Penicillins* (e.g., penicillin G) are most active against Gram-positive organisms, Gram-negative cocci, and anaerobes. They are poorly active against Gram-negative rods and are susceptible to hydrolysis by β-lactamases. *Antistaphylococcal penicillins* (e.g., nafcillin) are resistant to staphylococcal β-lactamases and are active against staphylococci and streptococci. They have no useful activity against enterococci, most anaerobic species, and Gram-negative organisms. *Extended-spectrum penicillins* (e.g., ampicillin, ticarcillin, and piperacillin) have improved activity against Gram-negative organisms, but they are destroyed by β-lactamases. Many extended-spectrum penicillins have enhanced activity against *P. aeruginosa.*

Cephalosporins are classified into four major groups or "generations," depending mainly on the spectrum of antimicrobial activity. As a general rule, first-generation compounds (e.g., cefazolin) have better activity against Gram-positive organisms, and the later generation compounds exhibit improved activity against Gram-negative aerobic organisms. Anaerobic cocci (e.g., *Peptostreptococcus*) are sensitive to most cephalosporins. Cephalosporins are more β-lactamase stable than penicillins and, therefore, usually have a broader spectrum of activity. The cephamycin group of second-generation compounds (cefoxitin, cefotetan, and cefmetazole) are active against anaerobes (including many *B. fragilis*). Third-generation cepahalsporins have improved Gram-negative coverage and most (an exception being ceftizoxime) achieve high levels in the cerebrospinal fluid. Cephalosporins are not active against enterococci, *Listeria monocytogenes*, or methicillin-resistant staphylococci. Cephalosporins are rarely the drugs of choice for a specific organism but, because of their broad spectra, they are used widely for empirical therapy. Third-generation cephalosporins, in particular, exert a strong selective pressure favoring colonization by multidrug-resistant organisms and fungi.

Imipenem and meropenem, are *carbapenems* that have very broad spectra of activity, including Gram-negative rods, Gram-positive organisms, and anaerobes. These compounds are resistant to most β-lactamases. However, *Enterococcus faecium*, methicillin-resistant strains of staphylococci, *Clostridium difficile*, *Burkholderia cepacia*, and *Stenotrophomonas maltophila* are resistant to carbapenems. Carbapenems are indicated for infections caused by multidrug-resistant organisms. They are effective as single agents for treatment of febrile, neutropenic patients, and they are an antibiotic of choice for treatment of *Enterobacter* infections. Seizures may occur with high doses of imipenem in patients with renal failure.

Monobactams (aztreonam is the only one available in the United States) are active only against Gram-negative organisms. The antimicrobial spectrum resembles that of aminoglycosides. Patients with serious allergic reactions to penicillins or other β-lactams can be safely treated with monbactams, which do not cross-react with other β-lactams.

β-*lactamase inhibitors* are β-lactam molecules with weak antibacterial activity that inhibit many bacterial β-lactamases. Plasmid-encoded β-lactamases, such as those produced by staphylococci, *Haemophilus influenzae*, *Neisseria gonorrhoea*, *Salmonella* organisms, *Shigella* organisms, *E. coli*, and *Klebciella pneumoniae*, are most susceptible to inhibition, as are the chromosomal β-lactamases of *Bacteroides and Moraxella* spp. The three inhibitors on the market, clavulanate, sulbactam, and tazobactam, are therapeutically similar. Inhibitors are available only in fixed combinations with specific penicillins: ampicillin/sulbactam, piperacillin/ tazobactam, and ticarcillin/clavulanate. The spectrum of the combination is determined by the companion penicillin. The activity of the companion penicillin is improved with the addition of an inhibitor only if resistance is caused by β-lactamase production and the inhibitor is active against the β-lactamase produced.

Vancomycin is a glycopeptide antibiotic that inhibits cell-wall synthesis by binding to the terminal D-alanyl–D-alanine of peptidoglycan precursor. Resistance to vancomycin in enterococci results from modification of the precursor by replacement of D-alanine with D-lactate, which eliminates a hydrogen bond critical for binding vancomycin. Vancomycin is bactericidal for Gram-positive bacteria, both aerobic and anaerobic. Vancomycin is administered orally only for the treatment of antibiotic-associated enterocolitis caused by *C. difficile*. However, because of the potential for selection of vancomycin-resistant enterococci, this use of oral vancomycin has fallen into disfavor. Parenteral doses must be administered intravenously. Vancomycin is eliminated by glomerular filtration. In functionally anephric patients, the half-life of vancomycin is

6–10 days. The drug is not removed by conventional hemodialysis but is partly removed by high-flux dialysis. The main indication for parenteral vancomycin is bacteremia caused by methicillin-resistant staphylococci. However, vancomycin is *less effective* than an antistaphylococcal penicillin for treatment of serious infections, such as endocarditis, caused by methicillin-susceptible strains (Chapter 71). Other indications are empiric or definitive therapy for infections (e.g., meningitis) caused by highly penicillin-resistant strains of pneumococcus or Gram-positive infections in patients with serious allergy to β-lactams.

Metronidazole is a nitroimidazole with potent antibacterial activity against most anaerobes, including *Bacteroides* and *Clostridia* spp. Resistance is uncommon among strict anaerobes. The drug has excellent oral bioavailability, achieving serum concentrations equivalent to those following intravenous administration. Metronidazole is indicated for treatment of anaerobic or mixed intra-abdominal infections. It is not active against streptococci and is less active than clindamycin against Gram-positive anaerobes.

Macrolides are bacteriostatic inhibitors of protein synthesis. They are a group of closely related compounds characterized by a 14- to 16-member cyclic lactone ring. Clarithromycin and azithromycin are semisynthetic derivatives of erythromycin. Clarithromycin is virtually identical to erythromycin with respect to antibacterial activity, except that clarithromycin is more active against atypical mycobacteria and *Haemophilus* spp. Compared with erythromycin and clarithromycin, azithromycin is slightly less active *in vitro* against staphylococci and streptococci and slightly more active against *H. influenzae*. Besides azithromycin's enhanced activity against *Chlamydia* spp., the clinical significance of these differences is unclear. These agents are very active for infections caused by *Legionella* organisms. Because of frequent resistance in pneumococci (15%–20%), group A streptococci (20%–40%), and staphylococci (46%–60%), macrolides should not be used as initial, single therapy in severely ill patients if these organisms are suspected. However, macrolides are effective for the outpatient treatment of community-acquired pneumonia (Chapter 65).

Clindamycin is a chlorine-substituted derivative of lincomycin, an antibiotic that resembles erythromycin in activity. Streptococci, staphylococci, and pneumococci are inhibited by clindamycin. Enterococci and Gram-negative aerobes are resistant. *Bacteroides* species and other anaerobes are usually susceptible. Clindamycin penetrates well into abscesses. The most important indication for clindamycin is in the treatment of serious mixed or anaerobic infections caused by *Bacteroides* organisms and other anaerobes. It is probably the antibiotic of choice for lung abscesses. *C. difficile* is resistant, and antibiotic-associated colitis caused by this organism is an important complication of clindamycin therapy.

Tetracyclines are broad-spectrum bacteriostatic inhibitors of protein synthesis. Their spectrum includes Gram-positive and Gram-negative bacteria, anaerobes, and *Rickettsia, Chlamydia,* and *Mycoplasma* organisms. Resistance results primarily from an efflux pump. Widespread and indiscriminate use of tetracyclines (including use in animal feed) has promoted resistance. Thus, tetracyclines have fallen into disuse for treatment of many serious bacterial infections. Tetracyclines are still among the drugs of choice for brucellosis, plague, tularemia, and infections with chlamydiae and rickettsiae. Doxycycline can be used alone for outpatient therapy of community-acquired pneumonia or for inpatient therapy in conjunction with other antibiotics (Chapter 65). Tetracyclines deposit in growing bones and teeth and should be avoided in pregnant women and children under age 8.

Trimethoprim-sulfamethoxazole blocks sequential steps in the bacterial folate synthetic pathway, inhibiting growth because bacteria are unable to take up exogenous folate. This combination is active against both Gram-positive organisms (although activity against β-hemolytic streptococci is weak) and Gram-negative aerobes including enteric organisms (such as *E. coli* and *Klebsiella, Salmonella, Shigella,* and *Enterobacter* organisms), *Nocardia* spp., and *Chlamydia trachomatis.* It is active against many respiratory tract pathogens, including the pneumococci, *Haemophilus* spp., *Moraxella catarrhalis,* and *Klebsiella pneumonia* (but not *Chlamydia pneumoniae, Chlamydia psittaci,* or *Mycoplasma* spp.), making it an alternative to β-lactams for treatment of less serious respiratory infections. However, the high prevalence of strains of penicillin-nonsusceptible pneumococci (PNSP) and *E. coli* (up to 30% or more) that are resistant to trimethoprim-sulfamethoxazole no longer permits this combination to be used for empirical therapy of pneumonia or upper urinary tract infection. Trimethoprim-sulfamethoxazole has no activity against anaerobes.

Fluoroquinolones are synthetic, fluorinated analogues of nalidixic acid. They are active against numerous Gram-positive and Gram-negative bacteria. Newer compounds (e.g., gatifloxacin and moxifloxacin) have similar or slightly less activity than ciprofloxacin against Gram-negative organisms but enhanced activity against Gram-positive organisms and anaerobes. Because of reports of hepatic toxicity, trovafloxacin use is now restricted to inpatients for whom no safe and effective alternative exists. Intracellular pathogens, including *Legionella* and *Chlamydia* organisms and mycobacteria, are inhibited. Resistance results from selection of mutants producing altered drug target. Fluoroquinolones are effective for serious infections caused by multidrug-resistant bacteria, such as *Pseudomonas* and *Enterobacter* organisms. However, increasing use of fluoroquinolones for nosocomial infections has resulted in steadily increasing resistance in formerly susceptible organisms. In addition, the extensive use of fluoroquinolones in the outpatient setting has led to an increase in fluoro-quinolone-resistant pneumococci. While this resistance is still uncommon, treatment failures have been reported, particularly in patients who previously received fluoroquinolones (2). The safety of fluoroquinolones is unknown during pregnancy, and these drugs may damage growing cartilage. Thus, they are relatively contraindicated in patients under age 18, during pregnancy, and for nursing mothers.

Quinupristin/dalfopristin is a streptogramin antibiotic which combines two semisynthetic derivatives of pristinamycin. The two components act synergistically at the site of the bacterial ribosome to inhibit protein synthesis. Although quinupristin/dalfopristin is effective against a number of Gram-positive organisms, including *S. aureus* and *Streptococcus pyogenes,* it is used mainly for infections with vancomycin-resistant *Enterococcus faecium,* against which it is one of the few active drugs. Note that it is not active against vancomycin-resistant *Enterococcus faecalis.* Use of this drug is limited by side effects, including phlebitis, myalgia, and arthralgia.

Linezolid is the first approved antibiotic of the oxazolidinone class. It is a protein synthesis inhibitor that has activity against staphylocci, streptococci, and enterococci. This drug is useful for infection with resistant Gram-positive organisms, especially vancomycin-resistant enterococci and, in some cases, methicillin-resistant *S. aureus.* Concerns about rapid development of resistance warrant prudent prescribing of linezolid (3). Linezolid is highly bioavailable and can be given orally or intravenously at the same dosage. Thrombocytopenia has been reported, and platelet counts should be monitored, especially with extended use.

Problem Organisms

Multidrug-Resistant Gram-Negative Rods

Pseudomonas aeruginosa frequently causes infections in patients who have been treated previously with antibiotics, patients with loss of skin integrity (e.g., burn victims), neutropenic patients, and patients with cystic fibrosis. It is often isolated from the skin and respiratory tract of hospitalized patients, and respiratory colonization is especially common in intubated patients. Therefore, a positive culture (unless from a sterile site) does not necessarily imply that an infection is present. However, invasive *Pseudomonas* infections are associated with a high mortality rate. Accordingly, patients with suspected serious infection should be treated with antipseudomonal therapy if *Pseudomonas* organisms are isolated from a corresponding site, such as sputum or tracheal aspirate samples, and are predominant in the sample. In addition to pneumonia in the hospitalized patient, *P. aeruginosa* may cause urinary tract infection, skin and soft-tissue infection, osteomyelitis, endocarditis, and bacteremia.

P. aeruginosa is intrinsically resistant to a variety of antibiotics because of its outer-membrane barrier and efflux-pump mechanisms. During therapy with a number of penicillins and cephalosporins, chromosomal β-lactamases, which are not inactivated by currently available β-lactamase inhibitors, may be induced and degrade these drugs. *P. aeruginosa* also has acquired plasmid-encoded resistance to many drugs. Because the development of resistance during therapy has been well documented, the use of combination chemotherapy in severe *P. aeruginosa* infections has been advocated. This recommendation is based on studies suggesting that patients receiving combination therapy, usually an antipseudomonal penicillin and an aminoglycoside, have better outcomes than patients receiving single-drug therapy (4, 5). Because synergism between these two classes often can be demonstrated *in vitro*, it has been postulated that synergism is at least partially responsible for improved outcomes. However, clinical studies have yielded conflicting results, with single agents often equivalent to combination therapy, except perhaps in neutropenic patients (6). Recent studies have demonstrated acceptable outcomes with use of a single, potent agent such as a quinolone (7). Optimal treatment of invasive infection remains controversial (Table 64.1).

In selecting agents to cover invasive infections of *P. aeruginosa*, several factors should be taken into account. If combination chemotherapy is selected, an anti-pseudomonal β-lactam antibiotic and an aminoglycoside are most likely to be synergistic in vitro. Synergy sometimes occurs between β-lactam and fluoroquinolone antibiotics, but it does not occur with fluoroquinolone-aminoglycoside combinations. Combinations of two antipseudomonal β-lactam antibiotics should be avoided; these combinations are not synergistic and may even be antagonistic. For example, one β-lactam antibiotic may induce a β-lactamase that degrades the other. As with all infections with a known organism, the antibiotic susceptibilities of the pathogen should be taken into account as soon as they are available.

Enterobacter spp., and the related organisms *Klebsiella*, *Citrobacter*, and *Serratia* spp., also frequently cause infections in the hospital setting. These organisms often are resistant to multiple drugs. They may cause bacteremia, pneumonia, intraabdominal infections, wound infections, and urinary-tract infections. *Enterobacter* spp. produce an inducible β-lactamase that slowly degrades second- and third-generation cephalosporins. With *in vitro* testing of cephalosporins, strains may appear susceptible. However, if there is a high inoculum infection, mutants producing large amounts of β-lactamase proliferate because of their selective advantage. The emergence of resistance during therapy appears to be associated with an increased mortality rate (8). Cefepime, which is referred to as a fourth-generation cephalosporin, is less susceptible to degradation by the *Enterobacter* β-lactamase than are second- and third-generation cephalosporins; therefore,

resistance may be less likely to emerge during treatment with this agent. The addition of a second antibiotic (aminoglycosides have been studied most extensively) does not seem to prevent the emergence of resistance or improve clinical outcomes. Therefore, second- and third-generation cephalosporins are not recommended for treatment of *Enterobacter* infections. Second- and third-generation cephalosporins have been used successfully for infections with *Citrobacter* and *Serratia* spp., but some caution is warranted. The drugs of choice for such infections are trimethoprim-sulfamethoxazole, a fluoroquinolone, or a carbapenem. *Klebsiella* spp. are reliably susceptible to fluoroquinolones, aminoglycosides, and carbapenems and are usually susceptible to third-generation cephalosporins. Extended spectrum β-lactamases (ESBLs) are increasingly common in *Klebsiella* and other aerobic Gram-negative rods. If the presence of this enzyme is known or suspected, cephalosporins should be avoided.

E. coli is the most frequently isolated enteric pathogen. Antibiotic resistance in *E. coli* has surfaced over the past several years. *Ampicillin can no longer be used as initial therapy*, because more than 50% of community strains are resistant to this drug. Similarly, *trimethoprim-sulfamethoxazole is no longer recommended as initial therapy for upper urinary tract infections* because of the recent emergence of resistance (Chapter 68).

Penicillin-Nonsusceptible Pneumococci

S. pneumoniae has been recognized for many years as the most common bacterial pathogen in community-acquired pneumonia, meningitis, otitis media, and sinusitis. PNSP are becoming increasingly prevalent worldwide. Resistance is mediated by mutations in penicillin-binding proteins, with which all β-lactam antibiotics must interact; therefore, PNSP are cross-resistant to many other penicillins and cephalosporins. PNSP also frequently are resistant to multiple unrelated antibiotics, including erythromycin, tetracycline, and trimethoprim-sulfamethoxazole. Strains in which the minimum inhibitory concentration (MIC) of penicillin is 0.1 to 1.0 mg/mL have "intermediate resistance," and strains with MICs of 2 mg/ml or greater are designated "highly resistant." This distinction is important because strains with intermediate resistance can, in most instances, be treated like susceptible pneumococci. Special considerations exist in the treatment of pneumococcal meningitis, which is covered in Chapter 70.

If given intravenously for invasive pneumococcal infections other than meningitis, β-lactam antibiotics produce serum levels that are much greater than the MIC for intermediately resistant PNSP and usually exceed the MIC of highly resistant PNSP. Therefore, penicillin and other β-lactam antibiotics remain the mainstay of initial therapy for pneumococcal pneumonia and bacteremia. However, concerns about potential treatment failures have led to the recommendation that a third-generation cephalosporin,

TABLE 64.1

SUGGESTED INITIAL THERAPY FOR COMMON HOSPITAL PATHOGENS IN WHICH DRUG RESISTANCE IS A PROBLEM

Organism	Initial therapy	Resistance common	Resistance emerging
Escherichia coli	Cephalosporin β-lactam/β-lactamase inhibitor combination Fluoroquinolone Aminoglycoside	Ampicillin Extended-spectrum penicillins Trimethoprim-sulfamethoxazole	Fluoroquinolones Cephalosporins
Klebsiella spp.	Fluoroquinolone Aminoglycoside Cephalosporin	Extended-spectrum penicillins	β-lactam/β-lactamase inhibitor combinations Cephalosporins
Pseudomonas aeruginosa	Antipseudomonal penicillin or Ceftazidime or Imipenem or meropenem or Cefepime Plus amikacin or tobramycin[a]	Antipseudomonal penicillins β-lactam/β-lactamase inhibitor combinations Ceftazidime Fluoroquinolones	Imipenem or meropenem
Enterobacter spp.	Trimethoprim–sulfamethoxazole Fluoroquinolone Imipenem or meropenem Cefepime	2nd- and 3rd-generation cephalosporins	Fluoroquinolones
Streptococcus pneumoniae[b]	2nd- or 3rd-generation cephalosporin Ampicillin or penicillin G (high doses)	Intermediate resistance to penicillin G and ampicillin Erythromycin Trimethoprim–sulfamethoxazole	High-level resistance to penicillin G and ampicillin 2nd- and 3rd-generation cephalosporins
Enterococci	Ampicillin or penicillin G +/− gentamicin[c]	Amikacin Streptomycin Tobramycin Tetracyclines Macrolides	Vancomycin Penicillin G Ampicillin Gentamicin Fluoroquinolones
Staphylococcus aureus[d]	Antistaphylococcal penicillin Vancomycin	Antistaphylococcal penicillins 1st-generation cephalosporins Fluoroquinolones	Vancomycin

Note: In some cases, there is significant resistance to the recommended initial regimen. Therefore, antibiotic therapy should be modified based on the results of *in vitro* susceptibility testing as soon as the results become available. Narrow-spectrum antibiotics should be substituted for broad-spectrum antibiotics whenever the resistance profile permits.

[a] Most authorities recommend β-lactam–aminoglycoside combinations for serious infections, except those of the urinary tract.

[b] For invasive infections other than meningitis, β-lactam antibiotics remain the initial treatment of choice. If high level resistance is identified, vancomycin, a 3rd-generation cephalosporin, or imipenem are commonly recommended, although high doses of ampicillin or penicillin G still may be effective.

[c] Gentamicin should be added in cases of endocarditis and meningitis.

[d] Vancomycin is recommended for initial treatment if the local prevalence of methicillin-resistant *Staphylococcus aureus* (MRSA) is >5%. Methicillin-susceptible strains usually are susceptible to 1st-generation cephalosporins and fluoroquinolones. However, MRSA strains usually are *not susceptible* to 1st-generation cephalosporins. More than half of MRSA strains are resistant to ciprofloxacin. Although the newer fluoroquinolones are more potent antistaphylococcal agents, resistance develops easily and may emerge during therapy.

imipenem, or vancomycin be used for invasive infections caused by known highly resistant PNSP. Studies to date have not demonstrated poorer outcomes associated with invasive PNSP versus sensitive strains (9).

Methicillin and Vancomycin-Resistant Staphylococci

S. aureus causes serious community-acquired and nosocomial infections. It is an important cause of skin and soft-tissue infections, bacteremia, endocarditis, osteomyelitis, and septic arthritis. *S. aureus* bacteremia is a particular problem because the organism has a tendency to seed deep tissue sites, which may lead to relapse. *S. aureus* produces several toxins that may lead to staphylococcal toxic shock syndrome (Chapter 25) or staphylococcal scalded-skin syndrome. Most hospital strains and the majority of community strains are resistant to penicillin because of the production of β-lactamases.

Methicillin-resistant *S. aureus* (MRSA) is a significant pathogen in hospitalized patients and residents of long-term care facilities, and is increasingly common in the community. Approximately 35% of *S. aureus* isolates in the United States are methicillin-resistant, but local rates vary considerably. MRSA are resistant to all β-lactam antibiotics, as well as multiple other antibiotics. Vancomycin has emerged as the most reliable agent for treating invasive MRSA infections. Unfortunately, vancomycin has relatively poor tissue penetration and slow bactericidal activity, which may lead to treatment failures. A number of agents have been tried in conjunction with vancomycin, but in most cases the combination has not proved superior to vancomycin alone. Many MRSA strains are resistant to fluoroquinolones, so these agents should not be used unless *in vitro* susceptibility is confirmed. Thus, with the increasing prevalence of MRSA, vancomycin use has dramatically increased, contributing to the development of vancomycin-resistant enterococci and the newly described strains of *Staphylococcus aureus* with reduced susceptibility or frank resistance to vancomycin Although vancomycin is the drug of choice for established infections caused by MRSA, *its use should be severely restricted in other situations.* If one suspects an infection caused by *S. aureus* based on clinical criteria, or *S. aureus* has been isolated but antimicrobial susceptibilities are not yet known, vancomycin often is used empirically. However, *it should be stopped within 48–72 hours if MRSA is not detected.* (See Chapter 72 for a discussion of catheter infections caused by coagulase-negative staphylococci.)

S. aureus with intermediate susceptiblity to vancomycin (MIC = 8–16 mcg/mL) were first identified in 1996 and have now been reported from the United States, Asia, and Europe (10). In 2002, *S. aureus* isolates with high level resistance to vancomycin were identified in the United States (11). Unlike the organisms with intermediate susceptibility, those with high level resistance appear to have acquired one of the resistance mechanisms found in vancomycin-resistant enterococci. Intermediately resistant and resistant isolates appear to evolve from methicillin-resistant strains but remain susceptible to certain other antimicrobials, including trimethoprim-sulfamethoxazole, tetracyclines, quinupristin-dalfopristin, linezolid, and rifampin. In the cases described thus far, patients generally received vancomycin prior to isolation of resistant organisms. Although these organisms remain uncommon, their emergence has generated great concern. The Centers for Disease Control and Prevention have recommended close monitoring for these strains and strict isolation precautions for patients who are colonized or infected.

Vancomycin-Resistant Enterococci

Enterococci, even those considered to be "sensitive," are intrinsically resistant to a number of antibiotics. For example, although penicillin (or ampicillin) has long been the preferred treatment, enterococci usually have only moderate susceptibility because of penicillin-binding proteins with low affinity. A cell-wall inhibitor (penicillin, ampicillin, or vancomycin) and an aminoglycoside (streptomycin or gentamicin) are required to kill the enterococcus; such killing is usually necessary to cure endocarditis and meningitis. Enterococci are part of the normal gut flora. Because of their intrinsic drug resistance, these organisms proliferate when patients are treated with antimicrobial therapy. Enterococci are among the most common nosocomial pathogens, and debilitated patients with serious underlying diseases are at greatest risk. Use of urinary or vascular catheters and ICU admission also increase a patient's risk of enterococcal infection. Enterococci cause a number of infections, including urinary tract infection, bacteremia, endocarditis, and intraabdominal infection.

Vancomycin-resistant enterococci (VRE) emerged in the 1990s as difficult-to-treat pathogens that do not possess the same virulence as organisms such as *S. aureus*. Although outcomes appear to be worse in vancomycin-resistant enterococcal bacteremia compared with bacteremia because of sensitive enterococci, the difference is modest and has not been demonstrated in all studies (12). For those rare organisms that do not have high-level ampicillin or aminoglycoside resistance, these agents remain the drugs of choice. Quinupristin-dalfopristin is one option for treating infections caused by vancomycin-resistant *E. faecium*, which accounts for about 80% of VRE infections. Linezolid, given orally or intravenously, appears to be active against vancomycin-resistant *E. faecium* and *E. faecalis*, although experience with species other than *E. faecium* is limited. Efforts have focused on preventing the development and spread of VRE. Treatment with vancomycin, third-generation cephalosporins, and other antibiotics, especially those with anaerobic activity, is a strong risk factor for colonization or infection with VRE. Avoiding overuse of antibiotics is a critical part of combatting the increasing prevalence of VRE. Current Centers for Disease Control guidelines recommend contact isolation and use of gloves and gowns for examining patients with VRE, although this approach is not efficacious in all settings.

Prevention of Resistance

As previously discussed, antibiotic selection pressure is the primary mechanism by which resistance develops. Using antibiotics in appropriately high doses if indicated also helps prevent the emergence of resistance. The goal of antibiotic dosing is to achieve a sustained antibiotic level that is greater than the organism's MIC. In addition, therapy should be given for the shortest period known to be effective, and empirical antibiotics should be discontinued promptly if an infection is not identified.

Patient-to-patient transmission is also an important consideration. Health care workers frequently are colonized with resistant organisms and may facilitate spread of resistant bacteria. *Strict adherence to hand cleansing after touching patients or the contents of the hospital room is essential.* Recent data support the superiority of using alcohol-based hand rubs over traditional handwashing for this purpose (13). Contaminated objects, such as thermometers, also can transmit bacteria from one patient to another. Therefore, rigorous attention must be paid to appropriate disposal of such items, or to adequate sterilization if they are to be reused. This approach must be adopted in all patients, not just those known to be colonized or infected (analogous to "universal precautions" for handling bodily fluids). If this infection-control practice is applied only to patients at known risk, transmission will probably occur prior to the detection of resistant organisms, even in hospitals with vigilant surveillance in place.

In outbreak situations, the use of barrier devices (e.g., gowns) and isolating infected or colonized patients may be effective. Treating carriers of some organisms, such as MRSA, has been investigated as a means of reducing infection and preventing the spread of resistant organisms. Mupirocin and other agents have been shown to be effective at reducing MRSA colonization in the oropharynx and nares and may reduce the incidence of MRSA pneumonia in patients in the ICU. However, recolonization is common, as is the development of resistance. Another strategy, which may be more helpful in the future, is vaccination against organisms with a propensity for antimicrobial resistance. Administration of pneumococcal vaccine has efficacy in preventing invasive pneumococcal disease.

CONCLUSIONS

The threat of multidrug-resistant bacteria is one of the world's greatest medical challenges. At this point, it seems unlikely that the development of effective new agents will keep pace with the ability of bacteria to evade them. The potential future consequences are enormous, with some experts predicting a return to the conditions last seen in the preantibiotic era. Controlled use of antibiotics is the key to stemming this accelerating phenomenon. A reasonable compromise must be struck by taking resistance into account in prescribing antibiotics, yet not compounding the problem through the overzealous use of broad-spectrum antibiotics. Knowing the common pathogens in clinical syndromes, along with local resistance patterns, allows one to take a rational approach.

KEY POINTS

- Resistance is a consequence of antimicrobial exposure.
- Always choose drugs with a narrow spectrum of action, if possible; if initial coverage is broad, switch to a narrower-spectrum antibiotic once a pathogen is isolated.
- Always attempt to make a microbiologic diagnosis.
- Therapy should be continued for the shortest duration known to be effective.
- Except in a few instances, there is little evidence supporting the "double coverage" of organisms.

REFERENCES

1. Steinman MA, Landefeld CS, Gonzales R. Predictors of broad-spectrum antibiotic prescribing for acute respiratory tract infections in adult primary care. *JAMA* 2003;289:719–725.
2. Davidson R, Cavalcanti R, Brunton JL, et al. Resistance to levofloxacin and failure of treatment of pneumococcal pneumonia. *N Engl J Med* 2002;346:747–750.
3. Tsiodras S, Gold HS, Sakoulas G. Linezolid resistance in a clinical isolate of *Staphylococcus aureus*. *Lancet* 2001;358:207–208.
4. Leibovici L, Paul M, Poznanski O, et al. Monotherapy versus beta-lactam-aminoglycoside combination treatment for gram-negative bacteremia: a prospective, observational study. *Antimicrob Agents Chemother* 1997;41:1127–1133.
5. Hilf M, Yu VL, Sharp J, et al. Antibiotic therapy for Pseudomonas aeruginosa bacteremia: outcome correlations in a prospective study of 200 patients. *Am J Med* 1989;87:540–546.
6. Vidal F, Mensa J, Almela M, et al. Epidemiology and outcome of *Pseudomonas aeruginosa* bacteremia, with special emphasis on the influence of antibiotic treatment: analysis of 189 episodes. *Arch Intern Med* 1996;156:2121–2126.
7. Torres A, Bauer TT, Leon-Gil C, et al. Treatment of severe nosocomial pneumonia: a prospective randomised comparison of intravenous ciprofloxacin with imipenem/cilastatin. *Thorax* 2000;55: 1033–1039.
8. Chow JW, Fine MJ, Shlaes DM, et al. Enterobacter bacteremia: clinical features and emergence of antibiotic resistance during therapy. *Ann Intern Med* 1991;115:585–590.
9. Feiken DR, Schuchat A, Kolczak M, et al. Mortality from invasive pneumococcal pneumonia in the era of antibiotic resistance, 1995–1997. *Am J Public Health* 2000;90:223–229.
10. *Staphylococcus aureus* with reduced susceptibility to vancomycin—Illinois, 1999. *MMWR Morb Mortal Wkly Rep* 2000;48:1165–1167.
11. *Staphylococcus aureus* resistant to vancomycin—United States, 2002. *MMWR Morb Mortal Wkly Rep* 2002;51:565–567.
12. Vergis EN, Hayden MK, Chow JW, et al. Determinants of vancomycin resistance and mortality rates in enterococcal bacteremia. *Ann Intern Med* 2001;135:484–492.
13. Pittet D. Hand hygiene: improved standards and practice for hospital care. *Curr Opin Infect Dis* 2003;16:327–335.

ADDITIONAL READING

Cassell GH, Mekalanos J. Development of antimicrobial agents in the era of new and reemerging infectious diseases and increasing antibiotic resistance. *JAMA* 2001;285:601–605.

Cooper BS, Stone SP, Kibbler CC, et al. Isolation measures in the hospital management of methicillin–resistant *Staphylococcus aureus*: systematic review of the literature. *BMJ* 2004;329:533–538.

Enright MC, Robinson DA, Randle G. The evolutionary history of methicillin-resistant *Staphylococcus aureus* (MRSA). *Proc Natl Acad Sci* 2002;99:7687–7692.

Hoban DJ, Doern GV, Fluit AC, et al. Worldwide prevalence of antimicrobial resistance in *Streptococcus pneumoniae, Haemophilus influenzae,* and *Moraxella catarrhalis* in the SENTRY antimicrobial surveillance program, 1997–1999. *Clin Infect Dis* 2001;32(Suppl 2):S81–S93.

Hooper DC. Emerging mechanisms of fluoroquinolone resistance. *Emerg Infect Dis* 2001;7:337–341.

Jacobs MR. *Streptococcus pneumoniae*: epidemiology and patterns of resistance. *Am J Med* 2004;117(Suppl 3A):3S–15S.

Resistance of *Streptococcus pneumoniae* to fluoroquinolones—United States, 1995–1999. *MMWR Morb Mortal Wkly Rep* 2001; 50:800–804.

Community-Acquired Pneumonia

65

Ethan A. Halm   Michael J. Fine

INTRODUCTION

There are approximately 4 million cases of community-acquired pneumonia (CAP) per year in the United States, resulting in more than 1 million hospitalizations. Thus, CAP is one of the most common inpatient medical conditions in both university and community hospitals, accounting for 2% of all hospital discharges. It is the most common infectious cause of death and is the sixth leading cause of death overall in the United States. The aggregate cost of hospitalization for the disease approaches $9 billion per year. Wide variations in rates of hospitalization, intensive care, length of hospital stay, choice and duration of antibiotic therapy, and performance of key processes of care for pneumonia have been well documented within different geographic regions, different hospitals in the same area, and even within the same hospital. Substantial differences in hospitalization rates and length of stay for pneumonia persist even after adjusting for disease severity, comorbid conditions, and hospital characteristics.

The traditional approach to managing CAP has been oriented primarily toward inpatient care, with considerable effort expended to determine the specific microbiologic etiology. This often involves repeated diagnostic studies of sputum and blood. The heterogeneity of bacterial and viral causes of CAP has long been recognized. Traditionally, pathogens are classified as "typical," referring to *Streptococcus pneumoniae* (the most common organism), *Haemophilus influenzae*, *Moraxella catarrhalis*, *Klebsiella pneumoniae*, other Gram-negative bacteria, and *Staphylococcus aureus*, among others. Atypical pathogens include *Mycoplasma pneumoniae*, *Legionella* spp., *Chlamydia pneumoniae* (TWAR), *Chlamydia psittaci*, and respiratory viruses.

There are several limitations to an etiology-oriented approach. First, microbiologic studies emphasize the difficulty of establishing a definitive, etiologic diagnosis in most cases of CAP, even when comprehensive microbiologic and serologic testing is performed. Second, contemporary series have highlighted broad geographic and seasonal differences in the relative incidence of various pneumonia pathogens. Finally, it is not possible to distinguish "typical" from "atypical" pathogens on the basis of the initial history, physical exam, and laboratory studies chapter (1–4).

This chapter describes a cost-effective, outcomes-oriented approach that de-emphasizes reliance on sputum studies in antibiotic selection and advocates the performance of key processes of care, such as the early institution of empiric, broad-spectrum antibiotics active against the most common pathogens. It also presents validated algorithms for risk-stratifying patients on presentation and outlines objective criteria for determining clinical stability so that patients can be safely converted to oral antibiotics and discharged in a timely fashion.

ISSUES AT THE TIME OF ADMISSION

Clinical Presentation

The overall prevalence of CAP among unselected patients presenting with respiratory complaints ranges from about 3%–10%, depending on the setting. Unfortunately, there are no individual (or combination of) findings on the history, physical examination, or laboratory examination that can rule in or exclude the diagnosis of pneumonia with adequate accuracy (4). Therefore, the diagnosis of CAP requires both the presence of *symptoms and signs of acute pulmonary infection and evidence of a new radiographic infiltrate*. Patients with pneumonia classically present with several days of fever, chills, sweats, shortness of breath, productive cough with purulent sputum, and pleuritic chest pain. Physical examination also reveals findings of lung consolidation, such as crackles, egophony, and increased fremitus. Unfortunately, the frequency and severity of these various signs and symptoms are highly variable. Nearly all patients (>90%) complain of cough and fatigue, two-thirds have dyspnea and sputum production, and about half have pleuritic chest pain. Nonrespiratory symptoms are present in 10%–30% of patients, including: headache, nausea and vomiting, abdominal pain, diarrhea, myalgias, arthralgias, and mental confusion. Older patients with pneumonia have significantly fewer symptoms than the non-elderly. Because of this phenomenon, the chest radiograph is an integral part of any workup of an elderly patient presenting with fever, constitutional symptoms, or mental status changes, even in the absence of respiratory complaints.

Fever is present in more than 80% of patients presenting with pneumonia, whereas hypothermia is present in 1%. Hypothermia is more frequent in elderly patients and those in nursing homes. Many patients also present with tachypnea, tachycardia, and diminished oxygen saturation. Approximately 80% of patients have crackles on auscultation, although classic physical findings of pulmonary consolidation are present in only 30% or fewer cases.

Differential Diagnosis and Initial Evaluation

The initial evaluation of patients presenting with suspected CAP should be aimed at confirming the diagnosis. Information from the history and physical examination is crucial in distinguishing patients with uncomplicated CAP from those with other pneumonia syndromes. A history of aspiration pneumonia or cerebrovascular disease, an impaired gag reflex, altered mental status, poor dentition, or foul-smelling sputum increases the likelihood of aspiration pneumonia. Post-obstructive pneumonia may present as recurrent episodes of pneumonia, particularly in those with a longstanding history of smoking. Patients who are immunosuppressed because of medications or HIV infection are at risk for opportunistic pathogens in addition to the organisms described previously.

Other noninfectious processes that should be part of the differential diagnosis include congestive heart failure, noncardiogenic pulmonary edema, pulmonary embolism, pulmonary hemorrhage, malignancy, collagen vascular disease or vasculitis, pulmonary-renal syndromes, and hypersensitivity pneumonitis. A careful clinical history and physical examination can usually define the likelihood of most of these nonpneumonia processes. Because of the high prevalence of congestive heart failure, a thorough cardiac history

and examination should be part of the initial evaluation of all patients suspected of having pneumonia.

Given the limited sensitivity and specificity of the history and physical examination, a chest radiograph is essential to confirm the diagnosis of pneumonia. Although the presence of a new pulmonary infiltrate is the gold standard for the diagnosis of pneumonia, it is important to recognize the limitations of chest radiography. There is some evidence that chest radiography might miss more subtle evidence of pulmonary consolidation compared to high-resolution computed tomography. False negative findings have also been reported in patients with dehydration on admission. Contrary to traditional teaching, radiographic appearance cannot accurately predict the etiology of pneumonia, nor does it differentiate bacterial from nonbacterial causes. Furthermore, agreement between radiologists interpreting the same chest radiographs is modest.

The chest radiograph can provide useful information about effusions, air-fluid levels (consistent with lung abscess), masses, and pulmonary vascular congestion. Pleural effusions are present in approximately 10% of patients with CAP. Bilateral effusions indicate more serious pneumonia with a higher risk of death during the short-term. Unusual findings of cavitation or miliary opacities can be helpful in suggesting other diseases. Characteristics of the radiographic infiltrate can be affected by a variety of features including underlying lung architecture, concomitant diseases (e.g., congestive heart failure or neutropenia), radiographic technique, and dehydration. In addition, both alveolar and interstitial opacities on chest radiograph may result from a variety of causes.

Although not necessary in the majority of patients with pneumonia, computed tomography of the chest may be useful in evaluating unusual cases or further characterizing pleural disease, cavitation, lymphadenopathy, or interstitial abnormalities. The absence of a pulmonary infiltrate in a patient suspected of having pneumonia should prompt strong consideration of alternative diagnoses.

There are no features of the history, physical examination, laboratory exam, or chest radiograph that are consistently predictive of a microbiological cause. Furthermore, there are no clinical or radiographic findings that allow one to accurately differentiate typical from atypical bacterial pathogens or bacterial from viral causes. Thus, the terms *typical* and *atypical* are misleading.

The usefulness of routine *sputum Gram stain and culture* is controversial. High-quality, uncontaminated sputum studies can help identify the causative organism and facilitate pathogen-tailored antibiotic therapy. However, sputum Gram's stain and culture tend to have low sensitivity, specificity, and predictive values. For example, the positive predictive value of finding *S. pneumoniae* on Gram's stain is about 30%–50%. The utility of sputum studies is further limited by the fact that about 30% of patients cannot produce an adequate sputum specimen, and 30% have received antibiotics prior to microbiologic testing. Even when studies are positive, it is often hard to know whether the organism originated in the lung or oropharynx. The diagnostic yield of sputum studies is further limited by the fact that many common pathogens, including *Mycoplasma pneumoniae* and *Chlamydia pneumoniae*, are not seen on Gram stain and are difficult to culture from sputum. Thus, sputum studies generally add little clinically useful information in the initial selection of antibiotics for an individual patient. The antibiotic-susceptibility information generated by sputum cultures is probably their most valuable feature both in terms of assuring appropriate antibiotic sensitivity for an individual patient and for monitoring resistance patterns in a given hospital or community.

Blood cultures are positive in only 5%–10% of patients hospitalized with CAP. About one-half of positive cultures are thought to be contaminants. *Streptococcus pneumoniae* is the most common cause of true positive blood cultures (accounting for about 50% of confirmed bacteremias) followed by *Haemophilus influenzae*, Gram-negative rods, and *Staphylococcus* spp. Patients who are ill enough to be hospitalized should have two sets of blood cultures drawn prior to the initiation of parenteral antibiotics. In one large study, the standard use of blood cultures within 24 hours of presentation was associated with decreased case fatality rates (5). Thus, blood cultures are increasingly viewed as a key process of care in the treatment of this disease. Monitoring antibiotic susceptibility from blood isolates is also a key factor in tracking the progression of drug resistant organisms. However, the clinical utility of subsequent sputum or blood cultures, especially once antibiotics have begun, is extremely limited. Other normally sterile sites such as pleural fluid and cerebrospinal fluid may yield definitive microbiologic data, but these fluids are not routinely obtained unless there are specific clinical indications.

For patients in whom infection by *Legionella* organisms is a concern, radioimmunoassay tests for urinary *Legionella* antigen have demonstrated sensitivity of 75%–99% and specificity of 99%. These tests only detect *Legionella pneumophila* serotype I, which accounts for about 70%–90% of all pneumonia resulting from *Legionella* organisms. *Legionella* infection can also be diagnosed rapidly by examination of pulmonary secretions with direct fluorescent antibody assays or specialized culture medium, though sensitivity of these tests tends to be lower (25%–80% and 50%–70%, respectively). Unfortunately, there are currently no rapid, commercially available tests for detecting *Mycoplasma pneumoniae*, *Chlamydia pneumoniae*, *Chlamydia psittaci*, or most respiratory viruses.

Although an early attempt at identifying a pathogen should be made in all patients, it is important to recognize that definitive microbial etiology is never found in 50%–70% of patients in usual practice, or in 30%–50% of patients in research studies. When an organism is recovered, it is increasingly common to find evidence of mixed infection. Fewer than 8% of patients have antibiotics changed because of the results of microbiological testing.

Because a definitive microbial diagnosis is not available in the vast majority of patients, antibiotic selection is usually empiric. Because of this, one should strongly consider covering potentially life-threatening pathogens such as *Legionella* spp., which are not covered by β-lactam antibiotics, especially in moderate- and high-risk cases. Though traditional teaching has emphasized *Legionella* spp. as the cause of severe pneumonia among the elderly and immunosuppressed, more recent data found that nearly half of patients with confirmed *Legionella* pneumonia had mild or moderate pneumonia and many patients had no major comorbidities or history of immunosuppression. Mixed infection with *Legionella* and other bacterial pathogens was also seen.

Indications for Hospitalization

The hospitalization decision should focus on three main factors: (1) the risk of short-term mortality and complications, (2) the patient's clinical stability, and (3) mitigating medical or psychosocial problems. The overall 30-day mortality rate from systematic reviews of CAP patients was 13.7%, ranging from 5.1% for cohorts that included ambulatory and hospitalized patients to 36.5% for a series of intensive care unit patients (4, 5). A *validated prediction rule* for quantitation of risk for persons with CAP is presented in Figure 65.1. This Pneumonia Severity Index (PSI) prediction rule relies on information readily available at the time of initial presentation and can be used to stratify patients into five risk classes with mortality rates ranging from 0.1%–27% (6). Use of this prediction rule to aid the admission decision has been endorsed by recent U.S. and Canadian national subspecialty practice guidelines for CAP (1–3, 7). Figure 65.2 outlines an algorithm for using the PSI risk-stratification information in combination with other key clinical data to determine whether a patient should be admitted or treated as an outpatient (8). Patients with contraindications to outpatient treatment caused by hypoxemia (room-air oxygen saturation less than 90% or PaO_2 less than 60 mm Hg), hemodynamic instability (shock or hypotension not responsive to initial fluid resuscitation), or active coexisting conditions requiring hospitalization should be admitted independent of their PSI Risk Class. Absent these acute features, patients should be risk-stratified using the PSI prediction rule depicted in Figure 65.1. Patients in Risk Classes I through III can be considered low risk, with a cumulative 30-day mortality rate of less than 1%, and can be managed as outpatients. Some patients in Risk Classes I through III may have other mitigating factors such as frail physical condition, poor response to oral therapy, substance abuse, or other psychosocial issues that may be relative contraindications to initial outpatient management. For these patients, alternatives to standard inpatient admission include brief inpatient admission, 23 hours of observation, admission to a sub-acute or intermediate care facility, "enhanced" home care (initial home parenteral antibiotic therapy with visiting nurse monitoring), and close outpatient follow-up.

Algorithm

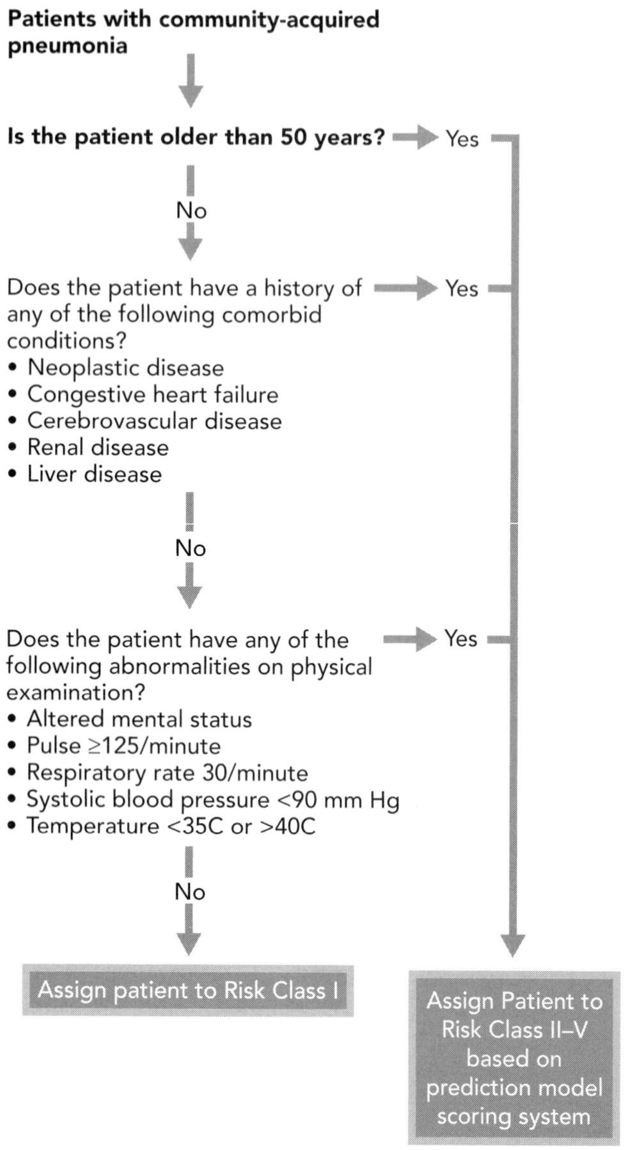

Patients with community-acquired pneumonia

↓

Is the patient older than 50 years? → Yes ┐

↓ No

Does the patient have a history of → Yes ┤
any of the following comorbid
conditions?
• Neoplastic disease
• Congestive heart failure
• Cerebrovascular disease
• Renal disease
• Liver disease

↓ No

Does the patient have any of the → Yes ┤
following abnormalities on physical
examination?
• Altered mental status
• Pulse ≥125/minute
• Respiratory rate 30/minute
• Systolic blood pressure <90 mm Hg
• Temperature <35C or >40C

↓ No

Assign patient to Risk Class I

Assign Patient to
Risk Class II–V
based on
prediction model
scoring system

Scoring System

Patient Characteristics	Points Assigned[a]
Demographic Factors	
Age: Males	age (y)
Females	age (y) – 10
Nursing home resident	+10
Comorbid Illnesses	
Neoplastic disease	+10
Liver disease	+20
Congestive heart failure	+10
Cerebrovascular disease	+10
Renal disease	+10
Physical Examination Findings	
Altered mental status	+20
Respiratory rate ≥30/minute	+20
Systolic blood pressure <90 mm Hg	+20
Temperature <35 or ≥40C	+15
Pulse ≥125/minute	+10
Laboratory Findings	
pH <7.35	+30
BUN >30 mg/dL	+20
Sodium <130 mEq/L	+20
Glucose >250 mg/dL	+10
Hematocrit <30%	+10
pO$_2$ <60 mm Hg[b]	+10
Pleural effusion	+10

[a]A risk score (total point score) for a given patient is obtained by summing the patient age in years (age – 10 for females) and the points for each applicable patient characteristic.

[b]Oxygen saturation <90% also was considered abnormal.

Stratification of Risk Score

Risk	Risk Class	Based on	Mortality
Low	I	Algorithm	0.1%
Low	II	≥70 total points	0.6%
Low	III	71-90 total points	0.9%
Moderate	IV	91-130 total points	9.3%
High	V	>130 total points	27.0%

Figure 65.1 Prediction model for identification of patient risk for persons with community-acquired pneumonia. (Adapted from Fine MJ, Auble TE, Yealy DM, et al. Improving the appropriateness of hospital care in community-acquired pneumonia: a prediction rule to identify patients at low risk for mortality and other adverse medical outcomes. *N Engl J Med*, 1997;336:243–250, with permission.)

This choice depends on the needed level of clinical monitoring, patient frailty, requirements for functional assistance, and patient and family preferences, as well as the local availability of these options. One implication of the algorithm is that age greater than 65 alone is not sufficient reason for hospitalization.

All patients in Risk Classes IV and V should be admitted to the hospital, given their significantly higher mortality and complication rates unless there are extenuating circumstances (e.g., terminal care). Other indications for admission include suspected or confirmed suppurative or metastatic complication (empyema, lung abscess, endocarditis, meningitis, or osteomyelitis) or the presence of high risk pathogens (e.g., *S. aureus*, anaerobes, and Gram-negative rods). For patients in Risk Classes I through III who are admitted because of nonmedical factors, consideration should be given to lower cost alternatives of care if such options are available.

A large multicenter, randomized controlled trial of a critical pathway for the treatment of pneumonia provides strong evidence that a PSI-based admission decision algo-

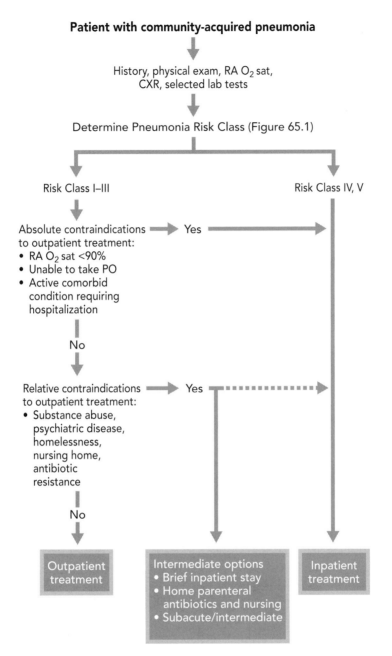

Figure 65.2 Hospitalization decision tree. CXR, chest radiograph; RA, room air.

rithm is safe and effective (9). Compared to control sites, hospitals randomized to implement the pneumonia pathway admitted significantly fewer low risk patients (defined as PSI Risk Class I through III, 31% vs. 49%). There were no changes in admission rates among moderate- or high-risk cases (Risk Classes IV through V) for whom the protocol recommended hospitalization. Although use of the hospital decreased, there were no differences between the two groups in ICU use, mortality, readmissions, complications or health-related quality of life at 2 and 6 weeks. This study confirms the results of an earlier single institution intervention trial that found that a PSI-based emergency department guideline reduced admissions among low-risk patients from 58%–43% without adverse effects on

mortality, symptom resolution, functional recovery or patient satisfaction (10). It is worth noting that in both studies approximately 30%–40% of low risk patients still required hospitalization because of clinical severity, other active clinical problems, psychosocial circumstances, or patient preferences.

Indications for Initial Intensive Care Unit Admission

In a large, multicenter CAP study, 9.2% of inpatients were admitted to an ICU, including 11.4% of class IV patients and 17.3% of class V patients (6). Clear indications for ICU admission include hemodynamic instability resulting from sepsis syndrome or hypovolemia, respiratory failure requiring mechanical ventilation, and severe hypoxemia or respiratory distress meriting close observation and frequent monitoring of clinical status or arterial blood gases. Given the high anticipated mortality rate, ICU care is appropriate for many patients in Risk Class V. Patients with coexisting exacerbations of comorbid conditions or with severe metabolic derangements may also benefit from a higher level of monitoring and treatment.

Initial Therapy

Because the responsible pneumonia pathogen is not known in the majority of cases in usual practice, the early initiation of empiric, broad-spectrum antibiotic therapy is strongly recommended. Our recommendations for first-line parenteral therapy in patients hospitalized with CAP are: (1) a second-generation or third-generation cephalosporin (e.g., cefuroxime, ceftriaxone, ceftizoxime, or cefotaxime) plus a macrolide or doxycycline, or (2) an anti-pneumococcal fluoroquinolone (e.g., gatifloxacin, levofloxacin, or moxifloxacin) (1–3, 8). These antimicrobial regimens were associated with 30% lower risk–adjusted odds of death within 30 days compared with therapy with a third-generation cephalosporin alone (11). Combination β-lactam and β-lactamase inhibitors with a macrolide (or doxycycline) is another alternative, although these regimens have not appeared to be as clinically effective in recent outcome studies. Antibiotic regimens that cover both typical and atypical pathogens have also been associated with shorter lengths of stay. Older fluoroquinolones (ciprofloxacin and ofloxacin) have been associated with treatment failure in some patients with pneumococcal disease. The newer fluoroquinolones (levofloxacin, gatifloxacin, moxifloxacin, sparfloxacin, and gemifloxacin) have greater activity against *S. pneumoniae* and *S. aureus*, and provide excellent coverage against atypical bacterial pathogens, including *Legionella* spp. As of January 2005, gatifloxacin, levofloxacin, and moxifloxacin were the primary anti-pneumococcal fluoroquinolones available as intravenous and oral preparations. Because of reports of severe hepatotoxicity, the use of alatrofloxacin/trovafloxacin is restricted to use on inpatients with no other safe and effective alternatives.

As suggested by the most recent American Thoracic Society guidelines, parenteral azithromycin alone may also be appropriate for empiric treatment of selected, low-risk patients (non-ICU patients without underlying cardiopulmonary disease who do not have risk factors for Gram-negative rods or drug-resistant *S. pneumoniae* [2]). However, the Infectious Disease Society of America guidelines do not recommend macrolide monotherapy as first-line therapy (1). Uncertainty about growing resistance to macrolides among drug-resistant pneumococcal isolates may explain some of the descrepancy among the different subspecialty recommendations. For individuals with

β-lactam allergy, an anti-pneumococcal fluoroquinolone (or azithromycin for a low-risk patient) would be a safe, broad-spectrum alternative.

Antibiotic recommendations for the treatment of confirmed cases of *Legionella* pneumonia have changed over the last few years. A fluoroquinolone or azithromycin are now considered to be first line choices, replacing the traditional regimen of high dose erythromycin (1 gram every 6 hours) because of their greater penetration into lung tissue, in vitro activity, and lower toxicity profile. Other acceptable alternatives include tetracycline, doxycycline, or clarithromycin. For severe cases of *Legionella*, many experts recommend adding rifampin to a fluoroquinolone or azithromycin.

Empiric treatment of patients requiring ICU admission should include two drugs to cover the increased risk of *S. aureus*, *Legionella*, drug-resistant pneumococci, *Pseudomonas aeruginosa*, and other Gram-negative bacteria. Patients with no increased risk for *Pseudomonas aeruginosa* or other resistant Gram-negative rod infection should receive one of the following combination regimens: (1) a third-generation cephalosporin plus an anti-pneumococcal fluroquinolone or macrolide or (2) β-lactam/β-lactamase inhibitor plus an anti-pneumococcal fluoroquinolone or macrolide (1–3). Observational data suggest that dual therapy is associated with lower mortality rates for patients with bacteremic pneumococcal pneumonia. Those at increased risk for *Pseudomonas aeruginosa* or other resistant Gram-negative rod infection should be treated with an anti-pseudomonal β-lactam plus an aminoglycoside plus an anti-pneumococcal fluoroquinolone or macrolide. Administration of two anti-pseudomonal agents is recommended for synergy until culture and sensitivities can rule out the possibility of resistance. If a definitive diagnosis becomes available, antimicrobial coverage should be narrowed according to the specific drug sensitivities.

There are some situations in which these antibiotic recommendations may not be optimal. Residents of institutional settings such as nursing homes have higher rates of methicillin-resistant staphylococcal pneumonia and may require coverage with vancomycin until culture results and sensitivities are known. Patients with aspiration pneumonia should be treated with an antimicrobial agent with activity against oropharyngeal anaerobes (e.g., clindamycin or β-lactam/β-lactamase inhibitor). Cases with a more protracted clinical presentation, hemoptysis, significant weight loss, or anemia should raise suspicion of more indolent pulmonary infections such as tuberculosis or fungal disease. In these instances, respiratory isolation should be immediately instituted until tuberculosis can be ruled out.

Increasing rates of drug-resistant *S. pneumoniae* (DRSP) and reduced susceptibility to a growing number of agents make generic antibiotic selection recommendations challenging. While penicillin resistance among DRSP isolates is often of greatest concern, high levels of cross-resistance to macrolides, tetracyclines, and amoxillin/clavulanic acid have also been documented (12). Therefore, clinicians need to be cognizant of local antibiotic resistance patterns. Reduced susceptibility of DRSP to the antipneumococcal fluoroquinolones (gatifloxacin, levofloxacin, and moxifloxacin) is uncommon, but is likely to grow given their widespread use.

The laboratory and clinical definitions of drug resistance are also in flux and not always the same. The historical MIC cutpoints for DRSP were based on data regarding the treatment of meningitis, not pneumonia, sinusitis, or otitis media. The Drug-Resistant *Streptococcus pneumoniae* Therapeutic Working Group recommends that the break points for interpreting penicillin susceptibility of *S. pneumoniae* isolates in patients with pneumonia be revised upward (12) to define susceptibility of pulmonary isolates as an MIC ≤1 mcg/mL, intermediate ≤2 mcg/mL, and resistant ≥4 mcg/mL. The clinical significance of intermediate-level resistance in terms of altering antimicrobial therapy for pneumococcal pneumonia is unknown and is an area of active investigation. However, for confirmed, high-level penicillin-resistant *Pneumococcus* spp. (MIC ≥4.0 mcg/mL), a highly active anti-pneumococcal fluoroquinolone, vancomycin, or possibly clindamycin are the drugs of choice. Because of concerns about the overuse of vancomycin increasing resistance, empiric use of vancomycin for patients with CAP is not recommended unless there is suspicion or documentation of accompanying penicillin-resistant pneumococcal meningitis (Chapter 70) (2–4).

Indications for Early Consultation

Between 80%–90% of cases of pneumonia are cared for by generalist physicians. There are no data to support the routine use of pulmonary or infectious disease consultation for most uncomplicated cases of CAP. However, early infectious disease consultation should be considered if unusual or highly resistant pathogens are identified. Early pulmonary consultation is indicated when diagnostic bronchoscopy is needed. If pneumonia is complicated by empyema, a surgeon or interventional radiologist should be consulted for placement of a chest tube for pleural drainage. Consultation with a pulmonary specialist also may be helpful for patients with respiratory failure requiring mechanical ventilation or when noninfectious pulmonary processes are suspected. Specialty consultation is also recommended for patients with CAP who fail to improve according to the timeline described below or who are getting worse.

ISSUES DURING THE COURSE OF HOSPITALIZATION

Figure 65.3 shows a sample critical pathway for CAP that delineates the multidisciplinary processes of care during the hospital stay. The initiation of parenteral antibiotics as early as possible should be a high priority. Patients who receive intravenous antibiotics within the first 8 hours of presentation have higher rates of survival compared with those in whom antimicrobial therapy was delayed (5). Recent data suggest that the receipt of antibiotics within 4 hours of arrival confers an additional survival benefit (13). Practically, this means that a patient needs to receive his or her first dose of antibiotics in the emergency department. All patients should have room-air oxygen saturation assessed, and supplemental oxygen should be administered to those individuals with oxygen saturation less than 90%–92%. The correlation between oxygen saturation measurements by pulse oximetry and the actual PaO_2 may differ at altitude and vary according to the degree of skin pigmentation. Patients with chronic hypoxemia should have oxygen therapy titrated to achieve their normal baseline PaO_2 or oxygen saturation. Intravenous fluids should be administered for volume depletion or inability to take fluids by mouth. Bronchospasm should be treated with bronchodilators delivered by metered-dose inhalers or by nebulizer. If the patient is not ambulatory and is likely to be bedridden for several days, prophylactic administration of subcutaneous heparin should be considered to prevent the development of deep vein thrombosis. Fever and pleuritic chest pain can be treated with acetaminophen or nonsteroidal anti-inflammatory drugs if there are no contraindications.

The risk of clinical deterioration is greatest during the first 2 days of hospitalization (14). Nearly two-thirds of ICU, CCU, or telemetry unit admissions in patients with pneumonia occur on the day of admission. Another 15% occur on the day after admission. Therefore, close monitoring of vital signs, oxygen saturation, need for supplemental oxygen, mental status, and clinical stability is imperative and ought to be performed a minimum of three to four times a day in the first two days. In addition, a nursing assessment of the patient's home situation, activities of daily living, and cognitive abilities should be done in the first 24 hours of hospitalization to help anticipate major problems that may delay hospital discharge significantly once a patient is medically stable. Because the average patient will become clinically stable on days 3 or 4, laying the groundwork to facilitate timely discharge must begin shortly after admission (14).

On day 2, microbiology results should be checked and the antibiotic regimen adjusted as appropriate if a definitive pathogen is identified. The official interpretation of the initial chest radiograph should also be verified, because preliminary readings may be revised or alternative causes for pulmonary opacities suggested. By day 2, most patients should be euvolemic. If the patient is able to take fluids by mouth, supplemental intravenous fluids can be discontinued. Vital signs should continue to be monitored regularly and supplemental oxygen titrated to the oxygen saturation.

	Day 1: 1st 4 hours of Stay	Day 1: Additional Tasks	Day 2:	Day 3:	Avg. Discharge Day: Days 3–4
Tests	• CXR • CBC/Diff, Chem-7, UA • Blood cultures • Room air O$_2$ Sat • ABG if O$_2$ Sat <90% • Consider sputum for AFB if upper lobe or cavitary disease • Determine pneumonia risk class (Figure 65.1)	• Notify PMD • Assess gag reflex (R/O aspiration)	• Check official CXR interpretation • Check culture result • D/C labs if normal	*If not improving:* • Consider CXR • R/O effusion-tap? • Check culture result • ?Uncovered or resistant organism • ?Nonpulmonary causes of infiltrates • ?Specialty consult	Notify PMD of patient discharge and F/U plans
Medications and Therapeutics	*Early Antibiotics:* • Begin after blood cx • IV ABX within 2–4 hours (in ED if possible) • 2nd or 3rd gen. Cephalosporin plus macrolide *Consider:* • Resp. isolation if R/O TB • O$_2$ if RA Sat<92% • IV fluids if unable to take PO or if dehydrated • If bronchospasm, bronchodilator • MDIs per RT protocol	• SQ Heparin if non-ambulatory • IV to saline lock if no hypovolemia and able to take PO	• Adjust ABX if C+S result • D/C IV fluids if appropriate • Titrate O$_2$ to keep Sat >92%	• Switch to PO ABX when clinical stability criteria are fulfilled • Adjust ABX to C+S results • D/C IV fluids if appropriate • Wean O$_2$ as tolerated	• Discharge criteria met? • Tolerates PO ABX? • Consider influenza or pneumonoccal vaccine before discharge
Nursing/ Assessment	• Vitals/Temp • RA O$_2$ Sat (if not done) • I's & O's • Orthostatics (if indicated) • Admit weight	• Vitals/Temp • RA O$_2$ Sat • Assess ADLs • I's & O's • RN assessment completed • Falls/cog. screen	• Vitals/Temp • RA O$_2$ Sat • I's & O's as needed • Assist w/ ADLs	• Vitals/Temp • RA O$_2$ Sat • Increase ADLs • D/C I's & O's	• Vitals/Temp • RA O$_2$ Sat • Patient/family can perform ADLs
Activity	• Bedrest with BR privileges	• Activity ad lib	• Increase activity as tolerated • PT consult if needed	• Increase activity as tolerated • SOB w/ activity?	• Ambulate or ADLs with no more than mild SOB
Nutrition	• Diet as tolerated • Encourage PO fluids unless contraindicated	• Encourage fluids • Nutritional screen	• Encourage fluids	• Encourage fluids	• PO intake adequate or plan for supplementation
Discharge Planning		• Discuss expected LOS w/ SW & pt/family (avg. 4 days) • Review home situation	• PMD/RN/SW communication re: patient status • Continue plan for discharge care	• PMD/RN/SW communication re: patient status • Continue plan for discharge care	• Discharge needs met (home O$_2$, DME, VNA, transportation) • F/U appt made • Patient instruction sheet given
Patient Education		• Orient to unit	• Discharge teaching (meds, MDIs)	• Discharge teaching (meds, MDIs)	*Review w/pt & family:* • Meds/MDIs • D/C plan • F/U appt • Return signs & Sx

Figure 65.3 Critical pathway: community-acquired pneumonia. *ABG,* arterial blood gas; *ABX,* antibiotics; *ADLs,* activities of daily living; *BR,* bathroom; *C + S,* culture and sensitivity; *CBC,* complete blood count; *CX,* culture; *CXR,* chest radiograph; *D/C,* discontinue; *DME,* durable medical equipment; *F/U,* follow-up; *I's & O's,* intake and output; *IV,* intravenous; *LOS,* length of stay; *MDI,* metered-dose inhaler; *PMD,* primary physician; *RA,* room air; *RN,* registered nurse; *R/O,* rule-out; *RT,* respiratory therapy; *SAT,* saturation; *SOB,* shortness of breath; *SW,* social work; *SX,* symptoms; *TB,* tuberculosis; *UA,* urinalysis; *VNA,* visiting nurse.

Patients who are clinically stable should be encouraged to increase their activity level as tolerated to avoid the deconditioning that can occur with bedrest. Physical therapy should be consulted as appropriate. Discharge planning and patient education about pneumonia should continue.

The time to clinical stability in patients hospitalized with CAP is much more rapid than previously appreciated. Among patients with vital sign abnormalities on presentation, the median time to stabilization of the heart rate ($\leq$100 beats/min) and systolic blood pressure ($\geq$90 mm Hg) is 2 days. Hospital day 3 is the median day that respiratory rate ($\leq$24 breaths/min), oxygen saturation ($\geq$92%), and temperature ($\leq$99° F [37.2° C]) abnormalities stabilize. By hospital day four, over 75% of all heart rate, blood pressure, respiratory, and temperature abnormalities resolve, as do 65% of all oxygenation deficits. The time to overall clinical stability, defined as stable vital signs, baseline mental status, and ability to eat, varies depending on the pneumonia severity on presentation. The median time to clinical stability is three days for low-risk patients (Risk Class I through III), four days for moderate-risk patients (Risk Class IV), and six days for high-risk patients (Risk Class V) (14).

For patients without metabolic or hematologic derangements or other active comorbid conditions on presentation, the utility of daily laboratory testing is low. Repetition of sputum studies or blood cultures is rarely indicated in uncomplicated cases because the diagnostic yield of such studies is very low once parenteral antibiotic therapy has been initiated. Similarly, repeat chest radiographs are rarely needed and should be reserved for patients who are not improving as expected or who are getting worse.

Administration of a 7- to 10-day course of intravenous antibiotics was once a central tenet of managing patients hospitalized with CAP. Many studies now indicate that early conversion from parenteral to oral antibiotic therapy is safe, clinically effective, and less expensive. Other potential advantages of streamlined antibiotic therapy include decreased incidence of phlebitis and line sepsis, and earlier return to usual activities. Table 65.1 describes criteria for deciding when patients are stable and can be converted from parenteral to oral antibiotics (14, 15). Randomized trial data support the safety of converting patients from intravenous to oral antibiotics shortly after they become stable, often after just a few days of parenteral therapy (15). In addition, newer agents (e.g., fluoroquinolones) can achieve high serum drug levels with oral administration, suggesting the possibility of initial oral therapy in certain uncomplicated patients with a functioning gastrointestinal system.

A variety of clinical characteristics, including initial disease severity, comorbidities, and response to treatment influence when an individual patient reaches clinical stability. However, once a patient reaches stability according to the criteria listed in Table 65.1, the risk of clinical deterioration serious enough to require admission to an ICU, CCU, or telemetry unit is 1% or less, even among the sickest subset of patients (14). Therefore, the use of explicit,

TABLE 65.1

CRITERIA FOR IDENTIFYING IF PATIENTS ARE CLINICALLY STABLE AND READY TO BE CONVERTED FROM PARENTERAL TO ORAL ANTIBIOTIC THERAPY

Patient with stable vital signs for $\geq$24 hours, defined as:

Temperature $\leq$37.8°C (100°F)
Heart rate $\leq$100 beats/min
Spontaneous respiratory rate $\leq$24 breaths/minute
Systolic blood pressure $\geq$90 mm hg (without vasopressor support)
Normal oxygenation on room air (O_2 saturation $\geq$90%)
Patient able to ingest and digest tablets, capsules, or liquids
No evidence of a metastatic infection site

physiologic criteria for defining appropriateness for conversion to oral antibiotics is more clinically sensible than practice guidelines, critical pathways, or utilization rules that rigidly prespecify days on which certain actions should occur. From an epidemiological standpoint, hospital days three and four appear to be a critical point of inflection in recovery from pneumonia for most uncomplicated cases. Patients who have not met vital sign stability criteria, have suppurative complications, or have *S. aureus* or Gram-negative bacteremia should receive longer courses of intravenous antibiotics.

There are no data to support the traditional practice of observing patients on oral therapy for 24 hours or requiring all temperature measurements to be absolutely normal prior to discharge. Patients can be discharged within 24 hours of stability and antibiotic conversion without any adverse effects on patient outcomes and recovery. Chest physical therapy should not be part of routine care, because randomized controlled trials in patients with pneumonia have found no clinical benefits.

It is important to recognize when a patient is failing to improve as anticipated (as described previously) or is getting worse. Warning signs include persistent heart rate, blood pressure, and respiratory rate abnormalities beyond day four and continued fever spikes or abnormal oxygen saturation beyond day six. Symptoms of worsening dyspnea, wheezing, chest pain, or mental status are also of grave concern. There are several diagnostic and therapeutic issues to consider if patients appear to be off the usual trajectory for recovery (Table 65.2). First, a repeat chest radiograph should be obtained to assess the possibility of a new or increasing pleural effusion. If a new pleural effusion is present, thoracentesis should be performed to determine the presence of empyema or to provide symptomatic relief. Second, culture and sensitivity data should be reviewed, and resistant or unusual infectious pathogens considered. Third, the possibility of a metastatic source of infection should be readdressed. Fourth, the possibility of a noninfectious pulmonary process should be entertained. Finally, an infectious disease or pulmonary

TABLE 65.2

CONSIDERATIONS FOR PATIENTS FAILING TO IMPROVE OR GETTING WORSE AFTER EMPIRIC THERAPY FOR PRESUMED COMMUNITY-ACQUIRED PNEUMONIA

Reasons for failure to improve or worsening	Recommended approach
Uncovered bacterial pathogen (e.g., *Legionella*)	Additional microbiologic testing Broaden antibiotic regimen to cover atypical bacterial organisms Consider infectious disease consultation
Uncovered nonbacterial pathogen (e.g., virus, tuberculosis, fungus)	Additional microbiologic testing Broaden antibiotic regimen Consider infectious disease consultation
Resistant bacterial pathogen (e.g., highly resistant *Streptococcus pneumoniae*)	Check drug sensitivities Switch to/add vancomycin or highly active anti-pneumococcal fluoroquinolone Obtain infectious disease consultation Notify hospital infection control
Nosocomial or opportunistic infection	Reconsider possibility of hospital-acquired or opportunistic infection (e.g., HIV disease) Targeted laboratory testing for immunosuppression
Airway obstruction by mass	Especially if history of recurrent pneumonia, smoking, cancer, or chest radiograph indicates volume loss or adenopathy Consider chest computed tomography, pulmonary consultation, or bronchoscopy
Development of empyema	Repeat chest radiograph, with lateral decubitus films if effusion is present Diagnostic thoracocentesis Chest tube drainage if empyema present
Metastatic source of infection (abscess, endocarditis, osteomyelitis, septic arthritis)	Thorough examination and workup looking for evidence of seeding of other organs Repeat chest radiograph, urinalysis, blood cultures, etc. Obtain appropriate fluid samples from normally sterile sites that may be infected
Noninfectious pulmonary process	Consider possibility of pulmonary edema, embolism, hemorrhage, vasculitis, pulmonary-renal syndromes, hypersensitivity pneumonitis, neoplasm, etc. Targeted imaging and laboratory studies

medicine consultation should be considered to assist in subsequent diagnosis and treatment.

DISCHARGE ISSUES

Criteria for identifying when patients are clinically stable and ready to be discharged from the hospital are listed in Table 65.3. The risk of adverse outcomes once clinical stability has been attained is quite low. Conversely, patients who are discharged prior to becoming stable have higher risk-adjusted rates of death or readmission and slower return to usual activities (16). Furthermore, the safety of these types of discharge criteria has been confirmed by several randomized controlled trials and observational studies (9,15).

TABLE 65.3

CRITERIA FOR IDENTIFYING WHETHER PATIENTS ARE CLINICALLY STABLE AND READY TO BE DISCHARGED FROM THE HOSPITAL

Patients should meet all criteria in Table 65.1 for conversion to oral antibiotics and should also:

Be tolerating oral antibiotics (give first dose in hospital, but no need to observe for 24 hours on oral antibiotics)

Have returned to normal (or baseline) mental status

Have no evidence of acute comorbid condition that necessitates continued inpatient management or close observation (such as active cardiovascular, pulmonary, renal, hepatic, or endocrine disease)

Most patients with pneumonia are ready to be converted to oral therapy on the day they reach stability and to be discharged shortly thereafter. At the time of discharge, patients should have stable vital signs, adequate room-air oxygen saturation, baseline mental status, and be able to tolerate oral medicines and fluids. The presence of other active comorbid conditions that themselves require hospitalization may also delay discharge. Although most patients have a fever curve on a downward trend, it is not imperative that patients have completely normal temperatures prior to discharge. The natural history of pneumonia symptoms can be quite prolonged. More than 80% of all ambulatory and hospitalized patients experience persistent fatigue and cough, and more than 50% complain of dyspnea and sputum production at day 7. Remarkably, prolonged fatigue and cough are present in 65% and 53% of patients, respectively, 30 days after presentation. Though these symptoms are not reasons in themselves for continued hospitalization, it is important that patients be told that it may take a few weeks before their symptoms are fully resolved and they will be able to return to their usual activities.

There may be special circumstances in which patients with poor functional status appear stable but still require low-flow supplemental oxygen, parenteral antibiotics, periodic nursing, physical therapy, or other services not related to their pneumonia. Several alternatives to continued acute care hospitalization can be considered. Some patients may be appropriate candidates for transfer to a sub-acute or intermediate care facility for continued treatment (intravenous antibiotics), monitoring, and rehabilitation. Use of once-a-day parenteral antibiotics (e.g., ceftriaxone, levofloxacin, or gatifloxacin) can minimize the frequency and intensity of visiting nurse services. Low-flow oxygen by nasal cannula can be safely administered at home. Patients who require more intensive oxygen therapy should be treated in postacute care facilities.

Although the optimal duration of antibiotic therapy has not been extensively studied, most experts recommend a total course of 10–14 days. Patients with documented *Legionella* pneumonia should receive 14–21 total days of antibiotics, with the longer courses used in immunosuppressed patients or those with severe pneumonia. The selection of oral antibiotics to finish the course of treatment should be guided by the desired microbial coverage, previous intravenous regimen, patient tolerance, and cost. Culture and sensitivity data, if available, should be reviewed to help guide selection of the narrowest spectrum, most cost-effective agent. Because no definitive pathogen will be identified in 50%–70% of cases, the choice of oral agent will most often be empiric. Options for empiric oral monotherapy (in no particular order) include a macrolide (azithromycin, clarithromycin, erythromycin), an anti-pneumoccocal fluoroquinolone, or doxycycline. Doxycycline is the least costly regimen. Among macrolides, azithromycin and clarithromycin are preferred if *H. influenzae* is suspected. These two agents may also result in better

patient compliance compared to erythromycin because of less frequent dosing and fewer gastrointestinal side effects. Other appropriate, but slightly more complicated alternatives are a β-lactam plus a macrolide or a β-lactam and doxycycline. Trimethoprim-sulfamethoxazole can no longer be recommended as a first-line oral agent in pneumonia because of the high rates of pneumococcocal drug resistance.

Other opportunities to improve the quality of care and patient health at the time of discharge are *pneumococcal vaccination* and *smoking-cessation counseling*. Hospital-based vaccination of patients with CAP is safe and effective, particularly because it targets patients who have proven to be truly at risk. Patients who are smokers should be strongly advised to quit, and smoking cessation strategies and medications should be discussed. Educational, resource, and motivational information to support smoking cessation are readily available from the American Cancer Society and the American Lung Association.

All patients should have arrangements made for outpatient follow-up to assure compliance with oral therapy and complete disease resolution. It generally is recommended that patients who smoke should have a chest radiograph repeated 4–6 weeks after discharge to exclude the possibility of postobstructive pneumonia caused by lung cancer. It is important to recognize, however, that only 50% of pulmonary infiltrates clear radiographically by 6 weeks.

COST CONSIDERATIONS AND RESOURCE USE

The hospitalization decision is the most important issue from the perspective of reducing the costs of treating patients with CAP. Hospital care for pneumonia is 10–20 times more expensive than outpatient management. The risk-stratification prediction rule outlined previously helps rationalize this critical triage decision. Implementation of this admission decision guideline in two studies resulted in a 25% and 37% relative decrease in hospitalization rates among low-risk patients without any adverse effects on patient outcomes or recovery (9, 10).

Among inpatients, the duration of hospital stay is the single best determinant of total resource use. Thus, optimizing the discharge decision so that patients are converted from parenteral to oral antibiotics soon after reaching stability and are discharged shortly thereafter, as appropriate, should have the second greatest impact on resource use. Adopting this streamlined approach to decision making has been estimated to potentially reduce the total number of hospital days for pneumonia by 60% (14). The early transition to oral antibiotics and the use of less expensive agents is another means of reducing medication costs. Avoiding standard ordering of multiple sputum studies, repeat chest radiographs, and daily blood tests, which have low diagnostic yield and rarely change management, also may reduce inpatient costs.

KEY POINTS

- Evidence-based practice guidelines and critical pathways can greatly reduce practice variation and improve the quality and efficiency of treatment for this common condition.

- By utilizing an admission decision algorithm based on readily available clinical data, clinicians can identify a subset of patients who may be safely managed as outpatients, thereby decreasing the admission rates of low-risk patients.

- Low-risk patients with contraindications to outpatient therapy and moderate- or high-risk patients should be admitted.

- A simple attempt at microbiological diagnosis, with blood cultures, should be performed early, prior to the initiation of parenteral antibiotics. Because there are no features of the history, physical exam, laboratory studies, or chest radiograph that are useful for determining microbial etiology, patients should be quickly started on an empirically guided, broad-spectrum antibiotic regimen covering common "typical" and "atypical" bacterial pathogens.

- Patients who are severely ill should be rapidly stabilized in an ICU or other monitored setting.

- Patients can be converted to oral antibiotics and discharged shortly thereafter once clinical stability criteria have been met, most often by days three or four.

- Shorter courses of parenteral antibiotics can lead to significantly shorter, less expensive hospital stays with excellent clinical outcomes.

REFERENCES

1. Mandell LA, Dowell SF, Bartlett JG, et al. Update of practice guidelines for the management of community-acquired pneumonia in immunocompetent adults *Clin Infect Dis* 2003;37:1405–1433.
2. Niederman MS, Mandell LA, Anzueto A, et al. Guidelines for the management of adults with community-acquired pneumonia: diagnosis, assessment of severity, antimicrobial therapy and prevention. *Am J Resp Crit Care Med* 2001;163:1730–1754.
3. Mandell LA, Marrie TJ, Grossman RF, et al. Canadian guidelines for the initial management of community-acquired pneumonia: an evidence-based update by the Canadian Infectious Diseases Society and the Canadian Thoracic Society. The Canadian Community-Acquired Pneumonia Working Group. *Clin Infect Dis* 2000;31:383–421.
4. Metlay JP, Fine MJ. Testing strategies in the initial management of patients with community-acquired pneumonia. *Ann Intern Med* 2003;138:109–118.
5. Meehan TP, Fine MJ, Krumholz HM, et al. Quality of care, process, and outcomes in elderly patients with pneumonia. *JAMA* 1997;278:2080–2084.
6. Fine MJ, Auble TE, Yealy DM, et al. Improving the appropriateness of hospital care in community-acquired pneumonia: a prediction rule to identify patients at low risk for mortality and other adverse medical outcomes. *N Engl J Med* 1997;336:243–250.
7. American College of Emergency Physicians. Clinical policy for the management and risk stratification of community-acquired pneumonia in adults in the emergency department. *Ann Emerg Med* 2001;38:107–113.
8. Halm EA, Teirstein AS. Management of community-acquired pneumonia. *N Engl J Med* 2002;347:2039–2045.
9. Marrie TJ, Lau CY, Wheeler SL, et al. A controlled trial of a critical pathway for treatment of community-acquired pneumonia. *JAMA* 2000;283:749–755.
10. Atlas SJ, Benzer TI, Borowsky LH, et al. Safely increasing the proportion of patients with community-acquired pneumonia treated as outpatients: an interventional trial. *Arch Intern Med* 1998; 158:1350–1356.
11. Gleason PP, Meehan TP, Fine JM, et al. Associations between initial antimicrobial therapy and medical outcomes for hospitalized elderly patients with pneumonia. *Arch Intern Med* 1999; 159:2562–2572.
12. Heffelfinger JD, Dowell SF, Jorgensen JH, et al. Management of community-acquired pneumonia in the era of pneumococcal resistance: a report from Drug-Resistant Streptococcus pneumoniae Therapeutic Working Group. *Arch Intern Med* 2000;160: 1399–1408.
13. Houck PM, Bratzler DW, Nsa W, et al. Timing of antibiotic administration and outcomes for Medicare patients with community-acquired pneumonia. *Arch Intern Med* 2004;164:637–644.
14. Halm EA, Fine MJ, Coley CM, et al. The time to clinical stability in patients hospitalized with community-acquired pneumonia: implications for practice guidelines. *JAMA* 1998;279: 1452–1457.
15. Rhew DC, Tu GS, Ofman J, et al. Early switch and early discharge strategies in patients with community-acquired pneumonia: a meta-analysis. *Arch Intern Med* 2001;161:722–727.
16. Halm EA, Fine MJ, Kapoor WN, et al. Instability on hospital discharge and the risk of adverse outcomes in patients with pneumonia. *Arch Intern Med* 2002;162:1278–1284.

ADDITIONAL READING

Battleman DS, Callahan M, Thaler HT. Rapid antibiotic delivery and appropriate antibiotic selection reduce length of stay of patients with community-acquired pneumonia. *Arch Intern Med* 2002; 162:682–688.

File TM. Community-acquired pneumonia. *Lancet* 2003;362: 1991–2001.

Musher DM, Barlett JG, Doern GV. A fresh look at the definition of susceptibility of *Streptococcus pneumoniae* to β-lactam antibiotics. *Arch Intern Med* 2001;161:2538–2544.

Niederman MS. Review of treatment guidelines for community-acquired pneumonia. *Am J Med* 2004;117(Suppl 3):51S–57S.

Rhew DC, Hackner D, Henderson L, et al. The clinical benefit of in-hospital observation in "low-risk" pneumonia patients after conversion from parenteral to oral antimicrobial therapy. *Chest* 1998;113:142–146.

Waterer GW, Somes GW, Wunderink RG. Monotherapy may be suboptimal for severe bacteremic pneumococcal pneumonia. *Arch Intern Med* 2001;161:1837–1842.

Hospital-Acquired Pneumonia

66

Donald E. Craven   *Catherine A. Fleming*   *Kathleen A. Steger Craven*

INTRODUCTION

Hospital-acquired pneumonia (HAP) (or nosocomial pneumonia) is defined as an infection of lung parenchyma not present at the time of hospital admission. Although HAP is the second most common nosocomial infection in the United States, it is the most serious in terms of mortality and morbidity rates (1–4). Crude mortality rates range from 10% to 40% and are highest in elderly, mechanically ventilated patients and those with serious underlying disease, bacteremia, or infection with more virulent organisms such as *Pseudomonas aeruginosa*. In case-control studies, the mortality rate directly attributed to pneumonia has been estimated to be 30% (1–4).

Aspiration of bacteria colonizing the oropharynx is the most common route of pulmonary infection. In nonventilated patients, increased sedation, change in mental status, and vomiting are important risk factors for aspiration. In mechanically ventilated patients, aspiration may occur during intubation or from leakage of secretions around the endotracheal tube. HAP may be caused by a variety of bacteria, and most infections are caused by more than one pathogen (1–4) (Table 66.1). Early-onset HAP occurs during the first four to seven days of hospitalization and is usually caused by "community-acquired pathogens" such as *Streptococcus pneumoniae* or *Haemophilus influenzae*. By comparison, late-onset disease is more often caused by more antibiotic-resistant or multidrug-resistant (MDR) nosocomial pathogens, such as *P. aeruginosa*, *Acinetobacter* spp., or methicillin-resistant *Staphylococcus aureus (MRSA)*. Patients who have been in health care facilities, received antibiotics during the previous 90 days, have organ failure or structural lung disease, are immunosuppressed, or are receiving immunosuppressive therapy or dialysis are also at risk for infections because of MDR pathogens (1–4) (Chapter 64).

ISSUES AT THE TIME OF DIAGNOSIS

Clinical Features and Diagnosis

Despite its poor specificity, most clinicians continue to rely on a clinical diagnosis of pneumonia, which is based on presenting symptoms of fever, cough, and shortness of breath, along with a new infiltrate on chest radiograph and the analysis of expectorated sputum or endotracheal aspirates. One can increase the specificity for the diagnosis of ventilator-associated pneumonia (VAP) by using quantitative analysis and Gram stains of endotracheal aspirates or bronchoalveolar lavage fluid, although these methods are not universally available in hospitals (3–6).

The initial evaluation of patients with suspected HAP is shown in Figure 66.1 and involves confirming the presence of an intrapulmonary process, establishing the presence and severity of infection, and ruling out alternative diagnoses such as atelectasis, pulmonary embolus, or congestive heart failure. Symptoms suggesting HAP include fever, cough, purulent sputum production, dyspnea, change in mental status, and pleuritic chest pain. For mechanically ventilated patients, pneumonia is often heralded by a change in secretions, increased oxygen requirements, new or increased infiltrate on chest radiograph, leukocytosis, or fever.

Physical examination may reveal fever, tachycardia, and tachypnea, with cyanosis and respiratory distress in severe cases. Additional signs may include lung consolidation, pleuritis, effusion, and changes in oxygenation requirements. Alternative causes of persistent fever and

TABLE 66.1

ETIOLOGY OF HOSPITAL-ACQUIRED PNEUMONIA (HAP)/VENTILATOR-ASSOCIATED PNEUMONIA (VAP) BY LOCATION AND FREQUENCY OF ISOLATION OF MULTI-DRUG RESISTANCE (MDR) PATHOGENS

Major HAP pathogens	Frequency	ICU or VAP pathogens	MDR strains
Gram-negative pathogens			
Pseudomonas aeruginosa	Common	+++	+++
Escherichia coli	Common	++	+
Klebsiella pneumoniae (ESBL+/−)	Variable	+	+/−
Enterobacter species	Variable	+	No
Serratia marcesens	Variable	+	No
Acinetobacter species	Variable	++	+++
Stenotrophomonas maltophilia	Uncommon	+	+++
Haemophilus influenzae	Variable	+	No
Legionella pneumophila	Variable	+	No
Gram-positive pathogens			
Staphylococcus aureus, methicillin sensitive (MSSA) & methicillin-resistant (MRSA)	Common	+++	+++
Streptococcus pneumoniae	Variable	+	+/−
Anaerobic pathogens	Rare	Rare	No
Fungal pathogens			
Candida species	Rare	Rare	+/−
Aspergillus fumigatus	Variable	Rare	No
Viruses (RSV, influenza, CMV)	Rare	Rare	No

+ = uncommon, ++ = common, +++ = frequent
CMV, cytomegalovirus; *ESBL*, extended spectrum β-lactamase; *RSV*, respiratory syncytial virus.
See Table 66.2 defining risk factors for MDR pathogens and Table 66.3 for effective antibiotics.

HAP (Including VAP) Suspected

Obtain appropriate cultures
Begin empiric antimicrobial therapy
based on most likely pathogens
and local microbiologic data

Check cultures and assess clinical response:
Temperature, WBC, CXR, PaO$_2$/FiO$_2$,
hemodynamic changes and organ function

Clinical improvement at 48–72 hours

No ——————— Yes

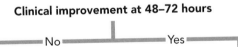

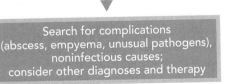

Search for complications
(abscess, empyema, unusual pathogens),
noninfectious causes;
consider other diagnoses and therapy

De-escalate antibiotics
based on microbiology results.
For uncomplicated HAP
(including VAP), treat for 7 days

Figure 66.1 Algorithm for managing hospital-acquired pneumonia (HAP). *CXR*, chest radiograph; *VAP*, ventilator-associated pneumonia; *WBC*, white blood cell count.

their evaluation in hospitalized patients are discussed in Chapter 62.

Chest Radiography

The finding of a new infiltrate on chest radiograph is necessary but not sufficient to make the diagnosis of HAP. Noninfectious causes of a new radiographic infiltrate in hospitalized patients include congestive heart failure, atelectasis, pulmonary embolus with infarction, and chemical pneumonitis caused by aspiration. In some patients, better assessment of the infiltrate can be made by a computerized axial tomographic (CAT) scan. Adult Respiratory Distress Syndrome (ARDS) and pulmonary hemorrhage also should be considered in critically ill patients. A false negative chest radiograph is rare but may occur in patients with neutropenia, early infection, and pneumonia due to *Pneumocystis jirovecii* (formerly *P. carinii*). Patients with symptoms of pneumonia and a negative chest radiograph may have purulent tracheobronchitis. Multilobar changes, rapid progression of pulmonary infiltrates, or the presence of cavitation all suggest a particularly severe case of HAP. In patients with a significant parapneumonic effusion, diagnostic thoracentesis should be performed to rule out empyema.

Laboratory Tests

Laboratory investigations are essential for definitively diagnosing HAP, assessing the severity of illness, and identifying the cause. Recommended routine laboratory tests in patients with HAP include a complete blood count, two sets of blood cultures, and a sputum Gram stain and culture. Blood cultures identify the infecting organism in 10%–20% of cases and a positive blood culture may predict a more complicated course with a higher risk of death. A properly prepared Gram stain of purulent sputum, the endotracheal aspirate, or bronchoalveolar lavage (BAL) fluid may provide initial clues to the infecting bacteria and important data for correlation with the sputum culture result. Sputum smears that have white blood cells but no bacteria raise suspicion for atypical organisms such as *Legionella*, mycobacterial species, or respiratory viruses. Sputum culture is useful for detecting the presence of resistant organisms, but has low specificity. Additional tests for *Legionella* urinary antigen should be obtained, as guided by institutional epidemiology.

Oxygenation should be assessed by pulse oximetry, with subsequent arterial blood gas determination in those with oxygen saturation less than 92%. Testing for HIV as well as appropriate evaluation for other causes of immunosuppression should be considered when risk factors or the clinical presentation dictate.

A clinical diagnosis of HAP in mechanically ventilated patients with a new infiltrate, fever, sputum production, leukocytosis (usually with a shift to greater numbers of polymorphonuclear leukocytes and band forms), and impaired oxygenation is sensitive but not specific (3–6). The use of the modified Clinical Pulmonary Infection Score (CPIS), which quantifies temperature, level of leukocytosis, oxygenation, changes on chest radiograph, and purlence of respiratory secretions, has been used to classify patients with HAP and predict outcomes from HAP (7–9). In one study, patients with mild HAP who had a low initial Clinical Pulmonary Infection Score (≤6) or a low likelihood of HAP were randomized to treatment with a short course (3 days) of ciprofloxacin versus "standard" therapy (multiple antibiotics for a longer periods of time) (8). Although the number of study patients was small, the group randomized to ciprofloxacin monotherapy had significantly shorter stays in the intensive care unit, fewer superinfections and drug resistant pathogens, and a trend toward decreased mortality.

If sputum is available, it should be cultured before starting antibiotics. In all intubated patients with suspected HAP, an endotracheal aspirate should be obtained for Gram stain and culture and, if available, for quantitative culture. The use of quantitative sputum cultures from blind bronchoalveolar lavage (BAL) or quantitative endotracheal aspirates increases the diagnostic specificity of *ventilator-associated pneumonia* (VAP) and correlates well with specimens obtained from bronchoscopy with bronchoalveolar lavage (BAL), but quantitative techniques for diagnosing VAP are not widely used in the United States (3–6). Data collected from one large randomized trial of patients with suspected VAP found that patients randomized to diagnosis by bronchoscopy with quantitative bronchoalveolar lavage (BAL) or protected specimen brush samples had significantly lower use of antibiotics and decreased mortality than those managed by clinical diagnosis and non-quantitative endotracheal aspirates (4). Bronchoscopy with BAL should be considered for patients who do not respond to initial, empiric antibiotic therapy.

Criteria for ICU Admission

Indications for ICU monitoring in patients with HAP include hemodynamic instability, respiratory failure, or obtundation sufficient to impede airway protection (3, 4). Manifestations of the Systemic Inflammatory Response Syndrome also may indicate the need for intensive care. Possible indications include advanced age, comorbid illnesses, and the need for higher levels of nursing care required for airway management.

Initial Antibiotic Therapy

Because it is difficult to establish a clear diagnosis of HAP and because aspiration predisposes to multiple pathogens, *we strongly recommend early, empiric, intravenous broad-spectrum antimicrobial coverage based on time of onset and risk factors for MDR bacteria* (3). Clearly, the prevalence of MDR pathogens varies by hospital, intensive care units within a

TABLE 66.2

MDR PATHOGEN RISK FACTORS

Prior antibiotics (<90 days)
Prior hospitalization, chronic care
Dialysis or organ failure
Immunosuppressive disease or therapy
Structural lung disease
Late onset HAP or VAP

HAP, hospital-acquired pneumonia; *VAP*, ventilator-associated pneumonia.

single hospital, and with time (3) (Tables 66.2, 66.3, and 66.4). Intravenous antibiotics, in appropriate doses, must be initiated promptly after appropriate blood and sputum cultures are obtained to limit progression of disease, improve patient outcomes, and decrease hospital costs (3).

Patients with HAP (early onset and without risk factors for MDR pathogens) should be treated with a 2nd- or 3rd-generation cephalosporin (cefuroxime 1.5 gms q8h or ceftriaxone 2 gms/day); a high-dose quinolone (such as levofloxacin 750 mg/day IV or ciprofloxacin 400 mg IV q8h); or a β-lactam, β-lactamase inhibitor (ampicillin/sulbactam 3 gms IV q6h), as shown in Table 66.3 (1, 3). With the emergence of penicillin-resistant and MDR strains of *S. pneumoniae*, the use of ceftriaxone or extended-spectrum quinolones (such as levofloxacin) may be preferable to earlier generation quinolones, such as ciprofloxacin. In contrast to the β-lactam regimens, quinolones also have activity against atypical pathogens such as *Legionella pneumophila*.

Broader-spectrum antibiotic therapy of HAP and VAP is recommended for patients with risk factors for MDR pathogens, and for those with late onset disease (1, 3) (as shown in Table 66.4). Initial selection of antibiotic coverage may depend on the prevalence and species, and antibiotic sensitivity of the specific MDR pathogens. Doses should be adjusted for impaired renal function. For Gram-negative bacilli, the following doses are recommended: antipseudomonal cephalosporins (ceftazidime 2 gm q8h IV or cefipime 2 gm q12h IV); β-lactam/ β-lactamase inhibitor (piperacillin-tazobactam 4.5 g q6h); carbepenems (imipenem 500 mg q6h or meropenem 1g q8h); fluoroquinolones (ciprofloxacin 400 mg q8h IV or levofloxacin 750 mg/day IV); aminoglycosides (gentamicin 7 mg/kg/d); tobramycin (7 mg/kg/d); or amikacin (20 mg/kg/d) with serum levels checked. For MRSA, the recommended doses are vancomycin 15 mg/kg q12h IV with doses monitored by serum levels, or linezolid 600 mg bid IV (10). If *Klebsiella pneumoniae* with extended spectrum β-lactamase is suspected, carbipenems should be used instead of cephalosporins. If *Legionella pneumophila* is suspected, the regimen should include a quinolone. A discussion of all possible regimens is beyond the scope of this chapter.

TABLE 66.3

TREATMENT RECOMMENDATIONS FOR PATIENTS WITH MILD-TO-MODERATE HOSPITAL-ACQUIRED PNEUMONIA (HAP), EARLY ONSET, AND NO KNOWN RISK FACTORS FOR MDR PATHOGENS[a]

Potential pathogens	Recommended antibiotics

Streptococcus pneumoniae[b]
 Haemophilus influenzae
 Methicillin-sensitive
   Staphylococcus aureus[c]
 Antibiotic-sensitive enteric
   gram-negative bacilli
     Escherichia coli
     Klebsiella pneumoniae
     Enterobacter species
     Proteus species
     Serratia marcescens
	2nd/3rd generation cephalosporin
	 (cefotaxime, ceftriaxone)
	 OR
	 3rd generation quinolone
	 (levofloxacin)
	 OR
	 β-lactam, β-lactamase inhibitor
	 (ampicillin/sulbactam)

[a] For risk factors, see Table 66.2.
[b] Frequency of penicillin-resistant *S. pneumonae* (PRSP) and multidrug resistant (MDR) *S. pneumoniae* strains increasing
[c] Reports of community-acquired methicillin-resistant *S. aureus* (CA-MRSA) are emerging in different geographic areas.
Adapted from American Thoracic Society and Infectious Diseases Society of America. Guidelines for the management of adults with hospital-acquired, ventilator-associated, and healthcare-associated pneumonia. *Am J Respir Crit Care Med* 2005;171: in press.

ISSUES DURING THE COURSE OF THE HOSPITALIZATION

Monitoring clinical response to initial therapy, adjusting or streamlining antibiotics based on clinical and microbiologic data, and checking for possible complications are of paramount importance. A critical pathway for the management of HAP is shown in Figure 66.3.

Day 1

The highest priority during the first 2–4 hours after suspicion of HAP is the rapid initiation of appropriate intravenous antibiotics following completion of initial assessments and collection of cultures (1, 3). The patient's room-air oxygen saturation should be measured; if it is below 92%, supplemental oxygen should be given. The need for ICU transfer, respiratory therapy, or intubation should be evaluated regularly during the first 12–24 hours, and thereafter as needed.

The patient's requirements for hydration and nutritional support should be assessed. Unless contraindicated, the head of the bed should be maintained at a 30 degree upright position (1, 3, 11). If resistant organisms or tuberculosis are suspected, the patient should be placed

TABLE 66.4

INITIAL EMPIRIC THERAPY FOR PATIENTS WITH HOSPITAL-ACQUIRED PNEUMONIA (HAP), INCLUDING VAP, AND RISK FACTORS FOR MULTIDRUG-RESISTANT (MDR) PATHOGENS OR LATE-ONSET DISEASE

Potential MDR pathogens[a]	Combination antibiotic therapy[e]
• *Pseudomonas aeruginosa*[a] • *Acinetobacter* species[a] • *Klebsiella pneumoniae*[a,c] • *Escherichia coli* • *Enterobacter aerogenes* • Methicillin-resistant *Staphylococcus aureus (MRSA)*[d,g]	3rd/4th generation antipseudomonal cephalosporin (ceftazidime, cefepime) OR carbepenem (antipseudomonal) (imipenem, meropenem) OR β-lactam, β-lactamase inhibitor (pipercillin-tazobactam) *PLUS* fluoroquinolone[b] (levofloxacin, ciprofloxacin)[f] OR aminoglycoside[b,h] (gentamicin, tobramycin, amikacin) *PLUS* linezolid or vancomycin (if MRSA is prevalent)[i]

[a] Sensitivities vary for gram-negative bacilli. Initial antibiotic therapy should be adjusted or streamlined based on subsequent microbiologic data and clinical response to therapy.
[b] If *Legionella pneumophila* is suspected, the combination antibiotic regimen should include a fluoroquinolone rather than an aminoglycoside.
[c] For ESBL+ isolates, imipenem or meropenem should be used instead of ceftazidime or cefepime.
[d] Outcomes for patients with HAP due to MRSA may be better for linezolid than vancomycin (12).
[e] Suggested regimens—equivalent substitutions are appropriate.
[f] Levofloxacin at higher dose (750 mg IV qd) approved for the treatment of nosocomial pneumonia has excellent activity against MDR *Streptococcus pneumoniae*. Ciprofloxacin at higher dose (400 mg q8h IV) has also been used to treat HAP, but has decreased activity against *Streptococcus pneumoniae* (which may cause early onset HAP).
[g] Rates of methicillin-reisistant *S. aureus* (MRSA) have increased in health care facilities, in the community and in persons who have received recent antibiotics.
[h] Aminoglycosides do not penetrate well into lung tissue and have renal and ototoxicity. Aminoglycosides should be dosed daily. Initial doses of gentamicin and tobramycin (7 mg/kg/day) and amikacin (20 mg/kg/day) are recommended along with monitoring of serum peak and trough levels along with renal function. Their use should generally be limited to 3–5 days.
[i] In patients with HAP due to MRSA, linezolid (600 mg bid) may provide better coverage than vancomycin (12). Doses of vancomycin should be 10–15 mg/kg q12 hrs. Trough levels of 15–20 mcg/mL should be maintained for treating HAP due to MRSA.

on respiratory isolation pending microbiological results. If the patient has restricted mobility, subcutaneous heparin or other appropriate prophylaxis should be administered (Chapter 52). Vital signs and oxygen saturation should be followed closely during the first 12–24 hours.

Day 2

On day two, culture results should be checked and antibiotics should be adjusted to cover the infecting pathogens and stopped if there is no evidence of HAP. The duration of therapy for uncomplicated HAP should be targeted for seven days, especially in patients who demonstrate prompt

clinical improvement (1, 3, 12). If the patient appears to be improving, extubation, transfer from the ICU, a switch to oral antibiotics, and advanced diet and activity can be considered. Although the course of HAP may vary, signs of clinical response should be evident within 48 hours after therapy is initiated. Lack of response to treatment may result from either an incorrect initial diagnosis of pneumonia or inadequate evaluation and therapy, as outlined in Table 66.5. To guide further management, a comprehensive evaluation should be performed and infectious disease and pulmonary consultations should be obtained. At this point, invasive microbiologic sampling to look for resistant or unusual pathogens is usually appropriate (1, 3). Negative cultures should raise the possibility of a noninfectious

	Day 1: Initial 4 hours	Day 1: Additional considerations	Day 2: If stable or improving	Day 2: If NOT stable or improving	Once stable, until discharge
Tests	• Physical examination • Chest radiograph • Sputum culture & Gram stain • CBC/diff, Chem-7, urinalysis • Blood cultures • O$_2$ sat; ABG if <92% • Sputum AFB if at risk for TB • Consider unusual pathogens (PCP, *Legionella*) if patient at risk • Consider quantitative tests: QEA, BAL, PSB +/– bronchscopy • Assess relevant hx: aspiration, chronic illnesses • ID consult & HIV testing as appropriate		• Check official chest radiograph report & culture results • Repeat O$_2$ sat, adjust O$_2$ if needed	• Repeat chest radiograph & culture • R/O effusion, empyema, abscess • Consider other diagnoses • Consider pulmonary/ID consults • Consider quantitative tests – QEA, BAL, PSB by bronchoscopy • Evaluate need for regimen changes • Assess O$_2$ sat	• Continue to monitor response to therapy
Medications and Therapeutics	• Early initiation of intravenous (IV) antibiotics (ABX) within 2–4 hours but after cultures (check ABX allergies). See Tables 66.2 and 66.3. • Consider respiratory isolation if TB or MDR strain suspected • Consider transfer to ICU if patient unstable or for severe HAP; intubate as needed • Respiratory therapy as needed	• Subcutaneous heparin if indicated • Assess need for IV fluids	• Consider oral regimen +/– narrow spectrum based on culture results • If stable, assess ongoing need for mechanical ventilation • If stable, consider transfer from ICU • Assess need for ongoing respiratory therapy	• Continue to monitor response to therapy, making necessary adjustments	• Begin patient education regarding medications • Document plan including expected date of discharge & disposition
Nursing/ Assessment	• Vital signs (VS), temp, I&O, O$_2$ sat, weight • Update code status & health care proxy as needed	• Continue to monitor VS, temp, I&O, O$_2$ sat as indicated	• Continue to monitor VS, temp, I&O, O$_2$ sat as indicated	• Continue to monitor VS, temp, I&O, O$_2$ sat as indicated	• Assess need for smoking cessation program & vaccination (pneumococcal & influenza)
Activity	• As tolerated, consider lateral bed for immobility • Elevate head of bed 30° unless contraindicated	• Encourage activity as tolerated	• Increase activity as appropriate; assess dyspnea on exertion; consider physical therapy consult	• Activity as tolerated	• Assess limitations in activities and incorporate intervention in discharge plan
Nutrition	• Baseline assessment with appropriate plan	• Consider need for IV hydration +/– enteral feeding	• Increase diet as tolerated	• Increase diet as tolerated	• Nutritional counseling as needed
Discharge Planning		• Notify primary care provider • Notify family	• Review home situation and needs, determine anticipated length of hospitalization	• Review discharge plan with family as needed	• Update patient status and continue to develop plan • Implement discharge plan • Include appropriate vaccination plans
Patient Education	• Orient to unit as soon as possible		• Begin discharge planning teaching (medications, return symptoms) as soon	• Reinforce patient education as needed; involve family if necessary	• Provide written & oral instructions of follow-up plan

Figure 66.2   Critical pathway: hospital-acquired pneumonia (HAP). *ABG*, arterial blood gas; *AFB*, acid-fast bacillus; *BAL*, bronchoalveolar lavage; *Chem-7*, chemical profile; *diff*, differential; *HIV*, human immunodeficiency virus; *hx*, history; *ICU*, intensive care unit; *ID*, infectious disease; *I&O*, intake and output; *MDR*, multidrug resistant; *O₂*, oxygen; *PCP*, *pneumocystis jirovecii* pneumonia; *PSB*, protected specimen brush; *QEA*, quantitative endotracheal aspirates; *R/O*, rule out; *sat*, saturation; *TB*, tuberculosis.

pulmonary process. In the patient who has not improved, further radiographic evaluation (including lateral decubitus films, ultrasound, or a computerized tomograpic scan) is also indicated at this time to rule out empyema, cavitation, or a post-obstructive process. A spiral computerized tomograpic scan or ventilation-perfusion scan should be considered in patients in whom an infectious process is not identified.

Remainder of Hospitalization and Discharge Planning

The most common pulmonary complication of HAP is *empyema.* Thoracocentesis is indicated in all patients with a sizable pleural effusion (defined as >10mm on lateral decubitus films) in whom pneumonia is suspected. Empyema is suggested by persistent fevers or leukocytosis associated with a parapneumonic effusion or the finding of a locu-

lated effusion, and the diagnosis is confirmed by thoracentesis. Early diagnosis and prompt drainage of the infected pleural space by needle aspiration, chest tube, or thoracotomy are crucial (Chapter 60). Lung abscess is a relatively uncommon complication of HAP and may be diagnosed by chest radiograph or computerized tomographic scan in patients who are not responding to otherwise appropriate therapy. Extrapulmonary complications may result from the appropriate interventions and treatment. These include *Clostridium difficile* colitis, central venous catheter infections, drug reactions or toxicity, venous thromboembolism, and respiratory-tract superinfection, seen most frequently in intubated patients. These complications may present as a failure to respond to antibiotic therapy (Table 66.5).

The duration of therapy for uncomplicated HAP is usually seven days (3, 12). Some patients with more severe underlying disease, impaired immune systems, or infection with antibiotic-resistant organisms who do not respond may need longer courses of antibiotics. Patients with complications such as empyema or lung abscess may require four to eight weeks of antibiotic therapy along with other therapeutic interventions. If the patient has a rapid response to antibiotic therapy for HAP, the duration of therapy may be shortened. Once the patient's condition has stabilized, the prescribed course may be completed at home or in step-down facilities. Nosocomial pathogens, such as *P. aeruginosa* and *S. aureus,* may persist in sputum after the patient's clinical parameters have returned to normal. This invariably represents colonization rather than infection and does not require further antibiotic therapy. Nevertheless, patients should be carefully monitored for relapse (3, 12).

Once the patient is responding to therapy, a nursing assessment should be done. This assessment should attempt to identify risk factors for pneumonia and aspiration, and address the condition of the patient's teeth, as well as the need for smoking cessation and other patient education. Pneumococcal and influenza vaccination status also should be ascertained. All patients with *Aspergillus,* tuberculosis, *Legionella pneumophila,* or MDR nosocomial pathogens should be reported to the infection-control staff (1, 3). In addition, cases of atypical or resistant organisms should be reported back to referring facilities from which the patient was transferred.

COST CONSIDERATIONS AND RESOURCE USE

Nosocomial pneumonia increases the duration of hospitalization two- to threefold compared with patients without pneumonia. When comparing infection rates across facilities, patients should be stratified by severity of pneumonia, presence of risk factors, and admission to the ICU, and comparisons should be based on incidence density

---

TABLE 66.5

DIFFERENTIAL DIAGNOSIS OF PATIENTS WHO FAIL TO RESPOND OR WHO DETERIORATE FOLLOWING INITIAL THERAPY, CLASSIFIED ACCORDING TO THE ACCURACY OF THE ORIGINAL DIAGNOSIS

Correct diagnosis	Incorrect diagnosis
Wrong organism	Atelectasis
Bacterial/legionella/	Neoplasm
mycobacteria	Pulmonary embolism
Viral	Congestive heart failure
Fungal/*Pneumocystis carinii*	Acute Respiratory
Resistant organism	Distress Syndrome
Methicillin-resistant	Pulmonary hemorrhage
Staphylococcus aureus	Pulmonary contusion
Multidrug-resistant	Chemical pneumonitis
Gram-negative[a]	

Complication

Empyema
Lung abscess
Clostridium difficile colitis
Central line infection
Drug fever

Inadequate antibiotic

  Wrong dose
  Poor absorption
Poor prognostic factors
  Age/underlying disease
  Postobstruction

[a] Common examples of multidrug-resistant Gram-negatives include *Pseudomonas aeriginosa, Acinetobacter baumanni, Klebsiella* pneumoniae (extended β-lactamase +).

(rates per 1,000 ICU or hospital days or, in ventilated patients, rates per 1,000 days on mechanical ventilator).

Appropriate prevention strategies can significantly decrease the incidence of HAP (1–3, 11). Such strategies can be divided into host factors, medications, and devices that facilitate patient colonization and environmental factors. Infection-control measures are aimed at preventing cross-infection or colonization with nosocomial pathogens from other patients and staff. Table 66.6 reviews recommendations that either have been proven in clinical trials or epidemiologic studies, or have been recommended by consensus panels convened by the Centers for Disease Control and more recent reviews by experts (1–3, 11). Clearly, some of the most effective prevention strategies are low technologic approaches, most of which are widely available, inexpensive, and noninvasive. For these reasons, their potential contribution to preventing cases of HAP may be underappreciated.

Further studies are needed to assess streamlined therapeutic approaches, such as the use of oral regimens or short courses of antibiotics. The time from diagnosis to discharge, length of ICU stay, and days of mechanical ventilation should be monitored, along with other outcome variables such as the numbers of patients requiring tracheostomy. Although most clinical outcomes for pneumo-

TABLE 66.6

PROPHYLAXIS OF HOSPITAL-ACQUIRED PNEUMONIA IN MECHANICALLY VENTILATED PATIENTS AND NONVENTILATED PATIENTS

Risk factor	Intervention	Recommended	
		Mechanically ventilated	Nonventilated
Host factors			
Aspiration/reflux	Elevate patient's head 30°	X	X
Chronic obstructive pulmonary disease/postoperative patient	Incentive spirometry		X
Comorbidity, age over 50 years (pneumococcal, influenza)	Appropriate vaccinations	X	X
Medications			
Emergence of resistance	Judicious use of antibiotics	X	X
Stress bleeding prophylaxis	Use of sucralfate vs. histamine-2 receptor blockers for stress bleeding prophylaxis	X	
Infection control			
Cross-infection	Proper isolation handwashing, and use of barriers	X	X
Spread of multidrug-resistant Gram-negative bacilli and methicillin-resistant *Staphylococcus aureus*	Use of barrier precautions	X	X
Environmental risk factors	Use of appropriate air filtration for high-risk patients to prevent aspergillosis	X	X
Devices			
Aspiration of subglottic secretions around the endotracheal tube	Maintain adequate cuff pressure	X	
Reflux of circuit condensate	Use heat-moisture exchanger; drain condensate away from patient	X	
Cross-infection	Use aseptic technique and proper disinfection or O_2 sensors/monitors, and resuscitation bags	X	X
Aspiration	Verify feeding tube placement; manage residuals	X	X

nia have focused on mortality rate as the primary endpoint, the use of other outcome measures (such as quality-of-life measures, hospital costs, antibiotic days, days of mechanical ventilation, hospital days, and length of convalescence) should be considered. New data are needed regarding the cost effectiveness of specific clinical strategies for diagnosis, treatment, and prevention of HAP.

KEY POINTS

- Despite an increased understanding of the pathogenesis of pneumonia, HAP continues to occur at disturbing rates and is associated with significant morbidity and mortality.
- The use of quantitiative sputum cultures increases the specificity of diagnosis for ventilator-associated pneumonia (VAP) and may reduce antibiotic use and improve patient outcomes, but is not widely available.
- Initial effective therapy of HAP should be based on the stratification of patients by severity of disease, time of onset, and the presence of risk factors for MDR pathogens that necessitate broader empiric antibiotic coverage.
- Early institution of broad-spectrum appropriate antibiotic therapy targeted to all suspected pathogens decreases mortality and morbidity.
- Antibiotic therapy should be streamlined or de-escalated based on the identification and antibiotic sensitivity of the pathogens isolated and the clinical response of the patient.
- The duration of antibiotic therapy for patients with uncomplicated HAP who respond to treatment should be seven days.
- Patients who do not respond to initial therapy, or have evidence of progressive disease, should have a prompt infectious disease or pulmonary consultation to reassess the diagnosis and the need for further diagnostic studies or additional therapy.
- Short-term and long-term prevention strategies for HAP and the emergence and spread of MDR pathogens are strongly recommended to reduce patient mortality, morbidity, and health care costs.

REFERENCES

1. Craven DE, Palladino R, McQuillen DP. Healthcare-associated pneumonia in adults: management principles to improve outcomes. *Infect Dis Clin North Am* 2004;18:939–962.
2. Weinstein R, CDC/HICPAC. Guideline for prevention of health care–associated pneumonia, 2004. *Infect Control Hosp Epidemiol* In press, 2005.
3. The American Thoracic Society and Infectious Diseases Society of America. Guidelines for the management of adults with hospital-acquired, ventilator-associated, and healthcare-associated pneumonia. *Am J Respir Crit Care Med* 2005;171: in press.
4. Fagon J-Y, Chastre J, Wolff M, et al. Invasive and noninvasive strategies for management of suspected ventilator-associated pneumonia: a randomized trial. *Ann Intern Med* 2000;132:621–630.
5. Chastre J, Fagon JY. Ventilator-associated pneumonia. *Am J Respir Crit Care Med* 2002;165:867–903.
6. Sanchez-Nieto JM, Torres A, Garcia-Cordoba F, et al. Impact of invasive and noninvasive quantitative culture sampling on outcome of ventilator-associated pneumonia: a pilot study [published erratum appears in *Am J Respir Crit Care Med* 1998 Mar;157:1005]. *Am J Respir Crit Care Med* 1998;157:371–376.
7. Pugin J, Auckenthaler R, Mili N, et al. Diagnosis of ventilator associated pneumonia by bacteriologic analysis of bronchoscopic and nonbronchoscopic blind bronchoalveolar lavage fluid. *Am Rev Respir Dis* 1988;138:117–120.
8. Singh N, Rogers P, Atwood CW, et al. Short-course empiric antibiotic therapy for patients with pulmonary infiltrates in the intensive care unit: a proposed solution for indiscriminate antibiotic prescription. *Am J Respir Crit Care Med* 2000;162:505–511.
9. Luna CM, Blanzaco D, NiedermanMS, et al. Resolution of ventilator-associated pneumonia: prospective evaluation of the clinical pulmonary infection score as an early clinical predictor or outcome. *Crit Care Med* 2003;31:576–582.
10. Wunderink RG, Rello J, Cammarata SK, et al. Linezolid vs Vancomycin: analysis of two double-blind studies of patients with methicillin-resistant *Staphylococcus aureus* nosocomial pneumonia. *Chest* 2003;124:1789–1797.
11. Kollef MH. Prevention of ventilator-associated pneumonia. *N Engl J Med* 1999;340:627–634.
12. Chastre J, Wolff M, Fagon JY, et al. Comparison of 8 vs 15 days of antibiotic therapy for ventilator-associated pneumonia in adults: a randomized trial. *JAMA* 2003;290:2588–2598.

ADDITIONAL READING

Cook DJ, Kollef MH. Risk factors for ICU-acquired pneumonia. *JAMA* 1998;279:1605–1606.
De Rosa FG, Craven DE. Management of nosocomial pneumonia. *Infections in Medicine* 2003;20:248–258.
Kollef MH. Inadequate antimicrobial treatment: an important determinant of outcome for hospitalized patients. *Clin Infect Dis* 2000; 31:S131–138.
McEachern R, Campbell GD Jr. Hospital-acquired pneumonia: epidemiology, etiology, and treatment. *Infect Dis Clin North Am* 1998; 12:761–779.

Tuberculosis

67

Charles L. Daley   Philip C. Hopewell

INTRODUCTION

Despite the decline in tuberculosis cases in the United States, tuberculosis continues to be a common reason for admission in many hospitals. Hospitalization may be necessary because of the disease's severe effects, for invasive diagnostic tests when tuberculosis is suspected but not proven, or for initiation of potentially toxic treatment regimens in patients with tuberculosis caused by multidrug-resistant organisms. Tuberculosis may also be diagnosed in patients who are hospitalized for other diseases, such as HIV disease, chronic renal failure, or another immunosuppressive condition. In addition to the considerations that apply to individual patients with or suspected of having this disease, tuberculosis in the hospital setting raises important issues of infection control. Consequently, the disease has implications for the hospital environment and health care worker safety, as well as for specific patients. Because of the need for rapid diagnosis of tuberculosis in hospitalized patients, there are also important implications for the microbiology laboratory.

This discussion will focus on management of the hospitalized patient with known or suspected tuberculosis. However, the separation of inpatient from outpatient management is artificial, and the care of patients with tuberculosis must be provided as a coordinated continuum in order to ensure that therapy is completed successfully. Additionally, there must be communication and coordination with local public health tuberculosis control programs. In many areas such programs provide ongoing patient care following hospital discharge. In addition, tuberculosis control personnel conduct epidemiologic investigations centered on each newly reported case. Promptly notifying the tuberculosis control program of a newly identified case will expedite the investigation of contacts and minimize the effects of secondary spread of *mycobacterium tuberculosis*.

TUBERCULOSIS IN NON-HIV-INFECTED PATIENTS

Issues at the Time of Admission

Clinical and Radiographic Presentation

The clinical presentation of tuberculosis varies greatly depending on a number of factors, including the site of involvement, extent of disease, and immunocompetence of the host. Most people with tuberculosis present with a subacute or chronic illness with symptoms that have been present for several weeks to months. Although it is traditionally taught that patients with pulmonary tuberculosis present with cough, fever, night sweats, weight loss, and, occasionally, hemoptysis, a recent study found that only 52% of patients had a cough at the time of diagnosis (1). Extrapulmonary manifestations of disease depend on the site of involvement. For example, tuberculous meningitis may present with headache and altered mental status, whereas tuberculous lymphadenitis presents with local swelling of lymph nodes, usually in the neck. Fifteen to 20% of patients with pulmonary tuberculosis will be asymptomatic at the time of diagnosis. Thus, a high index of suspicion should be maintained in high-risk populations.

The characteristic radiographic findings of tuberculosis vary depending on the underlying pathogenetic mechanism of disease. Patients who present with post-primary or reactivation disease usually have upper lobe radiographic opacities, often with cavitation. The most commonly involved lung segments include the apical and posterior segments of the right upper lobe and apical-posterior segment of the left upper lobe. Reactivation tuberculosis in immunocompetent adults does not typically cause intrathoracic lymphadenopathy. In primary tuberculosis, the chest radiograph may demonstrate lower lung zone opacities, usually without cavitation, and in some cases with associated intrathoracic lymphadenopathy. Miliary tuberculosis, characterized radiographically by diffuse small nodules, can occur with either primary or post-primary disease. Similarly, pleural effusions may occur with primary or post-primary disease, and the effusion may occur with or without evidence of pulmonary parenchymal disease.

Differential Diagnosis and Initial Evaluation

People suspected of having tuberculosis, based on clinical signs and symptoms, should have a chest radiograph performed. If the findings on the chest radiograph are consistent with tuberculosis and/or the patient has respiratory symptoms, three consecutive morning sputum specimens should be obtained for microscopic examination for the presence of acid fast bacilli (AFB) and mycobacterial culture. If the patient is unable to produce sputum spontaneously, sputum induction should be performed using ultrasonic nebulization of hypertonic saline. The sensitivity of AFB sputum smears is approximately 50%, although in some studies more than 70% of patients with pulmonary tuberculosis have had positive smears (2). Among patients with pulmonary tuberculosis, the sensitivity of mycobacterial cultures is around 80%–85%. The yields of sputum microscopy and culture increase in patients with cavitary disease.

Mycobacterial cultures may require days-to-weeks to become positive, depending on the method used. With liquid culture systems, growth can be detected within one or two weeks depending on the number of bacilli in the specimen. The combination of liquid culture systems and specific nucleic acid probes can enable species identification within two weeks. Drug susceptibility tests should be performed for the first-line agents on all initial isolates of *M. tuberculosis*. Regardless of the culture method used, decisions regarding treatment and further diagnostic testing must be made early in the course of the evaluation, without the benefit of drug susceptibility results. Antituberculosis therapy should be started when the clinical suspicion of disease is high, even if the sputum specimens are AFB smear-negative.

Two direct nucleic acid amplification tests (Amplicor, Roche and MTD, Genprobe) have been approved by the FDA for use in AFB smear-positive specimens. Additionally, the MTD test is approved for use in smear-negative specimens. Studies have demonstrated positive predictive values for direct amplification tests in AFB smear-positive specimens of approximately 100%, and negative predictive values of 86%–90% (3). However, the predictive values vary depending on the prevalence of disease in the population studied. When using the tests on smear-negative specimens, the results should be interpreted with caution because the positive predictive value will be low when the clinical suspicion for active tuberculosis is low (Chapter 6). On the other hand, when the clinical suspicion is high, the positive predictive value remains high, even when used with smear-negative specimens.

Fiberoptic bronchoscopy with transbronchial biopsy has been reported to yield a rapid diagnosis in 48% of suspected tuberculosis cases who have negative sputum smears for AFB (4). In this study, transbronchial biopsy provided the only specimens in which AFB were seen on stained specimens in 26% of the cases, although it did not increase the yield of culture. It is important to note that 60%–90% of pre-bronchoscopy sputum specimens eventually yield positive culture results. Therefore, unless a rapid diagnosis is needed, bronchoalveolar lavage with transbronchial biopsy is usually not necessary in the diagnostic evaluation of persons suspected of having pulmonary tuberculosis. If bronchoscopy is undertaken, transbronchial biopsies should be performed and post-bronchoscopy sputum specimens should be obtained because 35%–70% of post-bronchoscopy specimens will yield positive cultures. In the evaluation of miliary disease, if the initial sputum smears are negative, fiberoptic bronchoscopy with transbronchial biopsy should be performed to exclude other diseases such as fungal infections and malignancies, which can produce a miliary pattern on the chest radiograph (Chapter 63). In all instances, both bronchoalveolar lavage fluid and biopsy tissue should be cultured for mycobacteria and fungi.

The benefits of a rapid diagnosis provided by bronchoscopy must be weighed against the risk and costs of the invasive procedure as well as the potential exposure to health care workers. The authors favor empiric therapy over bronchoscopy in HIV-uninfected individuals in whom there is a moderate-to-high prior probability of tuberculosis, unless a malignancy or other disease is suspected. In San Francisco, of patients with suspected tuberculosis who were smear-negative and who were started on empiric therapy, approximately 50% were eventually found to have tuberculosis (5).

People with suspected extrapulmonary tuberculosis should have appropriate tissue and/or fluids obtained for AFB smear and culture. Patients with suspected tuberculous meningitis should have a lumbar puncture performed. Findings in the cerebrospinal fluid (CSF) that are consistent with tuberculosis include high protein concentration, low glucose concentration, and lymphocytic pleocytosis (2). AFB smears are positive in 10%–20% of cases and cultures are positive in 55%–80%, depending on whether or not multiple specimens are obtained.

Pleuritis with effusion is a common extrapulmonary manifestation of tuberculosis (Chapter 60). Findings in the pleural fluid that are consistent with tuberculosis include a lymphocytic exudate, often with a low glucose concentration. AFB smears of the pleural fluid are rarely positive, except in the setting of tuberculous empyema, and *M. tuberculosis* is isolated by culture in only 20%–35% of patients with proved pleural tuberculosis. Sputum cultures may be positive in 5%–40% of cases (6). The yield can be increased by performing a pleural biopsy, usually done under direct visualization. The combination of pleural tissue histopathology and culture is diagnostic of tuberculosis in approximately 90% of cases.

Neither the clinical presentation nor the radiographic manifestations of tuberculosis are specific for the disease. Other infectious diseases, such as bacterial pneumonias, *Pneumocystis carinii* (now renamed as *Pneumocystis jirovecii*), and other fungal pathogens, may be associated with an upper lobe radiographic infiltrates. Noninfectious causes of upper lobe densities include sarcoidosis, hypersensitivity pneumonitis, and ankylosing spondylitis. Ipsilateral hilar enlargement may occur in the setting of primary tuberculosis, but this finding in adults is highly suspicious for a malignancy, as is a mass-like lesion (Chapter 61).

Indications for Hospital Admission

Most people who have or are suspected of having tuberculosis can be treated effectively in the outpatient setting. Some patients, however, will require hospitalization because of the severity of their illness or for social reasons. Medical indications for hospitalization include severe extrapulmonary disease, pulmonary disease with respiratory compromise or hemoptysis, or, occasionally, a need for further diagnostic tests. Social indications usually relate to the potential for transmitting the infection to others with whom the patient may come in contact. Effective therapy, especially given under direct observation, rapidly reduces infectiousness, thereby decreasing or eliminating the need for hospitalization for isolation. Occasionally, patients with tuberculosis caused by multidrug-resistant organisms will require hospitalization for initiation of a treatment regimen that includes toxic or intravenously administered agents.

Infection Control

Patients with suspected pulmonary and/or laryngeal tuberculosis should be placed in respiratory isolation immediately. Once in isolation, it is important for the patient to remain in the room as much as possible. When the patient leaves the room, he/she should wear an unfitted surgical mask in order to minimize potential transmission of *M. tuberculosis* to others in the environment. Health care workers entering the room should wear a N95 respirator. Hospitalized patients with proven tuberculosis should remain in respiratory isolation until three consecutive AFB smears are negative and there has been clinical improvement with antituberculosis therapy (7). Patients who have smear-negative tuberculosis also pose some risk of transmission, although the risk is less than that in smear-positive cases. Smear-negative patients who have a high probability of tuberculosis should also be kept in isolation for several days or until an effective treatment regimen has been established.

Early identification and isolation of patients at high risk for tuberculosis is very important in preventing nosocomial transmission of *M. tuberculosis*. Unfortunately, the ability to quickly identify those patients who have tuberculosis is relatively poor, and thus the use of isolation rooms is generally inefficient. In one study, isolation of all patients with suspected tuberculosis would have resulted in a 92-fold overuse of isolation rooms (8). In a study examining the prediction of pulmonary tuberculosis, predictor variables were upper zone infiltrates on chest radiograph, a history of fever or weight loss, and low CD4 lymphocyte count (9). Using these predictors, the investigators developed a model that had a sensitivity of 100%, a specificity of 48%, and a negative predictive value of 100%. The investigators estimated that applying their model could have reduced the number of patients requiring isolation by more than 40% without increasing the risk of transmission. This model and others will need to be validated in other areas with different patient populations and prevalences of tuberculosis before they can be utilized routinely.

Because of the importance of rapid and accurate diagnosis of tuberculosis—both for the benefit of the patient and for efficient infection control—it is essential that hospitals have rapid access to high-quality mycobacteriology services, ether on-site or through arrangements with off-site facilities. The industry standard for return of AFB smear results is no longer than 24 hours. The time required for definitive identification of *M. tuberculosis* varies depending on the methods used, but most acute care hospitals should at least be using a liquid culture system to increase the speed of identification. Tests for speciation of any mycobacterium that is isolated and other tests for drug susceptibility can be referred to more specialized laboratories.

Initial Therapy

Individuals with suspected tuberculosis should be given a multidrug regimen as soon as possible to prevent the transmission of *M. tuberculosis*. There are four basic treatment regimens for adults (Table 67.1) (10). Each regimen has an initial phase of two months followed by a continuation phase of 4–7 months. The minimally acceptable duration of therapy for patients with culture-positive tuberculosis is 6 months. The initial phase of therapy should consist of a 2-month period of isoniazid, rifampin, pyrazinamide, and ethambutol. Once the patient has been determined to have tuberculosis caused by drug-susceptible organisms, ethambutol can be discontinued. The continuation phase of therapy should consist of isoniazid and rifampin given for 4 months. With appropriate dose adjustments (Table 67.2), the continuation phase can be given daily, or two or three times a week. Patients who are HIV-negative, have no evidence of cavitation on a chest radiograph, and who have negative smears after 2 months of therapy, can be treated with once weekly isoniazid and rifapentine in the continuation phase. However, if the patient has cavitation evident on a chest radiograph and a positive smear after 2 months of therapy, the once-weekly regimen is not recommended.

In patients who are suspected of having multidrug-resistant tuberculosis, six or more antituberculosis drugs may be appropriate for initial therapy. The composition and duration of regimens for patients with drug-resistant organ-

TABLE 67.1

DRUG REGIMENS FOR CULTURE-POSITIVE PULMONARY TUBERCULOSIS CAUSED BY DRUG-SUSCEPTIBLE ORGANISMS

		Initial Phase			Continuation Phase	Rating[a] (Evidence[b])	
Regimen	Drugs	Interval and doses[c] (minimum duration)	Regimen	Drugs	Interval and doses[cd] (minimum duration)	HIV −	HIV +
1	INH RIF PZA EMB	Daily for 56 doses (8 wk)	1a	INH/RIF	Daily for 126 doses (18 wk)	A (1)	A (II)
			1b	INH/RIF	2 times weekly for 36 doses (18 wk)	A (I)	A (II)[e]
			1c[f]	INH/RPT	1 time weekly for 18 doses (18 wk)	B (I)	E (I)
2	INH RIF PZA EMB	Daily for 14 doses (2 wk) and then 2 times/wk for 12 doses (6 wk)	2a	INH/RIF	2 times weekly for 36 doses (18 wk)	A (II)	B (II)[e]
			2b[f]	INH/RPT	1 time weekly for 18 doses (18 wk)	B (I)	E (I)
3	INH RIF PZA EMB	3 times/wk 24 doses (8 wk)	3a	INH/RIF	3 times weekly for 54 doses (18 wk)	B (I)	B (II)
4	INH RIF EMB	Daily for 56 doses (8 wk)	4a	INH/RIF	Daily for 217 doses (31 wk)	C (I)	C (II)
			4b	INH/RIF	2 times weekly for 62 doses (31 wk)	C (I)	C (II)

EMB, ethambutol; INH, isoniazid; PZA, pyrazinamide; RIF, rifampin; RPT, rifapentine.
[a] Definitions of ratings: A = preferred, B = acceptable alternative, C = offer when A and B cannot be given, E = should never be given.
[b] Definitions of ratings: I = randomized clinical trial, II = data from clinical trials that were not randomized or were conducted in other populations, III = expert opinion.
[c] When DOT is used, drugs may be given 5 days/week and doses adjusted accordingly. Five day a week dosing is rated AIII.
[d] Patients with cavitation on the initial chest radiograph and positive cultures at completion of 2 months of therapy should receive a 7-month continuation phase.
[e] Not recommended for HIV-infected patients with CD4 cell counts <100 cells/μl.
[f] Options 1c and 2b should be used only with HIV-negative patients who have negative sputum smears at the time of completion of 2 months of therapy and who do not have cavitation on initial chest radiograph (see text). For patients started on this regimen and found to have a positive culture from the 2-month specimen, treatment should be extended an extra 3 months.
Source: Treatment of Tuberculosis. *Morbidity and Mortality Weekly Report* 2003;52:1–77.

isms must be tailored individually, based on known or presumed drug susceptibility and the history of prior therapy.

Nine-month regimens using isoniazid and rifampin are also effective. As with 6-month regimens, ethambutol should be included in the initial phase of therapy. Shorter treatment regimens may be used in patients with sputum AFB smear-negative and culture-negative pulmonary tuberculosis. Four months of isoniazid and rifampin, preferably along with pyrazinamide for the first two months, is as successful as longer treatment regimens.

The most frequent cause of treatment failure or relapse is non-adherence to the treatment regimen. Therefore, all hospitalized patients should be treated with *directly observed therapy* (DOT). Arrangements should be made prior to discharge to continue DOT. Additionally, combination tablets such as Rifamate (isoniazid and rifampin) and Rifater (isoniazid, rifampin, and pyrazinamide) should be used whenever possible.

Treatment in Special Circumstances

Pregnancy

Antituberculosis therapy should not be withheld from pregnant women who are suspected of having tuberculosis because untreated tuberculosis represents a greater risk to the mother and fetus than does treatment itself. Antituberculosis therapy should be initiated in pregnant women who have a moderate to high suspicion of tuberculosis. Many clinicians do not start pyrazinamide in pregnant women because of the lack of teratogenicity data related to the drug. However, the World Health Organization and the International Union Against Tuberculosis and Lung Disease recommend its use, and in most countries, pyrazinamide is used during pregnancy (10). If pyrazinamide is not used in the initial phase of treatment, the duration of therapy must be increased from 6 to 9 months.

Renal Failure. Some antituberculosis medications are cleared by the kidneys, and some are removed via hemodialysis. Of the first-line antituberculosis drugs, only pyrazinamide and ethambutol are cleared significantly by the kidneys, and thus alterations in dosing may be required in patients with renal insufficiency and those with end-stage renal disease who are receiving hemodialysis (10). Ethambutol and pyrazinamide should be given in standard daily doses but given intermittently, generally three times a week after hemodialysis. Only pyrazinamide (and its metabolites) is cleared to any significant degree by hemodialysis, but if the drug is given after hemodialysis, supplemental dosing is not required. Isoniazid and rifampin are metabolized by the liver and are not removed via hemodialysis, so no dosage adjustments are necessary. Although pyrazinamide can be used in patients with renal failure, it increases the hyperuricemia that is common in such patients. It is important to monitor blood levels of ethambutol and the aminogylycoside/polypeptide antituberculosis drugs when they are being given to patients with renal insufficiency and those receiving hemodialysis.

Hepatic Disease. Most patients with underlying chronic liver disease will tolerate the standard antituberculosis treatment regimen, despite the fact that isoniazid, rifampin, and pyrazinamide are hepatotoxic (Table 67.2). If the serum aminotransferase levels are more than five times the upper limit of normal at baseline, a non-hepatoxic regimen should be initiated. One such regimen consists of ethambutol, streptomycin, cycloserine, and a fluoroquinolone. If and when the liver function tests return to normal, the standard regimen can be attempted as long as there is close monitoring of liver function tests. If the provider would prefer to use only two hepatotoxic medications instead of three, pyrazinamide can be withheld. This change in the initial treatment regimen will result in no loss of efficacy as long as the duration of therapy is increased to 9 months. A rifamycin should be used in all regimens unless there is a strong contraindication.

Drug Interactions. Several of the antituberculosis drugs are known to interact with other medications (10). The interaction of isoniazid and phenytoin increases the serum concentration of both drugs. When given together, the serum level of phenytoin should be monitored carefully and the dosage adjusted as necessary. Rifampin is a potent inducer of the hepatic cytochrome P450 enzyme system and may accelerate the clearance of drugs such as methadone, coumadin, glucocorticoids, estrogen, oral hypoglycemic agents, digitoxin, antiarrythmic agents, anticonvulsants, ketoconazole, theophylline, and cyclosporine. Rifabutin is a less potent inducer of the hepatic cytochrome enzyme system; thus, it may be used in circumstances where rifampin cannot be used.

Concurrent use of fluoroquinolones with theophylline may prolong the half-life of theophylline. Antacids with aluminum, magnesium, or calcium and ferrous sulfate may interfere with the absorption of quinolones. Cycloserine interferes with the elimination of phenytoin, particularly when taken with isoniazid. Thus, the dose of phenytoin should generally be reduced.

Extrapulmonary Tuberculosis. In general, the treatment for extrapulmonary tuberculosis is the same as for pulmonary disease. However, when tuberculosis involves the central nervous system or bones and joints, a longer course of therapy may be indicated (10). Additionally, surgery or corticosteroids are more likely to be necessary in extrapulmonary disease.

Because of the potential lethality of central nervous system (CNS) tuberculosis and the severity of neurologic sequelae, antituberculosis therapy should begin immediately whenever CNS tuberculosis is suspected. Isoniazid and pyrazinamide penetrate the blood-brain barrier well, but the aminoglycosides, rifampin, and, to some extent, ethambutol penetrate well only in the setting of inflamed meninges (10). Of the second-line agents, cycloserine and ethionamide penetrate the meninges even in the absence of inflammation. The continuation phase of therapy may be extended from 6 to 12 months, depending on the severity of illness and response to therapy. Adjunctive therapy with corticosteroids is generally indicated in patients with CNS involvement (see below). Monitoring the effectiveness of therapy requires frequent, careful clinical neurologic assessment and repeat examinations of spinal fluid.

Studies have demonstrated that bone and joint tuberculosis can be treated with 6- to 9-month regimens, although in some cases, surgery may be necessary. Surgery should be considered if there is instability of the bones, a large ileopsoas abscess is present, or the patient is not responding to medical therapy. The success of therapy should be judged by clinical and radiographic evaluations.

Other extrapulmonary sites of disease usually respond well to short-course chemotherapy. Of note, with tuberculous lymphadenitis, lymph nodes may enlarge, new nodes may appear, and nodes may spontaneously drain and create fistulas. These changes are seldom a sign of failure, but represent a vigorous immunological reaction. Similarly, pleural effusions may enlarge or even develop during the early stages of therapy.

Management of Tuberculosis Caused by Drug-Resistant Organisms. A detailed discussion of the management of patients with tuberculosis caused by drug-resistant organisms is beyond the scope of this text. However, there are a few critical points regarding the care of these patients. First, all patients who are suspected or known to have drug-resistant tuberculosis should be treated by or in consultation with a specialist with experience in such situations. Second, at least 3 drugs to which the organism is susceptible should be used. Third, the clinical and bacteriologic response to therapy may be delayed in patients with

TABLE 67.2

DOSES AND ADVERSE DRUG REACTIONS FOR FIRST-LINE ANTITUBERCULOSIS DRUGS

Drugs	Dose, in mg/kg (maximum dose)				Adverse reactions
	Daily	1 time/wk	2 times/wk	3 times/wk	
Isoniazid	5 (300 mg)	15 (900 mg)	15 (900 mg)	15 (900 mg)	Hepatic enzyme elevation Clinical hepatitis Peripheral neuropathy Central nervous system Lupus-like reaction Rash Drug interactions
Rifampin	10 (600 mg)	—	10 (600 mg)	10 (600 mg)	Gastrointestinal upset Hepatitis Hematologic problems Flu-like symptoms Rash Orange discoloration of bodily fluids Drug interactions
Rifabutin	5 (300 mg)	—	5 (300 mg)	5 (300 mg)	Gastrointestinal upset Hepatitis Hematologic problems Flu-like symptoms Rash Uveitis Orange discoloration of bodily fluids Drug interactions
Rifapentine[a]		10 mg/kg (600 mg)	—	—	Gastrointestinal upset Hepatitis Hematologic problems Flu-like symptoms Rash Orange discoloration of bodily fluids Drug interactions
Pyrazinamide	15–30 mg/kg (2 gm)	—	35–50 mg/kg (2 gm)	30–40 mg/kg (2 gm)	Hepatitis Rash Gastrointestinal upset Transient morbilliform rash Arthralgias Hyperuricemia Gout (rare)
Ethambutol	15–20 mg/kg (1gm)	—	40–50 mg/kg (2.5 gm)	20–35 mg/kg (2.5 gm)	Optic neuritis Rash Peripheral neuropathy (rare)

[a] Rifapentine should only be used in the continuation phase of therapy.
From American Thoracic Society/Centers for Disease Control and Prevention/Infectious Diseases Society of America. Treatment of tuberculosis. *Morbidity and Mortality Weekly Report* 2003;52:1–77.

multidrug-resistant tuberculosis. Fourth, second-line agents (Table 67.3) are associated with frequent side effects and, thus, close monitoring is necessary. Fifth, although the optimum duration of treatment is not known, regimens must be prolonged, generally to 18–24 months, depending on the regimen and the severity of the disease. Finally, surgical intervention may be indicated in some cases.

Adjunctive Therapy. Corticosteroids are indicated as adjunctive therapy in certain forms of tuberculosis. The administration of corticosteroids in patients with tuberculous meningitis reduces neurological sequelae and mortality. Adjunctive corticosteroid therapy is also used for documented tuberculous pericarditis, where it has been shown to reduce the size of the effusion, the need for drainage procedures,

TABLE 67.3

DOSES AND ADVERSE DRUG REACTIONS FOR SECOND-LINE ANTITUBERCULOSIS DRUGS

Drugs	Daily dose (maximum dose)	Adverse reactions	Monitoring	Comments
Streptomycin	15–30 mg/kg (1 g)	Hearing loss Vestibular dysfunction Renal toxicity	Vestibular/hearing function Measure BUN and creatinine	After bacteriologic conversion, may switch to intermittent dosing[a]
Amikacin	15–30 mg/kg (1 g)	Hearing loss Vestibular dysfunction Renal toxicity	Vestibular/hearing function Measure BUN and creatinine	After bacteriologic conversion, may switch to intermittent dosing[a]
Kanamycin	15–30 mg/kg (1 g)	Hearing loss Vestibular dysfunction Renal toxicity	Vestibular/hearing function Measure BUN and creatinine	After bacteriologic conversion, may switch to intermittent dosing[a]
Capreomycin	15–30 mg/kg (1 g)	Hearing loss Vestibular dysfunction Renal toxicity	Vestibular/hearing function Measure BUN and creatinine	After bacteriologic conversion, may switch to intermittent dosing[a]
Ethionamide	15–20 mg/kg (1 g)	Gastrointestinal upset Metallic taste Hepatotoxicity Hypersensitivity	Measure hepatic enzymes	Start with low dose and increase as tolerated May cause hypothyroidism, especially if used with PAS
Para-aminosalicylic acid (PAS)	150 mg/kg (12 gm)	Gastrointestinal upset Hypersensitivity Hepatotoxicity Sodium load	Measure hepatic enzymes Assess volume status	Start with low dose and increase as tolerated Monitor cardiac patients for sodium load
Cycloserine	10–15 mg/kg (1 g)	Psychosis Seizures Depresssion	Assess mental status Measure serum drug concentrations	Start with low dosage and increase as tolerated Pyridoxine may decrease central nervous system effects
Levofloxacin	500–1000 mg	Gastrointestinal upset Headaches Hypersensitivity Restlessness	Clinical	Avoid antacids, zinc, iron, sucralfate. Do not use in patients taking drugs that prolong the QT interval.
Moxifloxacin	400 mg	Gastrointestinal upset Headaches Hypersensitivity Restlessness	Clinical	Avoid antacids, zinc, iron, sucralfate. Do not use in patients taking drugs that prolong the QT interval.
Gatifloxacin	400 mg	Gastrointestinal upset Headaches Hypersensitivity Restlessness	Clinical	Avoid antacids, zinc, iron, sucralfate. Do not use in patients taking drugs that prolong the QT interval.

[a] Twice weekly dosing, 15–30 mg (1.5 g); three times weekly, 15–30 mg (1.5 g)
From American Thoracic Society/Centers for Disease Control and Prevention/Infectious Diseases Society of America. Treatment of tuberculosis. *Morbidity and Mortality Weekly Report* 2003;52:1–77.

and mortality. On occasion, corticosteroid treatment may be used in the setting of tuberculous pleuritis to speed the resolution of pain, fever, and the effusion itself. However, corticosteroid treatment does not reduce the likelihood of pleural fibrosis with consequent lung restriction. Patients with pulmonary tuberculosis resulting in respiratory failure may receive some acute benefit from corticosteroid treatment, although no long-term benefits have been demonstrated.

The vast majority of patients with pulmonary tuberculosis caused by drug-susceptible organisms will respond to a 6-month treatment regimen. However, in patients with underlying multidrug-resistant disease, the response rate is much lower and, in some cases, surgery may be necessary. In patients who have localized multidrug-resistant

tuberculosis and adequate pulmonary reserve, where a poor outcome is anticipated on medical therapy alone, surgical resection may offer some benefit. Surgery (or an interventional radiographic procedure) may also be necessary in patients with severe hemoptysis associated with either active tuberculosis or the residual of previous disease ("Rasmussen's Aneurysm").

Indications for Early Consultation

Clinicians should seek expert consultation in managing any patient who has severe pulmonary or extrapulmonary tuberculosis. Additionally, all patients with tuberculosis caused by drug-resistant organisms, particularly multidrug-resistance, should receive expert consultation. Patients who develop drug toxicity or who are not responding to medical therapy may require a change in therapeutic regimen. These decisions are often complicated and may alter the overall duration of therapy and efficacy of the regimen. Consequently, an expert should be consulted before any change in therapy.

Issues During the Course of Hospitalization

Patients who have begun antituberculosis therapy must be monitored closely for evidence of drug toxicity and for response to therapy. The most common toxicities associated with the first- and second-line agents are described in Tables 67.2 and 67.3. Baseline measurements of serum aminotransferases, total bilirubin, alkaline phosphatase, serum creatinine and glucose, complete blood count with differential cell count and platelet count should be obtained for all patients. Patients receiving ethambutol should have baseline measurements of visual acuity and red/green color discrimination, and patients receiving pyrazinamide should have a measurement of serum uric acid. Repeat laboratory measurements should be made if there are abnormal baseline values or indications of possible toxicity.

Patients should also be monitored for clinical and bacteriologic improvement. Most patients will be afebrile within 2 weeks of initiation of therapy. However, patients with extensive tuberculosis may have prolonged fever despite adequate therapy. Repeat sputum specimens should be obtained at weekly intervals in patients whose initial AFB smears are positive in order to judge the response to therapy. Cultures should be obtained at 1-month intervals until specimens for 2 consecutive months have been negative.

Approximately 85%–90% of patients being treated with an isoniazid- and rifampin-containing regimen will be culture-negative by 2–3 months (10). For patients who do not convert the sputum AFB cultures to negative by 2 months of treatment and who have evidence of cavitation on a chest radiograph, the continuation phase of therapy should be extended from 4 to 7 months in order to complete a total of 9 months of therapy. In addition, the patient's adherence to the treatment regimen should be questioned and measurement of serum drug levels considered. Repeat drug susceptibility testing should be performed if the cultures are still positive after 3 months of therapy. If the patient is clinically deteriorating, two new drugs should be added to the treatment regimen, preferably drugs that the patient has never taken. If the patient is clinically stable, the clinician may wait for the results of drug susceptibility testing before changing the treatment regimen.

Discharge Issues

Most patients with tuberculosis may be discharged when their clinical condition allows or when it is determined that they are no longer infectious. The local department of public health (DPH) should be notified before discharge so that plans can be made for outpatient therapy including DOT. In addition, in some areas the public health department may be able to provide housing and other incentives to encourage adherence with therapy.

Patients who are discharged to their home while still considered infectious should be asked to limit their contact with others. If they must leave their residence, they should be instructed to wear a mask and cover their mouth when coughing.

TUBERCULOSIS IN HIV-INFECTED PATIENTS

Issues at the Time of Admission

Clinical Presentation

The clinical manifestations of tuberculosis in HIV-infected patients will vary depending on the level of immunosuppression. As the CD4 lymphocyte count decreases, extrapulmonary disease and atypical findings on chest radiographs are increasingly likely. Early in the course of HIV disease, the findings on chest radiographs are not different from typical post-primary disease. However, as the CD4 lymphocyte count decreases, the chest radiograph is more likely to be atypical, with lower zone opacities, absence of cavitation, and the presence of intrathoracic lymphadenopathy, often mimicking primary tuberculosis.

Differential Diagnosis and Initial Evaluation

The variation in the clinical and radiographic presentation of tuberculosis in the setting of HIV-infection described above can result in a lowered clinical suspicion of tuberculosis. Therefore, clinicians should maintain a low threshold for including tests designed to diagnose tuberculosis in HIV-infected individuals who have lung disease and/or fever of unknown etiology. The initial diagnostic approach, however, is the same as discussed above. Fiberoptic bronchoscopy should be performed in HIV-infected individuals whose sputum specimens, including induced specimens, are AFB smear-negative and in whom no other diagnosis has been identified. In one study, bronchoscopy with transbronchial biopsy provided an early diagnosis (positive AFB smear or granulomata on biopsy) in 23 (34%) of 67 HIV-infected patients whose AFB smears were negative or not available (7). Pre-bronchoscopy sputum cultures were positive in 89% of the subjects. Transbronchial biopsy provided the exclusive means for an early diagnosis of tuberculosis in 10% of the patients (11). Therefore, when an HIV-infected patient is undergoing bronchoscopy as part of an evaluation for suspected tuberculosis, a transbronchial biopsy should be performed with bronchoalveolar lavage. Additionally, post-bronchoscopy sputum specimens should be obtained for AFB smear and culture.

Nontuberculous mycobacteria (NTM) also are a common cause of disease in patients with advanced HIV infection; the two most common are *Mycobacterium avium* complex (MAC) and *Mycobacterium kansasii*. *M. kansasii* may present with symptoms and findings exactly like those caused by *M. tuberculosis*. MAC usually presents as a disseminated disease in patients with CD4 lymphocyte counts less than 50 cells/μL. However, MAC complex occasionally causes focal pulmonary disease in patients with higher CD4 lymphocyte counts.

The predictive value for *M. tuberculosis* using a positive AFB sputum smear will vary depending on the relative prevalence of the different mycobacterial species in a given population. Individuals who have AFB seen on microscopic examination of a respiratory specimen should be assumed to have tuberculosis and treated accordingly until the cultures are final and/or the species is identified. For patients in whom MAC is highly likely, azithromycin or clarithromycin can be added to the standard antituberculosis treatment regimen.

Indications for Admission and Isolation

In addition to the indications for admission noted earlier for people who are not infected with HIV, all HIV-infected patients with lung disease of unknown etiology should be considered for admission to the hospital (Chapter 75). Because of the difficulty in distinguishing tuberculosis from other opportunistic pathogens, clinicians should have a low threshold for isolating HIV-infected patients with lung disease of unknown etiology. Although this practice is costly, in some centers all HIV-infected patients with pulmonary disease of unknown etiology are isolated until they are demonstrated to have 3 negative AFB sputum smears.

Initial Therapy

Despite being immunocompromised, HIV-infected individuals with tuberculosis respond well to regimens containing isoniazid and rifampin. Thus, the current recommendations are to begin the same antituberculosis regimens as used in HIV-seronegative patients, with two exceptions (10). On the basis of data demonstrating an increased frequency of rifamycin resistance among patients having CD4 cell counts <100/μL, it is recommended that patients with <100 cells/μL be treated with daily or 3-times weekly therapy in the continuation phase. Twice weekly therapy should not be used in patients with CD4 counts <100 cells/μL. Once weekly administration of isoniazid-rifapentine should not be used in any HIV-infected patient.

Therapy should be initiated as soon as tuberculosis is suspected because delays in treatment have been associated with a high mortality (9). The duration of therapy for most

HIV-infected patients should be 6 months. However, when breaks in therapy are frequent or prolonged, the duration of therapy should be prolonged to nine months, particularly in patients who are slow to respond to therapy. As with HIV-negative patients, the duration of treatment should be prolonged in patients who remain AFB smear-positive after two months of therapy and who have cavitation on a chest radiograph.

The treatment of tuberculosis in HIV-infected individuals is complicated by the frequency of drug interactions and the possibility of paradoxical reactions. Highly effective antiretroviral agents, such as the protease inhibitors (PIs) and non-nucleoside reverse transcriptase inhibitors (NNRTIs) have pharmacokinetic interactions with rifamycin derivatives, such as rifampin, rifapentine, and rifabutin. The rifamycin derivatives (rifampin > rifapentine > rifabutin) are inducers of the cytochrome P450 enzyme pathway. The PIs and NNRTIs are metabolized via this pathway, so when these drugs are given concurrently with a rifamycin, the serum concentration is decreased, possibly to subtherapeutic levels. To further complicate the situation, certain NNRTIs and PIs are inhibitors of the cytochrome P450 through which rifabutin is metabolized. Consequently, serum concentrations of rifabutin will be increased, sometimes to toxic levels. Fortunately, dosage adjustments in rifabutin and/or the PIs and NNRTIs can enable safe and effective dosing of each class of drug. The reader is referred to reviews (12) of this subject and a new CDC website (www.cdc.gov/nchstp/tb) and encouraged to obtain expert consultation because of the complexity of some of the dosage adjustments and the rapidly changing recommendations in this area.

In some patients, suspected tuberculosis turns out to be another mycobacterial infection such as *M. kansasii* or MAC. The current recommendation for the treatment of pulmonary disease caused by *M. kansasii* is the regimen of isoniazid, rifampin (rifabutin), and ethambutol given daily for 18 months, with at least 12 months of negative sputum cultures (13). For patients who do not tolerate one of these medications, clarithromycin or azithromycin are reasonable alternatives. Disseminated MAC should be treated with daily clarithromycin (500 mg twice a day) or azithromycin (250–500 mg once a day), plus ethambutol (15 mg/kg/day). A third drug, preferably rifabutin, should be added if possible (13). Therapy should be continued for life unless immune resconstitution occurs as a consequence of antiretroviral therapy. Secondary prophylaxis can be discontinued if the patient has received a completed course of at least 12 months of treatment for MAC, is asymptomatic with respect to MAC infection, and has a sustained increase (e.g., over at least 6 months) in the CD4 lymphocyte count to >100 cells/μL after antiretroviral therapy (14).

Clinicians should seek early expert consultation in the evaluation of HIV-infected patients with new lung disease or febrile illness. Invasive diagnostic procedures are much more likely to be necessary in the workup of HIV-infected patients than in seronegative individuals. In addition, HIV-infected patients, particularly those receiving antiretroviral therapy, may not tolerate standard regimens, as described above.

Issues During the Course of Hospitalization

HIV-infected patients with tuberculosis should be followed closely for signs of drug toxicity and for response to therapy. Whether or not HIV-infected patients have an increased frequency of side effects is not clear. However, because patients with HIV infection are frequently taking many different medications, the possibility of drug interactions is increased.

The HIV-infected patient should also be monitored carefully for signs of clinical and bacteriologic improvement. Repeat sputum specimens should be obtained in persons who have AFB smear-positive tuberculosis. Studies have demonstrated that sputum conversion rates are similar, regardless of HIV serostatus.

In some patients, clinical and/or radiographic findings worsen during the course of therapy. This is referred to as a "paradoxical reaction" and is thought to be the result of reconstitution of immune responsiveness, owing to either antiretroviral treatment or treatment of tuberculosis. Paradoxical reactions have been reported in 6%–36% of HIV-infected patients with tuberculosis, and the reactions appear to be more common in patients receiving antiretroviral drugs. When the reaction is severe and life threatening, corticosteroids are indicated.

Discharge Issues

It is very important to contact the local public health department well in advance of discharge. Generally, HIV-infected patients with tuberculosis should be treated with DOT. Because many HIV-infected patients may be returning to an institutional or congregate living facility, the rules of each facility must be ascertained before discharge. Most facilities require that patients have three consecutive negative AFB smears before returning.

COST CONSIDERATIONS AND RESOURCE USE

Most patients with suspected tuberculosis do not require hospitalization. The cost of treatment increases significantly if the patient is hospitalized. In fact, inpatient treatment of tuberculosis accounts for 60% of the total costs of tuberculosis treatment in the United States (15). If patients do not require hospitalization for clinical reasons, preventing unnecessary hospitalization would significantly reduce the overall costs of treatment. Most patients, even those with conditions likely to interfere with treatment compliance, can be treated as outpatients using DOT. Thus, hospitalization simply to ensure treatment is rarely neces-

sary. In persons who are hospitalized, enhanced ability to predict who does or does not have tuberculosis (such as with more rapid testing) would also save money by preventing the unnecessary isolation of many patients.

KEY POINTS

- The best way to prevent nosocomial transmission of tuberculosis is to not hospitalize patients unnecessarily.
- When hospitalization is necessary, patients should be isolated immediately and treatment begun as soon as possible in cases in which the clinical suspicion is moderate to high, even if the initial AFB smears are negative.
- Patients with suspect pulmonary tuberculosis may be safely removed from isolation after three negative AFB smears have been obtained and the patient is improving on therapy.
- Suspected cases of tuberculosis should be reported promptly to the local department of public health.
- The current 6-month tuberculosis treatment regimen is highly effective in both HIV-seronegative and seropositive cases, particularly when given under direct supervision.
- In HIV-infected individuals who are taking antiretroviral regimens, the tuberculosis treatment and/or antiretroviral regimen may need to be modified. Expert consultation should be obtained.

REFERENCES

1. Miller LG, Asch SM, Yu EI, et al. A population-based survey of tuberculosis symptoms: how atypical are atypical presentations? *Clin Infect Dis* 2000;30:293–299.
2. American Thoracic Society. Diagnostic standards and classification of tuberculosis in adults and children. *Am J Respir Crit Care Med* 2000;161:1376–1395.
3. American Thoracic Society. Rapid diagnostic tests for tuberculosis. *Am J Respir Crit Care Med* 1997;155:1804–1814.
4. Wallace JM, Deutsch AL, Harrell JH, et al. Bronchoscopy and transbronchial biopsy in evaluation of patients with suspected active tuberculosis. *Am J Med* 1981;70:1189–1194.
5. Gordin FM, Slutkin G, Schecter G, et al. Presumptive diagnosis and treatment of pulmonary tuberculosis based on radiographic findings. *Am Rev Respir Dis* 1989;139:1090–1093.
6. Conde MB, Loivos AC, Rezende VM, et al. Yield of sputum induction in the diagnosis of pleural tuberculosis. *Am J Respir Crit Care Med* 2003;167:723–725.
7. Centers for Disease Control and Prevention. Guidelines for preventing the transmission of *Myocobacterium tuberculosis* in healthcare facilities, 1994. *MMWR* 1994;43:1–132.
8. Scott B, Schmid M, Nettleman MD. Early identification and isolation of inpatients at high risk for tuberculosis. *Arch Intern Med* 1994;154:326–330.
9. El-Solh A, Mylotte J, Sherif S, et al. Validity of a decision tree for predicting active pulmonary tuberculosis. *Am J Respir Crit Care Med* 1997;155:1711–1716.
10. American Thoracic Society/Centers for Disease Control and Prevention/Infectious Diseases Society of America. Treatment of tuberculosis. *MMWR* 2003;52:1–77.
11. Kennedy DJ, Lewis WP, Barnes PF. Yield of bronchoscopy for the diagnosis of tuberculosis in patients with human immunodeficiency virus infection. *Chest* 1992;102:1040–1044.
12. Burman WJ, Jones BE. Treatment of HIV-related tuberculosis in the era of effective antiretroviral therapy. *Am J Respir Crit Care Med* 2001;164:7–12.

13. American Thoracic Society. Diagnosis and treatment of disease caused by nontuberculous mycobacteria. *Am J Respir Crit Care Med* 1997;156:S1–S25.

14. Recommendations of the U.S. Public Health Service and the Infectious Diseases Society of America. Guidelines for preventing opportunistic infections among HIV-infected persons, 2002. *Ann Intern Med* 2002;137:435–477.

15. Brown RE, Miller B, Taylor WR, et al. Health-care expenditures for tuberculosis in the United States. *Arch Intern Med* 1995;155: 1595–1600.

ADDITIONAL READING

Iseman E. *A Clinician's Guide to Tuberculosis.* 1st ed. Philadephia: Lippincot Williams & Wilkins, 2000.

Institute of Medicine. *Ending Neglect: The Elimination of Tuberculosis in the United States.* Geiter L, ed. Washington D.C.: National Academy Press, 2000.

Thwaites GE, Nguyen, DB, Nguyen HD, et al. Dexamethasone for the treatment of tuberculous meningitis in adolescents and adults. *N Engl J Med* 2004;351:1741–1751.

Urinary Tract Infection

68

Thomas M. Hooton

INTRODUCTION

Most urinary tract infections (UTIs) are diagnosed and treated in the outpatient setting, but many patients with community-acquired UTIs require hospitalization. Moreover, UTIs are the most common type of nosocomial infections in the United States, resulting in more than 1 million nosocomial UTIs annually, with urinary catheter-associated infections accounting for 88% of the infections (1). Catheter-associated bacteriuria is the most common source of Gram-negative bacteremia in hospitalized patients. Asymptomatic bacteriuria occurs in up to 53% of elderly women and 37% of elderly men who are institutionalized.

UTIs in hospitalized patients are either community-acquired or hospital-acquired and may be limited to the lower urinary tract (cystitis, asymptomatic bacteriuria, or prostatitis) or involve the upper urinary tract (including pyelonephritis and renal or perirenal abscess). It is unusual for patients with community-acquired cystitis or prostatitis to require admission to the hospital. UTI in hospitalized patients, therefore, generally consists of community-acquired acute uncomplicated pyelonephritis in young women, community-acquired complicated upper-tract infection in patients with functional or anatomically abnormal urinary tracts, and nosocomial lower or upper UTIs. Nosocomial UTIs are considered (by definition) complicated, and almost all occur in the setting of obstruction of the urinary tract, vesicoureteral reflux, neurogenic bladder, diabetes, or urologic instrumentation, especially urethral catheterization. A complicated UTI is one that is associated with a condition that increases the risk of treatment failure or serious complications (Table 68.1).

The approach to hospitalized patients with UTI is generally to (a) obtain a urine specimen to confirm the presence of pyuria, (b) make a definitive microbiologic diagnosis and determine the antimicrobial susceptibility profile of the causative uropathogen, (c) start empiric antibiotics, (d) determine whether there are complicating factors that might compromise antimicrobial management, (e) correct such factors if deemed appropriate, and (f) observe the patient carefully on therapy. *Escherichia coli* is the most common causative uropathogen, but the profile of uropathogens causing complicated UTI, especially nosocomial UTI, is broad (Table 68.2), and antimicrobial resistance is common. Resistance to commonly used antimicrobials appears to be increasing in prevalence even in the setting of uncomplicated UTI (2). Therefore, empiric therapy for a patient ill enough to be hospitalized should be broad-spectrum. The usual duration of therapy is approximately 7–14 days, but therapy might be for a longer or shorter period depending on the patient's underlying complicating factors, site of infection, and clinical response.

LOWER URINARY TRACT INFECTIONS (CYSTITIS, PROSTATITIS, ASYMPTOMATIC BACTERIURIA)

Issues at the Time of Diagnosis

Clinical Presentation

The presentation of hospitalized patients with UTI varies according to the clinical setting. Cystitis, prostatitis, and asymptomatic bacteriuria in the hospitalized patient are likely to have been acquired during the patient's hospitalization. Patients with community-acquired lower UTIs, on the other hand, usually do not require hospitalization. Patients with *acute cystitis*, whether community- or hospital-acquired, generally present with acute onset of dysuria, frequency, urgency, or suprapubic pain in the absence of fever or costovertebral angle tenderness. Symptoms and signs of patients with UTI at the extremes of age or with neurologic disease are often subtle and nonspecific and may be limited to symptoms such as fatigue, irritability, malaise, nausea, headache, abdominal or back pain, or

TABLE 68.1

SELECTED CONDITIONS COMPLICATING URINARY TRACT INFECTION IN ADULTS

Structural or functional abnormalities

Urolithiasis
Malignancies
Strictures
Fistulae
Ileal conduits and other urinary diversions
Neurogenic bladder
Vesicoureteral reflux

Foreign bodies

Indwelling catheter
Ureteral stent
Nephrostomy tube

Other conditions

Renal failure
Renal transplantation
Immunosuppression
Multidrug-resistant uropathogens
Hospital-acquired infection
Prostatitis
Pregnancy
Diabetes

Some factors complicate urinary tract infection through several mechanisms.

other vague symptoms. Men with *acute bacterial prostatitis* usually present with a UTI syndrome manifested by dysuria, frequency, urgency, obstructive voiding symptoms, fever, chills, and myalgias. The prostate also is tender and swollen. *Asymptomatic bacteriuria*, by definition (see later in this chapter), occurs in the asymptomatic patient and is detected by urine culture. Screening cultures for asymptomatic bacteriuria are recommended only in selected patients, as discussed below.

Differential Diagnosis and Initial Evaluation

The differential diagnosis for cystitis includes urethritis and vaginitis, and for prostatitis includes cystitis and obstructive uropathy. The clinician usually is alerted to the urinary tract as the source of the patient's symptoms because of the constellation of dysuria, frequency, and urgency in the presence of pyuria. Pyuria often is present in a catheterized patient and may lead the clinician to wrongly conclude that UTI is the cause of the patient's symptoms. Patients should undergo a complete history, physical examination, and laboratory evaluation to make sure that UTI is the correct diagnosis and that other intra-abdominal or genitourinary conditions are not present. A prostate examination is recommended in men in whom the diagnosis of acute

prostatitis is being considered, but *massage is contraindicated* because of the risk of precipitating bacteremia.

In patients with a suspected UTI, a urinalysis to look for pyuria and hematuria should be performed. Pyuria is present in almost all patients with acutely symptomatic UTI, and the absence of pyuria suggests a diagnosis other than UTI. Pyuria is not specific for UTI, however, especially in the catheterized patient. Microscopic evaluation of the urine for bacteriuria is an insensitive test, because pathogens in low quantities ($<10^4$ colonies per milliliter) are difficult to find on the wet mount or Gram stain, even on a spun specimen. A urine Gram stain may be particularly useful because distinction between Gram-positive and Gram-negative infections can influence empiric therapy. The presence of hematuria should be assessed in the noncatheterized patient because it is frequently present in persons with UTI but not in persons with urethritis or vaginitis.

Urine cultures and antimicrobial susceptibility testing of uropathogens should be performed routinely in all hospitalized patients with suspected UTI. The definitive diagnosis of UTI is made in the presence of significant bacteriuria, generally defined as more than 10^5 uropathogens per milliliter of voided midstream urine. Several recent studies have shown that this is an insensitive standard if applied to patients with acutely symptomatic UTI. The Infectious Disease Society of America has defined significant colony counts for acute *uncomplicated* cystitis in women as at least 10^3 colonies per milliliter, for *complicated* cystitis as at least 10^3 colonies per milliliter (except if urine cultures are obtained through a catheter, in which case a level of at least 10^2 colonies per milliliter is considered evidence of infection), and for *cystitis* in men as at least 10^4 colonies per milliliter (3). *Asymptomatic bacteriuria* is identified as the presence of two consecutive clean-voided urine specimens with at least 10^5 colonies per milliliter of the same uropathogen in the absence of symptoms.

TABLE 68.2

BACTERIAL ETIOLOGY OF URINARY TRACT INFECTION

Uncomplicated	Complicated
Escherichia coli	*Escherichia coli*
Staphylococcus saprophyticus	Enterococci
Klebsiella spp.	*Klebsiella* spp.
Proteus mirabilis	*Proteus mirabilis*
Enterococci	*Enterobacter* spp.
Other	*Pseudomonas aeruginosa*
	Citrobacter spp.
	Staphylococcus aureus
	Other

From Gupta K, Hooton TM, Stamm WE. Increasing antimicrobial resistance and the management of uncomplicated community-aquired urinary tract infections. *Ann Intern Med* 2001;135:41–50, and Nicolle LE. A practical guide to the management of complicated urinary tract infection. *Drugs* 1997;53:583–592.

Indications for Hospitalization and ICU Admission

Patients with community-acquired lower UTI usually do not require hospitalization. Indications for admission of patients with UTI to the hospital include the inability to maintain oral hydration or take medications, the need to relieve obstruction of the urinary tract or manage another complicating factor, uncertain social situation or concern about compliance, the need for parenteral antibiotics that cannot be arranged for on an outpatient basis, uncertainty about the diagnosis, and severe illness with high fevers, severe pain, and marked debility. Patients with lower UTIs rarely require ICU care, although ICU patients are at high risk for developing cystitis or asymptomatic bacteriuria because most of them require indwelling catheterization.

Initial Therapy

Cystitis

By definition, *cystitis requiring hospitalization or occurring in the hospital is complicated.* Unlike the narrow and predictable spectrum of causative agents in uncomplicated infection, a broad range of bacteria can cause complicated infections, and many are resistant to multiple antimicrobial agents. Although *E. coli* is the predominant uropathogen in complicated UTI, uropathogens other than *E. coli* account for a relatively higher proportion of cases compared with uncomplicated UTIs; these uropathogens include *Citrobacter* spp., *Enterobacter* spp., *Pseudomonas aeruginosa*, enterococci, *Staphylococcus aureus*, and fungi (Table 68.2) (4). Patients with chronic conditions, such as spinal cord injury and neurogenic bladder, are relatively more likely to have polymicrobial and multidrug-resistant infections.

Therapy of patients with complicated UTI must be guided by the results of urine cultures, which provide information on the responsible organism and antimicrobial susceptibility patterns. Any known underlying structural or functional urologic abnormalities related to the UTI must be corrected if possible to decrease the risk of severe complications, persistence, or recurrence of UTI. An ultrasound examination or other imaging procedure should be performed and a urinary catheter placed in a patient who has obstructive symptoms or who does not urinate appropriately under observation.

For empiric therapy in patients with mild-to-moderate cystitis who can be treated with oral medication, the fluoroquinolones provide the broadest spectrum of antimicrobial activity, covering most expected pathogens and achieving high levels in the urine and urinary tract tissue. In contrast to other fluoroquinolones, moxifloxacin and trovafloxacin may not achieve high enough concentrations in urine to be effective for complicated UTI and are not recommended for this indication. If the infecting pathogen is

known to be susceptible, other agents listed in Table 68.3 are reasonable therapeutic choices. β-lactam antibiotics and nitrofurantoin are generally considered to be safe in pregnancy, but a broad-spectrum parenteral agent other than a fluoroquinolone, such as ceftriaxone, should be used empirically in pregnant women for all symptomatic infections other than mild cystitis until susceptibility data are available. Nitrofurantoin should otherwise be avoided in the treatment of complicated UTI.

Fungal UTI is most often caused by *Candida* spp. and usually is associated with diabetes, advanced age, renal transplantation, or the use of indwelling catheters or stents, corticosteroids, or broad-spectrum antibiotics (5). The presence of pyuria and fungal quantification in urine culture may not distinguish colonization from invasive infection, and direct visualization or biopsy may be warranted. An ultrasound or other imaging study should be performed to rule out the possibility of predisposing factors or bladder or renal fungus balls, which may require surgical intervention. The urinary catheter, if present, should be changed or removed if possible. Symptomatic candidal cystitis should be treated with oral fluconazole 200 mg on day 1 followed by 100 mg once daily for 4 days, or local instillation of amphotericin-B 50 mg in 1 L of sterile water at 40 mL/h for 2–5 days. The optimal duration of therapy is not known, and shorter or longer courses are advised by some authorities.

Asymptomatic candiduria usually resolves spontaneously after catheter removal, although it may persist for months. Although the risk of symptomatic infection, especially upper

TABLE 68.3

ORAL REGIMENS FOR THERAPY OF ACUTE UNCOMPLICATED PYELONEPHRITIS AND COMPLICATED CYSTITIS

Drug	Dose	Interval
Ciprofloxacin	500 mg[a]	q 12 h
Ciprofloxacin XR	1 g[a]	q 24 h
Gatifloxacin	400 mg[a]	q 24 h
Levofloxacin	250–500 mg[a]	q 24 h
Ofloxacin	200–300 mg[a]	q 12 h
Trimethoprim–sulfamethoxazole	160/800 mg[b]	q 12 h
Amoxicillin	500 mg[c]	q 8 h
Amoxicillin	875 mg[c]	q 12 h
Amoxicillin-clavulanate	875/125 mg[c]	q 12 h
Nitrofurantoin monohydrate/ macrocrystals (Macrobid®)	100 mg[d]	q 12 h

[a] Fluoroquinolones are the agents of choice for empiric therapy, but should be avoided in pregnancy if possible.
[b] Trimethoprim-sulfamethoxazole should be used only if the causative uropathogen is known to be susceptible.
[c] Amoxicillin or amoxicillin-clavulanate should be used only if the causative uropathogen is known to be susceptible or in addition to a broad-spectrum agent if empiric coverage against enterococci is desirable.
[d] Nitrofurantoin should be used only for mild cystitis in pregnant women.

tract infection, appears to be low, persistent asymptomatic candiduria probably should be treated in patients with diabetes, neutropenia, or obstruction or those who have received a renal transplant or are about to undergo invasive urologic surgery. Oral fluconazole or amphotericin B irrigation can be used in such situations.

Asymptomatic Bacteriuria

Screening and treatment of the hospitalized patient for asymptomatic bacteriuria generally is not warranted, although recommendations vary according to the clinical setting. Patients with asymptomatic bacteriuria who may be at high risk for serious complications (and thus warrant a more aggressive approach to diagnosis and treatment) include pregnant women, patients undergoing traumatic genitourinary surgery, and renal transplant patients (6). The choice of antimicrobial agent should be based on the susceptibility of the uropathogen and the safety of the patient. Pregnant women with asymptomatic bacteriuria should be treated with agents considered to be safe in pregnancy, such as amoxicillin, cephalosporins, or nitrofurantoin.

There are some situations in which screening for and treatment of asymptomatic bacteriuria is not indicated and may in fact result in adverse effects and increased antimicrobial resistance. These situations include asymptomatic bacteriuria associated with bladder catheterization or neurogenic bladder, and asymptomatic bacteriuria in individuals older than 65 years.

Prostatitis

The most common organisms causing community-acquired acute bacterial prostatitis are Gram-negative bacilli and, less commonly, enterococci and *S. aureus*. Like complicated UTI, nosocomial prostatitis may be caused by a wider spectrum of bacteria, many of which are multidrug-resistant. Oral or parenteral fluoroquinolones are the antibiotics of choice for treatment of prostatitis because of their broad spectra of activity and excellent penetration into the prostate gland (7). Parenteral agents appropriate for the treatment of hospitalized patients with acute bacterial prostatitis are the same as those for complicated pyelonephritis (Table 68.4). If the urine Gram stain suggests the presence of Gram-positive cocci, a regimen with activity against *S. aureus* and enterococci as well as Gram-negative bacilli (e.g., piperacillin-tazobactam) should be considered. Empiric coverage should include vancomycin if methicillin-resistant *Staph aureus* (MRSA) is a concern. Nitrofurantoin should not be used for the treatment of prostatitis, because it does not achieve reliable tissue levels.

Indications for Early Consultation

A urologic evaluation is indicated at the time of admission if the patient presents with strong evidence of a complicating factor. For example, if the patient has renal colic in the setting of a UTI, an ultrasound or computed tomography

TABLE 68.4

PARENTERAL REGIMENS FOR THERAPY OF ACUTE UNCOMPLICATED PYELONEPHRITIS AND COMPLICATED UPPER TRACT INFECTION

Drug	Dose	Interval
Ceftriaxone	1–2 g	q 24 h
Cefepime	1 g[a]	q 12 h
Ciprofloxacin	200–400 mg[b]	q 12 h
Gatifloxacin	400 mg[b]	q 24 h
Levofloxacin	250–500 mg[b]	q 24 h
Ofloxacin	200–400 mg[b]	q 12 h
Gentamicin	3–5 mg/kg body weight (+/− ampicillin)[a] or	q 24 h
	1 mg/kg (+/− ampicillin)[a]	q 8 h
Ampicillin	1 g (+ gentamicin)	q 6 h
Trimethoprim–sulfamethoxazole	160/800 mg	q 12 h
Ampicillin–sulbactam	1.5 g	q 6 h
Ticarcillin–clavulanate	3.2 g[a]	q 8 h
Piperacillin–tazobactam	3.375 g[a]	q 6–8 h
Imipenem–cilastatin	250–500 mg[a]	q 6–8 h
Ertapenem	1 g	q 24 h

[a] Recommended for serious complicated pyelonephritis.
[b] Avoid fluoroquinolones in pregnancy if possible.

study should be performed to rule out the presence of a stone or obstruction. A urology consultation should be considered if the patient complains of obstructive symptoms, a large postvoid residual urine volume is found by catheterization or ultrasound, or there is radiographic evidence of an abscess or other complicating factor that may require surgical intervention. An infectious disease consultation should be considered if the diagnosis is in question after an initial evaluation of a febrile patient, the patient is very ill, or the antibiotic choice is complicated by multiple drug allergies, multidrug-resistant uropathogens, multiple sites of infection, young age, or pregnancy.

Issues During the Course of Hospitalization

Intravenous fluids are administered for volume depletion or for inability to take fluids orally. Phenazopyridine, 200 mg orally three times daily, is recommended for patients with severe dysuria. Opiates occasionally may be needed for severe pain, but it is important to make sure that the patient does not have a suppurative complication warranting drainage as the source of the discomfort.

Patients with lower UTI who are treated with antibiotics appropriate for the causative uropathogens usually demonstrate marked improvement in 24–48 hours. The antimicrobial regimen should be tailored once the infecting strain has been identified and antimicrobial susceptibilities are known. This information usually is available within 48–72 hours after the culture is taken. Those on parenteral therapy can be switched to oral treatment after clinical improvement occurs if the patient can tolerate oral hydration and medications.

Discharge Issues

Most individuals with lower UTIs are ready for discharge if they are able to tolerate oral medications. By the time of discharge, urinary signs and symptoms should be improved markedly, although they may not have resolved. The recommended duration of therapy for complicated cystitis ranges from 7–14 days, but longer therapy may be indicated in patients who have a delayed clinical response. Regimens of antibiotics for 3–7 days can be used if treatment of asymptomatic bacteriuria is indicated. The recommended duration of treatment for acute bacterial prostatitis is 10–14 days.

Patients being treated for cystitis or prostatitis should be instructed to contact their primary physicians or return to the emergency department if there is development, worsening, or recurrence of urinary symptoms, fever, or obstructive symptoms. Following treatment of UTI in pregnancy, a culture should be obtained one week after therapy to ensure bacteriologic cure. If the post-treatment culture is positive, a longer course with an antibiotic to which the causative uropathogen is susceptible should be used. A follow-up urine culture also generally is recommended in the nonpregnant patient, although it has not been established that treatment of asymptomatic bacteriuria in such populations is beneficial. Patients do not necessarily need to be seen for an office visit if their symptoms have resolved. If a follow-up urine culture is desired, patients can drop it off at the laboratory or office.

Prophylaxis may be indicated in some patients who have frequent recurrences of cystitis or pregnant women who have recurrences of asymptomatic bacteriuria.

UPPER URINARY TRACT INFECTION (PYELONEPHRITIS, PERIRENAL ABSCESS)

Issues at the Time of Diagnosis

Clinical Presentation

Acute uncomplicated pyelonephritis in young healthy women is suggested by fever, chills, flank pain, nausea or vomiting, and costovertebral-angle tenderness. Cystitis symptoms are variably present. Although acute pyelonephritis may present as a mild illness, it also may present as a catastrophic illness with sepsis syndrome, shock, and multiple organ system dysfunction (Chapters 25 and 26). Patients with *complicated pyelonephritis* present with similar symptoms and signs, but symptoms associated with the underlying complicating factor, such as nephrolithiasis, may obscure

the diagnosis. Patients with *renal or perirenal abscesses* usually present with fever, chills, back or abdominal pain, and costovertebral-angle tenderness. The pain may be referred to the groin or leg if there is extension of a perirenal abscess. Such patients may have no urinary symptoms or findings if the abscess does not communicate with the collecting system (as is often the case with a cortical abscess). Bacteremia is common in patients with upper UTI, especially those with an abscess.

Differential Diagnosis and Initial Evaluation

Even in patients presenting with classic pyelonephritis symptoms and signs, the clinician must consider other abdominal conditions in the differential diagnosis. Many conditions can be confused with UTI. The differential diagnosis includes appendicitis, cholelithiasis, diverticulitis, gastroenteritis, pelvic inflammatory disease, ectopic pregnancy, and other intra-abdominal or retroperitoneal conditions. Patients should undergo a complete history, physical examination, and laboratory evaluation to make sure that UTI is the correct diagnosis and that other serious conditions do not coexist. An evaluation of the patient's hemodynamic status is warranted because urosepsis is a serious complication of UTI.

A pretreatment urinalysis, urine Gram stain, and urine culture as described previously should be performed for all patients hospitalized with presumptive upper UTI. It is reasonable to obtain blood cultures in moderately-to-severely ill hospitalized patients with UTI to help stage the severity of the infection. A urologic evaluation is warranted at the time of diagnosis if the patient has symptoms or signs suggestive of obstructive uropathy, nephrolithiasis, or another potentially serious complicating factor. Computed tomography is recommended if an abscess is suspected to establish the diagnosis and location. It is sometimes necessary to aspirate fluid collections in order to confirm the diagnosis and to obtain cultures to direct therapy.

Indications for Hospitalization and ICU Admission

Outpatient treatment of UTI is considerably less expensive than inpatient treatment. The availability of broad-spectrum oral fluoroquinolones and once-daily dosing of ceftriaxone, ertapenem, and aminoglycosides allows for the effective outpatient treatment of many patients with upper UTIs, including many complicated infections, resulting in great cost savings. Outpatient therapy has been shown to be safe and effective for selected patients who can be stabilized with parenteral fluids and antibiotics in an urgent care facility and sent home on oral antibiotics under close supervision (8). In general, however, outpatient therapy should be reserved for nonpregnant individuals with mild-to-moderate acute cystitis (uncomplicated or complicated) or acute uncomplicated pyelonephritis, who are compliant and can be reached easily by telephone for early follow-up, and are likely to return to care in a timely fashion if symptoms do not resolve rapidly. Indications for admission of patients with upper tract infection include the factors mentioned previously for cystitis. In addition, patients with pyelonephritis who have underlying conditions such as pregnancy and diabetes that greatly increase the risk of serious complications generally should be admitted for close observation.

Clear indications for ICU admission or transfer include hemodynamic instability caused by the sepsis syndrome or hypovolemia. Rarely, pyelonephritis is complicated by Acute Respiratory Distress Syndrome and warrants ICU management.

Initial Therapy

Acute Uncomplicated Pyelonephritis

The spectrum of agents responsible for acute uncomplicated pyelonephritis is similar to that in uncomplicated cystitis, with *E. coli* the causative pathogen in approximately 70%–95% of cases and *Staphylococcus saprophyticus* in 5% to more than 20%. The antimicrobial susceptibility of causative uropathogens likewise is similar to that of uropathogens causing uncomplicated cystitis.

Women with uncomplicated pyelonephritis who are ill enough to be hospitalized should receive parenteral therapy with one of several broad-spectrum regimens (Table 68.4). For patients in whom the Gram stain is not suggestive of enterococcal infection, it is reasonable to initiate empiric treatment with ceftriaxone, 1 g per 24 hours. Aminoglycosides given once daily, parenteral fluoroquinolones, and penicillin/β-lactamase inhibitor combinations are also effective for the treatment of uncomplicated pyelonephritis. As noted previously, certain fluoroquinolones (moxifloxacin and trovafloxacin) may attain suboptimal levels in the urine and should not be used for renal infection. If enterococci are suspected based on the Gram stain, ampicillin plus gentamicin, ampicillin-sulbactam, or piperacillin-tazobactam are reasonable broad-spectrum empiric choices. Trimethoprim-sulfamethoxazole should not be used alone for empiric therapy in areas with a high prevalence of resistance to this agent. Nitrofurantoin should not be used for pyelonephritis.

Complicated Pyelonephritis

As noted in the previous section, complicated UTIs are caused by a broad range of bacteria (Table 68.2), many of which are resistant to multiple antimicrobial agents. Empiric therapy of patients with complicated pyelonephritis must be guided by the results of the urine Gram stain and subsequent culture and susceptibility data. Any known underlying structural or functional complications must be corrected, if possible. For initial empiric treatment, a broad-spectrum parenteral antimicrobial regimen should be used (Table 68.4). Empiric therapy should cover *S. aureus* until the possibility of infection with this organism can be excluded; this coverage should be active against MRSA (e.g., vancomycin) in areas with a high prevalence of MRSA. For patients with limited vascular access, oral ciprofloxacin, gatifloxacin, levofloxacin, or ofloxacin can be considered because of their excellent bioavailability. If the infecting pathogen is known to be susceptible, trimethoprim-sulfamethoxazole or other agents are also reasonable therapeutic choices. Linezolid 600 mg twice daily can be used orally or parenterally for documented infection with enterococci resistant to vancomycin or methicillin-resistant *S. aureus*.

Fungal infection of the upper urinary tract usually is caused by *Candida* spp. and may be caused by ascending infection or, much more commonly, hematogenous spread (5). Fungus balls in the ureter and renal pelvis are a complication of ascending infection; they may cause hematuria or obstruction. Most patients with renal infection from hematogenous spread do not have symptoms referable to the kidney. Systemic amphotericin B for a total dose of 1–2 g over a course of 4–6 weeks is recommended for renal fungal infection and other simultaneously infected sites (5). Fluconazole also may be effective. Surgery may be indicated for the treatment of fungus balls or complicating conditions.

Perirenal Abscess

A *renal cortical abscess* (renal carbuncle) is usually caused by *S. aureus*, which reaches the kidney through the hematogenous route. Treatment with antibiotics that cover *S. aureus* and other uropathogens causing complicated UTI (Table 68.2) is usually effective, and drainage usually is not required unless the patient is slow to respond. In contrast, a *renal corticomedullary (perinephric) abscess* usually results from ascending UTI in association with an underlying urinary tract abnormality such as obstructive uropathy or vesicoureteral reflux. It is usually caused by common uropathogenic species such as *E. coli* and other coliforms. Treatment with broad-spectrum antimicrobial agents without drainage is usually effective if the abscess is not very large and if the underlying urinary tract abnormality can be corrected. Aspiration of the abscess may be necessary in some cases, and nephrectomy may be required occasionally in patients with diffuse renal involvement or severe sepsis. Perinephric abscesses usually occur in the setting of obstruction or other complicating factors (Table 68.1) and result from ruptured intrarenal abscesses, hematogenous spread, or spread from a contiguous infection. Causative uropathogens are those commonly found in complicated UTIs (e.g., Gram-negative bacilli, *S. aureus*, and enterococci) (Table 68.2), and polymicrobial infections are common. In contrast to the other types of renal abscesses, drainage of pus is the cornerstone of therapy, and nephrectomy is sometimes indicated.

Indications for Early Consultation

A urologic evaluation or consultation with a urologist or infectious disease specialist is indicated for the same reasons as outlined for lower UTI. Moreover, any patient with a known anatomic or functional abnormality of the urinary tract who presents with clinical evidence of upper UTI should have an ultrasound or computed tomography performed to determine the need for surgery or other intervention.

Issues During the Course of Hospitalization

Intravenous fluids and analgesia may be warranted as noted in the previous section. The antimicrobial regimen should be tailored as soon as possible once the infecting strain has been identified and antimicrobial susceptibilities are known. The patient who has clinically improved and can tolerate oral hydration and medications may be switched to oral treatment with an agent to which the causative uropathogen is susceptible. Patients with acute uncomplicated pyelonephritis often can be switched to oral therapy within 72 hours (if susceptibility data are available), although longer intervals of parenteral therapy occasionally are indicated depending on the clinical response. Patients with complicated pyelonephritis or with an abscess respond more slowly.

If there has been little or no improvement in fever and symptoms by 72 hours, a repeat urine culture and an imaging study may be indicated to rule out persistent infection, obstruction, abscess, or other unrecognized urologic abnormalities. Patients whose conditions worsen after initiation of therapy may warrant an earlier evaluation. Conversely, many patients who have no detectable urologic abnormality remain febrile longer than 72 hours, and a urologic evaluation may be reasonably postponed if the patient is otherwise improving. Computed tomography is markedly superior to intravenous urography and ultrasound in demonstrating the parenchymal abnormalities caused by renal infection and in delineating the extent of the disease (9).

Discharge Issues

Most individuals with UTI are ready for discharge when they are able to tolerate oral medications. However, in a patient with multiple medical problems and an extended hospitalization, treatment of a nosocomial UTI may have little impact on the timing of discharge. By the time of discharge, urinary signs and symptoms should be markedly improved, although they may not be resolved. The presence of a low-grade temperature or mild abdominal or back tenderness is not a contraindication to discharge. It is important to make sure that the patient can tolerate the switch to an oral regimen for a few hours before discharge, but *it is not necessary to routinely observe the patient overnight* in the hospital after the switch. When patients are discharged depends on a number of issues including their social situation, support network, medical condition, insurance, and need for parenteral therapy.

Recommended treatment durations vary from one to three weeks or even longer. For acute uncomplicated pyelonephritis, 6-week regimens are no more effective than 14-day regimens and cause more side effects (10). In those mildly to moderately ill patients who have a rapid response with resolution of fever and symptoms soon after initiating treatment, treatment usually can be discontinued at 7–10 days (11). Of note, however, is that β-lactam regimens shorter than 14 days have been associated with unacceptably high failure rates. Patients with complicated pyelonephritis should be treated for 14–21 days or longer if symptoms and fever have not fully resolved.

Patients should be instructed to contact their primary care physicians or return to the emergency department if there is development, worsening, or recurrence of fever or of urinary or obstructive symptoms. A follow-up urine culture 1 or 2 weeks after treatment is recommended although, as noted previously for lower tract infection, it has not been established that treatment of asymptomatic bacteriuria in such populations is beneficial. Pregnant women should have follow-up urine cultures and be managed as described previously. Patients who have undergone urologic procedures may need to be seen by the urologist after discharge.

COST CONSIDERATIONS AND RESOURCE USE

Several developments in the past decade have resulted in cost-saving strategies in the management of UTI. Most importantly, the availability of the new oral fluoroquinolones and extended interval dosing of certain parenteral antibiotics have had tremendous impact on the cost of treatment of UTI. Thus, many patients with mild-to-moderately complicated UTIs caused by multidrug-resistant uropathogens now can be managed in the outpatient setting. Likewise, hospitalized patients can be discharged from the hospital after an early switch to broad-spectrum oral antibiotics or home parenteral antibiotic therapy. Earlier discharge from the hospital also has been facilitated by the wider availability and decreasing cost of sophisticated imaging studies and less invasive interventional techniques, both of which have allowed for more rapid diagnosis and management of disorders previously requiring surgical therapy.

Because the vast majority of nosocomial UTIs is associated with catheter use, prevention of catheter-associated infections should be given high priority in hospital settings. Effective strategies include avoidance of catheter placement if possible and, if catheter use is necessary, sterile insertion, prompt removal, and strict adherence to a closed collecting system (12). Silver alloy-coated urinary catheters appear to reduce catheter-associated bacteriuria (12). Intermittent catheterization and, in men, condom catheterization appear to result in lower rates of bacteriuria compared with long-term indwelling catheterization. Other approaches that have been effective in some (but not other) studies include the use of preconnected catheter-collecting tube units, the use of disinfectants in collecting bags, and the regular periurethral application of antimicrobial creams. Treatment of asymptomatic bacteriuria in catheterized patients is not recommended (6).

KEY POINTS

- Because the vast majority of nosocomial UTIs are associated with catheter use, prevention of catheter-associated infections should be given high priority in hospital settings.
- Unlike the narrow and predictable spectrum of causative agents in uncomplicated infection, a broad range of bacteria can cause complicated infections, and many are resistant to multiple antimicrobial agents.
- Therapy of patients with complicated UTIs must be guided by the results of urine culture and antimicrobial susceptibility test results.
- Screening and treatment of the hospitalized patient for asymptomatic bacteriuria generally is not warranted but should be performed in selected populations.
- A urologic evaluation should be considered in patients who have not had marked clinical improvement after 72 hours of therapy.
- Several developments in the past decade have resulted in huge cost-saving strategies in the management of UTI, including the availability of new oral fluoroquinolone antibiotics and extended interval dosing of certain parenteral antibiotics. These agents may obviate the need for hospitalization or may facilitate early discharge in those patients requiring an inpatient stay.

REFERENCES

1. Bronsema DA, Adams JR, Pallares R, et al. Secular trends in rates and etiology of nosocomial urinary tract infections at a university hospital. *J Urol* 1993;150:414–416.
2. Gupta K, Hooton TM, Stamm WE. Increasing antimicrobial resistance and the management of uncomplicated community-acquired urinary tract infections. *Ann Intern Med* 2001;135:41–50.
3. Rubin UH, Shapiro ED, Andriole VT, et al. Evaluation of new anti-infective drugs for the treatment of urinary tract infection. *Clin Infect Dis* 1992;15:S216–S227.
4. Nicolle LE. A practical guide to the management of complicated urinary tract infection. *Drugs* 1997;53:583–592.
5. Sobel JD, Vazquez JA. Urinary tract infections due to *Candida* species. In Mobley HLT, Warren JW, eds. *UTIs: Molecular Pathogenesis and Clinical Management.* Washington, DC: ASM Press, 1996:119.
6. Nicolle LE. Asymptomatic bacteriuria: when to screen and when to treat. *Infect Dis Clin N Am* 2003;17:367–394.
7. Krieger JN. Prostatitis revisited: new definitions, new approaches. *Infect Dis Clin N Am* 2003;17:395–409.
8. Israel RS, Lowenstein SR, Marx JA, et al. Management of acute pyelonephritis in an emergency department observation unit. *Ann Emerg Med* 1991;20:253.
9. Kawashima A, LeRoy AJ. Radiologic evaluation of patients with renal infections. *Infect Dis Clin N Am* 2003;17:433–456.
10. Stamm WE, McKevitt M, Counts GW. Acute renal infection in women: treatment with trimethoprim-sulfamethoxazole or ampicillin for two or six weeks: a randomized trial. *Ann Intern Med* 1987;106:341–345.
11. Talan DA, Stamm WE, Hooton TM, et al. Comparison of ciprofloxacin (7 days) and trimethoprim-sulfamethoxazole (14 days) for acute uncomplicated pyelonephritis in women: a randomized trial. *JAMA* 2000;283:1583–1590.
12. Saint S, Chenoweth CE. Biofilms and catheter-asssociated urinary tract infections. *Infect Dis Clin N Am* 2003;17:411–432.

ADDITIONAL READING

Carson C, Naber KG. Role of flouroquinolones in the treatment of serious bacterial urinary tract infections. *Drugs* 2004;64:1359–1373.

Hooton TM. The current management strategies for community-acquired urinary tract infection. *Infect Dis Clin N Am* 2003;17:303–332.

Ronald AR, Harding GKM. Complicated urinary tract infections. *Infect Dis Clin North Am* 1997;11:583–592.

Warren JW, Abrutyn E, Hebel JR, et al. Guidelines for antimicrobial treatment of uncomplicated acute bacterial cystitis and acute pyelonephritis in women. *Clin Infect Dis* 1999;29:745–758.

Cellulitis and Necrotizing Fasciitis

69

Dennis L. Stevens

INTRODUCTION

While many types of skin and soft tissue infection exist, this review focuses on cellulitis and necrotizing fasciitis (NF). Cellulitis is a common disease that is rarely life threatening and usually can be managed without hospital admission. It is most commonly caused by group A (GAS), B, C, or G streptococci or *Staphylococcus aureus*. Cellulitis may also be secondary to animal or human bites. NF is a rare but often life-threatening, necrotizing infection of subcutaneous tissue and fascia with relative sparing of the underlying muscle. Progression of necrosis can be alarmingly rapid, and shock and multiorgan failure is common. Despite the availability of highly active antibiotics, the morbidity and mortality rates of NF remain high. This is, in part, because of the failure of treatment strategies to alter the physiologic processes responsible for the local tissue destruction and systemic toxicity.

NF encompasses two microbiologic entities. Type I disease is polymicrobial in etiology, typically being caused by mixed anaerobes (e.g., *Clostridium*, *Bacteroides*, *Prevotella*, and *Peptostreptococcus* organisms), streptococci, and enteric Gram-negative bacilli (e.g., *Escherichia coli*, *Klebsiella*, and *Proteus* organisms). Infection often complicates deep wounds (including surgical wounds) when the vascular supply is compromised, as in severe traumatic injury or diabetes. Type II disease is typically a monomicrobial infection, most commonly caused by GAS (hemolytic streptococcal gangrene), *Clostridium perfringens* (traumatic gas gangrene), *Clostridium septicum* (spontaneous gas gangrene), *Aeromonas hydrophilia* (associated with injuries occurring in fresh water), and *Vibrio vulnificus* (associated with injuries exposed to salt water). In the case of GAS NF, infection may occur following bites or burns, postoperatively (postpartum sepsis), or spontaneously in the absence of a defined portal of entry.

Both cellulitis and NF present important challenges in diagnosis and management. In patients with cellulitis, several clinical conditions and responsible agents can be associated with an adverse outcome if not recognized. The most important challenge for the management of NF is early recognition. In its early stages, NF is difficult to distinguish from cellulitis and may not even be recognized as an infectious process.

CELLULITIS

Issues at the Time of Admission

Clinical Presentation

Prominent features of cellulitis tend to be local, with cutaneous pain, edema, warmth, erythema, and tenderness. The erythematous margins tend to be indistinct because the process is deep, involving the subcutaneous tissues in addition to the dermis. Regional lymphadenopathy and constitutional symptoms of fever, chills, and malaise are uncommon. Cellulitis most frequently involves the extremities, where it is associated with fungal infection of the toes, chronic stasis dermatitis, and chronic lymphedema following radical lymph node dissection. Cellulitis associated with these conditions is most commonly caused by Group A, C, or G streptococci. Recurrent cellulitis is most commonly caused by streptococci in association with chronic lymphedema or prior saphenous vein bypass grafts. Cellulitis associated with *Staphylococcus aureus* usually occurs with a defined focus of infection such as a suture line infection, carbuncle, sliver, or other foreign body. Cellulitis caused by *S. aureus* may also be associated with infected joints, olecranon bursitis, osteomyelitis, and a variety of prosthetic devices such as intravenous catheters and prosthetic joints. *Erysipelas* is a distinctive type of superficial cellulitis caused by group A streptococci that is associated with early systemic toxicity, prominent lymphatic involvement, and superficial spread with a raised, well-demarcated margin of brilliant red or salmon-colored erythema. Cellulitis can also be associated with animal bites caused by a variety of organisms that colonize the animals' mucous membranes (i.e., *Pasteurella multocida, Prevotella, Porphyromonas, Fusobacterium,* and *Staphylococcus*) and with organisms colonizing the human mouth (i.e., *Eikenella corrodens* and group A streptococcus).

Differential Diagnosis and Initial Evaluation

When an obvious portal of entry is evident or when symptoms appear in a distal extremity with lymphadenitis tracking proximally, the clinical diagnosis of cellulitis usually is obvious. However, irritation or allergic reactions to wound dressings, venous thrombosis, inflammatory skin lesions such as erythema nodosum, eosinophilic cellulitis or fasciitis, or fixed hypersensitivity reactions may cause similar local signs and symptoms. If inflammation is near joints, it may be important to consider gout or other inflammatory arthritides, olecranon bursitis, or a ruptured Baker's cyst.

In patients who have diffuse cellulitis without a defined portal of entry, establishing a specific diagnosis may be difficult. Superficial cultures of skin sites have low sensitivity and specificity for identifying the responsible agent. In contrast, a defined etiology can be established from Gram stain and culture in patients with a defined portal of entry, a localized area of carbuncle or abscess, or obvious draining pus or an animal bite. If the patient is immunocompromised or toxic or if the process is aggressive, establishing an etiologic diagnosis becomes more important and may require blood cultures, aspiration, biopsy, or surgical assistance. Blood cultures are rarely positive in patients with uncomplicated cellulitis but may be useful in the latter clinical situations. Aspiration can be performed by using a 21- or 22-gauge needle and injecting and aspirating 1.0 mL of preservative-free sterile saline (1). Unfortunately, punch biopsies and aspirates have relatively low-to-moderate sensitivity (5%–40%), partly because of sampling error and partly because of the fact that low numbers of bacteria may be present, suggesting that potent toxins or the host response to toxins mediate the signs of acute inflammation. Patients ill enough to require parenteral antibiotics should have a complete blood count. The need for other tests is dictated by the presence of specific underlying illness.

Outlining the margins of inflammation is useful to assess the progression of disease. This assessment is done with a pen at the initial assessment and periodically thereafter. Patients with any type of soft tissue infection who appear toxic should be evaluated carefully for under-lying deep or metastatic infections and for the possibility of NF. Clues for NF include pain that is out of proportion to the clinical findings, blisters or bullae, and subcutaneous necrosis. Patients with cellulitis over a joint should have a careful physical examination to rule out concomitant infectious bursitis or arthritis. Septic arthritis also may occur in distant joints, and all joints should be evaluated (Chapter 113).

Indications for Hospitalization and Intensive Care Unit Admission

Most patients with uncomplicated cellulitis can be managed in an outpatient setting, even if they require parenteral therapy (2–4). Admission is indicated if patients have clinical signs or laboratory tests suggesting systemic toxicity or if the possibility exists of NF, septic arthritis, or an abscess that may require surgical drainage.

ICU admission generally is necessary in patients who have evidence of septic shock. *Patients with necrotizing fasciitis can deteriorate quickly.* Thus, if the physician has a clinical suspicion of NF, admission to the ICU, aggressive fluid management, and assessment of markers of organ function should be the standard of care (even if the patient is initially stable). One useful marker of a high risk of deterioration is a normal or low white blood cell count. If deep necrotizing infection is suspected, an elevated creatine kinase may also be supportive evidence.

Initial Therapy

In general, cellulitis is caused by staphylococci or streptococci, and a variety of cephalosporins, nafcillin, clindamycin, or newer fluoroquinolones have been useful (Table 69.1). Empiric choices have become more difficult during the past three to four years because of evolving staphylococcal resistance (Chapter 64). For example, 10%–15% of methicillin-sensitive *S. aureus* organisms are now resistant to erythromycin and clindamycin. The prevalence of both hospital-acquired and community-acquired methicillin-resistant *S. aureus* (MRSA) infections is also increasing dramatically in the western world. In addition, aggressive soft tissue infections caused by MRSA have been described in communities across the United States, Australia, and Japan (5). With the prevalence of MRSA approaching 50% in many communities, empiric treatment of *S. aureus* infections must now be based on the clinician's judgment of severity. Specifically, suspected staphylococcal infections in patients who are toxic should be treated with vancomycin, linezolid, or daptomycin. Once susceptibility results are known, antibiotics can step down to more conventional agents. In contrast, in the patient with localized staphylococcal infections who is not toxic, cephalosporins or penicillinase-resistant penicillins can be used, along with careful monitoring for evidence of failure. GAS cellulitis can be treated with penicillin, a cephalosporin, or a penicillinase-resistant penicillin. In penicillin-allergic

TABLE 69.1

PRIMARY AND ALTERNATIVE THERAPEUTIC CHOICES FOR SOFT TISSUE INFECTIONS

Disease entity	Primary therapeutic agent	Alternative
Erysipelas	Penicillin	Macrolides
		Clindamycin
Cellulitis		
Localized, mild infection	Cephalosporin	Trimethoprim-sulfamethoxazole
	Nafcillin	Fluoroquinolones
	Dicloxacillin	Clindamycin
Localized, severe infection or MRSA	Vancomycin	None
	Linezolid	
	Daptomycin	
Diffuse, mild, no portal (Groups A, C, or G streptococci)	Penicillin	Clindamycin
		Cephalosporin
Diffuse, toxic	Clindamycin	
Animal bite	Ampicillin/sulbactam	Cefoxitin
	Amoxicillin/clavulanate	Cefotetan
		Doxycycline
		Carbapenem
Human bite	Ampicillin/sulbactam	Cefoxitin
		Cefotetan
		Fluoroquinolone + clindamycin
Necrotizing fasciitis		
Mixed aerobic/anaerobic	Ampicillin/sulbactam + ciprofloxacin + clindamycin or metronidazole	Carbapenem
		Piperacillin/tazobactam
Group A streptococcus	Clindamycin	

patients, clindamycin is a reasonable choice because erythromycin resistance has become more prevalent.

Issues During the Course of Hospitalization

Early administration of antibiotics is the most important immediate management concern. Patients may deteriorate systemically during the first 8–12 hours of antibiotic administration, and potentially septic patients should be monitored closely over this time. NF also may become evident only after hospital admission (see the earlier section on clinical presentation).

Most patients will have less pain and feel better within 24 hours of antibiotic treatment (3). After 3 days, improvement should be evident in virtually all patients, but some degree of fever may persist for several more days. Expansion of the margins of cellulitis almost invariably occurs in the first 24–36 hours after administration of antibiotics. In streptococcal infections in particular, such expansion may be dramatic over the first day. After this, the rate of increase should slow, but margins may continue to expand for 2–3 days. Inflammation in the area may persist for 1–2 weeks, and improvement may be especially slow in diabetic patients or in poorly vascularized limbs.

Elevation of the involved extremity helps reduce the swelling and pain. If it becomes apparent that the degree of pain and swelling requires immobilization of the limb for more than a few days, prophylaxis for deep venous thrombosis should be considered (Chapter 52).

Initial blood culture results should be reviewed to ensure that therapy is appropriate and to determine whether the spectrum of antibiotics chosen can be narrowed. Chronic wounds may become colonized with a variety of bacteria, including enterococci, enteric Gram-negative bacilli, and *Pseudomonas* organisms. In this setting, results of superficial cultures do not necessarily reflect the pathogens causing the initial infection.

As noted previously, the presence of *S. aureus* in blood cultures means that patients should be monitored carefully for the presence or development of signs of endocarditis. These patients should also have an echocardiogram (Chapter 71). In severely immunocompromised patients, skin flora such as coagulase-negative staphylococci or diphtheroids may cause intravenous site cellulitis. However, in other settings, the isolation of these organisms from blood is almost invariably a result of sample contamination at the time the blood culture was taken, and antibiotic therapy should not be modified in response to such a report.

By the second to fourth day of hospitalization, fever and pain should be improving, the area of cellulitis should be stable or regressing, and the patient should be feeling better. If such improvement is not evident, the initial diagnosis should be reassessed, and possible reasons for failure should be considered (Table 69.2). If a deep abscess

TABLE 69.2

CONSIDERATIONS IF PATIENT IS NOT RESPONDING TO THERAPY BY HOSPITAL DAY 4

Scenario	Considerations				
Alternate or concomitant diagnosis	Immune-mediated soft tissue inflammation (e.g., vasculitis or erythema nodosum)	Underlying deep infection (e.g., osteomyelitis or pyomyositis)	Deep venous thrombosis	Gout, pseudogout or other monoarthritis (or periarthritis)	Ruptured Baker's cyst (for leg cellulitis only)
Correct diagnosis but incorrect antimicrobial agent	See Table 69.1	Consider drug-resistant organism			
Correct diagnosis and antimicrobial agent	Drug not being administered	Oral medication not being absorbed (consider gastric pH)	Ineffective drug dosing (e.g., dosing too low or too infrequent, or drug interactions)		

is suspected, the use of imaging techniques, such as computed tomography (CT) and magnetic resonance imaging (MRI), may guide therapy (6,7).

In patients with uncomplicated cellulitis who are afebrile by the fourth or fifth hospital day, a switch may be made from parenteral to oral antibiotics. Patients with *S. aureus* bacteremia require parenteral therapy for at least 2 weeks if no evidence of an endovascular infection is seen and 4 weeks if it is. Neutropenic patients should be continued on therapy until their neutrophil count recovers or the cellulitis has completely resolved.

Discharge Issues

Patients may be discharged as soon as their infections are stable or improving. In the absence of septic shock, NF, or a requirement for surgery or therapy for serious intercurrent illness, a hospital stay longer than 3–4 days rarely should be required.

Patients should be told at discharge that, depending on the initial severity of the cellulitis, the signs and symptoms may remain for days and even weeks, especially if the cellulitis involves the lower extremities. Slowly improving residual swelling may be present for weeks. Limb elevation and support hose should generally be recommended.

Patients with erysipelas or streptococcal cellulitis who have required hospitalization are at risk of recurrent infection, especially if they have chronic underlying skin lesions (i.e., psoriasis) or impaired lymphatic or venous drainage (i.e., radical mastectomy or saphenous vein stripping). Such patients should be warned of the risk and the need for prompt treatment if cellulitis recurs. They should also be counseled about preventive foot or hand care (e.g., prompt treatment of tinea pedis and prevention of damage around nails).

NECROTIZING FASCIITIS

Issues at the Time of Admission

Clinical Presentation

The early diagnosis of necrotizing fasciitis may be difficult because patients may manifest only severe pain in a limb, along with malaise, chills, and fever (8). Later the area of intense pain may become red, hot, shiny, swollen, and exquisitely tender. Subsequently, there may be blue–black discoloration indicative of superficial necrosis near the center, blistering or bullae formation, and edema that extends beyond the margins of skin erythema. Crepitus may be palpable in patients with NF resulting from gas-forming organisms such as the *Clostridium* spp. (gas gangrene) or mixed aerobic/anaerobic bacteria (necrotizing fasciitis type 1) (7). In contrast, group A streptococcus does not produce gas.

Group A streptococcus causes two types of presentations with necrotizing fasciitis. Approximately 50% of patients with NF caused by group A streptococci may have only fever, chills, and severe pain. In many, hypotension and evidence of renal impairment precede the skin manifestations of NF. In these patients, elevated serum creatinine, hypotension, marked tachycardia, and severe pain should prompt surgical consultation to inspect the deep tissues and to obtain culture material (8,9). While plain radiographs, CT scans, and MRI may demonstrate swelling and edema in NF, they do not provide a definitive diagnosis. An elevation of serum creatinine kinase (CK) may provide additional clues facilitating surgical intervention.

The remaining 50% of patients with necrotizing fasciitis caused by group A streptococcus have an obvious portal of entry, such as a surgical incision, episiotomy, laceration, insect bite, or chicken pox lesion. These patients initially have cutaneous evidence of local infection and drainage. They then go on to develop toxicity or rapid localized spread and evolution to bullae formation, sloughing of skin, and ecchymosis. All this may occur despite antibiotic treatment, and this progression requires emergent surgical consultation.

Differential Diagnosis and Initial Evaluation

Fever and severe pain should lead to consideration of NF. In 50% of patients, the severe pain is at the exact site of recent, nonpenetrating trauma. *There may not be cutaneous evidence of soft tissue infection.* Depending on the location of the infection, patients who have NF without signs of cellulitis may be incorrectly diagnosed as having muscle strain, gout (or other arthritides), early herpes zoster reactivation, acute myocardial infarction, pulmonary embolus, or deep venous thrombosis.

Laboratory clues to NF include elevated CK, a marked left shift in the differential white blood cell count (8,9), elevated serum creatinine in patients who are not yet hypotensive, low serum albumin, low serum calcium, and markedly elevated C-reactive protein (8,10). Plain radiographs demonstrating tissue gas suggest necrotizing fasciitis type 1 or gas gangrene. CT and MRI scans will demonstrate the level of infection but are not specific for necrotizing fasciitis unless gas is present in the tissue. Because group A streptococcus does not form gas in the tissue, and because necrotizing fasciitis caused by this microbe occurs following nonpenetrating trauma in half the cases of NF, CT and MRI may not distinguish trauma from infection. This dilemma is most evident in women with postpartum group A streptococcal intrauterine infection, in whom the uterus is still swollen and enlarged from the birthing process.

Etiologic diagnosis is important in NF. The presence of soft tissue gas and foul smell suggests anaerobic organisms. Gram stain and cultures from aspiration of bullae or necrotic tissue often yield the responsible pathogens, and blood cultures are positive in approximately 50% of patients (7,8,11,12). Culture of surgical specimens also demonstrates the etiologic pathogen.

Indications for Hospitalization and ICU Admission

All patients in whom the diagnosis of NF has been entertained should be admitted to hospital for *supportive therapy, antimicrobials,* and *surgical debridement* if appropriate. Patients with NF can deteriorate rapidly, with development of sepsis and progression of the necrosis. Patients with concomitant sepsis syndrome (Chapter 26) require ICU admission. Patients not admitted to the ICU should have vital signs checked and a clinical assessment of the affected area made frequently until the diagnosis of NF is ruled out, surgery is performed, or the margins have stabilized.

Initial Therapy

If it is available immediately, the Gram stain result of an aspirate or biopsy may be used to guide therapy. Mixed Gram-positive and Gram-negative bacteria indicate type I disease, and broad-spectrum coverage for Gram-negative and anaerobic organisms is needed (Tables 69.1 and 69.3). Because of the risk of antimicrobial resistance in Gram-negative organisms, using at least two antibiotics active against enteric Gram-negative bacilli is recommended until culture results are obtained. A carbapenem or a third generation or fourth generation cephalosporin with metronidazole, in combination with ciprofloxacin or an aminoglycoside, is a reasonable option. In the absence of a Gram stain, patients should receive treatment for type II disease until a diagnosis is made. All persons with traumatic wounds or infections associated with the gastrointestinal tract require assessment for tetanus immunization status. Patients with NF caused by group A streptococcus should receive clindamycin. Clindamycin inhibits toxin production by bacteria, and animal studies (6) as well as one retrospective human study (13) support its use.

Surgical debridement is the mainstay of therapy for NF of all types, and the appropriate surgical team should be consulted early when NF is suspected (14,15). Surgical consultation also should be considered for infections of the hand, particularly infected cat, dog, or human bite wounds, and for patients with a history of intravenous drug abuse. The use of *hyperbaric oxygen* for the treatment of NF is controversial. Its use is not indicated in the treatment of GAS (type I) NF. It still is being advocated for the treatment of Fournier's gangrene (a life-threatening necrotizing polymicrobial infection of the genitals and perineum) and is indicated in gas gangrene.

A recommendation to use intravenous immunoglobulin (IVIg) to treat streptococcal toxic shock syndrome cannot be made with certainty. While ample evidence exists for the role of extracellular streptococcal toxins in shock, organ failure, and tissue destruction, IVIg contains variable quantities of neutralizing antibodies to some of these toxins, and definitive clinical efficacy data are lacking (16). One observational study demonstrated better outcomes in patients receiving IVIg, but these patients were more likely to have had surgery and were more likely to have received clindamycin than the historical controls (17). A second study, which was double blinded and placebo controlled, showed no significant difference in mortality and no change in the "time to no further progression of necrotizing fasciitis" (18).

Issues During the Course of Hospitalization

On day 2, definitive culture results should be available, and the antibiotic regimen can be adjusted appropriately (Table 69.3). Most patients require more than one procedure for debridement. Until day 5, clinical assessment of the

TABLE 69.3

MANAGEMENT OF NECROTIZING FASCIITIS

1. Admit to the ICU
2. Emergent consultation to infectious disease and general surgery
3. Establish an etiologic diagnosis
   a. Gram stain and culture of drainage, bullous fluid
   b. Gram stain and culture of surgical tissue samples
4. Emergent empiric antibiotics administration based upon Gram stain material
5. Aggressive, goal-directed intravenous fluid resuscitation
   a. Crystalloid/normal saline (20–30 cc/kg bolus) (19)
   b. Colloid (albumin/fresh frozen plasma). Note: Patients with necrotizing fasciitis frequently have profound hypoalbuminemia due to capillary leak.
6. Transfusion. Note: Acute anemia evolves rapidly because of absorbed toxins that are also hemolysins.
7. Calcium replacement. Profound hypocalcemia is a common finding in patients with necrotizing fasciitis, particularly those with staphylococcal or streptococcal TSS.
8. Surgical debridement. The extent of surgical debridement of nonviable tissue varies but will be apparent from the surgical consultation obtained under item 2 above.
9. Renal dialysis. Renal failure occurs early in necrotizing fasciitis, particularly in those infected with group A streptococcus and *Clostridium perfringens* or in association with staphylococcal TSS.
10. Ventilator support. ARDS develops in 60% of patients with some types of necrotizing fasciitis, particularly those caused by group A streptococcus.
11. Echocardiogram for persistent hypotension
12. Invasive monitoring for persistent hypotension or low cardiac output
13. Vasopressors for high-output hypotension. Note: Avoid pressors in low cardiac output hypotension because of the risk of symmetrical gangrene
14. Intravenous gamma globulin (IVIg). See the discussion on necrotizing fasciitis ("Initial Therapy").
15. Consider the use of activated protein C. However, there are no data to support its use in this setting, and it may be contraindicated in patients undergoing surgery.

ARDS, acute respiratory distress syndrome; *TSS*, toxic shock syndrome.

patient's pain and well-being and of the involved area should be performed every four to six hours. In patients with extensive disease, general anesthesia may be required daily for dressing changes and examination. Surgical re-exploration is indicated if new areas of necrosis are apparent, if the rate of extension of erythema does not slow or begins to increase, or if patients complain of increasing pain or malaise. Repeated operative debridement should be performed until the infection is controlled.

Between days 5 and 10, continued progression of NF becomes less likely. However, in patients who have required extensive surgery, superinfection is possible. Extension of infection during this time should prompt reculture of tissue. Skin grafting can be performed once the wound base is granulating well, at which time physical therapy should be consulted regarding rehabilitation. A nursing assessment should then be carried out, the home situation should be reviewed, and the anticipated length of stay and rehabilitation should be discussed with the patient and family members.

Issues of systemic management and duration of antibiotic therapy are the same as those for cellulitis. No clear guidelines have been formulated for the duration of antibiotic therapy. Ten days is a reasonable minimum, but a longer duration may be advisable if fever has persisted beyond the fifth day or the wound is still not healthy at day 10.

Because GAS are transmitted in families and secondary cases of streptococcal GAS have occurred, some public health jurisdictions require reporting of streptococcal toxic shock syndrome, and some physicians now recommend treating household contacts of cases with 10 days of cefazolin or a macrolide (7,20,21). Reporting those patients who are readmitted with erysipelas or surgical-site GAS cellulitis to the infection-control service is also important, as surgical-site infections of GAS are extremely rare and often are associated with outbreaks of serious nosocomial infection.

Discharge Issues

Timing of discharge largely depends on surgical issues surrounding skin grafting and the management of dressings. The main disease-related issues are wound care and rehabilitation. Home care for dressing changes and physiotherapy are nearly always required. Patients should be warned that pain may persist for weeks or months but should not worsen, and the risks for and appropriate response to surgical-site infections should be discussed. Recurrent NF is not a risk, but cellulitis in a limb with damaged vascular supply is, so skin care and nail care issues should be discussed as appropriate once the patient has recovered sufficiently.

COST CONSIDERATIONS AND RESOURCE USE

Physicians increasingly recognize that few patients with uncomplicated cellulitis require hospitalization. Guidelines for the management of skin and soft tissue infections are not available but will soon be published by the Infectious Disease Society of America. Currently, no guidelines exist to assist in determining whether hospitalization is indicated.

The prompt recognition of patients at risk for pathogens other than GAS and *S. aureus* (who may require broad-spectrum antimicrobial therapy or an antimicrobial other than those used to treat these pathogens) may hasten recovery. Once the patient with cellulitis has been stabilized and shows no evidence of disease progression, oral antimicrobials can be instituted, and the patient can be discharged.

In patients with NF, early surgical intervention can facilitate a definitive diagnosis and prompt surgical debridement, both of which can hasten recovery and discharge. The use of hyperbaric oxygen therapy is costly and has a questionable role in the management of necrotizing soft tissue infections. The only possible indication is for clostridial myonecrosis.

KEY POINTS

- During the past 20 years, invasive group A streptococcal infections such as necrotizing fasciitis have increased in incidence and severity.
- Diagnosis of severe GAS soft tissue infections may be difficult early in the course. Initially, patients may have only severe pain, flu-like symptoms, and fever.
- Most cases of cellulitis are caused by GAS or *S. aureus*. However, a meticulous history must be performed to specifically ask about exposure to fish and other animals, recent travel, trauma, recent surgery, insect bites, animal bites, human bites, exposure to salt water or fresh water, and presence of underlying immunocompromising conditions.
- Patients with systemic toxicity out of proportion to the physical findings of soft tissue infection require aggressive diagnostic and therapeutic efforts, primarily focused on ruling out necrotizing fasciitis.
- Methicillin-resistant *S. aureus* strains have increased dramatically throughout the world and cause a variety of soft tissue infections, including impetigo, abscesses, necrotizing soft tissue infections, and toxic shock syndrome.

REFERENCES

1. Kielhofner MA, Brown B, Dall L. Influence of underlying disease process on the utility of cellulitis needle aspirates. *Arch Intern Med* 1988;148:2451–2452.
2. Poretz DM. Treatment of skin and soft-tissue infections utilizing an outpatient parenteral drug delivery device: a multicenter trial. HIAT Study Group. *Am J Med* 1994;97:23–27.
3. Montalto M, Dunt D. Home and hospital intravenous therapy for two acute infections: an early study. *Aust N Z J Med* 1997;27:19–23.
4. Swartz MN. Clinical practice. Cellulitis. *N Engl J Med* 2004;350:904–912.
5. Stevens DL. Community-acquired *Staphylococcus aureus* infections: increasing virulence and emerging methicillin resistance in the new millennium. *Curr Opin Infect Dis* 2003;16:189–191.
6. Stevens DL. Group A streptococcal sepsis. *Curr Infect Dis Rep* 2003;5:379–386.
7. Stevens DL. Necrotizing soft tissue infections. *Current Treatment Options in Infectious Diseases* 2000;2:359–368.
8. Stevens DL, Tanner MH, Winship J, et al. Severe group A streptococcal infections associated with a toxic shock-like syndrome and scarlet fever toxin A. *N Eng J Med* 1989;321:1–7.
9. Bisno AL, Stevens DL. Streptococcal infections in skin and soft tissues. *N Engl J Med* 1996;334:240–245.
10. Chelsom J, Halstensen A, Haga T, Hoiby EA. Necrotising fasciitis due to group A streptococci in western Norway: incidence and clinical features. *Lancet* 1994;344:1111–1115.
11. Davies HD, McGeer A, Schwartz B, et al. Invasive group A streptococcal infections in Ontario, Canada. *N Engl J Med* 1996;335:547–554.
12. Kaul R, McGeer A, Low DE, Green K, Schwartz B. Population-based surveillance for group A streptococcal necrotizing fasciitis: clinical features, prognostic indicators, and microbiologic analysis of seventy-seven cases. Ontario Group A Streptococcal Study. *Am J Med* 1997;103:18–24.
13. Zimbelman J, Palmer A, Todd J. Improved outcome of clindamycin compared with β-lactam antibiotic treatment for invasive Streptococcus pyogenes infection. *Pediatr Infect Dis J.* 1999;18:1096–1100.
14. Majeski J, Majeski E. Necrotizing fasciitis: improved survival with early recognition by tissue biopsy and aggressive surgical treatment. *South Med J* 1997;90:1065–1068.
15. Bilton BD, Zibari GB, McMillan RW, Aultman DF, Dunn G, McDonald JC. Aggressive surgical management of necrotizing fasciitis serves to decrease mortality: a retrospective study. *Am Surg* 1998;64:397–400.
16. Stevens DL. Dilemmas in the treatment of invasive Streptococcus pyogenes infections. *Clin Infect Dis* 2003;37:341–343.
17. Kaul R, McGeer A, Norrby-Teglund A, et al. Intravenous immunoglobulin therapy for streptococcal toxic shock syndrome—a comparative observational study. *Clin Infect Dis* 1999;28:800–807.
18. Darenberg J, Ihendyane N, Sjolin J, et al. Intravenous immunoglobulin G therapy in streptococcal toxic shock syndrome: a European randomized, double-blind, placebo-controlled trial. *Clin Infect Dis* 2003;37:333–340.
19. Rivers E, Nguyen B, Havstad S, et al. Early goal-directed therapy in the treatment of severe sepsis and septic shock. *N Engl J Med* 2001;345:1368–1377.
20. The Prevention of Invasive Group A Streptococcal Infections Workshop Participants. Prevention of invasive group A streptococcal disease among household contacts of case patients and among postpartum and postsurgical patients: recommendations from the Centers for Disease Control and Prevention. *Clin Infect Dis* 2002;35:950–959.
21. Kakis A, Gibbs L, Eguia J, et al. An outbreak of group A streptococcal infection among health care workers. *Clin Infect Dis* 2002;35:1353–1359.

ADDITIONAL READING

Chapnick EK, Abter EI. Necrotizing soft-tissue infections. *Infect Dis Clin North Am* 1996;10:835–855.
Stevens DL. Infections of the skin, muscle and soft tissues. In: Braunwald E, Fauci AS, Kasper DL, Hauser SL, eds. *Harrison's Principles of Internal Medicine.* New York: McGraw-Hill, 2001:821–825.

Meningitis

70

Allan R. Tunkel   Michael Scheld

INTRODUCTION

Meningitis is defined as inflammation of the meninges identified by an abnormal number of white blood cells in cerebrospinal fluid (CSF). Meningitis may be caused by a variety of infectious agents (viruses, bacteria, fungi, and protozoa) as well as by a manifestation of various noninfectious disorders (e.g., collagen vascular disorders, malignancies, and medications). In patients who present with the meningitis syndrome, it is incumbent upon the physician to strongly consider the diagnosis of acute bacterial meningitis and to initiate an appropriate diagnostic plan and management for this disorder. This chapter focuses on the approach to the patient with presumed *acute bacterial meningitis* and considers other entities in the differential diagnosis.

The epidemiology of bacterial meningitis has changed in recent years. In the 1980s, *Haemophilus influenzae, Neisseria meningitidis,* and *Streptococcus pneumoniae* accounted for more than 80% of cases, most caused by *H. influenzae* type b. Recently, however, the incidence of invasive infections caused by *H. influenzae* type b has been dramatically reduced by the widespread use of conjugate vaccines against *H. influenzae* type b in children (1). In contrast, the incidence of *S. pneumoniae* meningitis is unchanged. This, too, may change in the future with the introduction of the heptavalent pneumococcal conjugate vaccine, which is now recommended for all infants and children in the United States (2).

ISSUES AT THE TIME OF ADMISSION

Clinical Presentation

More than 80% of patients with acute bacterial meningitis present with fever, headache, meningismus, and signs of cerebral dysfunction (3). The meningismus may be subtle or marked and may be accompanied by the Kernig or Brudzinski sign. These signs, however, are elicited in only about 5% of adult patients with acute bacterial meningitis. Other findings include cranial nerve palsies and focal cerebral signs (10%–20% of cases) and seizures (30% of cases). Papilledema is seen in fewer than 5% of patients early in infection, and its presence should suggest an alternative diagnosis. Some patients may not manifest many of the classic symptoms or signs of bacterial meningitis. For example, elderly patients may present insidiously with lethargy or obtundation, no fever, and variable signs of meningeal irritation. A high index of suspicion must be maintained for the diagnosis of bacterial meningitis in an elderly or alcoholic patient with altered mental status.

The etiologic diagnosis of bacterial meningitis may be suggested in patients with certain symptoms, signs, or underlying conditions. Patients with meningitis caused by *S. pneumoniae* often have contiguous or distant foci of infection such as pneumonia, otitis media, mastoiditis, sinusitis, or (rarely) endocarditis; serious infection also may be observed in asplenic patients and in those with multiple myeloma, hypogammaglobulinemia, alcoholism, malnutrition, chronic liver or renal disease, malignancy, diabetes mellitus, or basilar skull fracture. Meningitis caused by *N. meningitidis* may occur in epidemics and in patients with deficiencies in the terminal complement components (C5 through C9). About 50% of patients with meningococcemia, with or without meningitis, also present with a prominent rash located principally on the extremities. Early in the course of illness, the rash is typically erythematous and macular, but it quickly evolves into a petechial phase with further coalescence into a purpuric form.

Patients susceptible to *Listeria monocytogenes* meningitis include neonates, the elderly, alcoholics, cancer patients, immunosuppressed adults, and those with diabetes mellitus, liver disease, chronic renal disease, collagen vascular disorders, and conditions associated with iron overload. Outbreaks have been associated with consumption of contaminated food. Patients with *L. monocytogenes* meningitis may experience seizures and focal neurologic deficits early in the course of infection, and some patients may present with ataxia, cranial nerve palsies, or nystagmus.

Differential Diagnosis and Initial Evaluation

The diagnosis of bacterial meningitis rests on examination of CSF following lumbar puncture. Table 70.1 shows typical CSF findings and a comparison with other microorganisms that can produce the meningitis syndrome. There may be considerable overlap in CSF findings in cases of meningitis caused by various agents, necessitating use of other specialized tests to establish the correct diagnosis (see later in this chapter). Performance of a CSF Gram stain is a rapid, inexpensive, and accurate method to identify the causative microorganism in 60%–90% of patients with bacterial meningitis; the specificity is nearly 100%. The probability of identifying the organism may decrease in patients who have received prior antimicrobial therapy. If the Gram stain is negative, a CSF latex agglutination test to detect antigens of common meningeal pathogens can be considered. Unfortunately, the overall sensitivity of the latex agglutination test ranges from only 50%–100%; the sensitivity is lower for *N. meningitidis*. The routine use of CSF bacterial antigen tests has been questioned. They are currently not being performed in most clinical laboratories because positive results usually have not modified therapy and false-positive and false-negative results may occur.

Many other infectious agents can cause the meningitis syndrome and should be considered in the differential diagnosis (3). Viruses are the major cause of the *acute aseptic meningitis syndrome,* defined as any meningitis for which a cause is not apparent after initial evaluation and routine stains and cultures of CSF. Most of these cases (80%–85%) are caused by enteroviruses. These viruses are worldwide in distribution and are spread by the fecal–oral route, usually during periods of warm weather. Other viruses causing this syndrome include arboviruses, mumps virus, lymphocytic choriomeningitis virus, several herpesviruses, and HIV. Enteroviral meningitis is usually an acute illness, with fever in over 75% of patients. Headache is nearly always present in adults, photophobia is common, and more than half of patients have nuchal rigidity. The duration of illness is usually less than one week, and many patients report improvement after lumbar puncture, probably as a result of reduction of intracranial pressure. Currently, etiologic diagnosis is problematic, although recent advances in polymerase chain reaction technology should facilitate the diagnosis of enteroviral meningitis.

Meningitis caused by *Mycobacterium tuberculosis* accounts for approximately 0.7% of all cases of clinical tuberculosis in the United States (Chapter 67). The clinical presentation of tuberculous meningitis in adults is usually indolent, but patients also may present acutely, with a rapidly progressive meningitis syndrome indistinguishable from acute bacterial meningitis. On examination, fever is an inconstant finding, and signs of meningeal irritation are absent in 25%–40% of cases. Up to 30% of patients have focal neurologic signs on presentation, most frequently consisting of cranial nerve palsies. Identification of tuberculous organisms in CSF is difficult because of the small population of organisms present. Generally, fewer than 15%–25% of specimens are smear-positive, and up to 20% of patients have persistently negative CSF cultures, even if as many as four CSF specimens are cultured. Use of polymerase chain reaction testing to detect the fragments of mycobacterial DNA in CSF appears to be the most promising technique for the rapid diagnosis of tuberculous meningitis.

Spirochetes also can produce meningitis, with most cases caused by *Treponema pallidum* and *Borrelia burgdorferi*. The incidence of *syphilitic meningitis* is greatest in the first two years following initial infection, occurring in 0.3%–2.4% of untreated patients. Patients with syphilitic

TABLE 70.1

TYPICAL CEREBROSPINAL FLUID FINDINGS IN PATIENTS WITH VARIOUS INFECTIOUS CAUSES OF MENINGITIS

Cause	White blood cells, cells/mm³	Primary cell type	Glucose, mg/dL	Protein, mg/dL
Bacterial	1,000–5,000[a]	Neutrophilic[b]	<40[c]	100–500
Viral	50–1,000	Mononuclear[d]	>45	<200
Tuberculous	50–300	Mononuclear[e]	<45	50–300
Syphilitic	10–500	Mononuclear	35–75	30–300
Cryptococcal	20–500[f]	Mononuclear	<40	>45

[a] Range from <100 to >10,000 cells/mm³.
[b] About 10% of patients have a lymphocyte predominance on presentation.
[c] Should always be compared with a simultaneous serum glucose; ratio of CSF:serum ≤0.4 in most cases.
[d] May be neutrophilic early in infection.
[e] May see "therapeutic paradox" in which a mononuclear predominance becomes neutrophilic during therapy.
[f] More than 75% of AIDS patients have <20 cells/μL.

meningitis usually present with headache, nausea, and vomiting; meningismus and fever are seen in approximately one-half of cases. In contrast, meningovascular syphilis is found in 10%–20% of individuals with central nervous system involvement and occurs months-to-years after syphilis acquisition. If untreated, focal deficits may progress and become irreversible. No single routine laboratory test is definitive for the diagnosis of neurosyphilis. Although the specificity of the CSF VDRL test is generally high, blood contamination may lead to a false-positive serologic result. More problematically, the sensitivity is low, with reactive tests in only 50%–85% of patients. Therefore, a reactive CSF VDRL test in the absence of blood contamination is sufficient to diagnose neurosyphilis, but a nonreactive test does not exclude the diagnosis. The CSF fluorescent treponomal antibody (FTA-ABS) also has been examined as a possible diagnostic test for neurosyphilis; a nonreactive test effectively rules out the diagnosis. Polymerase chain reaction testing has been utilized, although further large-scale studies are needed to determine the sensitivity and specificity of this technique.

The nervous system is involved clinically in at least 10%–15% of patients with Lyme disease. Headache is the single most common symptom, followed by photophobia, nausea, and vomiting; neck stiffness is seen in only 10%–20% of cases. About one-half of patients have mild cerebral symptoms such as somnolence, emotional lability, depression, impaired memory and concentration, and behavioral changes. Approximately 50% of patients have cranial neuropathies, most commonly facial nerve palsy. The best currently available test for the diagnosis of Lyme disease is specific serum antibody to *B. burgdorferi*; a positive test in a patient with a compatible neurologic abnormality is strong evidence for the diagnosis. However, currently available serologic tests are not standardized, and there is marked variability between laboratories. Specific *B. burgdorferi* antibody also appears in CSF, and demonstration of intrathecal production of antibody suggests neurologic involvement. The technique of polymerase chain reaction for identifying *B. burgdorferi* DNA in CSF has been used successfully in some preliminary studies.

Many *fungal pathogens* have been reported to invade the central nervous system, although meningitis is seen most frequently with only a few of the species. Meningitis caused by *Cryptococcus neoformans* is usually seen in patients who are immunocompromised (Chapters 63 and 76). The most important diagnostic test is the CSF latex agglutination test for detection of cryptococcal polysaccharide antigen. A presumptive diagnosis is indicated by a CSF titer of at least 1:8. A serum cryptococcal polysaccharide antigen also may be detected in severely immunocompromised patients. *Coccidioides immitis* is endemic in the semiarid regions and desert areas of the southwestern United States, where approximately one-third of the population is infected. Less than 1% of patients develop dis-

seminated disease, usually within the first six months following infection, with one-third to one-half of those having meningeal involvement. Dissemination of infection has been associated with extremes of age, male gender, nonwhite race, pregnancy, and immunosuppression. Meningeal infection usually follows a subacute-to-chronic course, although it may present acutely. Common complaints include headache, low-grade fever, weight loss, and mental status changes. Signs of meningeal irritation are usually absent. CSF examination typically reveals a pleocytosis, often with a prominent eosinophilia. Only 25%–50% of patients have positive CSF cultures. CSF complement-fixing antibodies are present in at least 70% of cases of early meningitis and in virtually all patients as the disease progresses.

Primary *amebic meningoencephalitis* most often is caused by the protozoan *Naegleria fowleri*. Sporadic cases occur if persons swim or play in water containing the amebae, or if swimming pools or water supplies have become contaminated. Following an incubation period of 3–8 days, there is the sudden onset of high fever, photophobia, headache, and progression to stupor or coma. This presentation is usually indistinguishable from that of acute bacterial meningitis. Early symptoms of abnormal smell or taste may be reported because of involvement of the olfactory area. CSF examination reveals a neutrophilic pleocytosis, low glucose, elevated protein, and red blood cells. The Gram stain is negative, although examination of fresh, warm specimens of CSF can reveal the ameboid movements of the motile trophozoites. Death generally occurs within two or three days of the onset of symptoms in untreated patients.

In addition to the infectious causes described here, numerous noninfectious diseases also may produce the meningitis syndrome (Table 70.2). These entities also must be considered in the differential diagnosis.

Indications for Hospitalization and Initial Intensive Care Unit Admission

All patients with a suspected or confirmed diagnosis of acute bacterial meningitis should be hospitalized. Admission to the ICU is indicated by the presence of sepsis or neurologic compromise (Chapters 26 and 115). Patients should be admitted to the ICU if there is clinical evidence of increased intracranial pressure (obtundation, coma, hypertension, bradycardia, palsy of cranial nerve III; see Chapter 117), other cranial nerve palsies, focal cerebral signs, or seizures.

In patients with the acute meningitis syndrome, it is critical to distinguish between acute bacterial meningitis and the acute aseptic meningitis syndrome, the latter caused primarily by viruses (as described previously). Although the patient's general appearance and laboratory studies may be helpful in making this distinction, examination of the CSF profile is most important (Table 70.1). One study found that

TABLE 70.2

IMPORTANT NONINFECTIOUS CAUSES AND DISEASES OF UNKNOWN CAUSE LEADING TO THE MENINGITIS SYNDROME

Systemic illnesses
    Systemic lupus erythematosus
    Sarcoidosis
    Behçet's disease
    Granulomatous angiitis
Medications
    Antimicrobial agents (trimethoprim–sulfamethoxazole,
        ciprofloxacin, penicillin, isoniazid)
    Nonsteroidal anti-inflammatory agents
    Muromonab-CD3 (OKT3)
    Cytosine arabinoside (high-dose)
    Immunoglobulin
Procedure-related
    Postneurosurgery
    Spinal anesthesia
    Intrathecal injections
Malignancies
    Lymphomatous meningitis
    Carcinomatous meningitis
    Leukemia
Tumors and cysts
    Craniopharyngioma
    Dermoid or epidermoid cyst
Miscellaneous
    Seizures
    Migraine or migraine-like syndromes
    Mollaret's meningitis

any of the following findings—a CSF glucose concentration less than 34 mg/dL, a CSF:blood glucose ratio less than 0.23, a CSF protein concentration greater than 220 mg/dL, or more than 2,000 leukocytes or 1,180 neutrophils per cubic millimeter in CSF—predicted bacterial rather than viral meningitis with 99% certainty. However, considerable overlap exists in the CSF findings in patients with these disorders. For example, in enteroviral meningitis, a neutrophil predominance may be seen early in up to two-thirds of cases, with a tendency toward a shift to a lymphocyte predominance on follow-up lumbar puncture performed within 6–48 hours. Several authorities have suggested that in patients with a clinical diagnosis of viral meningitis and a neutrophil predominance on initial CSF analysis, a shift to a mononuclear predominance within 6–8 hours (in patients who have not received antimicrobial therapy) suggests a viral cause. Other studies have contradicted these findings. If the decision is made to withhold initial antibiotics in the patient who appears to have viral meningitis, the patient should be observed carefully, and antimicrobial therapy should be administered if there is evidence of clinical deterioration or if a repeat CSF analysis fails to reveal the typical lymphocyte predominance. Measurement of serum C-reactive protein (CRP) or procalcitonin may also be useful in discriminating between bacterial and viral meningitis, as they tend to be elevated in patients

with acute bacterial meningitis (4). In patients with acute meningitis in whom the CSF Gram stain is negative, serum concentrations of CRP or procalcitonin that are normal or below the limit of detection have a high negative predictive value for the diagnosis of bacterial meningitis. These patients can be carefully observed without initiation of antimicrobial therapy. However, the decision regarding hospital admission must be individualized and depend upon the clinical presentation, the level of concern by the clinician for the diag-

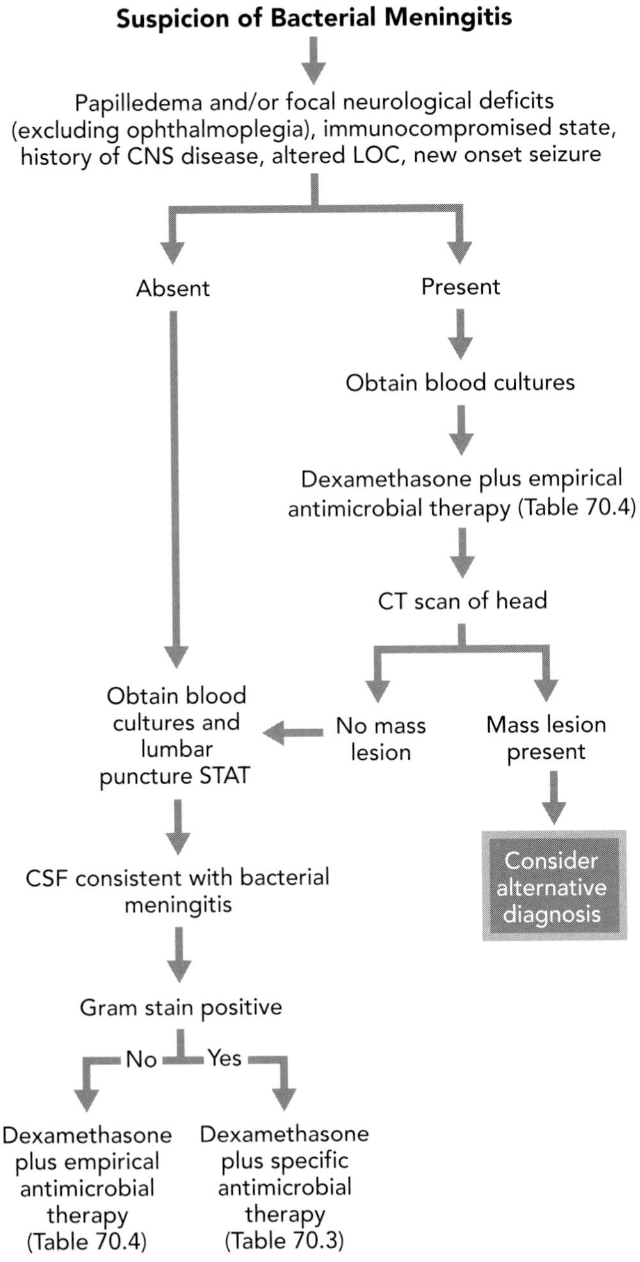

Suspicion of Bacterial Meningitis

Figure 70.1. Algorithm for initial management of patients with acute bacterial meningitis. See text for specific recommendations on use of adjunctive dexamethasone. *CNS*, central nervous system; *CSF*, cerebrospinal fluid; *LOC*, level of consciousness.

TABLE 70.3

SPECIFIC ANTIMICROBIAL THERAPY FOR BACTERIAL MENINGITIS

Microorganism	Standard therapy	Alternative therapies
Streptococcus pneumoniae		
Penicillin MIC < 0.1 mcg/mL	Penicillin G or ampicillin	3rd-generation cephalosporin[a]; chloramphenicol
Penicillin MIC 0.1–1.0 mcg/mL	3rd-generation cephalosporin[a]	Meropenem, cefepime
Penicillin MIC ≥ 2.0 mcg/mL	Vancomycin plus 3rd-generation cephalosporin[a,b]	Meropenem; 3rd-generation cephalosporin[b] plus rifampin; fluoroquinolone[d]
Neisseria meningitidis	Penicillin G or ampicillin[c] or 3rd-generation cephalosporin[a]	Chloramphenicol; fluoroquinolone
Haemophilus influenzae		
β-lactamase-negative	Ampicillin	3rd-generation cephalosporin[a]; chloramphenicol; aztreonam
β-lactamase-positive	3rd-generation cephalosporin[a]	Chloramphenicol; aztreonam; fluoroquinolone
Enterobacteriaceae	3rd-generation cephalosporin[a]	Meropenem; aztreonam; fluoroquinolone; trimethoprim–sulfamethoxazole
Pseudomonas aeruginosa	Ceftazidime[c] or cefepime[c]	Meropenem[c]; aztreonam[c]; fluoroquinolone[c]
Listeria monocytogenes	Ampicillin or penicillin G[c]	Trimethoprim–sulfamethoxazole
Streptococcus agalactiae (Group B)	Ampicillin or penicillin G[c]	3rd-generation cephalosporin[a]
Staphylococcus aureus		
Methicillin-sensitive	Nafcillin or oxacillin	Vancomycin; meropenem
Methicillin-resistant	Vancomycin	Linezolid
Staphylococcus epidermidis	Vancomycin[b]	Linezolid

[a] Cefotaxime or ceftriaxone.
[b] Addition of rifampin should be considered.
[c] Addition of an aminoglycoside should be considered.
Gatifloxacin or moxifloxacin: no data available for clinical use in patients with meningitis.
MIC, minimum inhibitory concentration.

nosis of bacterial meningitis, and the ability to carefully observe the patient and ensure close follow-up.

Initial Therapy

Figure 70.1 shows the initial approach to management in the patient with presumed bacterial meningitis. Patients without focal neurologic deficits or papilledema should undergo rapid lumbar puncture to determine whether the CSF formula is consistent with that diagnosis. If purulent meningitis is present, targeted antimicrobial therapy should be initiated based on results of the Gram stain (Table 70.3). However, if these means can identify no causative agent or if performance of the lumbar puncture is delayed, empiric antimicrobial therapy should be initiated based on the patient's age and underlying disease status (Table 70.4). In patients who present with a focal neurologic examination or papilledema and in whom bacterial meningitis is suspected, a computed tomography (CT) scan of the head should be performed prior to lumbar puncture to rule out the presence of an intracranial mass lesion. However, because the time involved in waiting for a CT scan significantly delays performance of lumbar puncture and initiation of appropriate therapy, emergent empiric antimicrobial therapy, after obtaining blood cultures, must be initiated before sending the patient to the CT scanner (Table 70.5). Although empiric antimicrobial therapy prior

to lumbar puncture may decrease the yield of subsequent CSF cultures, the CSF formula, Gram stain, and/or measurement of serum concentrations of CRP or procalcitonin likely will provide evidence for or against the diagnosis of bacterial meningitis. Some clinicians routinely order CT scans of the head before performing a lumbar puncture in adult patients with suspected bacterial meningitis. In a study of 301 patients with bacterial meningitis (5), the baseline clinical features associated with an abnormal finding on CT scan were an age of at least 60 years, immunocompromise, a history of central nervous system disease, a history of seizure in the week before presentation, and the following neurologic abnormalities: an abnormal level of consciousness, an inability to answer two consecutive questions correctly or to follow two consecutive commands, gaze palsy, abnormal visual fields, facial palsy, arm drift, leg drift, and abnormal language. Although the decision to perform a CT scan prior to lumbar puncture must be individualized, these are useful guidelines in determining specific groups that are unlikely to have abnormal findings on neuroimaging studies.

In addition, many patients presenting with suspected or proven bacterial meningitis should receive *adjunctive dexamethasone therapy* (6,7). Several clinical trials in infants and children with predominantly *H. influenzae* type b meningitis demonstrated that adjunctive dexamethasone decreases morbidity, with a lower incidence of neurologic and

TABLE 70.4

EMPIRIC THERAPY OF PURULENT MENINGITIS

Predisposing factor	Common bacterial pathogens	Antimicrobial therapy
Age		
1–23 months	Haemophilus influenzae, Neisseria meningitidis, Streptococcus pneumoniae, Streptococcus agalactiae, Escherichia coli	Vancomycin plus a 3rd-generation cephalosporin[a], or vancomycin plus ampicillin plus chloramphenicol
2–50 y	Streptococcus pneumoniae, Neisseria meningitidis	Vancomycin plus a 3rd-generation cephalosporin[a]
Older than 50 y	Streptococcus pneumoniae, Neisseria meningitidis, Listeria monocytogenes, aerobic Gram-negative bacilli	Vancomycin plus ampicillin plus a 3rd-generation cephalosporin[a]
Basilar skull fracture	Streptococcus pneumoniae, Haemophilus influenzae, group A streptococci	Vancomycin plus a 3rd-generation cephalosporin[a]
Head trauma; postneurosurgery	Staphylococcus aureus, Staphylococcus epidermidis, aerobic Gram-negative bacilli (including Pseudomonas aeruginosa)	Vancomycin + either ceftazidime or cefepime
Cerebrospinal fluid shunt	Staphylococcus epidermidis, Staphylococcus aureus, aerobic Gram-negative bacilli (including Pseudomonas aeruginosa), diphtheroids	Vancomycin + either ceftazidime or cefepime

[a] Cefotaxime or ceftriaxone.

TABLE 70.5

MAXIMAL RECOMMENDED DOSAGES OF ANTIMICROBIAL AGENTS FOR BACTERIAL MENINGITIS IN ADULTS WITH NORMAL RENAL AND HEPATIC FUNCTION

Antimicrobial agent	Total daily dose	Dosing interval, h
Amikacin[a]	15 mg/kg	8
Ampicillin	12 g	4
Aztreonam	6–8 g	6–8
Cefepime	6 g	8
Cefotaxime	8–12 g	4–6
Ceftazidime	6 g	8
Ceftriaxone	4 g	12–24
Chloramphenicol[b]	4–6 g	6
Ciprofloxacin	800–1200 mg	8–12
Gentamicin[a]	5 mg/kg	8
Meropenem	6 g	8
Nafcillin	9–12 g	4
Oxacillin	9–12 g	4
Penicillin G	24 million units	4
Rifampin[c]	600 mg	24
Tobramycin[a]	5 mg/kg	8
Trimethoprim–sulfamethoxazole[d]	10–20 mg/kg	6–12
Vancomycin[a,e]	30–45 mg/kg	8–12

Unless indicated, therapy is administered intravenously.
[a] Need to monitor peak and trough serum concentrations.
[b] Higher dose recommended for pneumococcal meningitis.
[c] Oral administration.
[d] Dosage based on trimethoprim component.
[e] May need to monitor cerebrospinal fluid concentrations in severely ill patients.

audiologic sequelae. Thus, adjunctive dexamethasone should be used routinely in all infants and children with *H. influenzae* type b meningitis at a dosage of 0.15 mg/kg every 6 hours for 2–4 days. If it can be given with or before antimicrobial therapy, dexamethasone should also be used in children with pneumococcal meningitis. In adult patients with bacterial meningitis, the routine use of adjunctive dexamethasone has been controversial until recently. In a prospective, randomized, double-blind trial in 301 adults with bacterial meningitis, adjunctive dexamethasone was associated with a reduction in the proportion of patients with unfavorable outcomes, including death (8). The benefits were most striking in the subgroup of patients with pneumococcal meningitis and in those with moderate-to-severe disease, as assessed by the score on the Glasgow Coma Scale at the time of admission. On the basis of these data and the apparent absence of serious adverse outcomes in patients who received dexamethasone, *the routine use of adjunctive dexamethasone is warranted in most adults with pneumococcal meningitis;* dexamethasone can be given with or just before the first dose of an antimicrobial agent (9). Adjunctive dexamethasone should not be used in patients who have already received antimicrobial therapy. If the etiology of meningitis is subsequently found not to be *S. pneumoniae,* dexamethasone therapy should be discontinued. The use of adjunctive dexamethasone is of particular concern, however, in patients with pneumococcal meningitis caused by penicillin-resistant or cephalosporin-resistant strains who are treated with vancomycin, as a diminished CSF inflammatory response may significantly reduce CSF vancomycin penetration and potentially delay CSF sterilization. In the study cited above, only 78 of 108 CSF cultures that were positive for *S. pneumoniae* were submitted for in vitro susceptibility testing, and all were susceptible to penicillin, a finding that is unusual in many areas of the world. In patients with pneumococcal meningitis caused by strains that are highly resistant to penicillin or cephalosporins and who do receive corticosteroids, careful observation and follow-up are critical.

Indications for Early Consultation

All patients with suspected bacterial meningitis should receive infectious diseases consultation to assist with antimicrobial therapy, especially in view of recent trends in the susceptibility of meningeal pathogens to standard antimicrobial therapy (see later in this chapter). The infectious diseases consultant also can assist with ensuring adequate antimicrobial dosages and dosing intervals, which are generally different from those for treating infections outside the central nervous system.

In patients with bacterial meningitis who have evidence of focal neurologic signs, seizures, or signs of increased intracranial pressure, neurology or neurosurgery consultation is recommended. Status epilepticus that is continuous for 90 minutes or longer can cause permanent neurologic sequelae (Chapter 118). Early termination of seizure activity usually can be accomplished using a short-acting anticonvulsant with a rapid onset of action (e.g., lorazepam or diazepam). A long-acting anticonvulsant then should be administered immediately. If this approach fails to control seizure activity, the patient should be intubated, mechanically ventilated, and treated with phenobarbital.

Patients with elevated intracranial pressure may benefit from neurosurgical insertion of an intracranial pressure monitoring device (Chapter 117). Pressures exceeding 20 mm Hg are abnormal and should be treated; there is also rationale for treating smaller pressure elevations (i.e., above 15 mm Hg) to avoid larger elevations, or so-called plateau waves, that can lead to cerebral herniation and irreversible brain-stem injury. Methods available to reduce elevated intracranial pressure include elevation of the head of the bed to 30°, hyperventilation to maintain the partial carbon dioxide pressure ($PaCO_2$) between 27 and 30 mm Hg, use of hyperosmolar agents, and use of corticosteroids (for details, see Chapter 117). Some experts have questioned the routine use of hyperventilation to reduce intracranial pressure in patients with bacterial meningitis. In infants and children with bacterial meningitis and evidence of cerebral edema on CT scan, hyperventilation may reduce intracranial pressure at the expense of significant reductions in cerebral blood flow. However, a controlled trial exploring this issue has yet to be performed. Patients whose intracranial pressure continues to be elevated despite these measures may be treated with high-dosage pentobarbital therapy, with appropriate intracranial, electroencephalographic, and hemodynamic monitoring. Pentobarbital is

administered until the intracranial pressure is reduced below 20 mm Hg or the electroencephalogram demonstrates a burst-suppression pattern. This mode of treatment for elevated intracranial pressure in bacterial meningitis is of unproven benefit and must be considered experimental.

ISSUES DURING THE COURSE OF HOSPITALIZATION

Following definitive identification and susceptibility testing of the pathogen causing meningitis, antimicrobial therapy should be modified for optimal treatment. Table 70.3 shows the recommendations for therapy of causative microorganisms of bacterial meningitis; recommended dosages in adults with normal renal and hepatic function are in Table 70.5 (3).

One microorganism deserves special comment. The therapy of meningitis caused by *S. pneumoniae* recently has been modified based upon current pneumococcal susceptibility patterns, with emergence of strains that are both relatively and highly resistant to penicillin G (3,10). Based upon these antimicrobial susceptibility trends and because sufficient CSF concentrations of penicillin are difficult to achieve with standard high parenteral dosages, *penicillin can no longer be recommended as empiric antimicrobial therapy if* S. pneumoniae *is considered a likely pathogen in a patient with purulent meningitis.* Patients with pneumococcal meningitis should be considered to have a highly resistant strain upon organism identification and treated with the combination of vancomycin plus a third-generation cephalosporin (either cefotaxime or ceftriaxone). If the physician determines that the organism is susceptible to penicillin (minimum inhibitory concentration [MIC] <0.1 mcg/mL), penicillin G or ampicillin can be used. If the organism is relatively resistant to penicillin (MIC between 0.1 and 1.0 mcg/mL), a third-generation cephalosporin (cefotaxime or ceftriaxone) is recommended. However, if the organism is highly resistant to penicillin (MIC ≥2.0 mcg/mL), the combination of vancomycin plus the third-generation cephalosporin should be continued for the full treatment course. This is based on anecdotal reports of vancomycin treatment failure in pneumococcal meningitis and from experimental data in which the combination of vancomycin and the third-generation cephalosporin was synergistic in the therapy of meningitis caused by highly penicillin-resistant pneumococci. The addition of rifampin or use of the combination of a third-generation cephalosporin plus rifampin should be considered in patients with documented infection caused by penicillin-resistant or cephalosporin-resistant *S. pneumoniae,* especially if dexamethasone is administered. Meropenem, a carbapenem with less proconvulsive activity than imipenem, yields microbiologic and clinical outcomes similar to either cefotaxime or ceftriaxone. The newer fluoroquinolones (e.g., levofloxacin, moxifloxacin, gatifloxacin) are active *in vitro* against resistant pneumococci;

one study found trovafloxacin to be therapeutically equivalent to ceftriaxone with or without vancomycin for treatment of bacterial meningitis (11). However, more clinical trials are needed before these agents can be recommended for use in patients with pneumococcal meningitis.

Strains of *N. meningitidis* with intermediate resistance to penicillin have been reported, accounting for about 3% of isolates in the United States (12). The clinical significance of these isolates is unclear because most patients with meningitis caused by these organisms have recovered with standard penicillin therapy. However, isolated reports of penicillin treatment failure have been described. Based on these data, some authorities would treat patients who have meningococcal meningitis with a third-generation cephalosporin (either cefotaxime or ceftriaxone) pending results of *in vitro* susceptibility testing.

Following the initiation of appropriate antimicrobial therapy in patients with acute bacterial meningitis, evidence of clinical improvement (represented by increased responsiveness) is usually seen within 2–4 days, with most patients becoming afebrile within 4–5 days (2–3 days for meningococcal meningitis). Table 70.6 shows the approach to patients who fail to improve or who develop complications.

Unfortunately, many patients with bacterial meningitis develop complications. The major central nervous system complications include cerebrovascular involvement, brain swelling, hydrocephalus, and intracerebral hemorrhage. In addition, systemic complications include septic shock, acute respiratory distress syndrome, and disseminated intravascular coagulation. Patients with bacterial meningitis must be monitored carefully for these complications, and appropriate therapeutic measures must be taken.

DISCHARGE ISSUES AND COST CONSIDERATIONS

Patients with acute bacterial meningitis must be treated with appropriate dosages of intravenous antimicrobial therapy for a full duration of therapy (Table 70.7) (3,10). Oral antimicrobial therapy is not recommended, and the intramuscular mode of administration is also discouraged because CSF penetration of antimicrobial therapy diminishes with reduction of meningeal inflammation. Traditionally, patients with bacterial meningitis have been hospitalized for the duration of parenteral antimicrobial therapy. Several recent studies have suggested that outpatient therapy is appropriate for selected cases of pediatric meningitis, based on data that the complications of meningitis occur most frequently within the first 2–3 days and that serious adverse complications are exceedingly rare after 3–4 days of antimicrobial therapy. The advantages of home therapy include decreased costs of hospitalization and decreased risk of development of nosocomial infections, as well as the psychologic, physical, and nutritional benefits. Basic criteria have been suggested for use of outpatient antimicrobial therapy in pediatric patients with bacterial meningitis (3). These guidelines advocate outpatient therapy for patients who have received inpatient therapy for at least 6 days and have no significant neurologic dysfunction, focal findings, or seizure activity; are clinically stable and taking fluids by mouth; have received at least one dose of the outpatient antimicrobial agent in the hospital; have access to home health nursing for the administration of the antimicrobial; have a daily examination by a physician; and have reliable parents with transportation and a telephone. Although not validated, these guidelines

TABLE 70.6

APPROACH TO COMPLICATIONS DURING HOSPITALIZATION IN PATIENTS WITH BACTERIAL MENINGITIS

Problem/complication	Recommended approach
Seizures	Close observation in ICU; administration of anticonvulsants; neuroimaging (CT or MR)
New focal neurologic deficit	Neuroimaging (CT or MR); neurologic consultation
Increased intracranial pressure (ICP)/ Hydrocephalus	Neurosurgical consultation
Subdural effusion	Observe; aspirate if patient develops focal neurologic findings and/or increased ICP or if clinical suspicion of empyema exists
Inappropriate secretion of antidiuretic hormone	Fluid restriction; nephrology consultation
Fever beyond 5 d	Evaluate for subdural effusion, disease at other foci, and nosocomial infection; repeat CSF analysis if clinically indicated; consider drug fever if patient has clinically improved

TABLE 70.7

DURATION OF THERAPY OF BACTERIAL MENINGITIS

Microorganism	Duration of therapy, d[a]
Streptococcus pneumoniae	10–14
Neisseria meningitidis	7
Haemophilus influenzae type b	7
Enteric Gram-negative bacilli	21
Listeria monocytogenes	≥21
Streptococcus agalactiae	14–21

[a] These are general recommendations; individual therapy may be different based upon clinical response.

also may be appropriate for adult patients, provided that compliance can be assured and the patient is in a safe environment, with access to a telephone, utilities, food, and a refrigerator (13). In addition, completion of antimicrobial therapy in a skilled nursing facility may be appropriate for selected patients who need continued care but do not require acute hospitalization.

Despite the availability of effective antimicrobial therapy, the morbidity and mortality rates from bacterial meningitis remain unacceptably high. In a review of almost 500 cases of acute bacterial meningitis in adults, the overall case fatality rate was 25% and did not vary significantly over the 27-year period of the study (14). Among patients with single episodes of bacterial meningitis, the in-hospital mortality rate was 25% in those with community-acquired meningitis and 35% in those with nosocomial meningitis. The three factors associated with a higher overall mortality rate were age older than 60 years, obtunded mental state on presentation, and onset of seizures within 24 hours of admission.

Furthermore, patients must be monitored carefully for long-term complications of bacterial meningitis. Persistent neurologic sequelae in infants and children with bacterial meningitis have included sensorineural hearing loss, seizure disorder, hemiplegia, and mental retardation. In a recent study that assessed neuropsychological outcome in 51 adults with bacterial meningitis and otherwise good recovery, a cognitive disorder was found in 27% of the patients with pneumococcal meningitis (15). Further studies are needed, however, to make decisions about planning neuropsychological follow-up in patients with bacterial meningitis to determine who is at risk for these complications.

KEY POINTS

- The epidemiology of bacterial meningitis has changed significantly in the past several years following introduction of *H. influenzae* type b conjugate vaccines, dramatically reducing the threat of *H. influenzae* type b meningitis in infants and children.

- Targeted or empiric antimicrobial therapy, based on the patient's age and underlying disease status, should be initiated as soon as possible in patients with presumed bacterial meningitis.

- Antimicrobial therapy should never be delayed while awaiting tests such as CT scans.

- Adjunctive dexamethasone therapy has been shown to reduce morbidity in infants and children with acute *H. influenzae* type b and *S. pneumoniae* meningitis. Adjunctive dexamethasone, administered concomitant with or immediately prior to the first dose of antimicrobial therapy, should also be used in adult patients with suspected pneumococcal meningitis.

- Empiric antimicrobial therapy for meningitis caused by *S. pneumoniae* should consist of vancomycin plus a third-generation cephalosporin (either cefotaxime or ceftriaxone), pending results of susceptibility testing.

- Complications of bacterial meningitis, including seizures and increased intracranial pressure, must be recognized and treated aggressively.

- Selected patients with bacterial meningitis may be considered for outpatient antimicrobial therapy.

REFERENCES

1. Schuchat A, Robinson K, Wenger JD, et al. Bacterial meningitis in the United States in 1995. *N Engl J Med* 1997;337:970–976.
2. American Academy of Pediatrics, Committee on Infectious Diseases. Policy statement: recommendations for the prevention of pneumococcal infections, including use of pneumococcal conjugate vaccine (Prevnar), pneumococcal polysaccharide vaccine, and antibiotic prophylaxis. *Pediatrics* 2000;106:362–366.
3. Tunkel AR, Scheld WM. Central nervous system infections. In: Betts RF, Chapman SW, Penn RL, eds. *A Practical Approach to Infectious Diseases.* 5th ed. Philadelphia: Lippincott Williams & Wilkins, 2003:173–221.
4. Nathan BR, Scheld WM. The potential roles of C-reactive protein and procalcitonin concentrations in the serum and cerebrospinal fluid in the diagnosis of bacterial meningitis. In: Remington JS, Swartz MN, eds. *Current Clinical Topics in Infectious Diseases.* Oxford: Blackwell Science, 2002;22:155–165.
5. Hasbun R, Abrahams J, Jekel J, Quagliarello VJ. Computed tomography of the head before lumbar puncture in adults with suspected meningitis. *N Engl J Med* 2001;345:1727–1733.
6. McIntyre PB, Berkey CS, King SM, et al. Dexamethasone as adjunctive therapy in bacterial meningitis: a meta-analysis of randomized clinical trials since 1988. *JAMA* 1997;278:925–931.
7. Saez-Llorens X, McCracken GH Jr. Bacterial meningitis in children. *Lancet* 2003;361:2139–2148.
8. de Gans J, van de Beek D. Dexamethasone in adults with bacterial meningitis. *N Engl J Med* 2002;347:1549–1556.
9. Tunkel AR, Scheld WM. Corticosteroids for everyone with meningitis? *N Engl J Med* 2002;347:1613–1615.
10. Tunkel AR, Scheld WM. Treatment of bacterial meningitis. *Curr Infect Dis Rep* 2002;4:7–16.
11. Saez-Llorens X, McCoig C, Feris JM, et al. Quinolone treatment for pediatric bacterial meningitis: a comparative study of trovafloxacin and ceftriaxone with or without vancomycin. *Pediatr Infect Dis J* 2002;21:14–22.
12. Rosenstein NE, Stocker SA, Popovic T, Tenover FC, Perkins BA. Antimicrobial resistance of *Neisseria meningitidis* in the United States, 1997. *Clin Infect Dis* 2000;30:212–213.
13. Tice AD, Strait K, Ramey R, Hoaglund PA. Outpatient parenteral antimicrobial therapy for central nervous system infections. *Clin Infect Dis* 1999;29:1394–1399.
14. Durand ML, Calderwood SB, Weber DJ, et al. Acute bacterial meningitis in adults: a review of 493 episodes. *N Engl J Med* 1993;328:21–28.
15. van de Beek D, Schmand B, de Gans J, et al. Cognitive impairment in adults with good recovery after bacterial meningitis. *Clin Infect Dis* 2002;186:1047–1052.

ADDITIONAL READING

Tunkel AR. *Bacterial Meningitis.* Philadelphia: Lippincott Williams & Wilkins, 2001.
Tunkel AR, Hartman BJ, Kaplan SL. Practice guidelines for the management of bacterial meningitis. *Clin Infect Dis* 2004;39:1267–1284.
Tunkel AR, Scheld WM. Acute meningitis. In: Mandell GL, Bennett JE, Dolin R, eds. *Principles and Practice of Infectious Diseases.* 5th ed. Philadelphia: Elsevier Churchill-Livingstone, 2005:1083–1126.

Endocarditis

71

Paul M. Sullam

INTRODUCTION

Despite long-standing research interest, improved diagnostic modalities, and the use of antimicrobial agents for prophylaxis, infective endocarditis remains an important medical problem. The overall incidence of this disease has not changed over several decades (1.8–11.6 cases per 100,000 population). Endocarditis is still associated with mortality rates of 16%–30%, even with the prompt initiation of therapy. In addition, the management of patients with endocardial infection has become increasingly complicated because of the emergence of new populations at risk, the application of echocardiography to stage the infection, and the increasing prevalence of drug-resistant microbes.

In view of these issues, the evaluation and treatment of individuals with endocardial infection requires considerable expertise in a variety of disciplines. This chapter provides an overview of the key aspects of managing such patients. Prosthetic valve endocarditis is reviewed in Chapter 41, and antibiotic prophylaxis is discussed in Chapter 30 (Tables 30.6 and 30.7).

ISSUES AT THE TIME OF ADMISSION

Clinical Presentation

Endocarditis is a relatively uncommon disease, with an estimated 10,000–15,000 cases per year in the United States. Patients with underlying structural heart abnormalities are at markedly increased risk for infection (Table 71.1), and such defects can often be identified retrospectively in many patients with endocardial infection. Increasingly, however, patients are being diagnosed in whom no predisposing condition can be implicated. In fact, given that in approximately 50% of cases no underlying cardiac abnormality can be detected (1), the absence of a detectable underlying abnormality does not exclude the possibility of infection.

The clinical manifestations of endocarditis are highly variable. Most patients have generalized *constitutional symptoms*, suggesting infection or chronic illness (Table 71.2). In some patients, the predominant manifestations of endocarditis stem from systemic embolization, presenting as a stroke, splenic pain, or sudden loss of limb perfusion. Intravenous drug users tend to develop tricuspid valve endocarditis, which may produce pulmonary emboli, often multiple. Signs of *cardiac involvement* may predominate, presenting as progressive congestive heart failure or palpitations. Although findings such as Osler nodes or Janeway lesions strongly indicate the presence of endocarditis, these symptoms are distinctly unusual (5%–10% of patients). Murmurs are present in 80% or more of patients, but these are mainly preexisting systolic murmurs. A changing or pathologic murmur was found in only 5% of patients in older series, but some more recent studies report a frequency of 35%–59% (2).

Differential Diagnosis and Initial Evaluation

Because the clinical manifestations of infective endocarditis are protean and usually not pathognomonic, the differential diagnosis of this disease is quite broad. A patient who presents with fever, malaise, and other generalized signs may appear to have rheumatic fever, influenza, tuberculosis, osteomyelitis, occult abscess, underlying malignancy, or collagen vascular disease. Local findings, such as stroke, may lead to an initial diagnosis of atherosclerotic thromboembolic disease. Occasionally, patients are diagnosed after an initial evaluation for anemia or hematuria.

Thus, the diagnosis of endocarditis requires the presence of a constellation of symptoms in conjunction with microbiologic or echocardiographic findings. Infective endocarditis should be considered in any patient with unexplained fever for longer than one week, especially if an

TABLE 71.1

CONDITIONS PREDISPOSING TO ENDOCARDITIS: INCIDENCE AND RELATIVE RISK OF INFECTION

Cardiac lesion	Cases/100,000/y	Relative risk
Prosthetic valve	450	100
Previous endocarditis	450	100
Rheumatic heart disease	350	75
Ventricular septal defect	220	48
Ventricular septal defect—repaired	60	13
Aortic stenosis (congenital)	180	39
Pulmonic stenosis	20	4
Mitral-valve prolapse and murmur	30	7
Mitral-valve prolapse, no murmur	4.6	1
Normal valve	4.6	1

underlying cardiac abnormality is present. Endocarditis also should be suspected in persons with unexplained embolic phenomena, splenomegaly, or cardiac valve dysfunction. In addition, the diagnosis should be entertained in patients with idiopathic bacteremia, especially if caused by Gram-positive cocci. In fact, studies suggest that endocarditis should be considered in all patients with bacteremia due to *Staphylococcus aureus*, even if this occurs within a nosocomial setting or if an infected intravascular device is present (3).

Role of the Microbiology Laboratory

Blood cultures have remained an essential aspect of managing patients with infective endocarditis. Because patients

TABLE 71.2

SIGNS AND SYMPTOMS OF ENDOCARDITIS

Sign	Prevalence, %
Fever	60–91
Malaise	40–92
Arthralgias/myalgias	16–70
Back pain	0–13
Weight loss	17–63
Murmur (any)	80–90
Murmur: new or changing	6–59
Splenomegaly	20–60
Congestive heart failure	18–52
Central nervous system manifestations	12–26
Osler nodes	5–15
Janeway lesions	4–10
Roth spots	0–11

Ranges shown compiled from clinical series.

with endocarditis usually have sustained bacteremia, the presence of multiple positive blood cultures is strongly indicative of endocardial infection. Recovery of a specific pathogen also allows testing *in vitro* for antimicrobial sensitivities, which facilitates the selection of effective antimicrobial therapy. In addition, blood cultures are valuable for monitoring the response of the patient to therapy (see later in this chapter). Thus, blood cultures should be obtained in all patients with suspected endocarditis.

The exact number needed depends in part on the underlying pathogen. For viridans-group streptococci, a single 10-mL blood sample is positive in 90% of patients, and, if three specimens are obtained, at least one is positive in 98% of cases. Similar high rates of recovery have been reported for staphylococci. Thus, for endocarditis caused by the most prevalent organisms, three blood cultures obtained one hour or more apart should be adequate. The detection of fastidious organisms, such as *Legionella* or *Bartonella* species, may require a larger number of blood samples or specialized culture techniques. Blood cultures also may be falsely negative in patients already receiving antibiotics. In such cases, specialized blood-collection systems that remove antibiotics can be used to improve recovery. For some pathogens, such as *Coxiella burnetti* (the agent of Q fever), diagnosis typically involves serologic methods.

Role of Echocardiography

In patients with native valve endocarditis, transthoracic echocardiography (TTE) can detect vegetations in about 50% of cases (range: 32%–71%) (3–5). The sensitivity of TTE is much lower for prosthetic valve infections (15%–30%). If a vegetation *is* detected by TTE, the specificity is 99% for both native valve and prosthetic infections. Compared with TTE, transesophageal echocardiography (TEE) is superior for evaluating patients with endocarditis. In native valve infection, the sensitivity is at least 85%, with more recent series reporting values of 95%–100%. In patients with prosthetic valve infection, the sensitivity is reduced only slightly (85%). The specificity of TEE is also excellent for both native and prosthetic valve infection (99%–100% in most series).

In addition to its ability to diagnose endocarditis by revealing vegetations, echocardiography can provide valuable structural, hemodynamic, and prognostic information (Chapter 36). TEE is especially good at detecting complications such as myocardial abscesses, ruptured chordae tendinae, perforated leaflets, or prosthetic dysfunction. Echocardiography also can be used to quantify valve regurgitation or degree of cardiac failure. Such complications, even if subclinical, may provide strong evidence in favor of prompt surgical replacement of the infected valve. Vegetations greater than 10 mm in diameter are associated with a significantly higher risk of embolization (6). Moreover, vegetations that fail to regress with antimicrobial therapy are also associated with embolic phenomena.

Guidelines from the American College of Cardiology and the American Heart Association summarize clinical settings in which echocardiography is definitely or possibly warranted (Table 71.3) (7). At a minimum, echocardiography should be considered for patients in whom the diagnosis of infective endocarditis remains uncertain and in patients in whom an intracardiac complication is suspected. Whether TTE or TEE should be the initial mode of evaluation remains controversial. In one cost-benefit analysis, employing TEE as the initial echocardiographic test was more cost effective than using TEE only in selected cases that had been first evaluated by TTE (8). TEE is associated with a complication rate of 0.5%–1.5%; complications can include serious events, such as esophageal rupture. For this reason, the noninvasive TTE remains the preferred initial procedure. In patients for whom this evaluation is nondiagnostic, TEE should be considered.

Duke Criteria

In an attempt to standardize the case definition of endocarditis, a group of investigators at Duke University developed a set of major and minor criteria for diagnosing endovascular infection (9) (Tables 71.4 and 71.5). Using this scoring system, patients can be stratified into categories of *definite, possible,* or *rejected* (no endocarditis). Several independent studies have confirmed the validity of the Duke criteria, which have sensitivity rates of 80%–89% and specificity rates of nearly 100%, with higher values reflecting recent refinements in the criteria.

Although the Duke criteria provide a useful diagnostic framework, not all patients with suspected endocarditis need to be formally evaluated by these standards. In many patients, the clinical presentation, in combination with blood culture results, is sufficient to support the diagnosis. Moreover, in over 50% of cases identified by these guidelines, echocardiography provided unequivocal evidence of endocardial infection, obviating the need for further diagnostic assessment. Aside from its value in a research setting, therefore, the Duke criteria are probably best used in selected cases, such as when the echocardiogram is equivocal, technically inadequate, or not feasible.

Indications for Hospitalization

Patients with infective endocarditis generally are hospitalized, for several reasons. First, hospitalization may facilitate the rapid and intensive evaluation of patients required during the first few days of management. Second, antimicrobial therapy is usually given intravenously, which, until recently, could be done only in an inpatient setting. Third, hospitalization permits close monitoring for the embolic and hemodynamic complications that may occur, particularly during the two weeks of treatment. Notwithstanding these advantages, several groups have proved the feasibility of outpatient therapy, either following a few days of hospitalization or from the onset of treatment. In most studies, outpatient therapy was generally reserved for individuals with the best chance of an uncomplicated course; nearly all had streptococcal endocarditis, which has the highest rate of successful medical treatment. Patients with

TABLE 71.3

AMERICAN COLLEGE OF CARDIOLOGY/AMERICAN HEART ASSOCIATION GUIDELINES FOR ECHOCARDIOGRAPHY IN ENDOCARDITIS

Indication	Class[a] (native/prosthetic valve)
1. Detection and characterization of valvular lesions, their hemodynamic severity, or ventricular compensation[b]	I/I
2. Detection of vegetations and characterization of lesions in patients with congenital heart disease	I/I
3. Detection of associated abnormalities (e.g., abscesses, shunts, etc.)[b]	I/I
4. Reevaluation studies in complex endocarditis (e.g., virulent organisms, severe hemodynamic lesion, aortic valve involvement, persistent fever or bacteremia clinical change, or symptomatic deterioration)	I/I
5. Evaluation of patients with high clinical suspicion of culture-negative endocarditis[b]	I/I
6. Evaluation of bacteremia without a known source[b]	IIa/I
7. Risk stratification in established endocarditis[b]	IIa/IIa
8. Routine re-evaluation in uncomplicated endocarditis during antibiotic therapy	IIb/IIb
9. Evaluation of fever and nonpathological murmur without evidence of bacteremia	III/(II–III)[c]

[a] Class I: evidence and/or general agreement that an echocardiography is useful; Class IIa: conflicting evidence or divergence of opinion about usefulness, but weight of evidence/opinion favors it; Class IIb: usefulness is less well established; Class III: evidence or general opinion that echocardiography is not useful.
[b] Transesophageal echocardiography (TEE) may provide incremental value in addition to information obtained by transthoracic echocardiography (TTE). The role of TEE in first-line examination awaits further study.
[c] Prosthetic valves—IIa: for persistent bacteremia; III: for transient bacteremia.

TABLE 71.4

MODIFIED DUKE CRITERIA: DEFINITIONS

Major criteria

1. Positive blood culture for infective endocarditis (IE)
   A. Typical microorganism for endocarditis from two separate blood cultures: viridans-group streptococci, *Streptococcus bovis*, HACEK group, *Staphylococcus aureus*; or community-acquired enterococci, in the absence of a primary focus; or
   B. Microorganisms consistent with IE, from persistently positive blood cultures, defined as follows: At least two positive cultures of blood samples drawn more than 12 h apart, or All of three or a majority of four or more separate blood cultures, with first and last drawn at least one h apart
   C. Single positive blood culture for *Coxiella burnetti* or antiphase I IgG antibody >1:800
2. Evidence of endocardial involvement
3. Positive echocardiogram for infective endocarditis (TEE recommended in patients with prosthetic valves, rated at least "possible IE" by clinical criteria, or complicated IE [paravalvular abscess]; TTE as first test in other patients), defined as follows:
   i. Oscillating intracardiac mass on valve or supporting structures, or in the path of regurgitant jets or on implanted material, in the absence of an alternative anatomic explanation, or
   ii. Abscess, or
   iii. New partial dehiscence of prosthetic valve
4. New valvular regurgitation (increase or change in preexisting not sufficient)

Minor criteria

1. Predisposing heart condition or intravenous drug use
2. Fever: ≥38.0° C
3. Vascular phenomena: arterial embolisms, septic pulmonary infarcts, mycotic aneurysm, intracranial hemorrhage, Janeway lesions
4. Immunologic phenomena: glomerulonephritis, Osler nodes, Roth spots, and rheumatoid factor
5. Microbiologic evidence: positive blood culture but not meeting a major criterion as noted above, or serologic evidence of active infection with organism consistent with endocarditis

HACEK, Haemophilus, Actinobacillus, Cardiobacterium, Eikenella, Kingella; TEE, transesophageal echocardiography; TTE, transthoracic echocardiography. See Table 71.5 for application of these findings.

complications of endocarditis at the onset of treatment were excluded, as were patients with underlying renal or eighth nerve impairment who required aminoglycosides. Under these conditions, outpatient treatment can achieve cure rates comparable with those seen in inpatient therapy.

If ambulatory management is chosen, patients must be carefully monitored for complications and drug toxicity. In addition, these patients must be able to aseptically manage long-term indwelling intravenous catheters. Finally, there should be a high level of confidence that antimicrobials will be administered properly, either by the patient or by a skilled infusion service. As for when to initiate outpatient therapy, recent guidelines recommend that most patients receive two weeks of inpatient therapy prior to initiating outpatient treatment (10). This approach permits close monitoring for complications and prompt intervention if needed.

Initiation of Antimicrobial Therapy

The selection of antibiotics for treating infective endocarditis should be based on the identification of a specific pathogen from blood cultures and *in vitro* assays for sensitivity. Because such information may not be immediately available at the time of diagnosis, combination therapy directly against the most likely organisms should be initiated once blood cultures have been obtained. Empiric therapy should be tailored to the underlying risk factors for infection (Table 71.6). Thus, patients with native valve endocarditis should receive treatment directed against streptococci, enterococci, and *Staphylococcus aureus*; that is, penicillin, nafcillin, and gentamicin. The same regimen should be adequate for endocarditis in intravenous drug users unless methicillin-resistant *Staphylococcus aureus* (MRSA) strains are likely to be present. Infection with MRSA should be considered in intravenous drug users who have been hospitalized recently or in geographic regions with a high prevalence of resistant strains (Chapter 64). If MRSA infection is suspected, vancomycin combined with gentamicin should be used until blood culture results and antimicrobial sensitivities are available. For patients with prosthetic valve infection, vancomycin should be used in combination with an aminoglycoside and rifampin pending microbiologic results.

TABLE 71.5

DUKE CRITERIA

Definite endocarditis

Pathologic criteria
  (1) Microorganisms: demonstrated by culture or histology in a vegetation, embolus, or intracardiac abscess or
  (2) Pathologic lesions: vegetations or intracardiac abscess present, confirmed by histology showing active endocarditis
Clinical criteria (as defined in Table 71.4)
  (1) Two major criteria, or
  (2) One major + three minor criteria, or
  (3) Five minor criteria

Possible infective endocarditis

  (1) One major criterion and one minor criterion, or
  (2) Three minor criteria

Rejected

  (1) Firm alternative diagnosis explaining evidence of infective endocarditis, or
  (2) Resolution of manifestations with antibiotic therapy for four d or less, or
  (3) No pathologic evidence of infective endocarditis at surgery or autopsy, after antibiotic therapy of four d or less, or
  (4) Does not meet criteria for possible infective endocarditis, as above

Once a pathogen is recovered from blood cultures, antimicrobial therapy should be targeted to that specific organism. The optimal regimen depends on *in vitro* sensitivities, whether a native or prosthetic valve is involved, and the patient's underlying medical condition. A detailed discussion of all possible regimens for every endocardial pathogen is beyond the scope of this chapter. However, recommended regimens for native valve endocarditis caused by the most common organisms are shown in Table 71.7. Because prosthetic valve endocarditis is more difficult to eradicate, this infection requires multidrug therapy for 4–6 weeks.

ISSUES DURING THE COURSE OF HOSPITALIZATION

Role of Consultants

The management of patients with endocarditis is complex. Selection of the correct antimicrobial regimen is often not straightforward because it must be tailored to each specific pathogen and its *in vitro* susceptibilities. In addition, considerable expertise is needed to manage the numerous complications associated with this disease as well as the adverse effects that can result from treatment. It is not surprising, therefore, that errors in the management of endocarditis are common, ranging from failure to obtain blood cultures to inappropriate delay in surgical treatment (11). Although the impact of an infectious diseases consultant on the outcome of such cases has not been formally addressed, patients with *S. aureus* bacteremia have been shown to benefit significantly by this intervention. In particular, patients who were treated according to the recommendations of an infectious diseases specialist had a higher rate of cure as well as lower rates of complications and relapses (12). Because it is likely that expert guidance has a similar beneficial effect on the management of infective endocarditis, all patients with this disease should be evaluated by an infectious diseases specialist.

Patients with evidence of mechanical complications or congestive heart failure should be evaluated promptly by a cardiologist. Relevant issues include the need for hemodynamic monitoring, temporary pacing, and valve replacement. Patients with prosthetic valve infection are more likely to develop complications requiring valve replacement and thus should be seen by both a cardiologist and a surgeon. These specialists can also help obtain previous data from invasive and noninvasive studies or observations from the time of surgery. Such information can be critical in determining whether there has been a change in valve function over time.

TABLE 71.6

MICROBIOLOGY OF INFECTIVE ENDOCARDITIS IN DIFFERENT RISK GROUPS

Microorganism recovered (% of cases)	Native valve endocarditis	Intravenous drug users	Prosthetic valve endocarditis	
			Early	Late
Viridans-group streptococci	50	20	7	30
Staphylococcus aureus	19	67	17	12
Coagulase-negative staphylococci	4	9	33	26
Enterococci	8	7	2	6
Miscellaneous	19	7	41	26

TABLE 71.7

TREATMENT REGIMENS FOR INFECTIVE ENDOCARDITIS

Organism	Regimens	Comments
Viridans-group streptococci		Prosthetic valves: 6 wks penicillin + 2 wks of gentamicin initially
Penicillin MIC ≤0.1 mcg/mL	1) Penicillin (2–3 × 10⁶ U IV Q4 h) × 4 wks 2) Ceftriaxone (2 g IV QD) × 4 wks 3) Penicillin + gentamicin (1 mg/kg Q8 h) × 2 weeks	Vancomycin (1 g Q12 h) × 4 wks for patients with hypersensitivity to β-lactam antibiotics
Penicillin MIC ≥0.1 to 0.5 mcg/mL	Penicillin × 4 wks + gentamicin (1 mg/kg Q8 h) × 2 weeks	
Penicillin MIC ≥0.5 mcg/mL	Penicillin + gentamicin × 4–6 weeks	
Staphylococcus aureus	1) Nafcillin (1.5–2 gms Q4 h) × 4–6 wks + gentamicin × 3–5 d 2) Nafcillin + gentamicin × 2 wks 3) Vancomycin × 4 wks + gentamicin × 3–5 d	Uncomplicated right-sided disease only Vancomycin should be used only in MRSA infections or if serious penicillin allergy is present. Combination therapy is recommended for prosthetic valves
Enterococci	1) Penicillin + gentamicin × 4–6 wks 2) Vancomycin + gentamicin × 4–6 wks	6 wk therapy if symptoms >3 mo
Coagulase negative staphylococci (*S. epidermidis*, etc.)	1) Vancomycin + rifampin (300 mg PO Q8 h) × 4–6 wks + gentamicin (1 mg/kg Q8 h) × 2 wks 2) Nafcillin × 4–6 wks	Add rifampin and gentamicin for prosthetic valves; ?native valves Most strains are resistant to nafcillin: check MICs/MBCs
Gram-negative enterics (e.g., *Pseudomonas*)	Gentamicin (5 mg/kg/d) + ureidopenicillin × 4–6 wks + surgical consultation	Response to medical treatment alone is variable
HACEK group	1) Ceftriaxone × 4 wks 2) Ampicillin (2 g Q4 h) + gentamicin (5 mg/kg/d) × 4 wks	Check *in vitro* sensitivities
Fungi	Amphotericin B (0.6–1.0 mg/kg/d) + surgery	
Culture negative	1) Ampicillin + nafcillin × 4 wks + gentamicin × 2 wks 2) Vancomycin + gentamicin × 4–6 wks	Native valves Prosthetic valves

HACEK, *Haemophilus, Actinobacillus, Cardiobacterium, Eikenella, Kingella.*

Monitoring Response to Therapy

Day 1

On the first day of hospitalization, patients should be carefully evaluated for evidence of *endocarditis-associated complications*. In particular, signs of valve dysfunction, congestive heart failure, conduction abnormalities, and peripheral embolization should be sought. If such signs are present, the patient may be a candidate for surgical valve replacement (see later in this chapter). Intravenous antibiotic therapy should be initiated immediately after collecting three sets of blood cultures. Additional routine tests, such as a complete blood count, electrocardiogram, and chest radiograph, should be obtained.

Days 2 Through 7

During the first week of hospitalization, patients should be evaluated daily for a *response to therapy*. Fever usually resolves after one or two days of treatment in cases of streptococcal endocarditis and by day 7 in patients with endocarditis caused by *Staphylococcus aureus*. Patients also should be examined daily for signs of embolization and other complications because these occur predominantly during the first week of treatment. Complications occur frequently during this period (9), even if patients are diagnosed and treated promptly (Table 71.8). Serum concen-

TABLE 71.8

COMPLICATIONS OF ENDOCARDITIS

Complication	Incidence, %
Congestive heart failure	17–41
Aortic insufficiency	6–21
Myocardial abscess	2–10
Stroke	17–43
Mycotic aneurysm	1–6
Peripheral embolization	8–10
Renal involvement	7–27

trations of aminoglycosides should be measured if these agents are to be used for more than a week. In selected patients, vancomycin levels help to confirm that therapeutic concentrations have been achieved or to avoid toxicity.

Week 2

The second week of therapy is an important time point for assessing *response to antimicrobials*. Fever lasting longer than 7–9 days suggests myocardial abscess formation, embolization, or metastatic foci of infection. Such patients should undergo echocardiography to look for structural complications. When clinical or laboratory findings indicate a site of embolization (e.g., the brain), computed tomography or magnetic resonance imaging may be warranted. Because blood cultures usually are sterile by the second week of successful therapy, all patients should have repeat blood cultures obtained in week 2. Persistent bacteremia is indicitive of complications and requires further evaluation. Additional parameters to be followed during this period are liver and renal function, and antibiotic levels. Moreover, patients should continue to be monitored for evidence of valve dysfunction.

The second week of therapy is also a useful time to *identify potential sources of bacteremia* that led to endocardial infection. The anatomic sites to be evaluated should be directed by the organism recovered from the initial blood cultures. Patients with streptococcal endocarditis should be examined for dental disease. Patients with endocarditis due to *Streptococcus bovis* are at increased risk for occult bowel pathology and therefore should be evaluated for lesions such as colonic carcinoma.

For some patients, therapy is completed at the end of 14 days. At the time of discharge, these patients should be evaluated as described below. Patients receiving 4–6 weeks of total therapy should continue to be evaluated for the onset of complications or drug-related toxicities until the completion of therapy. Issues for these patients at the end of therapy are identical to those receiving short-course treatment.

Indications for Valve Replacement

Despite prompt antimicrobial treatment, 14%–49% of patients with infective endocarditis require cardiac surgery. Indications for surgery include infection with an untreatable organism (e.g., fungi), development of congestive heart failure, mechanical complications (e.g., cusp fenestration or papillary muscle rupture), myocardial abscess formation, repeated large or critical vessel embolization (e.g., cerebral or coronary), and persistent bacteremia (13). *Once these indications have become apparent, surgery should be performed promptly.* This is because delay may increase the risk for further complications (which may be catastrophic), and valve surgery in patients with endocarditis is not intrinsically more risky than the same procedure in uninfected individuals. In fact, stratified by degree of congestive heart failure, patients undergoing valve replacement for active endocarditis have rates of survival comparable to those undergoing elective valve surgery. Moreover, the incidence of subsequent prosthetic valve infection is not increased in patients having valve replacement for active endocarditis.

ISSUES AT THE TIME OF DISCHARGE OR COMPLETION OF THERAPY

Although patients with endocarditis traditionally received therapy exclusively in the hospital, many inpatients now successfully complete treatment in other settings, such as skilled nursing facilities, infusion centers, or home. To be eligible for discharge before completion of therapy, several criteria should be met. First, the patient should be free of complications that might require prompt surgical intervention, such as significant valve dysfunction. Second, the antimicrobial regimen selected should be unlikely to require intensive monitoring or dosage changes resulting from adverse events or toxicities. Third, the agents chosen should have pharmacokinetic and chemical properties well suited to nonhospital settings. In cases in which nursing resources are limited, for example, drugs that can be administered once daily, such as ceftriaxone, are preferable to those requiring multiple daily doses. For patients receiving home intravenous therapy via an electronic multidose infusion pump, the antibiotics must be stable at room temperature for at least 24 hours. Because of restricted reservoir capacity, other infusion devices require that the drug remain soluble at high concentrations. Thus, the proper matching of antimicrobial regimens with infusion devices and therapeutic setting can be complicated. For this reason, many centers have an infusion team that actively participates in the discharge planning of patients selected for antimicrobial therapy in the nonhospital setting.

By the end of treatment, the patient should be afebrile, hemodynamically stable, and free of new complications. In some patients, an evaluation for underlying sites of bacteremia will have been either initiated or completed by this time. To confirm that endocardial infection has resolved, one or two additional blood cultures should be obtained 7–14 days after completing antimicrobial treatment.

Endocarditis is a destructive process, producing permanent deformities of the cardiac valves that leave patients with a *100-fold increased risk of recurrent disease.* Thus, all patients with a history of infective endocarditis should receive antimicrobial prophylaxis when indicated, such as prior to certain dental procedures (Tables 30.6 and 30.7). Despite long-standing guidelines, such recommendations are often not followed. Common errors include failure to recognize the need for prophylaxis, failure by physicians to inform the patient of the lifetime risk for endocarditis, not warning the patient's dentist about the medical history, and incorrect selection or dosage of antimicrobial agents.

To enhance the likelihood that patients will receive adequate prophylaxis in the future, they should be informed about their risk for reinfection and instructed about their lifetime need for antibiotic prophylaxis. It is important to emphasize the need for patients to alert their dentists or physicians of their high risk for recurrent infection. The American Heart Association produces a wallet card that can be carried by patients to document their medical histories. This card also details the recommended prophylactic regimen for specific procedures, which can be used by physicians or dentists as a reference. Good oral hygiene and regular dental care should also be encouraged because they are associated with a reduced risk of recurrent endocarditis (14).

In addition to problems with recurrent infection, patients with endocarditis are at increased risk for progressive valvular dysfunction, leading to hemodynamic impairment and the need for valve replacement. In a 15-year prospective follow-up of patients with native valve endocarditis, 47% required valve replacement during the period of observation. Patients with aortic valve involvement were at particular risk, with 55% undergoing valve surgery. For approximately two-thirds of patients, hemodynamic deterioration and valve replacement occurred within the first two years after having endocarditis. These results indicate that patients with a history of endocardial infection need to be monitored periodically for signs of valve dysfunction and congestive heart failure. Echocardiography may be indicated in some patients to detail the sites and extent of valvular involvement as well as to examine overall cardiac function.

COST CONSIDERATIONS AND RESOURCE USE

Few studies have attempted to analyze the costs associated with managing endocarditis. A decade ago, medical and surgical management were estimated to cost approximately $18,000 and $60,000 per case, respectively (15). Costs for medical management were based on expenses for inpatient therapy, so it is likely that outpatient treatment would be considerably less expensive. However, no systematic analysis of the relative savings associated with this approach has been published.

KEY POINTS

- Infective endocarditis is a relatively uncommon disease associated with a significant mortality rate. Many patients require surgical treatment, either at the time of infection or in the subsequent years.
- The management of patients with this infection requires expertise in areas of microbiology, infectious diseases, and cardiology.

- Patients suspected of having endocarditis need a prompt and definitive diagnostic evaluation followed by the rapid initiation of appropriate therapy.
- Selection of specific antimicrobial agents requires knowledge of the underlying risk factors for infection coupled with results from in vitro assays of antimicrobial sensitivity.
- In addition to choosing antibiotics, proper management entails careful monitoring for complications, identifying patients in need of surgery, and posttreatment follow-up for long-term valvular dysfunction.
- The physician managing such patients also should be certain that both the patient and his or her primary care physician are aware of the patient's lifelong need for antimicrobial prophylaxis in conjunction with certain dental or invasive procedures.

REFERENCES

1. Hoen B, Alla F, Selton-Suty C, et al. Changing profile of infective endocarditis: results of a 1-year survey in France. *JAMA* 2002; 288:75–81.
2. Bouza E, Menasalvas A, Munoz P, Vasallo FJ, del Mar Moreno M, Garcia Fernandez MA. Infective endocarditis—a prospective study at the end of the twentieth century: new predisposing conditions, new etiologic agents, and still a high mortality. *Medicine* (Baltimore) 2001;80:298–307.
3. Fowler VG Jr., Li J, Corey GR, et al. Role of echocardiography in evaluation of patients with *Staphylococcus aureus* bacteremia: experience in 103 patients. *J Am Coll Cardiol* 1997;30:1072–1078.
4. Sachdev M, Peterson GE, Jollis JG. Imaging techniques for diagnosis of infective endocarditis. *Infect Dis Clin North Am* 2002;16: 319–337.
5. Schulz R, Werner GS, Fuchs JB, et al. Clinical outcome and echocardiographic findings of native and prosthetic valve endocarditis in the 1990's. *Eur Heart J* 1996;17:281–288.
6. Tischler MD, Vaitkus PT. The ability of vegetation size on echocardiography to predict clinical complications: a meta-analysis. *J Am Soc Echocardiogr* 1997;10:562–568.
7. Cheitlin MD, Alpert JS, Armstrong WF, et al. ACC/AHA guidelines for the clinical application of echocardiography: executive summary. A report of the American College of Cardiology/American Heart Association Task Force on practice guidelines (Committee on Clinical Application of Echocardiography). Developed in collaboration with the American Society of Echocardiography. *J Am Coll Cardiol* 1997;29:862–879.
8. Rosen AB, Fowler VG Jr, Corey GR, et al. Cost-effectiveness of transesophageal echocardiography to determine the duration of therapy for intravascular catheter-associated *Staphylococcus aureus* bacteremia. *Ann Intern Med* 1999;130:810–820.
9. Li JS, Sexton DJ, Mick N, et al. Proposed modifications to the Duke criteria for the diagnosis of infective endocarditis. *Clin Infect Dis* 2000;30:633–638.
10. Andrews MM, von Reyn CF. Patient selection criteria and management guidelines for outpatient parenteral antibiotic therapy for native valve infective endocarditis. *Clin Infect Dis* 2001;33:203–209.
11. Delahaye F, Rial MO, de Gevigney G, Ecochard R, Delaye J. A critical appraisal of the quality of the management of infective endocarditis. *J Am Coll Cardiol* 1999;33:788–793.
12. Fowler VG, Jr., Sanders LL, Sexton DJ, et al. Outcome of *Staphylococcus aureus* bacteremia according to compliance with recommendations of infectious diseases specialists: experience with 244 patients. *Clin Infect Dis* 1998;27:478–486.
13. Olaison L, Pettersson G. Current best practices and guidelines indications for surgical intervention in infective endocarditis. *Infect Dis Clin North Am* 2002;16:453–475.

14. Strom BL, Abrutyn E, Berlin JA, et al. Risk factors for infective endocarditis: oral hygiene and nondental exposures. *Circulation* 2000;102:2842–2848.

15. Caro JJ, Migliaccio-Walle K, O'Brien JA. The cost of treating heart valve related complications. *J Heart Valve Dis* 1996;5:122–127.

ADDITIONAL READING

Houpikian P, Raoult D. Diagnostic methods current best practices and guidelines for identification of difficult-to-culture pathogens in infective endocarditis. *Infect Dis Clin North Am* 2002;16: 377–392.

Le T, Bayer AS. Combination antibiotic therapy for infective endocarditis. *Clin Infect Dis* 2003;36:615–621.

Moreillon P, Que YA. Infective endocarditis. *Lancet* 2004;363:139–149.

Mylonakis E, Calderwood SB. Infective endocarditis in adults. *N Engl J Med* 2001;345:1318–1330.

Seto TB, Thomas L, Baden LR, Manning WJ. Specialty and training differences in the reported use of endocarditis prophylaxis at an academic medical center. *Am J Med* 2001;111:657–660.

Weed HG. Antimicrobial prophylaxis in the surgical patient. *Med Clin North Am* 2003;87:59–75.

Wilson WR, Karchmer AW, Dajani AS, et al. Antibiotic treatment of adults with infective endocarditis due to streptococci, enterococci, staphylococci, and HACEK microorganisms. American Heart Association. *JAMA* 1995;274:1706–1713.

Catheter-Associated Infection and Bacteremia

72

Isaam I. Raad   Hend A. Hanna

INTRODUCTION

Each year, approximately 150 million intravascular catheters are placed in 30 million patients in the United States. These devices allow the provision of medications, transfusion of blood products, parenteral nutrition, and hemodynamic monitoring. Unfortunately, intravascular devices are also the source of many infections. Local infections at the insertion site, bacteremia, septic thrombophlebitis, endocarditis, and metastatic complications of hematogenous spread from the catheter to bone, joints, ocular tissues, or solid organs are the most common infectious complications. Overall, an estimated 850,000 *catheter-associated infections* (CAIs) and 250,000 *catheter-associated bacteremias* (CABs) occur annually in the United States. Of these, approximately 80,000 CABs occur in the intensive care units (ICUs). CABs are associated with significant increases in mortality (12%–25%), morbidity, duration of hospitalization (mean, additional seven days), antibiotic use, and additional costs to the health care system of about $25,000 per episode (1–3).

Today, many options are available for intravascular access (Table 72.1). The incidence and management of infectious complications vary with the type of device, the quality of infection control practices, and, most importantly, the condition of the patient. This chapter focuses on those CAIs attributable to intravenous access devices that are most often seen among adult patients in acute care settings.

ISSUES AT THE TIME OF ADMISSION

Clinical Presentation

Catheter-related infection should be suspected whenever evidence of local infection develops at the catheter insertion/exit site or cutaneous tunnel in a patient with a current or recent intravascular catheter or when unexplained fever or other evidence of systemic infection is noted. The type of catheter is a major factor affecting the probability and site of infection and the clinical presentation (4, 5).

Short-Term Catheters

The use of short-term peripheral venous catheters is only rarely complicated by infection. When infection does occur, it is usually confined to the insertion site; bacteremia is present in 0.1%–0.3% of cases. Although these catheters are not used for outpatient treatment or home infusion therapy, they are often used to treat patients in long-term care facilities. These catheters remain in place for an average of 48–72 hours. Such patients may be referred for evaluation of suspected CAI. Infection may be inapparent until after the peripheral catheter has been removed, so a diagnosis of CAI should be considered when unexplained fever or focal signs of infection at a prior catheter site develop after discharge.

Nontunneled short-term central venous catheters (CVCs) are usually made of polyurethane and remain in place for an average of one week. These catheters are often

TABLE 72.1

INTRAVENOUS CATHETERS ASSOCIATED WITH INFECTION

Type of catheter	Site	Expected duration of use
Short peripheral catheter	Forearm or hand	Days
Nontunneled polyurethane CVC	Subclavian, internal jugular, or femoral veins	Days
Nontunneled silicone CVC	Subclavian	Weeks to months
Midline catheters	Proximal basilic or cephalic veins	Days to weeks, sometimes months
Peripherally inserted CVC (PICC)	Basilic, cephalic, or brachial veins	Weeks to months
Tunneled CVC	Subclavian, internal jugular, or femoral veins	Months
Totally implantable port	Subclavian or internal jugular veins	Months

CVC, central venous catheter.

placed in critically ill patients. Local pain, erythema, phlebitis, and purulence are clues to infection at the catheter insertion site. Fever is unusual in uncomplicated infection at the insertion site and suggests a more serious local condition (e.g., abscess, cellulitis, or septic thrombophlebitis), bacteremia, or metastatic suppurative complications. However, the absence of fever does not exclude a diagnosis of complicating bacteremia, especially among elderly patients and in cases of sepsis or immunosuppression. CAB should be suspected when staphylococcal or fungal bloodstream infection is detected in the absence of an obvious source for the bacteremia or fungemia other than the intravenous catheter.

Long-Term Catheters

The most common types of catheters likely to be encountered among outpatients are those intended for long-term use: peripherally inserted central venous catheters (PICC), tunneled central venous catheters, and totally implantable intravascular devices (ports). Midline catheters are also sometimes included in this category, although they were originally intended for short-term use. Overall, totally implantable intravascular devices have the lowest rate of infection among long-term catheters, probably because there is no portal of entry for bacteria. A *"pocket" infection* should be suspected in the presence of erythema or necrosis of the skin over the reservoir of a totally implantable intravascular device or when a purulent exudate is found in the subcutaneous tissue containing the reservoir. Tunneled catheters also have a low infection risk. Infection should be suspected when pain or local signs of inflammation are evident in the tissues overlying a tunneled catheter or within 2 centimeters of the exit site.

The absence of local signs of infection does not exclude a long-term catheter infection. In fact, it is extremely difficult to make a clinical diagnosis of infection involving the intravascular portion of a long-term catheter because local signs are usually not present. Fever is the most common clue but is not always found or may be intermittent. As with

short-term catheters, CAB should be suspected when unexplained staphylococcal or fungal bloodstream infection, endocarditis, abscesses, or other evidence of hematogenous spread are observed (6).

Differential Diagnosis and Initial Evaluation

Diagnosing CAB is often based on the interplay between clinical and microbiological findings. Local signs at the insertion site are almost always present in patients with short-term peripheral catheter infections, except in neutropenic patients. If a purulent exudate is present, a Gram stain of an aspirated specimen should be obtained to help guide initial treatment. Cultures are also important to determine the causal organism and its microbial susceptibility when systemic antibiotic treatment is planned. For peripheral catheters (short venous or PICC), aseptic phlebitis may produce tenderness, swelling, and erythema and can easily be confused with local infection. A palpable venous cord is not as common as other signs of phlebitis. When a tender, palpable cord is present in a febrile patient, especially with overlying cellulitis or exudate, *septic thrombophlebitis* may be present (Chapter 52). Purulent material found in association with local insertion site or exit site infection, complicating long-term catheter use, should always be cultured for fungi in addition to bacteria.

Fever is the hallmark of CAB, but an outpatient with a vascular catheter is likely to have an underlying illness and to have received therapies that may increase the risk for fever, such as chemotherapeutic agents. A thorough history, examination, and targeted laboratory and radiographic studies are necessary to exclude other potential causes of fever. However, unless another source is apparent, CAB should be suspected. In the absence of local signs, the diagnosis depends on a high index of suspicion and the results of blood cultures (1).

Performance of *two percutaneous blood cultures* is the best method for diagnosing bacteremia. These cultures should be obtained before antibiotic treatment is initiated. However, the skin must be properly cleaned before blood cultures are obtained (1); failure to do so increases the potential for blood culture contamination. Blood cultures obtained in an emergency department, where other urgent matters often take precedence over appropriate culturing technique, are often contaminated. As a corollary, intravascular catheters placed in an emergency department or during other patient emergencies should be replaced within 24 hours to reduce the risk for infection (1).

Cleaning the skin with soap will remove dirt and surface lipids and improve the efficacy of whatever antiseptic is used. Alcohol preparations, tincture of iodine, povidone-iodine, or chlorhexidine solutions are effective antiseptics, but only when properly applied to clean skin. Alcohols have an immediate onset of action and broad-spectrum activity but are ineffective when the skin is not clean. Tincture of iodine also has a rapid onset of action but has the disadvantage of staining the skin and producing serious allergic reactions in some patients. Povidone-iodine has a slower onset of action and must be in contact with the skin for three to five minutes to achieve antisepsis, a time requirement that is not often met. A 2% tincture of chlorhexidine preparation is now recommended by the Centers for Disease Control (CDC) guidelines for the prevention of catheter-related infections (1). Proper hand cleansing, gloving of the health care personnel who obtain the blood cultures, and good practices in the clinical laboratory are also important to prevent contamination.

Blood culture contamination should be suspected if only one blood specimen demonstrates microbial growth, especially when skin commensals, such as coagulase-negative staphylococci, are found. When two blood samples obtained from different sites grow the same organism, true bacteremia is more likely. However, when coagulase-negative staphylococci are found in both specimens, the isolates should be identified at the species level and their antibiograms compared to ensure that they are, in fact, identical. Blood samples drawn through catheters should also be obtained aseptically after cleansing the hub with alcohol. When local infection is present, bacteremia without another source is sufficient to establish the diagnosis of CAB, especially if the same organism is isolated from the two sites. When evidence of insertion or exit site infection is not present, implicating the intravascular catheter as the source of infection is more difficult. The two main methods used are culturing the catheter and culturing the blood, but neither is ideal, and no "gold standard" is universally accepted (1).

Culturing the Catheter

The *roll-plate semiquantitative catheter culture technique* is the most commonly used method to culture a suspected catheter. With this method, the catheter is removed and its distal 2-centimeter segment is rolled on an agar plate, which is then incubated. The presence of 15 or more colonies of bacteria is taken as presumptive evidence of catheter colonization sufficient to cause bacteremia or fungemia. The roll-plate method cultures only the external surface of the catheter. Therefore, it is less sensitive when the infection arises from intraluminal colonization that is introduced through the catheter hub, which is particularly common with long-term catheters. The sensitivity may also be reduced when antibiotic-impregnated catheters are used. Hence, the utility of the roll-plate technique for diagnosing or excluding CAB is controversial.

Quantitative catheter culture by sonication technique improves the detection of intraluminal colonization. By sonication, a catheter is considered colonized if at least 1,000 colonies of bacteria are isolated from the catheter segment. Other alternative methods for culturing the catheter include flush techniques, vortex, and centrifugation methods. Like the roll-plate technique, all these methods have one major disadvantage—a requirement for catheter removal.

Culturing the Blood

Blood culture techniques to diagnose CAB rest on the assumption that the quantity of bacteria in blood drawn from an infected catheter will exceed the quantity obtained from a peripheral blood sample. A ratio of 5:1 (catheter blood colony count per milliliter to peripheral blood colony count per milliliter) is used as the cutoff for implicating the catheter as the source. Differential time to positivity (DTP) is defined as the time necessary for simultaneous blood cultures, taken through the catheter and via a peripheral puncture, to become positive. When DTP was 120 minutes or more, it was found to be highly sensitive and specific in diagnosing CAB (7). Two disadvantages of these methods are the laboratory time and expense needed to perform the quantitative cultures as well as the lack of routine reporting of DTP by most laboratories.

The single most important diagnostic step in diagnosing CAB is the demonstration of microbial growth in two or more percutaneous blood cultures of a catheterized patient with no other obvious source of infection. *Catheter tip cultures and quantitative blood cultures should not be performed unless their results would change the treatment plan.* Whether or not the catheter is removed, all CRI should be treated with appropriate antibiotics, administered parenterally (8).

Indications for Hospitalization and Initial Management

The management of CAI depends on at least four factors: (a) the severity of the infection (local or systemic), (b) the condition of the patient, (c) the known or suspected organism, and (d) the type of catheter (6) (Table 72.2). *Uncomplicated local infections of short-term peripheral venous catheters* usually can be treated by removing the catheter and administering a short course (3–5 days) of an oral

TABLE 72.2

MANAGEMENT OF CATHETERS WHEN CATHETER-ASSOCIATED INFECTION IS SUSPECTED OR DIAGNOSED

	Short-term peripheral intravenous catheter	Short-term central venous catheter	Long-term catheter
Routine replacement	Every 48–72 h	No recommendation	Not indicated
Local insertion or exit site tunnel infection	Remove catheter	Remove catheter, replace at new site (if needed)	Removal not usually required unless infection is present
Catheter-associated bacteremia known or suspected; uncomplicated	Remove catheter	• If patient is septic, remove catheter; replace at new site (if needed) • If patient is not septic, change catheter over guidewire; replace if catheter culture is positive	• Immediate removal not usually required unless patient is septic • If bacteremia persists >48 h on antibiotics or patient fails to respond, always remove catheter • If coagulase-negative staphylococcal bacteremia, treat with antibiotics 5–7 d; if early relapse occurs, remove catheter • If catheter need is long-term, consider elective replacement • If *Staphylococcus aureus*, Enterobacteriaceae, or *Candida* species bacteremia, catheter removal is indicated as soon as feasible
Catheter-associated bacteremia with complications[a]	Remove catheter	Remove catheter	Remove catheter

[a] Complications include septic thrombophlebitis and endocarditis or evidence of hematogenous spread.

antibiotic with antistaphylococcal activity. Such patients do not require hospitalization. Blood cultures should be obtained if the patient is febrile or has other evidence of systemic infection. If the index of suspicion for bacteremia is high or if evidence of septic thrombophlebitis is present, the patient should be admitted and treated with parenteral antibiotics.

Uncomplicated insertion or exit site infections of long-term catheters can usually be treated without removing the catheter (Table 72.2) unless caused by *Staphylococcus aureus*, Gram-negative bacilli, or *Candida* species (9). Obvious soft-tissue abscesses should be drained. Parenteral antibiotics can be administered through the catheter, so hospitalization is not mandatory if the patient is stable. Percutaneous blood cultures should be obtained before treatment is started. Tunnel infections are more serious; they require catheter removal and are best treated, at least initially, in the hospital.

All patients with known or suspected *complicated bacteremia* should be admitted to the hospital. Such complications include septic thrombophlebitis, endocarditis, or evidence of hematogenous spread of infection, and catheter removal is always required, in addition to appropriate antibiotic therapy (Table 72.2). Complicated bacteremia also should be suspected when bacteremia persists for more than 48 hours after catheter removal and initia-

tion of appropriate antibiotic treatment (Table 72.3). In these situations, additional investigations should be done, such as venogram to rule out septic thrombosis and transesophageal echocardiography to detect valvular vegetations in cases of endocarditis (Chapter 71) (9).

Patients with *uncomplicated bacteremia* always require parenteral antibiotic treatment, but catheter removal may not be necessary, depending on the causal organism (Table 72.2). Because the organism is usually not known at the time of initial evaluation, patients should generally be admitted to begin empiric antibiotic treatment. If the decision is made to retain the catheter in a clinically stable patient who is not neutropenic and who has access to supervised outpatient treatment, hospitalization can sometimes be brief or even avoided entirely. Persistent bacteremia (or fungemia) for more than 48 hours on appropriate parenteral therapy is an indication for catheter removal and a search for infectious complications, regardless of the etiologic agent (10).

When coagulase-negative staphylococci are the cause of long-term catheter infection, removal of the catheter has little impact on the acute outcome of the bacteremia. However, the risk of recurrent bacteremia is decreased if the catheter is removed, so elective replacement is usually indicated if the catheter is needed for long-term management. When *Staphylococcus aureus* is involved, immediate catheter removal is necessary because the acute mortality rate, complication rate, and relapse rate are higher when the catheter is retained (9). All patients with catheter-related candidemia should be treated, either with amphotericin B, an azole (e.g., voriconazole), or an echinocandin (e.g., caspafungin) based on the susceptibility of the organisms. Antifungal therapy should be given for 14 days after the last positive blood culture (9). Catheters should be removed in cases of catheter-related candidemia because salvage rates with systemic antifungal therapy are only in the 30% range (9). Gram-negative bacillary infections, especially those caused by *Pseudomonas* species, are difficult to cure without catheter removal.

Initial Antimicrobial Treatment

As with all infections, the goal of empiric antibiotic treatment of CAB is to provide a drug regimen with bactericidal activity against the most likely pathogens until culture data are available to guide definitive treatment decisions. Factors affecting the decision include the severity of illness, the extent of infection, the prevalence of organisms associated with CAB in the institution or among comparable patients (e.g., bone marrow transplant recipients), the prevalence of antimicrobial resistance among these organisms, and the recent history of infections and antibiotic treatment in the individual patient (9). Treatment must be individualized, and no single empiric regimen is appropriate for all patients. Most importantly, the treatment regimen should promptly be narrowed once the causative organism is identified.

Coagulase-negative staphylococci, most of which are resistant to nafcillin and other β-lactam antibiotics, are the most common pathogens associated with CAB. However, *empiric vancomycin treatment is not essential* unless the patient is neutropenic or profoundly immunosuppressed, because these infections are usually indolent and the treatment outcome is not better when vancomycin is included in the initial treatment regimen (10).

S. aureus is the most common pathogen associated with morbidity and mortality from CAB. Knowledge of the local prevalence of methicillin resistance among nosocomial staphylococcal bloodstream infections is helpful in determining the need for empiric use of vancomycin when CAB is suspected. Even where the prevalence is low, vancomycin should be included in the empiric treatment regimen if the patient is septic or has a prior history of infection or colonization with methicillin-resistant *S. aureus*. For vancomycin-resistant *S. aureus* or in patients colonized with vancomycin-resistant enterococci or allergy to vancomycin, linezolid or quinupristin/dalfopristin should be used (9). Otherwise, treatment with nafcillin plus an aminoglycoside is usually adequate. However, in the absence of methicillin-resistant organisms, penicillinase-resistant penicillins, such as nafcillin or oxacillin, should be used to avoid the unnecessary use of vancomycin (9).

Additional empirical coverage for Gram-negative bacilli and *Pseudomonas aeruginosa* with ceftazidime or cefepime should be considered for severely ill or immunocompromised patients when CAB is suspected, as well as in institutions where pseudomonas infections are not uncommon (Chapter 64).

Indications for Early Consultation

Surgical consultation should be obtained when septic thrombophlebitis is suspected, deep tissue metastatic

TABLE 72.3

DIAGNOSTIC CONSIDERATIONS IN PATIENTS WHO CONTINUE TO HAVE PERSISTENT BACTEREMIA OR FEVER AFTER EMPIRIC TREATMENT FOR CATHETER-ASSOCIATED BACTEREMIA

Reason for failure to improve	Recommended approach
Infected catheter remains	Remove catheter
Resistant bacterial organism (e.g., methicillin-resistant *Staphylococcus aureus, Enterococcus faecium*)	Evaluate susceptibility; broaden coverage; obtain infectious diseases consultation
Nonbacterial pathogen (e.g., *Candida* species, atypical pathogens)	Perform additional microbiological cultures to exclude these agents and mycobacteria
Inadequate treatment regimen	Check drug dosage, route, interval; consider measuring serum concentrations if vancomycin or aminoglycosides are being used
Complicated bacteremia (e.g., endocarditis, septic thrombophlebitis, septic pulmonary emboli, mycotic aneurysm)	Repeat physical examination and selected laboratory and imaging studies to diagnose these entities; obtain echocardiogram; obtain infectious diseases consultation; consider surgical consultation
Seeding of organs, abscess formation	Repeat physical examination and selected laboratory and imaging studies to diagnose these entities; obtain ophthalmology consultation; obtain infectious diseases consultation; consider surgical consultation
Other processes	Repeat physical examination and targeted laboratory and imaging studies to identify other causes of fever; consider drug fever, venous thrombosis, pulmonary embolism

abscesses are detected, endocarditis is diagnosed, or surgically implanted catheters require removal. Consultation with an orthopedic surgeon should be sought when complicating bone or joint infection is present. Early and serial retinal examinations are important for all patients with CAB, and consultation with an ophthalmologist can be helpful in detecting early retinal changes, especially when *S. aureus* or *Candida* species are the cause of bloodstream infection. Most cases of uncomplicated CAB do not require consultation with infectious disease specialists, but consultation is warranted when prolonged antibiotic treatment is being considered and when complicated infection is present.

ISSUES DURING THE COURSE OF HOSPITALIZATION

Catheter Infections Developing After Admission

Most infections attributable to intravascular catheters develop in the acute care setting. When short-term peripheral catheters and long-term catheters become infected during hospitalization, the presentation and evaluation are the same as at the time of admission, described in the preceding section. The most important CAIs that develop during hospitalization are related to short-term central venous catheters. These catheters are associated with an increased risk for local infection at the insertion site.

Short-term central venous catheters are frequently used in ICU patients, most of whom are seriously ill and at high risk for fever and infection from a variety of sources. Hence, diagnosing CAB is extremely difficult. When bacteremia is suspected, two simultaneous blood cultures should be obtained from the CVC and percutaneous sites. The quantitative blood culture method may be employed to help establish the diagnosis of CAB; otherwise, differential time to positivity could be useful. The diagnosis of CAB would be established when the blood culture drawn through the CVC becomes positive at least two hours before a simultaneously drawn peripheral blood culture (7).

Suspected short-term central venous CAB is initially managed according to the same principles that apply to long-term CAB, with one additional consideration: the possible role of *guidewire exchange* (Table 72.2). Replacing central catheters over a guidewire reduces the potentially serious risks associated with new insertion at an alternate site and is the preferred method of catheter replacement when infection is not suspected and catheter tip culture is required to rule out CAB. The procedure is contraindicated if evidence of infection at the insertion site is present (pain, purulence, erythema) and if the patient is septic. In a febrile patient without these contraindications in whom CAB is suspected, replacement over a guidewire is

reasonable, and culturing the tip of the removed catheter aids in the diagnosis of the suspected CAB. Guidelines from the Centers for Disease Control and Prevention (CDC)/Hospital Infection Control Practices Advisory Committee (HICPAC) recommend that a quantitative or semiquantitative culture of the catheter be obtained at the time of removal. If the culture is positive, then subsequent replacement of the catheter at a new site is also recommended (1).

Expected Response to Therapy

Uncomplicated infections at the insertion site should resolve quickly. If the patient's condition does not improve after 48 hours or if a fever develops or worsens, the site should be carefully examined to identify cellulitis, an undrained abscess, septic thrombophlebitis, or other local complications (Table 72.3). In addition, blood cultures should be obtained to exclude the possibility of a secondary bacteremia.

Likewise, among patients with CAB, blood cultures should be negative after 48 hours of initiating appropriate antibiotic treatment. If bacteremia persists beyond 48 hours, a comprehensive evaluation and consultation with an infectious diseases clinician are indicated to determine whether the patient has developed a deep-seated infection (10) (Table 72.3). If the implicated catheter was not removed when the problem first appeared, immediate removal is now necessary. The treatment regimen should be evaluated to determine whether the proper antibiotics were administered at the appropriate time and whether the dosage was adequate to achieve bactericidal activity against the pathogen. Additional studies to identify endovascular complications of CAB should also be initiated, especially if the original infection was caused by *S. aureus*. Septic thrombosis, endocarditis, and septic pulmonary emboli are relatively rare but life-threatening complications in this setting. Transesophageal echocardiogram, chest radiographs, venous Doppler studies, and, rarely, a peripheral or central venogram should be considered.

If the patient remains febrile more than five days, other complications of CAB should be considered, even in the face of sterile blood cultures. When *S. aureus* or *Candida* species cause CAB, hematogenous spread can produce metastatic abscesses and other infections in the retina, solid organs, soft tissues, bones, and joints. Detecting these complications is difficult, especially in severely ill patients who cannot provide information about localizing symptoms. The retina should always be examined, and ophthalmologic consultation is warranted. Abdominal ultrasonography will aid in the detection of occult splenic, hepatic, and renal abscesses. Additional studies that are sometimes needed include bone scans, computed tomography or magnetic resonance imaging, and white blood cell scans. Of course, patients with CAB are usually at risk for many other causes of fever, and these should not be overlooked when a diagnosis is being pursued.

DISCHARGE ISSUES

The duration of parenteral treatment required to cure CAB is variable, and clinical data have not completely elucidated the optimal duration (9). Uncomplicated infections caused by coagulase-negative staphylococci usually do not require treatment for more than five to seven days, even when the catheter is not removed. Uncomplicated Gram-negative bacillary CAIs should be treated for 10–14 days with appropriate antimicrobial therapy, and the catheter should be removed (9).

Antifungal therapy for 14 days after the last positive blood culture is recommended for uncomplicated CAI caused by *Candida* species (9). Most experts also recommend a 10-day to 14-day course of treatment for uncomplicated *S. aureus* CAB (10,11). However, the risk for hematogenous seeding, which potentially leads to serious endovascular infections, is high with both of these organisms. Failure to diagnose these complications and extend the duration of treatment accordingly accounts for a large proportion of the relatively high rates of delayed morbidity and mortality associated with CAB. The required duration of antifungal therapy for complicated CAB depends on the specific problem (e.g., endocarditis) and the need for surgical intervention. Treatment of CAB caused by *S. aureus* should be extended to 4–6 weeks when complications are diagnosed. If the blood cultures are not sterile after 48 hours or the patient's condition does not improve, treatment should also be continued for at least four weeks unless an alternate diagnosis is found (10,11).

No data are available to define the optimum duration of hospitalization for CAB. However, experience with outpatient and home infusion programs suggests that completion of therapy outside the hospital is a good option for many patients (12). Criteria for discharge include (a) clinical improvement and resolution of fever, (b) sterilization of blood cultures, (c) establishment of reliable venous access for parenteral treatment, and (d) access to supervised outpatient or home infusion therapy. Patients who meet the first three criteria but cannot be managed as outpatients might be transferred to step-down units or skilled nursing facilities until treatment is completed.

Patients who are able to participate in their own catheter care should be trained to do so before discharge. Essential information should cover dressing care, how to avoid contamination of the insertion site or hub, and which symptoms and signs should prompt medical evaluation. In addition, gloves and instructions for safe needle handling and an impervious needle disposal container should be provided if the patient or caregivers will be at risk for needle injury or blood exposure.

COST CONSIDERATIONS AND RESOURCE USE

The most important strategy for improving resource utilization relevant to CAB is to *reduce the nonessential use of intravascular catheters.* Decreasing the number of catheters used, the number of catheter lumens, and the total days of catheterization decreases infection rates. This can be accomplished through judicious use of parenteral treatments and changing to oral regimens when the patient's condition warrants the switch. It is important to choose the type of catheter with the lowest incidence of infection that is appropriate for the expected duration of catheterization. The use of *antimicrobial or antiseptic impregnated catheters* in adults whose catheter is expected to remain in place longer than five days is recommended if, after implementing a comprehensive strategy to reduce rates of CAB, the CAB rate remains above the goal set by the individual institution, based on benchmark rates (10). Catheters impregnated with minocycline and rifampin were shown to be highly effective in preventing CAB, even more so than antiseptic catheters coated with chlorhexidine gluconate and silver sulfadiazine. This was particularly true for catheters with an expected dwell time of longer than seven days (13). In addition, CAI can be prevented by adherence to CDC guidelines for catheter placement, care and replacement, and removal (1). The use of maximum sterile barriers during CVC insertion is particularly cost-effective (14).

For patients who do acquire CAI, significant resources can be saved by early discharge to a lower level of care for parenteral treatment, provided that adequate support services to ensure uninterrupted therapy and observation for new complications are available.

KEY POINTS

- Many cases of catheter-associated infection can be avoided by judicious use of intravascular catheters, proper placement and care of catheters, and removal as soon as intravenous access is no longer indicated. Antimicrobial or antiseptic-impregnated catheters can also lower infection rates in patients expected to have prolonged catheterization.
- Attention to antisepsis and infection control practices can reduce the number of false-positive blood cultures when catheter-associated bacteremia is suspected and decrease unnecessary use of vancomycin and other antimicrobial agents.
- Immediate long-term catheter removal is not always required, depending on the etiologic agent. However, to avoid relapse, elective replacement is advised if ongoing venous access is needed.
- Patients with catheter-associated bacteremia usually do not require hospitalization once they are clinically stable, have negative blood cultures, and have been

evaluated to exclude complications that increase morbidity and mortality and mandate a longer course of treatment.

REFERENCES

1. O'Grady NP, Alexander M, Dellinger EP, et al. Guidelines for the prevention of intravascular catheter-related infections. *MMWR Recomm Rep* 2002;51(RR-10):1–29.
2. Mermel LA. Prevention of intravascular catheter-related infections. *Ann Intern Med* 2000;132:391–402.
3. Mermel LA. Preventing intravascular catheter-related infections. *Ann Intern Med* 2000;133:395.
4. Crnich CJ, Maki DG. The promise of novel technology for the prevention of intravascular device-related bloodstream infection. I Pathogenesis and short-term devices. *Clin Infect Dis* 2002; 34:1232–1242.
5. Crnich CJ, Maki DG. The promise of novel technology for the prevention of intravascular device-related bloodstream infection. II Long-term devices. *Clin Infect Dis* 2002;34:1362–1368.
6. Raad II, Hanna HA. Intravascular catheter-related infections: new horizons and recent advances. *Arch Intern Med* 2002; 162:871–878.
7. Blot F, Nitenberg G, Chachaty E, Raynard B, Germann N, Antoun S, Laplanche A, Brun-Buisson C, Tancrede C. Diagnosis of catheter-related bacteremia: a prospective comparison of the time to positivity of hub-blood versus peripheral-blood cultures. *Lancet* 1999;354:1071–1077.
8. Paiva JA, Pereira JM. Treatment of the afebrile patient after catheter withdrawal: drugs and duration. *Clin Microbiol Infect* 2002;8:290–294.
9. Mermel LA, Farr BM, Sherertz RJ, et al. Guidelines for the management of intravascular catheter-related infections. *Clin Infect Dis* 2001;32:1249–1272.
10. Raad II, Bodey GP. Infectious complications of indwelling vascular catheters. *Clin Infect Dis* 1992;15:197–210.
11. Fowler VG, Olsen MK, Corey GR, et al. Clinical identifiers of complicated *Staphylococcus aureus* bacteremias. *Arch Intern Med* 2003;163:2066–2072.
12. Johansson E, Bjorkholm M, Wredling R, Kalin M, Engervall P. Outpatient parenteral antibiotic therapy in patients with haematological malignancies. A pilot study of an early discharge strategy. *Supportive Care in Cancer* 2001;9:619–624.
13. Darouiche RO, Raad II, Heard SO, et al. A comparison of two antimicrobial-impregnated central venous catheters. Catheter Study Group. *N Engl J Med* 1999;340:1–8.
14. Hu KK, Veenstra DL, Lipsky BA, Saint S. Use of maximum sterile barriers during central venous catheter insertion: clinical and economic outcomes. *Clin Infect Dis* 2004;39:1441–1445.

ADDITIONAL READING

Safdar N, Kluger DM, Maki DG. A review of risk factors for catheter-related bloodstream infection caused by percutaneously inserted, noncuffed central venous catheters: implications for preventive strategies. *Medicine* 2002;81:466–479.

Seifert H, Cornely O, Seggewiss K, et al. Bloodstream infection in neutropenic cancer patients related to short-term nontunneled catheters determined by quantitative blood cultures, differential time to positivity, and molecular epidemiological typing with pulsed-field gel electrophoresis. *J Clin Microbiol* 2003;41: 118–123.

Walshe LJ, Malak SF, Eagan J, Sepkowitz KA. Complication rates among cancer patients with peripherally inserted central catheters. *J Clin Oncol* 2002;20:3276–3281.

Bioterrorism

73

Thomas E. Terndrup   *Sarah D. Nafziger*

INTRODUCTION

The concept of using naturally occurring organisms as weapons is not new. History has documented numerous attempts at biological warfare (Table 73.1). Only in the past several years, however, has the health care community become aware of the growing threat of a biological weapons attack. For many, the first notice came with the October 2001 bioterrorism attack, in which anthrax was spread through the U.S. postal system, resulting in 18 cases of anthrax with five fatalities. This attack, along with the 2003 outbreak of severe acute respiratory syndrome (SARS), further demonstrated the underpreparedness of the United States health care system to respond not only to bioterror attacks, but also to other highly transmissible emerging infections.

THE CURRENT STATE OF HOSPITAL PREPAREDNESS

Limited data indicate that most hospitals are inadequately prepared to deal with attacks by weapons of mass destruction, including bioterrorism. A large-scale bioterrorism drill performed in Denver, Colorado, simulating aerosolized plague attacks resulted in over 3,000 simulated casualties within 4 days (1). One of the most valuable insights from this drill was that the systems and resources currently in place are inadequate to manage the stress of a large-scale bioweapons attack.

Fortunately, much of what should be done in anticipation of a biological attack is also applicable to any public health disaster or infectious disease outbreak, making these expensive but necessary preparations "dual-use" in nature. In contrast to preparation for chemical spills or terrorism (where preparation relies largely on prehospital hazardous material teams and equipment, immediate treatment in the streets, and cordoned-off crime scenes), preparation for biological terrorism relies much more on

education, a robust public health system, and broad interagency collaboration.

Not only must hospitals prepare to deal with the consequences of bioterrorism, they must also take measures to reduce their vulnerability as terrorist targets. As the epicenter of community emergency response, hospitals are valuable and often extremely vulnerable assets. While many public buildings have secure perimeters and require visitor searches, most hospitals have no such security measures. Hospital security is challenged by the appropriate desire to maintain ready access for patients, family members, and staff. To would-be perpetrators, these entryways may represent a tempting access point.

Today, rapid progress in the development and enrichment of our public health infrastructure is ongoing, but the system is not yet where it needs to be. Currently, no unified surveillance system is in place. The complexities of disease reporting and the lack of consistent feedback lead to physician frustration and poor compliance with current public health reporting mechanisms. Because our surveillance systems and response networks are underprepared, an even greater burden is placed upon the individual clinician to be alert to the possibility of biological warfare. Clinicians must be able to make an accurate diagnosis, to begin treatment of affected patients, and to notify and coordinate care with responsible public health authorities.

Simulation exercises and experience with disasters have taught us that communication during a crisis is often limited. Planning activities—such as mini-simulations (tabletop exercises) and disseminating contact information of key authorities—appear to significantly enhance local abilities to respond to true crises.

GENERAL CONSIDERATIONS FOR DIAGNOSIS AND TREATMENT

Because biological agents introduced by humans may cause disease syndromes nearly indistinguishable from

TABLE 73.1

HISTORICAL TIMELINE OF BIOTERRORISM

Year	Incident
190 BCE	Hannibal hurls venomous snakes onto enemy ships
400 BCE	Scythian archers use arrows dipped in blood and manure or decomposing bodies
1346	Mongols hurl plague-infected corpses over enemy walls
1405	Spanish contaminate wine drunk by French soldiers with blood of leprosy patients
1650	Polish soldiers place saliva from rabid dogs into hollow shell casings
1710	Russians invading Estonia hurl plague-infected corpses over enemy walls
1763	British officers give blankets used by smallpox victims to American Indians in Pennsylvania, resulting in a devastating smallpox outbreak
1860s	Confederate sympathizers during the American Civil War attempt to ship garments and bedding used by yellow fever victims to New York
1863	Confederate soldiers during the American Civil War leave dead animals in wells and ponds to contaminate Union soldiers' water supply
1972	Ratification of Biological and Toxin Weapons Convention outlawing offensive bioweapons
1992	Dr. Ken Alibek flees former USSR; debriefing indicates substantial bioweapons program
1984	Salad bars in 10 Oregon restaurants contaminated with *Salmonella*, sickening 750 people
2001	*Bacillus anthracis* attacks via the U.S. Postal System

naturally occurring illnesses, and because patients may not fall ill until days after exposure, bioterrorism may be difficult to distinguish from naturally occurring disease. Therefore, distinguishing the results of intentional release of a disease agent from a naturally occurring illness often requires the clinician to think "epidemiologically." Disease patterns with unusual organisms, large numbers of victims at the same stage of illness, unusual antibiotic resistances, or unusual seasonal presentations should all raise the question of bioterrorism (Table 73.2). For example, one case of rapidly progressive influenza-like illness may not herald a bioterrorist attack, but a pattern of several patients with the same syndrome should certainly raise the specter of bioterrorism. High risk biological agents have been identified and hospital-based physicians should be familiar enough with them to rapidly assess patients and begin treatment.

Biological attacks may either be overtly announced, or covert, with the first signs of attack being mildly symptomatic, minimally ill patients or hundreds of critically ill ones. In either case, early recognition of the disease outbreak and identification of the disease agent are critical to minimizing the number of casualties. Epidemiologic models have demonstrated that *rapid implementation of a post-attack prophylaxis program is the single most important means of reducing losses following a bioterrorist attack*. However, before prophylaxis can be initiated, the disease agent must be identified.

SPECIFIC BIOLOGICAL AGENTS

The Centers for Disease Control and Prevention (CDC) have issued a list of high-likelihood, potential bioterrorist agents. These have been prioritized according to ease of dissemination, transmissibility, mortality, potential for major public health impact, potential to cause public fear and social disruption, and requirement of special action for public health preparedness (Table 73.3) (2). Category A agents

TABLE 73.2

CHARACTERISTICS DISTINGUISHING A NATURAL DISEASE OUTBREAK FROM A BIOTERRORIST ATTACK

Natural outbreak	Bioterrorist attack
Gradual presentation of victims with no readily identifiable common exposure	Sudden presentation of large numbers of victims with a similar disease or syndrome (e.g., many cases of rapidly progressive pneumonia) who may have a readily identifiable common exposure
Cases present at varying stages of disease progression	Many cases present at similar stage in disease progression because of common source of exposure
Expected disease course for that specific pathogen with appropriate response to standard therapy	More severe disease than is usually expected for that specific pathogen or failure to respond to standard therapy
Slowly progressive disease with prodromal symptoms (e.g., natural progression of bubonic plague to pneumonic plague)	Rapidly progressive disease suggesting an unusual form of disease transmission (e.g., primary pneumonic plague with rapidly progressive fulminant pneumonia and no prodromal bubonic form of the disease)
Normal antibiotic sensitivities	Highly virulent strains possibly with antibiotic resistance
No announcement of attack	Possible announcement of bioterrorist attack
Presentation of common illnesses (such as influenza)	Presentation of a single case of any disease caused by CDC Category A, B, or C agent (Table 73.3)
Presentation of disease in the usual geographic area during the usual transmission season	Presentation of disease in an unusual geographic area or transmission season

TABLE 73.3
CRITICAL BIOLOGICAL AGENTS

Category A. High-priority agents include organisms that pose a risk to national security because they can be easily disseminated or transmitted person to person; cause high mortality with potential for major public health impact; might cause public panic and social disruption; and require special action for public health preparedness.

Variola major (smallpox)
Bacillus anthracis (anthrax)
Yersinia pestis (plague)
Clostridium botulinum toxin (botulism)
Francisella tularensis (tularemia)
Filoviruses
    Ebola virus (Ebola hemorrhagic fever)
    Marburg virus (Marburg hemorrhagic fever)
Arenaviruses
    Lassa fever virus (Lassa fever)
    Junin virus (Argentine hemorrhagic fever) and related viruses

Category B. Second-highest priority agents include those that are moderately easy to disseminate; cause moderate morbidity and low mortality; and require specific enhancements of CDC's diagnostic capacity and enhanced disease surveillance.

Coxiella burnetti (Q fever)
Brucella species (brucellosis)
Burkholderia mallei (glanders)
Alphaviruses
    VEE virus (Venezuelan encephalomyelitis)
    EEE and WEE viruses (eastern and western equine encephalo-
      myelitis)
    Ricin toxin from *Ricinus communis* (castor beans)
    Epsilon toxin of *Clostridium perfringens*
Staphylococcus enterotoxin B
A subset of List B agents includes pathogens that are foodborne or
    waterborne. These pathogens include but are not limited to:
    Salmonella species
    Shigella dysenteriae
    Escherichia coli O157:H7
    Vibrio cholerae
    Cryptosporidium parvum

Category C. Third-highest priority agents include emerging pathogens that could be engineered for mass dissemination in the future because of availability; ease of production and dissemination; and potential for high morbidity and mortality and major health impact.

Nipah virus
Hantaviruses
Tick-borne hemorrhagic fever viruses
Tick-borne encephalitis viruses
Yellow fever
Multidrug-resistant tuberculosis

are most likely to cause mass casualties if deliberately disseminated as small-particle aerosols and require broad-based public health preparedness. These agents, therefore, are a priority for preparation and training and will be discussed further here.

Because many of these diseases have been functionally eradicated and are very rare in the developed world, the medical literature often provides few data upon which to base clinical decisions. Consequently, public health experts have formed consensus-based guidelines to aid clinicians in making such decisions. Bioterrorism web sites at the CDC (www.bt.cdc.gov), the Agency for Healthcare Research and Quality (AHRQ) (www.bioterrorism-uab.ahrq.gov), and at various other institutions (for example, www.bioterrorism. uab.edu) are extremely useful as frequently updated sources of such information.

Anthrax

Clinical Presentation and Course

Classically, inhalational anthrax is a biphasic illness. After 0–6 days of incubation, the first phase appears as a nonspecific influenza-like illness characterized by mild fever, malaise, myalgias, nonproductive cough, and occasional chest or abdominal pain. Rhinorrhea and nasal congestion are uncommon with inhalational anthrax; the presence of these symptoms may indicate an etiology other than anthrax in patients presenting with influenza-like symptoms. The second phase of the illness appears 2–3 days later and is characterized by the abrupt onset of high fever, dyspnea, chest or abdominal pain, diaphoresis, cyanosis, and shock. Recent inhalational cases in the United States have manifested with sweats and gastrointestinal symptoms. Hemorrhagic meningitis and altered mental status are seen in up to 50% of cases as the disease spreads to the central nervous system. Death occurs within 24–36 hours (Table 73.4) (3).

TABLE 73.4
DISTINGUISHING INHALATIONAL ANTHRAX FROM INFLUENZA

Sign or symptom	Anthrax	Influenza or other influenza-like illness
Fever or chills	+++++	+++
Fatigue or malaise	+++++	+++++
Cough	++++	++++
Shortness of breath	++++	0
Chest discomfort or pleuritic chest pain	+++	+
Headache	++	++++
Myalgias	++	++++
Sore throat	0	++++
Rhinorrhea	0	++++
Nausea or vomiting	++++	+
Abdominal pain	+	+

Adapted from Centers for Disease Control and Prevention. Considerations for distinguishing influenza-like illness from inhalational anthrax. *Morb Mortal Wkly Rep* 2001;50:984–986.

Diagnostic Evaluation

Basic laboratory evaluation may show hemoconcentration or leukocytosis but is generally not helpful in making the diagnosis of anthrax. Gram stain and culture of fluid from cutaneous vesicles, blood, or cerebrospinal fluid will often show Gram-positive bacilli.

Rapid influenza tests may be useful in differentiating influenza from other influenza-like illnesses, including anthrax. However, the sensitivity of rapid influenza tests is relatively low (45%–90%). When the rapid influenza test is not positive, viral culture may be helpful in identifying true cases of influenza.

In asymptomatic patients with suspected exposure to inhalational anthrax, public health authorities have used nasal swab culture as an epidemiologic screening tool to confirm exposure to *B. anthracis*. The predictive value of this tool is not known, and, at present, the CDC does not recommend routine use of swab culture to rule out infection with *B. anthracis*.

Chest radiography in patients with inhalational anthrax often exhibits mediastinal widening and occasionally infiltrates or pleural effusion. In contrast, most cases of influenza are not associated with chest radiographic abnormalities. Computed tomography of the chest should be strongly considered in any patient with an influenza-like illness who presents with chest radiographic abnormalities. Computed tomography of the chest in cases of inhalational anthrax was first reported during the outbreak in October 2001. Findings included prominent mediastinal lymphadenopathy, pleural effusion, mediastinal edema, and basilar air space disease (4).

Prophylaxis and Treatment

In any suspected case of inhalational anthrax or in cases of cutaneous anthrax with signs of systemic involvement, extensive edema, or head and neck lesions, intravenous multidrug antimicrobial therapy should be started immediately. Based on animal and *in vitro* studies, the recommended agents include ciprofloxacin 400 mg every 12 hours or doxycycline 100 mg every 12 hours *plus* one of the following drugs: rifampin, vancomycin, penicillin, ampicillin, chloramphenicol, imipenem, clindamycin, or clarithromycin. For uncomplicated cases of cutaneous anthrax that do not involve the head or neck, oral ciprofloxacin 500 mg every 12 hours or doxycycline 100 mg every 12 hours alone are sufficient therapy. Because the major complications of systemic anthrax are caused by toxins released from the bacteria, it has been suggested that corticosteroid therapy could be of some benefit in treating cases of inhalational anthrax, but there are no controlled trials to inform this decision (5).

Prophylactic therapy for patients with confirmed exposure to *B. anthracis* must be promptly initiated. Again, oral ciprofloxacin (500 mg every 12 hours) or doxycyline (100 mg every 12 hours) is sufficient prophylactic therapy. Children or breastfeeding mothers may take amoxicillin at the appropriate dosage for prophylaxis only, but confirmed cases should be treated with ciprofloxacin or doxycycline, despite their known adverse effects in children (6). In any suspected or confirmed exposure to anthrax, public health authorities should be notified and involved in case management in order to assist with epidemiologic investigation. Currently, there is no vaccine for *B. anthracis* available to the public.

Infection Control

Anthrax is not transmissible through person-to-person contact. Universal precautions are generally sufficient to protect contacts from exposure to the disease. Decontamination with a soap and water bath is sufficient for gross exposures.

Smallpox

Clinical Presentation and Course

Infection occurs through direct contact with mucous membranes or through aerosol exposure. After an incubation period of 12–14 days, variola viremia causes a prodromal illness characterized by high fever, malaise, vomiting, headache, and myalgias, followed 2–3 days later by a characteristic macular rash of the face, hands, and forearms. As the rash spreads, the macules change to papules and eventually to pustular vesicles. Lesions are most prominent about the extremities and face and tend to develop synchronously, a characteristic that helps discriminate variola from varicella infection. Within 7–10 days, the rash begins to form scabs, leaving depressed pigmented scars when they heal. Scabs contain readily recoverable virus throughout the entire healing period; therefore, all patients should be considered infectious until all scabs are shed.

Diagnostic Evaluation

There is no widely available laboratory test to confirm smallpox infection. Thus, clinical presentation is the key to early diagnosis. The presence of a centrifugal, synchronous rash in the appropriate clinical setting must lead to consideration of the diagnosis of smallpox. If a case of smallpox is suspected, the patient must be placed in isolation until appropriate assessment is completed by public health authorities. Pustular fluid should be sampled only by persons recently vaccinated against smallpox. Samples should be handled by a Biosafety Level 4 (BSL-4) laboratory.

Prophylaxis and Treatment

Although animal trials with cidofovir are promising, there is currently no antiviral treatment for smallpox. In the United States, routine smallpox vaccination ceased in 1972.

Those vaccinated prior to 1972 retain partial immunity to the virus. Currently, vaccination of military personnel and civilian volunteers is ongoing. An emergency supply of smallpox vaccine and a limited supply of vaccina immune globulin (VIG) are under the control of the CDC and state health departments (7). Efforts are underway to increase the national stockpile of smallpox vaccine as well as to develop safer and more effective cell culture–derived vaccines.

Infection Control

Smallpox victims must be immediately isolated. All household and face-to-face contacts should be vaccinated and placed under surveillance. Because smallpox is rapidly spread via aerosol transmission, it poses a particular threat in hospitals, which have a limited number of negative pressure isolation facilities. Given the serious nature of this disease, home care and quarantine is a likely and reasonable alternative to inpatient hospital treatment.

Plague

Clinical Presentation and Course

Yersinia pestis, a Gram-negative coccobacillus, is the causative agent of plague. Microscopically, the bacteria have a characteristic bipolar appearance that is commonly referred to as "safety pin" pattern. When a human is infected by the bite of an infected flea, symptoms of bubonic plague develop 2–8 days later. These include sudden onset of influenza-like symptoms and the development of acutely swollen, painful lymphadenopathy, typically in the groin, axilla, or cervical regions. Septicemic plague is characterized by disseminated intravascular coagulation, necrosis of small blood vessels, purpuric skin lesions, and gangrene of acral regions such as the digits and nose.

Pneumonic plague can develop secondarily from bubonic or septicemic plague or can develop primarily when aerosolized bacilli are inhaled. After a 2–4 day incubation period, the first symptoms are fever, hemoptysis, and dyspnea. Other symptoms include nausea, vomiting, abdominal pain, and diarrhea. As the disease progresses, a fulminant pneumonia develops, with lobar consolidation, respiratory failure, sepsis, and death. Primary pneumonic plague, which results from aerosolized release of *Y. pestis*, typically does not cause the cutaneous lesions that are seen with the naturally occurring form of the disease.

Diagnostic Evaluation

Gram stain and culture of blood, cerebrospinal fluid, sputum, or lymph node aspirate may reveal the organism. Giemsa staining reveals bipolar "safety pin"-appearing bacilli. Cultures demonstrate growth within 24–48 hours.

Definitive laboratory diagnosis of *Y. pestis* can be made via antigen detection, immunoassay, immunostaining, or polymerase chain reaction performed at the CDC and other government-operated laboratories.

Prophylaxis and Treatment

Currently, no vaccine is available for plague. In the past, antibiotic therapy with streptomycin 15 mg/kg intramuscularly twice a day for 10 days was considered first-line therapy for pneumonic plague. Small numbers of human cases and animal data suggest that intravenous gentamicin or doxycycline are also effective treatments. Quinolones may also be efficacious, but no human data exist for this class of drugs. Laboratory and animal studies indicate that doxycycline or fluoroquinolone antibiotics given orally for seven days are adequate prophylaxis for those potentially exposed to plague (8).

Infection Control

Because plague is readily transmissible via aerosolized particles, strict isolation for the first 48 hours of treatment is required to prevent secondary spread of the disease. Patients with the pneumonic form of the disease must remain in isolation for four days after initiation of antibiotic therapy.

Botulism

Clinical Presentation and Course

Botulinum toxin blocks acetylcholine release, and ultimately neurotransmission, by binding to the presynaptic nerve terminal at the neuromuscular junction and at cholinergic autonomic sites. Within 24 hours and up to several days after inhalational exposure, symptoms develop, beginning with bulbar palsies characterized by dysarthria, dysphagia, blurred vision, and ptosis. With progression of disease, skeletal muscle is affected, manifested by descending, symmetrical, flaccid paralysis that may culminate in respiratory failure.

Diagnostic Evaluation

Physical examination reveals an afebrile, alert, and oriented patient. Bulbar palsies and flaccid paralysis are present while sensation remains intact. Laboratory tests are not generally useful in the early diagnosis of botulism intoxication. Definitive toxin testing is available through the Centers for Disease Control.

Prophylaxis and Treatment

Respiratory failure is the most common cause of death due to botulinum toxin (9). Therefore, supportive care with mechanical ventilation is the most important treatment for botulism intoxication. Because recovery may take weeks or months, this may require intensive nursing care for a prolonged period of time. A limited supply of antitoxin is available through government agencies. Recombinant vaccines are currently being developed.

Infection Control

Botulism is not transmissible from person to person; therefore, no special isolation procedures are required for affected patients.

Viral Hemorrhagic Fevers (VHFs)

Clinical Presentation and Course

Infection with VHF is characterized by high fever, headache, fatigue, myalgias, abdominal pain, and malaise following a 2–21 day incubation period. The VHFs are a group of disorders caused by filoviruses (Marburg, Ebola), arenaviruses (Lassa fever), and other related viruses. As the diseases progress, increased vascular permeability underlies many of the clinical findings. These findings include gastrointestinal bleeding, generalized mucous membrane hemorrhage, petechial or ecchymotic rash, conjunctival injection, nondependent edema, and hypotension. These diseases may progress rapidly to shock and death (10).

Diagnostic Evaluation

Routine laboratory testing may indicate leukopenia, thrombocytopenia, elevated hepatic aminotransferases, and prolonged prothrombin time (PT) and activated partial thromboplastin time (aPTT). No widely available rapid testing is available for the viruses responsible for VHFs. Definitive serologic diagnostic testing is available through government laboratories. Because of the highly contagious nature of these diseases, great care should be taken in handling all body fluid specimens.

Prophylaxis and Treatment

There is no widely available vaccine for VHFs. In limited studies, ribavirin administered intravenously has been effective in treating some cases of Lassa fever and Argentine hemorrhagic fever. Postexposure prophylaxis with orally administered ribavirin also seems to be effective. Otherwise, treatment is supportive and includes administration of crystalloids, blood products, and pressors as indicated.

Infection Control

Contact and droplet precautions, including the use of HEPA filter masks, should be employed when caring for patients with VHFs, particularly in cases with respiratory involvement. In patients with prominent cough, vomiting, diarrhea, or hemorrhage, a negative pressure room is recommended to prevent aerosol transmission of the disease. Decontamination of infected materials with household bleach is adequate (10).

ISSUES AT THE TIME OF ADMISSION OR PRESENTATION

Perhaps the most difficult problem at the time of initial hospitalization is how to best utilize limited resources. The use of an emergency management organizational plan, such as the Hospital Emergency Incident Command System (HEICS), is critical in a mass casualty situation. HEICS utilizes a standardized organizational chart with predefined job roles and task checklists, which are widely adopted by other responding agencies. Job titles with specific roles and color-coded vests or armbands help delineate individual functionality to other staff members. Systems such as this can be tailored to the specific organization or situation and are critical in management of limited resources during crises.

Another critical issue at the time of initial contact is determining whether patients need to be hospitalized. Patients mildly affected by a highly contagious disease agent for which only supportive care is available may be better served with home isolation and quarantine rather than hospitalization. Patients who are hemodynamically unstable or require aggressive supportive care should be admitted to intensive care units, preferably with contained air-handling or negative pressure capabilities when an aerosolizable pathogen may be involved. Patients who are concerned that they may have been exposed and have no findings of disease should receive appropriate prophylaxis and be followed on an outpatient basis.

During a bioterrorism incident, people seeking medical evaluation can be expected to overwhelm hospitals. Significant numbers may be suffering from anxiety and stress-induced physical symptoms that may mimic the effects of exposure. Thus, hospital staff dealing with a bioterrorism incident will be challenged by the need to triage patients who show signs of having been infected by an agent and others whose symptoms are psychogenic in origin. Coupling appropriate triage protocols with the availability of psychological support staff is vital. When dealing with patients who have mild symptoms, an observation area may help facilitate recovery of the "worried well" and identification of those who are truly ill. Hospital organizations should have an alternative site identified and equipped (e.g., ambulatory clinics, physical therapy area), with personnel trained in assisting the ED, for when large numbers of casualties arrive or are expected.

ISSUES DURING THE COURSE OF HOSPITALIZATION

Dealing with a bioterrorism or large-scale infectious disease outbreak can also be expected to subject hospital personnel to high levels of sustained physical and psychological stress. Staff members will be working long hours under additional stressors and will be exposed to infectious agents. Under these circumstances, health care workers can be expected to fall ill, as occurred in the SARS outbreak of 2003 (11). In addition to fatigue, health care workers will have to cope with additional personal protective equipment, prophylactic medications, and concerns for their own health and that of their family members. With this in mind, some health care workers may choose not to come to work, further diminishing the capacity of the health care system. Appropriate education and planning efforts may increase the confidence of staff and physicians in maintaining personal safety while carrying out their professional roles.

In addition to potential staffing issues, hospitals must address equipment and supply issues. For most hospitals, even small numbers of additional patients requiring isolation or mechanical ventilation could prove to be overwhelming. Personal protective gear, medications, disinfectant supplies, and other disposable equipment may be consumed rapidly. While bioterrorism "push packs" of medications and other supplies are readily available from the Strategic National Stockpile managed by the CDC, it is important that hospitals make efforts to assess their needs for additional supplies and equipment from other resources in order to maintain the appropriate readiness for mass casualties. For urban hospitals, interactions with the Metropolitan Medical Response System and their local or state Emergency Management Association provide a source of community-based supplies for disasters.

Early communication with government and public health authorities at the local, regional, state, and national level is vital. Because of the importance of establishing causality and isolating perpetrators, hospital personnel must work with public health and public safety to preserve and maintain a chain of evidence. A hospital-based command center will help coordinate the appropriate dissemination of public information with local authorities, medical staff, hospital administration, and the public information officer. This coordination enables public health authorities to assist with triage, supplies, and diagnosis, while enabling law enforcement to assist with crowd control and quarantine or isolation.

ISSUES AT THE TIME OF HOSPITAL DISCHARGE

As with any patient who recovers from a grave illness, follow-up is vitally important, not only to ensure the patient's well-being, but also for public health surveillance. Any patient who survives a bioterrorist attack should be closely monitored after discharge for signs of disease recurrence or long-term sequelae from the disease or its treatment. In addition, patients may suffer psychological consequences, including anxiety, paranoia, and posttraumatic stress disorder. Appropriate counseling should be provided.

KEY POINTS

- Recent concerns over bioterrorism have exposed our underpreparedness for both bioterror attacks and large-scale casualties from naturally occurring emerging infections.
- A clear communication plan must be coupled with vigorous planning and simulations to adequately prepare hospitals for bioterrorism attacks.
- The rapid implementation of a post-attack prophylaxis program is the most important strategy to limit losses following a bioterrorism attack.
- Evidence-based guidelines for managing emerging infections (including those potentially spread by bioterror) are maintained by federal agencies such as the Centers for Disease Control and the Agency for Healthcare Research and Quality.
- At the time of a large bioterror attack, hospitals must be prepared to triage, communicate (within their walls and with appropriate authorities), and deal with the psychological issues of patients, the "worried well," and providers.

REFERENCES

1. Inglesby TV, Grossman R, O'Toole T. A plague on your city: observations from TOPOFF. *Biodefense Quarterly* 2000;2:1–10.
2. Centers for Disease Control and Prevention. Biological and chemical terrorism: strategic plan for preparedness and response. *Morb Mortal Wkly Rep* 2000;49(RR-4):4–7.
3. Centers for Disease Control and Prevention. Notice to readers: considerations for distinguishing influenza-like illness from inhalational anthrax. *Morb Mortal Wkly Rep* 2001;50:984–986.
4. Jernigan JA, Stephens DS, Ashford DA, et al. Bioterrorism-related inhalational anthrax: the first 10 cases reported in the United States. *Emerg Inf Dis* 2001;7:933–944.
5. Centers for Disease Control and Prevention. Update: investigation of bioterrorism-related anthrax and interim guidelines for exposure management and antimicrobial therapy. *Morb Mortal Wkly Rep* 2001;50:909–919.
6. Centers for Disease Control and Prevention. Update: interim recommendations for antimicrobial prophylaxis for children and breastfeeding mothers and treatment of children with anthrax. *Morb Mortal Wkly Rep* 2001;50:1014–1016.
7. Guharoy R, Panzik R, Noviasky JA, Krenzelok EP, Blair DC. Smallpox: clinical features, prevention and management. *Ann Pharmacother* 2004;38:440–447.
8. Whitby M, Ruff TA, Street AC, Fenner FJ. Biological agents as weapons 2: anthrax and plague. *Med J Aust* 2002;176:605–608.
9. Josko D. Botulin toxin: a weapon in terrorism. *Clin lab Sci* 2004;17:30–34.
10. Peters CJ, LeDuc JW: Ebola: the virus and the disease. *J Infect Dis* 1999;179(suppl 1):ix–xvi.
11. Lee N, Hui D, Wu A, et al. A major outbreak of severe acute respiratory syndrome in Hong Kong. *NEJM* 2003;348:1986–1994.

ADDITIONAL READING

Alibek K, Handelman S. *Biohazard*. New York: Dell Publishing, 1999.

Becker SM. Meeting the threat of weapons of mass destruction terrorism: toward a broader conception of consequence management. *Military Medicine* 2001;166,S2:13–1613.

Bravata DM, McDonald KM, Smith WM, et al. Systematic review: surveillance systems for early detection of bioterrorism-related diseases. *Ann Intern Med* 2004;140:910–922.

Treat KN, Williams JM, Furbee PM, Manley WG, Russell FK, Stamper CD Jr. Hospital preparedness for weapons of mass destruction incidents: an initial assessment. *Ann Emerg Med* 2001;38: 562–565.

Wang JT, Chang SC. Severe acute respiratory syndrome. *Curr Opin Infect Dis* 2004;17:143–148.

Zajtchuk R, Bellamy RF, eds. *Medical Aspects of Chemical and Biological Warfare*. Bethesda: Office of the Surgeon General, Department of the Army, USA, 1997.

HIV Disease

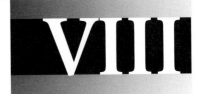

Signs, Symptoms, and Laboratory Abnormalities in HIV Disease

74

Harry Hollander

TOPICS COVERED IN CHAPTER

■ Fever 723
■ Lymphadenopathy 724
■ Rash 724
■ Hepatosplenomegaly 725
■ Abnormal Liver Enzymes 725
■ Elevated Creatinine 726
■ Anemia 726

INTRODUCTION

The global pandemic of HIV infection continues 25 years after the recognition of the first cases of AIDS in North America. In the United States, an increasing number of cases are attributed to sexual transmission between heterosexuals or injection drug use. In urban settings, minority populations are disproportionately affected. The incidence of HIV infection has increased in rural regions and parts of the country, such as the southeastern states, that had formerly been spared, and women now account for more than 25% of Americans living with HIV infection.

Before the era of prophylaxis and treatment of opportunistic infections, the course of HIV disease was often biphasic. Years of indolent immunologic decline and rela-tive paucity of symptoms were followed by rapidly progressive immunodeficiency, complicated by malignancies and multiple bouts of infection, which often proved fatal. The risk for certain infections rises markedly as the number of CD4 lymphocytes (normal >500/μL) declines below key levels (Table 74.1).

The use of prophylactic antibiotic therapy appropriate for the stage of disease led to significant declines in the incidence of *Pneumocystis jirovecii* pneumonia (formerly *P. carinii*, though still abbreviated "PCP") and *Mycobacterium avium* complex (MAC) infection, but patients continued to be hospitalized and die of other complications of advanced immunodeficiency, such as dementia, wasting, and high-grade non-Hodgkin's lymphoma.

The development of zidovudine (AZT) and other nucleoside reverse transcriptase inhibitors marked the beginning of the era of *antiretroviral therapy*. Administration of this first generation of drugs, alone or in combination with other drugs, resulted in modest prolongation of life but did not prevent progression of the underlying immunodeficiency. The face of antiretroviral therapy changed markedly in the mid-1990s. A better understanding of the pathogenesis of HIV disease and the introduction of two more classes of agents (*non-nucleoside reverse transcriptase inhibitors* and *HIV protease inhibitors*) allowed the design of combination

TABLE 74.1

RISK FOR OPPORTUNISTIC INFECTIONS BY CD4 STRATUM

CD4 cell count (per cubic millimeter)	Infections
200–500	Bacterial pneumonia, herpesvirus infection, mucosal candidiasis, oral hairy leukoplakia, tuberculosis
50–200	*Pneumocystis jirovecii* pneumonia (PCP), cryptococcal meningitis, toxoplasmosis
<50	Cytomegalovirus (CMV), *Mycobacterium avium* complex (MAC), progressive multifocal leukoencephalopathy

regimens that resulted in more potent suppression of viral replication. The paradigm shift was catalyzed by the recognition that active viral replication in blood, lymphoid tissue, and other compartments is continuous from the time of initial HIV infection and accounts for the progressive loss of immune function during the presymptomatic phase of illness. Furthermore, sensitive tests were developed that measured serum HIV RNA levels, and these measurements were found to be the *single best predictors of disease progression and death* in patients who had not received antiretroviral therapy (1). For example, persons with a baseline value of 5,000 copies per milliliter have a cumulative risk for disease progression of 30% if followed off therapy for nine years; this risk is 75% if the count is 50,000 copies per milliliter. When antiretroviral therapy is used, it is always given as a combination of at least three drugs at full dosage, with the goal of reducing viral load to below detectable limits and thereby minimizing the chance of development of drug-resistant mutations. When patients on antiretroviral combinations are hospitalized, every effort should be made to continue the drugs. Should dose interruption become necessary, the entire regimen should be stopped rather than risking the development of drug resistance by administering a partial, suboptimally effective combination. Because several of these agents induce or inhibit one of the cytochrome P-450 enzymes, drug interactions may occur with many classes of agents used in the hospital, including antiarrhythmics, sedative/hypnotics, anticonvulsants, and calcium channel blockers. Some of the most important interactions are shown in Table 74.2 (2).

Many patients who have tolerated and adhered to regimens of *highly active antiretroviral therapy* (HAART) have had extraordinarily gratifying responses, achieving clinical stability and partial immunologic reconstitution reflected by increases in the CD4 lymphocyte count. This has accounted for a marked decrease in hospitalization and mortality rates for HIV-related complications among patients receiving this therapy (3). However, the enthusiasm for HAART has been somewhat tempered by the recognition of long-term toxic-

ity of these regimens, including mitochondrial toxicity leading to lactic acidosis, and metabolic pertubations including glucose intolerance and hyperlipidemia. The latter two problems have raised concerns that patients receiving this therapy might be at increased risk for premature atherosclerosis. Finally, physicians must recognize that successful antiretroviral therapy may alter the natural history of opportunistic complications of HIV infection. *The immune reconstitution syndrome* may be observed within several months of initiation of HAART and is manifested as paradoxical worsening of undiagnosed or partially treated infections such as CMV or tuberculosis (4).

TABLE 74.2

DRUG INTERACTIONS WITH HIV PROTEASE INHIBITORS

Drug levels raised to toxic range by indinavir, nelfinavir, and ritonavir: do not coadminister

Amiodarone	Midazolam
Astemizole	Quinidine
Ergot alkaloids	Triazolam

Drug levels raised to toxic range by ritonavir: do not coadminister

Alprazolam	Flecainide
Bupropion	Flurazepam
Clonazipine	Meperidine
Clorazepate	Piroxicam
Diazepam	Propafenone
Encainide	Zolpidine

Drug levels raised 1.5-fold to 3-fold by ritonavir: coadminister with caution and close monitoring

Amlodipine	Nifedipine
Carbamazepine	Nimodipine
Dexamethasone	Ondansetron
Diltiazem	Pravastatin
Dronabinol	Prednisone
Erythromycin	Quinine
Fentanyl	Sertraline
Felodipine	Tamoxifen
Lidocaine	Trazodone
Lovastatin	Verapamil
Nicardipine	Warfarin

Drugs that affect concentration of HIV protease inhibitors

Carbamazepine	Decreases nelfinavir levels; avoid coadministration.
Ketoconazole	Increases indinavir, nelfinavir levels; reduce dose of protease inhibitor.
Phenobarbital	Decreases nelfinavir levels; avoid coadministration.
Phenytoin	Decreases nelfinavir levels; avoid coadministration.
Rifampin	Decreases indinavir levels; avoid coadministration.

Patients admitted to the hospital with complications of HIV infection discussed below and in the chapters that follow may have previously been unaware of their HIV infection, had little or no access to ongoing medical care, or been unable to cope with the significant toxicity and adherence demands of combination antiretroviral therapy. In contrast, patients who have benefited from aggressive therapy and monitoring are living longer and becoming increasingly likely to be hospitalized for unrelated medical problems (3).

SYMPTOMS, SIGNS, AND LABORATORY ABNORMALITIES

Fever

When Presenting at the Time of Admission

Fever, either alone or in combination with other findings, is a common symptom and sign in HIV-infected adults. Because fever is ubiquitous during the course of HIV infection and the differential diagnosis is broad, the evaluation should take into consideration acuity versus chronicity, risk for opportunistic infection given disease status (see above and Table 74.1), and the presence or absence of other localizing findings or laboratory abnormalities.

The initial consideration in a patient who presents with acute or subacute onset of fever is *bacterial infection*, which occurs at increased frequency during all stages of HIV disease. Common sources include the lower respiratory tract and sinuses. Endocarditis should be considered in persons actively injecting drugs (Chapter 71), and catheter-associated infections should be suspected in patients with indwelling catheters (Chapter 72). The presence of diarrhea raises the question of enteric pathogens, and headache and altered mental status make it imperative to exclude bacterial meningitis. The history and examination should focus on attempting to define possible sources of bacterial infection. Laboratory evaluation follows the prototypical approach to fever (Chapter 62), with acquisition of blood and other cultures as clinically indicated. Note that the sensitivity of cultures in patients on antimicrobial agents for opportunistic infection prophylaxis may be decreased. Because pneumonia secondary to unusual pathogens such as *Nocardia* and *Pseudomonas aeruginosa* can develop in HIV-infected adults, sputum culture may be more useful in these patients than in immunocompetent patients with community-acquired pneumonia (Chapter 65).

Once the evaluation is complete, patients with known sources are treated accordingly with antimicrobials. Although there are no data about immediate treatment versus observation for those without a clear source, the treatment threshold for hospitalized patients in general should be low, particularly because the incidence of bacteremia with invasive infection caused by certain organisms

(e.g., pneumococci) is high. HIV-infected patients with fever and neutropenia secondary to cytotoxic chemotherapy should always receive empiric antibiotics, and those with neutropenia secondary to other medications, such as AZT or ganciclovir, may also be at increased risk for bacterial infection.

When fever at the time of presentation is more chronic in nature, the prior probability of bacterial infection (with the notable exception of sinusitis) decreases, and opportunistic infections and other complications become more likely. Importantly, clinical series studying unexplained fevers in HIV-positive patients suggest that an etiology can be found approximately 90% of the time (5); the corollary to this is that a "diagnosis" of "fever due to HIV" should be regarded with suspicion. The most common diagnoses in HIV-infected patients presenting with chronic fever are occult *PCP* and *disseminated MAC*. Various clinical and laboratory findings may suggest other diagnoses (Table 74.3).

A cost-effective diagnostic evaluation will consider epidemiologic information in addition to the clinical data already discussed. For example, the probability of *Bartonella* infection rises in the patient who owns kittens, as does the probability of histoplasmosis in the patient from the midwestern United States. Judicious use of the microbiology laboratory in advanced disease, especially to detect serum cryptococcal antigen and MAC in blood cultures, is appropriate, but extensive and repeated culturing adds little to the diagnostic yield in most cases. Similarly, no data support the routine use of imaging studies such as computed tomography of the central nervous system or abdomen if localizing signs or symptoms are absent. More invasive testing is guided by initial diagnostic results.

Specific therapy is initiated if a treatable diagnosis is established. If no explanation for fever is obtained during the hospitalization, observation (with or without the administration of antipyretics) is reasonable for stable patients. Empiric antimicrobial trials may be considered when suspicion for a given underlying opportunistic infection is

TABLE 74.3
CHRONIC FEVER IN HIV-INFECTED PERSONS

Symptom/finding	Associated diagnoses
Skin lesions	Herpes virus, *Bartonella*, *Mycobacterium haemophilum*, drug fever
Lymphadenopathy	Mycobacteria, lymphoma
Hepatosplenomegaly	Mycobacteria, *Bartonella*, histoplasmosis, lymphoma
Abdominal pain	*Mycobacterium avium* complex, cytomegalovirus, lymphoma
Visual complaints	Cytomegalovirus
Headache/neurologic findings	Cryptococcal meningitis, toxoplasmosis
New hematologic abnormalities	Mycobacteria, histoplasmosis, lymphoma

reasonably high. For example, a trial of agents effective against MAC may be justified in a patient with chronic fever, anemia, and a CD4 cell count below 50/μL whose evaluation is otherwise unrevealing and whose MAC blood culture results are pending (Chapter 67).

When Presenting During the Hospitalization

When fever supervenes during the course of hospitalization, nosocomial bacterial infections are the greatest concern, and the evaluation and therapeutic approach should proceed as in other patient populations (Chapter 62). Because HIV-infected persons are also predisposed to allergy to multiple classes of drugs (especially antibiotics), this is the other important consideration in the differential diagnosis. As is the case with other forms of drug fever, patients may have isolated fever or fever with additional findings, such as rash, hematologic cytopenias, and liver enzyme abnormalities. A typical time course is the development of fever 7–10 days after initiation of therapy (e.g., trimethoprim-sulfamethoxazole for PCP). Given this differential diagnosis, costly evaluation for new opportunistic processes is not initially indicated when fever occurs as a new issue during hospitalization.

Lymphadenopathy

The significance of and approach to lympadenopathy in an HIV-positive person are guided by the pattern of nodal enlargement and stage of HIV disease. Persistent isolated or asymmetric lymphadenopathy should always be assumed to represent a secondary infectious or neoplastic process. The most frequent pathogens are *Mycobacterium tuberculosis* and MAC, although fungal infections and bartonellosis may also present with localized lymphadenopathy. Necrotizing adenitis caused by MAC is a common manifestation of immune reconstitution in individuals started on HAART when CD4 cell counts are below 50/μL. Kaposi's sarcoma (KS), lymphoma, and other lymphoproliferative lesions, such as Castleman's disease, are the most likely neoplasms. The diagnostic utility of noninvasive tests is limited; lymph node sampling must be performed for diagnosis. Cytologic examination and microbiologic staining and culture of a fine-needle aspirate may be sufficient to establish the diagnosis, but this procedure should be followed by excisional lymph node biopsy if it is nondiagnostic.

Generalized lymphadenopathy presents a different set of considerations. Syphilis can manifest this way and is always important to exclude, as many HIV-infected adults are at risk for exposure to other sexually transmitted diseases. Some patients with early HIV disease and preserved immune function have persistent generalized adenopathy, which reflects active HIV replication in lymphoid tissue. Lymph node sampling will reveal only reactive lymphoid hyperplasia in these cases; thus, generalized adenopathy does not require further evaluation in an asymptomatic person with a preserved CD4 cell count and a normal complete blood cell count. Interestingly, adenopathy usually wanes as immunodeficiency progresses. Therefore, the presence of new or progressive generalized adenopathy in a patient with advanced immunodeficiency should prompt lymph node sampling to investigate the diagnoses mentioned above.

Rash

A wide array of inflammatory, allergic, infectious, and neoplastic skin lesions can develop in HIV-infected persons, and a full discussion of these is beyond the scope of this chapter. The constellation of fever and rash in general is discussed in Chapter 62. This section reviews several cutaneous eruptions that may be particularly important in the hospitalized HIV-infected patient.

Raised red or purple lesions may represent KS or bacillary angiomatosis caused by *Bartonella* species. Although some morphologic features may be more suggestive of one lesion than another, punch biopsy with silver staining for organisms is often necessary for definitive diagnosis. Recognition of cutaneous KS may provide important clues in patients with unexplained pulmonary or gastrointestinal complaints or lymphadenopathy. Similarly, cutaneous bacillary angiomatosis, which must be treated in its own right, may also be an important indicator of systemic disease with bacteremia, in addition to skeletal, hepatic, and lymphatic involvement.

A diffuse maculopapular exanthem most often represents a drug reaction to antimicrobial agents, antiretroviral drugs, anticonvulsants, or other classes of drugs. Patients with this finding should be carefully examined for desquamation and involvement of conjunctiva and oral mucosa that indicate Stevens-Johnson syndrome. A small number of HIV-infected patients with recurrent staphylococcal toxic shock syndrome have also been described, so it is important to search for other clinical and laboratory criteria (Chapter 25) for this diagnosis in patients who present with a generalized exanthem.

Vesicles are most commonly indicative of *herpes simplex* or *herpes zoster*, but they may also be seen with other opportunistic infections. If lesions do not clearly follow a dermatomal pattern, establishment of the specific viral agent may affect dose and duration of antiviral therapy (herpes zoster requires higher dosing than does herpes simplex). Currently, this is most rapidly accomplished by scraping the base of a fresh vesicle and swabbing a slide, which is then air-dried and stained for viral antigen.

Finally, a petechial or purpuric rash in an afebrile patient may imply significant thrombocytopenia that is a consequence of either HIV-related immune-mediated platelet destruction, drug toxicity, or thrombotic microangiopathy. This finding warrants checking platelet count, performing coagulation studies, and examining the peripheral blood smear for findings of microangiopathy.

Hepatosplenomegaly

Enlargement of the liver, spleen, or both may be caused by HIV-related processes or by unrelated comorbidities. Patients who have acquired HIV through sexual exposure are clearly at higher risk for hepatitis B and probably also have a slightly elevated risk for hepatitis C infection. Needle-sharing injection drug users are at risk for both hepatitis B and hepatitis C. Alcoholic liver disease is common in HIV-infected adults, as alcohol abuse is a frequent comorbidity. In general, these hepatic diseases are more likely than HIV-specific processes to lead to complications of portal hypertension and liver failure. In immunodeficient persons with HIV infection, hepatitis C can have a more aggressive course because viral replication and hepatic injury occur more rapidly.

The infections and malignancies that secondarily involve the liver and spleen generally do so during the course of widespread systemic involvement. Thus, symptoms such as weight loss and fever are common. Common infiltrative infections include mycobacterial disease, fungal disease (particularly histoplasmosis and cryptococcosis), and bartonellosis, which leads to a distinctive picture of *hepatosplenic peliosis*. In Africa and the Mediterranean region, visceral leishmaniasis is an important diagnostic consideration. Lymphoma and metastatic malignancy account for the majority of neoplastic hepatic lesions, whereas KS may involve the spleen and extrahepatic bile ducts but rarely involves the liver. Nonspecific laboratory findings (e.g., anemia, elevated alkaline phosphatase) are commonly seen with all these diagnoses, but their predictive value is poor. Marked pancytopenia may be more suggestive of histoplasmosis or leishmaniasis, whereas marked elevation of lactate dehydrogenase is characteristic (but not diagnostic) of high-grade lymphoma. Microbiologic studies of blood in the evaluation of hepatosplenomegaly often obviate the need for liver biopsy. Appropriate studies include fungal and mycobacterial blood cultures and determination of the serum cryptococcal antigen titer. If the patient has resided in an area endemic for histoplasmosis, a urine antigen test should also be ordered.

Liver biopsy should be performed only if these less invasive studies are unrevealing.

Abnormal Liver Enzymes

Elevated hepatic aminotransferases should first and foremost prompt the usual considerations of underlying viral hepatitis or alcoholic liver disease in an HIV-infected patient (Chapter 82). Of the opportunistic infections, only cytomegalovirus (CMV) infection causes prominent hepatocellular injury, and mild aminotransferases rises are commonly noted during active CMV infection of other organs. When newly elevated aminotransferases are observed in HIV-infected persons, drug-related hepatotoxicity should also be considered. Common offenders include ritonavir, nevirapine, antituberculous agents (isoniazid, rifampin, pyrazinamide), trimethoprim-sulfamethoxazole, fluconazole, and didanosine (DDI). Flares of underlying hepatitis B or C may occur with immune reconstitution. When possible, potentially hepatotoxic drugs should be discontinued and other agents substituted to assess the potential contribution to abnormal enzymes. The HIV protease inhibitor indinavir commonly causes isolated hyperbilirubinemia without aminotransferase elevation; this finding should not provoke dose interruption.

Rises in hepatobiliary alkaline phosphatase are common in patients with advanced HIV disease. Abdominal imaging should be performed to differentiate between obstructive and nonobstructive etiologies (Chapter 84). Because gallstone disease is less likely in this setting than in the general population, computed tomography is preferred over ultrasonography as the initial imaging study because of the anatomic detail of the liver and surrounding structures it provides. When variable intrahepatic and extrahepatic biliary obstruction is demonstrated and no mass lesion is seen, the most likely diagnosis is *AIDS cholangiopathy*, a fibrosing process sometimes seen in association with CMV, *Cryptosporidium*, or microsporidial infection of the biliary tree. Diffuse abdominal or right upper quadrant pain is common with this syndrome, and rarely bacterial cholangitis may supervene. Endoscopic retrograde cholangiopancreatography may be considered because sphincterotomy provides symptomatic benefit to about half those patients with pain. However, the symptoms commonly recur. Antimicrobial therapy of associated opportunistic infections has not resulted in any improvement in the progressive course of AIDS cholangiopathy.

If biliary obstruction is excluded by right upper quadrant imaging, the differential diagnosis in the presence of elevated alkaline phosphatase shifts to cholestatic and infiltrative disorders. Medications especially likely to cause cholestasis are trimethoprim-sulfamethoxazole, antituberculous drugs, and phenothiazines. Occasionally, hepatic involvement with CMV disease manifests with a cholestatic pattern. All the infiltrative opportunistic infections and neoplasms listed above in the differential diagnosis of hepatomegaly may be accompanied by a rise in alkaline phosphatase. Computed tomography may show homogeneous enlargement of the liver, multiple inflammatory lesions, or a smaller number of space-occupying lesions; the presence of large mass lesions points toward lymphoma, but the ability of imaging studies to distinguish between this neoplasm and infections is limited. As was previously discussed for the evaluation of hepatomegaly, the yield of liver aspiration and biopsy is low for treatable diagnoses, and so these procedures are reserved for situations in which less invasive tests and biopsy of tissue from other sites fail to establish a diagnosis. In patients with advanced disease, MAC infection is statistically the most likely explanation for multiple liver lesions and alkaline phosphatase elevation.

Elevated Creatinine

The approach to azotemia in a person with underlying HIV infection must be broadly based because *a significant proportion of cases of renal failure are a consequence not of HIV-specific renal pathology but rather of a variety of problems common to all hospitalized patients* (Chapter 100). Thus, hypovolemia, hypotension, sepsis, and the nephrotoxicity of drugs such as aminoglycosides and nonsteroidal anti-inflammmatory agents all may play important roles.

With this caveat, several HIV-related renal problems do deserve consideration in the setting of increasing creatinine levels (6). Several of the antimicrobial agents used to treat opportunistic infections may cause renal failure. Trimethoprim-sulfamethoxazole can lead to an acute interstitial nephritis; the urine sediment often shows leukocytes with or without cellular casts. This drug may also cause isolated hyperkalemia via inhibition of potassium tubular secretion, but it is unusual for this to be a dose-limiting toxicity. Another sulfa drug, sulfadiazine, may cause obstructive renal failure through deposition in the distal tubules because of its poor solubility. Thus, if patients are being treated with high doses of sulfadiazine for toxoplasmosis, vigorous hydration is necessary to prevent this complication. Pentamidine, which is used for the treatment of PCP, may also cause tubular injury that leads to hyperkalemia or acute renal failure. Tenofovir, a nucleotide antiviral drug, may rarely cause proximal tubular dysfunction and hypokalemia. The HIV protease inhibitor indinavir may crystallize in urine and cause clinically apparent nephrolithiasis in 15% of patients taking this drug; cases of acute and chronic renal failure from interstitial nephritis are also reported.

The incidence of thrombotic thrombocytopenic purpura is also increased in HIV-seropositive patients; it can be triggered by intercurrent infection. In this case, other clinical findings, such as fever and altered mental status, accompany the renal failure. Laboratory abnormalities include thrombocytopenia and marked elevation of lactate dehydrogenase in addition to azotemia and microscopic hematuria. Obstructive uropathy should always be considered in patients with known lymphoma because of the possibility of retroperitoneal involvement. Finally, *HIV nephropathy* refers to several different histologic abnormalities that may lead to acute renal failure or, more commonly, progressive renal dysfunction and end-stage renal disease. Focal sclerosing glomerulonephritis is the most common pathologic pattern and tends to present with nephrotic-range proteinuria before the onset of renal failure. Patients who present with the nephrotic syndrome may be candidates for renal biopsy to exclude other potentially treatable glomerular lesions. Aggressive antiretroviral therapy may prevent or attenuate the course of HIV nephropathy.

Anemia

Mild anemia with hematocrits in the range of 30%–35% is common as a result of both HIV disease and

its treatment, and in general it does not warrant extensive evaluation. Patients with advanced HIV infection often have a component of anemia of chronic disease with inappropriately low reticulocyte counts. Another common contributor to chronic anemia is AZT therapy, which leads to macrocytosis and anemia. Mean corpuscular volume may reach 130 fL as a result of AZT administration alone, without signifying one of the common causes of megaloblastic anemia. However, the presence of megaloblastic changes in polymorphonuclear leukocytes does warrant the exclusion of vitamin B_{12} or folate deficiency. More than 50% of patients with the nonspecific anemia of HIV infection or AZT-associated anemia have low circulating levels of endogenous erythropoietin; if so, they will usually respond to recombinant erythropoietin therapy. The mean dose required for response in these patients is 25,000 units per week, administered subcutaneously in three divided doses. In general, this therapy is reserved for patients who have symptoms related to moderate or severe anemia. Responders show a trend toward normalization of the hematocrit within two to four weeks of the start of therapy.

Patients who may require more detailed evaluation of anemia include those with more severe anemia (hematocrit less than 25%–27%), rapid onset of anemia (which is atypical of the etiologies mentioned above), or coexistent abnormalities of other blood cell lines. The diagnosis of hemolysis or blood loss may be obscured by the inability of chronically ill patients to mount an appropriate reticulocytosis. Acute blood loss should always be considered in the hospitalized patient with a hematocrit drop. *Gastrointestinal bleeding is more likely to result from one of its usual etiologies than from HIV-related complications of the gastrointestinal tract* (Chapter 78). HIV-specific lesions that may rarely present with frank gastrointestinal bleeding include lymphoma, KS, and CMV colitis.

Although many patients have a positive microscopic direct antiglobulin (Coombs') test result as a consequence of the hyperglobulinemia caused by HIV, clinically important autoimmune hemolytic anemia is very uncommon. Hemolytic processes that deserve consideration include thrombotic thrombocytopenic purpura (see "Elevated Creatinine") and unrecognized glucose 6-phosphate dehydrogenase deficiency in African-American or Mediterranean patients receiving drugs such as dapsone or trimethoprim-sulfamethoxazole.

Severe anemia resulting from bone marrow failure can be an isolated hematologic abnormality or can be accompanied by other depressed cell lines. Although any of the infiltrative disorders that involve marrow can cause anemia alone, the development of a hypoproliferative normochromic, normocytic anemia makes several diagnoses more likely. An uncommon pattern of antiretroviral hematologic toxicity is AZT-induced pure red cell aplasia. Patients who experience this toxicity typically have profound suppression of hematopoiesis and a dramatic fall of the hematocrit within weeks of beginning AZT therapy. The time course and absence of macrocytosis differentiate this response from the more common hematologic effects of this drug mentioned above. Hematopoiesis generally recovers when AZT is discontinued. Red cell aplasia can also occur as a result of parvovirus B19 infection. In contrast to immunocompetent children, in whom fever, rash, or arthritis often develop during this infection, HIV-infected adults most frequently have bone marrow suppression as the predominant or sole clinical manifestation of parvovirus infection. Rapid diagnosis can be established by examining the serum for viral genome with a polymerase chain reaction assay, a highly sensitive test in this setting because of the intensity and duration of viremia in these immunocompromised hosts. If parvovirus B19 is diagnosed, the therapy of choice is infusion of pooled immunoglobulin, which contains adequate neutralizing antibody to clear the infection and thereby resolve the red cell aplasia. In patients with advanced disease and CD4 cell counts of less than 50/μL, the most common etiology of isolated severe hypoproliferative anemia is disseminated MAC infection. As is the case when MAC infection presents in the liver, other symptoms and signs of widespread infection are often present. The diagnosis is usually established by blood cultures with use of appropriate media.

When multiple cell line abnormalities are present, other marrow infiltrative processes deserve consideration. Because splenic infiltration also occurs with these diseases, the etiology of cytopenias may be multifactorial, with hypersplenism playing a role. Non-Hodgkin's lymphoma, tuberculosis, and cryptococcosis can all present with prominent hematologic abnormalities, and other signs and laboratory findings that accompany these diseases should be elicited. An important diagnostic point is that *only one-third of HIV-related lymphomas present with lymphadenopathy;* thus, the absence of this finding does not exclude the diagnosis. Pancytopenia is particularly common in HIV-infected patients with disseminated histoplasmosis. This endemic opportunistic infection may have protean manifestations, including acute or chronic fever, systemic inflammatory response syndrome, interstitial pulmonary infiltrates, acute renal failure, and disseminated intravascular coagulation. A urine polysaccharide antigen assay has a sensitivity of 97% in cases of extrapulmonary histoplasmosis in HIV-positive patients; false-positive results have been reported only with other invasive fungal infections, such as coccidioidomycosis and blastomycosis (7).

Nonspecific bone marrow abnormalities are common in HIV-infected patients, but the likelihood of finding previously undiagnosed treatable lesions via bone marrow sampling is very low. All the etiologies of anemia discussed above can be diagnosed by alternative means. Before the availability of urine antigen testing, bone marrow aspiration and biopsy were useful for the diagnosis of histoplasmosis, but the antigen test has obviated the need for marrow sampling to establish this diagnosis. Studies reviewing the evaluation of HIV-infected patients for fever of unknown etiology generally confirm the poor diagnostic utility of this test (8). Thus, bone marrow sampling should rarely be used in this population, except as a staging procedure for systemic lymphoma.

KEY POINTS

- The prognosis of HIV infection has improved with effective antiretroviral therapy.
- Disease stage is an important determinant of whether acute medical problems are HIV-related or incidental (i.e., the more advanced the disease, the more likely a complication is to be HIV-related).
- In the hospital, antiretroviral drugs should be continued when possible, but beware of drug interactions.
- Fever should be evaluated based on the company that it keeps (disease stage, signs, symptoms, and laboratory abnormalities).
- In the hospitalized patient, new fever more likely represents nosocomial infection or drug reaction than a new opportunistic infection.
- Several rash morphologies provide important diagnostic clues for systemic disease.
- Hepatosplenomegaly and hematologic abnormalities often signify disseminated infection or neoplasm, but biopsy of liver or marrow is rarely helpful diagnostically.
- Acute renal failure is more likely to be secondary to factors that are not HIV-specific than to be attributable to HIV nephropathy.

REFERENCES

1. Mellors JW, Munoz A, Giorgi JV, et al. Plasma viral load and CD4+ lymphocytes as prognostic markers of HIV-1 infection. *Ann Intern Med* 1997;126:946–954.
2. Drugs for HIV infection. *Med Lett Drugs Ther* 1997;39:111–116.
3. Cohen MH, French AL, Benning L, et al. Causes of death among women with human immunodeficiency virus infection in the era of combination antiretroviral therapy. *Am J Med* 2002;113: 91–98.
4. Sempowski GD, Haynes BF. Immune reconstitution in patients with HIV infection. *Ann Rev Med* 2002;53:269–284.
5. Sepkowitz KA, Telzak EE, Carrow M, Armstrong D. Fever among outpatients with advanced human immunodeficiency virus infection. *Arch Intern Med* 1993;153:1909–1912.
6. Herman ES, Klotman PE. HIV-associated nephropathy: epidemiology, pathogenesis, and treatment. *Semin Nephrol* 2003;23: 200–208.
7. Wheat J. Histoplasmosis: recognition and treatment. *Clin Infect Dis* 1994;19 (Suppl 1):S19–S27.
8. Volk EE, Miller ML, Kirkley BA, Washington JA. The diagnostic usefulness of bone marrow cultures in patients with fever of unknown origin. *Am J Clin Pathol* 1998;110:150–153.

75

Pulmonary Manifestations of HIV Infection

Laurence Huang   *Philip C. Hopewell*

INTRODUCTION

Pulmonary disease is a common reason for hospital admission among persons with HIV infection. The spectrum of pulmonary disease is broad and includes HIV-associated as well as non–HIV-associated disorders. As a result, the diagnostic approach to respiratory symptoms in an HIV-infected person can be challenging. However, knowledge of the spectrum of pulmonary disease and of the characteristic presentations of the most common diseases often enables the differential diagnosis to be narrowed. This chapter offers an overview of the spectrum of pulmonary disease in HIV-infected persons and describes a diagnostic approach to the patient with respiratory symptoms. A detailed discussion of *Pneumocystis jirovecii* pneumonia (formerly known as P. carinii, though still abbreviated "PCP") and community-acquired bacterial pneumonia, the two most common pneumonias seen in this population, is presented. Pulmonary tuberculosis in HIV-infected patients is discussed in Chapter 67.

SPECTRUM OF PULMONARY DISEASE

The spectrum of pulmonary disease in persons with HIV infection is broad, and illness can range in severity from self-limited (e.g., upper respiratory tract infection) to life threatening (e.g., PCP). The relative frequencies of the diseases depend on a number of factors. Overall, the most common cause of respiratory complaints among HIV-infected patients presenting to an outpatient facility is upper respiratory tract infections or acute bronchitis. However, PCP or bacterial pneumonia are more likely causes of severe illness that requires hospital admission. Table 75.1 summarizes common infectious and noninfectious causes of pulmonary complications in hospitalized patients.

DIAGNOSTIC APPROACH

The clinical presentations of HIV-associated pulmonary diseases vary and overlap. Thus, no symptom, sign, or combination of findings is diagnostic of a particular disease. The goals of the history and physical examination are to establish a basic differential diagnosis and to assess the need for and the approach to further evaluation. The history should also provide a subjective assessment of the severity of the disorder.

The cardinal respiratory symptoms in persons with HIV infection are the same as in those without HIV infection (1). The occurrence of specific respiratory symptoms, especially cough, should be taken seriously and evaluated appropriately. On the other hand, it is extremely unusual for patients with HIV infection to have asymptomatic respiratory disease; thus, screening for the presence of a respiratory process in a patient without symptoms is rarely indicated (2).

The approach to the medical history should be the same as in a person without HIV infection, but there should be an

TABLE 75.1

SPECTRUM OF PULMONARY DISEASE IN SEVERELY ILL HIV-INFECTED PATIENTS

Infections (most frequently identified organisms)

Bacteria
  Streptococcus pneumoniae
  Haemophilus influenzae
  Staphylococcus aureus
  Gram-negative bacilli (*Pseudomonas aeruginosa*, *Klebsiella pneumoniae*)

Mycobacteria
  Mycobacterium tuberculosis
  Mycobacterium avium complex
  Mycobacterium kansasii

Fungi
  Pneumocystis jirovecii (formerly *P. carinii*)
  Cryptococcus neoformans
  Histoplasma capsulatum
  Coccidioides immitis
  Aspergillus species

Virus
  Cytomegalovirus (CMV)

Parasite
  Toxoplasma gondii

Neoplasms
  Kaposi's sarcoma (KS)
  Non-Hodgkin's lymphoma (NHL)
  Bronchogenic carcinoma

Other Respiratory Diseases
  Lymphocytic interstitial pneumonitis (LIP)
  Nonspecific interstitial pneumonitis (NIP)
  Airways disease (asthma, emphysema, bronchitis, bronchiectasis)
  Primary pulmonary hypertension
  Illicit drug-induced lung disease

emphasis on identification of possible exposures to infectious diseases. The history should seek to identify any possible exposure to persons with or suspected of having tuberculosis, or to environmental fungi, such as *Coccidioides immitis* or *Histoplasma capsulatum*. Any history of prior respiratory diseases, such as asthma, should be sought. A focused review of the past medical history can provide important clues to the etiology of the current respiratory symptoms. For example, bacterial pneumonia and tuberculosis are more common among HIV-infected patients who are injection drug users. Bronchitis and bacterial pneumonia are more common in HIV-infected cigarette smokers than in nonsmokers or former smokers. Moreover, patients with a long history of cigarette use may have chronic obstructive lung disease as the etiology of their respiratory symptoms, rather than an HIV-associated opportunistic infection or neoplasm (3). Traveling to or living in a region where the endemic fungi are found are strong determinants of the risk for infection and subsequent disease caused by these organisms. In addition, tuberculosis is more common in certain geographic areas and populations (4).

A number of the HIV-related opportunistic infections frequently recur. PCP is an example. PCP prophylaxis decreases the recurrence rate of PCP, but breakthroughs can occur, especially at low CD4 cell counts. Similarly, patients who have had cryptococcosis, coccidioidomycosis, or histoplasmosis are at high risk for relapse. Fluconazole (cryptococcosis, coccidioidomycosis) and itraconazole (histoplasmosis) decrease the relapse rate, but prophylaxis does not preclude their occurrence. In many institutions, the two major diagnostic considerations for respiratory complaints in hospitalized HIV-infected patients are PCP and bacterial pneumonia. Thus, distinguishing between the two pneumonias is often the focus of the diagnostic approach (Table 75.2). PCP characteristically presents with a dry, nonproductive cough accompanied by fever and dyspnea. Symptoms are usually subacute. In contrast, pneumonia caused by *Streptococcus pneumoniae* or *Haemophilus influenzae* characteristically presents with acute symptoms of fever, shaking chills, dyspnea, pleuritic chest pain, and a cough productive of purulent sputum. The presence of purulent sputum is a strong negative predictor for PCP; its presence in a patient who has documented PCP nearly always indicates a concurrent bacterial infection.

The physical examination should emphasize the lungs and potential extrapulmonary sites of involvement. At least 50% of patients with PCP will have an unremarkable lung examination, and many patients with bacterial pneumonia will have focal lung findings (Table 75.2). Extrapulmonary findings may provide important clues to the risk for and nature of the pulmonary disorder. For example, the finding of oral candidiasis is indicative of severe immunocompromise and, therefore, of the risk of opportunistic disorders. An altered mental status in a patient whose CD4 cell count is $200/\mu L$ or less may suggest *Cryptococcus neoformans* as the cause of both the neurologic and pulmonary problems. Cutaneous lesions may suggest disseminated fungal disease, whereas lymphadenopathy or organomegaly may suggest either disseminated mycobacterial or fungal disease, or non-Hodgkin's lymphoma (5). Pulmonary involvement can develop in patients with mucocutaneous Kaposi's sarcoma (KS); however, the absence of mucocutaneous involvement does not preclude the possibility of significant pulmonary KS.

Although no laboratory abnormality is specific for a particular pulmonary disease, tests that can be useful include the complete blood cell count and measurement of the serum lactate dehydrogenase (LDH) and arterial blood gases. HIV-infected patients with neutropenia are at higher risk for bacterial and *Aspergillus* species infections. The white blood cell count is frequently elevated relative to the baseline value in persons with bacterial pneumonia. In contrast, the white blood cell count varies in persons with PCP (Table 75.2). The serum LDH is frequently elevated in persons with PCP; the sensitivity of an elevated serum LDH for PCP is in the range of 83%–100%. However, the serum LDH is relatively non-specific and it may be elevated in

TABLE 75.2

**CLINICAL PRESENTATION OF PNEUMOCYSTIS PNEUMONIA AND
BACTERIAL PNEUMONIA**

	Pneumocystis	Bacteria
CD4 cell count	200/μL	Any
Symptoms	Fever	Fever, chills, or rigors
	Dyspnea	Dyspnea
	Nonproductive cough	Pleuritic chest pain
		Productive cough
		Purulent sputum
Symptom duration	Typically 2–4 wk	Typically 3–5 d
Signs	Unremarkable lung examination	Focal findings on lung examination
Laboratory tests	WBC count varies	WBC count frequently elevated (relatively)
	LDH frequently elevated	LDH varies
	ABG nonspecific[a]	ABG nonspecific
Chest radiograph		
Distribution	Diffuse > focal	Patchy, focal > multifocal > diffuse
Location	Bilateral	Unilateral, segmental/lobar
Pattern	Reticular–granular	Consolidation
Associated findings		
Cysts	15%–20%	Rarely
Pleural effusions	Very rarely	25%–30%
Adenopathy	Very rarely	Very rarely
Pneumothorax	Occasionally	Rarely
Normal radiograph	Occasionally	Never
Chest computed tomography[b]		
Distribution	Patchy	Focal
Location	Bilateral	Unilateral, segmental/lobar
Pattern	Ground glass	Consolidation
Associated findings		
Cysts	Frequent	Rarely
Normal tomograph	Never	Never

[a] Used to determine severity of disease and whether adjunctive corticosteroids are indicated.
[b] If chest radiograph unremarkable.
ABG, arterial blood gas; *LDH*, lactate dehydrogenase; *WBC*, white blood cell.

many pulmonary and nonpulmonary conditions. The arterial blood gas values are also nonspecific. However, in persons with PCP, an arterial blood gas determination is essential in determining the severity of disease and the need for adjunctive corticosteroid therapy.

The CD4 cell count is an essential piece of laboratory data and many patients who have a previous diagnosis of HIV infection will know their CD4 count. It is an excellent indicator of the risk for development of specific conditions (Chapter 74) (6). Some pulmonary complications, such as bacterial pneumonia, tuberculosis, and non-Hodgkin's lymphoma, may occur at any CD4 cell count. However, the incidence of these diseases increases as the CD4 cell count declines. When it is 200/μL or less, bacterial pneumonia is often recurrent and *Mycobacterium tuberculosis* infection is often disseminated. In addition, PCP and pneumonia caused by fungal pathogens (*C. neoformans)* become signif-

icant considerations. When the CD4 cell count is 100/μL or less, *Pseudomonas aeruginosa* infection and pulmonary involvement with KS are increasingly common. Finally, diseases caused by endemic fungi (*H. capsulatum, C. immitis*), cytomegalovirus, nontuberculous mycobacteria, and *Aspergillus* species almost always occur at the lowest CD4 cell count ranges (below 50/μL).

The radiographic manifestations of HIV-associated pulmonary diseases also vary and overlap. To complicate matters, multiple diseases can present concurrently. Nevertheless, each disease has a characteristic radiographic presentation that, combined with clinical data, can suggest a diagnosis. Classically, PCP presents with diffuse bilateral reticular or granular opacities (Figure 75.1). Thin-walled cysts or pneumatoceles are seen in approximately 15%–20% of patients with PCP. Pneumatoceles may predispose patients to the development of pneumothorax,

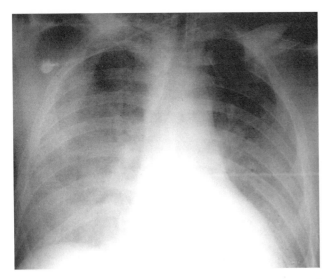

Figure 75.1 Pneumocystis pneumonia. Chest radiograph of an HIV-infected patient demonstrating diffuse bilateral granular opacities.

another radiographic finding suggestive of PCP. Less typical patterns include focal opacities, miliary infiltrates, nodules, and cavities. Intrathoracic adenopathy and pleural effusions are very rarely associated with PCP. In a patient with confirmed PCP, these radiographic findings usually represent a concurrent process. In mild cases of PCP, the chest radiograph may be normal. Patients with suspected PCP and a normal radiograph require additional evaluation (Figure 75.2).

Bacterial pneumonia caused by *S. pneumoniae* characteristically presents with patchy or focal consolidation in a segmental or lobar distribution, similar to what is seen in an immunocompetent person. An associated pleural effusion is seen in approximately 25%–30% of patients with bacterial pneumonia. In severe cases of pneumonia, the abnormalities may be diffuse. Bacterial pneumonia caused by *H. influenzae* may present with diffuse opacities similar to those of PCP, although it may also present with patchy or focal consolidation. The presentation of tuberculosis depends on the relative degree of immunosuppression (Chapter 67).

ISSUES AT THE TIME OF ADMISSION

Pneumocystis pneumonia and community-acquired bacterial pneumonia are the two most common pulmonary diseases leading to hospital admission of HIV-infected patients. Many of the issues arising at the time of admission, during the course of hospitalization, and after discharge are also relevant to other HIV-related pulmonary processes. This section addresses some of these issues in addition to specific concerns related to PCP and community-acquired pneumonia.

Clinical Presentation and Initial Evaluation

The characteristic clinical presentations of PCP and bacterial pneumonia have been described (Table 75.2). In a patient with respiratory symptoms and known or suspected HIV infection, an algorithm that utilizes the chest radiograph and the presence or absence of purulent sputum can often lead to an efficient diagnostic and treatment plan (Figure 75.2).

Indications for Hospitalization and Intensive Care

There are no specific admission criteria developed and validated for HIV-infected patients with pulmonary disease. The admission decision should therefore rely on an assessment of the severity of pulmonary disease, the patient's general health, and patient and clinician resources (Table 75.3). Outpatient management requires that patients have access to medical follow-up should their condition deteriorate or should side effects of the treatment develop. In settings where this is limited, it may be more prudent to hospitalize a patient than to attempt outpatient therapy.

Clear indications for ICU admission or transfer include respiratory failure requiring mechanical ventilation, hemodynamic instability or compromise requiring intravenous fluids and vasopressors, and altered mentation compromising the ability to protect adequately against aspiration. In settings without the resources to monitor patients closely outside the ICU (e.g., a "close observation" unit), patients who do not have these indications but who have severe respiratory impairment, rapidly progressive pulmonary disease, hypotension, or multiple organ system failure should also be considered candidates for ICU admission. In the setting of advanced HIV disease, patients may choose not to be intubated or receive certain other types of medical care. In these instances, intensive care may not be desired or warranted (Chapters 17 and 19).

Indications for Respiratory Isolation

Hospitalized HIV-infected patients with a clinical or radiographic presentation that is suggestive of tuberculosis or with known tuberculosis should be placed in respiratory isolation (7). If hospitalization continues to be necessary, isolation should be continued until tuberculosis is excluded or the patient has been on effective therapy for at least 2 weeks.

Numerous reports of clusters of PCP cases among different immunocompromised populations support the theories that PCP can result from person-to-person transmission and that *de novo* infection can occur in the setting of immunosuppression (8). However, the USPHS/IDSA guidelines for preventing opportunistic infections state that

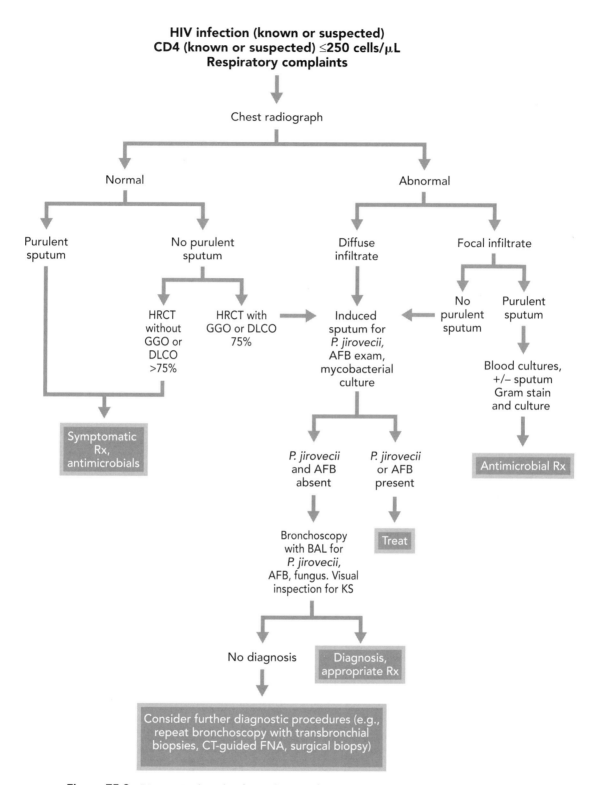

Figure 75.2 Diagnostic algorithm for evaluation of respiratory symptoms in an HIV-infected patient at risk for *Pneumocystis* pneumonia and bacterial pneumonia. *P. carinii* has recently been renamed *P. jirovecii*. *AFB*, acid-fast bacilli; *BAL*, bronchoalveolar lavage; *CT*, computed tomogram; *DLCO*, diffusing capacity for carbon monoxide; *FNA*, fine-needle aspirate; *GGO*, ground glass opacities; *HIV*, human immunodeficiency virus; *HRCT*, high-resolution computed tomogram; *KS*, Kaposi's sarcoma; *Rx*, treatment.

TABLE 75.3

INDICATIONS FOR HOSPITAL ADMISSION OF HIV-INFECTED PATIENTS WITH PULMONARY DISEASE

Pulmonary

Respiratory rate
  Elevated respiratory rate ≥30 breaths per minute
Arterial oxygenation
  Decreased PaO_2, elevated alveolar–arterial O_2 gradient requiring oxygen
Exercise tolerance and cardiopulmonary reserve
  Decreased exercise tolerance limiting ability to carry out daily activities
  Decreased cardiopulmonary reserve from underlying condition (e.g., COPD, CHF)
Chest radiograph
  Suspected tuberculosis and concern for transmission to other immunocompromised persons at place of residence
  Diffuse parenchymal disease and concern for progression
  Pneumothorax and concern for progression, need for observation/chest tube

General health

General appearance and vital signs
  Altered mental status
  Ill-appearing
  Temperature ≤35°C or ≥40°C
  Heart rate ≥125 beats/min
  Systolic blood pressure ≤90 mm Hg
Coexisting disease(s)[a]
  Neurologic
  Psychiatric
  Gastrointestinal
  Liver
  Renal
  Hematologic
Coexisting condition(s)[a]
  Illicit drug use
  Alcohol use

Patient resources

Homeless or unstable housing
No family or friends to assist patient with daily activities

Clinician resources

Inability to provide appropriate follow-up

[a] If compromises outpatient therapy and medication adherence.
CHF, congestive heart failure; *COPD,* chronic obstructive pulmonary disease.

"although certain authorities might recommend that HIV-infected persons who are at risk for PCP avoid sharing a hospital room with a patient who has PCP, data are insufficient to support this recommendation as standard practice" (6).

Empiric Therapy Versus Definitive Diagnosis

The diagnostic evaluation of an HIV-infected patient with suspected bacterial pneumonia may include sputum Gram stain and culture and should include two blood cultures. However, in the majority of patients with bacterial pneumonia, no etiological diagnosis will be made and empiric therapy will be necessary. Because *Pneumocystis* cannot be cultured, the diagnostic evaluation of a patient with suspected PCP involves microscopic examination of stained respiratory specimens obtained by sputum induction or bronchoscopy. These tests are sensitive (reported range of sensitivities for sputum induction, 55%–95%; for bronchoscopy, 89%–98%) and specific for the diagnosis. However, they may not always be available and, in the case of bronchoscopy, are invasive and require the presence of a bronchoscopist. For patients who present with "classic" PCP, an argument can be made for initiating empiric PCP therapy and reserving diagnostic procedures for the subset of patients who fail to respond to 5–7 days of therapy. An equally compelling argument can be made for establishing a diagnosis in all HIV-infected patients with pulmonary disease severe enough to require hospitalization so as to optimize therapy and follow-up. Should the promising results reporting the use of non-invasive specimens (e.g., oropharyngeal washing) combined with sensitive polymerase chain reaction (PCR)-based assays for the diagnosis of PCP be confirmed, then the diagnosis will be made non-invasively (without sputum induction or bronchoscopy) much more often (9).

Treatment Regimens

The considerations in choosing a specific treatment for community-acquired bacterial pneumonia in an HIV-infected patient should be similar to those in an immunocompetent host (Chapter 65) (10). In addition, coverage for *P. aeruginosa* and *Staphylococcus aureus* should be considered when the CD4 cell count is below 50/µL, there has been recent injection drug or antibiotic use, or there is cavitation seen on the chest radiograph.

The choices of specific treatment for PCP depend on the severity of disease, as determined by arterial blood gas measurement (Table 75.4). The regimens for mild disease are of comparable efficacy, and the decision about which regimen to use depends on the clinician's preference, in addition to consideration of potential adverse effects. Patients with moderate-to-severe PCP should be treated with trimethoprim-sulfamethoxazole (unless there is a history of a severe reaction) and adjunctive corticosteroids. *Corticosteroids* should be initiated at the time that PCP therapy is begun. In a patient with suspected PCP, the decision of whether or not to use corticosteroids must be based on the severity of disease (PaO_2 ≤70 mm Hg or alveolar-arterial O_2 gradient >35 mm Hg), not on the management approach chosen (e.g., definitive diagnosis versus empiric therapy). Empiric PCP therapy (including corticosteroids) may be initiated while the diagnostic evaluation is in progress. If the diagnosis of PCP is excluded, corticosteroids should be discontinued promptly. Patients with moderate-to-severe pulmonary disease who are

TABLE 75.4

PNEUMOCYSTIS PNEUMONIA TREATMENT REGIMENS FOR MILD AND MODERATE–SEVERE DISEASE[a]

PCP treatment regimen	Dose(s), route, frequency	Major side effects
Mild disease (PaO$_2$ >70 mm Hg AND alveolar–arterial O$_2$ gradient <35 mm Hg)		
TMP/SMX	15 mg/kg (TMP) PO daily (q6–8h)	Fever, dermatologic, gastrointestinal, hematologic
TMP + dapsone	15 mg/kg PO daily (q6–8h) + 100 mg PO once daily	Dermatologic, gastrointestinal, hematologic
Clindamycin + primaquine	1,800 mg PO daily (q6–8h) + 30 mg (base) PO once daily	Dermatologic, gastrointestinal, hematologic
Atovaquone	750 mg PO twice–thrice daily	Dermatologic, gastrointestinal
Moderate–severe disease[b] (PaO$_2$ ≤70 mm Hg OR alveolar–arterial O$_2$ gradient ≥35 mm Hg)		
TMP/SMX	15 mg/kg (TMP) IV daily (q6–8h)	See above
Pentamidine	3–4 mg/kg IV once daily	Renal, pancreatic
Clindamycin + primaquine	1,800 mg IV daily (q6–8h) + 30 mg (base) PO once daily	See above
Trimetrexate + leucovorin ± dapsone	45 mg/m^2 IV once daily + 20 mg/m^2 PO q6h ± 100 mg PO once daily	Hematologic, dermatologic, fever

[a] Recommended duration of therapy is 21 days.
[b] Adjunctive corticosteroids (prednisone 40 mg PO twice daily for 5 days, then 40 mg PO once daily for 5 days, then 20 mg PO once daily for 11 days; or IV equivalent of methylprednisolone) should also be administered.
TMP/SMX, trimethoprim-sulfamethoxazole.

treated with empiric PCP therapy and corticosteroids must be closely followed; in these patients, there should be a low threshold for pursuing a definitive diagnosis. Patients intolerant to trimethoprim-sulfamethoxazole may be started on one of the other regimens listed. No direct comparison of these regimens has been conducted. Whichever therapy is chosen, the recommended duration of therapy is 21 days.

ISSUES DURING THE COURSE OF HOSPITALIZATION

Time Course for Resolution

The time course for resolution of clinical symptoms and signs depends on the specific cause of pneumonia, severity of the pulmonary disease, and overall health of the patient. The typical time course for resolution of community-acquired bacterial pneumonia in an HIV-infected patient is similar to that in an immunocompetent person (Chapter 65). Usually, clear signs of clinical improvement should be evident within 2–5 days. The time course for resolution of PCP is generally longer. With successful therapy, fever, tachypnea, and oxygen requirements may persist or worsen for several days before improving. Thus, patients whose condition is neither improving nor significantly worsening may be treated for 7–10 days before a change in therapy is considered. However, if the patient's condition significantly

worsens, a number of considerations must be addressed promptly (Table 75.5). If the diagnosis is in doubt or if there is concern regarding a subsequent pulmonary disease, additional diagnostic evaluation is warranted. In these difficult cases, expert consultation is often helpful.

Initiation of Antiretroviral Therapy

Retrospective studies suggest that critically ill HIV-infected patients who receive antiretroviral therapy during their hospitalization have an improved survival compared to patients who do not receive this therapy (11). However, prospective studies are needed before firm recommendations can be made. In general, the potential benefits of antiretroviral therapy (e.g., rise in the CD4 cell count, decline in the HIV RNA level) must be balanced against the potential risks of these therapies (e.g., toxicity, drug interactions, immune reconstitution syndrome/paradoxical worsening) (12).

Prognosis of Patients with Respiratory Failure

The outcomes and mortality from PCP-associated respiratory failure have changed during the course of the AIDS epidemic. From 1981 to 1985, only 14% of patients with PCP who were admitted to an ICU survived to hospital discharge. This percentage improved to 40% between 1986

TABLE 75.5

CONSIDERATIONS IN A PATIENT FAILING TO IMPROVE AS EXPECTED

Problem	Main diagnoses	Diagnostic approach	Action(s)
Worsening dyspnea and/or hypoxemia[a]	Progressive pneumonia	Chest radiograph	Change treatment
	Pleural effusion/empyema	Chest radiograph	Thoracentesis (diagnostic and therapeutic)
	Superimposed pneumonia	Chest radiograph	Evaluate and add treatment for new process
	Pneumothorax	Chest radiograph	Consult specialist for chest tube placement
	Pulmonary embolism	Chest radiograph–if unchanged, then spiral chest CT or ventilation-perfusion scan	Evaluation for source and anticoagulation
Worsening cough	Progressive pneumonia	Chest radiograph	Change treatment
	Superimposed pneumonia	Chest radiograph	Evaluate and add treatment for new process
	Airways disease	Chest radiograph	Trial of nebulized bronchodilators
Persistent, new fever	Progressive pneumonia	Chest radiograph	Change treatment
	Pleural effusion/empyema	Chest radiograph	Thoracentesis (at least diagnostic)
	Superimposed pneumonia	Chest radiograph	Evaluate and add treatment for new process
	Drug fever	Chest radiograph	Switch treatment
New chest pain	Pneumothorax	Chest radiograph	Consult specialist for chest tube placement
	Pulmonary embolism	Chest radiograph–if unchanged, then spiral chest CT or ventilation-perfusion scan	Evaluation for source and anticoagulation
	Progressive pneumonia	Chest radiograph	Change treatment
	Superimposed pneumonia	Chest radiograph	Evaluate and add treatment for new process

[a] Also consider nonpulmonary etiologies (e.g., cardiac).
CT, computed tomography.

and 1988 but declined again to 24% from 1989 to 1991. The exact reasons for these changes are unclear. More recently, studies at multiple institutions have indicated that the survival of patients with PCP-associated respiratory failure may again be improving (13). Up-to-date outcomes data will be needed to help patients make decisions about life-sustaining treatments.

DISCHARGE ISSUES

Many drug toxicities first appear after 7–10 days of therapy. In patients who are discharged before this time, clinicians should describe the possible side effects to the patient and should ensure an adequate means of follow-up in the event that adverse effects do develop.

There are no published guidelines outlining when to discharge an HIV-infected patient with pneumonia. Each patient should be evaluated individually. In general, pulmonary disease should have improved to the point at which the patient can carry out daily activities (with supplemental oxygen if necessary), and other medical conditions should not pose significant risks to the completion of successful outpatient therapy. In certain instances, resources may permit the patient to complete a full course of intravenous therapy as an outpatient, either by returning to an outpatient infusion center or receiving home infusion

therapy supervised by a visiting nurse. Alternatively, some patients may complete their treatment course with oral medications, although the efficacy and timing of such a change have not been extensively studied.

PREVENTION OF PCP AND BACTERIAL PNEUMONIA

Patients with a CD4 cell count of 200/μL or less or a prior history of PCP should be given prophylaxis (6). The first-line prophylaxis regimen is trimethoprim-sulfamethoxazole (one double-strength tablet daily or thrice weekly, or one single-strength tablet daily). Alternative prophylaxis regimens include dapsone (100 mg daily), atovaquone (1,500 mg daily), and aerosolized pentamidine (300 mg via nebulizer monthly). Patients who are receiving trimethoprim-sulfamethoxazole for PCP prophylaxis may have a lower incidence of bacterial infections, although there may be an increased risk for development of drug-resistant bacteria. Patients with bacterial pneumonia are at risk for recurrent disease and patients who are cigarette smokers or injection drug users should be encouraged to quit. Ideally, the decision to quit will have been made during hospitalization, and appropriate referrals will have been made before discharge (14). In addition, pneumococcal vaccine is recommended if it has not been previously administered (6, 15).

COST CONSIDERATIONS AND RESOURCE USE

A number of cost–benefit analyses have examined the optimal approach to the management of patients with suspected PCP (empiric therapy vs. definitive diagnosis, sputum induction vs. bronchoscopy as the initial diagnostic procedure). There is no clear benefit of one approach over another. The choice of approach depends on a number of factors, including the availability of diagnostic procedures and their diagnostic sensitivity, the prevalence of PCP in a particular setting, and the prevalence of other pulmonary diseases that might also be diagnosed by one of the procedures.

KEY POINTS

- When evaluating an HIV patient with lung disease, recognize that the spectrum of illness is broad and includes both HIV-associated and non–HIV-associated conditions.
- Respiratory complaints are frequent in HIV-infected persons and increase in frequency as the CD4 cell count declines.
- The CD4 cell count is an essential piece of information. Each of the HIV-related pulmonary diseases usually develops at or below a characteristic range of CD4 cell counts.
- In many institutions, the most frequent pulmonary diseases seen are PCP and bacterial pneumonia. A careful history, physical examination, and review of the chest radiograph are often sufficient to differentiate between these two pneumonias.
- Specific guidelines for hospitalization and discharge of HIV-infected patients with pneumonia have not been developed and validated. In general, practical medical judgment is essential.

REFERENCES

1. Diaz PT, Wewers MD, Pacht E, Drake J, Nagaraja HN, Clanton TL. Respiratory symptoms among HIV-seropositive individuals. *Chest* 2003;123:1977–1982.
2. Gold JA, Rom WN, Harkin TJ. Significance of abnormal chest radiograph findings in patients with HIV-1 infection without respiratory symptoms. *Chest* 2002;121:1472–1477.
3. Diaz PT, King MA, Pacht ER, et al. Increased susceptibility to pulmonary emphysema among HIV-seropositive smokers. *Ann Intern Med* 2000;132:369–372.
4. Jasmer RM, Nahid P, Hopewell PC. Clinical practice. Latent tuberculosis infection. *N Engl J Med* 2002;347:1860–1866.
5. Ong A, Creasman J, Hopewell PC, et al. A molecular epidemiological assessment of extrapulmonary tuberculosis in San Francisco. *Clin Infect Dis* 2004;38:25–31.
6. Kaplan JE, Masur H, Holmes KK. Guidelines for preventing opportunistic infections among HIV-infected persons—2002. Recommendations of the U.S. Public Health Service and the Infectious Diseases Society of America. *MMWR Recomm Rep* 2002;51:1–52.
7. Blumberg HM, Burman WJ, Chaisson RE, et al. American Thoracic Society/Centers for Disease Control and Prevention/Infectious Diseases Society of America: treatment of tuberculosis. *Am J Respir Crit Care Med* 2003;167:603–662.
8. Kovacs JA, Gill VJ, Meshnick S, Masur H. New insights into transmission, diagnosis, and drug treatment of *Pneumocystis carinii* pneumonia. *JAMA* 2001;286:2450–2460.
9. Larsen HH, Huang L, Kovacs JA, et al. A prospective, blinded study of quantitative touch-down polymerase chain reaction using oral-wash samples for diagnosis of Pneumocystis pneumonia in HIV-infected patients. *J Infect Dis* 2004;189:1679–1683.
10. Niederman MS, Mandell LA, Anzueto A, et al. Guidelines for the management of adults with community-acquired pneumonia. Diagnosis, assessment of severity, antimicrobial therapy, and prevention. *Am J Respir Crit Care Med* 2001;163:1730–1754.
11. Morris A, Creasman J, Turner J, Luce JM, Wachter RM, Huang L. Intensive care of human immunodeficiency virus-infected patients during the era of highly active antiretroviral therapy. *Am J Respir Crit Care Med* 2002;166:262–267.
12. DeSimone JA, Pomerantz RJ, Babinchak TJ. Inflammatory reactions in HIV-1-infected persons after initiation of highly active antiretroviral therapy. *Ann Intern Med* 2000;133:447–454.
13. Morris A, Wachter RM, Luce J, Turner J, Huang L. Improved survival with highly active antiretroviral therapy in HIV-infected patients with severe *Pneumocystis carinii* pneumonia. *AIDS* 2003;17:73–80.
14. Niaura R, Shadel WG, Morrow K, Tashima K, Flanigan T, Abrams DB. Human immunodeficiency virus infection, AIDS, and smoking cessation: the time is now. *Clin Infect Dis* 2000;31:808–812.
15. Dworkin MS, Ward JW, Hanson DL, Jones JL, Kaplan JE. Pneumococcal disease among human immunodeficiency virus-infected persons: incidence, risk factors, and impact of vaccination. *Clin Infect Dis* 2001;32:794–800.

ADDITIONAL READING

HIV/AIDS Surveillance Report. Available at: http://www.cdc.gov/hiv/dhap.htm. Accessed March 8, 2005.
AIDS Epidemic Update: 2004. Available at: http://www.unaids.org/wad2004/report.html. Accessed March 8, 2005.
Guidelines for the Use of Antiretroviral Agents in HIV-1-Infected Adults and Adolescents. Available at: http://AIDSinfo.nih.gov. Accessed March 8, 2005.
Piscitelli SC, Gallicano KD. Interactions among drugs for HIV and opportunistic infections. *N Engl J Med* 2001;344:984–996.
Thomas CF, Limper AH. Pneumocystis pneumonia. *N Engl J Med* 2004;350:2487–2498.

Neurologic Complications of HIV Disease

76

Christina M. Marra

INTRODUCTION

Prior to the advent of potent antiretroviral therapy, central nervous system (CNS) complications of HIV infection were seen in about 40% of infected patients in the developed world. Neurological complications of HIV are now less common but still occur. A working knowledge of the clinical manifestations, diagnosis, and therapy of these disorders is important for any physician who cares for HIV-infected persons. Although a bewildering array of possibilities is included in the differential diagnosis, *HIV-associated dementia, cryptococcal meningitis, toxoplasmosis, and progressive multifocal leukoencephalopathy (PML)* are the most common CNS complications. These typically occur in the setting of advanced immunosuppression, when the peripheral blood CD4 cell count is less than 200/μL. Patients with acute meningitis, including cryptococcal meningitis, and with acute CNS mass lesions, including those due to toxoplasmosis, may be ill enough to warrant hospital admission. Alternatively, HIV-associated dementia and PML are generally subacute progressive illnesses that can be diagnosed and managed on an outpatient basis. This chapter uses a generic algorithm (Figure 76.1) to outline the approach to meningitis, CNS mass lesions, and other causes of acute change in mental status in HIV-infected patients. A differential diagnosis is provided for each problem, with a focus on the most common entities that require hospital care.

MENINGITIS IN THE HIV-INFECTED PATIENT

Issues at the Time of Admission

Clinical Presentation

Although HIV-infected patients with acute meningitis may present with the typical symptoms and signs of fever, headache, stiff neck, vomiting, and clouding of consciousness (Chapter 70), they may also have less typical presentations. For example, patients with cryptococcal meningitis may lack meningeal signs and present primarily with fever or clouding of consciousness. Alternately, the symptoms and signs of meningitis in patients infected with bacteria such as *Streptococcus pneumoniae* or *Salmonella* species may be overshadowed by signs and symptoms of systemic infection.

Differential Diagnosis and Initial Evaluation

Many pathogens can cause meningitis in patients infected with HIV; the more common entities are listed in Table 76.1. By far, the most common are *Cryptococcus neoformans* and *Mycobacterium tuberculosis*. The diagnosis and management of cryptococcal meningitis present special challenges and considerations in the HIV-infected person. On the other hand, the diagnosis and management of tuberculous

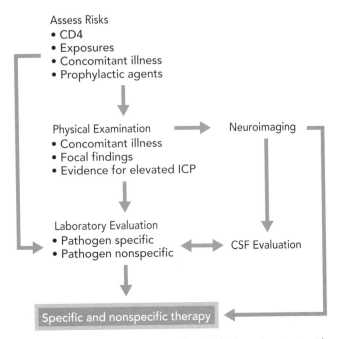

Figure 76.1 Diagnostic approach to HIV-infected patients with neurologic disorders. *ICP*, intracranial pressure.

meningitis do not differ significantly in HIV-infected and uninfected persons (1).

The first step in evaluating an HIV-infected patient with meningitis is to assess risk status. Risk assessment is based primarily on peripheral blood CD4 cell count but should also take into consideration PPD (purified protein derivative) status, exposure history, and any prophylactic therapies. Patients with CD4 cell counts below 200/μL are at greatest risk for opportunistic infections, such as crypto-

TABLE 76.1

MOST COMMON ETIOLOGIES OF MENINGITIS IN HIV-INFECTED PATIENTS

Category of pathogen	Specific etiologies
Bacteria	*Mycobacterium tuberculosis*
	Treponema pallidum
	Listeria monocytogenes
	Salmonella species
	Streptococcus pneumoniae
	Nocardia species
Fungi	*Cryptococcus neoformans*
	Coccidioides immitis
	Histoplasma capsulatum
	Candida species
	Aspergillus fumigatus
Viruses	HIV
	Cytomegalovirus
	Herpes simplex type 2
	Varicella-zoster virus
Noninfectious	Lymphomatous meningitis
	Drug-induced meningitis

coccal meningitis. Meningitis caused by more aggressive pathogens, such as *M. tuberculosis,* can occur with less advanced immunosuppression. Patients with a positive PPD or who are currently being treated for pulmonary tuberculosis are at greatest risk for tuberculous meningitis. Traveling or living in the southwestern United States increases the risk for *Coccidioides* meningitis, and traveling or living in the midwestern United States increases the likelihood of *Histoplasma* meningitis. Finally, fluconazole for prevention of oral candidiasis is also effective in preventing cryptococcal meningitis, and prophylactic trimethoprim-sulfamethoxazole may decrease the risk for conventional bacterial infections.

The next step is to perform a directed physical examination that focuses on identification of extrameningeal sites of concomitant disease, and identification of focal neurologic abnormalities or evidence of raised intracranial pressure (Chapters 70 and 117). Patients with either of the latter two findings should undergo neuroimaging to evaluate the possibility of a focal brain lesion. Contrast-enhanced magnetic resonance imaging (MRI) is the study of choice, but if it is not available, contrast-enhanced computed tomography (CT) is usually adequate. The presence of a brain lesion may still be compatible with a diagnosis of meningitis. For example, cryptococcomas are relatively common in HIV-infected patients with cryptococcal meningitis. Tuberculomas may be found in patients with tuberculous meningitis or may develop during the course of therapy, and gummas or infarcts may be seen in patients with syphilitic meningitis. Cryptococcomas, tuberculomas, and gummas resolve with medical therapy and generally do not require surgical intervention. Findings on neuroimaging determine whether a patient can safely undergo lumbar puncture. Shift of brain structures away from the midline and compression of the fourth ventricle are contraindications to this procedure. Cisternal or sulcal effacement and loss of gray matter/white matter distinction are less absolute contraindications that require individualized assessment.

Every effort should be made to obtain cerebrospinal fluid (CSF) in HIV-infected patients with suspected meningitis so that appropriate therapy can be administered. The CSF profile of patients with bacterial meningitis is discussed in Chapter 70, and with tuberculous meningitis in Chapter 67. The CSF profile is similar in HIV-infected and uninfected patients who have conventional bacterial meningitis or tuberculous meningitis, but this is not the case with cryptococcal meningitis. HIV-infected patients with cryptococcal meningitis are more likely to have a CSF white blood cell count of less than 20/μL and are more likely to have a positive CSF culture. In general, CSF evaluation should always include bacterial, mycobacterial, and fungal cultures. CSF cryptococcal antigen should be assessed if the serum cryptococcal antigen test is reactive or the result is unknown, and the CSF VDRL test should be performed if the serum syphilis serologic tests are reactive or the results are unknown (p. 741). The need for CSF cytologic examination, polymerase chain reaction (PCR) assays for viruses, and specific antigen

(*Histoplasma, Candida*) or antibody (*Coccidioides*) tests should be individualized.

The initial laboratory evaluation of HIV-infected patients with suspected meningitis should always include blood cultures and testing for serum cryptococcal antigen. The serum cryptococcal antigen is sensitive but not specific for the diagnosis of cryptococcal meningitis. Similarly, a nonreactive serum fluorescent treponemal antibody absorption test (FTA-ABS) or *Treponema pallidum* particle agglutination test (TP PA) effectively rules out the diagnosis of syphilitic meningitis. A chest radiograph should be obtained; in some instances, the etiology of meningitis can be presumptively established from the findings on pulmonary evaluation.

Indications for Hospitalization

Hospital admission is generally required for all HIV-infected patients with acute meningitis. It is particularly appropriate for those with evidence of acute hydrocephalus, increased intracranial pressure, new seizures or new focal neurologic abnormalities, significant change in mental status, or hemodynamic instability. Patients with a more subacute or chronic presentation, normal neurologic examination findings, normal lumbar puncture opening pressure, and mild lymphocytic pleocytosis can often be managed as outpatients if they do not live alone. As for all neurologic presentations, the goals of hospitalization are to establish the correct diagnosis, initiate appropriate therapy, and stabilize the patient. In the absence of complications, this can usually be accomplished within 2–5 days for HIV-infected patients with meningitis.

Indications for Initial Intensive Care Unit Admission

Hemodynamic instability and increased intracranial pressure are indications for admission to the ICU. Some experts recommend ICU admission for all patients with suspected bacterial meningitis. Elevated intracranial pressure is an important cause of morbidity and mortality in HIV-infected persons with cryptococcal meningitis and may require serial lumbar punctures or continuous lumbar or ventricular drainage (2). Similarly, hydrocephalus can complicate the course of tuberculous meningitis and may require continuous ventricular drainage.

Initial Therapy

The choice of initial therapy is based on the results of initial CSF and laboratory analysis. If the CSF cryptococcal antigen test is reactive, therapy with intravenous (IV) amphotericin (0.7 mg/kg daily), with or without oral flucytosine (100 mg/kg daily in four divided doses), should be initiated (3). Similarly, if the CSF Gram stain or formula suggest bacterial meningitis, appropriate antibiotics should be administered

(see Tables 70.3 and 70.4 for antibiotic regimens). In many instances, the etiology of meningitis will not be known immediately, and empiric treatment must be instituted based on the most likely diagnosis. Once the etiology is determined, therapy can be tailored. Appropriate empiric therapy for suspected bacterial meningitis should be given as soon as possible and should neither be delayed by the need to obtain neuroimaging nor by the time required to obtain the results of CSF testing. The use of dexamethasone in HIV-infected patients with bacterial meningitis has not been studied but is reasonable in patients who are suspected to have pneumococcal meningitis (4). Dexamethasone should be given before or with the first dose of antibiotics (Chapter 70). Empiric therapy for tuberculous meningitis is appropriate when the likelihood of disease is high and no other etiology is apparent (see Chapter 67 for recommendations). A recent study shows that adjunctive treatment with dexamethasone improves survival in HIV-uninfected patients with tuberculous meningitis, but does not decrease disability (5). No benefit was demonstrated in HIV-infected patients in this study (5). Generally, empiric antifungal therapy is not administered when cryptococcal meningitis has been excluded.

Indications for Early Consultation

Neurologic or neurosurgical consultation is appropriate for assistance in managing patients with elevated intracranial pressure. Infectious diseases consultation should be considered for patients in whom the etiology of meningitis remains elusive, or for patients with less common etiologies, such as *Coccidioides, Histoplasma,* or *Candida.*

Issues During the Course of Hospitalization

The first hours of hospitalization should be devoted to beginning appropriate, often empiric, therapy and to completing necessary diagnostic tests. Therapy for presumed bacterial meningitis should be initiated in the emergency department. Therapy for presumed *M. tuberculosis* meningitis or for cryptococcal meningitis can generally be delayed until the results of diagnostic tests, such as the CSF profile, CSF cryptococcal antigen test, and chest radiograph, are available. Adjunctive therapies, such as antipyretics, antiemetics, and pain medications, and correction of electrolyte abnormalities or volume depletion should be tailored to the individual patient. Although volume overload should be avoided, there is no role for iatrogenic dehydration to treat elevated intracranial pressure because this could potentially increase the possibility of cerebral infarction, which can result from infectious arteritis or venous sinus thrombosis. Empiric anticonvulsants are indicated if there is increased intracranial pressure, because a seizure could further elevate pressure.

Vital signs should be assessed three to four times daily; the assessment should include determination of the level of consciousness and screening for focal abnormalities. A nursing assessment and a home assessment should be performed in the first 24 hours after admission. Antibiotic regimens should be modified, if necessary, to cover organisms recovered from blood or CSF bacterial cultures. In most cases, antibiotic coverage for conventional bacteria can be discontinued at 48 hours if the cultures are negative. Patients who fail to improve or worsen by day 2 or 3 of hospitalization should be evaluated as outlined in Table 76.2.

Discharge Issues

By the third hospital day, patients who are neurologically stable or improving, are hemodynamically stable, can meet their fluid and nutritional needs by mouth, and can tolerate their antimicrobial therapy may be able to be discharged to complete their treatment at home or in a skilled nursing facility. The decision to discharge to home versus a more supervised setting depends on the frequency with which medication is administered, the degree of supervision required, and the patient's home situation. Generally, patients completing a course of therapy for acute meningitis should not be sent home if they live alone. Physician follow-up should be scheduled within the first week after discharge, and caregivers should be cautioned to contact the health care provider for worsening of symptoms and signs or development of new symptoms and signs, particularly focal neurologic abnormalities.

FOCAL CENTRAL NERVOUS SYSTEM LESIONS

Issues at the Time of Admission

Clinical Presentation

HIV-infected patients with focal CNS lesions typically present with mental status changes or focal neurologic findings, including weakness and clumsiness. Seizures may occur in as many as one-third of patients. The clinical findings are generally not helpful in distinguishing one etiology from another, although there are a few caveats. Patients with CNS toxoplasmosis may be more likely to have fever. Patients with primary CNS lymphoma may be less likely to have focal findings because of the predominance of frontal lobe involvement. Patients with PML may be more likely to have visual field deficits because occipital lobe involvement is common.

Differential Diagnosis and Initial Evaluation

Central nervous system lesions associated with neuroimaging evidence of brain edema, mass effect, and contrast enhancement in patients infected with HIV are most commonly caused by toxoplasmosis or primary CNS lymphoma. Tuberculomas may be more common than primary CNS lymphoma in specific risk groups, such as IV drug users and persons from countries where tuberculosis is prevalent. Focal CNS lesions not associated with brain edema, mass effect, or contrast enhancement are most commonly due to PML; less commonly, these lesions may be associated with varicella-zoster encephalitis, stroke, or, rarely, an atypical primary CNS lymphoma. A CSF PCR that is positive for JC virus in this setting increases the likelihood of PML from 68%–99% (6). The diagnosis of PML may be more difficult to establish in patients who are receiving potent antiretroviral therapy. Such patients may have enhancing lesions on MR because of improved immune competence or an "immune reconstitution syndrome" (7). In addition, potent antiretrovial therapy decreases the amount of JC virus DNA in CSF, thus decreasing the diagnostic sensitivity of this test (8).

As in the case of meningitis, the first step in evaluating an HIV-infected patient with a focal brain lesion is to assess risk status. Patients with CNS toxoplasmosis typically have CD4 cell counts below 200/μL, whereas patients with pri-

---

TABLE 76.2

DIAGNOSTIC CONSIDERATIONS IN HIV-INFECTED PATIENTS WITH MENINGITIS WHO FAIL TO IMPROVE ON THERAPY

Reason	Diagnostic approach
Diagnosis incorrect; patient does not have meningitis or presumed etiology incorrect	Repeat neuroimaging and cerebrospinal fluid evaluation. Look carefully for other sources of infection.
Increased intracranial pressure	Repeat neuroimaging and lumbar puncture with measurement of opening pressure.
Hydrocephalus	Repeat neuroimaging.
Stroke	Repeat neuroimaging.
Metabolic derangement	Check appropriate laboratory values such as electrolytes, calcium, magnesium, and serum liver chemistries.
Iatrogenic	Check drug administration records.

mary CNS lymphoma or PML usually have lower CD4 cell counts, generally below $100/\mu L$. Although there are no routine laboratory features that can predict the likelihood of primary CNS lymphoma or PML, 95% of patients with CNS toxoplasmosis have reactive serum anti-*Toxoplasma* immunoglobulin G. A nonreactive serology decreases the likelihood of CNS toxoplasmosis in a patient with a focal brain lesion from 78%–6% (6). Prior use of trimethoprim-sulfamethoxazole to prevent *Pneumocystis jirovecii* pneumonia (formerly *P. carinii*) also lowers the likelihood of CNS toxoplasmosis twofold to threefold (9).

Neuroimaging characteristics tailor the differential diagnosis. Contrast-enhanced CT is adequate for lesions associated with edema, mass effect, and enhancement, but MRI is superior for lesions that lack these characteristics. Because it is difficult to predict neuroimaging characteristics from clinical findings, proceeding directly to MRI is a more cost-effective approach. For patients who have lesions associated with edema, mass effect, and enhancement but a low likelihood of CNS toxoplasmosis, CSF should be examined if lumbar puncture can be performed safely. The PCR test for Epstein-Barr virus DNA in CSF is sensitive and specific for the diagnosis of primary CNS lymphoma. For patients who have nonreactive anti-*Toxoplasma* serology, the likelihood of lymphoma when a CSF PCR is positive for Epstein-Barr virus is 96%–98% (6).

Indications for Hospitalization

Patients with PML typically have a more subacute or chronic course than do patients with CNS toxoplasmosis or primary CNS lymphoma, and they can often be evaluated and managed as outpatients. Hospital admission is generally required for patients with suspected CNS toxoplasmosis or primary CNS lymphoma who have a depressed level of consciousness, significant mass effect, are too impaired to care for themselves safely, or do not have adequate living assistance. In the absence of complications, hospital stays of 2–5 days are typical for patients with mass lesions.

Indications for Initial Intensive Care Unit Admission

Obtundation, significant mass effect on neuroimaging, or frequent seizures are indications for admission to the ICU. These patients are at particular risk for brain herniation, which is the most acute risk of CNS toxoplasmosis and primary CNS lymphoma. They require frequent neurologic monitoring and may need neurosurgical intervention (see below).

Initial Therapy

In the past, an HIV-infected person who had a brain lesion associated with edema, mass effect, and enhancement had at least a 70% chance of having CNS toxoplasmosis. Be-

cause the prevalence of CNS toxoplasmosis was high, an HIV-infected patient with such a lesion was given a 2-week trial of toxoplasmosis treatment. The clinical and neuroimaging response to empiric therapy confirmed the diagnosis of CNS toxoplasmosis, and brain biopsy was reserved for patients who did not respond to the treatment trial. In recent years, the likelihood of CNS toxoplasmosis has decreased in patients with mass lesions associated with edema, mass effect, and enhancement, even when the anti-*Toxoplasma* serology is reactive (10).

An empiric treatment trial is now less appropriate for all HIV-infected patients with brain lesions associated with edema, mass effect, and enhancement. Patients appropriate for a toxoplasmosis treatment trial are those with a high likelihood of disease based on neuroimaging findings, reactive serum anti-*Toxoplasma* immunoglobulin G, and no prior use of trimethoprim-sulfamethoxazole for *Pneumocystis jirovecii* pneumonia (formerly *P. carinii*) prophylaxis. The results of PCR analysis of CSF can further define the likelihood of CNS toxoplasmosis. Initial therapy for toxoplasmosis includes pyrimethamine (100–200 mg PO load followed by 75–100 mg PO daily) and sulfadiazine (1.5–2.0 g PO four times daily). Adequate hydration must be maintained to avoid tubular crystallization of sulfadiazine with subsequent renal dysfunction. In patients who are allergic to sulfa medications, clindamycin (600–900 mg PO or IV) can be substituted for sulfadiazine. All treated patients should receive folinic acid (10–50 mg PO daily) to avert the marrow suppression caused by pyrimethamine.

In general, steroids should not be used in conjunction with a treatment trial because they can induce nonspecific clinical and neuroimaging improvement. However, a short course of steroids can be used in some instances to decrease edema and mass effect and thereby allow lumbar puncture to be performed safely. Empiric anticonvulsants should be given if there is significant brain edema or other evidence of elevated intracranial pressure. Patients with a low likelihood of CNS toxoplasmosis should not undergo a treatment trial. They should be referred for brain biopsy or, when the CSF PCR is positive for Epstein-Barr virus, for empiric radiation therapy.

In the era before the availability of potent antiretroviral therapy, the survival of HIV-infected patients with primary CNS lymphoma who have a good performance status and were treated with radiation therapy was 3–4 months. Today, patients with primary CNS lymphoma who respond to potent antiretroviral therapy may have prolonged survival (11). Figure 76.2 is a decision algorithm that addresses the diagnosis of focal CNS lesions.

Indications for Early Consultation

Patients admitted to the ICU because of concerns regarding brain herniation should undergo evaluation by neurosurgery for placement of an intracranial pressure monitor, a

Focal CNS lesion

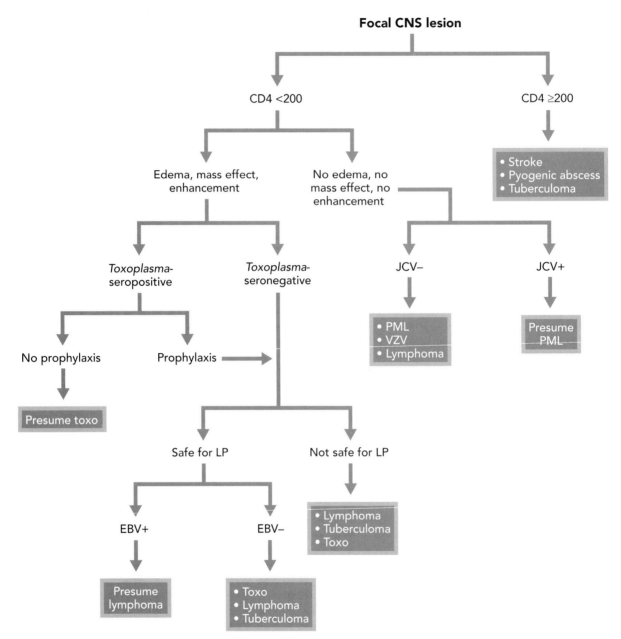

Figure 76.2 Suggested algorithm for the evaluation of HIV-infected patients with focal central nervous system lesions. *CD4*, peripheral blood CD4 lymphocyte count in cells per microliter; *CNS*, central nervous system; *EBV−*, Epstein-Barr virus DNA not identified in CSF by polymerase chain reaction; *EBV+*, Epstein-Barr virus DNA identified in CSF by polymerase chain reaction; *Edema, mass effect, enhancement*: lesion has edema, mass effect, and enhancement on neuroimaging; *JCV−*, JC virus DNA not identified in cerebrospinal fluid (*CSF*) by polymerase chain reaction; *JCV+*, JC virus DNA identified in CSF by polymerase chain reaction; *LP*, lumbar puncture; *No edema, mass effect, enhancement*: lesion does not have edema, mass effect, and enhancement on neuroimaging; *No prophylaxis*, patient is not taking trimethroprim-sulfamethoxazole; *PML*, progressive multifocal leukoencephalopathy; *Prophylaxis*, patient is taking trimethoprim-sulfamethoxazole; *Toxo*, CNS toxoplasmosis; VZV, varicella-zoster virus encephalitis.

CSF drainage procedure, or surgical resection (Chapter 117). A neurology consultation is appropriate for management of recurrent seizures (Chapter 118). An infectious disease consultation should be obtained to help devise an alternate treatment regimen if the patient is unable to tolerate the recommended therapy for CNS toxoplasmosis.

Issues During the Course of Hospitalization

The first hours of hospitalization should be devoted to completing the patient evaluation outlined above and initiating empiric therapy for CNS toxoplasmosis if this is determined to be the most appropriate course. As for patients with meningitis, an assessment of vital signs, including directed neurologic evaluations, should be performed 3–4 times per day, and a nursing and home assessment should be obtained in the first 24 hours after admission. During the hospitalization, patients with focal neurologic abnormalities should have physical and occupational therapy assessments; speech therapy assessment is appropriate for patients with swallowing difficulties or speech deficits. Although a CNS toxoplasmosis treatment trial is usually continued for 10–14 days before efficacy is assessed, half of the patients with CNS toxoplasmosis improve clinically by day three of therapy, and most improve by day 7 (12). Failure to improve within the first week of treatment increases the likelihood of an alternative diagnosis, such as primary CNS lymphoma.

Discharge Issues

By the third hospital day, patients who are neurologically stable or improving and can tolerate their therapy may be able to be discharged to home or a skilled nursing or rehabilitation unit provided that continued neurologic follow-up is available. The decision to discharge to home versus a more supervised setting depends on the factors mentioned previously. Physician follow-up should be scheduled within the first one to two weeks after discharge, and caregivers should be cautioned to contact the health care provider in case of worsening of symptoms and signs, or the development of new symptoms and signs, particularly a change in the level of consciousness.

OTHER CAUSES OF ALTERED MENTAL STATUS

Issues at the Time of Admission

Clinical Presentation

The term *altered mental status* includes a spectrum of cognitive changes that range from confusion to delirium and dementia. Dementia does not cause acute changes in mental status and, as noted in the introductory section, HIV-associated dementia is a subacute disorder that can be diagnosed and managed on an outpatient basis. Not uncommonly, HIV-infected patients present with acute changes in mental status. They may be confused, with disorientation and misinterpretation of external stimuli or clouding of consciousness. Patients who are delirious may be disoriented and have hallucinations, illusions, or delusions. These symptoms often fluctuate.

Differential Diagnosis and Initial Evaluation

The differential diagnosis of an acute change in mental status includes infectious, structural, toxic, metabolic, and

other disorders (Table 76.3). Patients with underlying cognitive impairment may be more susceptible to changes in mental status caused by these problems. The suggested evaluations for meningitis and focal CNS lesions are provided above. Encephalitis in HIV-infected patients is relatively uncommon. Before the advent of potent antiretroviral therapy, a common cause of encephalitis in HIV-infected patients was cytomegalovirus (CMV). CMV encephalitis is now quite rare but should be considered in patients with CD4 cell counts below 75/μL who are not receiving antiretrovirals. The remaining entities are listed in Table 76.3; none is unique to HIV-infected patients (Chapter 115). The exception to this statement may be that HIV-infected patients are particularly susceptible to the toxic effects of medications, and because they may be taking many different medications at the same time, they are at increased risk for drug–drug interactions.

Again, the first step in evaluating an HIV-infected patient with acute change in mental status is to assess risk status in terms of the degree of immunosuppression. Consideration should also be given to any history of trauma, use of recreational drugs and prescription medications, and history of previous neurologic disease, including seizures. The physical examination should include a formal assessment of mental status—for example, the Short Portable Mental Status Questionnaire (Table 16.3) or the Mental Alternation Test (13). The Glasgow Coma Scale (Table 117.1) can be used for obtunded or comatose patients. Because the differential diagnosis for acute change in mental status is extensive, most patients, particularly those with a CD4 cell count below 200/μL, should undergo neuroimaging.

TABLE 76.3

MOST COMMON CAUSES OF ACUTE CHANGE IN MENTAL STATUS IN HIV-INFECTED PATIENTS

Category of process	Specific etiologies
Non-CNS infection	Pneumonia Bacteremia
CNS infection	Meningitis Cerebritis Abscess *Herpes simplex* encephalitis Varicella encephalitis
Structural	Head trauma Hemorrhage Tumor
Toxic encephalopathy	Recreational drugs Prescription medications
Metabolic encephalopathy	Electrolyte abnormalities Hepatic dysfunction Hypoxemia
Other	Seizure Psychiatric disease

CNS, central nervous system.

Cranial CT with and without contrast is the study of choice in this setting to exclude quickly a focal lesion such as abscess or hemorrhage, and to determine the safety of lumbar puncture. Lumbar puncture should be performed to evaluate the possibility of CNS infection in patients at greatest risk based on clinical presentation or a low CD4 cell count. CSF studies should include a cell count and determination of glucose and protein levels. The use of PCR to detect CMV in CSF is appropriate if the patient is at risk for CMV encephalitis (see earlier in this chapter). *Herpes simplex virus* (HSV) encephalitis has been uncommonly described in HIV-infected patients and may have fewer focal features than in immunocompetent patients. Encephalitis due to HSV type 2, rather than type 1, may be more common in HIV-infected patients. PCR to detect HSV DNA in CSF is 98% sensitive and 94% specific for the diagnosis of HSV encephalitis. Blood should be sent for assessment of electrolytes and renal and hepatic function. A urine toxicology screen and determination of blood levels of psychoactive medications can be helpful. In particularly perplexing situations, it is useful to have a family member or friend bring all the patient's medications to the hospital for review.

Indications for Hospitalization and Intensive Care Unit Admission

Hospital admission is generally required for all patients with acute onset of significant change in mental status. Patients who are completely alert but confused or delusional, or in whom symptoms are slowly evolving, may be able to be evaluated on an outpatient basis. Because the differential diagnosis is so extensive, an estimate of the usual duration of hospitalization cannot be provided. In addition to the criteria for ICU admission listed above, patients who do not open their eyes to voice or who are comatose should be admitted to an ICU.

Initial Therapy

The choice of initial therapy is based on the results of initial neuroimaging and of CSF and other laboratory analyses. Patients with HSV encephalitis should be treated with acyclovir (10 mg/kg IV every 8 hours). Neurosurgical consultation is appropriate for assistance in managing patients with intracranial hemorrhage or contusion who may require treatment to decrease intracranial pressure or surgical excision. Metabolic abnormalities should be corrected. Medication toxicity can be treated by withdrawal of the offending agent or in some cases (benzodiazepines or opiates) by administering a reversing agent.

Issues During the Course of Hospitalization

The first hours of hospitalization should be devoted to beginning appropriate therapy and completing the necessary diagnostic evaluation. Therapy for presumed HSV encephalitis will often need to be initiated before the results of confirmatory tests are available. Assessment of vital signs and directed neurologic evaluations should be performed 3–4 times daily. As for most hospitalized patients, a nursing and a home assessment should be obtained in the first 24 hours after admission.

Discharge Issues

Because the differential diagnosis of acute change in mental status is so extensive, generalizations regarding expected hospital course are difficult to make. Broadly speaking, patients with reversible causes of toxic or metabolic encephalopathy can be expected to recover within 1–3 days and be discharged home. Patients with structural abnormalities or with encephalitis would be expected to have a more protracted course and to require rehabilitation, either in a skilled nursing facility or a rehabilitation unit, before eventual discharge home.

COST CONSIDERATIONS AND RESOURCE USE

Neurologic disease increases the length of stay and hospital costs for HIV-infected patients (14). The time required to establish a diagnosis is a likely contributor to increased costs. In addition, neurologic disease is more likely to result in discharge to an extended care facility, which suggests that HIV-infected patients with neurologic disease may be more severely ill than those without neurologic disease and thus require a longer length of stay. Given this information, means to increase the diagnostic accuracy of HIV-associated neurologic disorders could decrease the cost of hospital care. Neuroimaging is often considered to be a major contributor to the cost of neurologic care. Although the cost of cranial MRI can be as much as twice that of cranial CT, proceeding directly to the cranial MRI in selected patients may ultimately reduce costs because MRI often provides information that CT does not and thereby reduces the duration of hospitalization.

KEY POINTS

- HIV-associated dementia, cryptococcal meningitis, toxoplasmosis, and progressive multifocal leukoencephalopathy are the most common central nervous system disorders associated with HIV infection. All typically occur in the setting of advanced immunosuppression.
- The first step in evaluating an HIV-infected patient with a neurologic disorder is to assess the risk status of the patient based primarily on peripheral blood CD4 cell count, but also on the results of other laboratory tests, presence of concomitant illnesses, and administration of prophylactic therapies.

- Although HIV-infected patients with acute meningitis may present with the typical symptoms and signs of fever, headache, stiff neck, vomiting, and clouding of consciousness, they may also have less typical presentations. The most common causes of meningitis are *Cryptococcus neoformans* and *Mycobacterium tuberculosis*.

- Elevated intracranial pressure is an important cause of morbidity and mortality in HIV-infected patients with cryptococcal meningitis.

- Clinical findings are generally not very helpful in distinguishing one etiology of focal central nervous system lesions in HIV-infected patients from another.

- Central nervous system lesions associated with neuroimaging evidence of brain edema, mass effect, and contrast enhancement in patients infected with HIV are most commonly caused by toxoplasmosis and primary central nervous system lymphoma.

- Focal central nervous system lesions not associated with neuroimaging evidence of brain edema, mass effect, or contrast enhancement are most commonly caused by progressive multifocal leukoencephalopathy. However, mass effect and contrast enhancement may be seen in patients who develop PML shortly after beginning potent antiretroviral therapy as part of an "immune reconstitution syndrome."

- The differential diagnosis of acute change in mental status in HIV-infected patients includes infectious, structural, toxic, metabolic, and other disorders.

REFERENCES

1. Berenguer J, Moreno S, Laguna F, et al. Tuberculous meningitis in patients infected with the human immunodeficiency virus. *N Engl J Med* 1992;326:668–72.
2. Graybill JR, Sobel J, Saag M, et al. Diagnosis and management of increased intracranial pressure in patients with AIDS and cryptococcal meningitis. The NIAID Mycoses Study Group and AIDS Cooperative Treatment Groups. *Clin Infect Dis* 2000;30:47–54.
3. Brouwer AE, Rajanuwong A, Chierakul W, et al. Combination antifungal therapies for HIV-associated cryptococcal meningitis: a randomised trial. *Lancet* 2004;363:1764–1767.
4. de Gans J, van de Beek D. Dexamethasone in adults with bacterial meningitis. *N Engl J Med* 2002;347:1549–1556.
5. Quagliarello V. Adjunctive steroids for tuberculous meningitis—more evidence, more questions. *N Engl J Med* 2004;351:1792–1794.
6. Antinori A, Ammassari A, De Luca A, et al. Diagnosis of AIDS-related focal brain lesions: a decision-making analysis based on clinical and neuroradiologic characteristics combined with polymerase chain reaction assays in CSF. *Neurology* 1997;48:687–694.
7. Miralles P, Berenguer J, Lacruz C, et al. Inflammatory reactions in progressive multifocal leukoencephalopathy after highly active antiretroviral therapy. *AIDS* 2001;15:1900–1902.
8. De Luca A, Giancola ML, Ammassari A, et al. The effect of potent antiretroviral therapy and JC virus load in cerebrospinal fluid on clinical outcome of patients with AIDS-associated progressive multifocal leukoencephalopathy. *J Infect Dis* 2000;182:1077–1083.
9. Marra CM, Krone MR, Koutsky LA, Holmes KK. Diagnostic accuracy of HIV-associated central nervous system toxoplasmosis. *Int J STD AIDS* 1998;9:761–764.
10. Ammassari A, Cingolani A, Pezzotti P, et al. AIDS-related focal brain lesions in the era of highly active antiretroviral therapy. *Neurology* 2000;55:1194–1200.
11. Hoffmann C, Tabrizian S, Wolf E, et al. Survival of AIDS patients with primary central nervous system lymphoma is dramatically improved by HAART-induced immune recovery. *AIDS* 2001;15:2119–2127.
12. Luft BJ, Hafner R, Korzun AH, et al. Toxoplasmic encephalitis in patients with the acquired immunodeficiency syndrome. Members of the ACTG 077p/ANRS 009 Study Team. *N Engl J Med* 1993;329:995–1000.
13. Jones BN, Teng EL, Folstein MF, Harrison KS. A new bedside test of cognition for patients with HIV infection. *Ann Intern Med* 1993;119:1001–1004.
14. Dal Pan GJ, Skolasky RL, Moore RD. The impact of neurologic disease on hospitalizations related to human immunodeficiency virus infection in Maryland, 1991–1992. *Arch Neurol* 1997;54:846–852.

ADDITIONAL READING

Berenguer J, Miralles P, Arrizabalaga J, et al. Clinical course and prognostic factors of progressive multifocal leukoencephalopathy in patients treated with highly active antiretroviral therapy. *Clin Infect Dis* 2003;36:1047–52.

Sacktor N, Lyles RH, Skolasky R, et al. HIV-associated neurologic disease incidence changes: multicenter AIDS Cohort Study, 1990–1998. *Neurology* 2001;56:257–260.

Gastroenterology

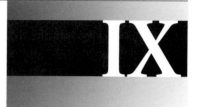

Signs, Symptoms, and Laboratory Abnormalities in Gastrointestinal Disease

77

Kenneth McQuaid

INTRODUCTION

Gastrointestinal symptoms and signs are common in the hospitalized patient. They are sometimes attributable to problems intrinsic to the gastrointestinal tract or may be indicative of a systemic disorder. When they are present on admission, the differential diagnosis of these symptoms and signs is lengthy. However, a complete history and physical examination focus on the diagnostic evaluation. Gastrointestinal symptoms that arise during hospitalization most commonly are caused by problems intrinsic to hospital treatment: medications, chemotherapy, nosocomial infections, and invasive procedures or surgery. In approaching hospitalized patients, physicians should first consider these nosocomial and iatrogenic factors while also keeping in mind that "outpatient disorders" may arise in the inpatient setting. In this chapter, the approaches to several common signs, symptoms, and laboratory abnormalities are addressed. The differential diagnosis, diagnostic considerations, evaluation, and management for patients presenting to the hospital are discussed and contrasted with those for patients whose problems arise during a hospitalization.

ABDOMINAL PAIN OCCURRING DURING THE COURSE OF HOSPITALIZATION

Description and Differential Diagnosis

Common disorders resulting in abdominal pain that lead to hospitalization are discussed in the subsequent chapters of the gastroenterology section (e.g., acute pancreatitis in Chapter 86, and bowel obstruction in Chapter 88). The patient in whom abdominal pain develops *after* hospitalization presents a difficult challenge. In many instances, such patients are critically ill with a major medical problem or are in a postoperative recovery period. They may be unable to provide a history of their symptoms because of alterations in mental status or the need for assisted ventilation.

Abdominal pain presenting in the hospitalized patient can generally be assigned to one of the following categories.

Conditions Overlooked or Misdiagnosed on Hospital Admission

Patients who are elderly, have a psychiatric illness or altered mental status, have multiple comorbid medical illnesses, or are taking long-term analgesics or corticosteroids may not manifest typical symptoms or signs of acute surgical disease on admission and may be admitted to a nonsurgical service. The admitting diagnoses of "fever," "gastroenteritis," "sepsis," "altered mental status," "obstipation," or "failure to thrive" may stem from undiagnosed intraabdominal conditions such as a perforated peptic ulcer, cholecystitis or cholangitis, diverticulitis, or appendicitis in patients reporting little or no initial abdominal pain. Significant pain may not become apparent until the disease progresses and complications (e.g., peritonitis or abscess) arise. In such cases, initial physical findings may be minimal, or the atypical location may confound the diagnostic impression.

Unrelated Conditions First Arising in the Hospital

Because physicians are trained to look for a "unifying diagnosis," the possibility of a second, unrelated problem arising anew in the hospitalized patient often is not even considered. The presentation of common causes of abdominal pain such as acute cholecystitis, acute appendicitis, and perforated peptic ulcer may be atypical in the hospitalized patient. This may lead to a delayed diagnosis and complications.

Conditions Arising as a Direct Consequence of Problems Related to Critical Illness

A host of problems may arise in the gastrointestinal tract that are a direct consequence of critical illness (Table 77.1), such as the following:

Mucosal Ischemia
As a consequence of severe physiological stress, shunting of splanchnic blood flow may give rise to ischemic damage throughout the gastrointestinal tract. Patients at greatest risk are those with sepsis, shock, coagulopathy, major trauma, major central nervous system events, multiple organ failure, or those who are undergoing mechanical ventilation or major surgery. Many critically ill patients are unable to report abdominal symptoms because of altered mental status or sedation. Hence, these conditions commonly are overlooked until complications supersede. *Acalculous cholecystitis* may manifest with any combination of right upper quadrant pain or tenderness, fever, and leukocytosis in the postoperative or ICU patient. Symptoms or signs referable to the right upper quadrant com-

TABLE 77.1

CAUSES OF ABDOMINAL PAIN IN THE HOSPITALIZED PATIENT

Problems arising from physiological stress
Stress-related gastric or duodenal ulcers
Mesenteric ischemia
Ischemic colitis
Acalculous cholecystitis
Pancreatitis
Ileus
Acute colonic pseudo-obstruction (Ogilvie's syndrome)
Acute adrenal insufficiency

Complications secondary to hospitalization
Postsurgical complications
Postprocedural complications
Clostridium difficile colitis
Medication-induced abdominal pain
Constipation
Pneumonia
Coronary ischemia

monly are not apparent or are overlooked until sepsis or cholangitis develops (Chapter 84). *Nonocclusive mesenteric ischemia* and *ischemic colitis* most commonly arise in patients with cardiogenic or hypovolemic shock that results in vasoconstriction or other compromise of the mesenteric arteries (Chapter 87).

Disruption of Intestinal Motility
Ileus and *acute colonic pseudo-obstruction (Ogilvie's syndrome)* are due to reversible inhibition of intestinal motility that develops in patients who are critically ill or in a postoperative state. They are characterized by diffuse abdominal pain and distention (Chapter 88).

Acute Pancreatitis
Acute pancreatitis may occur in the hospitalized patient for a number of reasons. The medication list must be carefully reviewed for potential causative agents. Fasting patients are predisposed to the development of biliary sludge and small gallstones, which can cause acute pancreatitis. Ischemic injury to the pancreas may occur in patients who have had shock. Up to 8% of patients sustain overt pancreatitis after cardiopulmonary bypass, and significantly more have subclinical injury. Finally, acute pancreatitis may occur after other abdominal surgeries, even when the pancreas is not directly manipulated (Chapter 86).

Acute Adrenal Insufficiency
Adrenal crisis may occur in hospitalized patients with latent adrenal disease due to the stress of surgery, trauma, infections, or prolonged fasting. It may also occur in patients taking chronic adrenocorticoids if these medications are not continued in the hospital. Acute adrenal

insufficiency (Chapter 109) may also occur following injury to adrenals by hemorrhage, thrombosis, or infection. Patients may complain of nausea, vomiting, abdominal pain, and diarrhea. Signs of adrenal crisis include fever, hypotension, hypoglycemia, and hyponatremia.

Complications Arising as a Consequence of Hospitalization Or Intervention

Postprocedural Complications

In the hospital setting, patients may undergo a variety of abdominal procedures. Any patient complaining of abdominal pain within 24–48 hours of an invasive procedure should be presumed to have a complication until proved otherwise. A full description of these complications is beyond the scope of this discussion, but three broad categories should be considered: (a) bleeding (intraperitoneal, retroperitoneal, within solid organs, or within the bowel wall); (b) perforation of a hollow viscus; or (c) infection.

Inflammatory Colitis

Clostridium difficile-associated colitis develops in 1% of patients receiving antibiotics (see the section on "Diarrhea" later in this chapter). Some patients present with fever, abdominal distention, pain, tenderness, and leukocytosis with minimal or no diarrhea. Such cases may be confused with ileus or Ogilvie's syndrome. *Neutropenic typhlitis* is an inflammatory process involving the cecum, ascending colon, and terminal ileum that occurs in some patients with profound neutropenia (<1,000 cells μL) after they receive cytotoxic drugs. It may lead to bacterial invasion, perforation, and shock, and carries a mortality of 50%. Right lower quadrant cramping pain, fever, and watery or bloody diarrhea usually are present.

Abdominal Pain Induced by Medication

A host of medications can cause dyspepsia, including nonsteroidal antiinflammatory drugs (NSAIDs), iron, niacin, corticosteroids, oral antibiotics, lactulose, sorbitol, acarbose, theophylline, digoxin, and L-dopa. Acute opiate withdrawal should be considered in high-risk patients with cramping abdominal pain and diarrhea. Anticoagulation may be associated with spontaneous or post-procedure hemorrhage in the liver, spleen, bowel wall, peritoneal cavity, retroperitoneum, or abdominal wall, resulting in acute, often dramatic, abdominal pain.

Constipation

Constipation is common in the hospital setting because of alterations in diet, bed rest, medications, postoperative pain, and restricted access to private facilities. It may go unnoticed until abdominal distention and pain develop.

Other Medical Conditions

Pneumonia and *coronary ischemia* may present with pain in the epigastrium or upper quadrants. Pursuit of abdominal causes of pain in these cases may lead to serious delay in diagnosis and appropriate treatment.

Evaluation

The initial approach to the hospitalized patient with abdominal pain is similar to that in the outpatient setting. When possible, a history and physical examination should be repeated, with emphasis on the presence of abdominal symptoms that preceded hospital admission. The findings of abdominal distention, recent incision or puncture sites, hematomas, and the presence or absence of bowel sounds should be noted. Tympany and tenderness are suggestive of ileus or perforation. Attention should be paid to the presence of tenderness in the right upper quadrant (cholecystitis), right lower quadrant (Ogilvie's syndrome or appendicitis), or left lower quadrant (ischemic colitis or diverticulitis). The finding of gross blood on digital rectal examination is suggestive of mesenteric ischemia or ischemic colitis.

Reports of all diagnostic and therapeutic procedures should be reviewed, and any complications noted. The medication list should be reviewed for antibiotics or other drugs that might cause abdominal pain. Anticoagulants increase the likelihood of an intra-abdominal or retroperitoneal hemorrhage.

Abdominal pain that develops in the hospitalized patient warrants further investigation. A complete blood cell count with differential, a urinalysis, and values for electrolytes, liver chemistries, and amylase should be obtained. A recent drop in hematocrit suggests intra-abdominal hemorrhage. Leukocytosis is nonspecific in the hospitalized patient, but a recent or continued rise suggests a serious cause of abdominal pain. The presence of an anion gap acidosis is worrisome for lactic acidosis caused by intra-abdominal abscess, sepsis, or ischemic bowel. Changes in liver chemistries, sometimes quite minor, may be indicative of calculous or acalculous cholecystitis, cholangitis, or both. Hyperamylasemia may point to acute pancreatitis.

A flat and upright or right lateral decubitus abdominal radiograph should be obtained in all hospitalized patients with abdominal pain to look for the presence of free intra-abdominal air. Increased gas throughout the small and large bowel suggests ileus. Acute obstruction of the large or small bowel can be distinguished from ileus by auscultation and abdominal radiographs. When the colon is predominantly dilated, Ogilvie's syndrome, *C. difficile* colitis, and (in immunosuppressed patients) typhlitis should be considered. The presence of gas in the rectum helps to distinguish these from a distal large-bowel obstruction. Hypaque enema or colonoscopy is sometimes necessary to exclude mechanical large-bowel obstruction

(Chapter 88). Significant thickening of the colonic wall may be evident with ischemic colitis, pseudomembranous colitis, or typhlitis. Sigmoidoscopy or colonoscopy may be indicated when ischemic colitis or *C. difficile* pseudomembranous colitis is suspected. Constipation is evidenced by a large, stool-filled rectum and descending colon.

When the above fail to indicate the cause of abdominal pain, further imaging is required. For suspected cholecystitis, ultrasonography is preferred. In most other patients, abdominal computed tomography (CT) is the optimal study to evaluate the presence of small amounts of intraperitoneal air, intraabdominal abscess, retroperitoneal hemorrhage, intestinal ischemia, cholecystitis, pancreatitis, and appendicitis. In patients with suspected complications of an invasive procedure, it is also the study of choice.

Management

The appropriate management of the hospitalized patient with abdominal pain depends on the suspected etiology. If there is any question of a complication related to a procedure, the service that performed that procedure should be contacted. The patient should be aggressively volume-resuscitated as needed. Patients with sepsis or suspected intra-abdominal infection should be treated with broad aerobic and anaerobic antibiotic coverage (Chapter 64). Placement of a nasogastric tube is indicated for the patient with vomiting, ileus, acute colonic pseudo-obstruction, or bowel obstruction. For specific management of stress ulceration (Chapter 80), acalculous cholecystitis (Chapter 84), acute pancreatitis (Chapter 86), ileus and Ogilvie's syndrome (Chapter 88), and surgical emergencies (Chapter 87), refer to the chapter indicated.

NAUSEA AND VOMITING

When Presenting at the Time of Admission

Description and Differential Diagnosis

The medullary vomiting center receives stimulatory input from (a) vagal and splanchnic fibers from the gastrointestinal tract, (b) the vestibular system, (c) the chemoreceptor trigger zone (rich in serotonin and dopamine receptors), and (d) higher central nervous system centers. The causes of acute vomiting can be subsumed under these general categories (Table 77.2).

Chronic vomiting may be a consequence of gastroparesis, gastric outlet obstruction, intestinal dysmotility, central nervous system disorders, systemic disorders, psychogenic factors, and pregnancy. It is important to distinguish mechanical causes (which may require surgical therapy) from other causes. Vomiting immediately after meals may represent bulimia or other psychogenic factors, but it also occurs in patients with pyloric stenosis from peptic ulcer disease. The vomiting of undigested food between one and several hours after meals suggests gastroparesis, gastric outlet obstruction, or proximal small-bowel obstruction. Morning vomiting is typical of alcoholic gastritis, pregnancy, uremia, and increased intracranial pressure.

Evaluation

In patients with acute vomiting, the goal is to distinguish "surgical" from "medical" conditions. The acute onset of vomiting without significant abdominal pain is commonly

---

TABLE 77.2

CAUSES OF ACUTE NAUSEA AND VOMITING

Visceral afferent sensation	Hyperglycemia
Infections	Adrenal crisis
Viral gastroenteritis	Radiation therapy
Toxin-mediated food poisoning	
Acute systemic infections	**Vestibular disorders**
Mechanical obstruction	
Extrinsic small bowel obstruction	**CNS stimulation**
Intrinsic small bowel obstruction	Increased intracranial pressure
Ileus	CNS tumors
Visceral pain or peritoneal irritation	Subarachnoid hemorrhage
Medications/irritants	Subdural hemorrhage
	Meningitis
Stimulation of CTZ	Encephalitis
Chemotherapy agents	Psychogenic
Other medications	
Opioids	**Other systemic conditions**
L-dopa	Myocardial infarction
Systemic disorders	Hypercalcemia
Uremia	Pregnancy
Diabetic ketoacidosis	Acute fatty liver of pregnancy

CNS, central nervous system; *CTZ*, chemoreceptor trigger zone.

caused by "medical" conditions, such as infectious gastroenteritis, food poisoning, myocardial infarction, or medications. The acute onset of abdominal pain that is accompanied or followed by vomiting is typical of "surgical" conditions, such as acute pancreatitis, cholecystitis, appendicitis, perforated viscus, renal colic, or intestinal obstruction. Patients should be asked about recent changes in medications, food ingestion, viral symptoms, or similar illnesses in family members.

On physical examination, evidence of volume depletion should be sought. Abdominal distention suggests ileus or intestinal obstruction. A succussion splash may be present with gastric outlet obstruction or gastroparesis. The presence of severe abdominal pain or tenderness or signs of peritoneal irritation is indicative of a surgical condition and warrants urgent attention (Chapter 87). Hernial orifices and surgical scars should be carefully examined. Neurologic and funduscopic examinations are mandatory to screen for increased intracranial pressure.

A complete blood cell count and values for electrolytes, glucose, liver chemistries, blood urea nitrogen, creatinine, and amylase should be obtained. Leukocytosis may suggest a "surgical" cause of vomiting but is also seen with viral gastroenteritis. Elevated liver chemistries or amylase may indicate hepatitis, cholecystitis, choledocholithiasis, or pancreatitis. A metabolic acidosis may be caused by renal insufficiency, adrenal insufficiency, and diabetic or alcoholic ketoacidosis. Prolonged vomiting may result in hypokalemia, metabolic alkalosis, hyponatremia or hypernatremia, and prerenal azotemia. In menstruating women, levels of urinary or serum β-HCG (human chorionic gonadotropin) should be determined.

A flat and upright abdominal radiograph should be obtained in patients with severe pain or in whom mechanical obstruction is suspected to look for free intraperitoneal air or dilated loops of small bowel. Aspiration of more than 200 mL of residual material via nasogastric tube in a fasting patient suggests gastric outlet obstruction, proximal small-bowel obstruction, or gastroparesis. The cause of gastric outlet obstruction is best determined by upper gastrointestinal endoscopy. In patients in whom mechanical obstruction is excluded by endoscopy or upper gastrointestinal series, gastroparesis can be demonstrated by a nuclear scintigraphic study showing delayed gastric emptying. Suspected pancreaticobiliary disease can be investigated with abdominal ultrasonography, CT, or endoscopic retrograde cholangiopancreatography (ERCP). Central nervous system symptoms warrant evaluation with magnetic resonance imaging (MRI) of the head.

Management

Management of the patient with vomiting is directed at the underlying disorder. Most cases of acute vomiting caused by infections or food poisoning are mild and self-limited, and they require no specific treatment. In patients with severe vomiting, metabolic alkalosis and hypokalemia can develop. Intravenous (IV) 0.45% saline solution with potassium chloride (20 mEq/L) can be given to maintain hydration. A nasogastric tube for gastric decompression improves patient comfort and permits monitoring of fluid loss.

Medications that inhibit different neural inputs into the vomiting center may be given to control vomiting. Combinations of agents from several drug classes provide greater efficacy with less toxicity (Table 77.3).

When Nausea and Vomiting Appear During Hospitalization

Description and Differential Diagnosis

Vomiting in hospitalized patients has a limited differential diagnosis. The most common cause is ileus, a nonspecific condition associated with a number of medical and surgical conditions (Chapter 88). Most cases resolve within 3–5 days, and persistent symptoms should prompt evaluation for an undrained abscess or systemic infection. A number of medications can cause nausea (Table 77.2 and Chapter 80). Although nausea and vomiting are common in patients receiving chemotherapy or radiation therapy, other causes of vomiting related to malignancy should be considered, including brain metastases, malignant bowel obstruction, and electrolyte imbalances (especially hypercalcemia). Nausea and vomiting can be early symptoms of acute veno-occlusive disease or graft-versus-host disease in transplant recipients (Chapter 96). In immunocompromised patients, vomiting can reflect hepatic or gastrointestinal involvement with opportunistic infections; the presence of headache or central nervous system symptoms suggests meningitis or brain abscesses caused by opportunistic pathogens (Chapter 70).

Evaluation

The hospital course should be reviewed, with particular attention paid to the medication record. A temporal relationship between the initiation of medications and the onset of nausea and vomiting is noteworthy. Physical examination should note the presence of distention, bowel sounds, and focal or diffuse abdominal tenderness. Ileus and mechanical obstruction can be difficult to differentiate in patients in the postoperative period (Chapter 88).

Further evaluation includes complete blood cell count and determination of values for electrolytes, calcium, liver chemistries, and amylase. A flat and upright abdominal plain film helps distinguish ileus from mechanical obstruction. When the diagnosis is in question, a limited barium radiographic study or abdominal CT may be helpful. Imaging with abdominal ultrasonography or CT is also indicated in patients with suspected acalculous cholecystitis or intraabdominal infection. Upper gastrointestinal endoscopy

TABLE 77.3

COMMON ANTIEMETIC REGIMENS

	Dosage	Route
Serotonin (5-HT3) antagonists		
Ondansetron	Postoperative: 8 mg or 0.15 mg/kg once daily	IV
	Before chemotherapy: 32 mg	IV
	8 mg twice daily	PO
Granisetron	1 mg or 0.01 mg/kg	IV
	2 mg once daily	PO
Dolasetron	100 mg or 1.8 mg/kg once daily	IV
	100–200 mg once daily	PO
Dopamine antagonists		
Prochlorperazine	5–10 mg q4–6h	PO, IM, IV
	25 mg suppository every 6–8 hrs	PR
Metoclopramide	10–20 mg q6h	PO
	0.5–2 mg/kg q6–8h	IV
Trimethobenzamide	250 mg every 6–8 hrs	PO
	200 mg every 6–8 hrs	PR, IM
Antihistamines and anticholinergics		
Diphenhydramine	25–50 mg q4–6h	PO, IM, IV
Scopolamine	1.5 mg q3d	Patch
Sedatives		
Lorazepam	1–2 mg q4–6h	PO, IV
Dronabinol	5 mg/m^2 q2–4h	PO

5-HT3, 5-hydroxytryptamine.

is sometimes performed to exclude peptic ulcer disease and to diagnose opportunistic infections in immunocompromised patients and acute graft-versus-host disease.

Management

The management of vomiting in the hospitalized patient is similar to that for the patient presenting this symptom. The management of intestinal ileus is discussed in Chapter 88.

DIARRHEA

When Presenting at the Time of Admission

Description and Differential Diagnosis

Diarrhea is a common symptom that ranges in severity from a self-limited annoyance to a life-threatening illness. In sorting among the myriad causes, it is helpful to distinguish acute from chronic diarrhea, as the differential diagnosis, evaluation, and treatment are entirely different. With rare exceptions, chronic diarrhea is evaluated on an outpatient basis and therefore is not discussed in this section.

Diarrhea that is acute in onset and persists less than three weeks is most commonly caused by viral or bacterial infections, bacterial toxins ("food poisoning"), parasites, or medications (Table 77.4). Similar illness in family members suggests an infectious origin. Recent ingestion of improperly stored or prepared food implicates food poisoning, especially if others have been similarly affected. Antibiotic use within the prior 1–2 months increases the likelihood of *C. difficile* colitis. All current medications (including over-the-counter medications), illicit drugs, nutritional and herbal supplements, alcohol, and caffeine should be reviewed, especially those started within the last 8 weeks. A careful travel history should be obtained. In elderly patients, acute cramping abdominal pain followed by bloody stools suggests ischemic colitis. Fecal impaction leading to pseudo-diarrhea should be considered in institutionalized or bedridden patients.

The nature of diarrhea helps to distinguish among different causes.

Noninflammatory Diarrhea

Watery, nonbloody diarrhea associated with periumbilical cramps, bloating, nausea, or vomiting suggests an enteritis caused by either a toxin-producing bacterium or other noninvasive agents that disrupt intestinal absorption or secretion. Prominent vomiting suggests viral enteritis or *Staphylococcus aureus* food poisoning. Although in most cases noninflammatory diarrhea in adults is mild, in some cases (e.g., infection with *Vibrio cholerae*) it leads to volu-

TABLE 77.4

MAJOR CAUSES OF ACUTE DIARRHEA (LESS THAN 3 WEEKS DURATION)

Infections
  Viral: rotavirus, Norwalk virus
  Toxin-producing bacteria
  —Preformed (ingested) toxin: *Staphylococcus aureus, Clostridium perfringens*
  —Secretory enterotoxin: *Bacillus cereus,* enterotoxigenic *Escherichia coli, Aeromonas, Vibrio cholerae*
  —Cytoxin: enterohemorrhagic *E. coli* O157:H7, *V. parahaemolyticus, C. difficile*
  Invasive bacteria: *Salmonella, Shigella, Campylobacter, Listeria monocytogenes, Yersinia enterocolitica*
  Parasitic/protozoal: *Giardia,* amebiasis
  Immunosuppression and HIV disease: cytomegalovirus, MAC, *Cryptosporidium,* microsporidia, *Isospora,* fungal
Medications
Ulcerative colitis
Ischemic colitis
Fecal impaction

MAC, *Mycobacterium avium* complex.

minous fluid loss and electrolyte imbalance. Because tissue invasion does not occur, fecal leukocytes are not present.

Inflammatory Diarrhea

The presence of fever and bloody diarrhea indicates colonic mucosal disruption as a consequence of direct bacterial invasion or cytotoxin production, inflammatory bowel disease, or ischemic colitis. Because such processes primarily involve the colon, diarrheal volume is small (<1 L/d) and is associated with lower abdominal cramps, urgency, and tenesmus. Although fecal leukocytes commonly are present, they may be absent (Table 77.5). *Escherichia coli* O157:H7, a toxigenic, noninvasive organism that can be acquired from contaminated beef or unpasteurized juice, has caused outbreaks of acute, often severe hemorrhagic colitis. It is the most common cause of infectious bloody diarrhea in adults and the most common cause of hemolytic uremic syndrome in children. In patients who have AIDS or are otherwise immunocompromised, cytomegalovirus infection can result in intestinal ulceration with watery or bloody diarrhea.

Enteric Fever

A severe systemic illness manifested by high fevers, confusion, and respiratory symptoms followed by abdominal tenderness, diarrhea, and rash can be caused by infection with *Salmonella typhi* or *S. paratyphi* and result in bacteremia and multiple organ dysfunction.

Evaluation

More than 90% of cases of acute diarrheal illness are mild and self-limited, responding within 5 days to simple rehy-

dration therapy or antidiarrheal drugs. In such cases, laboratory investigation is unnecessary because it usually is unrevealing and does not affect outcome. The isolation rate of pathogens from stool cultures is less than 3%. The goal is to distinguish patients with mild self-limited disease from those with serious illness. Patients with mild illness at presentation can be treated symptomatically without further stool studies or culture. If diarrhea persists or fails to improve within 10 days, stool should be sent for culture and ova and parasite evaluation.

Patients with signs of more severe illness manifested by any of the following require more aggressive evaluation: high fever ($\geq38.5°C$), bloody diarrhea, significant abdominal pain, and signs of volume depletion, tenesmus, or prolonged illness. Hospitalization is required for severe dehydration, abnormal mental status, suspected bacteremia, or marked abdominal pain. Peritoneal findings may signify the presence of enterohemorrhagic *E. coli* O157:H7 infection (patients are usually afebrile), enteric fever, or fulminant ulcerative colitis. An abdominal radiograph should be obtained in such patients to look for evidence of megacolon, perforation, or colonic thickening. Approximately 50% of patients with bloody or severe diarrhea requiring hospital admission have positive stool cultures for bacterial or parasitic pathogens.

Microscopic examination of the stool for *fecal leukocytes* is an easy, inexpensive test that helps distinguish inflammatory from noninflammatory diarrhea (Table 77.5). The presence of fecal leukocytes suggests an infectious diarrhea that warrants stool bacterial culture and ova and parasite determination, although results are sometimes positive in inflammatory bowel disease or ischemic colitis. Patients with mild-to-moderate diarrhea whose stool is negative for fecal leukocytes can be treated symptomatically.

TABLE 77.5

FECAL LEUKOCYTES IN ACUTE DIARRHEAL DISORDERS

Noninflammatory diarrheas: fecal WBCs absent
  Viral: rotavirus, Norwalk agent
  Protozoal: *Giardia, Cryptosporidium, Cyclospora, Isospora*
  Bacterial: *Staphylococcus aureus, Bacillus cereus, Clostridium perfringens,* enterotoxigenic *Escherichia coli, Vibrio cholerae*

Inflammatory diarrheas
  1. Fecal WBCs usually present
     Bacterial: *Shigella, Campylobacter jejuni*
     Noninfectious: ulcerative colitis, Crohn's disease, radiation or ischemic colitis
  2. Fecal WBCs variably present
     Bacterial: *Salmonella, Yersinia enterocolitica, Vibrio parahaemolyticus, Aeromonas, Listeria monocytogenes, E. coli* O157:H7, *C. difficile*
  3. Fecal WBCs absent: amebiasis, cytomegalovirus

WBC, white blood cell.

In most patients with severe acute diarrhea, the findings of flexible or rigid sigmoidoscopy are nonspecific and add little to the initial assessment. Infectious colitis cannot be distinguished from ulcerative colitis by sigmoidoscopy. In suspected ischemic colitis, the presence of sigmoid colitis with a normal-appearing rectum (rectal sparing) confirms the diagnosis. Sigmoidoscopy also can be helpful in assessing patients with symptoms of proctitis (tenesmus, rectal pain, bloody discharge), in which mucosal abnormalities are confined to the anorectum.

Management

Fluids and Diet

The majority of patients with mild acute diarrhea can be treated conservatively with oral fluids containing carbohydrates and electrolytes. Patients generally find it more comfortable to rest the bowel by avoiding high-fiber foods, fats, milk products, caffeine, and alcohol. However, oral intake of fluids and soft foods should be encouraged. In severe diarrhea, volume depletion can occur quickly, especially in children and the elderly. Oral rehydration is preferred to IV fluids because it is inexpensive, safe, and highly effective. Oral electrolyte solutions (e.g., Pedialyte) are commercially available. Fluids should be given at a rate of 50–200 mL/kg daily depending on hydration status. IV solutions may be necessary initially in patients with severe dehydration.

Symptomatic Therapies

Antidiarrheal agents can be used safely in mild diarrheal illness. Opioids reduce stool number and liquidity and control rectal urgency. They should not be used in patients with signs of severe colitis (high fever, severe pain, significant bleeding, tenderness) because of the possibility of exacerbating the illness. Loperamide is preferred because it does not cross the blood–brain barrier (4 mg initially, then 2 mg after each bowel movement; maximum, 16 mg/24 h). Bismuth subsalicylate (two tablets or 30 mL four times daily) is an effective treatment for diarrhea because of its antiinflammatory and antibacterial actions. Anticholinergics are contraindicated in acute diarrhea because they may (rarely) cause megacolon.

Antibiotic Therapy

Because more than 90% of patients with acute diarrhea have self-limited disease, empiric antibiotic treatment of all patients with acute diarrhea is not warranted. The exception to this is *traveler's diarrhea*, in which empiric treatment with loperamide and an antibiotic (trimethoprim-sulfamethoxazole or a fluoroquinolone) for 3–5 days markedly curtails the period of diarrhea. However, in patients with moderate-to-severe fever, bloody stools, or severe diarrhea, empiric treatment is recommended while stool bacterial cultures are pending. The choice of antibiotics depends on known local sensitivity patterns. The duration of treatment has not been

well defined, but five days is adequate in most cases. For patients with diarrhea and positive stool cultures, antibiotics are not recommended for nontyphoidal *Salmonella*, *Campylobacter*, *Aeromonas*, *E. coli* O157:H7, or *Yersinia* infection (except in severe or prolonged disease) because such therapy has not been shown to hasten recovery or reduce the period of fecal bacterial excretion.

When Diarrhea Appears During the Hospitalization

Description and Differential Diagnosis

Diarrhea is a common problem in hospitalized patients, occurring in up to 40% of patients in the ICU setting. Although many cases are mild, diarrhea can complicate nursing care, compromise nutrition by interfering with the administration of enteral feeds, and disturb fluid and electrolyte balance. Nosocomial diarrhea is associated with an increased incidence of other nosocomial infections, increased mortality, longer hospital stays, and higher hospital costs.

Diarrhea developing within the first three hospital days may be caused by any of the factors previously discussed. Thereafter, infectious diarrheas (other than those associated with *C. difficile*) are rare except in immunocompromised patients. The most common causes of diarrhea in the hospitalized patient are the following:

Antibiotic-Associated Diarrhea

Antibiotics account for more than half the cases of nosocomial diarrhea. In the majority of these cases, no pathogen can be identified. Alterations in colonic flora caused by antibiotics can lead to a decrease in colonic bacterial fermentation of fecal carbohydrates, resulting in an osmotic diarrhea, or to an increase in luminal fatty acids, resulting in secretory diarrhea.

Approximately 20% of cases of antibiotic-associated diarrhea are attributable to infection with *C. difficile*. It is estimated that 20% of hospitalized patients become colonized with *C. difficile*, and most remain asymptomatic. Standard infection control procedures, with hand washing between examinations and enteric precautions for patients with known infection, are important in preventing the nosocomial spread of *C. difficile*. Although most antibiotics have been associated with *C. difficile* disease, third-generation cephalosporins, ampicillin, and clindamycin are most commonly implicated. *C. difficile* is the major cause of nosocomial diarrhea, affecting between 1 in 100 and 1 in 1,000 persons receiving parenteral antibiotics. Most have mild-to-moderate watery diarrhea with lower abdominal cramps or tenderness. In a subset of patients, more severe colitis develops. The serum white blood cell count may be extremely high. Although some blood may be present, grossly bloody stools are unusual. Fulminant, life-threatening colitis characterized by lethargy, fever, tachycardia, abdominal pain, and distention occurs in a small number of patients. Complications include hypovolemia, hypoalbuminemia from mucosal protein loss, and toxic megacolon. The development of toxic megacolon with paralytic ileus can result in a paradoxical decrease in diarrhea.

Enteral Feedings

Diarrhea occurs in more than one-fourth of patients receiving enteral feedings. Causes include high osmolality of the solution, rapid rate of infusion, intestinal ileus with rapid transit, intestinal villous atrophy with malabsorption, hypoalbuminemia, and bacterial contamination.

Other Infections

In immunosuppressed patients, diarrhea can be caused by infection with cytomegalovirus, fungi, or *Cryptosporidium*.

Other Causes

Milk is included routinely in hospital diets, despite a high prevalence of lactose intolerance. Medications administered in the hospital can cause diarrhea. Fecal impaction with pseudo-diarrhea occurs in patients with prolonged constipation. The acute onset of cramping abdominal pain followed by bloody stools should suggest the possibility of ischemic colitis in elderly patients. Chemotherapy may result in diarrhea beginning within 3–10 days of treatment. Acute graft-versus-host disease occurs after allogeneic bone marrow transplants and is manifested by skin rash, jaundice, abdominal pain, and profuse diarrhea.

Evaluation

A stool assay for *C. difficile* cytotoxin and an assessment of fecal leukocytes should be performed in all patients. Fecal leukocytes are present in more than half of patients infected with *C. difficile*, especially those with severe or pseudomembranous colitis. One negative cytotoxin test result does not exclude the diagnosis, as the sensitivity is only 80% when the first stool sample is examined.

Sigmoidoscopy is not helpful in most patients with nosocomial diarrhea. In patients with mild *C. difficile*-associated diarrhea, the mucosal appearance is usually normal. However, in cases of severe disease, there is a patchy or diffuse colitis with or without pseudomembranes. Therefore, in a patient who has profuse diarrhea or signs of toxicity but whose stool test result is negative for *C. difficile*, flexible sigmoidoscopy should be performed and the patient treated presumptively for *C. difficile* infection if colitis is found. In 10% of cases of severe *C. difficile*-associated colitis, mucosal changes are confined to the proximal colon and are missed by sigmoidoscopy. Sigmoidoscopy also helps diagnose ischemic colitis or cytomegalovirus colitis.

Evaluation for other causes of nosocomial diarrhea should be pursued after *C. difficile* infection has been excluded. Routine stool cultures should be performed in patients with immunosuppression, AIDS, or persistent diarrhea when fecal leukocytes are present. The medication list must be reviewed and possible offending agents discontinued. Diarrhea caused by enteral feedings is suggested by the presence of an increased stool osmolality gap (>100 mOsm/L).

Management

Treatment of nosocomial diarrhea is directed at the underlying cause. In mild cases of antibiotic-associated diarrhea, symptoms usually improve without therapy within 2–3 days after discontinuation of the antibiotic. When *C. difficile*-associated diarrhea is persistent or severe, specific therapy is indicated. Metronidazole (250 mg orally four times daily for 10 days) is the drug of choice because of its high efficacy (>95%) and low cost. Diarrhea and fever begin to respond within 24–48 hours and resolve within 5–10 days. Failure to respond may be a consequence of ileus, perforation, or underlying colonic diseases, such as malignancy, inflammatory bowel disease, or ischemic colitis. Although vancomycin (125 mg orally four times daily) is equally effective, its use is discouraged because it is expensive and promotes the development of vancomycin-resistant organisms. It should be restricted to patients who fail initial treatment with metronidazole. Patients unable to take oral medications because of ileus and patients with severe colitis should be treated with IV metronidazole (500 mg every 6 hours) or with vancomycin given via nasogastric tube or retention enema (500 mg in 500 mL of saline solution every 8 hours). Seriously ill patients with fulminant or intractable symptoms may require colectomy for progressive deterioration, peritonitis, or perforation. After initial resolution, symptoms recur in 20% of cases. Most relapses respond to a second course of treatment. With recurrent relapses, prolonged antibiotic treatment with gradual tapering during 1–2 months may be successful.

Diarrhea associated with enteral feedings usually improves after a reduction in the rate of delivery of the enteral solution (Chapter 15). Iso-osmolar feeding solutions may be better tolerated than hyperosmolar formulations; however, further dilution of the enteral formulation is seldom helpful. Although no clear advantage has been demonstrated with formulations that contain extra fiber, they may benefit some patients. No clear benefit has been demonstrated for elemental or short-peptide enteral formulations. Opioids (loperamide or paregoric) can be useful, but should be avoided in patients with *C. difficile* colitis.

HEPATOMEGALY

The best means of determining liver size is ultrasonography or CT. Physical examination is neither sensitive nor specific in the detection of true enlargement. Half of the livers believed to be enlarged on physical examination are of normal size on ultrasonography. A nonpalpable liver with a percussion span of less than 12 cm in the midclavicular line makes hepatomegaly unlikely. The liver edge is palpable 1–2 cm below the costal margin in approximately one-third of normal adults.

Description and Differential Diagnosis

It is important to distinguish true hepatomegaly from inferior displacement by the right hemidiaphragm. True hepatomegaly can be caused by either focal or diffuse liver disorders. Although this distinction is not always appreciated on physical examination, it is readily established with imaging studies.

Among patients with *diffuse enlargement,* the acute onset of right upper quadrant discomfort is suggestive of hepatic venous congestion or acute hepatitis. Hepatic venous thrombosis (*Budd-Chiari syndrome*) occurs most commonly with hypercoaguable states, renal or hepatocellular carcinoma, and collagen vascular disorders. It can present acutely with right upper quadrant pain and hepatomegaly, or subacutely-to-chronically with hepatomegaly, ascites, and portal hypertension. The presence of hepatomegaly in patients with active alcoholism suggests fatty liver, active hepatitis, or the development of hepatocellular carcinoma. Fatty liver also occurs with obesity or diabetes mellitus. The presence of renal insufficiency and congestive heart failure may suggest amyloidosis. Hemochromatosis can be associated with diabetes and congestive heart failure.

Focal hepatic lesions are caused by cysts, abscesses, and benign and malignant tumors. The presence of fever, right upper quadrant pain, and tender hepatomegaly suggests hepatic abscess. However, some patients present with nonspecific malaise, weight loss, and hepatomegaly. Many abscesses are secondary to biliary disease, intraabdominal infection, or bacteremia, but half have no obvious cause. Amebic abscesses occur in patients with a history of travel to endemic areas. Echinococcosis is rare in the United States, occurring principally in people from sheep-raising regions. Peliosis hepatis is associated with the use of anabolic steroids or with HIV infection and bacillary angiomatosis.

Cavernous hemangiomas, which occur in up to 7% of the population and are almost always asymptomatic, are the most common type of hepatic tumor. Hepatic adenomas occur predominantly in women using birth control pills. Most remain asymptomatic unless complicated by hemorrhage, which can cause a tender right upper quadrant mass or hemoperitoneum. The majority of patients with malignant hepatic tumors lose weight. More than 90% of cases of hepatocellular carcinoma occur in patients with underlying cirrhosis or chronic hepatitis B or C, and in immigrants from Africa or Southeast Asia. Metastatic disease should be suspected in patients with a history of malignancy.

Evaluation

Patients with diffuse hepatomegaly should be asked about any history, symptoms, or signs of liver disease. Comorbid medical illnesses associated with diffuse hepatomegaly should be considered, including congestive heart failure, obesity, diabetes mellitus, and myeloproliferative disorders. Alcohol intake should be carefully assessed. Medication use should be determined.

Patients with focal hepatic lesions should be asked about fevers or chills and about travel history. A review of systems may suggest malignancy with possible hepatic metastases.

Physical examination should include a careful cardiac examination with a search for evidence of right-sided congestive heart failure. The degree of chest inflation and diaphragmatic excursion should be evaluated to exclude a low-lying liver caused by lung hyperinflation. Diffuse lymphadenopathy suggests lymphoma; regional lymph node enlargement suggests malignant disease with nodal and hepatic metastases. Signs of chronic liver disease should be carefully sought. Evidence of weight loss may point to chronic liver disease or metastatic malignancy. Feces positive for occult blood may indicate underlying gastrointestinal malignancy with hepatic metastases.

The liver size, contour, and texture and the presence of tenderness should be determined. Most diffuse liver disorders result in generalized enlargement. Significant tenderness indicates acute inflammation or acute distention (e.g., hepatic venous congestion). A tender, pulsatile liver is seen in tricuspid insufficiency. Cirrhosis leads to a firm, nontender liver with an irregular, nodular consistency. Depending on their size and location, focal liver lesions may or may not be palpable. Hepatic rubs or bruits occur in fewer than 10% of patients with hepatic tumors. The presence of concomitant spleen enlargement narrows the diagnostic considerations. *Hepatosplenomegaly* is most commonly caused by increased portal venous pressures but is also caused by infections and infiltrative disorders.

The extent of evaluation for hepatomegaly depends on the likelihood of underlying disease. It is reasonable to obtain a complete blood cell count and values for liver chemistries, prothrombin time, albumin, ferritin, iron, and transferrin saturation. When diffuse hepatomegaly is present, hemochromatosis is suggested by transferrin saturation above 50% and elevated ferritin levels. The evaluation of focal liver lesions must first distinguish cystic from solid tumors by means of ultrasonography or CT. Uncomplicated cysts require no further evaluation or treatment. In patients with hepatic abscesses, clinicians must distinguish between pyogenic and amebic infection. More than 90% of patients with amebic abscesses have positive serologic tests for *Entamoeba histolytica.* With pyogenic abscesses, diagnostic aspiration for culture under ultrasonographic or CT guidance is recommended before antibiotics are begun. Most benign liver tumors do not cause any significant abnormalities in liver chemistries. The vast majority of hemangiomas are asymptomatic and identified as incidental findings during the evaluation of abnormal liver chemistries by ultrasonography or CT. In such circumstances, they are problematic simply because they must be distinguished from malignant tumors. With metastatic liver disease or hepatocellular carcinoma, elevated alkaline phosphatase is common; however, liver chemistries are normal in half the cases, even in the presence of extensive liver involvement. A marked elevation in lactate dehydrogenase suggests hepatic infiltration by lymphoma or leukemia. Elevated levels of α-fetoprotein are seen in more than 70% of cases of hepatocellular carcinoma, but low levels do not exclude this cancer.

When hepatomegaly is thought to be secondary to hepatic venous congestion or other diffuse liver diseases, ultrasonography is an excellent means of evaluating liver size and excluding focal lesions. It also provides information about the presence of ascites, intra-abdominal varices, and splenomegaly. Ultrasonography with Doppler flow assessment is the preferred screening study to evaluate for hepatic venous thrombosis, and it is also the best study to distinguish cystic from solid liver lesions. Ultrasonography and CT are highly accurate in the diagnosis of hepatic abscess. Abdominal CT has an important role in the evaluation of focal benign or malignant liver lesions. In suspected metastatic disease, chest and abdominal CT may also identify the primary neoplasm. Based on the clinical history and CT or ultrasonographic appearance, most common hepatic focal lesions can be initially and reliably characterized as benign or malignant.

Percutaneous or transjugular liver biopsy is indicated in the evaluation of patients with unexplained diffuse hepatomegaly when the diagnosis cannot be established by other laboratory or imaging tests. Biopsies are particularly helpful in the diagnosis of diseases with diffuse hepatic involvement, such as non-alcoholic steatohepatitis, hemochromatosis, amyloidosis, or Wilson's disease. It also is helpful in the evaluation of patients with unexplained fever (especially the immunocompromised), suspected drug-induced hepatitis, and granulomatous liver disease. Fine-needle biopsy guided by ultrasonography or CT is useful in the evaluation of focal liver lesions.

Management

The extent of further evaluation and management depends on the initial findings and is beyond the scope of this chapter.

ABDOMINAL MASS

When Presenting at the Time of Admission

Description and Differential Diagnosis

An abdominal mass may be noted by the patient or the examining physician. Although the differential diagnosis for such lesions is lengthy, the etiology is determined readily by history, examination, and imaging with CT or ultrasonography. It is important to distinguish masses within the abdominal wall from those that are intra-abdominal. Causes of abdominal wall masses include hernias, lymph nodes, lipomas, hematomas, and abscesses. Intra-abdominal masses include abscesses, hematomas, aneurysms, enlarged solid organs, and feces.

The following questions help to discriminate among abdominal masses. *How long has the mass been present?* A mass that suddenly appears is suggestive of a hernia, hematoma, or abscess. Hematomas are most common in patients with recent trauma or those who are using anticoagulants. A mass that is increasing in size is worrisome for malignancy, abscess, or pseudocyst. Conversely, one that is unchanged over months-to-years is likely to be benign. *Is tenderness or pain present?* Pain or tenderness suggests an infectious or inflammatory process or distention of a hollow viscus, such as the gallbladder or urinary bladder. Severe pain in the epigastrium or back suggests a ruptured aortic aneurysm. *Is there fever?* If so, an intra-abdominal abscess should be considered. *Are there other constitutional symptoms?* Most patients with a palpable malignancy or abscess report fatigue, malaise, and weight loss. *Are there other gastrointestinal symptoms?* Dysphagia, early satiety, or postprandial vomiting suggests a gastric malignancy. Jaundice may be a sign of malignant biliary obstruction caused by pancreatic carcinoma or cholangiocarcinoma. Chronic diarrhea may be caused by Crohn's disease, or it may be pseudo-diarrhea resulting from a nearly obstructing colonic carcinoma. Severe constipation can cause bulky, pliable abdominal masses.

Evaluation

Abdominal examination should include inspection for bulges, asymmetry, and surgical scars. Masses should be characterized by their location, size, consistency, mobility, pulsation, and the presence of tenderness. Masses within the abdominal wall are superficial and best palpated with a light touch. The linea alba, umbilicus, inguinal and femoral canals, and all surgical scars should be palpated carefully with the abdomen relaxed first and then tensed to look for evidence of hernias. Uncomplicated hernias are minimally tender; significant tenderness is worrisome for incarceration with strangulation. For abdominal wall masses, imaging studies typically are not needed. When uncertainty remains, abdominal ultrasonography or CT definitively characterizes the location.

Examination of intra-abdominal masses is best performed with deep palpation. In patients with a right upper quadrant mass, proper examination can distinguish hepatomegaly (discussed in the previous section) from a dilated gallbladder or renal mass. A soft, palpable, nontender gallbladder is noted with malignant obstruction of the biliary tract by pancreatic carcinoma or cholangiocarcinoma, which results in "painless" jaundice. Epigastric masses may be gastric carcinoma, pancreatic carcinoma, or pancreatic pseudocyst. Left upper quadrant masses are caused by splenomegaly or renal disorders.

In the left lower abdomen, a nontender, doughy mass suggests a stool-filled colon. A tender mass in either the right or left lower abdomen is suggestive of an abscess from appendicitis or diverticulitis, especially if accompanied by fever. With Crohn's disease, a right lower quadrant mass may be an inflammatory reaction or abscess. Colonic malignancies are seldom palpable or tender upon abdominal examination unless extracolonic invasion is present. A distended urinary bladder may be confused with other abdominal masses; when in doubt, a catheter should be placed to ensure complete urinary drainage. A rectal examination should be performed to look for evidence of tenderness or fluctuance suggestive of abscess. Bimanual pelvic examination is required in all women to examine the uterus, adnexa, and pelvis. Large ovarian cysts may be palpable on abdominal examination and can be confused with an enlarged bladder. On pelvic examination, most ovarian tumors or cysts and uterine fibroids are nontender. The presence of adnexal pain and tenderness points toward a tubo-ovarian abscess or a hemorrhagic cyst. Abscesses felt on pelvic or rectal examination may also be caused by appendicitis or diverticulitis.

Most intra-abdominal masses warrant further evaluation. Laboratory studies should include a complete blood cell count and liver chemistries. A leukocytosis may indicate intra-abdominal abscess. Iron-deficiency anemia points toward a gastrointestinal malignancy with chronic intestinal blood loss. Elevated alkaline phosphatase and bilirubin indicate cholestasis, which can be caused by pancreatic or biliary cancer or metastatic liver disease. For a mass suspected to be stool, an abdominal radiograph confirms the diagnosis, and the mass should disappear after bowel cleansing. In most other patients, imaging with ultrasonography or CT of the abdomen is needed. Ultrasonography is excellent to screen for gallbladder and biliary tract distention, hepatomegaly or splenomegaly, renal cysts, ovarian or uterine cysts or masses, pancreatic pseudocysts, and abdominal aortic aneurysm. In patients in whom an abdominal mass is unequivocally present on examination, abdominal CT is the study of first choice, as it can distinguish between organomegaly, solid tumor, cyst, and abscess.

Management

The management of abdominal masses depends on the etiology and is beyond the scope of this discussion.

When an Abdominal Mass Appears During the Hospitalization

Description and Differential Diagnosis

The majority of abdominal masses that "appear" during hospitalization were present on admission but overlooked.

Therefore, the differential diagnosis is the same as in the patient presenting an abdominal mass. True masses arising *de novo* are unusual. Hematoma of the rectus sheath should be considered in patients receiving anticoagulants or subcutaneous injections. Intra-abdominal abscess should be suspected in patients with tenderness, fever, or leukocytosis. A large bladder secondary to acute urinary retention and a fecal mass secondary to constipation are common occurrences in the hospitalized patient.

Evaluation and Management

The evaluation and management of the hospitalized patient with an abdominal mass are the same as for the patient presenting at the time of diagnosis.

ABNORMAL LIVER CHEMISTRIES

When Presenting at the Time of Admission

Description and Differential Diagnosis

In the evaluation of the patient with possible liver disease, the history and physical examination are routinely supplemented by determination of liver chemistries. Although liver chemistry abnormalities are nonspecific, different types of hepatic and biliary disorders are associated with certain patterns of abnormalities (Table 77.6). By aiding the initial diagnostic impression, these patterns guide the course of subsequent evaluation with laboratory tests, imaging studies, and liver biopsy.

TABLE 77.6

CAUSES OF LIVER CHEMISTRY ABNORMALITIES

Hepatocellular pattern: aminotransferases >8 times normal; alkaline phosphatase <3 times normal (Chapter 82)

Cholestasis pattern: AST <3 times normal; alkaline phosphatase >2–3 times normal

1. **Infiltrative liver disorders**
   Hepatic malignancy, metastatic or primary
   Primary biliary cirrhosis
   Infections: TB, MAC, *Candida*, other fungal infections, bacillary angiomatosis
   Granulomatous hepatitis (drugs, infections, sarcoidosis)
2. **Intrahepatic and extrahepatic biliary obstruction** (Chapter 84)
   Choledocholithiasis
   Malignant biliary obstruction: pancreas, ampullary, cholangiocarcinoma
   Benign postoperative stricture
   Oriental cholangiohepatitis
   Primary sclerosing cholangitis

AST, aspartate aminotransferase; *MAC*, *Mycobacterium avium complex*; *TB*, tuberculosis.

Indicators of Hepatocellular Damage

Aspartate aminotransferase (AST) and alanine aminotransferase (ALT) are enzymes contained within hepatocytes. Normal serum values of AST and ALT are below 45 IU/L. Although AST can be released from other tissue, such as muscle, ALT is specific for liver injury. An elevation in AST or ALT reflects hepatocellular injury by factors such as viruses, toxins, ischemia, autoimmune disease, and drugs. An enzyme pattern in which the aminotransferase levels are increased to more than eight times normal and the alkaline phosphatase level to less than three times normal is indicative of significant hepatocellular damage. However, many serious causes of chronic hepatocellular injury cause only mild aminotransferase elevation.

The causes of a hepatocellular pattern may be considered according to the level of rise of AST and ALT. A more extensive discussion of the causes and management of acute hepatitis can be found in Chapter 82.

Indicators of Cholestasis

In response to stasis of bile flow, bile duct cells and canaliculi increase the production of alkaline phosphatase, leading to a rise in serum levels. Because alkaline phosphatase also may arise from bone and other organs, γ-glutamyl transpeptidase or 5′-nucleotidase levels are sometimes obtained to confirm the hepatic origin of an increased alkaline phosphatase. A small rise of serum alkaline phosphatase to less than 2–3 times normal is a nonspecific finding that can occur with almost any acute or chronic hepatic or biliary disorder. An increase to more than 2–3 times normal reflects significant cholestasis resulting from extrahepatic biliary tract obstruction, intrahepatic biliary tract obstruction, or infiltrative disorders (see below). The level of rise cannot be used to distinguish among these. Aminotransferase levels also are increased in cholestasis, but usually to less than three times normal.

Bilirubin

Unconjugated ("indirect") bilirubin is the normal end product of the degradation of heme derived from hemoglobin and liver hemoproteins. Circulating unconjugated bilirubin is taken up by hepatocytes through a carrier-mediated mechanism, conjugated in the endoplasmic reticulum to a glucuronide, and secreted across the canalicular membrane into bile, the rate-limiting step in metabolism.

The serum bilirubin level reflects the amount of bilirubin delivered to the liver, the efficiency of hepatocyte bilirubin clearance, and biliary drainage. In normal persons, the serum bilirubin level is less than 1.2 g/dL, and 95% is unconjugated. An increase in pigment production from hemolysis or a resorbing hematoma leads to an increase in serum unconjugated bilirubin. Conditions that affect hepatocyte function, such as hepatitis, may decrease clearance, so that serum direct bilirubin is significantly increased. Obstruction of one hepatic duct or the presence of infiltrative disorders results in a minimal increase of serum conjugated ("direct") bilirubin because of increased excretion by the unobstructed portion of the liver, whereas obstruction of the common bile duct or diffuse hepatic infiltration cause a dramatic rise in bilirubin. With either hepatocellular dysfunction or cholestasis, both direct and indirect bilirubin increase, although the increase in direct bilirubin usually predominates. The levels of direct versus indirect bilirubin are of no value in distinguishing hepatocellular dysfunction from intrahepatic or extrahepatic cholestasis.

Typical Patterns of Alkaline Phosphatase and Bilirubin in Various Conditions

- *More than twofold to threefold rise in alkaline phosphatase with minimal increase in bilirubin:* This pattern is typical of partial biliary tract obstruction, infiltrative liver disorders, or partial biliary tract obstruction.
- *Increase of alkaline phosphatase and bilirubin:* This is most commonly caused by extrahepatic obstruction of the common bile duct by malignancy, postoperative strictures, choledocholithiasis, or sclerosing cholangitis. With choledocholithiasis, the bilirubin level may fluctuate but usually remains below 5 mg/dL; a level above 10 mg/dL is uncommon. Advanced infiltrative liver disorders also may cause a combined increase in alkaline phosphatase and bilirubin.
- *Increase in bilirubin with normal alkaline phosphatase:* An isolated increase in indirect bilirubin may be caused by increased pigment load in cases of hemolysis, recent transfusion, or resorbing hematoma. Gilbert's disease is an autosomal dominant condition affecting 4% of the population; it is characterized by a mild increase in indirect bilirubin (<5 mg/dL), especially during fasting, sleep deprivation, or illness. Some drugs, such as HIV protease inhibitors, can cause isolated rises in either indirect or direct bilirubin through inhibition of bilirubin uptake or metabolism.

Evaluation

The evaluation of the patient with abnormal liver chemistries begins with a detailed assessment of risk factors for liver disease, including alcohol, intravenous drug use, blood transfusions, and prior hepatitis or jaundice. A record of all medications should be obtained, with special attention given to any started during the previous six months. Obesity and adult-onset diabetes mellitus are significant risk factors for steatohepatitis. A history of inflammatory bowel disease raises suspicion for sclerosing cholangitis. A benign stricture may develop after biliary tract surgery. A family history may raise suspicion of hemochromatosis (diabetes, heart failure), α_1-antitrypsin deficiency (early-onset chronic obstructive pulmonary disease), or Wilson's disease (neurologic, psychiatric disease).

Physical examination should note the presence of jaundice and icterus. The acute onset of jaundice with hepatic tenderness in a patient without a prior history of liver disease suggests acute viral hepatitis A or B, alcoholic hepatitis, toxin exposure, or drugs. The presence of jaundice, right upper quadrant pain, and fever suggests acute cholangitis. An indolent onset of jaundice points toward chronic liver disorders, such as cirrhosis, or extrahepatic duct obstruction by malignancy. Physical findings of chronic liver disease suggest advanced disease, most commonly caused by alcohol or chronic viral hepatitis. Such findings include spider angiomas, palmar erythema, gynecomastia, muscle wasting, asterixis, and evidence of portal hypertension (Chapter 83). Evidence of right-sided congestive heart failure suggests hepatic congestion.

In patients with acute liver disease, a rise in the prothrombin time is an ominous finding indicating significant hepatic failure. Because of the long half-life of albumin (20 days), serum albumin is not a useful indicator of hepatic function in patients with acute hepatitis. In patients with chronic liver disease, an increase in the prothrombin time of more than three seconds above normal or a serum albumin level below 3 g/dL reflects significant liver dysfunction.

The evaluation of the patient with acute hepatitis is reviewed in Chapter 82. In patients with elevated aminotransferases, viral serologies for hepatitis B and C (and hepatitis A, if acute) and iron studies should be ordered. Alcohol, potentially hepatotoxic drugs, and toxins should be discontinued. If the etiology remains in doubt, other serologic tests, including those for antinuclear antibody, α_1-antitrypsin, and ceruloplasmin, should be obtained. In patients with persistent aminotransferase abnormalities of uncertain etiology or whose physical examination suggests chronic liver disease, an imaging study is appropriate to look for evidence of chronic liver disease and to screen for primary or metastatic malignancy. α-fetoprotein should be determined in all patients with cirrhosis or chronic viral hepatitis to screen for hepatocellular carcinoma. Liver biopsy is indicated to evaluate the severity of chronic viral hepatitis, look for evidence of drug- or toxin-induced hepatitis, confirm alcoholic liver disease, and diagnose autoimmune hepatitis, hemochromatosis, or Wilson's disease.

The first goal in the evaluation of cholestasis is to distinguish, by means of abdominal ultrasonography, infiltrative liver disorders from disorders causing biliary obstruction (Chapter 84). The presence of dilation of the intrahepatic or extrahepatic biliary ducts confirms biliary obstruction. Biliary dilation may not be present in up to 20% of patients with acute biliary obstruction, especially those with cirrhosis. Therefore, if suspicion of an obstructive lesion is high (especially in patients with suspected cholangitis), ERCP should be performed to establish a definitive diagnosis even if ultrasonography does not demonstrate biliary dilation. In patients in whom there is no evidence of biliary obstruction, infiltrative disorders should be considered. Potential toxic medications should

be discontinued. An anti-mitochondrial antibody determination should be obtained if primary biliary cirrhosis is suspected. A liver biopsy usually is required for definitive diagnosis.

Management

The management of patients with liver chemistry abnormalities depends on the underlying etiology. The management of acute hepatitis is reviewed in Chapter 82. Either ERCP or biliary surgery is necessary to relieve extrahepatic biliary obstruction (Chapter 84).

When Liver Chemistry Abnormalities Appear During the Hospitalization

Description and Differential Diagnosis

The development of liver chemistry abnormalities in the hospitalized patient is a common event. Patients with chronic liver disease are susceptible to worsening of hepatic function in response to illness or major surgery. However, most hospitalized patients in whom liver chemistry abnormalities develop do not have underlying liver disease. The differential diagnosis of liver chemistry abnormalities in the hospitalized setting is limited.

Jaundice

The principal causes of jaundice in the hospitalized setting are increased pigment load, postoperative jaundice, multiple organ failure, total parenteral nutrition (TPN), acalculous cholecystitis, and veno-occlusive disease. Jaundice may follow massive transfusion, resorption of large hematomas after surgery, or severe trauma. Provided there is no intrinsic hepatic dysfunction, the serum indirect bilirubin level is increased but other liver chemistry values remain normal. In the patient with chronic liver disease, both direct and indirect bilirubin levels may rise because of the inability of hepatocytes to handle the need for increased bilirubin conjugation and secretion. Another cause of isolated hyperbilirubinemia is Gilbert's syndrome, which may develop in the setting of fasting or physiologic stress.

Jaundice may develop 2–10 days after a prolonged surgical procedure, especially when it has been complicated by hypotension or the need for transfusions. Bilirubin levels may rise from 10–30 mg/dL, with variable increases in alkaline phosphatase or aminotransferase levels. The etiology of postoperative jaundice is multifactorial. Hepatic ischemia caused by abdominal surgery, hypotension, or hepatic congestion associated with congestive heart failure may "stun" hepatocyte function. In the presence of this postoperative dysfunction, an increased pigment load resulting from transfusions or hematomas can cause profound jaundice. Postoperative infections, sepsis, or TPN can contribute to hepatocyte dysfunction and impaired bilirubin metabolism. Although halothane can cause hepatitis, it now is seldom used, and problems with other inhalational anesthetics are rare. The evaluation of jaundice in the liver transplant patient is discussed in Chapter 85.

Cholestatic jaundice with hyperbilirubinemia and elevated alkaline phosphatase are common in multiple organ system failure and may precede other signs of organ dysfunction, such as acute respiratory distress syndrome (ARDS), hypotension, renal failure, and coagulopathy (Chapter 25). With improved techniques for the administration of TPN, acute hepatic toxicity is unusual in adults. Aminotransferase elevations are common within the first 1–2 weeks of TPN, but these episodes are usually mild and self-limited and require no specific therapy. A rise in alkaline phosphatase and bilirubin occasionally seen after 3–4 weeks of TPN may be attributable to excess total calorie administration or an improper ratio of glucose versus fat (Chapter 15).

Aminotransferase Elevation

Mild-to-moderate rises in aminotransferases in the hospitalized patient usually are caused by medications. The majority of drug reactions are idiosyncratic toxicities that may not develop for weeks to months after initiation of a drug. A causal relationship is often difficult to establish. Hypersensitivity reactions become apparent within 2–10 weeks and are accompanied by fever, eosinophilia, and rash. Marked aminotransferase elevations may be caused by ischemic hepatitis ("*shock liver*") and usually normalize within one week.

Alkaline Phosphatase Elevation

The most common causes of increase are medications or TPN (discussed on p. 763).

Evaluation

Because chronic liver disease increases the risk for hepatic problems in the hospitalized setting, the prior medical history and risk factors for liver disease should be reviewed. A review of liver chemistries before hospitalization may reveal chronic abnormalities suggesting chronic hepatitis from drugs, alcohol, or virus. All medications taken before and during the hospitalization should be reviewed. The use of TPN should be noted and anesthesia records should be reviewed for episodes of hypotension, intraoperative blood loss, and type of anesthetic used. Review of the hospital record should note episodes of hypotension, sepsis, or arrhythmias that may have precipitated hepatic ischemia, and also the number of blood transfusions.

Physical examination should look for findings of chronic liver disease. Fever and right upper quadrant tenderness may indicate acalculous cholecystitis or sludge-induced cholangitis. In patients with congestive heart failure, tender hepatomegaly may suggest hepatic congestion. Fever with hepatomegaly may indicate infiltrative

fungal or bacterial infections, veno-occlusive disease, or graft-versus-host disease.

In the hospitalized patient with jaundice, the paramount goal is to distinguish "medical jaundice" from obstructive jaundice or acalculous cholecystitis. The former is treated with supportive medical care; the latter requires emergent drainage to preclude cholangitis. Therefore, in patients with an elevated direct bilirubin or alkaline phosphatase level, or in patients with nonspecific liver chemistry abnormalities and fever or leukocytosis, abdominal ultrasonography is vital to look for evidence of acalculous cholecystitis, biliary sludge, or choledocholithiasis. In patients with a cholestatic profile suggestive of infiltrative infection, a liver biopsy may be necessary.

Management

For patients with jaundice resulting from transfusions, surgery, or multiple organ failure, therapy is supportive. The jaundice *per se* is of no consequence and resolves gradually. When possible, TPN should be discontinued and enteral feedings begun at the earliest opportunity. Acalculous cholecystitis is discussed in Chapter 84. The management of drug-induced hepatitis associated with hypersensitivity or idiosyncratic reactions depends on the particular drug and the severity of the reaction. The drug should be discontinued in the presence of a hypersensitivity reaction (fever, eosinophilia), symptomatic hepatitis (malaise, fatigue, nausea, vomiting, jaundice), or aminotransferase levels persistently above three times normal values.

KEY POINTS

- Abdominal pain in the hospitalized patient is usually caused by physiologic stress (e.g., mesenteric ischemia), postsurgical or procedural complications, or *Clostridium difficile* colitis.
- In patients with acute vomiting, it is important to distinguish between "medical" and "surgical" causes.
- The fecal leukocyte test often helps separate noninflammatory from inflammatory causes of diarrhea.
- The physical examination for hepatomegaly is unreliable. Imaging studies may be needed to confirm the finding and to differentiate focal from diffuse hepatomegaly.
- Abnormal liver chemistries should be categorized as indicative of hepatocellular damage or of cholestasis.

ADDITIONAL READING

Apfel CC, Korttila K, Abdalla M, et al. A factorial trial of six interventions in the prevention of postoperative nausea and vomiting. *N Engl J Med* 2004;350:2441–2451.

Bartlett JG. Antibiotic-associated diarrhea. *N Engl J Med* 2002; 346:334–339.

Benson AB, Ajani JA, Catalano RB, et al. Recommended guidelines for the treatment of cancer treatment-induced diarrhea. *J Clin Oncol* 2003;22:2918–2926.

Bricker E, Garg R, Nelson R, et al. Antibiotic treatment for *Clostridium difficile*-associated diarrhea in adults. *Cochrane Database Syst Rev* 2005;1:CD004610.

Burke MD. Liver function: test selection and interpretation of results. *Clin Lab Med* 2002;22:377–390.

Faust TW, Reddy KR. Postoperative jaundice. *Clin Liver Dis* 2004;8:151–166.

Gan TJ. Postoperative nausea and vomiting—can it be eliminated? *JAMA* 2002;287:1233–1236.

Hasler WL, Chey WD. Nausea and vomiting. *Gastroenterology* 2003;125:1860–1867.

Hendrickson M, Naparst TR. Abdominal surgical emergencies in the elderly. *Emerg Med Clin North Am* 2003;21:937–969.

Kamin RA, Nowicki TA, Courtney DS, et al. Pearls and pitfalls in the emergency department evaluation of abdominal pain. *Emerg Med Clin North Am* 2003;21:61–72.

Limdi JK, Hyde GM. Evaluation of abnormal liver function tests. *Postgrad Med J* 2003;79:307–312.

Manatsathit S, Dupont HL, Farthing M, et al. Guidelines for the management of diarrhea in adults. *J Gastroenterol Hepatol* 2002;17(suppl):S54–S71.

Musher DM, Musher BL. Contagious acute gastrointestinal infections. *N Engl J Med* 2004;350:2417–2427.

Newton E, Mandavia S. Surgical complications of selected gastrointestinal emergencies: pitfalls in management of the acute abdomen. *Emerg Med Clin North Am* 2003;21:873–907.

Thielman NM, Guerrant RL. Clinical practice. Acute infectious diarrhea. *N Engl J Med* 2004;350:38–47.

Acute Gastrointestinal Bleeding

78

Jonathan P. Terdiman   Peter K. Lindenauer

INTRODUCTION

Acute gastrointestinal bleeding is a common medical condition, accounting for some 350,000–500,000 admissions to acute care hospitals in the United States each year. Overall hospitalization rates and mortality rates for gastrointestinal bleeding have not changed over the past decade. Bleeding can occur in the upper or lower gastrointestinal tract. *Upper gastrointestinal bleeding* is defined as bleeding from the esophagus, stomach, and duodenum. *Lower gastrointestinal bleeding* occurs from a site distal to the duodenum, the most common being the colon. The majority of patients with gastrointestinal bleeding have a self-limited illness and uncomplicated hospital stay. Many patients are admitted to or remain in the hospital despite this very low risk for a poor outcome. However, a sizable minority of patients have further bleeding and complications. Rapidly distinguishing between low- and high-risk patients is essential if care is to be appropriate and cost-effective.

The annual incidence of upper gastrointestinal bleeding is approximately 150 per 100,000 adults in Western populations, affecting twice as many men as women. Upper gastrointestinal bleeding is very common in the elderly; a 20–30 fold increase in incidence is seen between the third and ninth decades of life. Likely as a consequence of this, most patients who present with upper gastrointestinal bleeding are found to have comorbid medical conditions that can play a key role in determining outcome. Between 5%–25% of patients with acute upper gastrointestinal bleeding are already hospitalized for the treatment of another illness.

Lower gastrointestinal bleeding requiring hospitalization is becoming more common, although it is still not as common as upper gastrointestinal bleeding. The annual incidence has previously been reported at approximately 20 per 100,000 adults, but more recent reports place the figure at upwards of 100 per 100,000. Lower gastrointestinal bleeding is slightly more common in men and is overwhelmingly a disease of the elderly. The incidence of lower gastrointestinal bleeding increases more than 200-fold from the third to the ninth decade of life. In approximately 5% of cases, lower gastrointestinal bleeding occurs after hospital admission for another diagnosis.

Gastrointestinal bleeding stops spontaneously in approximately 80% of patients. However, both upper and lower gastrointestinal bleeding can result in considerable morbidity and mortality. The majority of patients with gastrointestinal bleeding require blood transfusions, and 2%–10% of patients require urgent surgery to arrest uncontrolled hemorrhage. The average length of stay varies but in general is approximately 4–7 days. Mortality rates between 2%–10% have recently been reported for patients admitted with gastrointestinal bleeding, translating into an overall mortality rate of approximately 20 per 100,000 in the general population. The mortality rate of patients in whom bleeding develops after admission to the hospital for another reason is over 20%.

Average hospital costs for gastrointestinal bleeding are more than $5,000, with an estimated annual expenditure of more than $2 billion in the United States. Most of the costs incurred are for hospital or ICU stays rather than for physician fees, blood products, medications, or diagnostic tests. Thus, a reduction in the rate of hospital admissions and length of stay has the greatest potential to reduce costs related to gastrointestinal bleeding.

DIAGNOSTIC AND THERAPEUTIC MODALITIES

A great deal of information about diagnosis and prognosis in patients with gastrointestinal bleeding can be obtained by a rapid and directed medical history, physical examination (including a rectal examination), nasogastric tube lavage, and simple laboratory evaluation. The information obtained from these simple steps can determine, with good accuracy, whether the source of bleeding is in the upper or lower gastrointestinal tract; it can also be used to gauge the severity of the event and to guide triage and the use of diagnostic tests and therapies. Key diagnostic tests employed in the patient with gastrointestinal bleeding are endoscopy, including esophagogastroduodenoscopy (EGD), sigmoidoscopy, and colonoscopy; technetium (Tc) 99m red blood cell scintigraphy (RBC scan); and mesenteric angiography. Other, less commonly employed diagnostic tools include barium radiographs, computed tomography (CT), magnetic resonance imaging (MRI), small-bowel endoscopy (enteroscopy), capsule endoscopy, and sodium pertechnetate (Tc) 99m scintigraphy (Meckel's scan).

A number of therapeutic modalities are also available. Ongoing bleeding can be terminated by a variety of invasive techniques, the most common of which involves the endoscopic delivery of hemostatic therapy. In nonvariceal hemorrhage, endoscopic therapy can be accomplished by thermal contact methods (heater probe, multipolar electrocoagulation) or by injection of the site of bleeding with a variety of substances, including dilute epinephrine and sclerosing agents such as alcohol. Less common forms of endoscopic therapy include injection of thrombin or fibrin glue, placement of hemostatic clips, argon plasma coagulation, or laser coagulation of bleeding lesions. Therapy is delivered to actively bleeding lesions, but prophylactic therapy is also delivered to nonbleeding lesions at high risk for rebleeding. In variceal hemorrhage, endoscopic therapy involves the injection of bleeding varices with sclerosing agents such as ethanolamine oleate, tetradecyl sulfate, or sodium morrhuate (sclerotherapy), or the ligation of varices with rubber bands. New forms of endoscopic therapy of variceal bleeding are being developed and include the injection of cyanoacrylate glue. Non-endoscopic therapies for nonvariceal gastrointestinal bleeding include directed intraarterial infusion of vasopressin after diagnostic angiography, embolization of bleeding lesions at angiography, surgical resection, or oversew of sites of bleeding. Refractory variceal hemorrhage can be terminated by the creation of a *transjugular intrahepatic portosystemic shunt* (TIPS). Surgical portosystemic shunting and liver transplant also terminate variceal bleeding, although emergency surgery for portal hypertension is rarely undertaken. Occasionally, balloon tamponade is used to treat ongoing variceal hemorrhage. Until recently, medical therapy was disappointing in its ability to stop ongoing gastrointestinal bleeding or prevent rebleeding. Several recent reports have demonstrated the efficacy of proton pump inhibitors, and possibly octreotide (a synthetic analog of somatostatin), in the control of nonvariceal bleeding, and the use of somatostatin or octreotide is well established in the treatment of variceal bleeding.

UPPER GASTROINTESTINAL BLEEDING

Issues at the Time of Admission

Upper gastrointestinal bleeding can present in a variety of ways. *Hematemesis,* the vomiting of either red blood or material resembling "coffee grounds," is observed in approximately one-fourth of patients. Another fourth present with *melena* alone, and a combination of the two is seen in the remaining half. *Hematochezia,* the passage of red stool, generally signifies a source of bleeding distal to the duodenum but is observed in as many as 15% of cases with upper gastrointestinal pathology, typically in the setting of massive hemorrhage. Most patients seek medical attention after witnessing blood in their vomitus or stool, but in some cases bleeding may be discovered only as part of an evaluation of syncope, chest pain, or fatigue.

Before the diagnosis of upper gastrointestinal bleeding can be made, it is important to exclude other causes of hematemesis or melena. These include bleeding from lesions of the oronasopharynx or respiratory tract. A directed history should focus on features that have been shown to predict etiology or influence outcome. Because peptic ulcer disease is the most common cause of upper gastrointestinal bleeding, a prior history of ulcers or dyspepsia should be sought. Other important historical features include portal hypertension, which predisposes patients to esophageal varices; and a history of coughing or retching, which is reported in as many as 50% of patients later found to have Mallory-Weiss tears. Medications and drugs that predispose to bleeding, such as nonsteroidal antiinflammatory agents (NSAIDs), anticoagulants, and alcohol, warrant review.

Other important historical items to review include the character of the bleeding and the presence of active comorbidities. *"Red blood" hematemesis* is a sign of active bleeding, and studies of prognosis have shown that the risk for rebleeding and death is higher among patients with this presentation than among those who present with "coffee grounds." Cirrhosis is the most important comorbidity to identify because it influences the differential diagnosis and identifies patients more likely to have a poor outcome. Other comorbidities shown to affect outcome adversely include renal failure, disseminated malignancy, cardiac ischemia, congestive heart failure, and sepsis.

Measurement of the vital signs is the most powerful way to evaluate severity of bleeding and lay a framework for appropriate risk stratification. Patients with shock and tachycardia benefit from aggressive resuscitation and early endoscopy. The remainder of the physical examination is of relatively limited diagnostic value but can identify the presence and severity of comorbid conditions. The patient's overall appearance should be observed for signs of hypoperfusion or stigmata of chronic liver disease. An altered level of consciousness in the setting of upper gastrointestinal bleeding is associated with a high risk for aspiration, and the airway should be protected before endoscopy is performed. However, routine endotracheal intubation for airway protection during endoscopy for severe upper gastrointestinal bleeding does not lower mortality or cardiopulmonary complication rates (including aspiration pneumonia). A brief examination of the oronasopharynx can sometimes disclose a previously unsuspected source of bleeding, and examination of the heart and lungs will identify signs of congestive heart failure, pneumonia, or obstructive lung disease. The abdominal examination should note any focal tenderness, peritoneal irritation, or signs of advanced liver disease, such as ascites, splenomegaly, or caput medusae. The patient's stool should be classified as brown, black, or red. Brown stool can be observed early in the course of upper gastrointestinal bleeding, but as little as 50–100 mL of fresh blood will rapidly render it melenic. Hematochezia, although typically a marker of lower gastrointestinal bleeding, can be observed when intestinal transit times are increased, as in the setting of brisk bleeding.

In patients who present with gross rectal bleeding or melena, but no hematemesis, a nasogastric tube should be placed. The finding of a bloody nasogastric aspirate confirms an upper gastrointestinal source of bleeding and can help identify high-risk patients who might benefit from early endoscopy. A nonbloody aspirate does not rule out an upper gastrointestinal source; as many as 15% of patients have this finding. Nevertheless, the presence of a clear aspirate in a patient with melena is a marker of lower risk.

Resuscitation with isotonic fluids (0.9% saline solution or lactated Ringer's solution), infused at a rate proportional to the degree of hemodynamic instability, should begin as soon as the patient arrives in the emergency department. Patients with any high-risk clinical features, even those who do not require immediate volume replacement or transfusion, should have two peripheral intravenous catheters ($\geq$18 gauge) placed in anticipation of rebleeding. Patients who present in shock should receive fluids as rapidly as possible until their hemodynamic status has improved or until complications of volume overload develop. Because cardiac ischemia is a common complication of hemorrhage, the hematocrit should generally be maintained above 25%. Patients with a history of coronary artery disease typically are transfused to maintain the hematocrit above 30%.

Initial laboratory evaluation includes a complete blood cell count, measurement of blood urea nitrogen and creatinine, serum liver chemistries and coagulation studies, and a complete set of serum electrolytes. An additional sample of blood should be sent for typing and cross-matching. Because the initial hematocrit can underestimate the magnitude of blood loss, management decisions should not be unduly influenced by its value. In the face of active bleeding, the clinician should anticipate rather than observe the nadir hematocrit and transfuse accordingly. In the setting of acute gastrointestinal bleeding, an elevated prothrombin time usually indicates advanced liver disease and should immediately raise the possibility of variceal hemorrhage. The utility of the routine chest radiograph is limited but may help identify patients with congestive heart failure or those with free air under the diaphragm. Abdominal films should be limited to patients with pain or distention. Because of the high incidence of ischemic complications, all patients 40 years of age or older and those with a history of coronary heart disease or congestive heart failure should undergo electrocardiography.

Indications for Hospitalization and Intensive Care

Historically, all patients with acute upper gastrointestinal bleeding have been admitted to the hospital for observation. Triage decisions have traditionally been based on clinical factors such as age, degree of hemodynamic instability, and character of the bleeding. Diagnostic/therapeutic endoscopy is carried out in the large majority of patients, usually on the day of or day after admission. Recently, this approach has been challenged by several studies in which clinical and endoscopic risk stratification was completed before admission (1, 2). By using such a strategy, it is possible to distinguish between patients who are likely to rebleed and require hospitalization, and those in whom the risk for rebleeding is negligible and who may be eligible for immediate or early discharge. Important clinical risk factors include advanced age, hemodynamic instability (shock or tachycardia), active red blood hematemesis, and major comorbidities such as congestive heart failure, cirrhosis, and end-stage renal disease. Endoscopic markers of high risk include actively bleeding ulcers, ulcers with visible arterial vessels, ulcers with adherent clots, and esophageal varices. Low-risk lesions include ulcers with a clean base, mucosal erosive disorders such as gastritis or duodenitis, and Mallory-Weiss tears (Table 78.1).

In one prospective study, a combination of similar clinical and endoscopic criteria was used to identify patients at low risk for further bleeding who could be safely managed in the outpatient setting. Approximately one-fourth of patients met the criteria and were discharged from the emergency department, and clinically significant rebleeding developed in less than 3% of patients managed in this way (1). An analysis of data from a nationwide audit of upper gastrointestinal bleeding in the United Kingdom estimated that the same strategy might have eliminated the need for admission in as many as 29% of patients (3), and subsequent studies from the United States have confirmed this finding (4). Thus, an initial strategy of immediate endoscopy for all clinically stable patients is warranted whenever this is available.

TABLE 78.1

PREDICTORS OF OUTCOME IN UPPER GASTROINTESTINAL BLEEDING

Clinical predictors of outcome	Endoscopic predictors of outcome
• Age >60 y	• Low-risk endoscopic findings
• Hemodynamic instability	Esophagitis
Tachycardia	Gastritis
Shock (SBP <100 mm Hg)	Duodenitis
• Comorbidities	Mallory-Weiss tears
Cirrhosis	Clean-based ulcers
Renal failure	• High-risk endoscopic findings
Metastatic cancer	Active bleeding of any lesion
Congestive heart failure	Peptic ulcers with visible
Cardiac ischemia	vessel or clot
Sepsis	Esophageal/gastric varices
Encephalopathy	
• Hematemesis	
• Coagulopathy	

SBP, systolic blood pressure.

Advanced age, persistent tachycardia, severe anemia, and significant comorbidities all warrant admission to an acute care bed. Where immediate endoscopy is not available to complete risk stratification, admission for all patients with acute gastrointestinal bleeding is recommended. Patients with shock or unstable major comorbidities, especially advanced liver disease, renal failure, congestive heart failure, or cardiac ischemia, and those who require intubation for airway protection should be initially managed in the ICU. Therapeutic endoscopy should be performed when the patient has been fully resuscitated and when life-threatening conditions have been stabilized.

Initial Therapy

Endoscopy is the diagnostic "gold standard" and has been shown to be an effective method of achieving hemostasis and reducing mortality for patients with nonvariceal upper gastrointestinal bleeding (5) (Table 78.2). Endoscopic therapeutic techniques are able to achieve initial hemostasis in 80% of actively bleeding, nonvariceal lesions. Injection and thermal therapies have similar rates of success; a combination of the two modalities may be superior than either alone for patients with spurting hemorrhage.

Newer endoscopic therapies, such as hemostatic clipping, have not yet been convincingly demonstrated to be superior to the standard techniques. With endoscopic sclerotherapy or band ligation, it is also possible to achieve hemostasis in as many as 75%–80% of patients with variceal bleeding. In addition to performing therapeutic functions, endoscopy provides prognostic information that can be used to estimate a patient's likelihood of rebleeding and mortality (Table 78.3) and assign an appropriate level of care. Population-based studies suggest that the clinical

TABLE 78.2

THERAPEUTIC ENDOSCOPY AND OUTCOME IN UPPER GASTROINTESTINAL BLEEDING

Therapy	Rebleeding odds ratio	Surgery odds ratio	Death odds ratio
Thermal	0.32	0.31	0.67
Laser	0.58	0.58	0.49
Injection	0.23	0.18	0.50
All	0.38	0.36	0.55

Odds ratios refer to the risk for rebleeding, requiring surgery, or dying, when the reference group (i.e., odds ratio of 1 for these negative outcomes) is drawn from similar patients who did not receive therapeutic endoscopy.
Adapted from Cook DJ, Guyatt GH, Salena BJ, et al. Endoscopic therapy for acute nonvariceal upper gastrointestinal hemorrhage: a meta-analysis. *Gastroenterology* 1992;102:139–148, with permission.

outcomes of high-risk patients who undergo endoscopy within 24 hours of admission are superior to those of patients in whom endoscopy is delayed, in great part because of the delivery of endoscopic therapy (6).

In addition, routine performance of a "second look" endoscopy in high-risk patients, may improve outcomes by detecting and treating persistent non-bleeding visible vessels. For patients at lower risk, early endoscopy can reduce the total duration of hospitalization by over 30% (Figure 78.1). This reduction is attributable to the delineation of low-risk features that allow for safe early discharge of patients (7).

Because endoscopy plays a central role in the diagnosis, treatment, and risk stratification of patients with upper gastrointestinal bleeding, early consultation with a skilled endoscopist is recommended for all patients. Consultation should be obtained after the initial resuscitation and evaluation have been completed. In many cases, patients will be found to be suitable candidates for immediate or early endoscopy.

Effective pharmacologic therapy for acute upper gastrointestinal bleeding has been challenging to identify. In recent years, the somatostatin analog octreotide has proved successful in controlling *variceal bleeding*, and may be as

TABLE 78.3

ULCER APPEARANCE AND PROGNOSIS IN PEPTIC ULCER DISEASE

Appearance	Prevalence (%)	Rebleed (%)	Mortality (%)
Clean base	42	5	2
Flat spot	20	10	3
Clot	17	22	7
Visible vessel	17	43	11
Active bleeding	18	55	11

Adapted from Laine L, Peterson WL. Bleeding peptic ulcer. *N Engl J Med* 1994;331:717–727, with permission.

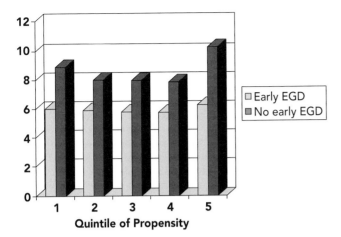

Figure 78.1 Unadjusted length of stay in patients who underwent endoscopy within 1 day of admission and those who did not, stratified by quintile of propensity of undergoing early endoscopy. Within each quintile of patients, length of stay was lower in patients who underwent endsocopy (p <0.0001). (Adapted from Cooper GS, Chak A, Connors AF, et al. The effectiveness of early endoscopy for upper gastrointestinal hemorrhage, a commmunity analysis. *Medical Care* 1998;36:462–474, with permission.)

good as or better than emergency endoscopic therapy for the initial control of bleeding. Its early and empiric use should be considered in patients with known cirrhosis or evidence of advanced liver disease. The combination of endoscopic therapy and octreotide has been demonstrated to reduce rebleeding rates better than either modality alone (8). The standard dose of octreotide is a 50-mg intravenous bolus followed by a continuous infusion at 50 mg/h. All patients found to have a variceal source of bleeding at endoscopy should remain on octreotide for 48–72 hours. The benefits of octreotide may extend beyond patients with varices to all those with nonvariceal upper gastrointestinal bleeding. In a meta-analysis, it appeared that the use of octreotide reduced rates of rebleeding by 27%–47% (9). These findings have not yet translated into widespread changes in clinical practice.

Despite numerous randomized controlled trials attesting to their ineffectiveness in the management of acute bleeding, H$_2$ receptor antagonists continue to be commonly used in this setting. *The use of these agents is not warranted.* However, proton pump inhibitors (PPIs) have become standard therapy for patients with high-risk upper gastrointestinal bleeding. Recent studies have demonstrated that the use of intravenous, or high dose oral, PPIs is effective at reducing rates of rebleeding, decreasing the need for blood transfusions, and decreasing length of hospital stay. Moreover, PPIs are cost-effective when used in patients that have received endoscopic therapy for nonvariceal bleeding (10, 11).

Both freshly frozen plasma and platelet concentrates are commonly used in the management of selected patients with upper gastrointestinal bleeding, but their efficacy is unproven. In general, patients with active bleeding and a significant coagulopathy should receive vitamin K and

freshly frozen plasma to reduce the prothrombin time to less than 1.5 times the midpoint of the institutional control. Patients with coagulopathy in the setting of advanced liver disease should receive vitamin K parenterally. Platelet transfusions should be reserved for actively bleeding patients who have platelet counts of less than 50,000/μL or have taken irreversible platelet inhibitors within three days of the bleeding episode. For details of managing coagulopathy, see Chapter 98.

Issues During the Course of Hospitalization

Determining the Need for Continued Hospitalization

Bleeding ceases spontaneously in 70%–80% of patients, but rebleeding remains a serious problem for a significant minority. Determining the need for continued hospitalization after the resolution of the initial episode of bleeding should be based on the patient's expected probability of rebleeding or death and on the management of any active comorbid conditions. A simplified scoring system based on clinical and endoscopic variables that can be used to predict rebleeding and mortality has been developed (Table 78.4 and Figure 78.2).

TABLE 78.4

SCORING SYSTEM FOR PREDICTING REBLEEDING AND MORTALITY

Variable	Score
Age (y)	
<60	0
60–79	1
≥80	2
Shock	
None	0
Tachycardia	1
Hypotension (SBP <100 mm Hg)	2
Comorbidity	
None	0
CAD, CHF, other major comorbidity	2
Renal failure, liver failure, malignancy	3
Diagnosis	
Mallory-Weiss tear or no lesion observed	0
All other diagnoses	1
Malignant lesions	2
Stigmas of recent hemorrhage	
None or spot in ulcer base	0
Blood in the GI tract, clot, visible or spurting vessel in ulcer base	2

CAD, coronary artery disease; *CHF,* congestive heart failure; *GI,* gastrointestinal; *SBP,* systolic blood pressure.
Adapted from Rockall TA, Logan RF, Devlin HB, et al. Risk assessment after acute upper gastrointestinal haemorrhage. *Gut* 1996;38: 316–321, with permission.

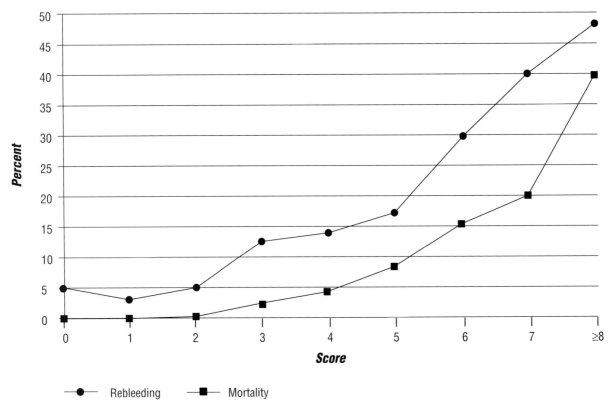

Figure 78.2 Rebleeding and mortality rates, in percentages, by risk score. (Adapted from Rockhall TA, Logan RF, Devlin HB, et al. Selection of patients for early discharge or outpatient care after acute upper gastrointestinal haemorrhage. National Audit of Acute Upper Gastrointestinal Haemorrhage. *Lancet* 1996;347:1138–1140, with permission.)

A growing body of literature has shown that treatment guidelines or clinical care pathways that incorporate the early discharge of stable patients with a low risk for rebleeding significantly reduce length of stay, save money, and do not lead to increased adverse outcomes (12, 13). An example of a guideline that combines local expertise and an evidence-based approach is shown in Table 78.5.

Refeeding

Patients should receive nothing by mouth until an endoscopy has been performed. Those found to have low-risk lesions can resume a normal diet immediately, whereas patients with moderate- or high-risk lesions should continue to have nothing by mouth for 24–48 hours.

Identification and Management of Rebleeding

A high degree of vigilance is required to detect rebleeding, because there may be a long delay between its onset and the appearance of overt blood. New hematemesis always indicates rebleeding and should prompt immediate action. In contrast, melena may persist for several days following an initial episode of bleeding. Marked changes in blood pressure, the development of tachycardia, or an unanticipated decline in the hematocrit should prompt repeat nasogastric aspiration and generally a repeat endoscopy. The effectiveness of repeat endoscopy in patients with rebleeding peptic ulcers has been demonstrated, with repeat endoscopy leading to durable hemostasis in 75% of patients, reduced need for surgery, and reduced complication rates compared with an operation at the first episode of rebleeding. Nevertheless, surgical intervention is required in 2%–10% of patients with gastrointestinal bleeding. Surgical consultation is mandatory whenever rebleeding has been detected because of the high risk for serious complications.

Discharge Issues

Most patients with acute gastrointestinal bleeding will be suitable for discharge within 1–4 days following admission. Rebleeding and cardiopulmonary complications of bleeding, such as myocardial infarction or aspiration pneumonia, can significantly prolong the hospital course. Once bleeding has resolved, hemodynamic status has returned to normal, and the risk for rebleeding has fallen to an acceptable level, patients can be safely discharged provided that other comorbidities are stable. Melena in the absence of other signs of rebleeding is not an indication for continued hospitalization.

TABLE 78.5

CLINICAL AND ENDOSCOPIC RISK STRATIFICATION AND TRIAGE FOLLOWING ENDOSCOPY

RISK ASSESSMENT: CLINICAL AND ENDOSCOPIC

Low	Moderate	High
CLINICAL FINDINGS		
Age <60 y	Age ≥60 y	—
Initial SBP ≥100 mm Hg; vital signs now normal	SBP ≥100 mm Hg on admission and/or mild ongoing tachycardia	Current SPB <100 mm Hg and/or severe ongoing tachycardia
Transfusion requirement <2 U	Transfusion requirement ≥2 U	Transfusion requirement ≥5 U
No active major comorbid disease[a]	Stable major comorbid disease[a]	Unstable major comorbid disease[a]
No liver disease	Liver disease—no coagulopathy or encephalopathy	Decompensated liver disease
No moderate- or high-risk clinical features	No high-risk clinical features	—
ENDOSCOPIC FINDINGS		
Clean ulcer <2 cm	Clean ulcer ≥2 cm	Bleeding ulcer
	Ulcer with spot or clot	Visible vessel
Nonbleeding Mallory-Weiss tear	Bleeding Mallory-Weiss tear successfully treated	Variceal bleeding
Esophagitis		Any lesion with bleeding that was not controlled at endoscopy
Gastritis duodenitis	Bleeding AVM successfully treated	
	No lesion identified and no fresh blood seen	Portal gastropathy without esophageal varices
	Neoplasm	

TRIAGE GUIDELINES

		CLINICAL		
		Low	**Moderate**	**High**
E N D O S C O P I C	**Low**	Immediate discharge	23 h observation[b]	ICU observation (48–72 h hospitalization)
	Moderate	48 h observation[c]	48–72 h observation[c]	ICU observation (48–72 h hospitalization)
	High	ICU observation (72 h hospitalization)	ICU observation (72 h hospitalization)	ICU observation (72 h hospitalization)

AVM, arteriovenous malformation.
[a] Major comorbid diseases include ischemic heart disease, CHF, acute renal failure, sepsis, disseminated malignancy, altered mental status, pneumonia, COPD/asthma.
[b] Patients may be discharged following 23 hours of observation if there is no evidence of rebleeding, vital signs are normal, there is no further need for transfusion, and the hematocrit has remained stable at the target range.
[c] In general, the same criteria for discharge as noted above hold true. Given the moderate risk for rebleeding, current standard of practice is to observe these patients for a period longer than 24 hours.

Most patients are able to return home following acute gastrointestinal hemorrhage and can resume normal activities as tolerated. Patients discharged with anemia should be advised that they may experience fatigue and dyspnea on exertion for several weeks following discharge and may benefit from iron replacement. Patients should be instructed to contact their primary care physician or return to an emergency department if hematemesis recurs or if they notice hematochezia or melena. Routine follow-up with the primary care physician should be scheduled within 1–2 weeks, depending on the patient's overall functional status.

Measures to prevent recurrent variceal bleeding and treat peptic ulcers and erosive mucosal disorders should be addressed at the time of discharge. Both nonselective β-blockers and a combination of β-blockers with long-acting nitrates have proved effective for the secondary prevention of variceal bleeding. Patients with documented peptic ulcers should undergo biopsy or serologic testing for *Helicobacter pylori* infection and should be treated according to current regimens, since this has been demonstrated to reduce rates of future bleeding (Chapter 80). Patients should be counseled to avoid NSAIDs and aspirin-containing compounds and to abstain from alcohol. Proton pump inhibitors or misoprostol should be given to patients who must resume NSAIDs or aspirin to prevent ulcer recurrence, although neither therapy is entirely effective. Alternatively, NSAIDs that selectively inhibit cyclooxygenase-2 (COX-2) (e.g., celecoxib, rofecoxib) appear to cause fewer gastrointestinal problems than do traditional NSAIDs, but their use can still lead to gastrointestinal hemorrhage. Recent concerns about cardiac toxicity should also be factored into decision-making regarding COX-2 inhibitors (14).

LOWER GASTROINTESTINAL BLEEDING

Issues at the Time of Admission

Hematochezia is characteristic of lower gastrointestinal bleeding. Unfortunately, the presence or absence of hematochezia cannot be used to distinguish upper from lower gastrointestinal bleeding with certainty (see p. 768). Although melena usually implies a source of bleeding in the upper tract, it can occur when the source of bleeding is in the small bowel and occasionally when the source is in the right side of the colon.

The majority of episodes of lower gastrointestinal bleeding are painless, though mild lower abdominal cramps may accompany the passage of bloody stool. Painless bleeding is the norm with diverticula, vascular ectasias, neoplasms, and hemorrhoids. Marked abdominal pain and tenderness can occur when bleeding occurs in the setting of ischemia, as in ischemic colitis, or in association with bowel inflammation, as in an infectious colitis or inflammatory bowel disease.

Because the distinction between upper and lower gastrointestinal bleeding is not always possible at initial presentation, the initial approach to management is the same for all patients. Rapid evaluation of hemodynamic status is mandatory, and prompt volume replacement is essential. Patients with abnormal vital signs or with evidence of ongoing blood loss based on the continuing passage of blood per rectum require placement of a minimum of two large-bore peripheral intravenous catheters. As with upper bleeding, volume replacement with isotonic crystalloid solutions should commence immediately, and blood products should be infused as soon as they become available to correct any significant laboratory abnormalities. Recommendations with respect to the appropriate use of blood products are the same as for upper gastrointestinal bleeding.

During the initial resuscitation of the patient, a directed medical history should be taken and physical examination performed. The initial vital signs and the response of the vital signs to the initial resuscitative efforts are the most important determinants of the severity of the bleed. The patient should be asked about hematemesis, the location of any abdominal pain, and any previous history of gastrointestinal disease or hemorrhage, as this information may suggest the diagnosis and lead to a consideration of bleeding in the upper tract. It is important to inquire about past abdominal operations, especially previous repair of an abdominal aneurysm, as *aortoenteric fistula* is a rare but often fatal cause of lower gastrointestinal bleeding. As in patients with bleeding from the upper tract, the remainder of the history should be directed toward identifying active comorbid conditions that can complicate the hospital course. A complete list of medications should be obtained. During the physical examination, the clinician should look for evidence of decompensated cardiopulmonary and liver disease, and the abdomen should be observed to determine if any significant focal tenderness or other abnormalities are present. Initial laboratory evaluation should be the same as for the patient with upper gastrointestinal bleeding, and a specimen should be sent to the blood bank for typing and cross-match. Bleeding caused by an inflammatory process is often associated with an elevated leukocyte count. Abdominal radiographs are not needed unless significant abdominal tenderness is present on physical examination.

A nasogastric tube aspirate should be obtained in all patients with clinically important bleeding in an attempt to distinguish upper from lower tract bleeding, even if the only overt manifestation of bleeding is hematochezia. A positive nasogastric aspirate for blood should trigger an endoscopic evaluation of the upper gastrointestinal tract. A negative nasogastric aspirate does not rule out an upper gastrointestinal bleed, although the presence of bile (without blood) makes an upper source very unlikely. Many experts support the rapid performance of upper gastrointestinal endoscopy in patients presenting with shock regardless of the results of nasogastric tube aspiration, especially in circumstances in which an operation is planned to treat lower tract bleeding when the site of bleeding has not been definitively identified.

In a patient presenting with hematochezia, careful inspection of the anorectum by digital examination and anoscopy is important. The examination may demonstrate a bleeding lesion, such as hemorrhoids or an anal fissure, which often can be treated at the bedside. Even if an anorectal source of bleeding is identified, most experts still recommend a complete evaluation of the lower gastrointestinal tract, although this may be performed electively.

Use of a flexible sigmoidoscope as part of the initial evaluation of patients presenting with clinically important hematochezia is widely recommended but is practiced routinely at few hospitals. It is unclear if the routine performance of urgent sigmoidoscopy at presentation would reduce admission rates and otherwise alter outcomes.

The list of possible sources of lower gastrointestinal bleeding is long, but colonic diverticulosis is the most common source and accounts for 20%–50% of cases. Other common sources of bleeding are colonic vascular ectasias, colonic neoplasms, colonic ulcers, colitis, and hemorrhoids. Small-bowel sources of bleeding are rare, accounting for fewer than 10% of cases of lower gastrointestinal bleeding.

Indications for Hospitalization and Intensive Care

Clinical risk stratification for patients with lower gastrointestinal bleeding is not as well defined as it is for those with upper gastrointestinal bleeding. A recent study identified seven clinical features that were predictive of severe lower gastrointestinal bleeding; tachycardia, low systolic blood pressure, syncope, nontender abdominal examination, bleeding per rectum during the first four hours of evaluation, aspirin use, and more than two active comorbid conditions (15). In up to 80% of cases of bleeding from the lower tract, the bleeding stops spontaneously and does not recur. Outpatient evaluation of patients with self-limited hematochezia is possible if there is no evidence of hypovolemia. Anemia alone does not necessitate hospitalization if it seems likely that the blood loss has been chronic and the present transfusion requirement is not great. All patients with abnormal vital signs or who continue to pass blood per rectum require hospitalization. Hospitalization also is appropriate for patients with significant abdominal pain, tenderness, or fever, and for patients with active comorbid medical conditions. All patients with a history of previous aortic surgery should be hospitalized, even if it appears that the bleeding has stopped, as an aortoenteric fistula may present with a self-limited "herald" bleed before an exsanguinating hemorrhage. The indications for hospitalization in patients with hematochezia are summarized in Table 78.6.

A subset of patients with lower gastrointestinal bleeding requires ICU admission. Patients in shock and or with massive hematochezia should be admitted to the ICU initially. The severity of other comorbid conditions should be taken into account during triage decisions.

Diagnosis

In light of the possible difficulties of distinguishing upper from lower gastrointestinal bleeding on clinical grounds, upper gastrointestinal endoscopy should be performed if any doubt remains, especially in the setting of a clinically severe bleed. Unfortunately, there is presently no standardized diagnostic and therapeutic approach to the patient with clinically important lower gastrointestinal bleeding. The specific diagnostic sequence is determined in part by the clinical status of the patient and the rate and pattern of bleeding, but also by local experience and expertise of the treating physicians. Massive bleeding often starts and stops

---

TABLE 78.6

INDICATIONS FOR HOSPITALIZATION IN PATIENTS WITH HEMATOCHEZIA

Abnormal vital signs
Continued passage of blood per rectum
Severe anemia (i.e., Hb <8 g/dL)
Fever, leukocytosis
Abdominal pain, tenderness
Unstable comorbid conditions
Suspicion of upper tract bleeding
Previous aortic surgery

Hb, hemoglobin.

spontaneously, thereby frustrating diagnostic efforts. In up to 20% of patients with clinically important lower gastrointestinal bleeding, a definitive diagnosis is never established.

Colonoscopy, technetium (Tc) 99m red blood cell scintigraphy, and selective mesenteric angiography are the most commonly employed diagnostic tests in the evaluation of lower gastrointestinal bleeding. *Colonoscopy* is the procedure of choice whenever bleeding has stopped. At colonoscopy, diverticula, vascular ectasias, neoplasms, ulcers, and areas of inflammation can be seen with good sensitivity. Because many of these lesions are common in the population at large, establishing the causal bleeding site in the absence of active bleeding may be difficult. The diagnostic evaluation of patients with ongoing or recurrent lower gastrointestinal bleeding remains controversial. Some experts support the performance of an RBC scan as the first test, whereas others recommend mesenteric angiography. Still other experts favor emergency colonoscopy after a rapid colonic purge as the initial test of choice. *RBC scintigraphy* can localize a site of gastrointestinal bleeding when rates of bleeding are as low as approximately 1 unit every 2–4 hours. Ideally, scintigraphy can detect and localize the site of bleeding with sensitivity five times greater than that of angiography. Scintigraphy cannot establish a specific diagnosis and has no therapeutic potential, but it can direct further diagnostic and therapeutic interventions, such as angiography or surgery, should they become necessary. In clinical practice, a great deal of controversy exists regarding the value of the RBC scan. *Selective visceral angiography* can localize the site of bleeding when the rate of bleeding is approximately 1 unit hourly. Even when angiography does not show extravasation of contrast into the bowel lumen, it may be diagnostic of abnormalities suggestive of a site of bleeding, such as a vascular ectasia.

Mesenteric angiography also has therapeutic potential (e.g., embolization of bleeding vessels and intraarterial infusion of vasoconstrictors such as vasopressin). Unfortunately, angiography has an associated morbidity of approximately 10%, including arterial thrombosis and dye-induced acute renal failure. Although angiography can be both diagnostic and therapeutic in patients with lower gastrointestinal bleeding, its precise role and value have not been established clearly. Some investigators argue that colonoscopy should be the test of choice for lower gastrointestinal bleeding, even when the bleeding is ongoing. In their hands, colonoscopy is technically possible in this setting after a rapid purge, and the diagnostic yield of this approach is far greater than that of angiography (>80% vs. <20%). In addition, colonoscopy does permit the delivery of endoscopic therapy to selected lesions, including actively bleeding diverticula, or those with a visible vessel (16). However, precise identification of the bleeding diverticulum remains uncommon, even with early colonoscopy. In one study, colonoscopy reduced rates of angiography from 50% to less than 5%, and the need for emergency surgery from 20% to less than 5%. Length of stay in the ICU was reduced by a mean of two days and the total hospital stay by at least three days, which resulted in a large reduction in the cost of services (17). Early colonoscopy (within 24 hours) also has been associated with a shorter length of hospitalization, primarily attributable to earlier delineation of low-risk stigmata rather than to the delivery of endoscopic therapy to high-risk lesions (18).

Other diagnostic tests are occasionally used in patients with lower gastrointestinal bleeding. Those with significant abdominal pain or tenderness may benefit from abdominal and pelvic CT. In patients with a previous history of aortic aneurysm or aortic surgery, the combination of CT and endoscopy beyond the duodenum is the best method of diagnosing an aortoenteric fistula. Aortogram is not as useful a test for this diagnosis. If a site of bleeding is suspected in the small bowel based on scintigraphy or angiography, an endoscopic examination of the small bowel with an

enteroscope is appropriate. The newest generation of scopes can examine the small intestine to approximately 100 cm beyond the ligament of Treitz. Lesions such as vascular ectasias and ulcers can be detected and, if need be, treated. Recently video capsule endoscopy has been introduced as a new method of detecting bleeding lesions in the small intestine beyond the reach of the enteroscope (19). If bleeding has stopped, a *small-bowel contrast study*, such as an enteroclysis, can be used to look for small-bowel pathology, such as ulcers, diverticula, Crohn's disease, or neoplasms. In young patients with lower gastrointestinal bleeding of obscure origin, a *Meckel's scan* should be performed.

A recommended diagnostic algorithm for patients with hematochezia is presented in Figure 78.3.

Therapy

As more than 80% of episodes of lower gastrointestinal bleeding spontaneously stop and do not recur, specific

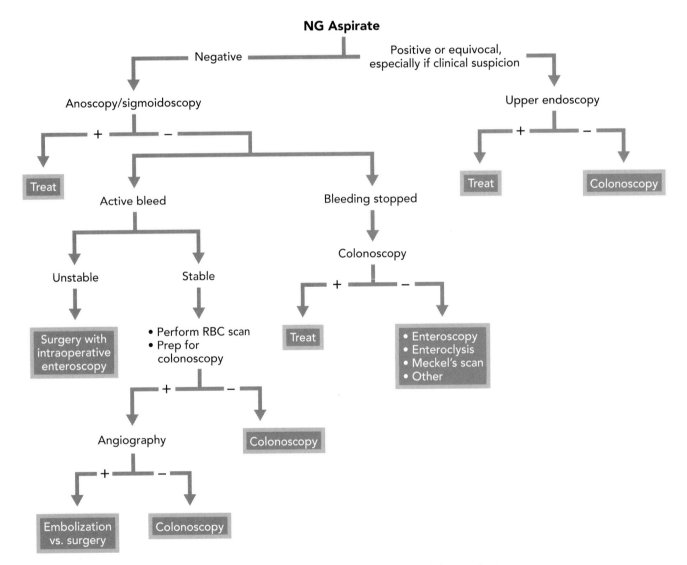

Figure 78.3 Diagnostic algorithm for patients with hematochezia.

therapy to arrest hemorrhage is generally not needed. Therapeutic maneuvers primarily are supportive. Medical therapy has been disappointing in its ability to arrest ongoing bleeding, prevent recurrent bleeding, and improve outcomes.

Endoscopic therapy is preferable to angiographic or surgical therapy if it is possible, and it may be possible in a significant fraction of cases of lower gastrointestinal bleeding. However, large controlled trials to evaluate the use of endoscopic therapy in lower gastrointestinal bleeding and define patients who would benefit from such therapy have not been performed. The type of therapy chosen depends on the lesion encountered. For bleeding vascular ectasias, thermal contact methods are the treatment of choice, whereas for ulcers and bleeding after polypectomy, either thermal contact methods or injection therapy can be employed. Bleeding polyps can be removed endoscopically, and bleeding from larger neoplasms can sometimes be stopped temporarily by epinephrine injection until definitive surgical therapy can be undertaken. Investigators have reported successful endoscopic treatment of bleeding diverticula with epinephrine injection or thermal contact methods (16).

Angiographic treatment of lower gastrointestinal bleeding is possible. Intraarterial infusion of vasopressin can arrest bleeding in up to 90% of cases, although bleeding will recur in as many as 50%–70% of cases on withdrawal of therapy. Small studies have demonstrated the efficacy and safety of subselective embolization of bleeding vessels, although concerns about the risks for intestinal infarction remain.

Surgical resection of bleeding lesions remains a viable therapeutic approach for patients with persistent lower gastrointestinal hemorrhage. Rarely, patients present with massive hematochezia, and attempts to fully resuscitate the patient and establish the location of the site of bleeding are impossible. Such patients require urgent surgical intervention to control the bleeding and prevent exsanguination. Intraoperative endoscopy can be attempted to localize the bleeding site if it is not obvious at laparotomy. Total abdominal colectomy is often undertaken if no site of bleeding can be localized in the operating room. Complication and rebleeding rates following this procedure are significant. Fortunately, this form of intervention is rarely required.

Much more commonly, patients have bleeding that starts, stops, and then starts again. The site of bleeding may or may not have been documented by previous diagnostic studies. The role of surgery in the management of these patients is not defined. Decisions about the need for and timing of surgical intervention are based on factors such as the number of episodes of rebleeding, total volume of blood transfused, clinical severity of each episode, and the patient's operative risk. Because the management of clinically important lower gastrointestinal bleeding is complex, gastroenterologic and surgical consultation should be obtained at the time of hospitalization in all patients.

Issues During the Course of Hospitalization

In the majority of cases, lower gastrointestinal bleeding stops and does not recur, and the hospital course is uncomplicated. Many patients may be eligible for early discharge once they are resuscitated. Risk assessment in lower gastrointestinal bleeding is based mostly on expert opinion, as large prospective studies exploring the relationship of clinical presentation, medical history, and endoscopic diagnosis to outcome have not been undertaken.

In our opinion, assessment of the clinical history and endoscopic diagnosis can be used to predict outcome and determine the need for ongoing hospitalization in patients with lower gastrointestinal bleeding (Table 78.7). Patients with high-risk features should be observed in the ICU for at least 24 hours and should remain in the hospital for at least 72 hours. Moderate-risk endoscopic findings include nonbleeding colonic ulcers, vascular ectasias that can be endoscopically treated, and bleeding polyps that can be endoscopically resected. Patients with these endoscopic findings and without high-risk clinical features should be observed in the hospital but can be given a regular diet. The optimal duration of inpatient observation is unclear, but it probably is safe to discharge these patients if there has been no sign of active bleeding for more than 24 hours. Low-risk endoscopic findings include bleeding hemorrhoids and mild colitis. In the absence of high-risk clinical features, such patients are appropriate for immediate discharge.

A difficult situation arises when no diagnosis can be established after conventional endoscopy of the upper and lower tract. A small bowel source of bleeding should be suspected, and these patients should remain in the hospital for further diagnostic evaluation. If no diagnosis is established, patients should be observed in the hospital for a minimum of 48–72 hours for rebleeding.

TABLE 78.7

CRITERIA THAT HELP IDENTIFY HIGH-RISK PATIENTS WITH LOWER GASTROINTESTINAL BLEEDING WHO REQUIRE ONGOING HOSPITAL OBSERVATION

Clinical criteria
  Presentation with shock
  Ongoing abnormality of vital signs
  Transfusion requirement of >3–4 units of blood on a single day
  Recurrent episodes of bleeding during hospital stay
  Persistent fever, abdominal pain or tenderness, leukocytosis
  Unstable comorbid conditions

Endoscopic criteria
  Diverticulum with active bleeding, visible vessel, or adherent clot
  Severe ischemic colitis
  Cancer
  Colonic ulcer with active bleeding, visible vessel, or adherent clot

During hospital observation, clinicians should be watching carefully for an exacerbation of comorbid medical conditions and for evidence of rebleeding. Passage of dark blood or melena per rectum does not necessarily indicate rebleeding. An assessment of the vital signs and the hematocrit will aid in the diagnosis of rebleeding. Passage of bright red blood indicates that bleeding has resumed. Appropriate management for an episode of rebleeding is not well defined and requires a case-by-case approach.

Discharge Issues

Patients are eligible for discharge after an appropriate interval of observation if bleeding has not recurred, the vital signs are normal, further transfusion is not required, and any comorbid medical conditions are stable. During a follow-up period of several years, a significant minority of patients requires readmission for further bleeding and a significant minority die, although death is rarely related to acute lower gastrointestinal bleeding. Of cases of diverticular bleeding in which surgical resection is not performed, bleeding recurs in approximately 10% by one year and in 25% by four years. Of patients admitted for their second diverticular bleed, approximately 50% have further bleeding after discharge. The rate of rebleeding requiring readmission for other diagnoses has not been well defined.

No ongoing medical therapy after discharge has been demonstrated to reduce rates of rebleeding or to improve long-term outcomes. Lower gastrointestinal bleeding is associated with aspirin and NSAID use. Whenever possible, these medications should be discontinued permanently or resumed in the lowest possible dose after an interval of several months. The risk associated with resumption of anticoagulants is unclear and must be determined on an individual basis.

GASTROINTESTINAL BLEEDING DEVELOPING IN THE HOSPITALIZED PATIENT

Gastrointestinal bleeding is a frequent and morbid complication of hospitalization. Patients in whom nosocomial bleeding develops are at very high risk for poor outcome and have a mortality rate upward of 30%. Most of this mortality is secondary to a deterioration of the patient's overall medical condition rather than to uncontrolled bleeding. Bleeding tends to occur after a prolonged hospital stay and is more likely to occur in patients with more severe underlying illnesses. Risk factors include ICU admission during the hospital stay, the need for mechanical ventilation, and coagulopathy. However, the majority of patients with nosocomial gastrointestinal bleeding are not in the ICU at the onset of bleeding. Duodenal ulcer disease is the most common source of this bleeding (Chapter 80). Preventive medical therapy (such as administration of intravenous proton pump inhibitors) is imperfect, as the majority of patients in whom bleeding develops have been receiving some form of prophylaxis. In general, the approach to the diagnosis and management of patients with nosocomial gastrointestinal bleeding is the same as for patients admitted with primary gastrointestinal bleeding.

COST CONSIDERATIONS AND RESOURCE USE

Evidence-based guidelines, management algorithms, and clinical care pathways show great promise in directing appropriate resource utilization for patients with gastrointestinal bleeding. Risk stratification data are available that will permit a more rational approach to admission decisions. It is estimated that up to 25% of admissions for upper gastrointestinal bleeding can be averted and care delivered in the outpatient setting without sacrificing safety. Several prospective studies basing admission decisions on clinical criteria and results of upper gastrointestinal endoscopy performed before hospital admission have validated this approach to care. Routine risk reassessment during the course of the hospital stay also aids in the early discharge of admitted patients, once again without compromising safety. Implementation of a risk assessment guideline at one institution decreased the mean length of stay for upper gastrointestinal bleeding from 4.6–2.9 days without any differences noted in complications, patient health status, or patient satisfaction measured one month after discharge (12). Similarly, in another study, implementation of a clinical care pathway for both upper and lower gastrointestinal bleeding reduced length of stay from 5.3–3.5 days without an increase in adverse outcomes (13).

KEY POINTS

- Gastrointestinal bleeding is a common medical condition, accounting for some 500,000 hospitalizations annually in the United States. Despite advances in medical and endoscopic therapy, mortality rates remain in the range of 2%–10%.
- Initial resuscitation should consist of prompt and adequate volume replacement and careful attention to airway management.
- Triage from the emergency department should be guided by an assessment of the patient's risk for further bleeding or death based on clinical risk assessment.
- Early endoscopy is recommended for all patients with acute upper gastrointestinal bleeding. Patients judged to be at low clinical risk may be suitable for immediate endoscopy and may be candidates for outpatient management.

- High-dose proton pump inhibitors are beneficial in high-risk upper gastrointestinal bleeding. Octreotide has been shown to improve short-term outcomes in patients with variceal hemorrhage.
- Clinical and endoscopic information can be combined to predict outcome and suggest an optimal length of stay for patients with upper gastrointestinal bleeding. The use of clinical practice guidelines or clinical care pathways based on these criteria has been shown to reduce length of stay without compromising clinical outcomes.
- In comparison with the approach to patients with upper gastrointestinal bleeding, the diagnostic and therapeutic approach to patients with lower gastrointestinal bleeding is not well standardized. Early colonoscopy may prove to be the best strategy to improve outcome and reduce costs.
- The likelihood of recurrent bleeding after discharge can be reduced by measures such as eradication of *Helicobacter pylori* in peptic ulcer disease, administration of nonselective β-blockers in patients with esophageal varices, and avoidance of aspirin and nonsteroidal anti-inflammatory drugs in all patients.

REFERENCES

1. Longstreth GF, Feitelberg SP. Outpatient care of selected patients with acute non-variceal upper gastrointestinal hemorrhage. *Lancet* 1995;345:108–111.
2. Almera P, Benages A, Peiro S, et al. Outpatient management of upper digestive hemorrhage not associated with portal hypertension: a large prospective cohort. *Am J Gastroenterol* 2001;96:2341–2348.
3. Rockall TA, Logan RF, Devlin HB, et al. Selection of patients for early discharge or outpatient care after acute upper gastrointestinal haemorrhage. National Audit of Acute Upper Gastrointestinal Haemorrhage. *Lancet* 1996;347:1138–1140.
4. Dulai GS, Gralnek IM, Oei TT, et al. Ultilization of health care resources for low-risk patients with acute, non-variceal upper GI hemorrhage: an historical cohort study. *Gastrointest Endosc* 2002;55:321–327.
5. Laine L. Endoscopic therapy for bleeding ulcers: room for improvement? *Gastrointest Endosc* 2003;57:557–560.
6. Chak A, Cooper GS, Lloyd LE, et al. Effectiveness of endoscopy in patients admitted to the intensive care unit with upper GI hemorrhage. *Gastrointest Endosc* 2001;53:6–13.
7. Cooper GS, Chak A, Way LE, et al. Early endoscopy in upper gastrointestinal hemorrhage: associations with recurrent bleeding, surgery, and length of hospital stay. *Gastrointest Endosc* 1999;49:145–142.
8. Banares R, Albillos A, Rincon D, et al. Endoscopic treatment versus endoscopic plus pharmacologic treatment for acute variceal bleeding: a meta-analysis. *Hepatology* 2002;35:609–615.
9. Imperiale TF, Birgisson S. Somatostatin or octreotide compared with H_2 antagonists and placebo in the management of acute nonvariceal upper gastrointestinal hemorrhage: a meta-analysis. *Ann Intern Med* 1997;127:1062–1071.
10. Lau JYW, Sung JJY, Lee KKC, et al. Effect of intravenous omeprazole on recurrent bleeding after endoscopic treatment of bleeding peptic ulcers. *N Eng J Med* 2000;343:310–316.
11. Javid G, Masoodi I, Zargar SA, et al. Oral omeprazole improves outcomes in ulcer bleeding. *Am J Med* 2001;111:280–284.
12. Hay JA, Maldonado L, Weingarten SR, et al. Prospective evaluation of a clinical guideline recommending hospital length of stay in upper gastrointestinal tract hemorrhage. *JAMA* 1997;278:2151–2156.
13. Podila PV, Ben-Menachem T, Batra SK, et al. Managing patients with acute, nonvariceal gastrointetinal hemorrhage: development and effectiveness of a clinical care pathway. *Am J Gastroenterol* 2001;96:208–219.
14. Finckh A, Aronson MD. Cardiovascular risks of cyclooxygenase-2 inhibitors: where we stand now. *Ann Intern Med* 2005;142:212–214.
15. Strate LL, Orav J, Syngal S. Early predictors of severity in acute lower intestinal tract bleeding. *Arch Intern Med* 2003;163:838–843.
16. Jensen DM, Machicado GA, Jutabha R, et al. Urgent colonoscopy for the diagnosis and treatment of severe diverticular hemorrhage. *N Engl J Med* 2000;342:78–82.
17. Jensen DM, Machicado GA. Colonoscopy for diagnosis and treatment of severe lower gastrointestinal bleeding. Routine outcomes and cost analysis. *Gastrointest Endosc Clin North Am* 1997;7:477–498.
18. Strate LL, Syngal S. Timing of colonoscopy: impact on length of hospital stay in patients with acute lower intestinal bleeding. *Am J Gastroenterol* 2003;98:317–322.
19. Arnott ID, Lo SK. The clinical utility of wireless capsule endoscopy. *Dig Dis Sci* 2004;49:893–901.

ADDITIONAL READING

Chung IK, Kim EJ, Lee MS, et al. Endoscopic factors predisposing to rebleeding following endoscopic hemostasis in bleeding peptic ulcers. *Endoscopy* 2001;33:969–975.

Khuroo MS, Khuroo MS, Farahat KL, Kagevi IE. Treatment with proton pump inhibitors in acute non-variceal upper gastrointestinal bleeding: a meta-analysis. *J Gastroenterol Hepatol* 2005;20:11–25.

Lau JYW, Sung JJY, Lam Y, et al. Endoscopic retreatment compared with surgery in patients with recurrent bleeding after initial endoscopic control of bleeding ulcers. *N Engl J Med* 1999;340:751–756.

Lee JG, Turnipseed S, Romano PS, et al. Endoscopy-based triage significantly reduces hospitalization rates and costs of treating upper GI bleeding: a randomized controlled trial. *Gastrointest Endosc* 1999;50:755–761.

Lewis JD, Bilker WB, Brensinger C, et al. Hospitalization and mortality rates from peptic ulcer disease and GI bleeding in the 1990s: relationship to sales of nonsteroidal antiinflammatory drugs and acid supression medications. *Am J Gastroenterol* 2002;97:2540–2549.

Ofman J, Wallace J, Badamgarav E, et al. The cost-effectiveness of competing strategies for the prevention of recurrent peptic ulcer hemorrhage. *Am J Gastroenterol* 2002;97:1941–1950.

Spiegel BMR, Ofman JJ, Woods K, et al. Minimizing recurrent peptic ulcer hemorrhage after endoscopic hemostasis: the cost-effectiveness of competing strategies. *Am J Gastroenterol* 2003;98:86–97.

Sung JJ, Chan FK, Lau JY, et al. The effect of endoscopic therapy in patients receiving omeprazole for bleeding ulcers with non-bleeding visible vessels or adherent clots: a randomized comparison. *Ann Intern Med* 2003;139:237–243.

Esophageal Disorders

79

Asyia Ahmad   James C. Reynolds

INTRODUCTION

Despite the relatively simple function of the esophagus, disorders involving it are a common source of patient symptoms, morbidity and mortality. The main function of the esophagus is the movement of an oral bolus into the stomach without allowing significant regurgitation back into the esophagus. Swallowing, the essential function of the esophagus, can be divided into three main phases. In the oral phase, food is masticated, lubricated with saliva, and passed to the back of the mouth. In the pharyngeal phase, food is passed to the pharynx and subsequently across the upper esophageal sphincter into the cervical esophagus. As the bolus is rapidly propelled to the pharynx, the nasal cavity and the trachea are protected by the soft palate and vocal cords, respectively. In the esophageal phase, food is propelled down the esophagus and through the gastroesophageal junction as the lower esophageal sphincter relaxes. A variety of esophageal disorders can occur if any part of this swallowing process is disrupted.

Most esophageal disorders present with symptoms of dysphagia, odynophagia or atypical chest pain. An outpatient evaluation is generally sufficient, and a thorough history and examination often suggest a diagnosis and aid the diagnostic strategy. Hospitalization is rarely required for acute esophageal disease, but complaints due to the esophagus are common among hospitalized patients. This chapter describes diagnostic and therapeutic strategies for a variety of esophageal conditions that are commonly encountered in the hospitalized patient.

DYSPHAGIA

Dysphagia is the sensation of food sticking as it passes from the mouth to the stomach. Dysphagia can be differentiated into two distinct clinical syndromes. *Oropharyngeal dysphagia* is the inability to adequately transfer food from the oropharynx into the cervical esophagus. Oropharyngeal dysphagia is the result of dysfunction of the upper esophageal sphincter or the oropharyngeal muscles and is commonly referred to as "transfer dysphagia." *Esophageal dysphagia* is a disturbance in the function of the esophagus itself. The differential diagnosis of this type of dysphagia is diverse and largely depends on differentiating mechanical causes from those related to motility disorders.

History is an important part of the evaluation of dysphagia. Patients will often point to the sternal notch as the site where food "gets stuck." While this may accurately describe the location in oropharyngeal dysphagia, patients with esophageal disorders often incorrectly localize their symptoms to this location. In contrast, patients who identify their symptoms as originating lower in the substernal region are usually accurate in pointing to the site of the pathology. Nasal regurgitation, coughing, or aspiration strongly suggest transfer dysphagia. Disorders of the oropharynx and proximal esophagus are often due to neuromuscular disorders of striated muscles. Symptoms of esophageal dysphagia are more varied and depend on the underlying etiology. For example, chronic heartburn suggests a benign cause such as a stricture. Advanced age, a history of weight loss, or heavy tobacco or alcohol use increase the risk of a malignant cause for the dysphagia. Dysphagia to solids suggests a mechanical obstruction, while dysphagia to both solids and liquids implies a functional or motility impairment as the cause. The constant sensation of a lump in the throat that is unaffected by swallowing is not dysphagia but "globus." Globus is most often due to GERD (gastroesophageal reflux disease, which is discussed later in this chapter), not hysteria (as had been taught for years). In summary, although characterization of symptoms is helpful, this assessment alone lacks adequate sensitivity or specificity in determining the cause of dysphagia.

The initial evaluation should be based on symptoms (Figure 79.1). A patient with oropharyngeal dysphagia should have a thorough evaluation for underlying abnormalities of the central nervous system, peripheral nerves and muscles. In addition, anatomical investigation

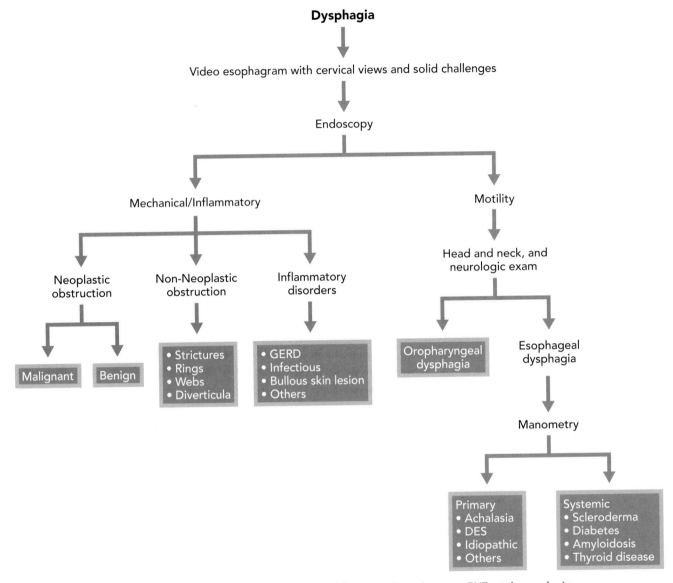

Figure 79.1 Approach to dysphagia. *DES*, diffuse esophageal spasm; *ENT*, otolaryngologic; *GERD*, gastroesophageal reflux disease.

of the hypopharynx and cervical esophagus, as well as a radiographic study of swallowing, should be completed. Causes of esophageal dysphagia can be divided into two categories. The evaluation of patients with symptoms implicating a mechanical cause for dysphagia should begin with a barium study to delineate the anatomy of the esophagus. Most will also require an upper endoscopy. Endoscopy provides a means to obtain biopsies for definitive diagnosis and for therapeutic maneuvers, including esophageal dilation. Patients with symptoms suggesting a functional cause for dysphagia should also undergo endoscopy. When endoscopy is negative, an esophageal manometry study should be performed to assess the adequacy of esophageal peristalsis and lower esophageal function.

Benign Esophageal Stricture

The majority of benign esophageal strictures are peptic in origin. The remainder occur as a complication of surgery (or from caustic toxin ingestion), pill esophagitis, infection, or radiation esophagitis. Another cause of a narrowed esophagus, a *Schatzki's ring,* is a fixed circumferential mucosal fold located at the squamocolumnar junction. Patients with strictures usually complain of progressive dysphagia to solid food and have a long-standing history of heartburn and/or ingestion of antacids. Barium swallow or upper endoscopy may reveal a smooth tapered narrowing, usually within the lower third of the esophagus. Biopsy and brush cytology of the strictured area can rule out underlying cancer.

The mainstay of treatment is esophageal dilation. In addition, an aggressive antireflux regimen with a proton pump inhibitor is warranted and has been shown to decrease the need for recurrent dilations (1). Unlike Schatzi's ring, in which quick disruption of the ring is required, gradual stretching is needed in peptic stricture. Stretching is usually accomplished by beginning with dilators of a diameter matching the size of the stricture. Patients may be dilated up to three successive sizes in one session and may have to return for further dilations (2).

Esophageal Carcinoma

Over 90% of all esophageal cancers are either adenocarcinoma or squamous cell carcinoma. Adenocarcinoma is more commonly diagnosed in Caucasian males with a long-standing history of GERD. These patients may have underlying Barrett's mucosa in which the carcinoma develops. The incidence of esophageal adenocarcinoma has risen since the 1970s; during the 1990s, it surpassed the incidence of squamous cell cancer (3). Squamous cell esophageal cancer is more likely to develop in African Americans who may have other risk factors such as tobacco and alcohol use, previous achalasia, or lye ingestion (4). Symptoms of esophageal cancer include progressive dysphagia to solids and rapid weight loss. A barium swallow that shows an ulcerated, irregular mass in the esophagus suggests esophageal cancer, and an upper endoscopy with biopsy is diagnostic. Staging of the tumor includes CT scanning of the chest. Endoscopic ultrasound can identify approximately 25% of patients who would otherwise be inaccurately staged (5). Surgery with esophagectomy remains the standard of care for localized tumors, while tumors with lymph node invasion or distant metastasis are treated with a regimen of chemotherapy and radiation. In aggressive obstructing tumors, esophageal stents can be placed for palliation, allowing oral intake to continue. Despite recent advances in surgical techniques and chemoradiation, prognosis in cases of esophageal cancer remains poor, with fewer than 25% of patients surviving 5 years (6).

Achalasia

Achalasia is an esophageal motility disorder characterized by loss of peristalsis in the esophagus and failure of the lower esophageal sphincter to relax. Although the cause is unknown, viruses, environmental factors and autoimmune mechanisms have been implicated as playing a role. Presentation of this disorder occurs equally in both genders and usually manifests with symptoms of dysphagia to both solids and liquids. Although dysphagia is the most common complaint, nocturnal regurgitation, chest pain with eating, and pulmonary complications are also seen. Long-term esophageal complications such as *Candida* esophagitis and squamous cell carcinoma may complicate the course. With advancing disease, dietary restrictions, social isolation, and malnutrition affect this population. Evaluation for achalasia includes barium studies, chest radiographs, upper endoscopy, and esophageal manometry. A barium swallow may reveal delayed esophageal transit or a dilated esophagus which tapers distally to give a "bird beak" appearance (7). There may be evidence of an air-fluid level in the mediastinum or signs of chronic aspiration on chest radiographs. Endoscopy may suggest achalasia in a patient with a tight lower esophageal sphincter (LES) and a dilated esophagus, but a definitive diagnosis can only be made by esophageal manometry. Characteristic findings on manometry include simultaneous esophageal contractions, a LES that fails to relax, and intraesophageal pressures that exceed gastric pressure. When simultaneous contractions are of high amplitude and associated with chest pain, the descriptive term "vigorous achalasia" is used.

Once the diagnosis is made, it is important to distinguish primary achalasia from secondary achalasia or pseudoachalasia. Secondary achalasia can be caused by malignancy, either by direct extension into the lower esophagus, as seen in cancer of the gastric cardia, or as a paraneoplastic phenomenon. An unusual cause is Chagas disease, an infection caused by *Trypanosoma cruzi*. Finally, extrinsic compression on the lower esophagus can mimic achalasia.

In primary achalasia, there is no treatment to reverse the degeneration of the neurons, so treatment merely aims to improve symptoms. Medications such as nitrates or calcium channel blockers have been used with limited success. Endoscopic treatment consists of botulinum injection or pneumatic dilation of the lower esophageal sphincter. Botulinum injection is a safe procedure than can relieve symptoms of dysphagia, but its effects are short-lived, with a mean duration of response of 16 months, at most (8). Patients generally require repeat injections, making this a costly procedure. Thus, botulinum injection is reserved for patients who cannot undergo pneumatic dilation. In contrast, a single pneumatic dilation can provide effective therapy in most patients. After a second dilation, 85%–90% of patients will enjoy long-term relief (9). The complications associated with pneumatic dilation include local bleeding, hematoma formation, and esophageal perforation, which occur in approximately 5% of patients. Despite these risks, pneumatic dilation is the most cost-effective treatment in healthy patients (10). Those patients who have a poor response to medical and endoscopic treatment may benefit from a surgical myotomy, with which up to 90% of patients achieve good results (11).

In secondary achalasia, treatment with dilation may be inappropriate, and it is important to determine the true cause for the abnormality. Clues that are helpful in recognizing secondary achalasia include an ulcerated or asymmetric lower esophageal sphincter seen on endoscopy or radiographic studies, significant weight loss, rapid onset of symptoms, and older age of onset.

Esophageal Spasm

Esophageal spasm is an intermittent, simultaneous, non-peristatic contraction of the esophagus that occurs during more than 10%, but less than 100%, of swallows. Symptoms can include intermittent dysphagia to either liquids or solids or chest pain with eating. Diagnosis is difficult since spasm occurs intermittently and may not be visualized by diagnostic studies. Barium studies may show a corkscrew-shaped esophagus or tertiary contractions, but these findings are only suggestive. Manometry confirms spasm in fewer than 5% of patients (12). Provocation studies with edrophonium or other acetylcholinesterase inhibitors may reproduce the symptoms of chest pain and suggest the diagnosis. If chest pain coincides with spasms, a definitive diagnosis of diffuse esophageal spasm (DES) can be made.

Treatment of these patients is often difficult. It is important to ensure that the patient does not have underlying cardiac disease as the cause of the symptoms. For symptoms related to esophageal spasm, agents such as nitrates, calcium channel blockers, anticholinergic drugs, and antidepressants can be tried. Anticholinergic agents, including hyoscyamine, provide relief in patients with spasm; however, they do have side effects such as dry mouth, constipation, and blurred vision. Side effects can be reduced by prescribing short-acting sublingual hyoscyamine products. Antidepressants improve symptoms in approximately 50% of patients, regardless of motility findings (13). In refractory DES, pneumatic dilation or surgical myotomy may provide relief but is rarely used.

Systemic Diseases with Esophageal Involvement

Many systemic diseases that cause multi-organ dysfunction and lead to hospitalization also involve the esophagus. These are listed in Table 79.1. One systemic disease with frequent esophageal involvement is scleroderma. The condition is most common in women in their 20s to 40s; gastrointestinal involvement may occur in up to 90% of these patients (14). Esophageal involvement is characterized by decreased lower esophageal pressures and low-amplitude peristalsis, which causes symptoms of dysphagia to solids and liquids, as well as severe reflux. Peptic strictures and Barrett's esophagus are dangerous complications that may occur in these patients. Treatment is based on behavioral modifications and an aggressive antireflux regimen. In addition, patients should be taught to eat slowly to compensate for the absence of ordered peristalsis.

ODYNOPHAGIA

Odynophagia is the sensation of pain during swallowing. It almost always results from a disorder that leads to mucosal disruption. The etiology of odynophagia is diverse. In immunocompromised patients, infectious etiologies such as *Candida, Herpes simplex* virus (*HSV*) and cytomegalovirus (*CMV*) must be considered. In some patient populations, other causes such as chronic reflux, radiation, and pill-induced damage are more commonly seen.

Infectious Esophagitis

Patients with organ transplants, neutropenia, cancer, and AIDS are particularly susceptible to infectious esophagitis. However, patients with diabetes, motility disorders such as achalasia, those on steroids, and alcoholics are also at increased risk. The most common infectious causes of esophagitis is *Candida*. Patients with *Candida* esophagitis usually present with dysphagia, but they may also complain of severe chest pain and odynophagia. On examination, oral thrush may be present, but *its absence does not exclude Candida* as the cause for the symptoms. Barium studies may reveal an esophagus with a foamy or shaggy appearance. Ulceration or masses are unusual, and their presence should suggest another etiology. Endoscopy is often performed in patients who fail to appropriately respond to empiric therapy; when performed, it may reveal characteristic white plaques. Diagnosis can be confirmed

---

TABLE 79.1

SYSTEMIC DISEASES WITH ESOPHAGEAL INVOLVEMENT

Rheumatologic
 Systemic lupus erythematosus (SLE)
 Polymyositis and dermatomyositis
 Mixed connective tissue disease
 Sjogren's syndrome
 Behçet's syndrome
 Inflammatory myopathies

Endocrine
 Hypothyroidism
 Diabetes mellitus

Infiltrative/Inflammatory
 Amyloidosis
 Sarcoidosis
 Crohn's disease

Neurologic
 Myasthenia gravis
 Amyotrophic lateral sclerosis
 Parkinson's disease
 Muscular dystrophies

by esophageal brushings with cytology or biopsies with histology. The latter is also helpful in ruling out other opportunistic infections. Treatment is with fluconazole 100 mg orally daily, or other appropriate anti-fungal agents, for 14 days. Patients with severe dysphagia, or those who fail initial therapy, need to be hospitalized for intravenous antifungal therapy with fluconazole, caspofungin, or amphotericin B.

Viruses such as cytomegalovirus (CMV) and *Herpes simplex* (HSV) are also important causes of infectious esophagitis. HSV esophagitis is seen in both the HIV and organ transplant population, and much less commonly in the immunocompetent host. Patients generally present with odynophagia. Barium studies reveal small discrete mucosal ulcerations without surrounding mucosal involvement. Endoscopy is necessary to confirm the presence of HSV. Treatment in patients who can tolerate oral medications consists of acyclovir 400 mg three times a day. In patients who cannot tolerate oral medications, intravenous acyclovir at 5–10 mg/kg every 8 hours can be used.

CMV esophagitis is more common than HSV in the AIDS population. Symptoms mainly consist of odynophagia. Barium studies may reveal deep ulcerations. Endoscopy with biopsy is needed for diagnosis. Treatment consists of ganciclovir intravenously, with an induction dose of 5 mg/kg every 12 hours for 2 weeks followed by a maintenance dose. Foscarnet can also be used in to treat CMV esophagitis; however, side effects such as electrolyte abnormalities and nephrotoxicity can occur. For patients with mild disease, oral valganciclovir at a starting dose of 900 mg twice daily is an option.

Other Causes of Odynophagia and Esophagitis

An often overlooked cause of odynophagia is *pill esophagitis*. Patients with pill-induced ulceration usually present with severe odynophagia or chest pain. It is important to obtain a thorough history, since patients with acute odynophagia may have received only one dose of the offending medication. Agents most commonly responsible include alendronate, tetracycline, quinidine, NSAIDs, and potassium. Pills may become temporarily lodged above the aortic indentation or at a stricture of the esophagus. Endoscopy may reveal circumferential ulceration in the mid- or distal-esophagus. Treatment is symptomatic, the offending agent is discontinued, and patients are instructed to take medications while in the upright position, drinking a 4- to–8-ounce glass of fluid both before and after taking the medication.

Radiation esophagitis may also cause odynophagia in patients undergoing radiation for head and neck cancers. Esophageal damage occurs in 40%–50% of patients, despite adequate shielding. In patients receiving concomitant chemotherapy, radiation injury to the esophagus may be more severe. Treatment may include sucralfate or a mixture of Mylanta and viscous lidocaine; both regimens appear to have similar efficacy. If odynophagia is severe, radiation treatment may have to be postponed and intravenous nutrition may be required.

GASTROESOPHAGEAL REFLUX DISEASE

Gastroesophageal reflux disease (GERD) results when the passage of stomach contents back into the esophagus causes symptoms or mucosal disease. Heartburn is a burning sensation behind the sternum after meals, especially when recumbent. This symptom alone has a high predictive value for diagnosing GERD. Symptoms such as a bitter taste in the back of the mouth, belching, nausea, dysphagia, and regurgitation are also common. Complaints such as chronic laryngitis, cough, hoarseness, and asthma can also be attributed to chronic GERD. Cohort studies reveal that GERD symptoms occur in almost 50% of patients at least once a month and approximately 20% at least once a week (15). Overall, Americans spend billions of dollars each year for medications to treat GERD.

Although transient reflux episodes occur normally, GERD leads to symptoms or mucosal injury as a result of impairment of normal esophageal defenses. Peptic stricture is a costly sequela of severe GERD (particularly if not treated with effective anti-reflux therapy). It may cause extensive esophageal narrowing and the need for repeat esophageal dilations. In addition, chronic GERD may lead to the development of Barrett's metaplasia or dysplasia. Once Barrett's is detected, patients need to undergo regular endoscopic surveillance in order to detect esophageal adenocarcinoma, which develops in approximately 0.5% of Barrett's patients per year (16).

Although GERD can cause erosive esophagitis, non-erosive GERD is a common cause of symptoms and can lead to an impaired quality of life. Patients with non-erosive esophagitis have the same severity of symptoms, reduction in quality of life, and utilize equal amounts of antireflux medications as patients with erosive esophagitis. Surprisingly, some patients with severe erosive esophagitis seen on endoscopy have minimal symptoms of heartburn and are only diagnosed incidentally.

Treatment Options for Gastroesophageal Reflux Disease

Nonpharmacologic Treatments

Lifestyle modifications are often recommended as the first step in treating reflux symptoms. These are listed in Table 79.2. Elevation of the head of the bed has been shown in prospective trials to be an effective maneuver. Avoidance of foods high in fat content or that may affect lower esophageal sphincter relaxation can be helpful. Lastly,

TABLE 79.2
NONPHARMACOLOGIC TREATMENTS OF GASTROESOPHAGEAL REFLUX

Avoidance of injurious medications
Agents that impair sphincter tone
   Anticholinergics
   Progestins
   Calcium channel antagonists
   Nicotine
   Theophylline
Agents that cause mucosal injury
   Aspirin
   Alendronate
   Nonsteroidal antiinflammatory agents
   Tetracycline
   Potassium supplements

Dietary measures
Reduce fat intake
Reduce meal size
Limit foods that impair sphincter function
   Caffeine
   Chocolate
   Peppermint

Life-style modifications
Stop smoking
Limit alcohol intake
Avoid tight garments
Remain upright after eating
Elevate head of bed

medications that reduce esophageal contractile force or that irritate the esophageal mucosa should be avoided if possible. If these medications cannot be avoided, they should be taken with an adequate amount of fluid to prevent injury to the esophagus.

Pharmacologic Therapy

There are three main approaches to the initial treatment of reflux. The *step-up approach* starts with the least costly measures. In patients who do not respond to initial treatment or who have breakthrough symptoms, medications of increasing efficacy are recommended until symptoms are relieved. This approach is appropriate only in patients with uncomplicated mild-to-moderate GERD.

The first step in this approach consists of lifestyle modifications and the nonpharmacologic interventions listed in Table 79.2. Patients should limit excess fat intake and lose weight if necessary. Smoking cessation is another important component of therapy. It not only improves GERD symptoms but decreases the incidence of peptic ulcer disease and various cancers. Concurrent medications should be carefully scrutinized, since specific medications known to reduce lower esophageal sphincter pressure can worsen GERD. Even with strict compliance with the above guidelines, most patients will remain symptomatic and need to proceed to step two. At this point, pharmacologic therapy with a histamine-2 receptor blocker (H₂RA) is initiated. Additionally, the prokinetic agent metoclopramide has been helpful in patients with mild GERD and symptoms of dyspepsia and bloating. If symptoms persist despite the above measures, step three consists of discontinuing the H₂RA and starting a proton pump inhibitor (PPI). While this *step-up approach* is commonly used, it has been shown to be the most costly due to repeated office visits and unnecessary testing. For this reason, clinicians increasingly favor the *step-down approach*.

The *step-down approach* begins with the use of a PPI, the best acid-suppression medication for GERD. This enhanced acid suppression leads to faster symptom relief, improved quality of life, and a greater percentage of patients achieving mucosal healing. In addition, this class of medications is the treatment of choice for GERD-related complications such as esophageal ulceration and strictures. PPIs may also play a substantial role in improving poorly controlled asthma, chronic cough, and laryngitis due to GERD. Once symptoms have been controlled for several months, patients may be switched to a less expensive, less potent medication such as a prokinetic agent or H₂RA. Although the step-down approach may reduce costs, 60%–80% of patients will require PPI maintenance therapy to remain symptom free.

Finally, the *on-demand approach* provides PPI therapy on an as needed basis. This approach is appropriate and cost-effective for patients who do not have esophagitis or esophageal ulcers. Studies using omeprazole have demonstrated only a 29% failure rate at 6 months in patients following this routine (17). Patients who do not respond to medical therapy may choose to undergo surgical fundoplication. Recommendation for surgery must be made after careful evaluation as recent studies show limited long-term benefit of this intervention. Furthermore, cost analysis reveals medical therapy to be more cost-effective (18).

SPONTANEOUS ESOPHAGEAL RUPTURE (BOERHAAVE'S SYNDROME)

Boerhaave's syndrome (or spontaneous esophageal rupture) is a full-thickness tear of the esophagus in the absence of prior instrumentation. Patients often have a preceding history of retching or vomiting, although any maneuver that increases intraabdominal pressure can precipitate esophageal rupture. The most common site for rupture is in the distal posterolateral esophagus. The patient may complain of chest, back, or abdominal pain; while others have symptoms of odynophagia, dysphagia or nausea. On physical examination, patients may appear acutely ill, with hypotension, tachcardia or fever. Signs of a pleural rub or decreased breath sounds should be sought. Chest or abdominal radiographs usually suggest the diagnosis by revealing pneumomediastinum or a left-sided pleural effusion.

Treatment of this syndrome is primarily surgical. Patients should be adequately resuscitated and promptly placed on intravenous antibiotics. Individuals with small tears in the esophagus which are not associated with complete perforation can be treated conservatively with antibiotics and close in-hospital observation.

COST-EFFECTIVENESS AND RESOURCE UTILIZATION

Esophageal disorders rarely require hospitalization. Exceptions include chest discomfort where cardiac causes must be ruled out. In this case, early PPI therapy may relieve symptoms of reflux esophagitis, allowing for shorter hospitalization stays. In addition, patients with poor oral intake secondary to radiation or infectious esophagitis may need to be hospitalized for intravenous fluids and antibiotics. Patients with esophageal rupture usually require urgent hospitalization for intravenous resuscitation, antibiotics, and emergency surgery.

Other esophageal conditions can be adequately evaluated and treated in the office. Patients with peptic stricture and achalasia may need repeat dilation. This can normally be done on an outpatient basis. Rarely do complications from these procedures require hospitalization. Early recognition of symptoms of esophageal cancer may lead to early diagnosis and shorter hospitalization stays if surgery is required. Lastly, suspected motility disorders should be thoroughly evaluated with barium studies, endoscopy, and esophageal manometry before complications develop. By following these recommendations, early treatment strategies can be implemented in a cost-effective manner.

KEY POINTS

■ Gastroesophageal reflux disease (GERD) is the most common esophageal disorder in hospitalized patients. It is a cause of esophageal cancer, atypical chest pain, asthma, chronic cough, chronic laryngitis, and tracheal stenosis.

■ All patients with GERD should be counseled in lifestyle modification, avoiding precipitating medications, and dietary measures. Most will also benefit from the use of a proton pump inhibitor.

■ Odynophagia is most commonly caused by reflux or infections, both of which can be effectively treated once a specific diagnosis is made.

■ Achalasia is an important treatable cause of dysphagia, angina-like chest pain, and recurrent aspiration. Botulinum toxin is an important new treatment of achalasia, but pneumatic dilation is generally more effective over the long term.

■ Dysphagia should be promptly evaluated to identify treatable causes and recognize cancer at its earliest stages.

REFERENCES

1. Richter JE. Peptic strictures of the esophagus. *Gastroenterol Clin North Am* 1999;28:875.
2. Pereira-Lima JC, Ramires RP, Zamin I, et al. Endoscopic dilation of benign strictures: report on 1043 procedures. *Am J Gastroenterol* 1999;94:1497–1501.
3. Brown LM, Devesa SS. Epidemiologic trends in esophageal and gastric cancer in the United States. *Surg Oncol Clin N Am* 2002;11:235–256.
4. Crew KD, Neugut AI. Epidemiology of upper gastrointestinal malignancies. *Semin Oncol* 2004;31:450–464.
5. Shumaker DA, deGarmo P, Gaigel DO. Potential impact of preoperative EUS on esophageal cancer management and cost. *Gastrointestinal Endoscopy* 2002;56:391–396.
6. Hofstetter W, Swisher SG, Correa AM, et al. Treatment outcome of resected esophageal cancer. *Ann Surg* 2002;236:376–385.
7. Nellermann H, Aksglaede K, Funch-Jensen P, et al. Bread and barium. Diagnostic value in patients with suspected primary esophageal motility disorders. *Acta Radiologica* 2000;41:145–150.
8. Kaufman JA, Oelschlager BK. Treatment of achalasia. *Curr Treat Options Gastroenterol* 2005;8:59–69.
9. Katz PO, Gilbert J, Castell DO. Pneumatic dilatation is effective long-term treatment for achalasia. *Dig Dis Sci* 1998;43:1973–1977.
10. O'Connor JB, Singer ME, Imperiale TF, et al. The cost-effectiveness of treatment strategies for achalasia. *Dig Dis & Sci* 2002;47:1516–1525.
11. Zaninotto G, Costanlini M, Portale G, et al. Etiology, diagnosis & treatment of failures after laparoscopic Heller myotomy for achalasia. *Ann Surg* 2002;235:186–192.
12. Dalton CB, Castell DO, Hewson EG, et al. Diffuse esophageal spasm: a rare motility disorder not characterized by high-amplitude contractions. *Dig Dis Sci* 1991;36:1025–1028.
13. Handa M, Mine K, Yamamoto H, et al. Antidepressant treatment of patient with diffuse esophageal spasm: a psychosomatic approach. *J Clin Gastroenterol* 1999;28:228–232.
14. Rose S, Young MA, Reynolds JC. Gastrointestinal manifestations of scleroderma. *Gastroenterol Clin North America* 1998;27:563–594.
15. Shaheen N, Ransohoff DF. Gastroesophageal reflux, barrett esophagus, and esophageal cancer: scientific review. *JAMA* 2002;287:1972–1981.
16. Reynolds JC, Rahimi P, Hirschl D. Barrett's esophagus: clinical characteristics. *Gastroenterol Clin North America* 2002;13:441–460.
17. Vakil N. Review article: cost-effectiveness of different GERD management strategies. *Alimentary Pharmacol & Therapeutics* 2002;16:4:79–82.
18. Myrvold HE, Lundell L, Liedman B, et al. The cost of omeprazole versus open anti-reflux surgery in the long-term management of reflux esophagitis. *Gastroenterology* 1998;114:A238.

ADDITIONAL READING

Spechler SJ. Clinical practice. Barrett's Esophagus. *New Engl J Med* 2002;346:836–842.
Ramakrishnan A, Katz PO. Overview of medical therapy for gastroesophageal disease. *Gastrointestinal Endoscopy Clin North America* 2003;13:57–68.
Richter JE. Oesophageal motility disorders. *Lancet* 2001;358:823–828.

Peptic Ulcer Disease and Stress-Related Mucosal Disease

80

Brennan M. R. Spiegel   *Gareth S. Dulai*

INTRODUCTION

Epidemiology

Peptic ulcer disease (PUD) and gastritis are two of the most commonly reported gastroenterologic disorders in hospitalized patients, accounting for more than 600,000 hospitalizations per year in the United States. PUD alone is the primary diagnosis in more than 450,000 hospitalizations per year, with an average hospital stay of four days and an annual mortality rate of 1.74 per 100,000 persons. Gastritis is the primary diagnosis for nearly 200,000 hospitalized patients per year, with an average hospital stay of four days and an annual mortality rate below 1 per 100,000 persons (1, 2).

Infection of the gastric mucosa with the Gram-negative bacillus *Helicobacter pylori* and the use of nonsteroidal anti-inflammatory drugs (NSAIDs) are the two most important causes of PUD. As many as 33 million people in the United States consume prescription and over-the-counter NSAIDs on a long-term basis, and the prevalence of NSAID use is increasing in lockstep with the aging of the American population. Epidemiologic data indicate that NSAID consumption increases the odds of developing an ulcer or ulcer-related complication by 3–6 times, depending on age. The prevalence of *H. pylori* infection in the population varies by age, but more than 50% of Americans older than 60 years are infected. Thus, millions are at risk for PUD and its complications. However, most endoscopic ulcers do not lead to clinically significant complications such as dyspep-

sia, ulcer hemorrhage, or ulcer perforation. In fact, data indicate that fewer than one-third of endoscopic ulcers lead to these relevant outcomes (3). The lifetime risk for symptomatic ulceration in those with chronic *H. pylori* infection is estimated to be 15% (3), and the annual risk for clinically significant ulceration in long-term users of NSAIDs is 1%–3% (4–6).

A number of factors associated with increased risk for PUD have been identified. In particular, the risk of developing NSAID-related GI complications is highest in patients using concurrent aspirin, coumadin, or steroids; patients with a previous history of an ulcer hemorrhage; and patients over 65 (7). Bacterial factors, such as the degree of cytotoxin A expression, and host factors, including the age at infection, genetic background, and degree of gastric acid secretion, may play a role in determining the risk for subsequent PUD among persons with *H. pylori* infection.

Accumulating data indicate that there may be a synergistic effect between NSAID use and *H. pylori* status. Specifically, meta-analysis reveals that *H. pylori* infection increases the risk of endoscopically detected ulcers in NSAID users by three and one-half fold compared to *H. pylori*-negative NSAID users. In addition, the risk of ulcer hemorrhage increases six-fold when both factors are present (8). In contrast, at least two case-control studies have found no evidence of an interaction between these risk factors (9, 10), and additional data indicate a protective effect of *H. pylori* on PUD in NSAID users (11). It is difficult to generalize these findings because the studies are limited by significant variations between study populations, definitions of NSAID use, and evaluated outcomes. Although data are conflicting, the weight of the evidence appears to support the notion that *H. pylori* and NSAIDs are likely to be at least additive, and possibly synergistic, risk factors for PUD (8).

Definition of Syndromes

Peptic ulcer disease and gastritis represent patterns of mucosal response to injury. *Peptic ulcers* are breaks in the gastroduodenal mucosa that occur as a result of an imbalance between mucosal defense mechanisms and mucosal irritants. Whereas the diagnosis of PUD is made by endoscopic or radiographic visualization, the diagnosis of gastritis is, by strict definition, based on the histologic finding of gastric mucosal inflammation. In practice, however, the term gastritis has been used to refer to a variety of endoscopic appearances, such as erythema of the stomach, that correlate poorly with actual histologic findings. Of the three major types of gastritis (erosive and hemorrhagic, nonerosive or chronic, and distinctive), it is primarily the erosive and hemorrhagic variety that are of any immediate clinical consequence in the hospitalized patient. The principal clinical consequence of erosive and hemorrhagic gastritis is upper gastrointestinal hemorrhage.

Because the diagnosis of erosive and hemorrhagic "gastritis" is most often made on the basis of endoscopic visualization without biopsy, and because the biopsy when performed does not show prominent inflammation, the preferred terms for this disease entity are either erosive and hemorrhagic "gastropathy" or simply subepithelial hemorrhage. Erosive and hemorrhagic gastropathy occurs primarily in response to stress, use of NSAIDs, and alcohol. *Stress-related gastropathy* is the most important type of gastropathy in hospitalized patients and is therefore the only type considered in this chapter.

Duodenal ulcers are more than twice as common as gastric ulcers. Among patients with PUD who are not taking NSAIDs, 90%–100% of those with duodenal ulcers and 60%–90% of those with gastric ulcers are infected with *H. pylori*. NSAID use is a more frequent cause of gastric ulcers but may cause duodenal ulcers as well. Both types of ulcers occur more commonly in the elderly, reflecting the increasing prevalence of NSAID use and *H. pylori* infection with increasing age. Erosive and hemorrhagic gastropathy, in contrast, tends to occur diffusely in the stomach without any known age-specific trend in prevalence.

Current Trends

Within the past two decades, a paradigm shift has occurred in the approach to the diagnosis and therapy of PUD. It is now recognized that most PUD is not caused primarily by oversecretion of acid, but rather by *H. pylori* infection, the

consumption of NSAIDs, or both. Management of PUD, therefore, has shifted from maintenance of remission with antisecretory therapy, to cure through identification and elimination of *H. pylori* infection and discontinuation of NSAIDs, use of co-therapy, or use of anti-inflammatory/analgesic agents with decreased ulcerogenic potential.

This chapter presents a rational approach to therapeutic decision making in hospitalized patients with uncomplicated PUD, with an emphasis on recent developments in care. Because gastropathy is a relatively uncommon cause of morbidity in the hospitalized patient, a short section is devoted to strategies for prophylaxis.

ISSUES AT THE TIME OF ADMISSION

Clinical Presentation and Differential Diagnosis

The most common symptom associated with uncomplicated PUD is chronic or recurrent pain or discomfort in the upper abdomen, referred to as *dyspepsia*. Dyspepsia affects more than 25% of the general population but rarely results in hospitalization. Although only 10%–30% of patients with dyspepsia who present for medical evaluation have PUD, a history of dyspepsia can be elicited in up to 50%–70% of patients with uncomplicated PUD. The remaining patients present with atypical symptoms or with "silent ulcers." The latter, who may present with complications of PUD, are commonly the elderly and those with NSAID-associated PUD. In numerous studies, discrimination of symptoms and symptom complexes has not been shown to be sensitive or specific for the presence of uncomplicated PUD. However, the presence of "alarm" features, such as weight loss, anemia, and dysphagia, are associated with a high probability of serious underlying pathology.

Complicated ulcer disease may present with acute, severe abdominal pain with guarding and rebound tenderness that suggest posterior penetration or perforation. Weight loss, early satiety, recurrent emesis, and a succussion splash on examination may indicate gastric outlet obstruction. A history of melena, hematochezia, or hematemesis may indicate acute or subacute gastrointestinal hemorrhage.

A wide range of disorders can present with dyspepsia or severe abdominal pain. Unfortunately, studies of dyspepsia are largely limited to the outpatient population and may not be directly applicable to hospitalized patients. Of outpatients presenting with dyspepsia, only one-third are found to have an underlying organic etiology, including erosive esophagitis, peptic ulcers, or, rarely, gastric cancer. In contrast, two-thirds of patients with dyspepsia have no discernible organic pathology and are said to have "functional dyspepsia." A subset of these patients may have undiagnosed non-erosive reflux disease.

Occasionally, biliary or pancreatic disease can mimic PUD. However, both entities tend to have classic presentations that are readily distinguishable from those of PUD. Classic cholecystitis (Chapter 84) causes episodes of acute, severe pain that often localize to the right upper quadrant. Pancreatitis (Chapter 86) tends to be associated with episodes of acute, severe pain in the left upper quadrant that radiates to the back. Rare causes of dyspepsia may include Crohn's disease, medications, systemic metabolic abnormalities, celiac disease, and intestinal ischemia. Intestinal ischemia (Chapter 87) should always be considered given its significant consequences, especially in patients with severe cardiovascular disease. In the "typical" case, however, intestinal ischemia presents with one or more warning signs, such as intestinal angina or weight loss.

Risk Stratification and Indications for Hospitalization

Patients presenting with symptoms suggestive of PUD may be divided into two groups: (1) those suspected of having uncomplicated PUD, and (2) those suspected of having complicated PUD. Patients with uncomplicated PUD require hospitalization mainly for debilitating symptoms that cannot be controlled on an outpatient basis, such as pain or inability to maintain adequate nutrient intake. The decision to admit the patient with suspected uncomplicated PUD hinges on the patient's nutritional status, comorbidities, reliability, and on the provider's clinical judgment.

In contrast, hospitalization of the patient with complicated PUD is generally straightforward. Patients with suspected perforation or penetration require prompt surgical evaluation and admission to an ICU. Those with suspected obstruction, or who have evidence of dehydration or are at risk for further complications such as aspiration should be admitted for observation and diagnostic evaluation. The triage of patients with upper gastrointestinal hemorrhage is addressed in Chapter 78.

Diagnostic Evaluation

Complicated Peptic Ulcer Disease

Patients with suspected complicated PUD require rapid evaluation. Important historical risk factors include the patient's age, prior history of PUD, active comorbid conditions, and use of NSAIDs, alcohol, anticoagulants, tobacco, or corticosteroids. A complete physical examination should include an assessment of vital signs, with particular attention paid to evidence of volume depletion. Laboratory tests to obtain a complete blood cell count and values for coagulation parameters, liver chemistries, electrolytes,

amylase, blood urea nitrogen, and serum creatinine should be routine. Elderly patients and those with pre-existing cardiovascular morbidities should receive a baseline electrocardiogram, especially if gastrointestinal hemorrhage is suspected. Patients with suspected perforation require both supine and upright radiographs of the abdomen to rule out pneumoperitoneum. If an "acute abdomen" is present or if perforation is suspected clinically, early surgical consultation is mandatory. Those with suspected hemorrhage should be managed according to the strategies outlined in Chapter 78. In particular, data indicate that early endoscopy within 12–24 hours improves patient outcomes and reduces length of stay *versus* delayed endoscopy, suggesting that early endoscopy should be a routine component of care for patients admitted with suspected ulcer complications (12). Patients with suspected gastric outlet obstruction require upright or decubitus radiographs of the abdomen to rule out distal small-bowel obstruction and placement of a nasogastric tube for decompression.

Uncomplicated Peptic Ulcer Disease as a Primary Diagnostic Consideration

The management of patients hospitalized principally for the evaluation of uncomplicated PUD has not been extensively evaluated, and current guidelines or decision aids are not available. Given the high physical, mental, and financial burden of continued medical uncertainty in the hospitalized patient, rapid and definitive diagnosis and treatment are warranted. A suggested algorithmic approach to diagnose patients hospitalized primarily for evaluation and treatment of suspected uncomplicated PUD begins with a referral for early upper gastrointestinal panendoscopy (Figure 80.1).

Endoscopy is a safe and accurate means of confirming or excluding the major organic causes of dyspepsia, including PUD, reflux esophagitis, and cancer, by direct visualization and biopsy of the gastrointestinal mucosa. With an experienced endoscopist, the procedure has a sensitivity and specificity for PUD of nearly 100%. Endoscopy allows further diagnostic evaluation with gastric biopsy to rule out *H. pylori* infection and cancer, and a number of studies have shown that patients prefer upper gastrointestinal endoscopy to upper gastrointestinal radiography.

Double-contrast upper gastrointestinal radiography is an acceptable, although much less sensitive (50%–60%) and slightly less specific (90%–100%), alternative when endoscopy is not readily available (13). Although the direct cost of radiography may be less than that of endoscopy, radiography does not allow targeted biopsy of gastric ulcers to rule out cancer, nor does it facilitate invasive testing for *H. pylori* or accurately exclude reflux esophagitis. Moreover, whereas endoscopy can be performed at the bedside of

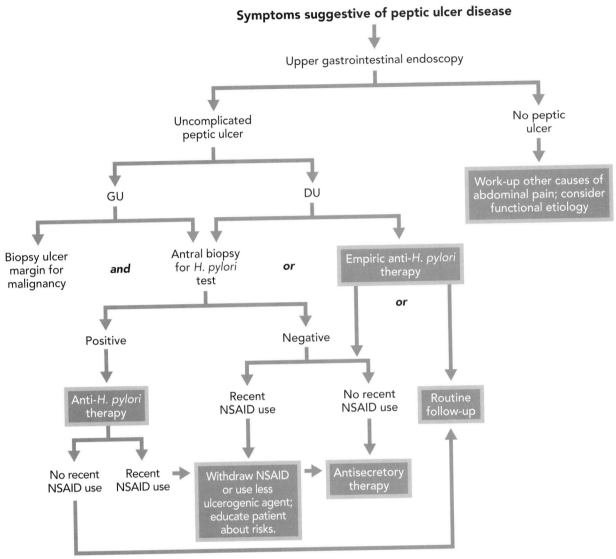

Figure 80.1 Algorithm for the management of patients with suspected peptic ulcer disease. *DU,* duodenal ulcer; *GU,* gastric ulcer; *NSAID,* nonsteroidal anti-inflammatory drug.

critically ill patients, radiography requires that the patient be able to cooperate with simple maneuvers and be suitable for transfer to the radiology suite. Finally, endoscopy may be precluded for days after radiography because of retained contrast, which also may damage the endoscope. For all of these reasons, endoscopy is the initial study of choice for the diagnosis of uncomplicated PUD in hospitalized patients.

Once PUD is confirmed by direct endoscopic visualization (preferably performed within the first 12–24 hours of admission), biopsy specimens should be taken from the antrum and midbody along the greater curvature to exclude *H. pylori* infection. Cost-effective analysis suggests that anti-*H. pylori* therapy may be given empirically without *H. pylori* testing, given the high pretest probability of *H. pylori* infection in patients with uncomplicated duodenal ulcers who deny NSAID use. Under these circumstances, treatment might still be warranted even in the presence of a negative

diagnostic test because the pre-test likelihood of *H. pylori* is very high (Chapter 6). If a gastric ulcer is present, biopsy specimens should be taken for *H. pylori,* as above, and also from the ulcer margin to exclude malignancy. A rapid urease test for *H. pylori* should be performed with antral biopsy specimens. The remaining specimens should be mounted and fixed for confirmatory histologic review in the event that the rapid urease test result is negative. If PUD is confirmed by radiography instead of endoscopy, a noninvasive test for *H. pylori* infection should be performed.

Diagnostic Tests for *Helicobacter pylori*

Determining which *H. pylori* testing method to employ is critical to implementing any evidence-based algorithm for PUD management. In patients with simple dyspepsia, noninvasive tests such as serology, carbon-labeled breath tests, and stool antigen tests have been shown to be more cost-effective than invasive tests requiring endoscopy (e.g., the rapid urease test or histology), and these are recommended for the diagnosis of *H. pylori* infection in ambulatory patients with dyspepsia. The stool antigen test, in particular, is an effective means of confirming cure following anti-*H. pylori* therapy (14). Deciding which noninvasive test to use may depend on variable local factors, such as availability, institutional test characteristics, and costs (15). In patients with a low prevalence (30%–50%) of *H. pylori* infection, such as a young ambulatory patient with simple dyspepsia, non-invasive testing should be undertaken only if it is decided *a priori* to treat in the event of positive test results (because the false-positive rate may be up to 21%). In patients hospitalized for evaluation of possible PUD, gastric biopsy with rapid urease test or histological evaluation is an accepted means of testing for *H. pylor* because they are already committed to early endoscopic evaluation.

Peptic ulcer disease in the absence of *H. pylori* infection and NSAID consumption presents a diagnostic challenge. The most common causes include false-negative *H. pylori* test results and surreptitious NSAID use. The clinician must also be cognizant of other medications that contain NSAID ingredients, including various herbal preparations, Alka Seltzer®, Anacin®, Bufferin®, Pepto Bismol® liquid, Darvon®, and Percodan®. Recent use of antibiotics, bismuth, or antisecretory agents, or recent upper gastrointestinal hemorrhage may cause false-negative results when tests for *H. pylori* that rely on the load of organisms are used, such as the carbon-labeled breath test or rapid urease test of biopsy specimens. Serology may be the test of choice in these situations. Given the high pretest probability of *H. pylori* infection in PUD patients who deny NSAID use, an initial negative test result for *H. pylori* has a low negative predictive value. Therefore, a second confirmatory test or empiric anti-*H. pylori* therapy may be warranted, especially in the case of recurrent or complicated PUD.

Biopsy specimens from *H. pylori*-negative and NSAID-negative PUD patients should be reviewed for evidence of malignancy, Crohn's disease, sarcoidosis, eosinophilic gastroenteritis, or viral infection. A history of recent radiation therapy, chemotherapy, or "crack" cocaine use may provide clues to other specific etiologies. In an appropriate setting, such as the presence of multiple ulcers in unusual locations, fasting serum gastrin levels should be ordered to rule out Zollinger-Ellison syndrome. Serum calcium should be checked to exclude hyperparathyroidism. Further workup for exceptional cases is beyond the scope of this chapter.

ISSUES DURING THE COURSE OF HOSPITALIZATION

Initial Therapy and Monitoring

The general management of patients with uncomplicated PUD should include intravenous administration of fluids for those who are unable to tolerate oral intake or who show evidence of intravascular volume depletion. There is little evidence to support the efficacy of routine antisecretory therapy before a definitive diagnosis has been made.

Vital signs should be monitored routinely every 6–12 hours. A daily assessment of symptoms and abdominal examination should be performed. Patients with dyspepsia in the setting of uncomplicated PUD may not become asymptomatic once antisecretory therapy is initiated. Scant data exist to define the appropriate length of in-hospital therapy before discharge. Medicare data from 2002 reveal an average hospital stay of four days for patients with a discharge diagnosis of PUD (2). However, a hospital stay of one to two days after the diagnosis is made should not be considered unusual in patients without significant comorbidity. We recommend that patients be discharged once their symptoms can be controlled on an outpatient basis. Patients whose symptoms increase in severity or who develop new symptoms or signs of complication will require longer hospitalization with gastroenterologic or surgical consultation.

Specific Therapy

This section emphasizes the management of uncomplicated PUD. A discussion of specific endoscopic and surgical therapeutic strategies employed in the management of complicated PUD is beyond the scope of this chapter.

Conventional Ulcer Therapy

Although more than 50% of ulcers heal spontaneously within 8 weeks, the addition of acid-inhibitory therapy with either H_2-receptor antagonists (H_2RAs) or proton pump inhibitors (PPIs) increases the speed of healing and the absolute percentage of healed ulcers at 8 weeks. PPI therapy for 8 weeks results in healing rates above 90%. However, an ulcer recurs within 1 year in 10% of those who continue on maintenance antisecretory therapy and in 80% of those who withdraw from therapy (3). Conventional ulcer-healing doses of H_2RAs (daily or in divided doses) include 800–1,200 mg of cimetidine, 300 mg of ranitidine, 40 mg of famotidine, or 300 mg of nizatidine for 4–8 weeks. Ulcer-healing doses of PPIs are 20 mg daily of omeprazole or esomeprazole, 30 mg daily of lansoprazole, 20 mg daily of rabeprazole, or 40 mg daily of pantoprazole for 4–8 weeks. Gastric ulcers may require 12 weeks for complete healing.

Anti-*Helicobacter pylori* Therapy

Curing *H. pylori* infection reduces the recurrence rate of PUD to less than 10% at one year, without the need for maintenance antisecretory therapy. The re-infection rate after successful eradication of *H. pylori* is less than 1% annually, though it is higher in patients with concurrently infected family members or other ongoing environmental exposures. National guidelines currently recommend anti-*H. pylori* therapy for all infected patients with PUD (3). Adequate eradication requires combination therapy that includes at least two antibiotics and an antisecretory agent. Issues that may influence the choice of therapy for the individual patient include efficacy, cost, compliance, and antibiotic resistance. There are several 10–14 day anti-*H. pylori* regimens that have been approved by the U.S. Food and Drug Administration (Table 80.1). In addition, recent data indicate that regimens lasting only 3–5 days may achieve eradication rates equivalent to longer regimens (16). Because there are only limited data supporting these foreshortened regimens, they have not yet become standard care.

Given adequate compliance and limited metronidazole resistance, a bismuth-based regimen improves outcomes at a lowest cost. However, because compliance is often poor, a PPI-based regimen may be the preferred choice because it requires taking fewer pills at less frequent intervals for a shorter period of time. In patients who have previously received metronidazole or clarithromycin therapy, or in geographic regions with known metronidazole or clarithromycin resistance, a regimen utilizing amoxicillin or tetracycline is preferred.

Despite initial concern, prior treatment with a PPI does not appear to influence the success or failure of subsequent antibiotic therapy. The principal benefit of *H. pylori* eradication for these patients lies in preventing recurrence of PUD, since *H. pylori*-associated ulcers heal on antisecretory therapy alone. Therefore, eradication regimens need not be instituted immediately.

Management of Peptic Ulcer Disease Induced by Nonsteroidal Antiinflammatory Agents

Patients with PUD who have been taking NSAIDs should discontinue these drugs if possible. Acetaminophen should be substituted for NSAIDs if only analgesia is required. The patient who discontinues NSAIDs should receive a standard course of healing antisecretory therapy with an H_2RA or a PPI. Although the degree of interaction between *H. pylori* and NSAIDs in PUD pathogenesis remains unclear, routine testing for *H. pylori* infection is recommended in patients with NSAID-associated PUD. All patients with documented *H. pylori* infection should receive a course of eradication therapy.

Management options for patients with NSAID-associated PUD who require chronic NSAID therapy include use of either a cyclooxygenase-2 (cox-2) selective inhibitor (known as a "coxib"), or a traditional non-selective NSAID with a co-prescribed PPI. Emerging data suggest that the latter option may be preferred in the majority of patients at high-risk for gastrointestinal complications of NSAID (17). First, despite the significant relative risk reduction in GI complications afforded by coxibs, their absolute risk reduction (compared with NSAIDs) is less than 1% for clinically-significant ulcer complications—an absolute reduction that does not offset their increased costs versus generic NSAIDs (17). Second, prospective studies in high-risk patients indicate that coxibs do not provide additional risk reduction for ulcer complications when compared with the NSAID + PPI combination. Third, cost-effectiveness analysis reveals that the coxib strategy is more expensive, yet less effective, than the NSAID + PPI

TABLE 80.1

FDA APPROVED ANTI-*H. PYLORI* REGIMENS

Regimen	Duration (d)	Efficacy (%)
Omeprazole 40 mg qd + clarithromycin 500 mg tid for 14 d, then omeprazole 20 mg qd for 14 d	28	88–94
Ranitidine bismuth citrate (RBC) 400 mg bid + clarithromycin 500 mg tid for 14 d, then RBC 400 mg bid for 14 d	28	71–75
Bismuth subsalicylate 525 mg qid + metronidazole 250 mg qid + tetracycline (TCN)[a] 500 mg qid for 14 d; + H_2RA for 28 d	28	77–82
Lansoprazole 30 mg bid + amoxicillin 1 g bid + clarithromycin 500 mg bid for 14 d	14	73–83
Lansoprazole 30 mg tid + amoxicillin 1 g tid for 14 d[b]	14	35–67
Omeprazole 20 mg bid + clarithromycin 500 mg bid + Amoxicillin 1 g bid for 10d	10	83–91
Lansoprazole 30 mg bid + Clarithroymycin 500 mg bid + Amoxicillin 1g bid for 10 d	10	81–84
Esomeprazole 40 mg bid + Clarithroymycin 500 mg bid + Amoxicillin 1 g bid for 10d	10	77–85

[a] Amoxicillin may be substituted for TCN when TCN is contraindicated.
[b] Restricted labeling: intolerant or allergic to clarithromycin or for infections with known or suspected clarithromycin resistance.
H_2RA, histamine$_2$ receptor antagonist.

strategy in high-risk patients. Fourth, whereas data reveal that the use of concurrent aspirin attenuates the relative gastrointestinal protective effects of coxibs, PPIs are highly effective in minimizing aspirin and other NSAID-related gastropathy. These data, combined with increasing concerns about cardiovascular safety of coxibs (18) (which led to the withdrawal of rofecoxib from the market), suggest that the purported gastrointestinal benefits of coxibs may not offset their additional risks and higher cost compared to the NSAID + PPI combination. Misoprostol may be an acceptable alternative to PPI co-therapy in selected patients. If possible, patients found to have an NSAID-related ulcer should receive a full healing course of anti-secretory therapy before initiating further NSAID therapy.

Patients with NSAID-negative and *H. pylori*-negative ulcers in whom no other etiology is immediately discernible should receive a course of healing antisecretory therapy. Consideration should be given to repeated *H. pylori* testing versus an empiric course of *H. pylori* eradication therapy. Those patients with complicated or recurrent disease should continue to receive maintenance antisecretory therapy indefinitely.

Prophylactic Therapy for Stress-related Mucosal Disease

There is an increasing consensus that stress-related erosive and hemorrhagic gastropathy, or "gastritis," is a less common cause of significant hemorrhage in hospitalized patients than previously thought. This trend possibly reflects the improved classification and identification of other endoscopic entities that can account for upper gastrointestinal hemorrhage. It may also reflect a decrease in the incidence and severity of gastropathy as a consequence of improved care for high-risk patients, such as the widespread use of rapid resuscitation, early enteral nutrition, and stress gastropathy prophylaxis. In this regard, the most significant recent change in the management of gastropathy has been the recognition that prophylactic therapy should be targeted to specific high-risk populations.

Although uncommon, clinically significant gastrointestinal hemorrhage from stress-related mucosal disease in a critically ill patient is associated with a 50% mortality rate when it occurs. Clinically significant upper gastrointestinal hemorrhage will develop in approximately 1%–2% of critically ill patients. Risk factors for clinically significant hemorrhage include mechanical ventilation, coagulopathy, head trauma, burns over more than 30% of the body, a history of recent PUD or gastrointestinal bleeding, and organ transplants. Of these, *48 hours of mechanical ventilation* and the presence of a *coagulopathy* are independent risk factors. The best available evidence suggests that the incidence of significant bleeding in patients without these factors is only 0.1% (19).

Multiple studies have demonstrated the efficacy of prophylactic therapy in decreasing the risk for bleeding, although an effect on mortality has not been convincingly demonstrated. H₂RAs, antacids, sucralfate, PPIs, and misoprostol have all been evaluated as prophylactic therapy. Initial studies suggested that prophylaxis with sucralfate reduced the rate of nosocomial pneumonia and death. Although the results of various studies are conflicting, the best available evidence suggests that, in comparison with sucralfate, H₂RAs provide a greater reduction in the risk for clinically significant bleeding, with no difference in mortality (20). The best candidates for prophylactic therapy may include ICU patients with uncorrected coagulapathies and those requiring sustained mechanical ventilation. H₂RAs are currently the preferred form of prophylactic therapy.

Recently, intravenous (IV) PPIs (pantoprazole, esomeprazole) have become available for inpatient use. Although IV PPIs have shown effectiveness in minimizing recurrent hemorrhage following endoscopic hemostasis of bleeding peptic ulcers, there are limited data regarding their use in stress ulcer prophylaxis. Physiologic data clearly indicate that IV PPIs produce more potent and longer-lasting acid inhibition than H₂RAs, and this finding suggests that IV PPIs might provide equal or superior clinical outcomes in stress ulcer prophylaxis than H₂RAs. In particular, recent data indicate that IV PPIs are capable of rapidly raising and maintaining intragastric pH in critically ill patients who cannot receive enteral feedings (21). Despite these suggestive physiologic data, there are currently no randomized trials that have demonstrated a benefit in clinically relevant outcomes for IV PPIs over IV H₂RAs for stress ulcer prophylaxis. In light of this shortcoming, H₂RAs may remain the agents of choice for many practitioners.

ISSUES AT DISCHARGE

Clinicians should be aware of several of the more common drug interactions and side effects of ulcer therapy. Potentially significant drug interactions include those of PPIs and clarithromycin with other drugs metabolized by cytochrome P-450 pathways. Cimetidine can act as an anti-androgen, has well-known effects on the metabolism of warfarin and phenytoin, and can decrease renal excretion of theophylline, lidocaine, and other cationic drugs. Sucralfate can decrease the absorption of a variety of drugs, cause hypophosphatemia, and result in constipation. Antisecretory therapy of any type can decrease absorption of itraconazole and ketoconazole, and may increase the risk for nosocomial pneumonia in ICU patients. Misoprostol is an abortifacient and should not be given to women of childbearing age. In addition, it may cause crampy abdominal pain, nausea, and diarrhea in a dose-related fashion. Antibiotic therapy may result in gastrointestinal symptoms such as nausea, diarrhea, or, rarely, pseudomembranous colitis. Metronidazole can cause a disulfiram-like reaction to alcohol, and clarithromycin can cause dysgeusia. Bismuth subsalicylate results in reversible darkening of the tongue and stool.

Patients should be educated about expected side effects of therapy, the importance of compliance, and specific symptoms that might warrant a phone call to the physician or an office visit. A list of NSAIDs and common over-the-counter preparations that contain NSAIDs should be given to patients, along with specific education about the ulcer risks of NSAIDs. Symptoms worthy of evaluation include the "warning symptoms" of potentially complicated PUD, in addition to uncontrolled or increasing pain.

Patients with complicated PUD require office follow-up in 1–2 weeks, followed by repeat endoscopy in 8–12 weeks to document healing and confirm *H. pylori* eradication. Patients with uncomplicated PUD may be seen within 2–4 weeks. Repeat endoscopy for confirmation of *H. pylori* eradication is not recommended in uncomplicated PUD.

QUALITY-OF-CARE CONSIDERATIONS AND RESOURCE UTILIZATION

Clinical practice guidelines already exist for the management of hospitalized patients with bleeding PUD (Chapter 78) and for ambulatory patients with dyspepsia. Similar strategies must be designed for the management of hospitalized patients with uncomplicated PUD. Such approaches should favor early endoscopy as the key step in diagnosis and disposition (15). Patients with uncomplicated PUD based on initial evaluation might fall into a low-risk category of patients who could be safely discharged from the emergency department or shortly after admission. Rapid diagnosis and institution of appropriate therapy should result in good, cost-effective outcomes.

KEY POINTS

- Most peptic ulcers are caused by *H. pylori* infection or nonsteroidal anti-inflammatory drug use and can be cured by eradicating *H. pylori* or eliminating the use of these drugs, respectively.
- Clinical practice guidelines and pathways for uncomplicated PUD require further development, evaluation, and implementation if the quality of care provided to patients hospitalized with this common condition is to improve.
- Strategies that utilize early endoscopy facilitate rapid diagnosis and therapy and should result in efficient, cost-effective care with improved outcomes.
- Gastritis, better referred to as gastropathy, is a relatively unusual cause of significant morbidity in hospitalized patients.
- Patients at high risk for the development of stress-related gastropathy (particularly those with coagulopathy or who are receiving prolonged mechanical ventilation) should receive appropriate prophylactic therapy.

REFERENCES

1. American Gastroenterological Association. Acid-related gastrointestinal diseases. In: *The Burden of Gastrointestinal Diseases.* Bethesda, MD: American Gastroenterological Association Press, 2001.
2. Center for Medicare and Medicaid Services. Medicare provider analysis and review (MEDPAR) of short-stay hospitals. Available at: www.cms.hhs.gov/statistics/medpar. Accessed April, 2004.
3. NIH Consensus Conference. *Helicobacter pylori* in peptic ulcer disease. *JAMA* 1994;272:65–69.
4. Silverstein FE, Graham DY, Senior JR, et al. Misoprostol reduces serious gastrointestinal complications in patients with rheumatoid arthritis receiving nonsteroidal antiinflammatory drugs: a randomized, double-blind, placebo-controlled trial. *Ann Intern Med* 1995;123:241–249.
5. Bombardier C, Laine L, Reicin A, et al. Comparison of upper gastrointestinal toxicity of rofecoxib and naproxen in patients with rheumatoid arthritis. *N Engl J Med* 2000;343:1520–1528.
6. Silverstein FE, Faich G, Goldstein JL, et al. Gastrointestinal toxicity with celecoxib vs nonsteroidal anti-inflammatory drugs for osteoarthritis and rheumatoid arthritis. The CLASS study: a randomized controlled trial. *JAMA* 2000;284:1247–1255.
7. Laine L, Bombardier C, Hawkey CJ, et al. Stratifying the risk of NSAID-related upper gastrointestinal clinical events: results of a double-blind outcomes study in patients with rheumatoid arthritis. *Gastroenterology* 2002;123:1006–1012.
8. Huang J, Sridhar S, Hunt RH. Role of *Helicobacter pylori* infection and non-steroidal anti-inflammatory drugs in peptic-ulcer disease: a meta-analysis. *Lancet* 2002;359:14–22.
9. Cullen DJE, Hawkey GM, Greenwood DC, et al. Peptic ulcer bleeding in the elderly: relative roles of *Helicobacter pylori* and non-steroidal anti-inflammatory drugs. *Gut* 1997;41:459–462.
10. Wu CY, Poon SK, Chen GH, et al. Interaction between *Helicobacter pylori* and non-steroidal anti-inflammatory drugs in peptic ulcer bleeding. *Scand J Gastroenterol* 1998;33:234–237.
11. Santolaria S, Lanas A, Benito R, et al. *Helicobacter pylori* infection is a protective factor for bleeding gastric ulcers but not for bleeding duodenal ulcers in NSAID users. *Alimen Pharmacol Ther* 1999;13:1511–1518.
12. Spiegel BM, Vakil NB, Ofman JJ. Endoscopy for acute non-variceal upper gastrointestinal tract hemorrhage: is sooner better? A systematic review. *Arch Intern Med* 2001;161:1393–1404.
13. Talley NJ, Silverstein MD, Agreus L, et al. AGA technical review: evaluation of dyspepsia. *Gastroenterology* 1998;114:582–595.
14. Vaira D, Vakil N, Menegatti M, et al. The stool antigen test for detection of *Helicobacter pylori* after eradication therapy. *Ann Intern Med* 2002;136:280–287.
15. Vakil N, Rhew D, Soll A, et al. The cost-effectiveness of diagnostic testing strategies for *Helicobacter pylori*. *Am J Gastroenterol* 2000;95:1691–1698.
16. Treiber G, Wittig J, Ammon S, et al. Clinical outcome and influencing factors of a new short-term quadruple therapy for *Helicobacter pylori* eradication: a randomized controlled trial (MACLOR Study). *Arch Intern Med* 2002;162:153–160.
17. Spiegel BM, Targownik LE, Dulai GS, et al. The cost-effectiveness of cyclooxygenase-2 selective inhibitors in the management of chronic arthritis. *Ann Intern Med* 2003;138:795–806.
18. Finckh A, Aronson MD. Cardiovascular risks of cyclooxygenase-2 inhibitors: where we stand now. *Ann Intern Med* 2005;142:212–214.
19. Cook DJ, Fuller HD, Guyatt GH, et al. Risk factors for gastrointestinal bleeding in critically ill patients. Canadian Critical Care Trials Group. *N Engl J Med* 1994;330:377–381.
20. Cook D, Guyatt G, Marshall J, et al. A comparison of sucralfate and ranitidine for the prevention of upper gastrointestinal bleeding in patients requiring mechanical ventilation. Canadian Critical Care Trials Group. *N Engl J Med* 1998;338:791–797.
21. Aris R, Karlstadt R, Paoletti V, et al. Intermittent intravenous pantoprazole achieves a similar onset time to pH>4.0 in ICU patients as continuous infusion H$_2$-receptor antagonist, without tolerance. *Am J Gastroenterol* 2001;96:S48.

ADDITIONAL READING

Chan FK, Chung SC, Suen BY, et al. Preventing recurrent upper gastrointestinal bleeding in patients with *Helicobacter pylori* infection who are taking low-dose aspirin or naproxen. *N Engl J Med* 2001;344:967–973.

Lee EL, Feldman M. Gastritis and gastropathies. In: Feldman M, Friedman LS, Sleisenger MH, eds. *Gastrointestinal and Liver Disease: Pathophysiology, Diagnosis, Management.* 7th ed. Philadelphia: WB Saunders, 2002:810–827.

Peura DA. Prevention of nonsteroidal anti-inflammatory drug-associated gastrointestinal symptoms and ulcer complications. *Am J Med* 2004;117(Suppl 5A):63S–71S.

Inflammatory Bowel Disease

81

Stephen B. Hanauer   *Sunanda V. Kane*

INTRODUCTION

The group of (idiopathic) inflammatory bowel diseases (IBDs) includes four disorders: ulcerative colitis (UC), Crohn's disease (CD), microscopic colitis, and collagenous colitis. This discussion is limited to the first two diagnoses. Ulcerative colitis and Crohn's disease are identified by a composite of non-specific clinical, endoscopic, and histologic characteristics (Table 81.1). There is no pathognomonic feature for either, and these diseases need to be distinguished from inflammatory disease caused by infections, ischemia, or drugs.

Ulcerative colitis was first described in 1859; by 1909, a detailed account of the disease and its natural history had been published. Crohn's disease is more recently known. It was first described as ileitis in 1913. In the late 1950s to 1960s, the potential for panenteric involvement or confinement to the colon became recognized. IBD is found worldwide, with the highest incidence in the United States, United Kingdom, Northern Europe, and Australia. The overall incidence of ulcerative colitis has remained steady during the past few decades: 3–15 cases per 100,000 annually, with a prevalence ranging from 50–80 cases per 100,000. The incidence and prevalence for Crohn's disease are similar, although the incidence has risen during the past 20 years. Any age group may be affected by IBD, with the peak incidence in the second and third decades and another peak in the elderly. The male-to-female ratio is near unity, and whites with IBD outnumber African-Americans and Asians four-fold. Risk for the development of IBD increases in people who have a family member affected with ulcerative colitis or Crohn's disease.

The specific etiologies of ulcerative colitis and Crohn's disease are unknown. Current theories implicate a genetic predisposition, with numerous potential environmental triggers initiating an overly exuberant mucosal immuno-inflammatory response. Neither specific pathogens nor consistent luminal factors have been identified. To date, the only differentiating etiologic factor in IBD is the smoking history; cigarette smoking is protective against the development of ulcerative colitis and is detrimental to the course of Crohn's disease. Eighty percent of adult patients with ulcerative colitis are nonsmokers, and 80% of adults with Crohn's disease smoke cigarettes. Recently, two independent teams of researchers described the first candidate gene in Crohn's disease, but it will be years before this discovery has direct clinical impact.

Ulcerative colitis is an idiopathic disorder primarily involving the superficial mucosal layer of the large intestine. The inflammatory process begins in the rectum and extends to a proximal margin that varies between persons. Approximately 30% of patients have disease limited to the rectum and another third to the left side of the colon; only about 20% have extensive disease involving the entire colon (pan-colitis). The extent of inflammation does not necessarily correlate with the severity and course of the disease. The primary symptom of ulcerative colitis is rectal bleeding, because the rectum is involved in all patients. The severity of disease depends on the extent of colon involved. Many patients with ulcerative proctitis present with constipation but frequent or urgent passage of blood or mucopus. Abdominal pain is uncommon. In severe colitis, the inflammation extends to deeper layers, with serosal inflammation and destruction of the circular and longitudinal muscles. This thinning of the colonic wall may lead to colonic dilation and toxic megacolon.

Eighty percent of patients have intermittent attacks throughout their lifetime, and 10%–15% experience a

TABLE 81.1

DIFFERENTIATING CHARACTERISTICS FOR ULCERATIVE COLITIS (UC) VS. CROHN'S DISEASE (CD)

	Clinical presentation	Endoscopic features	Radiologic findings	Histologic changes
UC	Bloody diarrhea Tenesmus Cramping	Diffuse pattern Circumferential Small ulcers	Extends proximally Fine ulcerations	Crypt abscesses Mucosal infiltrate
CD	Watery diarrhea Abdominal pain Perianal disease	Rectal sparing Skip lesions Linear ulcers	Segmental fistulas Strictures Small bowel involved	Focal inflammation Submucosal infiltrate Granulomas

chronic, continuous course. Only about 10% present with fulminant colitis necessitating colectomy during the first attack. With current medical therapies, life expectancy is normal. Long-term disease does, however, increase the risk for colorectal cancer. This increased risk begins after 10 years of disease, and the risk is higher for patients with more extensive disease. The increased risk is the rational for colonoscopic surveillance beginning 10 years after the onset of colitis, with multiple biopsy specimens taken from throughout the colon to identify epithelial dysplasia.

At endoscopy, the colonic mucosa is diffusely edematous and granular (instead of glistening), and it displays a spectrum of vascular changes ranging from a loss of the normal pattern to frank hemorrhage. Microscopic changes include an inflammatory infiltrate within the mucosa and neutrophilic infiltration of the epithelium, particularly the crypts. This inflammatory infiltration may lead to cryptitis, microabscesses, and architectural distortion of the glands.

Crohn's disease differs from ulcerative colitis in that the inflammatory changes are transmural (rather than superficial) and can involve any part of the alimentary tract, from the mouth to the anus. Crohn's disease typically affects the ileum, colon, and perianal region. Approximately 30%–40% of patients have isolated small bowel involvement, 40%–55% both small bowel and colonic involvement, and 15%–25% have isolated colitis.

Crohn's disease exhibits two predominant patterns: fibrostenotic-obstructing and penetrating-fistulizing. Macroscopically superficial ulcers (aphthae) may enlarge and coalesce into linear or irregularly shaped ulcers outlining areas of normal mucosa ("cobblestone" appearance). Because the disease is transmural, the bowel wall thickens and becomes fibrotic, stiff, and stenotic. Deep ulcers penetrate serosa, with development of fistulous tracking to adjacent loops of bowel, urinary bladder, vagina, or perineum. Symptoms of Crohn's disease are diverse and are determined by the disease location and severity within the involved segments. Because of its transmural nature, Crohn's disease often is associated with abdominal pain, obstruction, fevers, and malabsorption.

This chapter outlines the management issues for both acute ulcerative colitis and Crohn's disease. Despite significant overlap between the presentation and therapeutic principles, there is sufficient dissimilarity to warrant separate discussions. Most patients can be managed on an outpatient basis, and transitions between outpatient and inpatient status and vice versa are important milestones for patients with these diseases. Appropriate outpatient follow-up once the acute attack is resolved is important and will be addressed.

ULCERATIVE COLITIS

Issues at the Time of Admission

Clinical Presentation

Most patients with mild-to-moderate ulcerative colitis have had chronic symptoms with gradual progression and are managed as outpatients (1). Patients who have more than 6–10 urgent, bloody, or liquid stools, including nocturnal bowel movements, with mucopus and cramping require hospitalization. Such patients often have anorexia, nausea, vomiting (particularly with severe cramping during bowel movements), fever, dehydration (tachycardia, orthostasis) and prostration.

Patients with moderate ulcerative colitis who fail to improve with outpatient management also should be hospitalized. These patients may be less acutely ill but present with persistent diarrhea and rectal bleeding. They may have additional complications of colitis, including iron-deficiency anemia, anemia of chronic disease, hypoalbuminemia, and osteoporosis.

Important aspects of the physical examination include assessment of hemodynamics and volume status, and the abdominal examination. Patients are usually pale and orthostatic. Unusual patients may be febrile or toxic. Abdominal tenderness, especially rebound tenderness, implies transmural extension of superficial colitis to the

TABLE 81.2

EXTRAINTESTINAL MANIFESTATIONS OF INFLAMMATORY BOWEL DISEASE

Related to Activity[a]	Usually Related to Activity	Unrelated
Peripheral Neuropathy	Pyoderma gangrenosum	Sacroiliitis
Erythema nodosum	Anterior uveitis	Ankylosing spondylitis
Oral apthous ulcers	Primary sclerosing cholangitis	
Fatty liver		

[a] In terms of intestinal manifestations.

serosa. Bowel sounds are usually hyperactive, but colonic dilatation may result in distention and hypoactive or high-pitched bowel sounds. There usually is no significant perianal disease, even in patients with a history of prolonged diarrhea and straining. Extraintestinal manifestations can include ocular inflammation (episcleritis or iritis), large joint arthritis, erythema nodosum, or pyoderma gangrenosum (Table 81.2).

Differential Diagnosis and Initial Evaluation

The differential diagnosis of bloody diarrhea includes enteric infections, ischemia, radiation, other forms of IBD, and drugs (including nonsteroidal anti-inflammatory agents, gold, penicillamine, and chemotherapy). Most infectious colitis is acute and self-limited, but some cases may be fulminant and associated with systemic complications (e.g., Escherichia coli 0157:H7 infection with thrombotic thrombocytopenic purpura and renal failure). It is worth noting that in patients with a known diagnosis of ulcerative colitis, an exacerbation can be precipitated by an intercurrent infection, food poisoning, or antibiotic-associated diarrhea. Stool cultures for *Salmonella, Shigella, Campylobacter, Clostridium difficile,* amoebae, *E coli,* and, in the proper context, *Schistosoma,* cytomegalovirus, and atypical mycobacteria must be considered. It is important to alert the laboratory that the diarrhea is bloody, so that appropriate media can be used to identify *E. coli* 0157:H7. *C. difficile* infection is particularly common and should be sought by cytotoxin assay (Chapter 77).

Laboratory tests include a complete blood count with differential and platelets, coagulation studies, and a basic metabolic profile including liver chemistries. The erythrocyte sedimentation rate is nonspecific but can be useful to follow patients through the hospital course. Assessment of protein (albumin), calcium, and iron stores is important to define the overall nutritional status and replacement needs. A flat and upright abdominal radiograph is essential to rule out free air or dilatation of colon or small intestine. The proximal extension of colitis can be estimated by the absence of feces and haustra distal to the margin of disease (or

throughout the colon). If the transverse colon is dilated to more than 6 cm, *toxic megacolon* is considered to be present (Table 81.3). Contrast barium studies are contraindicated in acute colitis, as the insufflation can cause perforation. Likewise, aggressive attempts at colonoscopy are contraindicated. A limited proctoscopic or flexible sigmoidoscopic examination can define the presence of colitis, and a subsequent abdominal radiograph will outline the proximal extension of colonic wall involvement. If necessary in an acute presentation, labeled white blood cell scans may help define the extent of colonic inflammation and exclude small-bowel disease.

Indications for Initial Intensive Care Unit Admission

Patients presenting with hypotension, profuse bleeding requiring multiple transfusions, an acute abdomen, or altered mental status should be admitted to an intensive care setting. Patients with concurrent liver failure secondary to primary sclerosing cholangitis also require admission to the ICU.

TABLE 81.3

CRITERIA FOR DIAGNOSIS OF TOXIC MEGACOLON

Colonic distention of >6 cm with 3 of 4 of the following:

Fever >38.6° C
Tachycardia >120 bpm
[a]WBC >10.5
Anemia

In addition, 1 of the following:

Dehydration
Hypotension
Mental status changes
Electrolyte abnormalities

[a] WBC, White blood cell count

Initial Therapy

Patients presenting with evidence of volume depletion require intravenous (IV) fluid resuscitation until the pulse and blood pressure stabilize. It is important to include extra potassium (20–40 mEq/L) to replete losses from diarrhea and corticosteroid therapy. Other electrolyte disturbances, such as hypomagnesemia and hypophosphatemia, should be corrected with IV (not oral) supplements. Transfusions of packed red blood cells are indicated when the hematocrit is below 25% and bleeding is persistent. Administration of fresh frozen plasma is essential if there is evidence of clotting dysfunction.

The mainstay of pharmacologic therapy for the patient with a severe case of ulcerative colitis is IV steroids. Appropriate regimens include hydrocortisone (100 mg every 6 hours), methylprednisolone (16 mg every 6 hours), or dexamethasone (6–8 mg twice a day). The authors prefer a continuous infusion of 40 mg of methylprednisolone during a 24-hour period because this provides constant delivery of steroids. Doses higher than 60 mg of prednisone (or equivalent) have no added efficacy and can contribute to complications. In the setting of severe acute colitis, no oral therapy for colitis (i.e., aminosalicylates, azathioprine, 6-mercaptopurine) has been shown to add any benefit as an adjunct to corticosteroids. Rectal administration of hydrocortisone enemas can be helpful for patients with tenesmus if they are able to retain the small (60 mL) volume.

Analgesics are limited to acetaminophen and tramadol. Antispasmodics or antidiarrheal agents may be prescribed for patients with stable or improving colitis, but they should be avoided in the acute setting because they reduce peristalsis. Opiates are contraindicated because they can paralyze colonic musculature and precipitate toxic megacolon. Nonsteroidal anti-inflammatory drugs worsen colitis and should also be avoided. Low doses of benzodiazepines at bedtime may help the patient sleep.

The role of antibiotics in acute ulcerative colitis is controversial. In severe colitis, antibiotics have no additional value over steroids. However, in fulminant colitis or toxic megacolon, antibiotics are advocated to prevent transmigration and systemic bacteremia. Thus, in the presence of peritoneal findings, fever, tenderness, profound leukocytosis, or colonic dilation, we recommend broad-spectrum coverage with a combination of a second-generation cephalosporin, metronidazole, or a fluoroquinolone, in addition to an aminoglycoside. This regimen will also cover the patient for possible emergent surgery. The antibiotics are discontinued after 48 hours except when an infectious complication has been confirmed or surgery is pending.

Many patients are anorectic and do not wish to eat (fearing postprandial tenesmus or cramping). If patients are not vomiting and desire food, they may be allowed to consume liquids or a low-residue diet. Patients who present with toxic manifestations, high fever, or abdominal tenderness should have nothing by mouth until they improve. Patients with persistent vomiting and evidence of an ileus should be treated with nasogastric suction. Most patients with severe fulminant ulcerative colitis require parenteral nutritional support until they begin ingesting a full diet. Even those who are able to eat are often unable to consume the calories necessary to meet the additional catabolic demands associated with acute inflammation, corticosteroids, and protein exudation from the colon. Either peripheral or parenteral nutrition should supplement the oral intake to meet protein and caloric needs (Chapter 15).

Indications for Early Consultation

It is reasonable to request a gastroenterologic consultation for any patient hospitalized for the treatment of ulcerative colitis (2). The disease is relatively rare, and few patients are hospitalized with severe cases. Furthermore, the morbidity and mortality of ulcerative colitis can be greatly minimized by expert management. Despite the contraindication for full colonoscopy in the acute setting, a limited endoscopic study can assess the nature of intestinal bleeding. Finally, if the diagnosis is in question, a gastroenterologist can help define and then narrow the differential diagnosis. Surgical consultation at admission is warranted for patients presenting with fulminant colitis or toxic megacolon and for patients who fail to improve or who deteriorate within the first days of treatment (3).

Issues During the Hospital Course

The highest priority is to resuscitate an acutely ill, volume-depleted patient and rule out acute toxic megacolon and perforation (4). Frequent monitoring of vital signs and physical examinations during the first 24–48 hours are essential to detect early signs of deterioration. High doses of steroids can mask abdominal signs and fever. Tachycardia or a change in mental status may be the only signs of perforation. It is important to remember that acute perforation, which tends to involve the left side of the colon, can occur without being preceded by toxic megacolon.

In the absence of toxic megacolon, bowel movements should become less frequent within the first 36–48 hours. Each bowel movement may still be bloody and of liquid consistency. By the third full hospital day, the patient should be demonstrating improvement, with few bowel movements, less blood and urgency, and less anorexia. The therapeutic goal is for the patient, within 5–7 days, to have fewer than five movements a day and no fever, cramping, urgency, or nocturnal bowel movements. When a patient reaches this goal, the clinician can switch to 10 mg of oral prednisone four times daily to simulate the continuous delivery of IV steroids. At this point, the patient can be advanced to a low-residue diet with no limit on the number of calories consumed.

For patients who do not respond to 5–7 days of IV steroids, *cyclosporine* can be used as adjunctive therapy (5,

6). Initial dosing is 2–4 mg/kg over 24 hours as a continuous infusion. It is imperative that the patient's serum cholesterol is documented first because cyclosporine binds to cholesterol, and a cholesterol level below 120 mg/dL can lead to higher cyclosporine serum levels and increase the risk for toxicity (grand mal seizure). Blood levels should be monitored every 2–3 days and kept in a range of 200–400 mg/dL. Dosing adjustments should be based on either serum levels or patient side effects.

The therapeutic goals for IV cyclosporine are the same as those cited above. Patients can be switched from parenteral to oral cyclosporine when they are having formed bowel movements without blood or rectal urgency (this usually takes 5–10 days). The oral dose is twice the final IV dose in two doses. For example, a 70-kg patient with normal cholesterol who required 140 mg IV over 24 hours in the acute setting would be converted to 140 mg twice daily as an oral regimen.

If the patient has not improved within the first 2–3 days of cyclosporine therapy, another abdominal film should be obtained. If a megacolon is present, patients should receive nasogastric suction for decompression and frequent turning to aid in mobilization of air (patients should not spend more than two hours at a time in the prone position). If the findings on the repeated film are unremarkable, consider alternate diagnoses (Table 81.4). If the patient is on antibiotics, send stools for C. *difficile* toxin assay. Make certain that the patient has not been given any nonsteroidal agents for headache, fever, or pain, and that all electrolyte abnormalities have been corrected.

TABLE 81.4
CONDITIONS TO CONSIDER IF THE PATIENT FAILS TO IMPROVE

Inflammatory bowel disease-related

New fistula formation
Abscess formation
Obstruction
Perforation
Premature feeding challenge

Medication-related

Opiate withdrawal
Nonsteroidal anti-inflammatory agent use
Clostridium difficile infection secondary to antibiotics
Opportunistic infection secondary to immunosuppressants

Miscellaneous

Ischemia
Catheter infection
Thromboembolic event
Premenstrual syndrome or menses
Alternate etiologies of diarrhea: fat malabsorption, bile salt-induced colonic secretion, bacterial overgrowth, or factitious diarrhea

If the colitis symptoms are improving yet the patient is not doing well clinically, consider manifestations of immunosuppression: oral candidiasis or herpes simplex lesions can cause odynophagia, and fevers can be caused by opportunistic infection. Leukocytosis with a left shift is expected because of the steroids, but the presence of more than 20% immature cells is worrisome. If a gastroenterologist was not initially consulted, one should be when the patient has not improved and IV cyclosporine is being considered.

Continued bleeding or a blood transfusion requirement of more than 6 units within a 48-hour period is a poor prognostic sign; surgery should seriously be considered and is clearly indicated for the patient who worsens despite 24–48 hours of steroids and cyclosporine. Other poor prognostic signs after 48 hours of therapy include more than nine bowel movements a day, persistent tachycardia, fevers above 38°C, and abnormal radiographic findings. It should be pointed out that the option of surgical intervention ought to be discussed with patients who have severe ulcerative colitis even before it becomes necessary because of deterioration.

Discharge Issues

At discharge, the patient should be tolerating a low-residue diet and oral medications, have a stable hematocrit, and have no further need for transfusions. There should be adequate home support for the patient to engage in basic activities of daily living. The follow-up appointment should be about 1 week after discharge, with appropriate contact numbers in case of relapsing symptoms. The patient should be counseled about the risks of overexertion, dietary indiscretion, and medication non-adherence (Figure 81.1).

Oral prednisone should be continued at stable doses from discharge until the outpatient follow-up visit. If the patient was treated with cyclosporine, oral cyclosporine is continued along with trimethoprim-sulfamethoxazole three times weekly to prevent pneumocystis infection. Maintenance therapy with an aminosalicylate can be added at discharge (7). Additional education regarding the importance of adherence with maintenance therapy, follow-up, and drug monitoring are essential. The patient should be informed about the risk of nonsteroidal anti-inflammatory agents exacerbating colitis. At the first outpatient visit, the drug regimen is reviewed and, if cyclosporine has been used, trough blood levels are obtained. Many of these patients will be treated subsequently with long-term azathioprine or 6-mercaptopurine as supplemental maintenance therapy, in addition to an aminosalicylate. Over several months, first corticosteroids are tapered, then cyclosporine. The patient should be maintained on a long-term aminosalicylate (and azathioprine/6-mercaptopurine if cyclosporine has been used).

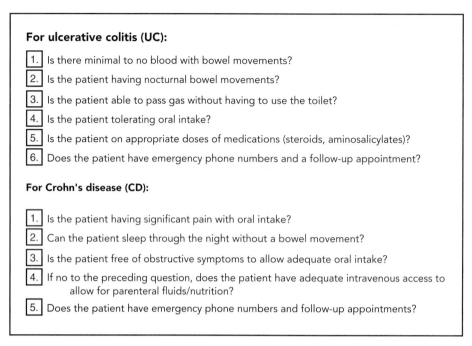

For ulcerative colitis (UC):

1. Is there minimal to no blood with bowel movements?
2. Is the patient having nocturnal bowel movements?
3. Is the patient able to pass gas without having to use the toilet?
4. Is the patient tolerating oral intake?
5. Is the patient on appropriate doses of medications (steroids, aminosalicylates)?
6. Does the patient have emergency phone numbers and a follow-up appointment?

For Crohn's disease (CD):

1. Is the patient having significant pain with oral intake?
2. Can the patient sleep through the night without a bowel movement?
3. Is the patient free of obstructive symptoms to allow adequate oral intake?
4. If no to the preceding question, does the patient have adequate intravenous access to allow for parenteral fluids/nutrition?
5. Does the patient have emergency phone numbers and follow-up appointments?

Figure 81.1 Checklist for hospital discharge

CROHN'S DISEASE

Issues at the Time of Admission

Clinical Presentation

Crohn's disease requiring hospitalization can present in several ways: refractory diarrhea, abdominal pain, bleeding, abdominal abscess, or obstruction. Volume depletion is common in the setting of nausea and vomiting resulting from obstruction or diarrhea. Fever, anorexia, and malnutrition are also common. On examination, abdominal tenderness may be localized or diffuse. There may be evidence of distention, an inflammatory mass, or frank abdominal or perianal abscess.

Differential Diagnosis and Initial Evaluation

The differential diagnosis for an acute flare of Crohn's colitis, like that for ulcerative colitis, includes infectious colitis, the use of nonsteroidal anti-inflammatory agents, antibiotic-related diarrhea, acute diverticulitis, and ischemia. Other acute processes such as appendicitis, pelvic inflammatory disease, lower lobe pneumonia, or acute hepatitis must be distinguished from a flare of Crohn's disease with small bowel involvement. Free perforation is uncommon and is more likely to occur as the first presentation of Crohn's disease than as a complication of an exacerbation. This is because transmural inflammation results in a "sticky" serosa, and the patient's own omentum usually will patch any chronic serosal leak. The transmural extension then results in thickened mesentery, an inflammatory mass of bowel wall

and mesentery, or localized fistula formation (e.g., entero-enteric, enterocolonic, or enterovesicular). In the patient with bowel obstruction, the differential diagnosis is between inflammatory obstruction secondary to a narrowed lumen and mechanical obstruction from a fibrotic stricture or adhesions from previous surgery. The acuity of the obstruction preceding inflammatory symptoms (abdominal pain, fevers, weight loss, diarrhea) and recent dietary history (consumption of hard roughage, such as nuts, celery, mushrooms) will assist in the differential diagnosis. Initial evaluation requires a thorough history to differentiate acute versus chronic symptoms. A complete physical examination should include a rectal examination and close inspection of the perianal region to rule out fistula or abscess. If the patient has diarrhea, the stool should be examined for fecal leukocytes, enteric pathogens, and *C. difficile*. Blood work should include a complete blood count with differential, chemistry panel, and cultures if the patient is febrile.

Flat and upright abdominal radiographs will rule out acute obstruction or ileus. In the presence of an abdominal mass and fever, ultrasonography or computed tomography of the abdomen and pelvis are indicated to rule out an abscess necessitating surgical consultation or percutaneous drainage.

Indications for Hospitalization

Hospitalization is indicated if the patient is unable to maintain adequate hydration or nutrition because of protracted diarrhea. It is also indicated for acute hemorrhage and severe abdominal pain or vomiting. Finally, patients presenting with fever, a tender abdominal mass, or evidence of an abdominal, pelvic, or perianal abscess should be admitted.

Indication for Intensive Care Unit Admission

Admissions to the ICU for Crohn's disease are rare and related to complications such as septic shock, intractable hemorrhage, or profound metabolic derangement.

Initial Therapy

Repletion of intravascular volume and electrolytes with IV fluids and blood products is paramount. Patients already receiving steroid therapy should receive stress doses of IV steroids (e.g., 200–400 mg of hydrocortisone or 40–60 mg of prednisone) to overcome relative adrenal insufficiency. In patients without prior steroids, glucocorticoids are withheld until infectious complications (abscess, perforation) have been ruled out. The initial distinction between fever secondary to the disease or to complications may be difficult until blood cultures and imaging studies are completed. Once infection has been excluded, it is safe to begin IV glucocorticoids (e.g., 16 mg of methylprednisolone every six hours, 100 mg hydrocortisone every 6 hours, or 6–8 mg of dexamethasone every 12 hours). *Sulfasalazine has no role in the treatment of a severe flare of Crohn's disease.* Antibiotics play more of a role in acute Crohn's disease than in ulcerative colitis. They are employed to treat the inflammatory disease or as an adjunct to prevent systemic seeding from an infectious focus (e.g., abscess). After appropriate cultures of blood, urine, and aspirates of fluid collections, broad-spectrum antibiotics (e.g., a second generation cephalosporin, a combination of an aminoglycoside and metronidazole, or a fluoroquinolone and metronidazole) are commonly employed for patients with abdominal pain and tenderness.

Once acute infection has been ruled out, an infusion with *infliximab* to treat severe inflammatory disease may be considered (8). Infliximab is administered as a 5 mg/kg IV infusion given over two hours. If the patient has received infliximab previously but not in the last eight weeks, premedication with acetaminophen 650 mg orally and 50 mg IV diphenhydramine to prevent an acute infusion reaction is warranted.

Pain is more prevalent in Crohn's disease than in ulcerative colitis because of transmural inflammation that involves pain receptors on the serosa and peritoneum. Patients presenting with pain should receive nothing by mouth and be placed on bowel rest. The pain of Crohn's disease usually abates when the patient is not eating. Opiate tolerance and seeking are not infrequent in patients with chronic Crohn's disease and should be considered when pain is the predominant symptom in the absence of inflammatory components (e.g., fever, leukocytosis, abdominal mass). If the patient has been receiving opiate analgesia before admission, gradual tapering may be necessary to avoid withdrawal symptoms. If the patient

is not able to eat, parenteral nutrition should be initiated and later tapered when the patient tolerates an advancing diet.

Indications for Early Consultation

Because of the complex and varied nature of Crohn's disease and its therapy, gastroenterologist consultation should be obtained for most patients. A surgical team should also be consulted for patients with obstructive symptoms, an inflammatory mass, an abscess, or profuse hemorrhage. Consultation from an anethesiologist or a pain service should be considered in patients receiving opiate analgesia outside the perioperative period. A nutritional support consultation is warranted for patients receiving parenteral nutrition or elemental diets, and for those with metabolic complications, short-bowel syndrome, or specific nutritional issues. Psychiatric or psychology/social work services can provide short-term emotional support, help manage acute psychosocial complications, and deliver ongoing outpatient counseling for adaptive problems related to chronic illness.

Issues During the Course of Hospitalization

The initial key management decision concerns whether the patient has an immediate indication for surgical intervention (9). If not, then the goal is to resolve acute inflammatory symptoms and work toward a stable maintenance regimen that minimizes the use of prolonged steroids and opiate analgesics. Indications for surgical exploration include the following: obstruction lasting more than 48 hours; unremitting fever; increasing abdominal pain, distention, rebound tenderness, or leukocytosis; and free intraperitoneal air. Likewise, an abscess that is not amenable to percutaneous drainage requires operative intervention.

In the absence of obstruction, ileus, or abscess, bowel rest and corticosteroids should alleviate abdominal pain and diarrhea. When the patient is pain-free after a period of bowel rest, then a trial of oral intake is initiated. An elemental diet is usually tolerated as well as total parenteral nutrition and represents a conservative approach to refeeding. Conversely, there is no advantage to a "clear liquid diet," which is commonly hyperosmotic and thus aggravates diarrhea. Patients can be advanced to low-residue diets with or without lactose, according to their history of milk intolerance. If lactose tolerance is an issue, lactose-free diets are started, with an evaluation of lactase deficiency deferred to a later date. Patients with significant ileal disease or who have had an ileal resection have an impaired ability to absorb fat and should be prescribed a low-fat diet to minimize diarrhea. At discharge, the patient should be able to tolerate sufficient calories from a low-residue diet to meet nutritional demands, and be able to perform most activities of daily life independently. There should be no need for opiates for pain control. Many patients may have "noninflammatory" symptoms of abdominal cramping or loose bowel movements that can be managed with anticholinergic antispasmodics or antidiarrheal agents (e.g., loperamide).

If the patient is not improving or is worsening, additional considerations include new fistula or abscess formation, opiate withdrawal, thromboembolic events, nonsteroidal drug-related diarrhea, *C. difficile* infection, and mechanical obstruction from adhesions or a fibrotic (rarely neoplastic) stricture. Fat malabsorption, bile salt-induced colonic secretion, or small bowel bacterial overgrowth can cause diarrhea in the absence of active inflammation of Crohn's disease. Persistent abdominal pain or distention, fever, or leukocytosis warrant repeated imaging with plain films or computed tomography, blood cultures, and a reassessment of the medication profile.

When patients with IBD are hospitalized for an unrelated problem, they should be maintained on their oral maintenance medication if possible. In the setting of other infectious illness, antibiotic or nonsteroidal drug exposure, or dietary alterations, it is not uncommon for inflammatory bowel symptoms to intensify. If the patient's disease remains stable, no gastroenterology consultation is necessary. If, however, the patient becomes symptomatic, must take nothing by mouth, has a new medical problem, or needs new medications, gastroenterology consultation is warranted.

Discharge Issues

The goal of inpatient management of Crohn's disease is to relieve pain, diarrhea, and inflammatory complications and allow resumption of a normal quality of life and social functioning with adequate oral intake to support metabolic demands. If the patient requires prolonged parenteral nutrition or antibiotics, appropriate IV access should be secured, and teaching and nursing arranged before discharge. At 7–10 days after discharge, follow-up should be coordinated with the primary treating physician (usually a gastroenterologist) and the requisite consultative teams (e.g., pain service, psychiatry, social work). If a patient has become deconditioned or requires specific rehabilitation services, then transfer to a short-term rehabilitation facility should be considered.

COST CONSIDERATIONS AND RESOURCE USE

A single study looking at the cost issues in inflammatory bowel disease estimated that in 1990, national health care expenditures were $1.2 billion to $1.4 billion (10). The primary component driving the cost of care was hospitalization. In Crohn's disease particularly, surgical costs are the main driver of overall hospital costs (11). Therefore, the optimal means of reducing the costs of IBD is to minimize the need for hospitalization, and in Crohn's disease, surgery. Early flares should be recognized and treated aggressively

before the patient's condition deteriorates. A patient should be educated regarding the importance of maintenance therapy to avoid disease exacerbations, the exogenous factors that aggravate disease activity (nonsteroidal agents, antibiotics, cigarette smoking), and the role of diet in controlling symptoms. The use of home nursing to administer parenteral nutrition, iron, or antibiotics can decrease the number of hospital days. Another key management tool is an "integrated approach" (sometimes referred to as "disease management") to outpatient care (12).

KEY POINTS

- Frequent physical exams within the first few days are essential for patients hospitalized with acute flares of ulcerative colitis or Crohn's disease.
- Crohn's disease can manifest in many ways, including diarrhea, bleeding, obstruction, severe abdominal pain, and abscess or fistula formation.
- Early gastroenterology and surgical consultation for either diagnosis is appropriate.
- If the patient is not responding to standard therapy, consider alternate diagnoses, such as infectious colitis or a complication of inflammatory bowel disease, such as abscess formation.
- If the patient is not responding to initial therapy, stop and redirect management. Patients with ulcerative colitis may benefit from adjunctive cyclosporine in addition to steroids, and patients with Crohn's disease may require antibiotics, infliximab, or surgery.
- When a patient shows improvement, advances should be slow and methodical.

REFERENCES

1. Kornbluth A, Sachar DB. Ulcerative colitis practice guidelines in adults. American College of Gastroenterology, Practice Parameters Committee. *Am J Gastroenterol* 1997;92:204–211.
2. Rizzello F, Giochetti P, Venturi A, et al. Review article: medical treatment of severe ulcerative colitis. *Aliment Pharmacol Ther* 2003;17(Suppl 2):7–10.
3. Travis SP, Farrant JM, Ricketts C, et al. Predicting outcome in severe ulcerative colitis. *Gut* 1996;38:9905–9910.
4. Stein R, Hanauer SB. Life-threatening complications pf IBD: how to handle fulminant colitis and toxic megacolon. *J Crit Illness* 1998;13:518–525.
5. Kornbluth A, Farrant JM, Lichtiger S, et al. Cyclosporin for severe ulcerative colitis: a user's guide. *Am J Gastroenterol* 1997;92:1423–1428.
6. Van Assche G, D'Haens G, Noman M, et al. Randomized, double-blind comparison of 4 mg/kg versus 2 mg/kg intravenous cyclosporine in severe ulcerative colitis. *Gastroenterology* 2003;125:1025–1031.
7. Hanauer SB, Present DH. The state of the art in the management of inflammatory bowel disease. *Rev Gastroenterol Disord* 2003;3:81–92.
8. Sandborn WJ, Hanauer SB. Infliximab in the treatment of Crohn's diseaes: a user's guide for clinicians. *Am J Gastroenterol* 2002;97:2962–2972.
9. Hanauer SB, Meyers S. Management of Crohn's disease in adults. *Am J Gastroenterol* 1997;92:559–566.

10. Hay AR, Hay JW. Inflammatory bowel disease: medical cost algorithms. *J Clin Gastroenterol* 1992;14:318–327.
11. Cohen RD, Larson LR, Roth JM, et al. The cost of hospitalization in Crohn's disease. *Am J Gastroenterol* 2000;95:524–530.
12. Kennedy AP, Nelson E, Reeves D, et al. A randomised controlled trial to assess the effectiveness and cost of a patient-oriented, self-management approach to chronic inflammatory bowel disease. *Gut* 2004;53:1639–1645.

ADDITIONAL READING

Cheung O, Regueiro MD. Inflammatory bowel disease emergencies. *Gastroenterol Clin N Am* 2003;32:1269–1288.
Farthing MJ. Severe inflammatory bowel disease: medical management. *Dig Dis* 2003;21:46–53.
Feagan BG. Maintenance therapy in inflammatory bowel disease. *Am J Gastroenterol* 2003;98:516–517.

Acute Hepatitis and Liver Failure

82

Marina Berenguer   *Teresa L. Wright*

INTRODUCTION

Fulminant hepatic failure (FHF), the appearance of severe liver injury with rapid onset of encephalopathy and profound coagulopathy in a previously healthy individual, remains one of the most challenging conditions faced by hepatologists today (1, 2). Of the approximately 2,000 cases of FHF in the United States each year, acetaminophen overdose and idiosyncratic drug reactions are the most common causes, followed by infection with hepatitis A and B viruses, poisoning, and Wilson's disease. The cause remains unknown in approximately 20% of cases (3, 4). Although acute viral hepatitis accounts for a significant proportion of FHF cases in most industrialized countries, FHF is an uncommon complication of viral hepatitis (3).

Despite advances in medical treatment of complications, the mortality rate of FHF continues to be very high (50%–90%) (1, 2). Liver transplantation (Chapter 85) achieves survival rates averaging 65% (5) and has been used increasingly as an alternative to conservative medical management. Accurate early prognostication is crucial. Indeed, patients likely to recover spontaneously must be identified so that they are not subjected to the operative risk of and the long-term immunosuppression from an unnecessary liver transplant. On the other hand, patients in whom remission is unlikely should be transplanted before complications make surgical rescue impossible (6).

The principle challenges in the care of patients with FHF are making the correct diagnosis of severe acute hepatitis, accurately and promptly identifying patients at high risk for liver failure, and recognizing the major complications (7) that should prompt liver transplantation.

Fulminant hepatic failure was defined in 1970 as a potentially reversible condition caused by severe liver injury, in which there is no prior history of hepatic disease and in which encephalopathy develops within eight weeks of the onset of illness. Though widely used, this definition was limited by the difficulty in determining the onset of the illness and the lack of a standard measure of the severity of hepatic failure. Newer classifications (1, 2, 6) emphasize: (a) the development of encephalopathy (which portends a worse prognosis); (b) the severity of hepatic failure, assessed by the prothrombin time and factor V level (higher prothrombin time and lower factor V level indicate worse prognoses); (c) the interval between the onset of jaundice and the development of encephalopathy (worst is 8–28 days); and (d) age (worse if younger than 10 years or older than 40 years).

In addition to patients with FHF, another group of patients suffers liver failure 60 days to six months after the initial injury. The cause of this delayed presentation is often "non-A, non-B" hepatitis. This *late-onset hepatic failure* tends to occur in older patients and has a very high mortality rate despite a relatively low likelihood of cerebral edema (8). In contrast, the rapidly progressive liver failure associated with hepatitis A and B viruses and drugs frequently is associated with cerebral edema but carries a lower mortality rate.

Etiology

Causes of FHF are listed in Table 82.1. For years, the most frequently identified cause was *viral hepatitis*. Newer data highlight the increasing importance of acetaminophen overdose (4) (Chapter 121). When no obvious viral or toxic cause can be implicated (approximately 20% of cases), liver failure is thought to be multifactorial. "Mutant hepatitis B viruses," "occult hepatitis B," unusual hepatitis viruses such as togavirus, cytomegalovirus, Epstein-Barr

TABLE 82.1

CAUSES OF FULMINANT HEPATIC FAILURE

Viral Hepatitis	Drug-induced Hepatitis	Other Causes
Hepatitis A–G	Acetaminophen	Metabolic (Wilson's disease, Reye's syndrome, galactosemia, sickle-cell disease)
Hepatitis non-A, non-G	Halothane	
Herpes simplex virus	Isoniazid	
Herpesvirus 6	Methyldopa	Poisoning (*Amanita* mushroom, other)
Cytomegalovirus	Tetracycline	
Epstein-Barr virus	Valproic acid	Autoimmune hepatitis
Varicella zoster	Nicotinic acid	Budd-Chiari syndrome or veno-occlusive disease
Adenovirus	Phenytoin	
		Partial hepatectomy
		Jejuno-ileal bypass
		Massive neoplastic infiltration
		Hyperthermia
		Giant-cell hepatitis
		Primary graft non-function
		Acute fatty liver of pregnancy

virus, and the recently discovered hepatitis E, C, and G viruses all have been considered as potential causes.

Prognosis

Several models have been proposed to aid in the early identification of those patients with a very poor prognosis who require liver transplantation for survival (6) (Table 82.2). King's system, which separates patients with acetaminophen toxicity from all others, has been validated

TABLE 82.2

FULMINANT HEPATIC FAILURE: CRITERIA FOR LIVER TRANSPLANTATION

Patients with acetaminophen-induced fulminant hepatic failure

pH <7.30 (irrespective of stage of encephalopathy)

or

PT >100 s (INR > 6.5) and serum creatinine >3.4 mg/dL in patients with stages III or IV encephalopathy

Patients with other causes of fulminant hepatic failure

PT >100 sec (irrespective of stage of encephalopathy)

or

Three of the following (irrespective of stage of encephalopathy):
- Age <10 or >40 y
- Etiology: non-A non-B hepatitis, halothane hepatitis, idiosyncratic drug reactions
- Duration of jaundice before onset of encephalopathy >7 d
- PT >50 s (INR >3.5)
- Serum bilirubin >17.5 mg/dL

From O'Grady JG, Alexander GJM, Hayllar KM, et al. Early indicators of prognosis in fulminant hepatic failure. *Gastroenterology* 1989;97:439–445.
INR, International Normalized Ratio; *PT*, prothrombin time.

prospectively in a number of centers worldwide and is the most commonly used.

With the exception of some rare causes of severe acute liver failure (Table 82.3), no effective medical therapy is available, and the guiding principles in the care of patients with FHF include: (a) prevention of complications, (b) identification and avoidance of aggravating factors (Table 82.4), (c) supportive management in an intensive care unit, and (d) early transfer to a liver transplant center (5–7).

The severity of acute viral hepatitis is generally age-dependent. Patients over age 50 have the most severe disease, while infection in children is usually asymptomatic or, if symptomatic, non-icteric. Pregnancy is not associated with an increased severity of disease and there is no increase in fetal loss or fetal abnormalities.

ISSUES AT THE TIME OF ADMISSION

Typical Clinical Presentation

The course of acute viral hepatitis is similar regardless of the responsible agent (Table 82.5) and can be divided into four phases: incubation, prodromal, icteric, and convalescent (3). Nonspecific constitutional symptoms of the respiratory and gastrointestinal tracts may develop during the prodromal phase. These symptoms include malaise, fatigue, myalgia, anorexia, nausea, vomiting, diarrhea, and mild abdominal discomfort. Less common prodromal symptoms include fever, headache, and arthralgias.

Most patients seek medical attention with the development of *jaundice*. When jaundice begins, fever typically declines and systemic symptoms begin to subside. Physical examination may be unrevealing or may identify tender hepatomegaly (generally mild), splenomegaly, and

TABLE 82.3
SPECIFIC THERAPIES IN ACUTE HEPATITIS

Condition	Therapy	Doses
Hepatitis B	Lamivudine (controversial)	100 mg daily (adjusted for renal insufficiency)
Acetaminophen-induced hepatitis	N-acetylcysteine within 36 hours of ingestion[a] (Chapter 121)	140 mg/kg followed by 70 mg/kg every 4 h for 68 h, total of 17 doses
Budd-Chiari syndrome	Portal vein decompression	Emergency mesocaval or mesoatrial shunt, or transjugular intrahepatic portosystemic shunt
Veno-occlusive disease	Anticoagulation	See Chapter 98
Wilson's disease	D-penicillamine	300 mg/d (increase to 1,500–2,400 mg/d)
Autoimmune hepatitis	Steroids	Prednisolone: 1–2 mg/kg/d intravenous
Acute fatty liver of pregnancy	Early delivery	
Herpes simplex or cytomegalovirus hepatitis	Acyclovir or ganciclovir	Ganciclovir: 5 mg/kg every 8h intravenous; Acyclovir: 5–10 mg/kg/three times daily intravenous
Carbon Tetrachloride poisoning	N-acetylcysteine	
Amanita mushroom poisoning	Penicillin G and silymarine Early massive rehydration	Penicillin G: 40 × 10^6 units/day + silymarine: 50 mg/kg/day

[a] N-acetylcysteine may improve survival rate even when the administration is delayed 72 hours after overdose.

TABLE 82.4
COMPLICATIONS OF FULMINANT HEPATIC FAILURE

Complication	Management	Therapy
Encephalopathy	Head computed tomography scan to rule out brain complications Consider neurology consultation	Avoid sedative-hypnotics Recognize and treat potentially reversible factors Lactulose (30–120 mL/d orally/rectally) Flumazenil (still experimental therapy with transient benefits) Neomycin is not recommended
Cerebral edema	Intracranial pressure monitoring	Keep head elevated Avoid aggravating conditions (head motion, hypoxemia, hypercapnia, fluid overload) Mannitol Pentobarbital
Coagulopathy	Regular monitoring of prothrombin time, platelet count	Vitamin K Fresh frozen plasma and platelet transfusion therapy for active bleeding or before invasive procedures; do not give prophylactically simply for elevated fibrin degradation products
Infection	Surveillance cultures If ascites, diagnostic paracentesis Chest radiograph	Low threshold for antibiotics Change intravascular catheters every 72 h Pulmonary toilet
Stress ulcerations	Intragastric pH monitoring	Histamine₂ antagonist
Renal failure	Regular laboratory monitoring (creatinine, BUN, urinary sodium, glomerular filtration)	Combination loop diuretics and albumin Low-dosage dopamine Avoid nephrotoxic drugs Continuous or intermittent hemodialysis
Hypoglycemia	Glucose monitoring every 4 h until stabilization	5–10% dextrose solutions (occasionally 25–50% solutions) should be started on admission
Metabolic acidosis	Arterial blood-gas monitoring	Bicarbonate replacement or hemodialysis
Respiratory failure	Arterial blood-gas monitoring	Intubation if encephalopathy stages III and IV
Gastrointestinal bleeding	Intranasal/oral examination to rule out bleeding gums Endoscopy	Somatostatin (100 mg bolus followed by 50 mg/h); no β-blockers in the acute setting Sclerotherapy or banding of varices Balloon tamponade if uncontrolled bleeding
Multiorgan failure	Invasive hemodynamic monitoring	Supportive

BUN, blood urea nitrogen.

TABLE 82.5

MAIN FEATURES OF VIRAL HEPATITIS

	HAV	HBV	HCV	HDV	HEV
Transmission	Fecal-oral, outbreaks	Sexual, parenteral, vertical	Parenteral, sexual, vertical	Sexual, parenteral	Fecal-oral, outbreaks
Incubation (in days)	15–45	30–180	15–160	30–180	14–60
Symptoms					
Fever	Common	Uncommon	Uncommon	Common	Common
Nausea, vomiting	Common	Common	Uncommon	Common	Common
Arthralgia, rash	Uncommon	Common	Uncommon	Uncommon	Common
Jaundice	Common in adults	Variable	Uncommon	Common	Common
Severity of acute hepatitis	Mild (depends on age)	30% icteric	Very mild	Severe	Variable (severe in pregnancy)
Frequency of hepatic failure	0.1%	0.1–1%	0.1%	5% coinfection 20% superinfection	1–2% (10–20% during pregnancy)
Frequency of chronicity	Never	1–10% adults 90% newborns	80%	5% if coinfection with HBV 95% if superinfection	Never
Acute diagnosis	Anti-HAV IgM	HBsAg, anti-HBc IgM	Anti-HCV, HCV RNA	Anti-HDV IgM / IgG, HDV RNA	Anti-HEV IgM, HEV RNA

HAV, hepatitis A virus; *HBV*, hepatitis B virus; etc.

lymphadenopathy. In the icteric phase, jaundice may be associated with pruritus and skin excoriations. Suspicion of hepatic failure is based on identification of the triad of jaundice, dark urine, and systemic symptoms. Although there are no pathognomonic laboratory abnormalities associated with viral hepatitis, rising aminotransferase values identify the development of hepatocellular necrosis. Aminotransferase values, which start rising during the prodromal phase (before elevations in bilirubin and alkaline phosphatase levels), usually peak at levels greater than 1,000 unit/L. There appears to be little correlation between the degree of aminotransferase elevation and prognosis. Prolonged prothrombin time, however, does signify worsening hepatic function and a poor prognosis.

Atypical Clinical Presentation

Cholestatic Hepatitis

Cholestatic hepatitis is characterized by marked pruritus and chemical evidence of intrahepatic cholestasis, with elevations of serum alkaline phosphatase and serum bilirubin levels (usually in excess of 15 mg/dL), but no substantial hepatocellular disease. Despite their jaundice, these patients generally feel and do well.

Fulminant Hepatic Failure

FHF complicates viral hepatitis in less than 5% of the cases. Hepatitis A rarely may lead to FHF (0.1% of acute cases). The risk is higher in older patients and in those with underlying chronic liver disease (9). Hepatitis B is the most common viral cause of FHF (50%–70% of virus-related cases). The low risk of developing FHF with acute hepatitis B virus infection (0.1%–1.0% of acute hepatitis B cases) is increased by infection with mutant strains or coinfection with hepatitis delta virus. Hepatitis C alone is a rare cause of FHF, but hepatitis C virus infection may contribute to hepatic failure in association with other viruses. By definition, patients with FHF have some degree of *cerebral dysfunction*, which may range from subtle personality changes to deep coma (Table 83.4). Jaundice is generally present; its absence may lead to an erroneous diagnosis of a psychotic episode, drug overdose, or septicemia. Other disorders that may masquerade as hepatic encephalopathy must be excluded. Laboratory investigations usually clarify the diagnosis.

Differential Diagnosis and Initial Evaluation

In patients presenting with severe acute hepatitis, an in-depth history including questions to assess suicidal ideation or surreptitious ingestion of toxins (including mushrooms or unusual herbal medicines) must be obtained. A rigorous examination also should be performed to look for incipient encephalopathy, which may be an early indicator of liver failure. Thereafter, neurologic status should be assessed frequently. If mental status worsens, intubation for airway protection must be considered. The physician also should search for signs of underlying chronic liver disease (such as spider nevi or palmar erythema), which is a risk factor for a severe course of acute hepatitis.

Because of the considerable overlap in the clinical symptoms, signs, and biochemical laboratory tests, serologic testing is needed to establish a specific diagnosis (Table 82.5). Useful laboratory tests include measurement of aminotransferases, total bilirubin, alkaline phosphatase levels, and prothrombin time. Evidence of a prolonged prothrombin time (INR of 1.5 or greater or prothrombin time of 17 seconds or longer), should raise concern regarding the potential development of FHF and should prompt continuous monitoring. These laboratory tests should be followed every 12 hours initially and then daily. If a coagulopathy is present, neither vitamin K nor fresh frozen plasma should be administered unless there is overt bleeding, as no benefit has been proven from these interventions, and therapy could mask the progression of the coagulopathy. Other useful tests include arterial blood-gas, creatinine, and hematocrit measurements. Ultrasound may be used to exclude biliary pathology in cholestatic forms of hepatitis.

Assessing the severity of the episode is essential for prompt referral to a transplant center (Table 82.2). In patients with signs of severe disease, information that is useful to the transplant center includes (a) *patient characteristics*, with special emphasis on height and weight, other medical problems that might preclude liver transplantation, social and psychological profile, and information about substance abuse; (b) *basic laboratory tests and measurements*, including complete blood counts with differential, platelet counts, electrolytes, serum aminotransferases, alkaline phosphatase, bilirubin, albumin, amylase, blood type, prothrombin time, arterial blood gases, urinalysis, and urine output; (c) *bacteriologic and serologic data*, including blood, urine, and ascitic fluid cultures, hepatitis B surface antigen, hepatititis B core IgM antibody, hepatitis A virus IgM antibody, hepatitis C virus antibody, and HIV serology; and (d) *imaging information*, including abdominal Doppler ultrasound, chest radiograph, and brain imaging results if indicated, electrocardiogram, and electroencephalogram.

Indications for Hospitalization

In the vast majority of cases, acute viral hepatitis is self-limited and most patients do not require hospitalization. Simple advice includes elimination of alcohol intake and discontinuation of potentially hepatotoxic medications. There are no mandatory dietary modifications. Sedatives and opiates should be avoided. Cholestyramine is the drug of choice for pruritus. There are certain clinical and biochemical characteristics that suggest a more complicated course and should lead to hospitalization (Table 82.6).

Indications for Early Consultation

Virtually all patients whose hepatitis is severe enough to require admission would benefit from a consultation by a

TABLE 82.6

ACUTE SEVERE HEPATITIS: INDICATIONS FOR HOSPITALIZATION

Serious underlying medical condition
Advanced age
Pregnancy
Treatment with hepatotoxic medication or immunosuppressive drugs
Underlying chronic liver disease
Malnutrition
Severe vomiting precluding adequate oral intake
Features suggestive of fulminant liver failure such as hepatic encephalopathy
Patients presenting with ascites
Laboratory findings of prolonged PT (>50% over the normal range), low serum albumin, hypoglycemia, or serum bilirubin >20 mg/dL
Any sign of gastrointestinal bleeding

PT, Prothrombin time.

hepatologist. In addition, patients with acute viral hepatitis and elevated creatinine, recent surgery, pregnancy, and HIV infection should be seen by a specialist.

Indications for Intensive Care Unit Admission

Any patient suspected of having FHF should be admitted to an ICU for monitoring for and treatment of complications (Table 82.6).

ISSUES DURING THE COURSE OF HOSPITALIZATION

There are no specific treatments for severe acute viral hepatitis. The use of lamivudine in the patient with acute hepatitis B is controversial; there are no randomized trials to guide this decision. Those rare acute causes of hepatitis with effective treatment are listed in Table 82.5. The highest priority during a hospitalization for acute viral hepatitis is thus *early recognition of FHF*. Avoidance of potential aggravating factors (such as electrolyte imbalance, nosocomial infections, and use of sedatives) and treatment of any complications (Table 82.4) are the key elements of successful management. Treatments that should be continued in patients with acute severe hepatitis include insulin in those with insulin-dependent diabetes (lowering the daily dosage to maintain blood glucose levels above 200 mg/dL), IV quinine in patients in whom falciparium malaria is suspected (i.e., travelers returning from endemic areas), and appropriate hormonal therapy in those with adrenal or thyroid insufficiency. Periodic assessments of neurologic status should be performed. In addition, information that ultimately could contraindicate liver transplantation should be assessed (Table 82.7) in case trans-

TABLE 82.7

CONTRAINDICATIONS TO URGENT LIVER TRANSPLANTATION IN CASE OF FULMINANT HEPATIC FAILURE

Severe irreversible brain damage
Active alcohol/drug abuse
Septic shock (bacterial infection is not a contraindication)
Severe cardiopulmonary disease
Acquired immunodeficiency syndrome
Severe hemorrhagic pancreatitis
Severe adult respiratory distress syndrome
Widespread thrombosis of portal and mesenteric veins
Sustained elevation of ICP >50 mm Hg
Cerebral perfusion pressure <40 mm Hg for >2 h

ICP, Intracranial pressure.

plantation is necessitated by worsening FHF. Attempts should be made to determine the cause, if it is still unknown at admission. Daily blood and urine cultures should be performed and broad-spectrum antibiotic therapy begun if there is any reasonable suspicion of active infection. It is important to remember that in severe forms of acute hepatitis, the classic signs of infection (such as fever, leukocytosis, or positive blood cultures) may be absent. An unexplained decrease in blood pressure or in urinary output, worsening hepatic encephalopathy, or development of severe acidosis should suggest sepsis (Chapter 26) and prompt the initiation of antibiotics and ICU admission. Liver function should be assessed frequently—initially every 12 hours, then daily. If prothrombin time or factor V levels are altered 50% or more out of the normal range, a hepatologist should be consulted. Finally, renal and pulmonary function should be measured daily so that complications can be recognized early.

DISCHARGE ISSUES

Once the prothrombin time has reached a plateau and begun to decrease, medical status has normalized, and other complications have resolved, the patient may be discharged from the hospital. Jaundice will still be present at this time; it may persist for as long as 4–6 weeks. Within two weeks of the onset of jaundice, the enlarged liver and spleen begin to shrink, pruritus resolves, and a sense of well-being returns. *Chronicity*, characterized by persistently abnormal liver function, is a major feature of hepatitis C virus infection (>80%) and to a lesser extent (1%–10%) of hepatitis B virus infection.

There are no specific measures to initiate upon discharge. The primary physician should assess laboratory values for chronicity. Any potential hepatotoxic medication should be avoided, as should alcohol. Follow-up by a primary physician should be scheduled within 2–3 weeks of discharge, with an earlier visit scheduled for older patients or those with underlying comorbidities.

Precautions against percutaneous and sexual transmission are recommended for patients with hepatitis B or C for as long as there is virus present in the serum. Patients should abandon these precautions only if and when the virus clears from their sera (and virus is cleared only rarely in hepatitis C). By the time a patient with hepatitis A is discharged, no additional precautions are required, as the shedding of virus in feces precedes the development of acute disease.

SEVERE NONVIRAL ACUTE HEPATITIS

Although a viral agent is the most common cause of acute hepatitis, some cases are related to other causes, including drugs and metabolic or autoimmune disorders. Clinical symptoms at presentation are indistinguishable from acute viral hepatitis, with jaundice being the most prominent feature. Some features may point toward a particular cause (10–12) (Table 82.8). Criteria for admission are the same as for viral hepatitis, and efforts should be directed at detecting signs of liver failure and defining the cause (Figure 82.1).

Alcoholic Hepatitis

Most alcohol abusers remain asymptomatic and may develop cirrhosis silently if they continue drinking. A minority have episodes of acute alcoholic hepatitis. Although the course of alcoholic hepatitis is similar to that of viral hepatitis, some features help differentiate the two entities (Table 82.8). If, after initial evaluation, the clinician remains unable to distinguish between alcoholic hepatitis and a surgical process such as *cholecystitis*, a liver biopsy is preferable to laparotomy, which is associated with a high mortality rate among acutely ill patients. Typically, liver biopsy reveals swollen hepatocytes, inflammation with polymorphonuclear leukocytes, macrovesicular fat, and Mallory's bodies. In the patient at high risk for bleeding, liver biopsy may be performed via the transjugular route.

The management of patients with alcoholic hepatitis depends upon the severity of disease. Most patients with mild-to-moderate alcoholic hepatitis recover spontaneously following abstinence from alcohol and the provision of sufficient nutrition (Chapter 15) and vitamins (particularly folic acid). Patients with *severe alcoholic hepatitis*, defined by the presence of encephalopathy or a discriminant function (calculated as 4.6 [prothrombin time − control time in seconds] + serum bilirubin [in micromoles per liter] /17) greater than 32 and without gastrointestinal bleeding or bacterial infection derive a short-term benefit from treatment with corticosteroids (40 mg of methylprednisolone daily for four weeks) (13). Patients require intensive nutritional support, lactulose for encephalopathy, frequent checks of glucose, and close observation for infection

TABLE 82.8

FEATURES CHARACTERISTIC OF DIFFERENT CAUSES OF NONVIRAL ACUTE LIVER FAILURE

Disease	Main Characteristics
Acute fatty liver of pregnancy	Third trimester, associated with preeclampsia, hyperuricemia, hyperleukocytosis, mild increase of aminotransferase and bilirubin values
Alcoholic hepatitis	Consistent ingestion history, pain and tenderness, fever and hepatomegaly, AST higher than ALT with neither over about 600 International Units, normal ultrasound, leukocytosis and left shift, mild elevation of serum alkaline phophatase, signs of chronic alcoholism
Amanita mushroom poisoning	Consistent ingestion history (lethal dose is approximately three medium-sized mushrooms), prominent abdominal cramps, vomiting, and diarrhea after a symptom-free interval of at least five hours
Budd-Chiari syndrome, veno-occlusive disease	History of chemotherapy or irradiation, bone-marrow transplantation; rapid onset of ascites, abdominal pain
Drug-induced hepatitis	Consistent ingestion history, absence of any other cause, hypersensitivity syndrome (cutaneous rash, fever, eosinophilia)
Ischemic hepatitis	History of hypoxia (septic or hemorrhagic shock, myocardial infarction, arrhythmias), coexistent renal failure, profound increase of serum aminotransferase values (>100 times normal) with moderate increase of bilirubin, improvement with treatment of the cause
Wilson's disease	Age <30 years, family history, Kayser–Fleischer ring, Coombs-negative hemolytic anemia, high levels of urine copper, very low concentration of serum ceruloplasmin
Autoimmune hepatitis	Young people (particularly women), presence of antiorganelle (anti-smooth muscle, anti-liver and kidney microsome type 1, antinuclear) antibodies. Giant-cell hepatitis (syncytial cells) may be a histological feature.

ALT, alanine aminotransferase; *AST*, aspartate aminotransferase.

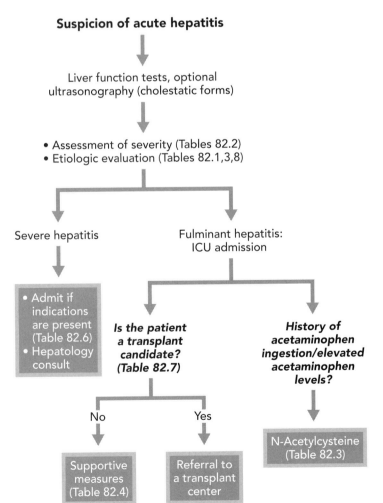

Figure 82.1 Management of acute hepatitis.

(including spontaneous bacterial peritonitis). These patients often benefit from the involvement of experienced hepatologists (Chapter 83).

Generally, serum bilirubin and albumin measurements and prothrombin time improve during the first 2–3 weeks of treatment, and patients may be discharged home to finish the six weeks of steroid therapy. Follow-up by a primary physician should be scheduled within one week of discharge.

The mortality rate among patients with severe alcoholic hepatitis is high, exceeding 60% in some series. The role of hepatic transplantation is still uncertain (Chapter 85). Although corticosteroids produce a short-term benefit in the small subset of severely ill patients with no bacterial infection or gastrointestinal bleeding, long-term survival is not improved. Because the prognosis of these patients is determined largely by their ability to remain abstinent from alcohol, careful long-term monitoring and appropriate counseling are important.

Acetaminophen Overdose

Acetaminophen is the most widely used nonprescription analgesic in the USA. If used according to package recommendations, there is very little risk of liver injury. However, it is a common putative cause of acute liver failure because of its recognized dose-related hepatotoxicity, its easy availability, and its frequent administration in the face of other cofactors, such as alcohol use, opiates, and starvation (5). Of all patients with FHF, those with acetaminophen-related liver failure have the best chances of spontaneous recovery with supportive care. However, clinicians should be aware of the rapidity with which liver injury evolves. Since outcome is unpredictable, early transfer to a transplantation unit should be considered. The monitoring should include repeated (twice daily) measurements of serum creatiniine and prothrombin time, two main prognostic factors. N-acetylcysteine (NAC) is the main antidote (Table 82.3), with survival rate being related to the rapidity of its administration (6). NAC may induce nausea and occasionally cardiac arrythmias.

COST CONSIDERATIONS AND RESOURCE USE

In considering the most cost-effective strategy for the management of acute liver failure, one needs to consider several variables, including the expected survival of patients with and without transplantation and the expected costs associated with transplantation. In 1996, the average charges for liver transplantation in the first year were $314,500, with an estimated annual follow-up charge of an additional $29,100. Because many transplant programs compete for contracts on the basis of both costs and outcomes, accept-

ing "difficult patients", such as those with severe acute liver failure, may provide a disadvantage to a program in the current health care marketplace.

KEY POINTS

- Acute viral hepatitis is, in the vast majority of cases, a self-limited and benign disease with complete recovery and restoration of liver function. Most patients do not require hospitalization.
- Because severe acute hepatitis can evolve into FHF, patients with features suggesting a more severe course and significantly impaired synthetic function should be hospitalized for monitoring.
- Fulminant hepatic failure (defined as spontaneous encephalopathy or biochemical evidence of advanced hepatocellular dysfunction) is an indication for ICU admission.
- The major markers of unfavorable outcome in patients with FHF include encephalopathy, a prolonged prothrombin time, or a diminished factor V level.
- Patients with severe alcoholic hepatitis without infection or bleeding derive a short-term benefit from corticosteroid therapy.
- Early contact with a liver-transplant program is mandatory if the disease follows a severe or atypical course. Liver transplantation remains the best therapeutic approach in patients with low likelihood of spontaneous recovery.

REFERENCES

1. Hoofnagle JH, Carithers RL, Shapiro C, et al. Fulminant hepatic failure: summary of a workshop. *Hepatology* 1995;21:240–252.
2. Mas A, Rodés J. Fulminant hepatic failure. *Lancet* 1997;349: 1081–1085.
3. Berenguer M, Wright TL. Viral hepatitis. In Feldman M, Friedman LS, Sleisenger MH, eds. *Gastrointestinal and Liver Disease.* 7th ed. Philadelphia: WB Saunders, 2002:1278–1342.
4. Ostapowicz G, Fontana RJ, Schiodt FV, et al. Results of a prospective study of acute liver failure at 17 tertiary care centers in the United States. *Ann Intern Med* 2002;137:947–954.
5. Castells A, Salmeron JM, Navasa M, et al. Liver transplantation for acute hepatic failure: analysis of applicability. *Gastroenterology* 1993;105:532–538.
6. Williams R. Classification, etiology, and considerations of outcome in acute liver failure. *Semin Liver Dis* 1996;16:343–348.
7. Muñoz SJ. Difficult management problems in fulminant hepatic failure. *Semin Liver Dis* 1993;13:395–446.
8. Ellis AJ, Saleh M, Smith H, et al. Late-onset hepatic failure: clinical features, serology and outcome following liver transplantation. *J Hepatol* 1995;23:363–372.
9. Vento S, Garofano T, Renzini C, et al. Fulminant hepatitis associated with hepatitis A virus superinfection in patients with chronic hepatitis C. *N Engl J Med* 1998;338:286–290.
10. Makin AJ, Wendon J, Williams R. A seven year experience of severe acetaminophen-induced hepatotoxicity 1987–1993. *Gastroenterology* 1995;108:1807–1818.
11. Berman DH, Leventhal RI, Gavaler JS, et al. Clinical differentiation of fulminant Wilsonian hepatitis from other causes of hepatic failure. *Gastroenterology* 1991;100:129.

12. Murphy EJ, Davern TJ, Shakil AO, et al. Troglitazone-induced fulminant hepatic failure. Acute Liver Failure Study Group. *Dig Dis Sci* 2000;45:549–553.
13. Ramond MJ, Poynard T, Rueff B, et al. A randomized trial of prednisolone in patients with severe alcoholic hepatitis. *N Engl J Med* 1992;326:507–512.

ADDITIONAL READING

Bailey B, Amre DK, Gaudreault P. Fulminant hepatic failure secondary to acetaminophen poisoning: a systematic review and meta-analysis of prognostic criteria determining the need for liver transplantation. *Crit Care Med* 2003;31:299–305.

Kjaergard LL, Liu J, Als-Nielsen B, et al. Artificial and bioartificial support systems for acute and acute-on-chronic liver failure: a systematic review. *JAMA* 2003;289:217–222.

Lee WM. Acute liver failure. *N Engl J Med* 1993;329:1862–1867.

Levitsky J, Mailliard ME. Diagnosis and therapy of alcoholic liver disease. *Semin Liver Dis* 2004;24:233–247.

Schmidt LE, Dalhoff K, Poulsen HE. Acute versus chronic alcohol consumption in acetaminophen-induced hepatotoxicity. *Hepatology* 2002;35:876–882.

Vaquero J, Blei AT. Etiology and management of fulminant hepatic failure. *Curr Gastroenterol Rep.* 2003;5:39–47.

Cirrhosis and Its Complications

83

Don C. Rockey

INTRODUCTION

Persistent liver injury leads to the clinical and pathologic entity known as cirrhosis. Although hepatic injury can be caused by a number of infectious or metabolic processes, the eventual clinical outcomes are identical, namely a histologic lesion consisting of bridging fibrosis with regenerative nodules. This scarring process leads to hepatocellular dysfunction and portal hypertension, each with attendant clinical sequelae and manifested as liver failure, hepatic encephalopathy, variceal hemorrhage, and ascites. Progressive hepatocellular dysfunction results in hepatic encephalopathy and liver failure; portal hypertension is the cause of ascites and variceal hemorrhage.

The complications of cirrhosis highlighted above are often life threatening. For example, the mortality rate of patients during the first episode of acute esophageal variceal hemorrhage is approximately 35%. Further, the 1-year mortality rate of patients with cirrhotic ascites approaches 50%. These poor outcomes underscore the severity of the underlying disease process. This chapter focuses on the major complications (ascites and spontaneous bacterial peritonitis [SBP], hepatic encephalopathy, and hepatorenal syndrome) in patients with known or presumed cirrhosis. Acute hepatitis, fulminant liver failure (Chapter 82), and acute variceal hemorrhage (Chapter 78) are reviewed elsewhere.

Portal Hypertension

Portal hypertension is the major complication of cirrhosis. The portal system is normally a low-pressure system. Portal hypertension occurs if the pressure in this system exceeds the pressure in the inferior vena cava by more than 5 mm Hg.

Collateral vessels (varices) form as the vascular system attempts to equalize the pressure between the portal and systemic circulation. The most common and clinically relevant sites in which collaterals form are in the esophagus and stomach. Elevated portal pressure results from increased intrahepatic resistance and/or increased flow through the portal venous system. Increased resistance probably occurs first and is followed by an increase in flow. Both increased resistance and flow are potential therapeutic targets.

Although portal hypertension most commonly results from cirrhosis (which leads to so-called "sinusoidal portal hypertension"), prehepatic portal hypertension (e.g., caused by portal or splenic vein thrombosis) and posthepatic portal hypertension (caused by cardiac disease or hepatic vein occlusion) must be considered in all patients. Altered portal hemodynamics contributes not only to varix formation but also to ascites formation. The mechanism of ascites formation is not entirely understood but is most likely related to derangement of the neurohumoral axis that regulates sodium and water excretion.

Practical Approach to the Patient with Cirrhosis

When approaching the patient with possible cirrhosis, it is important to search for evidence of chronic liver disease. Clinical signs of cirrhosis include the following: spider angiomata, distention of abdominal wall veins, ascites, splenomegaly, muscle wasting, Dupuytren's contractures (especially with ethanol-associated cirrhosis), gynecomastia and testicular atrophy in males, and palmar erythema. However, it is important to emphasize that even in patients with histologic cirrhosis, these physical signs may not always be present. Laboratory data provide further clues to the presence of cirrhosis as well as to the severity of the disease. In particular, the prothrombin time, bilirubin, albumin are important. These tests are important components of the Childs-Pugh classification (Table 85.1) and therefore are also used to help assess the severity of the liver disease. Additionally, the platelet count has proven to be a useful predictor of the presence of clinical portal hypertension (a low platelet count is caused by portal hypertension, splenomegaly, and sequestration of platelets in the spleen).

The cause of cirrhosis should be determined in all patients. An overview of initial evaluation is shown in Figure 83.1. The differential diagnosis of cirrhosis includes other diseases that may cause portal hypertension or ascites. All patients must have a careful cardiac examination, especially for constrictive pericarditis, because this disease easily can be mistaken for primary hepatic disease with portal hypertension. The nephrotic syndrome also can be misconstrued as cirrhosis. Ultrasound or computed tomography findings can suggest cirrhosis when portal hypertension is present. However, imaging tests are inadequate when an assessment of parenchymal architecture is required. Liver biopsy is the gold standard for assess-

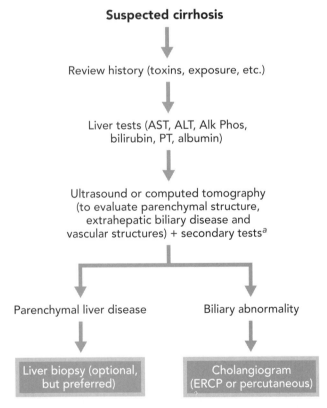

Figure 83.1. Evaluation of patients with suspected cirrhosis. Evaluation follows as outlined in the algorithm. ^aSecondary tests include the following: hepatitis serologies (B/C), iron studies (ferritin and iron saturation for hemochromatosis), copper studies (ceruloplasm, urinary copper excretion, or slit-lamp examination if the patient is young or has neuropsychiatric disease), antinuclear antibody (autoimmune hepatitis), antimitochondrial antibody (primary biliary cirrhosis). *Alk Phos*, alkaline phosphatase; *ALT*, alanine aminotransferase; *AST*, aspartate gaminotransferase; *ERCP*, endoscopic retrograde cholangiopancreatography; *PT*, prothrombin time.

ment of hepatic architecture and in some instances is required to document and assess the extent of hepatic disease. In situations in which the diagnosis is unclear, a hepatologist should be consulted.

Although many patients (up to 40%–50%) with cirrhosis are asymptomatic, once a complication of cirrhosis becomes clinically evident, an accelerated clinical course usually ensues. Generally, the underlying severity of liver disease dictates the clinical course. For this reason, it is imperative to assess the functional status of patients with liver disease early in their course. The presence of hepatic encephalopathy indicates severe hepatocellular dysfunction. Hepatocyte function is also judged by measurement of the prothrombin time, because hepatocytes synthesize clotting factors. An elevated prothrombin time in the absence of malnutrition or obstruction of the biliary system strongly suggests severe functional impairment. The serum albumin level also is used to judge hepatocellular function. In a patient with known liver disease, ascites strongly suggests portal hypertension and is also a sign of advanced disease. Such data allow a rapid assessment of the patient's clinical state and should be sought upon admission to the hospital. Child's classification, or the *Child-Pugh score* (Table 85.1), is a semiquantitative assessment of these and other factors that readily allows clinical ascertainment of the patient's clinical status, a discussion of prognosis with the patient, and a common ground for review of the literature. Recently, the *MELD (model for end-stage liver disease)* scoring system has been used to help assess the severity of liver disease. This quantitative scoring system calculates a single number based on the patient's bilirubin, prothrombin time, and creatitine and, unlike the Child-Pugh score, does not rely on subjective assessments, such as the degree of encephalopathy or the severity of ascites. Nonetheless, the Child-Pugh system remains useful for assessing the severity of the underlying liver disease. For example, the 1-year survival of patients with Child-Pugh class C disease is less than 50%.

Once a patient with cirrhosis presents with a complication, an assessment should be made as to patient's the suitability for liver transplantation (Chapter 85). This is because the prognosis of the cirrhotic patient in the face of one of the known complications of cirrhosis is generally very poor, and the 5-year survival rate with transplantation approaches 70%. Consultation with an experienced hepatologist should be pursued early.

ASCITES

Ascites is defined as an abnormal accumulation of fluid in the peritoneal cavity. The most common cause is portal hypertension, but primary peritoneal disease should be considered initially, at least once, in all patients. In patients with a tense collection of abdominal fluid, the diagnosis of ascites is straightforward. However, patients with small or moderate degrees of ascites often present a diagnostic dilemma. The physical examination is notoriously unreliable for detection of up to 5 L of fluid in the abdominal cavity. Thus, if there is any question as to the presence or absence of ascites, ultrasound should be performed because it is extremely reliable, relatively simple, and inexpensive.

Issues at the Time of Admission

An important consideration in the care of patients with ascites is determining whether admission is required. Patients should be considered strongly for admission if they present with fever, abdominal pain, volume depletion or severe volume overload, altered mental status, or severe hyponatremia (<115 mEq/L). These clinical features often suggest spontaneous bacterial peritonitis (see below).

Additionally, it is imperative to determine the cause of ascites. Although the majority of patients admitted to the hospital with ascites have liver disease and portal hypertension underlying their ascites, other causes must be excluded (Table 83.1). For this reason, all patients with new-onset ascites should undergo diagnostic paracentesis. Diagnostic paracentesis is performed with a large (16-gauge) catheter with or without local anesthesia. Paracentesis can be performed in either the lower quadrant or the midline; the left lower quadrant is probably the safest. In general, the measurement of the ascites fluid albumin level is mandatory in patients undergoing diagnostic paracentesis, and the result is used to measure the *serum-ascitic fluid albumin gradient*. Diseases with a portal hypertensive basis have a high gradient (>1.1 g/dL); those associated with primary peritoneal disease (e.g., tuberculous peritonitis or carcinomatosis) have a low gradient. It is important to emphasize that a high gradient is present in patients with mixed processes (i.e., portal hypertension and a peritoneal disorder). Ascitic fluid WBC has become the gold-standard test for the diagnosis of SBP (see later in this chapter) and, therefore, is required in all patients in whom this diagnosis is possible. The clinical situation dictates the use of other diagnostic tests. For example, amylase level may be useful in patients with a history of pancreatitis to exclude pancre-

atic ascites, triglyceride measurements should be obtained in those with cloudy fluid to exclude chylous ascites, and cytology is important if malignancy is a possibility.

Issues During the Course of Hospitalization

An algorithm for diagnosis and management of ascites is shown in Figure 83.2. Because sodium retention is a key element in cirrhotic ascites, sodium restriction is a highly effective—but poorly complied with—therapy for patients with ascites. Upon admission to the hospital, sodium intake initially should be restricted to 1,000 mg/d (44 mmol/d). Sodium can be restricted to as low as 250 mg/d; however, upon discharge, patients rarely comply with this degree of sodium restriction, and thus it is more realistic to institute a more lenient degree of restriction. Diuretics are used to promote additional sodium loss. Diuresis usually is begun with spironolactone (100 mg/d). If spironolactone alone is ineffective, furosemide usually is added (beginning at 20 mg/d). After diuresis has been induced (a target level is 500–1,000 mL/d in those with peripheral edema, and no more than 500 mL/d in those without edema), sodium restriction and diuretic dose may be tailored to appropriate outpatient levels. During sodium restriction and diuretic therapy, renal function and electrolyte levels should be monitored closely. All patients with elevated creatinine levels should have a careful analysis of urine and a formal creatinine clearance performed. Serum creatinine must be interpreted with caution, as it correlates poorly with renal function in cirrhotic patients. Patients with ascites often have impaired water excretion, and thus hyponatremia is common. Diuretics often compound the problem, although the pathogenesis of hyponatremia in this setting is unclear. Free water restriction is not always necessary in patients with ascites, particularly in those without hyponatremia. However, in patients with hyponatremia, free water restriction at a level of 1 to 1.5 L/d usually is required.

Approximately 20% of patients have ascites that is seemingly refractory to sodium restriction and diuretics. Although this is often because of poor compliance, these patients present difficult management problems. *Large-volume paracentesis* (5–10 L at a time) is effective for short-term removal of fluid and provides rapid symptomatic relief. Although large-volume paracentesis is generally safe, it is associated with functional changes in hemodynamics and plasma renin activity, and it can be complicated by renal impairment, dilutional hyponatremia, and hepatic encephalopathy. Controversy surrounds the use of volume expanders immediately after large-volume paracentesis. Use of intravenous albumin (8 g per liter of ascitic fluid removed) prevents many of the hemodynamic alterations associated with paracentesis and represents a sensible adjunct to large-volume paracentesis. Unfortunately, intravenous albumin is extremely expensive and, moreover, does not alter outcome compared with other less effective volume expanders such as dextran-70 or polygeline (1). If volume expansion is deemed essential, albumin is still the preferred agent despite its cost.

TABLE 83.1

CAUSES OF ASCITES

Cirrhosis (any cause)[a]
Congestive heart failure[a]
Renal failure
Pancreatic ascites
Chylous ascites
Tuberculosis
Metastatic peritoneal carcinomatosis
Myxedema
Connective tissue disease
Eosinophilic gastroenteritis
Bilious ascites
Primary peritoneal carcinomatosis

[a] high serum-albumin ascites gradient

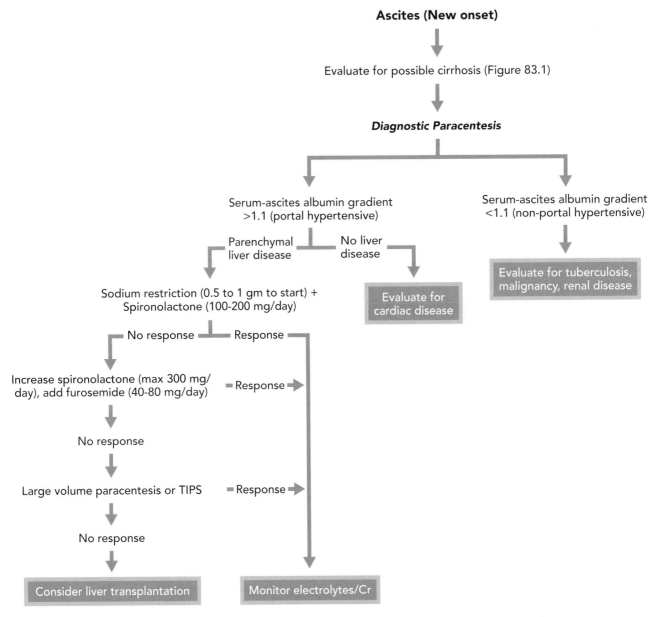

Figure 83.2 Evaluation and treatment of ascites. *Cr*, creatinine; *TIPS*, transjugular intrahepatic portosystemic shunt.

Peritoneovenous shunting can be highly effective for treatment of refractory ascites. This intervention leads to increases in glomerular filtration rate and decreases in serum aldosterone and plasma renin activity. However, frequent complications, including shunt occlusion, low-grade disseminated intravascular coagulopathy, and sepsis, have dampened enthusiasm for this procedure. Moreover, in a randomized controlled trial, peritoneovenous shunting did not result in increased survival compared with large-volume paracentesis or standard diuretic therapy (2). Finally, because peritoneovenous shunting may lead to recurrent SBP, venous thrombosis, and peritoneal fibrosis, the use of peritoneovenous shunting is not recommended in patients who are or may become candidates for liver transplantation.

The *transjugular intrahepatic portosystemic shunt* (TIPS) is an effective management strategy for some patients with refractory ascites (3). TIPS is performed via a transjugular approach and creates a shunt from the portal vein to the central venous system (Figure 83.3). A TIPS behaves like a side-to-side portocaval shunt. In selected patients, a TIPS results in resolution of ascites or a significant reduction in diuretic requirements, and appears to be associated with an apparent improvement in nutritional status (4). However, complications are common (Table 83.2). Additionally, patients undergoing a TIPS require careful follow-up because of the high incidence of shunt stenosis. Finally, in randomized trials of TIPS versus medical management in patients with refractory ascites, results have varied, but the consensus view is that TIPS does not improve the mortality rate compared with large-volume paracentesis (5, 6). Thus, although TIPS can be highly effective therapy for certain patients with refractory ascites, caution is required, and a

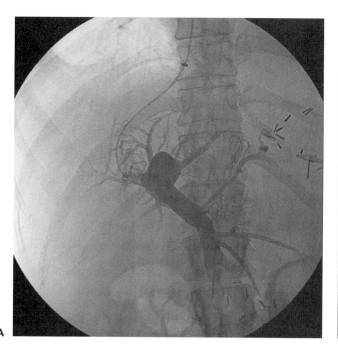

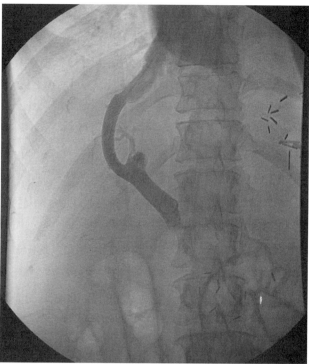

A   B

Figure 83.3 Radiographic example of TIPS. A TIPS is by creating a tract from the portal vein to the central venous drainage of the liver. Panel **A.** shows the portal venous anatomy in a patient with clinical portal hypertension and ascites prior to TIPS; prior to TIPS placement, varices are prominent. In **B.** varices are absent after the shunt is sucessfully created and portal pressure is dramatically reduced. Placement of a sucessful shunt results in correction of the hepatic venous pressure gradient. *TIPS*, transjugular intrahepatic portosystemic shunt. (Images courtesy of Paul Suhocki, M.D., Duke University Medical Center).

hepatologist should be involved in all cases prior to this intervention for patients with refractory ascites. TIPS is not recommended in certain patients with advanced liver disease, such as those with elevated bilirubin (greater than 5 mg/dL) or elevated prothrombin time (INR >2.5). The use of TIPS in patients with varices is covered in Chapter 78.

TABLE 83.2

COMPLICATIONS OF TRANSJUGULAR INTRAHEPATIC PORTOSYSTEMIC SHUNT (TIPS)

Procedure-related

Perihepatic hemorrhage
Sepsis
Cardiac arrhythmia
Puncture of hepatic vein/inferior vena cava
Neck hematoma

Portosystemic shunting–related

Hepatic encephalopathy
Hyperbilirubinemia
Rapidly progressive deterioration in liver or renal function

Other

TIPS hemolysis

Liver transplantation (Chapter 85) is highly effective for treatment of ascites. However, this therapy generally is reserved for patients who are severely incapacitated or who have had serious complications such as recurrent spontaneous bacterial peritonitis, hepatic hydrothorax, or functional renal impairment caused by diuretics. Hepatology input is required for consideration of liver transplantation.

The length of hospitalization generally depends on the severity of the ascites, and often the degree to which electrolyte or renal abnormalities dominate the clinical picture. Because continued hospitalization often is mandated by such renal and electrolyte problems, hospital stays are usually long, on the order of 3–5 days.

In summary, most patients with cirrhotic ascites can be managed with a combination of sodium restriction and diuretics. Given the poor long-term prognosis of patients once they have developed ascites, a decision should be made as to whether the patient is a liver-transplant candidate. If the patient is a transplantation candidate, treatment should focus on minimizing complications that might preclude transplantation. Large-volume paracentesis is probably the best initial approach. However, in patients with preserved renal function and without encephalopathy, a TIPS should be considered early. Unlike surgical shunting, this procedure does not alter the later ability to perform transplantation. The cost of TIPS maintenance in this situation also is minimized by the finite time period for which it is required. In patients who are not transplant candidates, management is much more difficult, but therapeutic options remain the same.

Discharge Issues

The most critical aspect of care for the patient with ascites is optimization of sodium balance, fluid intake, diuretics, electrolytes, and renal function. Overly aggressive diuresis may contribute to development of hepatorenal syndrome in some patients. Therefore, electrolytes and volume status must be monitored carefully as patients make the transition from the inpatient to the outpatient setting. It is imperative that patients be discharged on a reasonable diuretic regimen, and that they have follow-up within 1 week after discharge. Significant changes in the diuretic regimen close to the time of discharge are strongly discouraged.

Chronic oral antibiotic therapy should be considered for all patients with ascites, as this intervention reduces the risk of subsequent SBP (7). Several regimens exist, the best of which appear to be trimethoprim-sulfamethoxazole or ciprofloxacin given as a single daily dose or 3 times per week. All patients with cirrhosis should receive vaccination against hepatitis A. They should also be vaccinated against hepatitis B, if hepatitis B is not the cause of their disease and they are not already immune.

SPONTANEOUS BACTERIAL PERITONITIS (SBP)

SBP is a common complication in patients with liver disease and ascites. SBP is defined as infection of preexisting ascitic fluid in the absence of an intraabdominal primary infection. The diagnosis of SBP rests upon analysis of ascitic fluid. The diagnosis is established in the setting of an elevated polymorphonuclear leukocyte (PMN) count (>250 PMNs per cubic millimeter) in the presence of a positive culture for bacteria. Variants of SBP include "neutrocytic" ascites, in which a high PMN count is present but bacteria are not identified, and "bacterascites," in which the PMN count is low but bacteria are isolated from ascitic fluid.

Issues at the Time of Admission

The clinical presentation of SBP is highly variable. The classic presentation is with fever or abdominal pain. Some patients may be minimally symptomatic, at least initially, and any abrupt clinical change (e.g., worsening encephalopathy) in the patient with liver disease should raise suspicion for SBP. Furthermore, approximately 33% of patients with infected ascites present to the hospital without symptoms or signs of SBP; the prevalence of SBP at the time of hospital admission of patients with ascites is about 25%. Thus, a high index of suspicion for all patients with cirrhosis and

ascites is required to make this diagnosis, and those with ascites who require hospitalization should probably undergo diagnostic paracentesis.

A positive ascitic fluid culture is required to make a definitive diagnosis of SBP. However, the culture is imperfect because of its low sensitivity (which can be improved by innoculating 10 mL of ascitic fluid into blood-culture bottles) and the long lag time before results are known. Thus, the PMN count in ascitic fluid has become used widely for the diagnosis of SBP. The differential diagnosis of SBP is relatively limited; the main alternative diagnosis is secondary peritonitis. An extremely high PMN count (>5,000/μL) should raise the possibility of secondary peritonitis caused by a perforated viscus or other intraabdominal process. Further diagnostic studies (including abdominal computed tomography scan) are required in this setting.

Although most patients with SBP require hospitalization, there is a small subgroup of patients who may be able to be managed in the outpatient setting. These patients usually are relatively well compensated clinically, compliant, and present without evidence of sepsis. Consultation with a specialist and assurance of close follow-up are required if outpatient management is being contemplated.

Issues During the Course of Hospitalization

Without appropriate therapy, the mortality rate of SBP is high. Antibiotics are the cornerstone of therapy. Recent studies have suggested that selected patients can be treated with short courses of antibiotics and even with outpatient regimens (see above). Antibiotics are tailored to the specific organisms typically isolated from ascitic fluid. Because this process appears to result from translocation of bacteria from bowel to ascitic fluid, the most frequently isolated organisms are enterobactericiae. Gram-positive cocci, including *Streptococcus pneumoniae* and *Enterococcus* species, are also common. Anaerobes are rarely isolated.

The best initial antibiotic choice is a parenteral third-generation cephalosporin, such as ceftriaxone or cefotaxime. β-lactam/β-lactamase combinations also provide excellent coverage with little toxicity. Aminoglycosides should be avoided because of renal toxicity. The clinical response to antibiotics is usually good. If patients do not respond within 48 hours, other processes (Table 83.3) should be considered. If specific culture results are available, antibiotic coverage should be changed accordingly. The optimal duration of therapy for SBP is unknown but should be tailored to the individual clinical scenario. Generally, a 5-day course is adequate, some of which may be in the form of oral antibiotics. Repeat paracentesis may be an important tool in determining the length of antibiotic therapy. In patients with definite clinical improvement, a repeat paracentesis is usually not necessary, although some clinicians prefer to switch to oral antibiotics after the PMN count is below 250/μL. On the other hand, repeat paracentesis is essential in patients with an atypical course or in

TABLE 83.3

CONSIDERATIONS IN PATIENTS FAILING TO IMPROVE AFTER EMPIRIC THERAPY FOR SPONTANEOUS BACTERIAL PERITONITIS (SBP)

Did patient really have SBP?	Reason for failure	Recommended approach
Yes	Resistant organism (*Enterococcus, Pseudomonas*)	Microbiologic tests, change coverage
Yes	Nonbacterial pathogen (tuberculosis, fungus)	Repeat history for risk factors, microbiologic tests
Yes	Concomitant other infection	Further examination, urinalysis, chest radiograph, blood cultures
No	Secondary peritonitis (perforation)	Abdominal computed tomography, colon evaluation, surgical consultation
No	Other process (malignancy)	Review history and physical, specific tests

those who have persistent symptoms or signs. It is also helpful in those with bacterascites (a positive culture, with low PMN count) and a benign clinical course. In general, repeat paracentesis should be performed liberally in patients with SBP because it can help assess response to therapy. Intravenous albumin (1.5 mg/kg at the time of diagnosis, followed by 1.0 mg/kg daily) is an expensive intervention but does improve renal function and mortality in patients with SBP, and should be considered (8).

The length of hospitalization depends on the severity of illness. In patients with uncomplicated SBP, hospitalization is generally short (2–3 days). In patients with severe SBP or those with SBP and another problem such as variceal hemorrhage or hepatic encephalopathy, hospitalization is often much longer (5–7 days).

Discharge Issues

A complete course of appropriate antibiotics should be completed or planned at the time of discharge. Patients with SBP usually should receive chronic prophylactic antibiotics because one episode of SBP identifies the patient who is at risk for further episodes. If appropriate, vaccination against hepatitis A and B should be provided.

HEPATIC ENCEPHALOPATHY

Hepatic encephalopathy is common in patients with chronic liver disease and is a frequent indication for hospital admission. Its diagnosis is based on the presence of specific neurologic symptoms and signs in patients with advanced liver disease (Table 83.4). Importantly, the diagnosis of hepatic encephalopathy also requires exclusion of other causes of encephalopathy.

Issues at the Time of Admission

Although the diagnosis of encephalopathy as a clinical entity is straightforward, a differential diagnosis of the cause of encephalopathy in patients with known liver disease must be formulated in all cases. It is critical to consider metabolic encephalopathy (i.e., Wernicke-Korsakoff syndrome, hypoglycemia, electrolyte disturbances, ethanol intoxication), central nervous system infection, and structural lesions such as subdural hematoma. An ammonia level may be helpful in patients with a previous history of abnormal ammonia levels. However, this test must be interpreted with caution because its sensitivity and specificity are imperfect. In contrast, *cerebrospinal fluid glutamine levels*

TABLE 83.4

STAGES OF ENCEPHALOPATHY

Stage	Symptoms	Signs
Subclinical	Impaired work, personality changes	Impaired psychomotor testing
I	Mild confusion, agitation, apathy	Fine tremor, asterixis
II	Drowsiness, lethargy, disorientation	Asterixis, dysarthria
III	Sleepy but arousable, marked confusion	Hyperreflexia, hyperventilation
IV	Coma	Decerebrate posturing, oculocephalic reflexes intact

have a high sensitivity and specificity for hepatic encephalopathy.

Reversible predisposing factors, such as gastrointestinal bleeding, infection, increased dietary protein level, use of sedative drugs, and renal failure, also must be identified and corrected in patients with hepatic encephalopathy. In the majority of patients, hepatic encephalopathy results from noncompliance with a prescribed medical regimen. In patients with ascites, diagnostic paracentesis is essential. Head computed tomography (to exclude subdural hematoma) and lumbar puncture should be considered strongly in patients with atypical symptoms or signs.

Issues During the Course of Hospitalization

The management of hepatic encephalopathy centers on correction of factors that precipitate or induce the altered mentation and decreasing production of toxins that result from enteric bacterial metabolism of nitrogenous compounds. Thus, sedative drugs should be discontinued, and infection, bleeding, and electrolyte abnormalities should be corrected. To remove toxins, dietary protein is restricted and enteric bacteria are killed or their products purged. In patients with mild encephalopathy, dietary protein should be restricted to less than 40 g/d; in those with severe encephalopathy, dietary protein should be eliminated. In patients with severe encephalopathy, treatment entails aggressive lactulose therapy. Lactulose is given at a dose of 30 mL every two hours until diarrhea begins. If patients cannot take oral medications because of disorientation, a nasogastric tube is recommended. Once diarrhea occurs, the lactulose schedule should be modified based on response and stool output. Two to four loose stools per day are optimal, and profuse diarrhea should be avoided. Neomycin can be added (1–2 g every 6 hours) or may be used as a substitute for lactulose; it is unknown whether the combination of lactulose plus neomycin is more effective than either alone. Patients who do not respond to lactulose or neomycin within 24 hours must be reassessed carefully, and the issues raised in Table 83.5 should be readdressed.

The length of hospital stay for patients with hepatic encephalopathy often depends on the underlying cause. In patients hospitalized because of simple noncompliance, hospital stays are short (1–2 days). In those with severe underlying processes, however, hospital stays are longer (5–7 days).

Discharge Issues

Patients should be discharged only after their mental status has cleared and after a stable dosage of lactulose (or neomycin) has been achieved. Patient education is essential: all patients should be seen by a dietitian with expertise in liver-related diseases and placed on an appropriate diet. Follow-up and compliance are important. Thus, precise discharge instructions to the patient and care providers are essential. If appropriate, patients with cirrhosis should receive vaccination against hepatitis A and B.

HEPATORENAL SYNDROME

The hepatorenal syndrome is a common and extremely problematic complication of cirrhosis. It is characterized by intense activation of the renin-angiotensin-aldosterone system, with pronounced vasoconstriction of the renal circulation, which results in marked reduction of renal blood flow and glomerular filtration rate. The hepatorenal syndrome has been subtyped into two categories, which are likely to differ mechanistically and require divergent therapies. Type I is characterized by rapidly progressive deterioration in renal function, defined by a doubling of the serum creatinine to a value of more than 2.5 mg/dL or a 50% reduction of creatinine clearance to a level less than 20 mL/min in less than two weeks. Type II is characterized by a more moderate and slowly progressive reduction of glomerular filtration rate. One common thread in both forms of hepatorenal syndrome is the presence of vasoconstrictive compounds (including endothelin 1 and angiotensin II) in the afferent renal circulation.

Issues at the Time of Admission

The diagnosis of hepatorenal syndrome is established in the patient with rising creatinine and oliguria by documen-

TABLE 83.5

CONSIDERATIONS IN PATIENTS FAILING TO IMPROVE AFTER EMPIRIC THERAPY FOR HEPATIC ENCEPHALOPATHY

Does the patient really have hepatic encephalopathy?	Reason for failure	Recommended approach
Yes	Inadequate treatment	Increase lactulose, add neomycin
Yes	Worsening liver function	Evaluate for transplantation, specialist consultation
No	Electrolyte abnormalities	Check sodium, calcium; correct abnormalities
No	Subdural hematoma or other structural lesion	Careful examination and/or head computed tomography
No	Meningitis	Review history and physical, lumbar puncture

tation of low urinary sodium (<10 mEq/L) in the absence of intravascular volume depletion. Acute tubular necrosis (Chapter 100) resulting from contrast dye, nonsteroidal anti-inflammatory agents, or aminoglycosides is important to exclude; such patients often have high urine sodium levels. Because hypovolemia is often difficult to differentiate from hepatorenal syndrome, a volume challenge of at least 1 L of colloid is required, and in some instances central pressure monitoring is indicated. Obstruction and intrinsic renal disease also must be excluded; therefore, ultrasound and examination of the urine sediment are also important.

Issues During the Course of Hospitalization

Treatment is generally unsatisfactory, and prognosis is extremely poor. It is imperative to identify and discontinue potentially nephrotoxic compounds. Attention to volume is the most critical aspect of management. Intravascular volume depletion should be reversed if present; volume repletion is often best performed in an intensive care unit setting with central venous pressure monitoring. Medical therapy is generally ineffective, although there are some data indicating that the combination of prolonged ornipressin (a vasopressin-like peripheral vasoconstrictive substance) and plasma volume expansion with albumin may result in suppression of vasoconstrictor activity, improvement in glomerular filtration rate, and reversal of the hepatorenal syndrome (9). Another report suggested that the combination of midodrine and octreotide may reverse type I hepatorenal syndrome (10). TIPS, hemodialysis, and portocaval shunts have been reported to lead to reversal of hepatorenal syndrome in some cases, but controlled data to support their use are not available. Although liver transplantation may be appropriate in some instances, and the 3-year survival approaches 60% in patients with hepatorenal syndrome who undergo transplantation, many of these patients have extremely difficult postoperative courses. Hepatology and nephrology input is essential.

Discharge Issues

Unfortunately, the vast majority of patients with type I hepatorenal syndrome who do not undergo liver transplantation die. For those with type II hepatorenal syndrome, careful attention to volume status and electrolytes is essential. Consultation with a palliative care service is appropriate for patients who do not improve and who are not transplant candidates (Chapter 19).

COST CONSIDERATIONS AND RESOURCE USE

Care of patients with cirrhosis is extremely costly because of the severity of the underlying disease process. Complications requiring hospitalization in this patient population lend themselves to long and often complicated stays. In-

deed, a number of clinical findings preclude discharge (Table 83.6). Because of the degree of chronic debilitation in many of these patients, efforts to encourage ambulation and improve nutrition early in the hospital course are imperative. Patient education is particularly critical in all patients with cirrhosis and its complications. Because these disorders are chronic and generally not reversible, patient education (Figure 83.4) improves compliance and reduces cost by decreasing the need for future hospitalization.

In patients with esophageal varices or ascites, hospitalizations and cost can be reduced by prophylactic therapy. For example, *prophylactic antibiotics* in patients with ascites reduce the risk of SBP and thus of hospitalization. Additionally, *β-blockers* reduce the risk of future variceal hemorrhage and should be considered in all patients, especially those with large varices (Chapter 78). A detailed discussion of the prophylactic management of varices is beyond the scope of this chapter, but options include sclerotherapy, banding, and TIPS. Each technique has important advantages and disadvantages. In patients randomized to TIPS or sclerotherapy, TIPS is associated with a lower rate of rebleeding but no mortality advantage. Banding appears to be safer and more effective than sclerotherapy, but this technique has not been directly compared to TIPS.

Finally, a recent study found that, in patients with chronic hepatitis B and advanced liver disease, continuous treatment with lamivudine significantly reduced the rate of hepatic decompensation and progression to hepatocellular carcinoma (11).

TABLE 83.6

HIGH-RISK CRITERIA THAT HELP IDENTIFY PATIENTS *NOT* READY FOR DISCHARGE

Ascites

Sodium <120 meq/L
Fever or abdominal pain
BUN:creatinine >25:1 ratio
Rising creatinine or declining urine output
Major changes in diuretic regimen within previous 24 h
Altered mental status
Deteriorating liver function
Persistent tense ascites

Variceal hemorrhage

Persistent melena
Systolic blood pressure <90 mmHg, heart rate >120/min
Altered mental status
Deteriorating liver function

Hepatic encephalopathy

Persistent alteration in mental status
Unstable lactulose or neomycin regimen
Deteriorating liver function

BUN, blood urea nitrogen.

Cirrhosis

Your doctor has diagnosed you with cirrhosis. Cirrhosis is a scarring process of the liver caused by many years of injury to the liver (this can be caused by a virus, alcohol, too much iron or copper, an autoimmune disease, or a disease of the bile ducts). You may also have one of the many complications of cirrhosis which include ascites, intestinal bleeding, or encephalopathy. Ascites is a condition in which too much fluid accumulates in the abdomen. This can make you uncomfortable and/or can lead to infections. Treatment for this is usually done by removing fluid either with fluid pills or a needle. Intestinal bleeding occurs when veins in your stomach or esophagus rupture. This can be prevented by putting small bands on the veins or by taking medication that reduces the pressure in them. Encephalopathy refers to clouded thinking or confusion. This is caused because the liver can not clear out bad toxins from the system. It is treated by removing toxins from the intestinal tract with medicine (usually lactulose).

Follow-up Care

Follow-up with your physician is essential to your ongoing care. An appointment has been scheduled with:

Dr._____

Phone number_____

Date_____ Time_____

If you develop fever, shaking chills, vomiting, confusion, black stools, or abdominal pain or redness, you should call your doctor or go to the clinic or emergency room. Because your doctors are trying to control your liver disease with medicines, it is imperative that you take your medicine exactly as prescribed. If your doctor has advised you to avoid salt and water, it is also important that you follow this advice.

Figure 83.4 Sample patient discharge instructions for cirrhosis and its complications.

KEY POINTS

- Development of complications of portal hypertension or evidence of hepatocellular dysfunction herald an accelerated course that typically is associated with substantial morbidity and mortality rates.
- Ascitic fluid albumin and white count with differential are required in those undergoing diagnostic paracentesis.
- The cornerstone of management of ascites is careful adjustment of diuretics, fluid, and electrolytes. Most cases do not require other interventions such as TIPS.
- The diagnosis of spontaneous bacterial peritonitis is often subtle and may be manifested by low-grade

fever, change in mental status, or general clinical deterioration.
- Spontaneous bacterial peritonitis and gastrointestinal bleeding must be excluded in the patient with new or worsening hepatic encephalopathy.
- Aminoglycosides and all potential nephrotoxins should be avoided in cirrhotic patients.
- Patients with a new diagnosis of cirrhosis or any of its complications should be referred early for consideration of liver transplantation.

REFERENCES

1. Gines A, Fernandez-Esparrach G, Monescillo A, et al. Randomized trial comparing albumin, dextran 70, and polygeline in cirrhotic patients with ascites treated by paracentesis. *Gastroenterology* 1996;111:1002–1010.
2. Gines P, Arroyo V, Vargas V, et al. Paracentesis with intravenous infusion of albumin as compared with peritoneovenous shunting in cirrhosis with refractory ascites. *N Engl J Med* 1991;325:829–835.
3. Saadeh S, Davis GL. Management of ascites in patients with end-stage liver disease. *Rev Gastroenterol Disord* 2004;4:175–185.
4. Trotter J, Suhocki P, Rockey DC. Transjugular intrahepatic shunt for patients with refractory ascites: effect on body weight and Child-Pugh score. *Am J Gastroenterol* 1998;93:1891–1894.
5. Lebrec D, Giuily N, Hadengue A, et al. Transjugular intrahepatic portosystemic shunts: comparison with paracentesis in patients with cirrhosis and refractory ascites. A randomized trial. *J Hepatol* 1996;25:135–144.
6. Sanyal AJ, Genning C, Reddy KR, et al. The North American study for the treatment of refractory ascites. *Gastroenterology* 2003;124:634–641.
7. Singh N, Gayowski T, Yu VL, et al. Trimethoprim-sulfamethoxazole for the prevention of spontaneous bacterial peritonitis in cirrhosis: a randomized trial. *Ann Intern Med* 1995;122:595–598.
8. Sort P, Navasa M, Arroyo V, et al. Effect of intravenous albumin on renal impairment and mortality in patients with cirrhosis and spontaneous bacterial peritonitis. *N Engl J Med* 1999;341:403–409.
9. Guevara M, Gines P, Fernandez-Esparrach G, et al. Reversibility of hepatorenal syndrome by prolonged administration of ornipressin and plasma volume expansion. *Hepatology* 1998;27:35–41.
10. Angeli P, Volpin R, Gerunda G. Reversal of type 1 hepatorenal syndrome with the administration of midodrine and octreotide. *Hepatology* 1999;29:1690–1697.
11. Liaw YF, Sung JJ, Chow WC, et al. Lamivudine for patients with chronic hepatitis B and advanced liver disease. *N Engl J Med* 2004;351:1567–1570.

ADDITIONAL READING

Gines P, Guevara M, Arroyo V, Rodes J. Hepatorenal syndrome. *Lancet* 2003;362:1819–1827.
Kaplowitz N, ed. *Liver and Biliary Diseases.* 2nd ed. Baltimore: Williams and Wilkins, 1996.
Moore KP, Wong F, Gines P, et al. The management of ascites in cirrhosis: report on the consensus conference of the International Ascites Club. *Hepatology* 2003;38:258–266.
Sharara A, Rockey DC. Esophageal variceal hemorrhage. *N Engl J Med* 2001;345:669–681.

Disorders of the Biliary System

84

Douglas B. Nelson   **Paul Druck**   **Martin L. Freeman**

INTRODUCTION

Extrahepatic biliary-tract disease is most commonly associated with gallstones or neoplasia. Less common causes include inflammatory conditions such as primary sclerosing cholangitis, chronic pancreatitis, trauma or surgical injury, congenital anomalies, parasitoses, and primary infectious diseases such as HIV. Gallstone disease is by far the most common cause; it is estimated that 20 million adults in the United States have gallstone disease, and approximately 600,000 cholecystectomies are performed annually (1). Gallstones are composed primarily of cholesterol, as a result of cholesterol supersaturation of bile (75% of cases), or pigment, as a result of excessive secretion of bilirubin coupled with bacterial deconjugation of soluble glucuronides (25% of cases). In the absence of bile-duct abnormalities, the majority of gallstones form in the gallbladder. Epidemiologic correlates of cholesterol gallstones include advancing age, gender (female predominance prior to menopause), obesity, and race (increasing prevalence from African-American to Caucasian to Native-American). Pigment stones are associated predominantly with advancing age, cirrhosis, chronic hemolytic states, and chronic biliary-tract infections and are relatively more common in Asians (2).

Disorders of the biliary system most commonly become manifest as a result of obstruction, and the clinical presentation varies with the level of the obstruction. Figure 84.1 shows the relevant anatomy of the biliary tract. Bile cannaliculi join to form progressively larger bile ductules and then bile ducts. Anatomically, segmental bile ducts coalesce into the right and left hepatic ducts, which then unite to form the common hepatic duct. The junction of the cystic duct, communicating with the gallbladder and the common hepatic duct, forms the common bile duct. The pancreatic duct merges for a short but variable distance with the common bile duct at its terminus to empty into the duodenum at the ampulla of Vater.

Most gallstones reside in the gallbladder without causing symptoms (approximately 20% of patients develop symptoms within 15–20 years). However, stones that impact at any point from the cystic duct to the pancreaticobiliary junction can produce a variety of clinical symptoms and syndromes (Figure 84.1). The pathophysiology of gallstone-associated biliary-tract disease may involve contractile dysfunction of the gallbladder or cystic duct obstruction (*biliary colic*), cystic duct obstruction with infection of gallbladder or its contents (*acute cholecystitis*), common bile-duct obstruction (*pain, obstructive jaundice, or pancreatitis*), or bile-duct obstruction with superimposed infection (*acute cholangitis*). The pathophysiology of *acalculous cholecystitis* has not been elucidated fully.

Traditionally, *biliary colic* (episodic right upper quadrant or epigastric visceral-type pain with radiation to the subscapular area, often accompanied by nausea) has been attributed to transient obstruction of the cystic duct or neck of the gallbladder by a gallstone. This generally occurs postprandially and is relieved after a few hours when the obstructing stone returns to the gallbladder or passes into the common bile duct. Less commonly, the syndrome may be produced by transient common bile-duct obstruction or by gallbladder dysfunction as demonstrated by gallbladder emptying studies.

If the stones persist in obstructing the gallbladder, *acute cholecystitis* may occur. Acute cholecystitis is characterized pathologically by an acute inflammatory infiltrate of the gallbladder wall with thickening, arterial and venous dilation and engorgement, and occasionally areas of ischemic necrosis. Such necrotic foci may cause gallbladder

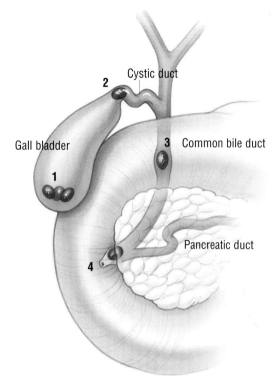

Figure 84.1 Illustration of biliary-tract anatomy, with obstruction caused by gallstones at various sites and their associated clinical manifestations. **1.** Gallstones in gallbladder; asymptomatic in most cases, unless impacted in neck or cystic duct. **2.** Gallstone in cystic duct; biliary colic if transiently obstructed; acute cholecystitis if impacted and infected. **3.** Gallstone in common bile duct; pain, jaundice, or abnormal liver chemistries, with or without cholangitis, if obstructing; may be minor or no symptoms if nonobstructing. **4.** Gallstone in distal bile duct (common channel with pancreatic duct); gallstone pancreatitis in some cases; may impact transiently, or pass into duodenum asymptomatically.

perforations, which usually are contained by adjacent adherent viscera and omentum to produce pericholecystic abscesses. Uncommonly, the perforations may be free (uncontained) and produce generalized peritonitis. In 40%–60% of cases, the bile is infected with enteric organisms. If there is progression to frank suppuration, *empyema of the gallbladder* occurs. Necrosis of the gallbladder may occur (*gangrenous cholecystitis*), and if the gallbladder is infected with gas-producing organisms, air may be visible within its wall on abdominal film, computed tomography (CT), or ultrasound (*emphysematous cholecystitis*). Longstanding obstruction may lead to reabsorption or degradation of bilirubin, producing colorless bile (*hydrops of the gallbladder*). Pathogenetic mechanisms of cholecystitis include bacterial invasion of the gallbladder wall, irritation caused by lysolecithin produced by action of phospholipase on bile phospholipids, and mucosal ischemia secondary to gallbladder distention.

Total parenteral nutrition (TPN)–associated cholecystitis is not a consequence of TPN administration but of the underlying fasting state that precipitates the use of TPN. Fast-

ing has been shown to rapidly lead to the development or progression of gallbladder sludge and stones, which may result in calculous (obstructive) cholecystitis. When this occurs in a postoperative or critically ill patient, the classic signs and symptoms of cholecystitis may be obscured by the underlying disorder(s), leading to a delay in diagnosis. TPN-associated cholecystitis is distinct from acalculous cholecystitis, which also may occur in a critically ill patient.

In postoperative, post-trauma, and other critically ill patients, *"acute acalculous cholecystitis"* may occur in the absence of stones or obstruction of the cystic duct. This condition is distinguished pathologically from acute calculous cholecystitis by arterial occlusions, lack of venous filling, and widespread necrosis of gallbladder wall and vessels. These findings, when combined with the strong association with hypotension, use of vasoconstrictor agents, Gram-negative sepsis, and positive pressure ventilation, support the role of splanchnic ischemia as the precipitating cause. Because of this pathophysiology, acalculous cholecystitis may occur in the absence or presence of gallstones. If stones pass into or form within the common bile duct, obstruction to bile outflow may occur, and this may lead in turn to *acute cholangitis*. The pathophysiology of acute cholangitis requires two components: bacterial colonization of biliary tract and increased pressure within the biliary tract because of obstruction. Bacterial colonization of the normally sterile biliary tract is thought to occur through one of three pathways: from duodenal reflux through an incompetent sphincter of Oddi, from an infected gallbladder, or from the portal venous system. The similarity between the microbiology of acute bacterial cholangitis and that of normal colonic bacterial flora suggests the latter as the most likely source. Bacteria entering the portal venous system from the intestine gain access to the biliary tree through the hepatic parenchyma. Under normal circumstances, flow of bile prevents colonization; however, obstruction caused by stones, strictures, or tumors may result in bacterial proliferation and infection. With increased bile-duct pressure resulting from obstruction, large quantities of bacteria can enter the systemic venous circulation, resulting in the clinical syndrome of sepsis.

Biliary tract obstruction is most commonly caused by *choledocholithiasis*, which accounts for 60%–80% of cases. Malignant biliary strictures can lead to obstruction at various levels of the extrahepatic and intrahepatic biliary tree, but they rarely cause cholangitis. However, in patients with malignant biliary obstruction, occlusion of endoscopically- or percutaneously-placed biliary stents and stenosis of surgical bypass anastomoses often do result in cholangitis. Other principal causes of biliary obstruction include benign strictures from inflammatory conditions, extrinsic obstruction caused by chronic pancreatitis, bile-duct injury resulting from biliary-tract surgery, or stenosis of surgical biliary-enteric anastomoses. Uncommon causes of obstruction include congenital choledochal cysts, pancreatic pseudocyst, chronic parasitic infestation, and AIDS cholangiopathy.

ACUTE CHOLECYSTITIS

Issues at the Time of Admission

Approximately 15% of patients harboring gallstones develop acute cholecystitis. The syndrome often begins with symptoms indistiguishable from ordinary biliary colic, which precedes the acute episode in 60%–70% of cases. Unlike biliary colic, which rarely lasts for more than a few hours, the symptoms of acute cholecystitis are unrelenting. As many as 70% of patients are afebrile on presentation; the remainder have low-grade fever. Marked right upper quadrant tenderness is almost always present and helps distinguish acute cholecystitis from biliary colic. *Murphy's sign* (inspiratory arrest during right upper quadrant palpation) is typical but not pathognomonic. With more advanced disease and development of peritonitis in the right upper quadrant, there may be pain on light palpation, movement, or coughing. A mass may be palpable, representing a distended gallbladder or a phlegmon. Diffuse abdominal tenderness or high fever are more consistent with other abdominal pathologies. Only 60% of patients present with leukocytosis, generally between 12,000 and 15,000 white blood cells/μL (3). Mild elevation of the serum bilirubin concentrations in the range of 2–5 mg/dL may occur, although levels above 3 mg/dL suggest the presence of common bile duct stones. Mild asymptomatic hyperamylasemia in the absence of pancreatitis accompanies cholecystitis in approximately 15% of cases (4).

The differential diagnosis of acute cholecystitis includes all conditions that cause right upper quadrant or right hypochondrium pain and tenderness. This includes acute cholangitis or bile-duct obstruction caused by common bile duct stones. Clinical distinction between cholecystitis and choledocholithiasis can be quite difficult, and rarely do they coexist in the same patient. The distinction is important because, in general, stone disease of the gallbladder is treated surgically, while common bile duct stones are treated primarily endoscopically, if expertise is available. Common bile duct stones generally are suggested by elevations of liver enzyme levels and by ductal dilation on imaging studies. Perforated gastric or duodenal ulcers (Chapter 80) typically cause very abrupt onset of symptoms, are associated with more diffuse upper abdominal tenderness, and cause pneumoperitoneum visible on upright chest films. Acute viral hepatitis (Chapter 82) generally has a gradual onset, often with nongastrointestinal prodromal symptoms, and usually is associated with dramatic rises (10- to 20-fold) in serum aminotransferases. Acute pancreatitis (Chapter 86) is distinguished by more tenderness to the left of midline than in acute cholecystitis, and by marked elevations in serum amylase and lipase. Other

diagnoses to consider include appendicitis, pyelonephritis, gonococcal perihepatitis, and acute hepatomegaly from right ventricular failure.

The two principal diagnostic imaging studies for suspected acute cholecystitis are ultrasound and radionuclide cholescintigraphy. Sonographic findings consistent with acute cholecystitis include gallbladder wall thickening or edema, pericholecystic fluid, gallstones impacted in the neck of the gallbladder or cystic duct, and air in the gallbladder wall. The absence of these findings does not rule out cholecystitis, nor does the simple presence of gallstones indicate gallbladder inflammation. Ultrasound has approximately 90% sensitivity and 80% specificity for acute cholecystitis (5). The so-called "sonographic Murphy's sign" (point tenderness over the sonographically visualized gallbladder fundus) may be more useful; it has approximately 90% overall diagnostic accuracy if gallstones are present. Ultrasound is the preferred initial study in patients with upper abdominal pain suspected of having biliary-tract disease, because it is easily performed, readily available, and inexpensive. In addition, it can provide useful information about the common bile duct, pancreas, and right kidney.

Radionuclide imaging may be required if ultrasound is nondiagnostic. Radionuclide cholescintigraphy can demonstrate cystic duct occlusion, present in almost all cases of acute calculous cholecystitis. Sensitivity and specificity have been reported to be as high as 97% and 95%, respectively (5). False positives (nonvisualizing gallbladder) are more frequent with prolonged fasting, chronic alcoholism, severe chronic cholecystitis, and unsuspected prior cholecystectomy. False negatives (visualized gallbladder in the presence of acute cholecystitis) may be seen in acalculous cholecystitis. The key principle is that *radionuclide imaging assesses the patency of the cystic duct, not the presence or absence of inflammation.*

CT scanning has comparable sensitivity and specificity to ultrasound for the signs of acute cholecystitis but is substantially less sensitive for the detection of gallstones in the gallbladder. In addition, CT is more expensive and requires intravenous contrast. The utility of CT scanning lies primarily in excluding other intra-abdominal pathology when ultrasound and cholescintigraphy are nondiagnostic.

Indications for Hospitalization and ICU Admission

Acute cholecystitis requires inpatient treatment. If the diagnosis remains in question, hospitalization is still appropriate, as most of the other conditions that can be confused with acute cholecystitis also require hospitalization. ICU admission is appropriate for monitoring and resuscitation of hemodynamically unstable patients. Patients with severe or destabilized comorbid conditions, especially coronary artery disease, left ventricular failure, or pulmonary impairment, also may require intensive care.

Initial Therapy

During evaluation for suspected acute cholecystitis, intravenous fluids should be administered to correct hypovolemia, if present, and to provide maintenance volume thereafter. The patient should be given nothing by mouth, and if abdominal distention or vomiting occur, nasogastric suction should be initiated. Surgical consultation should be obtained within 24 hours of making the diagnosis, or sooner if there is diagnostic uncertainty, presence of severe symptoms (either of sepsis or local inflammation), or progressive or diffuse peritonitis. Finally, analgesics should be administered if necessary, once the diagnosis has been confirmed. Morphine should be avoided as it causes sphincter of Oddi spasm. Intravenous antibiotic therapy should be started and selected for activity against the organisms typically implicated (i.e., Gram-negative rods, anaerobes, and enterococci) (Chapter 64). Patients who are severely ill, diabetic, or immunosuppressed or have failed initial therapy should receive either broader-spectrum single-agent therapy, such as piperacillin-tazobactam or imipenem, or multiagent regimens, such as ampicillin-gentamicin-

metronidazole. Third-generation cephalosporins and aztreonam lack activity against enterococci, and their use as single agents is controversial.

Issues During the Course of Hospitalization and Discharge Issues

Approximately 75% of patients improve significantly with the therapy previously described; the remainder have persistent symptoms or suffer recurrence within the first 6–8 weeks (Table 84.1). Of those who intially resolve, more than half will experience recurrences within the subsequent five years. Accordingly, *cholecystectomy is definitive therapy.* Several randomized prospective trials have demonstrated that prompt cholecystectomy performed during the initial admission has equivalent risk and long-term outcome as an "interval cholecystectomy" (performed a few weeks later). Early cholecystectomy avoids recurrences during the interval of observation, results in a shorter total length of hospital stay, and incurs lower costs (6). Preoperative preparation with antibiotics has been

TABLE 84.1

DIAGNOSTIC CONSIDERATION IN PATIENTS FAILING TO IMPROVE AFTER HOSPITALIZATION FOR ACUTE CHOLECYSTITIS

If the patient is being medically managed *prior to* cholecystectomy

Complication	Action
Persistent or worsening sepsis, development of peritonits	Proceed to cholecystectomy
Empyema	Proceed to cholecystectomy
Perforation or cholecystoenteric fistula/gallstone ileus	Proceed to cholecystectomy
Suspicion of common bile duct obstruction	Consider ERCP

If patient is *post–surgical cholecystectomy*

Complication	Action
Prolonged ileus	Obtain plain films of abdomen
Bile leak	Obtain RUQ ultrasound or computed tomography to detect biloma
	Obtain radionuclide cholescintigraphy to detect bile leak
	Perform ERCP to confirm diagnosis and perform sphincterotomy/place biliary stent to close bile leak
	Percutaneous drainage of biloma if collection is large or infected
	Surgery occasionally necessary to treat severe leak
Bile-duct stricture	Perform ERCP to diagnose and stent stricture
	Surgical choledochojejunostomy may be required
Bleeding	Obtain computed tomography scan or angiography
	Consider reexploration or angiographic therapy
Wound infection	Antibiotics
	Consider re-exploration, debridement for severe cases

ERCP, endoscopic retrograde cholangiopancreatography; *RUQ*, right upper quadrant.

shown to reduce septic complications of cholecystitis. Thus, optimal management of acute cholecystitis consists of prompt diagnosis, stabilization, and amelioration of fever and septicemia with intravenous antibiotics, followed by prompt cholecystectomy. Emergency cholecystectomy is rarely indicated, but is appropriate for diffuse peritonitis, severe or unimproving sepsis without concomitant common bile duct obstruction, or gas in the gallbladder wall (i.e., emphysematous cholecystitis suggesting gangrene of the gallbladder). *Laparoscopic cholecystectomy* has become the preferred approach, although there are cases in which contraindications to laparoscopy, technical difficulties, or limited local experience require laparotomy.

Specific postoperative complications of cholecystectomy include intra-abdominal fluid collections, bile-duct or adjacent viscus injury, retained common bile duct stones, and wound infection or dehiscence. The incidence of all complications after elective open cholecystectomy is approximately 20%, compared with 8% for laparoscopy. Severe complications (<1% incidence) are comparable. For acute cholecystitis, the complication rates are slightly higher, primarily because of an increase in septic complications.

After cholecystectomy, the occurrence of jaundice, sepsis, increasing or diffuse abdominal pain or tenderness, purulent or bilious wound drainage, unexplained tachycardia, or respiratory compromise strongly suggests a local abdominal complication and should be investigated thoroughly. Abdominal ultrasound and CT are appropriate initial studies and permit directed percutaneous drainage of intra-abdominal collections. Endoscopic retrograde cholangiopancreatography (ERCP) or percutaneous transhepatic cholangiography are usually required for diagnosis of bile-duct injury and, in some cases, may provide definitive therapy. When bile leakage from the cystic duct stump or other sites occurs, endoscopic stenting or biliary sphincterotomy is usually definitive in closing the leak.

The average hospital stay, including preoperative and postoperative recovery, is about 4 days for elective cholecystectomy with open technique versus 1–2 days for the laparoscopic technique. For acute cholecystitis, postoperative hospital stays average 5–7 days for open cholecystectomy and generally less for the laparoscopic technique, but the extent of right upper quadrant inflammation is often the critical factor.

Acute Cholecystitis in the Critically Ill

Acute cholecystitis may complicate the course of unrelated medical or surgical illness in approximately 1.5% of critically ill patients. In a postoperative setting, cholecystitis is acalculous in approximately 50% of cases; in post-trauma or burn patients this figure exceeds 90% (7). Often the etiology of cholecystitis in a critically ill patient is unclear preoperatively, and it may remain so postoperatively if

gallbladder necrosis is advanced. Mortality rates for cholecystitis in the critically ill exceed 50% in some series, because of the compromised condition of the susceptible patients as well as possible delays in diagnosis due to the absence or lack of specificity of classic signs of cholecystitis.

Ultrasound is the preferred initial test to evaluate suspected cholecystitis in critically ill patients. Positive findings include gallbladder wall thickening or edema, pericholecystic fluid, and intramural gas. Ascites or biliary sludge can contribute to exaggerated estimates of gallbladder wall thickening, however. The presence or absence of gallstones is only of marginal diagnostic significance. CT has comparable accuracy for detecting these abnormalities but requires transport of the patient to the radiology department. Radionuclide scanning is of limited utility, as negative results (i.e., visualization of the gallbladder) are common in acute acalculous cholecystitis, and positive results are not diagnostic in patients after prolonged lack of oral intake.

Ultrasound-guided *percutaneous cholecystostomy* is an important diagnostic and therapeutic tool. For the patient strongly suspected of having acute cholecystitis but at excessive risk for general anesthesia or surgery, bedside percutaneous cholecystostomy produces clinical improvement in 56%–94% of patients, with fewer than 10% having serious complications (bleeding, leakage of purulent bile with peritonitis, and catheter dislodgement) (8). Endoscopic transpapillary stenting of the cystic duct has been described as a potential alternative to percutaneous cholecystostomy, particularly in patients with coagulopathy or ascites in whom percutaneous approaches carry substantial morbidity (9). After nonsurgical drainage and recovery from the critical illness, cholecystectomy can be performed with more acceptable risk.

ACUTE CHOLANGITIS

Issues at the Time of Admission

The initial presentation of cholangitis can be variable, ranging from mild abdominal pain and fever to septic shock. The classic clinical presentation of cholangitis (commonly known as *Charcot's triad*) is comprised of right upper quadrant abdominal pain, fever, and jaundice. However, these findings are present in only 20%–70% of cases (10). The additional findings of hypotension and mental status changes have been described as *Reynold's pentad*, which is associated with a grave prognosis. Elderly patients are more likely to present with severe cholangitis and often with atypical features. Abdominal pain usually is present (80%–90%), although this can be absent in the elderly or the critically ill. Fever is present in 90%–100% of cases.

Laboratory examination can be variable in patients with acute cholangitis. Leukocytosis is present in 90% of cases;

however, with overwhelming sepsis the leukocyte count can be low. Although clinical jaundice is seen 60%–90% of the time, serum liver chemistry test results almost always are elevated. The pattern of liver enzyme abnormalities is to some degree dependent on the cause and chronicity of the obstructive process. The level of hyperbilirubinemia is generally greater in cases of cholangitis complicating malignant biliary obstruction (because of a gradual onset of high-grade obstruction) than in cases of calculous disease. Serum alkaline phosphatase levels usually are elevated in chronically obstructed patients but may be normal or near-normal in patients with acute obstruction caused by impacted stones. Aminotransferase levels also usually are elevated, but to varying degrees. In most instances, aminotransferase levels are less than two times the upper limits of normal. On occasion, patients presenting with acute common bile duct obstruction caused by gallstones may have dramatic elevation in aminotransferases (500–1,000 IU), which can be confused with viral hepatitis. However, the acute nature and severity of the pain should raise the concern of biliary-tract obstruction, and the markedly elevated aminotransferase levels rapidly fall within 24 hours. In general, the clinical presentation of acute right upper quadrant pain, fever, and abnormal liver chemistry tests, especially in older patients and in those without epidemiologic risk factors for acute viral or alcoholic hepatitis, strongly suggests the presence of extrahepatic biliary-tract disease.

The differential diagnosis of acute right upper quadrant abdominal pain, fever, and abnormal liver chemistries includes penetrating or perforating peptic ulcer disease (Chapter 80), pancreatitis (Chapter 86), appendicitis (Chapter 87), pyelonephritis (Chapter 68), gonococcal perihepatitis (Fitz-Hugh-Curtis syndrome), and conditions of acute liver enlargement resulting in painful stretching of the hepatic capsule (Chapter 82), including acute viral hepatitis, acute alcoholic hepatitis, and right heart failure. As mentioned previously, a common clinical error is the confusion of acute cholangitis with acute cholecystitis. At times, the distinction can be difficult and, rarely, these conditions may occur simultaneously. Both can present with fever and right upper quadrant abdominal pain. Although mild hyperbilirubinemia can occur with acute cholecystitis, it rarely exceeds 3 mg/dL. In general, elevated bilirubin levels should trigger suspicion of common bile duct obstruction. Although dilatation of the common bile duct on an ultrasound or CT scan supports the diagnosis of bile-duct obstruction, it is absent in up to one-third of patients with documented common bile duct stones.

Although not diagnostic of cholangitis, approximately 15% of gallstones are calcified and are apparent on plain films, raising the level of suspicion for calculous disease of the biliary tract. An ileus may be present on plain films, although it is nonspecific. Acute suppurative cholangitis is not associated with the presence of free intraperitoneal air, and this finding should point to another diagnosis. Air in the gallbladder wall may indicate emphysematous cholecystitis.

The most useful initial study is ultrasonography because it provides substantial information, is easily obtained (even at the bedside in critically ill patients), and is relatively inexpensive. Gallbladder stones are detected with a high degree of sensitivity and specificity, and the presence of calculous disease suggests a possible cause. However, ultrasound is much less accurate in identifying stones within the common bile duct. Because of overlying bowel gas, the distal duct is poorly visualized, and as a result ultrasound is able to visualize stones in the common bile duct in only about 10% of cases. Dilatation of the common bile duct suggests biliary obstruction but is present in only approximately 75% of cases of confirmed choledocholithiasis.

Radionuclide cholescintigraphy is rarely helpful in the setting of suspected common bile-duct obstruction; its value lies in the diagnosis of cystic-duct obstruction. There are few specific CT scan features of cholangitis because bile-duct stones and gallbladder stones seldom can be imaged directly, and biliary dilation is less reliably identified than by ultrasound. However, CT may be of value in excluding alternative causes of sepsis, such as suppurative cholecystitis, and may provide other evidence as to the cause of biliary obstruction and sepsis, such as malignant-appearing masses in the pancreas, porta hepatis, or liver.

Recent and promising alternatives for diagnosis of biliary obstruction include endoscopic ultrasound and magnetic resonance cholangiopancreatography (11). The role of these diagnostic modalities in the setting of acute cholangitis is limited, but they may be of value in high-risk patients in whom more traditional diagnostic tests fail to reveal the cause of the patient's illness.

ERCP is the procedure of choice both for diagnosis and therapy of bile-duct obstruction. Once the bile duct is cannulated selectively, removal of stones or drainage of other obstructing lesions can be performed. *Percutaneous transhepatic cholangiography* is an alternative in patients with dilated bile ducts in whom ERCP is technically unsuccessful because of surgical anatomy, or if available endoscopic expertise is limited.

Indications for Hospitalization and ICU Admission

All patients with suspected biliary obstruction and fever should be admitted promptly to the hospital. Indications for hospitalization and ICU admission are similar to those for acute cholecystitis.

Initial Therapy

Initial measures are aimed at stabilizing the patient until the biliary tract can be definitively decompressed. The patient should be given nothing by mouth. Intravenous fluids are administered for volume resuscitation and to correct any electrolyte imbalance, and central venous access is established for patients in shock. Approximately one-third of patients presenting with cholangitis have coagulopathy, and correction of this should be initiated promptly in anticipation of a procedure (Chapter 98). Severely ill patients may require ventilatory support prior to definitive therapy.

Medical therapy does not substitute for drainage of an obstructed biliary tree but can stabilize a patient to allow a safer, more elective decompression procedure. Broad-spectrum antibiotic therapy should be initiated after blood cultures have been drawn. The microbiology is similar to that for acute cholecystitis. In severely ill patients or those with prior biliary-tract surgery, definitive coverage for anaerobes is recommended (12) (Chapter 64).

Urgent decompression of the biliary tract is indicated for treatment of cholangitis and should be performed as soon as is feasible. Seventy to 85 percent of patients with cholangitis respond to appropriate intravenous antibiotics with improvement in fever and abdominal pain, such that the decompression procedure can be done semi-electively within 72 hours. If complicated by hypotension or mental-status changes, decompression should be performed emergently, although not before vigorous medical resuscitation is performed. Endoscopic drainage of the obstructed biliary tract is the treatment of choice for cholangitis, depending upon local expertise and availability (13). ERCP involves endoscopic cannulation of the common bile duct and re-

moval of stones with baskets or balloon catheters (Figure 84.2), or internal stenting to bypass and relieve the obstruction. Alternatives for stone removal in patients with severe coaguloapthy include extraction after balloon dilation of the sphincter or temporary decompression by stenting alone. Biliary drainage for obstructing stones or strictures can be established quickly by placing one or more internal stents above the level of obstruction, with more definitive endoscopic or other procedures deferred until the patient is more stable. For many patients, the initial endoscopic procedure is definitive. Procedural success rates range from 80%–98%, with complete duct clearance of stones at the first procedure in 80%–95% of cases, depending on local expertise, technical complexity, and comorbidity. The procedural morbidity rate, including cardiorespiratory events, bleeding, pancreatitis, perforation, or worsened sepsis in the event of a failed procedure, is approximately 5%–10%, with a direct procedure-related mortality rate of less than 1% (14). Gastric surgery or intestinal strictures may make ERCP difficult or impossible.

Percutaneous transhepatic drainage involves placement of a percutaneous catheter through the hepatic parenchyma into the dilated biliary tree. The procedural morbidity rate ranges from 7%–35%, with complications including sepsis, bleeding, bile leak, and fistula. The mortality rate from percutaneous transhepatic drainage in the setting of

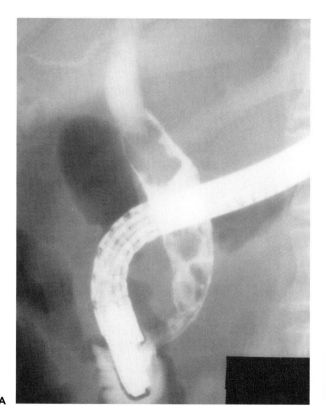
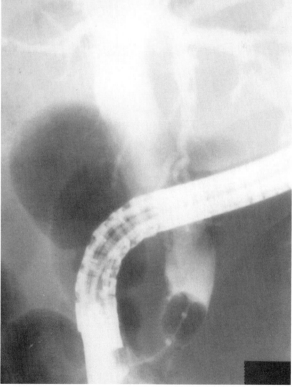

A   **B**

Figure 84.2. Endoscopic retrograde cholangiograms showing multiple stones in a dilated common bile duct **A.** and a cleared duct after endoscopic biliary sphincterotomy and subsequent stone extraction with a balloon catheter **B.**

cholangitis has been reported as high as 5%–16%. Unlike ERCP, the procedure is contraindicated in the presence of coagulopathy, and it often requires subsequent surgery or ERCP for definitive therapy in the setting of choledocholithiasis. The absence of ductal dilatation may make percutaneous transhepatic drainage difficult or impossible. Surgical decompression usually is reserved for those patients failing the procedures previously described. The morbidity rate ranges from 40%–60%, and the mortality rate from 10%–40%.

In general, the initial approach to suspected cholangitis and other biliary obstruction should involve ERCP. A randomized, controlled trial of endoscopic versus surgical management of acute suppurative cholangitis showed that endoscopic drainage was significantly safer (approximately three-fold lower mortality rate) (13). For malignant obstruction, a randomized controlled trial showed that endoscopic drainage is safer than percutaneous drainage (15).

Issues During the Course of Hospitalization

Table 84.2 shows a critical pathway for acute cholangitis. After successful decompression of the common bile duct, many patients experience an immediate and dramatic clinical improvement, occasionally by the end of the proce-

dure. Abdominal pain usually resolves within 24 hours. Not uncommonly, patients experience an elevated temperature after instrumentation of the biliary tract in acute cholangitis, even after successful drainage and stone extraction. However, this usually resolves within 24–48 hours. Improvement in leukocytosis usually occurs within 2–4 days. After successful decompression of an obstructed biliary tree, elevated serum bilirubin levels should begin to improve within 24 hours, but may take up to a week or more to completely normalize. Patients with marked elevation and particularly those with malignant obstruction may take even longer to normalize their bilirubin levels.

Failure of clinical parameters to improve suggests a number of possible causes. Failure of the bilirubin level to fall, or of signs of sepsis to improve, suggests incomplete drainage resulting from residual bile-duct stones, edema at the site of the biliary sphincterotomy due to manipulation or local thrombus, malfunctioning of an endoprosthesis, or a separate cause such as concomitant cholecystitis or intrahepatic cholestasis resulting from sepsis. Complications after ERCP may result in deterioration as well. These include cardiorespiratory problems, such as aspiration pneumonia, cholangitis, pancreatitis, perforation, or hemorrhage from the sphincterotomy site. Hemorrhage usually presents as upper gastrointestinal bleeding but is sometimes delayed up to a week or more after the procedure,

TABLE 84.2
CRITICAL PATHWAY: ACUTE CHOLANGITIS

	Admission	Post–ERCP/PTBD day one (usually hospital day 2–4)	Post–ERCP/PTBD day two (usually hospital day 3–5)
Tests	Abdominal radiograph RUQ ultrasound CBC/differential Electrolytes Liver panel Coagulation studies Blood cultures	CBC Liver panel Check blood culture results	CBC Liver panel
Medical Therapy	Intravenous antibiotics Intravenous fluids Correct coagulopathy Gastroenterology consultation to perform prompt biliary decompression after stabilization[a]	Discontinue intravenous fluids If not improving, consider: Repeat ERCP Surgical consultation Nongastrointestinal source	Convert to oral antibiotics
Nursing	Vital signs Oxygen saturation	Vital signs Assist with activities of daily living	Vital signs Assist patient with activities of daily living and begin counseling family
Nutrition	NPO	Clear liquids if pain-free	Advance as tolerated
Discharge planning	Begin addressing	Discuss cholecystectomy	Make follow-up appointment

[a] Septic patients should undergo *immediate* biliary drainage after stabilization.
CBC, complete blood count; *ERCP*, endoscopic retrograde cholangiopancreatography; *NPO*, nothing by mouth; *PTBD*, percutaneous transhepatic biliary drainage; *RUQ*, right upper quadrant.

especially in patients with coagulopathy or those placed on anticoagulation after the procedure. Trauma to the sphincterotomy site from multiple stone extractions during ERCP or localized thrombus can lead to edema, resulting in biliary obstruction and recurrent bacteremia. In instances in which a biliary stricture or incomplete clearance of bile-duct stones has required placement of a stent or nasobiliary tube, recurrence of symptoms may signal obstruction, malfunction, or dislodgement of the stent. Failure to improve within a reasonable period of time may force a repeat procedure to assess adequacy of decompression. In those cases in which the findings of ERCP were not suggestive of cholangitis, consideration should be given to nongastrointestinal sources of fever. In addition, the possibility of postprocedural aspiration pneumonia should be considered. Post-ERCP pancreatitis also can be a complication, and its onset can be delayed over 24 hours.

Discharge Issues

The optimal duration of antibiotic therapy for bacteremia associated with cholangitis has not been determined. Commonly, intravenous antibiotics are continued until the patient has become afebrile, and sometimes for an additional 1–2 days. Conversion to an oral antibiotic with suitable spectrum then can be instituted for a total duration of 7–10 days. One recent study has suggested that even shorter durations of post-procedure antibiotic therapy (3 days) may be appropriate after successful endoscopic drainage of the biliary tract (16).

Although endoscopic sphincterotomy and clearance of common bile duct stones represents definitive treatment of the index episode of cholangitis, cholecystectomy commonly is recommended for most patients who have intact gallbadders containing stones because of the risk of susbsequent cholecystitis. However, in elderly patients, or those whose comorbid medical conditions place them at high risk for surgery, the gallbladder may be left intact after endoscopic treatment of common bile duct stones. The natural history of gallbladders containing stones and left *in situ* after endoscopic sphincterotomy for bile-duct stones is variable. A large review suggested a subsequent requirement for cholecystectomy in this group of approximately 2%–3% per year, with the majority occurring within the first two years (17). Several randomized controlled trials comparing strategies of cholecystectomy and "watchful waiting" have suggested that, while a significant proportion of patients managed expectantly may ultimately require cholecystectomy, the non-surgical approach results in no increase in significant complications or mortality (18, 19). Discussions among the patient, primary care physician, gastroenterologist, and surgeon are appropriate at this time or at follow-up appointments regarding the risks and benefits of elective cholecystectomy.

COST CONSIDERATION AND RESOURCE USE

Important determinants of cost and resource use in the management of acute cholecystitis are the number of diagnostic modalities utilized, the choice among various antibiotic regimens, the use of the ICU, the promptness of surgical consultation and possible cholecystectomy, and the length of the postoperative stay. A strategy of delayed cholecystectomy offers no clinical advantages over prompt cholecystectomy (after resuscitation) and is more expensive.

In general, the most cost-effective approach to acute cholangitis involves rapid resuscitation and early definitive procedural intervention without unnecessary delays for additional imaging studies such as CT scans, especially if the diagnosis is clear on clinical grounds.

KEY POINTS

- With few exceptions, treatment is not indicated for asymptomatic cholelithiasis.
- Acute cholecystitis is a serious intra-abdominal infection, which can be life-threatening if not treated. Diagnosis is made utilizing clinical, ultrasound, or radionuclide scan data.
- Appropriate treatment of acute cholecystitis includes intravenous fluids, antibiotics, and prompt cholecystectomy. Prolonged treatment with antibiotics followed by discharge and interval cholecystectomy offers no clinical advantages and is more costly.
- Acute cholecystitis complicating critical illness may be calculous or acalculous in etiology, is associated with a high mortality rate, and may be treated by cholecystectomy, percutaneous cholecystostomy, or endoscopic transpapillary gallbladder drainage.
- Cholecystitis must be differentiated from cholangitis. In patients with right upper quadrant pain and fever, elevated serum bilirubin levels should suggest cholangitis rather than cholecystitis.
- Patients with cholangitis should be stablized with intravenous fluids, antibiotics, and correction of electrolyte and coagulation disturbances.
- ERCP is the procedure of choice for diagnosis and treatment of cholangitis.

REFERENCES

1. Everhart JE, Khare M, Hill M, et al. Prevalence and ethnic differences in gallbladder disease in the United States. *Gastroenterology* 1999;117:632–639.
2. Diehl AK, Schwesinger WH, Holleman DR Jr., et al. Clinical correlates of gallstone composition: distinguishing pigment from cholesterol stones. *Am J Gastroenterol* 1995;90:967–972.
3. Singer AJ, McCracken G, Thode HC Jr., et al. Correlation among clinical, laboratory, and hepatobiliary scanning findings in

patients with suspected acute cholecystitis. *Ann Emerg Med* 1996; 28:267–272.

4. Kurzweil SM, Shapiro MJ, Andrus CH, et al. Hyperbilirubinemia without common bile duct abnormalities and hyperamylasemia without pancreatitis in patients with gallbladder disease. *Arch Surg* 1994;129:829–833.

5. Shea JA, Berlin JA, Escarce JJ, et al. Revised estimates of diagnostic test sensitivity and specificity in suspected biliary tract disease. *Arch Intern Med* 1994;154:2573–2581.

6. Papi C, Catarci M, D'Ambrosio L, et al. Timing of cholecystectomy for acute calculous cholecystitis: a meta-analysis. *Am J Gastroenterol* 2004;99:147–155.

7. Barie PS, Eachempati SR. Acute acalculous cholecystitis. *Curr Gasteroenterol Rep* 2003;5:302–309.

8. Patel M, Miedema BW, James MA, et al. Percutaneous cholecystostomy is an effective treatment for high-risk patients with acute cholecystitis. *Am Surg* 2000;66:33–37.

9. Gaglio PJ, Buniak B, Leevy CB. Primary endoscopic retrograde cholecystoenoprosthesis: a nonsurgical modality for symptomatic cholelithiasis in cirrhotic patients. *Gastrointest Endosc* 1996;44: 339–342.

10. Csendes A, Diaz JC, Burdiles P, et al. Risk factors and classification of acute suppurative cholangitis. *Br J Surg* 1992;79:655–658.

11. Mark DH, Flamm CR, Aronson N. Evidence-based assessment of diagnostic modalities for common bile duct stones. *Gastrointest Endosc* 2002;56(Suppl):S190–S194.

12. van den Hazel SJ, Speelman P, Tytgat GNJ, et al. Role of antibiotics in the treatment and prevention of acute and recurrent cholangitis. *Clin Infect Dis* 1994;19:279–286.

13. Lai ECS, Mok FPT, Tan ESY, et al. Endoscopic drainage for severe acute cholangitis. *N Engl J Med* 1992;326:1582–1586.

14. Freeman ML, Nelson DB, Sherman S, et al. Complications of endoscopic biliary sphincterotomy. *N Engl J Med* 1996;335:909–918.

15. Speer AG, Cotton PB, Russell RCG, et al. Randomised trial of endoscopic versus percutaneous stent insertion in malignant obstructive jaundice. *Lancet* 1987;2:57–62.

16. van Lent AU, Bartelsman JF, Tytgat GN, et al. Duration of antibiotic therapy for cholangitis after successful endoscopic drainage of the biliary tract. *Gastrointest Endosc* 2002;55:518–522.

17. Silvis SE. Endoscopic sphincterotomy with an intact gallbladder. *Gastrointest Endosc Clin North Am* 1991;1:65–77.

18. Boerma D, Rauws EA, Keulemans YCA, et al. Wait-and-see policy or laparoscopic cholecystectomy after endoscopic sphincterotomy for bile-duct stones: a randomised trial. *Lancet* 2002;360:761–765.

19. Vetrhus M, Søreide O, Solhaug JH, et al. Symptomatic, non-complicated gallbladder stone disease: operation or observation? A randomized clinical study. *Scand J Gastroenterol* 2002;37:834–839.

ADDITIONAL READING

Baron RL, Tublin ME, Peterson MS. Imaging the spectrum of biliary tract disease. *Radiol Clin North Am* 2002;40:1325–1354.

Trowbridge RL, Rutkowski NK, Shojania KG. Does this patient have acute cholecystitis? *JAMA* 2003;289:80–86.

Yusoff IF, Barkun JS, Barkun AN. Diagnosis and management of cholecystitis and cholangitis. *Gastroenterol Clin North Am* 2003;32: 1145–1168.

Liver Transplantation

85

Raphael B. Merriman

INTRODUCTION

Liver transplantation has revolutionized the management of end-stage liver disease and acute liver failure since its inception more than four decades ago (1). Data from the United Network for Organ Sharing (UNOS) registry, which operates the Organ Procurement and Transplantatation Network (http://www.optn.org), reports that in 2003, patients had a 1-year survival rate of 88.1% and a 5-year survival rate of 74.3%. Improvements in patient survival reflect advances in surgical and anesthetic techniques, patient selection, and pre- and post-operative management, including the development of more effective immunosuppressive and antimicrobial agents. Liver transplantation (LT) continues to be challenged by organ shortages and prolonged waiting list times. The most significant recent development in liver transplantation in the United States was the 2002 implementation of an allocation policy based on the Model for End-stage Liver Disease (MELD) and the Pediatric End-stage Liver Disease score (PELD). This policy now preferentially directs livers to patients with the most imminent risk of death.

This chapter provides a review of general surgical principles, indications for transplantation, and the evaluation of patients for liver transplantation. The management of the patient after liver transplantation will be outlined and the common complications will also be reviewed.

SURGICAL PRINCIPLES

A suitable donor organ is matched to a recipient with a compatible ABO blood type. Typically, the surgical procedure is divided into the hepatectomy phase, the anhepatic phase, and the reperfusion phase. The typical biliary reconstruction involves a direct duct-to-duct reanastomosis (choledochocholedochostomy), although occasionally, when the recipent duct is diseased (e.g., primary sclerosing

cholangitis) or unsuitable, a choledochoduodenostomy is performed using a Roux-en-Y anastomosis. Stenting of the biliary anatomosis with externalization of bile via a T tube is now infrequently employed.

Modern liver surgery is based upon the functional segmental anatomy of the liver (Figure 85.1); the eight segments are based on the distribution of the portal veins. This is especially relevant when segmental grafts are employed, as in adult and pediatric living liver donation and split liver transplantation. For example, a right hepatectomy involves the resection of segments V, VI, VII, and VIII. Hepatic venous drainage begins as the central veins join to form the right, middle, and left hepatic veins, which empty into the suprahepatic inferior vena cava. Donor organ preservation has been enhanced by the use of Univeristy of Wisconsin (UW) cold storage solution. Knowledge of the common anatomic variations in the hepatic artery is essential, especially for successful donor hepatectomy. Radiologic determination of portal vein patency is important for operative planning because an obstructed portal vein will require a venous graft to bypass or reconstruct the occluded portal vein segment.

PATIENT SELECTION FOR LIVER TRANSPLANTATION

Prognostic Models and Prioritization for Organ Allocation

Policies related to organ allocation significantly impact patient selection for transplantation and have recently undergone major changes. The success of LT led to a marked disparity between the number of patients on the LT waiting list and the number of donor livers available for transplantation in the United States. The most common indications for LT are hepatitis C, alcoholic liver disease, and hepatocellular carcinoma (HCC). As of February 2005,

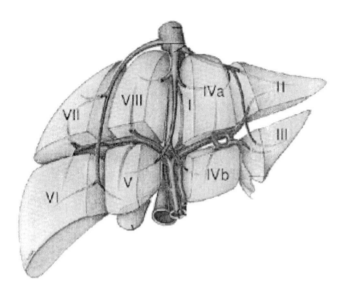

Figure 85.1 Functional anatomy of the liver.

nostic score was initially developed to predict short-term prognosis after transjugular intrahepatic portosystemic shunt (TIPS). Subsequently, the score was validated as an accurate predictor of pretransplantation short-term mortality from end-stage liver disease. The MELD score has the advantage of relying on objective and readily available standardized laboratory tests: serum creatinine, bilirubin, and INR (2). The PELD score has been adapted for organ allocation in children; it also accounts for age and growth failure. Policy developers recognized that the MELD score would not serve all candidates equally well and, therefore, introduced exceptions for certain conditions (e.g., HCC, hepato-pulmonary syndrome, portopulmonary hypertension, and familial amyloidosis) by assigning a higher initial score. Since the introduction of the MELD/PELD scores, the number of patients waiting for LT has decreased, with an increase in the number of patients who undergo LT for HCC (3). Unfortunately, the MELD/PELD system has its own shortcomings that will require further modifications over time.

17,678 patients were on the liver transplantation waiting list, while the total number of liver transplants in 2004 was only 5,136. *The Child-Turcotte-Pugh (CTP) score* (Table 85.1) is still used by UNOS to determine a patient's eligibility to be listed for LT. A CTP score of at least 7 is the minimum needed to be listed; this score reflects a predicted 1-year risk of death of at least 10%. Patients with fulminant hepatic failure (Chapter 82) who are highest risk for short-term mortality are classified separately and listed with the highest priority (Status I).

For patients without fulminant hepatic failure, the criteria for transplantation have changed. Prior to February 2002, the two major determinants of liver allocation were waiting time and CTP score. The former often did not reflect the medical need for transplantation, while the latter has subjective components that can be overestimated. In response to the clear need for an improved allocation policy, in March 2002 UNOS began using the MELD score as the basis for prioritizing organ allocation (1). Interestingly, the MELD prog-

Contraindications and Controversies

The contraindications to LT are generally not evidence-based, and it should therefore not be surprising that they are controversial, reflect local practice and culture, and constantly evolving. Broadly, they can be divided into two categories (Table 85.2). *Absolute contraindications* are conditions for which the results of LT are so poor that it is difficult to justify the use of the limited donor organ pool. *Relative contraindications* negatively affect survival, but not to such a degree that LT should never be considered. Many of these relative contraindications, in particular, are controversial. For example, early reports on the outcome of LT in patients with HCC were unfavorable because of a high incidence of tumor recurrence. However, data emerged indicating that patients with early stage HCC (stage I and II) have excellent results following LT, comparable to patients with non-HCC disease (4). In HIV-infected patients on highly active anti-retroviral therapy (HAART),

TABLE 85.1

CHILD-TURCOTTE-PUGH CLASSIFICATION

Feature	Points		
	1	2	3
Hepatic encephalopathy	None	Controlled	Not controlled
Ascites	None	Controlled	Not controlled
Total bilirubin (mg/dL)	<2	2–3	>3
Prothrombin time (secs prolonged)	0–3	3–6	>6
Albumin (gm/dL)	>3.5	2.8–3.5	<2.8
Childs Class A:	5–6 points		
Childs Class B:	7–9 points		
Childs Class C:	10–15 points		

TABLE 85.2

CONTRAINDICATIONS TO LIVER TRANSPLANTATION

Absolute Contraindications

Severe, irreversible comorbidities
Severe portopulmonary hypertension (mean pulmonary arterial pressure (PAP) ≥45 mmHg)
Extrahepatic malignancy (excluding some skin cancers)
Extensive hepatocellular carcinoma (including vascular invasion and lymph node involvement)
Severe and uncontrolled systemic infection
Multiorgan failure
Active alcohol or substance abuse
Advanced cardiac disease
Severe, uncontrolled psychiatric disease
Noncompliance
Extensive portal vein and mesenteric vein thromboses

Relative Contraindications

HIV seropositivity
Moderate portopulmonary hypertension (mean PAP ≥35 mmHg)
Severe hepatopulmonary syndrome (PaO_2 ≤50 mmHg)
Cholangiocarcinoma
Morbid obesity (Body Mass Index ≥40kg/m²)
Advanced age (≥70 years)
Recurrent hepatits C in a transplanted liver

end-stage liver disease related to hepatitis C and B is the most common cause of death. Preliminary data suggest that solid organ transplantation in such patients, if well selected and performed in experienced centers, is both feasible and effective (5). Transplantation for cholangiocarcinoma has also been performed in selected centers employing experimental treatment protocols. Severe obesity may be associated with cirrhosis related to non-alcoholic fatty liver disease, and LT in this increasingly prevalent patient population presents unique surgical and postoperative management challenges. The allocation of organs to patients with alcoholic liver disease was once frowned upon, but is now less controversial. Survival rates after LT in patients with this history are second highest, trailing only patients with cholestatic liver disease. Rates of rejection, disease recurrence, and re-transplantation are generally lower in patients with isolated alcoholic liver disease than for other etiologies. Rates of recidivism or relapse are highly variable, depending on method of evaluation. Most programs report an alcohol use relapse rate of 15%–30% over the first 2–3 years. A minimum of six months of documented sobriety with proven rehabilitation is required by most transplant programs.

Evaluation of the LT Candidate

Evaluation of potential LT recipients involves a multidisciplinary approach, typically including evaluation by a transplant hepatologist and surgeon, an addiction specialist, social-services personnel, nurse coordinators, financial counselors, and other specialist consultants according to patient needs (Table 85.3). Although usually occurring in the outpatient setting, rapidly deteriorating end-stage liver disease or acute liver failure will demand an expedited inpatient evaluation. The initial assessment involves a thorough history and physical examination, with an emphasis on the presence of complications related to chronic liver disease, assessment of co-morbidities and possible contraindications to transplantation, the potential recipient's current functional status, any history of ongoing or prior substance abuse, duration and reliability of abstinence, and risk of recidivism. The past medical and surgical history (especially hepatobiliary surgery or TIPS) guide further evaluation of surgical and postoperative risk. The patient meets with experienced transplant social workers, who evaluate the current and likely post-transplant level of family and other social support. The candidate also undergoes liver imaging (either ultrasonography with Doppler interrogation, multiple phase thin-cut spiral CT, or magnetic resonance imaging) that includes assessment of patency of the portal vein and other vascular structures and screening for HCC. The laboratory evaluation includes ABO typing and measurements of the serum albumin, total bilirubin levels, and prothrombin time. Other disease-specific assays are obtained if not previously performed. If no absolute contraindications are identified and the patient meets the minimal criteria for LT listing, the patient is listed. Many institutions make listing decisions at a multidisciplinary evaluation conference. Subsequently, a second phase of more invasive testing is initiated, often directed by symptoms or comorbidity. It includes a battery of infectious disease serologies, gynecologic evaluation and mammography for women, and screening tests for cardiopulmonary and renal disorders.

Evaluation of the Living Donor

Until 1989, all LTs used a cadaveric donor organ. Since the introduction of living donor transplants that year, the proportion of living donor transplants has grown steadily, from 1% in 1993 to 6% in 2004. Some of the unique features of the evaluation of a living liver donor deserve particular mention.

Transplantation of part of a liver from an adult into a child has been practiced for more than 15 years. The basic operation (a left lateral segmentectomy) is relatively predictable and has a low risk when done at experienced centers. In contrast, adult-to-adult living donation, which began about a decade ago, usually involves a more substantial operation, usually consisting of a right hepatectomy in the donor (6). Typically, potential donors are between 21 and 55 years of age, have a compatible blood

TABLE 85.3

EVALUATION OF THE LIVER-TRANSPLANT CANDIDATE

Consultations	Hepatologist
	Liver transplant surgeon
	Cardiologist, for recipients >50 years old
	Gynecologist (Pap test [all], mammography [recipients >40 years old])
	Addiction specialist, if history of substance abuse
	Anesthesiologist, if needed
	Medical social worker evaluation
	Transplant coordinator
	Financial counselor
Pathology	Review biopsy, if available
Radiology	Liver imaging with sonography or CT and assessment of portal vein patency
Cardiopulmonary	Arterial blood gas
	Electrocardiogram
	Echocardiogram
	Cardiac stress test, when appropriate
	Chest radiograph, posteroanterior and lateral
Laboratory tests	ABO blood type, antibody screen
	HIV serology
	Chronic hepatitis panel: HBsAg, HBcAb, and anti-HCV; HBV-DNA and HBeAg for patients who are HBsAg-positive
	Hepatitis B immunity (HBsAb)
	Hepatitis C genotype and viral load (using an amplified, PCR-based assay) if anti-HCV positive
	Cytomegalovirus antibody, RPR
	Alpha fetoprotein
	Iron, transferrin saturation, and ferritin
	Thyroid function tests
	Prostate specific antigen assay for men ≥ 50 years old
	Complete blood cell count, electrolytes, creatinine, blood urea nitrogen, alkaline phosphatase, total bilirubin, aminotransferases, albumin, prothrombin time, creatinine clearance estimate, if indicated
	Urinalysis and microscopy
	Random urine/blood toxicology screening (where appropriate)

Anti-HCV, antibody against hepatitis C virus; *HBcAb*, hepatitis B core antibody; *HBeAg*, hepatitis B e antigen; *HBsAb*, hepatitis B surface antibody; *HBsAg*, hepatitis B surface antigen; *HBV-DNA*, hepatitis B virus DNA; *HIV*, human immunodeficiency virus; *RPR*, rapid plasma reagin.

type, and are free of comorbid diseases. Currently, there is little standardization in the evaluation of donors and in the operative procedure, making it very difficult to assess the risks of complications and death to donors. However, the morbidity attributable to surgical resection in donors of grafts for adult recipients has been reported to be as high as 50% (6), substantially higher than that of donors of grafts for children. The most serious potential consequence is death caused by an intra-operative complication or postoperative liver failure. The donor should provide detailed informed consent and must be offered an opportunity to decline. In many programs, potential donors see a physician who is not part of the transplantation team, and in some programs, the potential donor is also evaluated by an ethicist. The evaluation places special emphasis on accurate determination of acceptable hepatic, biliary, and vascular anatomy; it may involve selective use of invasive procedures such as liver biopsy, cholangiography, and arteriography.

Evaluation of Selected Organ Systems

Pulmonary Evaluation

The differential diagnosis of pulmonary symptoms and gas-exchange abnormalities in patients with chronic liver disease is broad; efforts should focus on determining whether the severity of pulmonary dysfunction precludes LT and identifying conditions (such as hepatopulmonary syndrome and some cases of portopulmonary hypertension) that may reverse with transplantation. *Hepatopulmonary syndrome* (HPS), characterized by arterial hypoxemia (PaO_2 ≤70 mmHg or alveolar-arterial gradient of >20 mmHg), occurs in as many as 15% of patients with chronic liver disease. It is caused by intrapulmonary vasodilation, and it results in impaired oxygenation (7). Symptoms include dyspnea and platypnea. An examination may reveal orthodeoxia and central cyanosis. Pulmonary function testing is usually unhelpful; arterial blood gases confirm hypoxia.

Contrast-enhanced echocardiography following the injection of agitated saline is a sensitive method to detect intrapulmonary shunting; bubbles detected early within the left atrium correlate well with the presence of pulmonary arteriovenous communications. Technetium[99]-macroaggregated albumin scintigraphy is definitive but rarely required to confirm the diagnosis. Measuring the PaO_2 on 100% oxygen also provides useful information, as it usually normalizes in patients with HPS. Failure to exceed a PaO_2 of 200 mmHg on 100% oxygen implies the likely presence of significant true shunts and precludes LT at most centers, unless gas exchange can be improved by embolization of those larger true shunts. HPS is associated with increased postoperative morbidity and need for mechanical ventilation, with substantially increased mortality (>30%) when the HPS is severe and the PaO_2 is <50 mmHg. Consequently, patients with a diagnosis of HPS are usually awarded a higher MELD exception score to facilitate earlier transplantation.

Portopulmonary hypertension, defined by a mean pulmonary arterial pressure (mPAP) >25 mmHg, occurs in up to 2% of patients with cirrhosis and portal hypertension (7). Patients may be asymptomatic or present with exertional dyspnea. Chest pain and syncope are late features. Contrast-enhanced echocardiography assesses right and left heart function and anatomy and usually provides noninvasive estimates of pulmonary artery pressures. Other common causes of pulmonary hypertension must be excluded (Chapter 59). Echocardiographic features suggestive of right-ventricular compromise may be sufficient to exclude a patient from consideration for LT. If a borderline, uncertain, or elevated pulmonary artery pressure (mean PAP ≥25 mmHg or systolic PAP ≥40 mmHg) is demonstrated, patients should undergo right-heart catheterization for direct pulmonary pressure measurement and assessment of the effect of vasodilator therapy. Prostacyclin vasodilator therapy improves survival in primary pulmonary hypertension, but the longer term effect on portopulmonary hypertension is less clear and may be dose limited by the associated thrombocytopenia. Experience with bosentan, an endothelin-1 receptor antagonist, is limited and uncertain in portopulmonary hypertension, in part related to reports of associated hepatotoxicity.

Cardiac Evaluation

Cardiac evaluation of the LT candidate should include directed history (specifically assessing the risk factors for atherosclerosis) and physical examination, electrocardiography, and echocardiography. These tests screen for potential ischemic cardiac disease, arrhythmias, left-ventricular dysfunction, and the consequences of hepatopulmonary syndrome and portopulmonary hypertension. High cardiac output associated with a low systemic vascular resistance is common among patients with decompensated chronic liver disease. Thus, the presence of an ejection fraction <60% suggests underlying ventricular dysfunction and warrants further investigation. All men over age 35 and

women over age 45 should undergo noninvasive coronary artery disease evaluation (dobutamine echocardiography or dipyridamole-thallium testing). Candidates with abnormal noninvasive studies, multiple ischemic heart disease risk factors, or an ejection fraction of less than 60% should undergo coronary angiography (Chapter 36).

CARE OF THE HOSPITALIZED PATIENT

First Four Days Following Liver Transplantation

Surgery and the Immediate Perioperative Period

Initial assessment of hepatic function begins in the operating room. Prompt and homogenous reperfusion and a soft allograft texture correlate with good function, whereas a poorly functioning graft may reperfuse slowly or become hard and edematous. During the immediate postoperative period, metabolic recovery of the liver, as measured by clearance of acid (lactate) and the associated metabolic acidosis and glucose production, serves as a gauge of allograft function. Typically, the recipient with a well-functioning graft develops a mild metabolic alkalosis. Prompt recovery from anesthesia, as well as normalization of the hepatic dependent coagulations factors (II, VII, IX, and X), as reflected in normalization of prothrombin time, are additional measures of successful engraftment. However, use of fresh frozen plasma and recombinant Factor VIIA may be necessary in the immediate postoperative period, especially if difficulty is encountered in achieving hemostasis. Patients with severe preoperative hepatic encephalopathy may take days to improve, even with a well-functioning graft. With successful engraftment, serum aspartate aminotransferase and alanine aminotransferase activities usually peak within the first 24–48 hours and decline to levels within four times normal by seven days after LT. As discussed later in this chapter, persistent elevation of the serum aminotransferases after LT is often an ominous marker for allograft dysfunction.

Complications arising in the immediate postoperative period may be categorized into three types: (a) *technical problems* related to the recipient operation, such as intra-abdominal hemorrhage and hepatic artery thrombosis, (b) *primary nonfunction of the allograft,* including primary nonfunction, preservation injury, and acute rejection, and (c) *medical complications,* such as fever, altered mental status, and renal insufficiency.

Technical Postoperative Problems

Intra-abdominal hemorrhage in the early postoperative period is characterized by hypotension, tachycardia, abdominal distension with high-output bloody abdominal drainage, decreasing urine output, and a falling hematocrit level. Coagulopathy should be corrected and patients should be transfused to keep the hematocrit above 25%. Approximately 10% of recipients require early reoperation for control of hemorrhage. Hemodynamic instability or a transfusion requirement of more than 5–8 units of packed red blood cells in the first 24 hours are the usual indications for early operative reintervention.

Hepatic artery thrombosis (HAT) occurs in 7% of all adult transplants, usually within the first 30 days. Risk factors include small hepatic artery size, complex anatomy, the use of extension grafts for arterial anatomosis, prolonged ischemia time, and a hypercoagulable state. A marked elevation of levels of the serum aminotransferases (>1,000 IU/L), accompanied by evidence of hepatic allograft dysfunction, should prompt urgent abdominal Doppler ultrasonography and direct arteriography to confirm hepatic artery occlusion. If HAT is identified very early after LT, immediate angioplasty or reanastomosis may avoid the long term sequelae. The benefit of thrombolysis as a sole therapy or in conjunction with revascularization is unclear. Established HAT is associated with later ischemic biliary stricturing (as the bile ducts are supplied exclusively by this vessel), almost invariably necessitating later retransplantation. Once HAT is excluded in the patient with postoperative dysfunction, liver biopsy may be useful (Figure 85.2).

Primary Nonfunction of the Graft

Primary nonfunction of the hepatic allograft reflects a variety of insults, including damage inflicted by donor-related disease, harvesting (donor hepatectomy), or cold preservation, as well as reperfusion injury. Primary nonfunction is characterized by rapid and marked elevations of the serum aminotransferases (>2,000 IU/L), rapid development of severe metabolic acidosis, hepatic synthetic failure, and ultimately multiorgan failure. The diagnosis is made on clinical grounds after exclusion of HAT. Urgent retransplantation (and even hepatectomy while awaiting a suitable graft) is the only treatment; without this, death generally follows within 72–96 hours. Patients with primary nonfunction of the allograft require ICU-level care; management is similar to that for a patient with acute liver failure (Chapter 82). Patients with severe allograft dysfunction typically require ventilatory support until retransplantation is feasible. Prophylactic broad-spectrum antibiotic therapy is warranted to prevent sepsis. If retransplanted in time, patient recovery is rapid and similar to that of patients transplanted for fulminant hepatic failure.

Postoperative Medical Complications

Fever in the immediate postoperative period should be approached in the same manner as fever in any postsurgical patient, with a few exceptions. More than 50% of LT recipients will experience one or more episodes of infection in the postoperative period. The most common infections in the first days after orthoptic LT are bacterial (8). Risk factors include prolonged anesthesia and anhepatic time, duration of surgery, and amount of blood products given. These

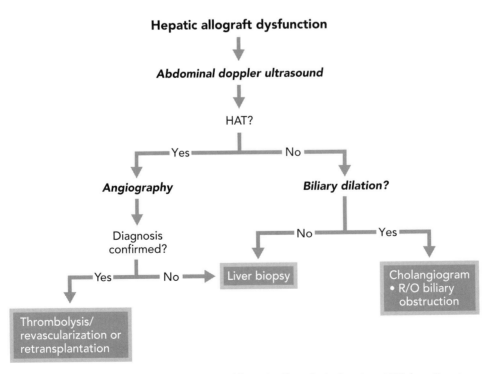

Figure 85.2 Algorithm for the evaluation of hepatic allograft dysfunction. *HAT*, hepatic artery thrombosis; *R/O*, rule out.

infections often are related to technical complications during the recipient operation and include pneumonia, liver abscess, and cholangitis. Vancomycin-resistant *Enterococcus* has emerged as an important nosocomial pathogen in LT patients.

Altered mental status in the immediate postoperative period is common and may result from residual or ongoing hepatic encephalopathy, poor clearance of analgesic or anesthetic medications, perioperative stroke, electrolyte and metabolic abnormalities, or drug toxicity. Central nervous system infections are rare during this time; therefore, lumbar puncture is not routinely indicated. Initial evaluation should include CT or magnetic resonance imaging, and possibly electroencephalography, to exclude seizure activity. Metabolic and electrolyte abnormalities should be corrected and may require temporary renal replacement therapy; potentially contributing psychotropic drugs should be discontinued. Central pontine myelinolysis may occur and should be included in the differential diagnosis. Idiosyncratic immunosuppressive-related neurotoxicity, especially caused by cyclosporine and tacrolimus, can result in a spectrum of neurologic deficits including seizures or coma (9). Predisposing factors include hypomagnesemia and hypocholesterolemia. Magnetic resonance imaging of the brain reveals a variety of changes, from reversible T2 prolongation in the occipital white matter to hemorrhagic infarcts. Treatment includes discontinuation of the medication and supportive care, including physical and speech therapy, as needed. Residual motor and speech impairments may result.

Renal insufficiency occurs frequently after orthoptic LT, may be either acute or chronic, and is usually multifactorial. It often requires hemodialysis (10). Pretransplant

renal impairent caused by hepatorenal syndrome, acute tubular necrosis precipitated by excessive diuresis or gastrointestinal bleeding, or specific disease-related conditions such as glomerulonephritis may all contribute to postopertive renal dysfunction. Pretransplant renal failure requiring dialysis (except hepatorenal syndrome) or associated with sepsis appear to be associated with a worse posttransplant outcome. Direct calcineurin inhibitor (e.g., cyclosporin or tacrolimus) vascular toxicity is the most common cause of renal insufficiency; primary allograft nonfunction, and hypovolemia resulting from intraoperative or postoperative hemorrhage and hypotension, also contribute. The routine use of low-dosage dopamine (1–3 mcg/kg/min) intraoperatively has not been shown to reduce the incidence of renal insufficiency after LT. The need for hemodialysis in the postoperative period has been associated with an increased mortality rate. Maintaining an adequate volume status, avoiding nephrotoxic antibiotics, withholding cyclosporine and tacrolimus early in the postoperative course, and closely monitoring serum drug levels may facilitate recovery of renal function.

Five to Thirty Days After Orthotopic Liver Transplantation

Presentations with Fever and/or Graft Dysfunction

Fever

Fever (Figure 85.3) occurring during this time frame warrants an inpatient evaluation. In the absence of liver function test abnormalities, an investigation for opportunistic

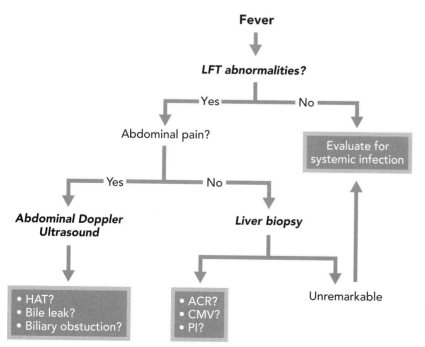

Figure 85.3 Algorithm for the evaluation of fever following liver transplantation. *ACR*, acute cellular rejection; *CMV*, cytomegalovirus infection; *HAT*, hepatic artery thrombosis; *LFT*, liver function test; *PI*, preservation injury.

infection should be initiated (Chapter 63). If liver tests are abnormal, it is important to determine whether the patient has localizing symptoms or signs. Differentiating fever and jaundice caused by biliary tract disorders from that caused by acute cellular rejection or viral infection may be challenging. Doppler ultrasonography enables evaluation of hepatic artery patency as well as identification of biliary dilatation and intra-abdominal bile collections (*bilomas*). If ultrasonography does not reveal biliary or vascular abnormalities, a liver biopsy should be performed, with an assessment of the biopsy specimen for acute cellular rejection or cytomegalovirus (CMV) infection.

Bile Leak

Abdominal or shoulder pain in the setting of fever and jaundice may indicate the presence of a *bile leak*, the most common biliary complication occurring during the first postoperative month. It may occur in up to 10% of recipients (11). Bile leaks are particularly common after adult-to-adult living donor transplantation, either in the recipient or the donor (7). Once a bile leak is suspected, cholangiography is indicated to identify the site of leakage. The mode of cholangiography will depend on the type of bile duct anastomosis. Most leaks can be managed successfully by the placement of a stent across the site of leakage (12). Nonanastomotic leaks, such as may occur from the cut surface of a living donor or split graft, may require endoscopic or surgical correction, depending upon the anatomy. It is also important to drain any intra-abdominal bile collections; this usually can be accomplished nonsurgically with a percutaneous catheter. *Biliary strictures* are usually anastomotic and may be related to local edema or ischemia. They are usually managed by stent placement, with or without balloon dilation.

Acute Cellular Rejection

The clinical presentation of *acute cellular rejection* (ACR) is variable. Patients may present with constitutional symptoms, such as fever associated with aminotransferase elevation, or with asymptomatic aminotransferase elevation. Abnormal aminotransferases within the first postoperative month should prompt a liver biopsy to determine the presence of ACR (13), which has a peak incidence on the 10th day following LT. ACR is treated by increasing the level of immunosuppression, initially with additional corticosteroid therapy, and may be managed in the outpatient setting. This approach is successful in >85% of cases. Patients with steroid-refractory ACR either have their maintenance immunosuppression changed or are treated with OKT3 (a murine monoclonal antibody to the CD3 receptor on T lymphocytes) or anti-thymocyte rabbit immunoglobulin. Both yield a 75% response rate. Treatment with such antilymphocyte antibody therapy requires hospitalization because of the potential adverse effects, including a cytokine release syndrome, aseptic

meningitis, capillary leak syndrome presenting as pulmonary edema, and gastrointestinal, renal, and dermatologic toxicities. The incidence of steroid-refractory rejection appears to have diminished with the implementation of tacrolimus-based immunosuppressive regimens. Newer immunosuppressive agents with less toxicity have recently been introduced. Mycophenolate mofetil is a reverse inhibitor of inosine monophosphate dehydrogenase and has gastrointestinal toxicity and bone marrow suppression as the main side effects. Sirolimus inhibits the response of lymphocytes to cytokine stimulation and inhibits antibody production by B cells. Because of its lack of nephrotoxicity, it may be used as an alternative to calcineurin inhibitors.

Cytomegalovirus and Other Viral Infections

Cytomegalovirus (and to a lesser extent *Herpes simplex* virus) may cause hepatitis within the first 6 weeks following LT (14). The clinical presentation includes fever and elevated serum aminotransferase levels. The routine use of prophylactic acyclovir or ganciclovir following LT has almost eliminated post-LT *Herpes simplex* virus hepatitis. Unfortunately, symptomatic CMV disease continues to occur relatively frequently after LT, especially with greater immunosuppression; this may result from reactivation or via primary acquisition from blood products or the hepatic allograft in a seronegative recipient. Seronegative LT recipients who receive seropositive organs are at greatest risk and should receive prophylaxis with ganciclovir. CMV hepatitis must be considered in patients with allograft dysfunction 21 days–3 months after LT (peak incidence, 30 days). Associated findings include fever and leukopenia. The diagnosis is confirmed by direct viral culture, the more rapid shell vial culture technique, or by the histologic documentation of cytopathic effects and microabscesses. Treatment is with intravenous ganciclovir or valganciclovir.

Jaundice Without Fever

Postoperative jaundice not attributable to a specific vascular, biliary, or hepatocellular process is termed *preservation injury*. The contributing causes are similar to those for primary nonfunction. Preservation injury is characterized by a rapid rise and decline of the serum aminotransferase levels followed by a progressive increase in the serum bilirubin. Although the general trend is one of improvement unless an additional insult occurs, preservation injury may take weeks to months to resolve and may be associated with later bile duct sequelae.

Recurrent Portal Hypertension

Portal vein thrombosis may occur in the first postoperative month and most commonly is manifested as recurrent gastrointestinal hemorrhage or ascites. Risk factors for portal vein thrombosis include preoperative portacaval shunt, hypercoagulable states, and intraoperative interposition or graft use. Doppler ultrasound is diagnostic. If thrombosis is detected early, balloon dilation and stenting may prevent the need for reoperation with reconstruction or clot removal, although both are usually followed by the need for anticoagulation.

Beyond 30 Days After Orthotopic Liver Transplantation

Fever with Jaundice

The differential diagnosis of fever with jaundice after the first postoperative month includes ACR, CMV hepatitis, and biliary obstruction. ACR is less common during this window, and its occurrence usually reflects a reduction in immunosuppression because of either decreased absorption, drug-drug interactions, or poor compliance. CMV hepatitis may occur as late as three months following transplantation.

Biliary obstruction occurs in 12%–15% of patients after LT (11). Cholangitis suggests the presence of a biliary stricture with obstruction caused by sludge or stones. Ultrasonography may reveal biliary dilation but is not a reliable finding in this setting. Cholangiography confirms the diagnosis and identifies the site of obstruction, which can be relieved by dilitation and stenting in 70%–80% of cases. Diffuse bile duct stricturing occurs in four settings: late HAT, ABO incompatibility, prolonged cold ischemia, and recurrence of sclerosing cholangitis. The long-term outcome of diffuse biliary stricturing is uncertain, and these patients often require retransplantation.

Fever

The differential diagnosis includes opportunistic infections (including fungal infections), post-transplant lymphoproliferative disease, and, in recipients more than six months post-LT, community-acquired infection. *Post-transplant lymphoproliferative disease* (PTLD) develops in 2% of LT recipients and may present as fever of unknown origin. Associated symptoms and signs include lymphadenopathy, unexplained graft dysfunction, gastrointestinal bleeding, hepatitis, weight loss, and night sweats. Epstein-Barr virus infection has been clearly implicated in PTLD pathogenesis (15). Both polyclonal reactive lymphoid hyperplasia and monoclonal large-cell lymphomas have been described. Risk factors for the development of PTLD include a greater degree of immunosuppression (e.g., use of OKT3) and lack of previous exposure to Epstein-Barr virus. Primary sites of disease may include the lymph nodes and tonsillar regions, hepatic allograft, and gastrointestinal tract. The diagnosis is suggested by radiographic imaging studies and confirmed histologically. The cornerstone of management is a reduction of immunosuppression and high-dosage antiviral therapy with ganciclovir. Occasionally, chemotherapy may be of benefit.

Jaundice

Chronic ductopenic rejection affects up to 10% of LT recipients, but its incidence seems to be decreasing. It rarely occurs during the first two months after LT, and it is usually preceded by multiple bouts of ACR. The diagnosis is based upon histologic criteria, with a progressive loss of interlobular bile ducts in at least 50% of portal tracts and an obliterative arteriopathy (14). Ductopenic rejection commonly leads to irreversible graft failure and may necessitate retransplantation.

Disease Recurrence

With the improved 5-year survival rate following LT, recurrence of native disease has become an important issue in the long-term management of the LT recipient. Recurrence of hepatitis C (HCV) is the greatest challenge and is almost universal. The rate of recurrence is highly variable, and the average time to cirrhosis is 9–12 years. Treatment of recurrent viral infection is complicated and usually unsuccessful. Risk factors for hepatitis C recurrence include high HCV RNA pretransplant levels, episodes of acute rejection, increased donor age, and use of more potent immunosuppression (16). An accelerated variant, known as fibrosing cholestatic hepatitis, may result in cirrhosis within one year. Graft reinfection with hepatitis B has been greatly reduced through the use of hepatitis B immune globulin (HBIg), often in combination with lamivudine. Primary biliary cirrhosis, autoimmune hepatitis, and primary sclerosing cholangitis may also recur. The evaluation and management of these patients and the controversy surrounding the role of retransplantation for recurrent disease is beyond the scope of this discussion.

KEY POINTS

- Liver transplantation is the treatment of choice for patients with decompensated cirrhosis, early stage hepatocellular carcinoma, or fulminant hepatic failure.
- Patients with a Child-Turcotte-Pugh score of 7 or higher (Class B or above) or criteria that potentially meet MELD exception criteria (e.g., HCC) should be referred to a transplant hepatologist for liver transplantation evaluation.
- Assessment of the potential liver-transplant recipient should focus on the identification of factors that may preclude transplantation or increase surgical and postoperative risk.
- Hepatic allograft function in the immediate postoperative period may be monitored by glucose production, resolution of metabolic acidosis, and normalization of coagulation parameters and aminotransaminases.
- Evaluation of hepatic allograft dysfunction may include abdominal Doppler ultrasonography, liver biopsy, cholangiography, or angiography.

■ Acute cellular rejection is one of the most common problems after LT and, after histologic confirmation, is treated by judiciously increasing the level of immunosuppression, adjusting the maintenance immunosuppressive regimen, and occasionally administering antilymphocyte antibody therapy.

■ Suspicion of biliary leaks and strictures should prompt cholangiography as well as Doppler ultrasonography to assess for hepatic artery thrombosis. Management includes antibiotics and endoscopic therapy and drainage of associated fluid collections.

■ The burden of recurrent hepatitis C with cirrhosis is increasing and presents unique challenges and dilemmas, particularly in the context of suboptimal treatment options and a limited donor organ pool.

REFERENCES

1. Wiesner R, Edwards E, Freeman R, et al. Model for end-stage liver disease (MELD) and allocation of donor livers. *Gastroenterology* 2003;12:91–96.
2. Available at www.unos.org (MELD/PELD Score). Accessed, February 3, 2005.
3. Freeman RB, Wiesner RH, Edwards E, et al. Results of the first year of the new liver allocation plan. *Liver Transpl* 2004;10:7–15.
4. Mazzaferro V, Regalia E, Doci R, et al. Liver transplantation for the treatment of small hepatocellular carcinomas in patients with cirrhosis. *N Engl J Med* 1996;334:693–699.
5. Roland ME, Stock PG. Review of solid-organ transplantation in HIV-infected patients. *Transplantation* 2003;75:425–429.
6. Trotter JF, Wachs M, Everson GT, et al. Adult-to-adult transplantation of the right hepatic lobe from a living donor. *N Engl J Med* 2002;346:1074–1082.
7. Hoeper MM, Krowka MJ, Strassburg CP. Portopulmonary hypertension and hepatopulmonary syndrome. *Lancet* 2004;363:1461–1468.
8. Fishman JA, Rubin RH. Infection in organ-transplant recipients. *N Engl J Med* 1998;338:1741–1751.
9. Bronster DJ, Emre S, Boccagni P, et al. Central nervous system complications in liver transplant recipients—incidence, timing, and long-term follow-up. *Clin Transplant* 2000;14:1–7.
10. Pham PT, Pham PC, Wilkinson AH. The kidney in liver transplantation. *Clin Liver Dis* 2000;4:567–590.
11. Greif F, Bronsther OL, Van Thiel DH, et al. The incidence, timing, and management of biliary tract complications after orthotopic liver transplantation. *Ann Surg* 1994;219:40–45.
12. Park JS, Kim MH, Lee SK, et al. Efficacy of endoscopic and percutaneous treatments for biliary complications after cadaveric and living donor liver transplantation. *Gastrointest Endosc* 2003;57:78–85.
13. Jones KD, Ferrell LD. Interpretation of biopsy findings in the transplant liver. *Semin Diagn Pathol* 1998;15:306–317.
14. Rubin RH, Schaffner A, Speich R. Introduction to the Immunocompromised Host Society consensus conference on epidemiology, prevention, diagnosis, and management of infections in solid-organ transplant patients. *Clin Infect Dis* 2001;33 (Suppl 1):S1–S4.
15. Randhawa PS, Jaffe R, Demetris AJ, et al. Expression of Epstein-Barr virus-encoded small RNA (by the EBER-1 gene) in liver specimens from transplant recipients with post-transplantation lymphoproliferative disease. *N Engl J Med* 1992;327:1710–1714.
16. Berenguer M, Crippin J, Gish R, et al. A model to predict severe HCV-related disease following liver transplantation. *Hepatology* 2003;38:34–41.

ADDITIONAL READING

Brown RS. A survey of liver transplantation *N Engl J Med* 2003;348:818–825.

Maddrey WC, Schiff ER, Sorrell MF, eds. *Transplantation of the Liver,* 3rd ed. Philadelphia, PA: Lippincott Williams & Wilkins, 2001.

Neuberger J. Developments in liver transplantation. *Gut* 2004;5:759–768.

Acute Pancreatitis

86

Douglas A. Corley

INTRODUCTION

Acute pancreatitis (AP) is a common inpatient diagnosis, accounting for approximately 100,000 hospital admissions per year in the United States. The overall incidence varies among populations, but one study from Olmsted County, Minnesota, estimated 17 episodes per 100,000 people per year. Patients with AP have high levels of resource utilization, with median hospital stays of nine days for mild pancreatitis to 17 days for severe pancreatitis, and a frequent need for ICU-level care and interventional procedures. Patients with complicated pancreatitis may require parenteral nutrition and surgery, with average ICU stays of 4–14 days. Variations in management strategies between centers suggest that a unified, evidence-based approach to care may improve patient outcomes, decrease the length of hospital stays, and lower the utilization of health care resources.

This chapter presents an evidence-based approach to the management of AP. Information from risk-stratification and treatment trials is combined to present an overall pathway for the initial triage and management of patients with pancreatitis, combined with considerations for postdischarge management.

ISSUES AT THE TIME OF ADMISSION

Clinical Presentation and Differential Diagnosis

The diagnosis of AP typically requires a combination of physical symptoms and laboratory abnormalities and can be elusive in some patients. The evaluation of diagnostic tests is hampered by the lack of an adequate gold standard.

The classic symptom of AP is *upper abdominal pain, often radiating to the back* and sometimes accompanied by nausea or vomiting. The pain is typically steady, dull, and of gradual onset over several hours. Although frequently severe, *the abdominal pain can be mild or absent.* Back pain or nausea and vomiting may be the only presenting symptoms. A small number of patients have no pain or vomiting and present with shock or coma. Pancreatitis can be asymptomatic, discovered incidentally on laboratory and radiologic tests obtained for other reasons.

Physical findings of patients with AP are not specific for this disorder. Patients typically have abdominal tenderness that is most pronounced in the epigastrium. Because of the retroperitoneal location of the pancreas, initial signs of peritonitis such as rebound tenderness, shake tenderness, and abdominal wall rigidity are less prominent than in patients with other causes of true peritonitis (Chapter 87). Peritoneal signs can develop with some of the late complications discussed subsequently. Patients with peritoneal signs on initial presentation should be evaluated carefully for a perforated viscus and other causes of peritonitis with the appropriate radiologic studies. Bowel sounds frequently are hypoactive because of an accompanying ileus (Chapter 88), and mild-to-moderate abdominal distension may be present. Purple or brown discolorations around the umbilicus (Cullen's sign) or on the flanks (Grey Turner's sign) are seen infrequently; these findings suggest fat necrosis and subcutaneous bleeding and may develop over the first few days in patients with necrotizing pancreatitis.

Evaluation of vital signs demonstrates nonspecific findings of inflammation and hypovolemia. Many patients have tachycardia, secondary to both pain and volume depletion. Patients may be orthostatic or frankly hypotensive secondary to volume depletion. Although the presence of fever requires evaluation for infectious causes (e.g., cholangitis), fever also can be secondary to underlying pancreatic inflammation in the absence of infection.

The differential diagnosis of AP is broad and includes peptic ulcer disease, perforated viscus, cholecystitis, cholangitis, mesenteric ischemia, abdominal aortic aneurysm, and intestinal obstruction; all these entities can be associated with abdominal pain and elevations of the serum amylase.

Plain radiographs of the abdomen usually differentiate pancreatitis from intestinal obstruction or free perforation of a viscus. Cholecystitis patients typically have pain that is more prominent in the right upper abdomen but can present almost identically to patients with AP. However, abdominal ultrasound in cholecystitis patients usually demonstrates the gallbladder wall thickening, gallstones, pericholecystic fluid, or "ultrasonographic Murphy's sign" characteristic of this disorder (Chapter 84). Although cholecystitis can coexist with pancreatitis, in patients with cholecystitis but without AP, the elevation of amylase level is typically mild and unaccompanied by an elevation of lipase.

Table 86.1 lists the primary causes of pancreatitis. The most common etiologies of AP are chronic alcohol ingestion(40%–60%) and gallstone pancreatitis (30%–50%). An additional 10%–20% of patients have idiopathic pancreatitis; the majority of these patients appear to have microlithiasis (biliary crystals or "sludge") or a motility abnormality of the ampulla, known as sphincter of Oddi dysfunction.

TABLE 86.1
MAJOR CAUSES OF PANCREATITIS[a]

Presumed mechanical obstruction
  Cholelithiasis/choledocholithiasis[b]
  Pancreatic tumors
  Sphincter of Oddi dysfunction
  Pancreas divisum
Direct injury
  Endoscopic retrograde cholangiopancreatography (ERCP)
  Trauma
Drugs/toxins[c]
  Alcohol[b]
  6-Mercaptopurine/azathioprine
  L-asparaginase
  Hydrochlorothiazide
  Sulfonamides
  Estrogens
  Pentamidine
  Furosemide
  Nonsteroidal anti-inflammatory drugs
  Tetracycline
  5-aminosalicylic acid
  Angiotensin-converting enzyme inhibitors
  Dideoxyinosine (ddI)
Metabolic/intrinsic
  Idiopathic[b]
  Hypertriglyceridemia
  Hypercalcemia
  Pregnancy
  Familial pancreatitis
  Hypoperfusion (shock, embolus, vasculitis)
Infections
  Viral (Coxsackievirus, mumps, cytomegalovirus)
  Bacterial (*Campylobacter*, *Mycoplasma pneumoniae*)
  Parasites (*Cryptosporidium*, *Ascaris*, *Clonorchis*)

[a] Definite and probable associations.
[b] Major cause (>5% of cases).
[c] Partial list of reported drugs, most are from case reports.

AP that develops during hospitalization for another condition has presenting symptoms, differential diagnosis, and causes similar to "outpatient pancreatitis". Although not extensively studied, inpatient pancreatitis is less often related to alcohol and more commonly related to drugs, the perioperative state, ischemia from hypoperfusion or embolism, or microlithiasis. The evaluation and management of inpatient and outpatient pancreatitis are similar and thus are discussed together.

Role of Diagnostic Tests

Laboratory Tests

The effective use of many common laboratory tests in AP has not been studied, but laboratory evaluation should include those tests found useful for AP diagnosis, risk stratification, and evaluation of complications and causes.

Admission tests should include amylase and lipase levels for diagnosis; total bilirubin, alkaline phosphatase, alanine aminotransferase (ALT), and aspartate aminotransferase (AST) levels for evaluation of cholangitis and biliary obstruction; and calcium, albumin, complete blood cell count, lactate dehydrogenase, and an electrolyte panel including blood-urea nitrogen and creatinine measurements for evaluation of volume status and risk stratification. Direct measurement of arterial PO_2 and base deficit is an integral part of initial risk stratification. Until validated data on the utility of peripheral saturations are available, an arterial blood gas should be obtained initially in patients demonstrating a room-air oxygen saturation of less than 93%. For patients without a known cause of the pancreatitis, serum triglycerides should be obtained to evaluate for hypertriglyceridemia as a cause. Patients with fever should receive blood cultures to search for the bacteremia that commonly accompanies cholangitis.

The *serum amylase* is the most frequently used test for diagnosing AP; its advantages include simplicity, availability, and good performance characteristics, with an overall sensitivity of 80%–90% and a specificity of approximately 70%. The magnitude of amylase elevation correlates poorly with the severity of pancreatitis and its subsequent clinical course. *Fatal episodes of pancreatitis have been reported without elevations of the amylase level.* The serum amylase rises within 2–12 hours of symptom onset and typically remains elevated for 3–5 days; it returns to normal more rapidly than the serum lipase. Normal amylase levels with elevated lipase levels and a clinical picture consistent with pancreatitis have been reported with delayed presentations, with alcoholic pancreatitis, and with acute exacerbations of chronic pancreatitis. Finally, lipemic serum can falsely depress laboratory determination of both amylase and lipase. Falsely elevated levels of serum amylase can be seen with renal failure, intestinal obstruction or perforation, mesenteric ischemia, pancreatic ascites, salivary gland abnormalities, and other conditions. *Macroamylasemia,* an uncommon condition consisting of poorly cleared aggregated amylase molecules, can cause a persistently elevated amylase level with a normal lipase level. These other sources of hyperamylasemia can usually be differentiated from pancreatitis by evaluating the serum lipase, by measuring the urinary levels of amylase (which are normal in renal failure or macroamylasemia despite high serum amylase levels), or by fractionating the amylase for the pancreatic subtype.

The *serum lipase* is about as sensitive as and is more specific (90%) than the serum amylase for diagnosing AP. It is not produced by the salivary glands; thus, false-positives are less frequent. *Combining the serum amylase and lipase is the most sensitive and specific strategy for diagnosing AP* (1). Elevation of either enzyme provides a sensitivity of approximately 95%, with a specificity of 90% provided by elevations of both enzymes. Urine tests, such as urinary trypsinogen-2, offer advantages in speed but not in accuracy of diagnosis compared with serum assays.

Laboratory evaluation facilitates the diagnosis of gallstone pancreatitis and cholangitis. A two-fold to three-fold elevation of any liver test (ALT, AST, alkaline phosphatase, or total bilirubin) is highly associated with gallstone pancreatitis (2). Overall, the most predictive tests are the ALT and AST. An ALT of more than 150 IU/L has a positive predictive value of 95% and a specificity of 96% but a sensitivity of only 48%; the AST performs similarly. Elevations of the alkaline phosphatase (>300 IU/L) and bilirubin (>2.9 mg/dL) have specificities greater than 90% but are very insensitive (<40%). These tests are thus relatively specific for gallstone pancreatitis if elevated; however, normal results do not exclude gallstones as the cause. Cholangitis is suggested by elevated liver tests accompanied by fever and leukocytosis.

Imaging Studies

Imaging tests in pancreatitis include plain radiographs, ultrasound, and computed tomography (CT). The appropriate use and cost effectiveness of these tests have not been well evaluated. Data support early use of some radiographic studies for diagnosis, triage, and guidance of therapy. Plain films of the abdomen are primarily helpful in diagnosing other causes of abdominal pain (see earlier in this chapter); a dilated "sentinel loop" of small bowel over the inflamed pancreas is a nonspecific finding of pancreatitis. A chest radiograph should be obtained in patients with impaired oxygen saturation to evaluate for evidence of acute respiratory distress syndrome (ARDS).

Abdominal ultrasound examination should be obtained within the first 24–48 hours in all patients with a first attack of pancreatitis and in any patient in whom there is no clear explanation for pancreatitis. Ultrasound effectively evaluates for the presence of cholelithiasis, cholecystitis, and common bile duct dilation in patients with potential gallstone pancreatitis. Ultrasound's shortcomings include its limited ability to evaluate pancreatic anatomy (due to interference from overlying bowel gas) and its poor sensitivity (<50%) for detecting common bile duct stones; the absence of ductal stones on ultrasound or CT does not exclude the presence of choledocholithiasis. Although it is often employed in patients with AP, validated risk-stratification protocols using ultrasonographic findings exist.

The *abdominal CT scan* provides clear visualization of the pancreas and its surrounding structures, and has implications for risk stratification (Table 86.2) (3). It also may facilitate diagnosis of AP in the small subset of patients with falsely normal amylase and lipase levels. Specific protocols ("pancreatic protocol") using rapid injection of intravenous contrast increase the accuracy of CT for detecting

TABLE 86.2

COMPUTED TOMOGRAPHY (CT) GRADING OF ACUTE PANCREATITIS

Category	CT findings	CT score	Necrosis present	Necrosis score
A	Normal	0	No	0
B	Focal or diffuse enlargement; irregular contour; inhomogeneous attenuation	1	<30% of pancreas	3
C	Findings of B plus peripancreatic haziness, streaky densities	2	50% of pancreas	4
D	Finding of B/C plus one ill-defined prepancreatic fluid collection	3	>50% of pancreas	6
E	Findings of B/C plus two or more ill-defined fluid collections	4		

Total score[a]	Morbidity, %	Mortality, %
0–3	8	3
4–6	35	6
7–10	92	17

[a] Total score is the sum of the CT score and the Necrosis score.
Adapted from Balthazar EJ, Robinson DL, Megibow AJ, Ranson JH. Acute pancreatitis: value of CT in establishing prognosis. *Radiology* 1990;174:331–336.

pancreatic necrosis. In one study, patients without pancreatic necrosis on any CT scans throughout their hospitalizations had no deaths and only a 6% complication rate; however, 22% of patients without necrosis on the initial CT scan subsequently developed complications. Therefore, a benign CT scan on admission does not preclude a complicated clinical course. In addition, the combination of early CT scans and clinical risk scores (see the following section) does not markedly improve the ability to predict which patients will require ICU admission beyond the clinical risk scores alone (4). *Currently, the routine use of early CT scans in all patients with AP is unnecessary.* If effective agents for altering the natural history of pancreatitis become available, early CT scans may be helpful to stratify patients for risk and guide appropriate therapy. In addition, patients with severe pancreatitis by clinical criteria may benefit from an early CT scan if the detection of extensive necrosis would prompt the initiation of prophylactic antibiotics. Magnetic resonance imaging may be useful in patients who cannot have CT scans performed (due to contrast allergy or renal insufficiency); its utility in evaluating for choledocholithiasis is unproved in this patient population.

Prognostic Factors

Several risk factor scoring systems can predict the risk of severe pancreatitis with moderate accuracy. However, these systems typically do not reach their peak prognostic value until 48 hours after admission (5). The development of new disease-modifying agents that are effective if given early in the clinical course will increase the need for prompt prognostication. The most commonly used scoring systems are the Ranson criteria, the Glasgow criteria, and APACHE scores (5). Table 86.3 outlines the Ranson and Glasgow criteria. A modification of the Ranson criteria to improve its performance for gallstone pancreatitis has been proposed but has not been extensively evaluated. The presence of more than three Ranson criteria at any time within the first 48 hours has the highest sensitivity (86%), specificity (98%), and positive predictive value (86%) for a severe clinical course in patients with alcohol-induced pancreatitis. The peak APACHE-II score and Glasgow criteria are more accurate for gallstone pancreatitis. APACHE-II scores on admission do not perform as well as the other multiple-factor criteria and are more cumbersome to calculate.

As a single scale, *the Glasgow criteria have the best overall performance characteristics for correctly predicting the development of complicated pancreatitis* (defined as the presence of infection, organ failure, pancreatic necrosis, or pseudocyst or the development of a major complication such as myocardial infarction or pulmonary embolism). The scoring systems predict complicated pancreatitis more accurately than clinical acumen alone, particularly in patients with gallstone pancreatitis. Clinicians correctly predict a severe course in approximately 19% of patients with gallstone pancreatitis and in 55% of patients with alcohol-induced pancreatitis. This compares with correct predictions of ap-

TABLE 86.3

CLINICAL RISK-STRATIFICATION CRITERIA

Modified Glasgow Criteria[a]
  Room-air arterial PO_2 <60 mm Hg
  Serum albumin <3.2 g/dL
  Serum calcium <8 mg/dL
  White blood cell count >15,000/μL
  Aspartate or alanine aminotransferase >200 IU/L
  Lactate dehydrogenase >600 U/L
  Serum glucose[b] >180 mg/dL
  Blood urea nitrogen >45 mg/dL
Ranson Criteria
  On admission
    Age >55 y
    White blood cell count >16,000/μL
    Serum glucose >200 mg/dL
    Lactate dehydrogenase >350 IU/L
    Aspartate aminotransferase >250 IU/L
  During the first 48 hrs
    Fall in hematocrit of >10 points
    Serum calcium <8 mg/dL
    Base deficit >4 mEq/L
    Increase in blood urea nitrogen >5 mg/dL
    Fluid sequestration >6 L
    Arterial PO_2 <60 mm Hg

---

[a] Predominantly useful in gallstone pancreatitis.
[b] Predominantly useful in alcoholic pancreatitis.
From Blamey SL, Imrie CW, O'Neill J, Gilmour WH, Carter DC. Prognostic factors in acute pancreatitis. *Gut* 1984;25:1340–1346; and Wilson C, Heath DI, Imrie CW. Prediction of outcome in acute pancreatitis: a comparative study of APACHE II, clinical assessment and multiple factor scoring systems. *Br J Surg* 1990;77:1260–1264; and Ranson JH, Rifkind KM, Roses DF, Fink SD, Eng K, Spencer FC. Prognostic signs and the role of operative management in acute pancreatitis. *Surg Gynecol Obstet* 1974;139:69–81; and Ranson JH. The timing of biliary surgery in acute pancreatitis. *Ann Surg* 1979;189:654–663.

proximately 65% and 70%, respectively, for the presence of at least three factors from the Glasgow criteria (6). The presence of at least three Glasgow criteria corresponds to a mortality rate of 25%, compared with 4% in patients with fewer than three criteria (6). These scoring systems thus can guide initial triage decisions, but modifications in the level of care frequently are necessary as the patient's clinical course evolves. Numerous laboratory tests (such as urinary trypsinogen activation peptide and C-reactive protein) have been evaluated, but none markedly enhances early prognostication beyond standard risk scores.

Indications for Intensive Care Unit Admission

Indications for admission to the ICU include hypoxemia and persistent hypotension or oliguria despite aggressive initial volume resuscitation. In addition, the presence of three or more Ranson or Glasgow criteria within the first 48 hours, or a peak APACHE-II score of greater than 9 in the first 72 hours, are highly associated with complicated pancreatitis and death. Although validated guidelines for AP do not exist, data suggest that patients with these features have a more severe clinical course and higher rates of ICU admission. In these patients, intensive or step-down care can facilitate vital-sign monitoring and access to equipment for rapid fluid resuscitation, intubation, and dialysis.

Initial Management

The principal goals of therapy in AP are controlling pain, treating reversible causes, preventing organ failure, and minimizing peripancreatic complications such as infection and complicated fluid collections. Figure 86.1 provides a suggested clinical pathway.

Supportive care with intravenous fluids, electrolyte replacement, and blood glucose monitoring with insulin (if needed) are standard clinical practices. Because pancreatic stimulation may aggravate pancreatitis symptoms, patients initially should not receive oral nutrition. Nasogastric suction may be employed for symptomatic relief in patients with vomiting or ileus; its routine use does not hasten recovery from AP.

Patients with inadequate volume resuscitation are at risk for hypovolemic shock, and experimental data support the role of adequate volume replacement as a primary initial intervention for AP. Volume replacement should be titrated to the patient's blood pressure, pulse rate, and urine output. Patients with persistent hypotension, tachycardia, and low urine outputs likely require vigorous ongoing fluid resuscitation; *patients with severe pancreatitis may require 8–12 liters of fluid over the first 24 hours.* The optimal fluid type for resuscitating AP patients is unknown, and the advantages and disadvantages of different types (e.g., crystalloids vs. colloids) are discussed in Chapter 25.

Pain control typically includes opiate analgesics. Although morphine has a theoretical advantage over meperidine in that it causes less spasm of the sphincter of Oddi, there is no evidence that this translates into a clinical advantage. Patient-controlled analgesia is associated with improved pain control and lower resource utilization.

Finally, reversible causes should be treated. Patients without a clear explanation for their pancreatitis should discontinue nonessential suspect medications and receive an evaluation for secondary causes such as gallstone pancreatitis (see the Diagnostic Tests section).

Despite extensive investigation, few therapies currently improve the outcome or symptoms of AP (Table 86.4). Although the trypsin inhibitor gabexate or somatostatin may decrease the incidence and severity of pancreatitis induced by endoscopic retrograde cholangiopancreatography (ERCP) (7), studies conflict, and neither agent is effective for treating AP. The platelet activation factor antagonist lexipafant decreased morbidity and mortality rates in initial trials, but subsequent investigations have not confirmed this observation (8). If proven to be effective, such agents may offer the potential for effective early pharmacologic intervention in AP.

Indications for Early Consultation

Management of pancreatitis varies markedly among institutions. Admission services include internal medicine, gastroenterology, and general surgery dependent upon institutional practices and expertise. No studies exist evaluating differences in outcome based on admitting service. For patients admitted to surgery or medicine services, early gastroenterology consultation for possible ERCP should be considered in patients with evidence of cholangitis, biliary pancreatitis, traumatic pancreatitis, evidence of pancreatic duct disruption, or severe, unremitting idiopathic pancreatitis. For patients admitted to medical services, early surgical consultation should be considered in patients with pancreatic necrosis, particularly if potential infection is indicated (i.e., fever, elevated white blood cell count). The management of complicated pancreatitis frequently requires a team approach with a medical intensivist, general surgeon, gastroenterologist, and interventional radiologist.

ISSUES DURING THE COURSE OF HOSPITALIZATION

Laboratory Monitoring

The need for ongoing laboratory monitoring is dictated by the severity of the pancreatitis. Daily measurements of serum amylase or lipase have no demonstrated prognostic value. Follow-up measurements may be helpful in confirming normalization of the amylase; additional measurements on day 2 or 3 and on day 5 or 6 provide sufficient information in an uncomplicated patient. Persistent elevations are associated with ongoing pancreatitis, pancreatic ascites, and the development of pseudocysts. Because of the potential for large fluid and electrolyte shifts, initial daily monitoring of electrolytes is advisable. Additional monitoring for signs of organ failure includes determination of blood-urea nitrogen, creatinine, bicarbonate, and oxygen saturation levels. Calcium monitoring is an integral part of some risk-stratification criteria. AP may cause hyperglycemia; thus, monitoring of serum glucose, accompanied by appropriate insulin administration, is required.

Nutrition

The initial withholding of enteral nutrition in AP patients is standard practice. The delivery of fats and proteins to the duodenum results in stimulation of pancreatic secretion, which may be harmful in the acute setting. In the absence of clinical trial data, this practice is supported by observations that patients with early pancreatitis may have increases of pain with eating, and there is no known detriment caused by brief periods of minimal nutrition.

Patients with peripancreatic fluid collections, pancreatic infections, and other complications of pancreatitis

	Day 1: First 4 hours of stay	Day 1: Additional Tasks	Day 2	Day 3	Day 4	Day 5-10: Uncomplicated course	Complicated Pancreatitis
Tests	Amylase, lipase, Chem-7, CBC, calcium, albumin, LDH, triglycerides, ALT, AST, total bilirubin. Blood cultures if fever. ABG and CXR if room air saturation < 93%. Determine clinical risk stratification, other appropriate tests to establish diagnosis (e.g. abdominal film, CT)	Abdominal ultrasound for index presentation or unexplained pancreatitis Notify PMD. Consider CT for severe pancreatitis or if patient unstable	Chem-7, CBC, calcium, albumin; recheck ALT, AST, bili if initially abnormal, ABG if severe pancreatitis. Check blood cultures if obtained. Confirm official ultrasound interpretation	Amylase or lipase, Chem-7, CBC, calcium, albumin Check final culture results	Recheck unstable laboratory values (e.g., electrolytes)	Recheck unstable laboratory values (e.g., electrolytes)	If not improving after 4–5 days, consider abdominal CT, amylase or lipase, Chem-7, CBC, calcium, LFTs ?Specialty consult
Medications and Theraputics	Intravenous fluid Opiate analgesics. IV antibiotics if possible cholangitis. Discontinue potentially offending medications. Glucose monitoring with insulin as needed	Intravenous fluid Opiate analgesics. Glucose monitoring with insulin as needed *Consider:* ERCP for complicated gallstone pancreatitis	Intravenous fluid Opiate analgesics *Consider:* ERCP for complicated gallstone pancreatitis	Intravenous fluid as needed Taper analgesics as tolerated	Intravenous fluid as needed Taper analgesics as tolerated	Intravenous fluid as needed Taper analgesics as tolerated, consider change to p.o. pain medications for mild residual pain in stable patients	*Consider:* Prophylactic antibiotics if CT shows severe necrosis
Nursing Assessment	Vitals/Temp Room Air O_2 sat I&O's Admission weight	Vitals/Temp Room Air O_2 sat I&O's	Vitals/Temp Room Air O_2 sat I&O's	Vitals/Temp Room Air O_2 sat I&O's Weight	Vitals/Temp	Vitals/Temp	Vitals/Temp Continue I&O's and daily weights if not improving to monitor volume
Activity	As tolerated	As tolerated	As tolerated	As tolerated	As tolerated	As tolerated	
Nutrition	NPO except simple fluids as tolerated	NPO except simple fluids as tolerated	NPO except simple fluids as tolerated	Advance diet if AP resolving	Advance diet if AP resolving	Advance diet if AP resolving	Consider supplemental nutrition
Discharge Planning		Discuss expected LOS with SW & pt/family (avg. 8–10 days for mild, 2–3 weeks for severe AP); Review home situation, alcohol use	MD/RN/SW communication re: pt status, plan for discharge care, need for alcohol rehabilitation	MD/RN/SW communication re: pt status, plan for discharge care	MD/RN/SW communication re: pt status, plan for discharge care	Discharge needs met: meds, VNA, transportation, risk reduction (e.g. alcohol rehab, change in meds, etc.), F/U appt made, Pt instruction sheet	
Patient Education		Orient to unit		Discharge teaching (meds)	Discharge teaching (meds)	Review with pt & family: Meds, D/C plan, F/U appt, return signs & sx	

Figure 86.1 Critical pathway: acute pancreatitis. ABG, arterial blood gas; ALT, alanine aminotransferase; AP, acute pancreatitis; AST, aspartate aminotransferase; CBC, complete blood count; CT, computed tomography; CXR, chest radiograph; D/C, discharge; ERCP, endoscopic retrograde cholangiopancreatography; F/U, follow-up; I&O's, intake and outputs; IV, intravenous; LDH, lactate dehydrogenase; LFTs, liver function tests; NPO, nothing by mouth; O_2 sat, oxygen saturation; PMD, primary care physician.

TABLE 86.4

MEDICAL THERAPIES IN ACUTE PANCREATITIS

Effective therapies[a]
  ERCP for patients with pancreatitis and cholangitis
  Analgesics for pain relief
  Antibiotics in patients with severe pancreatitis and risk factors
    for/clinical signs of cholangitis/pancreatic necrosis
Probably effective therapies[b]
  Correction of electrolyte abnormalities
  Volume replacement
  Initially holding oral nutrition
  Debridement or drainage of infected necrosis
  Lexipafant administration within 48 h of initial symptoms
  Gabexate or somatostatin for prophylaxis of ERCP-induced
    pancreatitis
  Nasogastric suction for symptoms related to ileus
Probably ineffective therapies[c]
  Pharmacologic inhibition of pancreatic secretion (e.g., octreotide)
  Trypsin inhibition after initiation of pancreatitis
  Peritoneal lavage
  Nasogastric suction

---

[a] Demonstrated in randomized clinical trials without significant
conflicting data.
[b] Large clinical experience or generally supported by experimental
studies.
[c] No benefit in randomized trials.
ERCP, endoscopic retrograde cholangiopancreatography.

frequently require prolonged hospitalization; the optimal route of nutrition in these patients has changed in recent years. Traditionally, patients with complications received parenteral nutrition. Most late complications of AP, however, are secondary to peripancreatic damage and infection rather than from ongoing active pancreatitis. Recent small randomized trials of AP patients found that patients receiving enteral nutrition had fewer total complications, fewer infections, and lower overall hospital costs than patients receiving parenteral nutrition (9). These findings are consistent with trials of enteral versus parenteral nutrition for other gastrointestinal disorders (Chapter 15). Thus, *patients who lack contraindications to enteral feeding and who are unable to initiate oral nutrition after 5–7 days should receive enteral nutrition via nasoenteric tube rather than parenteral nutrition.* If pancreatitis recurs after starting enteral nutrition, patients are intolerant of enteral feeding, or other contraindications to enteral feeding exist, parenteral nutrition should be considered.

Antibiotics

Prophylactic antibiotic use in patients with severe pancreatitis is beneficial in reducing infectious complications but has not been clearly demonstrated to improve the overall survival rate. Septic complications are the most frequent late cause of death in AP. Thus, the use of prophylactic antibiotics in pancreatitis patients has been the subject of several randomized controlled trials. Early trials suggested no benefit from prophylactic antibiotics. More recent trials using antibiotics with better pancreatic penetration (e.g., quinolones and imipenem) demonstrated significantly fewer infectious complications in treated patients than in placebo-treated control subjects (10), but concerns about the development of antibiotic resistance and fungal superinfections have tempered widespread use of prophylactic antibiotics in patients with AP.

The best current evidence supports prophylactic antibiotic use in patients with evidence of cholangitis or severe necrotizing pancreatitis. Patients with clinical evidence of severe pancreatitis should receive an early CT scan to look for pancreatic necrosis; patients without necrosis or fluid collections appear unlikely to benefit from prophylactic antibiotics. In other patients who develop clinical signs of infection, early antibiotic use should be considered. Patients may benefit from needle aspiration of necrotic tissue to guide antibiotic therapy (see the section on pancreatic necrosis). Further research (evaluating both mortality and nonlethal endpoints) will be needed to determine precisely which patients benefit from antibiotics.

Endoscopic Retrograde Cholangiopancreatography

ERCP with sphincterotomy improves outcomes in a subgroup of AP patients with gallstone pancreatitis. This technique uses endoscopic guidance to open the sphincter of Oddi using an electrocautery wire, with removal of common bile duct stones and "biliary sludge." The primary benefit occurred in patients with severe pancreatitis and evidence of cholangitis or biliary obstruction (11,12). The only study demonstrating no morbidity-rate benefit excluded patients who were febrile or who had a total bilirubin level greater than 5 mg/dL. In studies of endoscopic sphincterotomy performed for any reason, complications (bleeding, perforation, pancreatitis, and death) occurred in approximately 10% of all patients and were usually managed conservatively. However, the overall complication rate appears lower in patients with AP, with a 2.3% rate noted in a recent trial. Because of the risk of complications and the apparent lack of efficacy in patients with mild pancreatitis, *endoscopic sphincterotomy should be reserved for patients with presumed gallstone pancreatitis and evidence of cholangitis, persistent biliary obstruction, or unremitting pancreatitis.* Patients without evidence of cholangitis and those with elevated liver tests that rapidly normalize typically do not require emergent sphincterotomy. Patients with severe idiopathic pancreatitis also may benefit given the substantial proportion of these patients having microlithiasis (see later in this chapter). Magnetic resonance cholangiopancreatography recently has been evaluated for diagnosing abnormalities of the pancreas and biliary tree. Although it is noninvasive, it is also expensive and does not offer a therapeutic potential. Its role in acutely diagnosing common bile-duct stones in this patient population is unclear.

Complications of Pancreatitis

Early Complications

Complications in the first 48 hours usually are related to hypovolemia, shock, intra-abdominal hemorrhage, ARDS, renal failure, and electrolyte abnormalities. Pancreatitis can result in massive volume shifts, with subsequent hypovolemic shock. ARDS and other severe pulmonary complications occur in approximately 15% of patients.

The management of early complications is primarily supportive. Patients require aggressive early hydration, as discussed for initial management. Serum electrolytes should be assayed at least daily for the first few days, with appropriate replacement. Hypocalcemia frequently develops; it is usually asymptomatic. Renal failure may require dialysis, and respiratory failure may require intubation. Patients with persistent hypotension after initial volume resuscitation, oliguria, or ARDS may benefit from hemodynamic monitoring to guide volume replacement.

Late Complications

Complications occurring after 5–7 days are primarily infectious. The principal one is *infected necrosis,* occurring in approximately 5% of patients. Although the majority of infections occur within the first two weeks, delayed presentations are not uncommon. In one series, almost 50% of infections occurred more than 2 weeks after presentation. Pancreatic infection is associated with a high mortality rate, accounting for up to half of all deaths in necrotizing pancreatitis. If pancreatic infection is suspected because of fever or an elevated white blood cell count, radiologically guided percutaneous aspiration should be performed. This method permits reasonable discrimination between infected and sterile necrosis and may allow isolation of a pathogen for culture and antibiotic sensitivities. Indications for CT scans in the setting of AP include failure to respond to conservative therapy after the first 5–7 days, persistent pain or elevations of serum amylase, fever beyond the first 5–7 days, or progressive abdominal distension. Under these conditions, the presence of necrosis, large peripancreatic fluid collections, or significant ascites suggestive of pancreatic duct disruption with resultant pancreatic ascites alters clinical management.

The management of pancreatic infection is primarily surgical. The traditional approach has been open debridement of the necrotic tissue. Because the devitalized tissue is typically neither liquefied nor vascularized, it would seem that nonsurgical drainage would be unlikely to successfully evacuate the infected tissue, and antibiotics would have limited penetrance. Nevertheless, percutaneous drainage, endoscopic drainage, and antibiotics alone all have been used successfully in selected patients with infected necrosis (there are no trials comparing these methods). For example, a pancreatic abscess consisting largely of infected fluid rather than pancreatic tissue may be treated adequately with antibiotics and percutaneous drainage. It frequently is difficult, however, to distinguish between infected fluid and infected necrosis by CT. *The weight of the evidence suggests that patients with extensive areas of infected necrosis should be treated surgically.* Consultation with a general surgeon experienced in pancreatic surgery and an interventional radiologist trained in percutaneous drainage is advisable in patients with pancreatic infection to discriminate between available therapies. Studies indicate that the treatment of *limited sterile necrosis* with surgery, peritoneal lavage, or percutaneous evacuation is ineffective or even harmful.

Pancreatic Duct Disruption

A less common complication is pancreatic duct disruption. Pancreatic disruption can occur at any time. If localized, this disruption can lead to an expanding pseudocyst; if the leak is not contained, disrupted ducts may cause pancreatic ascites. Fluid in pancreatic ascites is high in amylase (approximately fivefold more than serum amylase), usually has a white blood cell count of more than 500 per cubic millimeter, and can lead to pancreatic hydrothorax. Treatments attempted for pancreatic duct disruption include octreotide to decrease pancreatic secretion, stenting of the pancreatic duct via ERCP to bypass the sphincter, percutaneous catheter drainage of pseudocysts, and surgical repair. No comparative trials exist, but these strategies appear equally efficacious (60%–90% in small series). The majority of duct disruptions resolve slowly with conservative therapy over 4–6 weeks. Initially, octreotide should be used as primary therapy or in conjunction with endoscopic or percutaneous drainage. Available data suggest a dose of at least 150 mg subcutaneously every eight hours. Critically ill inpatients may receive an intravenous infusion of 25–50 mg per hour. Patients who fail these therapies should be evaluated for surgical correction of the disrupted duct.

The majority of peripancreatic fluid collections resolve by six weeks after presentation; the remainder may develop into organized collections known as *pseudocysts* that are surrounded by adjacent organs and inflammatory material. Asymptomatic pseudocysts can be observed safely (13); infected, markedly symptomatic, or enlarging pseudocysts require drainage. Even large pseudocysts (>6 cm) can be followed, with interventions performed only for complications.

The optimal means of pseudocyst drainage is unknown and likely varies with the location of the fluid collection and whether it communicates with the pancreatic duct. Surgical techniques typically create a communication between the pseudocyst and adjacent bowel. Radiologic methods utilize continuous or intermittent drainage with percutaneous catheters. Endoscopic techniques either create a communication with adjacent stomach or duodenum or place a stent across the ampulla through the pancreatic duct and into the pseudocyst. All these methods appear to have similar efficacy, and the optimal technique in a given patient should be decided with the appropriate consultants, considering the pseudocyst's anatomic location and local expertise.

DISCHARGE ISSUES

Patients with mild pancreatitis typically have an uncomplicated course characterized by a rapid improvement in symptoms over 3–5 days and are able to restart oral intake by days 3–6. The amylase rapidly returns to normal, and the average hospital stay is 8–10 days. In contrast, protracted pain, fever, abdominal distension, or pain upon refeeding suggest a complicated course. Criteria for discharge include the ability to take adequate oral nutrition without symptoms or signs of recurrent pancreatitis, and appropriate recognition and treatment of any complications. Patients with large asymptomatic pseudocysts, for example, do not require ongoing hospitalization; however, they do require close outpatient monitoring for the development of pain or fever. In addition, a follow-up CT scan or ultrasound should be obtained 1–3 weeks after discharge to confirm that the pseudocyst is not enlarging. Permanent pancreatic endocrine or exocrine insufficiency is uncommon in the absence of chronic pancreatitis. Patients requiring insulin during the hospitalization should be instructed in insulin administration and glucose monitoring; their insulin requirement frequently decreases or is eliminated as the pancreas recovers.

Important discharge issues include evaluation of the cause of pancreatitis and prevention of future episodes. Follow-up management should include cessation of alcohol use in patients with alcoholic pancreatitis, cholecystectomy in patients with gallstone pancreatitis, and further evaluation of patients with idiopathic pancreatitis.

Patients with gallstone pancreatitis should have a cholecystectomy as soon as the pancreatitis and its immediate complications resolve. More than 30% of patients with gallstone pancreatitis and uncorrected cholelithiasis have a recurrent episode, many within the next several months. Significant delays in surgery do not appear to improve surgical outcomes for patients with *mild-to-moderate pancreatitis;* thus, cholecystectomy should be performed prior to or soon after discharge from the index hospitalization in these patients. Patients with *severe pancreatitis* are at a higher risk of surgical complications; in this population, the risk of recurrent pancreatitis may be less than the risk of early surgery performed prior to the improvement of pancreatic necrosis and fluid collections. Selected patients with primarily biliary tract disease, particularly those at high risk for surgery, may require only an endoscopic biliary sphincterotomy.

Approximately one-third of patients with AP have "idiopathic pancreatitis," without any potential causes found on history or laboratory examination. The likelihood of recurrent episodes of pancreatitis in these patients is controversial, and the appropriate evaluation is unknown. However, numerous small series suggest that microlithiasis ("biliary sludge") frequently is responsible (14). Microlithiasis is detected by aspirating bile percutaneously or during ERCP, or by ultrasonographic detection of sludge in an acute or convalescent patient. Nearly three out of four patients with idiopathic pancreatitis (without a prior cholecystectomy) will be found at ERCP to have either microlithiasis or common bile duct stones. Microlithiasis patients treated with cholecystectomy or biliary sphincterotomy have a lower recurrence rate of pancreatitis (10%) than patients treated conservatively (73%), in nonrandomized series. Patients with evidence of biliary sludge by ultrasonography or ERCP, therefore, should undergo cholecystectomy or biliary sphincterotomy.

An uncommon but potentially serious cause of idiopathic pancreatitis is a pancreatic or periampullary neoplasm. Although survival from most pancreatic neoplasms is poor, detection significantly alters management decisions. If not obtained during the attack of pancreatitis, patients with idiopathic pancreatitis should have an abdominal CT scan to rule out a pancreatic mass once the index episode of pancreatitis resolves.

If these investigations are unrevealing, the patient may be observed. Randomized studies suggest that anatomic or functional biliary obstruction is a frequent cause of idiopathic pancreatitis. Thus, if pancreatitis recurs, ERCP should be performed to evaluate the pancreatic anatomy. Based on its findings, sphincterotomy, aspiration of bile for crystal analysis, and/or biliary manometry should be considered.

COST CONSIDERATIONS AND RESOURCE USE

The vast majority of patients with AP require management and observation in the inpatient setting. The average hospital costs associated with complicated pancreatitis are estimated at more than 10 times those of mild pancreatitis. The serious complication rate is approximately 25%, with a total mortality rate of 2%–10%. The most important issue from the perspective of reducing the costs for AP patients is managing the use of the ICU and invasive procedures. The appropriate triage of patients to the ICU, identification of patients likely to have a complicated course, and initiation of appropriate individualized therapies are the principal determinants of hospital stay. The impact of a directed guideline on total cost is unknown. Avoiding daily blood tests once patients have stabilized, minimizing CT scans in patients with mild pancreatitis, and using enteral (rather than parenteral) nutrition in appropriate patients likely would reduce inpatient costs without adversely affecting patient outcomes.

KEY POINTS

- All patients with AP should be evaluated for possible admission.
- A combination of amylase and lipase levels is most sensitive and specific for diagnosis.
- Persistent hypotension or oliguria despite resuscitation, or the presence of several clinical risk-stratification criteria (Ranson or Glasgow score >3 or an APACHE-II score >9) identifies a subset of patients at greater need for ICU admission and at higher risk of subsequent complications.
- Patients with adverse prognostic indicators should be stabilized rapidly in an ICU and monitored for complications (e.g., renal failure, ARDS, and hypotension).
- Evaluation for the etiology of an index episode of pancreatitis includes a careful history for alcohol, medication, and toxin exposure; evaluation of serum aminotransferases and an abdominal ultrasound for gallstone pancreatitis; acute and convalescent evaluation for hyperlipidemia and hypercalcemia; and an abdominal CT to evaluate for a pancreatic neoplasm.
- ERCP with sphincterotomy improves outcomes in patients with gallstone pancreatitis and evidence of cholangitis or ongoing biliary obstruction.
- Use of prophylactic antibiotics in patients with severe pancreatitis may improve outcomes.
- For most patients requiring supplemental nutrition, enteral nutrition improves outcomes and decreases costs compared with parenteral nutrition.
- Identifiable causes of pancreatitis require in-hospital or posthospital interventions to decrease the risk of recurrent pancreatitis.
- Patients with more than one episode of unexplained pancreatitis should undergo ERCP for evaluation (and potential treatment) of biliary microlithiasis, functional disorders of the ampulla, and structural abnormalities of the pancreatic duct.

REFERENCES

1. Agarwal N, Pitchumoni CS, Sivaprasad AV. Evaluating tests for acute pancreatitis. *Am J Gastroenterol* 1990;85:356–366.
2. Tenner S, Dubner H, Steinberg W. Predicting gallstone pancreatitis with laboratory parameters: a meta-analysis. *Am J Gastroenterol* 1994;89:1863–1866.
3. Balthazar EJ, Robinson DL, Megibow AJ, Ranson JH. Acute pancreatitis: value of CT in establishing prognosis. *Radiology* 1990;174:331–336.
4. De Sanctis JT, Lee MJ, Gazelle GS, et al. Prognostic indicators in acute pancreatitis: CT vs APACHE II. *Clin Radiol* 1997;52:842–848.
5. Wilson C, Heath DI, Imrie CW. Prediction of outcome in acute pancreatitis: a comparative study of APACHE II, clinical assessment and multiple factor scoring systems. *Br J Surg* 1990;77:1260–1264.
6. Corfield AP, Cooper MJ, Williamson RC, et al. Prediction of severity in acute pancreatitis: prospective comparison of three prognostic indices. *Lancet* 1985;2:403–407.
7. Andriulli A, Leandro G, Niro G, et al. Pharmacologic treatment can prevent pancreatic injury after ERCP: a meta-analysis. *Gastrointest Endosc* 2000;51:1–7.
8. Johnson CD, Kingsnorth AN, Imrie CW, et al. Double blind, randomised, placebo controlled study of a platelet activating factor antagonist, lexipafant, in the treatment and prevention of organ failure in predicted severe acute pancreatitis. *Gut* 2001;48:62–69.
9. Abou-Assi S, Craig K, O'Keefe SJ. Hypocaloric jejunal feeding is better than total parenteral nutrition in acute pancreatitis: results of a randomized comparative study. *Am J Gastroenterol* 2002;97:2255–2262.
10. Sharma VK, Howden CW. Prophylactic antibiotic administration reduces sepsis and mortality in acute necrotizing pancreatitis: a meta-analysis. *Pancreas* 2001;22:28–31.
11. Neoptolemos JP, Carr-Locke DL, London NJ, Bailey IA, James D, Fossard DP. Controlled trial of urgent endoscopic retrograde cholangiopancreatography and endoscopic sphincterotomy versus conservative treatment for acute pancreatitis due to gallstones. *Lancet* 1988;2:979–983.
12. Folsch UR, Nitsche R, Ludtke R, Hilgers RA, Creutzfeldt W. Early ERCP and papillotomy compared with conservative treatment for acute biliary pancreatitis. The German Study Group on Acute Biliary Pancreatitis. *N Engl J Med* 1997;336:237–242.
13. Yeo CJ, Bastidas JA, Lynch-Nyhan A, Fishman EK, Zinner MJ, Cameron JL. The natural history of pancreatic pseudocysts documented by computed tomography. *Surg Gynecol Obstet* 1990;170:411–417.
14. Ko CW, Sekijima JH, Lee SP. Biliary sludge. *Ann Intern Med* 1999;130(4 Pt 1):301–311.

ADDITIONAL READING

Banks PA. Practice guidelines in acute pancreatitis. *Am J Gastroenterol* 1997;92:377–386.
Baron TH, Morgan DE. Acute necrotizing pancreatitis. *N Engl J Med.* 1999;340:1412–1417.
Bradley EL. A clinically based classification system for acute pancreatitis: summary of the International Symposium on Acute Pancreatitis, Atlanta, Ga, September 11 through 13, 1992. *Arch Surg* 1993;128:586–590.
Nathens AB, Curtis JR, Beale RJ, et al. Management of the critically ill patient with severe acute pancreatitis. *Crit Care Med* 2004;32:2524–2536.
Shankar S, van Sonnenberg E, Silverman SG, Tuncali K, Banks PA. Imaging and percutaneous management of acute complicated pancreatitis. *Cardiovasc Intervent Radiol* 2004;27:567–580.
Yadav D, Agarwal N, Pitchumoni CS. A critical evaluation of laboratory tests in acute pancreatitis. *Am J Gastroenterol* 2002;97:1309–1318.

Other Abdominal Emergencies: Appendicitis, Diverticulitis, and Ischemic Bowel

87

Lily C. Chang   E. Patchen Dellinger

INTRODUCTION

This chapter discusses the evaluation of patients with acute abdominal pain. We have chosen three clinical conditions to highlight this process, but several principles apply to the evaluation of all patients with acute abdominal pain. The first of these principles is the importance of shifting the initial focus from making a diagnosis to caring for the acute needs of the patient. In addition to gathering information that elucidates a diagnosis, the physician should also initiate immediate resuscitative measures; sometimes these will reverse or alleviate the symptoms associated with the disease process. These initial resuscitation measures are based on an assessment of the standard "ABCs" of basic life support. In the setting of abdominal pain, the "C" in "ABC" should serve as a reminder to establish large-bore intravenous access for volume resuscitation and administration of medications. The risks incurred during resuscitation need to be weighed against the risks from inaction. For example, a patient with a history of congestive heart failure might develop pulmonary edema from volume repletion but may also be at risk for myocardial infarction or renal complications as a result of inadequate fluid resuscitation.

Following the "ABCs," the next three steps are employed variably but should be considered in each case.

"D, E, and F" represent nasogastric decompression, physical examination, and Foley catheterization. *Nasogastric decompression* is often necessary in a patient with nausea, vomiting, and abdominal pain. Decompressing the stomach reveals the nature of its contents and diminishes the risk of aspiration. *Foley catheterization* is integral to assessing the adequacy of resuscitation. A patient with an acute abdomen often requires large volumes of intravenous fluids before urine output begins. The fluid shifts that accompany diffuse peritonitis can approximate those seen with a 50% body surface area burn. In general, fluid resuscitation should be pursued vigorously until urine output is adequate or rales are auscultated on pulmonary examination. The initial *physical examination* is critical for establishing the pace and focus of the workup. A patient with mild vague abdominal tenderness can be evaluated with a thorough history and repeat physical examinations, whereas a patient with signs of diffuse peritoneal inflammation requires immediate surgical consultation.

Once a patient is stabilized, a thorough history and physical examination are two of the most valuable pieces of information for accurately diagnosing the cause for abdominal pain. The history should elucidate the onset, nature, location, and duration of the pain as well as alleviating and aggravating factors. The onset may be discrete and memorable, as in the case of perforated viscus, but more often is insidious and difficult to define. Pain can be progressive (e.g., appendicitis), episodic (e.g., biliary colic), or sudden and severe (e.g., acute mesenteric ischemia). The origin, current location, and shift in pain help identify the location and status of the disease process.

Although not always feasible, physical examination should be performed early and often by the same examiner. A complete examination that assesses the heart, lungs, kidneys, and reproductive systems is essential to define potential nongastrointestinal sources of abdominal pain such as myocardial infarction, pneumonia, nephrolithiasis, or pelvic inflammatory disease. The abdominal examination should be directed to the point of maximum tenderness last. Tenderness upon light palpation is significant, especially if it persists while the patient is distracted. Pain elicited with the release of deep palpation ("rebound tenderness") does not necessarily differentiate among gastroenteritis, constipation, ileus, or more serious causes of abdominal pain. *The technique of eliciting rebound tenderness is crude and unnecessarily painful for a patient with peritoneal inflammation.* The same information can be obtained by detecting direct and referred percussion tenderness in the same manner as percussing the chest. This can be performed with only enough force to elicit a minimal response, and graded accordingly. Rectal and pelvic examinations are essential and further localize tenderness. By adhering to this initial approach, one can initiate rational diagnostic testing and therapy for the patient with abdominal pain regardless of the cause. The remainder of this chapter discusses three different causes of abdominal pain requiring surgical evaluation: acute appendicitis, diverticulitis, and ischemic bowel. Other causes of acute abdominal pain are covered elsewhere in this section of this book (e.g., cholecystitis, Chapter 84; pancreatitis, Chapter 86).

ACUTE APPENDICITIS

The appendix arises from the cecum and generally lies within the right lower quadrant of the abdomen. However, anatomic variation is common, and this can lead to an unusual presentation and delay in the diagnosis of acute appendicitis. Appendicitis may result from luminal obstruction secondary to fecaliths, lymphoid hyperplasia, parasites, or tumors. Venous engorgement, with resultant

impairment in arterial flow, leads to ischemia, then necrosis, first of the mucosa and subsequently of the muscular wall. Mucosal erosions or ischemia allows bacterial invasion and a subsequent local inflammatory response. The incidence of acute appendicitis is approximately 11 cases per year per 10,000 population. Appendectomy is the most common surgical procedure performed because of abdominal pain, resulting in approximately 300,000 yearly appendectomies in the United States (1).

Issues at the Time of Admission

Clinical Presentation

The clinical presentation of acute appendicitis is highly variable. Classically, the sequence of events begins with vague epigastric or periumbilical abdominal pain, followed by anorexia, nausea, and vomiting. This symptom complex is usually but not always associated with low-grade fever. Within 24 hours the pain migrates to the right lower quadrant, and there is discomfort on walking, coughing, or moving. Pain is usually constant and unremitting. Variation of this sequence is common, but the symptoms and signs are generally progressive. If perforation occurs, there may be temporary relief from pain until symptoms of peritonitis become evident.

The key to diagnosis is often the physical examination. Over 95% of patients have abdominal tenderness, often localized to one-finger palpation over McBurney's point. There may be mild muscular rigidity and localized peritoneal signs. Other signs include pain in the right lower quadrant with palpation of the left lower quadrant (Rovsing's sign). In less than 10% of patients, the psoas sign (pain in right hip with extension associated with retrocecal appendix) or obturator sign (pain with internal hip rotation associated with pelvic appendix) are also present. Rectal and pelvic examinations may help differentiate appendicitis from gynecologic problems.

Differential Diagnosis and Initial Evaluation

Acute appendicitis may mimic almost any acute abdominal illness. Conversely, most acute abdominal problems may resemble appendicitis. The differential diagnosis varies with the age and the gender of the patient (Table 87.1). The rate of incorrect (false-positive) diagnoses of appendicitis has been reported to be as high as 20% in males and 40% in females (2). *Perforated appendicitis* may have a different presentation, with higher fevers, longer duration of symptoms (2–5 days), and a history of pain that suddenly improves. A periappendiceal abscess or phlegmon may be palpable on physical examination.

If a patient presents with typical symptoms and signs, few diagnostic studies are needed. If the presentation is atypical, several studies may be helpful. The white blood cell count is greater than 10,000/μL, with neutrophilia in

TABLE 87.1

DIFFERENTIAL DIAGNOSIS OF ACUTE APPENDICITIS IN ADULTS

Abdominal pain of unknown origin
Gastroenteritis
Colonic diverticulitis
Perforated peptic ulcer
Gallbladder disease
Incarcerated hernia
Inflammatory bowel disease
Testicular or ovarian torsion
Mittelschmerz
Ruptured ovarian cyst
Ectopic pregnancy
Pelvic inflammatory disease
Urinary tract disease or infection
Pneumonia
Pancreatitis
Perforated neoplasm[a]
Mesenteric vascular insufficiency[a]
Aortic or iliac artery aneurysm[a]

[a] Especially in elderly patients.

70%–90% of cases. A normal white count does not rule out appendicitis, and in immunocompromised patients the count is often normal. Serial white blood cell counts usually demonstrate an elevation over the course of 4–8 hours. This finding has been shown to be associated with a 92% diagnostic sensitivity. Urinalysis may be abnormal with appendicitis, but marked elevations of the urinary cell counts suggest urinary tract disease (Chapter 68). Microscopic hematuria is more suggestive of nephrolithiasis, which can often mimic appendicitis. A pregnancy test in all women of childbearing age is mandatory.

Plain-film examinations are nonspecific but occasionally may show small-bowel obstruction, ileus, an appendicolith, or a gas-containing abscess. Rarely, perforated appendicitis may present with free intraperitoneal air. Chest radiograph may demonstrate right lower lobe pneumonia as an alternative diagnosis. *Graded compression ultrasonography* can be a useful tool in the diagnosis of appendicitis if a highly experienced ultrasonographer is available. An inflamed appendix is characterized by an outer diameter greater than 7 millimeters and noncompressability. Appendicoliths, loss of normal appendiceal wall architecture, or periappendiceal fluid also may be seen. Although the reported sensitivity in selected series is 75%–95% and the specificity 85%–95%, this modality is limited by its dependence on the experience of the ultrasonographer. Nonvisualization of the appendix is common and does not exclude appendicitis. Even if nonvisualization occurs, ultrasonography may be helpful by identifying pelvic or biliary disease.

Computed tomography (CT) has been shown to be 94%–100% accurate in confirming or ruling out appendicitis (3). Like ultrasonography, CT is useful in diagnosing causes of abdominal pain other than appendicitis. CT has the advantage of less interobserver variability and increased sensitivity, but adequate oral contrast is essential. However, a focused appendiceal CT with rectal (but not oral) contrast has demonstrated sensitivity of 95% in the pediatric population (4). Findings on CT scan considered to be diagnostic of acute appendicitis include appendiceal distension, wall thickening, or peri-appendiceal inflammation. A series utilizing routine "appendiceal" CT suggested improved diagnostic accuracy, along with cost savings attributable to a decreased incidence of negative appendectomies and shorter average hospital stays (5). Confirmation of these findings and of their generalizability to the community setting needs to be documented prior to the adoption of appendiceal CT as the standard of care in evaluating patients with possible acute appendicitis. A recent report suggests that the widespread availability of CT examinations has not resulted in a reduction in the rate of negative appendectomy (6). If a periappendiceal abscess or phlegmon is suspected based on physical examination, CT should be performed to direct surgical or radiologic intervention.

Indications for Hospitalization and Intensive Care Unit Admission

Patients with a clear diagnosis of appendicitis require admission to the hospital and prompt surgical consultation for operative management. If the history and physical examination are equivocal and the etiology of abdominal pain is uncertain, then further evaluation is essential. This may be performed on either an inpatient or outpatient basis, depending on the patient's presentation and modifying circumstances. Missed or delayed diagnosis of appendicitis can result in serious complications, whereas early diagnosis and treatment allows for a brief hospitalization and rapid recovery. Perforation is associated with a marked increase (from 8% to 40%) in the rate of postoperative complications and a prolonged hospital stay. Thus, the threshold for admission to the hospital and observation should be low for suspected appendicitis. This is especially true for pediatric, geriatric, and pregnant patients.

Appendicitis alone is generally not an indication for ICU admission. However, patients may require ICU care for other comorbid medical conditions, sepsis syndrome, or rare complications, such as *suppurative phlebitis* of the portal vein. Patients with this complication experience fever, chills, right upper quadrant abdominal pain and tenderness, malaise, mild jaundice, and anorexia. It is associated with late development of hepatic abscesses and has a 50% mortality rate. Acute appendicitis at the extremes of age has a higher incidence of delayed diagnosis and is associated with perforation in 50% of cases. These patients are more likely to be severely ill and require aggressive resuscitation in the ICU.

Initial Therapy

During the hospitalization, patients admitted for abdominal pain should have serial evaluations in the same manner as when they were evaluated in the office or emergency room. The symptoms and signs of acute appendicitis usually progress in the first 24 hours unless perforation has occurred. It is essential that the patient continue to be resuscitated, receive intravenous hydration, and have nothing by mouth during this time. Volume depletion and electrolyte abnormalities should be corrected. During this period, no antimicrobial agents should be given until a diagnosis is made.

If a patient does not prove to have acute appendicitis, the evaluation should be continued to determine the cause of pain. The patient should continue to receive nothing by mouth and receive intravenous hydration. Persistent or worsening unexplained tenderness is usually an indication for ultrasound or CT scan. Rising temperature, leukocytosis with migration of the pain to the right lower quadrant, and development of focal right lower quadrant tenderness are surgical indications. If an alternative diagnosis is made, the patient should be treated accordingly.

Once appendicitis is suspected or diagnosed, surgery is indicated. Patients should be resuscitated adequately prior to the administration of anesthesia and surgery. Any reversible coagulopathy should be corrected. An electrocardiogram and chest radiograph should be obtained in patients older than 40 years of age (Chapter 30). Preoperative antibiotic therapy should initially be directed against enteric Gram-negative rods and anaerobes (Chapter 64). Exploration and appendectomy generally are performed through a right lower quadrant muscle-splitting incision or laparoscopically. The advantage of the *open approach* is low cost and familiarity among surgeons and operating-room staff. *Laparoscopy* improves diagnostic accuracy (by sometimes discovering alternative causes in cases found to have a normal appendix, especially in female patients) and may be technically easier than the open approach in the obese patient. However, it has no proven advantage in recovery or hospitalization times. Because of the serious consequences of a delay in diagnosis, a 10%–30% "negative" appendectomy rate is the historic standard. If the appendix looks grossly normal, it is removed for microscopic analysis, and a careful exploration is performed to look for an alternative cause of pain.

Issues During the Course of Hospitalization

Figures 87.1 and 87.2 show critical pathways for uncomplicated and perforated appendicitis.

Following a routine appendectomy, antibiotics may be discontinued and the patient started on oral intake on the same or next postoperative day. If this is tolerated and the patient defervesces, discharge is appropriate. Persistent fevers often respond to pulmonary toilet, but a missed abscess or wound infection must also be considered.

	Day 0	**Post-op Day 1: Discharge home**
Tests	• Physical examination	• Examine wound • Notify primary MD
Medications and Therapeutics	• IV fluids • Preoperative antibiotics once diagnosis is made Aerobic and anaerobic coverage • **APPENDECTOMY**	• Discontinue IV fluids • No further antibiotic therapy
Nursing/ Assessment	• Vitals • Input/Output • Admission weight	• Vitals • Input/Output
Activity	• OOB with assist	• Ambulate
Nutrition	• NPO until surgery • Ice chips or sips of liquid as tolerated postoperatively	• Diet as tolerated
Discharge Planning	• Discuss plan for discharge on POD 1 • Review home situation and initiate referrals as needed	• Discharge needs met
Patient Education	• Pulmonary toilet	*Review with patient/family:* • Discharge plan • Follow-up appointment • Return signs/ symptoms • Activity/driving

Figure 87.1 Critical pathway for uncomplicated acute appendicitis. *IV*, intravenous; *NPO*, nothing by mouth; *OOB*, out of bed; *POD*, post-operative day.

If *perforation* is found, the appendix is removed, and, if contamination is minimal, the incision may be closed. Otherwise, the abdomen should be irrigated and the skin and subcutaneous tissue left open for healing by secondary intent or, in some cases, delayed primary closure on postoperative day 4. Antibiotics are continued postoperatively for 3–5 days. Oral intake is started when bowel function recovers, as evidenced by hunger or the passage of flatus.

Ideally, a *periappendiceal abscess* is diagnosed preoperatively; if so, it can be managed with antibiotics and percutaneous drainage by interventional radiologists. If an abscess is diagnosed at the time of appendectomy, it is evacuated, and drains are placed into the cavity. The appendix is removed if this can be done safely. If abscesses are drained without removal of the appendix, the colon must be evaluated to rule out other causes of perforation (such as diverticulitis or malignancy) prior to committing the patient to an interval appendectomy after 6–8 weeks. This may be done with colonoscopy or barium enema

	Day 0	*Post-op Day 1*	*Post-op Day 2*	*Post-op Day 3-5+: Discharge home*
Tests	• Physical Examination	• Examine wound • Monitor drainage		• If not improving by POD 7, CT abdomen/pelvis, assess for abscess • Colonoscopy prior to or after discharge if abscess was drained without appendectomy
Medications and Therapeutics	• IV fluids • Preop antibiotics once diagnosis is made • Aerobic and anerobic coverage • *APPENDECTOMY and/or DRAINAGE of abscess cavity*	• Continue antibiotics • Start wet to dry dressing changes if wound is open		• Discontinue antibiotics when clinically ready • Delayed primary closure of wound on POD 4 if wound clean and healthy
Nursing/ Assessment	• Vitals • Input/Output • Admission weight • Orthostatics (if indicated)	• Vitals • RN assessment • Record drain output	• Vitals/Temperature	• Vitals/Temperature
Activity	• Out of bed with assist	• Ambulate		
Nutrition	• NPO	• Start diet if anorexia resolved	• Start diet if anorexia resolved	• Advance diet as tolerated
Discharge Planning		• Review home situation and initiate referrals as needed	• MD/RN/SW communication regarding discharge • Plan for discharge care	• Discharge needs met (home care RN, transportation) • Follow-up appointment made
Patient Education	• Incentive spirometry		• Teach dressing changes/wound care	*Review with patient/family* • Discharge plan • Follow-up appointment • Return signs/symptoms • Activity/driving

Figure 87.2 Critical pathway: for acute appendicitis, perforated. *CT*, computed tomography scan; *NPO*, nothing by mouth; *POD*, post-operative day; *SW*, social worker.

prior to or shortly after discharge, once the acute inflammation has resolved. A periappendiceal abscess usually is accompanied by an ileus (Chapter 88). Once abdominal tenderness improves and bowel function returns, the patient may be started on oral intake. Patients usually defervesce after they are adequately drained, either percutaneously or surgically. Lack of improvement in serial physical examinations or fever curve suggests a persistent undrained collection, and a repeat imaging study such as CT or fluoroscopic sinography through the drain should be performed. Occasionally, definitive surgical drainage is required after an ineffective percutaneous attempt.

Discharge Issues

Following routine appendectomy without perforation, most patients are ready for discharge within 24 hours. Fevers and abdominal pain usually have resolved, and there is no rationale for continued oral antibiotic therapy.

Follow-up with the surgeon should be in 2–4 weeks. After appendectomy for perforated appendicitis, most patients are ready for discharge on postoperative day 3–5, depending on the degree of contamination, the fever curve, and the ability to tolerate oral intake. There is no need to continue antibiotics once the temperature and white blood cell (WBC) count are normal. Patients with wounds healing by secondary intent need to learn wound care and wet-to-dry dressing changes. A visit by a home care nurse followed by evaluation by the surgeon in 1–2 weeks ensures optimal wound management. Open wounds do not require antibiotic treatment.

Timing of discharge is variable following drainage of a periappendiceal abscess. It depends on the adequacy of drainage and is dictated by the clinical course, including the relief of pain, resolution of fever, and return of bowel function. The patient needs to learn to care for the drains, which can be removed by the surgeon when the output has tapered (which indicates obliteration of the abscess cavity). The presence of a drain alone is not an indication for antibiotic therapy. Antibiotics are usually continued until the patient defervesces and has a normal white blood cell count. These patients also need visiting nursing care and early follow-up with the surgeon. If patients are debilitated, transfer to a skilled nursing facility may be required for on-going wound care or rehabilitative therapy.

Patients should be encouraged to resume activities progressively as tolerated. Driving is safe when the patient is able to get in and out of the car and use the controls without discomfort. The diet should be advanced as tolerated. Patients should call their surgeons in case of fever, redness or drainage from the wound, or increase in pain.

DIVERTICULITIS

Diverticulitis is caused by a perforation of a diverticulum. In most cases, the perforation is microscopic, causing localized inflammation in the colonic wall or paracolic tissues. In more severe cases, an abscess may form, or the diverticulum may rupture freely into the peritoneal cavity, causing generalized peritonitis. The average age at presentation is in the early sixties; more than 90% of cases occur after 50 years of age. Fifty to 90% of cases in the United States occur in the left colon, particularly the sigmoid. However, among the Asian population, the incidence of right-sided disease is much higher (7). Fifty percent of patients have been symptomatic for less than one month before presentation; the duration of symptoms is inversely correlated with the severity of disease.

Issues at the Time of Admission

Clinical Presentation

Patients with acute diverticulitis can have a broad spectrum of symptoms but typically present with the gradual onset of left lower quadrant abdominal pain and low-grade fever. The pain tends to be constant and does not radiate. The localized inflammatory process may lead to irritation of the contiguous small bowel, colon, and bladder, which may subsequently cause anorexia, nausea, vomiting, diarrhea, constipation, dysuria, and urinary frequency or urgency. On physical examination, tenderness to palpation usually is present in the left lower quadrant or suprapubic region. A mass suggestive of a peridiverticular abscess or phlegmon also may be palpable. Rectal examination may reveal a boggy mass anteriorly if an abscess is present. Diffuse peritonitis is less common; when present, it usually represents frank perforation into the peritoneal cavity. Unlike diverticulosis (Chapter 78), acute diverticulitis usually is *not* associated with hemorrhage, although 30%–40% of cases have guaiac-positive stool. Pneumaturia or fecaluria suggests the presence of a colovesical fistula.

Differential Diagnosis and Initial Evaluation

A classic clinical presentation is often sufficient to establish the diagnosis without confirmatory testing. Laboratory studies are nonspecific and frequently unrevealing. Leukocytosis may be absent in up to one-half of cases. Urinalysis may be abnormal, with microscopic pyuria. An electrocardiogram should be considered in older patients with a history of coronary disease. In older individuals or immunocompromised patients, the presentation may be subtle, and immunocompromised patients are more likely to have complications of diverticulitis. The differential diagnosis is listed in Table 87.2.

When the diagnosis is unclear or complications of diverticulitis are suspected, further studies are necessary. Plain-film abdominal series, including an upright chest radiograph, should be obtained first to rule out free intraperitoneal air or a lower-lobe pneumonia. These studies may be normal or may demonstrate a distal large-bowel obstruction, localized ileus, or extracolonic air. *CT with intravenous and oral contrast is the study of choice.* Water-soluble rectal contrast may be used, but it carries the risk of perforation and should be carefully considered. CT scan is superior to barium enema in that it can directly demonstrate extraluminal complications of the disease such as abscess, phlegmon, free intraperitoneal air, or colovesical fistula and also can identify other causes of symptomatology.

If the results of the CT scan are equivocal or suggest an alternate diagnosis, contrast enema studies can be helpful in establishing the diagnosis and excluding cancer. *Barium should be avoided in the acute setting of diverticulitis* because of the risk of extravasation into the peritoneal cavity. Contrast studies can suggest the presence of an abscess in over 85% of cases but may underestimate the severity of extraluminal disease. Ultrasonography is up to 98% sensitive and 97%

TABLE 87.2

DIFFERENTIAL DIAGNOSIS OF ACUTE DIVERTICULITIS

Appendicitis
Carcinoma
Colonic spasm
Gastroenteritis
Infectious colitis
Ischemia
Irritable bowel
Inflammatory bowel disease
Pelvic inflammatory disease
Perforated peptic ulcer
Foreign-body perforation
Volvulus
Urosepsis
Pneumonia

specific in expert hands but is limited by higher false-negative rates in some series and greater interobserver variability.

Colonoscopy or sigmoidoscopy is generally contraindicated in the setting of acute diverticulitis. Limited examination with minimal or no air insufflation should be reserved for special situations in which the diagnosis of diverticulitis is uncertain and other diagnoses, such as ischemic bowel, obstructing carcinoma, or colitis, are being considered.

Indications for Hospitalization and Initial Intensive Care Unit Admission

Mild cases of acute diverticulitis in immunocompetent patients can be managed on an outpatient basis with clear liquids and oral antibiotics. Ideal patients for outpatient management are those who are able to tolerate a diet, have no systemic symptoms or diffuse peritoneal signs, and are reliable or have a reliable family. Immunocompromise, steroid therapy, and advanced age are contraindications to outpatient therapy. If outpatient therapy is elected, patients need to watch for systemic signs or progression of symptoms and should be instructed to return if these develop. Follow-up with the treating physician must occur within 48–72 hours after presentation to ensure resolution of symptoms. Patients who do not meet outpatient criteria or who fail outpatient management should be admitted to the hospital for total bowel rest, intravenous antibiotics, surgical consultation, and further evaluation as indicated. The decision for ICU admission should be based on the assessment of physiology and comorbidity as outlined at the start of this chapter. Patients with free perforation and peritonitis may need resuscitation in the ICU in preparation for urgent operative therapy.

Initial Therapy

Patients hospitalized for acute diverticulitis should be on complete bowel rest (NPO) and receive intravenous hydration and intravenous broad-spectrum antibiotics to provide coverage for Gram-negative organisms and anaerobes (Chapter 64). Figure 87.3 demonstrates an algorithm for the management of acute diverticulitis. Nasogastric decompression should be instituted for significant nausea, vomiting, or bowel obstruction. A Foley catheter may be placed for urinary retention. Appropriate analgesia should be administered. Enemas to treat constipation should be avoided. If the fever is greater than 38.5°C, a routine fever evaluation should be done (Chapter 62). As with any acute abdominal illness, patients must continue to be resuscitated during this time and have serial examinations performed to monitor the course of illness. Patients presenting with free perforation represent a surgical emergency and have a 6%–35% mortality rate. Aggressive resuscitation and cardiovascular support should be followed by prompt operative therapy. The same aggressive approach should be taken if a patient worsens on therapy.

Diverticulitis may be complicated by abscess, fistula, or bowel obstruction. These complications develop in about one-quarter of patients who present with symptomatic diverticulitis (7). Patients with recurrent diverticulitis have a 60% risk of a complicated course (8). In all types of diverticular complications, carcinoma must be ruled out as the cause. An *abscess* may resolve with conservative therapy if it is small and favorably located. It is preferable to drain a large abscess percutaneously prior to definitive therapy, because the presence of an abscess is a relative contraindication to primary anastomosis after colon resection. Seventy to 90% of abscesses can be percutaneously drained. *Fistulas* develop in only 2% of all patients with diverticulitis, but patients with fistulas represent 20% of all patients undergoing surgery for diverticulitis. Most commonly, fistulas occur between the colon and the bladder, but colovaginal, coloenteric, or colocutaneous fistulas also occur. A patient with a fistula should undergo an elective procedure to resect the affected bowel and close the fistula after the acute inflammation has resolved. *Bowel obstruction* from diverticular disease is an acute process, with perforation and bowel wall edema complicating a chronic response to previous inflammation. Obstruction is generally partial and usually is relieved as the edema from the acute inflammation resolves, leaving a fibrotic, strictured colon that can be resected electively. Patients with complete obstruction should undergo surgery expeditiously following acute resuscitation with hydration and nasogastric decompression (Chapter 88).

Indications for Early Consultation

Although most cases of diverticulitis are mild and resolve with medical management, prompt surgical consultation should be obtained for patients in whom significant systemic signs or peritonitis exist, and for those individuals presenting with a complication of diverticulitis such as abscess, fistula, obstruction, or free perforation. Consultation should be obtained at the onset of initial treatment in order to facilitate appropriate management.

Issues During the Course of Hospitalization

Most patients correctly diagnosed and treated for diverticulitis show significant improvement within the first 48 hours, denoted by decreased pain, less tenderness, and resolution of fever and leukocytosis. Bowel rest and antibiotics should be continued until the patient has improved subjectively and demonstrates return of bowel function. Nasogastric decompression is needed only in patients who present with nausea and vomiting; it can be discontinued as soon as the daily output decreases.

Worsening signs or symptoms or failure to improve during this period despite maximal medical therapy are indications for immediate reassessment. The diagnosis may be incorrect, or there may be unrecognized complications.

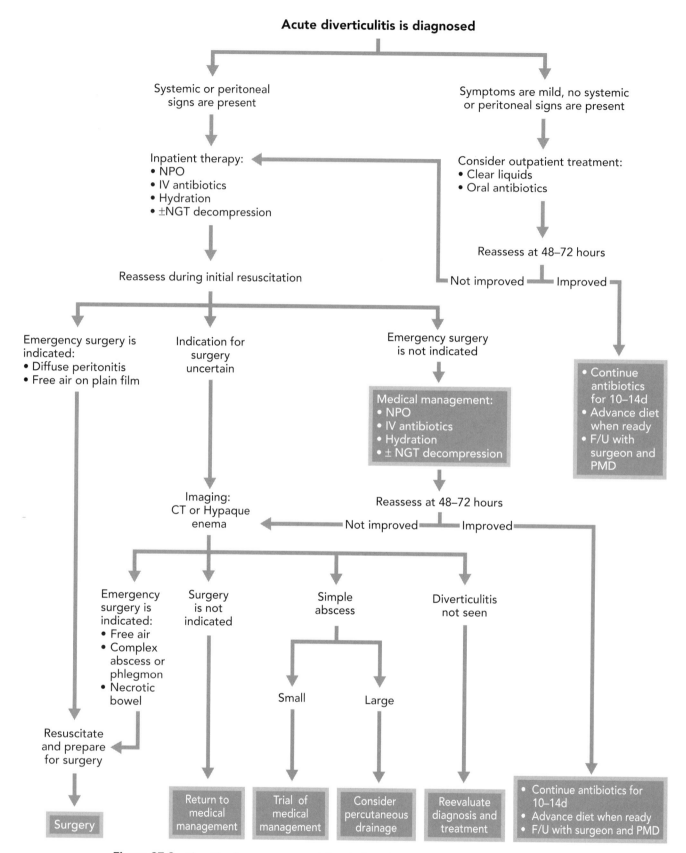

Figure 87.3 Algorithm for management of diverticulitis. *CT,* computerized tomography scan; *F/U,* follow-up; *IV,* intravenous; *NGT,* nasogastric tube; *NPO,* nothing by mouth; *PMD,* primary physician.

This occurs in 10%–25% of patients. In most cases, a CT scan should be obtained to seek an alternative diagnosis or to locate an abscess that might be drainable percutaneously. At this point, if no process amenable to medical management is identified, immediate surgical exploration is indicated. In preparation for surgery, an electrocardiogram and chest radiograph should be obtained in patients older than 40 years, and all comorbid conditions should be treated optimally (Chapter 30).

The exact nature of the surgical intervention depends on the severity of the disease and the nature of associated complications. Abscesses must be adequately drained. The diseased colonic segment should be resected if technically feasible. Under optimal circumstances, patients can undergo resection with primary colorectal anastomosis in a one-stage operation. A two-stage procedure is often required, with resection and colostomy formation followed later by re-anastomosis. There is now evidence suggesting that even in the presence of a pelvic abscess and focal peritonitis, a single-stage procedure can be performed with low risk of injury or death. This is preferable for most patients from both quality-of-life and cost standpoints. Rarely, patients who are critically ill may not be able to tolerate resection, in which case diversion and drainage may be the safest alternative.

Antibiotics should be continued after surgery for a duration determined by the patient's response to therapy. Five to seven days of intravenous antibiotics are usually sufficient. After the initial operation, an oral diet can be resumed when the patient feels hungry. This usually occurs on postoperative day 2 or 3, although it may take longer if significant contamination was present or ileus has developed.

If the patient has persistent high fevers, unimproving tenderness and pain, or persistent or worsening leukocytosis after surgical intervention, a recurrent abscess may be present. Alternatively, infection with resistant organisms is a possibility, and the antibiotic regimen should be reconsidered. Such a patient should be kept on bowel rest, and total parenteral nutrition should be considered. For patients with a primary anastomosis, anastomotic leak must also be ruled out. If present, it should be treated appropriately. If drain output has declined precipitously, the drain may be occluded, and a sinogram with catheter exchange may be helpful. Repeat imaging with CT may be helpful in directing further therapy.

Discharge Issues

Most patients with diverticulitis respond to medical therapy and are ready for discharge 5–7 days after initiation of therapy. By this time, the patient should have resolution of fever and marked improvement of abdominal pain, tenderness, and leukocytosis. Although it is not necessary that the patient tolerate a regular diet prior to discharge, he or she must be able to maintain oral hydration without an increase in abdominal pain. Oral antibiotics should be continued.

Usually a 10–14 day combined total course of therapy is adequate. Follow-up with the treating physician or surgeon should occur 2–4 weeks after discharge. Successful nonsurgical treatment of diverticulitis should always be followed by examination of the colon by colonoscopy or by flexible sigmoidoscopy with barium enema once the acute inflammation has resolved, to rule out carcinoma.

Approximately 10%–30% of patients who respond to medical therapy later go on to have another episode of diverticulitis. Age younger than 50 years and polycystic renal disease are risk factors for recurrent disease. Elective resection may be indicated. Patients with complications such as fistulas or strictures also ultimately require surgical intervention.

Following surgical intervention, the criteria for discharge are similar to those following other abdominal operations. Surgical follow-up should occur within 1–2 weeks for those with drains or open wounds and within 2–4 weeks for those with simple surgical resection without drains. Patients should be instructed to resume their diets gradually, as tolerated. Dietary changes should be directed at decreasing intraluminal pressure, which is thought to be partly responsible for diverticula formation. High fiber intake with generous fluid intake should be advised, as this appears to reduce complications in patients with diverticula.

ACUTE BOWEL ISCHEMIA AND ISCHEMIC COLITIS

Acute mesenteric ischemia results from insufficiency of the blood supply to the bowel resulting from embolic or thrombotic arterial occlusion, venous occlusion, or nonocclusive hypoperfusion. Although uncommon, acute mesenteric ischemia has a high mortality rate, with many series reporting rates over 60% (9). This is because diagnosis is difficult and patients often present late and have multiple comorbidities. Ischemic colitis usually follows a more benign clinical course. Untreated, however, it too can progress to transmural necrosis and systemic sepsis, with a high mortality rate. The watershed areas of the right and left colon are at particularly high risk. An important subset of patients develops colon ischemia following major operations such as abdominal aortic aneurysm repair or cardiac surgery involving cardiopulmonary bypass. Chronic mesenteric ischemia is not discussed here because it involves different pathophysiologic and therapeutic considerations.

Issues at the Time of Admission

Clinical Presentation

Acute intestinal ischemia, typically secondary to an embolus, is heralded by the sudden onset of poorly localized, severe, crampy abdominal pain, classically out of proportion to physical examination findings. Acute ischemia usually occurs in patients with cardiovascular comorbidities. Risk factors include arrhythmias, structural cardiac disease, hypotension, atherosclerosis, and hypercoagulable states. Nausea, vomiting, diarrhea, or hematochezia may be present and suggest evolving intestinal infarction. An abdominal bruit is present in 10%–25% of cases. With ischemia resulting from arterial thrombosis, venous occlusion, or ischemic colitis, the progression of symptoms is more insidious and starts with vague gastrointestinal symptoms of pain, bloating, changes in bowel habits, or nausea. Initially, peritoneal irritation may not be present, but the signs and symptoms progress as bowel infarction and necrosis begin. Later in the disease course, abdominal distention, guarding, rebound tenderness, or altered mental status with signs of systemic sepsis, renal failure, and cardiovascular compromise may occur. Not infrequently, the patient in whom acute bowel ischemia is being considered is already in critical condition, obtunded or intubated in the ICU. In this particular setting, the pathophysiology usually is related to nonocclusive ischemia or vasospasm.

Differential Diagnosis and Initial Evaluation

Diagnosis of ischemic bowel is often very difficult because the initial physical findings may be unremarkable. Thus, the differential diagnosis is vast. However, the absence of abnormal physical findings in the setting of severe, sudden abdominal pain is an important clue to the diagnosis of acute mesenteric occlusion. Diagnosis is often based on early suspicion and clinical intuition because no specific noninvasive diagnostic study can reliably diagnose or exclude mesenteric ischemia. Most abnormal findings occur late and are nonspecific. These include leukocytosis with a left shift; hemoconcentration; elevations in serum phosphate and amylase; and elevated lactate level with resultant metabolic acidosis.

Plain radiographs may be completely normal or show nonspecific findings. In more advanced cases of acute mesenteric ischemia, bowel-wall thickening, pneumatosis intestinalis, portal venous air, or free air may be seen. These late findings usually represent full-thickness necrosis and portend a poor prognosis. CT of the abdomen and pelvis with oral, rectal, and intravenous contrast may show bowel wall thickening, intramural or portal venous air, or thrombus within the mesenteric arteries or veins. Although less sensitive for arterial occlusions, CT is the diagnostic study of choice for mesenteric venous thrombosis, with reported sensitivities as high as 90%. Duplex ultrasound scanning also can be helpful in the diagnosis of either arterial or venous occlusion but is often technically difficult because of overlying bowel gas.

The definitive diagnostic study for arterial pathology is mesenteric angiography. It can differentiate occlusive from nonocclusive sources of ischemia and can direct intervention. Furthermore, it offers the opportunity for non-surgical interventions such as selective vasodilator or thrombolytic infusion. Emboli usually are seen impacted 3–10 cm from the origin of the superior mesenteric artery and distal to the origin of the middle colic branch. A meniscus sign often is seen at the point of occlusion. In contrast, superior mesenteric artery thrombosis usually occurs at the origin and may manifest as nonvisualization of the artery. Alternatively, nonocclusive mesenteric ischemia is seen as vasospasm, with multiple areas of narrowing of the mesenteric arteries without occlusion. In the setting of venous thrombosis, arteriography may demonstrate subtle signs such as delayed visualization of the venous phase, prolonged opacification of the bowel wall, or nonvisualization of the ischemic segments. Flexible colonoscopy can evaluate the mucosal viability of the colon and terminal ileum and is the procedure of choice to evaluate early ischemic colitis.

Indications for Hospitalization and Initial ICU Admission

All patients in whom acute mesenteric ischemia is suspected should be admitted to the hospital for observation and further evaluation. Many patients with mesenteric ischemia need initial ICU admission for resuscitation because of hemodynamic instability caused by hypovolemia or systemic sepsis. Mesenteric ischemia is also more likely to occur in patients with significant cardiovascular comorbidities, which themselves may need ICU management. The underlying cause of mesenteric ischemia must be evaluated and treated concurrently.

Initial Therapy

The goal of initial intervention is resuscitation, regardless of the cause of the ischemia. The loss of intravascular volume to surrounding tissues is typically massive, and volume should be aggressively replaced with crystalloid and colloid (Chapter 25). Acidosis caused by tissue hypoperfusion may not be fully corrected with volume alone, and the administration of sodium bicarbonate may be necessary (Chapter 105). Broad-spectrum intravenous antibiotics to cover aerobic and anaerobic intestinal flora should be given immediately (Chapter 64). Systemic sepsis arising from ischemic bowel may be especially difficult to manage and is recalcitrant to therapy unless the source of sepsis is removed.

If the history and clinical presentation strongly suggest acute visceral embolization, immediate laparotomy with embolectomy and resection of infarcted bowel should be performed after preoperative resuscitation. For patients with superior mesenteric artery (SMA) thrombosis, nonocclusive ischemia, or unclear diagnosis, mesenteric angiography with selective cannulation should be performed urgently to establish the diagnosis and plan further therapy. If an embolus or thrombosis is confirmed, the patient should be prepared immediately for embolectomy or thrombectomy as above. In selected cases, intra-arterial thrombolytics and vasodilators may be successful. Nonocclusive ischemia is the entity more commonly seen in ICU patients. The highest priority is reversal of any precipitating causes. Vasoconstricting agents should be discontinued if possible, and systemic vasodilators should be used in conjunction with positive inotropes to maintain splanchnic perfusion pressure. If the diagnosis is established angiographically, a catheter should be left in place and intra-arterial papaverine delivered continuously. Surgery is indicated only if there is evidence of bowel necrosis. Premature operative intervention in this setting may prove detrimental.

Patients with mesenteric venous occlusion should be anticoagulated with heparin, and a hypercoagulability evaluation should be undertaken (Chapter 98). Initial surgical intervention is reserved for evidence of bowel necrosis or perforation.

Flexible sigmoidoscopy or colonoscopy should be performed early for ischemic colitis. If ischemia is mild and there are no signs of peritonitis or sepsis, these patients sometimes can be managed with oral antibiotics and a clear liquid diet, but the cause of ischemia should be pursued and corrected if possible. If ischemic colitis progresses to full-thickness necrosis, operative intervention must be undertaken.

Indications for Early Consultation

The management of acute mesenteric ischemia requires a multidisciplinary approach involving surgeons and interventional radiologists. Early surgical consultation should be obtained whenever mesenteric ischemia is suspected. The interventional radiology team is also needed for urgent angiography unless immediate exploration is indicated.

Issues During the Course of Hospitalization

Approximately 25%–50% of cases of acute mesenteric ischemia are caused by *arterial embolus*, usually originating in the left atrium as a consequence of atrial fibrillation. The immediate definitive treatment is embolectomy with enterectomy if necessary. *Arterial thrombosis* accounts for another 25%–50% of acute ischemia. Thrombectomy alone is usually insufficient therapy, as the diseased vessel is likely to reocclude. Surgical treatment consists of revascularization with enterectomy as needed.

Operative therapy is usually performed through a midline incision so that the entire abdomen can be evaluated. Heparin is given to avoid additional thrombus formation. The primary goal is to restore blood flow to the intestine. Once the SMA is identified at the root of the mesentery, an embolectomy or thrombectomy can be performed. If thrombosis has occurred in a diseased artery, mesenteric bypass or endarterectomy may be necessary to establish adequate blood flow (10). After revascularization, the bowel viability must be assessed and areas of necrosis resected. There are often areas of the bowel in which viability is questionable. For these cases, a second-look laparotomy can be performed in 24–48 hours to re-assess viability.

Nonocclusive mesenteric ischemia occurs as a result of a low cardiac output state, and management can be challenging. In most cases, treatment of the underlying conditions with resuscitation and discontinuation of vasopressors results in resolution. However, if no improvement is seen in 24 hours, angiography should be performed and a continuous papaverine infusion (30–60 mg/h for 12–24 hours) into the mesenteric vessels initiated. Significant clinical deterioration often reflects bowel infarction and signals the need for laparotomy. If the patient remains stable or improves, the angiogram should be repeated.

Mesenteric venous thrombosis that has not progressed to bowel necrosis should be treated by immediate anticoagulation with heparin. Thrombectomy usually is contraindicated, as most patients have diffuse thrombosis. All patients with local or diffuse peritonitis should undergo immediate laparotomy with resection of clearly infarcted bowel. Peritonitis may become apparent after the patient has been fully anticoagulated. In this case, heparin should be continued throughout the perioperative period. Simultaneously, the underlying disorder that caused the thrombosis should be addressed. More than 80% of all cases of mesenteric venous thrombosis are secondary to hypercoagulable states; hematology consultation should be obtained (Chapter 98).

The primary therapy for *ischemic colitis* is supportive. In the hospital setting, intravenous hydration and antibiotics should be administered. Cautious colonoscopy may be performed early to document the extent and severity of the disease and may be repeated at 24- to 72-hour intervals to evaluate the progression or regression of disease. Necrosis or gangrene seen on colonoscopy or clinical evidence of peritonitis should prompt surgical intervention. Patients treated conservatively should show improvement within the first several days and resolution of symptoms by two weeks.

With all forms of bowel ischemia, the hospital course depends on multiple factors, including underlying systemic disorders and the severity of the ischemic disease. Generally, patients should have complete bowel rest and be started on oral intake slowly after they have demonstrated a trend toward improvement, as evidenced by stability in hemodynamic status, resolution of sepsis, and return of bowel activity.

Regardless of the precise nature of ischemia, the development of peritonitis or evidence of bowel necrosis should prompt surgical intervention. At the time of exploration, all infarcted bowel is resected. However, it is often difficult to reliably ascertain the viability of the bowel by visual inspection alone. A second-look laparotomy at 24–48 hours may be necessary. Bowel viability determines whether intraoperative management involves the creation of an enterostomy or a primary anastomosis. All patients need continued close monitoring for evidence of ongoing bowel infarction.

Discharge Issues

Patients are ready for discharge if they have become physiologically stable with the resolution of sepsis, improvement of pain, and return of bowel function. The timing of discharge is variable. Among the highest priorities at the time of discharge is the optimal treatment of underlying systemic diseases to minimize the likelihood of recurrent bowel ischemia. Early follow-up should be scheduled to ensure optimization of medical therapy and to monitor for recurrent disease. As is the case after any operation for an intra-abdominal source of sepsis, the patient may have enterostomies, drains, open wounds, parenteral nutrition, or antibiotics to manage at home. A visiting nurse is often helpful, and follow-up with the surgeon should occur within 1–2 weeks. Diet and activities should be resumed as tolerated. Driving can be resumed when the patient is off opiates and feels comfortable. There is no indication for routine antibiotics at discharge.

COST CONSIDERATIONS AND RESOURCE USE

Approximately 250,000 appendectomies are performed in the United States each year, at a total cost of about $1.5 billion. About 20% of the appendectomies performed find no pathology attributable to the appendix. This has led to efforts to improve the diagnostic accuracy of appendicitis with modalities such as ultrasound and limited abdominal CT scan. If accurate preoperative diagnosis could be achieved routinely without the need for extensive and expensive diagnostic studies, the cost of the "negative" appendectomy could be avoided.

Recent advances in surgical and interventional radiologic techniques have reduced the morbidity and cost resulting from treating complicated diverticulitis. Percutaneous drainage of a large peridiverticular abscess allows the surgeon to treat the disease definitively with a single operation in which the colon is resected and a primary anastomosis is created. This previously required two or three operations and a temporary colostomy. The resultant savings in the cost of multiple operations, hospitalizations, and patient morbidity are significant.

Despite advances in the treatment of mesenteric ischemia, there have been only small gains in patient survival. This reflects the difficulty of diagnosis and treatment. As the population ages, the incidence of mesenteric ischemia has increased, with a resultant increase in the cost of treating these patients. Early diagnosis and intervention, and increased focus on prevention, offer the only chance to decrease the mortality rate and cost.

KEY POINTS

General

- Although the causes of intra-abdominal emergencies are legion, unifying themes should guide the care of these acutely ill patients. Most importantly, attention should be directed to rapid and aggressive resuscitation of the patient before searching for the diagnosis.
- Physical examination performed early and often by the same examiner is the safest, most cost-effective tool in the evaluation of abdominal pain.
- Early surgical consultation and a multidisciplinary approach are important to ensure rapid intervention should the necessity for surgery arise or the patient's condition rapidly deteriorate.

Acute Appendicitis

- The classic presentation of acute appendicitis is vague periumbilical pain that shifts to become localized right lower quadrant pain, associated with anorexia.

Acute Diverticulitis

- Complete bowel rest, intravenous hydration, broad-spectrum antibiotic therapy, and serial physical examinations are the key elements of the management of diverticulitis.
- CT with intravenous and oral contrast is the study of choice in the evaluation of acute diverticulitis.
- Successful nonsurgical treatment of diverticulitis should be followed by examination of the colon to rule out carcinoma.

Ischemic Bowel

- Early recognition and intervention is the key to successful treatment of acute mesenteric ischemia.
- A paucity of abnormal physical findings in the setting of severe, sudden abdominal pain is an important clue to the diagnosis of acute mesenteric occlusion.

REFERENCES

1. Kozak LJ, Owings MF, Hall MJ. National Hospital Discharge Summary: 2001 annual summary with detailed diagnosis and procedure data. Ambulatory and inpatient procedures in the United States, 1996. *Vital Health Stat* 2004;156:1–198.
2. Hale DA, Molloy M, Pearl RH, Schutt DC, Jaques DP. Appendectomy: a contemporary appraisal. *Ann Surg* 1997;225:252–261.
3. Paulson EK, Kalady MF, Pappas TN. Clinical practice. Suspected appendicitis. *N Engl J Med* 2003;348:236–242.
4. Stephen AE, Segev DL, Ryan DP, et al. The diagnosis of acute appendicitis in a pediatric population: to CT or not to CT. *J Pediatr Surg* 2003;38:367–371.
5. Rao PM, Rhea JT, Novelline RA, Mostafavi AA, McCabe CJ. Effect of computed tomography of the appendix on treatment of patients and use of hospital resources. *N Engl J Med* 1998;338:141–146.

6. Flum DR, Morris A, Koepsell T, Dellinger EP. Has misdiagnosis of appendicitis decreased over time? A population-based analysis. *JAMA* 2001;286:1748–1753.

7. Farrell RJ, Farrell JJ, Morrin MM. Diverticular disease in the elderly. *Gastroenterol Clin North Am* 2001;30:475–496.

8. Wolff BG, Devine RM. Surgical management of diverticulitis. *Am Surg* 2000;66:153–156.

9. Park WM, Gloviczki P, Cherry KJ Jr, et al. Contemporary management of acute mesenteric ischemia: factors associated with survival. *J Vasc Surg* 2002;35:445–452.

10. Mansour MA. Management of acute mesenteric ischemia. *Arch Surg* 1999;134:328–331.

ADDITIONAL READING

Farthmann EH, Ruckauer KD, Haring RU. Evidence-based surgery: diverticulitis—a surgical disease? *Langenbecks Arch Surg* 2000; 385:143–151.

Greenwald DA, Brandt LJ, Reinus JF. Ischemic bowel disease in the elderly. *Gastroenterol Clin North Am* 2001;30:445–473.

Kraemer M, Franke C, Ohmann C, Yang Q, Acute Abdominal Pain Study Group. Acute appendicitis in late adulthood: incidence, presentation, and outcome. Results of a prospective multicenter acute abdominal pain study and a review of the literature. *Langenbecks Arch Surg* 2000;385:470–481.

Ileus and Obstruction of the Gastrointestinal Tract

88

Daniel T. Dempsey   *Sean P. Harbison*

INTRODUCTION

Bowel obstruction is defined as any mechanical or functional process that interferes with normal transportation of intestinal contents through the alimentary tube. Complete bowel obstruction implies total luminal compromise; partial obstruction implies otherwise. The cause of bowel obstruction usually is categorized as extrinsic, intrinsic, or luminal (Table 88.1). *Ileus* is defined as any functional or reflex abnormality of gut peristalsis that interferes with the passage of luminal contents. Ileus may be focal or generalized and is thought to be caused by dysfunction of the enteric nervous system or smooth muscle. Causes of ileus may be categorized as reflex, metabolic, drug induced, systemic, or other (Table 88.2). Bowel obstruction and ileus are important clinical entities because they are common and may result in death if not properly managed.

The care of the patient with ileus or bowel obstruction is guided by the following principles:

1. Patients with complete small-bowel obstruction require an urgent operation.
2. Patients with complete colon obstruction (except some with sigmoid volvulus) require an urgent operation.
3. Ileus is often an indication of a serious underlying medical or surgical problem.
4. Proximal decompression and fluid resuscitation are critically important in the management of patients with ileus and bowel obstruction.

This chapter emphasizes the importance of these simple principles. Gastric-outlet obstruction and gastroparesis are not discussed.

BOWEL OBSTRUCTION OR ILEUS AS A PRESENTING COMPLAINT

Issues at the Time of Admission

Clinical Presentation

Patients presenting with intestinal obstruction or ileus usually complain of abdominal discomfort or pain, nausea with or without vomiting, anorexia, decreased output of stool and flatus, and abdominal distension (1). The constellation of signs and symptoms depends on the degree and level of obstruction. *Proximal* small bowel obstruction typically produces crampy abdominal pain, frequent bilious vomiting, and variable amounts of abdominal distension. *Distal* small bowel obstruction causes impressive abdominal distension, less frequent (but often feculent) vomiting, and intermittent crampy abdominal pain. *Colon* obstruction may cause severe distension and little vomiting, especially if the ileocecal valve is competent. *Ileus* presents with distension and anorexia. Because ileus often is indicative of an intra-abdominal process (e.g., pancreatitis) or a systemic illness (e.g., pneumonia), accompanying symptoms can be myriad (2).

TABLE 88.1

CAUSES OF BOWEL OBSTRUCTION IN THE ADULT

Small bowel	Colon
Extrinsic	
Adhesions[a]	Volvulus[a]
Hernia[a]	
Neoplasm[a]	
Abscess	
Volvulus	
Intrinsic	
Crohn's disease	Neoplasm[a]
Neoplasm	Diverticulitis[a]
Ischemia	Ischemia
Stricture	Stricture
Radiation	IBD
Anastomotic	Anastomotic
	Ischemic
Luminal	
Intussusception	Intussusception
Gallstone ileus	Stool
	Foreign body

[a] Most common causes.
IBD, inflammatory bowel disease.

Differential Diagnosis and Initial Evaluation

A good physical examination is essential (see Table 88.3). The vital signs and the general appearance of the patient are important. Fever may indicate a strangulation obstruction or an abscess associated with obstruction or ileus (e.g., appendiceal abscess with distal small-bowel obstruction).

TABLE 88.2

CAUSES OF ILEUS

Reflex	Drug-induced
Spinal cord injury	Opiates
Retroperitoneal process	Anticholinergics
Hematoma	Antihistamines
Kidney stone	Systemic illness
Pyelonephritis	Sepsis
Pancreatitis	Cardiogenic shock
Peritonitis	Pneumonia
Postoperative ileus	Other
Metabolic	Intestinal ischemia
Hypokalemia	Inflammatory bowel disease
Hypothyroidism	Enterocolitis (e.g.,
Kidney or liver failure	*Clostridium difficile*)
	Pseudo-obstruction

TABLE 88.3

IMPORTANT PHYSICAL FINDINGS IN PATIENTS WITH BOWEL OBSTRUCTION

Sign or symptom	Possible causes
Hypotension/tachycardia	Intravascular volume depletion
	Sepsis (bowel gangrene or perforation)
Tachypnea, rhonchi	Pneumonia
Cachexia, lymphadenopathy	Advanced malignancy
Jaundice	Periampullary malignancy
	Gallstone ileus
Irregular heart rate/ heart murmur	Embolism with ischemic bowel
Bruit (abdominal/ carotid/femoral)	Thrombosis with ischemic bowel
Abdominal scars	Adhesive small bowel obstruction
Peritoneal signs	Strangulation, obstruction
	Acute abdomen causing bowel obstruction (e.g., appendiceal abscess)
Hernia (groin, abdominal)	Incarceration or strangulation
Guaiac–positive stool	Carcinoma
	Ischemia

Cachexia may suggest that the obstruction is caused by carcinoma (primary bowel or metastatic) or that the patient has intestinal ischemia presenting as ileus or obstruction. Tachycardia and hypotension may indicate septic shock from an abdominal catastrophe or urosepsis with reflex ileus. It is notoriously difficult for even the most experienced clinician to discern the presence of threatened or strangulated bowel in the patient with a small-bowel obstruction (2,3). Thus, if a complete obstruction is suspected (the situation in which most bowel strangulation occurs), an urgent operation is necessary.

More commonly, in the patient with bowel obstruction, tachycardia and hypotension reflect a fluid deficit. *The patient with bowel obstruction or ileus often has a profound deficit in extracellular fluid volume.* Thus, fluid resuscitation is an important part of initial clinical management (Figure 88.1; Chapter 87). Blood should be sent for determination of electrolyte, blood-urea nitrogen, glucose, calcium, and amylase levels and complete blood count (CBC) with differential count.

In every patient presenting with abdominal pain and distension, nausea or vomiting, and alteration in bowel function, *early surgical consultation is mandatory* (4). The following questions must be addressed:

- Does the patient have a small- or large-bowel obstruction?
- If so, is it a complete obstruction?

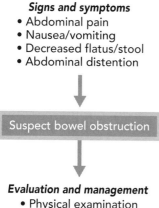

Signs and symptoms
- Abdominal pain
- Nausea/vomiting
- Decreased flatus/stool
- Abdominal distention

Suspect bowel obstruction

Evaluation and management
- Physical examination
- Isotonic IV fluid
- Urinary catheter
- Nasogastric tube
- Radiograph series
- Surgical consultation

Figure 88.1   Initial approach to bowel obstruction and ileus. *IV*, intravenous.

- If the patient has a partial obstruction, is early operation necessary?
- What is the likely cause of the obstruction?
- If the patient has ileus, why?

Upright chest and abdominal and supine abdominal radiographs constitute the standard "obstruction series;" they should be obtained in every patient with suspected bowel obstruction or ileus (Figure 88.2). Computed tomography (CT) or magnetic resonance imaging is not necessary routinely but may yield important information in selected patients (5,6). If the radiographs show distended small and large intestine, the diagnosis is either ileus or colonic obstruction, and a sigmoidoscopy or contrast enema is indicated. If there is small-bowel distension without colonic distension, the diagnosis is probably small-bowel obstruction. The presence or absence of air in the colon in this setting is an unreliable determinant of complete small-bowel obstruction. If the patient denies passage of stool or flatus, by definition the patient has a *complete* bowel obstruction. This is a surgical emergency because intestinal necrosis or perforation occurs frequently in this setting. Clinical judgment is notoriously poor in predicting bowel compromise in patients with bowel obstruction (3). If a lucid patient admits to passage of stool or flatus, the patient has a *partial* small-bowel obstruction. The patient with obvious partial small-bowel obstruction does not necessarily require operation if there is no tenderness, leukocytosis, fever, tachycardia, or physical signs of peritoneal irritation (after fluid resuscitation) (7). In patients with bowel obstruction in whom nonoperative therapy is contemplated, enteroclysis with water soluble contrast is a useful way to confirm a partial obstruction. At times, it may also be therapeutic (8).

The common causes of small-bowel obstruction in the adult are (in descending order of frequency) adhesions, hernia, and cancer (Table 88.1). Abscess (commonly appendiceal or diverticular) or ischemia are important but less common causes of small-bowel obstruction. The common causes of large-bowel obstruction in the adult are cancer, diverticulitis, and volvulus. Causes of ileus are myriad and include a variety of intra-abdominal and systemic conditions (Table 88.2).

All patients with a diagnosis of small- or large-bowel obstruction should have a nasogastric tube inserted for decompression. Distension of bowel loops with fluid and gas is important in the pathophysiology of bowel obstruction, and decompression via tube is an effective way to decrease the distension. Long intestinal nasoenteric tubes are rarely necessary and may increase the risk of aspiration. Nasogastric decompression also makes general anesthesia safer in patients requiring an operation because it lowers the risk of aspiration on induction.

An unusual but noteworthy disorder is *chronic intestinal pseudo-obstruction* (9). Patients with it (not to be confused with hospitalized patients who develop colonic pseudo-obstruction or Ogilvie's syndrome) are thought to have a diffuse motor disorder of the GI tract. The presentation may be very similar to that of mechanical bowel obstruction. In fact, many of these patients have had previous abdominal operations, and they can develop mechanical obstruction from adhesions and hernias, with an attendant risk of bowel strangulation or perforation. Management of this difficult subset of patients is best done in a referral center by surgeons and gastroenterologists experienced with this disease.

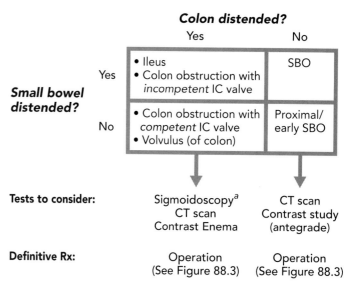

Figure 88.2   Differential diagnosis and treatment of small- and large-bowel distension. *ᵃ*May be therapeutic in sigmoid volvulus. *IC*, ileocecal; *SBO*, small-bowel obstruction.

Indications for Hospitalization and ICU Admission

All patients with the diagnosis of acute small- or large-bowel obstruction require hospitalization. Patients with complete obstruction require an urgent operation, usually within 6–12 hours. Patients with partial small-bowel obstruction may be treated nonoperatively, provided that they have no fever, tachycardia, leukocytosis, or pain or tenderness. Occasionally, patients with bowel obstruction and terminal disease who are not deemed candidates for an operation may be treated palliatively at home or in the hospital (Chapter 19) (10). Most patients with ileus severe enough to have caused a visit to an emergency department or whose symptoms have lasted more than 24 hours require hospitalization to treat the associated illness, dehydration, and underlying cause.

Patients with bowel obstruction should be admitted to the ICU if they have hemodynamic instability after the initial resuscitation or if invasive hemodynamic monitoring is required for safe fluid resuscitation. This usually includes patients with compromised cardiovascular, pulmonary, or renal status (Chapter 25). Patients with possible aspiration pneumonia, a frequent complication of bowel obstruction, also should be admitted to the ICU (Chapter 66). Patients with ileus may require admission to the ICU, depending on the severity of the primary disease causing the ileus.

Indications for Operation

Patients with complete small- or large-bowel obstruction require an *urgent operation* (Figure 88.3). This is because intestinal strangulation or perforation in this setting is a very real possibility (3). Patients with partial small-bowel obstruction who have unremitting abdominal pain, tenderness, fever, or leukocytosis also require surgery. Otherwise, the patient with partial obstruction may be treated with nasogastric tube suction and intravenous fluids with the hope that the partial obstruction resolves (7). If there is no sign of clinical or radiologic improvement in 48 hours, surgery should be considered. Patients with acute sigmoid volvulus can often be decompressed with a sigmoidoscope; an urgent operation is not required unless pain and peritoneal signs are present (11). Recurrence is common, and elective surgery should be considered. Treatment of partial colon obstruction depends upon the cause. If the patient has a partially obstructing colorectal carcinoma, early elective surgery should be performed. If the patient has acute diverticulitis, several days of antibiotic treatment usually result in improvement in gastrointestinal function. Patients with a colonic stricture from any cause who present with signs and symptoms of partial obstruction usually require elective surgery.

Patients with ileus may require an operation to treat the primary disease that has given rise to the ileus (e.g., pancreatic debridement in necrotizing pancreatitis, appendec-tomy for perforated appendicitis, or patch closure for perforated duodenal ulcer). Patients with primary colonic ileus (also called colonic pseudo-obstruction, or Ogilvie's syndrome) usually can be treated with colonoscopic decompression (12). If this is not possible, operative decompression may be necessary.

Obstructing Colon Carcinoma

Primary carcinoma of the colon may present with bowel obstruction. Colon cancers may involve the small bowel by direct extension and rarely also may cause symptoms of small-bowel obstruction. Metastatic colon carcinoma is a much more common cause of small-bowel obstruction (see later in this chapter). If the colon obstruction is deemed to be complete on clinical or radiologic grounds, an urgent operation is indicated (Figure 88.3). A diverting loop colostomy is the procedure of choice in debilitated or high-risk patients. Otherwise, the obstructing tumor may be removed at the initial operation. Because preoperative bowel preparation is impossible, primary colon anastomosis usually is contraindicated, and a double-barrel colostomy, or "Hartmann procedure" (proximal colostomy, distal closed defunctionalized segment), is performed. This is reversed with a second procedure at a later date (at least two months later) after the remaining colorectum is studied to rule out a synchronous lesion. If the primary tumor is resected with a proximal colectomy, a primary ileocolonic anastomosis is acceptable. Recently, some groups have practiced intraoperative colonic lavage and primary colonic anastomosis in patients with obstructing colon carcinoma, with acceptable results. If the primary colon tumor is not completely obstructing, it may be possible to cleanse the colon with a mechanical bowel preparation and perform a one-stage procedure (i.e., resection of tumor with primary anastomosis). Preoperative or intraoperative endoscopy is advisable to rule out other synchronous lesions when this technique is used (11).

Colon carcinoma frequently metastasizes to small intestine, omentum, mesentery, and peritoneum. Thus, in Western society, metastatic colon cancer is a fairly common cause of small-bowel obstruction. A more common cause of small-bowel obstruction in the patient who has undergone colon resection is adhesions. Thus, the primary differential diagnosis in the patient presenting with small-bowel obstruction months or years following a colon resection for carcinoma is adhesions vs. metastatic carcinoma. There is no completely accurate way of determining the cause preoperatively. Adhesions usually are treated with lysis; obstructing metastases are treated by resection, bypass, or enterostomy.

Initial Therapy

Early treatment of patients with bowel obstruction or ileus consists of nasogastric tube decompression and appropri-

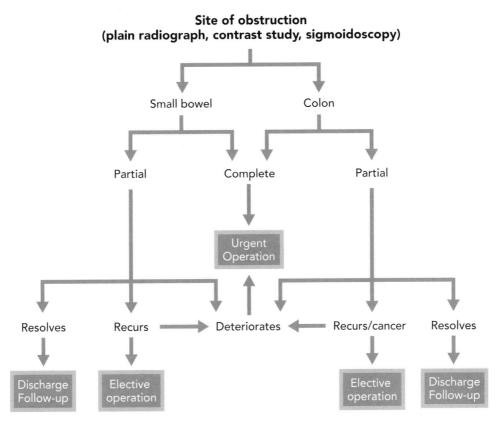

Figure 88.3 Management of bowel obstruction.

ate intravenous fluid resuscitation. Those with complete obstruction or peritonitis require early surgery. Patients with partial obstruction and those with ileus may be observed with frequent examinations and daily plain-film abdominal series if there is no sign of abdominal catastrophe. Patients with a colonic ileus may be helped with a rectal tube, but colonoscopic decompression is more effective.

Patients operated upon for bowel obstruction are given perioperative antibiotics. This may be extended to a therapeutic course if ischemic bowel is resected, if an abscess or peritonitis is encountered, or if spillage of gastrointestinal contents occurs. The use of antibiotics in patients with partial obstruction or ileus is controversial. Antibiotics should be given if the disease process that has contributed to the development of the ileus requires antibiotics (e.g., pneumonia); otherwise, there is no clear indication. Fever, tenderness, and leukocytosis should be regarded as indications for operation rather than as indications for antibiotics in most patients.

Indications for Early Consultation

A surgeon must see all patients with intestinal obstruction, preferably within 2 hours of presentation (4). Surgical consultation is also prudent in most patients with ileus. Gastroenterology consultation is usually unnecessary in patients with bowel obstruction or ileus but might be helpful

for colonoscopic decompression in patients with ileus and massive colonic distension (cecum greater than 10–12 cm in diameter).

Issues During the Course of Hospitalization

Fluid resuscitation and nasogastric tube decompression are important in all patients presenting with bowel obstruction or ileus. One of the most important issues after admission is to determine whether the patient has a complete bowel obstruction. Patients with partial obstruction who are not operated upon should be followed closely because they may develop complete obstruction or signs of bowel compromise during hospitalization. Most patients with partial small-bowel obstruction resolve with appropriate conservative management, but radiologic investigation or operation should be considered if no improvement occurs within 48 hours. Whether or not they undergo operations, hospitalized patients with bowel obstruction or ileus require close monitoring. The abdomen and chest must be examined by a physician at least twice daily, and vital signs, fluid balance, and nasogastric tube function assessed. Bowel strangulation or perforation and aspiration pneumonia are complications that can be prevented by aggressive gut decompression and early operation (3,13). Serum electrolytes and blood counts should be monitored daily until the nasogastric tube is removed and bowel function returns. Serial abdominal radiographs are important in patients who are treated nonoperatively or in postoperative patients who fail to improve clinically. Wound infection, fluid overload, pneumonia, and pulmonary embolism are not uncommon postoperative complications in patients operated on for bowel obstruction (14).

A variety of important issues must be considered if the patient with bowel obstruction or ileus fails to improve. These generally can be grouped as occurring in patients who have just been operated on for obstruction versus those inpatients with presumed partial obstruction or ileus who are being treated nonoperatively. In the patient who has been operated on for bowel obstruction, it is important to know the operative findings and what was done at the operation. What was the cause of the obstruction? Was the bowel completely viable? Was the bowel entered? (That is, was a bowel resection necessary? Was the bowel injured and repaired during a difficult dissection?) Generally, patients operated on for bowel obstruction have return of bowel function within 5 days of the operation. Patients with chronic obstruction or those with slow progressive development of bowel obstruction may require much more time postoperatively for bowel function to resume. If the patient is not progressing as expected, one should consider peritonitis, abscess, intestinal ischemia, persistent or recurrent obstruction, electrolyte disorders (e.g., hypokalemia), and "postoperative ileus" (15).

In the patient with partial obstruction or ileus who fails to improve, the main issue is whether the patient in fact has a complete obstruction or compromised bowel. Thus, patients with evidence of systemic toxicity or peritonitis should be operated on. Partial obstruction may progress to complete obstruction, and rarely, partial obstruction may be associated with bowel strangulation or perforation. Patients with ileus also may develop ischemic perforation of massively distended bowel, frequently the cecum.

Two difficult situations must be approached individually in consultation with a general surgeon. The first is the patient who requires multiple admissions for partial small-bowel obstruction that resolves with medical management (7). Most of these patients are best managed with an elective operation, although there may be relative contraindications to an operation (e.g., medical comorbidities or intra-abdominal scarring). The second problematic situation is the patient with bowel obstruction and advanced abdominal malignancy, in whom optimal palliation might or might not involve surgery (10).

Discharge Issues

The length of hospitalization varies depending on the primary disease. Patients requiring surgery are hospitalized for approximately 5–7 days. Patients who have resolution of partial obstruction without the need for surgery are often ready for discharge in three days. Patients with ileus generally have improvement in their gut motor function as the primary disease process resolves.

The patient with bowel obstruction or ileus may be discharged from the hospital when bowel function has returned and an oral diet is tolerated. Generally, distension and nausea have resolved at this point and the patient is passing flatus and has had a bowel movement. The patient should be tolerating a full liquid or regular diet. With earlier discharges in the modern era, postoperative complications that previously were recognized in the hospital may present after discharge (13). The patient should be instructed to contact the physician for fever, abdominal pain, nausea, or vomiting.

ILEUS OR OBSTRUCTION DEVELOPING IN THE HOSPITAL

Patients developing bowel obstruction or ileus in the hospital usually fall into two categories: those recovering from abdominal surgery, and those with other problems, usually medical. These patients are less likely to require an urgent operation, but the same principles discussed previously generally apply (15). Although most of these patients can be managed conservatively, the clinician must be vigilant for the possibility of bowel strangulation or perforation. These patients all should be managed in consultation with a general surgeon.

Issues During the Course of Hospitalization

The Patient Recovering from an Abdominal Operation

The patient recovering from an abdominal operation may develop progressive abdominal distension, hypoperistalsis, and obstipation (15). A functioning nasogastric tube should be placed (if not already present) and intravenous fluids given to maintain euvolemia. The patient should be examined and an obstruction series ordered. The differential diagnosis includes an abdominal catastrophe (leaking anastomosis with peritonitis, ischemic bowel, perforation), localized abscess, anastomotic obstruction, adhesions, internal or wound herniation, and postoperative ileus. The patient who has an abdominal disaster generally has systemic signs of toxicity as well as peritoneal signs. The plain films may show free intra-abdominal air (not pathognomonic, because this may persist for several days after laparotomy), and a CT scan may show pneumatosis intestinalis, pneumoperitoneum, a generous amount of free intraperitoneal fluid, or a fluid collection with air bubbles. Patients with these findings require an immediate operation. Broad-spectrum antibiotics are administered, and a functioning nasogastric tube must be in place to avoid pulmonary aspiration during the induction of general anesthesia.

A localized abdominal or pelvic abscess may be associated with mechanical obstruction or ileus postoperatively. There may be focal tenderness, fever, and leukocytosis. Rectal examination may reveal a tender bulge in the cul-de-sac, and the diagnosis can be confirmed with CT scan and needle aspiration. Percutaneous drainage usually is successful if a safe course to the collection can be charted without passing through distended bowel loops. Otherwise, operative drainage may be necessary. Transrectal drainage of pelvic abscesses remains a useful technique.

The patient who has had a bowel resection may develop mechanical or functional obstruction at the anastomotic site during the postoperative period. Common causes are edema, leaks, adhesions, and other technical problems. In the absence of signs of sepsis, these patients are usually managed expectantly, with nasogastric decompression and intravenous fluids. Serial radiographs are useful in monitoring the degree of distension and the progression of gas distally. If a small anastomotic leak is suspected, intravenous antibiotics are appropriate. These patients rarely develop ischemia or perforation unless they have a colorectal anastomosis and a competent ileocecal valve. In this case, massive colonic distension proximal to the anastomosis may result in a cecal perforation or a disruption of the anastomosis. Cecostomy or decompressing loop colostomy should be considered if cecal diameter exceeds 10–12 centimeters.

Postoperative adhesions form within days of an operation, and these may cause mechanical obstruction at any time. Postoperative mechanical small-bowel obstruction secondary to adhesions may be difficult to distinguish from postoperative ileus. This fact, coupled with the observation that bowel strangulation or perforation is unusual in this setting, make expectant nonoperative therapy the treatment of choice (15). Surgery is indicated for peritoneal signs or if the patient fails to improve by 10–14 days.

Internal herniation or volvulus should always be considered as a cause of bowel obstruction in a patient who has undergone a bowel resection. The bowel may herniate through the mesenteric defect of the resected bowel, and strangulation may occur. Rarely, during the course of intestinal resection the remaining bowel (usually small bowel) is inadvertently rotated on its axis, causing a *volvulus*, which results in ischemia. The patient presents with pain and acidosis within 24–48 hours of the index operation and requires an immediate operation. Massive bowel loss is the usual outcome. *Internal herniation* presents as a mechanical obstruction and should be suspected if localized distended bowel loops are seen on radiograph or CT scan. The loops may be located eccentrically within the abdomen. If this diagnosis is suspected, an urgent operation is also indicated.

Postoperative ileus is probably the most common cause of abdominal distension, nausea and vomiting, and obstipation seen in the patient recovering from an abdominal or pelvic operation. The pathophysiology is poorly understood, but the result is a disruption in normal peristalsis. In

patients recovering from laparotomy, effective peristalsis returns first to the small intestine, then to the stomach, and finally to the colon. In some patients, pain, medications (e.g., opiates), electrolyte disturbances, and other disease states may result in a prolonged delay in the return of bowel function. Progressive distension usually can be prevented by maintaining a functioning nasogastric tube. Rectal tube and colonoscopic decompression may be useful in patients with massive colonic dilatation, but should be used very cautiously, if at all, in patients who have just undergone colon resection. Early ambulation, decreasing the opiate dose, and correcting electrolyte disturbances helps in some patients. Enemas and suppositories may be useful in patients who do not have a left-sided colon anastomosis. Oral stimulants (bisacodyl, magnesium compounds) and promotility agents (cholinergic agonists, cisapride) may have a role in some patients but should be used cautiously and in consultation with the surgeon.

Opiate analgesia is thought to play an important role in ileus after abdominal surgery. Systemic opiates affect pain and splanchnic receptors equally, contributing to disrupted peristalsis. An investigational agent, ADL 8-2698 (Adalor) selectively reverses opioid inhibition of gastrointestinal motility without blocking systemic analgesia. The effectiveness of this agent is currently being determined.

Cisapride is a promotility agent that works through a cholinergic mechanism and commonly is used to treat gastroparesis, gastroesophageal reflux, and idiopathic constipation (16). It has been tried with more modest success in postoperative ileus, colonic inertia, and intestinal pseudo-obstruction. The usual adult dose is 10 mg orally 4 times daily. It is generally contraindicated in mechanical small-bowel obstruction because increased motor activity from the drug may lead to increased intraluminal intestinal pressure.

Intestinal distension and altered motility are important pathophysiologic components of both mechanical small-bowel obstruction and ileus. *Octreotide*, a long-acting somatostatin analog, has been tried in these diseases. Research in both animals and humans shows that this drug decreases luminal fluid accumulation in small-bowel obstruction and increases effective peristalsis in ileus. Patients with routine mechanical small-bowel obstruction or postoperative ileus should not be considered candidates for treatment with this agent because its effectiveness has not been shown in these settings. However, patients with terminal cancer and malignant bowel obstruction, or those with unusual causes of ileus (e.g., scleroderma, idiopathic pseudo-obstruction, small-bowel transplant), may get significant improvement in symptoms with octreotide in divided subcutaneous doses of 300–600 mg daily (17).

The Patient Hospitalized with Other Diagnoses

A hospitalized patient who develops abdominal distension while being treated for some seemingly unrelated problem may have an ileus or an intra-abdominal catastrophe. Such a patient should be evaluated and managed as outlined previously. The most important initial consideration is whether the patient has abdominal pain or tenderness. If so, the patient should be seen expeditiously by a surgeon. Unlike the patient discussed previously who comes to the hospital with abdominal pain and distension and has mechanical bowel obstruction, the patient who develops abdominal distension while being treated in the hospital for another problem is more likely to have an acute surgical condition of the abdomen or an ileus rather than simple mechanical obstruction. Other medical problems that have led to hospitalization may distract the managing team and delay recognition of a new problem, and they also make an operation more risky. These facts, together with the greater acuity of illness in modern hospitalized patients and the greater percentage of immunosuppressed patients, help explain the high mortality rate in patients requiring an urgent abdominal operation in this setting. Thus, the surgeon should be involved as early as possible.

If the patient is able to cooperate, a diagnosis usually can be reached by taking a history, performing an examination, reviewing the chart and recent laboratory data, and evaluating a plain radiograph series. Ileus may be suspected according to the algorithm in Figure 88.2. Ileus may be associated with other serious intra-abdominal pathology requiring an urgent operation. As a general rule, a CT scan can rule out such pathology, with the exception of ischemic bowel (Chapter 87). The diagnosis of intestinal ischemia should be pursued vigorously unless the lucid patient denies significant abdominal pain.

Colonic pseudo-obstruction (Ogilvie's syndrome) is not uncommon in the hospitalized, bedbound, elderly patient. It presents with abdominal distension, and radiographs show a distended air-filled colon with or without small-bowel distension. Although some patients respond to rectal tube insertion and frequent repositioning, colonoscopic decompression is the treatment of choice (12). If this is unsuccessful or if there is abdominal tenderness, laparotomy and operative decompression must be considered. Laparoscopic exploration (to rule out actual or impending perforation) and cecostomy are less invasive options.

Toxic megacolon is another important diagnostic consideration in the hospitalized patient. This occurs in the setting of inflammatory bowel disease or antibiotic-associated colitis (Chapters 81 and 77, respectively). Patients appear ill, with fever and tachycardia. There is abdominal distension, hypoperistalsis, and tenderness, frequently along the course of the colon. Plain radiographs show an air-filled, often featureless colon. CT scan shows a thick-walled colon. Clinical deterioration, increasing toxicity, worsening abdominal examination, and radiologic signs of impending or actual perforation all are indications for surgery. Abdominal colectomy and ileostomy is the procedure of choice, even though the colon may not appear compromised at the time of the operation.

Discharge Issues

The patient who has developed ileus or bowel obstruction while in the hospital for another problem may be discharged when gastrointestinal function has returned and the initial problems are under control. The patient should be tolerating at least a full liquid diet. If oral medications are required, there must be a means of assuring that the patient is taking and tolerating the medication. Follow-up and monitoring of nutritional status are important in many of these patients (13).

COST CONSIDERATIONS AND RESOURCE USE

Early surgery, avoidance of unnecessary tests, and judicious use of antibiotics all are part of good clinical care in the patient with bowel obstruction. Adequate and expeditious fluid resuscitation and nasogastric decompression are clinically important and help save resources.

The use of laparoscopy in the patient with bowel obstruction is controversial, and much of the controversy revolves around the safety and cost (14). The technique is safe in experienced hands and probably leads to some cost savings for patients in whom laparotomy is avoided (a small minority of patients with bowel obstruction or ileus). These patients can be discharged earlier and may return to work sooner (18). However, the technique may increase costs in the operating room. Minimizing these costs by the selective use of this technology by experienced surgeons might lead to an overall reduction in the cost of caring for small-bowel obstruction in selected patients (19).

KEY POINTS

- Patients presenting to the hospital with bowel obstruction or ileus should be seen promptly by a general surgeon. All patients with bowel obstruction or ileus require hospitalization.
- Careful fluid resuscitation and nasogastric decompression are important in all patients with bowel obstruction or a significant ileus. Selective use of specialized procedures such as CT scan, flexible colonoscopy, contrast radiography, and arteriography may be useful in some patients.
- The patient with complete obstruction requires an urgent operation. The patient with partial obstruction may require an urgent operation based on clinical or radiologic findings; those managed nonoperatively are best admitted to a surgical service for close monitoring.
- Patients with ileus often have a surgical problem causing the ileus (e.g., diverticulitis, appendicitis, perforated ulcer, ischemic bowel). Those patients without an obvious surgical problem still warrant careful monitoring, lest dangerous distension with ischemia and perforation supervene.

- Patients who develop bowel obstruction or ileus while in the hospital, including those recovering from an abdominal or pelvic operation, may have an acute surgical condition of the abdomen.
- Ischemia always must be considered as a possible cause of ileus or obstruction, and early arteriography should be performed in the appropriate circumstance.

REFERENCES

1. Richards WO, Williams LF Jr. Obstruction of the large and small intestine. *Surg Clin North Am* 1988;68:355–376.
2. Miller G, Boman J, Shrier I, Gordon PH. Etiology of small bowel obstruction. *Am J Surg* 2000;180:33–36.
3. Sarr MG, Bulkley GB, Zuidema GD. Preoperative recognition of intestinal strangulation obstruction: prospective evaluation of diagnostic capability. *Am J Surg* 1983;145:176–182.
4. Malangoni MA, Times ML, Kozik D, Merlino JI. Admitting service influences the outcome of patients with small bowel obstruction. *Surgery* 2001;130:706–711.
5. Maglinte DD, Kelvin FM, Rowe MG, Bender GN, Rouch DM. Small bowel obstruction: optimizing radiologic investigation and nonsurgical management. *Radiology* 2001;218:39–46.
6. Maglinte DD, Heitkamp DE, Howard TJ, Kelvin FM, Lappas JC. Current concepts in imaging of small bowel obstruction. *Radiol Clin North Am* 2003;41:263–283.
7. Seror D, Feigin E, Szold A, et al. How conservatively can postoperative small bowel obstruction be treated? *Am J Surg* 1993;165:121–126.
8. Choi HK, Chu KW, Law WL. Therapeutic value of gastrograffin in adhesive small bowel obstruction after unsuccessful conservative treatment: a prospective randomized trial. *Ann Surg* 2002;90:542–546.
9. Kamm MA. Intestinal pseudo-obstruction. *Gut* 2000;47:84–87.
10. Krouse RS, McCahill LE, Easson AM, Dunn GP. When the sun can set on an unoperated bowel obstruction: management of malignant bowel obstruction. *J Am Coll Surg* 2002;195:117–128.
11. Strodel WE, Nostrant TT, Eckhauser FE, Dent TL. Therapeutic and diagnostic colonoscopy in nonobstructive colonic dilatation. *Ann Surg* 1983;197:416.
12. Fielding LP, Shultz SM. Treatment of acute colonic pseudoobstruction. *J Am Coll Surg* 2001;192:422–423.
13. Landercasper J, Cogbill TH, Merry WH, Stolee RT, Strutt PJ. Long-term outcome after hospitalization for small bowel obstruction. *Arch Surg* 1993;128:765–771.
14. Wilson MS, Hawkswell J, McCloy RF. Natural history of adhesional small bowel obstruction: counting the cost. *Br J Surg* 1998;85:1294–1298.
15. Kehlet H, Holte K. Review of postoperative ileus. *Am J Surg* 2001;182(5 Suppl):3–10.
16. Tack J, Coremans G, Janssens J. A risk benefit assessment of cisapride in the treatment of gastrointestinal disorders. *Drug Safety* 1995;12:384–392.
17. Mangili G, Franchi M, Mariani A, et al. Octreotide in the management of bowel obstruction in terminal ovarian cancer. *Gynecol Onc* 1996;61:345–348.
18. Sato Y, Ido K, Kumagai M, et al. Laparoscopic adhesolysis for recurrent small bowel obstruction: long-term follow-up. *Gastrointest Endosc* 2001;195:117–128.
19. Leon EL, Metzger A, Tsiotos GG, Schlinkert RT, Sarr MG. Laparoscopic management of small bowel obstruction: indications and outcome. *J Gastrointest Surg* 1998;2:132–140.

ADDITIONAL READING

Bungard TJ, Kale-Pradhan PB. Prokinetic agents for the treatment of postoperative ileus in adults: a review of the literature. *Pharmacotherapy* 1999;19:416–423.

Mazzacco SL, Dempsey DT. Mechanical disorders of the stomach duodenum and intestine. In: Miller TA, ed. *Modern Surgical Care: Physiologic Foundations and Clinical Applications.* 2nd ed. St. Louis: Quality Medical Publishing, 1998.

Hematology–Oncology

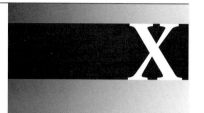

Signs, Symptoms, and Laboratory Abnormalities in Hematology–Oncology

89

Hope S. Rugo

TOPICS COVERED IN CHAPTER

- Splenomegaly 885
- Lymphadenopathy 887
- Anemia 889
- Neutropenia 893
- Leukocytosis 894
- Pancytopenia 895

INTRODUCTION

Nonspecific symptoms such as fatigue resulting from anemia, or signs such as splenomegaly or lymphadenopathy, are often the first clinical manifestations of serious underlying disease. Early recognition and evaluation are critical to patient management. Appropriate and timely therapy can maintain quality of life and function and in some cases prolong survival.

Abnormalities in the complete blood count are among the most common presenting laboratory findings on admission to the hospital. In addition, hospitalization commonly causes additional hematologic disorders, resulting from either the illness that led to admission or the treatments rendered during the inpatient stay. Careful review of

blood counts and the peripheral blood smear can result in earlier diagnosis and treatment of both hematologic and nonhematologic illnesses. Disorders of platelets and coagulation are discussed in Chapter 98, and polycythemia is covered in Chapter 95.

SIGNS AND LABORATORY ABNORMALITIES

Splenomegaly

Presenting at the Time of Admission

Examination of the left upper quadrant for splenomegaly may be difficult in an obese or uncooperative patient. Palpation with the patient in the left decubitus position or with the knees raised during deep inspiration may help circumvent these difficulties. Occasionally, dilated loops of bowel mimic an enlarged spleen. Confirmation of suspected splenomegaly is best obtained by ultrasound examination.

The differential diagnosis of splenomegaly is listed in Table 89.1. Patients may present with left upper quadrant fullness, anorexia, or early satiety resulting from a markedly

TABLE 89.1

DIFFERENTIAL DIAGNOSIS OF SPLENOMEGALY

Disease category	Examples	Specific blood-smear findings
Malignancy	Chronic myelogenous leukemia	Left shift and basophilia
Myeloproliferative/dysplastic	Myelofibrosis with agnogenic myeloid metaplasia	Nucleated red blood cells, tear drop-shaped red blood cells
	Myelodysplastic syndromes	Dysplastic neutrophils
	Chronic myelomonocytic leukemia	Dysplastic monocytes
	Acute myelogenous leukemia	Blasts with granules
Lymphoproliferative	Chronic lymphocytic leukemia	Lymphocytes and smudge cells
	Non-Hodgkin's lymphoma	
	Hodgkin's disease	
	Acute lymphocytic leukemia	Blasts with prominent nucleoli
	Hairy cell leukemia	Spiculated lymphocytes
Infection	Schistosomiasis	
	Leishmaniasis	
	Disseminated mycobacteria	
	Bacterial endocarditis	Dohle bodies, vacuoles
	Acute viral hepatitis	
	Malaria	Red cell inclusions on thick smear
Hemolytic anemia		
Hereditary	Hereditary spherocytosis	Spherocytes
	Sickle cell disease with splenic sequestration crisis	Sickled red cells
	Thalassemia (severe)	Microcytes, fragments
	Autoimmune hemolytic anemia, with (Evans' syndrome) or without ITP	Spherocytes
Acquired	Autoimmune neutropenia with rheumatoid arthritis (Felty's syndrome)	
Infiltrative disorders	Lipid storage disorders (Gaucher's disease)	
	Amyloid	
Portal vein obstruction	Cirrhosis	Target cells
(sequestration)	Portal vein thrombosis	Target cells

ITP, immune-mediated thrombocytopenic purpura.

enlarged spleen. The size and character of the enlarged spleen, as well as the presence of tenderness or left-sided pleuritic pain, help in the differential diagnosis. A massively enlarged and firm spleen is almost always caused by an underlying infiltrative malignancy such as a lymphoproliferative or myeloproliferative disorder (1). Marked enlargement of the spleen also may be seen in chronic infections such as malaria and from infiltrative processes such as Gaucher's disease. Splenic or pleuritic pain may be caused by splenic infarct; this pain is usually acute and lasts 2–3 days. Splenic infarcts generally are caused by emboli, acceleration of myeloproliferative or myelodysplastic diseases, or splenic abcesses.

Evaluation of splenomegaly should include a focused physical examination to look for the presence of lymphadenopathy or hepatomegaly. The evaluation of lymphadenopathy is discussed subsequently. The presence of both splenomegaly and significant lymphadenopathy is likely to result from a lymphoproliferative disease or a chronic infection. If hepatomegaly is found, evaluation should focus on disorders involving the liver (Chapter 77). The finding of lymphadenopathy or hepatomegaly should prompt a computed tomography scan to look for additional abdominal pathology. Positron emisson tomography (PET) scanning may be a useful way to distinguish benign from malignant lymphadenopathy. The physical examination also may reveal spider angiomata and other stigmata of liver disease, or ecchymoses and petechiae, suggesting coexistent marrow pathology or cellular sequestration.

A complete blood count and examination of the peripheral blood smear are essential. If the white cells are elevated and the blood smear shows a lymphocytosis, *chronic lymphocytic leukemia* is possible. The diagnosis is established by flow-cytometric analysis of the peripheral blood. Alternatively, if the white-cell count is elevated but the blood smear shows a "left shift," nucleated red blood cells and basophilia, a *myeloproliferative disease* such as chronic myelogenous leukemia is likely (2) (Chapter 95). The presence of blast cells on the peripheral smear suggests *acute leukemia* (Chapter 93). The diagnosis is made by bone-marrow evaluation with cytogenetics.

Malignant disease with splenomegaly often is accompanied by anemia. However, if anemia is the predominant abnormality and the blood smear shows abnormal red-cell morphology such as spherocytes (Table 89.2), then a hemolytic anemia is the likely cause of splenomegaly. The evaluation of hemolytic anemia is covered subsequently. Hemolytic anemia or immune thrombocytopenia may complicate the marked splenomegaly found in lymphoproliferative diseases such as chronic lymphocytic leukemia. A patient with a chronic hemolytic anemia such as sickle-cell disease may develop splenic sequestration crisis and present with splenomegaly, fever, and severe anemia (Chapter 97). This is because of marrow suppression from acute infection with parvovirus B19; it is usually self-limited.

Patients with *chronic infections* (e.g., malaria, tuberculosis, or endocarditis) may have splenomegaly associated with recurrent fevers. Diagnosis is made by examination of the blood smear for parasites, blood cultures, chest radiograph, and placement of a purified protein derivative (PPD) skin test. A biopsy of an enlarged lymph node or bone-marrow culture may be necessary to make the diagnosis of disseminated mycobacterial infection. Liver chemistry tests should be obtained to rule out acute viral hepatitis or portal vein obstruction caused by cirrhosis or thrombosis. Ultrasound with evaluation of blood flow can help evaluate the presence of *portal vein thrombosis*. Patients with portal vein thrombosis should undergo further testing for hypercoagulable states or myeloproliferative disease such as polycythemia vera (Chapters 95 and 98). Infiltrative disease and lipid-storage disorders usually are evaluated by bone-marrow aspiration and biopsy, as well as fat pad biopsy for amyloid.

Management of splenomegaly is entirely dependent on the underlying cause. Regardless of the cause, a massively enlarged spleen traps white blood cells, red blood cells, and platelets, leading to variable cytopenias. Patients with splenomegaly may not respond to transfusions of red blood cells and platelets; the latter can complicate plans for procedures. If a procedure is planned for a patient with splenomegaly and thrombocytopenia, it is important to check the response to transfused platelets immediately after the transfusion to ensure that the resulting count is adequate. Occasionally, patients with splenomegaly require splenectomy. This is usually beneficial in autoimmune hemolytic anemia and is curative in hereditary spherocytosis. In addition, patients with significant cytopenias from sequestration caused by chronic myeloproliferative or lymphoproliferative diseases that are unresponsive to chemotherapy may benefit from splenectomy. In general, splenectomy is not advisable for patients with significant

obstruction to portal vein blood flow. Splenic irradiation is a rarely used technique to manage massive splenomegaly associated with malignancy in a patient who is not a surgical candidate. Pain resulting from splenic infarcts is generally transient and responds to pain medications.

Presenting During Hospitalization

Mild or moderate splenomegaly may develop during hospitalization. The differential diagnosis is much narrower than for splenomegaly observed at presentation. Patients with chronic hemolytic anemia are at risk for *splenic sequestration crisis* resulting from infection with parvovirus B19 (see above). An already enlarged spleen resulting from myeloproliferative or lymphoproliferative disease may increase in size after multiple transfusions, because of sequestration of blood products.

Hospitalized patients often are given medications that can cause hemolytic anemia (see the section on "Anemia" later in this chapter). The development of a hyperproductive anemia with splenomegaly in a hospitalized patient should provoke an investigation into possible drug-induced hemolysis. Patients with acute presentations of autoimmune diseases may develop splenomegaly while hospitalized for evaluation of fever. The diagnosis may be elusive and is often one of exclusion. As with splenomegaly presenting on admission to the hospital, management is entirely dependent on the etiology of splenomegaly.

Lymphadenopathy

Presenting at the Time of Admission

The most common cause of lymphadenopathy on admission to the hospital is a contiguous infected area. However, both isolated nodal enlargement and generalized lymphadenopathy are associated with lymphoma, leukemia, HIV disease, other chronic infections, and autoimmune disease (3). The differential diagnosis of lymphadenopathy depends on the age of the patient, the time course, associated symptoms, the presence of localized or generalized adenopathy, consistency of the nodes, and the areas of involvement (Table 89.3). As with other symptoms and signs, an older patient is less likely to have a benign cause of adenopathy. Reactive lymph-node hyperplasia is most common in children. Acute, painful adenopathy is more likely associated with infection than are slowly progressive, nontender nodes. Associated symptoms such as weight loss, fevers, and night sweats may be seen with lymphoproliferative disease, chronic infections, and autoimmune disease.

Malignancy more often presents as a single nontender enlarged node rather than the generalized mild adenopathy seen in response to infection or autoimmune disease. A hard, fixed node usually represents involvement with

TABLE 89.2

APPROACH TO ANEMIA

Reticulocyte count	MCV	Blood smear	Diagnosis	Workup
Low	Low	Hypochromia, target cells, basophilic stippling, pencil cells, thrombocytosis	Iron deficiency	Iron, iron binding capacity, ferritin (and consider serum transferrin receptor)
		Target cells, basophilic stippling	Thalassemia trait	Hemoglobin electrophoresis
		Mixed population of red blood cells	Sideroblastic anemia or myelodysplasia	Bone marrow aspirate with iron stain to look for ringed sideroblasts
Low–normal	Low	Unremarkable	Anemia of chronic disease	
		Basophilic stippling	Lead poisoning	Occupational history, free erythrocyte protoporphyrin, lead levels
Low	Normal	Tear drops and red cell fragments in myelophthisic process (leukoerythroblastic), rouleaux in myeloma	*Primary marrow failure:* aplastic anemia, pure red cell aplasia, myelophthisic (infiltrative) process, myelodysplasia, leukemias, myeloma, early iron deficiency	Iron studies, bone marrow aspiration and biopsy with iron stain and cytogenetics
		Burr cells in renal disease, pencil cells in HIV	*Secondary marrow failure:* hypo- and hyperthyroidism, anemia of chronic disease, anemia of renal failure, HIV infection	Thyroid function tests, creatinine, HIV serology, erythropoietin level
		Normal	Splenomegaly with sequestration	
Low[a]	High	Macro-ovalocytes, hypersegmented neutrophils	*Megaloblastic anemia:* vitamin B_{12} or folate deficiency, myelodysplastic syndrome, drug-induced	B_{12} and folate level, LDH, Schilling test, bone marrow aspirate and biopsy with cytogenetics if normal levels found
		Acanthocytes, spur cells and target cells in liver disease, reticulocytes	*Nonmegaloblastic anemia:* liver disease, hypothyroidism, reticulocytosis	Liver function tests, thyroid function tests
High	Normal–high	Normal	Acute blood loss	
		Spherocytes (warm) or red-cell agglutination (cold)	*Acquired hemolytic anemia:* autoimmune or drug-induced hemolytic anemia (warm or cold)	Direct Coombs test (DAT), cold agglutinins, LDH, direct bilirubin
		Schistocytes	*Mechanical hemolysis:* valve or microangiopathic hemolytic anemia (TTP/HUS)	LDH, creatinine, coagulation tests to rule out DIC
		Red blood cell inclusions (malaria, babesiosis)	*Infection:* Clostridium, malaria, babesiosis, *Bartonella*, sepsis	Blood cultures, examination of thick smear
		Dysplastic neutrophils	Paroxysmal nocturnal hemoglobinuria	Urine hemosiderin, flow cytometry for CD 55/59
		Abnormal size and shape of red blood cells (hemoglobinopathy), bite cells (G6PD), spherocytes (HS)	*Hereditary hemolytic anemia:* hemoglobinopathies (e.g., sickle-cell disease), enzyme defects (e.g., G6PD deficiency) membrane defects (HS), unstable hemoglobins	Hemoglobin electrophoresis, G6PD level in nonacute setting, Heinz body prep, osmotic fragility testing
High	Low	Target cells, basophilic stippling, fragments	α- or β-thalassemia	Hemoglobin electrophoresis, family history

[a] Except when macrocytosis is due to hemolytic anemia and reticulocytosis.
DAT, direct antiglobulin test; *DIC,* disseminated intravascular coagulation; *G6PD,* glucose-6-phosphate dehydrogenase; *HIV,* human immunodeficiency virus; *HS,* hereditary spherocytosis; *HUS,* hemolytic uremic syndrome; *LDH,* lactate dehydrogenase; *TTP,* thrombotic thrombocytopenic purpura.

TABLE 89.3

DIFFERENTIAL DIAGNOSIS OF LYMPHADENOPATHY

Infection	Autoimmune
Epstein-Barr virus	Systemic lupus
Cytomegalovirus	erythematosus
HIV	Rheumatoid arthritis
Toxoplasmosis	Sarcoid
Tuberculosis	Pseudolymphoma
Histoplasmosis	Malignancy
Coccidioidomycosis	Hematologic (lymphoid and
Brucellosis	myeloid)
Bacterial endocarditis	Other
Viral hepatitis	Drug reaction
Secondary syphilis	Dilantin
Cat scratch disease	Hydralazine
Bacterial skin infections	Allopurinol

metastatic carcinoma or sarcoma. In contrast, rubbery, mobile, and matted nodes often are found in lymphoproliferative diseases. Soft, mobile nodes are more common in reactive adenopathy; the nodes associated with mycobacterial infection may be fluctuant. Firm or hard supraclavicular adenopathy often indicates underlying intrathoracic or intraabdominal carcinoma, although a single enlarged, rubbery supraclavicular node in a young adult is one of the most common presentations of Hodgkin's disease. Unilateral enlarged axillary nodes may indicate advanced breast cancer. An isolated hard periumbilical node (Sister Mary Joseph node) is associated with metastatic adenocarcinoma, usually of gastric origin. Intraabdominal lymphadenopathy may be palpated as an abdominal mass and be confused with colon or ovarian cancer. In contrast, occipital adenopathy rarely is associated with malignancy. Epitrochlear nodes may be seen with infection (e.g., cat scratch disease, cellulitis), sarcoidosis, or with lymphoproliferative disease.

Evaluation of lymphadenopathy should include a careful physical examination with digital rectal and bimanual examinations. A chest radiograph and appropriate scans also should be obtained. Computed tomography, magnetic resonance imaging, gallium, and positron emission tomography scans also may be indicated, depending on the circumstances. *Fine-needle aspiration* (FNA) of the enlarged node should be performed and the aspirate sent for microbiologic studies, cytology, and flow-cytometric analysis if indicated. If adenopathy is caused by carcinoma or sarcoma, fine-needle aspiration may allow diagnosis without invasive surgery to remove a biopsy sample from the primary tumor. *In general, a biopsy should be performed if the fine-needle aspiration is nondiagnostic or suggests lymphoma.* The tissue sections obtained with a biopsy allows the subtype of lymphoma to be determined, which significantly influences treatment recommendations and prognosis. If possible, it is prudent to avoid biopsy of an inguinal node, because of the

common occurrence of reactive hyperplasia that may confuse the diagnosis. If mediastinal and abdominal adenopathy are the only sites of disease, mediastinoscopy or laparoscopy with biopsy may be required.

Generalized lymphadenopathy is often a presenting sign of HIV disease (Chapter 74). Other infections should be evaluated with serologic tests, cultures, and node biopsy if necessary. Endocrinopathies such as thyrotoxicosis and adrenal insufficiency may be associated with mild lymphadenopathy.

Treatment of lymphadenopathy depends on the underlying diagnosis.

Presenting During Hospitalization

Lymphadenopathy presenting during hospitalization may be caused by a drug reaction or evolving autoimmune disease. A newly enlarged lymph node may indicate progression of an underlying malignancy. The most common cause of new lymphadenopathy during hospitalization is infection. This usually results from bacterial contamination of a peripheral or central line site. In addition, patients with untreated chronic infection may develop adenopathy if they are receiving corticosteroids.

Anemia

Anemia can be classified by the size of the red cell (mean corpuscular volume [MCV]) or by the response of the bone marrow (hyperproductive versus hypoproductive) to a decreased red cell mass. An MCV less than 70 fL is consistent with iron deficiency or thalassemia; an MCV over 125 fL is almost always diagnostic of megaloblastic anemia. The reticulocyte count helps differentiate a hypoproductive anemia from a hyperproductive anemia. The reticulocyte count may be expressed as a percentage of the red blood cell count, but this does not correct for the degree of anemia. A more useful number is the absolute reticulocyte count, which is calculated as follows: Absolute reticulocyte count = % reticulocytes $\times$ red blood cell count/μL^3.

A result greater than 100,000 per cubic millimeter indicates increased production of red cells. Reticulocytes are larger than mature red blood cells; a significant reticulocytosis increases the MCV. Review of the peripheral blood smear is a critical diagnostic procedure in the evaluation of anemia. The differential diagnosis of anemia based on the MCV, reticulocyte count, and review of the peripheral smear is shown in Table 89.2 (4).

Presenting at the Time of Admission

Anemia is the most common laboratory abnormality in the newly admitted patient. It may be the first sign of a serious systemic illness or may indicate reaction to medications, infection, or a primary bone-marrow process. A careful evaluation should include a detailed history with attention to diet, prescription and nonprescription medications, alternative therapies, occupation (e.g., lead exposure), menstrual history, recent travel (e.g., malaria, tuberculosis), hospitalizations or surgeries, prior history of anemia, and family history (of anemia, autoimmune disease, or infections). The duration of symptoms such as fatigue and shortness of breath, and the presence of pica or neurologic symptoms also can help narrow the differential diagnosis. Many patients with *hereditary hemolytic anemias* have a history of cholecystitis, with resulting cholecystectomy, caused by bilirubin gallstones. Physical examination should include a thorough examination of the skin (ecchymoses, spider angiomata, jaundice), oropharynx (glossitis and angular cheilosis in nutritional deficiencies, petechiae, gum swelling, telangiectasias), nails (spoon nails in iron deficiency), lymph nodes, and abdomen (hepatomegaly or splenomegaly), and a neurologic examination with attention to position and vibration sense (vitamin B_{12} deficiency).

The most common cause of anemia worldwide is *iron deficiency* (5). This microcytic, hypochromic, hypoproductive anemia may initially present as mild normocytic anemia. The most common causes of iron deficiency include blood loss from the gastrointestinal tract, menstruation, blood donation, and increased requirements with inadequate dietary iron (e.g., pregnancy and lactation). The cause of blood loss from the gastrointestinal tract always should be thoroughly investigated for serious pathology, although prolonged use of aspirin or other nonsteroidal antiinflammatory drugs may cause enough blood loss to result in iron deficiency. Blood loss also may be caused by significant hematuria or chronic intravascular hemolysis (e.g., mechanical heart valve or paroxysmal nocturnal hemoglobinuria).

It is important to evaluate microcytic anemia with appropriate iron studies before instituting therapy (6). Tests should include a serum iron level, transferrin level, percentage saturation, and ferritin level. A low ferritin level (<30 μg/L is a sensitive cut-off) may be the only way to detect early iron deficiency. As the depletion in iron stores progresses, the transferrin level rises as the iron level and saturation fall. Characteristic changes in red blood cell morphology may be found on the peripheral blood smear. As iron deficiency progresses, red blood cell abnormalities become more pronounced. If iron studies are normal, the most likely diagnosis is *thalassemia* or *anemia of chronic disease* (AOCD). With thalassemia, the MCV is usually very low for the degree of anemia, and the red blood cell morphology is abnormal (Table 89.2). One useful formula for differentiating pure thalassemia from iron deficiency is the *Mentzer index*: MCV/red blood cell count is usually less than 20 in thalassemia and more than 20 in iron deficiency. The hemoglobin electrophoresis can be diagnostic for severe α- and β-thalassemia but is normal in α-thalassemia minor. The most important reasons for diagnosing thalassemia are to avoid inappropriate iron supplementation (resulting in iron overload) and to facilitate genetic counseling.

AOCD may be microcytic or, more commonly, normocytic and is seen with malignancy, autoimmune disease, chronic infections, or other debilitating illnesses (7). It may be particularly difficult to differentiate the anemia of chronic disease from the anemia of iron deficiency. The *serum transferrin receptor* (sTfR) may help delineate these two disorders. Nutritional iron deficiency is associated with an increased level of sTfR; this level is not affected by AOCD. The sTfR results are affected by a number of other hematologic disorders (including erythropoeisis, thalassemia, hemolytic anemia, and megaloblastic anemia), limiting the specificity of this test for general hematologic evaluation. Elevation of this value appears to be relatively sensitive and specific for the diagnosis of iron deficiency (6), but lack of standardization for the assay limits its widespread use. A less expensive test that can be used as a quick screen for iron deficiency even in the absence of anemia is the erythrocyte zinc protoporphyrin/hemoglobin ratio; this ratio also is affected by other hematologic disorders.

Table 89.4 shows the key differences and similarities in laboratory studies. AOCD is associated with an inappropriately low erythropoietin level for the degree of anemia. The erythropoietin level is extremely low if anemia is caused by renal insufficiency. Other causes of a normocytic, hypoproductive anemia, such as hypothyroidism or a primary bone-marrow infiltrative process, should be considered. If other cell counts are abnormal, aplastic anemia, myelodysplasia, leukemia, myelofibrosis, and other infiltrative processes also should be considered. Splenic sequestration can lead to a hypoproductive anemia. The degree of anemia should correlate with the degree of splenomegaly (i.e., if the spleen is barely palpable, it is not the cause of significant anemia).

TABLE 89.4

DIFFERENTIATING IRON DEFICIENCY FROM ANEMIA OF CHRONIC DISEASE

Parameter	Anemia of chronic disease	Iron deficiency
Iron	Low	Low
Transferrin (TIBC)	Normal–low	High
Saturation	Low	Low
Ferritin	Normal–high	Low
Serum transferrin receptor	Normal	High
Erythropoietin	Low	High

TIBC, Total iron binding capacity.

The evaluation of a *hypoproductive, normocytic anemia* should include appropriate iron studies (Table 89.4) and review of the peripheral smear. A careful physical examination should be performed to look for signs of underlying malignancy that might cause AOCD or infiltrate the marrow. A chest radiograph is indicated. Additional laboratory studies (as indicated) and an erythropoietin level may help determine the cause of anemia. If a diagnosis is not readily apparent, a bone-marrow aspirate and biopsy are indicated.

Hypoproductive, macrocytic anemia is seen most commonly with folate or B_{12} deficiency or myelodysplastic syndromes. In addition, chronic drug therapy (e.g., cyclosporine, azathioprine, and hydroxyurea) can cause a megaloblastic anemia. B_{12} deficiency may be seen in patients with decreased absorption of dietary B_{12} resulting from decreased production of intrinsic factor (pernicious anemia, gastrectomy), abnormalities of the ileum (surgical resection, inflammatory bowel disease) or gastric mucosa (infection with *Helicobacter pylori*), or bacterial overgrowth (blind loop syndrome). Dietary B_{12} deficiency is very rare and is seen only in strict vegetarians who avoid all dairy products. Pernicious anemia is a hereditary autoimmune disease; signs of B_{12} deficiency are not usually evident before 35 years of age. Because of high body stores, deficiency of B_{12} resulting from malabsorption may not be evident for many years after gastric or ileal resection. Patients with a history of bowel surgery should be screened for deficiency before clinical symptoms develop. Folate deficiency is most often caused by inadequate dietary intake and may be exacerbated at times of increased requirements such as during pregnancy or in patients with hemolytic anemia. Deficient dietary intake of folate is seen in alcoholics, in elderly patients who do not eat fresh fruits and vegetables, and during starvation. Occasionally, medications, including phenytoin, trimethoprim–sulfamethoxazole, and sulfasalazine, may interfere with absorption of folate from the gasrtrointestinal tract. Patients with tropical sprue also may malabsorb folate. Nonmegaloblastic hypoproductive macrocytic anemia can be seen associated with liver disease and hypothyroidism.

The diagnostic approach to *macrocytic anemia* should begin with a careful history, a serum B_{12} level, a red-cell folate level, and review of the peripheral smear. Even if the red blood cells are normocytic, the presence of hypersegmented neutrophils (defined as more than one five-lobed or at least one six-lobed or more neutrophil) should instigate a workup for B_{12} or folate deficiency (8). A normocytic anemia might be seen, caused by thalassemia or iron deficiency, in addition to deficiencies of B_{12} or folate. A B_{12} level less than 100 pg/mL is diagnostic of overt deficiency; the lactate dehydrogenase (LDH) is also elevated. Further evaluation of B_{12} deficiency has included the Schilling test, which is performed after replacement of B_{12}. Several additional blood tests can now be used to confirm the diagnosis, and assess etiology. Methylmalonic acid is elevated

when cobalamin levels are low, and falls with replacement therapy. Antibodies to intrinsic factor are a highly specific but insensitive method of diagnosing pernicious anemia; only 50% of patients with pernicious anemia have elevated antibodies. A low red blood cell folate level (<150 mg/mL) is consistent with folate deficiency. Serum homocysteine levels will also be elevated. It is still important to rule out concurrent B_{12} deficiency, because the hematologic effects may be masked by folate replacement, leaving the resultant neurologic damage untreated.

Hyperproductive, normocytic anemias are caused by acute blood loss or hemolysis. The most common form of acquired immune hemolytic anemia is caused by warm (IgG) antibodies that adhere to the red blood cell surface, with subsequent destruction of the red cell by the spleen (extravascular hemolysis). Antibody production may be idiopathic, or associated with systemic autoimmune disease, lymphoproliferative disease, or medications (9). High-dosage penicillin, cephalosporins, and hydralazine are common offending agents. About 10% of patients with acquired immune hemolytic anemia have coexistent immune thrombocytopenia (Evans' syndrome). *Intravascular hemolysis* is seen with cold agglutinin disease, paroxysmal nocturnal hemoglobinuria (a myelodysplastic syndrome), and, rarely, toxins (e.g., snake venom, arsine). *Cold agglutinin disease* is caused by IgM antibodies that adhere to the red cell surface at temperatures lower than 37°C (e.g., in the peripheral circulation or in cold weather). The red cells are then susceptible to complement-induced lysis and sequestration. Cold agglutinin disease may be idiopathic in older patients or may be associated with lymphoproliferative or autoimmune diseases. Waldenstrom's macroglobulinemia is a B-cell malignancy in which a monoclonal IgM paraprotein is produced. Cold agglutinins also may be found following *Mycoplasma pneumoniae* infection or infectious mononucleosis. The hemolytic anemia associated with infections is usually mild.

Infection of the red blood cell with malarial or other parasites or direct action of a toxin (e.g., *Clostridium* spp.), as well as sepsis with or without disseminated intravascular coagulation (DIC), can cause acute hemolysis. Methemoglobinemia caused by medications or toxins causes hemolysis because of oxidation and subsequent precipitation of hemoglobin. *Microangiopathic hemolytic anemias* are a heterogeneous group of disorders associated with thrombocytopenia, elevated LDH, schistocytes on the peripheral blood smear, and variable neurologic and renal dysfunction (Chapter 98). The differential diagnosis includes thrombotic thrombocytopenic purpura, hemolytic uremic syndrome, malignant hypertension, microangiopathic hemolytic anemias associated with pregnancy, DIC, vasculitis, and hemolysis caused by a mechanical valve. A markedly elevated LDH in the absence of coagulopathy is consistent with microangiopathic hemolytic anemia. Urgent therapy with large-volume plasma exchange is indicated to avoid serious and life-threatening complications.

Inherited hemolytic anemia usually is caused by hemoglobinopathies (e.g., thalassemia, sickle cell disease) but also may result from defects in the red cell membrane (e.g., hereditary spherocytosis, elliptocytosis), reduced capability of the red cell to adapt to oxidative stress (G6PD deficiency), and abnormalities in the glycolytic pathway (pyruvate kinase deficiency). *Hereditary spherocytosis* is an autosomal dominant disease with variably severe extravascular hemolytic anemia that is not uncommonly diagnosed in adults. Patients usually have a lifelong history of anemia and may have splenomegaly on physical examination. *G6PD deficiency* is an X-linked recessive disorder seen in 10%–15% of African-American men (10). Women rarely are affected. G6PD is an enzyme that is critical to the production of reduced glutathione, which protects hemoglobin from oxidation. In the common form of this disease, older red cells lack adequate levels of G6PD and are therefore unusually sensitive to oxidative stress from drugs (see Table 89.5 for a list of common drugs causing oxidative hemolysis) or infection. Patients may present with jaundice and dark urine. Hemolysis is self-limited, even if the offending agent is continued. After the older G6PD-deficient red cells have been destroyed, the younger cells with adequate levels of the enzyme are able to resist the oxidative stress.

The evaluation of *hyperproductive anemias* begins with a direct antiglobulin test (DAT) and review of the peripheral smear. The indirect bilirubin and LDH are elevated with active hemolysis. If the DAT is positive for IgG with or without complement, acquired immune hemolytic anemia or drug-induced hemolysis is likely; the smear shows spherocytes. If the DAT is positive for complement and the smear shows clumping of red cells, cold agglutinins should be checked, as IgM is not identified by the DAT. If the DAT is negative and the smear shows spherocytes, hereditary spherocytosis should be suspected. An osmotic fragility test can establish this diagnosis. Intravascular hemolysis is associated with hemoglobinemia and filtration of hemoglobin through the glomerulus. The hemoglobin is absorbed by tubular cells and may be detected as hemosiderin in the urine.

Blood cultures and review of the thick smear should be performed if infection is suspected. A hemoglobin electrophoresis may be useful to diagnose underlying hemoglobinopathies. G6PD levels should not be measured immediately during or after an acute hemolytic episode, because the younger red blood cells that have survived the hemolysis and reticulocytes may have a normal level of the enzyme. Instead, levels should be measured about 3 months after the hemolytic event. Hemolytic anemia can be present without elevation of the reticulocyte count in the setting of coexistent nutritional deficiency, or if there is suppression of erythropoiesis by an infiltrative process or anemia of chronic disease.

Presenting During Hospitalization

Anemia presenting during hospitalization commonly is caused by frequent drawing of blood or gastrointestinal blood loss. AOCD may be exacerbated in ill, hospitalized patients. Drugs given during hospitalization (e.g., immunosuppressive or chemotherapeutic agents, high-dose antibiotics) may further suppress reticulocytosis. Hemolysis may be caused by therapy with drugs such as high-dosage penicillin or sulfonamides (with G6PD deficiency) or worsening of an autoimmune disease. Severe hypophosphatemia (resulting from use of medications or nutritional deficiency) is associated with hemolysis. Sepsis with DIC or microangiopathic hemolytic anemia also may develop during hospitalization. Mechanical hemolysis may be seen after cardiopulmonary bypass. The approach to diagnosing and managing anemia acquired during hospitalization is similar to anemia presenting on admission; a detailed review of events and medications given during the hospitalization is required for complete evaluation.

Treatment of Selected Causes

Treatment of iron deficiency with oral iron (325 mg three times daily) is usually adequate; gastrointestinal intolerance is reduced with coated formulations and absorption may be increased with concomitant vitamin C ingestion. The hemoglobin should begin to rise within 1 week of beginning therapy. Hemoglobin levels usually return to normal within 2 months after beginning replacement, but iron should be continued for 3–6 months to replete iron stores. Occasionally patients may not tolerate or cannot adequately absorb oral iron; these patients may require treatment with parenteral iron. The usual dose is 1.5 to 2.0 g. The infusion takes 4–6 hours and rarely can be complicated by severe hypersensitivity reactions. A test dose should be given, and the infusion must be carefully monitored, with medications for treating anaphylaxis available (Chapter 120).

AOCD is often mild and relatively asymptomatic; severe and symptomatic anemia may be treated with red cell transfusions or erythropoietin. Erythropoietin is given by

---

TABLE 89.5

COMMON DRUGS THAT CAN CAUSE OXIDATIVE HEMOLYSIS

Medications	Other
Sulfonamide drugs	Amyl nitrite
Sulfones	Moth balls (naphthalene)
Pyridium	Hydrogen peroxide
Nitrofurantoin	Fava beans
Quinidine	
Primaquine	
Phenylhydrazine	

subcutaneous injection three times a week; a larger dose (40,000 units) once a week is equally effective and much more convenient for the patient. A longer acting erythropoietin (darbopoietin) is now available and may be given every two (200 micrograms) or three (300 micrograms) weeks by subcutaneous injection. B_{12} deficiency has traditionally been treated with intramuscular B_{12} injections (100 mg) given daily for 1 week, weekly for 1 month, then monthly for life. An emerging and easier alternative is initial treatment with injections to treat acute symptoms, then chronic replacement with oral B_{12} at a dose of 1000 micrograms per day (11). There are insufficient data to treat severe neurologic symptoms with oral B_{12}. Initial replacement may be complicated by hypokalemia. B_{12} deficiency associated with *Helicobacter pylori* infection may improve with effective therapy for the infectious process. Folate deficiency is treated with 1 mg/d of oral folic acid. Patients with increased requirements for folate (as described previously) should receive regular supplementation with daily folic acid. Replacement of B_{12} and folate should result in reticulocytosis within 1 week and recovery of the hemoglobin to normal levels within 2 months. If reticulocytosis is not seen, either an alternative or coexistant diagnosis should be suspected and ruled out. In the absence of known iron deficiency, this would require a bone-marrow aspiration and biopsy. Transfusion generally is not indicated and can result in high-output congestive heart failure due to the increase in plasma volume associated with a chronic reduction in red cells. Neurologic effects of B_{12} deficiency improve slowly and may not completely resolve. Megaloblastic anemia associated with medications is usually mild (although the MCV may be dramatically elevated), and does not require specific therapy.

All patients with hemolysis should receive folate supplementation. Acquired immune hemolytic anemia is treated with prednisone, 1–2 mg/kg. In cases in which a rapid response is required for symptomatic severe anemia, intravenous immunoglobulin (2 mg/kg) or plasmapheresis to remove circulating antibodies can be effective. Transfusions should be given cautiously because of difficulty with cross-matching. Steroids are gradually tapered over 3 months, usually with recurrence or persistence of hemolysis. If the anemia is well compensated, no additional therapy is required. Most patients require splenectomy at some time for persistent and poorly compensated hemolysis. Immunosuppressive or cytotoxic therapy is used for continued anemia. If hemolysis is caused by medications, the offending agents should be discontinued if possible. Hemolysis resulting from lymphoproliferative disease is managed by treating the underlying malignancy; occasionally splenectomy is also required. Idiopathic cold agglutinin disease is treated by avoidance of cold temperatures and immunosuppressive and often cytotoxic therapy. Acute hemolysis may be treated with plasma exchange.

Hereditary hemolytic anemia caused by hereditary spherocytosis is treated with splenectomy. Although spherocytes remain, hemolysis ceases, as does the risk of parvovirus B19 aplastic crisis. Patients with G6PD deficiency do not generally require therapy in the acute setting other than folate supplementation, but should be counseled carefully regarding the risks of hemolysis from oxidative stress caused by infection, ketoacidosis, or the medications listed in Table 89.5.

Neutropenia

Presenting at the Time of Admission

Neutropenia is defined as an absolute neutrophil count less than 1,500 per microliter. However, certain population groups (e.g., African-Americans) and certain families may normally have neutrophil counts between 1,200 and 1,500 per microliter. The risk of infection is related both to the degree of neutropenia (higher if the absolute neutrophil count is less than 500 per microliter and very high if the count is less than 100 per microliter) and the functional properties of the neutrophils. Neutropenia with concomitant steroid use or associated with myelodysplastic syndromes results in a significantly higher risk of infection. In contrast, "benign" familial neutropenia is associated with a very low risk of infection.

The differential diagnosis of neutropenia can be divided into *decreased production, peripheral destruction, splenic sequestration, or a combination* of these causes. Causes of neutropenia include infections, medications, autoimmunity, and congenital or cyclic neutropenia. Any agent capable of causing aplastic anemia and pancytopenia also is capable of causing isolated neutropenia. Viral infections may cause neutropenia both by decreasing marrow production and by causing peripheral destruction. Infections that have been associated with neutropenia include varicella, measles, rubella, hepatitis A, B, or C, cytomegalovirus, influenza, and the Epstein-Barr virus. HIV infection causes neutropenia by peripheral destruction with production of autoantibodies; bone-marrow suppression and sequestration also may contribute. Significant neutropenia can occur in the setting of bacterial sepsis, resulting from a combination of suppression of marrow production and destruction of peripheral cells. Chronic infection can cause modest neutropenia.

Drug-induced neutropenia is one of the most common causes of "benign" neutropenia (12). Chemotherapeutic drugs (Chapter 90) cause direct marrow suppression; other agents cause immune neutropenia both from peripheral destruction and from destruction of marrow precursors by antibodies. Most drugs suppress the marrow in a dose-dependent manner. Common medications causing neutropenia include phenytoin, procainamide, antibiotics (sulfonamides, semisynthetic penicillins, and cephalosporins), antithyroid agents (methimazole and others), hypoglycemic agents (tolbutamide, chlorpropamide), phenothiazines (chlorpromazine), and antiretrovirals. Prolonged use of drugs such as azathioprine to prevent organ rejection following transplantation or to treat autoimmune disease can be associated with severe neutropenia.

Autoimmune neutropenia (12) usually is associated with underlying autoimmune disease but also may be idiopathic or caused by drugs or infections. Immune neutropenia can be associated with immune hemolytic anemia or immune thrombocytopenia. The severity of neutropenia is variable, but the risk of infection may be extremely high in severely neutropenic patients on chronic immunosuppression for autoimmune disease. Systemic lupus erythematosus (Chapter 112) is the autoimmune disease most frequently associated with neutropenia.

Patients with neutropenia may present with mouth ulcers, fever, and systemic infection. For a complete discussion of infectious complications, see Chapter 63. Physical examination may reveal signs of autoimmune disease such as rheumatoid arthritis or splenomegaly. The evaluation of neutropenia should begin with a review of the peripheral smear. The presence of morphologic abnormalities in the red cells or remaining white cells suggests a primary marrow process. A thorough medication history, including over-the-counter preparations, should be obtained. Laboratory studies should include viral serology for hepatitis and HIV. A positive antinuclear antibody (ANA) may be useful in establishing the diagnosis of immune neutropenia and also may be found in HIV-associated neutropenia; however, the test is neither sensitive nor specific. If a diagnosis such as viral infection or drug-mediated neutropenia is not readily apparent or the neutropenia is severe or fails to resolve, bone-marrow aspiration and biopsy should be done. In most cases, the aspirate shows maturation arrest with normal or increased cellularity.

Neutropenia resulting from medications should resolve within 1–2 weeks of stopping the offending agent. If neutropenia is mild and associated with a medication that is not easily replaced, careful monitoring while continuing the drug is possible. Treatment of neutropenia associated with infection includes antibiotics and support of significant neutropenia with myeloid growth factors (Chapters 63 and 90). Patients with asymptomatic, modest neutropenia and without sites of tissue breakdown can be managed as outpatients. Antibacterial mouthwashes decrease the risk of infection.

Severe neutropenia, or neutropenia with recurrent or serious infections associated with autoimmune disease, usually is treated with steroids and other cytotoxic therapy if necessary. Treatment with intravenous gamma globulin may improve the neutrophil count, but the effect is transient. Myeloid growth factors are usually effective, and prolonged use in severe neutropenia may allow reduction in immunosuppression. Splenectomy is controversial and should be reserved for patients with repeated bacterial infections or refractory neutropenia. Although the neutrophil count often responds, the effect may be transient and there

may be a subsequent increased risk of infection. Neutropenia associated with absent white cell progenitors is treated with antithymocyte globulin and cyclosporine.

Presenting During Hospitalization

Neutropenia presenting during hospitalization is likely caused by medications or severe infection. Any possible offending agent should be stopped and the possibility of infection should be investigated. Patients should be followed until the neutropenia resolves. Persistent neutropenia requires a more extensive evaluation, as outlined previously.

Leukocytosis

Presenting at the Time of Admission

An elevation in the white cell count may be caused by increased total neutrophils, lymphocytes, monocytes, or rarely eosinophils. Immature myeloid or lymphoid cells can cause leukocytosis in the setting of acute leukemia. By far the most common cause of leukocytosis is *neutrophilia* (13). Leukocytosis with neutrophilia is a common presenting abnormal laboratory value on admission to the hospital. The major differential is between primary and secondary causes (e.g., leukemoid reaction) (Table 89.6). A markedly elevated white blood cell count (>70,000/μL) is rarely associated with benign disease. Splenomegaly may be a sign of leukocytosis due to a defined systemic disorder such as a myeloproliferative disease. Chronic leukocytosis

TABLE 89.6

DIFFERENTIAL DIAGNOSIS OF LEUKOCYTOSIS WITH NEUTROPHILIA

Primary neutrophilia	Paraneoplastic:
Myeloproliferative disease	Nonhematopoietic
Chronic myelogenous	malignancy
leukemia	Drug-induced
Myelofibrosis	Steroids
Polycythemia vera	Lithium
Essential	β-agonists
thrombocythemia	Myeloid growth factors
Benign neutrophilia	Chronic marrow stimulation
Down syndrome	Hemolytic anemia
Familial or idiopathic	Immune
Secondary (reactive)	thrombocytopenia
neutrophilia	Recovery from marrow
Infection	suppression
Acute	Asplenia or hyposplenia
Chronic	
Stress	
Exercise, catecholamines	
Postictal state	
Chronic inflammation	
Tissue damage	

rarely can occur in patients who are otherwise well.

Lymphocytosis may be reactive in the setting of pertussis, viral infection, or a lymphoproliferative disorder such as chronic lymphocytic leukemia, hairy-cell leukemia, or leukemic phase of lymphoma. Viral infections usually are evident from fever, sore throat, and other symptoms. A diagnosis of chronic lymphocytic leukemia requires a sustained peripheral lymphocytosis of more than 5,000 per microliter. Lymphadenopathy and splenomegaly are common physical findings. Monocytosis may be reactive in the setting of chronic infections (e.g., tuberculosis, endocarditis), autoimmune disease, carcinomas or lymphomas, or postsplenectomy. Recovery from marrow injury or chronic neutropenia also may be associated with monocytosis. Malignant monocytosis is seen in chronic myelomonocytic leukemia and myelodysplastic syndromes.

The most common causes of *eosinophilia* are atopic disorders and helminthic infections. Other causes are autoimmune disorders, drug reactions, and paraneoplastic causes (most commonly, Hodgkin's disease). Eosinophilia caused by drugs is rarely symptomatic and usually resolves with withdrawal of the offending agent, although tissue damage can occur (e.g., hypersensitivity pneumonitis). One notable exception is the chronic *eosinophilia–myalgia syndrome* seen following the ingestion of contaminated tryptophan. Primary eosinophilic disorders include idiopathic hypereosinophilic syndrome, Churg–Strauss syndrome with vasculitis (Chapter 111), and diseases associated with infiltration of specific organs such as eosinophilic pneumonitis (Chapter 57).

Evaluation of leukocytosis should begin with a careful review of the peripheral blood smear. Leukemoid reactions and myeloproliferative disease (2) may be indistinguishable on the blood smear and are characterized by a "left" shift in the neutrophils with increased bands, as well as metamyelocytes, myelocytes, promyelocytes, and rare blasts. In the setting of infection or stress, neutrophils may show toxic granulations, cytoplasmic vacuoles, and Döhle's bodies. Hypogranular and increased basophils, and occasionally eosinophils, are found in myeloproliferative disease and may be the first clue to the diagnosis. The leukocyte alkaline phosphatase score may be useful in distinguishing a leukemoid reaction from chronic myelogenous leukemia. This score is high in secondary leukocytosis and low in chronic myelogenous leukemia. In contrast, blast cells and neutrophils on the peripheral smear ("leukemic hiatus") are characteristic of acute leukemia. Variably sized mature lymphocytes with "smudge" cells (crushed lymphocytes) are suggestive of chronic lymphocytic leukemia. Lymphocytes with an atypical appearance and hairy-like projections may be seen in some but not all cases of hairy-cell leukemia. The monocytes and neutrophils in chronic myelomonocytic leukemia are dysplastic; rare blasts also may be seen. If a myeloproliferative disease or leukemia is suspected, a bone-marrow aspirate and biopsy with cytogenetics, special stains, and flow cy-

tometry should be obtained. In an older or ill patient, or one in whom the bone marrow is inaspirable, peripheral blood may be sent for chromosome and DNA analysis, special stains, and flow cytometry.

A patient with eosinophilia should be asked about travel history, animal exposure, and personal or family history of atopy, eczema, or asthma, as well as for a detailed medication history. Serial stool samples should be examined for ova and parasites. The detection of *Strongyloides stercoralis* may be difficult and can require serologic testing. Review of the peripheral blood smear may show dysplastic features suggestive of a primary hematologic disorder.

The goal in secondary leukocytosis is to treat the underlying disorder. There are no untoward effects of benign leukocytosis; no specific therapy is required. However, leukocytosis that does not resolve following treatment of infection or resolution of stress should be investigated thoroughly, as it may represent early chronic myelogenous leukemia. Unlike the leukocytosis with acute leukemia, marked elevations of the white blood count caused by differentiated cells in chronic myelogenous leukemia are not usually dangerous. The treatment of leukocytosis resulting from myeloproliferative disease and leukemias is covered in Chapters 93 and 95.

Presenting During Hospitalization

Leukocytosis of any sort occurring during hospitalization is usually caused by infection or a reaction to medications. Leukocytosis may be the first sign of infection, especially in an immunocompromised patient. For further discussion, see Chapters 62 and 63.

Pancytopenia

Presenting at the Time of Admission

Pancytopenia is defined as a reduction in all three blood cell lines. The differential diagnosis is broad and includes toxin or immune suppression of marrow precursors, infiltration of the marrow, and splenic sequestration. *Aplastic anemia* is characterized by a hypocellular bone marrow with normal cytogenetics. The most common cause is thought to be autoimmune suppression of hematopoiesis by a T-cell-mediated mechanism. Aplastic anemia also may be caused by direct stem-cell injury from drugs, including phenytoin, sulfonamides, carbamazepine, tolbutamide, gold salts, and chloramphenicol, and from toxins including benzene, toluene, and some insecticides. Pancytopenia with an aplastic marrow has been seen following pregnancy and infection with hepatitis B or C. Treatment with chemotherapy or radiation therapy (especially to the pelvis) may result in aplasia. Autoimmune pancytopenia may be seen with systemic lupus; the marrow is cellular often without appreciable abnormalities. Nutritional deficiency in B_{12} or folate can result in marked pancytopenia.

Infiltration of the marrow may present as pancytopenia. Primary bone-marrow disorders include hairy-cell leukemia, myelodyplasia, myelofibrosis, and acute leukemia. Disseminated infections resulting from tuberculosis, brucellosis, leishmaniasis, and HIV can result in pancytopenia. Modest panycytopenia, caused by sequestration, is a frequent finding in patients with significant splenomegaly.

The symptoms of patients with pancytopenia usually result from the decrease in cell counts, with stomatitis and fever related to neutropenia, fatigue and dyspnea from anemia, and bleeding from thrombocytopenia. Fever also may be a sign of malignancy or infection. The evaluation of pancytopenia almost always includes bone-marrow aspiration and biopsy after a drug and toxin history, careful physical examination, and review of the peripheral smear.

Treatment of aplastic anemia depends on the underlying cause. Aplastic anemia caused by medications may resolve with cessation of the offending agent. "Idiopathic," or autoimmune, aplastic anemia may respond to immunosuppressive therapy with antithymocyte globulin and cyclosporine. Allogeneic bone-marrow transplantation (Chapter 96) is the only curative treatment for severe aplastic anemia or aplasia resulting from direct stem-cell injury by toxins. Androgen therapy has been used for refractory aplastic anemia in patients who are not candidates for bone-marrow transplantation with some response. Pancytopenia caused by deficiency of B_{12} or folate responds rapidly to replacement with recovery of counts within 7–14 days.

Presenting During Hospitalization

Like neutropenia, pancytopenia presenting during hospitalization is almost always caused by drug toxicity or infection. Treatment includes cessation of the offending drug, and transfusion and antibiotics as needed.

KEY POINTS

- Careful evaluation of the peripheral blood smear is essential for the evaluation of abnormal blood counts.
- Splenomegaly and lymphadenopathy are usually signs of underlying systemic illness and always require evaluation.
- Medications are a common cause of blood-count abnormalities in hospitalized patients.
- Nutritional deficiencies should be carefully screened for, particulary in elderly patients.

- Anemia may be classified by the size of the red blood cell, the reticulocyte count, and review of the peripheral blood smear.
- Leukocytosis is usually due to neutrophilia; the differential diagnosis is primarily between a reactive process and myeloproliferative disease.

REFERENCES

1. O'Reilly RA. Splenomegaly in 2,505 patients in a large university medical center from 1913 to 1995. *West J Med* 1998;169:78–87.
2. Spivak JL, Barosi G, Tognoni G, et al. Chronic myeloproliferative disorders. *Hematology* (Am Soc Hematol Educ Program). 2003:200–224.
3. Ferrer R. Lymphadenopathy: differential diagnosis and evaluation. *Am Fam Phys* 1998;58:1313–1320.
4. Carmel R. A focused approach to anemia. *Hosp Prac* 1999;34:71–78.
5. Beutler E, Hoffbrand AV, Cook JD. Iron deficiency and overload. *Hematology* (Am Soc Hematol Educ Program). 2003:40–61.
6. Brugnara C. Iron deficiency and erythropoiesis: new diagnostic approaches. *Clin Chem* 2003;49:1573–1578.
7. Spivak JL. Iron and the anemia of chronic disease. *Oncology* 2002;16:25–33.
8. Snow CF. Laboratory diagnosis of vitamin B12 and folate deficiency. *Arch Int Med* 1999;159:1289–1298.
9. Garratty G. Review: drug-induced immune hemolytic anemia—the last decade. *Immunohematol.* 2004;20:138–146.
10. Mehta A, Mason PJ, Vulliamy TJ. Glucose-6-phosphate dehydrogenase deficiency. *Baillieres Best Pract Res Clin Haematol* 2000;13:21–38.
11. Nyholm E, Turpin P, Swain D, et al. Oral vitamin B12 can change our practice. *Post Grad Med J* 2003;79:218–220.
12. Bhatt V, Saleem A. Review: drug-induced neutropenia–pathophysiology, clinical features, and management. *Ann Clin Lab Sci.* 2004;34:131–137.
13. Reding MT, Hibbs JR, Morrison VA, et al. Diagnosis and outcome of 100 consecutive patients with extreme granulocytic leukocytosis. *Am J Med* 1998;104:12–16.

ADDITIONAL READING

Andres E, Loukili NH, Noel E et al. Vitamin B12 (cobalamin) deficiency in elderly patients. *CMAJ* 2004;171:251–259.
Brokering KL, Qaqish RB. Management of anemia of chronic disease in patients with the human immunodeficiency virus. *Pharmacotherapy* 2003;23:1475–1485.
Bunn HF. Pathogenesis and treatment of sickle cell disease. *N Engl J Med* 1997;337:762–769.
Greer JP, ed. *Wintrobe's Clinical Hematology,* 11th ed. Philadelphia: Lippincott Williams & Wilkins, 2004.
Hoffman R, Benz EJ, Shattil SJ, et al., eds. *Hematology: Basic Principles and Practice,* 3rd ed. Edinburgh: Churchill Livingstone, 2000.
Iolascon A, Miraglia del Giudice E, Perrotta S, et al. Hereditary spherocytosis: from clinical to molecular defects. *Hematologica* 1998;83:240–257.
Katz SD, Mancini D, Androne AS et al. Treatment of anemia in patients with chronic heart failure. *J Card Fail* 2004;10:S13–S16.
Kis AM, Carnes M. Detecting iron defiency in anemic patients with concomitant medical problems. *J Gen Int Med* 1998;13:455–461.
Petz LD. Review: evaluation of patients with immune hemolysis. *Immunohematol* 2004;20:167–176.
Rothenberg ME. Eosinophilia. *N Engl J Med* 1998;338:1592–1600.

Principles of Chemotherapy

90

Robert J. Ignoffo

INTRODUCTION

History of Chemotherapy

Dr. Paul Erlich coined the term *chemotherapy* in the early 1900s as a result of his work in developing new antibiotics for use against parasitic organisms. However, it was not until 1945 when the alkylating agents were discovered and used successfully in the treatment of lymphomas and Hodgkin's disease. During the same era, Huggins and Hodges determined that androgens promoted the growth of prostate cancer cells and subsequently tested the concept of androgen deprivation, showing that castration and estrogens were effective in the treatment of prostate cancer. Today the term chemotherapy is used for both cytotoxic and hormonal therapy.

After the initial success of cytotoxic chemotherapy, other alkylating agents were developed, including cyclophosphamide, which was claimed to have a selective effect on tumor cells. Although toxicities were observed on normal cells, cyclophosphamide therapy became a mainstay in the treatment of many malignancies. Soon thereafter, antimetabolites (i.e., methotrexate and fluorouracil) were discovered to have anticancer activity. Preclinical studies demonstrated that combinations of multiple agents could produce synergistic activity when given in the appropriate schedule. In the late 1970s it was shown that chemotherapy was effective in early stages of responsive cancers, probably because of increased tumor sensitivity in the setting of small tumor size or fewer numbers of cancer cells. In the 1980s, the advent of platinum therapy heralded advances in the treatment of genitourinary and gynecologic tumors. This was followed in the 1990s by the maturing of important studies of adjuvant chemotherapy showing an improved survival for breast and colorectal cancer, and the emergence of the effective new drugs to prevent chemotherapy toxicities. These supportive care drugs included mesna to prevent ifosfamide uropathy, hematopoietic growth factors (G-CSF, GM-CSF, erythopoietin, and oprelvekin) to minimize myelosuppression, 5-HT3 antagonists (ondansetron, granisetron, and dolasetron) to prevent acute chemotherapy-induced nausea and vomiting, dexrazoxane to prevent anthracycline-induced cardiomyopathy, and amifostine to prevent cisplatin-induced nephrotoxicity and neurotoxicity. These supportive therapies could possibly enhance patient compliance and allow for improved dose intensity of chemotherapy. The burgeoning biotechnology revolution holds the promise of more selective therapies, some of which are already finding their way into clinical practice (1).

Current Strategies in the Use of Chemotherapy and Biologic Therapy

Chemotherapy may be used in a variety of ways to treat cancer: as induction chemotherapy for advanced disease; as adjuvant chemotherapy after initial surgical debulking of localized cancer; as neoadjuvant chemotherapy for large cancers given prior to primary surgery; and as site-directed chemotherapy via installation into sanctuaries (intrathecal or peritoneal) or regional perfusion of tumors (e.g. intra-arterial).

Induction chemotherapy is most often used in the treatment of hematologic malignancies such as acute leukemias or lymphoma, with the goal of producing a complete or partial remission. High-dose chemotherapy is usually given in the hospital setting and often requires bone marrow rescue either with bone marrow or peripheral stem cells (Chapter 96). Patients undergoing high-dose chemotherapy often develop severe bone marrow suppression. The resulting grade 4 neutropenia usually requires empiric antibiotic therapy with broad-spectrum agents.

Other strategies include adjuvant and neoadjuvant chemotherapy. The rationale of *adjuvant chemotherapy* is to eliminate small numbers of remaining cancer cells that may be present systemically after primary surgery or radiation therapy. Adjuvant chemotherapy uses drugs that are very active in an advanced stage of the same cancer. *Neoadjuvant chemotherapy* is systemic chemotherapy that is used for localized cancers that may not be surgically resectable initially. This therapy may completely eradicate the localized tumor or result in shrinkage of the tumor such that it becomes surgically resectable. This strategy also has the advantage of providing information on the tumor's sensitivity to postsurgical chemotherapy. *Regional therapies* are used to improve the therapeutic advantage of a cytotoxic drug by increasing intratumor drug concentration while minimizing systemic exposure of the drug. Examples of regional chemotherapy are intra-arterial perfusion, intraperitoneal (belly-bath) instillation, and intrathecal injection.

CLINICAL OUTCOMES IN EVALUATING THE RESPONSE FROM CHEMOTHERAPY

In its early years of development, chemotherapy was not expected to cure patients but rather to shrink tumors and provide palliation. Responses to chemotherapy were of short duration, and relapse was common and heralded the development of drug resistance. With the discovery of new drugs and combinations, however, a higher rate of tumor response and even cure became an increasing reality. Unfortunately, these advances affected a relatively small percentage of the total population of cancer patients, with about 90% of the cures being observed in only 10% of the known cancers.

Goals of Therapy

The goals of therapy are often determined on a case-by-case basis and should involve both the physician and patient. The most desirable response, of course, is cure. *Cure* comes when a therapy leads to total eradication of the cancer and allows the patient to live a normal life span. Similarly, *complete remission* is total eradication of measurable cancer or normalization of a tumor marker; it must

be obtained before cure can be achieved. The best way to monitor the quality of a complete remission is by assessing the duration of the disease-free survival. For acute leukemia, complete remission involves normalization of a patient's bone marrow and at least a 2-year disease-free survival.

Partial remission is the next most desirable outcome. It is defined as a decrease of measurable cancer by at least 50% of its original volume. Partial remissions are meaningful to patients if they result in either a prolonged survival or palliation of symptoms. Furthermore, partial responses may also be useful in determining the effectiveness of a new drug or new drug regimen. Outcomes such as median duration of remission and median overall survival are used for comparing the efficacy of new therapies. Improved quality of life and palliation of symptoms are considered as important, if not more so, as partial remission, especially in patients with advanced incurable cancer. The achievement of stable disease can be beneficial to a patient who has rapidly progressive cancer with worsening symptoms. Progressive disease is defined as the development of any new cancer lesion or an increase of cancer volume by 25% or more, and it may or may not be associated with worsening symptoms.

Some patients without measurable tumors may have a tumor marker that can be used as an indicator of response or recurrence of systemic cancer. Examples include testicular cancer or gestational trophoblastic tumor, both of which can be monitored with a serum test for the β-subunit of human chorionic gonadotropin (β-HCG). Similarly, the tumor marker CA-125 can be used to assess the response of ovarian cancer to treatment. As with a partial remission, a 50% decrease in a tumor marker usually corresponds to tumor response, while an increase indicates tumor progression.

In the setting of minimal residual disease, as in patients who have had initial debulking surgery, complete response is not a relevant clinical outcome because the primary tumor has been totally removed. Other response indicators must be used, such as freedom from recurrence or relapse-free survival. These indicators report the amount of time elapsed for the regrowth of tumor cells to a clinically detectable level of cancer.

Table 90.1 lists the response rate for several cancers over time. The improved cure rate for cancers such as acute leukemia, Hodgkin's disease, testicular carcinoma, and choriocarcinoma is primarily caused by the use of combination chemotherapy. Recent advances have also been observed with multimodal therapy, using surgery, radiation therapy, hormonal therapy, and adjuvant chemotherapy, for breast and colorectal cancer. Improvements in response and long-term survival have also been realized for previously highly resistant solid tumors such as malignant melanoma and ovarian carcinoma. Table 90.2 lists several of these cancers and regimens associated with improved response.

TABLE 90.1

CURABLE OR HIGHLY RESPONSIVE CANCERS AND COMMONLY USED CHEMOTHERAPY

Cancer	Chemotherapy regimen
Acute myelogenous leukemia	Daunorubicin + cytarabine; Idarubicin + cytarabine
Acute lymphoblastic leukemia	Vincristine + prednisone + thioguanine
Hodgkin's disease (stage III or IV)	Adriamycin + bleomycin + vinblastine + dacarbazine; Mechlorethamine + vincristine + procarbazine + prednisone
Non-Hodgkin's lymphoma (high-grade)	Cyclophosphamide + hydroxydaunorubicin (doxorubicin) + vincristine + prednisone
Neuroblastoma	Cyclophosphamide + doxorubicin + vincristine
Testicular carcinoma (nonseminoma)	Bleomycin + etoposide + cisplatin

PRINCIPLES OF SUCCESSFUL CHEMOTHERAPY

Several principles of chemotherapy have been associated with a positive outcome in cancer patients. These principles include the following:

1. *Use combinations of chemotherapeutic drugs.* With a few exceptions, combinations of drugs with synergistic activity produce higher response rates and more cures than monotherapy. Combinations with different mechanisms of action usually offer the best chance for optimal response and also delay the onset of drug resistance.
2. *Use combinations of chemotherapy drugs with nonoverlapping toxicities.* Most chemotherapeutic drugs affect rapidly dividing normal cell populations such as bone marrow, hair follicles, gonadal tissue, and mucosa. Thus, myelosuppression, sterility, alopecia, and mucositis are common side effects. The agents also produce a wide variety of other organ system toxicities. Thus, combination regimens are often developed that allow the maximally tolerated doses of each drug in the regimen.
3. *Use an optimal dose intensity or dose density of chemotherapy.* The effectiveness of a drug combination often depends on both the dose and the dose schedule prescribed. For example, the effectiveness of the combination of cyclophosphamide, methotrexate, and fluorouracil in breast cancer is optimal when the dose intensity is at least 75% of the ideal dosage. Recently,

the use of combination fluorouracil, epirubicin, and cyclophosphamide given in a dose-dense fashion (e.g. every 2 weeks) was shown to decrease the recurrence rate in patients with high-risk breast cancer.

4. *Use supportive care drugs and therapies to prevent or minimize grade III or IV chemotherapy-induced toxicity.* Supportive care drugs and therapies, including hematopoietic growth factors, antiemetics, cytoprotectants (mesna, dexrazoxane, amifostine, and mannitol), pre- and postchemotherapy hydration, and antidotes (leucovorin), can be used prophylactically for chemotherapy regimens that commonly cause significant toxicity. Such therapies improve a patient's quality of life and enhance patients' abilities to tolerate chemotherapy.
5. *Use strategies to overcome drug resistance.* Some tumor cells contain cell-membrane proteins that act as gatekeepers, denying entry of toxic substances into the cell as well as pumping substances through the cell membrane to the outside. This pump is referred to as P-glycoprotein or P-gp. It is found in several body sites, including the blood-brain barrier, the intestinal mucosa, the liver, and the kidney. P-gp is one of the mechanisms of tumor resistance and can be induced by some drugs. Another pump is the multidrug resistance gene (MDR-1), which is present in many normal tissues and also serves as a protective mechanism against toxic substances. Attempts to overcome tumor resistance has been the subject of recent intense research. One strategy has been the use of very high doses of chemotherapy with bone marrow rescue. This approach results in high concentrations of cytotoxic drugs and is often used in cases of tumor relapse. Unfortunately, the toxicities of high-dose therapy are substantial. More selective methods have been investigated recently and include developing drugs that block either the P-gp protein or MDR-1.

TABLE 90.2

CANCERS DEMONSTRATING IMPROVED RESPONSE TO CHEMOTHERAPY

Cancer	Chemotherapy
Colorectal cancer	Leucovorin + fluorouracil + irinotecan; Leucovorin + fluorouracil + oxaliplatin
Melanoma	Cisplatin + vinblastine + dacarbazine (or temozolamide) + α-interferon + interleukin 2
Soft-tissue sarcoma	High-dose ifosfamide
Ovarian cancer (stage III/IV)	Paclitaxel + cisplatin; Paclitaxel + carboplatin
Non-small cell lung cancer	Cisplatin or carboplatin + paclitaxel

PHARMACOLOGY OF ANTINEOPLASTICS AND BIOLOGIC DRUGS

Pharmacokinetics and Pharmacodynamics

Pharmacokinetic and pharmacodynamic studies are being increasingly utilized in oncology to characterize the absorption, distribution, metabolism, and excretion of chemotherapy drugs. Pharmacokinetic data provide clinicians with the means to design more effective administration schedules and dosage regimens. The most important pharmacokinetic parameters are the amount of free drug available for effect, the active metabolites, the routes of elimination, and the half-life. Metabolism is probably the most complex aspect of pharmacokinetics. Cytochrome P450 enzymes in the liver, especially the CYP3A4 isoenzymes, are involved in the metabolism of several cytotoxic drugs. Clinicians should be aware that many cancer patients take alternative medications (such as St John's Wort) that may alter the metabolism of chemotherapy drugs, particularly the taxanes. Drug interactions, along with the large variations in hepatic enzyme activity, are probably responsible for widely variable toxicities of and responses to chemotherapy. A complete description of these interactions is beyond the scope of this chapter.

The amount of free drug is inversely related to the degree of protein binding. Unfortunately, for most chemotherapeutic drugs, the degree of protein binding varies widely among patients. Thus, dosing the drug on the basis of body weight or body surface area may not correlate closely to drug clearance. Nevertheless, relative dosing using weight or body surface area remains the most common method of dosing chemotherapy.

Some chemotherapeutic drugs must be activated by hepatic enzymes. For example, cyclophosphamide is activated by hepatic CYP3A4 to two active metabolites. Patients may vary in their ability to activate the drug, which can result in fluctuating levels of active metabolites and variable responses to the treatment. Improving hepatic metabolism of cyclophosphamide can be accomplished with inducing drugs such as cimetidine or phenobarbital. In some cases, the ratio of metabolites in the body may explain a particular toxicity. For example, a high level of the metabolite of irinotecan (SN-38) is associated with a high incidence of severe diarrhea. Some patients with enhanced metabolism are at greater risk for severe diarrhea. Pharmacokinetic assessment may identify such patients.

The major routes of elimination for some chemotherapeutic drugs are the kidney and liver. Diminished liver or kidney function may lead to decreased drug clearance. The dose of chemotherapy should be reduced to account for the decreased clearance to minimize excessive organ-system toxicity. Patients with decreased drug clearance will have a prolonged drug half-life. Drugs that are affected by altered renal or hepatic clearance are listed in Table 90.3.

Side Effects of Chemotherapy

Table 90.4 lists side effects associated with chemotherapy drugs that are commonly used in the hospital setting.

CARE OF THE HOSPITALIZED PATIENT

Indications for Admission of the Oncology Patient

With the advent of better supportive care therapies and skilled oncology nurses, most chemotherapy is currently administered in the outpatient setting. However, many cancer patients are still admitted to the hospital for high-dose chemotherapy or complicated chemotherapy regimens. Other reasons for admission include the treatment of complications caused by chemotherapy, oncologic emergencies (Chapter 92), or pain control (Chapter 18).

Prescribing of Cancer Chemotherapy

Erroneous chemotherapy orders may have disastrous consequences. In one review, the most frequently observed errors were caused by poor handwriting or prescribing practices that lead to misinterpretation of the chemotherapy order by nurses and pharmacists (2). Computerized order sets and/or preprinted standardized chemotherapy order forms are recommended both for regimens that are used commonly in practice as well as for clinical studies (see also Chapter 21). The advantage of preprinted, standardized chemotherapy order forms are that they prompt the prescriber to enter the information necessary for all health care personnel to double check the order for accuracy. At the very least, to ensure that orders are written with utmost clarity, clinicians should follow order-writing guidelines that have been established by a collaborative practice committee at their institution or adopt guidelines of other institutions or organizations. The guidelines used at UCSF Medical Center are shown in Table 90.5. The use of computer software programs that compare the chemotherapy dose to existing protocols for the institution may further improve the chemotherapy ordering process. These software programs are in the early stages of development (Chapter 10).

Administration of Cancer Chemotherapy

Several classes of chemotherapy may be administered in the hospital setting. Some of the more commonly prescribed drugs include cytarabine, daunorubicin, cyclophosphamide, ifosfamide plus mesna uroprotection, high-dose methotrexate with leucovorin rescue, carboplatin, and cisplatin. Other agents include busulfan, etoposide, fluorouracil, paclitaxel, thiotepa, idarubicin, and doxorubicin. Continuous infusions are also monitored in the hospital setting, especially vesicant drugs such as daunorubicin,

TABLE 90.3

CONDITIONS ALTERING THE CLEARANCE OF SELECTED CHEMOTHERAPEUTIC DRUGS

Drug	Condition	Percentage of full dose
Bleomycin	Renal impairment: CrCl > 35 ml/min	100
	CrCl 10–50 ml/min	50
	CrCl < 10 ml/min	40
Carboplatin	Renal impairment	Dose (mg) = AUC × (CrCl + 25)[a]
Carmustine	Renal impairment CrCl: <10 ml/min	25–50
Cisplatin	Renal impairment CrCl: <50 ml/min	0
Cyclophosphamide	Renal impairment CrCl: <10 ml/min	50
Cytarabine	Renal impairment CrCl: 10–50 ml/min	50
	CrCl <10 ml/min	25
Daunorubicin	Hepatic dysfunction	
	Bili 1.2–3.0 mg/dL	75
	Bili >3.0 mg/dL	50
Doxorubicin	Hepatic dysfunction	
	Bili 1.2–3.0 mg/dL	50
	Bili >3.0 mg/dL	25
Epirubicin	Hepatic dysfunction	
	Bili 1.2–3.0 mg/dL	50
	Bili >3.0 mg/dL	25
Etoposide	Hepatic dysfunction	
	Bili 1.2–3.0 mg/dL	50
	Bili >3.0 mg/dL	0
Fluorouracil	Hepatic dysfunction	
	Bili 1.2–3.0 mg/dL	100
	Bili >3.0 mg/dL	50
Idarubicin	Hepatic dysfunction	
	Bili 2.5–5.0 mg/dL	50
	Bili >5.0 mg/dL	0
Ifosfamide	Renal impairment: CrCl 10–50 ml/min	75
	CrCl <10 ml/min	50
Lomustine	Renal impairment: CrCl 10 ml/min	25–50
Methotrexate	Renal impairment: CrCl 10–50 ml/min	25–50
	CrCl <10 ml/min	0
Mitoxantrone	Hepatic dysfunction	
	Bili 1.5–3.0 mg/dL	50
	Bili >3.0 mg/dL	25
Plicamycin	Renal impairment: CrCl 10–50 ml/min	50–75
	CrCl <10 ml/min	0
Streptozocin	Renal impairment: CrCl 10–50 ml/min	100
	CrCl <10 ml/min	25–50
Vinblastine	Hepatic dysfunction	
	Bili 1.2–3.0 mg/dL	50
	Bili >3.0 mg/dL	25
Vincristine	Hepatic dysfunction	
	Bili 1.2–3.0 mg/dL	50
	Bili >3.0 mg/dL	25
Vinorelbine	Hepatic dysfunction	
	Bili 1.2–3.0 mg/dL	50
	Bili >3.0 mg/dL	25

[a] This is the "Calvert formula."
AUC, area under the curve, in mg/mL × minutes; *bili*, total bilirubin; *CrCl*, creatinine clearance.

doxorubicin, vincristine, and vinblastine. When administered as a long infusion, these drugs should be given via a central venous access line to minimize the risk of local skin reactions. In addition to intravenous, other routes of administration include intraperitoneal (IP), intrapleural (IPl), intrathecal (IT), and intravesicle (bladder). These routes require special knowledge and clinician expertise for proper administration. Drugs given by the intraperitoneal route include cisplatin, carboplatin, etoposide, fluorouracil, and bleomycin. Drugs given by the intrathecal route include cytarabine, methotrexate, and thiotepa. BCG and mitomycin are frequently given by bladder instillation.

TABLE 90.4

SIDE EFFECTS OF CHEMOTHERAPY DRUGS COMMONLY USED IN THE HOSPITAL SETTING

Drug	Adverse effects
Asparaginase	Hypersensitivity, anaphylaxis, hepatic aminotransferase and alkaline phosphatase elevation, increased serum bilirubin, decreased clotting factor synthesis leading to elevated prothrombin time and bleeding, rare disseminated intravascular coagulation, CNS (lethargy and somnolence), pancreatitis
Bleomycin	Anaphylaxis, rash, pulmonary fibrosis (doses > 200 Units/m^2)
Busulfan	Myelosuppression, nausea, vomiting, hyperpigmentation, seizures after high doses (4 mg/kg/day), alopecia
Carboplatin (Paraplatin)	Myelosuppression, acute nausea and vomiting, peripheral neuropathy
Carmustine	Myelosuppression, acute nausea and vomiting, delayed pulmonary toxicity, encephalopathy and seizures, vasculitis along the vein used for drug injection
Cisplatin (Platinol)	Myelosuppression, acute emesis, delayed emesis (days 2–5), peripheral neuropathy, acute renal failure, chronic renal failure, hypomagnesemia, hypokalemia, fatigue and weakness, high-frequency hearing loss, hypersensitivity reactions, alopecia
Cyclophosphamide	Myelosuppression, acute emesis, delayed emesis, cystitis, SIADH within 48 hours, cardiomyopathy after high-dose therapy, alopecia
Cytarabine (Ara-C)	Myelosuppression, mucositis, stomatitis, CNS (lethargy, confusion, ataxia, seizures), conjunctivitis after high-dose therapy, nausea and vomiting
Dacarbazine (DTIC)	Myelosuppression, acute emesis, acute nausea, flulike syndrome (fever and chills), hypotension after rapid infusion, hepatic aminotransferase elevations, hypersensitivity reactions
Daunorubicin HCl (Cerubidine)	Myelosuppression, acute emesis, delayed emesis, fever, alopecia, cardiomyopathy (dose related), acute arrhythmias, mucositis, diarrhea, hyperpigmentation of nails, nail ridging, hepatic aminotransferase elevation, orange urinary coloration, **local skin necrosis upon extravasation**
Doxorubicin HCl (Adriamycin)	Myelosuppression, acute emesis, delayed emesis, fever, alopecia, cardiomyopathy (dose related), acute arrhythmias, mucositis, diarrhea, hyperpigmentation of nails, nail ridging, hepatic aminotransferase elevation, orange urinary coloration, **local skin necrosis upon extravasation**
Etoposide (VP-16)	Myelosuppression, acute emesis, hypotension during IV administration, alopecia, hypersensitivity reactions, CNS (lethargy, sedation) after high doses, metabolic acidosis after high doses
Fluorouracil	Myelosuppression, mucositis, stomatitis, diarrhea, ataxia, venous hyperpigmentation, dacrocystitis (tear duct inflammation and blockage), alopecia, nail changes
Idarubicin	Myelosuppression, acute emesis, delayed emesis, fever, alopecia, cardiomyopathy (dose related), acute arrhythmias, mucositis, diarrhea, hyperpigmentation of nails, nail ridging, hepatic aminotransferase elevation, orange urinary coloration, **local skin necrosis upon extravasation**
Ifosfamide/Mesna (IFEX/MESNEX)	Myelosuppression, acute emesis, delayed emesis, cystitis, SIADH within 48 hours, cardiomyopathy after high-dose therapy, alopecia, CNS (lethargy, confusion, ataxia, seizures), hepatic aminotransferases and alkaline phosphatase, rare nephrotoxicity
Interferon alfa (Intron, Roferon)	Myelosuppression, weakness, fever, chills, malaise, myalgia, anorexia, somnolence, depression, tremor, seizures
Melphalan	Myelosuppression, acute emesis, hypotension, alopecia, pulmonary fibrosis, hypersensitivity
Methotrexate	Myelosuppression, mucositis, stomatitis, hepatic aminotransferase elevation, moderate acute emesis after high doses, acute renal failure after very high doses in patients with inadequate prehydration and urinary alkalinization, rare acute pneumonitis
Mitoxantrone (Novantrone)	Myelosuppression, cardiomyopathy, CHF, mild nausea and vomiting, blue-green urinary discoloration, alopecia
Octreotide (Sandostatin)	Mild nausea, abdominal pain, local skin reactions at injection site
Paclitaxel (Taxol)	Myelosuppression, mild acute emesis, peripheral neuropathy, hypersensitivity reactions, rare bradycardia and hypotension, alopecia, local skin reactions upon extravasation but not necrosis
Streptozocin	Myelosuppression, renal dysfunction, acute emesis, hyperglycemia, hepatic aminotransferase elevation, venous irritation during IV administration

CHF, congestive heart failure; CNS, central nervous system; SIADH, syndrome of inappropriate antidiuretic hormone.

TABLE 90.5

CHEMOTHERAPY ORDER-WRITING GUIDELINES AT UCSF MEDICAL CENTER

1. All orders should contain the patient's name, height, weight, and BSA in order for nurse or pharmacist to double check the calculation.
2. No abbreviations or brand names should be allowed. (i.e., do not use "MTX" for "methotrexate" or "U" for "units").
3. The total daily dose should be written as "**X** mg/kg or mg/m^2 = **Y** mg on day 1" for single-day regimens. Indicate the duration of infusion if an IV infusion, i.e., 1 hour, 4 hours, etc. Multiday regimens should be written as "**X** mg/kg or mg/m^2 = **Y** mg daily for **Z** days."
4. Do not write a zero after a whole number (e.g., 2.0 mg). Leave off the decimal and zero (e.g., 2 mg). Decimal points are easily obliterated by the lines on order sheets and can lead to serious errors in dosage.
5. Continuous infusions of vesicant drugs should be given only via a central line.
6. A co-signature by an attending physician is required for all transplant protocol orders. A co-signature by the oncologist will be required within 24 hours if orders are faxed. Faxed orders *must* be written on an acceptable institutional order form.
7. For intravenous agents, write the method of drug administration as either "IV push" or "IV infusion."
8. The solution and volume may be specified for IV infusions of chemotherapy. If not specified, the solution and volume will be determined by the pharmacist or clinic nurse based on the appropriate guideline.
9. Whenever possible, order practical doses of chemotherapy. The pharmacist may confer with you regarding the acceptability of rounding certain drug doses to their most practical dose as long as it does not vary by more than 5% from the original dose. The exceptions are vincristine, in which exact dosing is required, and vinblastine, mitoxantrone, and idarubicin, which should be rounded to the nearest **mg**.
10. Leave a space between the number and its unit value, e.g., 100 mg, not 100mg.
11. Changes in chemotherapy must be written by the fellow or attending (verbal orders to nurses or house staff are not acceptable).
12. Orders should not contain Latin abbreviations. Specifically, do not use qd, bid, or qid. Use the term *daily* instead of *qd*, *q12h* instead of *bid*, etc.
13. Order anti-emetics, hydration, and other supportive care on the same chemotherapy order form.

BSA; body surface area.

Each of these drugs is absorbed systemically and may produce systemic side effects, especially myelosuppression.

It is desirable that patients receive their chemotherapy within a few hours of being admitted to the hospital. In order to enhance efficiency, clinicians should try to obtain all the preliminary data (e.g., labs, radiographs) the day before the patient is admitted. Hydration and premedications should be given promptly on the patient's arrival and soon followed by the first dose of chemotherapy. Patients receiving chemotherapy do not necessarily require daily laboratory tests. Exceptions are drugs specified on protocol or certain antineoplastics (cisplatin, ifosfamide, methotrexate, cytarabine, and aldesleukin), which can produce rapid changes in electrolytes or renal function or require prolonged postchemotherapy assessment.

High-Dose Chemotherapy

Recent advances in the role of supportive care and bone marrow rescue have allowed for dose intensification of chemotherapy for both hematologic and solid tumors. High-dose therapy is often given in the hospital setting because of the high incidence of acute side effects and major organ system toxicity. However, for some drugs, the initial doses may be administered in the outpatient setting with hospital admission 3–5 days later when severe bone marrow suppression is expected. Hematopoietic growth factors can be used to decrease the intensity and onset of life-threatening bone marrow suppression. Measures to prevent life-threatening bacterial infection include the use of prophylactic antibiotics during the period of severe neutropenia (Chapter 63). Thrombocytopenia and anemia are also

common and are treated with transfusions, erythropoietin, or oprelvekin. Severe mucositis and diarrhea are common after high-dose chemotherapy. They typically peak at the same time as the hematologic toxicity, and last for 3–5 days after recovery of the neutrophils. During this time period, patients may require parenteral nutrition. Use of the recently-approved agent palifermin (recombinant human keratinocyte growth factor) may decrease the severity and duration of severe oral mucositis (3). High-dose therapy may cause major organ system complications, including cardiomyopathy, pulmonary toxicity, vasculitis, and hepatic veno-occlusive disease.

Prevention of Chemotherapy-Induced Complications

Chemotherapy-Induced Nausea and Vomiting

Until recently, nausea and vomiting were the most feared side effects of chemotherapy. With the advent of 5-HT3 antagonists, 60%–90% of patients have complete protection from acute chemotherapy-induced emesis. The emetogenic potential of individual chemotherapy drugs tends to be severe in hospitalized patients because combinations that include cisplatin or high-dose chemotherapy are often given. Chemotherapy orders of highly emetogenic drugs (Table 90.6) should be accompanied by an antiemetic order for a 5-HT3 antagonist with or without dexamethasone (Table 90.7). This regimen should control acute emesis in about 60%–80% of patients, but not delayed nausea or emesis, which occurs in about 40%–60% of patients given cisplatin or high-dose chemotherapy. A

TABLE 90.6

EMETOGENIC POTENTIAL OF COMMONLY USED CHEMOTHERAPEUTIC AGENTS

Level IV–V (Moderately high to high 60–100%)	Level III (Moderate 30–60%)	Level II (Mod-low 10–30%)	Level I (Low <10%)
Busulfan (4 mg/kg/day)	Amifostine (≥740 mg/m²)	Asparaginase	Bleomycin
Carmustine	Azacitidine	Cytarabine	Busulfan
Cisplatin (≥50 mg/m²/day)	Carboplatin	(<250mg/m²/day)	Chlorambucil
Cyclophosphamide (≥750 mg/m²/day)	Cisplatin	Daunorubicin (Liposomal)	Cladribine (2-CdA)
Cytarabine (≥500 mg/m²/day)	(≤50 mg/m²/day)	Docetaxel	Cyclophosphamide (oral)
Dacarbazine	Cyclophosphamide	Etoposide	Cytarabine (<20 mg
Dactinomycin	(<750 mg/m²/day)	(<200 mg/m²/day)	IV or <50 mg IT)
Etoposide, high dose (≥400 mg/m²/day)	Cytarabine	Gemcitabine	Doxorubicin (Liposomal)
Ifosfamide (≥2,500 mg/m²/day)	(250–500 mg/m²/day)	Irinotecan	Floxuridine IA
Lomustine	Daunorubicin	Methotrexate	Fludarabine
Mechlorethamine	Doxorubicin	(≤250 mg/m²)	Hydroxyurea
Melphalan (≥100 mg/m²/day)	Etoposide	Mitomycin	Melphalan (oral)
Methotrexate, high-dose (>1,000 mg/m²/day)	(≤200–400 mg/m²/day)	Paclitaxel	Mercaptopurine
Paclitaxel (>250 mg/m²/day)	Estramustine phosphate	(<175 mg/m²/day)	Methotrexate
Pentostatin	Floxuridine IV	Thiotepa (≤12 mg/m²/day)	(<50 mg/m²/day)
Plicamycin	Flourouracil (>1000 mg)	Topotecan	Pegasparaginase
Streptozocin	Idarubicin		Tamoxifen
Thiotepa (>100 mg/m²/day)	Ifosfamide		Thioguanine
	(<2,500 mg/m²/day)		Tretinoin
	Melphalan		Vinblastine
	(50–100 mg/m²/day)		Vinorelbine
	Methotrexate		
	(250–1000 mg/m²/day)		
	Mitomycin		
	Mitoxantrone		
	(≤15 mg/m²/day)		
	Paclitaxel		
	(175–250 mg/m²/day)		
	Procarbazine		
	Teniposide		

IA, intra-arterial; IT, intrathecal; IV, intravenous.

regimen of oral dexamethasaone and ondansetron, both given 8 mg twice daily orally, often helps prevent delayed chemotherapy induced emesis (4). Although dexamethasone is effective in preventing emesis in patients with solid tumors treated with chemotherapy, some hematologists are concerned that this corticosteroid increases the risk of fungal infection in induction regimens for acute leukemia. While few studies implicate short courses of dexamethasone in causing fungal infection, further study is needed to establish its role in the setting of high-dose chemotherapy for acute leukemias.

Chemotherapy-Induced Neutropenia

One of the most common complications that may result in hospitalization of the chemotherapy patient is febrile neutropenia. The usual pattern of myelosuppression is the occurrence of neutrophil nadir between day 7 and 14

after chemotherapy. Severe neutropenia, defined as a neutrophil count of 500/μL or less with associated fever and shaking chills, should lead to a presumptive diagnosis of Gram-negative bacteremia. Mortality (about 3%) is associated with prolonged neutropenia (greater than seven days), especially below a neutrophil count of 100/μL and other high-risk features (e.g., expected long duration of neutropenia).

The hospital management of chemotherapy-induced febrile neutropenia involves appropriate cultures, followed by immediate prophylactic broad-spectrum antibiotic therapy to prevent progression to septic shock and death (also see Chapter 63) (5). Filgrastim and sargramostim have also been studied in the treatment of severe febrile neutropenia. Although several studies have demonstrated that these agents shorten the duration of severe neutropenia, mortality has not been affected. This is probably because of rapid neutrophil recovery (3–5 days) from the effects of

TABLE 90.7

AGENTS FOR THE PREVENTION OF CHEMOTHERAPY-INDUCED EMESIS

Level IV–V or Combinations including level III

Granisetron 2 mg PO or 1 mg PO (on each day of chemotherapy) prior to chemotherapy. If patients cannot tolerate oral granisetron, may use intravenous granisetron (10 mcg/kg IV q24h).
> OR

Granisetron 10 mcg/kg (round up to the nearest 50 mcg) IV over 5–15 minutes q24 hours (on each day of chemotherapy) or as IV push over 30 seconds.
> OR

Ondansetron 8 mg IV q8h or Ondansetron 8 to 16 mg IV over 15 minutes × 1 (on each day of chemotherapy).
> OR

Dolasetron 100 mg IV or PO prior to chemotherapy.
All of the above may continue up to 24 hours after the last dose of chemotherapy.
> **PLUS**

Dexamethasone 10–20 mg IV over 15–30 minutes prior to chemotherapy or 10 mg PO/IV bid on days of chemotherapy for 1–5 days (if not contraindicated).

Combinations of Level II or III

Ondansetron 16–24 mg PO qd (on each day of chemotherapy).
> OR

Granisetron 1 mg PO q12 hours (on each day of chemotherapy).
> OR

Ondansetron 8 mg IV over 15–30 minutes × 1 (for each day of chemotherapy).
All of the above may continue up to 24 hours after the last dose of chemotherapy.
> **PLUS**

Dexamethasone 10–20 mg IV over 15–30 minutes prior to chemotherapy or 10 mg PO/IV bid on days of chemotherapy for 1–5 days (if not contraindicated).

For levels see Table 90.6.
Oral agents should be administered at least 60 minutes prior to chemotherapy. Intravenous agents should be administered at least 30 minutes prior to chemotherapy. Ondansetron and Granisetron should be discontinued 12–24 hours after the completion of the last dose of chemotherapy.
IV, intravenous; *PO*, orally.

chemotherapy. Thus, the use of broad-spectrum antibiotics without concurrent hematopoietic growth factor is adequate to manage most uncomplicated patients. However, patients with shaking chills and ill appearance are at greater risk for life-threatening sepsis and may benefit from filgrastim or sargramostim to shorten the course of neutropenia. Some experts recommend using hematopoietic growth factors in the treatment of febrile neutropenia in the presence of constitutional symptoms and evidence for clinical infection (e.g. pneumonitis, cellulitis).

Patients who have developed life-threatening febrile neutropenia after chemotherapy should be treated prophylactically with a hematopoietic growth factor (filgrastim, pegfilgrastim, or sargramostim) to prevent future episodes of severe neutropenia. When using filgrastim in an adult, dose the drug by weight, and give full vial sizes. For those under 70 kilograms, use one 300 microgram vial. Pegfilgrastim, a longer-acting neutrophil stimulator, should be reserved for outpatient prevention of neutropenia (6). Its role in the acute management of chemotherapy-induced neturopenia is not well defined.

Other Oncologic Emergencies

Hypercalcemia, spinal cord compression, and superior vena cava syndrome are reviewed in Chapter 92. Tumor lysis syndrome is covered in Chapter 94. Pain management and palliative care are discussed in Chapters 18 and 19, respectively.

DISCHARGE ISSUES AND FOLLOW-UP CARE

Management of Infections as an Outpatient

Patients considered low-risk may be converted from intravenous to oral antibiotic therapy after initial response to antibiotics. A variety of antibiotics are available and should be chosen based upon site of infection, therapeutic response, and the typical antibiotic sensitivities for the particular institution (Chapter 63).

Delayed Emesis

Patients who have received cisplatin, cyclophosphamide, or high-dose chemotherapy may develop delayed nausea and vomiting 3–5 days after discharge. Patients should be discharged with antiemetics to manage delayed emesis. The most cost-effective therapy is a combination of ondansetron (or prochlorperazine or metoclopramide) plus dexamethasone (Table 90.7). The neurokinin-1 receptor antagonist aprepitant may be used for patients with severe delayed emesis (7). It must be given on day 1–3, in conjunction with a 5-HT3 antagonist and dexamethasone. The dose of dexamethasone should be decreased to a maximum of 12 mg.

Prevention of Hemorrhagic Cystitis

The cytotoxic drugs cyclophosphamide or ifosfamide can cause severe bladder and ureteral toxicity. Complete protection for cyclophosphamide toxicity is virtually assured by using hydration (eight 6-ounce glasses of water or liquid) over the 24 hours following chemotherapy. Ifosfamide requires a uroprotectant drug, mesna, plus hydration for 24 hours post-therapy. Mesna is given by the intravenous route during hospitalization but may be converted to oral mesna every 4 hours for 3 doses at discharge. It is critical that patients are compliant with this regimen.

Methotrexate Monitoring

Methotrexate is an important antimetabolite drug that requires the antidote leucovorin for rescue of methotrexate doses greater than 500 milligrams. Patients must be instructed to take their oral leucovorin exactly as prescribed. In addition, they must return to the clinic for follow-up serum samples of methotrexate to determine the duration of leucovorin rescue (usually 3 days).

KEY POINTS

- Although cancer patients are being treated more often in the ambulatory setting, many patients still are admitted to the hospital for a variety of reasons, including administration of high-dose chemotherapy and management of complications related to chemotherapy.
- More cancer patients are responding to chemotherapy than in the past because of newer strategies such as dose-intense chemotherapy, high-dose chemotherapy with bone marrow rescue, and improved supportive care.
- High-dose therapies usually necessitate admission to the hospital for close monitoring. However, newer supportive care therapies, especially antibiotics and antiemetics, allow the clinician to initially treat patients in the ambulatory setting.
- Hospitals should streamline the processing of chemotherapy orders. All information (laboratory data, premedications) relevant to the protocol should be obtained prior to hospitalization.
- The hospital physician should be familiar with the management of chemotherapy-induced complications, especially febrile neutropenia and emesis.
- Discharge issues that should be considered are prevention of delayed emesis, prevention of cyclophosphamide-induced cystitis, and monitoring of methotrexate serum levels.

REFERENCES

1. Kohn EC, Lu Y, Wang H, et al. Molecular therapeutics: promise and challenges. *Semin Oncol* 2004;31(1 Suppl 3):39–53.
2. Fischer DS, Alfano S, Knobf MT, Donovan C, Beaulieu N. Improving the cancer chemotherapy use process. *J Clin Oncol* 1996;14: 3148–3155.
3. Spielberger R, Stiff P, Bensinger W, et al. Palifermin for oral mucositis after intensive therapy for hematologic cancers. *N Engl J Med* 2004;351:2590–2598.
4. Dexamethasone alone or in combination with ondansetron for the prevention of delayed nausea and vomiting induced by chemotherapy: The Italian Group for Antiemetic Research. *N Engl J Med* 2000;342:1554–1559.
5. Klastersky J. Empirical treatment of sepsis in neutropenic patients. *Internat J Antimicrob Ag* 2000;16:131–133.
6. Waladkhani AR. Pegfilgrastim: a recent advance in the prophylaxis of chemotherapy-induced neutropenia. *Eur J Cancer Care* 2004;13: 371–379.
7. Dandon TM, Perry CM, Aprepitant: a review of its use in the prevention of chemotherapy-induced nausea and vomiting. *Drugs* 2004;64:777–794.

ADDITIONAL READING

ASHP Council on Professional Affairs. ASHP guidelines on preventing medication errors with antineoplastic drugs. *Am J Health-syst Pharm* 2002;59:1649–1669.

DeVita VT. Principles of cancer management chemotherapy. In: DeVita VT, Hellman S, Rosenberg SA, eds. *Cancer. Principles and Practice of Oncology.* 7th ed. Philadelphia: Lippincott Williams & Wilkins, 2004:333–348.

Dorr RT, Von Hoff DD, eds. *Cancer Chemotherapy Handbook.* 2nd ed. Norwalk, CT: Appleton and Lange, 1994.

Ignoffo RJ, Viele CS. Cancer chemotherapy drugs and prescribing guidelines. In: *Cancer Chemotherapy Pocket Guide.* Philadelphia: Lippincott Raven, 1997:1–225.

Lacy CF, Armstrong LL, Goldman MP. *Drug Information Handbook: 2004–2005.* Hudson, OH: Lexi-Comp, Inc., 2004.

Perry MC, Clay MA, Donehower RC. Chemotherapy. In: Abeloff MD, Armitage JO, Lichter AS, Neiderhuber JE, eds. *Clinical Oncology.* 2nd ed. New York: Churchill Livingstone, 2000:378–422.

Ratain MJ. Pharmacology of cancer chemotherapy Section 1. In: DeVita VT, Hellman S, Rosenberg SA, eds. *Cancer. The Principles and Practice of Oncology.* 7th ed. Philadelphia: Lippincott Williams & Wilkins, 2004:375–384.

Principles of Transfusion Medicine

91

Susan A. Galel   Edgar G. Engleman

INTRODUCTION

Various blood components—either fresh or commercially processed—are available for clinical use. The appropriate use of blood components depends on an understanding of their characteristics, therapeutic value, and risks.

FRESH BLOOD COMPONENTS

Blood Collection

Fresh blood components are obtained from healthy volunteer donors. These donors are extensively screened for potential exposure to infectious diseases. The standard blood donation consists of approximately 500-milliliter "units" of whole blood collected in a citrate anticoagulant. This volume represents approximately 10% of a donor's blood. Each unit of whole blood can then be separated by centrifugation into its components: red cells, plasma, and platelets. One hundred milliliters of a nutrient additive solution is usually added to each red cell product to prolong its shelf life. Each blood component derived from one donation of whole blood is referred to as a "unit" of that component and constitutes approximately 10% replacement therapy for an adult patient (1).

Apheresis

Apheresis is an alternative approach to blood collection, in which a donor's blood is drawn into an automated processor that centrifuges the blood into its components and selectively harvests the desired component(s). The remainder of the donor's blood is returned to the donor. By means of continuous flow and centrifugation, multiple unit-equivalents of a particular blood component can be harvested. This technology is a primary source of platelets and plasma. The product of an apheresis platelet collection is equivalent to approximately six whole blood-derived platelet units. Apheresis technology can also be used to collect two units of red cells from larger donors, returning plasma and saline to the donors to preserve their intravascular volume. Granulocyte concentrates can also be collected by apheresis. To obtain therapeutic doses of granulocytes, however, donors must be premedicated with steroids and/or granulocyte colony stimulating factor (G-CSF) to increase their predonation white blood cell count.

Table 91.1 summarizes the therapeutic value of the most commonly prepared components of fresh blood.

MODIFICATIONS OF COMPONENTS OF FRESH BLOOD

Leukocyte Reduction

During centrifugation and separation of whole blood into components, white blood cells are partitioned into both the red cell and platelet products. These white blood cells, up to 10^9 per product, may cause febrile transfusion reactions and can stimulate human leukocyte antigen (HLA) immunization in transfusion recipients. White cells can be removed from blood components by passing the components through special synthetic fiber filters, which reduces levels of white cells from approximately 10^9 per product to 10^5 per product. Some platelet apheresis technologies select blood components so specifically that the products are essentially leukocyte-reduced at collection. The U.S. Food and Drug Administration (FDA) defines leukocyte-reduced

TABLE 91.1

FRESH BLOOD COMPONENTS AND THEIR USE

Component	Approximate unit volume	Therapeutic indication	Therapeutic impact/unit[a]	Approximate dose[b]	Approximate preparation and/or compatibility testing time
Whole blood[c]	500 mL	Acute hypovolemia with anemia	↑ Hgb ~ 1 g/dL ↑ Blood vol ~ 10%	Determined by estimated volume deficit	Type and cross-match (60 min)
Red blood cells	325 mL[d]	Anemia	↑ Hgb ~ 1 g/dL ↑ Blood vol ~ 5%	Determined by degree of anemia	Type and cross-match (60 min)
Fresh frozen plasma	200 mL	Replacement of multiple coagulation factors Warfarin reversal Factor V deficiency	↑ Coagulation factors ~ 8% ↑ Blood vol ~ 4%	4 units (10–15 mL/kg)	Thawing (30 min)
Platelet concentrate a) single unit b) pheresis unit	a) 50 mL b) 250 mL	Thrombocytopenia	↑ Platelet count by a) 2–7,000/μL b) 15–40,000/μL	a) 6 units b) 1 pheresis unit	a) ±Pooling (15–30 min) b) None
Cryoprecipitate	15 mL	Hypofibrinogenemia Topical fibrin adhesive	↑ Fibrinogen ~ 5 mg/dL (also includes factors VIII, XIII, von Willebrand factor)	10–15 units (1 U/5 kg)	Thawing (30 min) ±pooling (15–30 min)

[a] Anticipated response expressed either as a directly measurable increment or as a percentage of normal blood volume replacement in an adult.
[b] Common empiric adult doses.
[c] Transfusion services do not routinely store whole blood.
[d] Volume includes 100 mL nutrient additive solution.

products as those that contain fewer than 5×10^6 white blood cells per product. Most red cell and platelet pheresis products produced today are leukocyte-reduced.

Frozen Red Blood Cells

Red blood cells can be preserved for up to 10 years by freezing. After thawing, the shelf life is limited to 24 hours unless freezing and thawing were carried out using new closed-processing systems. Frozen storage is most applicable to cells of rare phenotype and is typically a service of large regional blood suppliers. Most hospitals do not maintain their own frozen storage facilities.

Washed Blood Products

"Washing" refers to the removal of plasma from cellular products (red blood cells, platelets) by resuspending the product in saline solution. This practice is primarily indicated for patients with known sensitivity to plasma proteins, such as patients with immunoglobulin A (IgA) deficiency (who may be extremely sensitive to IgA). Washing has no role in leukocyte reduction.

Irradiated Blood Products

Cellular products, including leukocyte-reduced products, contain lymphocytes potentially capable of mediating graft-versus-host disease in susceptible patients. Gamma-irradiated (≥2,500 rads) blood products are recommended for such patients (see Adverse Effects of Transfusion).

Pathogen-Inactivated Products

Several processes to inactivate residual pathogens in fresh blood products have been the subject of clinical trials. Chemicals that can bind to nucleic acid are added to the blood component; in some cases, exposure to light is required to achieve covalent binding. This binding renders pathogens unable to replicate. Product shelf life or in vivo recovery may be mildly diminished by the treatment. Substantial incremental costs, reduced therapeutic effectiveness of the product, and potential toxicities raise questions regarding the appropriate application of these technologies. These processes may serve as a reasonable approach for reducing the risk of transmission of nucleic acid-containing pathogens for which there are currently no donor screening tests.

COMMERCIAL BLOOD PRODUCTS

Red Cell Substitutes

Effective red cell substitutes must bind oxygen at pulmonary oxygen pressures, release oxygen at tissue oxygen pressures, and have adequate intravascular retention and limited toxicity. Currently, no red cell substitutes are licensed for clinical use in the United States. For many years, trials of red cell substitutes were foiled by toxicity and difficulty in demonstrating efficacy. Several red cell substitutes have been evaluated in recent clinical trials. Some are perfluorocarbon emulsions, which actually dissolve oxygen and have linear oxygen-carrying characteristics. The vast majority of oxygen carriers in trials, however, are hemoglobin-based products, in which the hemoglobin molecules are cross-linked to reproduce the classic S-shaped cooperative oxygen-binding curve. Some of the products use recombinant hemoglobin and may ultimately be acceptable to Jehovah's Witnesses, but others are made from outdated human red cells or bovine red cells. Although hemoglobin solutions most accurately mimic natural red cell oxygen-carrying characteristics, concerns have been raised that the binding of hemoglobin to nitric oxide and the resultant vasoconstriction may limit the ability of these products to deliver oxygen to tissues. All these products have very limited intravascular retention, and it is doubtful that their safety profile will be better than that of fresh red cell products. The most appealing features of these products would be immediate availability and universal applicability. Therefore, the products are most likely to be useful in settings of acute trauma or surgery.

Commercial Plasma Protein Products

Relatively purified preparations of selected plasma proteins can be isolated from pooled human plasma by means of industrial techniques. Thousands of units of plasma are pooled, and the pool is subjected to various precipitation or affinity purification steps that separate different plasma proteins. The earliest products produced in this way had a high probability of carrying infectious agents because of the large numbers of donors represented in each pool. Thus, in the 1970s and 1980s, many patients with hemophilia became infected with hepatitis viruses and HIV through clotting factor products derived from pooled plasma.

Today, the U.S. FDA requires that most products derived from pooled plasma be further processed with heat, ultrafiltration, or chemicals (e.g., with organic solvents and detergents that inactivate lipid-coated viruses) to reduce viral infectivity. These processes essentially eliminate the risk for transmission of HIV, hepatitis B virus, and hepatitis C virus. However, some other infectious agents—in particular viruses that do not have lipid coats such as hepatitis A virus and the B19 parvovirus—may survive the usual inactivation processes, and transmission of these agents by some pooled plasma products has been documented. Given the fact that thousands of donors are represented in each plasma pool and not all infectious agents are inactivated, the theoretical risk of transmitting some infectious agents remains higher with pooled products than with fresh products from single donors. For example, concerns have been raised regarding the potential for transmitting prions (the causative agents of spongiform encephalopathies) via pooled plasma products, although there is no evidence that such transmissions have occurred. Because of persistent concerns regarding infectivity of pooled plasma products, several human plasma proteins have been produced by recombinant DNA techniques, including clotting factors VIII, IX, and VIIa. However, these products may be expensive.

Table 91.2 illustrates the variety of plasma protein products currently available.

ROLE OF TRANSFUSION IN THE CARE OF THE HOSPITALIZED PATIENT

Indications for Use of Blood Components

Intravascular Volume Replacement

The need for volume replacement must be distinguished from the need for specific blood components. Normal blood volume is approximately 70 mL per kilogram, or 3,500 mL for an average-size female adult and 5,000 mL for an average-size male adult. Acute volume losses of 500–750 mL (10%–15%) can be tolerated in otherwise healthy persons without replacement because of sympathetically mediated vasoconstriction and increased cardiac output. Larger losses result in hypotension when cardiac output is compromised by inadequate preload. Volume replacement is typically initiated with crystalloid or colloid solutions. Blood components should be used for volume replacement only if the specific components themselves are needed. In general, red cells are the first blood component for which replacement is considered.

Replacement of Red Cells

The role of red blood cells is to carry and deliver oxygen to the tissues. Oxygen delivery is a function of blood flow and the oxygen (O_2) content of blood, as follows:

$$O_2 \text{ Delivery} = \text{Cardiac Output} \times \text{Arterial } O_2 \text{ Content}$$

where O_2 content is defined by the hemoglobin level and the oxygen saturation (expressed as a percentage) of hemoglobin. As the hemoglobin content of the blood declines, oxygen delivery is maintained through an increase in cardiac output. As noted above, this increase in cardiac output is dependent on adequate intravascular volume.

TABLE 91.2

EXAMPLES OF COMMERCIAL PLASMA PROTEIN PRODUCTS

Products	Source	Therapeutic use
Plasma substitutes		
Albumin	Human[a]	Raise oncotic pressure
Immunoglobulins		
Immune serum globulin	Human	Mitigate exposure to viruses
Intravenous IgG	Human	Immunodeficiency, therapy of immune disorders
Rh immune globulin	Immune human	Mitigate exposure to RhD antigen; treatment of ITP
Coagulation factors		
Factor VIII	Human	Factor VIII deficiency, von Willebrand's disease
	Recombinant[b]	Factor VIII deficiency
	Porcine	Treatment of factor VIII inhibitors
Factor IX complex		
Factor IX (purified)	Human	Factor IX deficiency
	Recombinant	Factor IX deficiency
Partially purified	Human	Factor IX deficiency
		Deficiency of Vitamin K-dependent factors
Activated	Human	Treatment of factor VIII inhibitors
Fibrinogen	Human	Topical fibrin adhesives
Antithrombin III	Human	AT III deficiency
Factor VIIa	Recombinant	Treatment of factor VIII or factor IX inhibitors
		Uncontrolled bleeding[c]

[a] All human source products are derived from pools of plasma from thousands of donors. These donors may have been paid.
[b] Recombinant products may be stabilized in human source albumin.
[c] Not yet an approved indication, but anecdotally reported to be effective at times.
AT III, antithrombin III; *FFP,* fresh frozen plasma; *ITP,* idiopathic thrombocytopenic purpura; *RhD,* Rhesus D antigen.

When normal intravascular volume is maintained and the heart and lungs are healthy, increases in cardiac output alone have been shown to compensate for acute losses of up to three-fourths of red cells, or a reduction in hemoglobin levels to 3 g/dL. In the face of myocardial, pulmonary, or peripheral vascular disease, oxygen delivery to specific tissues becomes inadequate at hemoglobin levels well above 3 g/dL.

Several organizations have published guidelines for red cell replacement therapy (2–4). All these panels agree that reduced hemoglobin levels to 6–7 g/dL are well tolerated in otherwise healthy persons. Oxygen delivery to the myocardium becomes inadequate at hemoglobin levels between 3 and 6 g/dL. All the published practice guidelines suggest that transfusion should be given to patients with hemoglobin levels below 6 g/dL. At hemoglobin levels above 6 g/dL, the need for transfusion should be assessed on a case-by-case basis. Clinical signs, such as tachycardia or lightheadedness, may suggest the need for transfusion. In patients undergoing invasive monitoring, the finding of low levels of mixed venous oxygen (<25 mm Hg) or high levels of oxygen extraction (>50%) is objective evidence of inadequate oxygen delivery (2,3,5). However, even these measurements may not adequately assess oxygen delivery to key critical tissues, such as the myocardium. Concern has been raised that certain populations, particularly elderly patients and those with coronary artery, pulmonary, or peripheral vascular disease, may be at increased risk for adverse events with hemoglobin levels between 6 and 10 g/dL. There is some evidence that critically ill patients with ischemic heart disease may benefit from a hemoglobin of 10 or above (6, 7). However, the appropriate transfusion trigger for critically ill patients in general is not clear, as two large studies found an association of transfusion with *increased* mortality in some critically ill patients (8, 9). Thus, a more restrictive transfusion regimen (e.g., to maintain hemoglobin between 7 and 9) may be more appropriate for critically ill patients without ischemic heart disease. More studies are needed to define the risks and benefits of red cell transfusion in the critical care setting. *In summary, evidence suggests that replacement of red cells is unnecessary at hemoglobin levels above 10 g/dL and usually indicated at hemoglobin levels below 6 g/dL.* Between these levels, the need for replacement should be considered on a case-by-case basis. Red cells are usually replaced in the form of packed red blood cells. Although whole blood may be the product of choice in hypovolemic anemia, in practice it is not usually available.

Replacement of Platelets and Plasma

Table 91.2 lists available agents for the treatment of bleeding diatheses. Guidelines for the transfusion of platelets and clotting factors are discussed in detail in Chapter 98.

Granulocyte Transfusion

Granulocyte transfusion may be considered for patients with neutropenia and life-threatening infections that are not responding to antimicrobials. The therapeutic effectiveness of this treatment is controversial. Acquisition of these products is complicated by the need to prescreen donors for infectious diseases (because products must be infused immediately after collection) and the need to premedicate donors to increase their predonation white blood cell counts. Physicians considering this intervention should consult their transfusion service medical director.

Empiric Therapy of Acute Bleeding

In patients who have experienced an acute hemorrhage, the initial hemoglobin determination may not accurately reflect the degree of red cell deficiency. Empiric therapy can be based on estimated volumes lost. The general strategy is similar to that described above: the first goal should be intravascular volume replacement with crystalloid, colloid, or both. If blood loss continues after replacement of 1,500 to 2,000 mL of fluid (i.e., 30%–40% of blood volume), red cell replacement should be considered. The need for platelet and plasma transfusion should be guided by the results of laboratory testing if it is rapidly available. However, replacement of these components is generally not needed until one or two entire blood volumes have been replaced.

PRINCIPLES OF RED BLOOD CELL COMPATIBILITY

Compatibility testing is necessary for red blood cell and plasma transfusion to prevent hemolytic transfusion reactions. The most important component of compatibility testing is the determination of the ABO blood type.

ABO System

The ABO antigens are carbohydrate chains on large membrane-bound glycosphingolipid molecules, expressed on almost all tissues of the body. The A and B antigens are produced by genetically encoded glycosyltransferases that modify the terminal sugar of the precursor O substance. These A and B antigens are similar to carbohydrates found on common bacteria, and during the first year of life all people begin to produce antibodies that cross-react with the carbohydrate A and B antigens other than those expressed by their own cells. Thus, group O persons, who express neither the A nor B antigens, produce antibodies against both A and B; group A persons produce only anti-B, and group B persons produce anti-A. These antibodies are typically of the immunoglobulin M (IgM) class and are complement fixing. If red blood cells are infused bearing the A or B antigen that the recipient lacks, these naturally occurring IgM antibodies will cause a rapid, intravascular lysis of the transfused cells, activating complement and releasing hemoglobin into the bloodstream. This *acute hemolytic transfusion reaction* can result in disseminated intravascular coagulation, shock, renal failure, and death.

Thus, if red blood cells are to be transfused safely, it is essential to type patients for their A and B antigens and provide red cells compatible with their pre-existing anti-A or anti-B IgM antibodies. Group O cells, which express neither A nor B antigens, can be safely infused into patients of any ABO type. Plasma components must also be selected for ABO compatibility; these contain the anti-A or anti-B antibodies of the plasma donor, and infusion of plasma containing anti-A or anti-B would cause hemolysis of the red cells of a recipient expressing those antigens. Table 91.3 illustrates the selection of red cell and plasma products according to donor and recipient ABO type. ABO compatibility is the most essential aspect of blood transfusion, and infusion of ABO-incompatible blood is the most common cause of fatal transfusion reactions. Most of these events are a consequence of *human error,* as when a typing specimen is obtained from the wrong patient or a unit of blood is infused into the wrong patient (Chapter 20). Therefore, we cannot overemphasize the importance of verifying the identity of the patient at the time the specimen is drawn for typing and at the time the blood is administered.

TABLE 91.3

ABO COMPATIBILITY

Patient's blood type	Antigens on RBC	Antibodies in plasma	Compatible donors	
			RBC	Plasma
A	A	Anti-B	A or O	A or AB
B	B	Anti-A	B or O	B or AB
O	None	Anti-A, anti-B	O	O, A, B, or AB
AB	A and B	None	AB, A, B, or O	AB

RBC, red blood cell.

Rhesus and Other Non-ABO Red Cell Antigens

Whereas antibodies to the A and B carbohydrate antigens are produced spontaneously, antibodies to other red cell antigens, such as Rhesus (RhD) antigen, are produced only after specific exposure to foreign red cells, either through transfusion or pregnancy. Among the non-ABO red cell antigens, RhD is the most immunogenic. About 15% of people lack the RhD antigen and are said to be "Rh-negative." If these people are challenged with red cells bearing the RhD antigen ("Rh-positive blood"), there is a high likelihood that they will produce anti-RhD antibody. The other non-ABO red cell antigens are much less immunogenic, with antibodies produced in fewer than 5% of transfusion recipients. Antibodies to non-ABO antigens, including anti-RhD antibodies, are typically of the immunoglobulin G (IgG) class and do not fix complement. If red cells bearing the target antigen are transfused into a person who has produced one of these IgG antibodies, the antibodies bind to the transfused cells, and the survival of the antibody-coated cells is likely to be shortened because of accelerated destruction in the spleen. Non-ABO antibodies only rarely cause intravascular hemolysis. In women of childbearing age, these IgG antibodies may be of additional concern because they can cross the placenta and destroy fetal cells bearing the target antigen.

Compatibility Testing

The three components of routine compatibility testing are type, screen, and cross-match. ABO and Rh typing is performed by incubating patient red cells with anti-A, anti-B, or anti-RhD reagents, centrifuging specimens, and looking for agglutination. Because of the importance of ABO typing in transfusion, ABO type is confirmed by verifying the presence of the expected anti-A or anti-B antibodies in the patient's plasma by incubating patient plasma with reagent cells of known ABO type. ABO/Rh typing takes approximately 10 minutes to perform.

Antibody screening is performed to detect IgG non-ABO anti-red cell antibodies. The plasma of the transfusion recipient is incubated with a panel of group O cells selected for their expression of the clinically significant non-ABO antigens to which patients may become sensitized. The binding of patient IgG to the target cells is detected by adding an anti-IgG reagent. Anti-Rh and other non-ABO antibodies are detected by this process, which takes approximately 30–45 minutes.

In patients with negative results on antibody screens, ABO/Rh-compatible cells (Table 91.3) are provided for transfusion. The only "cross-match" performed is a final check on ABO compatibility between donor and recipient. The check can be performed either electronically (by computer verification of donor and recipient ABO types) or serologically, with an "immediate spin" (IS) cross-match.

IS cross-matching is performed by incubating the patient's plasma with donor red cells, centrifuging, and looking for agglutination. A positive IS cross-match would indicate the presence of IgM antibodies (i.e., anti-ABO) against donor cells. The completion of type, screen, and IS cross-match takes approximately one hour.

If the result of the antibody screen is positive, further testing is required to identify the specific non-ABO antigen(s) to which the patient's IgG antibody is directed. Donor red cells that lack the target antigen(s) must then be located. Finally, compatibility between the patient's antibodies and donor cells is verified with an "IgG serologic cross-match," performed by incubating patient plasma with donor cells, adding an anti-IgG reagent to detect binding, and looking for agglutination. Only antigen-negative, "IgG cross-match−compatible" cells should be transfused. Antibody identification and selection of IgG cross-match−compatible cells can take 2 hours or longer.

Selection of Red Cells for Transfusion in Emergencies

Except in emergencies, transfusion should be withheld until the antibody screen is performed and compatibility is verified. *In emergencies, selection of red cells on the basis of ABO compatibility alone* (Table 91.3) *is sufficient for avoidance of most acute intravascular hemolytic reactions.* When feasible, RhD-negative (Rh-negative) patients are also provided with Rh-negative cellular components because of the high likelihood that these patients will produce anti-Rh antibodies after transfusion. Avoidance of Rh immunization is of particular importance in women of childbearing age. A positive antibody screen often results in a delay in providing cells for transfusion because of the additional testing required. Clinicians are urged to communicate with the transfusion service physician regarding the clinical urgency of transfusion and to discuss the relative risks and benefits of transfusion before the completion of laboratory testing.

ADVERSE EFFECTS OF TRANSFUSION

Acute Complications

Hemolytic Reactions

Acute intravascular hemolysis occurs in approximately 1 in 30,000 transfusions. This is most frequently a consequence of infusion of ABO-incompatible blood and is the most common cause of fatal transfusion reaction. Symptoms may include fever, chills, chest or back pain, and hypotension. Laboratory tests reveal hemoglobinemia, hemoglobinuria, and possibly coagulopathy. Treatment is supportive, with particular attention to hydration and diuresis to prevent renal failure. Diagnosis is based on the presence in the recipient's plasma of free hemoglobin in addition to antibodies that bind to the red cells from the donor unit. The result of a post-transfusion direct antiglobulin test, a test for antibody bound to red cells circulating in the recipient, may be negative if the incompatible cells were immediately lysed.

Extravascular hemolysis is caused by non-ABO red cell antibodies, including most Rh antibodies. Extravascular hemolysis may be seen if a non-ABO antibody is not detected on the pre-transfusion antibody screen. More commonly, it is caused by IgG non-ABO antibodies produced following transfusion (*delayed transfusion reaction*). Although fever may be seen, often there are no symptoms at all. Destruction of the transfused cells is usually gradual. Splenic enlargement may occur if several units of transfused cells are destroyed. Laboratory testing demonstrates serologic incompatibility of recipient plasma with the donor red cells, a falling hematocrit, and hyperbilirubinemia; results of direct antiglobulin testing are positive.

Allergic Reactions

Allergic reactions occur in up to 1% of transfusions and typically reflect the recipient's reaction to plasma in the transfused product. Symptoms usually are limited to urticarial rash. Reactions may recur with subsequent transfusions, but the severity does not usually increase with time. Symptoms can often be reduced by pretreatment of the recipient with antihistamines. Rarely, systemic anaphylactic reactions can occur, often in patients with no prior history of reaction (Chapter 120). The majority of anaphylactic reactions have no identifiable cause, although some are caused by anti-IgA antibodies in patients with IgA deficiency. Transfusion of plasma should be avoided in patients with a history of anaphylactic transfusion reactions, and for these patients, red cell and platelet products should be thoroughly washed with saline solution to remove plasma before infusion.

Febrile Reactions

Fever occurring during or immediately after infusion may indicate an acute hemolytic reaction, but more often it reflects a nonhemolytic reaction mediated by white blood cells and their metabolic products. Febrile nonhemolytic reactions are associated with up to 1% of red cell transfusions and with a much higher proportion of platelet transfusions. Symptoms may include fever, chills, flushing, nausea and vomiting, hypertension, and, rarely, shortness of breath. Febrile nonhemolytic reactions are frequently caused by the binding of antibodies in the transfusion recipient to white blood cells in the transfused product. These reactions can be minimized by the use of leukocyte-reduced blood products. Febrile nonhemolytic reactions to platelet products may also be caused by cytokines produced *in vitro* by white blood cells in the platelet products. Leukocyte reduction of platelet products before storage or removal of product supernatant immediately before infusion may reduce the number of febrile nonhemolytic reactions associated with these products. Rarely, anti-white cell antibodies of donor origin, present in the plasma of a transfused product, can cause febrile nonhemolytic reactions or cytokine-mediated pulmonary edema (*transfusion-related acute lung injury*) in a transfusion recipient.

Bacterial Contamination

Fever at the time of, or shortly after, transfusion may indicate bacterial contamination of the blood product. The presence of asymptomatic bacteremia in a blood donor or of donor skin flora at the phlebotomy site can result in the contamination of blood products. Low-level contamination with bacteria, most commonly nonvirulent skin flora, is found in approximately 1 in 5,000 blood products. Rarely, contaminating organisms multiply to a significant extent during storage of the blood product, especially platelet products, which are stored at room temperature rather than in the refrigerator. Fever resulting from bacterial contamination is reported to occur with infusion of 1 in 10,000 platelet concentrates and 1 in 30,000 red cell units. Rarely, infusion of bacterially contaminated red cells or platelets can cause sepsis, endotoxin-mediated shock, or even death. The small numbers of bacteria that may be present in blood products on the day of collection cannot be detected by currently available technology. Recently implemented processes that detect bacteria in platelet products after 24 hours of storage can interdict at least some contaminated products.

Complications Related to Large or Rapid Transfusions

The infusion of multiple units of blood or plasma can result in volume overload and pulmonary edema. The rapid infusion of large volumes of blood can also cause acute metabolic complications, including transient hypocalcemia (a consequence of the binding of free calcium by the citrate anticoagulant), hyperkalemia (resulting from the presence of free potassium in the supernatant of stored red cells), and hypothermia (related to infusion of large volumes of refrigerated blood). These metabolic complications are not generally encountered except in the setting of trauma or surgery.

Other Immunologic Complications of Transfusion

Approximately 30% of multiply transfused patients become immunized to HLA antigens expressed on white cells and platelets. Anti-HLA antibodies may cause refractoriness to platelet transfusion and febrile nonhemolytic transfusion reactions. HLA allo-immunization can be prevented or delayed by the prophylactic use of leukocyte-reduced blood products. Other immunologic effects may include transfusion-related immunosuppression. Several authors have suggested an association between transfusion and an increased risk of cancer recurrence, postoperative infection, or activation of endogenous viruses such as HIV and cytomegalovirus. However, these effects have not been conclusively demonstrated. Rarely, white blood cells from the transfused product can engraft in the recipient and cause graft-versus-host disease.

Viral Infections Transmitted by Transfusion

HIV and Hepatitis

The risk for transmitting hepatitis or HIV viruses by transfusion is now extremely low. Blood donors are screened with explicit questioning to identify previous exposure to these viruses or a history of activities that increase their risk for exposure to blood-borne or sexually transmitted disease. Risk activities that blood banks must inquire about are defined by the U.S. Public Health Service and the FDA and are revised periodically based on epidemiologic investigation. Blood may be drawn only from persons who pass questioning. Questioning alone eliminates approximately 90% of virally infected potential donors. All blood that is collected then undergoes a panel of serologic tests mandated by the FDA. Table 91.4 shows a list of the tests currently performed on donated blood. Only blood that passes both questioning and testing can be used for transfusion.

The combined effectiveness of donor questioning and testing is so high that the risk for transmitting hepatitis virus or HIV by transfusion is too small to be measured accurately by prospective studies. Estimated risk has been calculated by using epidemiologic models (10, 11). The majority of disease transmissions are thought to be caused

TABLE 91.4

DONOR SCREENING TESTS FOR INFECTIOUS DISEASE (UNITED STATES)

Agent	Donors tested for
HIV	Antibody to HIV-1 and HIV-2[a]
	HIV-1 nucleic acid[b]
Hepatitis B	Antibody to hepatitis B core antigen[a]
	Hepatitis B surface antigen
Hepatitis C	Antibody to hepatitis C[c]
	HCV nucleic acid[b]
HTLV	Antibody to HTLV-I and HTLV-II[c]
Syphilis	RPR or anti-treponemal antibody

[a] Test detects both IgM and IgG antibodies.
[b] Test may be performed on pooled specimens from 16–24 donors.
[c] Test detects only IgG antibodies.
HTLV, human T-cell lymphotropic virus; *RPR*, rapid plasma reagin.

TABLE 91.5

RATES OF VIRAL TRANSMISSION BY TRANSFUSION OF SCREENED BLOOD

	Estimated risk of transmission (per unit transfused)
Human immunodeficiency virus	1/1,779,000
Hepatitis C virus	1/1,613,000
Hepatitis B virus	1/171,000
Human T-cell lymphotropic virus	1/428,000

Estimates are based on Dodd et al. (10), adjusted as recommended by Glynn et al. (11) to reflect a mix of 80% repeat donors and 20% first-time donors with a two-fold increased incidence of new infections in first-time donors.

when blood from donors recently exposed to infectious agents but whose test results have not yet become positive (so-called window-period donations) is transfused. Recent introduction of donor screening tests that detect HCV and HIV nucleic acid has shortened the estimated window period for these agents to 10–11 days. These highly sensitive donor screening tests, combined with the low incidence of infections in the blood donor population, are responsible for the extremely low estimated risks of transfusion-transmitted viral infection today (Table 91.5).

Cytomegalovirus

This common virus can cause severe morbidity in premature or unborn infants and in patients who are immunodeficient, immunosuppressed, or have had their spleens removed. Patients previously unexposed to this virus (CMV-seronegative) should be protected from transfusion transmission of the virus by the use of blood obtained from CMV antibody-negative blood donors. Extensive leukocyte reduction also appears effective in reducing the CMV infectivity of blood components.

Other Agents

Any agent found in the blood of an apparently healthy blood donor can be transmitted by transfusion. Parasites have only rarely been reported to be transmitted by transfusion in the United States, where there is currently no blood donor testing for parasitic infection. Up to three cases of transfusion-transmitted malaria occur in the United States each year. Recent studies show that approximately 1 in 10,000 U.S. blood donors is infected with *Trypanosoma cruzi*, the parasite that causes Chagas disease, but transfusion transmission of this infection appears to be rare. Transfusion transmission of the intraerythrocytic parasite *Babesia* may be much more common. Investigational testing for West Nile virus (WNV) RNA was implemented in 2003 following documented transmission of this agent during the 2002 epidemic. Concern about transmission of other infectious agents, such as new retroviruses or prions, has also been raised. The AIDS epidemic generated a heightened awareness of the importance of maintaining surveillance for new emerging pathogens and of continually assessing the need for additional donor testing or blood product processing. Additional nucleic acid-based donor screening tests and/or processes that inactivate residual pathogens in blood products are likely to be used in the future.

Transfusion Options

Autologous Blood

Autologous blood is blood collected from patients and retained for their own use. In general, this is the safest transfusion option because it eliminates the potential for transmission of viral infection and for most transfusion reactions. The benefits of autologous transfusion are limited by the extremely low risk for transmission of viral disease associated with allogeneic blood transfusions and by the high likelihood that many patients will die of their underlying disease before a transfusion-transmitted virus will become clinically manifest. The cost of autologous collection strategies must be weighed against the limited benefits. Analyses suggest that autologous transfusion is most cost effective in the youngest patients (12). In some patients, the risks of autologous collection and transfusion may outweigh the potential benefits; examples include patients who are too ill to tolerate the donation process safely or patients with bacterial infections whose products may be contaminated.

Designated (Directed) Donations

Some patients request that their friends or relatives donate blood products specifically for their use. These so-called designated or directed donors must pass all the same questions and tests that volunteer community donors do. The rates of infectious disease markers in directed donations are not lower than those in donations from volunteer community donors. On the contrary, there is a concern that directed donations are potentially *less* safe because such donors might be more reluctant to admit to risky behaviors that could result in the deferral of their donation. Patients who ask friends and relatives to donate may actually compromise their own safety if they put undue pressure on these people to donate. Blood components from designated donations are usually released for general transfusion if not needed by the intended recipient. All directed donations from blood relatives of the recipient must un-

dergo gamma irradiation to prevent transfusion-related graft-versus-host disease.

COST CONSIDERATIONS IN TRANSFUSION MEDICINE

Since the mid-1980s, public fears of transfusion-transmitted HIV have fueled an increase in government regulation of the blood industry, the application of many additional donor screening tests, and the commercial production of recombinant and virally inactivated plasma protein products. This has dramatically increased the safety of blood but also has raised the cost of blood products. Today, the acquisition cost of leukocyte-reduced red blood cells is $200–$300 per unit. Irradiation adds further costs to each product. Commercial products can cost thousands of dollars per dose. Blood products constitute a significant proportion of the total operating costs of hospitals. Therefore, cost containment considerations, as well as risk-versus-benefit concerns, often enter into discussions of transfusion guidelines. The general guideline of "using only what is necessary" is, of course, applicable. In addition, however, the cost effectiveness of expensive options such as autologous, designated, recombinant, or pathogen-inactivated products should be evaluated rationally.

CONCLUSIONS

Although blood transfusions continue to save many lives, the field of transfusion medicine has changed dramatically in recent years. Concern in the 1980s about transfusion-related infection led to stricter guidelines regarding indications for transfusion, such that transfusions are now recommended only when absolutely necessary. Similar safety concerns catalyzed the addition of a number of mandatory blood screening procedures, including assays for the presence of selected infectious agents, so that the incidence of life-threatening transfusion-related infections is now extremely low. New methods for preparing blood products, including genetic engineering and viral inactivation technologies, have led to the availability of numerous alternative forms of blood products with improved potency and safety, but almost all these products are substantially more expensive than standard blood components. Therefore, when considering transfusion alternatives, physicians must carefully weigh both benefits and costs.

KEY POINTS

- The need for volume replacement should be distinguished from the need for blood components.
- In cases of acute bleeding, red cells are the first blood component to be considered for replacement.

- Red cell transfusion is usually indicated in patients with hemoglobin levels below 6 g/dL and is usually not indicated in patients with hemoglobin levels above 10 g/dL. In patients with hemoglobin levels between 6 and 10 g/dL, the need for transfusion of red cells should be assessed on a case-by-case basis.
- The risk for transmission of known viral agents by fresh blood components is now extremely low.
- Recombinant plasma proteins may be safer than pooled plasma products but may also be extremely expensive.
- The cost effectiveness of transfusion options such as autologous donation is limited by the extremely low risk for transmission of viral disease by allogeneic blood components.

REFERENCES

1. Simon TL, Dzik WH, Snyder EL, Sowell C, Strauss R, eds. *Rossi's Principles of Transfusion Medicine.* 3rd ed. Philadelphia: Lippincott Williams & Wilkins, 2002.
2. Simon TL, Alverson DC, AuBuchon J, et al. Practice parameter for the use of red blood cell transfusions. *Arch Pathol Lab Med* 1998; 122:130–138.
3. Practice guidelines for blood component therapy. A report by the American Society of Anesthesiologists Task Force on Blood Component Therapy. *Anesthesiology* 1996;84:732–747.
4. Audet A-M, Goodnough LT. Practice strategies for elective red blood cell transfusion. *Ann Intern Med* 1992;116:403–406.
5. Spiess BD, Counts RB, Gould SA. *Perioperative Transfusion Medicine.* Baltimore: Williams & Wilkins, 1998.
6. Wu WC, Rathore SS, Wang Y, Radford MJ, Krumholz HM. Blood transfusion in elderly patients with acute myocardial infarction. *N Engl J Med* 2001;345:1230–1236.
7. Hebert PC, Yetisir E, Martin C, et al. Is a low transfusion threshold safe in critically ill patients with cardiovascular diseases? *Crit Care Med* 2001;29:227–234.
8. Vincent JL, Baron J-F, Reinhart K, et al. Anemia and blood transfusion in critically ill patients. *JAMA* 2002;288:1499–1507.
9. Hebert PC, Wells G, Blajchman MA, et al., and the Transfusion Requirements in Critical Care Investigators for the Canadian Critical Care Trials Group. A multicenter, randomized, controlled clinical trial of transfusion requirements in critical care. *N Engl J Med* 1999;340:409–417.
10. Dodd RY, Notari IV EP, Stramer SL. Current prevalence and incidence of infectious disease markers and estimated window-period risk in the American Red Cross blood donor population. *Transfusion* 2002;42:975–979.
11. Glynn SA, Kleinman SH, Wright DJ, Busch MP. International application of the incidence rate/window period model. *Transfusion* 2002;42:966–972.
12. Etchason J, Petz L, Keeler E, et al. The cost effectiveness of preoperative autologous blood donations. *N Engl J Med* 1995;332: 719–724.

ADDITIONAL READING

Galel SA, Malone JM III, Viele M. Transfusion medicine. In: Greer JP, Foerster J, Lukens JN, et al., eds. *Wintrobe's Clinical Hematology.* 11th ed. Philadelphia: Lippincott Williams & Wilkins, 2004:831–882.

Hébert PC. Clinical consequences of anemia and red cell transfusion in the critically ill. *Crit Care Clin* 2004;20:225–235.

Oncologic Emergencies

Judith A. Luce

92

INTRODUCTION

Cancer is a common disease and a common cause of hospitalization for adults. Health care expenses for patients having cancer are usually concentrated in the last few months of life, when quality of life is declining and the utility of hospital-based interventions may also be declining. Therefore, it is important that physicians evaluating cancer patients with acute, potentially life-threatening complications carefully consider the context in which these complications present. What is the patient's short and long-term prognosis? What are the patient's wishes for the final days of life? What alternatives remain for systemic and local treatment of the patient's problems? Is it medically appropriate to treat the problem or not? The optimum approach to these complex questions usually involves consultation with a multidisciplinary management team.

In most adult patients who present with oncologic emergencies, cancer has already been diagnosed. Initial presentations with the entities discussed in this chapter are relatively uncommon, however, the cancers most likely to cause these emergencies will be emphasized in order to guide the physician who needs to make a tissue diagnosis prior to initiating specific cancer-directed therapy. There is little cost-effectiveness and outcomes research regarding the treatment of oncologic emergencies. Therefore, implementing many of the recommendations made in this chapter depends on the status of individual patients. Ambulatory, well-supported patients with access to transportation and home care may receive treatment for many of these conditions with minimal or no hospitalization. Others require hospitalization to enforce bed rest or to ensure compliance with more complex therapies or observation of evolving problems such as neurologic symptoms. Clinical judgment is of paramount importance.

This chapter covers cancer-related neurologic conditions, pericardial effusion, superior vena cava syndrome, and hypercalcemia. Infections in the immunocompromised host are covered in Chapter 63, and the tumor lysis syndrome is reviewed in Chapter 94. When found early, these conditions are often not truly emergencies, and the evaluation and treatment can be carried out over several days. Even when discovered very late, they may not be emergencies. For example, neurologic injury may have progressed to the point at which no intervention can restore function. The patients for whom time is of the greatest importance are those whose symptoms are severe but of very brief duration. Rapid reversal within hours may result in an outcome that restores function, and delays may be critical.

NEUROLOGIC EMERGENCIES

Issues at the Time of Admission

Clinical Presentation

There are three cancer-related neurologic conditions that may be regarded as emergencies: metastases to the brain, spinal cord compression, and meningeal carcinomatosis. Cerebral metastases are common, occurring in up to half of all patients with cancer at the time of autopsy; the highest rates occur in hematogenously disseminated cancers. Breast cancer and lung cancer are the most common causes of central nervous system (CNS) metastases, but the diagnosis should also be considered in advanced melanoma, renal cell carcinoma, rectal cancer, and gastric cancer. As many as one-fourth of patients with advanced cancer develop symptomatic CNS disease.

Cerebral metastases may present with focal CNS deficits, with global changes in mentation or behavior, or with seizures. Headache, nausea, and dizziness are nonspecific symptoms; difficulties with memory and other subtle signs of CNS dysfunction may occur. Seizures are most common in patients having multiple metastases, particularly to the frontal lobe, and are rare in patients with lesions in the posterior fossa.

Meningeal carcinomatosis may similarly present non-specifically with nausea, headache, mentation difficulties, or with seizures. A classic presentation is the presence of asymmetric radiculopathy (lower motor neuron deficit) of the cranial nerves and peripheral nerves. This presentation may be quite rapid in onset and variable in severity. Meningeal carcinomatosis occurs most often in breast and lung cancer and in cancers with involvement of the vertebral bodies and retroperitoneum. Non-Hodgkin's lymphoma and leukemia may also involve the meninges, especially in advanced or relapsing disease. Meningeal carcinomatosis occurs in fewer than 5% of cancer patients.

Meningeal involvement must be distinguished from *spinal cord compression*, which may also present with radiculopathy that is asymmetric; however, spinal cord compression does not involve cranial nerves and may also be accompanied by a sensory deficit. The most florid manifestation of spinal cord compression is myelopathy, which consists of sensory and motor loss below a specific spinal level, accompanied by bowel and bladder dysfunction. Back pain is an almost universal feature of spinal cord compression, but is rare in meningeal carcinomatosis. Most spinal cord compression occurs in the thoracic spine (70%), but *cauda equina syndrome* may result when the compression occurs in the lumbar spine. The most common causes of spinal cord compression are breast cancer, prostate cancer, lung cancer, and lymphoma. Spinal cord compression may occur in as many as 8% of patients with prostate cancer, and slightly fewer with lung or breast cancer. Spinal cord compression develops in approximately 20% of patients with spread of cancer to the vertebral bodies.

Differential Diagnosis and Evaluation

Newly onset back pain in a patient having known metastatic cancer should trigger an evaluation for spinal cord compression. Evaluation of new back pain in patients with known vertebral metastases results in a diagnosis of cord compression in about 30% of patients with normal neurologic findings. If the neurologic examination is normal and the pain is not severe, investigation can take place on an outpatient basis, and should begin with a bone scan and spinal radiography. The positive predictive value of abnormal bone scan is at least 40%, and the positive predictive value of abnormal spine x-rays much higher.

The presence of *any* neurologic finding should prompt performance of an MRI of the entire spine. All regions should be imaged to rule out multiple synchronous metastases, which may occur in as many as half of patients with spinal cord compression. Benign fracture, disc disease, abscess, and hematoma may be in the differential diagnosis, and are usually readily distinguishable from cancer by an MRI. MRI imaging is also a critical prelude to radiation therapy treatment planning. Thus, this test must be performed even when the physical examination, bone scan, and plain radiographic findings are diagnostic.

Because of the overlap between the presentation of CNS metastases and meningeal carcinomatosis, patients with both presentations are usually first evaluated with an MRI, which is the evaluation of choice for patients for whom the suspicion is high for either condition. Computed tomography (CT) is insensitive for the detection of meningeal changes, and an MRI can detect CNS metastases smaller than those seen on CT, thus potentially altering the treatment plan.

The definitive diagnosis of meningeal carcinomatosis involves large-volume lumbar puncture and CSF cytology. Obtaining up to three large volume specimens (at least 5 mL) will provide a diagnosis in the vast majority of patients. Abnormalities such as low glucose and high protein levels may be seen but are not diagnostic; cell counts are not helpful unless other causes of meningitis are in the differential diagnosis.

Some patients who present with neurologic emergencies may require staging of the cancer in order to make therapy decisions. This is particularly true if this is the first sign of metastatic disease or the first diagnosis of cancer. Other patients may require formal evaluation of spinal stability by a neurosurgeon or orthopedic surgeon, or formal consideration of surgical intervention (Table 92.1).

Indications for Hospitalization

Clear indications for hospitalization are listed in Table 92.2. Patients with minimal neurologic injury who are capable of self-care and whose symptoms are not rapidly evolving may be evaluated and treated as outpatients, as long as the evaluation will take place rapidly and therapy is initiated within a few days. However, most patients are admitted because evaluation is usually faster in the inpa-

---

TABLE 92.1

WHEN TO CALL THE NEUROSURGEON IN NEUROLOGIC EMERGENCIES

No tissue diagnosis available: needs biopsy
Possible resection of *solitary* CNS metastasis
  Slow paced cancer
  Primary site controlled or readily controllable
  Low likelihood of significant neurologic injury due to resection
  No other contraindications to craniotomy
CNS metastases, treatable cancer, evidence of imminent herniation
Cord compression, treatable cancer, rapid onset of severe neurologic injury (within hours)
Cord compression, unstable spine with potential for good functional outcome
Progression during radiation therapy and otherwise good prognosis
Previous radiation therapy, local recurrence with otherwise good prognosis
Need for insertion of Ommaya reservoir for intrathecal therapy of meningeal disease

TABLE 92.2

INDICATIONS FOR HOSPITALIZATION FOR NEUROLOGIC EMERGENCIES

Rapidly evolving neurologic changes, including seizures
Severe neurologic injury of recent onset
Inability to perform self-care at home
Unstable spine

---

tient setting and the necessary consultations may be obtained rapidly. Intensive care unit admission is necessary for neurological monitoring if the neurologic status is evolving and the patient has not expressed wishes to the contrary.

Initial Therapy

The mainstay of therapy for patients with neurologic emergencies is bedrest and careful nursing observation. Patients who are not ambulatory will require precautions for thrombosis, urinary retention, decubitus ulcers, and contractures. Patients who are ambulatory but who have had rapid progression of symptoms may require frequent monitoring of neurologic vital signs. Patients who have known or suspected spinal cord compression must remain at bedrest until spinal stability has been established, symptoms are not worsening, and pain has been appropriately managed. All patients require evaluation by physical and occupational therapy for treatment of functional problems.

Steroids have been shown to be effective initial therapy of CNS metastases, which are often accompanied by considerable surrounding edema. The usual drug is dexamethasone at a dose of 4 mg either orally or intravenously every six hours. The utility of a loading dose or higher doses has not been proven by clinical trials, but higher doses may be necessary in patients on diphenylhydantoin because of the associated accelerated metabolism of dexamethasone.

One clinical trial found no additional efficacy for total dexamethasone doses above 4 mg daily (1). Dexamethasone can produce rapid neurologic improvement in up to half of patients; this is generally regarded as a favorable sign for potential neurologic recovery. The use of mannitol or other drugs aimed at reducing intracranial pressure has not been demonstrated to be beneficial. Management of patients without steroids is possible if there is little or no cerebral edema, but the preponderance of evidence suggests that steroid-treated patients have better neurologic outcomes.

Dexamethasone may be of benefit to patients with spinal cord compression, although this has not been proven (2). Dexamethasone is of no benefit to patients with meningeal carcinomatosis. Protracted dexamethasone therapy should be accompanied by chemoprophylaxis for *Pneumocystis jirovecii* (formerly *P. carinii*) pneumonia to prevent this opportunistic infection. All patients who present with seizures or who undergo resection of their CNS tumors should receive anti-seizure therapy, but prophylaxis for seizures is controversial, especially in low-risk patients.

Radiation therapy is the mainstay of treatment of patients with spinal cord compression and cerebral metastases. Spinal cord radiation is usually performed as multiple fractional doses to a wide area surrounding the site of compression. CNS radiation therapy may be administered as whole brain radiation in fractionated doses or as localized treatment of metastases (called stereotactic radiosurgery [or "gamma knife"]), either alone or combined with whole brain radiation. Patients who are eligible for the stereotactic approach are those with potential for longer survival (Table 92.3), and with less than 5–6 metastases, none larger than 3 cm in diameter. The indications for either approach have not yet been standardized, and controversy remains about whether the functional outcomes are better with one or the other (3, 4).

Some cases of spinal cord compression may be successfully treated with *systemic therapy*. Previously untreated small cell lung carcinoma and non-Hodgkin's lymphoma have been shown to respond well to chemotherapy as

TABLE 92.3

PROGNOSTIC INDICATORS AND SURVIVAL IN PATIENTS WITH CEREBRAL METASTASES TREATED WITH RADIATION THERAPY (6)

Class	Performance status[a]	Age	Primary tumor controlled?	Other mets?	Median survival, months
1	≥70%	<65	Yes	No	7–10 months
2	≥70%	>65	Or not controlled	No or yes	4–6 months
3a	≤70%	<65	Yes	No	6–8 months
3b months	≤70%	>65	Or not controlled	No or yes	1.5–3

[a]Performance status: >70% is out of bed, ambulatory, capable of self-care without assistance, though not working.
Mets, metastases.

initial treatment. As adjuncts to radiation therapy, hormone therapies may be used for breast and prostate cancer patients. Prostate cancer patients without prior hormone therapy benefit from treatment. However, only orchiectomy or high-dose ketoconazole (800–1200 mg orally per day) produce sufficiently rapid responses to help patients with acute cord compression. Primary CNS lymphoma is treated first with chemotherapy (the regimens usually include high-dose methotrexate) prior to considering irradiation. Oral chemotherapy with temozolomide may benefit certain patients with symptomatic CNS or meningeal metastases who have failed previous radiation therapy (5).

Meningeal carcinomatosis is treated with radiation therapy to the site of greatest involvement—the whole brain if cranial neuropathies are present, or on the spinal cord if peripheral radiculopathy is the presenting problem. Total cranial and spinal irradiation is not usually performed because of marrow suppression. In addition to radiation therapy, *intrathecal chemotherapy* is administered, usually through a ventricular Ommaya reservoir. Placement of this device by neurosurgeons through a burr hole in the skull is a low-risk procedure that is well tolerated by most patients. Chemotherapy is placed in the reservoir two or three times weekly until cytology of the CSF shows either no response or clearance of malignant cells. The complications of an Ommaya reservoir include infection and meningeal irritation. Although chemotherapy may also be administered through repeated lumbar punctures, this is less well tolerated and less likely to ensure even distribution of the cytotoxic drugs.

Indications for Early Consultation

Oncology consultation is essential to making the critical early decisions about whether and how to treat patients with neurologic emergencies. Many patients who are at risk for oncologic emergencies are already under the care of an oncologist, and the oncologist will order and administer chemotherapy for appropriate patients with neurologic emergencies. Radiation therapy consultation is appropriate for nearly all patients with neurologic emergencies, because even if surgical resection is undertaken, it will usually be followed by consolidation radiation therapy unless the patient has already received radiotherapy. The indications for neurosurgical intervention are listed in Table 92.1. Physical and occupational therapy consultations are also needed in most patients with neurologic signs and symptoms.

Issues During the Course of Hospitalization

Neurologic signs or symptoms may progress while patients are undergoing treatment. When the spinal cord is compressed, the most widely accepted surgical therapy is posterior decompression by laminectomy. This is usually well tolerated and successful if the underlying neurologic injury is mild or very recent. Neurosurgical intervention to decompress the brain in patients with threatened herniation or to relieve symptoms of hydrocephalus in patients with meningeal disease is controversial and much less likely to result in good quality of life. Hemorrhage into vascular CNS tumors may also occur during treatment, and is usually not treatable. During the early phases of treatment, the patient's neurologic status should be monitored. In the event of deterioration, patients should be promptly re-imaged.

The treatment of spine instability is another complex issue that may arise during hospitalization. If bony destruction by tumor has progressed to render ambulation unsafe, a procedure to stabilize the spine must be considered. Generally, one of two approaches is employed: definitive attempts to provide long-term stability with bone grafts and other mechanical devices, or less invasive surgeries using methacrylate and external appliances to attempt short term stabilization. Some procedures combine these strategies, and the precise procedure should be determined by the expertise of the consulting surgeon and the precise nature of the lesion. However, all of these surgeries are more complex than laminectomy for decompression. Stabilization requires an anterior approach; for the thoracic spine it requires thoracotomy. Whether these procedures are appropriate or will be tolerated by the patient is a decision that must be made by a multidisciplinary team in consultation with patients and their families.

Complications of steroid therapy and of bedrest, and loss of neurologic function and performance status, frequently arise during treatment of neurologic emergencies. Most of these should be treated the same as in a patient without cancer. One major exception might be the use of aggressive supportive measures such as feeding tubes, which requires discussion with patients and their families regarding the overall aims of end-of-life support (Chapter 19). Radiation therapy to the thoracic spine and cervical spine is usually accompanied by transient esophagitis; radiation therapy to the lumbar spine may be accompanied by nausea, diarrhea, and abdominal pain.

Discharge Issues

Patients with spinal stability and stable neurologic signs and symptoms may be discharged home to complete their radiation therapy as outpatients. Physical therapy, occupational therapy, and home nursing support may be offered to patients for whom the potential for rehabilitation is good. Hospice referral should be considered in appropriate patients. Ambulation status at the time of admission is the single most important predictor of post-discharge neurologic status. Those who are ambulatory at the time of diagnosis tend to remain that way, and those who are not have a varied, but markedly less favorable, outcome.

Survival following neurologic emergencies is generally short. Patients with previously untreated (but highly treatable) cancers have the best survival rates and neurologic outcomes. For spinal cord compression, these patients are those with newly diagnosed small cell lung cancer, breast cancer, and prostate cancer, as well as those with Hodgkin's or non-Hodgkin's lymphomas. Neurologic outcomes are good with chemotherapy alone in patients with small cell lung cancer and lymphomas, although radiation therapy may also be given. Pain relief should be achievable, even for less treatable cancers. Patients may have recurrence at a previously treated site if their cancer recurs. This occurs in about half of the patients with metastatic prostate cancer, at an average of approximately 2 years. Survival is shorter in patients with paraplegia and incontinence, and longer for ambulatory patients and patients with only a single site of vertebral metastasis.

Survival data for CNS metastases treated with radiation therapy, with or without surgery, have been reported in several large patient series (Table 92.3) (6). Patients with solitary (without systemic disease) cerebral metastases who have undergone resection and irradiation have a median survival of more than a year. Patients for whom surgery is not possible have an average survival of 6 months, and relatively high rates of recurrence of neurologic symptoms. The outcomes are very dependent on the age of the patient and the severity of neurologic symptoms. Less radiation-responsive tumors have the poorest survival, and there is little evidence that radiation therapy enhances survival in patients with such tumors.

Meningeal carcinomatosis has the worst prognosis of all: only a few months for patients with treatable malignancies, and a few weeks for patients with tumors that generally do not respond well to intrathecal chemotherapy. Patients with leukemia or lymphoma have the best outcomes, followed by patients with small cell lung cancer and breast cancer. Others have very poor short-term prognoses.

PERICARDIAL EFFUSION AND TAMPONADE

Issues at the Time of Admission

Clinical Presentation

The presentation of pericardial tamponade in cancer patients is quite varied (the entity of tamponade is described more fully in Chapter 46; this section focuses on malignant pericardial disease). The classic findings of Kussmaul's sign, narrow pulse pressure, pulsus paradoxus and ECG findings of low voltage may be present. However, tamponade in cancer patients may also present as left- or right-sided heart failure, or with more subtle findings including fatigue, dyspnea, failure to thrive, and hiccups. Chest pressure, anxiety, and dyspnea may lead to a suspicion of coronary ischemia. Patients may even complain of upper gastrointestinal symptoms. Suspicion may be raised only by an enlarging cardiac silhouette on a chest x-ray.

These protean manifestations are part of the reason that pericardial disease in cancer patients is diagnosed more often post-mortem than in life.

Differential Diagnosis

Patients who have received mediastinal radiation therapy have a significant risk of benign pericardial inflammation, especially if 4,000 or more cGy have been delivered to a considerable area of the heart. Pericarditis may be acute, appearing during or immediately after the treatment; or chronic, with a delay of a few months to many years. Viral and bacterial causes of pericarditis should be considered, especially in immunosuppressed patients. The possibility of constrictive pericarditis due to fungal or mycobacterial organisms should be entertained in the appropriate risk groups.

The initial step in the diagnosis of pericardial effusion and tamponade is echocardiography. This may demonstrate thickened pericardium and pericardial fluid. Signs of tamponade physiology, including paradoxical septal motion, right atrial collapse, and low stroke volumes, should be sought. Pericardiocentesis should be performed at the time of initial echocardiography, especially if the patient is hemodynamically compromised (see Chapter 46). CT or MRI scanning of the thorax may assist in the diagnosis but should not be done in preference to echocardiography (7).

The definitive diagnosis rests in part on the clinical circumstances and in part on the pericardial fluid cytology. Patients with bulky thoracic tumors or extensive mediastinal involvement who have not had previous irradiation and who lack evidence of infection are highly likely to have malignant pericardial effusion, even if the first fluid cytology is not diagnostic. The fluid in malignant pericardial disease is often bloody. Because cytology is relatively insensitive, if the first sample is negative and there is reason to question the diagnosis, repeat pericardiocentesis should be performed.

Indications for Early Consultation

Cardiology consultation should be part of the initial evaluation of patients with confirmed or suspected pericardial tamponade, while hemodynamically compromised patients require CCU admission. Thoracic surgery consultation may be necessary if patients have failed initial therapy or have evidence of pericardial constriction (see the section on "Treatment" below).

Issues During the Course of Hospitalization

Treatment

There are many choices for treatment of pericardial tamponade, as shown in Table 92.4. Needle drainage and catheter drainage are the most common initial steps, and are

TABLE 92.4
SURGICAL TECHNIQUES FOR TREATMENT OF MALIGNANT PERICARDIAL EFFUSION

Catheter drainage
  One-time; removed the same day
  Simple catheter drainage until "dry"
  Catheter drainage with sclerosis
  Catheter drainage with repeated sclerosis
Percutaneous balloon catheter pericardiotomy
Subxiphoid pericardiotomy
Thoracotomy with
  Pericardial "window"
  Pericardiectomy

generally successful in restoring hemodynamic function. For the majority of patients, a single drainage procedure is sufficient to resolve the problem, and it does not recur (8). Some clinicians routinely use a sclerosing agent, usually doxycycline, at the end of the initial drainage. However, sclerosis is quite painful and may not be necessary. Sclerosis with chemotherapy or radiopharmaceuticals is a great deal more expensive and has not been shown to be superior to no sclerosis or doxycycline. Pericardial catheters are usually not left in longer than about 72 hours because of the risk of infection. Drainage with or without sclerosis is the least costly approach to malignant pericardial effusion (8).

If more than 20–25 mL of fluid continue to drain from a pericardial catheter daily, or if the fluid reaccumulates rapidly, a more definitive drainage procedure should be considered. The most common of these is subxiphoid pericardiotomy, a surgical procedure in which the pericardium is opened inferiorly and drained into the peritoneal cavity through the membranous portion of the diaphragm. This procedure is minimally invasive; it is usually performed using a percutaneous balloon catheter, although a minimally invasive surgical technique is also available.

Thoracotomy and surgical "window" placement or pericardial stripping may be offered to selected patients who are not only able to tolerate a much more invasive procedure but who are also reasonably likely to have enough quality of life remaining to benefit from such surgery. Patients with constrictive pericarditis may be candidates for such a procedure. The rare patient who fails subxiphoid drainage may also benefit.

After the initial drainage procedure, local or systemic therapy may be used to resolve pericardial effusion and tamponade. Cancers for which effective therapy exists are usually treated in this manner. Radiation therapy may be used to a limited extent in previously untreated patients. Most healthy hearts will tolerate 1,800–2,500 cGy, and this dose may allow some patients with responsive diseases to remain asymptomatic. Other supportive measures are similar to those for patients having benign pericardial tamponade.

Discharge Issues

Patients who are hemodynamically stable and have undergone the final therapeutic maneuver may be discharged home. Those who are well enough to be sent home should be followed by visiting nurses until it is clear that pericardial fluid is not rapidly reaccumulating and hemodynamic compromise reoccurring. Nursing facility or hospice placement may be an option for patients who have no further intervention planned.

The prognosis of patients with pericardial effusion and tamponade depends on their underlying disease. Patients with treatable cancers such as lymphoma usually enjoy a relatively long survival. The exception is HIV-infected patients with primary effusion lymphomas who present with tamponade. Most solid tumors are bulky and at a terminal stage when tamponade occurs; survival times are very short, usually less than 6 months.

Appropriate follow-up of patients who have had an episode of tamponade is difficult. Since many of these patients are very close to the end of their lives, further testing for recurrence may not be appropriate. On the other hand, vigorous, active patients may wish to have echocardiographic follow-up in order to avoid emergency hospitalization. These decisions must be made individually, since there are few data to provide guidelines.

SUPERIOR VENA CAVA SYNDROME

Issues at the Time of Admission

Clinical Presentation

Superior vena cava syndrome (SVCS) is the oncologic emergency most likely to be the first symptom of cancer. As many as half of the patients with SVCS do not have a pre-existing cancer diagnosis. SVCS is a clinical diagnosis. Patients complain of dyspnea, and present with facial and upper extremity swelling. Occasionally, patients may complain of cough, chest tightness, or other symptoms caused by the tumor in the thorax. Physical findings typically consist of venous distention across the upper chest and neck, facial edema and plethora. Arm edema is present in approximately 15% of patients. Patients may have other physical findings caused by the mass within the thorax, including signs of airway obstruction, pleural effusion, or volume loss.

Differential Diagnosis

SVCS is usually due to cancer in the modern era, but nonmalignant causes are still found in about 15% of patients. Thrombosis around central lines is a common event that may cause SVCS. Histoplasmosis and other chronic inflammatory diseases cause the remainder of the benign cases.

Most cases of malignant SVCS are caused by lung cancer, usually small cell lung cancer. It has been estimated that SVCS occurs in more than 20% of patients with small cell lung cancer. Non-Hodgkin's lymphomas account for 7%–10% of cases of SVCS, and breast cancer for another 10%. Rare causes include germ cell tumors of the mediastinum, thymoma, and Hodgkin's disease.

Chest x-rays are abnormal in 85% of cases of SVCS. Superior mediastinal widening is seen in the majority of cases, and right hilar mass or pleural effusions are common findings. Anterior mediastinal mass should be a clue to thymoma, lymphoma, or germ cell tumor. Cardiomegaly is occasionally seen.

CT of the thorax is the most important diagnostic tool. In addition to demonstrating the anatomy of SVCS, it accurately guides both biopsy and radiation therapy. MRI is not clearly superior to CT for this purpose and is much less widely used.

Because SVCS is often the first sign of cancer, priority should be given to making a tissue diagnosis. Sputum cytology and fine needle aspiration are the most commonly used and highest yield techniques. The yield of sputum cytology in suspected lung cancer might be as high as 50%. Lymph nodes in the supraclavicular and axillary areas should be sought; fine needle aspiration biopsy of these is useful when they are present. If pleural effusion is present, thoracentesis may produce a histologic diagnosis. Bronchoscopy can be safely performed if the patient is suspected of having lung cancer, and has a high yield in SVCS (about 50%).

If these less invasive procedures are not helpful diagnostically, it may be necessary to obtain tissue from within the thorax. The safest technique is CT-guided fine needle aspiration biopsy. Either mediastinoscopy or limited anterior thoracotomy can be safe and highly effective ways to establish a diagnosis. Neither procedure is associated with a significant increase in serious complications in patients with SVCS, although rare patients do require additional surgical intervention.

Although as many as half of all patients with SVCS have some thrombus in association with the obstruction to blood flow, the identification of thrombus is of no clinical or therapeutic significance (see the section on "Issues During the Course of Hospitalization" below). Venography may be performed as part of the evaluation to identify candidates for vascular stenting.

Initial Therapy

Routine care of patients with SVCS includes bed rest with elevation of the head of the bed, oxygen therapy as indicated, and other comfort measures for relief of pain and cough. Steroids and diuretics have been used for symptom management, although no clear data support their benefit.

Anticoagulation is controversial. The routine use of heparin or warfarin anticoagulation has not been shown to hasten the relief of symptoms, and thrombolysis is risky and without proven benefits. Life threatening pulmonary embolization is highly unusual in patients with SVCS, and anticoagulation may delay efficient diagnosis and treatment. In contrast, when SVCS in cancer patients is caused by thrombosed central lines, this entity is quite effectively treated with local thrombolysis followed by heparin and warfarin. Removal of the catheter is necessary only if the clot fails to lyse. The use of angioplasty has been reported, although the expertise and experience necessary to safely perform this procedure is not widely available.

Vascular stenting as initial therapy for SVCS is also controversial. Insertion of a stent produces rapid relief of symptoms for 95% of patients with SVCS due to lung cancer (9). Long-term complications of stent placement, including rates of thrombosis or reocclusion rates, have not been well established. Whether cancer patients with superior vena cava stents should all receive anticoagulation remains an unanswered question. Most experts recommend that stents be the initial therapy when patients have recurred after radiation treatment of SVCS, when patients have SVCS due to cancers that are not likely to respond to radiation and chemotherapy, or when radiation therapy might be uniquely burdensome. There are no cost comparison studies and no long-term follow-up studies of stent placement.

SVCS caused by small cell lung cancer and by lymphoma is treated with chemotherapy, and clinical resolution occurs just as rapidly as with radiation therapy. Radiation therapy is the primary treatment for all other malignant causes, although chemotherapy is increasingly used concurrently for diseases such as non-small cell lung cancer. Radiation and/or chemotherapy of SVCS in non-small cell lung cancer results in relief of symptoms for more than 60% of patients. *The initiation of either chemotherapy or radiation therapy should be prompt, but SVCS is not so urgent as to mandate treatment immediately* (i.e., especially prior to making an accurate tissue diagnosis).

Issues During the Course of Hospitalization

The signs and symptoms of patients with SVCS begin to resolve in 5–7 days after the start of treatment. Resolution of symptoms is not necessarily accompanied by radiographic change; thus, there is no indication to follow the chest x-ray frequently. Complications of radiation therapy include esophagitis, bone marrow suppression, fatigue, and mild immunosuppression. These side effects are treated expectantly. Patients who have large lung cancers are at risk of developing bronchial obstruction or pneumonia during treatment. Clinically apparent pulmonary embolism as a complication of SVCS is rare, but should be treated conventionally if it occurs (Chapter 53). Most patients with SVCS should receive prophylaxis for deep venous thrombosis while they are at bedrest.

Patients may fail to respond to treatment because of formation of thrombus, refractoriness of the primary tumor, or hemorrhage or edema around the primary tumor that further occlude the vena cava. The assumption that treatment is failing should not be made until at least two weeks of radiation therapy has been delivered, since responses to radiation may still occur. The evaluation of patients with poor responses should include repeat chest CT and possibly venography.

Patients whose SVCS recurs after an initial response, and patients who have failed to respond to radiation, are candidates for vascular stent or surgical intervention. Several types of vascular stents have been developed. Stenting is clearly less invasive than surgical options (such as thoracotomy with vascular excision and grafting or SVC bypass), although individual anatomy may not always permit stent placement. Complications of stents and grafts include infection, stent migration, mediastinitis, graft failure, perforation, and thrombosis. Patients must be carefully selected, and the extent of institutional expertise considered.

Discharge Issues

Patients who are physiologically stable while being treated for SVCS may be discharged home. Outpatient radiation therapy and chemotherapy may be augmented by home nursing visits if necessary. The response to treatment is followed clinically. Repeated imaging of the tumor is planned as needed to evaluate further therapy. Analgesia for esophagitis should be offered prophylactically; the patient's oral intake and hydration may require monitoring once esophagitis occurs.

The prognosis of SVCS depends on the cause. Small cell lung cancer and lymphoma are highly responsive to initial therapy, potentially curable, and often accompanied by durable remissions. Non-small cell lung cancer is much less responsive, and relapse is common. Seventeen percent of small cell lung cancer patients and 19% of non-small cell lung cancer patients experienced recurrence of SVCS after treatment (9). SVCS caused by other cancers responds variably, depending on whether effective treatment is available. Thymoma has a variable natural history, and survival may be long even when treatment is relatively ineffective. Extragonadal germ cell tumors are treatment-responsive, but have a much worse prognosis than testicular germ cell tumors.

HYPERCALCEMIA

Issues at the Time of Hospitalization

Etiology

Hypercalcemia is the most common life-threatening metabolic emergency in cancer patients. Its incidence is highest in patients with breast cancer and multiple myeloma, 40% of whom may have hypercalcemia during the course of their illness. Hypercalcemia is less common in non-small cell lung cancer, squamous carcinomas of other sites, and renal cell carcinoma, and is rare in prostate cancer, pancreatic cancer, and other gastrointestinal cancers.

The most common cause of cancer-related hypercalcemia is *tumor production of parathormone-related protein (PTH-rp)*, a peptide that shares the N-terminal 8–13 residues with human parathormone, is abundant in many normal tissues, and has unknown physiologic function. Patients with measurable levels of PTH-rp may also display phosphaturia, hypophosphatemia, and other parathormone-related abnormalities. Other pathways that cause increased bone resorption and release of calcium may be important to the pathogenesis of hypercalcemia in malignancy. Tumors may produce mediators such as calcitriol (in Hodgkin's disease), prostaglandins, cytokines such as TGF-β, interleukin-6, and tumor necrosis factor, all of which may result in the hypercalcemia of malignancy.

Clinical Presentation

Patients with hypercalcemia have a wide range of presenting signs and symptoms, related to the severity of hypercalcemia. At low levels of hypercalcemia, patients may exhibit only fatigue, anorexia, constipation, mild nausea, and polyuria. Symptoms may be more progressive and severe if the hypercalcemia is more sudden in onset. As levels of calcium increase, CNS symptoms dominate, including lethargy, muscle weakness, confusion, psychosis or delirium, and coma. Volume depletion is a prominent feature of hypercalcemia, because of the combination of anorexia, isosthenuria, and nephrogenic diabetes insipidus. Hypotension and ECG changes are generally seen late in the illness.

Differential Diagnosis and Evaluation

Most patients hospitalized with symptomatic hypercalcemia have a known cancer diagnosis. The evaluation of patients who present with hypercalcemia and do not have a cancer diagnosis begins with a careful history and physical examination. Such often present with readily observable physical findings and symptoms to suggest the presence of cancer. Laboratory data should include complete blood count, differential and platelet counts, measures of renal function, a chest radiograph, urinalysis, and serum protein electrophoresis if other laboratory data are normal. Additional imaging studies should be chosen based on symptoms, signs, and laboratory abnormalities. Serum PTH and PTH-rp levels may be measured, but are rarely necessary to prove the source of malignant hypercalcemia.

Indications for Hospitalization

Patients with mild hypercalcemia may be treated as outpatients, provided that they are able to increase their intake of salt and water adequately and the diagnosis is clear. Most patients with moderate-to-severe hypercalcemia require hospitalization for adequate volume repletion and rapid correction of the problem. Any patient with significant elevation in serum creatinine or inability to hydrate themselves adequately must be admitted, regardless of the serum calcium level.

The most common acute problems in patients with altered mental status and hypercalcemia are complications of stupor, including aspiration pneumonitis and falls. These must be anticipated when deciding whether to admit. The processes that may trigger hypercalcemia in an otherwise stable outpatient include intercurrent illnesses, immobilization, use of diuretics (especially thiazides), and administration of hormonal therapy to breast cancer patients. The presence of any of these comorbidities should also be a factor in the decision to admit a patient.

Initial Therapy

Volume repletion with normal saline is the single most important therapy for hypercalcemia. Patients are usually moderately to severely volume depleted, and, because natriuresis increases calcium excretion, normal saline is the fluid of choice. *The early use of furosemide is contraindicated,* as it may actually reduce the amount of calcium that is excreted and worsen volume depletion. Close monitoring of patients with heart disease and renal insufficiency is necessary, at times in an ICU setting, but initial therapy must include vigorous volume resuscitation despite the risk for fluid overload.

Pharmacotherapy directed at reducing serum calcium levels is outlined in Table 92.5. *Calcitonin* is the drug of choice for very rapid reduction in calcium levels, because all other agents require about 48 hours to take effect.

Calcitonin use cannot be sustained due to the rapid development of tachyphylaxis. The *aminobisphosphonates zoledronate and pamidronate* are the most commonly used drugs for hypercalcemia because of their potency, long duration of action, and safety in the presence of mild renal failure. All of the drugs used for hypercalcemia have comparable costs. Plicamycin is the only drug that may be used in patients with severe renal failure. Steroids are potent inhibitors of calcitriol and should be employed for the treatment of hypercalcemia in patients with Hodgkin's disease. Steroids may have an anti-tumor effect in other hematologic malignancies and are useful when combined with other pharmacotherapy for hypercalcemia.

Patients hospitalized for hypercalcemia should receive close monitoring of their neurologic status, renal function, and urine output. Low calcium diets may be ordered, although patient acceptance is poor. However, milk and other very high calcium foods should be eliminated. Because bedrest increases mobilization of calcium from the skeleton, it is discouraged unless the patient's mental status is too depressed to safely allow sitting or ambulation.

Indications for Early Consultation

Severe hypercalcemia (greater than 15 mg/dL) is a potential indication for hemodialysis. Patients who have coma, severe renal failure, electrocardiographic changes, or who cannot receive aggressive hydration should be considered for dialysis. Patients who have hypercalcemia along with other standard indications for acute dialysis due to renal failure should be treated with hemodialysis. The effect of dialysis on calcium is transitory, and all such patients must also be treated aggressively with drugs to lower their calcium levels.

TABLE 92.5

DRUGS FOR TREATMENT OF HYPERCALCEMIA

Drug	Dose	Precautions/Comments
Zoledronate	4–8 mg IV over 15 min	Agent of choice due to greatest potency, most rapid action, longest duration, ease of use Use up to a creatinine of 4.5 Flu symptoms, myalgias, bone pain
Pamidronate	60 or 90 mg IV over 2–4 hours	Use up to a creatinine of about 3.0 Takes 48–72 hours Myalgias, arthralgias most common side effects
Calcitonin	4–8 units/kg sq every 6–12 hours	Tachyphylaxis at 48–72 hrs Mild nausea, rare hypersensitivity
Etidronate	7.5 mg/kg IV over 2–4 hrs qd for 3–5 days	Less potent than pamidronate; rarely used Oral may be used for maintenance
Plicamycin (mithramycin)	25 mcg/kg IV × 1 (repeat in 5–7 d)	Thrombocytopenia in some patients. Vesicant; requires careful administration.

Consultation for cancer diagnosis and management is likely to be needed during hospitalization. Effective long-term control of hypercalcemia is best achieved by effective treatment of the underlying cancer.

Issues During the Course of Hospitalization

Failure to respond to initial treatment of hypercalcemia is a common and potentially serious problem. The patient's volume status should be carefully reassessed to be sure that repletion has been adequate. Failure to correct volume depletion and produce natriuresis is the most common cause of unresponsiveness to treatment. Poor renal function can also decrease calcium excretion, and this is an indication for hemodialysis. Patients with clear evidence of volume overload should be treated with furosemide. The addition of calcitonin to an aminobisphosphonate-treated patient may improve early responses. In one large series, failure to respond to drug therapy was associated with a 100% in-hospital mortality (10).

Volume overload, hypokalemia and hypomagnesemia, and complications of stupor and coma are additional problems in patients treated for hypercalcemia. Careful monitoring of intake and output and electrolytes is important, and assessment of volume status is crucial during the first few days of treatment.

Treatment of the underlying malignancy may complicate the hospital course. Chemotherapy and hormone therapy may have an impact on the disease process. Studies of outcome in patients with hypercalcemia and cancer show conclusively that the only patients who enjoy long survival are those whose cancer is successfully treated (10).

Discharge Issues

Patients are ready for discharge when they are capable of being supported at home. Home nursing and home hospice are frequently needed. Further treatment of hypercalcemia may not be undertaken in hospice patients, and outpatient prescriptions should be directed at palliating other symptoms (Chapter 19).

Maintenance of normocalcemia is a goal for highly functional patients at discharge, and may be accomplished in a variety of ways. Patients who have chemotherapy-responsive disease may not need further treatment of their calcium, or may only need a single additional dose of a potent drug such as an aminobisphosphonate. Patients with mild hypercalcemia may be maintained with less potent agents such as steroids or non-steroidal anti-inflammatory agents, which may have a moderating effect on the hypercalcemia of squamous carcinomas. Intermittent outpatient dosing of aminobisphosphonates has been advocated for maintenance of normocalcemia, and has been shown to be cost-effective as maintenance therapy for patients with extensive osseous disease, especially those with multiple myeloma and breast cancer. Oral etidronate therapy has

also been proposed for maintenance, although there are no long-term studies of outcome.

Unfortunately, hypercalcemia of malignancy is often an end-stage event. The average survival of patients hospitalized for hypercalcemia is 30 days. The addition of systemic anti-cancer therapy only lengthens this survival to 135 days (10). About half of the patients discharged from the hospital have relief of their hypercalcemic symptoms.

KEY POINTS

- Magnetic resonance imaging is the method of choice for the evaluation of neurologic emergencies in patients with cancer.
- The urgency of therapy for neurologic complications of cancer is dependent on the duration and severity of the neurologic deficit.
- Treatment of neurologic emergencies may involve surgery, radiation therapy, and chemotherapy.
- Malignant pericardial effusion is treated most often with catheter drainage or subxiphoid pericardiotomy.
- Superior vena cava syndrome is recognizable clinically and most often occurs in the setting of lung cancer.
- Keys to successful treatment of hypercalcemia include use of aggressive hydration with saline solution and potent drugs such as aminobisphosphonates.

REFERENCES

1. Vecht C, Hovestadt A, Verbiest H. et al. Dose-effect relationship of dexamethasone on Karnovsky performance in metastatic brain tumors: a randomized study of doses of 4, 8, and 16 mg per day. *Neurology* 1994;44:675–680.
2. Maranzano E, Latini P, Beneventi S, et al. Radiotherapy without steroids in selected metastatic spinal cord compression patients. A phase II trial. *Am J Clin Oncol* 1996;19:179–183.
3. Sneed P, Suh J, Goetsch S, et al. A multi-institutional review of radiosurgery alone vs. radiosurgery with whole brain radiotherapy as the initial management of brain metastases. *Int J Radiat Oncol Biol Phys* 2002;53:519–526.
4. Kondziolka D, Patel A, Lunsford LD, et al. Stereotactic radiosurgery plus whole brain radiotherapy versus radiotherapy alone for patients with multiple brain metastases. *Int J Radiat Oncol Biol Phys* 1999;45:427–434.
5. Abray L, and Christodoulou C. Temozolomide for treating brain metastases. *Semin Oncol* 2001;38(suppl 13):34–43.
6. Gaspar L, Scott C, Rotman M, et al. Recursive partitioning analysis (RPA) of prognostic factors in three Radiation Therapy Oncology Group (RTOG) brain metastases trials. *Int J Radiat Oncol Biol Phys* 1997;37:745–751.
7. Wang ZJ, Reddy GP, Gotway MB, et al. CT and MR imaging of pericardial disease. *Radiographics* 2003;23:S167–180.
8. Anderson TM, Ray CW, Nwogu CE, et al. Pericardial catheter sclerosis versus surgical procedures for pericardial effusions in cancer patients. *J Cardiovasc Surg (Torino)* 2001;42:415–419.
9. Rowell N, and Gleeson F. Steroids, radiotherapy, chemotherapy, and stents for superior vena caval obstruction in carcinoma of the bronchus (Cochrane Review). *Cochrane Database Syst Rev* 2001;4: CD001316.
10. Ralston SH, Gallacher SJ, Patel U, et al. Cancer-associated hypercalcemia: morbidity and mortality. Clinical experience in 126 treated patients. *Ann Intern Med* 1990;112:499–504.

ADDITIONAL READING

Blair SL, Schwarz RE. Critical care of patients with cancer. Surgical considerations. *Crit Care Clin* 2001;17:721–742.

Krimsky WS, Behrens RJ, Kerkvliet GJ. Oncologic emergencies for the internist. *Cleve Clin J Med* 2002;69:209–210, 213–214, 216–217.

Kvale PA, Simoff M, Rakash UB. Lung Cancer. American College of Chest Physicians. *Chest* 2003;123:284S–311S.

Schiff D. Spinal cord compression. *Neurol Clin* 2003;21:67–86.

Stewart AF. Hypercalcemia associated with cancer. *N Engl J Med* 2005;352:373–379.

Warrell RP, Jr. Metabolic emergencies. In DeVita VT, Hellman S, Rosenberg SA, eds. *Cancer: Principles and Practice of Oncology.* 7th ed. Philadelphia: Lippincott Williams & Wilkins, 2004:2633–2644.

Leukemia

David A. Rizzieri   Gwynn D. Long   Nelson J. Chao

93

INTRODUCTION

The term *leukemia* encompasses a number of diseases characterized by the clonal proliferation of hematopoietic stem cells, which results in the accumulation of abnormal (leukemic) cells in the bone marrow and a decreased production of normal blood cells. The four most common types of leukemia are acute myelogenous leukemia, acute lymphoblastic leukemia, chronic myelogenous leukemia, and chronic lymphocytic leukemia. In general, patients with chronic leukemia are treated on an outpatient basis. The chronic leukemias, which are readily distinguished from the acute leukemias by the clinical presentation and blood smear findings (Table 93.1), are not extensively discussed in this chapter.

EPIDEMIOLOGY AND ETIOLOGY

Acute myelogenous leukemia (AML) is characterized by the proliferation of primitive hematopoietic cells of myeloid lineage, and acute lymphoblastic leukemia (ALL) by the proliferation of primitive lymphoid hematopoietic cells. The overall incidence of acute myeloid leukemia is 3.6 per 100,000 in the population, with a much greater incidence in older people. Acute lymphocytic leukemia has an overall incidence of 1.5 per 100,000 in the population, with a much higher incidence in young children than adults (1). Unfortunately, the majority of adults in whom acute leukemia is diagnosed ultimately die of the disease.

The etiology of acute leukemia is unknown and is undoubtedly complex, including genetic and environmental factors. Exposure to high levels of ionizing radiation is a well-established risk factor. Increased rates of leukemia have been observed in survivors of the atomic bombs and in workers in the radium industry. Previous chemotherapy with alkylating agents for other malignant diseases also increases the risk for acute leukemia, as does industrial over-

exposure to benzene, carbon tetrachloride, and carbon disulfide. The role of pesticide exposure is controversial, but a higher-than-expected incidence of acute leukemia has been observed in farmers and agricultural workers. A small increased risk is also probably associated with smoking. Several genetic syndromes, including Down syndrome, Bloom syndrome, Fanconi's anemia, and ataxia–telangiectasia, are associated with an increased risk for the development of acute leukemia. The risk associated with a family history of leukemia is uncertain, and although there is an increased risk for childhood leukemia in twins (especially during infancy), no increased risk has been documented in adult twins. Most patients, however, have no history of exposure to any known risk factor (2).

CLASSIFICATION

AML and ALL are each divided into multiple subtypes based on morphology, histochemistry, immunophenotyping by flow cytometry, and cytogenetics. However, cytogenetic description is replacing the French-American-British Cooperative Group (FAB) system of classification of Acute Leukemia (Table 93.2). Retrospective studies have found that a normal white blood cell count, younger age, and normal hemoglobin at presentation are favorable prognostic factors. Cytogenetic analyses have furthered these observations by allowing more in-depth risk assessment based on survival statistics. Individuals with t(15;17) have "FAB M3" or promyelocytic leukemia and do very well. Unfortunately, overall only 20% of patients with other types of AML survive long term. Leukemia patients with (t[8;21] or inv[16]) are felt to have a high chance for cure with standard therapy (55% 5-year survival with continuous remission). Those with normal cytogenetics or t(9;11) are at intermediate risk (24% 5-year survival in remission), and those with complex genetic changes or other single abnormalities are felt to be at a very high risk for

TABLE 93.1

SUMMARY OF CHARACTERISTICS OF THE TWO MOST COMMON CHRONIC LEUKEMIAS

Diagnosis	Clinical characteristics	Common laboratory abnormalities	Cellular characteristics	Median survival
CML	Median onset in fourth decade; fatigue, splenomegaly	Increased WBC, low LAP score, PB blasts (<30%), splenomegaly, hemolytic anemia, thrombocytopenia	Philadelphia chromosome-positive	~3–5 y
CLL	Median onset in seventh decade; adenopathy, splenomegaly, hepatomegaly	Lymphocytosis and smudge cells, >30% lymphocytes in BM, anemia, thrombocytopenia	CD5-positive B cells	10 y in early stage, 3 y in advanced stage

BM, bone marrow; *CLL*, chronic lymphocytic leukemia; *CML*, chronic myelogenous leukemia; *LAP*, leukocyte alkaline phosphatase; *PB*, peripheal blood; Philadelphia chromosome, [t(9;22)]; *WBC*, white blood cells.

relapse (5% survival in remission at five years) (3). For patients with ALL arising *de novo*, the overall long-term survival is approximately 20%. Important unfavorable prognostic factors in ALL include older age at onset, mature B-cell ALL, and a high white cell count at presentation. However, here too, cytogenetic analyses have further defined outcomes based on the abnormalities found in these patients. Adults with t(9;22) have less of a chance to attain a remission and poorer long-term survival than those with normal cytogentics or other changes. A slow response time (longer time to attain remission) is the worst prognostic factor (4).

GENERAL PRINCIPLES OF MANAGEMENT

The goals of therapy of acute leukemia are to *eliminate the neoplastic clone and restore normal hematopoiesis.* Therapy is generally divided into two phases: the *induction phase*, designed to achieve a complete remission; and *post-remission therapy*, to prevent relapse and achieve cure. Complete remission is defined as fewer than 5% blasts in the bone marrow and restoration of normal hematopoiesis with an absolute neutrophil count of at least 1,500/μL and a platelet count of 100,000/μL. The achievement of complete remission is the only clinically significant response to therapy and is a necessary first step toward cure. Post-remission therapy (consolidation) attempts to eradicate minimal residual disease. Patients with ALL are also treated with more prolonged courses of lower-dose maintenance chemotherapy. This chapter focuses on the issues involved in the administration of induction therapy to a patient with a newly diagnosed disease. The successful completion of induction therapy depends on the ability to support patients through the many attendant complications associated with a 2- to 5-week period of pancytopenia.

ACUTE MYELOGENOUS LEUKEMIA

Issues at the Time of Admission

Adult acute myeloid (or nonlymphoid) leukemias typically present after a few weeks of general decline in overall well being as a consequence of either the leukemia itself or associated neutropenia, anemia, and thrombocytopenia. Fatigue, malaise, bruising, and occasionally anorexia with weight loss are reported. Presenting signs typically reflect anemia (e.g., pallor of the skin), thrombocytopenia (e.g., petechiae or ecchymoses), or both. Adenopathy or fever may also be present. Hepatosplenomegaly and lymphadenopathy are more common with ALL. Neurologic symptoms are uncommon. A delay in diagnosis is common, but when symptoms persist and intensify or the above signs are noted, a blood cell count and qualitative review of the smear often reveal abnormalities that prompt further analysis.

By the time patients present to the hospital for evaluation and therapy, most will have some degree of anemia and many are also severely thrombocytopenic. The white blood cell count is variable, with approximately 20% of patients presenting with counts below 5,000/μL and fewer than 20% with counts above 100,000/μL. Leukemic blasts are nearly always found in the peripheral blood. The prothrombin and partial thromboplastin times may be prolonged, especially in some forms of AML. Chemistries are usually normal, although the uric acid may be elevated in patients with high white blood cell counts.

Because of the variable nature of the presenting blood cell counts, the differential diagnosis may remain broad (Table 93.3). Review of the blood film and bone marrow biopsy specimen from a patient with leukemia will show a hypercellular marrow, lack of heterogeneity, and lack of maturation with a significant increase in blast forms (>30%), in addition to a suppression of normal precursors.

TABLE 93.2

FAB COOPERATIVE GROUP CLASSIFICATION OF ACUTE LEUKEMIA

FAB subtype	Description	Morphology	Histochemistry	Immunophenotype	Cytogenetics
AML-M0	Undifferentiated	>30% agranular blasts	Negative	CD13, 33, 34 HLA-DR	
AML-M1	Myeloblastic without Differentiation	>90% blasts with rare granules and Auer rods	Sudan black Myeloperoxidase	CD13, 14, 15, 33, 34 HLA-DR	Occasional inv(3)
AML-M2	Myeloblastic with Differentiation	30%–90% blasts with granules and many Auer rods	Sudan black Myeloperoxidase Chloroacetate esterase	CD13, 15, 33, 34 HLA-DR	t(8;21)
AML-M3	Promyelocytic	>30% blasts with hypergranular promyelocytes	Myeloperoxidase (intensely positive)	CD13, 15, 33	t(15;17)
AML-M4	Myelomonocytic	>30% blasts with 20%–80% of monocytic lineage plus monocytosis in blood	α-naphthyl butyrate esterase	CD13, 14, 15, 33, 34 HLA-DR	inv(16) in eosinophilic variant
AML-M5	Monocytic	Large, often bizarre cells, >80% monocytic lineage	α-naphthyl butyrate esterase	CD13, 14, 33, 34 HLA-DR	abnormal 11q23
AML-M6	Erythroid	>50% of cells of erythroid lineage, often dysplastic; >30% of nonerythroid cells are blasts	Periodic acid Schiff	CD13, 33, 41, 71 HLA-DR Glycophorin A	del(5) del(7)
AML-M7	Megakaryocytic	>30% blasts of megakaryocytic origin	Platelet peroxidase by electron microscopy	CD41, 61	inv(3) t(3;3) trisomy 21
ALL-L1	Childhood form	Small cells with minimal cytoplasm, no granules, and rare nucleoli	TdT	B cell: CD10, 19, 20, 22, 34; HLA-DR; cytoplasmic immunoglobulin T cell: CD2, 5, 7, 10, 34	t(9;22) t(4;11) t(1;9)
ALL-L2	Adult form	Larger cells with moderate amount of cytoplasm and prominent nucleoli	TdT	B cell: CD10, 19, 20, 22, 34; HLA-DR; cytoplasmic immunoglobulin T cell: CD2, 5, 7, 10, 34	t(9;22) t(4;11) t(1;9)
ALL-L3	Burkitt's type	Large, round cells with basophilic cytoplasm and vacuoles		CD10, 19, 20, 21, 22 Surface immunoglobulin	t(8;14) t(2;8) t(8;22)

ALL, acute lymphoblastic leukemia; AML, acute myeloid leukemia; CD, clusters of differentiation; del, deletion; FAB, French-American-British; HLA, human leukocyte antigen; inv, inversion; M0–M7 and L1–L3 denote leukemia subtype; t, translocation; TdT, terminal deoxytransferase.

In contrast, the bone marrow specimens of patients with *aplastic anemia,* including those with an accompanying viral infection, are very hypocellular. Cultures and tests based on the polymerase chain reaction can rule out such viral infections. *Myelodysplasia,* a preleukemic condition, also is characterized by a hypocellular marrow with ringed sideroblasts and mildly increased blast counts, but not above the 30% required for a diagnosis of acute leukemia. The history is

very important in elucidating any potential *environmental or medication exposures* that might cause conditions that mimic leukemia. Typically, slightly more variability and maturation are found in the marrow and blood of these patients than in patients with leukemia. Sarcoidosis and tuberculosis are associated with the appearance of granulomas on biopsy specimens of the marrow. In patients presenting with high white blood cell counts, the differential diagnosis

TABLE 93.3

DIFFERENTIAL DIAGNOSIS OTHER THAN ACUTE LEUKEMIA BASED ON BLOOD CELL COUNTS

Pancytopenia (abnormally low counts of platelets, white cells, and red cells)
 Aplastic anemia
 Paroxysmal nocturnal hemoglobinuria
 Parvovirus B19 infection (typically limited to or affecting red cells most severely)
 Chronic infections (tuberculosis, cytomegalovirus, Epstein-Barr virus)
 Medications (trimethoprim-sulfamethoxazole, chlorambucil or other chemotherapeutic agents)
 Autoimmune illnesses (sarcoidosis)
 Myelodysplasia
Leukocytosis (abnormally elevated white cell count)
 Stress (extreme environments)
 Smoking
 Exercise
 Pregnancy
 Severe nausea or vomiting
 Chronic infections (parasites, fungus)
 Medications (prednisone, digitalis, heparin)
 Hemolysis/hemorrhage
 Post-splenectomy
 Metabolic conditions (gout, hyperthyroidism, ketoacidosis)
 Plasmacytosis
 Chronic myeloid leukemia
Lymphocytosis (abnormally elevated lymphocyte count)
 Viral infection
 Chronic lymphocytic leukemia
 Hairy cell leukemia
 Transformed lymphoma

is still broad (Table 93.3). However, a review of the history coupled with the peripheral blood film and marrow findings usually reveals the correct diagnosis.

The process of evaluation is outlined in Figure 93.1. An early hematologic consultation should be obtained for all patients in whom a diagnosis of acute leukemia is being considered. A Wright's-stained blood film revealing an increase in blast forms is essential for a diagnosis of acute leukemia. In addition, analysis of the peripheral blood or marrow cells by flow cytometry is required to support the diagnosis by proving monoclonality. Cytogenetic analysis is also important because it provides information related to prognosis and therapeutic decisions. Therefore, on admission, all patients should have a blood film prepared in addition to undergoing bone marrow aspiration and biopsy. Adequate samples can be obtained in the majority of patients with minimal discomfort from the posterior iliac crests. Sternal aspirates should be obtained only from patients in whom sampling from the posterior iliac crests is not possible because of their clinical condition or body habitus. The bone marrow should be evaluated with routine Wright's staining plus special lineage-specific stains.

In addition, flow cytometry of the aspirate (or of the peripheral blood if the number of circulating blasts is significant) and standard cytogenetics should be requested. Other initial laboratory studies should include a chemistry panel including values for electrolytes, renal function, serum liver chemistries, lactate dehydrogenase, calcium, phosphorus, and uric acid; coagulation studies; type and screen; and urinalysis. Blood and urine cultures should be obtained for all febrile patients. Lumbar puncture is usually not carried out as part of the initial workup. Rather, it is delayed until peripheral blood blasts have cleared to avoid confusing central nervous system involvement with a "bloody" tap. A chest radiograph should also be obtained for all patients. Peripheral blood for HLA typing (A/B/DR) should be taken from all patients at the time of diagnosis in anticipation of the need for HLA-matched platelets and the need to identify a potential bone marrow donor. This initial evaluation yields a combination of morphologic and cytogenetic data that allow one to predict the course of an individual patient's illness and determine appropriate therapy.

Initial Therapy

All patients with a new diagnosis of acute leukemia require hospitalization. Initial management should concentrate on stabilization of the patient and preparation for chemotherapy with placement of central venous access. If severe anemia (hematocrit <25 g/dL) or thrombocytopenia (platelets <10,000/μL) or symptoms referable to the cytopenias are present, then the patient should have a transfusion. Filtered blood products (to prevent transmission of cytomegalovirus and reduce the risk for allo-immunization and nonhemolytic, febrile transfusion reactions) and irradiated blood products (to prevent transfusion-associated graft-versus-host disease) should be used (Chapter 91).

If the patient is neutropenic (absolute neutrophil count <1,000/μL) and febrile, a standard infectious evaluation with blood cultures, urinalysis and culture, and chest radiography, should be undertaken and broad-spectrum antibiotics immediately begun (Chapters 63 and 64). A careful physical examination (ruling out oral and rectal abscesses) should also be included. All patients become neutropenic following chemotherapy. The risk for infection is influenced by the depth and duration of neutropenia and by other factors, such as the presence of mucositis and indwelling catheters. Although the definition of fever varies across studies, we favor the initiation of empiric antibiotic coverage in a patient with a temperature above 38.5°C or three or more temperatures above 38.0°C in a 24-hour period. Signs and symptoms of infection without fever should also prompt administration of antibiotics in neutropenic patients. The early use of antibiotics has reduced infection-related mortality to 5%–10%, with most deaths from infection occurring in patients with prolonged neutropenia. In the past, the primary goal of therapy was the treatment of Gram-negative bacterial infections. However, *Gram-positive organisms are also emerging as major causes of infection*

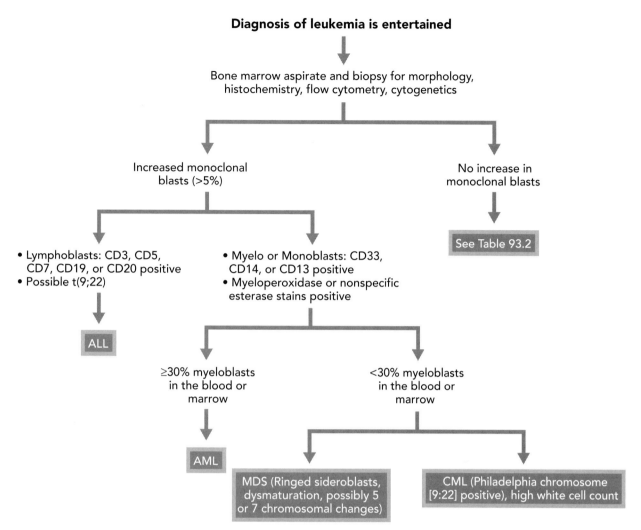

Figure 93.1 Algorithm for evaluation of a patient suspected of having acute leukemia. The initial steps require a bone marrow examination to prove whether or not there is an increase in monoclonal blast cells. If so, the subsequent steps entail defining the specific type of abnormal blasts to allow for proper classification of the illness. *ALL,* acute lymphoblastic leukemia; *AML,* acute myelogenous leukemia; *CML,* chronic myelocenous leukemia; *MDS,* myelodysplastic syndrome; *t,* translocation.

in neutropenic patients. Many reasonable options are available for single- or double-agent coverage, such as the third-generation cephalosporins, monobactams, or a broad-spectrum penicillin in combination with an aminoglycoside or a quinolone antibiotic (Chapter 63).

If the presenting white blood cell count is very high (>100,000/μL), the patient may be in danger of *tumor lysis* (Chapter 94). Aggressive hydration (at least 200 mL of fluid per hour) and 300 mg of allopurinol per day may be used to minimize this risk. Laboratory values should be followed every 6–8 hours until the white cell counts are nearly entering the neutropenic stage, which typically takes 4–5 days after induction therapy is initiated. Leukostasis may also develop in patients with blast counts above 100,000/μL, and with signs of end-organ compromise, such as changes in mental status or angina. Emergent leukapheresis should be considered, along with 500–1,000 mg of hydroxyurea every 6 hours until definitive chemotherapy can be initiated.

Subtypes of leukemia present certain special considerations. All leukemia patients, but particularly those with *promyelocytic leukemia,* are prone to *disseminated intravascular coagulation,* and coagulation parameters should be evaluated on admission and followed daily during induction therapy (Chapter 98). If laboratory abnormalities consistent with disseminated intravascular coagulation are present but the patient has no manifestation of bleeding or clotting, then it is appropriate to follow the patient closely with laboratory monitoring every 6–8 hours during therapy. If the patient has evidence of clotting or bleeding from disseminated intravascular coagulation, therapy may be very difficult, and the outcome is often poor.

Monocytic leukemia is often an invasive disease (into skin, joints, and visceral organs). Not uncommonly, patients present with a persistent cough and chest radiographic findings of diffuse bilateral infiltrates, which often leads to a delay in initiation of chemotherapy while antibiotics are administered for pneumonia. Patients in this situation should be carefully evaluated, cultures taken, and antibiotics started, but chemotherapy for the leukemia should not be delayed beyond 1–2 days, as the pulmonary infiltrates often clear with chemotherapy. Bronchoscopy for cultures, cytology, and even biopsy to rule out infection may be needed early in the evaluation so as not to delay appropriate therapy. Monocytic leukemia can also present with renal failure resulting from infiltration of the kidney, which can be seen on ultrasonography. The physical examination must attempt to identify reservoir sites of disease. Granulocytic sarcomas or chloromas (nodules of leukemia cells) may develop in multiple sites, including the skin, liver, lungs, bowel, and bone.

Various chemotherapy regimens are used for induction chemotherapy (Chapter 90). Typically, a nucleoside analog such as cytarabine (continuous infusion of 100–200 mg/m^2 daily for seven days) is combined with an anthracycline such as idarubicin (12 mg/m^2 daily for days one through three). Addition of a topoisomerase inhibitor such as etoposide is advocated by some to improve remission rates. A bone marrow examination is usually repeated 2 weeks after the start of chemotherapy, and, if residual blasts are identified, a second round of induction is immediately begun. This is typically slightly less intense than the first cycle (e.g., five days of cytarabine and two days of an anthracyline). It is important to note that those with t(15;17) FAB M3 cytogenics require a different initial therapy. In these patients, all-trans retinoic acid is delivered first to induce maturation of the leukemic blasts, with most patients achieving a remission within a 6-week period. This is followed with standard induction and consolidation chemotherapy to optimize the long-term outlook for the patients. One to three cycles of consolidation therapy are given. Patients are typically much more stable at the initiation of consolidation than during induction. High dose therapy with autologous or allogeneic hematopoietic stem cell support is advocated by some investigators, but this has not been proven to improve long-term survival when used as initial consolidation therapy.

Chronic myelogenous leukemia is typically managed on an outpatient basis until it progresses to a blast crisis, which is often indistinguishable from acute leukemia, presenting with extremely high white blood cell counts (often >200,000/μL). The prognosis for patients with chronic myelogenous leukemia in blast crisis is extremely poor, but an attempt should be made to induce younger patients into a second chronic phase and then proceed to allogeneic bone marrow transplantation (Chapter 96) if an appropriate donor can be identified.

Issues During the Course of Hospitalization

Febrile neutropenia should be treated aggressively. Daily physical examinations should rule out oral or perirectal abscesses, in addition to more common causes. Digital rectal examinations should not be performed on neutropenic patients. Prophylactic antibiotic therapy with a quinolone

started during induction or consolidation may decrease the numbers of episodes of fever and readmissions during consolidation. However, when a patient becomes febrile, these antibiotics are not sufficient, and broader coverage must be initiated. The treatment of the febrile neutropenic patient is discussed in detail in Chapter 63.

Transfusion support to maintain the platelet count above 10,000/μL and the hematocrit above 25 g/dL with filtered, irradiated blood products remains appropriate. If patients are febrile or actively bleeding, the platelet transfusion threshold is often increased to 20,000/μL (5). Transfusions of packed red blood cells are indicated to keep hemoglobin levels above 7–8 g/dL to maintain adequate oxygen-carrying capacity. Growth factor support may be effective in patients over 55 years of age and may hasten the recovery of granulocytes when it is started at some point after the completion of induction therapy (usually initiated between days 11 and 14).

Severe mucositis may require opiates for pain control. Attention must be paid during the daily oral examination to ensure that superinfection with *Candida* or herpes virus is not also involved. Empiric therapy with acyclovir, fluconazole, or both is often used. Colitis with severe abdominal cramping, bloating, and radiographic findings of distended loops of bowel are consistent with neutropenic colitis (typhlitis) as a side effect of chemotherapy, neutropenia, or secondary causes. *Clostridium difficile* infection must be excluded, and supportive care, often including nasogastric drainage, is required.

The side effects of chemotherapy are numerous and should be monitored by the hematologist, but a few bear mentioning. Cytarabine, a standard agent used in many regimens, at higher doses may cause cerebellar dysfunction that requires immediate discontinuation of the drug. All patients receiving doses of more than 1 g/m^2 should undergo a neurologic exam looking for cerebellar findings before each dose of the drug is administered. In addition, at doses above 1 g/m^2, steroid eye drops must be used to prevent severe conjunctivitis. Cyclophosphamide, which is sometimes used in consolidation therapy, can cause hemorrhagic cystitis (Chapter 90). The commonly used anthracycline agents cause cardiomyopathy at high cumulative doses. The use of all-trans retinoic acid has been a great advance in the therapy of promyelocytic leukemia, but the *"retinoid syndrome"* is seen in up to 40% of patients. This is a constellation of findings including high fevers with respiratory distress, pulmonary infiltrates and pleural effusions, weight gain, and leukocytosis. Early recognition and initiation of steroid therapy (10 mg of dexamethasone every 12 hours) usually allows for successful management.

Recovery and Discharge Issues

The bone marrow examination is repeated at recovery of white cells (absolute neutrophil count above 1,000/μL and platelet count above 100,000/μL, usually 3–4 weeks after the initiation of chemotherapy) to document whether remission has been attained. At discharge, important issues are nutrition (Chapter 15), which should include high-carbohydrate and caloric supplements if needed, and daily exercise to promote recovery from the long hospital stay and prepare for future chemotherapy. Oral electrolyte supplements such as potassium and magnesium may be required for a few weeks after chemotherapy. Antifungal and antiviral therapy can be discontinued at the same time as broad-spectrum antibiotics unless invasive fungal disease has been documented. The initial duration of hospitalization for induction is typically 4 weeks, with patients remaining hospitalized for the initial delivery of chemotherapy and the management of fevers (during the neutropenic phase) and chemotherapy side effects. These challenging phases are generally followed by the simultaneous recovery of blood cell counts and improvement in performance status. On recovery, patients can be discharged if they maintain adequate oral intake, ambulate with minimal assistance, and have any infections well controlled. The discharge decision must be made carefully after such intensive chemotherapy; premature discharge before the ability to perform activities of daily living has returned commonly leads to readmissions, prolonged requirements for recovery, delays of consolidation therapy, and increased total costs.

Depending on the clinical condition and remission status of the patient, consolidation therapy usually begins 2–3 weeks after recovery from induction. Consolidation often requires a 1-week hospitalization to deliver the chemotherapy in a supervised setting, and then discharge with close outpatient follow-up through the 3- to 4-week recovery period. When consolidation is complete, the approach to follow-up depends on the risk for relapse and the patient's clinical status. Typically, patients should be observed closely at 3-month intervals for approximately two years, with bone marrow examinations performed at the first sign of possible relapse.

ACUTE LYMPHOBLASTIC LEUKEMIA

Issues at the Time of Admission

The evaluation and stabilization of the patient with ALL are similar to those for patients with AML; however, the initial evaluation of ALL must take into account reservoirs of disease, including the testes and central nervous system. At presentation, a careful genital examination must be performed. A lumbar puncture for cell counts, chemistry, and cytology should be performed in all patients with ALL after peripheral blood blasts have cleared.

The treatment of ALL involves multiple-agent chemotherapy with prophylactic treatment of potential reservoirs, followed by prolonged administration of maintenance chemotherapy at regular intervals. Many regimens

continue therapy for up to two years, although some newer regimens, directed at L3 ALL or Burkitt's disease, provide a dose-dense approach with more intense alkylator support and shorter total duration of therapy (6, 7). The potential complications of therapy are the same as for AML. The agent L-asparaginase, which is utilized in the treatment of ALL, has the potential to cause severe pancreatitis. Serum amylase and lipase levels should be followed. This agent also inhibits the synthesis of proteins, including vitamin K-dependent coagulation factors and antithrombin III and proteins C and S, with the potential to cause both coagulopathies and thrombosis. Coagulation parameters and fibrinogen levels should be followed and fresh frozen plasma administered before L-asparaginase when the fibrinogen level falls below 100 mg/dL. Patients should also be monitored for hypersensitivity reactions during repeated doses of L-asparaginase. Unlike patients with AML, those with ALL receive prophylactic intrathecal chemotherapy, typically in the form of 8–10 doses of methotrexate weekly, depending on the regimen used. If the patient has active central nervous system disease, additional intrathecal chemotherapy is given and craniospinal radiation is commonly administered.

Issues During the Course of Hospitalization

See the preceding discussion of AML.

Recovery and Discharge Issues

The same issues that apply to ensuring a safe discharge for patients with AML also apply to those with ALL. Consolidation and maintenance therapy can generally be performed in an outpatient setting with close follow-up.

COST CONSIDERATIONS AND RESOURCE USE

The treatment of acute leukemia is expensive. Patients require prolonged hospitalizations, often with intensive care, and significant quantities of blood products and broad-spectrum antibiotics and other antimicrobial agents are administered. The average costs of induction therapy for patients with newly diagnosed AML range from $50,000 to more than $100,000. Opportunities to conserve resources, especially blood products, and contain costs have been identified and shown not to have a negative impact on outcome. Lowering the platelet transfusion threshold from 20,000/μL to 10,000/μL results in a decreased number of transfusions and lower costs without increased complications of bleeding (5). The use of filtered, leukocyte-depleted, ABO-compatible platelet products is associated with a decrease in allo-immunization and fewer platelet transfusions, which in turn results in a decrease in cost of approximately $14,000 per patient with acute leukemia (8).

The role of *hematopoietic growth factor support* in the management of acute leukemia remains controversial. In general, growth factor use results in fewer days of neutropenia and antibiotic use, but it does not necessarily reduce the number of days of hospitalization or improve overall survival. At the same time, growth factor use has not been associated with an increased relapse rate. Prospective trials assessing the cost effectiveness of growth factor use have yielded conflicting results. Some studies note significantly shorter durations of hospitalization and antibiotic use, while others do not (9–11) (Chapters 9 and 90). The routine use of growth factors in patients undergoing chemotherapy for acute leukemia cannot be strongly recommended, although the use is increasing, especially in patients over age 55.

Early discharge from the hospital may be an option for some patients. Those who have recovered from neutropenia and have a good performance status, but are still transfusion-dependent, can be supported with red blood cell and platelet transfusions on an outpatient basis. Prolonged therapy with antimicrobial agents can also be administered in the outpatient setting if patients are otherwise clinically stable.

KEY POINTS

- Acute leukemia remains a difficult problem for the patient and the hospital physician; patients often have protracted inpatient courses that require significant intensive care unit stays.
- Approximately 75% of treated patients attain a remission and are discharged home for further therapy.
- Pitfalls in the management of a patient with newly diagnosed acute leukemia include failure to recognize how quickly a patient can decompensate and delay in referral to a hematologist.
- A thorough initial evaluation and aggressive management of the consequences of both leukemia and its treatment (including coagulopathies, fevers, infections, and chemotherapy toxicity) will optimize a patient's chances for attaining a remission and potential cure of the disease.

REFERENCES

1. National Cancer Institute: surveillance, epidemiology and end-results 1995–1999. http://seer.cancer.gov/. Accessed February 5, 2005.
2. Sandler DP, Ross JA. Epidemiolgy of acute leukemia in children and adults. *Semin Oncol* 1997;24:3–16.
3. Byrd JC, Mrozek K, Dodge RK, et al. Pretreatment cytogenetic abnormalities are predictive of induction success, cumulative incidence of relapse, and overall survival in adult patients with de novo acute myeloid leulkemia: results from CALGB 8461. *Blood* 2002;100:4325–4336.
4. Ribera JM, Ortega JJ, Oriol A, et al. Prognositic value of karyotypic analysis in children and adults with high risk acute lymphoblastic leukemia included in the PETHEMA ALL-93 trial. *Haematologica* 2002;87:154–166.
5. Wandt H, Frank M, Ehninger G, et al. Safety and cost effectiveness of a 10 × 10(9)/l trigger for prophylactic platelet transfusions compared with the traditional 20 × 10(9)/l trigger: a prospective comparative trial in 105 patients with acute myeloid leukemia. *Blood* 1998;91:3601–3606.
6. Rizzieri DA, Johnson JL, Niedzwiecki D, et al. Intensive chemotherapy for lymphoma: final results of cancer and leukemia group B study 9251. *Cancer* 2004;100:1438–1448.
7. Annino L, Vegna ML, Camera A, et al. Treatment of adult acute lymphoblastic leukemia (ALL): long-term follow-up of the GIMEMA ALL 0288 randomized study. *Blood* 2002;99:863–871.
8. Blumberg N, Heal JM, Kirkley SA, et al. Leukodepleted ABO identical blood components in the treatment of hematologic malignancies: a cost analysis. *Am J Hematol* 1995;48:108–115.
9. Rowe JM, Anderson JW, Mazza JJ, et al. A randomized placebo-controlled phase II study of granulocyte macrophage colony stimulating factor in adult patients (>55 to 70 years of age) with acute myelogenous leukemia: a study of the Eastern Cooperative Oncology Group (E1490). *Blood* 1995;86:457–462.
10. Uylde Groot CA, Lowenberg B, Vellenga E, et al. Cost effectiveness and quality of life assessment of GM-CSF as an adjunct to intensive remission induction chemotherapy in elderly patients with acute myeloid leukemia. *Br J Haematol* 1998;100:629–636.
11. Alonzo TA, Kobrinsky NL, Aledo A, et al. Impact of granulocyte colony stimulating factor use during induction for acute myelogenous leukemia in children: a report from the Children's Cancer Group. *J Pediatric Hematol Oncol* 2002;24:627–635.

ADDITIONAL READING

Chanock SJ, Pizzo PA. Infectious complications of patients undergoing therapy for acute leukemia: current status and future prospects. *Semin Oncol* 1997;24:132–140.

Cheson BD, Bennett JM, Kopecky KJ, Buchner T, et al. International working group for diagnosis, standardization of response criteria, treatment outcomes, and reporting standards for therapeutic trials in acute myeloid leukemia. Revised recommendations of the international working group for diagnosis, standardization of response criteria, treatment outcomes, and reporting standards for therapeutic trials in acute myeloid leukemia. *J Clin Oncol* 2003; 21:4642–4649.

Laport GF, Larson RA. Treatment of adult acute lymphoblastic leukemia. *Semin Oncol* 1997;24:70–82.

Mollee P, Gupta V, Song K, Reddy V, et al. Long-term outcome after intensive therapy with etoposide, melphalan, total body irradiation and autotransplant for acute myeloid leukemia. *Bone Marrow Transplant* 2004 Apr 19 [epub ahead of print].

Rebulla P, Finazzi G, Marangoni F, et al. The threshold for prophylactic platelet transfusions in adults with acute myeloid leukemia. *N Engl J Med* 1997;337:1870–1875.

Soignet S, Fleischauer A, Polyk T, et al. All-trans retinoic acid significantly increases 5-year survival in patients with acute promyelocytic leukemia: long-term follow-up of the New York study. *Cancer Chemother Pharmacol* 1997;40[Suppl]:S25–S29.

Trial to Reduce Alloimmunization to Platelets Study Group. Leukocyte reduction and ultraviolet B irradiation of platelets to prevent alloimmunization and refractoriness to platelet transfusions. *N Engl J Med* 1997;337:1861–1869.

Yucebilgin MS, Cagirgan S, Donmez A, Ozkinay E, et al. Acute myeloblastic leukemia in pregnancy: a case report and review of the literature. *Eur J Gynaecol Oncol* 2004;25:126–128.

Lymphoma

94

Ranjana H. Advani   *Steven M. Horwitz*
Sandra J. Horning

INTRODUCTION

The non-Hodgkin's lymphomas and Hodgkin's disease comprise a heterogeneous group of lymphoid neoplasms with differing presenting features, natural histories, and responses to treatment. They also are among the most treatable and curable of all malignancies. The treatment goals guide the approach to specific problems.

Non-Hodgkin's lymphoma (NHL) is the sixth most common cause of cancer in the United States, with 54,000 new cases and as many as 24,000 deaths estimated in 2002. Whereas the overall incidence of cancer increased about 1% annually, the incidence of NHL rose 3%–4% annually, rising more than 50% between 1973 and 1990 (1). Some of this increase represented AIDS-related lymphomas in young men. However, significant increases have been observed in women and in all age groups except the very young. The incidence of NHL in the United States increases with advancing age, with 8.5 cases per 100,000 for people under age 65 and 68.8 per 100,000 for the group over 65. There is a slight male preponderance. Whites are affected more than African Americans and other minorities. The incidence of NHL is significantly higher in industrialized countries than in the developing world.

Hodgkin's disease is far less common than NHL, with an annual incidence in the United States of 7,000 cases and 1,500 deaths. Unlike NHL, the incidence of Hodgkin's disease has remained relatively stable. Hodgkin's disease has a bimodal distribution in developed countries, with most cases occurring in persons between the ages of 15 and 34, and a second, smaller peak in incidence observed in people over age 50. Like NHL, Hodgkin's disease is more common in whites than in blacks and more common in men than in women. Other epidemiologic features of Hodgkin's disease include increased risk with higher educational levels of patients or their mothers, fewer siblings, single-family homes, familial association, and history of mononucleosis. There is a small increase in the incidence of Hodgkin's disease among HIV-infected patients.

Risk Factors

Current evidence suggests that factors or conditions precipitating immunosuppression or chronic antigenic stimulation provide a milieu for the development of NHL. Congenital immunodeficiency states all confer a greatly increased risk for the development of lymphoma. In people with acquired immunodeficiency (e.g., after transplantation of a solid organ or HIV infection), the risk increases as much as 50- to 100-fold in comparison with a baseline population. NHL ultimately develops in as many as 5% of cardiac transplant patients (Chapter 40).

Several infectious agents have been implicated as causal in specific types of lymphomas. *Helicobacter pylori* infection is clearly involved in the development of mucosa-associated lymphoid tissue (MALT) lymphomas in the stomach. Eradication of the bacteria with antibiotics (Table 80.3) leads to regression of the lymphoma in cases limited to the mucosal surface. There are similar associations between Epstein-Barr virus (EBV) and African Burkitt lymphoma, and between HTLV-I (human T-cell lymphotropic virus type I) and cutaneous T-cell lymphoma, in which viral infection and integration into the malignant cells have been demonstrated. Both EBV infection and a history of infectious mononucleosis in young adults have been associated with many of the T-cell lymphomas.

TYPICAL PRESENTATION AND DIFFERENTIAL DIAGNOSIS

The typical presentation of lymphoma is painless lymphadenopathy. However, the differential diagnosis of an enlarged lymph node or nodes is extensive (Chapter 89). The most common causes of lymphadenopathy in one series were lymphoma, tuberculosis, toxoplasmosis, infectious mononucleosis, and Hodgkin's disease (2). Rarely, a rapidly enlarging lymph node containing lymphoma may be painful and associated with signs of inflammation. The adenopathy of lymphoma is often characterized by rounded nodules or groups of nodules clustered together, sometimes with adjacent groups of enlarged nodal sites. The neck, axillae, inguinal region, and mediastinum are the most common sites of enlarged nodes in lymphomas and Hodgkin's disease. Epitrochlear or femoral adenopathy strongly suggest NHL.

Constitutional (also known as "B") symptoms, although common in lymphomas and Hodgkin's disease, are often not helpful in distinguishing these neoplasms from infectious entities. Pruritus or pain at involved nodal sites after ingestion of alcohol more strongly suggests Hodgkin's disease. Other, less common presenting features of lymphomas and Hodgkin's disease include cytopenias, which result from bone marrow involvement or immune destruction, and extranodal lesions, which can involve the skin, gastrointestinal tract, Waldeyer's ring, testes, and other sites. Neurologic symptoms caused by enlarging masses can be seen in primary central nervous system (CNS) lymphomas, and peripheral neuropathy can be part of a paraneoplastic syndrome.

Nodal size has some predictive value, as most lymphadenopathy less than 1 cm^2 in size, especially when unaccompanied by systemic symptoms, is benign. Patients with persistent adenopathy (lasting longer than 2–3 weeks), enlarging adenopathy, constitutional symptoms, abnormal blood cell counts or serum chemistries, or underlying immune deficiency should be evaluated further with biopsy of abnormal tissue.

Diagnosis

The diagnosis of NHL requires examination of an adequate sample of representative tissue. Tissue can be obtained by fine-needle aspiration, core needle biopsy, or excisional lymph node biopsy. Although fine-needle aspiration may be adequate for cell type, it does not allow the examination of lymph node architecture to classify many lymphomas. In addition, the paucity of tissue makes a diagnosis of Hodgkin's disease difficult and does not allow for further immunophenotyping. In general, the greater amount of lymph tissue obtained with multiple core biopsies or lymph node excision is preferred. If infection is in the differential diagnosis, tissue should be processed for routine histology and microbiologic examination. Specimens that demonstrate NHL are studied by immunophenotyping to determine B or T cell lineage and for classification. In selected cases, classical cytogenetics or Fluorescence *in situ* Hybridization (FISH) may allow more precise diagnosis. Storage of frozen material for genotyping to determine monoclonality is encouraged in difficult cases. It may become more routine in the future as a means to measure gene expression quantitatively.

Classification

The classification of NHL has undergone several revisions over the last four decades. Two of the more important and commonly used classifications are described here. The older classification, known as the *Working Formulation*, was based on microscopic appearance and survival characteristics. The Working Formulation separated the lymphomas into low-, intermediate-, and high-grade categories. Simplistically, survival among untreated patients was considered to be measured in years for low-grade disease, months for intermediate-grade disease, and weeks for high-grade disease. Although it did not account for the subtle differences within each category, the Working Formulation provided a useful clinical framework to guide the approach to a complicated array of disorders.

The World Health Organization (WHO) classification (3) has now replaced the Working Formulation. The WHO classification is based on cell of origin, primarily B-cells or T-cells, and characterizes NHL entities as individual diseases. In addition to morphologic features, immunophenotypic and genetic markers and clinical characteristics are integrated into the current NHL classification (Table 94.1).

Staging

While classification systems have been frequently updated and modified, staging for lymphomas has remained static. The *Ann Arbor staging system*, initially proposed for Hodgkin's disease, is also used for NHL (4) (Table 94.2). It stages lymphomas according to the number of nodal sites involved, their relation to the diaphragm, and the extent of extranodal disease. The presence of "B" symptoms is indicated by adding a letter "B" to the Roman numeral stage. An "A" denotes the absence of "B" symptoms.

Although the Ann Arbor staging system provides important prognostic information for Hodgkin's disease, it remains inadequate for NHL, which does not follow the same orderly progression of contiguous disease sites. Systemic involvement is more common, which makes distinctions about the relationship of disease to the diaphragm less important. To provide better prognostic information for NHL, independent prognostic factors have been defined. Factors that are independently predictive of overall survival include age less than 60 (vs. 60 and older), stage I or II (vs. stage III or IV), number of extranodal sites of disease, performance status, and serum lactate dehydrogenase level (5). On the basis of these variables, patients can be divided into four risk groups ranging from low-risk (zero or one adverse prognostic factor) to high-risk (4–5 adverse prognostic factors). Overall, the 5-year survival is 78% in low-risk patients, but only 26% in the most unfavorable group. Staging evaluation should be guided by a hematologist/oncologist and include abdominal and chest computed tomography, bone marrow biopsy, and the routine laboratory determinations mentioned above. Fluorine-18 deoxyglucose positron emission tomography (FDG-PET) scanning is increasingly becoming an important imaging modality, especially when following up with patients in whom the initial presentation was bulky (6). Multiple studies have

---

TABLE 94.1

THE WORLD HEALTH ORGANIZATION CLASSIFICATION OF NEOPLASMS OF THE HEMATOPOIETIC AND LYMPHOID TISSUES

B-cell neoplasms

Precursor B-cell neoplasm
Precursor B-lymphoblastic leukemia/lymphoma

Peripheral B-cell neoplasms
1. B-cell CLL/PLL/SLL
2. Lymphoplasmacytic lymphoma
3. Mantle cell lymphoma
4. Folliclular lymphoma
5. Extra nodal marginal zone lymphoma
6. Nodal marginal zone lymphoma
7. Splenic marginal zone lymphoma
8. Hairy cell leukemia
9. Primary effusion lymphoma
10. Diffuse large B-cell lymphoma
11. Burkitt's lymphoma

T-cell and NK-cell neoplasms

Precursor T-cell neoplasm
Precursor T-lymphoblastic lymphoma/leukemia

Peripheral T-cell and NK-cell neoplasms
1. T-cell CLL/PLL
2. T cell granular lymphocytic leukemia
3. Aggressive NK cell leukemia
4. Mycosis fungoides/Sézary syndrome
5. Peripheral T-cell lymphomas, unspecified
6. Adult T-cell lymphoma/leukemia
7. Angioimmunoblastic T-cell lymphoma
8. Extranodal NK nasal/nasal type T cell lymphoma
9. Enteropathy type T-cell lymphoma
10. Anaplastic large cell lymphoma (systemic)
11. Anaplastic large cell lymphoma (cutaneous)
12. Hepatosplenic gamma delta lymphoma
13. Subcutaneous panniculitis-like lymphoma

Hodgkin's disease

1. Lymphocyte predominance
2. Nodular sclerosis
3. Mixed cellularity
4. Lymphocyte depletion
5. Lymphocyte-rich classic Hodgkin's disease

ALCL, anaplastic large cell lymphoma; *CLL,* chronic lymphocytic leukemia; *NK,* natural killer; *PLL,* prolymphocytic leukemia; *SLL,* small lymphocytic leukemia.

TABLE 94.2

ANN ARBOR STAGING SYSTEM

Stage	Characteristics
I	Involvement of a single lymphatic region (I), or localized involvement of a single extralymphatic organ or site (IE).
II	Involvement of two or more lymphatic regions on the same side of the diaphragm (II), or localized involvement of a single extralymphatic organ or site and one or more lymphatic regions on the same side of the diaphragm (IIE).
III	Involvement of lymphatic regions on both sides of the diaphragm (III), which may also be accompanied either by localized involvement of an extralymphatic organ or site (IIIE), or by involvement of the spleen (IIIS), or by both (IIIE+S).
IV	Diffuse or disseminated involvement of one or more extralymphatic organs with or without associated lymphatic involvement.

The absence or presence of unexplained fever, night sweats, and/or weight loss of more than 10% of the usual body weight in the six months before diagnosis is denoted by the suffix letters A (absence) or B (presence).

demonstrated better predictive accuracy with FDG-PET than with computed tomography in restaging of NHL patients after therapy.

SPECIFIC CATEGORIES OF LYMPHOMAS

Given the wide diversity of entities, clinical behaviors, and treatments, it is helpful to understand some basic concepts about the different types of lymphomas.

Diffuse Small Cell Lymphomas

Diffuse small cell lymphomas are a group of B-cell lymphomas that include the entities of small lymphocytic lymphoma, lymphoplasmacytoid lymphoma, marginal zone lymphoma, and mantle cell lymphoma. With the exception of mantle cell lymphoma, which can have a more aggressive course, the diffuse small cell lymphomas are categorized as indolent. Diffuse small cell lymphomas make up 10%–20% of all NHLs. Men are affected more than women, and the average age at diagnosis is 50 years. Diffuse small cell lymphomas typically present in advanced stages, with diffuse adenopathy and bone marrow involvement. Splenomegaly and other extranodal sites of involvement are common. Anemia and thrombocytopenia can result from splenic or marrow involvement, or both. Mantle cell lymphoma tends to follow a shorter, more aggressive course than that of the other diffuse small cell lymphomas, with median survival times of 3–5 years.

Although the other entities in this group are not thought to be curable, survival is measured in years; many patients are alive more than 10 years after diagnosis. Marginal zone lymphomas frequently involve extranodal sites alone at presentation, particularly in the gastrointestinal tract, and this subset is referred to as mucosa-associated lymphoid tissue (MALT) lymphoma.

Treatment may be reserved for symptomatic disease in selected patients, because early intervention has not been demonstrated to alter survival. Symptoms can take the form of discomfort from compression of extranodal structures by adenopathy and clinically significant anemia or thrombocytopenia. Most patients respond to therapy, with significant or complete regression of measurable disease during initial treatment. Unfortunately, relapses are characteristic. Remissions typically last 2–4 years. If symptoms are confined to one area of disease, such as a single mass or lymph node group, radiation can be used to control local problems when chemotherapy is contraindicated. Diffuse small cell lymphoma undergoes transformation to a higher grade lymphoma in up to 10% of patients.

Follicular Lymphomas

This group of mostly indolent lymphomas includes follicular center lymphoma of small cleaved cell type (grade I), follicular mixed small and large cell type (grade II), and follicular large cell type (grade III). Follicular lymphomas comprise 35%–40% of all NHLs. They affect men and women equally, and the mean age at diagnosis is 55 years. As with other indolent lymphomas, disease is usually advanced at presentation. Typical features include widespread adenopathy, often with bone marrow or splenic involvement. The follicular lymphomas have an indolent course in most patients, with median survival time varying from 6–10 years from diagnosis. Some patients have a more aggressive disease, whereas others live more than 20 years following diagnosis. Intermittent relapses are the rule. Because of this natural history, a watchful waiting strategy has been employed, with treatment delayed until symptoms caused by bulky adenopathy, organ compromise, or constitutional symptoms develop. The disease course is highly variable, but most patients require treatment within four years of diagnosis. Controversy exists regarding whether some patients with stage I or II disease are cured with local radiation therapy.

Historically, treatment has included alkylating agents such as cyclophosphamide or chlorambucil, alone or in combination with other chemotherapeutic drugs and steroids (Chapter 90). The pan-B-cell monoclonal antibody (rituximab) is approved for the re-treatment of follicular lymphomas based on a 50% response rate (7). Newer data indicate that rituximab alone is effective in previously untreated patients and prolongs time to treatment failure in combination with chemotherapy. In addition, monoclonal antibodies conjugated to radioisotopes have been approved for the treatment of recurrent follicular lymphoma (8, 9). Like other indolent lymphomas, most follicular lymphomas respond to treatment but repeatedly relapse. Histologic transformation to higher grade lymphoma is more common than in the diffuse low-grade lymphomas (up to 60% of patients). When diagnosed, this must be treated with intensive chemotherapy. Although transformation is often an ominous prognostic sign, transformed lymphoma is sometimes curable, and patients who respond completely to therapy may have a life expectancy similar to that of patients with the underlying low-grade lymphoma.

Diffuse Aggressive Lymphomas

The diffuse aggressive lymphomas include diffuse large B-cell lymphoma, which accounts for about one-third of all NHLs, and the rare peripheral T-cell lymphomas. Diffuse large B-cell lymphomas are characterized by aggressive growth leading to clinical consequences in weeks to months and the potential to be cured with current therapies. Diffuse aggressive lymphomas present with early-stage or localized disease in more than 30% of patients. Extranodal sites of disease are common, as in primary lymphomas of the CNS, testis, and stomach. Approximately 20% of patients present with classic "B" symptoms. Given the aggressive nature of these lymphomas, treatment should begin as soon as staging studies are complete. The new standard of treatment is combination chemotherapy plus rituximab, based upon superior efficacy in multiple clinical trials (10). Treatment is generally given for about six months; radiation therapy delivered after a shortened course of chemotherapy may be used for patients with favorable localized disease presentations. The peripheral T-cell lymphomas are a heterogeneous group of lymphoproliferative diseases with unique clinical and pathologic features. As a group, they are characterized by relatively poor response to or early relapse after treatment and brief survival times. An exception are the anaplastic large T-cell lymphomas that occur in younger patients; these are frequently cured with combination chemotherapy.

Other Important Non-Hodgkin's Lymphomas

Lymphoblastic lymphoma is a rare, aggressive T-cell lymphoma. It commonly presents with a rapidly enlarging mediastinal mass. Superior vena cava syndrome (Chapter 92), pleural or pericardial effusion, and bone marrow involvement with circulating lymphoma cells may be seen at presentation. Burkitt lymphoma is a high-grade B-cell lymphoma presenting with rapidly enlarging masses in the head and neck or abdominal regions, frequently with bone marrow and central nervous system involvement. Lymphoblastic lymphomas and Burkitt lymphomas have high proliferative rates and are exquisitely sensitive to chemotherapy induction with regimens used for acute leukemia. This combination of high tumor burden and high growth fraction make tumor lysis syndrome a frequent complication of therapy. Hospitalization during initial therapy is often required (see later in this chapter).

HIV-associated lymphomas usually occur as late manifestations of HIV disease, often after previous AIDS-defining illnesses. They are typically B-cell lymphomas of intermediate or high grade that present in extralymphatic sites, particularly the CNS, gastrointestinal tract, bone marrow, and liver. Constitutional symptoms are present in 80% of patients at diagnosis. The CD4 cell count at diagnosis is prognostically significant. The advent of highly active antiretroviral therapy has resulted in better therapeutic tolerance for therapy and improved overall outcomes (11).

Hodgkin's Disease

Hodgkin's disease is classified in the broad category of lymphoid malignancies but remains separate from the NHLs given its unique pathologic and clinical patterns. The *Reed-Sternberg cell*, the malignant cell in Hodgkin's disease, derives from a B-cell lineage. Hodgkin's disease is divided into classical (nodular sclerosis, mixed cellularity, lymphocyte-rich, and lymphocyte depletion) and lymphocyte predominant subtypes. Hodgkin's disease most commonly presents as asymptomatic lymph node enlargement, often in the neck, supraclavicular fossa, or axilla. Another common presentation is an anterior mediastinal mass incidentally discovered on chest radiograph. Lone abdominal or inguinal disease is uncommon. Other presenting features characteristic of Hodgkin's disease include pruritus and cyclic fevers.

The initial evaluation of the patient with Hodgkin's disease is similar to that for NHL. Most patients present with stage II or III disease. "B" symptoms are more common in patients with advanced disease. Although uniformly fatal if untreated, Hodgkin's disease is among the most curable of all malignancies, with approximately 75%–85% of patients surviving more than 10 years after diagnosis. More than 90% of patients with early stage disease are cured with primary or secondary treatment. Patients with localized disease are currently managed with brief chemotherapy and limited radiotherapy. Patients with widespread disease receive chemotherapy as the basis of treatment. The contribution of radiation therapy is debatable after a full course of chemotherapy in advanced disease. Recurrent disease is treated with high-dose chemotherapy and autologous stem cell transplantation, often with good results (Chapter 96). Given the long-term survival of the majority of patients with Hodgkin's disease, late complications of treatment are common and have become a major cause of morbidity and mortality. These complications include coronary artery disease, cardiomyopathy, cardiac valvular lesions, secondary cancers (associated with radiation therapy), and secondary acute leukemia (associated with chemotherapy containing alkylating agents). NHL is seen as a complication of either radiation therapy or chemotherapy. Other common long-term complications include hypothyroidism and infertility.

COMPLICATIONS REQUIRING HOSPITALIZATION

The diagnosis, staging, and treatment of lymphomas currently are performed entirely on an outpatient basis. With the exception of particularly dose-intensive treatments or chemotherapy regimens requiring continuous infusions over several days, hospital admissions rarely are planned as part of the management strategy. Therefore, the inpatient physician most often plays a role in the management of complications that arise from the disease or its treatment.

Tumor Lysis Syndrome

The tumor lysis syndrome is a series of metabolic derangements (hyperuricemia, hyperphosphatemia, hypocalcemia, and hyperkalemia) that can result in acute renal failure or death. The syndrome develops when induction therapy for sensitive malignancies leads to the sudden release of intracellular ions, nucleic acids, and proteins that overwhelm the kidneys' ability to excrete them. Although most clinical consequences occur after treatment, high cellular turnover in rapidly dividing tumors often leads to a degree of renal insufficiency before the initiation of therapy. Tumor lysis syndrome is most commonly observed with high-grade NHLs.

Hyperuricemia and *hyperuricosuria* are usually the earliest manifestations of the tumor lysis syndrome. The increased uric acid load leads to the deposition of uric acid crystals in the collecting ducts and distal tubules. Once the crystals are delivered to the distal tubules, the relatively acid environment renders the uric acid even less soluble. Further deposition takes place and impairs urine excretion. This results in a decreased glomerular filtration rate and, without treatment, acute renal failure. Any condition that predisposes to a decreased glomerular filtration rate or decreased urine flow can predispose to acute renal failure.

Hyperphosphatemia develops later than hyperuricemia, often 48 hours into treatment, peaking on the second and third days of therapy. As the serum phosphate rises, it can form complexes with serum calcium and precipitate, resulting in hypocalcemia. In the most severe circumstances, this can lead to cramping, tetany, and cardiac arrhythmias. Less common but potentially more life-threatening is hyperkalemia, which can develop with the release of intracellular potassium from the disrupted tumor cells. When this is superimposed on renal insufficiency, dramatic increases in potassium levels can occur. If not corrected, hyperkalemia can lead to cardiac arrhythmias and sudden death (Chapter 104).

Initial Therapy

The best management of tumor lysis syndrome is to prevent it through early recognition of patients at risk and prompt institution of prophylactic measures. Patients at highest risk for development of the syndrome include those who have tumors with high proliferative rates, high serum levels of lactate dehydrogenase, and elevated serum levels of uric acid before treatment. Patients at highest risk for the development of clinical consequences include those with underlying renal insufficiency and volume depletion.

Figure 94.1 shows a critical pathway for the management of tumor lysis syndrome. Whenever possible, patients at high risk for the development of tumor lysis syndrome should be admitted to the hospital 24–48 hours before the institution of therapy. Unfortunately, given the aggressive nature of these tumors, delaying treatment is often difficult. All supplemental potassium should be avoided, with a goal

	Day 1: 1–2 days before therapy if possible	**Day 2:** Day before therapy	**Day 3:** Initiate chemotherapy	**Days 4–5:** 1–2 days post-therapy	**Days 6–8:** 3–5 days post-therapy
Tests	• Serum chemistries • LDH • Uric acid • Calcium • Phosphorus • Urine pH	• Serum chemistries • LDH • Uric acid • Calcium • Phosphorus • Urine pH	• Serum chemistries q 12 hrs • LDH • Uric acid • Calcium • Phosphorus	• Serum chemistrires q 12 hrs • LDH • Uric acid • Calcium • Phosphorus	• Serum chemistries q 24 hrs If no evidence of lysis, can discontinue • LDH • Uric acid • Calcium • Phosphorus
Patient evaluation	• Weight • Vital signs incl. orthostatics • Volume status • I&Os q 8 hrs • Assess node size	• Weight • Vital signs • Volume status • I&Os q 8 hrs	• Weight • Vital signs • Volume status • I&Os q 8 hrs	• Weight • Vital signs • Volume status • I&Os q 8 hrs • Assess node size	• Weight • Vital signs • Volume status • I&Os q 8 hrs • Assess node size
Medications and theraputics	• IV fluid NS or 0.5 NS @4–5L/24 hr • Allopurinol 300–400mg/m²/day PO[a] *Consider:* • Add NaHCO3 to IV fluids (1 amp to 0.5 NS, 2 amps to 0.25 NS, 3 amps to D5W) • Acetazolamide 150–500 mg/m² PO • Aluminum hydroxide if phosphorus elevated	• IV fluids • Mannitol 200–500 mg/kg if volume overload or urine output <100mL/hr • Allopurinol[a] *Consider:* • Nephrology consult or ICU transfer if severe volume overload or oliguria	• IV fluids • Mannitol prn • Allopurinol[a] • D/C NaHCO3 *Consider:* • Nephrology consult or ICU transfer if severe volume overload or oliguria	• IV fluids • Mannitol prn • Allopurinol[a] • Treat hyperkalemia if develops • Treat hypocalcemia only if symptomatic • If oliguria or increased creatinine, or refractory electrolyte disturbances, consult nephrology for early hemodialysis, if necessary	*If no evidence of tumor lysis:* • Decrease IV fluids • Continue allopurinol • If ongoing tumor lysis, continue previous measures
Nutrition	• Low K⁺ diet • Low PO4 diet	• Low K⁺ diet • Low PO4 diet	• Low K⁺ diet • Low PO4 diet	• Low K⁺ diet • Low PO4 diet	• Encourage PO fluids
Discharge planning				• Begin if no evidence of tumor lysis	• F/U appt made
Patient education					• Discharge teaching • F/U appt

Figure 94.1 Critical pathway for tumor lysis syndrome. [a]Rasburicase may be used as a substitute for allopurinol (see text for details). *D/C*, discontinue; *F/U*, follow-up; *I&O*, fluid intake and output; *ICU*, intensive care unit; *IV*, intravenous; *LDH*, lactate dehydrogenase; *NS*, normal saline.

of attaining a low-to-normal serum level before therapy. As soon as possible, an *intravenous infusion of saline solution* should be started. In patients with underlying cardiac or renal dysfunction, this is accomplished most safely in an ICU setting. Aggressive hydration (up to 4 L/d) should be instituted before therapy and continued during and for several days after the treatment. Sometimes, as many as 5 or 6 L of saline solution may be necessary. *Allopurinol* has long been the mainstay in preventing tumor lysis syndrome. It should be given as long before the start of therapy as possible in patients at high risk for tumor lysis. The goal of treatment is to normalize or greatly reduce the serum uric acid level to minimize uric acid deposition in the kidney. Allopurinol can cause a syndrome of rash, hepatitis, eosinophilia, and worsening renal function in patients with underlying renal insufficiency. Lower doses should be used in these patients, and the drug should be discontinued at the first sign of rash. The role of alkalinazation of the urine remains controversial. Recombinant urate oxidase (rasburicase) is a new IV, once-a-day agent that produces a sharp and consistent decrease in uric acid levels in patients undergoing cytoreductive therapy. In a randomized study of patients at high risk of tumor lysis, rasburicase led to more rapid control and lower levels of plasma uric acid than allopurinol (12).

Even when mild hypocalcemia develops, calcium replacement should be avoided unless serious clinical consequences such as tetany or cardiac arrhythmias occur. Aluminum hydroxide should be used to minimize hyperphosphatemia. Hyperkalemia should be watched for closely and treated aggressively with standard treatments (Chapter 104).

Indications for Consultation

Despite aggressive preventive measures and management of electrolyte disturbances, oliguria and acute renal failure or very severe electrolyte disturbances develop in some patients. A nephrologist should be consulted in cases of oliguria, inability to hydrate adequately because of third spacing, or an electrolyte disturbance that does not readily respond to the measures described above. Hemodialysis is often required short-term and can be life-saving, as the renal impairments are most often reversible (Chapter 100).

Discharge Issues

Tumor lysis is an uncommon and life-threatening situation. The patient should be discharged only after the cycle of chemotherapy is completed and any electrolyte imbalances have been corrected. Good urine output should be maintained through this period. Stabilization of lactate dehydrogenase and uric acid beyond 48–72 hours suggests that further tumor lysis is not going to occur. The patient should not have uncontrolled nausea or vomiting, which might impair the ability to consume fluids by mouth. Allopurinol or rasburicase should be continued.

Hypercalcemia

Although hypercalcemia is common in many malignancies, it is unusual in NHL and Hodgkin's disease. HTLV-I–associated T-cell lymphoma is an exception. NHL patients with hypercalcemia usually have high tumor burdens and advanced disease. Their debilitation leads to inactivity and dehydration, which exacerbate the hypercalcemia. Acute hypercalcemia should be treated urgently, as described in Chapter 92. Corticosteroids can be quite effective in the treatment of hypercalcemia secondary to lymphoma.

Infections

Fever and neutropenia are the most common serious treatment-related complications. Because cure is the goal of treatment for many aggressive lymphomas, the therapeutic regimens are dose-intensive and often leave patients severely neutropenic and at high risk for infection and its sequelae. The general approach to fever and neutropenia is the same as in other immunocompromised hosts (Chapter 63). However, it is worth noting several points specific to lymphoma.

Issues at the Time of Admission

In addition to being neutropenic as a consequence of cytotoxic therapy, many lymphoma patients are otherwise immunodeficient from their disease process. Patients often have deficiencies in cell-mediated immunity that place them at increased risk for opportunistic, nonbacterial infections (Chapter 63). A particularly high incidence of these infections has been noted in NHL patients receiving purine analog agents such as 2-CDA and fludarabine. Prophylaxis against infection with *Pneumocystis jirovecii* (formerly *P. carinii*) and herpes viruses should be considered in this population. Additional sources of immune compromise include immunoglobulin deficiency (in patients with small lymphocytic lymphoma), impairment of phagocytic function, and previous splenectomy (secondary to staging or treatment). Despite the widespread use of rituximab, which depletes B-cells for many months, infectious complications of this therapy have rarely been reported.

Although the modern approach to fever in the immunocompromised host often includes outpatient treatment and oral antibiotics, lymphoma patients undergoing chemotherapy rarely fit into the low-risk group that can be safely managed on an outpatient basis. This is particularly true in the special cases listed above. Admission to the hospital for intravenous administration of broad-spectrum antibiotics and close observation is usually warranted.

Discharge Issues

Despite the frequent use of dose-intense therapy, the routine use of hematopoietic growth factors has not been shown to decrease mortality in lymphoma patients (with the exception of patients receiving high-dose therapy during bone marrow transplantation). However, the prophylactic use of growth factors can decrease the incidence of neutropenic fever and chemotherapy-induced anemia, and it often allows patients to stay on a therapeutic regimen without persistent delays in treatment because of low blood counts. Thus, growth factors are recommended for patients who have been hospitalized for fever and neutropenia during previous cycles of therapy, or for patients in whom potentially curative treatment is delayed because of neutropenia. Newer liposomal formulations of growth factors (pegfilgastrim and darbepoetin) have been approved (13, 14). These preparations allow for dosing intervals of 2–3 weeks, with an efficacy equivalent to the shorter acting preparations.

Syndromes of Organ Involvement or Compression

Non-Hodgkin's lymphoma can involve and compromise any organ system. Nodal disease can cause external compression of normal structures by extension, or disease can develop *de novo* in extranodal sites. This can occur at any time in the course of the disease and often presents challenging diagnostic and management problems.

Issues on Admission

Several general principles apply to lymphoma patients with growing masses and organ compromise. In patients without a diagnosis, a good sample of representative tissue must be obtained for diagnosis. Once a diagnosis is established, the goals of treatment can be defined. If the patient has a curable disease, local problems usually are best treated with systemic chemotherapy as part of the overall treatment plan. However, if the disease is incurable, local problems can be palliated with systemic chemotherapy or local radiation.

Patients with a known diagnosis and relapsed or progressive disease present complex issues. Many patients with a first relapse of aggressive NHL or Hodgkin's disease remain curable with measures such as high-dose chemotherapy and stem cell transplantation. In these patients, systemic treatment of local disease is usually indicated. In patients with indolent NHL, progressive disease should prompt consideration of *histologic transformation*. This requires repeated biopsy at times of changing disease manifestations, such as a rapid increase in size or development of new "B" symptoms. If histologic transformation is present, a more aggressive approach is warranted. Patients with multiple relapses and multiple prior treatments often lack the bone marrow reserve to tolerate intensive chemotherapy. In these instances, local radiotherapy can often palliate focal symptoms. Therefore, the approach to local acute problems must take into account the most ef-

fective immediate therapy as well as the patient's treatment history and prognosis.

Issues During Hospitalization—Specific Anatomic Sites

Chest

The mediastinum is one of the more common sites of NHL. Growing thoracic disease can extend to and compromise the adjacent great vessels, heart, lung, and thoracic duct. *Superior vena cava syndrome* (SVCS) is the clinical picture of dyspnea, cough, and edema of the face and upper extremities arising from obstruction of the superior vena cava. NHL is the second leading malignant cause of superior vena cava syndrome (after lung cancer). In NHL, superior vena cava syndrome is often a presenting feature of disease; it may also occur after a recurrence or histologic transformation of low-grade disease to a more aggressive type. The evaluation and management of SVCS is described in Chapter 92.

In patients without a diagnosis, a pathologic diagnosis should be obtained whenever possible before therapy is begun. In patients with previously diagnosed indolent lymphomas, biopsy of a new, rapidly growing mass should be performed to evaluate a histologic transformation. In NHL, careful physical examination often reveals an accessible peripheral node for biopsy, so that the need to obtain tissue from a mass obstructing the superior vena cava is avoided.

In contrast to lung cancer (where radiation therapy is generally preferred), chemotherapy is typically the initial treatment of choice and can provide equally prompt resolution of SVCS. However, both medical and radiation oncologists should be consulted urgently at the time of diagnosis of SVCS.

Other problems arising in the chest include pleural and pericardial effusions. They can develop in any type of NHL and can present at any time during the course of the disease. They may develop rapidly, presenting with acute dyspnea, or have a more insidious onset. *Pleural effusions* can develop either from obstruction of the thoracic duct by mediastinal adenopathy or by direct involvement of the pleura. Thoracentesis should be performed for diagnosis and symptomatic relief (Chapter 60). At times, lymphoma is not diagnosed by cytologic examination of the fluid; immunophenotyping may increase the diagnostic yield in such instances. The best treatment for this complication remains treating the underlying lymphoma. Effusions often respond to chemotherapy, which makes pleurodesis unnecessary. In slowly resolving effusions, several therapeutic thoracentesis procedures are required before systemic therapy takes effect. Pleurodesis should be reserved for palliation of patients with refractory effusions, unresponsive disease, or an inability to tolerate systemic treatment.

Less common but more immediately life-threatening are *pericardial effusions*. These most often result from direct extension of the disease to the pericardium from adjacent lymph nodes. Small effusions are easily demonstrated by computed tomography of the thorax. Patients with cough, orthopnea, dyspnea, or distended neck veins should undergo echocardiography to evaluate for cardiac tamponade (Chapter 46). Urgent drainage is necessary for symptomatic effusions. Chemotherapy is the preferred and most definitive treatment. In rare cases, an indwelling pericardial drain or window is required to prevent reaccumulation of fluid (Chapter 92).

Pulmonary nodules are occasionally seen with NHL or Hodgkin's disease. They are most common in patients with mediastinal disease. Biopsy is indicated in patients without mediastinal or widespread adenopathy or with lung nodules as the sole site of recurrence. Infections and primary lung carcinomas can develop in heavily treated patients and can mimic lymphoma (Chapter 61).

Abdomen

The gastrointestinal tract, primarily the stomach and small bowel, is involved in 16% of patients with NHL, most commonly Burkitt and diffuse large B-cell lymphomas. Large masses can cause obstruction. Lymphoma can occasionally erode through bowel walls. As lymphoma quickly regresses with treatment, the result can be *gastrointestinal bleeding* or a *perforated viscus*. Perforation can occur in 5%–15% of these patients, with mortality as high as 50% in patients in whom an acute abdomen develops. Surgery should be limited to patients with active bleeding or perforation. Patients at risk for perforation should be educated about the signs and symptoms of abdominal pain, bleeding, and fever. If perforation is suspected, the patient should be admitted to the hospital and abdominal radiography or computed tomography performed to evaluate for free air (Chapter 87). Urgent surgical consultation should be obtained. Early intervention with broad-spectrum antibiotics and, if necessary, surgical resection, are the best ways to minimize mortality from this infrequent complication. Gastrointestinal bleeding and perforation are most common shortly after the initial course of chemotherapy. However, these complications can still develop more than a month into treatment.

Extensive retroperitoneal and pelvic disease from NHL can lead to *ureteral obstruction*, resulting in hydronephrosis and renal insufficiency (Chapter 103). Often, nonspecific symptoms of back pain or intermittent abdominal cramping are present for weeks to months before the lymphoma is detected. In patients with known disease, a high degree of suspicion must be maintained. Abdominal ultrasonography or computed tomography can quickly rule out ureteral obstruction and hydronephrosis. Ureteral obstruction is best managed by systemic treatment in patients with newly diagnosed aggressive lymphomas. In patients with

extensive low-grade lymphoma, systemic chemotherapy also is often the best course. In patients with indolent disease who present with a local obstruction, or in patients who may not tolerate further chemotherapy, local radiation can alleviate the obstruction. If renal function is compromised or the patient is very symptomatic, stenting can often palliate the obstruction while definitive treatment is provided. Stenting does expose the patient to a risk for perforation and infection but is necessary at times to preserve renal function.

Hyperbilirubinemia can result from hepatic infiltration with lymphoma or extrinsic constriction of the biliary system by periportal lymphadenopathy (Chapters 77 and 84). As in other circumstances, this often responds promptly to systemic chemotherapy. As a result, biliary drainage or stenting is rarely indicated, except in patients with cholangitis or refractory disease. When patients with hyperbilirubinemia are treated, modification of the doses of drugs excreted in bile, such as adriamycin and vincristine, should be considered (Table 90.3).

Splenomegaly is frequently observed at presentation in patients with Hodgkin's disease or NHL, particularly diffuse small cell lymphomas. It may be discovered on physical examination or present symptomatically with pain or thrombocytopenia. In rare cases of "splenic lymphoma," the spleen is the primary or sole site of disease. Good responses have been observed with splenectomy, but cytotoxic chemotherapy can achieve equally good results and leave a functional spleen. In general, splenectomy should be reserved for patients with pancytopenia or thrombocytopenia that does not respond to systemic treatment of the lymphoma, or for palliation of symptoms such as pain in patients with refractory disease.

Nervous System

The CNS can be involved at initial presentation of advanced-stage disease, at relapse, or by primary CNS lymphoma. CNS disease is more common in high-grade lymphomas and diffuse histologies and is rare in follicular subtypes. Hodgkin's disease very rarely spreads to the CNS. Other risk factors for CNS disease include bone marrow involvement and epidural, testicular, and paranasal sinus disease. Potential CNS involvement in high-risk patients should be evaluated with cytologic analysis of cerebrospinal fluid.

Parenchymal brain involvement presents with symptoms of increased intracranial pressure or with focal neurologic deficits. *Leptomeningeal disease* often presents with cranial nerve palsies, mental status decline, or both. NHL of the brain is diagnosed by radiologic imaging. Magnetic resonance imaging can show greater detail, but computed tomography often suffices. Lymphoma appears as contrast-enhancing lesions on either study. Stereotactic biopsy is necessary to differentiate lymphoma from infection. Rapid disappearance of CNS mass lesions after initiation of corticosteroids has been described with these lymphomas. Leptomeningeal disease can be more difficult to diagnose; cerebrospinal fluid cytology can be positive in as few as 20% of patients. Immunophenotyping of cerebrospinal fluid can increase the yield.

Spinal cord compression is rare in NHL. It most often occurs by direct extension from extradural masses. Cord compression can develop with any histologic subtype and should be evaluated as an oncologic emergency, as described in Chapter 92. As in other instances of organ compromise from lymphoma, chemotherapy often achieves as rapid a response as radiation therapy while simultaneously treating systemic disease.

COST CONSIDERATIONS

Most of the presentation, diagnosis, and management of lymphomas takes place entirely on an outpatient basis. Preventing hospitalization is the main way to control costs in managing this disease. Most hospitalizations are for complications of the disease or its treatment. Few cost analyses have been performed in the management of lymphoma complications. However, the routine use of hematopoietic growth factors is expensive and has not been shown to improve outcome except in the specific circumstances listed above.

KEY POINTS

- Non-Hodgkin's lymphoma and Hodgkin's disease are among the most treatable and curable of all malignancies. The treatment goals guide the approach to specific problems.
- Most diagnosis and treatment can be performed on an outpatient basis.
- Tumor lysis syndrome is a constellation of life-threatening metabolic disturances that occur during the treatment of aggressive lymphomas and other malignancies. The best management is identification of patients at risk and institution of preventative measures, such as vigorous hydration and allopurinol.
- Acute renal failure in the setting of the tumor lysis syndrome is almost always reversible, even if a short course of hemodialysis is required.
- Infections in lymphoma patients undergoing treatment can be complicated by other immune deficiencies. Particular therapeutic urgency is required for splenectomized patients.
- Unlike other malignancies, non-Hodgkin's lymphoma or Hodgkin's disease causing obstruction or compression of normal structures can best be treated by chemotherapy.

- Gastrointestinal bleeding and perforation are uncommon but potentially fatal complications in the treatment of lymphoma of the gastrointestinal tract. Early surgical evaluation should be sought.

REFERENCES

1. Clarke CA, Glaser SL. Changing incidence of non-Hodgkin lymphomas in the United States. *Cancer* 2002;94:2015–2023.
2. Pangalis GA, Vacsilakopoulos TP, Boussiotis VA, et al. Clinical approach to lymphadenopathy. *Semin Oncol* 1993;20:570–575.
3. Harris NL, Jaffe ES, Diebold J, et al. The World Health Organization classification of neoplasms of the hematopoietic and lymphoid tissues: report of the Clinical Advisory Committee meeting—Airlie House, Virginia, November, 1997. *Hematol J* 2000;1:53–66.
4. Carbone PD, Kaplan HS, Musshoff K, et al. Report of the committee on Hodgkin's disease staging classification. *Cancer Res* 1971; 31:1860–1861.
5. The International Non-Hodgkin's Lymphoma Prognostic Factors Project. A predictive model for aggressive non-Hodgkin's lymphoma. *N Engl J Med* 1993;329:987–994.
6. Elstrom R, Guan L, Nakhoda K, et al. Utility of FDG-PET scanning in lymphoma by WHO classification. *Blood* 2003;101:3875–3876.
7. Maloney DG, Grillo-Lopez AJ, White CA, et al. IDEC-C2B8 (Rituximab) anti-CD20 monoclonal antibody therapy in patients with relapsed low-grade non-Hodgkin's lymphoma. *Blood* 1997; 90:2188–2195.
8. Witzig TE, White CA, Gordon LI, et al. Safety of Yttrium-90 Ibritumomab Tiuxetan radioimmunotherapy for relapsed low-grade, follicular, or transformed Non-Hodgkin's lymphoma. *J Clin Oncol* 2003;21:1263–1270.
9. Kaminski MS, Zelenetz AD, Press OW, et al. Pivotal study of iodine I 131 tositumomab for chemotherapy-refractory low-grade or transformed low-grade B-cell non-Hodgkin's lymphomas. *J Clin Oncol* 2001;19:3918–3928.
10. Coiffier B, Lepage E, Briere J, et al. CHOP chemotherapy plus rituximab compared with CHOP alone in elderly patients with diffuse large-B-cell lymphoma. *N Engl J Med* 2002;346:235–242.
11. Noy A. Update in HIV-associated lymphoma. *Curr Opin Oncol* 2004;16:450–454.
12. Goldman SC, Holcenberg JS, Finklestein JZ, et al. A randomized comparison between rasburicase and allopurinol in children with lymphoma or leukemia at high risk for tumor lysis. *Blood* 2001;97: 2998–3003.
13. Vose JM, Crump M, Lazarus H, et al. Randomized, multicenter, open-label study of pegfilgrastim compared with daily filgrastim after chemotherapy for lymphoma. *J Clin Oncol* 2003;21:514–519.
14. Glaspy JA, Tchekmedyian NS. Darbepoetin alfa administered every two weeks alleviates anemia in cancer patients receiving chemotherapy. *Oncology* 2002;(10 Suppl 11):23–29.

ADDITIONAL READING

Arrambie K, Toto RD. Tumor lysis syndrome. *Semin Nephrol* 1993;13: 273–280.

DeVita VT, Hellman S, Rosenberg SA, eds. *Cancer: Principles and Practice of Oncology,* 7th ed. Philadelphia: Lippincott Williams & Wilkins, 2004.

Ozer H, Armitage JO, Bennett CL, et al. American Society of Clinical Oncology. 2000 update of recommendations for the use of hematopoietic colony-stimulating factors: evidence-based, clinical practice guidelines. American Society of Clinical Oncology Growth Factors Expert Panel. *J Clin Oncol* 2000;18:3558–585.

Pui CH, Jeha S, Irwin D, et al. Recombinant urate oxidase (rasburicase) in the prevention and treatment of malignancy-associated hyperuricemia in pediatric and adult patients: results of a compassionate-use trial. *Leukemia* 2001;15:1505–1509.

Chronic Myeloproliferative Disorders

95

Ayalew Tefferi

INTRODUCTION

Hematologic malignancies are organized into lymphoid or myeloid disorders, depending on whether the clonal (neoplastic) process involves cells of the myeloid lineage (granulocytes, monocytes, erythrocytes, platelets) or lymphoid lineage (lymphocytes, plasma cells). Within each lineage, disease is classified as acute or chronic, depending on the percentage of blasts in the bone marrow; more than 20% defines acute leukemia. Accordingly, the chronic myeloid disorders represent relatively mature proliferative disorders of the myeloid lineage and are subdivided into four major categories, including chronic myeloid leukemia (CML), the myelodysplastic syndrome (MDS), the chronic myeloproliferative diseases (CMPD), and the atypical chronic myeloid disorders (ACMD). Among the chronic myeloid disorders, CML is the easiest to identify because of its specific association with the Philadelphia chromosome or its molecular equivalent (bcr/abl translocation). The morphologic demonstration of dyserythropoiesis strongly suggests MDS; it is also characterized by granulocyte and megakaryocyte dysplasia. In addition, patients with MDS often display peripheral blood cytopenia(s), while those with CML and CMPD display peripheral blood cytosis.

The current classification of the CMPD includes essential thrombocythemia (ET), polycythemia vera (PV), and agnogenic myeloid metaplasia (AMM). At present, there is not one specific diagnostic marker for any of these three clinico-pathologic entities, and a working diagnosis is formulated by a set of laboratory and clinical features. The fourth category of the chronic myeloid diorders, ACMD, is reserved for a miscellaneous group of myeloid disorders that do not fit into the other three categories. These include mast cell disease, hypereosinophilic syndrome, chronic neutrophilic leukemia, juvenile myelomonocytic leukemia, chronic myelomonocytic leukemia, and undifferentiated MDS/CMPD.

EPIDEMIOLOGY

In a population-based study from Olmsted County, Minn., annual incidence rates were 2.5/100,000 for ET, 2.3/100,000 for PV, and 1.3/100,000 for AMM (1–3). As is true for most hematologic malignancies, the incidence rates were significantly higher in the older age groups. However, as many as 20% of patients with ET and 7% of those with PV are younger than 40 years, and approximately 10% of those with AMM are younger than 50 years. Women are overrepresented (1.6:1) in ET, whereas men have a slight predominance in both PV and AMM. In all three disorders, the median age at diagnosis is approximately 60 years. In general, the connection between disease incidence and exposure to environmental factors has not been strong.

PATHOGENESIS

Studies based on analyses of glucose-6-phosphate dehydrogenase isoenzyme patterns and X-linked DNA analyses have supported the stem cell origin of the clonal process in the CMPD. New evidence suggests that both B and T lymphocytes may also be clonally involved in AMM (4). Recent studies have focused on the pathogenetic role of genes regulating the production and expression of lineage-specific growth factors (erythropoietin in PV and thrombopoietin in ET). So far, genetic lesions involving erythropoietin, thrombopoietin, or their receptors have not been recognized in either PV or ET. In all CMPD but primarily in PV, there is an abnormal growth factor response during in vitro myeloid colony growth including both growth factor-independence and hypersensitivity. Bone marrow fibrosis is often demonstrated in AMM and also may develop in the later stages of PV and ET. The process appears to be reactive; circumstantial evidence and animal experiments suggest the role of megakaryocyte- and/or monocyte-derived growth factors, including transforming growth factor-β, in its pathogenesis (5).

CLINICAL FEATURES AND PROGNOSIS

Essential Thrombocythemia

Essential thrombocythemia is a chronic state of increased platelet count. Although the disorder does not significantly compromise life expectancy during the first decade of the disease (1), the clinical course may be complicated by frequent vasomotor and thrombohemorrhagic events. Vasomotor symptoms result from platelet-mediated endothelial injury in small vessels and include headache, erythromelalgia (burning pain and erythema of the hands or feet), paresthesia, and visual symptoms. Although defective platelets are believed to contribute to the abnormal thrombosis and bleeding associated with ET, the risk has not been correlated with detectable qualitative or quantitative platelet abnormalities.

Most patients with ET are asymptomatic. Approximately one-third of patients have vasomotor symptoms, leukocytosis, or palpable splenomegaly. Bleeding complications are infrequent (5%) and usually inconsequential. Thrombotic complications are more frequent (15%) and can be life-threatening. The types of thrombotic complications are similar to those in PV (see later in this chapter). The risk for thrombosis is highest in patients with a prior history of thrombosis (31% per patient-year) and in those who are older than 60 years (15% per patient-year) (1). In the absence of these two risk factors, the risk for thrombosis is low (3%). It is important to note that the degree of thrombocytosis has not been correlated with thrombotic risk.

Polycythemia Vera

At presentation, patients may have symptoms and signs related to hyperviscosity and splenomegaly. These include headaches, dizziness, visual symptoms, paresthesias, fatigue, abdominal discomfort, weight loss, and night sweats. Pruritus after bathing is a frequent but poorly understood complaint (6). Clinical examination may reveal plethora (facial fullness and erythema), retinal vein distention, and palpable splenomegaly. More than half of all patients have associated leukocytosis or thrombocytosis. Microcytosis is frequent and indicates iron deficiency from phlebotomy or occult gastrointestinal blood loss. Nonspecific additional laboratory abnormalities include increases in the leukocyte alkaline phosphatase score and in the serum vitamin B_{12} and uric acid levels.

Thrombotic events are frequent (20%) in PV and include stroke, transient ischemic attack, retinal vein thrombosis, central retinal artery occlusion, myocardial infarction, angina, pulmonary embolism, hepatic and portal vein thrombosis, deep vein thrombosis, and peripheral arterial occlusion. Similar to the situation in ET, thrombotic risk correlates with advanced age and history of thrombosis (2). In addition, the increased blood viscosity associated with the increased red cell mass contributes to thrombosis. Bleeding in PV is less frequent than in ET, and tends to occur in the gastrointestinal system. In addition, patients may experience vasomotor disturbances. Compared with ET, PV is more likely to undergo transformation into acute leukemia and myelofibrosis.

Agnogenic Myeloid Metaplasia

The median survival in AMM may be as long as eight years or as short as one year, depending, respectively, on the absence or presence of anemia and leukocytosis (7). Causes of death include heart failure, infection, and leukemic transformation; the latter occurs in approximately 10% of patients. Most patients experience progressive anemia requiring frequent red blood cell transfusions, massive hepatosplenomegaly, and the hypercatabolic symptoms of profound fatigue, weight loss, night sweats, and low-grade fever. In addition, in some patients, extramedullary hematopoiesis may develop in the spinal cord, the pleural and peritoneal cavity, and various organs. At presentation, 45% of patients will have a hemoglobin level of less than 10 g/dL, and 25% have thrombocytopenia, thrombocytosis, or leukocytosis.

DIFFERENTIAL DIAGNOSIS AND INITIAL EVALUATION

Once a chronic myeloproliferative disease is suspected, the initial step is to exclude the possibility of reactive thrombocytosis in cases of ET (Table 95.1 and Figure

TABLE 95.1
CAUSES OF REACTIVE THROMBOCYTOSIS

Acute conditions

Immediate postsurgical period
Acute bleeding
Acute hemolysis
Infections
Tissue damage (acute pancreatitis, myocardial infarction, trauma, burns)
Coronary artery bypass procedure
Rebound effect from chemotherapy or immune thrombocytopenia

Chronic conditions

Iron-deficiency anemia
Surgical or functional asplenia
Metastatic cancer, lymphoma
Inflammatory disorders (rheumatoid arthritis, vasculitis, allergies)
Renal failure, nephrotic syndrome

TABLE 95.2
CAUSES OF ACQUIRED SECONDARY POLYCYTHEMIA

Appropriate erythropoietin response

Chronic lung disease
Arteriovenous or intracardiac shunts
High-altitude habitat
Continuous carbon monoxide exposure (smoking)

Pathologic erythropoietin production

Tumors (liver, kidney, cerebellum)
Uterine fibroids
After renal transplantation

95.1), apparent or secondary polycythemia in cases of PV (Table 95.2 and Figure 95.2), and other causes of bone marrow fibrosis in cases of AMM (Table 95.3). After the possibility of a reactive process is ruled out, the next step is to classify the chronic myeloproliferative disease accu-

rately. Accordingly, *all patients in whom a reactive process cannot be identified require a bone marrow examination with cytogenetic studies.*

With regards to the diagnosis of ET, one should first determine the duration of thrombocytosis; acute onset suggests reactive thrombocytosis while chronicity suggests ET. Initial laboratory tests should include measurement of serum ferritin and a peripheral blood smear examination (Figure 95.1). A low serum ferritin level is diagnostic of iron deficiency, which is associated with reactive thrombocytosis.

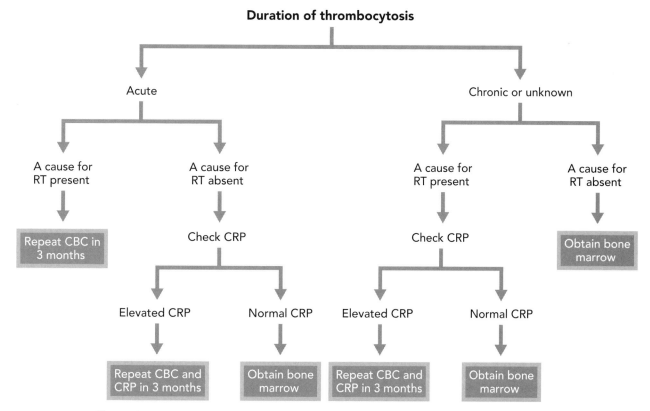

Figure 95.1 Diagnostic approach to the asymptomatic patient with thrombocytosis. *CBC,* complete blood cell count; *CRP,* C-reactive protein; *ET,* essential thrombocythemia; *RT,* reactive thrombocytosis.

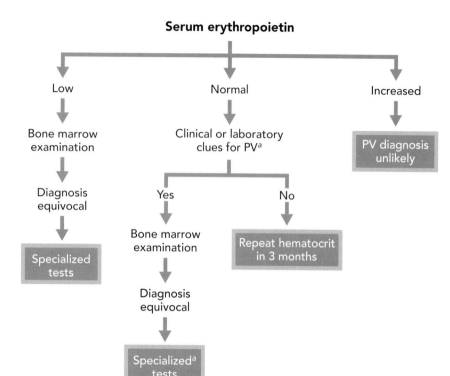

Figure 95.2 A practical algorithm for the diagnosis of polycythemia vera (PV). *aSpecialized testing includes bone marrow immunohistochemistry for the thrombopoietin receptor (c-Mpl), reverse transcriptase-polymerase chain reaction (RT-PCR) for neutrophil expression of polycythenia rubra vera (PRV)-1 gene, and spontaneous erythroid colony assay.

However, a low serum ferritin does not exclude the possibility of ET. Similarly, the demonstration of Howell-Jolly bodies in the peripheral blood smear suggests reactive thrombocytosis associated with functional or surgical hyposplenism. Measurement of the serum C-reactive protein level helps address the possibility of an underlying occult inflammatory or malignant process. C-reactive protein level should be normal in uncomplicated ET and increased in most cases of reactive thrombocytosis. If all of these tests are unrevealing, a bone marrow examination is indicated; the characteristic finding in ET is megakaryocyte clusters.

In regards to PV diagnosis, it is no longer necessary to perform red cell mass and plasma volume measurements in view of the current availability of PV-characteristic biologic tests. Similarly, the Polycythemia Vera Study Group criteria (which utilized measues of red cell mass, leukocyte alkaline phosphatase, and vitamin B_{12} levels) are neither essential nor accurate in the diagnosis of PV. Instead, it is much more practical to follow a diagnostic algorithm that utilizes clinical and bone marrow biopsy information in combination with one or more pertinent special laboratory tests (Figure 95.2).

The first step in the diagnostic evaluation of "polycythemia" is to determine whether or not PV should be suspected. PV should be suspected if the hemoglobin level in a male Caucasian is above 17.5 g/dL (or the corresponding sex- and race-adjusted value for females or African-American males). It should also be suspected if a high-normal hemoglobin is associated with either a PV-characteristic clinical feature or a documented increase from an individual's basline hemoglobin level. Otherwise, a repeat blood count in three months should suffice.

In the presence of one of the above mentioned criteria for suspecting PV, the next step is to measure the serum erythropoietin level. Unlike all other causes of erythrocytosis, the erythroid proliferation in PV is erythropoietin-independent, and therefore it down-regulates erythropoietin production. As a result, serum erythropoietin levels are usually low, occasionally normal, but *never increased* in PV (Figure 95.2). Accordingly, PV should remain in the differential diagnosis in the presence of either low or normal EPO level. The next step is bone marrow examination with cytogenetic studies. An experienced hematopathologist is able to identify the histologic features of CMPD in general and PV in particular in the majority of cases. Occassionally, the diagnosis remains uncertain despite the information from bone marrow biopsy. In such instances, depending on availability, specialized tests may be utilized for further clarification.

The presence of substantial bone marrow fibrosis requires that other causes of fibrosis be excluded before AMM is diagnosed (Table 95.3). In this regard, particular attention should be paid to the possibility of either CML or MDS, since their prognosis and treatment are substantially different. The rates of cytogenetic abnormalities are 12% in untreated PV, 6% in ET, and 30% in AMM.

TABLE 95.3
CAUSES OF BONE MARROW FIBROSIS

Myeloid disorders

Chronic myeloproliferative diseases
Myelodysplastic syndrome
Acute myelofibrosis
Acute myeloid leukemia
Mast cell disease
Malignant histiocytosis

Lymphoid disorders

Lymphomas
Hairy cell leukemia
Multiple myeloma

Non-hematologic disorders

Metastatic cancer
Connective tissue disease
Infections
Vitamin D-deficiency rickets
Renal osteodystrophy
Gray-platelet syndrome

LONG-TERM MANAGEMENT

Essential Thrombocythemia

The use of acetylsalicylic acid (aspirin) in low doses (81 mg/d) is effective in controlling vasomotor symptoms. The use of platelet-lowering (cytoreductive) agents is primarily for prevention of thrombosis. The risk for thrombosis is very low in patients less than 60 years of age who do not have a history of thrombosis. Therefore, these patients may not require cytoreductive therapy. The use of these drugs in low-risk women of childbearing age is particularly discouraged.

In high-risk patients (prior history of thrombosis or age >60 years), hydroxyurea has been shown to reduce thrombotic events significantly, when compared with no treatment (8), and therefore its use is reasonable in this population. There is no hard evidence that hydroxyurea is leukemogenic when used in ET. Two other drugs, oral anagrelide and subcutaneous interferon-α, might also be used to lower platelet counts in patients with ET. With anagrelide therapy, side effects occur in one-third of patients and include headache, fluid retention, dizziness, palpitations, tachycardia, diarrhea, and rarely congestive heart failure. The response rate is more than 90%, and response occurs at a median time of 3 weeks. Anagrelide does not significantly affect the leukocyte count, but may cause severe anemia in approximately 25% of treated patients (9).

Interferon-α controls thrombocytosis, splenomegaly, and disease-associated symptoms in approximately 80% of patients with ET. The average response time is 12 weeks. Side effects include a transient influenza-like syndrome associated with fever and chills, myalgias, headache, and arthralgias. Chronic side effects include fatigue, nausea, anorexia, weight loss, diarrhea, increase in liver transaminases, altered mental status, and depression. Currently, hydroxyurea is the first line choice of drug therapy in ET regardless of age unless in women of childbearing age. In this regard, a recent randomized study demonstrated a significantly better anti-thrombotic as well as anti-hemorrhagic effect with hydroxyurea than with anagrelide. Furthermore, patients treated with anagrelide had a higher risk of transformation into myelofibrosis (10). Regardless of the particular platelet-lowering agent used, it is recommended that the platelet count be kept below 400,000/μL (9).

Polycythemia Vera

Based on currently available information, recommendations for the management of patients with PV are as follows: all patients should undergo phlebotomy to keep the hematocrit below 45% in men and 42% in women. Approximately 500 mL of blood may be removed daily (in symptomatic patients) or weekly (in asymptomatic patients) until the target hematocrit level is reached. Thereafter, the frequency of phlebotomy is adjusted to maintain the required hematocrit level at all times. In addition, a recent randomized study has demonstrated the anti-thrombotic value of low-dose aspirin in all risk categories of PV (11). In patients at high risk, hydroxyurea can be used to supplement phlebotomy (2).

For patients who do not tolerate hydroxyurea because of either side effects or neutropenia, interferon-α is a reasonable alternative. Interferon-α may also be considered as an alternative to hydroxyurea in women of childbearing age. A recent study involving over 1,600 patients with PV did not show increased leukemogenicity associated with single agent use of hydroxyurea (12). Phosphorus-32 may be considered if a patient's life expectancy is less than 10 years and when compliance with medication is an issue. Low-dose acetylsalicylic acid (81 mg/d) is effective for alleviating vasomotor symptoms and can be used if other treatment indications are present.

Agnogenic Myeloid Metaplasia

In young patients with AMM, allogeneic bone marrow transplantation sometimes leads to durable remissions (Chapter 96). Otherwise, most patients are treated palliatively. The combination of an androgen preparation (fluoxymesterone, 20 mg/d) and a corticosteroid improves anemia in one-third of patients (7). After one month of therapy, fluoxymesterone is continued in responding patients and the corticosteroid is tapered. All patients treated with androgens should undergo periodic monitoring of serum liver chemistries, and male patients should be screened for prostate cancer before therapy is initiated. In addition, the virilizing side effects should be emphasized to female patients. Periodic red cell transfusion remains the major supportive therapy in AMM. Recent studies suggest that anemia in AMM may sometimes respond to either erythropoietin (13) or a combination of low-dose thalidomide and prednisone (14).

Splenectomy is considered for patients who have symptomatic splenomegaly (mechanical discomfort, refractory thrombocytopenia, hypercatabolic symptoms, or portal hypertension) (15). If laboratory evidence of disseminated intravascular coagulation is noted before splenectomy, the risk for perioperative bleeding may be increased, and it is recommended that the operation be postponed until the abnormalities are corrected. At experienced centers, the mortality rate for splenectomy should be less than 10%. Postsurgical complications include intraabdominal bleeding, subphrenic abscess, sepsis, thrombosis of large vessels, extreme thrombocytosis, and accelerated hepatomegaly. Thrombocytosis and hepatomegaly may be transiently controlled with hydroxyurea.

After splenectomy, almost all patients experience relief of hypercatabolic symptoms and portal hypertension. In addition, approximately one-third of the patients with refractory anemia benefit from splenectomy. In poor surgical candidates, the alternative to splenectomy is splenic irradiation, which usually provides a transient (3–6 months) benefit. Radiation therapy is most useful in the management of extramedullary hematopoiesis (16).

ISSUES DURING HOSPITALIZATION

The major indications for hospitalization of patients with PV and ET are thrombosis and bleeding. In AMM, indications for hospitalization include severe cachexia, extramedullary hematopoiesis involving the central nervous system, and scheduled splenectomy. Infrequent indications for hospitalization include acute leukemic transformation and life-threatening infections. Clinical situations that do not require hospitalization include asymptomatic thrombocytosis, erythrocytosis, leukocytosis, or marked hepatosplenomegaly. However, if these conditions are associated with bleeding, thrombosis, or severe pain (the latter may accompany splenic infarction), then hospitalization may facilitate prompt cytapheresis and pain control.

In the patient with thrombosis or bleeding, initial evaluation should include a complete blood cell count and determination of the prothrombin and activated partial thromboplastin times and bleeding time. (See Chapter 98 for a discussion of the more detailed evaluation of patients

with abnormal thrombosis or bleeding.) When a patient with myeloproliferative disease is bleeding or has prolonged prothrombin or partial thromboplastin times, measurement of coagulation factors may reveal an acquired factor V deficiency. In the patient being prepared for splenectomy, tests for disseminated intravascular coagulation are recommended because an elevated D-dimer level may be associated with increased perioperative bleeding. The imaging tests of choice are ultrasonography for suspected thrombosis of abdominal large vessels (portal and hepatic vein thrombosis), computed tomography for suspected central nervous system thrombosis or bleeding and for splenic infarcts, and magnetic resonance imaging for suspected extramedullary hematopoiesis involving the central nervous system.

Thrombosis

Patients with thrombosis should be anticoagulated unless there are contraindications (see Chapters 52 and 53 for general discussions regarding the initiation of heparin and warfarin therapy). Oral hydroxyurea should be started at the following dosages: 1 g four times a day for three days if the platelet count is more than 1 million/μL; 1 g two times a day if the count is 600,000/μL–1 million/μL; and 500 mg two times a day if the count is 400,000/μL–600,000/μL. In addition, the blood bank should be contacted for immediate platelet apheresis if the platelet count is more than 800,000/μL. In patients with PV, phlebotomy should be performed daily until the hematocrit is less than 45% in men and 42% in women. Oral allopurinol should be started at a dose of 300 mg/d (100 mg/d if the creatinine value is >2 mg/dL) if the leukocyte count is more than 30,000/μL.

Heparin therapy is discontinued after a 5 day overlap with warfarin. In general, thrombocytosis and erythrocytosis are considered reversible risk factors for thrombosis, and warfarin therapy is continued for three months (target international normalized ratio of between 2.0 and 3.0) after the thrombotic event. In the presence of additional prothrombotic traits, more prolonged warfarin therapy may be required. After the first three days, the dose of hydroxyurea is adjusted to keep the platelet count below 400,000/μL without reducing the leukocyte count to below 2,000/μL. If a low leukocyte count does not allow the use of hydroxyurea, oral anagrelide at a dosage of 0.5 mg four times a day may be used instead. A high leukocyte count not associated with a high blast percentage does not require cytapheresis.

Bleeding

The first step in the management of bleeding complications is to discontinue the use of any antiplatelet agent. If the platelet count is less than 10,000/μL, platelet transfusion is recommended. Initial laboratory evaluation should include an evaluation for disseminated intravascular coagulation and coagulation factor deficiency. Acquired factor V deficiency is treated with fresh frozen plasma infusion or platelet concentrates. Occasionally, extreme thrombocytosis is associated with acquired type II von Willebrand's disease because of abnormal platelet adsorption of circulating von Willebrand's factor multimers. As such, platelet apheresis is recommended for bleeding associated with thrombocytosis. Concomitantly, therapy with a platelet-lowering agent should be started. See Chapter 98 for a fuller discussion of the management of abnormal bleeding.

Extramedullary Hematopoiesis

Extramedullary hematopoiesis can occur at several locations, including the spleen, liver, lymph nodes, peritoneum (causing ascites), pleura (causing pleural effusions), lung, bladder, and paraspinal and epidural spaces (causing spinal cord and nerve root compression). A patient with new-onset back pain should be evaluated for possible spinal cord compression. Neurologic symptoms and signs of spinal cord compression include paresthesia, motor weakness, hyperreflexia, and bladder or bowel incontinence. Magnetic resonance imaging with gadolinium is the preferred initial diagnostic test. If the clinical data are highly suggestive of cord compression, the patient should receive 10 mg of oral dexamethasone even before imaging is performed. If the test supports the diagnosis, dexamethasone should be continued at 4 mg orally four times a day until definitive treatment with irradiation is started. The steroid dose should be tapered during the course of radiation therapy. Extramedullary hematopoiesis is best treated with low-dose irradiation (1,000 cGy) in 5 to 10 fractions. Occasionally, a laminectomy may be required.

COST CONSIDERATIONS

Patients with chronic myeloproliferative diseases are usually managed in the outpatient setting. Attention to laboratory details prevents inadequate disease control and reduces the incidence of complications requiring hospitalization and other costly measures such as emergency cytapheresis. In addition, anticoagulant therapy for thrombosis with subcutaneous low-molecular-weight heparin may be administered on an outpatient basis.

There are substantial cost differences among the currently available platelet-lowering agents. The three most frequently used agents (hydroxyurea, anagrelide, and interferon-α) are similar in their ability to lower platelet counts but differ significantly in their side effect profile and cost. At the time of this writing, the annual drug costs for the

usual doses of these agents are $1,700 for hydroxyurea, $6,300 for anagrelide, and $8,600 for interferon-α.

KEY POINTS

- The chronic myeloproliferative disorders represent relatively mature proliferative disorders. They include chronic myelogenous leukemia, essential thrombocythemia, polycythemia vera, and agnogenic myeloid metaplasia.
- Patients with essential thrombocythemia are usually asymptomatic but may have vasomotor symptoms, bleeding, or thrombosis. Patients with polycythemia vera are more commonly symptomatic and more often suffer thrombotic events. Patients with agnogenic myeloid metaplasia are often symptomatic; they usually have progressive, transfusion-dependent anemia.
- In general, chronic myeloproliferative disorders are diagnosed by bone marrow examination, performed after reactive disorders have been excluded.
- The following are key principles in the management of patients with essential thrombocythemia and polycythemia vera:
  —The patient should avoid smoking and using high doses of aspirin or nonsteroidal agents.
  —Aspirin (81 mg/d) is safe and effective for treating vasomotor symptoms.
  —Asymptomatic young women may not require platelet-lowering agents.
  —In patients older than 60 years and in those with a history of thrombosis, the platelet count should be kept below 400,000/μL in both essential thrombocythemia and polycythemia vera.
  —In patients with polycythemia vera, the hematocrit should be kept below 45% in men and 42% in women. This is accomplished by phlebotomy, supplemented by hydroxyurea in patients at high risk for thrombosis.

REFERENCES

1. Tefferi A, Murphy S. Current opinion in essential thrombocythemia: pathogenesis, diagnosis, and management. *Blood Rev* 2001;15:121–131.
2. Tefferi A. Polycythemia vera: a comprehensive review and clinical recommendations. *Mayo Clin Proc* 2003;78:174–194.
3. Tefferi A. Treatment approaches in myelofibrosis with myeloid metaplasia: the old and the new. *Semin Hematol* 2003;40:18–21.
4. Reeder TL, Bailey RJ, Dewald GW, Tefferi A. Both B and T lymphocytes may be clonally involved in myelofibrosis with myeloid metaplasia. *Blood* 2003;101:1981–1983.
5. Chagraoui H, Komura E, Tulliez M, et al. Prominent role of TGF-beta 1 in thrombopoietin-induced myelofibrosis in mice. *Blood* 2002;100:3495–3503.
6. Diehn F, Tefferi A. Pruritus in polycythaemia vera: prevalence, laboratory correlates, and management. *Br J Haematol* 2001;115:619–621.
7. Tefferi A. Myelofibrosis with Myeloid Metaplasia. *N Engl J Med* 2000;342:1255–1265.
8. Finazzi G, Ruggeri M, Rodeghiero F, Barbui T. Second malignancies in patients with essential thrombocythaemia treated with

busulphan and hydroxyurea: long-term follow-up of a randomized clinical trial. *Br J Haematol* 2000;110:577–583.

9. Storen EC, Tefferi A. Long-term use of anagrelide in young patients with essential thrombocythemia. *Blood* 2001;97:863–866.

10. Green AR, Campbell P, Buck G, et al. The medical research council PT1 trial in essential thrombocythemia. *Blood* 2004;104:Abstract #6.

11. Landolfi R, Marchioli R, Kutti J, et al. Efficacy and safety of low-dose aspirin in polycythemia vera. *N Engl J Med* 2004;350:114–124.

12. Finazzi G, Caruso V, Marchioli R, et al. Acute leukemia in polycythemia vera. An analysis of 1,638 patients enrolled in a prospective observational study. *Blood* 2005; in press.

13. Hasselbalch HC, Clausen NT, Jensen BA. Successful treatment of anemia in idiopathic myelofibrosis with recombinant human erythropoietin *Am J Hematol.* 2002;70:92–99.

14. Mesa RA, Steensma DP, Pardanani A, et al. A phase 2 trial of combination low-dose thalidomide and prednisone for the treatment of myelofibrosis with myeloid metaplasia. *Blood* 2003;101:2534–2541.

15. Tefferi A, Mesa RA, Nagorney DM, et al. Splenectomy in myelofibrosis with myeloid metaplasia: a single-institution experience with 223 patients. *Blood* 2000;95:2226–2233.

16. Steensma DP, Hook CC, Stafford SL, Tefferi A. Low-dose, single-fraction, whole-lung radiotherapy for pulmonary hypertension associated with myelofibrosis with myeloid metaplasia. *Br J Haematol* 2002;118:813–816.

ADDITIONAL READING

Barbui T, Barosi G, Grossi A, et al. Practice guidelines for the therapy of essential thrombocythemia. A statement from the Italian Society of Hematology, the Italian Society of Experimental Hematology, and the Italian Group for Bone Marrow Transplantation. *Haematologica* 2004;89:215–232.

Deeg HJ, Gooley TA, Flowers ME, et al. Allogeneic hematopoietic stem cell transplantation for myelofibrosis. *Blood* 2003;102:3912–3918.

Landolfi R, Marchioli R, Kutti J, et al. Efficacy and safety of low-dose aspirin in polycythemia vera. *N Engl J Med* 2004;350:114–124.

Tefferi A, Lasho TL, Wolanskyj AP, Mesa RA. Neutrophil PRV-1 expression across the chronic myeloproliferative disorders and in secondary or spurious polycythemia. *Blood* 2004;103:3547–3548.

Hematopoietic Cell Transplantation

96

Frederick R. Appelbaum

INTRODUCTION

Biology of Hematopoietic Cell Transplantation

Bone marrow transplantation was the generic term used to describe the collection and transplantation of hematopoietic stem cells for therapeutic purposes. With the increasing use of peripheral blood and umbilical cord blood as sources of stem cells, *hematopoietic cell transplantation* has now become the preferred generic term for this procedure. The basic technique of hematopoietic cell transplantation is relatively straightforward. Following an appropriate pretreatment evaluation and identification of a source of stem cells, patients are first treated with a high-dose "preparative" regimen. This serves to eradicate the disease being treated and induce a sufficient degree of immunosuppression for the patient to be able to adequately accept the marrow graft. Following the preparative regimen, hematopoietic stem cells from an appropriate donor or previously harvested from the patient, are administered intravenously. After transplantation, patients require intensive supportive care until marrow function has been restored. Although simple in concept, transplantation is a complex procedure and is best carried out at centers specializing in the approach.

Several characteristics of the hematopoietic stem cell make transplantation possible and broadly applicable. First, it is amenable to cryopreservation, a relatively straightforward freezing and rethawing process. Second, the hematopoietic stem cell has enormous regenerative capacity and gives rise to a wide variety of mature progeny. In humans, transplanting as little as a few million highly purified stem cells can result in complete and sustained engraftment.

This occurs with subsequent production of all of a patient's red cells, granulocytes, and T- and B-cells, in addition to pulmonary alveolar macrophages, Kupffer cells of the liver, osteoclasts, Langerhans cells of the skin, and microglial cells of the brain. Finally, the remarkable homing capacity of the hematopoietic stem cell greatly simplifies the process of transplantation. Following intravenous infusion, a substantial proportion of hematopoietic stem cells collect in the bone marrow.

The source of hematopoietic stem cells used for transplantation can be defined by the relationship between the donor and the recipient, and also according to their anatomic source.

Donor–Recipient Relationship

The three broad categories defined by the relationship between donor and recipient are *syngeneic* (identical twins), *autologous* (self-harvest), and *allogeneic* (genetically dissimilar individuals). The source of first choice is an identical twin (syngeneic transplant). In syngeneic transplantation, there is no risk that stem cells will be contaminated with tumor, as can happen in autologous transplantation, and there is no risk for the development of *graft-versus-host disease* (GVHD), as there is in allogeneic transplantation. Autologous transplantation may be appropriate if the primary purpose of the transplant is to administer higher doses of chemotherapy or systemic radiotherapy than would be possible without transplantation. Autologous transplantation also has the advantage of avoiding GVHD. Nonetheless, an autologous transplant carries the dual disadvantages of lacking a *graft-versus-tumor effect* and of possibly being contaminated with the patient's tumor. Allogeneic transplantation is considerably more complicated than syngeneic or autologous transplantation. It carries the related risks of graft rejection and GVHD. Because the donor and the recipient are genetically different, the immune system of the patient can reject the transplanted marrow. At the same time, the immune-competent cells developing from, or transplanted with, the stem cell inoculum can react against the new host, causing GVHD.

Matching

For an allogeneic transplant to be successful, a close, if not identical, match of HLAs (human leukocyte antigens) is necessary. With greater HLA disparity between donor and host, there is greater immunologic reactivity between the two. This immunologic reactivity is, for the most part, mediated by T-cells reacting with histocompatibility antigens encoded by genes of the major histocompatibility complex (MHC). The HLAs produced by the genes of the MHC are a group of molecules that bind endogenous or exogenous antigenic peptides and present them on the cell surface, an important step in mediating an immune response. The HLA molecules themselves are termed *major determinants*. If T-cells are exposed to cells of a different HLA type, they will react vigorously to the mismatched HLA antigens on the cell surface. T-cells exposed to cells from HLA-matched but nonsyngeneic individuals may also react, although less vigorously, because endogenous proteins presented by the HLA molecules differ. Such differences are termed *minor determinants*.

The probability of success in allogeneic transplants is greatest when siblings are HLA-identical. For any given patient, the likelihood that a specific sibling will be HLA-identical is one in four. Given the average size of American families, *approximately 35% of patients have an HLA-identical sibling*. The results when a transplant from a family member donor mismatched for a single antigen is used are nearly equivalent in terms of survival, although there is a higher incidence of GVHD. Results using matched unrelated donors are approaching those seen using matched or single antigen-mismatched family member donors, although the incidence of GVHD and graft rejection may be somewhat higher using unrelated donors (1). In most studies, the use of transplants from donors mismatched for two or more antigens has resulted in a substantially higher incidence of fatal GVHD or graft rejection and lower posttransplant survival. The HLA antigens are extremely polymorphic; therefore, the likelihood that any two unrelated persons would match is extremely low—less than 1 in 10,000. Finding an HLA-matched *unrelated* donor is possible because of the formation of various donor registries, through which more than 7 million normal persons have volunteered to provide stem cells for an unrelated patient. Currently, the odds of finding an HLA-matched unrelated donor are approximately 60%. On average, it requires three months from the time a search is initiated to identify a donor and schedule the transplant.

Location of Harvested Stem Cells

The source of stem cells can also be categorized according to their anatomic location. Traditionally, the source of stem cells has been the bone marrow. Marrow is usually obtained by multiple aspirations from the anterior and posterior iliac crests. Hematopoietic stem cells also circulate in the peripheral blood, although at very low numbers. The concentration of stem cells in peripheral blood increases dramatically during recovery from cytotoxic therapy or following administration of a hematopoietic growth factor, such as granulocyte colony-stimulating factor (G-CSF) or granulocyte-macrophage colony-stimulating factor (GM-CSF). With such pretreatment, sufficient stem cells for autologous or allogeneic engraftment can be obtained by leukapheresis. Use of *peripheral blood stem cells* is generally associated with a more rapid engraftment than is seen with the use of bone marrow. Umbilical cord blood contains a high concentration of hematopoietic stem cells, and cord blood can be used as a source of stem cells for transplantation (2). Cord blood is relatively devoid of mature T cells. As a consequence, the risk for GVHD is less with cord blood, but the risks of graft rejection tend to be higher. Because of the limited numbers of stem cells within cord blood, engraftment tends to be slower than when peripheral blood stem cells or marrow are used.

INDICATIONS FOR HEMATOPOIETIC CELL TRANSPLANTATION

As outlined in Table 96.1, hematopoietic cell transplantation can be used successfully in children with congenital immunodeficiency states. The technique is also widely used to provide a normal lymphohematopoietic system to patients with severe but nonmalignant disorders of hematopoiesis. *Aplastic anemia* is readily curable with marrow transplantation. With use of the optimal preparative regimen, cure rates of 90% have been reported following HLA-matched sibling transplantation. Hematopoietic cell transplantation is also used in the treatment of patients with *hemoglobinopathies*. Cure rates of 70%–90% have been reported in the treatment of thalassemia major, with the best results seen in patients undergoing transplantation before the development of hepatomegaly or portal fibrosis. Similar results have been reported in the treatment of *sickle cell anemia*, although fewer patients have been studied (3).

Hematopoietic cell transplantation plays a major role in treating a variety of malignant diseases by allowing for the administration of far higher doses of chemotherapy and systemic radiotherapy than would be possible without marrow support. In addition, in the allogeneic setting, cells derived from the transplant provide an immunologic graft-versus-tumor effect. Although the antitumor effects of the dose escalation and graft-versus-tumor reaction provided by the transplant are considerable, they are not sufficient to

TABLE 96.1

DISEASE-FREE SURVIVAL AFTER BONE MARROW TRANSPLANTATION

Disease	5-year disease-free survival (%)
Severe combined immunodeficiency disease	90
Aplastic anemia	90
Thalassemia major	70–90
Sickle cell disease	70–90
Fanconi's anemia	50–70
Acute myeloid leukemia	
First remission	40–70
Second remission	30
Acute lymphocytic leukemia	
First remission	40–70
Second remission	30–50
Chronic myeloid leukemia	
Chronic phase	60–70
Accelerated phase	30–40
Blast crisis	15–20
Myelodysplastic syndrome	45
Non-Hodgkin's lymphoma, first relapse	40–50
Hodgkin's disease, first relapse	40–60
Multiple myeloma	35
Breast cancer	
High-risk stage II	70
Chemotherapy-responsive stage IV	10–30

allow for meaningful responses in tumors that are completely refractory to standard-dose treatment. Thus, the major utility of transplantation has been in the treatment of hematologic malignancies and other chemotherapy-responsive tumors.

Hematopoietic cell transplantation is the only curative therapy for patients with *acute myeloid leukemia* who have failed initial induction chemotherapy, and it is generally considered to be the treatment of choice for patients who relapse after an initial complete response (Chapter 93). Whether patients should undergo transplantation while in first remission is a topic of considerable study. The bulk of recent evidence from randomized controlled trials favors allogeneic transplantation, especially for patients with high-risk AML as determined by cytogenetic risk factors. The evidence for autologous transplantation for AML in first remission is more equivocal (4). The indications for transplantation for adult acute lymphoblastic leukemia are similar to those noted above for AML, except that there is less evidence addressing the role of transplantation for adult patients with acute lymphoblastic leukemia in first remission (5).

Allogeneic and syngeneic transplantation are the only therapies capable of curing patients with *chronic myelogenous leukemia* (CML). Five-year disease-free survival rates of 60%–70% for patients who undergo transplantation during chronic phase, 30%–40% for transplantation during

accelerated phase, and 15%–20% for transplantation during blast crisis can be expected. The best results with transplantation have been obtained when the procedure is carried out within the two years of diagnosis. However, recommendations for early transplantation are complicated by the development of imatinib mesylate, a very effective, relatively nontoxic oral agent. Because imatinib does not generally result in complete molecular remissions in CML, allogeneic transplantation remains an important option for younger patients with matched donors. Older patients and those without matched donors should generally be treated initially with imatinib. Results of transplantation for the treatment of *myelodysplastic syndrome* in many ways mirror those seen in chronic myelogenous leukemia. Although transplantation is the only curative therapy for myelodysplastic syndrome, patients with refractory anemia can live with their disease for a long period, which makes recommendations about early versus delayed transplantation complex.

Patients with disseminated intermediate- or high-grade *non-Hodgkin's lymphoma* who fail to achieve an initial complete remission or who relapse after first remission should be considered for transplantation (Chapter 94). In one study, the 5-year disease-free survival of patients who underwent autologous transplantation for recurrent non-Hodgkin's lymphoma was 46%, compared with 12% for patients undergoing chemotherapy (6). The role of transplantation for patients with high-risk non-Hodgkin's lymphoma in first remission is unsettled. In general, the results with *Hodgkin's disease* mirror those seen in non-Hodgkin's lymphoma, but large randomized trials comparing results of transplantation with those seen with chemotherapy have not been reported.

Allogeneic transplantation results in approximately 35% survival for patients with *multiple myeloma* who have failed first-line therapy. Because of substantial morbidity and mortality associated with the procedure, most experts do not currently recommend allogeneic transplantation during first remission. Autologous transplantation provides less potential for cure but is considerably safer. In one large trial, autologous transplantation during first remission substantially improved disease-free and overall survival (7). A novel approach of autologous transplantation followed by nonmyeloablative allogeneic transplantation shows great promise in the treatment of myeloma.

The role of high-dose chemotherapy followed by autologous transplantation in the treatment of breast cancer is controversial. Although promising phase II results were reported both in patients with stage IV disease and in patients with high-risk stage II disease, the early results of randomized trials have been more equivocal. High-dose chemotherapy followed by autologous transplantation has also been studied in a variety of other chemotherapy-sensitive solid tumors, including neuroblastoma, testicular cancer, ovarian cancer, and pediatric sarcomas, but randomized trials have not yet been reported.

HOSPITAL CARE OF THE HEMATOPOIETIC CELL TRANSPLANT PATIENT

Preparative Phase and Early Posttransplant Issues

Chemotherapy, radiation therapy, or both are administered during the preparative phase of the pretransplant period. To optimize the safety and effectiveness of the preparative regimen, the physician must be aware of the unique features of each of the drugs used in the preparative regimen. Specific chemotherapy toxicities are discussed in Chapter 90. General guidelines relating to the care of patients in the preparative phase are presented in the following sections.

General Supportive Care

Nausea and vomiting are frequent immediate side effects of the chemotherapy and radiation used in most preparative regimens. Prevention of nausea and vomiting is far preferable to reacting to symptoms once they develop. High-dose cyclophosphamide and cisplatin are highly emetogenic, whereas melphalan, thiotepa, busulfan, paclitaxel (Taxol), etoposide, and total body irradiation (TBI) are moderately so. The use of intravenous antiemetics before and during the administration of highly emetogenic agents can control nausea and vomiting in 70%–90% of cases. Oral antiemetics are often sufficient if the agents used in the preparative regimen are of low-or-moderate emetogenic potential. See Chapter 90 for a discussion of therapeutic options.

Patients who began the transplant preparative regimen with hematologic malignancies in relapse are at risk for the development of the acute tumor lysis syndrome. See Chapter 94 for a complete discussion of the prevention and treatment of this entity.

Total Body Irradiation

Total body irradiation can be administered as a single dose, fractionated over several days with single fractions given daily, or hyperfractionated with multiple doses given two or more times a day for several days. TBI is generally administered at a slow rate (7–15 cGy/min), so that single-dose TBI may require 2–3 hours, whereas individual fractions may take 15–30 minutes. Single-dose TBI is more toxic and no more effective than fractionated TBI. Patients receiving fractionated TBI become nauseated later in the day if not given antiemetics. Parotitis and pancreatitis are rare early complications of TBI. Mucositis, diarrhea, alopecia, and severe pancytopenia are expected complications that develop during 1–2 weeks following TBI.

Stem Cell Collection and Infusion

Marrow is usually obtained by multiple aspirations from the donor's (or in the autologous setting, the patient's) anterior and posterior iliac crests. A total marrow volume of 10–15 mL/kg of donor weight is usually obtained. The number of marrow cells infused correlates with survival following allogeneic marrow transplantation, with a higher number of cells being associated with a more favorable outcome. Following donation, pain at the site of aspiration invariably occurs but is usually manageable with oral analgesics. Serious complications are uncommon and usually limited to local hematomas or infection. If peripheral blood stem cells are to be used, the donor is generally treated with a hematopoietic growth factor for 4–5 days. Following this, leukapheresis is performed over 1–3 days depending on the collection yield. The bone pain sometimes caused by the high doses of myeloid growth factors used for mobilization usually responds well to hydrocodone or similar oral analgesics (Chapter 18).

Stem cells are generally infused shortly after the preparative regimen has been completed, usually within 24–48 hours, depending on the amount of time needed to clear the last chemotherapeutic agent. In cases of ABO incompatibility, the red cells or plasma from the marrow may need to be removed before transplant to prevent transfusion reactions. Possible complications of fresh stem cell infusions include volume overload, mild transfusion reactions, and occasional allergic reactions to plasma proteins or other marrow components. Occasionally, a patient may complain of dyspnea, chest pain, and cough during marrow infusion. Slowing of the infusion and administration of oxygen usually relieve these symptoms. For autologous transplantation, the marrow or peripheral blood has been cryopreserved, usually with dimethylsulfoxide. Reactions are common following infusion of previously cryopreserved stem cells, both because many cells lyse during thawing and because some patients are sensitive to dimethylsulfoxide. Nausea, vomiting, and hypotension are the most frequently seen complications. To lessen these symptoms, premedication with diphenhydramine and dexamethasone is often given.

Prophylaxis for Graft-versus-Host Disease

Patients undergoing allogeneic transplantation generally require some form of GVHD prophylaxis. The most commonly used regimens have included a combination of methotrexate administered on post-transplant days 1, 3, 6, and 11, together with cyclosporine given daily from the time of transplant until day 50 and then tapered. Although it is sometimes difficult to administer methotrexate soon after transplant to patients with severe mucositis, studies have demonstrated that omission of methotrexate doses results in an increased incidence of GVHD. Cyclosporine is usually administered intravenously at a dose of 1.5 mg/kg every 12 hours, or orally at a dose of 6 mg/kg every

12 hours. Cyclosporine is a potent immunosuppressant and has a number of significant side effects (Chapter 102). If GVHD develops and a patient's blood levels of cyclosporine are low, increasing the cyclosporine dose is appropriate. Other agents sometimes used as GVHD prophylaxis include prednisone, tacrolimus and monoclonal antibodies directed at T-cells or T-cell subsets.

EARLY COMPLICATIONS (DAYS 1 TO 21 AFTER TRANSPLANT)

Figure 96.1 summarizes posttransplant complications in terms of time of onset.

Neutropenia

Virtually all patients become severely neutropenic following transplant. The duration of neutropenia is generally from 7–21 days, depending on the source of stem cells, whether methotrexate is used to prevent GVHD, and whether hematopoietic growth factors are used. Peripheral blood stem cells generally engraft most quickly, often by posttransplant day 10, whereas cells from cord blood take the longest, on average 25 days or more. Methotrexate delays engraftment by 3–5 days, and the use of hematopoietic growth factors accelerates engraftment by 4–6 days.

To reduce the risk for infection during the neutropenic period, patients are usually treated in some sort of protected environment, with either laminar air flow isolation or HEPA (high-efficiency particulate air) filtering. Careful hand washing and avoidance of contact with anyone having a communicable disease are absolutely necessary. Because the risk for bacterial infection is so great, most centers initiate antibiotic therapy once the granulocyte count falls below 500/μL. Fluconazole prophylaxis at a dose of 200–400 mg/d reduces the risk for candidal infections. In patients who are seropositive for *Herpes simplex* virus, severe local or disseminated disease can develop early after transplant, but this can be prevented in most patients by the use of acyclovir prophylaxis (either 250 mg/m^2 intravenously every 12 hours or 500 mg/m^2 orally twice daily). Despite the use of protected environments and various prophylactic regimens, most patients become febrile while neutropenic. See Chapter 63 for a complete discussion of the approach to this problem.

Thrombocytopenia

Platelet transfusions are routinely used to prevent bleeding in severely thrombocytopenic patients. In general, platelets

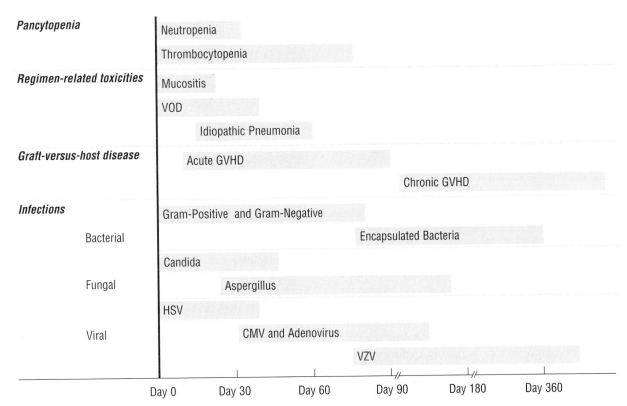

Figure 96.1 Major syndromes complicating marrow transplantation. An approximate time frame for some of the major complications occurring during the first year after transplant. *CMV*, cytomegalovirus; *GVHD*, graft-versus-host disease; *HSV*, *Herpes simplex* virus; *VOD*, veno-occlusive disease of the liver; *VZV*, varicella-zoster virus.

are transfused once the platelet count drops below 20,000/μL, but a lower threshold of 10,000/μL can be used for clinically stable afebrile patients without evidence of hemorrhage (Chapters 93 and 98). Attention must be paid to the cytomegalovirus (CMV) serologic status of the patient (see the "Infection" section later in this chapter). Platelets should be irradiated with 2,500 cGy before infusion to prevent accidental engraftment and the development of transfusion-induced GVHD.

Mucositis

Oropharyngeal mucositis is an almost invariable result of most preparative regimens and may range from mild to severe. The first signs of mucositis appear within the first week after completion of the preparative regimen and usually peak at about 2 weeks. Intensive management of mucositis can significantly lessen symptoms. Oral rinsing with 0.9% saline solution every hour while the patient is awake helps keep tissue clean and debrided. If mucous membranes are intact, topical analgesics like viscous lidocaine or a mixture of dicyclomine HCl and diphenhydramine may relieve local symptoms. Systemic analgesics, including opioids, are frequently needed to control the pain associated with mucositis.

Veno-Occlusive Disease of the Liver

The intensive cytoreductive chemotherapy and radiotherapy comprising the transplant preparative regimen can occasionally result in a syndrome of liver toxicity termed *veno-occlusive disease* (VOD), also sometimes called sinusoidal obstruction syndrome (SOS). VOD is characterized by tender hepatomegaly, weight gain, and jaundice. The first signs of VOD usually appear during the first 21 days after transplant. The overall incidence of VOD ranges from 10%–25% and is influenced by a number of factors. VOD is more commonly seen in patients with preexisting liver disease, those with fever and infection at the time they receive the preparative regimen, and in patients who are treated with more intensive preparative regimens. Although development of tender hepatomegaly with weight gain and jaundice during the first 3 weeks after transplant is usually secondary to VOD, occasionally hepatic infiltration by fungus or tumor, congestion resulting from right ventricular failure, or cholestatic jaundice secondary to cyclosporine toxicity or GVHD can contribute to the picture. The only way to differentiate these entities with certainty is by liver biopsy. Because of the risk for bleeding during the early posttransplant period, biopsy is usually performed via a transvenous approach. VOD is more likely to be severe if the onset is early (before posttransplant day five) and accompanied by a rapid rise in bilirubin levels and rapid weight gain.

The management of VOD requires careful attention to supportive care in addition to consideration of specific therapies. The primary objective of supportive care is to minimize fluid retention while maintaining renal perfusion. Careful monitoring of fluid and electrolyte balance is critical. If volume overload develops, the daily intake of sodium and fluids should be restricted, and attempts to increase sodium excretion by the use of diuretics should be carefully initiated. However, diuretics can deplete intravascular volume and reduce renal blood flow, which should be avoided. If diuresis is unsuccessful and the patient shows signs of severe volume excess (e.g., tense ascites, pleural effusions, hypoxemia), paracentesis of ascitic fluid, hemodialysis, or hemofiltration should be considered. Patients with severe VOD have increased platelet sequestration and are at an increased risk for bleeding complications. Efforts should be made to maintain platelet counts at higher levels, although this can be difficult.

No specific therapies have been unambiguously demonstrated to ameliorate the course of VOD, but several therapies have shown promise in preliminary studies. A combination of tissue plasminogen activator and heparin has been used, because microthrombi can be found in the walls of the central veins of the liver in VOD. Approximately 30% of patients with mild-to-moderate VOD appear to respond to tissue plasminogen activator and heparin, but this therapy increases the risk for severe bleeding. The dose of tissue plasminogen activator is 20 mg infused over 4 hours on each of 4 consecutive days. The activated partial thromboplastin time is generally kept at or just above the upper limit of normal by adjusting the heparin dose. Defibrotide is an experimental drug that, in an uncontrolled study, was associated with responses in 30%–40% of patients with moderate-to-severe VOD (8). Nephrotoxic and hepatotoxic drugs should be avoided in patients with VOD, and the pharmacology of drugs normally metabolized by the liver may be altered in these patients.

INTERMEDIATE COMPLICATIONS (DAYS 14 TO 80 AFTER TRANSPLANT)

Graft Failure

Although complete and sustained engraftment is seen in the large majority of transplant patients, marrow function occasionally does not return, nor is it lost after temporary engraftment. Graft failure occurring after autologous transplantation may be related to stem cell damage that occurred before stem cell collections, during the storage process, or after transplantation. A correlation has been found between poor graft function after autologous transplantation and prior exposure to extensive chemotherapy before marrow storage. Poor graft function has also been seen in recipients of highly purified stem cells. Exposure after transplant to potential marrow toxins, such as ganciclovir, and infection with CMV or human herpesvirus six have also been associated with graft failure.

Similarly, graft failure after allogeneic transplantation can be caused by exposure to marrow toxins or viral infections, but it may also be the result of graft rejection when host immune cells react against the new marrow graft. Graft rejection is more commonly seen in recipients of T-cell-depleted marrow, patients who receive HLA-mismatched or unrelated grafts, and those in whom less intensive preparative regimens are used. The approach to treating graft failure depends on its most likely cause. A reasonable first step in patients with poor graft function is to remove all potential myelosuppressive agents. The addition of a myeloid growth factor, such as GM-CSF, results in increased granulocytes in 40%–50% of patients. Immunologically-mediated graft rejection is demonstrated by the presence of a severely hypoplastic marrow and circulating host-derived lymphocytes in the peripheral blood of the patient. Occasional patients may recover host hematopoiesis with prolonged support. More often, however, patients remain severely hypoplastic, and it is necessary to consider a second transplant. Recent studies have shown that second grafts can be successful in the majority of patients when a combination of steroids and an anti-CD3 monoclonal antibody is used before the second marrow infusion.

Acute Graft-versus-Host Disease

Graft-versus-host disease results when allogeneic T-cells transfused with the graft, or developing from it, react with major or minor histocompatibility antigens on the genetically different host. Acute GVHD usually develops between days 14 and 28 after transplant and most often involves the skin, liver, and gastrointestinal tract. The skin rash is classically an erythematous maculopapular rash on the arms, legs, and trunk and involves the palms and soles. Liver disease is characterized by increases in bilirubin, transaminases, and alkaline phosphatase, but the weight gain and tender hepatomegaly generally associated with VOD are not usually seen. Gastrointestinal disease most commonly presents with diarrhea and abdominal pain, but anorexia and upper abdominal discomfort may predominate. Because the therapy of GVHD involves systemic immunosuppression, and because other diseases can mimic GVHD, a biopsy for definite diagnosis should be performed if possible. Pathologic features include lymphocytic and monocytic infiltration into perivascular spaces in the dermis and epidermal junction of the skin, into the base of the intestinal crypts in the small or large bowel, and into the periportal areas of the liver. Acute GVHD is usually staged and graded according to the Seattle criteria (Table 96.2). Most clinicians withhold therapy until grade 2 or higher acute GVHD develops. If the patient is on cyclosporine or tacrolimus, it is customary to continue that drug and add another immunosuppressive agent, usually 1 or 2 mg of prednisone per kilogram daily. Prednisone is normally continued for 2 weeks and then slowly tapered in responding patients. Other immunosuppressive agents that can be used instead of prednisone or in patients who fail to respond to prednisone include antithymocyte globulin, monoclonal antibodies against T-cells, mycophenolate mofetil or rapamycin.

Patients with significant gastrointestinal symptoms are generally given nothing by mouth until symptoms abate and then are carefully allowed to resume eating. Rash associated with GVHD can lead to significant skin breakdown. Cleansing excoriated areas and applying nystatin/polymyxin powders to skin folds may help. Aquaphor ointment or emollients can be used for flat surfaces or extremities. Severe rashes with bullae and desquamation should be treated like burns.

Infection

Infections in the neutropenic patient are considered above (see Early Complications). Even after engraftment, transplant patients remain severely immunosuppressed for months, and infectious complications are frequent (Chapter 63). The risk for bacterial infection diminishes after granulocyte recovery. Thus, patients are not normally kept on prophylactic systemic antibiotics once granulocyte counts recover to $500/\mu L$. However, a wide variety of bacterial infections is seen after engraftment, and any fever in the posttransplant patient requires intensive evaluation. Gram-positive infections associated with indwelling catheters are common, but a wide array of other organisms can also cause infection. The incidence of candidal infections can be lessened by the use of prophylactic fluconazole (200–400 mg/d through day 75) (9). With the use of fluconazole, aspergillosis has emerged as the most common

TABLE 96.2			
CLINICAL STAGING OF ACUTE GRAFT-VERSUS-HOST DISEASE			
Stage	Skin	Liver	Gut
I	Maculopapular rash <25% body surface	Bilirubin 2–3 mg/dL	Diarrhea 500–1,000 mL/d
II	Maculopapular rash 25–50% body surface	Bilirubin 3–6 mg/dL	Diarrhea 1,000–1,500 mL/d
III	Generalized erythroderma	Bilirubin 6–15 mg/dL	Diarrhea >1,500 mL/d
IV	Desquamation and bullae	Bilirubin >15 mg/dL	Pain and ileus

fungal infection in the posttransplant patient. *Aspergillus* infections are often fatal, and successful treatment, when it occurs, requires that infection be diagnosed while still relatively localized, so that it can be controlled with antifungals and, if possible, surgical excision. The preferred initial therapy of documented *Aspergillius* infection includes voriconazole plus caspofungin (10).

In the past, CMV infections involving the lungs and gastrointestinal tract were frequent and led to death in 10%–15% of allogeneic transplant patients. Currently, if the donor and recipient are CMV-seronegative at the time of transplant, CMV infections can be entirely prevented by avoiding exposure to blood products from CMV-seropositive donors. In patients who are CMV-seropositive at the outset of transplant, the incidence of CMV infection can be substantially reduced with the use of *prophylactic ganciclovir* (11). One strategy is to use ganciclovir prophylaxis in all seropositive patients beginning at the time of engraftment and continuing until day 100. Although ganciclovir is highly effective in preventing CMV disease when used this way, it is also associated with significant marrow suppression. In some patients, severe granulocytopenia and life-threatening infection can result. Other centers monitor patients for the development of CMV antigenemia and begin ganciclovir only when a positive result is observed. Ganciclovir prophylaxis can prevent CMV disease, but it also delays the recovery of immune responses to CMV. Thus, with ganciclovir prophylaxis, late CMV infections (after day 100) are occasionally seen in patients once prophylaxis is stopped. Foscarnet is effective for some patients in whom CMV antigenemia or infection develops despite the use of ganciclovir, or for patients who cannot tolerate the drug.

Pneumocystis jirovecii (formerly *P. carinii*) pneumonia, previously seen in 5%–10% of transplant patients, can be prevented by treatment with oral trimethoprim-sulfamethoxazole for one week before transplant and resumption of the treatment once engraftment has occurred. The usual dose is one double-strength tablet orally twice daily 2 days a week. Treatment is usually continued as long as patients are on immunosuppressive medications. If allergy to trimethoprim-sulfamethoxazole develops in a patient, desensitization is a reasonable course. Dapsone is an alternative, but must be avoided in patients with glucose-6-phosphate dehydrogenase (G6PD) deficiency.

Interstitial Pneumonia

Pneumonias that develop after transplant are frequently caused by bacterial, fungal, or viral organisms. In 5%–10% of cases, however, no infectious cause can be found, and biopsy reveals diffuse cellular damage with or without an additional interstitial component. This type of pneumonia, termed *idiopathic interstitial pneumonia*, is thought to be the result of direct toxicity of the preparative regimen to the lung, although evidence for a role of soluble cytokines is growing. Many infectious causes of posttransplant pneumonias can be identified by bronchoalveolar lavage. If no organism is found and idiopathic pneumonia is diagnosed, therapy with high-dose glucocorticoids is often tried, although no randomized trials have validated this approach.

LATE TOXICITIES (BEYOND DAY 80 AFTER TRANSPLANT)

Late Infections

Even more than 3 months after transplant, patients are still at risk for the development of significant, life-threatening infections. This risk is considerably less after autologous than after allogeneic transplantation, and it is increased in patients on immunosuppressive therapy for chronic GVHD. A wide variety of bacterial, viral, and fungal diseases have been reported in the late posttransplant period. Because the risk for bacterial infection is so high in patients with chronic GVHD, many centers place such patients on prophylaxis with trimethoprim-sulfamethoxazole, penicillin, or both. Herpes zoster is common; it usually presents as localized disease, but subsequent dissemination is noted in about one-third of infected patients. The case fatality rate of disseminated herpes zoster is high. Thus, some centers place all patients on acyclovir prophylaxis for one year to prevent reactivation. At a minimum, all patients in whom dermatomal disease develops within the first year of transplant should be treated with acyclovir to prevent dissemination. As discussed above, CMV infections developing after posttransplant day 100 are becoming more common. Patients typically present with fever, leukopenia, or interstitial pneumonia. Treatment is with ganciclovir and CMV-specific immunoglobulin, if available.

Chronic Graft-versus-Host Disease

Manifestations of the graft-versus-host reaction that occur more than three months after transplantation are termed *chronic GVHD*. Chronic GVHD differs markedly from the acute form in its manifestations and tempo. Chronic GVHD resembles a collagen vascular disease, with skin involvement (malar erythema, sclerodermatous changes, and cutaneous ulcers), alopecia, sicca syndrome, polyserositis, and liver dysfunction. Chronic GVHD develops in 20%–40% of matched sibling transplants, and it is more common in patients who have had a prior episode of acute GVHD, in older patients, and in recipients of mismatched or unrelated transplants. Prednisone, cyclosporine, or the two in combination are the usual treatments. Thalidomide and azathioprine have also been reported to be useful.

Immunosuppressive therapy is usually required for prolonged periods. Patients are generally treated for 9 months, after which the immunosuppression is gradually tapered if their chronic GVHD is in remission. In most patients, chronic GVHD eventually resolves and immunosuppression can be entirely withdrawn, but this may require 1–3 years of treatment. If corticosteroids are used as treatment, an alternate-day schedule after initial remission may help avoid late toxicities.

Second Malignancies

Survivors of marrow transplantation are at increased risk for the development of second malignancies. Patients who have been transplanted with T-cell-depleted marrow or who receive multiple cycles of immunosuppressive therapy to treat GVHD are at increased risk for the development of an aggressive lymphoproliferative disease associated with the Epstein-Barr virus. This syndrome often begins as a polyclonal disorder but evolves into an aggressive monoclonal B-cell malignancy. Infusion of Epstein-Barr virus-specific donor T cells can reverse the disease in some cases. Rituximab may also be effective.

A small increase in the incidence of solid tumors has been documented after marrow transplantation. At 10 years, the cumulative incidence is 2.9%, with a higher incidence seen in patients with chronic GVHD and those who have received extensive radiation. An incidence of myelodysplasia approaching 10% has been reported following autologous transplantation for malignant lymphomas. Whether this is caused directly by the transplant or is a long-term effect of previous chemotherapy before transplantation is unknown.

Relapse After Transplant

The risk for recurrence of malignancy is substantial after transplant, particularly when transplantation is performed for relapsed or refractory disease rather than for disease at an earlier stage. Management of posttransplant relapse is influenced by the transplant setting. Patients who relapse after autologous transplantation may respond to subsequent chemotherapy, and occasionally these responses can be complete and prolonged. Additional options are available to the patient who relapses following allogeneic transplantation, including discontinuation of immunosuppressive therapy and infusion of viable donor lymphocytes.

KEY POINTS

- Marrow transplantation, particularly allogeneic transplantation, is a complex undertaking and is best carried out at centers specializing in the procedure.

- It takes on average at least three months to identify a matched unrelated donor and schedule a transplant, which means that physicians and patients considering the procedure must provide the transplant center with sufficient lead time.
- Marrow transplantation is widely applicable in the treatment of hematologic malignancies and other chemotherapy-responsive tumors, but it has little role in the treatment of tumors completely refractory to standard-dose therapy.
- With appropriate prophylactic measures, most cases of early posttransplant cytomegalovirus and *Candida albicans* infection can be prevented.
- *Pneumocystis jirovecii* infection can be prevented with oral trimethoprim-sulfamethoxazole prophylaxis.
- Immunosuppression is profound in early posttransplant patients, and any infection can be lethal. Even after engraftment, patients are at substantial risk for the development of severe and life-threatening infection. Thus, patients must be followed closely and any potential infection pursued vigorously.
- Determining the cause of early posttransplant liver dysfunction is often difficult. A transvenous liver biopsy is often helpful in such patents and can usually be performed safely, even in patents requiring platelet support.
- Treatment of chronic graft-versus-host disease may require prolonged immunosuppressive therapy with cyclosporine and prednisone. Such patients are at high risk for a number of complications, including infections, aseptic necrosis, and cataracts.
- Posttransplant relapse can be treated successfully in some cases with further chemotherapy, a second transplant, or donor lymphocyte infusions.

REFERENCES

1. Hansen JA, Gooley TA, Martin PJ, et al. Bone marrow transplants from unrelated donors for patients with chronic myeloid leukemia. *N Engl J Med* 1998;338:962–968.
2. Laughlin MJ, Eapan M, Rubinstein P, et al. Outcomes after transplantation of cord blood or bone marrow from unrelated donors in adults with leukemia. *N Engl J Med* 2004;351:2265–2275.
3. Walters MC, Patience M, Leisenring W, et al. Bone marrow transplantation for sickle cell disease. *N Engl J Med* 1996;335:369–376.
4. Drobyski WR. The role of allogeneic transplantation in high-risk acute myelogenous leukemia. *Leukemia* 2004;18:1565–1568.
5. Popat U, Carrum G, Heslop HE. Haemopoietic stem cell transplantation for acute lymphoblastic leukaemia. *Cancer Treat Rev* 2003;29:3–10.
6. Philip T, Guglielmi C, Hagenbeek A, et al. Autologous bone marrow transplantation as compared with salvage chemotherapy in relapses of chemotherapy-sensitive non-Hodgkin's lymphoma. *N Engl J Med* 1995;333:1540–1545.
7. Attal M, Harousseau J-L, Stoppa A-M, et al. A prospective, randomized trial of autologous bone marrow transplantation and chemotherapy in multiple myeloma. *N Engl J Med* 1996;335:91–97.
8. Richardson PG, Elias AD, Krishnan A, et al. Treatment of severe veno-occlusive disease with defibrotide—compassionate use results in response without significant toxicity in a high-risk population. *Blood* 1998;92:737–744.

9. Wingard JR, Leather H. A new era of antifungal therapy. *Biol Blood Marrow Transplant* 2004;10:73–90.
10. Herbrecht R, Denning DW, Patterson TF, et al. Voriconazole versus amphotericin B for primary therapy of invasive aspergillosis. *N Engl J Med* 2002;347:408–415.
11. McGavin JK, Goa KL. Ganciclovir: an update of its use in the prevention of cytomegalovirus infection and disease in transplant recipients. *Drugs* 2001;61:1153–1183.

ADDITIONAL READING

Appelbaum FR. Haematopoietic cell transplantation as immunotherapy. *Nature* 2001;411:385–389.

Bensinger WI, Martin PJ, Storer B, et al. Transplantation of bone marrow as compared with peripheral-blood cells from HLA-identical relatives in patients with hematologic cancers. *N Engl J Med* 2001;344:175–181.

Davies SM, Kollman C, Anasetti C, et al. Engraftment and survival after unrelated-donor bone marrow transplantation: a report from the National Marrow Donor Program. *Blood* 2000;96: 4096–4102.

McSweeney PA, Niederwieser D, Shizuru JA, et al. Hematopoietic cell transplantation in older patients with hematologic malignancies: replacing high-dose cytotoxic therapy with graft-versus-tumor effects. *Blood* 2001;97:3390–3400.

Vogelsang GB, Lee L, Bensen-Kennedy DM. Pathogenesis and treatment of graft-versus-host disease after bone marrow transplant. *Ann Rev Med* 2003; 54:29–52.

Sickle Cell Disease

97

Martin H. Steinberg   Harrison W. Farber

INTRODUCTION

Sickle cell disease results from a mutation in the gene for β-globin, a subunit of adult hemoglobin (HbA). A point mutation in codon six of this gene encodes the synthesis of the sickle β-globin chain (β^s), which contains a valine residue in place of the glutamic acid normally found at this position. Sickle hemoglobin (HbS, $\alpha_2\beta_2^s$) has the unique property of polymerizing when deoxygenated. Sufficient HbS polymer within the erythrocyte evokes the cellular injury responsible for the phenotype of sickle cell disease (1).

Sickle cell disease is a phenotype with distinctive clinical and hematologic features, in which at least half the hemoglobin present is HbS. *Sickle cell trait*, the heterozygous carrier of an HbS gene, is present in about 8% of African-Americans. It is not considered a type of sickle cell disease because it is clinically benign. Among the common genotypes of sickle cell disease are homozygosity for the HbS mutation (*sickle cell anemia*), compound heterozygosity for HbS and HbC (*HbSC disease*), and compound heterozygosity for HbS and β-thalassemia (HbS–β-thalassemia) (Table 97.1). Whenever possible, a diagnosis of sickle cell disease should be assigned by the genotype of the patient because this designation allows the best assessment of prognosis. Accurate genetic counseling—an important aspect of patient management—is possible only when the genotypic diagnosis is known.

Pathophysiology

Sickle hemoglobin has the property of polymerizing when deoxygenated. The *vaso-occlusive features of sickle cell disease are unique among the hemolytic anemias.* Sickle cells cause vascular injury, occluding small and sometimes large blood vessels. No single mechanism explains sickle vaso-occlusion (Figure 97.1). Hemolysis is the other cardinal feature of sickle cell disease, but it causes fewer problems than the myriad vaso-occlusive events.

Erythrocyte heterogeneity in sickle cell anemia is dependent on the cellular content of fetal hemoglobin (HbF). Vaso-occlusion is initiated and sustained by interactions among sickle cells, endothelial cells, leukocytes, and plasma proteins. Sickle erythrocytes alone do not initiate vaso-occlusive disease. Activated neutrophils liberate harmful cytokines and interact with sickle and endothelial cells. Activated platelets release thrombospondin, which promotes adherence of sickle erythrocytes to endothelium. Young reticulocytes contain additional adhesive ligands that facilitate erythrocyte endothelium interactions.

Diagnosis

Diagnosing sickle cell disease is not difficult. Examining the parents or siblings of affected patients is the least costly way of establishing the genotype, and this can be accomplished with simple combinations of blood cell counts and quantitative studies of hemoglobin fractions (Table 97.1). Sickled cells are nearly always seen in sickle cell anemia and HbS–β^0-thalassemia, but are less common in other forms of sickle cell disease. Their presence does not help diagnose acute complications like painful episodes. In untreated adults with sickle cell anemia, HbS nearly always forms more than 80% of the hemolysate. Sickle cell anemia and HbS–β^0-thalassemia are very much alike hematologically and clinically, and the distinction between them requires genetic testing and cannot be made from hemoglobin studies or blood cell counts alone.

TABLE 97.1

LABORATORY DIFFERENTIATION OF SICKLE HEMOGLOBINOPATHIES

Diagnosis	Hemoglobin (g/dL)	Reticulocytes (%)	MCV (fl)	HbS (%)	HbA$_2$ (%)	HbF (%)
Sickle cell anemia	6–9	10	85–95	>90	2–3	7
HbSC disease	8–12	4	70–85	50	2–3	3
HbS–β^0 thalassemia	7–10	10	65–75	>90	4–6	8
HbS–β$^+$ thalassemia	10–12	2	60–70	70	4–6	2
Sickle cell trait	13–16	1	80–90	35	2–3	<1

These are average laboratory values in adults with stable disease. They may vary considerably in individual patients and also be affected by acute disease complications.
HbA$_2$, minor fraction of adult hemoglobin; HbF, fetal hemoglobin; HbS, sickle cell hemoglobin; HbSC, sickle cell hemoglobin C disease; MCV, mean corpuscular volume.

Clinical Features

Sickle cell anemia is present in 1 in 600 African-Americans, and the prevalence of sickle cell disease is about 1 in 300. Sickle cell disease is associated with acute, recurrent, and chronic complications, the most common of which are shown in Table 97.2. Vaso-occlusive disease can occur almost anywhere blood flows and is responsible for the unique features and the most severe complications of this disorder. Hemolysis, which is constantly present, explains why the temporary interruption of erythropoiesis can cause the rapid development of severe anemia (the so-called "aplastic crisis"), and why gallstones form in most patients.

Adults with sickle cell anemia or HbS–β^0-thalassemia are most frequently hospitalized for the treatment of severe painful episodes and acute chest syndrome, and for surgical procedures. Patients with HbSC disease and with HbS–β$^+$-thalassemia require hospitalization about half as often as those with sickle cell anemia and on average live about 20 years longer. Nevertheless, with the promising results of hydroxyurea treatment in patients with sickle cell anemia (see the section on "Discharge Issues" later in this chapter), patients with HbSC disease are beginning to

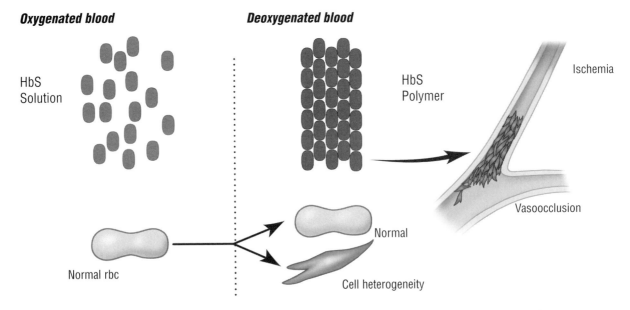

Figure 97.1 Pathophysiology of sickle cell disease. With deoxygenation, sickle hemoglobin polymerizes and eventually causes cell sickling and damage to the membrane. Red cells are heterogeneous, with a spectrum of densities, membrane injury, and fetal hemoglobin. Some cells adhere to the endothelium to cause vaso-occlusion.

TABLE 97.2

CLINICAL FEATURES OF SICKLE CELL DISEASE

	Features
Vaso-occlusive complications	
Painful episodes	>70% of patients affected; very frequent in some, rare in others
Stroke	~10% in childhood; two to three times more patients with "silent" MRI defects and cognitive impairment
Acute chest syndrome	50% of all patients; more common in children, more severe in adults
Priapism	10–40% of male patients; severe cases cause impotence
Hepatopathy	<2%; many causes; extreme bilirubin elevations
Splenic sequestration	Children <6 y; often preceded by infection
Spontaneous abortion	~6% in sickle cell anemia; much less in HbSC disease
Leg ulcers	~20% of adult sickle cell anemia; rare in HbSC disease
Osteonecrosis	10–15% of adults with sickle cell anemia and HbSC disease
Proliferative retinopathy	Rare in sickle cell anemia; 50% adults with HbSC disease
Renal insufficiency	5–20% of adults; severe anemia often present
Complications of hemolysis	
Anemia	PCV 15–30 in sickle cell anemia; greater in HbSC disease
Cholelithiasis	Present in most adults; often asymptomatic
Acute aplastic episodes	May be caused by parvovirus B19; rapidly occurring severe anemia
Infectious complications	
Streptococcus pneumoniae sepsis	10% of children <5 y with sickle cell anemia
Osteomyelitis	*Salmonella* spp. and *Staphylococcus aureus* are usual agents
Escherichia coli	In adults, usually initiated by UTI urinary sepsis
Chlamydia	May cause acute chest syndrome

HbSC, sickle cell hemoglobin C disease; *MRI*, magnetic resonance imaging; *PCV*, packed cell volume; *UTI*, urinary tract infection.
From Steinberg MH. Drug therapy: management of sickle cell disease. *N Engl J Med* 1999;340:1021–1030, with permission.

represent an increasing proportion of sickle cell disease patients who need hospital care.

PAINFUL EPISODES AND PRIAPISM

Issues at the Time of Admission

Acute painful episodes are the main cause of hospitalization in sickle cell disease. Although these are generally believed to be caused by vaso-occlusion by sickle erythrocytes, some authorities believe that they have a neurovascular basis, as blood is shunted away from involved regions. Whatever the physiology, the episodes are characterized by bouts of excruciating pain in the chest, back, abdomen, or extremities. Painful episodes often involve multiple areas simultaneously, symmetrically affect the extremities, and might last days or even weeks. Sickle cell pain is notorious for severity surpassing that of postsurgical pain and the pain of trauma. Some patients never describe a painful episode, whereas others seem to have them continuously. These discrete attacks of pain must be separated from the more chronic pain of osteoporosis and osteomalacia that usually affects the spine, the pain associated with osteonecrosis of the hips and shoulders, and the milder aches, pains, and soreness that frequently are present between severe episodes.

On average, patients with sickle cell anemia and HbS-β^0-thalassemia have twice as many episodes of pain yearly as do persons with HbSC disease and HbS-β^+ thalassemia. Clearly, some patients are more predisposed to painful episodes than others. Whereas about 5% of patients account for more than 30% of the crises, nearly 40% of patients with sickle cell anemia do not have a single episode of pain in a given year. Rates of pain are highest during the third and fourth decades of life (1). The rate of pain varies directly with the packed cell volume (PCV) and inversely with the HbF level. As the pain of a crisis intensifies, there is also a small decrease in PCV and a rise in reticulocytes, but this is insufficient to be diagnostically useful in an individual patient. Unfortunately, *no useful laboratory test can determine whether a vaso-occlusive pain crisis is occurring, and the history remains the best clue.*

Frequent episodes of pain portend increased mortality in adults. Patients with the highest PCVs and leukocyte counts and the lowest HbF levels are at the greatest risk. Often, death in adults is unexpected and occurs in the midst of an acute event—most often a pain episode—as a result of cardiovascular collapse. In the United States, the median age of death is about 45 years in sickle cell anemia and about 65 years in HbSC disease.

Painful episodes are often stereotypical, affecting each patient in the same manner from episode to episode. Patients usually know if the pain they are experiencing is different from their typical painful episode, and physicians should heed what patients say about the need for hospitalization or the likelihood that their pain can be explained by something other than a "pain crisis."

The pain of acute cholecystitis, splenic sequestration crisis, splenic infarction, and right upper quadrant syndrome can sometimes be mistaken for uncomplicated pain episodes. In splenic sequestration and right upper quadrant syndrome, the spleen and liver can be distended by blood that accumulates as the vasculature of these organs dilates. Usually, in splenic sequestration crisis, the hemoglobin concentration falls rapidly, whereas in right upper quadrant syndrome, parameters of liver function become grossly abnormal. Neither acute, severe anemia nor newly deranged liver functions are typical features of a painful episode. Acute painful episodes are often the heralding events in acute chest syndrome, discussed below. Occasionally, pain episodes end with multiple organ failure. No data allow one to foretell whether a "usual" pain episode will have a morbid or mortal outcome.

It has been estimated that nearly 40% of adult men with sickle cell anemia have had at least one episode of *priapism*. Recurrent attacks of priapism can last for several hours with tolerable discomfort and be self-limited. These episodes, which have been termed stuttering priapism, usually have a nocturnal onset. Erectile function is mostly preserved between these attacks, which can recur for years and number in the dozens. Major episodes of priapism often (not always) follow a history of stuttering attacks, last for days, and can be excruciatingly painful. They usually destroy sexual function by causing irreversible damage to the corporal bodies. Priapism has been considered one manifestation of severe vascular disease and has been associated with an increased chance of cerebrovascular accidents.

Indications for Hospitalization

Patients are generally quite "savvy" about the management of painful episodes. They know when the event is sufficiently minor that they can be cared for at home with rest, oral fluids, local measures such as heating pads, and oral analgesics. When the pain is beyond home treatment, patients will, depending on the resources available, visit a physician's office, a medical clinic, day hospitals that focus on the treatment of acute sickle cell pain episodes, or the emergency department. From these venues, after the duration and severity of pain and the history of response to pain treatment have been assessed, the decision regarding hospitalization can be made. It is important to consider whether or not complicating factors are present, such as excessive tachycardia, hypotension, temperature above 101°F, marked leukocytosis, a fall in hemoglobin level, reduced O_2 saturation, or evidence of pneumonia on examination or chest radiography. The presence of any of these factors argues for early admission.

If the pain episode appears to be uncomplicated, and if, after treatment in the emergency department or day hospital, pain has not diminished to the point at which the patient feels that it is manageable at home, hospitalization is warranted. Because of the pressures of their jobs and family life, the chronicity of their illness, or adverse experiences with pain management in the hospital, many patients are reluctant to be hospitalized. Conversely, some patients—a small minority—actively seek hospitalization because of their inability to cope psychologically with pain or because they are seeking opiates. It cannot be overemphasized that *this latter class of patients comprises only a small percentage of the population with sickle cell anemia*, although they may be responsible for a disproportionate amount of the monetary and medical resources expended on this disease.

Indications for Initial Intensive Care Unit Admission

Respiratory distress, reduced O_2 saturation, high-grade fever, rising serum creatinine, falling PCV and platelet count, and circulatory instability all suggest that acute chest syndrome may be present or multiple organ failure is developing. These findings should prompt consideration of ICU admission.

Initial Approach

A close and mutually satisfactory relationship between the patient and the treating physician is a major adjunct to the successful management of an acute painful episode. This provides the patient with confidence that his or her history of prior painful events and their effective treatment has been considered in the formulation of a treatment plan. Reliance on a succession of skeptical physicians as primary caregivers can compromise effective treatment. Most pain episodes do not have an identifiable precipitating cause, but this does not mean that one should not be diligently sought. Painful episodes are sometimes triggered by an infection, extremes of temperature, or physical and emotional stress. Pneumonia is the most prevalent infection associated with acute pain episodes and is caused by the organisms responsible for community-acquired pneumonia (Chapter 65).

More commonly, painful episodes begin with little warning. Physical examination is usually not helpful for determining if an acute pain episode is in progress, but sometimes localized swelling and pain are noted over an involved bone. A chest radiograph should be obtained in most patients sufficiently ill to be hospitalized to exclude acute chest syndrome or pneumonia. Most patients with sickle cell anemia have a leukocyte count between 12,000 and 14,000/μL in their basal state, so that mild leukocytosis does not signify infection. Elevation beyond the baseline may be a clue to an infectious process but also occurs with acute chest syndrome and severe painful episodes. Low-grade fever can accompany the acute painful episode, but higher elevations may point to infection or extensive tissue damage.

Table 97.3 outlines one approach to the treatment of painful events in sickle cell anemia. Administration of opiate analgesics in sufficient doses and frequency is the foundation of treatment. The choice of drug and the dose can be guided by the history of previous pain episodes. For severe pain, parenteral opiates are required. They must be given at frequent fixed intervals, not "as needed," until the pain has diminished, at which time they can be tapered, then stopped, and oral analgesics substituted (1) (Table 97.3). Breakthrough pain can be managed by giving one-half to one-fourth of the maintenance dose. Nonsteroidal antiinflammatory agents and other adjuvant drugs like hydroxyzine are useful in some patients. The use of pain measurement scales and frequent reassessment of pain, at 2- to 3-hour intervals if possible, help guide the intensity of treatment. Some patients prefer patient-controlled analgesia. (For further information on the general principles of pain management, see Chapter 18.)

The conundrum of managing priapism lies in determining when "conservative" treatment should be stopped and operative intervention initiated, a challenge made greater because of the lack of controlled clinical trials of any acute treatment modality (2). Pain should be relieved in the same manner as pain affecting other areas, and adequate fluids provided. If the episode differs from prior episodes of stuttering priapism according to the patient's history and physician's experience, aspiration and irrigation should be performed within a 12-hour window after the onset of erection. Simple or exchange transfusions may also be useful. Invasive treatment for priapism in sickle cell anemia is designed to evacuate stagnant blood within the corpora cavernosa

TABLE 97.3

MANAGEMENT OF ACUTE PAIN IN SICKLE CELL DISEASE

Treat cause if one is identified; begin analgesic treatment promptly.

Liberal fluid replacement, 3–4 L daily in adults

Orally, if possible.
Intravenously, if needed. Use 0.5 N saline solution.

Analgesics for acute pain

Morphine, hydromorphone (Dilaudid) or, if necessary, meperidine (Demerol), parenterally, at *full therapeutic doses*, at intervals of 2–4 h to relieve pain. Additional smaller doses for "breakthrough" pain. Reassess pain frequently.
Do not order as needed (prn) medication.
Consider use of adjunctive drugs like hydroxyzine, diphenhydramine, or promethazine, and nonsteroidal antiinflammatory drugs.
Consider patient-controlled analgesia if more frequent dosing is needed. Use pain scales (digital analog or 0–10, absent to worst possible [Chapter 18]) to gauge treatment effects and determine doses.

Analgesics for mild–moderate pain

Fentanyl patches for prolonged moderate–severe pain
Acetaminophen with codeine for mild–moderate pain not requiring physician visit
Nonsteroidal antiinflammatory agents for pain of osteonecrosis if not contraindicated because of renal disease or severe liver disease

Modified from Ballas SK. Neurobiology and treatment of pain. In Embury SH, Hebbel RP, Mohandas N, et al., eds. *Sickle Cell Disease: Basic Principles and Clinical Practice.* New York: Raven Press, 1997:745–772.

and prevent immediate recurrence of corporal expansion. While the simplest surgical procedure is aspiration of the corporal bodies with irrigation, aspiration of blood is usually difficult after a major episode of priapism has lasted for 24–48 hours. Operative intervention can be considered if detumescence is not achieved with aspiration and irrigation. When surgery is chosen, a Winter shunt between the glans penis and corpora cavernosa should be placed within 24 hours. This plan requires crucial decisions within 12 hours of the onset of priapism, and, because patients are often reluctant to visit the emergency department or clinic based on their experience with self-limited priapism, time for observation may be lacking. Urologists conversant with the management of priapism should be consulted when the patient with a severe episode is first seen.

Indications for Early Consultation

Patients who have very frequent pain episodes are the most difficult to manage. Early and continued consultations with therapists, psychiatrists, and experts in pain management may decrease their rate of hospitalization and emergency department visits, but the general effectiveness of this adjunctive treatment has not been critically evaluated. Priapism has a tendency to recur, until erectile function is lost. Efforts should be made to interrupt the episodes of stuttering priapism that presage a major event. However, the options available are imperfect and untested. These include pseudoephedrine, leuprolide, stilbesterol, and prophylactic transfusion. Penile prostheses may help some impotent patients.

Issues During the Course of Hospitalization

Painful episodes resolve with time, but their length varies considerably between patients and from episode to episode. On average, pain diminishes to the point at which oral analgesics are sufficient and discharge can be contemplated in 4–7 days, but persistence of pain far beyond this interval is common. In unusually prolonged pain episodes, the question of whether pain persists because of "organic" reasons versus psychological factors is often raised. With laboratory tests indicative of a painful episode lacking, this distinction is often impossible to resolve. Because acute painful episodes can be the sign of more ominous events, such as acute chest syndrome, the search for signs and symptoms of lung involvement must be vigilant.

Discharge Issues

Discharge is possible when pain has receded to the point at which it can be managed at home with oral analgesics and rest. Unless events during hospitalization warrant, such as deterioration in renal or liver function or a fall in PCV, a special clinic appointment for follow-up is not necessary. A telephone call will suffice, and regularly scheduled outpatient appointments can be kept. Perhaps because of the fluctuation in erythrocyte populations during the evolution of painful episodes, recurrence within weeks of an apparent resolution sometimes happens. This does not signify a treatment failure.

Now that an effective approach for the prevention of painful episodes is available, initiation of this therapy in selected hospitalized patients who qualify for this type of treatment should be considered (3). In adults with a history of several pain episodes yearly, *hydroxyurea* reduces by nearly half the incidence of pain crisis, acute chest syndrome, hospitalization, and blood transfusion. Treatment is also associated with a substantial reduction in mortality (4).

Hydroxyurea should be reserved for patients who average one or two pain episodes per year that require sustained treatment with parenteral opiates, who have had severe episodes of acute chest syndrome, or who have other severe vaso-occlusive events (Table 97.4). These patients must also be willing and able to comply with the treatment regimen. Therapy is initiated with 500 mg of hydroxyurea daily (10–15 mg/kg). Dose titration and continued monitoring of patients is carried out in the office or clinic.

Patients should be explicitly counseled regarding the following: responses differ among individuals; many months may be needed to find the best dose of the drug; medication must be taken exactly as directed, with frequent blood tests performed; and long-term toxicities and effects of treatment are unknown. It is not yet established if hydroxyurea is mutagenic, carcinogenic, or leukemogenic. Also unknown is whether hydroxyurea will prevent organ damage, or restore function to already injured organs. Finally, whether hydroxyurea can affect the course of HbSC disease is unknown.

ACUTE CHEST SYNDROME

Issues at the Time of Admission

Acute chest syndrome (ACS) is the most common form of acute pulmonary disease in patients with sickle cell disease. It occurs in almost one-half of all sickle cell patients (1). ACS is most common but less severe in children and, after the painful episode, is the second most frequent cause of hospitalization in sickle cell anemia. It is the most frequently reported cause of death in adults and is a risk factor for early mortality, particularly since recurrent events can end in chronic sickle cell lung disease characterized by pulmonary hypertension (see the section on "Pulmonary Hypertension" later in this chapter), cor pulmonale and eventual death. ACS is defined as the presence of the following signs and symptoms in a patient with sickle cell disease: (1) presence of a new pulmonary infiltrate, involving at least one complete lung segment (not atelectasis); (2)

TABLE 97.4

USE OF HYDROXYUREA IN SICKLE CELL ANEMIA

Indication for treatment

Adolescents or adults with frequent pain episodes, history of acute chest syndrome, other severe vaso-occlusive complications, severe symptomatic anemia

Baseline evaluation

Blood counts, red cell indices, HbF, serum chemistries, pregnancy test, willingness to adhere to all recommendations for treatment, absence of chronic transfusion program

Initiation of treatment

Hydroxyurea 500 mg (10–15 mg/kg) each morning for 6–8 wk, CBC q2wk

Treatment end points

Less pain, increase in HbF (or MCV), increased hemoglobin level if severely anemic, acceptable myelotoxicity (granulocytes >2,000/μL, platelets >80,000/μL)

Special caution should be exercised in patients with compromised renal or hepatic function or who are habituated to opiates. Contraception should be practiced by both men and women because the effects of hydroxyurea on pregnancy are not known. Granulocyte count should be >2,000/μL, platelet count >80,000/μL. A fall in hemoglobin level and absolute reticulocyte count should be carefully evaluated (in most patients who respond, the hemoglobin level increases slightly).
CBC, complete blood count; *HbF*, fetal hemoglobin; *MCV*, mean corpuscular volume.
From Steinberg MH. Drug therapy: management of sickle cell disease. *N Engl J Med* 1999;340:1021–1030, with permission.

chest pain; (3) temperature >38.5°C; (4) tachypnea, wheezing, or cough; and (5) hypoxemia. On examination, there may be splinting, signs of pulmonary consolidation, or scattered rales. Chest findings can change rapidly and dramatically, which highlights the need for continual reassessment.

The principal causes of ACS remain unclear. However, probable etiologic factors include: (1) Macrovascular or microvascular infarction within the pulmonary vasculature, most likely due to *in-situ* thrombosis; (2) pulmonary fat embolism, a result of bone marrow necrosis. Lipid-laden macrophages are found in 50%–60% of children and adults with ACS. Patients with fat emboli are more likely to complain of bone pain and may develop neurologic symptoms, a finding not seen in ACS without fat emboli; (3) rib and sternal infarctions, leading to hypoventilation. Splinting due to local pain results in atelectasis and hypoxemia, which furthers the development of ACS; (4) although bacterial pneumonia was once thought to be responsible for ACS in 50% of children, more recent culture-based studies have failed to demonstrate its role as a major etiologic factor in children or adults. Pulmonary edema may also contribute, either secondary to excessive hydration or to changes in pulmonary vascular permeability due to opioids. In a study of 671 episodes of ACS in 538 patients with sickle cell disease,

the following causes of ACS were identified: pulmonary infarction, 16%; fat embolism (with or without infection), 9%; *Chlamydia pneumoniae* infection, 7%; *Mycoplasma pneumoniae* infection, 7%; viral infection, 6%; mixed infection, 4%; other pathogens, 1%; unknown cause, 46% (5).

Differentiating among the various infectious and non-infectious causes of acute chest syndrome is difficult. However, with our current state of knowledge, this sorting probably does not change the course of treatment. No current laboratory or radiographic finding permits the differentiation of ACS from other acute pulmonary manifestations of sickle cell disease, including pneumonia and infarction.

Sputum and blood cultures should be obtained. General measures that improve symptoms in many patients include optimal hydration, administration of oxygen to maintain a PaO$_2$ of 70–100 mm Hg, incentive spirometry, and the use of bronchodilators. Pain usually accompanies acute chest syndrome and must be treated. However, excessive opiate use can suppress respiration and should be avoided. Although microbiologic data are rarely diagnostic, antibiotic regimens that include coverage for community-acquired and atypical organisms should be employed (Chapter 65). Exchange transfusion is recommended in the setting of progressive infiltrates and hypoxemia refractory to conventional therapy. Reduction of the HbS level to below 30% can lead to marked improvement in the majority of cases. These recommendations are based on observations that transfusions rapidly reverse hypoxia in some patients. However, no controlled clinical studies have documented the value of transfusion or have compared exchange transfusions with simple transfusions (6).

Indications for Initial Intensive Care Unit Admission

Hypoxia with respiratory distress, high-grade fever, circulatory instability, and acute respiratory distress syndrome (ARDS) are all adverse prognostic findings that should prompt consideration of ICU admission.

Issues During the Course of Hospitalization and at Discharge

Hypoxic patients should be closely monitored with frequent blood gas measurements (see Chapter 24 for management of respiratory failure). Serial assessments of blood cell counts and changes in chest radiograph, especially in the first few days of the episode, can be useful prognostically and suggest whether ICU transfer is advisable. It may take weeks for all signs of acute chest syndrome to resolve and hospitalization can last 1–2 weeks, depending on the cause and severity of the episode.

One or more documented episodes of acute chest syndrome may be an indication for initiating treatment with hydroxyurea. The rationale for this suggestion is the observation that acute chest syndrome tends to be a recurrent event that is associated with increased morbidity and early mortality in adults. Hydroxyurea can reduce by 50% the incidence of this complication.

Multiple acute chest episodes presage a poor prognosis. Sometimes, consideration of bone marrow transplantation in this situation is warranted (Chapter 96). Children below the age of 16 with an HLA-matched donor are presently the best candidates, but only 1% of sickle cell anemia patients meet these requirements. Of the approximately 200 patients who have undergone transplantation, more than 90% survived, 70%–85% had prolonged event-free survival, and 15% suffered graft rejection. Whether or not transplantation can reverse established organ damage has not been determined, but early reports suggest some improvement in chronic lung disease.

PULMONARY HYPERTENSION

Using echocardiography as the diagnostic tool, the estimated incidence of pulmonary hypertension in sickle cell anemia has been found to be between 8% and 30%. In a recent catheterization study of 34 adult patients with sickle cell disease, 20 patients (59%) were diagnosed with pulmonary hypertension (average mean pulmonary artery pressure 36 mm Hg). Several of these patients had elevated pulmonary capillary wedge pressures consistent with left ventricular diastolic dysfunction. Mean pulmonary artery pressure was inversely related to survival. Each increase of 10 mmHg in mean pulmonary artery pressure was associated with a 1.7-fold increase in the rate of death (7). Chapter 59 reviews the diagnosis and management of pulmonary hypertension.

BLOOD TRANSFUSIONS

Transfusions play a vital role in the treatment of some complications of sickle cell anemia, and there are singular considerations and discrete indications for their use (Table 97.5). Transfusions are not needed for the usual anemia or painful episode. Except for aplastic crises and precipitous falls in PCV that occasionally occur during acute events like chest syndrome or sepsis, the PCV remains quite constant over time. Some patients can be

TABLE 97.5
TRANSFUSIONS IN SICKLE CELL DISEASE

Indicated

Symptomatic acute anemic episodes
Severe symptomatic chronic anemia—for example, with renal failure
Prevention of first stroke and recurrent strokes in childhood
Acute chest syndrome with hypoxia[a]
Surgery with general anesthesia or eye surgery[b]

Perhaps useful

Complicated obstetric problems
Severe right upper quadrant syndrome with extreme hyperbilirubinemia
Refractory leg ulcers
Refractory and protracted painful episodes
Acute severe priapism, when given early in episode

Probably not indicated

Raising the customary hemoglobin level
Uncomplicated painful episode
Uncomplicated pregnancies
Minor surgery with local anesthesia

[a] Controlled studies of exchange versus simple transfusions in acute chest syndrome are lacking.
[b] Exchange transfusion appeared to increase the incidence of transfusion-related complications like allo-immunization. When possible, leukocyte-depleted, phenotypically matched packed red cells should be transfused.
From Steinberg MH. Drug therapy: management of sickle cell disease. *N Engl J Med* 1999;340:1021–1030, with permission.

active and symptom-free with PCVs of 16%–20%. Sudden severe anemia, which occurs in children when blood is sequestered in an enlarged spleen or when parvovirus B19 infection causes transient aplastic crisis, often requires urgent blood replacement. Symptomatic anemia occasionally accompanies renal failure, and some of these patients may require transfusion. Alternatively, the judicious use of erythropoietin can sometimes restore hemoglobin levels to pre-renal failure levels.

Recent clinical trials have evaluated the efficacy of transfusion in preventing some of the complications of sickle cell disease (8, 9). Measuring the velocity of cerebral blood by trans-cranial Doppler flow studies and placing individuals at high risk for stroke on prophylactic transfusions reduces the liklihood of an initial stroke (10). Long-term transfusion reduces the recurrence of stroke in children with sickle cell anemia with a prior stroke. The aim of exchange transfusion is to rapidly reduce the HbS level to less than 30% and maintain this level for 3–5 years. Stopping transfusions—even after many years—is often followed by recurrent stroke. Reducing the frequency of transfusion and permitting the HbS level to rise to 50% after four years of more intensive transfusion appears safe.

When general anesthesia is used, preoperative transfusion to a PCV of about 30% prevents postoperative complications as effectively as aggressive exchange transfusion, and is associated with half as many transfusion-related complications (5). Routine intrapartum transfusions are not indicated (8).

Among the general complications of transfusion, *alloimmunization* stands out as a special hazard for patients with sickle cell disease. Because of antigenic differences between the erythrocytes of a predominantly Caucasian blood donor pool and the African-American recipients, 20%–30% of patients with sickle cell anemia who undergo transfusion become allo-immunized. Therefore, red cells phenotypically matched for the antigenic determinants most often eliciting an immune response and depleted of leukocytes are the preferred transfusion product. Another consequence of repetitive transfusion is *iron storage disease*. When transfusions are utilized continually, iron chelation therapy should be planned. Presently, this can be accomplished only with desferrioxamine, given by prolonged subcutaneous or intravenous infusion 8–12 hours nightly, 5–6 days weekly, at doses of 2–6 g daily.

COST CONSIDERATIONS AND RESOURCE USE

Each hospital admission for treatment of a painful episode may last between 5 and 11 days and is associated with charges of $4,000–$16,500. Emergency department charges for treating the pain of sickle cell disease vary between $400 and $600. Treating acute chest syndrome is usually far more expensive. Treating patients with hydroxyurea appears to be associated with a reduction in medical costs (11). Regular clinic attendance has also been shown to reduce the health care costs of sickle cell disease.

KEY POINTS

- Frequent painful episodes and acute chest syndrome portend a poor, sometimes fatal, prognosis. Hydroxyurea reduces morbidity and mortality in these patients.
- Large amounts of opiates may be needed to relieve pain during an acute painful episode.
- Acute chest syndrome may develop in the course of a painful episode, even if it was not apparent on first presentation.
- Blood transfusions are indicated in acute chest syndrome with hypoxia.
- Blood transfusions are not indicated in uncomplicated pain episodes or to treat the usual level of anemia.
- Severe priapism must be evaluated early in its course and the decision made within 24 hours to move from conservative to invasive therapy.

REFERENCES

1. Steinberg MH, Forget BG, Higgs DR, Nagel RL. *Disorders of Hemoglobin: Genetics, Pathophysiology, and Clinical Management.* 1st ed. Cambridge: Cambridge University Press, 2001.
2. Mantadakis E, Ewalt DH, Cavender JD, et al. Outpatient penile aspiration and epinephrine irrigation for young patients with sickle cell anemia and prolonged priapism. *Blood* 2000;95:78–82.
3. Steinberg M.H., Rodgers G.P. Pharmacologic modulation of fetal hemoglobin. *Medicine* 2001;80:328–344.
4. Steinberg MH, Barton F, Castro O, et al. Effect of hydroxyurea on mortality and morbidity in adult sickle cell anemia: risks and benefits up to 9 years of treatment. *JAMA* 2003;289:1645–1651.
5. Vichinsky EP, Neumayr LD, Earles AN, Williams R. Causes and outcomes of the acute chest syndrome in sickle cell disease. National Acute Chest Syndrome Study Group. *N Engl J Med* 2000; 342:1855–1865.
6. Gladwin MT, Rodgers GP. Pathogenesis and treatment of acute chest syndrome of sickle cell anemia. *Lancet* 2000;355:1476–1478.
7. Castro O, Hoque M, Brown BD. Pulmonary hypertension in sickle cell disease: cardiac catheterization results and survival. *Blood* 2003;101:1257–1261.
8. Vichinsky EP, Haberkern CM, Neumayr L, et al. A comparison of conservative and aggressive transfusion regimens in the perioperative management of sickle cell disease. *N Engl J Med* 1995;333: 206–213.
9. Koshy M, Burd L, Wallace D, et al. Prophylactic red cell transfusions in pregnant patients with sickle cell disease. A randomized cooperative study [see comments]. *N Engl J Med* 1988;319:1447–1452.
10. Adams RJ. Stroke prevention and treatment in sickle cell disease. *Arch Neurol* 2001;58:565–568.
11. Moore RD, Charache S, Terrin ML, Barton FB, Ballas SK, Investigators of the Multicenter Study of Hydroxyurea in Sickle cell Anemia. Cost-effectiveness of hydroxyurea in sickle cell anemia. *Am J Hematol* 2000;64:26–31.

ADDITIONAL READING

Castro O, Brambilla DJ, Thorington B, et al. The acute chest syndrome in sickle cell disease: incidence and risk factors. *Blood* 1994;84:643–649.

Chui, DHK., Steinberg, MH. Laboratory Detection of Hemoglobinopathies and Thalassemias. In: Hoffman R, Benz EJ Jr, Shattil SJ, et al., eds. *Hematology. Basic Principles and Practice.* 4th ed. New York: Churchill-Livingstone, New York 2004.

Platt OS, Brambilla DJ, Rosse WF, et al. Mortality in sickle cell disease: life expectancy and risk factors for early death. *N Engl J Med* 1994;330:1639–1644.

Steinberg MH. Drug therapy: management of sickle cell disease. *N Engl J Med* 1999;340:1021–1030.

Hemorrhagic and Thrombotic Disorders

98

Julie Hambleton   Marc Shuman

INTRODUCTION

The hemostatic system is a finely balanced network of coagulation factors and endothelial and platelet components. Its normal function is either to rapidly arrest the bleeding associated with trauma or to terminate this process to prevent excessive clotting. Abnormalities in any of these components can lead to pathologic bleeding or thrombosis. The following general overview of hemorrhagic and thrombotic disorders includes a summary of our approach to evaluating and treating hospitalized patients with disorders of bleeding or thrombosis.

Pathologic Bleeding Caused by Platelet and Coagulation Disorders

A fundamental issue in patients presenting with a bleeding diathesis is to determine whether the bleeding is entirely the consequence of a structural problem, or whether a significant primary platelet or coagulation defect is present. This distinction is not always clear, and it may be necessary to exclude the latter possibilities by laboratory testing. Bleeding caused by a coagulation or platelet disorder frequently occurs at sites where a structural abnormality is present, such as one caused by peptic ulcer disease, a recent surgical procedure, or a traumatic injury.

When evaluating for a possible bleeding disorder, the patient's history may suggest whether a bleeding diathesis is congenital or acquired and, if the latter, the most likely category into which it falls. Moreover, careful physical examination may reveal signs that indicate a platelet or vascular defect vs. a coagulation defect. Based on this information, it frequently can be determined whether bleeding is secondary to a platelet or a coagulation disorder (Table 98.1).

The following historical information is useful in narrowing the diagnostic possibilities:

1. *Timing of the first manifestation of bleeding.* In severe hereditary bleeding disorders, the onset is frequently at birth or at the time of male circumcision. In milder congenital disorders, abnormal bleeding may present (as epistaxis) later in childhood when a child becomes more physically active, or at menarche in affected girls.
2. *Frequency and duration of bleeding.* A history of bleeding on some occasions but not others does not exclude the diagnosis of a primary bleeding disorder. Patients with mild von Willebrand disease or factor XI deficiency, for example, may have this type of history.
3. *Events frequently complicated by bleeding.* These include menorrhagia or postpartum bleeding in von Willebrand disease.
4. *Location of bleeding.* In platelet disorders, epistaxis, cutaneous bleeding, and excessive menstrual bleeding are common. In hemophilia, joint bleeding is typical.
5. *Medications.* See Table 98.2 for a list of drugs that alter platelet activity or coagulation.
6. *Family history.* Most coagulation and platelet disorders are autosomal recessive; the inheritance pattern of von Willebrand disease is autosomal dominant, and hemophilia A and B (Factor VIII and IX deficiency, respectively) are X-linked recessive disorders.

Examination findings provide important clues to the nature of bleeding disorders. In platelet abnormalities or vascular defects, hemorrhage is usually mucosal or cutaneous. Bleeding secondary to a clotting factor deficiency is often intramuscular or intra-articular. The presence of petechiae indicates a platelet or vascular defect rather than deficiencies of clotting factors. Quantitative platelet disorders are associated with petechiae only when the platelet count is

TABLE 98.1

DISTINGUISHING PLATELET-TYPE BLEEDING DISORDERS FROM COAGULATION DISORDERS

	Hereditary			
	Hemophilia	**von Willebrand disease**	**Qualitative platelet abnormalities**	**Blood vessel disorders**
Genetics	X-linked recessive	Autosomal dominant	Autosomal dominant Autosomal recessive	Autosomal dominant
Type of bleeding	Hemarthrosis Visceral CNS Soft tissues	Mucocutaneous	Mucocutaneous	Mucocutaneous Arterial rupture (connective tissue disorders)
Onset of bleeding after injury	Delayed	Immediate	Immediate	Immediate
Physical examination findings	Joint deformities Hematomas Ecchymoses	Ecchymoses	Petechiae Ecchymoses	Ecchymoses, telangiectasia (HHT), skin, joint, and eye abnormalities (connective tissue disorders)
Coagulation tests	aPTT: Abn	aPTT: Abn/N	N	N
Bleeding time	N	Abn/N	Abn/N	N/Abn

	Acquired		
	Coagulation	**Platelet**	**Blood vessel disorders**
Type of bleeding	Visceral Soft tissues	Mucocutaneous	Mucocutaneous
Onset of bleeding	Delayed	Immediate	Immediate
Physical examination findings	Hematomas Ecchymoses	Petechiae Ecchymoses	Ecchymoses Perifollicular hemorrhage (scurvy)
Coagulation tests	PT: Abn/N aPTT: Abn/N	N	N
Bleeding time	N	Abn	N/Abn

Abn, abnormal; *aPTT*, activated partial thromboplastin time; *CNS*, central nervous system; *HHT*, hereditary hemorrhagic telangiectasia; *N*, normal; *PT*, prothrombin time.

profoundly low. Purpura is found more commonly in platelet than in clotting factor disorders. Punctate telangiectases on the tongue, nasal mucosa, lips, or fingertips are diagnostic of hereditary hemorrhagic telangiectasia.

Laboratory evaluation is used to elucidate the underlying defect suggested by history and examination. Figure 98.1 provides a general algorithm for the evaluation of possible bleeding disorders. The platelet count can be obtained either by automated techniques or by estimating the number in the peripheral blood smear, a useful method for rapidly detecting low platelet counts. Normally, 3–10 platelets per high-power (oil immersion) field appear on the peripheral smear. The *bleeding time* is a crude measure of platelet function and is prolonged when the platelet count is below 90,000/μL or when a functional platelet abnormality is present. The platelet function analyzer (PFA-100®) is another tool available in some laboratories and may detect the presence of abnormal platelet function. While both the bleeding time and PFA-100® have varying sensitivities for platelet disorders and neither are predictive of surgical bleeding, the PFA-100 may

be the more sensitive assay. Platelet aggregometry measures temporal, semiquantitative, and qualitative parameters of platelet aggregation *in vitro*. This technique is of greatest value in diagnosing congenital qualitative platelet disorders.

The two most useful and commonly performed tests to assess the integrity of the coagulation system are the prothrombin time (PT) and activated partial thromboplastin time (aPTT). Whenever results of these tests are abnormal, they should be repeated on a fresh blood sample to be certain that the abnormality is not artifactual. The PT reflects the combined activity of clotting factors II, V, VII, and X and fibrinogen. The aPTT measures the combined activity of factors II, V, VIII, IX, X, XI, and XII and fibrinogen.

Other laboratory tests useful in pinpointing the diagnosis in coagulation disorders include the following:

1. *Fibrinogen* (quantitative). Decreased fibrinogen is seen most commonly in severe liver disease and disseminated intravascular coagulation (DIC). Heparin in the plasma sample may cause a falsely low value as a result of incomplete clotting.

TABLE 98.2

DRUGS THAT MAY ALTER HEMOSTASIS

Drugs reported to cause thrombocytopenia

Immune mechanisms proposed[a]

Quinine/quinidine	Ranitidine
Sulfa compounds	Cimetidine
Ampicillin	Danazol
Penicillin	Procainamide
Thiazide diuretics	Carbamazepine
Furosemide	Acetaminophen
Chlorthalidone	Phenylbutazone
Phenytoin	Aminosalicylate
α-Methyldopa	Rifampin
Heparin	Acetazolamide
Digitalis derivatives	Anazolene
Aspirin	Arsenicals
Valproic acid	

Nonimmune mechanisms (hemolytic-uremic syndrome)

Mitomycin C	
Cisplatin	Cyclosporine
	Ticlopidine

Mechanisms undefined
Gold compounds
Indomethacin

Drugs that alter platelet function

Primary antiplatelet agents

Aspirin	
Dextran	Sulfinpyrazone
Dipyridamole	Ticlopidine/clopidogrel
	Glycoprotein IIb/IIIa inhibitors

Drugs in which inhibition of platelet function is associated with prolongation of the bleeding time
Nonsteroidal antiinflammatory agents
β-lactam antibiotics
ε-Aminocaproic acid (>24 g/d)
Heparin
Plasminogen activators (streptokinase, urokinase, tissue plasminogen activator)

Drugs that affect coagulation factors

Induction of antibodies inhibiting function

Lupus anticoagulant[b]	Factor V antibodies
Phenothiazines	Aminoglycosides
Procainamide	Factor XIII antibodies
Factor VIII antibodies	Isoniazid
Penicillin	

Inhibitors of synthesis of vitamin K-dependent clotting factors (Factors II, VII, IX, X, proteins C and S)
Coumarin compounds
Moxalactam

Inhibitor of fibrinogen synthesis
L-asparaginase[c]

[a] List is limited to drugs for which there are multiple reports and *in vitro* or *in vivo* evidence of antiplatelet antibodies.
[b] Does not cause bleeding.
[c] May cause thrombosis.

2. *Specific factor assays.* Factor assays are performed by determining the extent to which the patient's plasma corrects the clotting time of plasma known to be deficient only in one particular clotting factor.

3. *Mixing tests* are used to detect inhibitors of clotting. When a plasma sample with a deficiency of one of the coagulation factors is mixed with an equal volume of normal plasma, the PT or aPTT is normalized. Conversely, if an inhibitor is present in the patient's plasma, the PT or aPTT will still be prolonged.

4. *Tests for fibrin degradation products.* Most tests measure plasmin degradation products of fibrin(ogen) by means of an antibody against fibrin. Fibrin degradation products are elevated in DIC and in liver and kidney failure, organs in which large and small fragments are cleared, respectively. Fibrin degradation products are also increased after major surgery and trauma. In the D-dimer test for intravascular clotting and fibrinolysis, a plasmin cleavage product of cross-linked fibrin, D, is measured. D-dimer is elevated in DIC, and venous thromboembolic disease, and after major surgery.

5. *Thrombin time* measures the ability of fibrin to form a clot. It is abnormal in the presence of a dysfibrinogenemia or heparin.

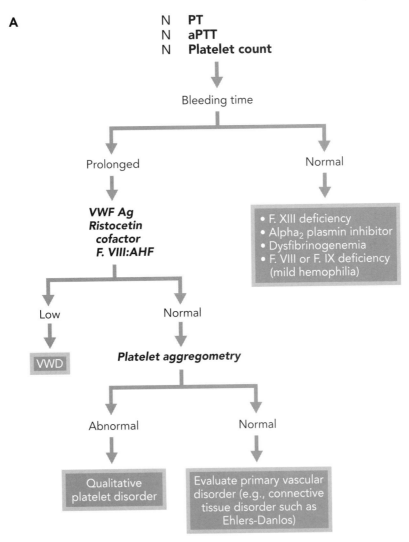

Figure 98.1A   A–E: Laboratory evaluation of clinical bleeding disorders. *A*, abnormal; *AHF*, antihemophilic factor; *aPTT*, activated partial thromboplastin time; *DIC*, disseminated intravascular coagulation; *FSP*, fibrin split products; *N*, normal; *PT*, prothrombin time; *RVV*, Russell viper venom test; *VWD*, von Willebrand disease; *VWF*, von Willebrand factor. ᵃAssumes patient is not receiving heparin. Consider checking aPTT on Hepasorb to rule out heparin effect if unsure. ᵇSupratherapeutic heparin or warfarin effect can result in elevations of both PT and aPTT.

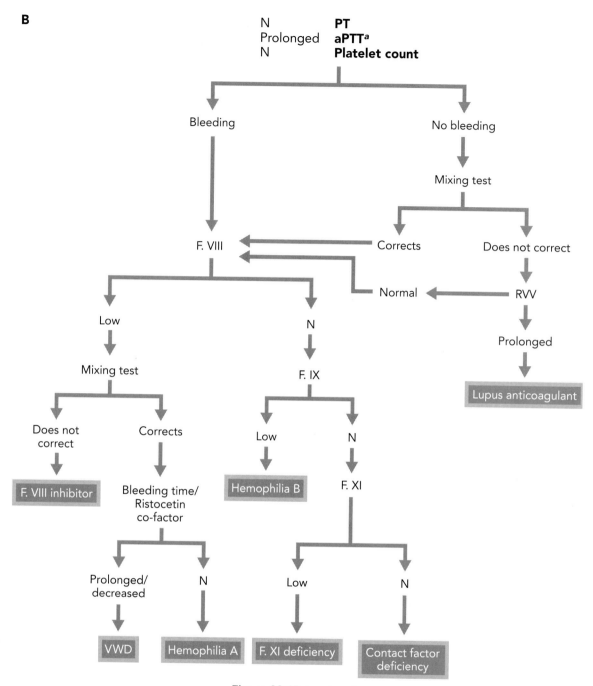

Figure 98.1B *(continued)*

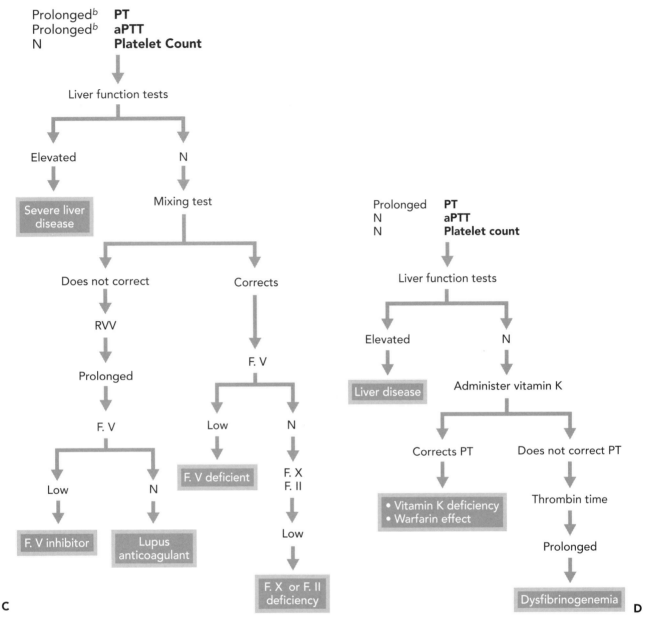

Figure 98.1C–D *(continued)*

Typical charges for the laboratory tests used in evaluating patients with disorders of bleeding (or clotting) are shown in Table 98.3.

Thrombotic Disorders

Acute venous thromboembolic (VTE) disease is diagnosed annually in approximately 250,000 patients; the major morbidity relates to recurrent disease, pulmonary embolism, and post-phlebitic syndrome. These patients and patients with thrombosis in an unusual location present some of the greatest medical challenges for treating physicians. When evaluating the patient presenting with thrombosis, it is necessary to define the nature and extent of thromboembolic disease

by addressing the following issues:

Does the disease involve the arterial or venous vasculature?

Is the clot located in the cerebral, peripheral, mesenteric, renal, or cardiopulmonary vessels?

Is there an underlying risk factor for thrombosis?

Should the patient undergo additional evaluation?

What type of anticoagulant should be used, and what is the optimal duration of therapy?

These questions will guide the treating physician in evaluating and treating the patient, and help determine if further hematologic consultation should be obtained.

The definition of *hypercoagulability* (also referred to as *thrombophilia*) is a clinical one (Table 98.4). No screening

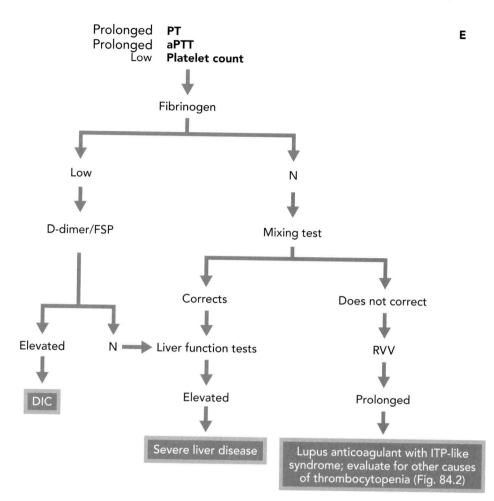

E

Figure 98.1E *(continued)*

TABLE 98.3

TYPICAL COSTS FOR TESTS USED IN THE LABORATORY EVALUATION OF BLEEDING AND THROMBOTIC DISORDERS[a]

PT	$9
aPTT	$13
Platelet count	$9
vWF disease panel	$95
Factor VIII activity	$25
Ristocetin cofactor	$89
vWF antigen	$71
Factor VIII (AHF) assay	$102
dRVVT	$23
Fibrinogen	$12
Bleeding time	$28
D-dimer	$20
Anticardiolipin antibody	$35
Antithrombin III	$26
Protein C	$56
Protein S	$56
Factor V Leiden and prothrombin 20210	$67
Homocysteine	$23

[a]Cost at a university hospital in 2004. Charges may be significantly higher.
AHF, antihemophilic factor; *aPTT*, activated partial thromboplastin time; *dRVVT*, dilute Russell viper venom time; *PT*, prothrombin time; *vWF*, von Willebrand factor.

test exists that identifies which patients have an underlying cause for their tendency to clot. In general, the hospital physician should try to determine whether the patient has elements of a primary or secondary form of thrombophilia (Table 98.5). It is important to distinguish whether the acute thrombosis arose in the arterial or venous vasculature, as the differential diagnosis differs for these two events.

The inherited disorders of thrombophilia pertain to either quantitative or qualitative abnormalities of the natural anticoagulant system. Deficiencies in the natural anticoagulants antithrombin (AT), protein C, and protein S account

TABLE 98.4

GENERAL CLINICAL FEATURES OF HYPERCOAGULABILITY

- Positive family history
- Recurrent thromboses
- Idiopathic thrombosis on trivial provocation, especially in a patient under age 65
- Unusual site of thrombosis (i.e., Visceral, cerebral, axillary, or cutaneous vessels)
- Recurrent thrombosis despite adequate anticoagulation

TABLE 98.5

CAUSES OF THROMBOEMBOLIC DISEASE

Primary (inherited)

Deficiencies of natural inhibitors or qualitative abnormalities of the clotting cascade
  Antithrombin deficiency
  Protein C deficiency
  Protein S deficiency
  Factor V Leiden mutation
  Prothrombin 20210
  Hyperhomocysteinemia
Qualitative abnormalities of fibrinogen
  Dysfibrinogenemia
Defects in the fibrinolytic system with impaired clot lysis

Secondary (acquired)

Abnormalities of coagulation and fibrinolysis
  Disseminated intravascular coagulation
  Malignancy
  Pregnancy, estrogen use
  Nephrotic syndrome
  Inflammatory bowel disease
  Lupus anticoagulant
  Anti-phospholipid antibody syndrome
Abnormalities of platelets
  Myeloproliferative disorders: essential thrombocytosis,
    polycythemia rubra vera
  Paroxysmal nocturnal hemoglobinuria
  Heparin-induced thrombocytopenia
Abnormalities of blood vessels and rheology
  Venous stasis—congestive heart failure, immobilization, obesity,
    age, postoperative state
  Artificial surfaces (grafts)
  Vasculitis
  Hyperviscosity syndromes (Waldenstrom's, leukostasis)
  Thrombotic thrombocytopenic purpura

TABLE 98.6

SUGGESTED LABORATORY WORKUP FOR PRIMARY HYPERCOAGULABILITY IN A PATIENT SUSPECTED OF HAVING A HYPERCOAGULABLE STATE[a]

Must be sent while patient is off anticoagulants[b]	Can be sent while patient is on anticoagulants
Protein C	DNA-based tests
Protein S	Factor V Leiden mutation
Antithrombin III	Prothrombin 20210 mutation
Lupus anticoagulant (dilute	Homocysteine level
Russell viper venom time)[c]	Antiphospholipid antibody assay

[a] For example, a young patient presenting with an idiopathic episode of thromboembolism. See Table 98.3 for typical charges for these tests. Also, see text for additional screening studies for hypercoagulable states (e.g., cancer workup).
[b] Either send before anticoagulation is initiated or send after a treatment course is completed. If an abnormal test result will lead to lifelong therapy, consider repeating test before acting on one abnormal result.
[c] Although the lupus anticoagulant is not a "primary" hypercoagulable state, a test for it should be included in the workup of a patient with an idiopathic thromboembolism because of its high rate of recurrent venous and arterial thromboembolic disease.

for only 15% of selected patients with juvenile or recurrent thrombosis and 5%–10% of unselected cases of acute venous thrombosis. Factor V Leiden mutation, hyperhomocysteinemia, and the prothrombin 20210 polymorphism account for a greater number of hypercoagulable patients (1).

An approach to the laboratory workup of patients suspected of having hypercoagulable blood is shown in Table 98.6. Note that certain tests can be interpreted only while patients are off anticoagulant medications.

Antithrombin Deficiency

Antithrombin inactivates thrombin and factors Xa, IXa, XIa, and XIIa. Its anticoagulant activity is enhanced by the presence of heparin, which forms a ternary complex with AT and the procoagulant factors. A deficiency of this natural anticoagulant results in recurrent VTE.

The inheritance pattern of AT deficiency is autosomal dominant. The frequency of symptomatic AT deficiency in the general population has been estimated to be between 1 in 2,000 and 1 in 5,000. In unselected patients with a history of VTE, the frequency is 1.1%; in selected patients with histories of recurrent VTE or a familial history, the frequency is approximately 2.4%. The majority of affected persons are heterozygotes with AT levels between 40%–70% of normal. Of the three types of AT deficiency, the majority is either type I or II and can be diagnosed by determining the functional AT level.

Deficiency of Proteins C and S

Proteins C and S are vitamin K-dependent glycoproteins that are involved in the inactivation of activated factors V and VIII. Protein C is slowly activated by thrombin to form activated protein C (APC). This activation is enhanced by the formation of complexes with thrombin and the endothelial receptor thrombomodulin. Protein S in and of itself has no intrinsic anticoagulant activity. Instead, it enhances the affinity of APC for negatively charged phospholipids, such as the platelet surface, by forming a membrane-bound APC–protein S complex that renders factors Va and VIIIa more easily accessible to APC-mediated cleavage.

Deficiencies in protein C and protein S are transmitted as autosomal dominant traits. Homozygous protein C deficiency is associated with neonatal purpura fulminans and warfarin-induced skin necrosis. The frequency of protein C and protein S deficiencies is 2.2%–3.2% in unselected patients with venous thrombosis and 3% to 3.8% in selected patients.

Factor V Leiden Mutation

The factor V Leiden mutation is represented by a single adenine-to-guanine point mutation in the gene encoding coagulation factor V. This results in the replacement of arginine by glutamine at a key proteolytic site on the activated factor V protein, such that the molecule cannot be cleaved by activated protein C—hence the so-called "APC resistance." Factor V clotting activity is normal in coagulation assays. Rather, factor V is resistant to inactivation *in vivo*. The factor V Leiden mutation is found in 2%–5% of the asymptomatic Caucasian population, and it accounts for approximately 40% of patients presenting with idiopathic VTE disease. It has also been associated with increased risks for recurrent venous thromboembolism, for venous thrombosis during use of oral contraceptives and pregnancy, and for thrombosis in the presence of other genetic and acquired abnormalities of anticoagulation, such as protein C and S deficiencies (2).

Prothrombin 20210

A polymorphism in the 3'-untranslated region of the prothrombin (factor II) gene is associated with mild increases in plasma prothrombin levels and in the risk for venous thrombosis. The factor II 20210A polymorphism may be found in 18% of selected patients with a personal and family history of venous thrombosis, in 6.2% of unselected consecutive patients presenting with their first idiopathic deep venous thrombosis, and in 2.3% of normal controls. Carriers of the 20210A allele have a 2.8-fold increased risk for VTE.

The clinical manifestations in patients with protein C, protein S, AT deficiencies, or the Leiden and prothrombin mutations are very similar. More than 90% of patients present with venous thrombosis of the lower extremity, with or without accompanying pulmonary embolus. A minority of patients (generally 5%) present with venous thrombosis in an unusual location, such as the sagittal sinus or mesenteric vessels. Rarely are these disorders associated with arterial thrombosis. VTE develops in 60%–80% of people heterozygous for AT, protein C, or protein S deficiency, typically before the age 40–45. About 50% of patients have recurrent disease. People with the Leiden and prothrombin mutations have a lesser tendency for thrombosis, and the first episode of thrombosis often occurs at a more advanced age. However, the concomitant occurrence of the factor V Leiden or prothrombin mutation and AT, protein C, or protein S deficiency greatly enhances a person's risk for thrombosis.

About 50% of patients with these thrombophilic defects have no inciting event as the cause of their deep venous thrombosis. In the remaining patients, thrombosis may be associated with minor trauma, pregnancy, use of oral contraceptives, recent surgery, or immobilization. The frequency of thrombosis during pregnancy and the peripartum period has been thought to be quite high (31% and 44%, respectively, for AT deficiency; 10% and 19%, respectively, for protein C and protein S deficiency; 28% for the Leiden mutation), although recent studies suggest a lower risk. Administration of estrogen to a woman with the factor V Leiden or Prothrombin mutation will increase her risk of developing cerebral vein thrombosis, and recurrent fetal loss has been associated with the presence of these genetic thrombophilic defects. The frequency of postoperative thrombosis has been shown to be high in patients with AT, protein C, or protein S deficiencies: 21% in patients undergoing abdominal surgery and 37% in patients undergoing high-risk orthopedic or cancer surgery. Patients with factor V Leiden mutation do not have an increased risk for thrombosis after joint replacement surgery if treated with appropriate anticoagulant prophylaxis.

Hyperhomocysteinemia

The early descriptions of hyperhomocysteinemia involved patients with homozygous mutations in genes encoding for enzymes of homocysteine metabolism. The classic disorder of hyperhomocysteinemia is associated with a mutation in cystathionine β-synthase that leads to fasting plasma homocysteine concentrations as high as 100–400 mmol/L (normal, <16 mmol/L). The clinical manifestations of this disorder include mental retardation, ectopic lens, skeletal abnormalities, premature arterial disease, and venous thrombosis. Severe elevations in plasma homocysteine are also associated with homozygous defects of the methylenetetrahydrofolate reductase (MTHFR) gene or of various enzymes that participate in the vitamin B_{12} cycle. However, these mutations are uncommon.

More common forms of hyperhomocysteinemia are subtle in presentation and may be caused by less severe defects in genes encoding for enzymes or by inadequate status of vitamins involved in homocysteine metabolism. Inadequate folate, vitamin B_{12}, or pyridoxine may result in a substantial increase in plasma homocysteine concentration. When present in the homozygous state, a common thermolabile polymorphism of the MTHFR gene has been found to be associated with elevated homocysteine levels in the setting of folate deficiency.

Mild (16–24 mmol/L) and moderate (25–100 mmol/L) hyperhomocysteinemia has been shown to be an independent risk factor for stroke, myocardial infarction, peripheral arterial disease, and extracranial carotid artery stenosis. It has also been shown to be a risk factor for VTE disease, and it augments the risk for VTE associated with oral contraceptive use, pregnancy, trauma and surgery, immobilization, and inherited disorders of thrombophilia, most notably factor V Leiden mutation and presence of lupus anticoagulant.

As the evaluation of inherited causes of hypercoagulability is both complex and expensive (Table 98.3), it is generally best directed by a hematologist or by a specialist knowledgeable in this area.

ISSUES IN THE HOSPITALIZED PATIENT

Approach to the Bleeding Patient

Thrombocytopenia

The most common causes of abnormal bleeding in hospitalized patients are acquired thrombocytopenia, an acquired qualitative platelet defect (e.g., associated with aspirin use), or the presence of a structural lesion. Thrombocytopenia can be caused by disturbances in production, distribution, or destruction (Figure 98.2). With splenic enlargement, platelet

pooling increases, which can cause thrombocytopenia. Platelet counts below 30,000–50,000/μL are unusual. Hypoplasia of hematopoietic stem cells can cause thrombocytopenia. Causes of hypoplasia include decreased numbers of megakaryoblasts following injury of the bone marrow by drugs, chemicals, or radiation, and replacement of bone marrow by abnormal tissue, most commonly cancer. Examination of the bone marrow reveals decreased numbers of megakaryocytes and either an overall decrease in cellularity or infiltration by abnormal cells.

Decreased production of platelets may also be a consequence of abnormal maturation of megakaryocytes. Deficiencies of either vitamin B_{12} or folate can cause ineffective thrombocytopoiesis leading to thrombocytopenia (Chapter 89). Similarly, abnormal platelet production is common in hematopoietic dysplasias. In both disorders, megakary-

Initial evaluation

Dilutional	Increased peripheral destruction		Sequestration
Cause	Cause	Laboratory findings	Cause
Massive transfusion	1. Sepsis	Leukocytosis	Hypersplenism (Check physical examination, liver-spleen scan)
	2. Disseminated intravascular coagulation	PT-Prolonged or N aPTT-Prolonged or N Schistocytes Fibrinogen-decreased D-dimer-increased	
	3. Thrombotic thrombocytopenic purpura/hemolytic-uremic syndrome	Anemia Schistocytes LDH-elevated BUN/creatinine-elevated PT/aPTT-N	
	4. Cardiac: Post-cardiac bypass, prosthetic heart valve	Anemia Schistocytes LDH-elevated	
	5. Platelet antibodies	Normal screening studies	

Secondary evaluation
(Negative initial evaluation or additional evidence necessary for diagnosis)

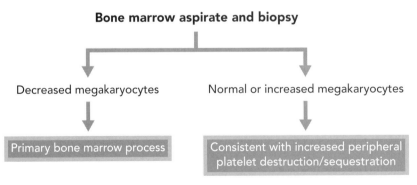

Bone marrow aspirate and biopsy

Decreased megakaryocytes → Primary bone marrow process

Normal or increased megakaryocytes → Consistent with increased peripheral platelet destruction/sequestration

Figure 98.2 Evaluation of thrombocytopenia. *aPTT*, activated partial thromboplastin time; *BUN*, blood urea nitrogen; *LDH*, lactate dehydrogenase; *N*, normal; *PT*, prothrombin time.

ocytes are usually increased. In hematopoietic dysplasia, megakaryocytes may be abnormal in appearance.

Increased peripheral destruction or decreased production of platelets as consequences of drug therapy are probably the most common causes of thrombocytopenia in hospitalized patients. The etiology of drug-induced thrombocytopenia is typically destruction of platelets by drug-induced antibodies (Table 98.2). More than 50 drugs have been reported to cause immune thrombocytopenia, but conclusive confirmation is rare (3, 4). In most instances, the drug must be present to cause antibody binding and thrombocytopenia, and the platelet count returns to normal within a few days after discontinuation. Glucocorticoids do not accelerate recovery. Platelet antibody tests, with and without the putative offending agent, are useful in determining the cause of thrombocytopenia, but they cannot be performed until the drug clears from the plasma. In addition, a drug metabolite, rather than the parent compound, may be responsible for antibody formation. Unless the metabolite is specifically tested, a negative result will be obtained.

Heparin therapy is associated with a transient decline in the platelet count that often resolves spontaneously despite continuation of the drug. This early thrombocytopenia (within five days of initial therapy) may be seen in more than 9% of patients. A more worrisome association of thrombocytopenia with heparin occurs after 5–10 days of initial heparin therapy. In 3%–5% of patients receiving unfractionated heparin therapy, platelet counts fall by more than 50%, or patients become frankly thrombocytopenic. This *heparin-induced thrombocytopenia* is mediated by the induction of an IgG antibody that binds the heparin-platelet factor 4 complex, which in turn binds the Fc receptor of an adjacent platelet, causing platelet aggregation and clearance. Heparin-induced thrombocytopenia is seen with both full-dose unfractionated heparin and low-dose therapy, and it occurs with the low-molecular-weight heparins, but to a lesser extent. Heparin-induced thrombocytopenia does not result in abnormal bleeding. Rather, in a subset of patients, arterial or venous thrombosis may ensue, posing a therapeutic challenge (see later in this chapter).

Idiopathic thrombocytopenic purpura (ITP) is an autoimmune bleeding disorder characterized by the development of antibodies to one's own platelets, which are then destroyed by phagocytosis in the spleen and liver. In adults, the onset is usually gradual, lacks a preceding illness, and runs a chronic course. In a small percentage of adult cases, the disease has an acute onset. Ninety percent of adults with ITP are under age 40, and the ratio of women to men is between 3:1 and 4:1. Petechiae, ecchymoses, and epistaxis develop, and menorrhagia may develop in women. Death from hemorrhage occurs in about 5% of patients with chronic ITP. Cerebral bleeding occurs in approximately 1% of cases. The diagnosis of ITP depends on excluding underlying systemic disorders that result in increased peripheral destruction or decreased production of platelets. On physical examination, the spleen is not enlarged. In ITP, the hemoglobin level is normal unless the patient has significant bleeding. Peripheral blood smears reveal normochromic, normocytic red blood cells. The value of antiplatelet antibody assays in diagnosing ITP is uncertain. In most cases of ITP, the diagnosis is clear, making it unnecessary to confirm the presence of antiplatelet antibodies. In complex cases, the antibody test may be helpful. If the clinical evaluation and blood tests do not identify any systemic disorder causing the thrombocytopenia, the bone marrow should be examined. In ITP, the marrow is normal, although megakaryocytes may be increased in number.

Patients with ITP and platelet counts below 20,000/μL are usually symptomatic and require treatment. Initially, bleeding associated with ITP is treated with prednisone or a similar corticosteroid at a dose of 1–2 mg/kg daily. In 80%–90% of patients, the platelet count rises to hemostatic levels within 2–3 weeks. Failure to respond to steroids is indicated by a platelet count below 50,000/μL after 4 weeks of treatment. A subnormal platelet count after 6 weeks of treatment also indicates steroid failure. Once the platelet count has reached its apex and is stable, steroids are tapered slowly. However, when the dose of prednisone is tapered, most patients (>90%) exhibit a recurrence of thrombocytopenia. Thus, the primary benefit of prednisone is in the acute management of bleeding.

Another effective approach to managing patients with ITP who are actively bleeding or for whom major surgery is necessary is the use of *intravenous gamma globulin*. IgG concentrate raises the platelet count within 3–5 days in most patients and is the most rapidly active agent. Unfortunately, the therapeutic effect is usually transient, with the platelet count falling to baseline levels during the next month. The dosage is 1 g/kg daily for two successive days. In 80% of patients, subsequent platelet counts rise above 50,000/μL. A slightly less expensive alternative is anti-Rh antibody (Winrho), which may be effective in Rh-positive patients with intact spleens (5).

Given the lack of a sustained remission in most patients with severe ITP treated with steroids or IgG, a more definitive approach is often necessary. *Splenectomy* improves the platelet count in 70% of patients with ITP and induces a sustained remission in approximately 60%, but no tests reliably predict which patients will respond. The platelet count rises within a few days after splenectomy, or at most in 1–2 weeks. A more recent approach to treating patients with ITP is the use of *Rituximab* (Rituxan®), an anti-CD20 antibody. CD-20 is present on the surface of B lymphocytes. Immunotherapy with an anti-CD20 antibody has resulted in clinical remissions of a number of malignant and benign lymphoproliferative disorders, including ITP.

The management of ITP in pregnancy is complicated by the additional risk for the development of thrombocytopenia in the fetus, secondary to maternal antibodies. Intraventricular hemorrhage, gastrointestinal bleeding, and death have been reported in such newborns. When ITP first develops during pregnancy, the risk for serious bleeding in the newborn is negligible. Conversely, neonates born to women with a history of ITP preceding pregnancy have a 20% risk for severe thrombocytopenia. In addition to treating the underlying ITP, some experts recommend cesarean delivery in this situation to decrease the risk for intracranial bleeding in the newborn, although this is controversial.

Antibodies directed against platelets may occur in several disorders other than ITP. Antibody-mediated destruction of platelets occurs in lymphoproliferative disorders, such as chronic lymphocytic leukemia and lymphoma. Generally, thrombocytopenia improves with treatment of the underlying malignancy. The platelet count improves with immunosuppressive therapy such as prednisone. Immune thrombocytopenia is also common in systemic lupus erythematosus (Chapter 112). The platelet count is usually mildly-to-moderately decreased. Other manifestations of the disease are present in most cases. Immune thrombocytopenia occurs less commonly in other systemic autoimmune disorders. Thrombocytopenia associated with antiplatelet antibodies has been reported in patients with infectious mononucleosis, HIV infection, and cytomegalovirus infection. In the case of infectious mononucleosis and cytomegalovirus infection, thrombocytopenia is usually self-limited, with recovery in 3–4 weeks. In patients with severe thrombocytopenia and bleeding, a short course of glucocorticoids may help raise the platelet count.

When packed erythrocytes or non-fresh whole blood is transfused to replace lost blood, thrombocytopenia may ensue (Chapter 91). Approximately 35%–40% of platelets remain in the circulation after replacement of 1 blood volume; microvascular bleeding from thrombocytopenia occurs rarely after replacement of 1–2 volumes. Platelets should be transfused only when thrombocytopenia and bleeding are present. Finally, microangiopathies associated with an increased consumption of platelets (as in DIC) are often the cause of thrombocytopenia in hospitalized patients (see later in this chapter).

Qualitative Disorders of Platelet Function

Drugs that inhibit platelet function include nonsteroidal anti-inflammatory agents, which inhibit platelet function by blocking platelet synthesis of prostaglandins. Aspirin permanently impairs platelet function. One aspirin tablet is sufficient to cause this effect. Fortunately, in most people, this does not result in excessive bleeding, but in patients with von Willebrand disease or with severe coagulation factor deficiency, serious bleeding can result. Therefore, aspirin is contraindicated in these disorders. High doses of β-lactam antibiotics induce an abnormality in platelet function that persists for 2–3 days after the drug is discontinued. The mechanism is unclear. The bleeding time is prolonged, and patients may have increased bleeding.

Platelets function abnormally in patients with renal failure. The uremic metabolites responsible for this dysfunction are uncertain. Thrombocytopenia is uncommon and usually mild, and it may be a consequence of the underlying cause of renal disease. Uremic bleeding is usually mucocutaneous and reflects abnormal platelet or vascular hemostasis. The bleeding time is commonly prolonged, but other causes of prolongation must be excluded. Hematocrits of <24% also prolong the bleeding time in uremia. Transfusion of packed red blood cells to elevate the hematocrit above 26% improves the bleeding time, and is thus a reasonable therapeutic approach for patients with acute bleeding or whose risk for bleeding is high. Administration of recombinant erythropoietin to raise the hematocrit above 26% is also effective as prophylaxis against bleeding before elective surgery or in cases of chronic blood loss.

When abnormal bleeding develops in a uremic patient, one must evaluate the possibilities of a structural lesion and other hemostatic abnormalities. Platelet abnormalities are seldom the sole cause. When the hemostatic defect of renal failure is believed to be a significant contributing factor to bleeding, the patient should undergo dialysis (Chapter 101). Both peritoneal dialysis and hemodialysis usually reverse the hemostatic defect. If the bleeding time remains prolonged and the patient is bleeding, other agents can be tried. In order of preference, these are low-dose conjugated estrogens, 1-deamino-8-D-arginine vasopressin (DDAVP), and cryoprecipitate. Their efficacy, however, has not been firmly established. Platelet transfusion usually has no benefit.

Platelet function is sometimes abnormal in liver disease, but the extent to which this contributes to bleeding is unclear. The bleeding time may be prolonged in moderately severe liver disease when the platelet count is <90,000/μL. DDAVP has been reported to improve the bleeding time in these circumstances. More commonly in hepatic failure, a bleeding diathesis is secondary to deficiencies of coagulation factors (Chapters 82 and 83).

The inherited disorders of platelet function are found in a minority of hospitalized patients, but the presence of these disorders should be suspected in those patients with a supportive history of bleeding. Patients may provide a lifelong history of easy bruising, epistaxis, and prolonged oozing after venipuncture, dental extractions, and menses. These disorders often are characterized by a prolonged bleeding time and by platelets that fail to aggregate normally when stimulated with specific agonists, the particular pattern depending on which disorder is present. The platelet count is normal in most of these disorders.

The most common congenital bleeding disorder is *von Willebrand disease*. An autosomal dominant disorder, it is characterized by a deficiency of von Willebrand factor, which is necessary for the adhesion of platelets to connective tissue. Because von Willebrand factor is a carrier protein for factor VIII, patients with von Willebrand disease can be deficient in both activities. In most patients, *von Willebrand disease causes a platelet-like bleeding diathesis.* The manifestations of disease differ from those of hemophilia in that bleeding is predominantly confined to the skin and mucous membranes; hemarthrosis is rare.

There are three general types of von Willebrand disease, based on whether the defect is quantitative (type I, the most common, and type III) or qualitative (type II). Measurement of the bleeding time is often the first screening test employed, but the bleeding time may be normal in some patients. A specific assay of von Willebrand factor is the measurement of the response of platelets to ristocetin. In the presence of ristocetin and von Willebrand factor, platelets agglutinate. Deficiency of factor VIII/von Willebrand factor can be quantified by measuring the extent of platelet agglutination in response to a standard concentration of ristocetin. The level of von Willebrand factor in plasma is also measured by immunologic techniques. However, the diagnosis of von Willebrand disease can be exceptionally difficult because the concentrations of von Willebrand factor and factor VIII in persons with and without von Willebrand disease can fluctuate considerably. Factors known to increase the concentrations of von Willebrand factor and factor VIII are stress, pregnancy, use of oral contraceptives, and estrogen replacement therapy in postmenopausal women.

Most types of von Willebrand disease are treated with administration of DDAVP, which is thought to increase endothelial cell release of stored von Willebrand factor. For those patients with severe quantitative defects of von Willebrand factor and qualitative defects, infusion of factor VIII concentrates enriched with von Willebrand factor may be necessary (6).

Treatment of Bleeding Patients with Platelet Disorders

The Role of Platelet Transfusions

When serious bleeding complicates thrombocytopenia, platelet transfusions are effective only if the cause is decreased production. Thrombocytopenia secondary to increased peripheral destruction or sequestration is usually refractory to platelet transfusion. Bleeding secondary to qualitative platelet disorders ordinarily responds to platelet transfusions, except when the bleeding diathesis is a consequence of uremia or hepatic failure or when an offending drug persists in the circulation. For patients with congenital platelet disorders, platelets must be transfused judiciously because repeated transfusions stimulate the production of allo-antibodies. Eventually, it may become impossible to raise the platelet count through transfusion. Accordingly, platelet transfusions should be reserved for serious bleeding or in preparation for surgery in patients with moderately severe platelet defects.

TABLE 98.7

RISK FOR BLEEDING IN PATIENTS WITH THROMBOCYTOPENIA, ACCORDING TO PLATELET COUNT[a]

Platelet count (#/μL)	Usual clinical consequences
>100,000	No abnormal bleeding, even with major surgery.
50,000–100,000	Patients may bleed longer than normal with severe trauma.
20,000–50,000	Bleeding occurs with minor trauma, but spontaneous bleeding is unusual.
<20,000	Patients may have spontaneous bleeding.
<10,000	Patients are at high risk for severe bleeding.

[a]Assumes normal platelet function.

The consequences of thrombocytopenia are entirely hemostatic. The risk for bleeding varies according to the platelet count (Table 98.7) (7).

Platelet transfusions are indicated for patients who are bleeding actively and have either a platelet count below 50,000/μL or a qualitative platelet abnormality manifested by a prolonged bleeding time. Platelet transfusions may also be indicated prophylactically before surgery or other invasive procedures. Before surgery, platelet counts should be above 50,000/μL in most cases, and above 90,000/μL for procedures such as neurosurgery or ophthalmologic surgery, in which any abnormal bleeding may cause excessive morbidity. For invasive procedures, such as kidney or liver biopsies, a platelet count above 50,000/μL is probably sufficient, provided platelet function is normal.

For patients who require platelet transfusions continually, platelets should be obtained from a single donor for each transfusion (generally 6–7 units) to reduce the risk for formation of multiple allo-antibodies (see later in this chapter). In a 70-kg patient, one unit of platelets usually raises the platelet count by approximately 10,000/μL. The count should be repeated 10–60 minutes after transfusion to assess the compatibility of the transfused platelets and to determine whether the desired count has been achieved. In actively bleeding patients, the platelet count should be maintained above 50,000/μL.

Allo-antibodies Against Platelets

In approximately 50%–60% of patients who become refractory to random donor platelets, anti-HLA (human leukocyte antigen) antibodies appear to be responsible. If this occurs, platelet cross-matching to find compatible donors is performed. Usually, a panel of platelets from 20–30 donors is tested. If a satisfactory response is not achieved with cross-matched platelets, HLA-compatible platelets are used because HLA antigens are the most important in determining allo-immunization. Antibodies against platelet-specific antigens probably represent fewer than 1% of allo-immunization problems. Cross-matched platelets are available immediately, whereas HLA-compatible platelets usually are not available for 24 hours. With cross-matching, a number of compatible units may be identified with one test, but HLA testing is performed one donor at a time. The two platelet products are equally effective. Only 50% of refractory patients are refractory on the basis of allo-immunization.

Eventually, it may become impossible to raise the platelet count through transfusion. Accordingly, platelet transfusions should be reserved for serious bleeding or in preparation for surgery in patients with moderately severe platelet defects. When patients are refractory to platelet transfusion, consultation with a hematologist (if not already obtained) should be requested.

Platelet Growth Factors

Recently, it was discovered that recombinant forms of the cytokine interleukin 11 (IL-11, also called Neumega) and the growth factor thrombopoietin have the ability to raise the platelet count in patients with bone marrow failure and thrombocytopenia secondary to chemotherapy. IL-11 has been approved for use by the U.S. Food and Drug Administration, and recombinant forms of thrombopoietin are in clinical trials. Because these agents work by stimulating platelet production, their utility in disorders characterized by platelet destruction is uncertain.

Coagulation Disorders Associated with Bleeding

Hospitalized patients may also have a known or previously undiagnosed coagulation disorder as a cause of their bleeding. With few exceptions, a clinically significant coagulation disorder will present with elevations in the PT, aPTT, or both (Figure 98.1).

In descending order of frequency, the differential diagnosis of isolated prolongation of the PT includes the following:

1. Early liver disease
2. Vitamin K deficiency
3. Early warfarin therapy
4. Factor VII deficiency in the early stage of any disorder in which multiple coagulation factors are depleted (e.g., DIC)

Sole prolongation of the PT without prolongation of the aPTT occurs when the coagulation disorder involves only factor VII. Any process that diminishes all coagulation factors will initially be manifested as an isolated prolongation of the PT, because factor VII has the shortest plasma half-life and becomes depleted first. Therefore, in early or mild liver disease, the PT is often prolonged (with a normal aPTT). However, as the disease progresses, eventually all coagulation factors are depleted, accompanied by prolon-

gations in both the PT and aPTT. Similarly, though vitamin K deficiency and warfarin can ultimately prolong both the PT and the aPTT, early vitamin K deficiency or early warfarin (Coumadin) therapy is generally associated with an isolated prolongation of the PT. Disorders such as DIC or dilutional coagulopathy (in which all coagulation factors are depleted) can also present in their early stages as an isolated prolongation of the PT.

Factors II, V, VII, VIII, IX, X, and XIII, fibrinogen, and probably factor XI are all synthesized in the liver. Moderately severe liver disease can lead to a deficiency of any combination of these factors and produce a bleeding diathesis. Liver disease can also increase a patient's risk for bleeding by causing thrombocytopenia secondary to congestive splenomegaly and increasing baseline fibrinolysis. Correction of the hemostatic defects in patients with liver failure and acute bleeding is difficult. Because of the short half-life of factor VII (6 hours), correction of the PT by transfusion of plasma is transient. With severe clotting factor deficiency, volume limitations necessitate the use of factor II/VII/IX/X concentrates (prothrombin complex) in addition to plasma. Hypofibrinogenemia is usually present in end-stage liver disease. When the fibrinogen level is <100 mg/dL, patients can be treated with cryoprecipitate. When significant thrombocytopenia secondary to portal hypertension is present, platelet transfusion is frequently ineffective because of splenic sequestration. Consequently, one can often improve but not completely correct the hemostatic defects associated with end-stage liver disease.

Vitamin K is required for calcium-dependent activation of factors II, VII, IX, and X. Consequently, vitamin K deficiency is associated with decreased activity of these factors and a hemorrhagic tendency. Vitamin K deficiency and consequent abnormalities in coagulation are not unusual in severely ill, hospitalized patients. Antibiotics that eliminate the intestinal bacteria that synthesize vitamin K are commonly used, and patients frequently have an inadequate dietary intake of vitamin K. Vitamin K deficiency as a cause of abnormal clotting is diagnosed empirically by assessing the results of administering vitamin K. Improvement of the PT should be seen within 6 hours, with total correction within 24 hours, if vitamin K deficiency was the culprit.

Severe bleeding can develop in patients given warfarin for anticoagulation, whether the international normalized ratio (INR) is in the target therapeutic range or excessively prolonged. When the INR is in a therapeutic range, the aPTT may be mildly prolonged or normal. A localized cause of bleeding should be sought under these circumstances. Depending on the severity of bleeding, patients can be treated with plasma replacement, or, in severe cases, prothrombin complex concentrates, recombinant activated factor VII (rFVIIa, Novo7®), and fresh frozen plasma. Vitamin K should also be administered in those patients with marked prolongation of the INR and major bleeding (8). The most common causes of an isolated elevation of the aPTT in a hospitalized patient are the presence of lupus anticoagulant, which is not associated with a bleeding diathesis, and unfractionated heparin therapy. Deficiencies of the factors that comprise the aPTT pathway and inhibitors of these factors are seen much less frequently, but they must be considered if the patient's bleeding is to be treated appropriately. Systemic administration of unfractionated heparin results in an elevated aPTT, or the aPTT can be increased artifactually when blood samples are drawn through intravenous lines containing heparin. Patients with the lupus anticoagulant and a prolonged aPTT are at increased risk for thrombosis. The remaining causes of an isolated, prolonged aPTT are relatively rare; they include hemophilia, other factor deficiencies, and inhibitors of clotting factors.

Patients in whom severe bleeding occurs while they are taking heparin usually have an underlying cause, such as a postoperative wound or a structural lesion (e.g., peptic ulcer, colonic polyp, recent trauma). Stopping the heparin is usually sufficient to stop the bleeding because heparin has a short half-life (about 1.5 hours). When life-threatening bleeding occurs and the aPTT is significantly prolonged by heparin, intravenous *protamine sulfate* can be given to reverse the effects of heparin. The amount given should be equivalent to the estimated dose of heparin given, with the short half-life of heparin taken into account (1 mg of protamine sulfate for approximately 90 units of heparin). If, for example, major bleeding occurs half an hour after a heparin bolus, the amount of protamine sulfate given should be equivalent to one-half the initial heparin dose. Protamine sulfate must administered cautiously—slowly over 10 minutes—as it can be associated with anaphylactic reactions. The anticoagulant effect of low-molecular-weight heparin is only partially neutralized by protamine sulfate.

The PT and aPTT are most likely to be prolonged together in clinical situations in which multiple clotting factors are diminished or altered in production (i.e., liver disease, vitamin K deficiency, warfarin therapy) or depleted through dilution or generalized consumption.

Hypercoagulability in the Hospitalized Patient

Secondary Thrombophilia

In the majority of patients admitted to the hospital with an idiopathic VTE event, an underlying cause is not diagnosed, and they are successfully treated with a standard regimen of heparin followed by warfarin. However, a minority of patients admitted to the hospital with thrombosis, and many patients in whom thrombosis develops while they are in the hospital, will be refractory to conventional treatment. Cancer patients with VTE, patients with chronic inflammatory bowel disease or a central line, patients undergoing revascularization procedures, and patients who have undergone transplantation of a solid organ are all at risk for the development of refractory thrombosis syndromes.

Hospitalized patients with thrombosis who have accompanying thrombocytopenia or coagulopathy are especially challenging. Anticoagulation in these patients must be approached with great caution.

The most common cause of hypercoagulability in hospitalized patients is secondary thrombosis associated with the postoperative state, prolonged immobilization, advanced age, or cancer. Thrombosis occurs after joint replacement surgery in more than 40%–60% of patients who do not receive prophylactic anticoagulation, and in approximately 30% of patients who do (5). Additionally, trauma, major abdominal surgery, and postoperative complications such as pneumonia, which prolong bed rest and immobilization, increase the risk for thrombosis.

The association of *thrombosis with cancer* is well documented, with or without accompanying DIC. In large series evaluating patients with deep venous thrombosis and pulmonary embolism (DVT/PE), more than 20% of patients had underlying cancer (9). In a cohort study of patients presenting with DVT/PE, the standardized incidence ratio for all types of cancer was 3 during the first 6 months of follow-up; at one year after the thrombotic event, it declined to one (10). The extent of an evaluation for cancer that should be performed in a patient presenting with DVT/PE is controversial, in that there is no evidence that early detection in this situation improves outcome. A reasonable approach would include a thorough physical examination, including breast and gynecologic examinations in a woman and a prostate examination in a man. Laboratory studies should determine the following: hematocrit, platelet count, PT, aPTT, fibrinogen level, and (in a man) possibly prostate-specific antigen level. Standard cancer screening techniques (such as colonoscopy or fecal occult blood testing and mammography) are appropriate, and chest radiography is also reasonable in this setting. Cancer patients with VTE are often refractory to warfarin treatment when it is given to achieve a standard target INR range of 2–3. Oftentimes, the thrombophilic disorder of these patients is best controlled by warfarin with an INR of 3–4 or with long-term low-molecular-weight heparin therapy, regardless of whether DIC complicates the picture (Chapter 52).

Heparin-induced thrombocytopenia should be considered in patients receiving heparin therapy when frank thrombocytopenia or a decrement of the platelet count by 50% occur. As discussed above, the exposure to heparin may not always be via a therapeutic heparin infusion. Patients with heparin-induced thrombocytopenia do not bleed; rather, they are at risk for the development of either arterial or venous thrombosis. These patients pose a great challenge because they cannot be treated with heparin (*either unfractionated or low-molecular-weight heparin*), and warfarin should not be used acutely as the sole anticoagulant. A hematology consultant should aid the treating physician in obtaining one of the newer thrombin inhibitor agents or heparinoids to treat these patients during episodes of acute thrombosis (11).

Central venous catheter-associated thrombosis is not uncommon, but it is often overlooked because of its initially subtle presentation. Neurology patients needing intermittent plasmapheresis, cancer patients receiving chemotherapy, patients with gastrointestinal disease who need nutrition or hydration, or patients with poor venous access often acquire some form of a central venous catheter while hospitalized. Central venous catheter-associated thrombosis may occur in 6%–60% of patients. The great variability in defining this complication is reflected in the broad range of definitions used in various clinical studies. The placement of central venous catheters is responsible for up to 60% of cases of superior vena cava syndrome in some series. The most common presentations of central venous catheter-associated thrombosis include a swollen, painful arm; facial swelling; breast swelling; overt superior vena cava syndrome (Chapter 92); evidence of an inferior vena caval clot associated with placement of a femoral vein line; or pulmonary embolus.

If these symptoms develop acutely while the patient is in the hospital and are severe, thrombolytic therapy, such as with tissue plasminogen activator (tPA), can be successfully administered (12), although rigorous studies proving its effectiveness are limited. Thrombolytic therapy should be administered in the ICU to allow close monitoring of laboratory test results and bleeding complications. Heparin therapy can be used concomitantly with and continued after the completion of the thrombolytic therapy. Bleeding commonly complicates the use of thrombolytic therapy in this setting. It typically manifests at the site of a large-bore venous catheter or any arterial puncture site, so caution should be exercised. Patients can then be treated for several months with warfarin (Chapter 52).

In very ill or medically complicated patients with significant pulmonary embolism, an inferior vena cava filter is often placed (Chapters 52 and 53). The presence of an inferior vena cava filter decreases the risk for subsequent pulmonary embolus acutely if the origin of the new clot is distal to the existing filter. However, placement of an inferior vena cava filter may be associated with recurrent VTE if the patient is not maintained on long-term anticoagulation (13).

Microangiopathies

The thrombotic microangiopathies are hematologic emergencies associated with abnormal clotting. They are characterized by the presence of microangiopathic hemolytic anemia, thrombocytopenia, microvascular thrombosis, and multiple organ dysfunction. Diagnosis of the microangiopathies is crucial to avoid the morbidity and mortality associated with these disorders.

Disseminated intravascular coagulation represents an imbalance of the clotting and fibrinolytic systems and is characterized by either clinical bleeding or clotting, thrombocytopenia, hypofibrinogenemia, and coagulopathy. It may be associated with an acute presentation of sepsis and clinical bleeding, or a subtle presentation with DVT or migrating thrombophlebitis. The classic *Trousseau's syndrome* is the syndrome of hypercoagulability associated with cancer, especially of the adenomucinous type, with or without DIC. In "well-compensated DIC", the patient presents with DIC characterized by a low-to-normal platelet count and a normal PT and aPTT. Once suspected, the diagnosis of DIC is confirmed by a review of the blood smear, which demonstrates the presence of schistocytes, and by laboratory findings of a low fibrinogen level and a positive D-dimer test result.

Patients with DIC and thrombosis can be treated both acutely and on a long-term basis with standard heparin therapy, although this is controversial. The patient with DIC who presents with bleeding presents a greater therapeutic challenge. Treatment of the underlying disorder is paramount, but not always feasible or successful. Patients can be supported with low-dose unfractionated heparin (300–500 units/h) in an attempt to control the consumptive thrombotic process. Platelet and cryoprecipitate transfusions may be necessary to treat the profound thrombocytopenia and hypofibrinogenemia, respectively. An antifibrinolytic agent (e.g., Amicar) is generally contraindicated unless the patient has excessive bleeding, in which case an antifibrinolytic agent may be a necessary addition to the heparin therapy. These complicated clinical scenarios are best handled with the active input of a hematologist who specializes in the clinical care of patients with coagulopathies.

Thrombotic thrombocytopenic purpura and *hemolytic uremic syndrome* are also thrombotic microangiopathies with overlapping clinical components. Hemolytic uremic syndrome is more common in children than in adults and is typically associated with a gastrointestinal illness caused by enterotoxigenic Gram-negative bacteria. Thrombotic thrombocytopenic purpura has been found to be an autoimmune disorder marked by the presence of an antibody directed against a metalloprotease responsible for cleaving large molecular weight forms of circulating von Willebrand factor (VWF). The TTP antibody inhibits the function of this protease, thereby inhibiting additional processing of VWF. The result is the presence of large multimeric forms of VWF in circulation, which are highly thrombogenic, leading to the widespread deposition of platelet microthrombi.

The classic presentation of thrombotic thrombocytopenic purpura includes the "pentad" of thrombocytopenia, microangiopathic hemolytic anemia, renal dysfunction, neurologic deficit, and fever. Hemolytic uremic syndrome, on the other hand, is characterized by only thrombocytopenia, anemia, and renal dysfunction. The clinical manifestations and systemic involvement of thrombotic thrombocytopenic purpura vary greatly, but the most consistent abnormalities include hemolytic anemia, with hematocrits in the 21%–26% range, and consumptive thrombocytopenia, with platelet counts in the range of 20,000–40,000/μL. In one review, only 34% of patients with the clinical diagnosis of thrombotic thrombocytopenic purpura had the classic pentad. Ninety-eight percent of patients had an elevated lactate dehydrogenase level, with a median value of 1,208 units/L (14).

The diagnosis of thrombotic thrombocytopenic purpura is crucial because untreated TTP is associated with a 90% mortality rate. Thrombosis of the microvasculature may involve the myocardial, cerebral, renal, or mesenteric vessels, resulting in marked dysfunction of the affected organs. Once the diagnosis is suspected, a hematologist should be consulted immediately to confirm the diagnosis and institute therapy. The mainstay of therapy is *plasmapheresis*, which is associated with a 56%–80% response rate. Salvage therapy for those patients refractory to plasmapheresis includes splenectomy, steroid therapy, and rituximab (15).

KEY POINTS

- Proper use and interpretation of screening tests—prothrombin time, activated partial thromboplastin time, and platelet count—will usually be sufficient to determine whether a patient has a bleeding disorder and to define it. A normal prothrombin time means that the patient does not have liver disease as a cause of bleeding; a normal bleeding time means that uremia-associated hemostatic abnormalities are not the cause of bleeding.
- Most causes of abnormal bleeding are acquired: drug-induced thrombocytopenia, sepsis, poor vitamin K intake, administration of antibiotics in the intensive care unit, anticoagulants, and liver and renal failure.
- Blood products should be used judiciously in patients with abnormal laboratory results. If the patient is not bleeding, or is bleeding with mild laboratory abnormalities, transfusion of fresh frozen plasma, platelets, or both is not likely to be indicated.
- A careful drug history is critical in evaluating thrombocytopenia in hospitalized patients. The diagnosis of thrombophilia, whether of primary or secondary cause, is often a clinical one that may affect the intensity and duration of anticoagulant therapy.
- Hypercoagulability in the hospitalized patient can result from the presence of an underlying disease, especially cancer, and the presence of central venous access catheters.
- Thrombophilia caused by heparin therapy or microangiopathies is rare but constitutes a medical emergency that necessitates consultation with a coagulation specialist.

REFERENCES

1. Joffe HV, Goldhaber SZ. Laboratory thrombophilias and venous thromboembolism. *Vasc Med* 2002;7:93–102.
2. Juul K, Tybjaerg-Hansen A, Schnohr P, et al. Factor V leiden and the risk for venous thromboembolism in the adult Danish population. *Ann Intern Med* 2004;140:330–337.
3. George JN, Raskob GE, Shah SR, et al. Drug-induced thrombocytopenia: a systematic review of published case reports. *Ann Inten Med* 1998;129:886–890.
4. Rizvi MA, Kojouri K, George JN. Drug-induced thrombocytopenia: an updated systematic review. *Ann Intern Med* 2001;134:346.
5. George JN. Initial management of adults with idiopathic (immune) thrombocytopenic purpura. *Blood Rev* 2002;16:37–38.
6. Cox Gill J. Diagnosis and treatment of von Willebrand disease. *Hematol Oncol Clin North Am* 2004;18:1277–1299.
7. Rebulla P. Revisitation of the clinical indications for the transfusion of platelet concentrates. *Rev Clin Exp Hematol* 2001;5:288–310; discussion 311–312.
8. Makris M. Management of excessive anticoagulation or bleeding. *Semin Vasc Med* 2003;3:279–284.
9. The Columbus Investigators. Low-molecular-weight heparin in the treatment of patients with venous thromboembolism. *N Engl J Med* 1997;337:557–562.
10. Sorenson HT, Mellemkjaer L, Steflensen FH, et al. The risk of a diagnosis of cancer after primary deep venous thrombosis or pulmonary embolism. *N Engl J Med* 1998;338:1169–1173.
11. Warkentin TE, Greinacher A. Heparin-induced thrombocytopenia: recognition, treatment, and prevention: the Seventh ACCP Conference on Antithrombotic and Thrombolytic Therapy. *Chest* 2004;126:311S–337S.
12. Bernardi E, Piccioli A, Marchiori A, et al. Upper extremity deep vein thrombosis: risk factors, diagnosis, and management. *Semin Vasc Med* 2001;1:105–110.
13. Decousus H, Leizorovicz A, Parent F, et al. A clinical trial of vena cava filters in the prevention of pulmonary embolism in patients with deep-vein thrombosis. Prévention du Risque d'Embolie Pulmonaire par Interruption Cave Study Group. *N Engl J Med* 1998;338:409–415.
14. Thompson CE, Damon LE, Ries CA, et al. Thrombotic microangiopathies in the 1980s. *Blood* 1992;80:1890–1895.
15. Lämmle B, George JN. Thrombotic thrombocytopenic purpura: advances in pathophysiology, diagnosis, and treatment. *Semin Hematol* 2004;41:60–67.

ADDITIONAL READING

Bauer KA. The thrombophilias: well-defined risk factors with uncertain therapeutic implications. *Ann Intern Med* 2001;135:367–373.
Dahlback B. Blood coagulation. *Lancet* 2000;355:1627–1632.
George JN. Platelets. *Lancet* 2000;55:1531–1539.
Greaves M, Cohen H, Machin SJ, et al. Guidelines on the investigation and management of the antiphospholipid syndrome. *Brit J Haematol* 2000;109:704–715.
Hambleton J. Diagnosis and incidence of von Willebrand disease. *Current Opinion Hematol* 2001;8:306–311.
Hayward CP. Inherited platelet disorders. *Curr Opin Hematol* 2003;10:362–368.
Heal JM, Blumberg N. Optimizing platelet transfusion therapy. *Blood Reviews* 2004;18:149–165.
Hirsh J, Albers GW, Guyatt GH, et al. eds. The Seventh ACCP Consensus Conference on Antithrombotic Therapy. *Chest* 2004;126 (Supplement).
Mannucci PM, Tuddenham EGD. The hemophilias—from royal genes to gene therapy. *New Eng J Med* 2001;344:1773–1779.
McKenna R. Abnormal coagulation in the postoperative period contributing to excessive bleeding. *Med Clin North Am* 2001;85:1277–1310.
Seligsohn U, Lubetsky A. Genetic susceptibility to venous thrombosis. *New Engl J Med* 2001;344:1222–1231.

Renal Disease

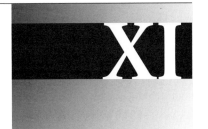

Signs, Symptoms, and Laboratory Abnormalities in Renal Disease

99

Rudolph A. Rodriguez   *Burl R. Don*

TOPICS COVERED IN CHAPTER
- Urinalysis 995
- Oliguria and Anuria 998
- Edema 1001
- Elevated BUN and Creatinine 1003

INTRODUCTION

The clinical presentation of renal disease varies from signs and symptoms caused directly by the kidney (hematuria, proteinuria, flank pain) to those caused by the systemic effects of kidney disease (hypertension, edema). However, many patients are asymptomatic despite significant renal disease. After the presence of significant renal disease is recognized, the primary goal of the history, physical examination, and laboratory assessment is to make a correct diagnosis of the cause. The proper interpretation of the urinalysis and diagnosis of the cause of oliguria, increasing blood urea nitrogen (BUN) and creatinine levels, or edema help guide therapy and predict prognosis.

RENAL SIGNS, SYMPTOMS, AND LABORATORY ABNORMALITIES

Urinalysis

Interpretation at Time of Admission

In deciding whether to hospitalize a patient, the urinalysis can serve as an invaluable tool in the initial evaluation. This is true regardless of whether the patient has renal disease or not. The urine dipstick provides a battery of tests, which can provide clues to liver disease, volume status, diabetic control, urinary tract infection or stones, acid-base derangements, multiple myeloma, and rhabdomyolysis. The urinalysis also serves as the first and most important diagnostic test in any patient with acute or chronic renal disease. There are no abnormalities of the urinalysis that in isolation would necessitate hospitalization, but abnormalities may support a diagnosis that requires hospitalization. Early attention to the urinalysis may expedite appropriate hospitalization, consultations, and treatment.

Specific Gravity

One of the common diagnostic dilemmas faced at the time of admission is determining fluid status. The urine specific gravity is a useful adjunct to the history and physical examination in indicating volume status and, more importantly, the *effective circulating volume*. Urine osmolality is an accurate reflection of antidiuretic hormone secretion. Urine osmolality ranges from a low of 50–100 mOsm/L in the absence of antidiuretic hormone, to 900–1200 mOsm/L in the presence of maximum arginine vasopressin (AVP) effect if there is normal renal function. Urine specific gravity correlates well with urine osmolality, and specific gravity increases by 0.001 for every increase in urine osmolality of 35–40 mOsm/L. Urine that is iso-osmolar with plasma has a urine osmolality of 280 mOsm/kg or a specific gravity of 1.008. However, osmolality is a measure of particles in solution, and specific gravity is a measure of the number of particles and weight expressed as weight compared with water. These differences may lead to situations in which specific gravity and urine osmolality do not correlate, such as if there are large amounts of large particles in the urine (e.g., contrast media, heavy proteinuria, glucosuria). This leads to a very high specific gravity (1.030–1.050); the urine osmolality may be much lower.

Urine pH

The urine pH is useful in evaluating patients with an anion-gap metabolic acidosis (Chapter 105) or monitoring the response to intravenous bicarbonate therapy. If alkali therapy is used to prevent acute renal failure from rhabdomyolysis or uric acid or sulfadiazine stone disease, the urine pH should be kept above 6.5–7.0. The urine pH loses its diagnostic value if the urine is infected with urease-producing bacteria such as *Proteus* or *Klebsiella* organisms, which raise the urine pH.

Leukocyte Esterase and Nitrites

Leukocyte esterase is released from neutrophils and normally is not found in urine. The urine leukocyte esterase test screens for more than 10 leukocytes per high-power field. Nitrate is reduced to nitrite by the enterobacteriaceae family of Gram-negative bacteria, which includes many of the common urinary pathogens. The urine nitrite test predicts the presence of more than 10^5 colonies of these bacteria. However, urinary tract infections caused by Gram-positive bacteria is missed by the nitrite test. Both tests have a sensitivity of 90% and a specificity of 75%, with a negative predictive value of 99%. The decision to admit the patient with pyelonephritis usually is made on clinical grounds (Chapter 68), but the presence of urinary tract infection is supported by these screening tests, along with urine microscopy and culture.

Occult Blood

Most commercially available urine dipsticks test for occult blood. This test is very sensitive in detecting more than three red cells per high power field, with a sensitivity of 80%–95% and specificity of more than 95%–99%. The presence of red cells should be confirmed with microscopy. On most occasions occult blood correlates with the red cells, but the occult-blood test also is positive in the presence of free hemoglobin or myoglobin. The presence of significant occult blood in the absence of red cells should raise the suspicion of rhabdomyolysis or massive intravascular hemolysis (1).

Ketones

In a patient with hyperglycemia and a high anion-gap metabolic acidosis, the diagnosis of diabetic ketoacidosis can be confirmed quickly with the urine dipstick, which confirms the presence of ketones. The urine dipstick detects the presence of acetoacetic acid and acetone but does not detect β-hydroxybutyric acid.

Bilirubin/Urobilinogen

Unconjugated bilirubin is protein-bound, water-insoluble, and not usually found in the urine. Thus, the urine dipstick test for bilirubin is negative if there is hemolytic anemia. Conjugated bilirubin is water-soluble and is detected readily by urine dipstick in clinical conditions such as biliary obstruction. Urine suspected of containing bilirubin should be tested quickly, because bilirubin breaks down quickly after exposure to light.

Intestinal bacteria convert bilirubin to urobilinogen, which is reabsorbed and may appear in the urine. Most conditions that cause increased bilirubin therefore also increase urinary urobilinogen levels. An important exception is biliary obstruction, which may prevent the entry of bilirubin into the intestine. Thus, patients with biliary obstruction may have a urine dipstick test that is positive for urine bilirubin but negative for urobilinogen.

Protein

The urine dipstick for protein detects urinary albumin. The test becomes positive if total albumin excretion is more than 300–500 mg/d. The result usually is reported from trace to "4+" protein, which corresponds to a range of between 15–30 and 500 mg/dL. Thus, the test result is a concentration that is influenced by both the total daily albumin excretion and the urine volume. The urine dipstick is not a sensitive test for proteinuria. In diabetic patients, a positive urine dipstick probably reflects macroalbuminuria and significant renal injury. The urine dipstick also is negative in patients excreting immunoglobulin light chains because of multiple myeloma. However, the sulfosalicylic acid test detects all urinary protein; this test should be performed in elderly patients presenting with unexplained renal failure, a negative urine sediment, and a negative dipstick test for protein.

Urine Microscopy

In the evaluation of renal disease, urine microscopy is the most important component of the urinalysis. The history and physical examination along with dipstick and microscopy results narrow the differential diagnosis, guide further evaluation, and help with decisions about need for urgent treatment (Figure 99.1). The urine is examined under low power (10x) and high power (40x) for the presence of cells, casts, and crystals. Polarizing light is valuable in identifying crystals and lipids in the urine, and phase-contrast microscopy is useful in providing more detail of red-cell morphology.

In addition to noting the numbers per high-power field of the three cell types, the *red cell morphology* should be described as dysmorphic if acanthocytes are seen; dysmorphic

red cells are characteristic markers for glomerular bleeding (2). They are best seen under phase-contrast microscopy. Significant acanthocyturia (defined as ≥5% of the excreted red cells) has a sensitivity of only 52% but a specificity of 98% for glomerular bleeding. Urine sometimes reveals lipid droplets, an abnormal finding that is diagnostic of glomerular disease.

The presence of *cellular casts* is extremely helpful in the evaluation of renal disease. Hyaline and granular casts are not abnormal findings in the urine sediment. However, *red cell casts* are virtually diagnostic of glomerulonephritis, with a specificity of 97% but a sensitivity of less than 25%

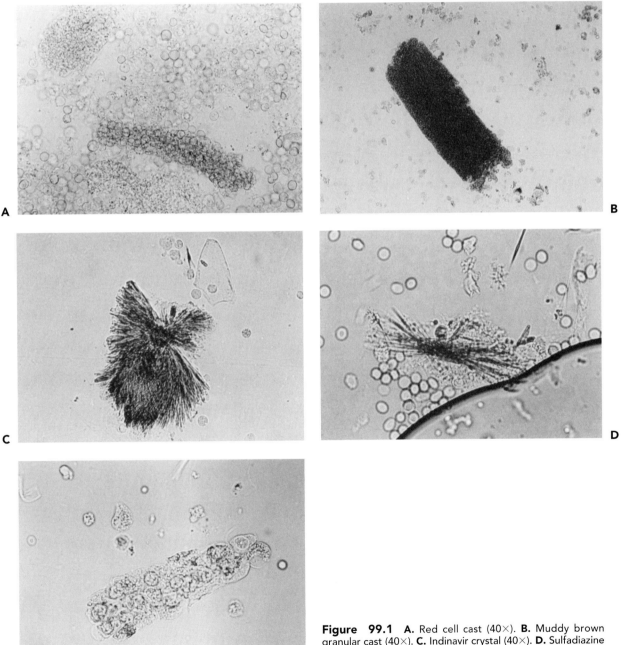

Figure 99.1 **A.** Red cell cast (40×). **B.** Muddy brown granular cast (40×). **C.** Indinavir crystal (40×). **D.** Sulfadiazine crystal (40×). **E.** Renal tubular epithelial cell cast (note eccentric nucleus; 40×).

(Figure 99.1A). In the absence of dysmorphic red cells or red cell casts, it is difficult to distinguish urologic from glomerular bleeding. More than 500 mg/d of proteinuria, "cola"-colored urine, and the absence of blood clots are all consistent with glomerular bleeding. The presence of red cells in the urine does not significantly increase urine protein concentration. Thus, significant proteinuria seen on the dipstick test should not be attributed to the presence of red cells. *White cell casts* indicate the presence of renal interstitial inflammation as seen in pyelonephritis or interstitial nephritis. The presence of white cell casts also helps differentiate pyelonephritis from cystitis.

The presence of muddy brown granular casts, free renal tubular cells, and renal tubular epithelial cell casts in the urine is indicative of tubular damage, and these findings support the diagnosis of *acute tubular necrosis* in a patient with acute renal failure (Figure 99.1 B, E). However, absence of these urinary findings does not exclude the diagnosis of acute tubular necrosis. Muddy brown granular casts and renal tubular cells also can be seen in patients with hyperbilirubinemia, normal renal function, and no tubular damage.

The presence of *crystalluria* is useful in the evaluation of renal disease in certain clinical situations. Many drugs can crystallize in the urine and can cause acute renal failure from bilateral ureteral drug stones or from intratubular crystal obstruction, nephrolithiasis, and dysuria. These drugs are used commonly in HIV-infected patients and include sulfadiazine, indinavir, and intravenous acyclovir (Figure 99.1 C, D). Some patients with normal renal function may have drug-induced crystalluria, which is not an abnormal finding. All patients with crystalluria and renal failure should be evaluated with a renal ultrasound study to exclude urinary tract obstruction. *Uric acid nephropathy* is the presence of acute renal failure caused by renal tubular obstruction by urate and uric acid crystals. The urine sediment may be normal but occasionally has amorphous material containing uric acid crystals, which appear as rhomboidal crystals or as microcrystallites. Crystalluria also is seen in ethylene glycol (automobile antifreeze) intoxication. In this case, the urinalysis typically reveals mild proteinuria, microscopic hematuria, pyuria, and calcium oxalate crystals.

Urinalysis Obtained During Hospitalization

The urinalysis is used in the same manner during hospitalization as at the time of admission. The main diagnostic dilemma in hospitalized patients is diagnosing the cause of acute renal failure (Chapter 100). The diagnosis of acute tubular necrosis can be confirmed with a urinalysis showing the presence of muddy brown granular casts and renal tubular cells. Allergic acute interstitial nephritis resulting from drugs given during the hospitalization should be suspected in patients developing acute renal failure; the presentation may include pyuria, white cell casts, fever, rash, and occasionally eosinophiluria. Glomerular diseases usually are present at the time of hospital admission and rarely develop *de novo* during hospitalization.

Oliguria and Anuria

Presenting at the Time of Admission

Description and Differential Diagnosis

The presence of oliguria or anuria is an important sign of impaired renal function that requires immediate evaluation, because early identification and treatment of potentially reversible causes of oliguria may restore normal renal function or prevent more prolonged renal dysfunction (3). The patient may relate a history of diminished or absent urine output over a variable period of time prior to admission. *Oliguria* usually is defined as a urine output of less than 20 mL/h, or 400–500 mL per 24 hours. This definition is based on the fact that an adult ingesting a normal diet is obliged to excrete approximately 600 mOsm of solute per day; because the urine can be maximally concentrated to 1200 mOsm/L, the minimum amount of urine needed to excrete this solute load is 0.5 L. Thus, any urine amount less than this results in the retention of solutes, including nitrogenous waste products. A subset of patients with oliguria may have negligible-to-absent urine output. This condition is referred to as *anuria*, defined as a urine output of less than 50 mL per 24 hours. The differential diagnosis for anuria is limited and includes urinary tract obstruction (the most common cause), renal cortical necrosis, necrotizing rapidly progressive glomerulonephritis, aortic aneurysm, and bilateral renal artery occlusion (4).

Oliguria is categorized as prerenal, renal, intrinsic (parenchymal) or postrenal (obstructive). The list of prerenal causes of oliguria includes conditions that result in decreased absolute intravascular volume or decreased effective circulating volume. Prerenal causes also include the use of drugs such as nonsteroidal anti-inflammatory drugs and angiotensin-converting enzyme (ACE) inhibitors that disrupt normal renal hemodynamics. The common denominator that underlies the prerenal causes of oliguria is decreased renal blood flow to normal, undamaged kidneys, resulting in decreased glomerular filtration rate (GFR) and subsequent reduction in urine output. Prompt restoration of renal blood flow in patients with prerenal oliguria usually results in rapid improvement in GFR and urine output.

Renal or intrinsic causes of oliguria result from damage to specific areas of the renal parenchyma resulting in decreased GFR. The renal causes can be subdivided based on the anatomic location of the renal lesion: tubular (most commonly, acute tubular necrosis), interstitial (acute interstitial nephritis), or glomerular (acute glomerulonephritis). Many of the prerenal causes of oliguria lead to ischemic injury to the tubules if not corrected. Thus, there is a continuum from prerenal events to intrinsic renal damage in the untreated patient. Moreover, patients frequently have both prerenal (volume depletion) and intrinsic renal (acute tubular necrosis) components to their decreased GFR and consequent oliguria.

Obstruction of the urinary tract sufficient to result in oliguria can occur anywhere along the urinary tract, from the renal pelvis to the urethral meatus, and can result from a wide spectrum of causes including neoplasms, strictures, stones, retroperitoneal fibrosis, blood clots, and prostatic disorders (Chapter 103). Urinary tract obstruction can be divided into upper or lower urinary tract (bladder outlet) causes. In order to cause oliguria, upper urinary tract obstruction must involve both kidneys or a solitary kidney. Lower urinary tract obstruction resulting from prostatic disease is probably the most common cause of oliguria or anuria in patients presenting to the hospital emergency department.

Evaluation

Oliguria requires prompt evaluation to identify the presence of either prerenal or postrenal (obstructive) causes that can be reversed quickly. Early identification and treatment of prerenal causes may prevent or attenuate renal tubular injury and a prolonged course of acute renal failure. Early detection and relief of urinary tract obstruction may prevent or minimize permanent renal damage and hasten recovery of viable renal function.

The initial assessment of a patient with oliguria begins with characterization of the intravascular volume status. This involves obtaining a history, performing a careful physical examination, and, if necessary, invasive hemodynamic monitoring. True volume depletion usually is readily apparent in patients presenting with a history of fluid or blood loss and the physical signs and symptoms of hypovolemia. It is more difficult to assess the effective circulating volume in patients with obvious extracellular volume overload, such as those with congestive heart failure or cirrhosis. In these situations, invasive hemodynamic monitoring, including a pulmonary artery catheter, may be necessary to provide insight into the effective circulating volume and the cardiac output. In addition, patients who develop oliguria after the initiation of ACE inhibitors should be evaluated for renal artery stenosis.

Urinary tract obstruction always should be considered early in the evaluation of a patient with oliguria, especially in patients without evidence of volume depletion. The patient may present with symptoms and signs of obstruction, including difficulty initiating or maintaining urinary flow, dysuria, and suprapubic or back pain. A history of alternating episodes of polyuria and oliguria is also suggestive of possible urinary tract obstruction. Physical examination should include an abdominal examination, a digital rectal examination in men to evaluate the prostate, and a bimanual pelvic examination in women to detect possible causes of lower-tract obstruction. A bladder catheter should be placed after a spontaneous urinary void to measure the postvoid residual urine volume. As part of the assessment of oliguria, a renal ultrasound should be performed to evaluate for evidence of hydronephrosis. Renal ultrasonography has a greater than 90% sensitivity and a 74%–92% specificity for detection of urinary tract obstruction. It may be falsely negative in the setting of conditions in which the calyces do not dilate despite the presence of obstruction. Such conditions include retroperitoneal malignancies, retroperitoneal fibrosis, volume depletion, and very early urinary tract obstruction. If urinary tract obstruction still is suspected despite lack of demonstrable hydronephrosis on ultrasound, a retrograde pyelogram should be performed.

The *urinalysis* is the first and most important laboratory test to be performed in the initial evaluation of the patient with oliguria. Prerenal causes of oliguria usually are associated with a bland urinary sediment, whereas intrinsic renal causes of oliguria usually result in abnormal sediment. Measurement of *serum BUN and creatinine* levels also are performed as part of the laboratory evaluation. Oliguria resulting from prerenal causes (and occasionally with obstructive causes) is usually associated with a BUN-to-creatinine ratio of greater than 20:1 because of enhanced urea reabsorption by the kidney. Oliguria caused by intrinsic renal disease is usually associated with a ratio less than 20:1. However, this ratio can be affected by other conditions. For example, increased catabolism or blood in the gastrointestinal tract augment urea production and increase the ratio, whereas a low-protein diet or liver disease reduce urea production and decrease the ratio.

Evaluation of *urinary sodium and water excretion* can be a helpful guide in the evaluation of a patient with oliguria, and serve as an indicator of the functional integrity of the renal tubules (Table 99.1). Patients with prerenal causes of oliguria intensely reabsorb sodium and water to maintain intravascular volume. Thus, in prerenal oliguria, the urinary sodium concentration and the fractional excretion of sodium ([urine/plasma Na] × [urine/plasma creatinine] × 100) are low, and the ratio of urine to plasma osmolality and creatinine is greater than 1. In the setting of intrinsic renal causes of oliguria, tubular function is impaired. The pattern of urinary indices in this setting reflects these defects, as manifested by high urinary sodium concentration and fractional excretion of sodium and urine osmolality that is equal or less than plasma osmolality. Similar urinary indices have been noted in acute interstitial nephritis. Not all intrinsic renal causes of oliguria show this pattern of urinary indices, however. For example, in acute glomerulonephritis, contrast- and myoglobin-induced acute tubular necrosis, and early urinary tract obstruction, the urinary indices may have a prerenal pattern. This probably results from intense renal vasoconstriction in the early stages of these disorders, which leads to avid sodium retention. In addition, the use of diuretics or dopamine and the presence of solutes in the urine such as glucose increase the urinary excretion of sodium. A recent study suggested that the fractional excretion of urea ([urine/plasma urea] × [urine/plasma creatinine] × 100) can help distinguish between prerenal azotemia versus acute tubular necrosis, especially when

TABLE 99.1

DIFFERENTIAL DIAGNOSIS OF OLIGURIA: URINALYSIS, WATER, AND SODIUM METABOLISM

Diagnosis	Urinalysis	Water Metabolism — Urine/plasma osmolality	Sodium handling — Urine Na, mEq/L	Sodium handling — Fractional excretion of Na (%)
Prerenal	Normal, or hyaline casts	≥1	<20	<1
Intrarenal				
• Tubular necrosis	Granular and epithelial cell casts	≤1	>20	≥1
• Interstitial nephritis	Pyuria, hematuria, mild proteinuria, granular and epithelial cell casts, eosinophils	≤1	>20	≥1
• Glomerulonephritis	Hematuria, marked proteinuria, red blood cell casts, granular casts	≥1	<20	<1
• Vascular disorders	Normal or hematuria, mild proteinuria	≥1	<20	<1
Postrenal	Normal or hematuria, granular casts, pyuria	≤1	Early, <20 Late, >20	Early, <1 Late, >1

Na, sodium.
Adapted from Toto RD. Approach to the patient with acute renal failure. In Greenberg A, ed. *Primer on Kidney Diseases.* San Diego: Academic Press, 1998:258.

diuretics have been administered (5). A low fractional excretion of urea (<35%) was found to be more sensitive and specific of an index of prerenal azotemia than was a low fractional excretion of sodium. Interpretation of the urinary indices should be done with caution. The diagnosis of the cause of oliguria should be based primarily on a thorough history and physical examination; the urinalysis and urinary indices should serve only as confirmatory data.

Management

Patients found to have true volume depletion should be hydrated with appropriate volume therapy (crystalloid, colloid, or blood products) to reestablish euvolemia (Chapter 25). In addition, drugs that cause volume depletion (diuretics), disrupt renal hemodynamics (ACE inhibitors, nonsteroidal anti-inflammatory drugs), or decrease vascular resistance (antihypertensive agents) should be discontinued. Lower urinary tract obstruction usually is relieved by placement of a bladder catheter, whereas upper-tract obstruction requires urologic or interventional radiologic intervention. Following relief of urinary tract obstruction, there can be a substantial postobstructive diuresis (often 500–1000 mL/h) resulting from excretion of the retained excess sodium and water and impaired tubular reabsorptive function. Patients with a brisk postobstructive diuresis may need intravenous fluids to avoid hypovolemia (Chapter 103).

Oliguria and azotemia caused by disorders associated with decreases in effective circulating volume such as congestive heart failure or cirrhosis can be therapeutic challenges, because the treatment must be directed at improving cardiac or hepatic function in patients with chronic irreversible damage of these organs (Chapters 39 and 83). The management of oliguria resulting from intrinsic renal disorders is discussed in Chapter 100.

Presenting During Hospitalization

Oliguria that develops in a hospitalized patient frequently is caused by multiple hemodynamic and nephrotoxic insults endured during the hospitalization (Chapter 100) (6, 7). This often is seen in the severely ill patient in the ICU with multi-organ system failure. Such insults include septicemia, volume contraction, surgery and anesthesia, nephrotoxic drugs, and radiocontrast agents. The majority of cases of oliguria in hospitalized patients are caused by iatrogenic factors. Classifying the cause of oliguria using the prerenal, intrinsic renal, and obstructive classes outlined previously is helpful in the hospitalized patient. Prerenal factors account for 30%–60% of the cases of oliguria. The major intrinsic renal cause for oliguria is acute tubular necrosis resulting from the various hemodynamic and nephrotoxic insults noted previously. Although acute interstitial nephritis resulting from administered drugs is a frequent cause of acute decrease in GFR in the hospitalized patient, this lesion usually does not cause oliguria. Urinary tract obstruction is encountered much less frequently in hospital-acquired oliguria, but patients with bladder catheters should be evaluated for possible occlusion of the catheter.

In evaluating a patient with acute oliguria, it is helpful to review the hemodynamic flow sheet for evidence of hypotension, especially hypotension during a perioperative period. In addition, the temporal relationship between the onset of oliguria and the use of drugs that are potentially nephrotoxic or alter renal hemodynamics should be noted. The physical examination and changes in body weight should help determine the patient's volume status. If there is uncertainty as to the volume status, invasive hemodynamic monitoring should be considered. The evaluation of oliguria should include the performance of a urinalysis and, if necessary, obtaining urinary indices.

The management of acute oliguria in the hospitalized patient follows the same approach as for the patient in whom it presents at admission. Drugs that are nephrotoxic or negatively alter renal hemodynamics should be discontinued.

Edema

Presenting at the Time of Admission

Description and Differential Diagnosis
Edema is defined as a palpable swelling produced by expansion of the interstitial fluid volume and results because the amount of fluid filtered exceeds the amount returned in the lymphatics. The differential diagnosis can be divided into four groups by primary mechanisms (8) (Table 99.2): (a) in-

creased capillary hydrostatic pressure, which is responsible for edema formation in heart failure, cirrhosis, and sodium retention caused by renal disease or drugs, pregnancy, or idiopathic edema; (b) hypoalbuminemia caused by protein loss or reduced synthesis, as occurs in nephrotic syndrome and liver disease, respectively; (c) increased capillary permeability caused by burns, sepsis, allergic reactions, trauma, or the adult respiratory distress syndrome; and (d) lymphatic obstruction or increased interstitial oncotic pressure, exemplified by lymph node enlargement or with hypothyroidism.

Evaluation
The first step in the evaluation of the patient with edema is to characterize the edema as localized or generalized (Table 99.2). Generalized edema reflects a widespread increase in extracellular fluid, and the location of edema reflects dependent forces. *Anasarca* is severe generalized edema that can be detected in virtually all body parts. Localized edema results from the local disturbance of the balance between fluid filtration and reabsorption. The differential diagnosis of localized edema includes inflammation, lymphatic obstruction, venous obstruction, and thrombophlebitis. Localized edema is easily differentiated from generalized edema by asymmetry and other associated findings such as redness, warmth, and pain. Cellulitis, lymphatic obstruction caused by tumor involvement of lymph nodes, and deep venous thrombosis all are causes of localized edema that usually require immediate attention and may require hospitalization.

Even in the absence of structural renal disease or renal insufficiency, the common derangement among the major causes of *generalized edema* is abnormal sodium retention by the kidney. In the patient with generalized edema, the goal is to identify the responsible disease process. The history, physical examination, and laboratory results should help the clinician differentiate among edema caused by congestive heart failure, cirrhosis, or renal diseases such as nephrotic syndrome, acute glomerulonephritis, or chronic renal insufficiency. Identifying patients with pulmonary edema is important independent of the cause of the generalized edema, because these patients need immediate attention and may require hospitalization (Chapter 39). Pulmonary edema is more likely to accompany congestive heart failure than cirrhosis or nephrotic syndrome. Isolated right ventricular dysfunction may present with peripheral edema, ascites, and edema of the abdominal wall without pulmonary edema. It may be confused with cirrhosis because of consequent liver dysfunction from hepatic congestion. However, right ventricular dysfunction causes elevation of the jugular venous pressure, while cirrhosis usually does not. Patients with generalized edema caused by hepatic cirrhosis are also more likely to give a history of developing ascites prior to developing peripheral edema.

Periorbital and peripheral edema (and at times ascites) characterize generalized edema resulting from nephrotic

TABLE 99.2

MAJOR CAUSES OF EDEMA, BY PRIMARY MECHANISM

Generalized	Localized
Increased capillary hydrostatic pressure	**Increased capillary hydrostatic pressure**
Heart failure	Venous obstruction
Cirrhosis	(e.g., deep venous
Renal sodium retention	thrombosis)
Pregnancy/premenstrual	
Idiopathic edema	
Hypoalbuminemia	
Nephrotic syndrome (protein loss)	
Liver disease (reduced synthesis)	
Increased capillary permeability	**Increased capillary permeability**
Burns, sepsis, allergic reactions	Infection
Trauma	
Lymphatic obstruction or increased interstitial oncotic pressure	**Lymphatic obstruction or increased pressure**
Hypothyroidism	Malignant nodal involvement

syndrome. Although the early stage of renal disease is usually asymptomatic, the history may provide some clues. A history of frothy urine, which is caused by proteinuria, may help delineate the time course of the nephrotic syndrome. Patients with chronic renal insufficiency may complain of nocturia and frequency because of the inability to concentrate their urine. Significant glomerular hematuria leads to a history of "cola"-colored urine. The presence of renal disease may be confirmed by elevated serum BUN and creatinine levels, or a urinalysis showing proteinuria with or without hematuria. Patients with nephrotic syndrome and normal renal function usually do not present with signs of true intravascular volume expansion. However, patients with severe chronic renal insufficiency, acute renal failure, diabetic nephropathy, or acute glomerulonephritis may have renal sodium retention leading to true intravascular volume expansion and pulmonary edema.

The cause of localized and generalized edema should be diagnosed quickly on presentation, aided by the history, examination, and minimal tests. Patients who may require hospital admission include those with the combination of generalized edema and pulmonary edema, those with localized edema caused by deep venous thrombosis or cellulitis, and possibly those with unexplained venous obstruction (who may have an undiagnosed malignancy). Patients with generalized edema caused by nephrotic syndrome or cirrhosis but with no pulmonary edema rarely require hospital admission because of edema. However, even these patients may require hospitalization for control of the edema if they fail to respond to outpatient treatment with diuretics or develop other edema-related complications, such as skin breakdown and cellulitis.

Patients with no evident cardiac, renal, or hepatic cause of edema may have idiopathic edema, a diagnosis of exclusion that most often occurs in young, menstruating women. The etiology is not well understood. Idiopathic edema should not be confused with premenstrual edema, which resolves shortly after the onset of menses.

Management

The treatment of localized edema is directed at the underlying cause (9) (Chapters 39, 52, 69, and 83). Patients with localized edema usually become volume-depleted if diuretics are used to treat the edema. However, patients with generalized edema and pulmonary edema require immediate therapy. If cardiac disease is present, the initial treatment of the edema should include treatment of the underlying cardiac disease that precipitated pulmonary edema (e.g., ischemia, infarction, arrhythmia). The mainstay of treatment of generalized edema accompanied by pulmonary edema is loop diuretics (10), the use of which should be guided by a few basic principles. The pharmacologic properties of all loop diuretics are very similar; thus, patients who do not respond to adequate doses of one loop diuretic probably will not respond to another. All commonly used loop diuretics are highly protein-bound, and hypoalbuminemia leads to a larger extravascular space and slower diuretic delivery to the kidney. Being protein-bound, diuretics do not enter the tubular fluid by glomerular filtration but by proximal tubule secretion. In addition, patients with significant proteinuria have filtered albumin, which can inactivate some of the diuretic in the nephron.

The first step in using loop diuretics is to determine the threshold dose. If a patient does not respond to the starting dose, the dose should be doubled until adequate natriuresis is achieved. Increasing the frequency of administration of the diuretic before the threshold dose is achieved does not lead to an improved natriuresis. The maximum effective dose of intravenous furosemide in patients with moderate renal insufficiency is 80–160 mg; severe renal insufficiency, 160–200 mg; nephrotic syndrome, 80–120 mg; cirrhosis, 40 mg; and congestive heart failure, 40–80 mg. The dose should be doubled when converting from intravenous to oral administration.

Ineffective natriuresis may occur for many reasons. Patients on a high sodium intake have an inadequate net natriuresis, and all patients started on diuretics for generalized edema should be placed on a low sodium diet (less than 100 mEq/d). Poor absorption of furosemide also should be considered. Patients with severe congestive heart failure may be prone to slower absorption and low bioavailability because of poor intestinal perfusion. Bumetanide or torsemide both have better bioavailability than furosemide and should be tried if oral doses of furosemide are not effective in patients with heart failure. If patients do not respond to maximal doses of loop diuretics, the addition of a thiazide diuretic usually increases natriuresis by blocking sodium absorption at a different nephron site. Spironolactone is usually a weak diuretic, but in patients with cirrhosis, it can be more effective than furosemide.

In the absence of cirrhosis, there is no limit to the rate of fluid removal in patients with generalized edema and pulmonary edema. Two to three liters per day can be removed safely in most patients. Rapidity of fluid removal is assured by maintaining an adequate effective circulating volume. The BUN and creatinine levels can serve as a monitor of this. The main exception to the safety of rapid fluid removal occurs in patients with cirrhosis and ascites, who do not have peripheral edema, and in whom diuresis should be slower (Chapter 83).

The main adverse reactions to diuretics include allergic reactions, ototoxicity, and fluid and electrolyte abnormalities. Ototoxicity is mostly associated with high doses of loop diuretics given in combination with other ototoxic drugs such as aminoglycosides. Most cases of deafness caused by loop diuretics are transient in nature. Continuous intravenous infusion of a loop diuretic may help minimize the risk of ototoxicity in hospitalized patients receiving high-dose diuretics. To maintain a constant diuresis, continuous intravenous infusion should be considered in ICU patients who have only a short-lived response to bolus therapy.

Edema Presenting During Hospitalization

The previous discussion also applies to patients who develop edema during hospitalization. Some patients with compensated heart failure, nephrotic syndrome, or cirrhosis develop edema during hospitalization because the underlying condition worsens. However, most patients develop edema because of iatrogenic reasons. Rigorous fluid resuscitation in the ICU may initiate edema formation, and many causative factors unique to the ICU may maintain the edema. Sodium retention is triggered by the following three factors: (1) mechanical ventilation with positive end-expiratory pressure, which decreases cardiac output; (2) reduced muscle-pump activity, which reduces venous return; and (3) cytokine release from sepsis, causing hypotension, cardiac depression, and increased capillary permeability. The edema usually resolves with improvement of the underlying illness that necessitated ICU admission. Diuretic therapy is indicated only in those patients with clinical signs of volume overload as evidenced by pulmonary edema, or abnormal invasive monitoring variables, such as a high pulmonary capillary wedge pressure.

Elevated BUN and Creatinine

Presenting at the Time of Admission

Description and Differential Diagnosis

Elevated BUN and creatinine levels in patients presenting to the hospital are usually indicative of decreases in GFR. The term *renal insufficiency* usually is applied to patients with mild-to-moderate decreases in GFR who do not require dialytic support. Decreases in GFR can be either acute or chronic. Chronic renal insufficiency or failure usually is a slowly progressive irreversible loss of renal function that results in end-stage renal disease.

Before assuming that elevated BUN and creatinine indicate renal dysfunction, the possibility of nonrenal factors should be considered. Because creatinine is freely filtered across the glomerulus and is not reabsorbed by the kidney, measurement of the serum creatinine concentration is a good endogenous indicator of GFR. However, there is some tubular secretion of creatinine (10%–40%); thus, the creatinine clearance may overestimate the true GFR by the same margin. Drugs such as trimethoprim and cimetidine that block the secretion of creatinine result in an increase in serum creatinine level unrelated to any changes in GFR. Similar to creatinine, urea is excreted primarily by glomerular filtration. Therefore, the BUN level tends to vary inversely with GFR. However, there are factors that can increase the BUN level without affecting the GFR. These conditions include a high-protein diet, hyperalimentation, gastrointestinal bleeding, severe catabolic states, and the administration of corticosteroids or tetracycline. Conversely, a low-protein diet or liver disease can result in a lower BUN concentration. The percentage of urea reabsorption increases during volume depletion, resulting in elevation of the BUN level without decreases in GFR.

Evaluation

The first question to consider in evaluating a patient presenting with elevated BUN and creatinine levels is whether renal insufficiency is acute or chronic (3). An important historical clue is prior measurements of serum creatinine concentration. Reviewing the medical record may reveal an abnormal urinalysis in the past, which may suggest a chronic process. Oliguria is an unusual finding in patients with chronic renal insufficiency and suggests that the process is acute. Serial measurements of serum creatinine may be helpful; a stable value is more consistent with a chronic process. The presence of anemia also is suggestive of chronic renal insufficiency. Determining the kidney size by ultrasound imaging is helpful, because small kidneys are more indicative of chronic renal insufficiency. Although normal- to large-sized kidneys in a patient with renal insufficiency usually are suggestive of an acute process, there are five chronic conditions associated with normal- to large-sized kidneys: diabetic nephropathy, amyloidosis, HIV-associated nephropathy, adult polycystic kidney disease, and, rarely, infiltrative disorders of the kidney (e.g., lymphoma, leukemia). Chapter 100 includes a complete discussion of acute renal failure.

For patients in whom it is established that renal insufficiency is chronic, the next question to consider is the cause of the renal disease. Table 99.3 lists the major causes of chronic renal insufficiency. After a careful history and physical examination, the first laboratory tests to be performed in evaluating a patient with chronic renal insufficiency are a urinalysis and a 24-hour urine collection for protein excretion. Figure 99.2 presents a differential diagnosis for the major causes of chronic renal insufficiency based on the results of these two tests (11). A renal ultrasound should be performed in the evaluation of all patients with either acute or chronic renal insufficiency to rule out urinary tract obstruction.

TABLE 99.3

MAJOR CAUSES OF CHRONIC RENAL INSUFFICIENCY

Cause	Prevalence
Diabetes mellitus	31%
Hypertension	27%
Cystic diseases (polycystic kidney disease)	14%
Glomerulonephritis	5%
Urologic diseases	5%
Others/unknown	18%

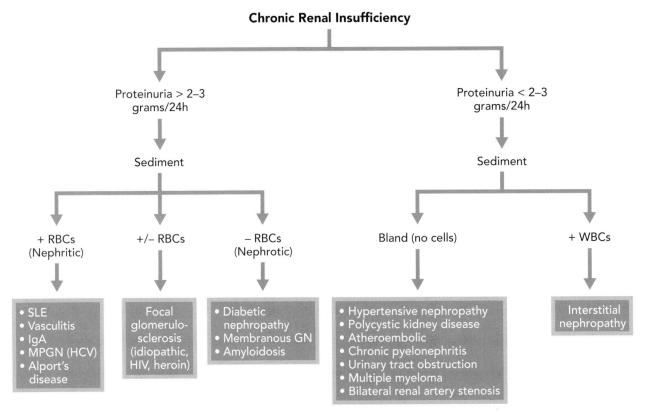

Figure 99.2 Diagnostic approach to chronic renal insufficiency. *GN,* glomerulonephritis; *HCV,* hepatitis C virus; *HIV,* human immunodeficiency virus; *MPGN,* membranoproliferative glomerulonephritis; *RBC,* red blood cells; *SLE,* systemic lupus erythematosus; *WBC,* white blood cells.

Management

Chapter 100 includes a discussion about managing acute renal failure and Chapter 101 discusses dialysis issues. For most patients with chronic renal insufficiency, renal function usually continues to deteriorate over time and progresses inexorably to end-stage renal disease. There is no specific therapy to reverse this progression for most causes of renal disease, but there are treatments that can slow the rate of renal function loss. Control of systemic hypertension is the most important therapeutic maneuver. Also, both experimental and clinical studies have suggested that ACE inhibitors may have a therapeutic advantage over conventional antihypertensive drugs in slowing the progression of many types of renal disease, especially if started early in the course of renal insufficiency. Similar results also have been achieved with the nondihydropyridine calcium channel blockers. Administering ACE inhibitors can produce some negative effects in patients with renal insufficiency, including acute deterioration in renal function, hypotension, hyperkalemia, and a nonproductive cough. Blood pressure, renal function, and serum potassium concentration should be monitored closely during initiation of ACE-inhibitor therapy. Dietary protein restriction also has been advocated as a therapeutic modality to slow progression of chronic renal insufficiency; one meta-analysis and a recent trial suggest that a low-protein diet slows the progression of renal disease (12, 13).

Increased BUN and Creatinine Presenting During Hospitalization

Chapter 100 covers the management of elevated BUN and creatinine levels presenting in hospitalized patients.

KEY POINTS

■ Urine microscopy is the most important tool in the evaluation of renal disease and can be invaluable in deciding whether to hospitalize a patient.

■ The presence of oliguria or anuria is a critical sign of impaired renal function. It requires immediate evaluation by the admitting physician, because early identification and treatment may restore normal renal function or prevent more prolonged renal dysfunction.

■ The cause of localized and generalized edema should be diagnosed quickly on presentation with history and physical examination and few tests. Patients that may require hospital admission include those with the combination of generalized edema and pulmonary edema and those with localized edema.

■ Once it is established that an increase in BUN and creatinine levels or the presence of oliguria or anuria in a patient is associated with renal insufficiency, prerenal, intrinsic renal, or obstructive causes should be considered.

REFERENCES

1. Zager RA. Rhabdomyolysis and myohemoglobinuric acute renal failure. *Kidney Int* 1996;49:314–326.
2. Kohler H, Wandel E, Brunck B. Acanthocyturia—a characteristic marker for glomerular bleeding. *Kidney Int* 1991;40:115–120.
3. Thadhani R, Pascual M, Bonventre JV. Acute renal failure. *N Engl J Med* 1996;334:1448–1460.
4. Klahr S, Miller SB. Acute oliguria. *N Engl J Med* 1998;338:671–675.
5. Carvounis CP, Nisar S, Guro-Rauzman S. Significance of the fractional excretion of urea in the differential diagnosis of acute renal failure. *Kidney Int* 2002;62:2223–2229.
6. Hou SB, Bushinsky DA, Wish JB, et al. Hospital-acquired renal insufficiency: a prospective study. *Am J Med* 1983;74:243–246.
7. Nolan CR, Anderson RJ. Hospital-acquired acute renal failure. *J Am Soc Nephrol* 1998;9:710–718.
8. Palmer BF, Alpern RJ. Pathogenesis of edema formation in the nephrotic syndrome. *Kidney Int* 1997;51(suppl 59):21–27.
9. Humphreys MH. Mechanisms and management of nephrotic edema. *Kidney Int* 1994;45:266–281.
10. Brater CD. Diuretic therapy. *N Engl J Med* 1998;339:387–395.
11. Hass M, Meehan SM, Karrison TG, et al. Changing etiologies of unexplained adult nephrotic syndrome: a comparison of renal biopsy findings from 1976–1979 and 1995–1997. *Am J Kidney Dis* 1997;30:621–631.
12. Pedrini MT, Levey AS, Lau J, et al. The effect of dietary protein restriction on the progression of diabetic and nondiabetic renal diseases: a meta-analysis. *Ann Intern Med* 1996;124:627–632.
13. Hansen HP, Tauber-Lassen E, Jensen BR, et al. Effects of dietary protein restriction on prognosis in patients with diabetic nephropathy. *Kidney Int* 2002;62:220–228.

ADDITIONAL READING

Don BR, Rodriguez RA, Humphreys MH. Acute renal failure associated with pigmenturia or crystal deposits. In: Schrier RW, Gottschalk, eds. *Diseases of the Kidney.* 6th ed. Boston: Little, Brown, and Co., 1997.

Hostetter TH. Prevention of the development and progression of renal disease. *J Am Soc Nephrol* 2003;14(7 Suppl 2):S144–S147.

Kellum JA, Decker J. Use of dopamine in acute renal failure: a meta-analysis. *Crit Care Med* 2001;29:1526–1531.

Acute Renal Failure

Ravindra L. Mehta   Frank Liu

100

INTRODUCTION

Although there is no consensus regarding a standard definition, acute renal failure (ARF) is most commonly defined as a recent decline in renal function resulting in a reduced ability to excrete nitrogenous waste products, often associated with fluid retention. Elevations in the serum levels of urea nitrogen and creatinine often are used to judge the severity of ARF. From a practical standpoint, ARF can occur *de novo* or be superimposed on previously impaired renal function, and can be community-acquired or develop in the hospital. It also may complicate the course of an ICU patient. The delineation of timing and setting of ARF is of some importance because the strategies for diagnosis and management, and the outcomes, are different (Table 100.1). Recent evidence suggests that ARF may increase the risk for developing nonrenal complications such as sepsis and bleeding. It is thus increasingly evident that early recognition and appropriate management of ARF are important goals. This chapter outlines the key principles for and a sequential approach to the diagnosis and management of ARF.

ACUTE RENAL FAILURE PRESENTING AT THE TIME OF ADMISSION

Community-acquired ARF in the absence of any other problem is a relatively infrequent cause for hospital admission and usually suggests a primary renal process that may have been unrecognized. More commonly, ARF may complicate the course of a patient presenting with other organ dysfunction (e.g., cardiac or hepatic failure, or sepsis). The main issues that require attention are recognition and diagnosis of ARF, initial management to correct reversible factors, and determining the need for and timing of dialytic intervention.

Issues at the Time of Admission

Diagnosis

Patients with ARF usually are identified from a laboratory result demonstrating an elevation in blood urea nitrogen and creatinine levels (most commonly a rise in serum creatinine from a known previous baseline by >1 mg/dL, or an absolute value of >2 mg/dL). This elevation may be associated with a decline in urine volume and symptoms of uremia (fatigue, fluid retention, easy bruising, and confusion). Often these findings are overshadowed by the clinical features of other organ failure. It is thus important to evaluate the setting in which ARF is identified and determine possible contributing factors.

Traditionally, causes of ARF have been delineated as *prerenal*, *renal*, and *postrenal*. This approach utilizes an anatomic separation of the possible factors responsible for ARF, permitting an easy method for considering the possible causes. However, an alternative and equally useful classification of ARF is based on the *anticipated course of the disease and the reversibility of the lesion* (Table 100.2). This approach suggests that initial efforts should be directed toward determining whether the process can be reversed easily, as is the case in many prerenal and postrenal conditions (e.g., volume depletion and obstructive uropathy). Similarly, it is equally important to ascertain if there is potentially irreversible damage to the kidney (e.g., vascular occlusion), which may leave a limited window of opportunity for reversal. For the remaining clinical entities, diagnostic strategies are currently helpful only in a limited way, because the therapeutic approaches are similar (except if ARF is caused by an aggressive acute glomerulonephritis, as discussed later).

A standardized approach to diagnosing ARF begins with a detailed history and chart review to determine recent clinical events and potential nephrotoxin exposure. Volume status should be assessed, as should changes in urinary vol-

TABLE 100.1

CLINICAL SETTING FOR ACUTE RENAL FAILURE

	Community-acquired	Hospital-acquired	ICU-acquired
Incidence	Low (<1%)	Moderate (2%–5%)	High (10%–20%)
Cause	Often single (pre > post > renal)	May be single or multiple	Often multifactorial (pre > renal)
Outcome (patient survival)	Good (70%–95%)	Moderate (30%–50%)	Poor (10%–30%)

Pre, prerenal; *Post*, postrenal.
Modified from Elasy TA, Anderson RJ. Changing demography of acute renal failure. *Semin Dial* 1996;9:438–443.

ume, color, and symptoms. Every attempt should be made to determine recent intake of prescription and over-the-counter drugs (particularly nonsteroidal anti-inflammatory agents, which are a common cause of renal function decline, especially in elderly patients and those with heart failure or cirrhosis). Evidence of pre-existing renal dysfunction always should be sought; the patient may or may not be aware of the dysfunction. A comprehensive physical examination looking for reversible factors responsible for decreased effective renal perfusion and renal obstruction is an important next step. In the elderly male patient, a rectal examination should be performed to evaluate for prostatic hypertrophy. Auscultation revealing an abdominal bruit may suggest an ischemic cause of ARF. Similarly, the presence of a cardiac arrhythmia such as atrial fibrillation may point to the possibility of embolic disease.

All patients with ARF should have a urinalysis, serum chemistry tests (including measurement of electrolytes, urea nitrogen, creatinine, calcium, phosphate, uric acid, and liver enzymes), and complete blood count with platelets. Evaluation of the anion gap (Chapter 105) can be an important clue to an underlying tubulointerstitial pro-

TABLE 100.2

CLASSIFICATION OF ACUTE RENAL FAILURE

Reversible

Decreased effective renal perfusion
Extrarenal obstruction to renal flow

Self-Limited

Acute tubular necrosis
Acute interstitial nephritis
Intrarenal obstruction secondary to drugs or uric acid
Acute glomerulonephritis

Irreversible

Cortical necrosis
Large vessel occlusion
Certain nephrotoxins (e.g., methoxyflurane)
Microvascular occlusions

cess (i.e., renal tubular acidosis) and may even point to the cause of ARF (e.g., myeloma associated with a low anion gap). Urine and serum chemistry tests can provide important clues to the underlying disorder, particularly the presence of prerenal factors. Urine electrolyte patterns associated with prerenal or renal profiles may be influenced by several factors, and their diagnostic utility may be somewhat limited. Nevertheless, tests that measure tubular reabsorption (i.e., fractional excretion) can help indicate whether the condition is caused by tubular (i.e., intrinsic renal) dysfunction or by prerenal factors. The fractional excretion of urea nitrogen ([urine/plasma urea nitrogen] $\times$ [plasma/urine creatinine] $\times$ 100) may be more accurate than the more commonly used fractional excretion of sodium ([urine/plasma sodium] $\times$ [urine/plasma creatinine] $\times$ 100) (1). Unlike the fractional excretion of sodium, the fractional excretion of urea nitrogen is relatively unaffected by prior diuretic use and metabolic alkalosis (both conditions may result in high fractional excretion of sodium in the presence of volume depletion). A cut-off of less than 35% is fairly discriminatory for prerenal conditions (the traditional cut-off for the fractional excretion of sodium is <1%) (2). Serum creatinine may be a poor surrogate for estimating the magnitude of decline in renal function, because it is influenced by the patient's age, gender, muscle mass, and volume status. Similarly, in the presence of hepatic failure, serum creatinine levels may be underestimated by chromogenic methods. Quantification of glomerular filtration rate by creatinine clearance is preferable but may not always be possible.

Abdominal ultrasound is usually indicated, and Doppler examination of the renal vasculature also may be useful in some circumstances. In the setting of ARF in the ICU, contrast studies should be avoided in the workup of renal failure. If the integrity of renal perfusion is in question, an isotope scan can provide useful information. If there is any doubt about the quality of the scan, however, a renal angiogram may be necessary.

In the presence of active urine sediment and other features suggestive of glomerulonephritis, immunologic tests for antineutrophilic antibodies, antiglomerular basement antibodies, and complement levels may be useful. Renal biopsy is generally the most definitive way of diagnosing ARF, but this test is often omitted because of fear of complications and/or confidence in the clinical diagnosis. However, in patients with intrinsic renal failure ultimately found to be caused by glomerular disease, biopsy has been shown to change management in more than half the cases (3). As newer therapeutic interventions become available, biopsy is likely to become increasingly important in establishing a specific diagnosis and guiding therapy.

Diagnostic Tests on the Horizon

Because the most commonly used clinical tools for diagnosing renal failure—rise in creatinine and decrease in urine output—are far from ideal, researchers have tried to identify other biomarkers that can quickly and accurately diagnose renal injury (and give a clue as to pathogenesis) at an early stage of ARF. For example, high urinary levels of cysteine-rich protein-61 (CYR61) have been shown in animal studies to distinguish between prerenal causes of ARF and acute tubular necrosis (4). Similarly, urinary levels of the Na-H+ antiporter isotype 3 (NHE3), which is the most abundant sodium transporter in the proximal tubule, and kidney injury molecule-1 (KIM-1), which is upregulated in the proximal tubule in response to ischemia, may eventually be used to distinguish between prerenal azotemia, ATN, and intrinsic ARF other than ATN (5, 6). If additional research supports these associations, such biomarkers may allow for more rapid and directed intervention in cases of potentially reversible renal failure.

Indications for Hospitalization and Intensive Care Unit Admission

When a patient presents with an abrupt decline in renal function associated with a marked decrease in urine output, hospitalization should always be considered, because rapid changes in electrolyte, acid-base, and volume status may occur (Table 100.3). Additionally, a prompt diagnosis of the nature of renal injury may require aggressive diagnostic testing, including renal biopsy, which is easier to perform in the hospital. If urine output is not compromised and renal function changes are gradual (e.g., an increase in serum creatinine of <0.5 mg/dL over 72–96 hours), and if there is no concern that the patient will be lost to follow-up, an initial outpatient evaluation can be initiated with follow-up in 1–2 days. Often, the decision to hospitalize a patient for ARF is influenced by knowledge of the event leading to renal function decline (e.g., exposure to contrast agents). If the nature and timing of a renal insult are well known, it is easier to be more confident in a decision to follow a patient as an outpatient. If the renal insult is unknown or if there is any doubt about the patient's ability to follow instructions, it is safer to hospitalize. If ARF complicates other organ dysfunction, it is always preferable to hospitalize the patient, because the presence of ARF worsens the prognosis of the primary illness and makes it more difficult to manage the patient. In the presence of preexisting renal dysfunction, an acute and significant decline in renal function should prompt hospitalization, because dialytic intervention may be necessary. Patients with severe ARF (blood urea nitrogen level >100 mg/dL or creatinine level >8 mg/dL with uremic complications such as pericarditis), marked electrolyte abnormalities (e.g., potassium >6.5 mEq/L), or marked acidosis (pH <7.33) should be admitted to a monitored floor or an ICU setting for closer observation.

Initial Management and Indications for Consultation

The treatment of ARF has the following goals: maintaining fluid and electrolyte, acid-base, and solute homeostasis; preventing further insults to the kidney; promoting

TABLE 100.3

INDICATIONS FOR HOSPITALIZATION FOR ACUTE RENAL FAILURE (ARF)

Description of case	Outpatient	Hospital	ICU	Nephrology consultation indicated?
New-onset ARF				
Oliguric, severe electrolyte and metabolic disturbances, volume overload		+	+	+
Nonoliguric, marked rapid changes in renal function, renal insult not known		+	±	+
Nonoliguric, mild changes in renal function, nature and timing of insult known	+			±
Preexisting ARF				
Marked rapid decline in renal function		+		+
Gradual decline in renal function	+			+
ARF complicating other illness				
Change in renal function with heart failure, pneumonia, gastroenteritis		+	±	+

healing and renal recovery; and permitting other support measures such as nutrition to proceed without delay. Therapeutic interventions should be designed to achieve these goals and take the clinical course into consideration. Classically, ARF is said to progress through three phases: (1) an *initiation phase*, (2) a *maintenance phase*, and (3) a *recovery phase*. A fourth phase, during which extension of the initial injury occurs, has also been proposed. Although these four phases are not always distinct, their recognition facilitates the development of a treatment plan because therapeutic strategies differ from one phase to another. For example, in the initiation phase, the major emphasis is on preventing and attenuating the severity of the renal dysfunction, whereas once ARF is established the emphasis is on maintaining homeostasis to allow recovery. The latter often requires renal replacement therapy with dialysis. It is often helpful to consult a nephrologist early in the course of the disease (Table 100.3) because appropriate intervention in each phase may influence the need for dialysis and the outcome. Patients with advanced renal dysfunction should always have a nephrology consultation, because dialytic intervention may be required emergently.

Initiation Phase

The initial phase of ARF represents the period of actual insult resulting in glomerular or tubular epithelial injury and resultant decline in renal function. In most circumstances, the effect of the injury is manifested over a few days, thus permitting interventions that may reverse or attenuate the effect of the insult. These interventions should be selected based on the clinical status of the patient; the goal is to correct any reversible contributing factors such as volume depletion and obstruction, to restore renal perfusion and urine output, and to minimize further tubular injury. Several agents, described below, are now available for this purpose; however, they should be used judiciously, because they all can cause deleterious side effects.

Volume Expanders Volume expanders should be considered early in the management of ARF, particularly if there is evidence of intravascular volume contraction. The use of volume expanders can be both diagnostic and therapeutic in potential prerenal states. Saline infusions have been shown to have a beneficial effect in experimental ARF and to attenuate the nephrotoxic potential of aminoglycosides and amphotericin. In the hypoalbuminemic patient, it is preferable to use a colloid solution. Although albumin has traditionally been used in this setting, recent data suggest ICU patients resuscitated with albumin do no better than those resuscitated with normal saline (7). As such, if colloid administration is deemed necessary because of presumed inadequate intravascular oncotic pressure, packed red blood cell transfusions may be preferable to albumin administration, because the former are likely to be retained in the intravascular compartment longer and theoretically should improve oxygen-carrying capacity as well.

The amount of volume and the rate of administration must be individualized depending on the patient's clinical status. Hemodynamic monitoring can help determine the rate of fluid replacement and reduce the potential for fluid overload in severely ill patients (Chapter 25). In general, in a volume-contracted patient with hemodynamic compromise, rapid volume expansion with 0.9% saline should be initiated at a rate of 250–500 mL/h for 1–3 hours, after which the volume status and urinary output should be reassessed. If the initial volume replacement results in an improvement in urinary output, volume expansion should continue, with the rate of infusion based on the clinical response. If there is no improvement in urinary output, a diuretic challenge can be employed (see later in this chapter). If this fails, the rate of fluid administered should be reduced to avoid volume overload.

Diuretics The use of diuretics in the initial phase of ARF is based on observations from experimental and clinical studies. In addition to improving urine flow, these agents may reduce smooth-muscle swelling and tubular obstruction (8). They also have a vasodilatory action, which is beneficial in maintaining renal perfusion. However, it is also apparent from several studies that there is a limited window of opportunity during which diuretics are efficacious. In animal models, the use of mannitol from a period beginning an hour before to 10–15 minutes after an acute ischemic insult prevents or attenuates ARF. Unfortunately, in clinical practice it is rarely possible to anticipate an insult.

An initial diuretic challenge should be undertaken only once the patient is volume replete. An intravenous bolus dose of a loop diuretic (40–80 mg of furosemide or 1–2 mg of bumetanide) is usually sufficient to elicit a response. If the urine output does not increase, it is unlikely that the patient will benefit from a continuous infusion of the diuretic. If an initial response is obtained (increase in urine output by 50–200 mL/h), the diuretic can be given as frequent bolus injections (every 4–6 hours) or as a continuous infusion (20–80 mg/h furosemide or 0.5—2.0 mg/h bumetanide). The effect of a loop diuretic can be enhanced by giving a thiazide diuretic (metolazone 5 mg or hydrodiuril 50–100 mg) about 30 minutes beforehand. However, sustained high-dose diuretic therapy to force urine from a relatively diuretic-resistant ICU patient (i.e., a patient who requires >1 mg furosemide per 1 ml urine output) is discouraged because diuretic use in this setting has been associated with higher mortality (9). Although this association may not be causal, the available evidence indicates that patients resistant to diuretics are unlikely to benefit from continued aggressive diuretic therapy, and more definitive therapy (i.e., dialysis) should be administered.

Vasoactive Agents Renal blood flow changes are a common feature of all forms of ARF. As a consequence, there has been a significant interest in use of renal vasodilators to improve the course of the disease. The use of "renal-dose dopamine" (0.5–3 mcg/kg/min) is based on the selective and specific effect of dopamine on DA1 receptors, resulting in renal vasodilatation without effects on the β- and α-receptors. Adding low-dose dopamine has been shown to increase urine flow rates in diuretic-resistant oliguric ARF. However, no large trials have demonstrated any benefit of renal-dose dopamine in ARF; there is no change in the requirement for dialysis or ultimate outcome (8, 10). Because of this absence of evidence, *the use of renal-dose dopamine to enhance urine output cannot be supported*, although it continues to be used widely in practice. Other vasoactive agents, such as norepinephrine or phenylephrine, are increasingly being used to improve hemodynamics and maximize oxygen delivery and cardiac output in septic patients, and this has been associated with improved outcomes (Chapter 26). It is likely, however, that improved urine output and renal outcomes are the result of enhanced cardiac performance rather than any specific effect on the renal vasculature. As such, the choice of inotropic therapy should be based on individual patient parameters and guided by right-heart catheterization, if necessary; it should not be instituted simply to influence renal perfusion (Chapter 25).

Natriuretic Peptides Atrial natriuretic peptide (ANP) increases glomerular filtration rate and renal blood flow in several forms of experimental renal failure and has also been shown to be effective in clinical studies. The increase in glomerular filtration rate occurs despite a decrease in systemic arterial pressure. It results from glomerular afferent arteriolar dilatation and efferent arteriolar constriction; the overall effect is to increase the intraglomerular pressure gradient. In animal models, ANP has been shown to be protective and also improves the recovery from established ARF. Combining this peptide with dopamine appears to attenuate the hypotensive effect. The biological half-life of ANP is short because it is cleared from the circulation by its receptor, filtered by the glomeruli, and metabolized by tubule cells. Initial clinical studies are promising but mixed. The recombinant form of ANP has been evaluated in two multi-center trials for treating ARF that results from acute tubular necrosis. While the first showed a reduced need for dialysis and improved 21-day mortality rate in oliguric patients (but not in nonoliguric patients) (11), subsequent trials failed to show any benefit of ANP (12). Currently, no other natriuretic peptide is available in the United States for treating ARF.

Calcium Channel Blockers Experimental evidence suggests that cellular damage in ARF results in an increase in cytosolic calcium, which can damage cellular integrity by several pathways. It, thus, has been proposed that calcium channel blockers may attenuate the injury. Although several studies have shown that calcium channel blockers may help preserve renal perfusion in the postischemic state if administered before the insult, they have been variably protective when given after the insult (8). Verapamil and diltiazem have been used to perfuse renal allografts before transplantation and have been shown to reduce the incidence of delayed graft function (Chapter 102). Human studies are limited, and there is insufficient evidence to support their general use for ARF.

Other Potentially Promising Agents Growth factors have shown some promising results in experimental models of ARF, particularly that caused by ischemia. However, there are no clinically available therapies in this class because many of the growth factors that appeared promising in experimental models have been less impressive in animal or human trials (e.g., insulin-like growth factor-1 [13], epidermal growth factor, transforming growth factors, and hepatocyte growth factor).

Oxygen-radical scavengers, such as glutathione, superoxide dismutase, and allopurinol, have been used to block the effects of free oxygen radicals in causing cellular injury, but the results are not consistent. Adenine nucleotides have shown a protective effect in experimental ARF and can be beneficial, even if administered several hours after ischemia. Human trials have suggested an improved survival rate from ARF (14), but hemodynamic effects (particularly hypotension) limit their use. Modulation of endothelin and endothelium-derived relaxing factor seemed promising, but trials in contrast nephropathy revealed a detrimental effect (15). Finally, in a mouse model of sepsis and acute renal failure, a single intravenous dose of ethyl pyruvate inhibited functional and histologic renal damage and other organ damage, even when given hours after the insult (16). Although none of these agents are currently available for general use, it is likely that some will be in the future.

Issues During the Course of Hospitalization

Prevention of Contrast-Induced Nephropathy

In addition to the obvious measures such as avoidance of known nephrotoxins and potential prerenal states, a special consideration should be given to prevention, or at least mitigation, of contrast-induced nephropathy. Given the ubiquity of imaging-based diagnosis, administration of radio-contrast media often cannot be avoided even in a patient at high risk for contrast nephropathy (i.e., diabetics, patients with acute or chronic kidney disease, etc.). Luckily, a variety of preventive therapies may lessen the chance for contrast-induced renal failure. These therapies include periprocedural ingestion of N-acetylcysteine and infusion of normal saline or sodium bicarbonate. One prominent study demonstrated a marked protective effect from N-acetylcysteine administered to patients with CRI undergoing contrast studies (17), presumably by scavenging free radicals. Although subsequent studies failed to confirm this benefit, use of this agent remains widespread because it has few side effects and is inexpensive. More recently, the infusion of sodium bicarbonate (given 3 ml/kg/hr for 1 hour prior to the procedure, 1 ml/kg/hr during, and for 6 hours after) was also found to significantly improve outcomes when compared with normal saline treatment in patients with mild renal insufficiency (creatinine 1.7–1.8) (18). Another study demonstrated benefit from periprocedural prophylactic continuous venovenous hemofiltration in high-risk patients; it is unclear whether the benefit was from tighter volume control or a reduction in contrast toxicity. We recommend the use of sodium bicarbonate as first-line prophylactic therapy, reserving dialytic support for patients with very low hemodynamic reserve. In addition, a nonionic, iso-osmolar contrast agent such as iodixanol should be used because it may be less nephrotoxic than ionic or higher osmolarity agents (19).

Extension Phase

Though not part of the classical description of the natural history of ARF, Molitoris and colleagues have proposed an *extension phase* (20), during which renal endothelial dysfunction and ischemia lead to vascular congestion, inflammation, and coagulopathy in the microvasculature of the corticomedullary junction, even after the initial tubular or glomerular insult has subsided. This poorly characterized and short-lived (likely <24 hours) phase may represent a future therapeutic window during which inhibitors of the inflammatory cascade might be administered and extension of ARF mitigated.

Maintenance Phase

Once ARF is established, fluid, electrolyte, and solute balance need to be maintained and new insults prevented. Attention to detail is crucial in this phase and is best assured with the help of a nephrologist.

Fluid and Electrolyte Balance

The development of ARF limits the kidney's ability to maintain fluid balance and electrolyte composition. Oliguric ARF is more limiting in this respect than nonoliguric states. The daily fluid requirement for patients with ARF should be equal to urine output, nonurinary losses (through the gastrointestinal tract, drains, etc.), and insensible water losses. This balance is often difficult to achieve because of obligate intakes necessary for drugs, transfusions, and nutrition. In this situation, clinicians sometimes restrict nutrition to reduce the volume deliv-

ered. It is better, however, to consider earlier intervention with dialysis to allow for both fluid removal and nutritional support. With the newer methods of continuous dialysis described in Chapter 101, it is possible to keep patients in fluid balance without compromising supportive measures. Fluid management is crucial in these patients, because volume overload has been associated with increased morbidity and mortality rates.

Acid-Base Abnormalities

Metabolic acidosis is common in ARF and is caused by the kidney's inability to excrete hydrogen ions. The retained acid is largely buffered by bicarbonate; some is excreted by the lungs as carbon dioxide. Both anion-gap and non-anion-gap acidosis can occur in ARF patients. The former is more likely in the hypotensive septic patient; the latter often can be seen if there are large losses of bicarbonate-rich intestinal secretions. Bicarbonate therapy for acidosis should be used with caution to avoid rebound metabolic alkalosis (Chapter 105). Dialysis may be required if the acidosis is profound and persistent. Metabolic alkalosis is also a common finding in ARF, especially if there are large nasogastric losses. Citrate load from blood-product transfusions also can contribute to alkalosis.

Medications

All renally excreted medications need to be dosage-adjusted in patients with ARF or those on dialysis. It is also important to limit the use of nephrotoxic antibiotics. Opiate doses should be modified; meperidine (Demerol) should be avoided because its metabolites are retained in renal failure, are not easily dialyzed, and may cause seizures. Injectable nonsteroidal anti-inflammatory drugs (e.g., ketorolac) block renal prostaglandin synthesis, which is required to maintain blood flow, and thus should also be avoided.

Dialysis

Dialytic intervention in ARF usually is considered if there is clinical evidence of uremic symptoms or biochemical features of solute and fluid imbalance (Table 100.4). Unfortunately, there is no consensus on the optimal timing of dialytic intervention. The strategy in treating ARF is to minimize and avoid uremic complications; thus, it is not necessary to wait for progressive uremia to initiate dialytic support. On the contrary, there is some evidence that "early" or "prophylactic" dialysis may improve outcome in this setting (21), although comprehensive data on this strategy is lacking. In critically ill patients, the need for dialysis may be dictated by volume overload rather than azotemia. In the ICU setting, dialysis should be viewed as an overall support modality whose use is not limited to replacement of renal function.

The choice of dialysis method influences the frequency of dialytic intervention. Several methods of dialysis are cur-

TABLE 100.4

COMMONLY USED INDICATIONS FOR DIALYSIS

Blood urea nitrogen >100 mg/dL
Hyperkalemia
Marked acidosis
Diuretic-unresponsive fluid overload
Uremic encephalopathy
Uremic pericarditis
Uremic bleeding (e.g., gastrointestinal hemorrhage)

rently available for renal replacement therapy and are discussed in detail in Chapter 101. *Intermittent hemodialysis* (IHD) has been used widely for the past four decades for patients with end-stage renal disease and ARF. It remains the standard form of therapy for treatment of ARF in both the ICU and non-ICU settings. Continuous dialysis modalities are increasingly in use, as well, especially in critically ill or otherwise hemodynamically unstable patients. *Peritoneal dialysis* (PD) has limited application for ARF in the ICU but can be used in some settings when ARF is isolated and the patient weighs less than 100 kg. Its advantages include possible cost savings and that it does not require specialized ICU staff to operate. However, its disadvantages include detrimental effects on respiratory status resulting from diaphragmatic splinting, technical limitations in patients with abdominal sepsis or abdominal surgery, relative inefficiency in removing waste products in catabolic patients, and association with a high incidence of peritonitis. It is inferior to continuous venovenous hemofiltration in ICU patients with ARF (22). The availability of highly permeable membranes has allowed development of *continuous renal replacement techniques* (CRRT) that gradually remove fluids and solutes from the vasculature, resulting in better hemodynamic stability and fluid and solute control. In addition, these modalities may ultimately provide the (as yet unrealized) potential to offer not only renal support but also therapy with sorbents and high-flux membranes that remove harmful inflammatory mediators in a way not previously possible. These methods are limited to the ICU setting, because they require close monitoring and frequent adjustment of fluid balance.

The choice of intermittent hemodialysis versus continuous renal replacement techniques currently is based largely on the local availability of these techniques and the familiarity of the nephrologist and other personnel (particularly ICU staff) with the procedures. Despite the intuitive notion that CRRT should produce better outcomes than IHD, clinical trials have not demonstrated a consistent benefit (23).

Determining the *frequency* of dialysis is a major issue in patients undergoing intermittent therapy. It usually is determined by the patient's clinical and biochemical status (particularly the blood urea nitrogen level and electrolyte and acid-base status). Whether there is benefit from dialyz-

ing patients beyond a given metabolic parameter using IHD is still a matter of contention, and studies on this question have yielded mixed results (24, 25). On the other hand, because CRRT by nature runs continuously, frequency of administered therapy is not an issue. As with intermittent dialysis, it remains controversial whether aggressive, high-dose CRRT improves the outcome of ARF. Recent data suggest a possible benefit to higher dose CRRT, especially in septic patients (26), but this practice is not universally followed.

The *duration* of dialysis for ARF is determined largely by the underlying renal disease and also by any additional insults to the kidney during the course of ARF. In most circumstances, dialysis is discontinued when renal function recovers. Traditional teaching suggests that most patients with reversible ARF improve within 4–6 weeks and that the need for dialysis beyond this period likely represents chronicity. Although this is true in most instances, two important factors need to be considered. First, some patients with ARF in the ICU setting may require prolonged dialysis support (>8 weeks) before recovering renal function, and recovery may be incomplete. Second, the duration of dialysis support may need to be limited (and sometimes predefined) in some patients with ARF if other organ-system failure accompanies ARF (Chapter 25). In this situation, the ultimate prognosis depends on the recovery of other organ systems, and dialytic support may serve only to prolong the dying process (Chapters 17 and 19).

Nutritional Considerations

Aggressive nutritional support is a key component in the management of the patient with ARF. Malnutrition is an independent risk factor for death. In general, nutritional support should take precedence over dialytic intervention, and nutrition should not be withheld to prevent dialysis (i.e., for fear of fluid overload). Rather, early dialysis should be instituted to allow adequate nutrition. Continuous renal replacement techniques offer an advantage over intermittent hemodialysis in this respect. The nutritional prescription should be based on the patient's energy needs. Protein goals should be established to achieve positive nitrogen balance, and carbohydrate and fat amounts prescribed should allow for an appropriate mix of substrates. The contribution of renal replacement therapy to protein and amino-acid losses and glucose absorption should be accounted for in the calculations. It is preferable to use the enteral route whenever possible (Chapter 15). If the parenteral route is used, however, specific renal formulas such as Nephramine or Travesol may be utilized.

Recovery Phase

The recovery phase is characterized by a gradual return of renal function to a level allowing discontinuation of dialysis. This phase often is prolonged, and renal function may not return to baseline levels. During this phase, the main strategy is to maintain adequate fluid and electrolyte balance and prevent further insults to the kidneys. The decision to discontinue dialysis is often difficult and may require gradual weaning with a progressive increase of time between dialysis treatments. Unfortunately, there currently are no specific agents that can speed the recovery phase.

ACUTE RENAL FAILURE DEVELOPING IN THE HOSPITAL

ARF that develops in the hospital carries a worse prognosis than ARF present at the time of admission. In a large study of more than 740 patients from 13 tertiary-care hospitals in Madrid, Spain, 45% of the cases of hospital-acquired ARF were caused by acute tubular necrosis, 21% by prerenal causes, 10% by postrenal causes, 3% by renal vascular disorders, 3% by glomerulonephritis, and 2% by acute interstitial nephritis (27). In a French multi-center study of severe ARF in the ICU (serum creatinine level >3.5 mg/dL), ischemic acute tubular necrosis was the most common reason identified for ARF, although the cause was often unknown or multifactorial (28). Patients who developed ARF during the course of their ICU stays had worse prognoses than those who had ARF at the time of ICU admission.

Recognition

The basic approach for diagnosing ARF in hospitalized patients is similar to that described earlier for ARF at the time of admission. In addition, it helps to remember a few settings in which ARF is particularly common, including the postoperative state and after solid organ and bone-marrow transplantation. In addition, patients with advanced cardiovascular disease, multiple organ failure, sepsis, malignancy, and HIV infection are predisposed to ARF in the hospital. Factors contributing to renal failure are volume depletion, hemodynamic instability, hypotension, and nephrotoxic agents. It should also be recognized that by the time sizable changes in the serum creatinine level occur in the high-risk patient, significant renal damage may have already occurred and the patient's prognosis dramatically affected. Indeed, a recent study suggests that even small, seemingly insignificant changes in creatinine are associated with adverse outcomes in postoperative cardiothoracic surgery patients (29). As such, careful attention to even small changes in renal function (e.g., increases or decreases of creatinine of >0.3 mg/dL) and to the context in which those changes occur is of paramount importance and may lead to improved outcomes if specific supportive therapy can be instituted before the situation deteriorates further. Unfortunately, it is often difficult to pinpoint a single factor, and in many instances there is no evidence of any specific precipitant. In those cases, it is important to utilize a systematic approach to diagnosing ARF.

Management

The initial management of ARF developing in the hospital is similar to that for ARF at the time of hospital admission with the following exception: The course preceding the decline in renal function can be assessed more easily and can be extremely helpful in determining the intervention required. A gradual decline in renal function without obvious evidence of fluid overload should prompt an initial limited volume and diuretic challenge, whereas a rapid elevation in serum creatinine, oliguric state, and fluid overload may require dialytic intervention. It is essential to utilize the information obtained from the patient's observed course to guide therapeutic interventions. Early consultation with a nephrologist may be beneficial, particularly if the exact cause is unclear and ARF complicates pre-existing renal dysfunction.

Outcome

It is well recognized that uncomplicated ARF usually can be managed outside the ICU setting and carries an excellent overall prognosis, with mortality rates usually less than 10%. In contrast, ARF complicating other organ failure in the ICU setting carries mortality rates of more than 50% (Table 100.1) (12, 30). Despite significant advances in the management of ARF during the past four decades, these mortality figures have not changed appreciably; the availability of dialysis has not led to an unequivocal improvement in survival. Although death is an important outcome from ARF, it should not be the only outcome considered, because it often is influenced by multiple factors. For example, renal function recovery is an independent outcome of interest but one that is conditioned by the final outcome of patient death. Survival with full renal recovery is the ideal outcome, but for some patients survival may come at the expense of chronic dialysis. The impact of ARF on the length of stay in the ICU and the resultant costs of care are of obvious additional interest.

There are multiple factors that influence outcomes from ARF. It is possible to broadly classify these as (a) patient characteristics contributing to the nature and severity of the underlying disease associated with ARF, (b) the effects of dialysis itself, and (c) other factors including practice variability and the impact of post-ARF interventions.

Patient Characteristics

The development of ARF is associated with an increase in mortality rate, and patients with ARF as part of multiorgan system failure have a higher mortality rate than those with limited ARF (12, 23). One study in four ICUs found that patients who received nephrology consultation within 48 hours had a lower mortality rate than those who had consultation after 48 hours, an effect that was independent of severity of illness (31). These data suggest that ARF compounds the effects of multiorgan failure and, if unrecognized, can affect outcome adversely.

There appears to be a relationship between the cause and type of ARF and outcome. Patients with ARF secondary to multisystem disorders (e.g., lupus nephritis) have the lowest mortality rate; the highest rate is seen in ischemic acute tubular necrosis. Nephrotoxic acute tubular necrosis has an intermediate mortality rate. Although nonoliguric ARF carries a better prognosis than oliguric ARF, recent data suggest that nonoliguric ARF may have a worse prognosis in ICU patients. A possible explanation is that nonoliguric states lead clinicians to overestimate renal function, leading to a delay in initiation of dialysis. In general, patients do better if the cause of renal dysfunction is quickly identified and specific treatment is instituted.

Dialysis Process Factors

The timing of renal replacement therapy, the amount and frequency of dialysis, and the duration of therapy all impact the eventual outcome. Because physician preferences and experience are variable and universal guidelines for dialysis are not followed, comparing outcomes between centers or patients is difficult. Further discussion of these issues is in Chapter 101.

Practice Variation and Post-Acute Renal Failure Interventions

The provision of ancillary support for ARF patients may also affect outcomes. Several studies in ICU patients suggest that malnutrition worsens outcome, and calorie deprivation has been associated with poor outcomes in dialyzed ARF patients. The importance of other interventions after ARF is established also should be considered. For instance, angiographic or surgical procedures and the use of nephrotoxic agents and antibiotics all may prolong the duration of ARF and increase the mortality rate.

DISCHARGE ISSUES

As described previously, the main goal in managing ARF is to provide supportive therapy to enable the patient to regain renal function. The nature and severity of renal injury and the interventions required to maintain homeostasis are key determinants of outcomes. Discharge planning should incorporate a strategy to monitor renal function at frequent intervals. Patients with new-onset ARF who do not undergo dialysis in the hospital and who regain renal function should have outpatient follow-up to ensure that the recovery is maintained, and they should be advised to avoid nephrotoxic agents and renal insults. If renal function recovery is incomplete, follow-up with a nephrologist may be indicated for periodic monitoring of renal function. Any medications prescribed should be adjusted for the level of

renal function, and patients should be cautioned not to take over-the-counter medications (particularly nonsteroidal anti-inflammatory agents) without checking with their physicians. Patients with pre-existing renal dysfunction who suffer an episode of ARF should have follow-up with a nephrologist because the recent insult may worsen the progression of renal failure and hasten the need for subsequent dialytic intervention. Specific strategies to reduce progression of renal disease may need to be instituted depending on the clinical circumstance (e.g., use of ACE inhibitors in diabetic nephropathy). For patients who require dialysis in the hospital, the continued need for dialytic support is an important consideration (32). If dialysis continues to be required at the time of hospital discharge, an outpatient dialysis regimen must be established. The consulting nephrologist who provides the dialytic support in the hospital can usually secure this follow-up. A major factor in this case is whether the patient is likely to recover enough function to discontinue dialysis or is likely to remain dialysis-dependent. In the latter circumstance, the diagnosis of end-stage renal disease permits the institution of long-term dialysis and establishes a payer (in the United States, Medicare) for the dialysis treatments. Often patients have to transition to a rehabilitation facility before returning home and may require dialysis at that or another facility.

COST CONSIDERATIONS AND RESOURCE UTILIZATION

The development of ARF adds to the overall cost of a patient's hospitalization, particularly if dialytic intervention is required (8, 12, 26). Early recognition, along with appropriate and timely intervention, can minimize the effect of ARF on other organ function. Timely consultation with a nephrologist may help in streamlining the management of the patient and facilitate early dialytic intervention. If dialysis is required, the choice of modality, frequency of intervention, and duration all affect the cost (Chapter 101). More importantly, the long-term costs from an episode of ARF are influenced by the recovery of renal function and need for chronic dialysis. All attempts should be made to prevent this complication in high-risk patients and situations. Resources can be monitored by evaluating the frequency with which patients require dialysis and the frequency of renal functional recovery.

KEY POINTS

- ARF is an important complication that has a variable frequency but is predictable in certain circumstances.
- Recognition of the risk for ARF should result in the initiation of strategies to prevent ARF and attenuate the insult.
- In the high-risk (i.e., postoperative) patient, even subtle changes in serum creatinine level can indicate a potentially worse outcome.

- Early recognition of renal dysfunction, understanding of the clinical context, and management are keys to ensuring a good outcome. Understanding the natural history of this disorder should permit appropriate and timely decisions for therapeutic intervention. Although ARF has been divided traditionally into prerenal, renal, and postrenal causes, an equally useful nosology is to divide cases into reversible, self-limited, and irreversible causes.

- Several therapeutic options are now available for the nondialytic and dialytic management of ARF. The former include the use of volume, diuretics, and vasoactive agents (although "renal-dose dopamine" has not been shown to be beneficial). The latter include intermittent or continuous hemodialysis, as well as peritoneal dialysis for a limited number of indications.

REFERENCES

1. Myers BD, Moran SM. Hemodynamically mediated acute renal failure. *N Engl J Med* 1986;314:94–105.
2. Carvounis CP, Nisar S, Guro-Razuman S. Significance of the fractional excretion of urea in the differential diagnosis of acute renal failure. *Kidney Int* 2002;62:2223–2229.
3. Prakash J, Tripathi K, Usha, Kumar P. Clinical significance of kidney biopsy in acute renal failure. *Indian J Med Science* 1992;46:328–331.
4. Muramatsu Y, Tsujie M, Star RA, et al. Early detection of cysteine rich protein 61 (CYR61, CCN1) in urine following renal ischemic reperfusion injury. *Kidney Int* 2002;62:1601–1610.
5. Han, WK, Bailly V, Bonventre JV, et al. Kidney Injury Molecule-1 (KIM-1): a novel biomarker for human renal proximal tubule injury. *Kidney Int* 2002;62:237–244.
6. Du Cheyron, D, Daubin, C, Poggioli J, et al. Urinary measurement of Na+/H+ exchanger isoform 3 (NHE3) protein as new marker of tubule injury in critically ill patients with ARF. *Am J Kidney Dis* 2003;42:497–506.
7. Finfer S, Bellomo R, Boyce N, et al. A comparison of albumin and saline for fluid resuscitation in the intensive care unit. *N Engl J Med* 2004;350:2247–2256.
8. Alkhunaizi AM, Schrier RW. Management of acute renal failure: new perspectives. *Am J Kidney Dis* 1996;28:315–328.
9. Mehta RL, Pascual MT, Soroko S, et al. Diuretics, mortality, and nonrecovery of renal function in acute renal failure. *JAMA* 2002;288:2547–2553.
10. Bellomo R, Chapman M, Finfer S, et al. Low-dose dopamine in patients with early renal dysfunction: a placebo-controlled randomised trial. Australian and New Zealand Intensive Care Society (ANZICS) Clinical Trials Group. *Lancet* 2000;356:2139–2143.
11. Allgren RL, Marbury TC, Rahman SN, et al. Anaritide in acute tubular necrosis: auriculin anaritide acute renal failure study group. *N Engl J Med* 1997;336:828–834.
12. Star RA. Treatment of acute renal failure. *Kidney Int* 1998;54:1817–1831.
13. Hirschberg R, Kopple J, Lipsett P, et al. Multicenter clinical trial of recombinant human insulin-like growth factor I in patients with acute renal failure. *Kidney Int* 1999;55:2423–2432.
14. Fischereder M, Trick W, Nath K. Therapeutic strategies in the prevention of acute renal failure. *Semin Nephrol* 1994;14:41–52.
15. Wang A, Holsclaw T, Bashore TM, et al. Exacerbation of radiocontrast nephrotoxicity by endothelin receptor antagonism. *Kidney Int* 2000;57:1675–1680.
16. Miyaji T, Hu X, Yuen PST, et al. Ethyl pyruvate decreases sepsis-induced acute renal failure and multiple organ damage in aged mice. *Kidney Int* 2003;64:1620–1631.
17. Tepel M, van der Giet M, Schwarzfeld C, et al. Prevention of radiographic-contrast-agent-induced reductions in renal function by acetylcysteine. *N Engl J Med* 2000;343:180–184.
18. Merten GJ, Burgess WP, Gray LV, et al. Prevention of contrast-induced nephropathy with bicarbonate. *JAMA* 2004;291:2328–2334.
19. Aspelin P, Aubrey P, Fransson SG, et al. Nephrotoxic effects in high-risk patients undergoing angiography. *N Engl J Med* 2003;348:491–499.
20. Sutton TA, Fisher CJ, Molitoris BA. Microvascular endothelial injury and dysfunction during ischemic acute renal failure. *Kidney Int* 2002:62:1539–1549.
21. Mehta RL. Therapeutic alternatives to renal replacement therapy for critically ill patients in acute renal failure. *Semin Nephrol* 1994;14:64–82.
22. Phu NH, Hien TT, Day N, et al. Hemofiltration and peritoneal dialysis in infection-associated acute renal failure in Vietnam. *New Engl J Med* 2002;347:895–902.
23. Kellum JA, Angus DC, Linde-Zwirble WT, et al. Continuous versus intermittent renal replacement therapy: a meta-analysis. *Intensive Care Med* 2002;28:29–37.
24. Schiffl H, Lang SM, Fischer R. Daily hemodialysis and the outcome of acute renal failure. *N Engl J Med* 2002;346:305–310.
25. Marshall MR, Ma T, Galler D, et al. Sustained low-efficiency daily diafiltration (SLEDD-f) for critically ill patients requiring renal replacement therapy: towards an adequate therapy. *Nephrol Dial Transplant* 2004;19:877–884.
26. Ronco C, Bellomo R, Homel P, et al. Effects of different doses in continuous venovenous hemofiltration on outcomes of acute renal failure: a prospective randomized trial. *Lancet* 2000;355:26–30.
27. Liaño F, Pascual J. Outcomes in acute renal failure. *Semin Nephrol* 1998;18:541–550.
28. Brivet FG, Kleinknecht DJ, Loirat P, et al. The French study group on acute renal failure: acute renal failure in intensive care units. Causes, outcome, and prognostic factors of hospital mortality. A prospective, multicenter study. *Crit Care Med* 1996;24:192–198.
29. Lassnigg A, Schmidlin D, Mouhieddine M, et al. Minimal changes of serum creatinine predict prognosis in patients after cardiothoracic surgery: a prospective cohort study. *J Am Soc Nephrol* 2004;15:1597–1605.
30. Nolan CR, Anderson RJ. Hospital acquired acute renal failure. *J Am Soc Nephrol* 1998;9:710–718.
31. Mehta RL, Farkas A, Pascual M, et al. Effect of delayed consultation on outcome from acute renal failure in the ICU. *J Am Soc Nephrol* 1995;6:471.
32. Firth JD. Acute irreversible renal failure. *Q J Med* 1996;89:397–399.

ADDITIONAL READING

Esson ML, Schrier RW. Diagnosis and treatment of acute tubular necrosis. *Ann Intern Med* 2002;137:744–752.

Leblanc M. Acid-base balance in acute renal failure and renal replacement therapy. *Best Pract Res Clin Anaesthesiol* 2004;18:113–127.

Luyckx VA, Bonventre JV. Dose of dialysis in acute renal failure. *Semin Dial* 2004;17:30–36.

Mehta RL. Outcomes research in acute renal failure. *Semin Nephrol* 2003;23:283–294.

Mehta RL, Chertow GM. Acute renal failure definitions and classification: time for change? *J Am Soc Nephrol* 2003;14:2178–2187.

Schrier RW, Wang W. Acute renal failure and sepsis. *N Engl J Med* 2004;351:159–169.

Schrier RW, Wang W, Poole B, et al. Acute renal failure: definitions, diagnosis, pathogenesis, and therapy. *J Clin Invest* 2004;114:5–14.

Yegenaga I, Hoste E, Van Biesen W, et al. Clinical characteristics of patients developing ARF due to sepsis/systemic inflammatory response syndrome: results of a prospective study. *Am J Kidney Dis* 2004;43:817–824.

Management of the Hospitalized Patient on Dialysis

101

Glenn M. Chertow

INTRODUCTION

In 2004, there were more than 325,000 patients being treated with hemodialysis and peritoneal dialysis in the United States (1). Given the myriad complications associated with end-stage renal disease (ESRD), it is not surprising that patients with ESRD are far more likely than the general population to be hospitalized, and that the length of hospital stay, compared with the general population, is significantly longer. ESRD can result in widespread organ dysfunction, either as a result of the disease processes that lead to chronic kidney disease, or because of uremia or the physiologic disturbances associated with renal replacement therapy itself. This chapter outlines the unique disease entities that must be considered in caring for the hospitalized patient on dialysis and management strategies to address these conditions.

DIALYSIS PRIMER

Renal replacement therapy is a term used frequently to describe the global approach to patients with ESRD. The kidneys perform four major functions: regulation of electrolyte and acid-base balance, disposition of metabolic byproducts and drugs, maintenance of volume status, and organ-specific endocrine and metabolic effects. Kidney transplantation can replace all four functions and is appropriately called renal replacement therapy (Chapter 102).

Dialysis can assist with the first three functions, and the fourth can be regulated with the help of exogenous hormone replacement, which is also discussed.

Hemodialysis

In the United States, hemodialysis is the dialytic modality prescribed for most patients. More than 80% of dialysis patients undergo hemodialysis, usually three times weekly in a hospital-affiliated or independent outpatient dialysis center (1). The key to successful provision of hemodialysis is the *vascular access*, because high blood flow rates ($\geq$300 mL/min) are required to perform solute clearance most efficiently. The most reliable vascular access is the native arteriovenous (Brescia-Cimino) fistula, usually an end-to-side anastomosis of the cephalic vein to radial artery at the wrist. Variations on the Brescia-Cimino fistula also are seen in the upper arm and, rarely, in the leg. The most common permanent vascular access for hemodialysis is the arteriovenous graft, usually constructed as a loop graft of polytetrafluroethylene in the forearm. For patients whose permanent vascular access has not matured (in the case of a fistula) or healed, a variety of percutaneous and tunneled central venous catheters are available, which can provide temporary access to the circulation for the dialysis procedure.

The duration of dialysis (typically 3–4 hours per session) depends on the needs of the patient and is typically driven by quantitative assessment of the adequacy of clearance, using urea as the marker solute. For a given dialyzer type, blood flow rate, dialysate flow rate, and vascular access, a longer treatment results in more efficient solute clearance. Longer dialysis times may also be required to facilitate ultrafiltration to "dry weight," because rapid ultrafiltration rates may exceed the body's vascular refill capacity.

In the outpatient setting, the net health-related benefits of prolonged dialysis times must be balanced against the potential effects on quality of life and convenience. In the inpatient setting, the constraints on the provision of dialysis are quite different, because dialysis competes with diagnostic tests and surgical procedures for precious time during daytime hours. It has been observed that patients with ESRD tend to receive a lower dose of dialysis when hospitalized, at precisely the time that more thorough treatments may be required because of stress (including cardiovascular dysfunction, inflammation, and sepsis, often accompanied by hypotension) and catabolism (promoting azotemia). It is important to ensure that sufficient dialysis time be provided to hospitalized patients by coordinating schedules at least 1 day in advance of the need for dialysis.

Peritoneal Dialysis

Peritoneal dialysis typically is provided in one of two ways: either with manual exchanges several times during the day (*continuous ambulatory peritoneal dialysis*) or with automated exchanges delivered by a device (a "cycler") usually for 10–12 hours at night (*continuous cyclic peritoneal dialysis*). Most patients have a flexible silastic catheter placed within the peritoneal cavity. The concentration of dextrose in the dialysate is the principal variable in therapy, with 1.5%, 2.5%, and 4.25% dextrose concentrations being the most common. It is the concentration of dextrose that drives ultrafiltration of plasma water, again by diffusion across the semipermeable membrane. Higher dextrose concentrations are associated with higher rates of ultrafiltration. Patients on peritoneal dialysis usually can continue their regular home dialysis schedule if hospitalized.

Table 101.1 lists the major complications of the dialysis procedure. In addition to hemodialysis and peritoneal dialysis, newer methods of dialysis have been developed principally to assist in the management of critically ill, hospitalized patients: the *continuous renal replacement therapies*. An outline of the methods and potential indications for these therapies is given in Table 101.2.

MANAGEMENT OF THE HOSPITALIZED DIALYSIS PATIENT

General Issues

Subsequent sections describe specific conditions that frequently result in hospitalizations for patients on dialysis. This section discusses several general inpatient management issues that require modification for dialysis patients.

Admission Orders

If a patient with ESRD is admitted to the hospital, several things should be done immediately. First, the dialysis unit and the nephrologist who care for the patient should be informed of the admission; the dialysis unit often maintains its own set of comprehensive medical records, and certain information relevant to the acute problem requiring hospitalization, including recent laboratory values, may be unavailable to the hospital staff. If the hospital has an inpatient dialysis program, that unit should be informed, as well, to assist in the organization of the dialysis schedule.

Blood pressure should be taken in the arm *contralateral* to the vascular access if an arteriovenous fistula or graft is present. Otherwise, repeated compression of the vascular access by the sphygmomanometer cuff can result in access thrombosis. Elderly patients with ESRD and patients with ESRD and diabetes tend to be unsteady in the few hours following dialysis treatment because of autonomic dysfunction and delayed vascular refill. Although bedrest may not be necessary, physical activity in the 2–4 hours following dialysis generally should be supervised. Routine placement of an intravenous catheter should be discouraged, unless clearly clinically indicated. Many medications and blood products can be administered during or just after the dialysis procedure with greater safety because of concurrent ultrafiltration. Furthermore, the puncture and subsequent scarring that often occurs if veins of the upper extremities are cannulated can result in the loss of potential venous sites for future permanent vascular access. Venous sclerosis is a particularly troublesome complication of therapy with nafcillin or oxacillin, drugs frequently prescribed to patients on dialysis with infectious complications. If an intravenous line is required, it should be placed distal to the arteriovenous fistula or graft, or in a vein of the contralateral arm, preferably in the hand.

Several *medications* routinely administered in hospitalized patients should be used with caution in ESRD patients. Antacids containing magnesium are relatively safe in small quantities but can lead to hypermagnesemia in patients treated with large doses over several days. Sedative drugs tend to be poorly tolerated in ESRD patients. The risks of delirium and other central nervous system effects increase in ESRD patients treated with anticholinergic drugs, such as diphenhydramine. Short-acting benzodiazepines can lead to a paradoxic agitated state.

The *diet order* requires careful thought in most patients with ESRD and should be individualized. The "renal diet" in most hospitals is typically low in protein (<60 g/d) and potassium (<2 g/d), and usually low in sodium (<2 g/d) and phosphorus (<1 g/d). The restrictions on sodium and potassium sometimes, but not always, are required, depending on the type of kidney disease and the effectiveness of medications, including diuretic agents and dialysis. There is little rationale for the restriction of dietary protein. Although over the long term there is some evidence that

TABLE 101.1

SELECTED MAJOR COMPLICATIONS OF THE DIALYSIS PROCEDURE AND METHODS OF PREVENTION

Complication	Preventive measures
Hemodialysis	
Hypotension	Extend dialysis time
	Perform sequential ultrafiltration-hemodialysis
	Discontinue antihypertensive (not antianginal) agents
	Decrease dialysate temperature
	Increase dialysate calcium concentration
	Increase hemoglobin concentration
	Consider administration of colloid
	Consider change in estimated dry weight
Arrhythmia	Increase dialysate potassium concentration
	Consider discontinuing digoxin and other antiarrhythmic agents
	Supplemental oxygen during dialysis
Muscle cramps	Extend dialysis time
	Consider hypertonic saline
	Consider vitamin E
	Consider quinine sulfate
Pyrogen reaction	Culture dialysate
	Immediate water testing for lipopolysaccharide
Dialysis disequilibrium	Attenuate clearance by limiting time, dialyzer surface area, blood flow, and dialysate flow
	Consider mannitol
Hypoxemia	Use noncellulosic dialyzer
	Supplemental oxygen during dialysis
Hemolysis	Examine blood lines
	Immediate water testing for chloramine
Peritoneal Dialysis	
Constipation	Regular administration of lactulose or other nonstimulant cathartic
	Consider changing phosphate binder
Early satiety	Consider change from continuous ambulatory peritoneal dialysis to continuous cyclic peritoneal dialysis
Hyperglycemia	Investigate for infection
	Consider adding (or increasing) insulin in dialysate
	Limit dextrose concentration
	Consider diuretics to augment ultrafiltration

protein restriction can attenuate the progression of certain types of renal disease (2), the net benefits are small and must be balanced against the potential for contributing to the development of protein malnutrition (3). Because protein-rich foods tend to be high in phosphorus content, the restriction of dietary phosphorus is counterproductive. The administration of phosphate binders is a better strategy for phosphorus control. Because malnutrition is an important contributing factor to hospitalization in patients undergoing dialysis, these individuals should be not be subjected to dietary restrictions while in the hospital (4). The exception is patients with vascular access failure or another reason for inefficient dialysis, because they tend to be hyperkalemic and cannot afford a diet high in potassium.

Laboratory tests that require venipuncture, including blood cultures, can be performed easily at the start of the hemodialysis session, and nonessential tests should be deferred on nondialysis days. The serum potassium concentration should not be checked for at least 4 hours following the dialysis procedure to allow for rebound of potassium from intracellular stores. This avoids the unnecessary and potentially unsafe practice of potassium supplementation when an early postdialysis potassium concentration returns in the range less than 4 mEq/L.

Examination and Laboratory Findings in Patients with End-Stage Renal Disease

Certain aspects of the general physical examination and laboratory profile are characteristic of this population. On initial observation, many dialysis patients appear thin, with overt muscle wasting. Depending on the nutritional assessment method used, 50%–90% of patients on dialysis have some evidence of malnutrition. If there is muscle

TABLE 101.2

ALTERNATIVE METHODS OF DIALYSIS FOR ACUTE RENAL FAILURE

Method	Intensity of nursing effort[b]	Cost[b]	Potential indications
Intermittent hemodialysis	+	++	Hyperkalemia Mild-to-moderate volume overload Hemodynamic stability ICU or non-ICU setting Poisoning
Peritoneal dialysis	++	+	No abdominal surgery or active issues Pregnancy Pediatrics ICU or non-ICU setting
Continuous renal replacement therapy[a]	++++	+++	Hemodynamic instability Large obligate fluid load (including blood products and parenteral nutrition) Moderate-to-massive volume overload Severe metabolic acidosis ICU setting

[a] Hemofiltration alone (continuous venovenous hemofiltration) or hemodiafiltration (continuous venovenous hemodiafiltration).
[b] Semi-quantitative scale, with "+" representing lowest and "++++" representing highest.

wasting and other overt signs of malnutrition, the risk of death or injury increases. Therefore, the lean dialysis patient should be considered at high risk. Hypertension is likewise extremely common in dialysis patients. Elevated blood pressure is often indicative of volume overload and should be managed with the patient's dialysis schedule and hospital presentation in mind. Physical examination should always include careful auscultation of the chest, in search of an uremic pericardial or pleural rub. Systolic flow murmurs are common, especially among patients with anemia. These should be carefully differentiated from sounds transmitted from an arteriovenous fistula, which tend to be harsher and often extend through systole and diastole. The abdomen should be carefully examined for signs of hepatic congestion. A detailed neurologic examination should be performed if uremia is implicated in a change in cognitive or functional status.

The laboratory profile of dialysis patients is characteristically abnormal. The degree of elevation of urea nitrogen and creatinine levels relative to the patient's overall condition and dialysis history is extremely important. A serum urea nitrogen that is extremely high (e.g., >150 mg/dL) might indicate gastrointestinal bleeding, glucocorticoid therapy, or an overwhelming catabolic process. An extremely low level of serum urea nitrogen (e.g., <30 mg/dL) might be expected several hours after the completion of dialysis but might indicate a marked reduction in dietary protein intake if obtained on a nondialysis day. The electrolytes are frequently abnormal, with a propensity for hyperkalemia and metabolic acidosis. Hyperphosphatemia, hyperuricemia, and an elevated anion gap are common findings in patients on dialysis. Liver enzymes, lactate de-

hydrogenase, and bilirubin concentrations should be normal. The alkaline phosphatase often is elevated, an indication of the effect of secondary hyperparathyroidism on bone. The serum albumin concentration is on average significantly lower in dialysis patients than in age-matched controls; hypoalbuminemia has been shown to predict markedly higher mortality and morbidity rates in these patients (5).

The most common finding on the complete blood count is a low hemoglobin concentration. The problem of "renal anemia" has been alleviated greatly with the introduction of recombinant erythorpoietin, which is now administered routinely to patients with chronic kidney disease, sometimes before the initiation of dialysis. Anemia has been further lessened with the more widespread prescription of intravenous iron compounds and better control of hyperparathyroidism. The platelet count and coagulation studies should be normal.

Cardiovascular Disease

Except for procedures related to the vascular access, cardiovascular complications, including congestive heart failure, and coronary, cerebral, and peripheral vascular disease, account for an overwhelming proportion of hospitalizations and considerable morbidity in patients with ESRD. The incidence of atherosclerotic vascular disease is markedly increased in patients with ESRD and accounts, at least in part, for a majority of deaths (6).

Chest pain in a dialysis patient must be taken seriously, given the high pretest probability of disease and the anticipated level of disease severity. Treatment of suspected ischemia should be similar to that in non-ESRD patients. All patients without other contraindications should receive aspirin. The long-acting β-adrenergic antagonists atenolol and nadolol are eliminated by the kidney and should have their dosages reduced, or alternative agents (e.g., metoprolol) should be used. Most angiotensin-converting enzyme inhibitors are eliminated by the kidney, and lower doses at less frequent intervals initially should be employed in dialysis patients. Parenteral opiate analgesics should be used with caution. Low-dose morphine or hydromorphone are acceptable options; meperidine should be avoided because its major metabolite (normeperidine) is epileptogenic and accumulates in ESRD. Calcium antagonists and nitrates do not require dose adjustment. Short-acting dihydropyridine calcium antagonists should be avoided.

Most if not all antianginal agents should be continued to the time of dialysis. The dialysis procedure is a stressful event, and dialysis patients with known coronary artery disease should be protected from developing tachycardia during dialysis. If hypotension develops during dialysis, ultrafiltration should cease temporarily, and the ultrafiltration rate should be reduced. Sequential ultrafiltration and hemodialysis or an additional treatment of ultrafiltration alone may be required in selected cases. Nonischemic causes of chest pain in patients on dialysis include pericarditis, esophagitis, and a variety of musculoskeletal disorders.

Pericarditis should be suspected in any patient who has not adhered faithfully to the dialysis schedule or who regularly terminates the dialysis session prematurely. The cause of pericarditis cannot easily be determined on clinical grounds. Hemodynamically insignificant posterior pericardial effusions may be present in 15%–20% of stable, asymptomatic dialysis patients. Larger effusions, especially if they are anterior and posterior, usually are related to pericarditis and reflect significant disease. Fever, leukocytosis, a large-sized effusion, and hemodynamic instability suggest a nonuremic cause. Regardless of the suspected cause of pericarditis, more frequent and intensive dialysis should be provided for at least 10–14 days if uremic pericarditis is a possibility. Pericardiocentesis is indicated urgently for tamponade physiology or if a large effusion persists after intensifying the dialysis regimen. Tamponade should be suspected from the usual physical findings (Chapter 46) or if the usual quantity of ultrafiltration at dialysis is not tolerated.

Pulmonary edema in the patient undergoing dialysis can be of cardiac or noncardiac origin. Dietary indiscretion can lead to pulmonary edema, because of the inability to excrete an increased load of salt and water with reduced or absent native kidney function. A pattern of previous episodes and the timing of the event can provide clues to this diagnosis. Another common scenario leading to pulmonary edema is a loss in body cell mass associated with either a period of reduced dietary intake or hypermetabolism. If the goal of postdialysis ("dry") weight remains the same and the amount of intracellular water decreases, extracellular fluid is retained in its place, often leading to hypertension and pulmonary edema. Although standard therapies for pulmonary edema can provide some symptomatic relief, mechanical ultrafiltration with or without dialysis is the treatment of choice. Some patients on dialysis maintain urine output for months-to-years following the development of ESRD (especially those on peritoneal dialysis) and may remain responsive to high-dosage diuretics (e.g., furosemide ≥160 mg intravenous). Topical and intravenous nitrates, selected opiate analgesics, nesiritide, and nitroprusside may each be useful in selected cases; the latter agent should not be used for >12 hours to avoid significant toxicity. High-output congestive heart failure also should be considered in patients with ESRD. Anemia can contribute to tachycardia and dyspnea, and the presence of an arteriovenous shunt can increase cardiac output significantly. Patients with ESRD and severe degrees of left ventricular hypertrophy tolerate anemia and tachycardia especially poorly. Hyperthyroidism should be considered; typical symptoms may be absent or masked by uremia or dialysis asthenia. Finally, beriberi should be considered as a possible cause of heart failure, especially if a metabolic acidosis is present. Frank thiamine deficiency can develop in dialysis patients with poor or marginal oral intake who fail to take water-soluble vitamin supplements.

Infectious Disease

Infectious complications are common in dialysis patients. The most important infectious complications relate to dialysis access: the arteriovenous graft or central venous catheter for hemodialysis (bacteremia) and the peritoneal catheter for peritoneal dialysis (peritonitis). *Protein-calorie malnutrition* can increase susceptibility to a wide variety of infections and is probably more responsible than uremia for the increased incidence of infection, particularly among patients receiving an adequate dialysis dose. Environmental exposures, the need for blood transfusion, and exposure to immunosuppressive agents following failed kidney transplantation also can increase the risk of infection.

Hemodialysis requires repetitive access to the blood stream. Despite efforts taken to sterilize the skin prior to needle placement, infections of the vascular access are extremely common. The overall rate of serious line infection is approximately one per patient per year (just less than 10% per month), an exceptionally high rate. Most often, the organism is a Gram-positive species, usually *Staphylococcus epidermidis* or *aureus*. Other Gram-positive cocci are frequently seen, including Vancomycin-resistant *Enterococcus* (VRE); Gram-positive rods such as *Bacillus* sp. may also be pathogenic. Gram-negative rods, including *E. Coli* and *Klebsiella* spp., are seen 10%–15% of the time, although their presence in blood cultures should prompt investigation elsewhere, such as the gastrointestinal and genitourinary tracts. Other Gram-negative rods, such as *Stenotrophomonas maltophilia* and *Acinetobacter* spp., have been observed with increasing frequency in recent years, related to the use of broad-spectrum antibiotics and, potentially, to contaminated environmental sites. Native arteriovenous fistulas are rarely the source of infection, although their repeated puncture may be an entry site for bacteremia. In contrast, a blood-borne infection may harbor at the graft site, an artificial endovascular device prone to seeding. Although parenteral antibiotics are clearly indicated for infection of the vascular graft, the likelihood of clearing grossly infected polytetrafluroethylene graft is extremely low. Thus, *in most circumstances, the graft should be removed promptly.* Infections in the setting of tunneled hemodialysis catheters should be approached with a similar degree of caution. Attempts to "treat through" line infections with bacteremia typically fail, as catheter "biofilm" serves to harbor bacteria that can cause relapsing infections after antibiotics have been discontinued. Such infections can lead to endocarditis, osteomyelitis, and other serious deep-tissue infections. In the setting of line-associated bacteremia, some advocate removal of all tunneled dialysis catheters followed by placement of temporary catheters until bacteremia has cleared. Others have found that catheter exchange over a wire (when there is no evidence of catheter tunnel infection) has yielded exceptionally low rates of treatment failure (i.e., relapse) and considerably less morbidity. Only in the case of *Staphylococcus epidermidis* infection do we recommend antibiotic therapy without line exchange. The duration of antibiotic therapy for an access-associated infection should be 3 weeks. If there is evidence of endovascular infection, 6 weeks of parenteral antibiotics are recommended. Empiric therapy for suspected infection of the vascular access should be based on the microbiologic epidemiology of the hospital and surrounding region (Chapter 72). Definitive therapy then should be based on microbiologic results.

Actual transmission of infection via dialysate has been reported but is rare, because the dialysate is not infused into the patient. It is clearly possible, however, for bacterial cell-wall products or bacterial fragments to be transmitted to the patient on dialysis, which can result in the *pyrogen reaction,* clinically indistinguishable from sepsis syndrome. Patients with pyrogen reactions typically require hospitalization because of high fever, rigors, and leukocytosis or severe leukopenia, and they must be evaluated and treated for sepsis syndrome (Chapter 26). The signs and symptoms usually resolve within 24 hours, and blood cultures are negative. A cluster of patients with fever and systemic symptoms from the same dialysis unit should raise suspicion that the dialysate may have been contaminated.

Peritonitis is probably the most important complication for peritoneal dialysis patients. It is the most frequent cause of hospitalization, and the principle reason for switching from peritoneal to hemodialysis. As with hemodialysis-associated line infections, skin organisms are the most common pathogens. *Staphylococcus epidermidis* and *aureus* lead the list of responsible pathogens. Gram-negative rods and fungi are especially troublesome, resulting in more frequent hospitalization, catheter removal, and change to hemodialysis. The most common clinical findings are fever, abdominal pain, and cloudy dialysate. *Many patients with peritonitis do not require hospitalization.* If the episode is addressed early, appropriate cell counts and cultures can be obtained and empiric parenteral antibiotic therapy begun, via either the intravenous or intraperitoneal route. Cefazolin and vancomycin are reasonable first-line therapies, and either can be safely administered in the peritoneal dialysate. Hospitalization, if necessary, should be brief (<72 hours). Usually, the patient's technique is as good as that of the nondialysis nursing staff, and the odds of contracting a resistant organism are lower in the home than in the hospital environment.

Blood-borne viral infections are more common in hemodialysis patients because of shared risk factors (e.g., hepatitis B and C viruses and HIV-associated kidney diseases) and the need for frequent hospitalization and transfusions. It is strongly recommended that all patients with advanced chronic kidney disease be vaccinated against hepatitis B, although the strength and durability of the antibody response are attenuated compared with other populations. Patients who are known to be positive for hepatitis B surface antibody are isolated. Hepatitis C infection should be suspected in any dialysis patient with a history of transfusion, injection drug abuse, or high-risk sexual behaviors.

Respiratory Disease

Pulmonary edema is the most common respiratory manifestation of the dialysis patient. Its management has been discussed previously. Pneumonia, though not specific to ESRD, is an extremely common reason for hospitalization. Pleural effusion is seen with higher frequency than in the population without ESRD, perhaps owing to subtle serosal inflammation or hypoalbuminemia. An increased frequency of pleuritis and hemorrhagic pleural effusion also has been noted. Except if more intensive dialysis and ultrafiltration are required, the management of these syndromes in ESRD is no different than in the general population (see Chapters 39, 65, and 60, respectively for pulmonary edema, pneumonia, and pleural effusion).

Sleep apnea has been reported in up to 60% of patients with ESRD, regardless of modality of dialysis, and can be central or obstructive in origin. Affected dialysis patients are at increased risk for systemic and pulmonary hypertension, as well as for a variety of atrial and ventricular arrhythmias, including sudden death. Acidemia and hyperkalemia induced by uncompensated respiratory acidosis may be the mechanism in many cases. Respiratory therapy with continuous positive airway pressure and supplemental oxygen may be required during hospitalization.

Gastrointestinal Disease

Patients with previously undetected, advanced chronic kidney disease usually seek medical attention (and often require hospitalization) because of the gastrointestinal manifestations of uremia. These include anorexia, dysgeusia, nausea and vomiting (characteristically upon awakening), gastrointestinal hemorrhage, and the nitrogenous fetor. A variety of gastrointestinal abnormalities persist in ESRD patients after the initiation of dialysis, and some prompt hospitalization. Gastritis and upper gastrointestinal bleeding are more common than in the general population; upper endoscopy is abnormal in approximately 50% of ESRD patients, depending on the severity of symptoms and the indication for study. Although most patients are found to have an inflammatory infiltrate in the gastric epithelium, 5%–15% of patients have evidence of atrophic gastritis. *Helicobacter pylori* infection may contribute to the development of peptic ulcer disease in dialysis patients, although it is not clear if the incidence of *H. pylori* infection increases in this population relative to the general population. Because dialysis patients without serious gastrointestinal disease may have blood loss and iron deficiency caused by increased bleeding tendencies and long-term anticoagulation, the interpretation of guaiac-positive stools or nasogastric aspirate must be tempered. Nevertheless, repeated positive tests should prompt investigation.

The treatment of *peptic ulcer disease* in dialysis patients is similar to that in patients with normal renal function (Chapter 80). If gastric lavage is deemed appropriate, 5% dextrose in water, rather than saline, should be used to avoid sodium overload. Antacids (containing magnesium and aluminum) and sucralfate (containing aluminum) should be used sparingly. Histamine-2 receptor blockers and proton pump inhibitors can be safely used in ESRD; the former should be dose reduced (e.g., daily rather than b.i.d.). Correction of the bleeding diathesis seen in some dialysis patients is described in Chapter 98. Heparinization should be limited during subsequent dialysis treatments.

Common lower gastrointestinal abnormalities in dialysis patients include colonic ulceration, diverticulosis, diverticulitis, spontaneous colonic perforation, and prolonged ileus (7). Diverticulosis is seen in more than 80% of patients who have polycystic kidney disease as a cause of ESRD. Ischemic enteritis and colitis are relatively common in dialysis patients, especially the elderly and diabetics, because of the severity of atherosclerosis (Chapter 87). Ischemic bowel disease should be suspected in patients whose pain is worsened during dialysis. Intestinal necrosis with bowel perforation has been observed following rectal administration of sorbitol with sodium polystyrene sulfonate. If required, sodium polystyrene sulfonate should be mixed with water or, preferentially, given enterally.

There is an increased frequency of acute and chronic *pancreatitis* in dialysis patients. Certain drugs used for kidney diseases should be considered in the differential diagnosis of pancreatitis, including corticosteroids, loop and thiazide diuretics, and a variety of antiretroviral drugs (Chapter 86). Hypercalcemia, hyperparathyroidism, and hypertriglyceridemia are additional risk factors. In general, amylase and lipase are elevated in ESRD because of reduced renal clearance and minimal clearance with dialysis. Specificity for the diagnosis of pancreatitis increases if the amylase level is greater than three times the upper limit of normal.

Hematologic Disease

In the hospitalized patient with ESRD, the hematologic problem of greatest importance is anemia. The etiology of anemia in ESRD is multifactorial, although the principal cause is related to a deficiency in *erythropoietin*, a growth factor primarily produced in the proximal tubule of the functioning kidney. Table 101.3 outlines other contributing causes to ESRD-related anemia and to potential resistance to the effects of erythropoietin. Most of these conditions are preventable or readily manageable in the outpatient setting.

In addition to correcting the anemia of ESRD, erythropoietin therapy has been shown to improve cardiac hemodynamics, improve oxygen-releasing capacity, and decrease the degree of intradialytic hypotension. These improvements in overall cardiac function have led to tangible improvements in physical activity, work capacity, sexual function, and quality of life. Furthermore, the associated decrease in transfusion requirements has decreased the frequency of hepatitis and presensitization before kidney transplantation. Therefore, it is prudent to continue erythropoietin in maintenance dialysis patients if they are admitted to the hospital. Clinical practice guidelines recommend maintaining hematocrit concentrations in the 33%–36% range, with the liberal use of intravenous iron compounds to maintain transferrin saturation greater than 20% and ferritin concentration greater than 100 mg/L.

TABLE 101.3

CAUSES (BEYOND ERYTHROPOIETIN DEFICIENCY) CONTRIBUTING TO ANEMIA IN END-STAGE RENAL DISEASE

Iron deficiency[a]
Excessive blood draws
Inflammatory disease[a]
Persistent uremia (underdialysis)[a]
Aluminum toxicity
Lead toxicity
Folate deficiency
Vitamin B_{12} deficiency
Multiple myeloma
Secondary hyperparathyroidism (osteitis fibrosa cystica)[a]
Hemolysis associated with primary disease (systemic lupus erythematosus)
Hemolysis related to mechanical factors, dialysate contamination, hyper-osmolality, hypo-osmolality, or severe hypophosphatemia

[a]Major causes of erythropoietin resistance.

Carefully conducted clinical trials are still necessary to determine the optimal hemoglobin concentration or hematocrit for maintenance dialysis patients. There are few side effects of erythropoietin therapy. Exacerbation of hypertension and seizures were observed in early studies with erythropoietin but seldom are seen today.

Uremia is associated with a *bleeding diathesis related to platelet dysfunction*. This usually is controlled with adequate dialysis. Nevertheless, there are several maneuvers that can help with the management of the dialysis patient who is bleeding. First, ensure that there has been no unrecognized or mistaken administration of heparin. Typically, central venous double-lumen catheters used for dialysis are instilled with 5,000–7,500 units of heparin in each port to prevent *in situ* catheter thrombosis. If excessive heparin has been administered, protamine or fresh frozen plasma can be given to counteract its effects. If the prothrombin and partial thromboplastin times are normal and there is active bleeding, the patient should be transfused to a hematocrit in excess of 30% to increase blood viscosity. The intensity of dialysis should be maximized, including daily dialysis if necessary. Desmopressin acetate and intravenous estrogens may be of some additional benefit (8) (Chapter 98).

Endocrine Disorders

More than 40% of all new dialysis patients have diabetes as a primary or contributing cause of ESRD or as an important comorbidity. People with diabetes and chronic kidney disease frequently exhibit a decreasing requirement for insulin as GFR declines, sometimes requiring no insulin after many years of insulin dependence. Insulin catabolism is decreased with reduced GFR, and an occult decrease in protein and calorie intake can further decrease the patient's insulin requirement. Hypoglycemia is a relatively common occurrence in patients with ESRD. Causes include alcohol abuse (which tends to be less frequent among dialysis patients than the general population), liver disease (including hepatitis C with minimal transaminitis), sepsis, metabolic acidosis, and especially malnutrition. Patients with reduced muscle mass and reduced glycogen stores are at highest risk for hypoglycemia.

The use of oral sulfonylurea agents can place patients at serious risk for hypoglycemia because of both the increased half-life of insulin and the retention of active metabolites of the sulfonylurea agent. First-generation sulfonylureas (e.g., chlorpropamide, tolazamide) should be avoided in patients with ESRD, and second-generation agents should be used with caution. Insulin therapy should be recommended to all dialysis patients who require glycemic control. *Metformin should not be used in patients with ESRD* because of the risk of serious lactic acidosis. If a sulfonylurea must be used, glipizide is preferred, because its retained metabolites are less active than those of glyburide. Peripherally acting agents that enhance insulin sensitivity (e.g., rosiglitazone, piogli-

tazone) are well tolerated, although long-term safety and efficacy data in patients with ESRD are lacking.

Hyperosmolar coma resulting from hyperglycemia occasionally complicates ESRD, and levels of blood glucose can be extremely high (500–1,000 mg/dL or more). In contrast to patients with nonketotic hyperosmolar syndrome and normal baseline renal function (Chapter 107), volume expansion does not correct the disorder in dialysis patients and should be avoided. Indeed, volume depletion rarely complicates the disorder because of the blunted or absent response to glucose as an osmotic diuretic. In dialysis patients, the most appropriate therapy for hyperglycemia with or without ketoacidosis is an intravenous insulin infusion. Ketoacidosis is an infrequent occurrence in long-term dialysis patients, in contrast to non-ESRD patients with diabetes. The unexplained occurrence of severe hyperglycemia or ketoacidosis in the dialysis patient should raise a strong suspicion for infection.

Some of the signs and symptoms of uremia or dialysis asthenia may be confused with hypothyroidism. Therefore, it is important to appropriately interpret thyroid function tests in this population (Chapter 106). In general, serum total thyroxine and tri-iodothyronine are reduced because of changes in binding protein metabolism and competitive inhibition of binding caused by accumulated organic acids. Free hormone levels, however, tend to be normal or slightly reduced. Thyroid-stimulating hormone levels are usually normal to slightly increased, and there is a blunted response to thryotropin-releasing hormone. The incidences of frank hypothyroidism and goiter are increased in ESRD, perhaps related to iodine retention secondary to reduced excretion.

Electrolytes, Acid-Base Balance, Metabolism, and Nutrition

Hyperkalemia is the most important electrolyte issue for the hospitalized ESRD patient (see Chapter 104 for a complete discussion). Metabolic acidosis is extremely common in ESRD. In the past, metabolic acidosis was an expected complication of ESRD and was rarely treated. More recently, it has been demonstrated that chronic metabolic acidosis can promote protein catabolism leading to a reduction in lean body mass, and it may accelerate the ill effects of metabolic bone disease. Although it is rarely urgent in the hospital setting, some experts recommend treating a metabolic acidosis (bicarbonate concentration <22 mEq/L) with oral sodium bicarbonate. Sodium citrate should be used sparingly and never in conjuction with aluminum-based compounds (see below).

The optimal management of calcium, phosphorus, parathyroid hormone, and vitamin D is one of the most complex issues in ESRD. In hospitalized patients, the most common abnormality is *hyperphosphatemia*. Hyperphosphatemia should be avoided to prevent complications related to its effects on bone and other tissues. Elevated phosphate concentrations have been associated with mortality and hospitalization because of cardiovascular disease and fracture (9). Elevated calcium concentrations have also been associated with mortality in ESRD patients; it can usually be avoided by judicious use of calcium-based binders and vitamin D, and with physiologic dialysate calcium concentrations. The best treatment for hyperphosphatemia in the hospital depends on the corresponding level of calcium and on whether or not the patient is eating. Although some phosphorus can be absorbed from the sloughed gut mucosa, the majority of phosphorus absorbed from the gastrointestinal tract is from food. As such, phosphate binders should be given with, rather than in between, meals.

Calcium carbonate and acetate are both effective as phosphate binders. If the levels of serum calcium and calcium-phosphate product are elevated, a short course of aluminum hydroxide can be given. Aluminum alone tends to be extremely constipating. Modest degrees of hyperphosphatemia (4.5–6.5 mg/dL) should be tolerated in the hospital to avert the complications of treatment. Aluminum hydroxide should never be given with citrate-based alkalinizing agents, because citrate markedly enhances aluminum absorption; nor should it be given with sodium polystyrene sulfonate, because intraluminal binding renders both drugs ineffective and often causes severe obstipation. Sevelamer is a polymeric phosphate binder that contains no aluminum or calcium and may prove to be useful in the hospital setting. As a hydrogel, sevelamer may expand within the lumen of feeding tubes; rapid flushing of sevelamer after instillation into feeding tubes is required to avoid mechanical complications.

Metabolic and nutritional abnormalities are extremely common in long-term dialysis patients. These abnormalities exert direct ill effects on organ function in dialysis patients and themselves contribute to the risks for death and injury. The subjective global assessment of nutritional status (Table 16.2), initially developed and validated in hospitalized surgical patients (10), is a simple, reproducible tool that can identify dialysis patients at nutritional risk. Nutrition support should be given to dialysis patients who are moderately or severely malnourished by subjective global assessment criteria, or who have serum albumin concentrations less than 3.5 g/dL. Enteral nutrition should be provided whenever possible. The choice of enteral supplements depends on individual patient factors, such as the need for sodium and potassium restriction and the degree of fluid overload. There are many commercially available products designed for patients on dialysis. Alternatively, total parenteral nutrition or intradialytic parenteral nutrition can be prescribed (Chapter 15).

Neurologic Disorders

Most of the central nervous system manifestations of advanced uremia, such as impaired mentation, lethargy, sleep disorders, asterixis, and multifocal myoclonus, are reversible with dialysis. In addition to uremic encephalopathy, two neurologic syndromes—dialysis dysequilibrium and dialysis dementia—are specific to patients with ESRD and often are confused, although they are quite distinct.

Dialysis dysequilibrium refers to a condition characterized by headache, confusion, disorientation, nausea, vomiting, and, rarely, seizures during or just after dialysis. It is thought to be related to the rapid shift of extracellular solutes during the dialysis procedure and the subsequent shift of water into cells of the brain. The risk of this reaction can be reduced by dialysis modifications. Some clinicians infuse mannitol, a substitute osmole that is not removed with dialysis, in an effort to limit fluid shifting. Dialysis against a high sodium bath (145–150 mEq/L) also may limit extracellular to intracellular water shifting. The risk of dialysis dysequilibrium is increased with more severe degrees of uremia. In addition to changes in the dialysate and the administration of mannitol, it is reasonable to use phenytoin in patients with a history of seizures or with a known structural brain injury that could serve as a seizure focus (Chapter 118).

Dialysis dementia is characterized by disorders of speech, such as dysarthria and dysphasia, along with dyscalculia, dyslexia, dyspraxia, dysgraphia, impaired memory, poor attention span, depression, paranoia, myoclonus, and seizures. The symptoms are initially intermittent and often most severe during or immediately after dialysis. Dialysis dementia is a progressive dementing disorder and, if untreated, usually progresses to death within 12–15 months. Aluminum was implicated in the pathogenesis of dialysis dementia after finding clusters of cases in dialysis units whose water-collection systems were contaminated with aluminum. The association with osteomalacia and microcytic anemia provided additional evidence, as did the high concentrations of aluminum in the plasma and brains of affected patients.

Although not specific to ESRD, stroke and subdural hematoma are two conditions seen more commonly in dialysis patients than in the general population and should be suspected in the setting of either focal neurologic deficits or nonspecific neurologic findings. Subdural hematoma in particular can present with indolent changes in behavior that may be attributed incorrectly to uremia. Because intermittent heparinization with dialysis can increase the risk of rebleeding, a CT scan of the head should be obtained if subdural hematoma is suspected in a patient with ESRD (Chapter 117).

Drug Disposition

The kidneys are responsible for much of the metabolism of drugs in the human body. Therefore, in caring for the hospitalized patient it is absolutely essential to appreciate not only the effects of drugs on the kidney (nephrotoxicity), but also the role of the kidney in the disposition of prescription drugs. Drug-related nephrotoxicity is covered in Chapter 100. An exhaustive listing of drugs that require dose and frequency modifications in patients with chronic kidney disease is beyond the scope of this chapter. A computerized order-entry system can considerably reduce excessive dosing and reduce pharmacy costs by more than 10%. Whether renal or other adverse drug events can be reduced, or whether other outcomes (e.g., length of hospital stay, level of renal function at discharge) can be influenced, remains to be determined (Chapter 21).

KEY POINTS

■ A nephrologist often functions as the primary or principal care physician for the dialysis patient. Consultation with the nephrologist and outpatient dialysis facility can provide vital information and facilitate effective and efficient inpatient care.

■ The most common reasons for hospitalization of the dialysis patient include thrombosis, infection of the vascular or peritoneal access, and a variety of cardiovascular diseases, including congestive heart failure and myocardial infarction.

■ Special attention should be paid to the serum potassium concentration. Sliding scales and other liberal methods of potassium repletion should be avoided.

■ Routine intravenous fluids should not be administered to patients on dialysis. Routine placement of intravenous lines also should be discouraged.

■ The majority of patients with ESRD are either malnourished or at nutritional risk. Physicians should routinely provide nutritional support to dialysis patients who are critically ill or taking nothing by mouth for extended periods.

■ Physicians should consider the role of kidney function on drug disposition when prescribing medications. Close attention to these issues may limit adverse drug events and reduce costs.

REFERENCES

1. US Renal Data System. *USRDS 2003 annual report.* Bethesda, MD: National Institutes of Health, National Institute of Diabetes and Digestive and Kidney Diseases.
2. Klahr S, Levey AS, Beck GJ, et al. The effects of dietary protein restriction and blood pressure control on the progression of chronic renal disease. Modification of Diet in Renal Disease Study Group. *N Engl J Med* 1994;330:877–884.
3. Kopple JD, Levey AS, Greene T, et al. Effect of dietary protein restriction on nutritional status in the Modification of Diet in Renal Disease Study. *Kidney Int* 1997;5:778–791.
4. Sanders HN, Narvarte J, Bittle PA, et al. Hospitalized dialysis patients have lower nutrient intakes on renal diet than on regular diet. *J Am Diet Assoc* 1991;91:1278–1280.
5. Lowrie EG, Lew NL. Death risk in hemodialysis patients: the predictive value of commonly measured variables and an evaluation of death rate differences between facilities. *Am J Kidney Dis* 1990;15:458–482.
6. Herzog CA, Ma JZ, Collins AJ. Poor long-term survival after acute myocardial infarction among patients on long-term dialysis. *N Engl J Med* 1998;339:799–805.
7. Adams PL, Rutsky EA, Rostrand SG, et al. Lower gastrointestinal tract dysfunction in patients receiving long-term hemodialysis. *Arch Intern Med* 1982;142:303–306.
8. Weigert AL, Schafer AI. Uremic bleeding: pathogenesis and therapy. *Am J Med Sci* 1998;316:94–104.
9. Block GA, Klassen PS, Lazarus JM, et al. Mineral metabolism, mortality and morbidity in maintenance hemodialysis. *J Am Soc Nephrol* 2004;80:2208–2218.
10. Detsky AS, Baker JP, O'Rourke K, et al. Predicting nutrition-associated complications for patients undergoing gastrointestinal surgery. *JPEN J Parenter Enteral Nutr* 1987;11:440–446.

ADDITIONAL READING

Eknoyan G, Beck GJ, Cheung AK, et al. Effect of dialysis dose and membrane flux in maintenance hemodialysis. *N Engl J Med* 2002;347:2010–2019.

Foley RN, Guo H, Snyder JJ, et al. Septicemia in the United States dialysis population, 1991–1999. *J Am Soc Nephrol* 2004;15:1038–1045.

Panigua R, Amato D, Voneshs E, et al. Effects of increased peritoneal clearances on mortality rates in peritoneal dialysis: ADEMEX, a prospective, randomized, controlled trial. *J Am Soc Nephrol* 2002;13:1307–1320.

Raggi P, Boulay A, Chasan-Taber S, et al. Cardiac calcification in adult hemodialysis patients. A link between end-stage renal disease and cardiovascular disease? *J Am Coll Cardiol* 2002;39:695–701.

Rubin HR, Fink NE, Plantinga LC, et al. Patient ratings of dialysis care with peritoneal dialysis vs. hemodialysis. *JAMA* 2004;291:697–703.

Renal Transplantation 102

William J.C. Amend, Jr.   Flavio Vincenti

INTRODUCTION

Renal transplantation had its successful beginnings in 1954 with the experience of identical-twin transplants at the Peter Bent Brigham Hospital in Boston. Over the next 50 years, there have been major advances in both surgical technique and medical management leading to improved outcomes. The clinician involved in immediate and post-transplant follow-up care should understand the particulars of the transplant implantation (Figure 102.1). It is vital that complete arterial circulation be supplied to both the transplanted kidney and the proximal-to-distal transplanted ureter. This is ensured through careful inspection of donor angiograms (in living donors) or of operative findings of either cadaver or living donors at the time of organ procurement. Multiple renal arteries occur in about 30% of donor kidneys.

For the renal-transplant recipient, inadequate or overlooked arterial supply vessels can lead to early postoperative bleeding, partial graft infarction, segmental acute tubular necrosis, or later ureteral ischemic complications (with a leak caused by necrosis or a transplant ureteral stricture). Currently, most renal transplants have an end-to-side anastomosis to the recipient's arteries, with a decreased incidence of later anastomotic transplant renal artery stenosis compared with an end-to-end arterial anastomosis. The transplanted ureter is implanted with either a tunneling antirefux technique or with an extravesicular re-implant procedure. The disadvantage of the former surgery is a prolonged initial hospital stay with two bladder incisions and the potential for early postoperative leaks. This surgery, however, is associated with less post-transplant ureteral reflux, which may be important in reducing later infections or secondary focal sclerosis in the transplanted kidney.

Careful dissection of the iliac fossa reduces the likelihood of peritransplant hematomas and excessive pooling of lymphatic drainage. The latter presents as a postoperative lymphocele that is usually medial to the transplanted kidney (between the transplant and bladder) (Figure 102.1). Lymphoceles can cause obstructive uropathy or obstructive lower-extremity venous thrombosis; they also can become infected. The incidence of lymphoceles is 3%–20% and varies by surgeon and transplant center. The recipient's diseased kidneys usually are left *in situ*. Indications for pretransplant unilateral or bilateral nephrectomy include infection, hemorrhage, renal-cell cancer, excessively morbid enlargement (as in the case of polycystic kidneys), refractory hypertension, and persistence of the nephrotic syndrome. If there is reflux present, native nephrectomies can be accomplished pre- or post-transplant if infections occur. Occasional ureteral implantation into an ileal loop or augmented bladder is accomplished in patients with urologic abnormalities. Bladders that have been in disuse for many years often are contracted and present post-transplant reconditioning challenges, with possible urologic complications of leak, retention, and infection.

Postoperatively, the donor and recipient solitary kidneys undergo compensatory hypertrophy or hypotrophy, if the recipient is much smaller than the donor. Hypertrophy is characterized by an increase in glomerular filtration rate, renal blood flow, and tubular function to 80% of normal "two-kidney" function. These physiologic recoveries are identical for both the donor and the recipient if immunosuppressives are not used and rejection does not occur. Most recipients who do not receive an identical-twin transplant recover substantial function, but full renal recovery (to 80% of normal) is unusual. There are several reasons for this partial recovery. Rejection and immunosuppressive drugs can cause important physiologic changes. Posturemic endocrinologic abnormalities such as ongoing secondary hyperparathyroidism also may affect post-transplant recipient renal physiology, causing proximal tubular reabsorbtive defects of phosphorpus and bicarbonate. The kidney donor's renal recovery (donor compensatory hypertrophy) is complete at 6–8 weeks, postdonor nephrectomy. On follow-up of donors for 10–20 years, there appears to be a slightly increased risk of later hypertension in those

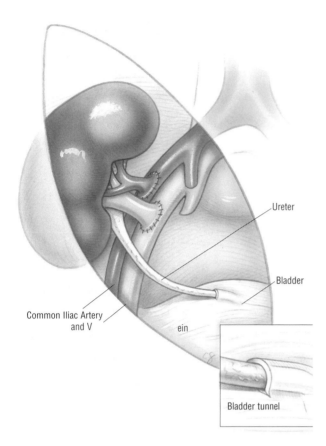

Figure 102.1 Renal transplant with end-to-side vascular anastomosis and bladder implant.

TABLE 102.1

STEPS IN LIVING KIDNEY DONOR EVALUATION

1. Education/information: review outcomes and risks
2. Immunologic testing
   (a) Human leukocyte antigen (HLA) typing
   (b) Donor lymphocyte-recipient sera cross-match
3. Physical examination
4. Multiphasic blood/urine/pulmonary and cardiovascular tests
5. Re-review expected outcomes and donor/recipient risks
6. Radiography
   (a) Donor intravenous pyelogram
   (b) Renal angiogram or magnetic resonance angiogram

with a family history of hypertension and of proteinuria. It is not yet known whether there is an excessive risk of impaired renal function in donors more than 20 years postnephrectomy.

Renal-transplant donor medical and surgical principles vary depending upon donor source. The surgical team coordinates renal-organ procurement with the *United Network for Organ Sharing (UNOS) system* and its local organ-donor network. If a living volunteer wishes to undergo evaluation, a systematic process is undertaken (Table 102.1)(1). If transplantation is done pre-emptively before dialysis is needed, there is often a more favorable prognosis (2).

Seventy percent of patients in end-stage renal failure lack available living donors and are dependent on cadaver organs for transplants. Many of the steps outlined in Table 102.1 obviously cannot be performed with cadaver donors. Cadaver donors are identified from patients at "low risk" for transmissible diseases who meet brain-death criteria. Because of procurement technique, frequent multiorgan donation, storage, preservation, and shipping to recipient hospitals, both warm and cold ischemic times tend to be longer for cadaveric kidneys than the surgical ischemic times for organs procured from living renal donors. This, along with cadaver donor preprocurement hemodynamic

instability, create an expectedly greater incidence of *delayed graft function*, which manifests itself as nonoliguric or oliguric acute tubular necrosis and, rarely, cortical necrosis. Delayed graft function is the primary cause of early postkidney transplant renal failure; its differential diagnosis and therapy are discussed later. With a relative scarcity of cadaver donors, recent emphasis has been placed on utilizing living unrelated donors; outcomes are comparable to those seen in partially matched related donors. "Marginal" cadaver donors (older, deceased donors with mild degrees of azotemia or with histories of hypertension) are also increasingly being used (3).

Recipient medical and surgical considerations are also important in assessing early and late post-transplant events. Immunologic predictors of outcome include the type of graft, the match grade, and rejection syndromes. *Isografts* (between identical twins) are rare; such recipients have no rejections and have no post-transplant need for immunosuppression but are at higher risk for certain recurrent diseases. The usual kidney transplant is an *allograft* and occurs between genetically disparate individuals. ABO blood group compatibility and a negative immediate pretransplant lymphocytotoxic cross-match are essential to reduce severe early rejections. Matching for the human leukocyte antigen system is performed; increasing degrees of matching correlate with improved post-transplant outcomes. The most common post-renal transplant organ complication continues to be rejection. The types of rejections include the following:

- *Hyperacute:* a nearly immediate graft loss through an undetected antidonor tissue antibody response with subsequent cortical necrosis.

- *Delayed hyperacute:* a severe cellular and humoral inflammatory response, often treatment-resistant, which likely represents an amnestic or secondary immune response.

- *Acute:* the most common form of rejection, occurring with post-transplant donor antigen-host responses, usually of a cellular variety.

■ *Chronic:* developing months-to-years post-transplant and thought to be either effects of cumulative injury from previous acute rejections or a slow vascular injury from antidonor enothelial responses.

Younger individuals, women, patients with lupus, African Americans, and noncompliant individuals are at higher risk of rejection. Conversely, patients with IgA nephropathy have a lower risk. If a patient who has rejected a first kidney receives a subsequent kidney transplant, the immunologic course of the first transplant often is repeated. Better cross-matching and newer immunosuppressive drugs may improve the outcomes for retransplanted patients.

In addition to the matching issues described previously, a patient awaiting transplant may be difficult to match to prospective living or cadaver donors because of increased *lymphocytotoxic antibodies.* These antibodies occur in response to pregnancies, blood transfusions, previous transplants, or other antigenic exposures. Currently, there are no therapies to reduce these tissue-reactive antibodies, so such patients simply must wait until an acceptable (and negative cross-match) donor is available. Cross-matching in such circumstances must be done carefully with multiple sera and sensitive technical methods to avoid early rejection and graft loss.

The recipient's past and immediate pretransplant medical condition needs thorough review. Table 102.2 gives an overview of various medical factors that are most important in determining a kidney transplant patient's candidacy (4). Elevated body mass index is associated with increased morbidity (5). These medical factors include both the presence of various systemic illnesses and features of the patient's primary renal disease. For example, patients with certain primary renal diseases such as idiopathic focal sclerosing glomerulonephritis, IgA nephropathy, and membranoproliferative glomerulonephritis can have kidney-transplant recurrence (6). The presence of hepatitis C in the potential recipient must be thoroughly evaluated, including with a liver biopsy (7). If cirrhosis is present, transplant is contraindicated. Based on these considerations and the patient's pretransplant immune status, estimates of patient and graft outcome can be provided. Overall renal-transplant graft and patient survival outcomes are given in Table 102.3. More precise prognostication can be

TABLE 102.2

IMPORTANT FACTORS TO KNOW ABOUT POTENTIAL KIDNEY-TRANSPLANT RECIPIENTS

Cause of chronic renal failure

Presence or absence of systemic illnesses
    Diabetes mellitus
    Vasculitis
    Genetic disorders

Obesity (body mass index ≥30)

Vascular disease

Pulmonary
    Chronic illnesses
    Acute illnesses (pretransplant)

Gastrointestinal
    Hepatitis B and C status
    Previous ulcer disease
    Diverticular disease
    Biliary/pancreas diseases

Preceding neoplastic illness
    May require a certain tumor-free interval and often needs tumor-board clearance

Neuropsychiatric
    Understanding and compliance issues (best screened with surrogate and social service inputs)

done on a case-by-case basis given the individual patient's surgical, medical, and immunologic status.

Evaluation of a prospective renal-transplant patient requires several steps. This evaluation is depicted in Figure 102.2. The evaluation is easier to complete if the transplant is from a living donor, because planned timing of the transplant means that the recipient's preoperative condition can be assessed and optimized. In contrast, the recipient on the renal-transplant cadaver waiting list may be transplanted several months or years (present average wait is 2–5 years) after this first evaluation. A repeat evaluation usually is recommended if the precadaver renal-transplant waiting period exceeds 2 years. This is in order to screen for later disease development while the patient remains on continued dialysis. This time lag is in contrast to liver (Chapter 85) or

TABLE 102.3

KIDNEY-TRANSPLANT OUTCOMES

Donor source	2-y patient survival, %	2-y graft survival, %	50% graft survival, y
Cadaver	92	78	8–11
Living donor	96		
Unrelated		88	12–15
Partial match		88	12–18
Full match (2-haplotype)		94	25–27

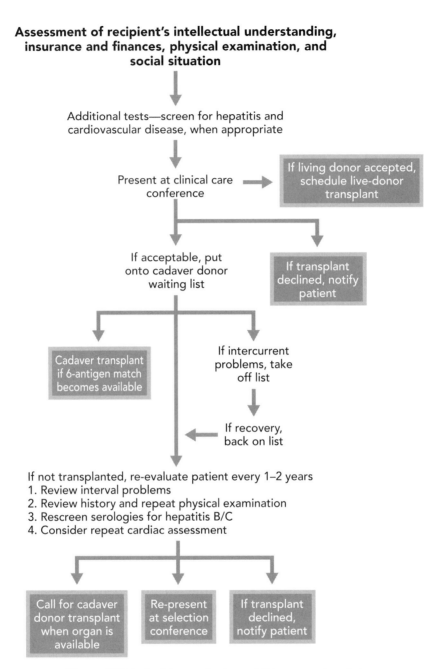

Figure 102.2 Recipient evaluation and kidney transplant timing.

heart and lung (Chapters 40 and 58) transplants, whose recipients are transplanted much closer to the time of their primary pretransplant evaluation. Of particular concern are the various neoplasms that can occur in the population undergoing renal dialysis. Patients should be screened for these neoplasms, because transplant immunosuppression may accelerate tumor growth.

Clinicians must understand the actions and toxicities of various immunosuppressive drugs in order to manage patients after renal and other organ transplantation (8–11). The types of postrenal transplant immunotherapy are shown in Table 102.4. These drugs have a variety of general and agent-specific side effects, all of which may vary among individuals. The major complications of this group of drugs are infections (of both usual and opportunistic types) and neoplasms. Neoplasms that occur more commonly after transplant include lymphomas and other hematologic malignancies, epithelial cancers, and Kaposi's sarcoma (12). These and other drug complications are reviewed specifically in the remainder of this chapter. A detailed discussion of infections in the immunocompromised host is contained in Chapter 63.

TABLE 102.4

IMMUNOSUPPRESSIVE AGENTS

Drug group	Drug name generic (brand) name	Mechanism of action	Drug interactions	Major side effects
Corticosteroid	Prednisone	Anti-inflammatory with immunosuppressive effects mediated by decreasing cytokine gene activation	Anticonvulsants decrease immunosuppressive effects	Osteopenia, aseptic necrosis, cataracts, hyperglycemia, cushingoid features
Antiproliferative	Azathioprine (Imuran)	Inhibits purine synthesis in both the *de novo* and the salvage pathway	Allopurinol potentiates effect	Leukopenia, hepatic dysfunction (hepatitis and cholestasis), pancreatitis, alopecia
	Mycophenolate mofetil (CellCept) (selective inhibition of T- and B-cell proliferation)	Inhibits purine synthesis in the *de novo* pathway	None	Leukopenia, diarrhea, duodenitis-gastritis, increased risk of cytomegalovirus infection
	Sirolimus (Rapamune)	Inhibits proliferative signal 1	Same as calcineurin inhibitors	Hyperlipidemia, diarrhea, leukopenia, thrombocytopenia interstitial pneumonia, has no nephrotoxicity
Calcineurin inhibitors	Cyclosporine (Sandimmune, Neoral)	Decreases cytokine gene activation by inhibiting calcineurin	Drugs that inhibit cytochrome P-450 (potentiate effects of nondihydropyridine calcium channel blockers, macrolide antibiotics)	Nephrotoxicity, hepatotoxicity, hirsutism, gingival hyperplasia, hyperlipidemia
	Tacrolimus (Prograf)	Same	Drugs that induce cytochrome P-450 reduce effects (isoniazid, rifampin, and anticonvulsants)	Nephrotoxicity, hepatotoxicity, neurotoxicity, hyperglycemia (especially in African-American and Hispanic patients), alopecia
Antilymphocyte agents	Antilymphocyte globulin (ATGAM)	Equine antilymphocyte polyclonal antibody	None	Leukopenia, thrombocytopenia, serum sickness
	Rabbit antithymocyte globulin (Thymoglobulin)	Rabbit antithymocyte polyclonal antibody	None	Leukopenia, thrombocytopenia, serum sickness
	OKT3 (Orthoclone)	Murine anti-CD3 monoclonal antibody	None	Cytokine-release syndrome (fever, chills, headache, rarely acute respiratory distress syndrome and aseptic meningitis after first dose), increased risk of opportunistic infections and lymphoma
Interleukin 2–receptor blockade	Basiliximab (Simulect)	Chimeric anti-interleukin 2α–receptor monoclonal antibody (half-life 7 d)	None	No drug-specific side effects
	Daclizumab (Zenapax)	Humanized anti-interleukin 2α–receptor monoclonal antibody (half-life 20 d)	None	No drug-specific side effects

CARE OF THE HOSPITALIZED PATIENT

Preoperative Management

Preoperatively, the prospective renal-transplant recipient must be examined carefully to be sure that there are no cardiorespiratory conditions precluding general anesthesia (Chapter 30) and high-dosage initial post-transplant immunosuppression. Patients with end-stage renal disease are at high risk for atherosclerotic complications and may have cardiac ischemia or dysrhythmia. Antilymphocyte immunosuppressives can be associated with post-transplant acute respiratory distress syndrome, so left ventricular function and volume status should be assessed carefully by an echocardiographic study. Because of autonomic dysfunction, many uremic patients cannot exercise to a maximum heart rate, so persantine thallium stress tests are utilized to screen for coronary artery disease. The recipient should receive pretransplant dialysis to optimize the preoperative electrolytes. Blood potassium levels below 5.5 mEq/L are mandatory for safe general anesthesia. In patients receiving peritoneal dialysis, peritoneal dialysate is tested for cell count and differential, and a concentrate is sent for Gram's stain and culture to exclude latent peritonitis. Assessment and treatment are coordinated closely with the transplant surgeons and anesthesiologists. This evaluation and care must be performed expeditiously in the case of cadaver donor renal transplantation. Outside records and periodic re-examinations by the transplant service help

with adequate and rapid preoperative assessments. The cadaver donor kidney must be implanted within 72 hours (preferably within 12–48 hours) after procurement, because prolonged preservation leads to severe delayed graft function and technical loss.

Initial Postoperative Renal-Transplant Care

Postoperative renal-transplant care is done in close collaboration with the transplant surgical staff. Medical and nephrology input is needed for management of a number of clinical problems, especially delayed graft function, hypertension, diabetes, respiratory distress, and cardiac ischemic events or arrhythmias. The usual post-transplant care of recipients for the first 7–14 days can be directed along a clinical pathway developed after input from both internists and transplant surgeons (Table 102.5). Superimposed complications, such as persistence of renal failure resulting from delayed graft function or a cardiac ischemic event, would alter the clinical pathway.

Before discharge, the patient's outpatient care is coordinated with the referring medical staff, home health agencies, payors, and post-transplant care clinics. Because most renal-transplant rejections occur in the first 3 months, it is vital that follow-up recommendations be addressed thoroughly at the time of post-transplant discharge. Patients with kidney transplants have an initial hospital stay of 7–10 days. An average of 5–10 days per year of hospitalization may be required for the first 2–5 years post-

TABLE 102.5

POST-TRANSPLANT CLINICAL PATHWAY (EXAMPLE)

Day	Surgical	Medical	Nursing
0	Surgical transplant Initiate immunosuppression	Postoperative recovery Floor vs. ICU	Fluid Pain management Monitor graft
1	Wound check Monitor immunosuppression	Monitor transplant function Dialyze, if needed	As above Ambulate
2	As above	As above Medical management (e.g., manage blood pressure, diabetes)	As above Start oral intake
3–4	As above Discontinue Foley catheter	As above	As above Discontinue intravenous fluids Educate Review social services
5–6	As above	As above If delayed function, arrange backup dialysis If normal, organize discharge	As above Patient and family self-medicate Patient takes a "care test"
7–10	Discharge Communicate with primary physician and ancillary services	Discharge Communicate with primary physician and ancillary services	Arrange clinic and local follow-up

If prolonged operative time, early graft dysfunction, or early rejection, the timing of this pathway may need to be extended.

transplant (typical problems are discussed below). Because patients are more independent after transplant than during dialysis, family conferences and instruction with the hospital-based staff are necessary so that patient understanding and adherence can be encouraged.

Acute Renal Failure

One of the most common problems following renal transplant is acute renal failure (ARF). Because recipients have a solitary functioning kidney, surgical and urologic causes of ARF must be excluded routinely. Occasionally, dialysis patients have normal urine outputs; these post-transplant patients may continue to have normal urine volumes despite having severe transplant ARF. In addition, several pathophysiologic processes may be superimposed (e.g., acute rejection during initial delayed graft function) so that diagnostic transplant biopsy may be indicated more frequently than in cases of ARF affecting the general medical patient population (Chapter 100). The overall approach to renal transplant ARF or delayed graft function is presented in Figure 102.3.

Immediate Post-Transplant Acute Renal Failure

If the grafted kidney fails to function post-transplant (a situation seen with 10%–40% of cadaver donors, and 1%–5% of living donors), early diagnostic tests must be done to exclude *obstruction, leak,* or *vascular thrombosis.* These usually include renal isotope scans or transplant ultrasound with Doppler flow studies. Abnormalities showing urologic or vascular problems dictate surgical re-exploration.

Hyperacute rejection occurs rarely, and graft thrombosis may occasionally develop in hypercoaguable patients, requiring that the infarcted allograft be removed. More commonly, delayed graft function is on the basis of initial *post-transplant acute tubular necrosis* and, in the case of cadaver donation, reflects procurement renal hemodynamic changes as well as injury during preservation time. Recipients of cadaver transplants from the same donor usually both develop delayed graft function, demonstrating the influence of cadaver-procurement issues on the probability of success.

Early Post-Transplant Acute Renal Failure (One Week to Three Months)

One week to three months is the most common time frame in which post-transplant ARF presents a diagnostic dilemma. ARF may be superimposed on delayed graft function or may occur after good initial graft function. Although change in serum creatinine is an imperfect measure of altered glomerular filtration rate, its use is standard because of its wide availability. Its utility can be maximized by having the blood tested at a similar time of day with steady-state degrees of exercise, activity, and diet.

Post-transplant pyelonephritis frequently causes a degree of ARF, because the infection is in a solitary kidney. The post-transplant patient with ARF secondary to pyelonephritis usually has both local and general symptoms.

After measuring cyclosporine or tacrolimus levels, testing should turn to evaluating the possibility of transplant prerenal and postrenal failure. Because of the solitary transplant kidney, imaging studies are ordered much more commonly than in native kidney settings of ARF. Surgical consultation is necessary if these studies show obstruction, urinary leak, or possible arterial stenosis. Many times, interventional radiologists can provide temporary relief with stents, but the therapeutic approach needs to be reviewed by the transplant surgical staff.

Most cases of early post-transplant ARF require either drug modification (lowering of cyclosporin or tacrolimus dosages) or alterations in immunotherapy. Sonographically directed renal-transplant biopsies are standard and clinically safe. Based upon the biopsy results (Figure 102.3), the diagnosis of post-transplant ARF may be made with precision, and appropriate therapy can be rendered.

Late Post-Transplant Acute Renal Failure (Longer Than Three Months)

Post-transplant acute renal failure occurring after 3 months usually is diagnosed by a confirmed change in serum creatinine. Of note, any significant change in the degree of physical exertion may elevate serum creatinine without necessarily representing ARF. The approach to ARF in this time frame initially may be carried out in the outpatient setting. Allografts in patients receiving cyclosporine or tacrolimus are very sensitive to renal blood flow alteration. Such grafts often develop prerenal azotemia in the setting of fluid losses and dehydration and recover well with intravenous volume resuscitation. In addition, late acute rejections may present as asymptomatic ARF in the setting of drug noncompliance or several weeks after a flu-like illness. Follow-up laboratory tests should be obtained after any viral illness. Recently, many cases of a BK polyomavirus infection of the renal graft have been observed, often progressing to full transplant failure (13). Patients have no systemic symptoms or signs. There is no known effective treatment.

Drug toxicity also can lead to ARF. Patients may be very sensitive to nonsteroidal anti-inflammatory drugs and develop ARF after their use. Post-transplant ARF may be caused by the use of angiotensin-converting enzyme inhibitors, especially if there is concurrent renal-transplant artery stenosis. Hospitalization becomes necessary to perform diagnostic biopsies or for urologic or vascular reconstructive procedures. Late postrenal transplant ARF can occur during hospitalization for transplant pyelonephritis, as a consequence of contrast dye used for angiographic studies (often needed because so many patients have atherosclerosis), or from significant sepsis or pancreatitis producing late post-transplant acute tubular necrosis.

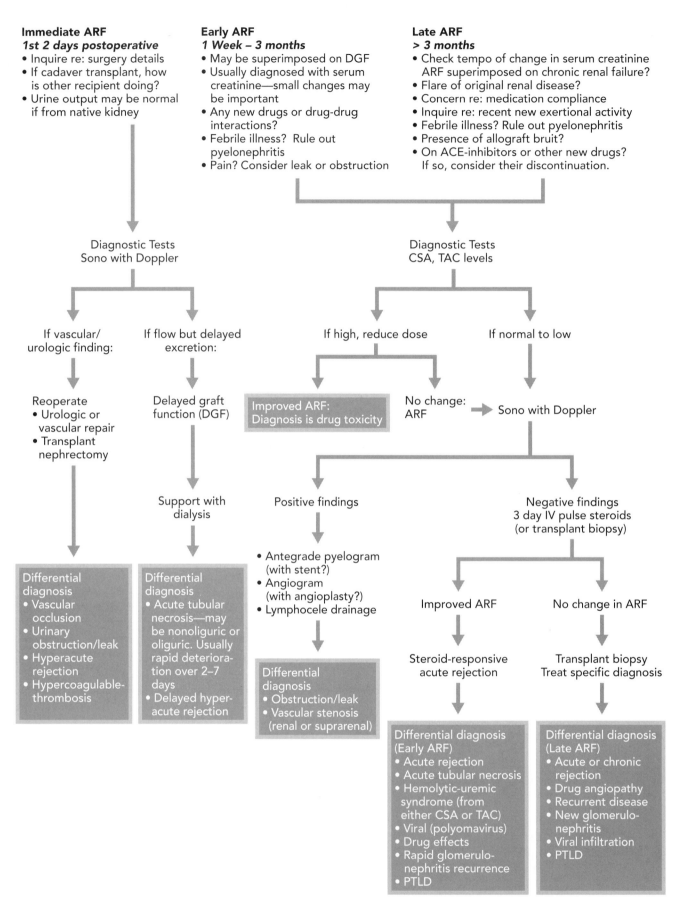

Figure 102.3 Approach to renal transplant patients with acute renal failure (ARF). *ACE,* angiotensin-converting enzyme; *CSA,* cyclosporine; *DGF,* delayed graft funtion; *IV,* intravenous; *PTLD,* post-transplant lymphoproliferative disease; *Sono,* renal sonogram; *TAC,* tacrolimus.

Fever

Certain features should be emphasized in considering fever in the renal-transplant recipient. First, uremic patients may not exhibit normal temperature curves; they may even be hypothermic if infected. Second, immunosuppression may reduce pyrexis, as well. Foremost among potential causes of fever in the hospitalized transplant patient is infection. In the first month, bacterial infections are most common. Thereafter, the most common infection causing fever is cytomegalovirus, either as an isolated febrile syndrome or with tissue site infection. Infection always must be considered in any ill renal transplant recipient; an approach is detailed in Chapter 63. A chest radiograph should be obtained, because there is often a paucity of auscultatory findings despite pneumonia. In addition, drugs and nosocomial infections are in the differential diagnosis of fever. Attention must be paid to *in situ* intravascular catheters or retained peritoneal dialysis catheters. If these are present, surgeons should be consulted for their removal, if possible.

With current immunosuppressive regimens, acute rejection rarely is associated with fever. More often, febrile patients with post-transplant ARF have transplant pyelonephritis. However, "end-stage" rejection that occurs after the patient has returned to dialysis can present with fever, cachexia, weight loss, anemia, hematuria, and graft discomfort. These patients require hospitalization, surgical consultation, and transplant nephrectomy, with medical and dialysis supportive management.

Abdominal Pain

Patients with abdominal pain require early surgical consultation because there may be a paucity of physical examination findings in the setting of immunosuppression. Some of the conditions causing abdominal pain are transplant-related and include urinary leak, pyelonephritis, perirenal trauma and hematoma, renal artery aneurysm, and internal hernia into the iliac fossa. Because kidney transplants are denervated, transplant renal stones are painless. Pain unrelated to the graft can be caused by biliary (Chapter 84) and pancreatic (Chapter 86) diseases (which occur at a higher incidence in this population), ulcer disorders (Chapter 80), acute reflux esophagitis (Chapter 79), and diverticulitis (Chapter 87). In the renal-transplant patient whose primary renal disease resulted from adult-onset polycystic kidney disease, pain may be caused by bleeding into native kidney or liver cysts. Finally, patients with preceding peritoneal dialysis are at higher risk for peritoneal adhesion and intestinal obstruction.

Respiratory Distress

Renal-transplant patients may be hospitalized with respiratory distress. In a high percentage of these cases, chest radiographs indicate either a diffuse, segmental, or nodular pattern providing clues to an infectious cause. Pulmonary consultation should be obtained. The diagnostic and therapeutic approach is detailed in Chapter 63. In addition, there is a higher incidence of pulmonary emboli in transplant patients, particularly if there is post-transplant erythrocytosis or if the patient has been inactive. The embolic source may be in the pelvic venous plexus. If so, the patient generally has no peripheral deep venous findings. The approach is the same as with other patients with pulmonary embolus (Chapter 53). If an inferior vena caval filter is indicated, the surgical transplant staff should be consulted along with interventional radiology. The filter should be placed via the femoral vein opposite the renal transplant if possible.

Altered Mental Status

Encephalopathy can occur soon after the transplant and usually is associated with high-dosage steroids or administration of OKT3. This is especially common in older recipients, in whom psychosis is accompanied by visual hallucinations. If there are profound post-transplant alterations in electrolytes (e.g., declines in serum calcium, phosphorous, or magnesium levels), lethargy can occur. Occasionally, either cyclosporine or tacrolimus can lead to early idiosyncratic central nervous system effects that are unrelated to drug levels. These psychotic responses are reversible over days after drug substitution. In addition, both drugs rarely are associated with central nervous symptoms in the late post-transplant period. These patients may have white matter changes on CT scan, which usually are discovered during evaluation of encephalopathy or other neurologic complaints.

New psychological or cognitive symptoms in the long-term transplant patient should be taken seriously. Important in the differential diagnosis are central nervous system neoplasms (especially lymphoma), infectious meningitides (fungal or parasitic), or progressive leukoencephalopathy. Urgent cerebral imaging study, lumbar puncture, and neurologic consultation all should be considered.

Hypertensive Emergency

Although hypertension is common post-transplant, only rarely do patients require hospitalization for a severe exacerbation of hypertension. It is important to inquire about cessation of or noncompliance with previously prescribed antihypertensive regimens (Chapter 48 discusses standard management). The patient's transplanted kidney should be auscultated for the presence of a bruit. In addition, ultrasonography may reveal the development of renal artery stenosis (which is more common if an end-to-end arterial anastomosis was performed) or the development of a urologic transplant obstruction. In either case, the transplant surgical staff should be consulted, and operative or percutaneous interventional therapy provided.

KEY POINTS

- Because of advances in immunosuppressive and surgical techniques, renal transplantation is becoming more common, and patients, therefore, are encountered more frequently in general clinical practice.
- Post-transplant patients all have solitary kidneys, so radiographic studies are often indicated to assess transplant complications.
- Transplant patients are highly sensitive to states of renal hypoperfusion, especially because of volume depletion or the use of concomitant nonsteroidal or angiotensin-converting enzyme inhibitor.
- Other problems may be associated with immunosuppressive drug side effects, systemic complications, or the patient's underlying renal disease.
- Close communication with the patient's transplant center is helpful because pre- and perioperative factors may be correlated with later events.

REFERENCES

1. Bia MJ, Ramos EL, Danovitch GM, et al. Evaluation of living renal donors. *Transplantation* 1995;60:322–327.
2. Mange KC, Joffe MM, Feldman HI. Effect of the use or nonuse of long-term dialysis on the subsequent survival of renal transplants from living donors. *N Engl J Med* 2001;344:726–731.
3. Ojo AO, Hanson JA, Meier-Kriesche H-U, et al. Survival in recipients of marginal cadaveric donor kidneys compared with other recipients and wait-listed transplant candidates. *J Am Soc Nephrol* 2001;12:589–597.
4. Kasiske BL, Ramos EL, Gaston RS, et al. The evaluation of renal transplant candidates: clinical practice guidelines. *J Am Soc Nephrol* 1995;6:1–34.
5. Meier-Kriesche H-U, Arndorfer JA, Kaplan B. The impact of body mass index on renal transplant outcomes: a significant independent risk factor for graft failure and patient death. *Transplantation* 2002;73:70–74.
6. Chadban SJ. Glomerulonephritis recurrence in the renal graft. *J Am Soc Nephrol* 2001;12:394–402.
7. Meier-Kriesche H-U, Ojo AO, Hanson JA, et al. Hepatitis C antibody status and outcomes in renal transplant recipients. *Transplantation* 2001;72:241–244.
8. Danovitch GM. Immunosuppressive medications for renal transplantation: a multiple choice question. *Kidney Int* 2001;59:388–402.
9. Vincenti F. What's in the pipeline? New immunosuppressive drugs in transplantation. *Am J Transplant* 2002;2:898–903.
10. Kahan BD, for the Rapamune U.S. Study Group. Efficacy of sirolimus compared with azathioprine for reduction of acute renal allograft rejection: a randomized multicenter study. *Lancet* 2000;356:194–202.
11. Gaber AO, First MR, Tesi RJ, et al. Results of the double-blind, randomized, multicenter, phase III clinical trial of Thymoglobulin versus ATGAM in the treatment of acute graft rejection episodes after renal transplantation. *Transplantation* 1998;66: 29–37.
12. Ojo AO, Hanson JA, Wolfe RA, et al. Long-term survival in renal transplant recipients with graft function. *Kidney Int* 2000;57:307–313.
13. Hirsch HH, Knowles W, Dickenmann M, et al. Prospective study of polyomavirus type BK replication and nephropathy in renal-transplant recipients. *N Engl J Med* 2002;347:488–496.

ADDITIONAL READING

Danovitch GM. *Handbook of Kidney Transplantation*, 3rd ed. Boston: Little, Brown and Company; 2001.
Halloran PF. Immunosuppressive drugs for kidney transplantation. *N Engl J Med* 2004;351:2715–2729.
Kasiske B, Vasquez MA, Harmon WE, et al. Recommendations for the outpatient surveillance of renal transplant recipients. *J Am Soc Nephrol* 2000;11:S15,51–586.
Pascual M, Theruvath T, Kawai T, et al. Strategies to improve long-term outcomes after renal transplantation. *N Engl J Med* 2002;346:580–589.

Renal Stone Disease and Obstruction

103

David S. Goldfarb   Fredric L. Coe

INTRODUCTION

The anatomy of the urinary tract can be divided into the upper tract, composed of the ureters and the kidneys, and the lower tract, composed of the bladder and the urethra. Obstruction by kidney stones tends to occur at sites of relative narrowing, where stones can become impacted. The renal calyces drain into the renal pelvis via a narrow infundibulum, and focal calyceal dilatation can occur if the infundibulum is obstructed. Beyond the calyces, common sites of stone impaction include the ureteropelvic junction, the distal third of the ureters (where they are crossed by large blood vessels), the ureterovesical junction, and the bladder neck or proximal urethra.

At least 80% of kidney stones contain calcium. Most of these are composed mostly of calcium oxalate, and a smaller proportion are predominantly calcium phosphate. Stones composed predominantly of calcium phosphate suggest the diagnoses of hyperparathyroidism and renal tubular acidosis. Uric acid, struvite, and cystine stones compose the rest. Stones occur more often in men than in women, at a ratio of 2:1. A synopsis of the pathophysiology of renal stone formation is presented in Table 103.1 (1).

The presentation of renal obstruction resulting from kidney stones is often relatively easy to diagnose. In fact, the patient often already has made the diagnosis at the time of presentation. Internists, emergency-room physicians, and urologists most frequently see the patient at that point and need to make decisions about the need for diagnostic testing, hospitalization, and requisite medications. Decisions about utilization of modalities to remove stones that do not pass spontaneously from the urinary tract are made most often by urologists. Stone disease today usually is managed in the outpatient setting. Renal obstruction resulting from causes other than stones generally is more insidious in onset and more likely to require admission for diagnosis and management. However, stones sometimes can cause painless obstruction that damages the kidney. Whatever the cause, the more rapidly obstruction is relieved, the more likely is complete recovery of the premorbid glomerular filtration rate. A delay in relief of obstruction, especially in the setting of infection, is likely to lead to irreversible loss of kidney function.

CLINICAL PRESENTATION

The vast majority of patients with obstructing kidney stones present with renal colic. This syndrome usually is characterized by sudden onset of flank pain that radiates anteriorly and downward into the scrotum or labia as the stone moves. At first the pain is usually modest; with continued ureteral contractions, it worsens and then remains steady after reaching a plateau of severity. The evolution from onset to plateau typically takes 30 minutes. The patient may describe the pain as the worst he or she has ever experienced. Nausea and vomiting may accompany the pain. When a stone passes, relief of pain is sudden and complete.

About 40% of patients have a family history of nephrolithiasis, so this specific history has some positive predictive value. Gross hematuria is noted in many cases, but microscopic hematuria is neither very sensitive nor specific for diagnosing ureteral obstruction caused by stones (2). If hematuria is defined as more than five red blood cells per high-power field, urinalysis has a sensitivity of 67% and a specificity of 66%. Using definitions of hematuria that require fewer red blood cells per high-power field increases sensitivity but significantly reduces the specificity

TABLE 103.1

CAUSES OF KIDNEY STONE FORMATION

Calcium stones

Low urine volume	Hyperoxaluria
	Idiopathic
Hypercalciuria	Dietary
With hypercalcemia	Primary (enzymatic
Primary hyperparathyroidism	defects)
Sarcoidosis	
	Hypocitraturia
Normal serum calcium	Idiopathic
Increased intestinal	Metabolic acidosis
absorption	Renal tubular acidosis
Decreased renal	Diarrhea/ileostomy (also
re-absorption	causes low urine volume)
Increased release from bone	Acid loads (e.g., protein
Metabolic acidosis	ingestion)
Increased protein and salt	
ingestion	
Decreased renal phosphate	
re-absorption	

Uric acid stones

Low urine pH	Hyperuricosuria
Idiopathic	Gout
Chronic intestinal disease	Increased purine ingestion
Associated with gout	
Renal insufficiency	Low urine volume
Hyporenin, hypoaldosteronism	
Diabetes mellitus	
Obesity	

Struvite stones

Infection with urease-producing organisms

Cystine stones

Cystinuria

Drugs (partial list)

Indinavir	Sulfonamides	Topiramate
Triamterene	Acyclovir	Felbamate

of the finding. Crystalluria is not specific for stone disease, although in the setting of proven stones, the nature of the crystals usually correlates with stone composition.

Obstruction by other causes rarely results in the syndrome of renal colic. These cases can be divided into obstruction of the lower and upper urinary tracts. Lower-tract obstruction refers to the bladder neck or urethra. Renal failure is an unusual manifestation of lower-tract cases, because symptoms of obstruction and bladder irritation usually lead to medical attention before the ureterovesical valves become incompetent. Patients almost always complain of acute urinary retention, diminished strength of urinary stream, dribbling, low-volume polyuria, and nocturia long before renal failure occurs. In men, benign prostatic hypertrophy and prostate cancer account for almost all such cases. In women, this syndrome is much less common on an anatomic basis but can be caused by large uterine fibroids, pelvic carcinomas, or occasionally urethral strictures. If renal failure does occur because of outflow obstruction, the bladder hypertrophies, and for a long interval the kidneys are protected by competent ureterovesical valves. As the bladder wall dilates, the valves become incompetent and renal damage occurs.

Renal failure as a result of lower-tract obstruction more commonly occurs in patients with loss of normal bladder sensation (e.g., in diabetes), bladder sphincter dysfunction (in Parkinson's disease or multiple sclerosis), or spinal cord injury affecting bladder motor segments. Overdistention and smooth muscle decompensation follow. Complete interruption of sensory and motor pathways to and from the spinal cord after trauma results in a reflex neurogenic bladder. In this case, the bladder empties well reflexively, and the ureterovesical valves are intact. Nevertheless, chronic catheterization is necessary because of incontinence and sphincteric dysfunction, and this leads to infection and struvite stones. Renal failure may ensue. Lower tract obstruction caused by unnoticed urinary retention also occurs in patients with moderate-to-severe dementia.

Upper urinary tract obstruction from lesions other than stones is often chronic and fails to evoke ureteral contractions. It is therefore most often, silent, without the pain and colic of stone disease. Most often, such patients present with vague discomfort or are diagnosed only when their other medical problems lead them to seek evaluation. Asymptomatic renal obstruction may be found in the patient being evaluated for any number of malignancies, particularly lymphoma, colon cancer, and bladder tumors. Renal failure is unusual because this requires obstruction of two kidneys. It tends to occur only with the bulkiest tumors, or with significant retroperitoneal lymphadenopathy or fibrosis. About 0.1% of people have only one kidney, either on a congenital basis or resulting from surgery. Such patients are at greater risk for renal failure caused by obstruction. Stone disease easily may cause renal failure in this setting.

Differential Diagnosis and Initial Evaluation

The differential diagnosis of flank pain and colic is detailed in Table 103.2. The classic syndrome of renal colic also may be the initial presentation of pyelonephritis (Chapter 68). Confusion can result from the ability of obstructing stones to lead to concomitant urinary tract infection. The key distinguishing feature is that neither fever nor pyuria are signs of stone disease unaccompanied by infection. Urine is sterile in the case of most stones, except for struvite stones, which arise after infection with urease-producing organisms such as *Proteus* spp. and are often associated with urine pH values greater than or equal to 8. However, these stones are less likely to produce the syndrome of acute renal colic. Although renal colic may cause leukocytosis, high white blood cell counts (>12,000 cells/μL) suggest infec-

TABLE 103.2

DIFFERENTIAL DIAGNOSIS OF FLANK PAIN/RENAL COLIC

Condition	Distinguishing diagnostic features
Common causes of flank pain	
Stones	Hematuria is common (but not invariable), normal-to-slightly high WBC, absence of fever; onset of pain is acute, not positional
At the ureteropelvic junction	Flank pain predominates
At the crossing iliac vessels	Flank pain with radiation to genitalia
At the ureterovesical junction	Voiding symptoms, radiation to genitalia
At the bladder neck	Anuria, suprapubic discomfort
Pyelonephritis	Fever, leukocytosis, pyuria; onset of pain is more subacute, more constant; WBC casts
Nephrolithiasis and infection	Features of both stones and pyelonephritis
Unusual causes of flank pain	
Renal infarction	In setting of atrial fibrillation, dilated cardiomyopathy, hypercoagulable states, polyarteritis nodosa, cocaine use
Acute interstitial nephritis	In setting of drug use associated with syndrome; rash, fever, pyuria, eosinophilia
Acute glomerulonephritis	In setting of streptococcal infection; hematuria, proteinuria, RBC casts
Renal vein thrombosis	In setting of nephrotic syndrome, especially membranous nephropathy; hypercoagulable states
Non-nephrologic/non-urologic causes	
Ovarian cysts, torsion	
Ectopic pregnancy	
Diverticulitis	
Intestinal obstruction	
Appendicitis	

RBC, red blood cell; *WBC*, white blood cell count.

tion. *Papillary necrosis* occurs with pyelonephritis (particularly in the setting of diabetes), analgesic nephropathy, and sickle-cell disease or trait. The syndrome may cause renal obstruction as papillae lodge at the ureterovesical junction. Without radiologic studies, this condition may not be readily distinguishable from stone disease causing obstruction. *Renal infarction* can present with flank pain and hematuria. This diagnosis should be suspected in patients with atrial fibrillation, hypercoagulability, cocaine use, or vasculitis, and is usually associated with elevated serum and urine lactate dehydrogenase levels, with isoenzyme one level greater than that of isoenzyme 2.

Diagnosing obstruction by stones is often straightforward in the patient with the appropriate history, hematuria, and a plain radiograph of the abdomen that demonstrates a radio-opaque stone. Even with a clear-cut diagnosis, management decisions still may require more elaborate imaging studies such as ultrasound, computed tomography, or intravenous pyelogram to define urinary-tract anatomy. These studies also are indicated if the history, examination, and laboratory data do not lead to an obvious diagnosis of nephrolithiasis. Plain radiographs

do not disclose radiolucent stones and cannot diagnose obstruction resulting from other causes besides stone disease.

The dominant test in diagnosing and managing stone disease has traditionally been the intravenous pyelogram. The risk of nephrotoxicity despite the use of nonionic contrast agents, and the relative ease and speed of helical computed tomography, have diminished the intravenous pyelogram's role (3). Helical, or spiral, computed tomography has the advantages of being much faster than other tests (it can be completed in 5 minutes) and not requiring intravenous or oral contrast. Both its sensitivity and specificity are superior to ultrasound and IVP. The cost of CT is falling and now approaching that of IVP. Radiolucent uric acid stones (which appear as filling defects in IVPs) can be visualized directly by helical computed tomography and distinguished from intraluminal clot, tumors, and other obstructing masses. Ultrasound may miss stones causing obstruction, especially in the lower ureter, but the test does detect hydronephrosis well.

For obstruction resulting from causes other than stones, the diagnosis of lower urinary tract obstruction

TABLE 103.3

DIFFERENTIAL DIAGNOSIS OF LOWER URINARY TRACT OBSTRUCTION

Lower-tract obstruction	Distinguishing diagnostic features
All causes	Suprapubic pain; voiding symptoms: low-volume polyuria, nocturia, diminished stream, dribbling, progressing to anuria
Specific disorders	
Prostatic hypertrophy	Smooth, symmetrical, firm gland
Prostatic cancer	Nodular, asymmetrical, hard gland
Cervical/uterine cancers	Appropriate pelvic examination
Bladder stones	History of stone, occasional hematuria, often associated with prostatic hypertrophy
Urethral stricture/bladder neck stenosis	Difficult passage of Foley catheter
Neurologic diseases (e.g., spinal-cord injury)	Appropriate neurologic history, examination
Pain	Postoperative or posttraumatic
Hysteria	

should be considered in patients with symptoms of voiding difficulties. The differential diagnosis is reviewed in Table 103.3. The physical examination should focus on the rectal examination in men, looking for prostatic hypertrophy and carcinoma. Women should undergo pelvic examination. The bladder may be distended and palpable as a large suprapubic mass. After the patient voids (assuming anuria is not present), suprapubic ultrasound can estimate the postvoiding residual volume. If this modality is not available, a Foley catheter should be placed and the postvoid residual volume estimated. If the residual volume is less than 250 ml, the catheter should be removed. Although volumes of less than 150 mL normally are expected, volumes less than 1 L are unlikely to be associated with renal failure.

Upper urinary tract obstruction is readily diagnosed by ultrasound. This is a safe, relatively inexpensive, and sensitive (98%) test for this diagnosis (3). False negative results, such as in cases of obstruction of such short duration that the finding of hydronephrosis is not evident, or in conditions such as retroperitoneal fibrosis, in which ureteral entrapment prevents the development of hydroureter despite obstruction, are highly unusual. The ability of ultrasound to disclose the exact cause and location of obstruction is limited by its poorer visualization of the ureters and pelvis. The test's specificity (78%–90%) also is diminished by hydronephrosis not caused by obstruction (e.g., pregnancy and diuresis) and lesions with similar radiographic presentation, such as renal sinus cysts (4). For all of these reasons, helical computed tomography may soon supplant the intravenous pyelogram and ultrasound in visualization of the urinary tract (5). Magnetic resonance imaging is expensive, of no proven utility in the diagnosis of urinary tract obstruction, and does not visualize stones well.

ISSUES AT THE TIME OF ADMISSION

Indications for Hospitalization

One review indicates that up to 98% of stones smaller than 5 mm in diameter, especially those in the distal ureter, pass spontaneously (6). Stones greater than 7–8 mm have less than a 20% chance of spontaneous passage. These figures should contribute to the decision regarding observation, hospitalization, or immediate intervention. Controlled trials have demonstrated that passage of distal ureteral stones can be facilitated by administration of steroids to reduce ureteral edema and nifedipine or tamsulosin to reduce ureteral spasm (7). These trials have been performed in outpatients; whether such regimens could reduce hospitalizations is not clear.

Patients with urinary tract infection and obstruction are at risk for renal parenchymal damage and urosepsis and, therefore, should be hospitalized. Relief of obstruction should be accomplished rapidly by urologic or interventional radiologic intervention, and parenteral antibiotics should be administered. Although renal colic often is manageable in outpatients with oral medication, intractable pain, accompanied by nausea and vomiting, also leads to hospitalization. Patients with higher grades of obstruction are more likely to lose renal function over time if obstruction is unrelieved. Larger stones are less likely to pass and more often lead to hospitalization. Anatomic anomalies, such as horseshoe kidneys or duplicated collecting systems, also impede spontaneous stone passage and may support the admission decision. Renal failure of a degree approaching the need for dialysis arising from bilateral obstruction, or from obstruction of a solitary kidney, is always an indication for admission.

Patients with urinary retention resulting from benign prostatic hypertrophy relieved by catheterization need not be admitted if adequately instructed regarding the use of a drainage bag. Definitive therapy can include immediate institution of α-blockers leading to a trial of catheter removal. If this fails, surgery or other ablative therapies for benign prostatic hypertrophy may be required.

Indications for Initial Intensive Care Unit Admission

Acute renal obstruction rarely requires ICU admission. ICU monitoring is prudent if the sepsis syndrome (Chapter 26) is present. Urinary tract infection proximal to an obstructed ureter can lead to pyonephrosis, which in turn is associated with pyelonephritis, papillary necrosis, and destruction of renal parenchyma, with progressive loss of kidney function. Renal failure resulting from bilateral obstruction, or obstruction of a single kidney, may be an indication for ICU admission if severe complications develop, such as refractory hyperkalemia, metabolic acidosis, circulatory congestion, or deteriorating mental status caused by uremia (Chapter 100). If such effects cannot be reversed rapidly by prompt relief of obstruction or by dialysis, ICU management of these complications may be needed.

Initial Therapy

The choices for pain relief of renal colic are nonsteroidal anti-inflammatory drugs (NSAIDs) or opiate agonists. Both have advantages and disadvantages (Chapter 18). One randomized trial demonstrated that ketorolac was slightly superior to morphine for renal colic, with better pain control and faster discharge from the emergency room (8). The sedative properties of opiates make them less desirable for patients who are not admitted or who are discharged with stones still in place. Opiates in general, and meperidine specifically, can cause nausea, vomiting, and constipation. Meperidine also is contraindicated in renal failure because accumulation of its renally-cleared metabolite normeperidine has been associated with seizures. Morphine also has a glucuronide metabolite that accumulates in renal insufficiency and can be toxic when it accumulates in neurons. NSAIDs such as ketorolac provide effective, nonsedating analgesia and diminish ureteral motility, but have the disadvantages of causing gastric irritation (particularly in the elderly) and diminished renal function (particularly in those with extracellular fluid volume depletion or other causes of renal insufficiency). They are also more expensive than opiates. Antibiotics should be administered in any patient with evidence or suspicion of infection. The most common organisms in patients who are not immunosuppressed and have not received multiple courses of antibiotics are Gram-negative rods, such as *Escherichia coli*, *Proteus* spp., and *Klebsiella* spp., and the enterococci. Chapter 68 suggests empiric antibiotic regimens.

Attention to repletion of intravascular volume in the patient with nausea and vomiting, and correction of electrolyte derangements associated with acute renal failure, are addressed in Chapters 100 and 104. Administration of saline and forced diuresis have not been shown to increase likelihood of spontaneous stone passage and may increase intra-ureteral pressure and pain.

Indications for Early Consultation

Most patients with small stones (5 mm or less) can be managed with analgesia as appropriate and without urologic consultation. Larger stones are associated with a progressively smaller likelihood of spontaneous passage. A urologist must evaluate such patients in anticipation of a definitive intervention. Any patient requiring hospitalization for a large stone, accompanying infection, renal failure, or with a solitary kidney should be seen by a urologist as quickly as possible. Urology consultation should also be sought for patients with urinary retention and significant postvoid residual volumes.

For patients with acute renal failure, consultation with a nephrologist in anticipation of possible dialysis is generally prudent, particularly in cases complicated by uremia and more severely deranged serum electrolyte concentrations. In many cases, dialysis may be obviated by prompt treatment to relieve obstruction, which produces an immediate improvement in renal function.

ISSUES DURING THE COURSE OF HOSPITALIZATION

The key decisions during the first hospital day involve choosing a means to relieve renal obstruction. In the case of lower-tract obstruction, it is easily relieved by placing a Foley catheter. Larger catheters (22 or 24 Fr) with coudé tips may allow passage past an enlarged prostate. If this is not possible, a urologist needs to perform suprapubic cystostomy. α-blockers (e.g., terazosin or tamsulosin) can be started immediately if prostatic obstruction is present. For upper-tract obstruction, options include passing a retrograde stent into the ureter via cystoscopy, passing a percutaneous nephrostomy tube with antegrade passage of a stent, or prompt removal of an obstructing stone by percutaneous nephrolithotomy, extracorporeal shock-wave lithotripsy (ESWL), or ureteroscopy. If a stent is passed via cystoscopy, pain and infection can occur and more definitive therapy can be scheduled in the outpatient setting. Open surgery for stone disease is almost never required. Long-term management of obstruction that cannot readily be relieved, such as bilateral obstruction caused by advanced carcinoma of the bladder, may require urinary diversion such as construction of an ileal conduit.

On day 2, after obstruction in patients with bilateral obstruction and renal failure is relieved, an immediate improvement in renal function should occur. A poor prognostic feature is if little recovery has occurred after 2–3 days. A postobstructive diuresis often accompanies the fall in creatinine. Extracellular fluid volume must be assessed carefully to ensure that the patient does not become volume-depleted. Though recommendations often are made to replace a certain proportion of the urine volume, it is preferable to monitor the patient's requirements by monitoring for signs of extracellular fluid volume depletion. If necessary, hypotonic fluid administration (e.g., 0.45% normal saline) can be used to replace some proportion of the urinary losses.

On subsequent days, diagnosis of specific causes of obstruction should be made if not previously established, and therapy instituted for the underlying disorder, if possible.

DISCHARGE ISSUES

Patients with stones still in place can be discharged if pain and obstruction are largely relieved and infection, if present, is under control (e.g., resolution of fever and leukocytosis). Definitive treatment of stones remaining in the urinary tract can be scheduled on an outpatient basis if these criteria are met. Mild pain still may be present but should be manageable with either NSAIDs or lower doses of oral opiates. The patient's ability to function normally and go to work or school on such a regimen should be taken into account before delaying definitive treatment. Patients with stents in place may be troubled by flank pain, because voiding causes urinary reflux, or by urinary frequency caused by bladder irritation. A string may be left exiting from the urethra to allow easy removal of the stent in the office without cystoscopy.

Patients should be given a strainer for screening urine for passed stones or fragments if none have been recovered by the time of discharge. This allows stone analysis to be done and confirms passage of stones and fragments. Stone analysis is very inexpensive and can produce insight into the patient's pathophysiology.

Dietary recommendations on discharge of patients with nephrolithiasis can await definitive evaluation of the urinary chemistries. However, certain dietary advice is always appropriate (9). Restriction of protein intake to 8 ounces each day should be stressed. This reduces urinary calcium, uric acid, and cystine excretion and increases urinary citrate excretion and urine pH. Restriction of salt intake also can reduce calcium, uric acid, and cystine excretion, and it reduces hypokalemia caused by thiazides. Dietary oxalate accounts for a variable proportion of urinary oxalate, but even small reductions may significantly reduce calcium oxalate supersaturation. Restriction of calcium intake has not been shown to prevent stone recurrence and may lead to bone demineralization. In patients with hypercalciuria, there is nearly a 50% reduction in stone recurrence when patients ingest 1200 mg of elemental calcium accompanied by decreased dietary salt, protein, and oxalate, compared with patients eating an oxalate-restricted diet containing only 400 mg of calcium per day (10).

Patients with benign prostatic hypertrophy may be treated with α-blockers. These drugs improve voiding symptoms but can be associated with orthostasis, particularly with the first dose. Patients should be instructed to take the first dose at night in bed to minimize the incidence of syncope. The drug can be started while a Foley catheter is still in place, and the patient can be discharged if voiding is then possible. If α-blockers are ineffective, transurethral resection of the prostate may be indicated.

Patients with obstructive renal failure may be discharged after nephrostomies are removed, if possible, and after internal stent placement. Alternatively, they may go home with the nephrostomy draining externally. This may be painful and require analgesia. Patients require instruction on the proper care and maintenance of the tube and site and may need assistance. Postobstructive diuresis may persist for several days. Patients should not be discharged if they still require intravenous fluids to replace inappropriate urinary sodium losses.

ASSESSMENT AND MANAGEMENT OF THE PATIENT PRESENTING WITH RENAL OBSTRUCTION DURING HOSPITALIZATION

Patients who develop acute renal failure while hospitalized most commonly have acute tubular necrosis, disorders of renal perfusion ("prerenal renal failure"), and nephrotoxic effects of radiocontrast, aminoglycosides, or NSAIDs (Chapter 100). If no other explanation is readily apparent, the possibility of obstruction is worth investigating. Most patients with other diagnoses may be oliguric or nonoliguric, but anuria is rare. Anuria does occur with complete obstruction. If voiding symptoms or a palpable bladder are detected, the postvoiding residual volume should be estimated by ultrasound or directly measured by a Foley catheter. The catheter should be left in only if a significant postvoiding residual volume is detected, because it otherwise constitutes a substantial risk for urinary tract infection. Ultrasound of the kidneys should be performed if a diagnosis still is not apparent.

Intratubular obstruction resulting from crystal formation in nephrons can cause renal failure often accompanied by bilateral flank pain. Hydronephrosis is absent in such cases. Urinalysis can disclose acid urine pH and uric-acid crystals associated with urate nephropathy. This most often occurs after chemotherapy for bulky lymphomas or chronic lymphocytic leukemia. Sulfa crystals can cause a similar syndrome, although usually this is seen if sulfadiazine is given in larger doses. Acyclovir causes renal dysfunction via a similar mechanism in patients receiving high doses intravenously. The protease inhibitor indinavir can also present with renal insufficiency, crystalluria, or stones; such stones are not visualized by CT scanning.

The underlying diagnosis for which the patient is hospitalized should be considered in formulating a differential diagnosis of acute renal failure. Cancer of the colon, cervix, prostate, and bladder, and lymphomas are the most common causes of extrinsic obstruction of the urinary tract. Inflammatory diseases such as Crohn's disease and endometriosis can cause obstruction, as can surgical complications and aneurysms of the aorta or iliac vessels. The evaluation should be similar to that in patients first seen as outpatients.

COST CONSIDERATIONS AND RESOURCE USE

Patients with symptomatic stones can be treated as outpatients once they are pain-free and obstruction has been relieved. In managing stone disease, the choice among ESWL, ureteroscopy, and percutaneous nephrolithotomy is based mostly on technical issues, reviewed in part in Table 103.4. ESWL initially may be less expensive if the procedure is successful. However, second-generation ESWL machines are somewhat less powerful than their predecessors, so that efficacy is lower, though less intense sedation is required. Calculation of expense then must take into account the possibility of multiple courses of therapy. On the other hand, use of these machines does not require much anesthesia and should allow outpatient therapy. Percutaneous nephrolithotomy and ureteroscopy both are more likely to be successful with a single course, though both require greater skill (11). ESWL also is more likely to leave stone fragments in the kidney, especially when used for treating lower pole stones. These may serve as the nidus for new stones. Again, more invasive procedures may allow more thorough removal of these fragments, ultimately resulting in lower costs.

Evaluation of the metabolic factors responsible for stone formation has been shown to lead to significant savings (12). Abnormalities are disclosed in more than 90% of patients. Classification of the specific causes of hypercalciuria, the most common abnormality, has no specific consequences for therapy. Thiazides are effective for idiopathic hypercalciuria, regardless of the specific cause (13). Increased fluid intake to achieve urine volumes of more than 2 L is especially useful for calcium oxalate and cystine stones. Potassium citrate is given for hypocitraturia and calcium stones, and also for urinary alkalinization for uric acid and cystine stones. Dietary therapy has been discussed previously. Allopurinol is useful if diet fails and calcium stones persist in the setting of hyperuricosuria. Surgery is indicated for primary hyperparathyroidism. All of these therapies are relatively inexpensive, and all are cost-effective.

KEY POINTS

- The diagnosis of urinary tract obstruction is most often suggested by history and physical examination.
- Modern imaging options make confirmation of the diagnosis relatively easy. The diagnosis of renal obstruction, from stones or other causes, therefore has been expedited dramatically.
- The advent of flexible ureteroscopy, ESWL, and smaller percutaneous nephrolithotomy instruments has also had a beneficial impact on management of obstruction and stone disease. These therapeutic options have made open surgery nearly obsolete and almost never indicated. The results of these advances are much lower hospitalization rates and minimally invasive outpatient surgery.
- Stones smaller than 5 mm most often pass spontaneously and often do not require intervention.
- Recent demonstrations of the efficacy and cost-effectiveness of metabolic evaluation and treatment for prevention of recurrent stone formation may shift attention to prophylaxis for a larger proportion of afflicted patients.

TABLE 103.4

TREATMENT RECOMMENDATIONS FOR MANAGEMENT OF SYMPTOMATIC URETERAL STONES

Condition	Recommended therapy	Comment
Stone with high probability of passage (<5 mm)	Observation	Intervention appropriate if symptoms demand
Stone <10 mm in proximal ureter	ESWL	PNL or USC if needed
Stone >10 mm in proximal ureter	ESWL, PNL, or USC	PNL becomes more appropriate with larger stones
Stones <10 mm in distal ureter	ESWL, USC	ESWL may require more procedures, cost more
Stones >10 mm in distal ureter	USC, ESWL	USC may be preferable with larger stones, lower pole stones

ESWL, extracorporeal shock-wave lithotripsy; PNL, percutaneous nephrolithotomy; USC, ureteroscopy.
Adapted from Segura JW, Preminger GM, Assimos DG, et al. Ureteral stones clinical guidelines panel summary report on the management of ureteral calculi. J Urol 1997;158:1915–1921.

REFERENCES

1. Scheinman SJ. New insights into causes and treatments of kidney stones. *Hosp Pract* 2000;35:49–63.
2. Bove P, Kaplan D, Dalrymple N, et al. Reexamining the value of hematuria testing in patients with acute flank pain. *J Urol* 1999;162:685–687.
3. Older RA, Jenkins AD. Stone disease. *Urol Clin North Am* 2000; 27:215–29.
4. Heidenreich A, Desgrandschamps F, Terrier F. Modern approach of diagnosis and management of acute flank pain: review of all imaging modalities. *Eur Urol* 2002;41:351–362.
5. Smith RC, Coll DM. Helical computed tomography in the diagnosis of ureteric colic. *BJU Int* 2000;(86 Suppl 1):33–41.
6. Segura JW, Preminger GM, Assimos DG, et al. Ureteral Stones Clinical Guidelines Panel summary report on the management of ureteral calculi. *J Urol* 1997;158:1915–1921.
7. Cooper JT, Stack GM, Cooper TP. Intensive medical management of ureteral calculi. *Urology* 2000;56:575–578.
8. Larkin GL, Peacock WF, Pearl SM, et al. Efficacy of ketorolac tromethamine versus meperidine in the ED treatment of acute renal colic. *Am J Emerg Med* 1999;17:6–10.
9. Assimos DG, Holmes RP. Role of diet in the therapy of urolithiasis. *Urol Clin North Am* 2000;27:255–268.
10. Borghi L, Schianchi T, Meschi T, et al. Comparison of two diets for the prevention of recurrent stones in idiopathic hypercalciuria. *N Engl J Med* 2002;346:77–84.
11. Albala DM, Assimos DG, Clayman RV, et al. Lower pole I: a prospective randomized trial of extracorporeal shock wave lithotripsy and percutaneous nephrostolithotomy for lower pole nephrolithiasis-initial results. *J Urol* 2001;166:2072–2080.
12. Parks JH, Coe FL. The financial effects of kidney stone prevention. *Kidney Int* 1996;50:1706–1712.
13. Pearle MS, Roehrborn CG, Pak CY. Meta-analysis of randomized trials for medical prevention of calcium oxalate nephrolithiasis. *J Endourol* 1999;13:679–685.

ADDITIONAL READING

Dellabella M, Milanese G, Muzzonigro G. Efficacy of tamsulosin in the medical management of juxtavesical ureteral stones. *J Urol* 2003;170:2202–2205.

Loughlin KR, Ker LA. The current management of urolithiasis during pregnancy. *Urol Clin North Am* 2002;29:701–704.

Miller OF, Kane CJ. Time to stone passage for observed ureteral calculi: a guide for patient education. *J Urol* 1999;162:688–690.

Shekarriz B, Stoller ML. Uric acid nephrolithiasis: current concepts and controversies. *J Urol* 2002;68:1307–1314.

Teichman, JM. Clinical practice: acute renal colic from ureteral calculus. *N Engl J Med* 2004;350:684–693.

Tiselius HG, Ackermann D, Alken P, et al. Guidelines on urolithiasis. *Eur Urol* 2001;40:362–371.

Common Electrolyte Disorders

104

Kerry C. Cho

INTRODUCTION

Disorders of sodium and potassium are the most common electrolyte disorders in hospital medicine. Electrolyte abnormalities may be incidental findings on routine laboratory tests and have few symptoms and little clinical significance. Severe disturbances, complicated by or resulting from other medical conditions, may require hospitalization or even intensive care monitoring. The diagnostic evaluations of potassium and sodium disorders in clinical practice are often incomplete and unfocused (1). Furthermore, therapy for electrolyte disorders can be overly aggressive and have disastrous results if basic pathophysiologic rules are violated. One fundamental rule guides the approach to common electrolyte disorders: *potassium disorders result from abnormal potassium handling, but sodium disorders result from abnormal water handling.*

SODIUM

Hyponatremia

Hyponatremia, defined as a plasma sodium concentration less than 135 mEq/L, is the most common electrolyte abnormality in hospitalized patients. The majority of cases reflect hypotonicity because sodium is the main solute that determines serum osmolality (Table 104.1). Hypertonic and isotonic forms of hyponatremia occur infrequently. Hypertonic hyponatremia occurs with hyperglycemia or mannitol infusion. The movement of water from the intracellular space driven by the hypertonicity of the extracellular compartment dilutes the sodium concentration and produces hyponatremia. The standard correction factor for hyperglycemic hyponatremia is a 1.6 mEq/L decrease in sodium concentration per 100 mg/dL increase in glucose (2). A revised correction factor of 2.4 mEq/L Na^+ per 100 mg/dL glucose has been proposed recently (3). The incidence of isotonic *pseudohyponatremia*, a laboratory artifact produced by hypertriglyceridemia or hyperproteinemia, has decreased with the direct measurement of sodium by ion-specific electrodes.

The total body sodium in hyponatremic patients may be low, normal, or high. Thus, patients may be hypovolemic, isovolemic, or hypervolemic. Although the serum sodium concentration does not reflect total body sodium or water, there is always a relative excess of water to sodium in all cases of hyponatremia. In general, hypotonic hyponatremia results from primary sodium loss (with secondary water gain), primary water gain (with secondary sodium loss), or primary sodium gain (with excessive water gain). The first category includes patients with sodium losses from either renal or nonrenal sources. Examples of renal sodium loss include the use of thiazide diuretics, osmotic diuresis, postobstructive diuresis, nonoliguric acute tubular necrosis, and salt-wasting nephropathy. Nonrenal sources of sodium loss include insensible losses from the respiratory tract or skin and gastrointestinal losses (vomiting, nasogastric suctioning, and diarrhea). Whether renal or nonrenal, the sodium loss produces contraction of the extracellular fluid volume, stimulation of thirst, increased fluid intake, and increased ADH release. The net result of increased water intake and decreased renal water excretion is hyponatremia.

The category of primary water gain includes the syndrome of inappropriate antidiuretic hormone release (SIADH), hormonal disorders, primary polydipsia, and chronic renal insufficiency. The main disturbance in these conditions is decreased renal water excretion (or water

TABLE 104.1

MAJOR CAUSES OF HYPONATREMIA

Pseudohyponatremia
  Hypertriglyceridemia
  Hyperproteinemia

Hypertonic hyponatremia
  Hyperglycemia
  Mannitol administration

Hypotonic hyponatremia
  Hypovolemic (primary sodium loss with secondary water gain): Thiazide diuretics and other renal losses, gastrointestinal losses, insensible losses
  Euvolemic (primary water gain with secondary sodium loss): Syndrome of inappropriate antidiuretic hormone, primary polydipsia, glucocorticoid deficiency, hypothyroidism, chronic renal disease
  Hypervolemic (primary sodium gain with excessive water gain): Congestive heart failure, cirrhosis, nephrotic syndrome

intake exceeding excretory capacity in the case of primary polydipsia). High levels of ADH alone are usually insufficient to produce hyponatremia; increased water intake or administration must also be present. SIADH is the most common cause of isovolemic, hypotonic hyponatremia. The ADH release is nonphysiologic ("inappropriate") in the absence of hypovolemia or hyperosmolality, the usual triggers for ADH. The numerous causes of SIADH can be classified into the following broad categories: malignancy, pulmonary disorders, central nervous system disorders, and medications. Deficiencies of cortisol and thyroid hormone can produce hyponatremia by directly or indirectly stimulating ADH release; these hormone deficiencies should be differentiated from SIADH for evaluation and treatment purposes.

In primary or psychogenic polydipsia, massive water intake overwhelms the renal water excretory capacity of 12 L/day. Increased water intake in psychiatric patients may be due to phenothiazines, which enhance thirst perception by causing dry mouth. In beer potomania, decreased dietary intake and cachexia limit the daily solute load. If the kidneys have a limited supply of solutes and the minimum urine osmolality is fixed at 50 mOsm/kg, then a moderately increased daily water intake can exceed the diminished renal water excretory capacity. For example, a beer drinker may have a daily solute load of only 250 mOsm, compared with the 600 mOsm/day generated by the metabolism of a normal diet. With a solute load of 250 mOsm/day, the renal excretory capacity is limited to 5 L/day at the minimum urine osmolality of 50 mOsm/kg.

Hypervolemic hyponatremia reflects primary sodium gain with excessive water gain, typified by the edematous states of heart failure, cirrhosis, and the nephrotic syndrome. Heart failure and cirrhosis are states with decreased effective circulating volume, due to either decreased cardiac output or decreased systemic vascular resistance (4). Activation of the renin-angiotensin-aldosterone system increases ADH release and sodium and water retention in an attempt to restore effective circulating volume, at the expense of hypo-osmolality and hyponatremia. The severity of hyponatremia in heart failure and cirrhosis has been shown to be an important predictor of survival.

Clinical Manifestations

Hyponatremia causes primarily neurologic manifestations. The severity and rate of change of the serum sodium concentration determine the extent of symptoms. Most patients with mild hyponatremia (sodium >125 mEq/L) are asymptomatic. Chronic, slowly developing hyponatremia is usually better tolerated because the brain decreases its intracellular tonicity, limiting cellular edema. Early symptoms of hyponatremic encephalopathy include headaches, nausea, malaise, lethargy, muscle cramps, and hyperreflexia. More severe symptoms include obtundation, bizarre behavior, hallucinations, asterixis, and incontinence. Advanced symptoms include seizures, coma, brain stem herniation, central diabetes insipidus, permanent brain injury, respiratory arrest, and death. Patients at increased risk for cerebral edema and hyponatremic encephalopathy include prepubertal children, postoperative patients, menstruant women, psychiatric patients with polydipsia, hypoxic patients, and elderly women recently started on thiazide diuretics (5,6). Figure 104.1 contains a diagnostic algorithm.

Therapy

Hospitalization should be considered for symptomatic patients, especially in the presence of significant medical comorbidities. Severe neurological symptoms require intensive care monitoring and frequent sodium measurements. The goals of therapy for hyponatremia include correction of the underlying disease (if possible), correction of sodium concentration by restricting free water intake and promoting water loss, and avoidance of overly rapid sodium correction. Medications that cause or contribute to hyponatremia should be stopped if possible; these include sedatives, hypnotics, analgesics, tranquilizers, oral hypoglycemics, opiates, antineoplastic drugs, antidepressants, and diuretics (5). Hypovolemic patients may require fluid resuscitation with normal saline, while hypervolemic patients may require diuretics and/or dialysis to correct volume overload.

Correction of the sodium concentration is potentially hazardous because serum tonicity may increase more quickly than brain tonicity, especially if the brain has adapted to chronic hyponatremia. *Overly rapid correction may lead to cerebral osmotic demyelination.* Originally called central pontine myelinolysis, this pathologic process can also occur in extrapontine sites. Demyelination is more

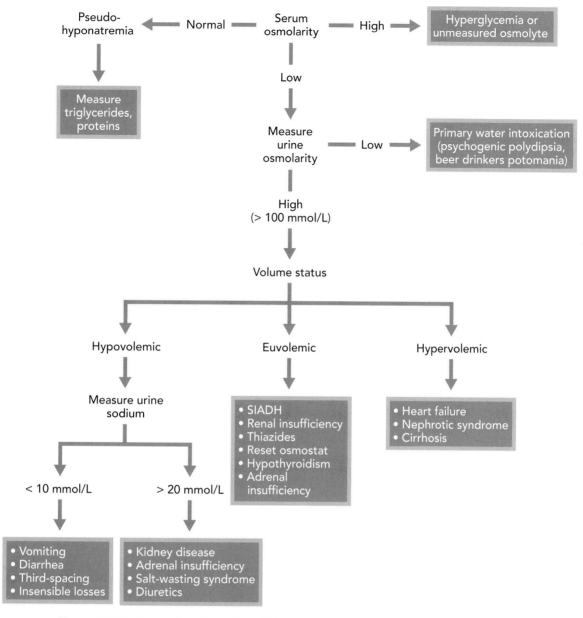

Figure 104.1 Approach to the patient with hyponatremia. *CHF*, congestive heart failure; *SIADH*, syndrome of inappropriate antiduretic hormone.

likely to occur with chronic hyponatremia (>48 hours) and in certain clinical settings: alcoholism, malnutrition, hypokalemia, burns, and thiazide diuretic use (6). Symptoms include mutism and dysarthria initially, followed by spastic quadriparesis and pseudobulbar palsy. Computed tomography and magnetic resonance imaging may not detect radiographic evidence of myelinolysis within the first 2 weeks. There is no specific therapy for myelinolysis.

When considering the appropriate management, physicians must weigh the risk of sodium correction and myelinolysis against the risks of hyponatremic encephalopathy. The chronicity of hyponatremia and the severity of symptoms are the major guides to appropriate therapy. Chronic hyponatremia is generally well tolerated and causes fewer

symptoms than acute hyponatremia, but it carries the highest risk of osmotic demyelination. Thus, in the absence of symptoms, management should be conservative. Free water restriction alone may be sufficient, although the rate of sodium correction may not exceed 1.5 mEq/L per day. Some patients with SIADH may require *demeclocycline* (150 mg four times daily) to antagonize ADH effect by inducing a nephrogenic diabetes insipidus, but its use may be complicated by nephrotoxicity.

Severely symptomatic patients generally require hypertonic saline (3% NaCl) at approximately 1–2 mL/kg/hr. Acute hyponatremia (<48 hours) can be corrected quickly (i.e. 2.0–2.5 mEq/L/hour), while chronic hyponatremia correction should not exceed 1.0–1.5 mEq/L/hr. There is likely no correction rate that is completely risk free, unfortunately. Many authorities have proposed correction rates ranging from 8–15 mEq/L/day (5–9). Loop diuretics may be required to augment free water excretion and prevent hypervolemia. Serum sodium levels should be checked as frequently as every 1–2 hours. Sodium correction should stop if the patient is no longer acutely symptomatic or if the serum sodium has been corrected to a mild level of hyponatremia (125–130 mEq/L).

Nephrology consultation should be considered for severely symptomatic patients, neurological or neurosurgical patients, obstetrical patients, or whenever hypertonic saline, hemodialysis, or demeclocycline are being considered.

Hypernatremia

Hypernatremia is defined as a plasma sodium concentration >145 mEq/L. Unlike hyponatremia, where osmolality may be decreased, normal, or increased, *hypernatremia always reflects a hyperosmolar state*. The hyperosmolality of the extracellular compartment moves fluid out of cells and causes intracellular fluid contraction. The appropriate physiologic response to hypernatremia is thirst, increased water intake, and excretion of a minimum volume (500 mL/day) of maximally concentrated urine (>800 mOsm/kg) caused by ADH release. Hypernatremia usually does not develop unless a defective thirst mechanism or limited access to water impairs the protective response. Common clinical settings include altered mental status, physical handicaps, the postoperative state, mechanical ventilation, and primary hypodipsia caused by hypothalamic disorders.

Most hypernatremia occurs with hypotonic fluid losses and inadequate intake of sodium and water (Table 104.2). These patients are either hypovolemic or euvolemic. Nonrenal sources of water loss include insensible losses from the skin and respiratory tract, gastrointestinal losses, or wound losses (including surgical drains). Fever, heat exposure, exercise, severe burns, and mechanical ventilation may increase insensible losses. Gastrointestinal losses are caused by vomiting, nasogastric suctioning, enterocutaneous fistulas, and diarrhea. Although any form of diarrhea can produce volume contraction, osmotic diarrheas (from lactulose, sorbitol, or carbohydrate malabsorption) and viral gastroenteritides are particularly likely to present with hypernatremia because of water losses in excess of sodium losses.

The kidney is also a potential source of hypotonic fluid losses. Osmotic diuresis from mannitol administration, hyperglycemia, or excessive protein loads can promote excess water loss, leading to hypernatremia and volume depletion. These patients have polyuria with submaximal urine osmolality. A dilute urine (urine osmolality <100 mOsm/L) is an inappropriate response to hypernatremia, raising the suspicion for either *central or nephrogenic diabetes insipidus (DI)*. Central DI results from trauma, surgery, infection, granulomatous disease, malignancy, and vascular events. Nephrogenic DI may result from drugs (most commonly lithium), hypercalcemia, hypokalemia, papillary necrosis, and pregnancy (because of increased amounts of vasopressinase by the placenta during the second and third trimester). There are also congenital forms of central and nephrogenic DI caused by mutations in genes for ADH, its V_2 receptor, or the aquaporin-2 water channel.

Hypernatremia may also (uncommonly) be caused by excess total body sodium. Examples include ingestion or administration of hypertonic sodium solutions (chloride or bicarbonate salts) and hypertonic feeding preparations. Primary hyperaldosteronism and Cushing syndrome are rare causes of hypertonic hypernatremia with hypervolemia. A review of seven patients with hospital-acquired hypernatremia and edema demonstrated that patients shared several key characteristics: medical comorbidities, isotonic fluid resuscitation, marked weight gain, hypoalbuminemia, and diminished glomerular filtration rate (10).

Clinical Manifestations

As with hyponatremia, the signs and symptoms of hypernatremia are mainly neurologic (11,12). Whether an individual develops symptoms depends on the rate of rise of the sodium concentration and the absolute value. Symptoms include thirst, irritability, lethargy, and weakness. As hypernatremia progresses, confusion, agitation, hyperreflexia, myoclonus, seizures, and coma can develop. In severe cases, brain shrinkage applies traction on the dural veins and venous sinuses, resulting in intracranial hemorrhage. Physical findings include tachycardia, poor skin turgor, dry mucous membranes, and warm, dry skin. Patients admitted with hypernatremia are usually elderly and often have coexisting fever or hyperglycemia. However, hospital-acquired hypernatremia is often iatrogenic and can occur in younger patients with restricted access to free water.

TABLE 104.2

MAJOR CAUSES OF HYPERNATREMIA

Water losses
  Gastrointestinal losses
  Diabetes insipidus, either central or nephrogenic
  Diuretics
  Increased insensible losses through respiration and skin
  Hypothalamic lesions with impaired thirst perception

Sodium overload
  Hypertonic sodium intravenous fluids
  Hypertonic feeding preparations
  Primary hyperaldosteronism
  Cushing syndrome

Therapy

The goals of hypernatremia management are to replace the free water deficit and to stop or decrease ongoing water losses if possible. The first step is to review iatrogenic factors: hypertonic solutions, feeding preparations, diuretics, and other medications. The next step is volume resuscitation of hypovolemic patients with isotonic saline. The free water deficit can be estimated from the following formula: free water deficit (liters) = 0.6 × body weight (in kg) × [(serum sodium/140) − 1]. As with hyponatremia, overly rapid correction of hypernatremia is potentially hazardous. *To avoid cerebral edema, the correction rate should not exceed 0.5 mEq/L/hr.* If mental status worsens during the correction of hypernatremia, cerebral edema may have occurred; free water administration should be stopped until symptoms improve. The preferred route of water administration is via oral intake or nasogastric tube; 5% dextrose is the intravenous equivalent. The fluid replacement rate should account for ongoing water losses. Patients with hypervolemic hypernatremia need slow free water replacement to avoid volume overload. Diuretics are used to maximize natriuresis, but hemodialysis may be required to correct the combined sodium and water imbalance.

Patients with central diabetes insipidus or partial nephrogenic DI may require desmopressin (ddAVP), the synthetic analogue of AVP. Complete nephrogenic DI is a therapeutic challenge. Most patients require large amounts of water intake because of obligate renal water losses, but the water requirement may decrease with judicious use of thiazide diuretics, nonsteroidal anti-inflammatory drugs, and dietary sodium restriction. Chlorpropamide, clofibrate, and carbamazepine have been used to stimulate AVP secretion or enhance its action.

Consultation for hypernatremia is generally not required unless diabetes insipidus is suspected. A nephrologist or endocrinologist should assist with the diagnosis of diabetes insipidus, its differentiation (nephrogenic versus central) via a water-deprivation test, and appropriate therapy. Patients with hypervolemic hypernatremia and concomitant chronic renal failure may require nephrology consultation for diuretic recommendations or hemodialysis.

Outcomes

Patients admitted with hypernatremia are often geriatric patients transferred from nursing homes, whereas hospital-acquired hypernatremia occurs in younger patients with an age distribution that resembles the overall hospital population (13). Hypernatremia carries a high mortality rate. A recent study of 116 patients admitted with hypernatremia (serum sodium >145 mEq/L) found that 77 (or 66%) expired (14). Another report noted hypernatremia (serum sodium >150 mEq/L) in 111 (3.46%) of 3,209 hospitalizations (15). Sixty-five patients were hypernatremic on admission, while 45 developed hypernatremia while hospitalized. Hospital mortality for all hypernatremic patients was 48.6%.

Hospital-acquired hypernatremia is often iatrogenic and/or preventable. In 85 patients with hospital-acquired hypernatremia, Palevsky et al. found that 86% lacked free access to water, 94% received less than 1 L/day of IV electrolyte-free water during the development of hypernatremia, and 49% received no supplemental electrolyte-free water during the first 24 hours of hypernatremia (13). One group has proposed using hypernatremia as an indicator of poor quality of care in the medical intensive care unit (16).

POTASSIUM

The normal plasma potassium concentration is 3.5 to 5.0 mEq/L, but extracellular potassium comprises only 2% of the total body potassium content of 4,000 mEq. At a concentration of 140 mEq/L, intracellular potassium is the major cation generating the membrane potential for normal neuromuscular function. The Na^+-K^+-ATPase pump maintains the ratio of intracellular-to-extracellular potassium concentrations. Hormones, acid-base status, osmolality, and cell turnover affect potassium distribution between the two compartments. Insulin increases Na^+-K^+-ATPase activity, increasing uptake of plasma K^+ into liver and skeletal muscle cells. Catecholamines have varied affects; β_2-adrenergic agonists increase Na^+-K^+-ATPase activity, while α-adrenergic agonists decrease activity. Metabolic acidosis promotes exchange of intracellular K^+ for extracellular H^+, resulting in hyperkalemia. Organic acidoses such as lactic acidosis or diabetic ketoacidosis may not produce hyperkalemia, because lactate and β-hydroxybutyrate anions can shift into cells along with H^+. Metabolic alkalosis produces hypokalemia as potassium moves into cells to buffer the outward shift of H^+.

The gastrointestinal tract absorbs 90% of dietary potassium, which is 40–120 mEq/day on an average western diet, an amount equivalent to that of extracellular potassium. Stimulated by insulin and catecholamines, intracellular potassium uptake prevents immediate postprandial hyperkalemia. Stool losses account for 10–20 mEq/day of potassium excretion, but this amount can increase with diarrhea and chronic renal insufficiency. The kidney regulates net potassium balance via the principal cells in the distal nephron. In response to hyperkalemia or high renin and angiotensin II levels, aldosterone increases potassium excretion by stimulation of the basolateral Na^+-K^+-ATPase pump.

Hypokalemia

Etiology and Differential Diagnosis

Defined as a plasma $[K^+]$ <3.5 mEq/L, hypokalemia results from decreased intake, increased loss, or intracellular redistribution (17,18). Pseudohypokalemia may occur rarely in leukemia patients when abnormal leukocytes take up extracellular potassium after phlebotomy. Rapid separation of the plasma after phlebotomy prevents this artifact. In an individual patient with true hypokalemia, one or more pathophysiological mechanisms may be implicated. Low dietary intake rarely produces hypokalemia because renal excretion can decrease to less than 15 mEq/day. Starvation may reduce total body potassium stores, but tissue catabolism will preserve serum [K$^+$]. Causes of increased potassium loss can be either renal, gastrointestinal, or dermal (via excessive sweating). Gastrointestinal losses result from diarrhea, fistulas, and cathartic use. Renal potassium losses fall into two categories: mineralocorticoid excess (either real or apparent) and impaired renal sodium-chloride transport (Bartter syndrome and Gitelman syndrome). The mineralocorticoid group includes primary hyperaldosteronism, adrenal hyperplasia, Cushing syndrome, Liddle syndrome, and others (18,19). Redistribution hypokalemia includes hyperthyroidism, familial hypokalemic periodic paralysis, delirium tremens, and increased cell production (treatment of anemia with vitamin B$_{12}$ or folate, granulocyte colony stimulating factor (GM-CSF) therapy, and parenteral nutrition).

Numerous medications cause hypokalemia (18). Excluding cathartic agents, drugs cause hypokalemia either by redistributing potassium into cells or by increasing renal potassium excretion (Table 104.3).

TABLE 104.3

MAJOR CAUSES OF HYPOKALEMIA

Pseudohypokalemia

Redistribution
  Hyperthyroidism
  Familial hypokalemic periodic paralysis
  Delirium tremens
  Increased cell production

Decreased intake

Gastrointestinal losses
  Diarrhea
  Fistulas

Renal losses
  Mineralocorticoid excess
  Bartter syndrome and Gitelman syndrome

Drugs that redistribute potassium into cells
  β$_2$-agonists (epinephrine, decongestants, bronchodilators, tocolytics)
  Xanthines (caffeine, theophylline)
  Verapamil
  Chloroquine
  Insulin

Drugs that increase renal potassium excretion
  Diuretics
  Mineralocorticoids
  High-dose glucocorticoids and antibiotics
  Magnesium-depleting drugs (aminoglycosides, cisplatin, foscarnet, and amphotericin B)

Clinical Manifestations

Hypokalemia is usually asymptomatic unless the plasma concentration falls below 3.0 mEq/L. In contrast to dysnatremias, where the symptoms are primarily neurologic, symptoms of potassium disorders are primarily muscular and cardiac. The first manifestations are fatigue, myalgias, and muscle weakness of the lower extremities. Severe hypokalemia may progress to respiratory muscle depression, hypoventilation, complete ascending paralysis, and death. Smooth muscle dysfunction may manifest as a paralytic ileus. Rhabdomyolysis with myoglobinuria and renal failure can also be seen. Electrocardiographic (ECG) changes are caused by delayed ventricular repolarization but do not correlate well with the severity of hypokalemia. Early changes include flattening or inversion of the T wave, a prominent U wave, ST-segment depression, and prolonged QT interval. Severe hypokalemia may result in PR-interval prolongation, widening of the QRS complex, and ventricular arrhythmias. Cardiac ischemia, heart failure, and left ventricular hypertrophy increase the likelihood of arrhythmias. Hypokalemia increases the risk of digoxin toxicity; both can cause ST-segment depression on ECG. Rapid changes in plasma [K$^+$] should be avoided during hemodialysis in patients taking digoxin. Hypokalemia can exacerbate hypertension, particularly in African-Americans. Hypokalemia promotes ammoniagenesis and may increase hepatic encephalopathy in susceptible patients.

Therapy

Therapeutic goals are correction of potassium level, avoidance of iatrogenic hyperkalemia, and correction of the underlying cause if possible. The plasma potassium concentration does not correlate well with total body stores in cases of redistribution. The classic example is diabetic ketoacidosis, where renal potassium losses from osmotic diuresis can be masked by insulin deficiency and extracellular redistribution of intracellular potassium. These patients may have intracellular hypokalemia and low total body potassium stores, with normal or high serum potassium levels. However, in the absence of potassium redistribution, each 1.0 mEq/L decrease in the serum concentration reflects a 200 to 300 mEq reduction in total body stores. Oral replacement is the preferred route because the slower absorption prevents hyperkalemia. Except in patients with metabolic acidosis, potassium chloride is preferred over bicarbonate or citrate-based formulations because chloride minimizes renal potassium losses. Potassium phosphate may be used in patients with concomitant hypophosphatemia. Intravenous replacement can be given at 10 mEq/hr through a peripheral IV, 20 mEq/hr via a central line, or 40 mEq/hr via a central line with continuous ECG monitoring. In nondiabetic patients, intravenous potassium in dextrose solution can paradoxically decrease plasma levels by causing redistribution of potassium into cells. Thus, intravenous potassium should be delivered in saline. Hypomagnesemia can produce renal potassium wasting and refractory hypokalemia. Patients with diuretic-induced hypokalemia may require chronic potassium supplementation, a high potassium diet, or the addition of a potassium-sparing diuretic (e.g., triamterene, amiloride, or spironolactone).

Criteria for hospitalization, ECG monitoring, and ICU admission are neither clearly defined nor universally accepted. Symptomatic hypokalemia requires aggressive replacement, frequent monitoring of plasma potassium, and possible hospitalization. Patients with ECG changes should be considered for continuous monitoring and ICU admission. Nephrology consultation may be required in cases of renal potassium wasting without an identifiable cause. Cases of surreptitious diuretic use, laxative use, and self-induced vomiting may benefit from social services or psychiatric consultation.

Outcomes

A recent retrospective analysis examined the management of inpatients with severe hypokalemia (defined as [K+] <3.0 mEq/L) in a university hospital (20). Hypokalemia was present in 2.6% of all patients; 28% were admitted with hypokalemia, while 72% developed hypokalemia during hospitalization. Hospital mortality was 20.4% in hypokalemic patients, compared with 1.9% for all patients. Mortality rates increased with the degree of hypokalemia. Thirty percent of patients were discharged with hypokalemia. A random sample of 100 medical records were reviewed for "appropriate management," defined as potassium replacement or initiation of potassium-sparing agents. In 76% of cases, medical management was considered adequate (20).

Hyperkalemia

Etiology and Differential Diagnosis

Defined as a plasma concentration greater than 5.0 mEq/L, hyperkalemia results from increased intake, redistribution, and impaired renal excretion (Table 104.4). Increased intake is rarely a cause of hyperkalemia unless there is impaired renal excretion. However, herbal supplements, salt substitutes, and blood transfusion are exogenous potassium sources that can cause hyperkalemia (21). Iatrogenic hyperkalemia may result from inappropriate potassium replacement. Pathological conditions such as intravascular hemolysis, rhabdomyolysis, and tumor lysis syndrome can produce hyperkalemia via redistribution and release of intracellular potassium. Redistribution hyperkalemia can also result from hyperglycemia, insulin deficiency, hypertonicity, and acidosis. Impaired renal excretion of potassium may involve decreased glomerular filtration (either acute or chronic) or an intrinsic

TABLE 104.4

MAJOR CAUSES OF HYPERKALEMIA

Pseudohyperkalemia
    Fist clenching
    Hemolysis
    Leukocytosis or thrombocytosis

Increased intake
    Herbal supplements
    Salt substitutes
    Blood transfusion
    Iatrogenic hyperkalemia

Redistribution
    Hyperglycemia
    Acidemia

Impaired renal excretion
    Renal failure, acute or chronic
    Renal tubular acidosis

Medications
    Potassium-sparing diuretics
    Nonsteroidal anti-inflammatory drugs
    ACE inhibitors and angiotensin-II receptor blockers
    β-blockers
    Trimethoprim
    Pentamidine
    Calcineurin inhibitors
    Heparin
    Digoxin

From Perazella MA. Drug-induced hyperkalemia: old culprits and new offenders. *Am J Med* 2000;109:307–314.

defect in excretion (e.g., a renal tubular acidosis). Medications can cause hyperkalemia through redistribution or impaired excretion. *Pseudohyperkalemia* results from release of intracellular potassium caused by fist clenching, prolonged tourniquet use, and marked leukocytosis or thrombocytosis. This diagnosis should be considered in any asymptomatic patient with an elevated serum potassium but no obvious cause of hyperkalemia.

A recent study in a tertiary care university hospital found that hyperkalemia was often multifactorial; 77% of patients had renal failure, 63% were on medications that can contribute to hyperkalemia, 49% were hyperglycemic, 17% were acidemic, and 15% were receiving potassium supplements or total parenteral nutrition (22).

Clinical Features

By increasing the resting membrane potential, hyperkalemia may cause prolonged depolarization, producing weakness, flaccid paralysis, and respiratory muscle weakness with hypoventilation. As with hypokalemia, ECG changes correlate poorly with the severity of hyperkalemia. Early signs include T-wave peaking and progress to PR-interval prolongation, widening of the QRS complex, and loss of P waves. Patients with left ventricular hypertrophy and/or congestive heart failure are more susceptible to malignant arrhythmias such as ventricular tachycardia, ventricular fibrillation, and sudden cardiac death. The cardiac effects of hyperkalemia are enhanced by hyponatremia, hypocalcemia, and acidemia.

Treatment

The degree of hyperkalemia, muscle weakness, and ECG changes determines the necessity for and rapidity of treatment. Emergent therapy for severe hyperkalemia has three components: minimizing membrane depolarization, shifting potassium into cells, and removing potassium from the body (23,24). Therapy should also include correcting the underlying cause if possible, stopping or avoiding offending medications, and removing all exogenous potassium sources. The initial therapy for patients with hyperkalemic ECG changes is intravenous calcium (e.g., 10 mL of 10% calcium gluconate), which decreases membrane excitability and reverses ECG changes within minutes. Its effect is short-lived (30–60 minutes). The transient hypercalcemia of calcium infusions may enhance the cardiac toxicity of digoxin; calcium should be given as a slow infusion over 30 minutes. Insulin (e.g., 10 units of regular insulin IV) shifts potassium into cells and will decrease [K+] by 0.5–1.5 mEq/L in 15–30 minutes. The effect may last for several hours. Glucose (25–50 grams IV) is given to prevent hypoglycemia but should be withheld in hyperglycemic patients. Nebulized albuterol, a β_2-adrenergic agonist, in doses of 10–20 mg (compared with 2.5 mg for bronchodilation) will have a similar onset of action and effect as insulin. Intravenous sodium bicarbonate (e.g., an isotonic solution of three ampules, or 150 mEq/L in D5W) should be reserved for patients with concomitant metabolic acidosis and may be ineffective in patients with end-stage renal disease. Patients with volume overload may not tolerate the additional sodium load.

Definitive therapy, potassium removal, can be achieved with diuretics, cation-exchange resin, or hemodialysis. Loop and thiazide diuretics increase potassium excretion if renal function is adequate. Sodium polystyrene sulfonate (Kayexalate) is a cation exchange resin that absorbs gastrointestinal potassium in exchange for sodium; each gram binds 1 mEq of potassium. Given orally or rectally in doses of 30–60 grams, the resin is usually delivered with sorbitol to prevent constipation. This mixture should be avoided in postoperative patients because of the risk of sorbitol-induced colonic necrosis, especially in renal transplantation patients. While effective, the resin has a delayed onset of action of 1–2 hours. Hemodialysis effectively and quickly removes potassium and corrects metabolic acidosis, but significant time may be required for nephrology consultation, catheter insertion, and dialysis preparation. Peritoneal dialysis and continuous renal replacement therapy correct potassium too slowly for treatment of acute hyperkalemia.

Criteria for hospitalization are poorly defined. A recent retrospective analysis compared patients hospitalized for hyperkalemia to those treated as outpatients; no significant differences in acid-base status, electrolyte levels, and renal function were found (25). Failure to discontinue use of all medications that promote hyperkalemia was common. The authors suggested hospitalization for severe hyperkalemia (≥ 8.0 mEq/L with ECG changes other than peaked T waves), acute worsening of renal function, and supervening medical problems (26). Patients with [K+] between 6.5 and 8.0 mEq/L and ECG changes limited to peaked T waves can be successfully treated in the emergency department. Patients with milder hyperkalemia can be treated as outpatients. Continuous electrocardiographic monitoring is indicated for patients with severe hyperkalemia and/or ECG changes, although there are no universally accepted criteria for monitoring. Nephrology consultation should be considered for patients with end-stage renal disease, hyperkalemia with ECG changes, and renal tubular acidosis.

Outcomes

Recent evidence suggests that physicians poorly manage in-hospital hyperkalemia. One study found that only 39% of episodes satisfied published criteria for diagnosis, treatment, and follow-up of hyperkalemia (22). Only 30% of patients had a 12-lead ECG, 46% of which had typical changes of hyperkalemia (despite the study threshold of [K+] >6.0 mEq/L). Computer ECG interpretations were not reliable; only one of 33 available interpretations was consistent with hyperkalemia (22). The mortality of patients hospitalized with hyperkalemia is difficult to estimate. One study reported a mortality rate of 17% among 35 adult inpatients with [K+] >5.5 mEq/L, although none died of hyperkalemic arrhythmias (25). Another study of 242 episodes reported no deaths from hyperkalemia and no significant morbid events from treatment (22).

KEY POINTS

- Many electrolyte abnormalities can be prevented by careful review of medications and proper fluid management.
- Potassium disorders reflect abnormal potassium handling, while sodium disorders reflect abnormal water handling.
- Dysnatremias lead to primarily neurologic symptoms, while dyskalemias are associated with muscular and cardiac symptoms.
- Treatment of hyponatremia may be more hazardous than the hyponatremia itself.
- Hypernatremia reflects a free water deficit and often occurs with decreased access to free water. It is frequently preventable or iatrogenic.
- ECG changes correlate poorly with the degree of potassium disturbance.
- Hyperkalemia is often multifactorial; renal failure is often implicated.

REFERENCES

1. Saeed BO, Beaumont D, Handley GH, Weaver JU. Severe hyponatraemia: investigation and management in a district general hospital. *J Clin Pathol* 2002;55:893–896.
2. Katz MA. Hyperglycemia-induced hyponatremia—calculation of expected serum sodium depression. *N Engl J Med* 1973;289: 843–844.
3. Hillier TA, Abbott RD, Barrett EJ. Hyponatremia: evaluating the correction factor for hyperglycemia. *Am J Med* 1999;106:399–403.
4. Schrier RW, Abraham WT. Hormones and hemodynamics in heart failure. *N Engl J Med* 1999;341:577–585.
5. Fraser CL, Arieff AI. Epidemiology, pathophysiology, and management of hyponatremic encephalopathy. *Am J Med* 1997;102: 67–77.
6. Lauriat SM, Berl T. The hyponatremic patient: practical focus on therapy. *J Am Soc Nephrol* 1997;8:1599–1607.
7. Adrogue HJ, Madias NE. Hyponatremia. *N Engl J Med* 2000;342: 1581–1589.
8. Laureno R, Karp BI. Myelinolysis after correction of hyponatremia. *Ann Intern Med* 1997;126:57–62.
9. Cadnapaphornchai MA, Schrier RW. Pathogenesis and management of hyponatremia. *Am J Med* 2000;109:688–692.
10. Kahn T. Hypernatremia with edema. *Arch Intern Med* 1999;159: 93–98.
11. Kumar S, Berl T. Sodium. *Lancet* 1998;352:220–228.
12. Adrogue HJ, Madias NE. Hypernatremia. *N Engl J Med* 2000; 342:1493–1499.
13. Palevsky PM, Bhagrath R, Greenberg A. Hypernatremia in hospitalized patients. *Ann Intern Med* 1996;124:197–203.
14. Mandal AK, Saklayen MG, Hillman NM, Markert RJ. Predictive factors for high mortality in hypernatremic patients. *Am J Emerg Med* 1997;15:130–132.
15. Borra SI, Beredo R, Kleinfeld M. Hypernatremia in the aging: causes, manifestations, and outcome. *J Natl Med Assoc* 1995;87: 220–224.
16. Polderman KH, Schreuder WO, Strack van Schijndel RJ, Thijs LG. Hypernatremia in the intensive care unit: an indicator of quality of care? *Crit Care Med* 1999;27:1105–1108.
17. Weiner ID, Wingo CS. Hypokalemia—consequences, causes, and correction. *J Am Soc Nephrol* 1997;8:1179–1188.
18. Gennari FJ. Hypokalemia. *N Engl J Med* 1998;339:451–458.
19. Halperin ML, Kamel KS. Potassium. *Lancet* 1998;352:135–140.
20. Paltiel O, Salakhov E, Ronen I, Berg D, Israeli A. Management of severe hypokalemia in hospitalized patients: a study of quality of care based on computerized databases. *Arch Intern Med* 2001;161:1089–1095.
21. Perazella MA. Drug-induced hyperkalemia: old culprits and new offenders. *Am J Med* 2000;109:307–314.
22. Acker CG, Johnson JP, Palevsky PM, Greenberg A. Hyperkalemia in hospitalized patients: causes, adequacy of treatment, and results of an attempt to improve physician compliance with published therapy guidelines. *Arch Intern Med* 1998; 158: 917–924.
23. Weiner ID, Wingo CS. Hyperkalemia: a potential silent killer. *J Am Soc Nephrol* 1998;9:1535–1543.
24. Greenberg A. Hyperkalemia: treatment options. *Semin Nephrol* 1998;18:46–57.
25. Stevens MS, Dunlay RW. Hyperkalemia in hospitalized patients. *Int Urol Nephrol* 2000;32:177–180.
26. Charytan D, Goldfarb DS. Indications for hospitalization of patients with hyperkalemia. *Arch Intern Med* 2000;160:1605–1611.

ADDITIONAL READING

Halperin ML, Goldstein MB. *Fluid, Electrolyte, and Acid-Base Physiology: A Problem-Based Approach.* 3rd ed. Philadelphia: WB Saunders, 1998.

Milionis HJ, Liamis GL, Elisaf MS. The hyponatremic patient: a systematic approach to laboratory diagnosis. *CMAJ* 2002;166: 1056–1062.

Common Acid–Base Disorders

105

Orson W. Moe   Daniel Fuster   Robert J. Alpern

INTRODUCTION

Acid–base disturbances represent a diverse group of disorders commonly encountered in patients presenting to the emergency room as well as in hospitalized patients. The identification of acid–base disorders per se does not establish an end point in the diagnostic process but rather serves to alert and direct the clinician to search for and address the underlying diseases that generated the disturbances. The treatment of acid–base disorders is largely directed at the underlying cause, although primary correction of the alkali or acid deficit also is indicated in certain situations. The spectrum of clinical outcomes of diseases associated with acid–base disturbances ranges from the completely benign to the imminently life-threatening. Therefore, the hospital physician must come rapidly to the correct diagnosis and initiate the appropriate treatment.

Although the body continually is faced with acid loads that are many orders of magnitude higher than the free hydrogen concentration in the plasma, normal individuals are able to maintain the plasma pH within a narrow range. Two defense mechanisms contribute to this homeostasis. First, buffers are present in all body compartments and cushion the effect of any acid or alkali assault. Second, external acid–base balance is maintained by eliminating acid (or alkali) in an amount commensurate to that added to the body. A mismatch between addition and excretion of acid (or alkali) constitutes the fundamental pathophysiology of all acid–base disorders. Volatile acids such as carbonic acid are excreted in the lungs; nonvolatile acids such as those derived from dietary proteins are excreted by the kidneys. Clinical disorders of acid–base balance are divided into those of *respiratory* and *metabolic* origin. In respiratory acid–base disorders, carbon dioxide accumulation or depletion results from primary abnormalities of lung function. In metabolic disorders, nonvolatile acid or alkali accumulates as a result of renal or extrarenal derangements.

Because acid–base disorders are largely laboratory diagnoses, several concepts deserve emphasis. One is the distinction between *acidemia* (or *alkalemia*) and *acidosis* (or *alkalosis*). Acidemia and alkalemia simply refer to deviations of blood pH from normal. Acidosis and alkalosis refer to processes that lead to an abnormal excess of acid or alkali. A patient with a well-compensated acidosis can have a near-normal blood pH; one with a mixed acid–base disorder can have a completely normal pH. The terms *acidosis* and *alkalosis* always indicate pathology and should not be used to describe a normal compensatory process. For example, a normal physiologic increase in ventilation and lowering of blood carbon dioxide tension (pCO_2) in response to a metabolic acidosis should not be referred to as respiratory alkalosis.

Although the interpretation of electrolytes alone is informative and often can reveal the correct acid–base diagnosis, *it is frequently necessary to obtain blood-gas measurements* to be certain of the diagnosis. For example, a patient with a high plasma bicarbonate concentration ($[HCO_3^-]$) is either suffering from a metabolic alkalosis or compensating for a respiratory acidosis. Likewise, a patient with a low plasma $[HCO_3^-]$ either has a metabolic acidosis or is compensating for a respiratory alkalosis. In each of these examples, the clinical history and a careful physical examination often can distinguish the two possibilities. However, blood gases yield additional and often critical information. For instance, no matter what the primary disorder is, one needs to know whether the secondary compensation is appropriate. Thus, blood-gas analysis may provide the sole indication of a mixed acid–base disorder. For primary respiratory acid–base disturbances, knowledge of the arterial oxygen tension and the calculated alveolar–arterial oxygen tension (pO_2) is an integral part of the laboratory interpretation and guides management of the patient.

Once these analyses have been completed, the physician should know whether he or she is dealing with an acidosis or an alkalosis, whether it is metabolic or respiratory in origin, and whether the appropriate compensations have occurred. In this chapter, a brief summary is presented for each of these disorders. Although these diagnoses are largely based on laboratory data, one must underscore the importance of the clinical history and examination in alerting the clinician to look for mixed disorders and in identifying the cause of the acid–base disturbances.

METABOLIC ACIDOSIS

In general, metabolic acidosis is rarely the sole reason for admission to the hospital, but *the presence of metabolic acidosis always necessitates a careful search for an underlying cause.* Patients with metabolic acidosis are admitted for conditions that may or may not be related causally to the acidosis. Metabolic acidosis is usually detected as a low serum [HCO_3^-]. It is important to remember that a low serum [HCO_3^-] associated with a normal to slightly increased anion gap may result from primary respiratory alkalosis with metabolic compensation. If the clinical setting suggests the cause of a primary metabolic acidosis, it may not be necessary to measure an arterial blood gas. The only finding on physical examination indicative of a metabolic acidosis is the slow, deep breathing pattern known as Kussmaul respirations.

Diagnostic Approach

After a primary metabolic acidosis is documented, the next step in the clinical approach is to assess the plasma or serum *anion gap* (Figure 105.1), the difference between unmeasured cations and unmeasured anions. This is calculated as: Anion gap = $Na^+ - (Cl^- + HCO_3^-)$.

A normal anion gap is 8 to 16 mEq/L. An increased anion gap can help pinpoint the underlying cause of metabolic acidosis. Because the normal range of the anion gap is rather broad, a mild elevation on a single laboratory sample should not be considered diagnostic.

Elevated Anion Gap

Conditions associated with an increased anion gap include ketoacidosis, lactic acidosis, ingestion of poisons, and advanced renal failure. With the possible exception of renal failure, all these conditions are medical emergencies that require rapid definitive diagnosis. The clinical effects of severe metabolic acidosis are myriad and affect multiple organs. In the acute setting, the most life-threatening

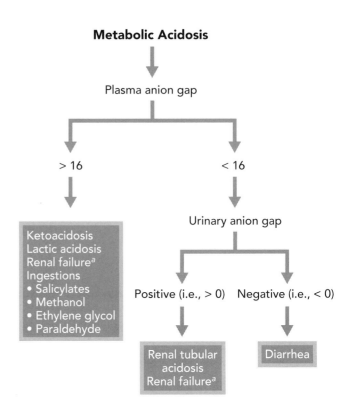

Figure 105.1 Approach to the patient with primary metabolic acidosis. *a* Renal insufficiency may be associated with a normal or increased anion gap.

sequelae are depressed cardiac contractility and vascular collapse. *Lactic acidosis* usually occurs secondary to tissue hypoxia. It should be suspected in a patient with low blood pressure or a known infection. *Ketoacidosis* occurs in conditions in which the body switches from carbohydrate to fat metabolism. Known diabetic and alcoholic patients who recently have stopped ingesting food are at risk for ketoacidosis. Measurement of serum lactate and ketones confirms the diagnosis of lactic acidosis and ketoacidosis, respectively. *Overdoses and ingestions* associated with anion-gap acidosis include salicylates (which can generate lactic and ketoacidosis) and methanol or ethylene glycol, which are metabolized to organic acids. Salicylate overdoses are suggested by a coexistent respiratory alkalosis and tinnitus. Methanol and ethylene glycol intoxication are associated with an increased osmolar gap; measured plasma osmolality is more than 10 mOsm/L greater than that calculated from the following formula: Plasma osmolality (calculated) = 2 Na^+ + glucose / 18 + blood urea nitrogen / 2.8.

Methanol intoxication is associated with retinal pallor and visual complaints; ethylene glycol intoxication causes renal failure, calcium oxalate crystalluria, and symptoms of hypocalcemia. These clinical features are often absent, in which case the only clue to these diagnoses is elevation of both the osmolar and anion gaps. Delays in the recognition and treatment of methanol or ethylene glycol poisoning result in poor outcomes; early recognition and management (including dialytic therapy) are highly effective (Chapter 121).

Normal Anion Gap

A significant proportion of regulated acid excretion is in the form of NH_4^+. For clinical purposes, urinary NH_4^+ level can be used to assess renal acid excretion. In anion gap acidoses such as ketoacidosis, lactic acidosis, or poisons, measuring renal acid excretion is of little relevance because the acid production rate is so high that even a perfect renal response would not be able to correct the acidosis. Renal acid excretion is of more clinical interest if there is a normal anion-gap metabolic acidosis. This form of metabolic acidosis can result from gastrointestinal bicarbonate loss (e.g., massive diarrhea) or failure of the kidneys to excrete acid (i.e., renal acidosis). The distinction between these two groups of disorders is based on the urinary NH_4^+ excretion. In extrarenal acidoses such as diarrhea, urinary NH_4^+ excretion is increased. In renal acidosis, the urinary NH_4^+ level is inappropriately low. Urinary NH_4^+ excretion is regulated by changes in NH_3 synthesis, as well as by H^+ secretion. Urinary pH is a poor indicator of acid excretion in the urine because the amount of acid (primarily NH_4^+) in the urine cannot be estimated from the urinary pH alone. In patients with chronic diarrhea, increased urinary NH_4^+ excretion is associated with a urinary pH greater than 5.5. Conversely, in acidosis of chronic renal disease, NH_3 synthesis is decreased and low levels of urinary NH_4^+ excretion are associated with a low urine pH (<5.5).

Clinically, the most readily available estimate of urinary ammonium excretion is based on the *urinary anion gap*, which is calculated as follows: urinary anion gap = urinary Na + urinary K − urinary Cl.

In the normal physiological steady state, when urinary NH_4^+ excretion is in the normal range, the urinary anion gap is positive (20–60 mmol/L). In patients with a chronic metabolic acidosis of extrarenal origin and normal renal function, urinary NH_4^+ excretion increases significantly. Because NH_4^+ is excreted as NH_4Cl, this leads to a significant increase in urinary $[Cl^-]$, causing the urinary anion gap to become more negative (<0 mmol/L). Patients with all forms of acidoses of renal origin fail to increase urinary NH_4^+ excretion appropriately for the level of acidosis and thus have a positive urinary anion gap (>0 mmol/L).

Patients with renal acidosis may have either renal insufficiency or a renal tubular acidosis. It is important to remember that renal insufficiency can be associated with a normal or increased plasma anion gap. The high anion gap results from a failure of the kidney to excrete unmeasured anions such as sulfate, while the generation of acidosis results from a failure of the kidney to excrete sufficient acid (NH_4^+) in the urine. Although these defects both frequently occur around a glomerular filtration rate of 20 mL/min, they can occur independent of each other.

Figure 105.2 shows the workup for a patient with renal tubular acidosis. Table 105.1 lists the causes of renal tubular acidosis. Hyperkalemic distal renal tubular acidosis is caused either by a decrease in mineralocorticoid activity or by an abnormal cortical collecting duct. These defects lead to defects in both K^+ and H^+ secretion, resulting in hyperkalemic acidosis (1). Low mineralocorticoid states can be associated with low renin and aldosterone levels (*hyporeninemic hypoaldosteronism*) or with isolated decreases in aldosterone secretion (*hypoaldosteronism*). Hypokalemic distal renal tubular acidosis is most commonly associated with hypergammaglobulinemic disorders, such as Sjögren syndrome in adults. It also can been seen with amphotericin B therapy. Proximal renal tubular acidosis and Fanconi syndrome (generalized proximal tubule dysfunction) occurring in adults is usually associated with dysproteinemic disorders such as multiple myeloma and monoclonal gammopathies. Regardless of the cause of the metabolic acidosis, the lung compensates for the low $[HCO_3^-]$ by

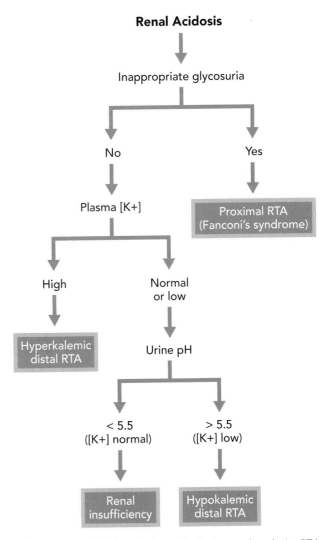

Figure 105.2 Workup of the patient with renal acidosis. *RTA*, renal tubular acidosis.

TABLE 105.1

CAUSES OF RENAL TUBULAR ACIDOSIS

Hyperkalemic distal
  Decreased mineralocorticoid activity
    Hyporeninemic hypoaldosteronism
      Glomerular and interstitial disease, e.g., diabetes
      Nonsteroidal anti-inflammatory drugs
  Hypoaldosteronism
    Adrenal insufficiency
    Heparin
    Angiotensin-converting enzyme inhibitor
  Abnormal cortical collecting duct
    Obstruction
    Systemic lupus erythematosus
    Diabetes
    Sickle-cell disease
Hypokalemic distal
  Hypergammaglobulinemic disorders: Sjögren syndrome
  Amphotericin B
  Congenital disorders of H^+ or HCO_3^- transporters
Proximal
  Dysproteinemias
  Multiple myeloma
  Monoclonal gammopathies
  Amyloidosis
  Congenital disorders of HCO_3^- transporter

increasing alveolar ventilation and lowering pCO_2. For every 10 mEq/L fall in serum $[HCO_3^-]$, one expects a fall in pCO_2 of 10 to 15 mm Hg. Deviation from the expected compensation should alert the clinician to look for superimposed respiratory acid–base disturbances.

Treatment Issues

The management of acute metabolic acidosis in the hospital usually is directed at the underlying disorder. Level of care and monitoring are dictated by the nature of the causative disorder. One key decision related to metabolic acidosis is whether to administer bicarbonate or to wait for other treatment to correct the acidosis. In general, it is not necessary to treat with alkali, because most levels of metabolic acidosis seen clinically are not immediately life threatening. However, if the plasma pH is less than 7.15 and reversal of the underlying disorder of acid generation is not imminent, alkali therapy can be administered. If one does treat metabolic acidosis, it is important to give enough bicarbonate to accomplish one's goal. Because metabolic acidosis is associated with increased acid–base buffering and an increased apparent volume of distribution of bicarbonate, one can use the following equation to guide the therapy: administered $HCO_3^- = \Delta HCO_3^-{}_{serum} \times$ body weight in kg (Example: 4 ampules of each 50 ml 8.4% $NaHCO_3^-$-solution [ampule $[HCO_3^-]$ concentration 1 mmol/mL] administered to a patient with a body weight of 100 kg would increase the patient's serum $[HCO_3^-]$ by 2 mmol/L).

It is important to note that this equation merely guides the initial dose of bicarbonate. As bicarbonate deficits vary tremendously among individuals with the same plasma bicarbonate concentration, modifications must be made based on response. It is imperative that one not neglect the reversal of the underlying disease simply because alkali therapy is correcting the plasma bicarbonate level transiently.

In adult ethylene glycol and methanol poisoning, metabolism of the poisons to their toxic metabolites can be inhibited by the administration of *fomepizole,* an alcohol dehydrogenase inhibitor (2,3). Fomepizole treatment can be combined with hemodialysis and has proven safe and effective. After initial loading of 15 mg/kg intravenously, 10 mg/kg q 12 hrs intravenously for four doses are administered, followed by 15 mg/kg q 12 hrs intravenously until methanol or ethylene glycol levels become undetectable. With simultaneous hemodialysis, dosage frequency needs to be increased to q 4 hrs.

Although alkali treatment of acute metabolic acidosis is usually unnecessary, the treatment of chronic metabolic acidosis is important. The sequelae of untreated chronic metabolic acidosis include muscle wasting, nephrocalcinosis, nephrolithiasis, and loss of bone density. Patients with this problem can be given either bicarbonate or citrate. Citrate is better tolerated but cannot be used in patients with renal insufficiency who are taking aluminum-containing phosphate binders, because it enhances aluminum absorption. Alkali can be administered as Na^+ or K^+ salts. K^+ salts are somewhat advantageous in that Na^+ administration increases urinary Ca^{2+} excretion and also can worsen hypertension. Such treatment regimens need not be started in the hospital but are most conveniently initiated before discharge.

METABOLIC ALKALOSIS

Again, patients are rarely admitted for the sole indication of metabolic alkalosis but generally are admitted for conditions either causative of or concurrent with metabolic alkalosis. This problem usually manifests as a high plasma HCO_3^- level. Elevated plasma $[HCO_3^-]$ can be caused by either a primary metabolic alkalosis or a primary respiratory acidosis with metabolic compensation. If the cause of metabolic alkalosis is obvious and hypoventilation is not suspected, arterial blood-gas measurements are not necessary. The finding of hypokalemia with a high serum $[HCO_3^-]$ also suggests metabolic alkalosis rather than respiratory acidosis. The respiratory compensation for metabolic alkalosis can be incomplete because the alkalemia-induced ventilatory suppression is overridden by secondary hypoxemia.

Diagnostic Approach

The differential diagnosis of metabolic alkalosis depends on the assessment of the effective arterial volume (Figure

105.3). In most patients with metabolic alkalosis, effective arterial volume is decreased, and the kidney attempts to compensate by retaining sodium bicarbonate. Metabolic alkalosis is not an invariant finding in all patients with a low effective arterial volume. However, once alkalosis is generated, a low effective arterial volume triggers the kidney to maintain the alkalosis. A low effective arterial volume is suggested by a constellation of findings, including postural changes in pulse or blood pressure, low central venous pressure, a low urinary [Na$^+$] or [Cl$^-$], and a high blood urea nitrogen or serum uric acid level.

The two most common conditions causing low effective arterial volume are vomiting and diuretic use. In vomiting, loss of hydrochloric acid (HCl) from the stomach generates an alkalosis, and low effective arterial volume maintains it. With diuretics, the kidney is responsible for both the generation and maintenance of the metabolic alkalosis. In patients with no apparent cause of metabolic alkalosis, magnesium deficiency should be considered because it also can lead to renal generation and maintenance of the alkalosis. *Posthypercapneic alkalosis* refers to chronic hypercapnia, leading to a compensatory increase in the serum [HCO$_3^-$]. Correction of the hypercapnia then should lead to correction of the alkalosis. However, if a patient is volume contracted, alkalosis fails to correct and there is a persistent posthypercapnic alkalosis.

Metabolic alkalosis also may be associated with an increased effective arterial volume and hypertension. In this setting, it is maintained by increased mineralocorticoid activity or level, which stimulates urinary acid excretion. These disorders represent the most common causes of curable secondary hypertension. Importantly, the triad of hypertension, metabolic alkalosis, and hypokalemia is not always present in hyperaldosterone states.

If volume depletion is absent in a patient with metabolic alkalosis, the next diagnostic step depends upon serum renin and aldosterone levels. Because there are wide ranges of normal plasma renin and aldosterone levels, random plasma levels should be interpreted cautiously, in the context of volume status and dietary NaCl intake. Simultaneous low renin and high aldosterone levels can be diagnostic regardless of volume status. As shown in Figure 105.3, renin and aldosterone levels may both be high (*primary hyperreninemia*), renin may be low and aldosterone high (*primary hyperaldosteronism*), or both renin and aldosterone levels may be low (*aldosterone-independent mineralocorticoid effect*). In the case of both high renin and high aldosterone levels, it is important to distinguish primary hyperreninism from low effective arterial volume. All causes of metabolic alkalosis associated with a low effective arterial volume are associated with high renin and aldosterone levels. If uncertainty exists about the effective arterial volume, it is useful

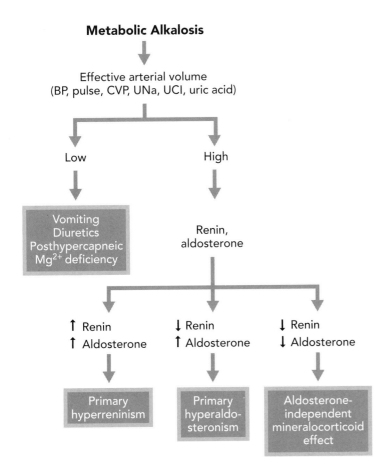

Figure 105.3 Approach to the patient with metabolic alkalosis. BP, blood pressure; *CVP*, central venous pressure; *UCl*, urine chloride; *UNa*, urine sodium.

to perform a saline-suppression test. The high renin and aldosterone levels secondary to hypovolemia normalize in response to saline infusion, whereas this response is not seen with primary hyperreninism.

Table 105.2 lists the more common causes of metabolic alkalosis associated with hypermineralocorticoid states. Primary hyperreninism is most frequently associated with *renovascular disease*, although a majority of patients with renovascular disease do not exhibit hypokalemic alkalosis. Renovascular disease can be diagnosed by renal angiography (Chapter 48). Primary hyperaldosteronism usually is caused either by an adrenal adenoma or a bilateral adrenocortical hyperplasia. The distinction between these disorders is extremely important, because aldosterone-secreting adenomas can be cured by unilateral adrenalectomy. In contrast, adrenalectomy is not recommended for bilateral adrenocortical hyperplasia. The distinction between these two disorders is based upon computed tomography results and adrenal vein sampling.

The combination of metabolic alkalosis, hypertension, and low renin and aldosterone levels frequently occurs in patients with *Cushing syndrome* (Chapter 106). The magnitude of the hypokalemia and alkalosis depend on the level of cortisol and typically are most severe in ectopic ACTH syndrome. Other possibilities to consider in this setting are licorice ingestion and Liddle syndrome, a rare familial disorder caused by a mutation in the cortical collecting duct luminal membrane Na^+ channel.

Treatment Issues

Clinical decisions regarding hospitalization or ICU admission are based on the associated disorders rather than the metabolic alkalosis per se. Metabolic alkalosis usually does not require treatment acutely. However, there are a few situations in which acute treatment is recommended. In patients with chronic obstructive lung disease, respiratory suppression caused by the metabolic alkalosis may be problematic. Also, in patients with cerebral or cardiac ischemia, tissue hypoxemia may occur secondary to an alkalosis-induced increase in the oxygen affinity of hemoglobin and vasoconstriction. In these settings, the alkalosis can be corrected by treating the cause responsible for maintenance of the alkalosis (decreased effective arterial volume, primary increase in mineralocorticoid). If one cannot treat the primary cause and if pH is greater than 7.55, metabolic alkalosis can be corrected with carbonic anhydrase inhibitors such as acetazolamide, 250 to 500 mg given orally every 8 hours with strict monitoring of electrolytes. Alternatively, 0.1-N hydrochloric acid can be administered via central line at a rate of 10 to 20 mEq/h; this is generally safe if administered slowly.

RESPIRATORY ACIDOSIS

In general, respiratory acid–base disturbances have less complex underlying pathophysiologies than the metabolic disorders described previously. Metabolic acidosis may result from increased acid production, reduced acid disposal, or both. *In respiratory acidosis, the acid load is always from metabolic carbon dioxide.* However, increased carbon dioxide production alone does not lead to carbon dioxide accumulation if the ventilatory system is intact. For example, plasma pCO_2 changes minimally when carbon dioxide production rises from 15,000 mmol/d at rest to 450,000 mmol/d with heavy exercise. This 30-fold increase in carbon dioxide production is compensated completely by an increase in carbon dioxide excretion. Respiratory acidosis is invariably caused by abnormal carbon dioxide clearance, not increased production. In other words, in respiratory acidosis, one is dealing exclusively with a ventilatory problem, and therefore, for clinical purposes, one can *equate respiratory acidosis with alveolar hypoventilation.* Causes of alveolar hypoventilation are reviewed subsequently.

Diagnostic Approach

The clinical presentation of respiratory acidosis reflects the underlying pulmonary disease (Chapter 24). Carbon dioxide retention can lead to lethargy and coma (*carbon dioxide narcosis*), increased intracranial pressure, cardiac dysrhythmias, and impaired myocardial contractility. These effects are more pronounced if the carbon dioxide retention is acute. Of note is that physiologic hypoventilation secondary to metabolic alkalosis never compromises arterial oxygenation. Respiratory acidosis should be considered if there is a high plasma pCO_2 level (hypercapnia). If arterial blood gases have not been drawn, respiratory acidosis may be suggested by an elevated plasma $[HCO_3^-]$, reflecting renal compensation. Therefore, in a patient with a high plasma $[HCO_3^-]$, respiratory acidosis always should be excluded by measurement of arterial blood gases before proceeding to a full workup of metabolic alkalosis. Figure 105.4 shows an algorithm for the evaluation of respiratory acidosis.

TABLE 105.2

METABOLIC ALKALOSIS ASSOCIATED WITH PRIMARY HYPERMINERALOCORTICOID STATE

Primary hyperreninism
   Renovascular disease
Primary hyperaldosteronism
   Adrenal adenoma
   Bilateral adrenal hyperplasia
Aldosterone-independent mineralocorticoid effect
   Cushing syndrome
   Licorice intoxication
   Liddle syndrome

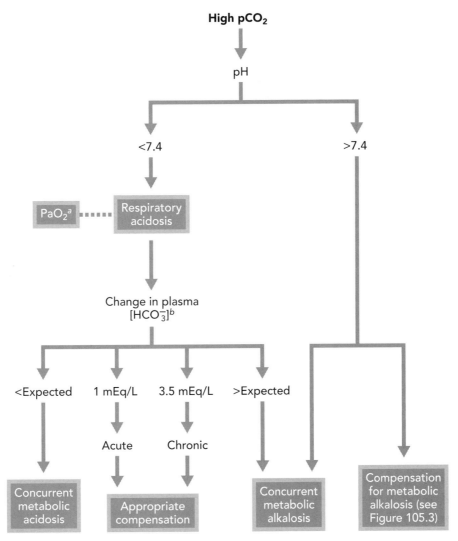

Figure 105.4 Approach to the patient with elevated pCO₂.
[a] Hypoxemia may pose the most acute threat to patients with alveolar hypoventilation; oxygenation should be checked and treated promptly. [b] For each 10 mm Hg increase in pCO₂, in primary respiratory acidosis one expects serum [HCO₃⁻] to increase (from 24 meq/L) by 1 meq/L (in acute respiratory acidosis) to 3.5 meq/L (in chronic respiratory acidosis). pCO₂, partial pressure of carbon dioxide; PaO₂, partial pressure of oxygen.

In a patient with hypercapnia, the clinician first should examine the blood pH. A high pCO₂ in the presence of alkalemia usually is caused by respiratory compensation for metabolic alkalosis. A high pCO₂ with acidemia secures the diagnosis of respiratory acidosis. There are then two further issues to consider. The first is the degree of rise in [HCO₃⁻] in response to carbon dioxide retention. The magnitude of the secondary change in serum [HCO₃⁻] may indicate superimposed metabolic disorders. For example, in a patient with chronic obstructive pulmonary disease and right-heart failure being treated with diuretics, a pCO₂ of 58 mm Hg and a pH of 7.36 would establish the diagnosis of respiratory acidosis. If the serum [HCO₃⁻] were 40 mmol/L, this would be inappropriately high for physiologic renal compensation (expected serum [HCO₃⁻] around 32 mmol/L) and would indicate a mixed disorder of respiratory acidosis and metabolic alkalosis.

The second issue after establishing the diagnosis of respiratory acidosis is to determine the cause of the alveolar hypoventilation (Table 105.3). The first two categories ("would not breathe" and "could not breathe") represent pathologic alveolar hypoventilation; the third represents physiologic hypoventilation. A discussion of the neuroanatomy and pulmonary mechanics of ventilatory control is beyond the scope of this chapter, but hypoventilation can result from lesions in the respiratory center, the peripheral nerves controlling the diaphragm, the thoracic cage, and the lower and upper airways.

TABLE 105.3

TABLE 105.3
CAUSES OF ALVEOLAR HYPOVENTILATION

"Would not breathe": pathologic decrease in central respiratory drive
- Pharmacologic respiratory depressants
  - Sedatives
  - Opiates
  - General anesthetics
- Primary central nervous system diseases
  - Neoplasm
  - Infection
  - Inflammatory
  - Hemorrhage
  - Idiopathic

"Could not breathe": impairment of ventilatory mechanisms
- Peripheral nerve
  - Pharmacologic: e.g., succinylcholine
  - Traumatic
  - Neoplastic invasion
  - Inflammatory: e.g., Guillain-Barré syndrome
- Diaphragm
  - Massive ascites
  - Myopathies
- Thoracic spine: kyphoscoliosis
- Chest wall/thorax
  - Flail chest
  - Malignant obesity
  - Pneumothorax
- Airway obstruction
  - Chronic obstructive pulmonary disease
  - Bronchospasm
  - Upper airway obstruction

"Should not breathe": physiologic decrease in central ventilatory drive
- Metabolic alkalosis

Treatment Issues

The management of respiratory acidosis is directed at the underlying cause. Indications for intubation and mechanical ventilation are covered in Chapter 23. Although the acidemia from hypercapnia may be dangerous, accompanying hypoxemia often poses the most immediate risk to survival. Two points regarding the acid–base aspects of hypoventilation management are key. The first concerns the rate of correction of the hypercapnia. If chronic respiratory acidosis is treated with mechanical ventilation, the compensatory metabolic changes persist after the normalization of pCO_2. If eucapnia is restored suddenly, formerly adaptive mechanisms can become detrimental. An example is the change that occurs in the affinity of hemoglobin for oxygen. Acidemia lowers the oxygen affinity of hemoglobin, which thereby enhances tissue oxygen delivery. During chronic respiratory acidosis, intraerythrocytic metabolic changes increase and restore the oxygen affinity of hemoglobin back toward normal. Upon sudden normalization of pCO_2, acidemia disappears, and the high serum $[HCO_3^-]$ greatly enhances the oxygen affinity of hemoglobin, impairing oxygen release to tissues. This may result in tissue hypoxia, despite the presence of well-oxygenated arterial blood. The sudden alkalemia and the vasoconstriction it induces further aggravate this situation. Thus, one should not immediately and completely correct pCO_2 in treating a hypercapnic patient.

Chronic respiratory acidosis is frequently associated with metabolic alkalosis, particularly if diuretic agents are used. Even if metabolic alkalosis is not initially present, it may develop as hypercapnia is being corrected (see later in this chapter). Alkalemia suppresses ventilatory drive and thus may delay and impair the ability to improve ventilation and oxygenation. Carbonic anhydrase inhibitors such as acetazolamide (250 mg orally twice or three times daily) induce sufficient bicarbonaturia to lower plasma $[HCO_3^-]$ toward normal. Use of acetazolamide should be considered daily, with continued assessment of the patient's clinical and laboratory status guiding dosage modification or cessation. Acetazolamide therapy can lead to life-threatening hypokalemia, "overshoot" metabolic acidosis, and aggravate extracellular fluid volume contraction. Concurrent NaCl and KCl supplementation are frequently necessary. An alternative way of lowering serum $[HCO_3^-]$ is to infuse dilute HCl through a central venous catheter or to administer it orally. Either of these maneuvers can be used to facilitate weaning from mechanical ventilation or to improve oxygenation after transfer from the ICU.

The outcome of respiratory acidosis depends on the underlying cause. One cannot overemphasize the frequency and lack of recognition of metabolic alkalosis in patients with chronic respiratory acidosis. Chronic diuretic use is a common culprit. In addition to metabolic alkalosis, the potassium depletion caused by diuretic therapy can lead to respiratory muscle weakness and worsened hypoventilation. Aggressive diuretic therapy, therefore, should be reserved for patients with severe pulmonary, gastrointestinal, or peripheral edema, those with anorexia or dyspnea from ascites, or those with hepatic congestion.

RESPIRATORY ALKALOSIS

A number of the pathophysiologic principles discussed previously can be applied to respiratory alkalosis. *Respiratory alkalosis is synonymous with alveolar hyperventilation.* If the cause of alveolar hyperventilation is hypoxemia, respiratory alkalosis is an appropriate compensation to maintain oxygen saturation at the expense of acid–base homeostasis. A patient presenting with pulmonary disease and respiratory alkalosis who "normalizes" the pCO_2 and pH may be tiring and on the verge of impending respiratory failure (Chapter 24).

The clinical presentation of respiratory alkalosis reflects the underlying disease. The clinical examination may reveal dyspnea; increased respiration rate and tidal volume; symptoms and signs of neuromuscular irritability such as acroparesthesia, carpopedal spasm, or seizures; and cardiac dysrhythmias. Hyperventilation is not pathognomonic for respiratory alkalosis because it may be a response to metabolic acidosis. Like respiratory acidosis, the diagnosis of respiratory alkalosis relies on laboratory data, especially arterial blood gases. Abnormalities in routine blood chemistries may be indistinguishable from those seen in the setting of normal anion gap metabolic acidosis. This confusion is compounded further by the fact that patients with metabolic acidosis usually have evidence of compensatory hyperventilation on physical examination. The reduced plasma [HCO₃⁻] level seen in patients with primary respiratory alkalosis may not be completely offset by an equivalent rise in Cl⁻; this results in a slight elevation of the anion gap. Therefore, it is imperative that arterial blood-gas measurements be used to evaluate the patient with respiratory alkalosis.

Diagnostic Approach

Figure 105.5 outlines the approach to a patient with a low pCO₂. The presence of acidemia suggests that the hyperventilation is secondary to metabolic acidosis; the evaluation of the patient should proceed as outlined in Figure 105.1. Hypocapnia and alkalemia establishes the diagnosis of respiratory alkalosis. As discussed in the preceding section, hypocapnia causes secondary changes in serum [HCO₃⁻]. Acute or chronic reduction in pCO₂ leads to lowering of the serum [HCO₃⁻], which minimizes the change in plasma pH. Because the renal response develops gradually, there is no sharp distinction between acute and chronic phases. An analysis of the serum [HCO₃⁻] helps identify possible superimposed metabolic disorders,

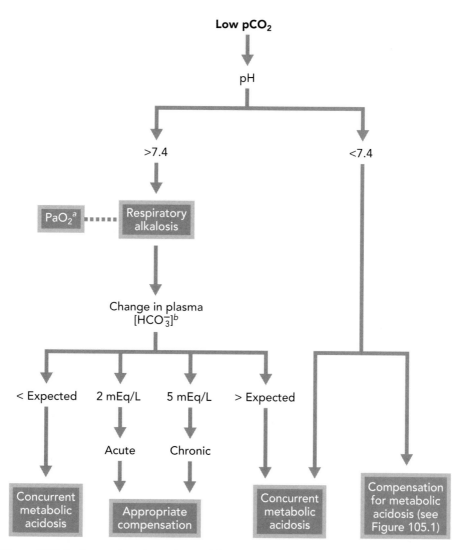

Figure 105.5 Approach to the patient with low pCO₂. *a* Use to determine etiology of respiratory alkalosis—see text and Table 105.4. *b* For each 10 mm Hg decrease in pCO₂, in primary respiratory alkalosis one expects serum [HCO₃⁻] to decrease (from 24 meq/L) by 2 meq/L (in acute respiratory alkalosis) to 5 meq/L (in chronic respiratory alkalosis). *PaO₂*, partial pressure of oxygen; *pCO₂*, partial pressure of carbon dioxide.

which is important because mixed acid–base disorders frequently are encountered. If the fall in serum [HCO_3^-] exceeds that predicted from the normal renal compensation, a superimposed metabolic acidosis should be considered. Common scenarios of *concurrent respiratory alkalosis and metabolic acidosis* include salicylate poisoning, sepsis, and advanced liver disease. If renal compensation for respiratory alkalosis appears to be inadequate, one should consider a superimposed metabolic alkalosis. For example, an individual who is hyperventilating from mountain sickness and begins to vomit may develop severe, life-threatening alkalemia.

Respiratory alkalosis can be divided into causes driven by hypoxemia, non–hypoxemia-related causes, or both (see Table 105.4). Arterial blood gases are absolutely essential in making this distinction. If tissue hypoxia is present, cardiopulmonary diseases most commonly are implicated. Although hyperventilation may be seen in patients with mild pulmonary diseases prior to the development of hypoxemia, hypoxemia is usually a more important factor. A number of disorders can produce hypoxemia through multiple mechanisms. For example, pulmonary edema resulting from left-heart failure lowers pO_2 by reducing the ventilation:perfusion ratio and increasing diffusion block, at the same time lowering venous oxygen concentration caused by low cardiac output and increased peripheral extraction (Chapter 39).

Conditions in which patients hyperventilate despite relatively normal pO_2 and tissue oxygenation include disorders with heightened ventilatory drive caused by factors other than pH, pCO_2, or pO_2. In *early septicemia*, respiratory alkalosis can precede the onset of fever, leuko-

cytosis, or hypotension (Chapter 26). Sudden onset of unexplained respiratory alkalosis in the hospitalized patient should prompt the clinician to consider sepsis. *Salicylate intoxication* also may cause respiratory alkalosis without hypoxemia (Chapter 121). Salicylates directly stimulate the central respiratory center, and respiratory alkalosis may be the only abnormality seen in early acute intoxication. In this instance, the alkalemia is protective against the central nervous system toxicity of salicylates because it increases the fraction of salicylate in its ionized, impermeable form. As salicylate intoxication evolves, the acid–base picture is compounded by a metabolic acidosis that aggravates the central nervous system toxicity of salicylates. Management includes general supportive measures plus alkaline diuresis and, in severe cases, hemodialysis (Chapter 121). Respiratory alkalosis also can be seen with rapid correction of chronic compensated metabolic acidosis. If the serum [HCO_3^-] suddenly is raised to normal and plasma pH rises, the peripheral acidemic ventilatory drive decreases, and pCO_2 transiently rises. The rise in peripheral [HCO_3^-] is followed by a slow rise in cerebrospinal fluid [HCO_3^-], but the rise in plasma pCO_2 is transmitted rapidly to the cerebrospinal fluid, providing a strong drive for ventilation. This is of particular concern if the acidosis is overcorrected rapidly; the combination of metabolic and respiratory alkalosis may generate severe alkalemia.

Treatment Issues

In addition to correcting hypoxemia (if present), the most important therapeutic consideration when respiratory alkalosis is present is to treat the underlying cause(s), as outlined above. Rarely does alkalemia warrant therapy unless a metabolic alkalosis is also present.

KEY POINTS

- The establishment of acid–base diagnoses often reveals previously unrecognized diseases and provides an index of their severity. Therapy is usually directed at the underlying condition.
- Plasma electrolytes alone often can establish an acid–base diagnosis. However, if there is any uncertainty, arterial blood-gas measurements are invaluable. Arterial blood-gas levels should be obtained in all situations in which a respiratory or mixed acid–base disorder is suspected.
- Metabolic acidosis should be approached in terms of whether there are accumulated unmeasured anions in the plasma. If the anion gap is not elevated, renal and extrarenal causes can be distinguished by measur-

---

TABLE 105.4

CAUSES OF RESPIRATORY ALKALOSIS

Associated with tissue hypoxia
  Decreased pO_2 of inspired gases: e.g., high-altitude exposure
  Reduced ventilation/perfusion ratio: e.g., pneumonia, pulmonary edema
  Shunt
    Anatomic: e.g., congenital heart disease
    Physiologic: e.g., pulmonary embolus with reperfusion
  Diffusion block: e.g., pulmonary fibrosis
  Decreased venous pO_2: low cardiac output, anemia
Not related to tissue hypoxia
  Anxiety-related psychogenic hyperventilation
  Primary central nervous system diseases: e.g., stroke, infection, malignancy
  Hormonally induced: e.g., progesterone in pregnancy
  Pharmacologic: e.g., salicylates
  Fever/septicemia
  Liver disease
  Rapid correction of metabolic acidosis

ing the urinary anion gap, which assesses renal acid excretion.

- Metabolic alkalosis can result from effective arterial volume contraction or heightened mineralocorticoid activity. The latter represents the most frequently encountered form of curable secondary hypertension and can be divided into primary disturbances in renin secretion, aldosterone secretion, and mineralocorticoid effect.

- Respiratory acidosis and alkalosis are disorders of alveolar hypoventilation and hyperventilation, respectively. Mixed acid–base disorders are common in patients with pulmonary disease.

- Chronic respiratory acidosis with stable renal compensation should not be corrected acutely. Always look for and correct concurrent metabolic alkalosis in patients with chronic respiratory acidosis.

- Respiratory alkalosis is usually secondary to tissue hypoxemia, and management should be directed at improving oxygenation. If alveolar hyperventilation is not associated with hypoxemia, it may be a harbinger of other important systemic diseases.

REFERENCES

1. Rodriguez Soriano J. Renal tubular acidosis: the clinical entity. *J Am Soc Nephrol* 2002;13:2160–2170.
2. Brent J, McMartin K, Phillips S, et al. Fomepizole for the treatment of ethylene glycol poisoning. Methylpyrazole for Toxic Alcohols Study Group. *N Engl J Med* 1999;340:832–838.
3. Brent J, McMartin K, Phillips S, et al. Fomepizole for the treatment of methanol poisoning. *N Engl J Med* 2001;344:424–429.

ADDITIONAL READING

Adrogué HJ, Madias NE. Medical progress: management of life-threatening acid-base disorders, parts I and II. *N Engl J Med* 1998;338:26–34,107–111.
Halperin ML, Goldstein MB. *Fluid, Electrolyte, and Acid-Base Physiology: A Problem-Based Approach.* 3rd ed. Philadelphia: WB Saunders, 1999.
Krapf R, Seldin DW, Alpern RJ. Clinical syndromes of metabolic acidosis. In: Seldin DW, Giebisch G, eds. *The Kidney: Physiology and Pathophysiology.* 3rd ed. New York: Raven Press, 2000:2073–2130.
Madias NE, Adrogué HJ. Respiratory alkalosis and acidosis. In: Seldin DW, Giebisch G, eds. *The Kidney: Physiology and Pathophysiology.* 3rd Ed. New York: Raven Press, 2000:2131–2166.
Wesson DE, Alpern RJ, Seldin DW. Clinical syndromes of metabolic alkalosis. In: Seldin DW, Giebisch G, eds. *The Kidney: Physiology and Pathophysiology.* 3rd ed. New York: Raven Press, 2000:2055–2072.

Endocrinology

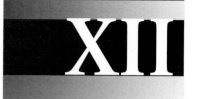

Signs, Symptoms, and Laboratory Abnormalities in Endocrinology

106

Kenneth A. Woeber

TOPICS COVERED IN CHAPTER
- Goiter 1069
- Clinical Signs of Cushing Syndrome 1071
- Abnormal Results of Thyroid Laboratory Tests 1073
- Laboratory Assessment of Hypopituitarism 1076

INTRODUCTION

Clinical endocrinology encompasses an extensive range of disorders. The majority of these begin insidiously and progress gradually, with the result that their evaluation and management are largely based in the ambulatory setting. Thus, endocrine disease is seldom the principal admitting diagnosis in the hospital setting. Rather, it either presents as a comorbid condition or is first detected clinically or through abnormal laboratory test findings as an ancillary disorder during hospitalization. On the other hand, non-endocrine disease and certain medications can lead to profound abnormalities in some laboratory values that might normally indicate the presence of endocrine disease.

This chapter addresses certain clinical signs that suggest endocrine disease and offers recommendations for their cost-effective evaluation and management. In addition, the chapter considers the interpretation of abnormal results of thyroid laboratory tests during acute illness and discusses some laboratory tests for assessing pituitary function.

GOITER

When Presenting at the Time of Admission

Description and Differential Diagnosis

The term *goiter* refers to enlargement of the thyroid gland (*thyromegaly*). The enlargement may involve the gland diffusely (*diffuse goiter*) or may comprise one or more nodules (*uninodular* or *multinodular goiter*). In a patient who presents with a goiter, the palpatory characteristics of the gland, such as size, consistency, nodularity, and the presence or absence of tenderness, should be determined, as they may shed light on the cause. Movement on swallowing should be assessed, as this is a characteristic feature of the thyroid gland, distinguishing it from other neck masses. Movement is lost when the gland is fixed to adjacent structures, such as may occur with thyroid carcinoma or Riedel thyroiditis. Auscultation of the goiter should be performed, as it may disclose a systolic or continuous bruit, usually signifying the hypervascular gland of Graves' disease. The presence of a retrosternal goiter may be revealed by the arm-raising test, which leads to further narrowing of the thoracic outlet and results in facial congestion and inspiratory stridor (*Pemberton's sign*).

Goiter may lead to hyperthyroidism, be associated with hypothyroidism, cause obstructive manifestations, or harbor a malignant neoplasm (Table 106.1). A diffuse goiter that is softer than normal and has a bruit is characteristic of *Graves' disease*, and the patient will be thyrotoxic and may display other features of Graves' disease, such as infiltrative ophthalmopathy. A diffuse goiter that is firmer than normal and has a finely irregular surface is highly suggestive of chronic autoimmune thyroiditis (*Hashimoto's thyroiditis*), and the patient may be hypothyroid. A multinodular goiter is found in older patients, has usually been present for many years, and may cause obstructive manifestations if it is very large or plunges retrosternally, or it may lead to hyperthyroidism, especially if the patient has received large quantities of iodine (*Jod-Basedow disease*). A dominant nodule in a multinodular goiter or a solitary nodule in a normal thyroid gland may be the seat of thyroid carcinoma, especially if it is hard or adherent to adjacent structures or if there is a history of radiation exposure, recent growth, or dysphonia. Tenderness of the thyroid gland indicates either acute or subacute thyroiditis or hemorrhage into a preexisting nodule.

Evaluation

The clinical characteristics of the goiter and the metabolic state of the patient should delimit the type and extent of evaluation. For example, a diffuse goiter in a patient with thyrotoxicosis, confirmed with an undetectable value for serum thyroid-stimulating hormone (TSH) and a high level of serum free thyroxine (FT_4) or free triiodothyronine (FT_3), requires no additional evaluation, as the patient almost certainly has Graves' disease. Similarly, a firm, diffuse goiter in a euthyroid or hypothyroid patient is in all likelihood a manifestation of chronic autoimmune thyroiditis, and this diagnosis can be confirmed by the demonstration of thyroperoxidase (antimicrosomal) antibody in serum. On the other hand, in a patient with a multinodular goiter, scintigraphic scanning with radioactive iodine should be undertaken, as it will define the functional nature of the nodules and may reveal retrosternal extension. Furthermore, it will serve to identify a hypofunctional, dominant nodule from which a specimen should be obtained by *fine-needle aspiration biopsy* (FNAB). In the evaluation of a solitary nodule in an otherwise palpably normal gland, FNAB is the only procedure that should be performed, as it will empty a cystic lesion and provide a cytologic diagnosis of a solid lesion with an overall diagnostic accuracy of approximately 95%. Ultrasonographic examination of the thyroid provides a very accurate assessment of goiter size and morphology and is sometimes needed to direct FNAB. However, its principal utility is to complement physical examination in monitoring goiter size and morphology over time.

Management

When goiter is accompanied by thyroid dysfunction, management is primarily directed at restoring the patient to a eumetabolic state. In the case of a thyrotoxic patient, endocrinologic consultation should be sought, as management entails various therapeutic considerations concerning antithyroid drugs, radioiodine, and surgery. Similarly, management of a goiter that is producing obstructive manifestations or a nodule that yields a malignant cytologic diagnosis on FNAB is the province of the endocrine surgeon. The management of a benign solitary nodule or multinodular goiter has customarily involved long-term suppression of TSH with levothyroxine, but prospective studies have not consistently demonstrated shrinkage (1). Moreover, the doses of levothyroxine required over the long term may be associated with reduced bone mineral density and an increased risk for atrial fibrillation.

TABLE 106.1

TYPES OF GOITER AND ASSOCIATED DISORDERS

Palpatory features	Cause	Clinical picture
Diffuse goiter	Graves' disease	Hyperthyroidism; infiltrative ophthalmopathy common
	Chronic autoimmune thyroiditis	Hypothyroidism common[a]
Multinodular goiter	Idiopathic, iodine deficiency, goitrogens, genetic defect	Hyperthyroidism common[b]; thoracic outlet syndrome uncommon
Uninodular goiter	Follicular adenoma	Hyperthyroidism uncommon
	Carcinoma[c]	Cervical lymphadenopathy common

[a] Spontaneous or induced by iodine excess or lithium.
[b] Spontaneous or induced by iodine excess.
[c] May also present as a dominant nodule in a multinodular goiter.

When Presenting During Hospitalization

Description and Differential Diagnosis

A goiter that is predominantly retrosternal in location may present during hospitalization with episodes of acute ventilatory insufficiency. These episodes are characterized by inspiratory stridor and are precipitated or aggravated by the supine position and promptly alleviated by endotracheal intubation.

Imaging of the neck for indications unrelated to the thyroid may reveal the presence of a *nonpalpable* thyroid nodule (*thyroid "incidentaloma"*).

Evaluation

Magnetic resonance imaging (MRI) or computed axial tomography (CT) of the mediastinum will reveal the presence of a retrosternal goiter. A thyroid "incidentaloma" should be subjected to FNAB under ultrasonographic guidance if the patient has a history of radiation exposure or a family history of thyroid carcinoma (as these are risk factors for thyroid carcinoma), or if it displays suspicious ultrasonographic features (2).

Management

A retrosternal goiter that is obstructing the airway or a thyroid "incidentaloma" that yields a malignant cytologic diagnosis on FNAB requires surgical excision. In the case of a thyroid "incidentaloma" that does not meet the criteria for ultrasonographically-guided FNAB or is benign, ultrasonographic surveillance is currently recommended.

CLINICAL SIGNS OF CUSHING SYNDROME

When Presenting at the Time of Admission

Description and Differential Diagnosis

Cushing syndrome is characterized by a constellation of clinical and biochemical manifestations that are caused by cortisol excess. Clinical signs that might suggest the presence of Cushing syndrome at the time of admission include facial rounding and plethora, truncal obesity with prominent dorsal cervical and supraclavicular fat deposition, thin skin with violaceous abdominal striae, and proximal muscle wasting in a patient with moderate hypertension. None of these physical signs is specific, but together they increase the likelihood of Cushing syndrome.

The causes of Cushing syndrome are manifold, but in the absence of exogenous glucocorticoid excess, pituitary adrenocorticotropin (ACTH)-dependent Cushing syndrome (*Cushing disease*) accounts for at least 70% of cases (3) (Table

TABLE 106.2

SPECTRUM OF CUSHING SYNDROME

Cause	Prevalence (%)[a]
ACTH-dependent	
Pituitary ACTH (Cushing disease)	70
Ectopic ACTH or, rarely, CRH	15
ACTH-independent	
Adrenal adenoma or carcinoma	15
Bilateral micronodular or macronodular hyperplasia	Rare
Pseudo-Cushing	
Alcohol-induced	Rare
Megestrol-induced	Rare

[a] In absence of exogenous glucocorticoid.
ACTH, adrenocorticotropic hormone; *CRH*, corticotropin-releasing hormone.

106.2). The underlying cause of Cushing syndrome may modify the clinical presentation greatly. For example, in contrast to Cushing disease, the *ectopic ACTH syndrome*, which is caused by a small-cell carcinoma of the lung or other neuroendocrine neoplasms and accounts for about 15% of cases, is usually found in older men rather than in women. Moreover, it is usually characterized by extreme elevations of ACTH and cortisol secretion. These lead to a much more rapid evolution of clinical manifestations, accompanied by hyperpigmentation (secondary to the extremely high ACTH concentration) and by features of mineralocorticoid excess, such as hypokalemia and metabolic alkalosis (secondary to the extreme cortisol excess). Similarly, in contrast to patients with Cushing disease, those with adrenal carcinoma often display the additional features of adrenal androgen excess, such as hirsutism, acne, and other signs of masculinization, in addition to mild polycythemia.

Several other conditions, apart from exogenous glucocorticoid excess, may mimic spontaneous Cushing syndrome. They include the rare alcohol-induced pseudo-Cushing syndrome and the pseudo-Cushing syndrome that can be associated with the use of megestrol acetate (Megace) (4), which has glucocorticoid-like activity, for the management of cancer or wasting states. In the alcohol-induced syndrome, liver function is deranged, and the syndrome resolves with abstinence.

Evaluation

The most reliable test for detecting Cushing syndrome is measurement of cortisol in a 24-hour urine collection (along with creatinine to assess completeness of collection) as it most closely reflects the cortisol secretion rate (5). A normal value essentially rules out Cushing syndrome, but mildly increased values for urinary cortisol may occur during major stress and in alcohol-induced pseudo-Cushing syndrome. A clearly increased value confirms the presence of Cushing syndrome but does not indicate its cause. Thus, the most efficient and cost-effective manner for evaluating the patient is to measure serum cortisol and ACTH during the evening of the 24-hour urine collection so as to exploit the normal circadian depression of both, which is lost in Cushing syndrome (Figure 106.1). Under these conditions, an increased serum ACTH level accompanying increased values for serum and 24-hour urinary cortisol would indicate ACTH-dependent Cushing syndrome, whereas a subnormal serum ACTH would indicate adrenal adenoma, carcinoma, or bilateral nodular hyperplasia. Moreover, patients with the ectopic ACTH syndrome usually display extremely high values for cortisol and ACTH. Tests based on the suppressibility of serum or urinary cortisol with large doses of dexamethasone have been used in an attempt to differentiate between Cushing disease, in which cortisol is usually suppressible, and the ectopic ACTH syndrome, in which it is usually not suppressible. However, these tests may give misleading results, as their overall diagnostic accuracy (~80%) is less than the pretest probability of Cushing disease (>90%) in patients with ACTH-dependent Cushing syndrome (5). Rather, the consideration of variables such as age, sex, rate of progression, presence of hypokalemia, and magnitude of elevation of urinary cortisol and serum ACTH together yield an overall diagnostic accuracy of 90% or greater in the differential diagnosis of ACTH-dependent Cushing syndrome. (In contrast to Cushing disease, the ectopic ACTH syndrome usually occurs in older men rather than in women and is characterized by a much higher cortisol secretion rate that leads to hypokalemia and metabolic alkalosis and to more rapid clinical progression.) This issue of differentiation is highly important, as both the pituitary adenoma causing Cushing disease and the ectopic ACTH-secreting neoplasm may be small and difficult to localize using imaging techniques. It is at this juncture in the patient's evaluation that endocrinologic consultation should be sought.

Once a functional diagnosis of Cushing syndrome has been established, localization of the cause needs to be undertaken. In ACTH-independent Cushing syndrome, thin-section CT of the abdomen will reveal an adrenal mass or bilateral hyperplasia. A pituitary-dedicated MRI study will detect a pituitary adenoma in most, but not all, patients with Cushing disease. The majority of patients with the

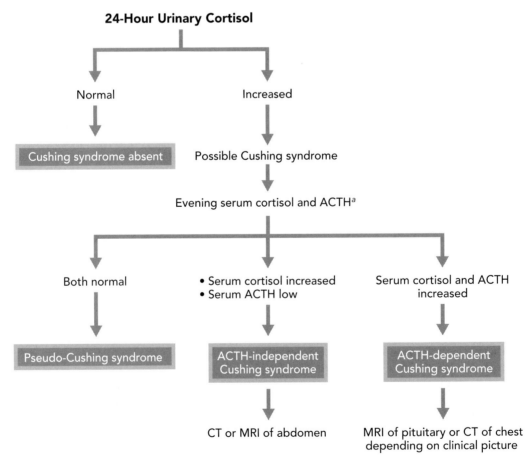

Figure 106.1 Laboratory investigation of Cushing syndrome. ^{a}Serum cortisol and adrenocorticotropic hormone (*ACTH*) should be measured during the evening of the 24-hour urine collection. *CT*, computed axial tomography; *MRI*, magnetic resonance imaging.

ectopic ACTH syndrome will harbor a small-cell carcinoma of the lung, and CT of the chest, therefore, will usually provide the necessary confirmation. If the aforementioned imaging studies are unrevealing and the functional diagnosis is not entirely consistent with Cushing disease, inferior petrosal venous sinus sampling with determination of central-to-peripheral serum ACTH ratios before and after intravenous administration of corticotropin-releasing hormone (CRH) is indicated, as Cushing disease is still the most likely cause.

Management

The treatment of choice for patients with Cushing disease is transsphenoidal pituitary microsurgery, which results in a 10-year remission rate of approximately 75%. For those patients in whom surgery is unsuccessful or who relapse, pituitary irradiation is indicated. In Cushing syndrome with an adrenal cause, unilateral or, in the rare case of bilateral nodular hyperplasia, bilateral adrenalectomy (which can now be performed through a laparoscope) is the appropriate treatment. The management of patients with the ectopic ACTH syndrome, which is usually caused by a small-cell or other neuroendocrine carcinoma or by an adrenal carcinoma, involves the use of adrenal enzyme inhibitors, such as ketoconazole or mitotane. Glucocorticoid replacement therapy will be required for a short time in some patients after pituitary surgery or unilateral adrenalectomy and permanently in all patients who have undergone bilateral adrenalectomy.

When Presenting During Hospitalization

Description and Differential Diagnosis

During hospitalization, the appearance of certain clinical signs should lead one to entertain a diagnosis of Cushing syndrome. Thin skin and an increased fragility of the tissues predispose to the formation of ecchymoses after phlebotomy and to decubitus ulceration, and these are especially noteworthy findings when they occur in a younger patient. A fracture with little or no antecedent trauma, reflecting the loss of bone mass in Cushing syndrome, may be the presenting manifestation and reason for admission. Difficulty in rising from the lying or sitting position may point to wasting and weakness of the limb-girdle musculature in Cushing syndrome. In a hypertensive patient, the presence of hypokalemia and metabolic alkalosis, suggesting a disorder of mineralocorticoid excess, may be the presenting manifestation of the ectopic ACTH syndrome, especially if there is a history of recent darkening of the skin.

Evaluation

This is undertaken in the same manner as described in the corresponding previous section.

Management

This is the same as described in the corresponding previous section.

ABNORMAL RESULTS OF THYROID LABORATORY TESTS

When Presenting at the Time of Admission

Description and Differential Diagnosis

Because of its sensitivity, measurement of serum TSH is the test used first to screen patients for thyroid dysfunction. This sensitivity resides in the approximate negative logarithmic–linear relationship between serum TSH and FT_4 concentrations, with the result that small changes in FT_4 result in large changes in serum TSH. Current second-generation (sensitive) and third-generation (ultrasensitive) TSH assays have approximate functional sensitivities of 0.1 and 0.01 mU/L, respectively, with an approximate normal range of 0.5–5.0 mU/L (6).

The finding of low or undetectable serum TSH in a patient at the time of admission suggests the presence of thyrotoxicosis. However, a low serum TSH may also be found in about 15% of patients with various systemic nonthyroid illnesses (*euthyroid sick syndrome*), in calorically-deprived patients, or in the occasional patient with hypopituitarism. In these circumstances, serum TSH, although low and sometimes undetectable with a sensitive assay, is rarely undetectable with an ultrasensitive assay. By contrast, in patients with thyrotoxicosis, serum TSH is virtually *always undetectable* (6).

The finding of an increased serum TSH in a patient at the time of admission is highly suggestive of primary hypothyroidism, especially if the value exceeds 10 mU/L. On the other hand, values between 5–10 mU/L may revert to normal on follow-up testing in some patients.

Evaluation

Measurement of serum FT_4 and sometimes FT_3 will provide the necessary discrimination among the various causes of an abnormal serum TSH (Figure 106.2). These measurements have replaced the older measurements of total T_4 and total T_3, which reflect alterations in hormone binding in serum in addition to alterations in hormone production.

In patients with nonthyroid illness, serum FT_4 is usually normal, even when serum total T_4 is reduced (7). A high serum FT_4 will confirm the diagnosis of thyrotoxicosis in a patient with an undetectable serum TSH. Uncommonly, an undetectable serum TSH with an ultrasensitive assay will be accompanied by a normal serum FT_4. In this circumstance, measurement of serum FT_3 should be

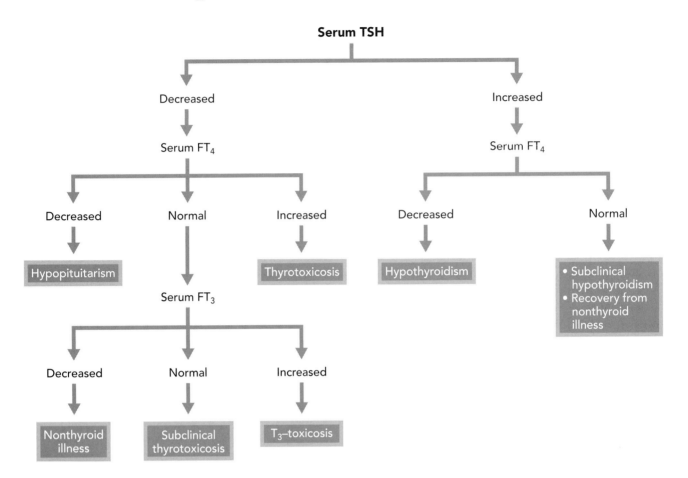

Figure 106.2 Evaluation of abnormal serum values of thyroid-stimulating hormone (*TSH*). *FT₄*, free thyroxine; *FT₃*, free triiodothyronine.

undertaken, as an increased value would establish a diagnosis of T_3 *toxicosis*, whereas a normal value would indicate the presence of *subclinical thyrotoxicosis*. A low serum FT_4 in conjunction with a subnormal serum TSH is virtually diagnostic of *hypopituitarism*. On the other hand, a low serum FT_3 is much less specific, as it is often found in patients with nonthyroid illness (7).

In a patient with a high serum TSH, a low serum FT_4 will establish the diagnosis of *primary hypothyroidism*. If the serum free T_4 is normal and the serum TSH is above 10 mU/L, the patient has *subclinical hypothyroidism*, and progression to overt hypothyroidism is very likely. In a patient with a serum TSH between 5–10 mU/L, measurement of serum thyroperoxidase (antimicrosomal) antibody should be undertaken because its presence, indicating chronic autoimmune thyroiditis, would be an independent risk factor for the eventual development of overt hypothyroidism (8).

Management

In patients with non-thyroid illness, a low value for serum TSH will eventually revert to normal during convalescence, and no specific treatment is indicated. In a patient with

clinical or subclinical thyrotoxicosis, endocrinologic consultation should be sought, as management will entail various considerations concerning choice of therapy. Similarly, endocrinologic consultation is required in a patient with suspected hypopituitarism, as assessment of the functional integrity of the pituitary–adrenal axis becomes critical.

In a patient with established primary hypothyroidism, replacement therapy with levothyroxine should be initiated, as hypothyroid patients tolerate anesthesia and surgery less well than euthyroid patients. In an elderly patient or a patient with pre-existing heart disease, treatment should be initiated with smaller than usual doses of levothyroxine (e.g., 25 mcg daily) and careful monitoring. As there are no outcome data to support therapeutic intervention in patients with subclinical hypothyroidism, management should consist of surveillance with monitoring of serum TSH.

When Presenting During Hospitalization

Description and Differential Diagnosis

The interpretation of abnormal values for thyroid laboratory tests in patients during hospitalization is the same as that described in the corresponding previous section, except that the potential confounding effects of certain drugs also need to be considered (Table 106.3).

Dopamine or pharmacologic doses of glucocorticoids acutely suppress pituitary TSH secretion and lead to decreases in serum TSH and FT_4 in patients with nonthyroid illness, resulting in a laboratory profile that might suggest hypopituitarism. Moreover, in a patient with primary hypothyroidism, these drugs, when administered concurrently, may suppress the serum TSH into the normal range, with the result that the diagnosis of hypothyroidism can be overlooked. By contrast, amiodarone acutely increases pituitary TSH secretion through inhibition of the conversion of T_4 to T_3 within the pituitary and reduces the peripheral uptake of T_4 and its conversion to T_3, thereby leading to increases in serum TSH and FT_4 and a decrease in serum FT_3. Sodium iopanoate and ipodate, which are non–water-soluble radiographic contrast agents, produce effects similar to those of amiodarone.

Drugs that increase the hepatic uptake and metabolism of T_4, such as phenytoin, rifampin, and carbamazepine, may lead to a decrease in serum FT_4 with little or no change in serum FT_3 or TSH. Lithium interferes with the secretion of hormone by the thyroid and may lead to an increase in serum TSH, sometimes accompanied by a decrease in serum FT_4, if the patient has an underlying chronic autoimmune thyroiditis that limits thyroid functional reserve.

During recovery from nonthyroid illness, serum TSH may rebound from a normal or suppressed value to a value as high as 20 mU/L in euthyroid patients, mimicking primary hypothyroidism, before reverting to normal levels over several days.

Evaluation

The evaluation of abnormal results of thyroid laboratory tests in hospitalized patients is the same as that described in the corresponding previous section, except that the interpretation of the values must take into account the potential confounding effects of certain drugs.

Management

In patients with nonthyroid illness who are being treated with any of the aforementioned drugs, abnormal values for thyroid laboratory tests will revert to normal after the drug has been discontinued during convalescence, and no specific treatment is indicated. With the long-term administration of amiodarone, even though the values return to normal, patients with chronic autoimmune thyroiditis or multinodular goiter are at risk for later development of iodine-induced hypothyroidism or iodine-induced thyrotoxicosis, respectively, as a result of the iodine released during the degradation of amiodarone. Similarly, the long-term administration of lithium may unmask hypothyroidism in some patients with chronic autoimmune thyroiditis. On the other hand, the long-term administration of phenytoin, carbamazepine, or rifampin, although accompanied by a decrease in serum FT_4, does not lead to hypothyroidism, because a normal serum TSH concentration is maintained. For patients in whom thyroid dysfunction has been established through an appropriate profile of abnormal laboratory values, management is the same as described in the corresponding previous section.

TABLE 106.3

NONTHYROID CAUSES OF ABNORMAL THYROID LABORATORY TEST RESULTS

	Serum TSH	Serum FT_4	Serum FT_3
Systemic illness	N/↓	N	N/↓
Recovery from illness	↑	N	N
Glucocorticoids	↓	N/↓	↓
Dopamine	↓	N/↓	N/↓
Amiodarone[a]	N/↑	N/↑	↓
Iopanoate, ipodate	N/↑	N/↑	N/↓
Phenytoin	N	↓	N
Rifampin	N	↓	N
Carbamazepine	N	↓	N
Lithium[a]	↑	N/↓	N/↓

[a] May cause clinical thyroid dysfunction when taken on a long-term basis by patients with intrinsic thyroid disease.

↓, decreased; ↑, increased; FT_4, free thyroxine; FT_3, free triiodothyronine; N, normal; TSH, thyroid-stimulating hormone.

LABORATORY ASSESSMENT OF HYPOPITUITARISM

When Presenting at the Time of Admission

Description and Differential Diagnosis

Prompt assessment of the functional integrity of the pituitary is critical in a patient with suspected hypopituitarism so as to avoid overlooking the secondary cortisol deficiency, which can lead to shock and death (9). The clinical presentation of hypopituitarism depends on the nature of the pituitary insult. Thus, hemorrhagic necrosis of a pituitary adenoma (*pituitary apoplexy*) presents dramatically with severe headache, visual field defects, oculomotor palsies, and hypotension. In contrast, more gradual destruction by a slowly growing adenoma or other infiltrative lesion or following radiation therapy for head and neck carcinoma presents with nonspecific manifestations, such as lethargy, pallor, loss of sexual hair, and orthostatic hypotension. In the presence of severe stress, however, ACTH deficiency may emerge as symptomatic hyponatremia, mimicking the syndrome of inappropriate antidiuretic hormone secretion (SIADH) (Chapter 104). Finally, hypoglycemia for which there is no ready explanation may be the presenting manifestation of hypopituitarism.

Measurement of serum cortisol under stressful conditions imposed by acute illness or during hypoglycemia is the single most helpful test because a serum cortisol level below 20 mcg/dL—that is, an inappropriately normal or low value—points to a defective pituitary–adrenal axis (9) (Chapter 109). Similarly, the absence of an increased serum growth hormone level in these circumstances also points to pituitary hypofunction. Measurement of serum follicle-stimulating hormone in a postmenopausal woman is helpful, as in this circumstance an increased value is expected, and consequently an inappropriately normal or low value suggests the presence of hypopituitarism. Finally, the finding of a low serum FT_4 that is accompanied by a subnormal serum TSH is characteristic of hypopituitarism (Table 106.4).

Evaluation

Functional evaluation of the pituitary–adrenal axis is of paramount importance in a patient with suspected hypo-pituitarism, and endocrinologic consultation should be sought. Although the absence of an increased serum ACTH level in a patient with a low serum cortisol level indicates pituitary ACTH deficiency, some patients with hypopituitarism display values for serum cortisol under basal conditions that are within the normal range. Accordingly, various tests have been devised to provoke the hypothalamic–pituitary–adrenal axis. Of these, the stimulation test with synthetic ACTH (Cortrosyn) is undertaken first; a normal serum cortisol response (i.e., a value exceeding 20 mcg/dL at 60 minutes following an intravenous bolus of 250 mcg of synthetic ACTH) excludes the presence of hypopituitarism unless it is of such recent onset that adrenocortical atrophy has not yet occurred (9). On the other hand, a subnormal serum cortisol response is also found in patients with primary adrenocortical insufficiency. Tests that evaluate pituitary ACTH secretion directly include the insulin-induced hypoglycemia test, the metyrapone tartrate stimulation test, and the CRH stimulation test. These tests are associated with some risks, and their selection, performance, and interpretation are the province of the consulting endocrinologist.

The most common cause of hypopituitarism is a *pituitary adenoma*, often a prolactin-secreting macroadenoma. Accordingly, measurement of serum prolactin and a pituitary-dedicated MRI study should be performed.

Management

Cortisol is essential for survival under stressful conditions. Accordingly, once hypopituitarism has been recognized, replacement therapy with hydrocortisone must be instituted promptly, in stress doses if indicated by the clinical circumstance (Chapter 109). Replacement therapy with levothyroxine should also be instituted, but *not before hydrocortisone*, as the increase in metabolic rate may aggravate the cortisol deficiency. At this juncture, treatment of a pituitary adenoma or other potentially remediable cause of hypopituitarism can be undertaken. Finally, replacement therapy with gonadal steroids, although not essential for survival, will preserve bone mass and restore vitality. With full hormone replacement therapy and appropriate surveillance, patients with hypopituitarism should be able to lead normal lives.

When Presenting During Hospitalization

Description and Differential Diagnosis

This is the same as described in the corresponding previous section.

Evaluation

This is undertaken in the same manner as described in the corresponding previous section.

TABLE 106.4

LABORATORY TEST RESULTS THAT SUGGEST HYPOPITUITARISM

- Normal or low serum cortisol during severe stress
- Normal serum FSH (<20 U/L) in a postmenopausal woman
- Low serum FT_4 in association with subnormal TSH

FSH, follicle-stimulating hormone; *FT₄*, free thyroxine; *TSH*, thyroid-stimulating hormone.

Management

This is the same as described in the corresponding previous section.

KEY POINTS

- In the evaluation of a solitary nodule in an otherwise palpably normal thyroid gland, or a dominant nodule in a multinodular thyroid gland, fine-needle aspiration biopsy is the initial procedure of choice, as it empties a cystic lesion and provides a cytologic diagnosis of a solid lesion with an overall diagnostic accuracy of 95%.

- A nonpalpable thyroid nodule discovered incidentally by nonthyroid imaging of the neck should be subjected to fine-needle aspiration biopsy under ultrasonographic guidance if the patient has a history of radiation exposure or a family history of thyroid carcinoma, or if the nodule displays suspicious ultrasonographic features.

- The overall diagnostic accuracy of the collective use of variables such as age, sex, rate of progression, presence of hypokalemia, and magnitude of elevation of urinary cortisol and serum ACTH exceeds that of high-dose dexamethasone suppression testing in differentiating between pituitary ACTH-dependent Cushing syndrome and the ectopic ACTH syndrome.

- In a hypertensive patient, the presence of hypokalemia and metabolic alkalosis, suggesting a disorder of mineralocorticoid excess, may be the presenting manifestation of the ectopic ACTH syndrome.

- In hospitalized patients, abnormal results of thyroid laboratory tests are more often the consequence of nonthyroid illness or the effects of drugs than of intrinsic thyroid disease.

- In nonthyroid illness, serum TSH may be low but is rarely undetectable with an ultrasensitive assay, whereas in thyrotoxicosis, serum TSH is virtually always undetectable.

- During recovery from nonthyroid illness, serum TSH may transiently increase to values as high as 20 mU/L in euthyroid patients, mimicking primary hypothyroidism.

- In severe illness or during hypoglycemia, a normal serum cortisol value is inappropriate and indicates a defective pituitary–adrenal axis.

REFERENCES

1. Castro MR, Caraballo PJ, Morris JC. Effectiveness of thyroid hormone suppressive therapy in benign solitary thyroid nodules: a meta-analysis. *J Clin Endocrinol Metab* 2002;87:4154–4159.
2. Ross DS. Editorial: nonpalpable thyroid nodules—managing an epidemic. *J Clin Endocrinol Metab* 2002;87:1938–1940.
3. Boscaro M, Barzon L, Fallo F, Sonino N. Cushing's syndrome. *Lancet* 2001;357:783–791.
4. Caparros GC, Zambrana JL, Delgado-Fernandez M, Diez F. Megestrol-induced Cushing syndrome. *Ann Pharmacother* 2001;35:1208–1210.
5. Raff H, Findling JW. A physiologic approach to diagnosis of the Cushing syndrome. *Ann Intern Med* 2003;138:980–981.
6. Ross DS. Serum thyroid-stimulating hormone measurement for assessment of thyroid function and disease. *Endocrinol Metab Clin N Am* 2001;30:245–264.
7. Langton JE, Brent GA. Nonthyroidal illness syndrome: evaluation of thyroid function in sick patients. *Endocrinol Metab Clin N Am* 2002;31:159–172.
8. Huber G, Staub J-J, Meier C, et al. Prospective study of the spontaneous course of subclinical hypothyroidism: prognostic value of thyrotropin, thyroid reserve, and thyroid antibodies. *J Clin Endocrinol Metab* 2002;87:3221–3226.
9. Marik PE, Zaloga GP. Adrenal insufficiency in the critically ill. A new look at an old problem. *Chest* 2002;122:1784–1796.

ADDITIONAL READING

Bogazzi F, Bartalena L, Gasperi M, Braverman LE, Martino E. The various effects of amiodarone on thyroid function. *Thyroid* 2001;11:511–519.

Cooper MS, Stewart PM. Current concepts: corticosteroid insufficiency in acutely ill patients. *New Engl J Med* 2003;348:727–734.

Hamrahian AH, Oseni TS, Arafah BM. Measurements of serum free cortisol in critically ill patients. *New Engl J Med* 2004;350:1629–1638.

Hegedus L. Clinical practice. The thyroid nodule. *New Engl J Med* 2004;351:1764–1771.

Woeber KA. Update on the management of hyperthyroidism and hypothyroidism. *Arch Intern Med* 2000;160;1067–1071.

The Management of Hyperglycemia and Diabetes Mellitus in Hospitalized Patients

Harold E. Lebovitz

INTRODUCTION

It has long been recognized that patients with diabetes mellitus are at increased risk for morbidity and mortality when they are stricken with an illness that requires hospitalization. Special attention must be paid to many aspects of their illnesses in order to maximize health care benefits and minimize health care costs. A relatively new area of concern is the hospitalized patient who does not have diabetes mellitus but presents with significant hyperglycemia during the acute phase of a general medical or surgical illness. Several major studies show that careful management of the hyperglycemia has profound effects in decreasing both morbidity and mortality. These findings mandate that physicians extend their intensive efforts to control metabolism from the diabetic hospitalized patient to the hyperglycemic, nondiabetic patient as well.

Diabetes mellitus encompasses many disorders, the phenotypic expression of which is hyperglycemia occurring in the fasting and/or postprandial state. Approximately 12.1 million patients in the United States (4.1% of the U.S. population) have clinically diagnosed diabetes mellitus. It is estimated that an additional 30%–40% have undiagnosed diabetes mellitus. Those clinically diagnosed diabetic patients consume 91.8 billion dollars per year in direct health care costs and an additional 40 billion dollars per year in indirect costs such as lost wages. The clinically diagnosed diabetic patient costs the health care system 2.4 times more per year than comparable nondiabetic patients, and their aggregate costs consume 10.1% of the entire U.S. health care budget. In 2002, patients with diabetes utilized 16.9 million inpatient hospital days (43.9% of direct costs) and 82.35 million nursing home bed days (15.1% of direct costs). It is noteworthy that 61% of diabetics' inpatient costs were for the management of general medical conditions, 24% were for cardiovascular disorders, and only 5% were for uncontrolled diabetes.

Newly diagnosed hyperglycemia in a patient hospitalized for an acute illness may represent stress-induced hyperglycemia or diabetes mellitus in a previously undiagnosed individual. Frequently it is not possible to make the differentiation at presentation, and the outcome appears to depend on the effectiveness of treating the hyperglycemia rather than its cause. In patients with acute myocardial infarction, admission plasma glucose level is an independent predictor of nonfatal reinfarction, hospitalization for heart failure, and death. In one large intensive care unit (ICU) study, 70% of patients presented with blood glucose >110 mg/dL, yet only 13% had a history of diabetes mellitus (1).

In such patients, morbidity and mortality are directly correlated to the extent of the increase in plasma glucose values above 110 mg/dL. Several randomized prospective studies indicate that treating hyperglycemia in hospitalized patients with acute illnesses by insulin infusion can reduce morbidity, mortality, and hospital costs by approximately 30%–50%. The treatable detrimental effects of excess hyperglycemia (>110 mg/dL) in acutely ill hospitalized patients has opened an important new therapeutic window for the hospital-based physician.

Rational management of hospitalized patients with diabetes or excessive hyperglycemia requires an understanding of the metabolic consequences of hyperglycemia. Hyperglycemia increases oxidative stress, alters the coagulation pathway, and activates the inflammatory cascade. Clinically, these derangements result in greater susceptibility to bacterial infections, poorer responses to treatment of bacterial infections, increases in thromboembolic events, weight loss and negative nitrogen balance, depressed tissue anabolism, and poor wound healing.

The impaired host resistance to infection in diabetes has been known for decades (2). One significant component of this impaired response is deficient polymorphonuclear leukocyte function. Polymorphonuclear leukocytes from patients with diabetes mellitus demonstrate impaired adherence, chemotaxis, phagocytosis, oxidative activity, and bactericidal activity (3). These disturbances become evident when plasma glucose levels exceed 130–175 mg/dL and become increasingly more severe as the plasma glucose rises to 300–400 mg/dL. Impaired function of polymorphonuclear leukocytes renders patients particularly susceptible to *Staphylococcus aureus* and *Escherichia coli* infections.

In a prospective, randomized, controlled clinical trial in a surgical ICU, patients admitted with a plasma glucose ≥140 mg/dL were randomized to standard insulin treatment (target glucose levels 180–220 mg/dL) or strict insulin therapy (target glucose levels 80–120 mg/dL) throughout their ICU stay (1). The "strict control" group (mean plasma glucose 125 ± 36 mg/dL) had significantly fewer bloodstream and surgical site infections than the standard treatment group (mean plasma glucose (179 ± 61 mg/dL). Another prospective study, the Portland Diabetic Project, assessed the effects of glycemic control of 4,864 patients with diabetes who underwent cardiovascular surgery (4). Tight perioperative diabetes control (150–200 mg/dL in the early years of the trial, later further tightened to 100–150 mg/dL) was achieved by continuous intravenous administration of insulin. In diabetic patients whose mean perioperative blood glucose averaged 175 mg/dL or less, deep sternal wound infections occurred in about 0.5%, comparable to the risk in the nondiabetic population. Diabetic patients whose mean blood glucoses exceeded 175 mg/dL had rates of 1.1%, while those with glucoses above 250 mg/dL had rates of 3.7%, a sevenfold increase over the base rate. Length of

hospital stay increased from 8.2 days in diabetic patients with tight control to 11.0 days in those with poorly controlled perioperative blood glucoses.

Short-term hyperglycemia increases the glycosylation of many proteins and may interfere with their function. Such effects have been demonstrated with circulating immunoglobins. Additionally, acute hyperglycemia has been shown to increase mediators of both coagulation and adhesion. Uncontrolled hyperglycemia is also associated with proteolysis and impaired protein synthesis (5). This leads to delay and deficiencies in tissue repair and regeneration. In an active wound, hyperglycemia increases collagenase activity and decreases collagen content. In diabetic patients with medical or surgical disease, these processes may prolong hospitalizations and impair recovery.

The above data suggest that these untoward acute and subacute consequences of hyperglycemia can be minimized by maintaining plasma glucose levels below 175 mg/dL. As will be discussed in subsequent sections, new data indicate that the glycemic target should probably be even tighter: *blood glucoses between 80 and 110 mg/dL in hospitalized acutely ill patients.*

The treatment goals for diabetic ketoacidosis and nonketotic hyperosmolar state are somewhat different because they change with the stage of treatment. Moreover, in such patients, clinicians must attend to the management of dehydration, acidosis, and electrolyte balance in addition to the glucose level.

HOSPITAL-BASED TREATMENT REGIMENS FOR GLYCEMIC CONTROL

Most hospitalized diabetic patients require some type of insulin regimen to maintain their glucose in the target range of 80–175 mg/dL. Acute illnesses are associated with a significant stress response, inadequate nutritional intake, and increased tissue requirements for energy. As a consequence, secretion of catecholamines, cortisol, growth hormone, and glucagon is increased. These hormonal changes both inhibit insulin secretion and increase insulin resistance, rendering oral antihyperglycemic agents ineffective in most hospitalized patients. Maintaining tight glycemic control (blood glucose 80–110 mg/dL) in hyperglycemic, acutely ill hospitalized patients who may or may not have diabetes mellitus generally requires continuous intravenous insulin with frequent blood glucose monitoring.

Table 107.1 outlines insulin treatment regimens that are effective for hospitalized diabetic patients. Diabetic or nondiabetic hyperglycemic patients who are severely ill and not taking oral nutrients are best managed with intravenous (IV) regular insulin. This includes virtually all patients admitted to an ICU and undergoing surgery and most patients in the first 48–72 hours following surgery or an acute myocardial infarction (5). The

TABLE 107.1

INSULIN TREATMENT REGIMENS FOR HOSPITALIZED DIABETIC PATIENTS

Patients	Insulin administration	Glucose administration	Monitoring and dose adjustments
Acute glucose regulation by intravenously administered regular insulin			
Acutely ill patients not on oral nutrition	Regular insulin is administered intravenously at 0.5 to 5.0 units/h by infusion pump.	Glucose is administered simultaneously through the same port, either by a separate glucose infusion ("piggyback") or by mixing glucose with insulin in the same solution but varying the ratio of glucose to insulin.	Blood glucose is monitored every 1–2 hours, with adjustments of insulin and glucose infusions based on results.
Subacute glucose regulation by subcutaneously administered regular and intermediate-acting insulin			
Hospitalized patients on oral nutrition	Regular and intermediate-acting insulins are administered subcutaneously 2–4 times a day (three times is preferable).	None	Blood glucose is monitored by finger-stick before meals and at 10 PM. Insulin doses are adjusted every 1–2 days based on results.

advantages of IV regular insulin are its immediate delivery to the tissues and its rapid disappearance from the plasma (half-life of five minutes). IV insulin delivery is independent of adipose tissue perfusion, which may greatly alter the uptake of subcutaneously administered insulin. Because the cellular effects of insulin are short-lived (20–60 minutes), changes in the delivery rate of IV insulin are reflected in the glucose concentration within 30–60 minutes. *IV insulin must be administered together with a glucose solution,* which can be independently regulated but is delivered through the same portal as the insulin. The glucose is not only necessary to prevent hypoglycemia but also essential to maintain caloric intake and reduce catabolism. The regular insulin and glucose infusions should not be administered through separate portals, as unrecognized infiltration of the glucose infusion can lead to severe hypoglycemia. Concurrent administration can be accomplished by "piggybacking" the glucose infusion into the insulin line or by administering the glucose and insulin from the same container but changing the glucose-to-insulin ratio as necessary. Monitoring of blood glucose and subsequent adjustment of the insulin and glucose infusion rates must always be performed frequently (every one, two, or four hours as dictated by the specific circumstances). Supplemental potassium is generally necessary because insulin and glucose administration facilitate the intracellular movement of potassium.

Hospitalized diabetic patients who are taking oral nutrition and are not in a rapidly fluctuating state can be managed with one of several subcutaneous insulin treatment programs (6), shown in Table 107.2.

The initial doses of insulin are determined by the body weight, severity of hyperglycemia, and knowledge of a previous history of diabetic treatment and its effectiveness. The calorie distribution among the meals will influence the amount of insulin given at each specific time. A general guideline is to start with a total daily insulin dose of approximately 0.50 units/kg, with about 75% of the dose used to

TABLE 107.2

SUBCUTANEOUS INSULIN MANAGEMENT PROGRAMS

Regimen 1

Regular insulin and intermediate-acting insulin before breakfast
Regular insulin before the evening meal
Intermediate-acting insulin at 10 PM

Regimen 2

Basal insulin (glargine insulin) once a day
Regular or rapid-acting insulin before each meal

Regimen 3

Regular insulin before each meal (breakfast, lunch, and evening meal)
Intermediate-acting insulin at 10 PM

Regimen 4

Regular and intermediate-acting insulin before breakfast
Regular and intermediate-acting insulin before the evening meal

1082 Section XII: Endocrinology

control meal-mediated glycemia and 25% to control the overnight plasma glucose. The initial insulin dose will need to be modified based on the patient's degree of insulin resistance. The insulin dose then is adjusted every day or two based on the results of blood glucose monitoring (which should be performed before breakfast, before lunch, before the evening meal, and at 10 PM). Table 107.3 presents the time courses of action of human insulin, and Table 107.4 details the use of finger-stick blood glucose monitoring to adjust the insulin. Many insulins are available for subcutaneous use. These include basal insulin (such as glargine insulin), intermediate-acting insulins (such as NPH and Lente insulin), and regular soluble insulin and rapid-acting synthetic insulin analogs (such as lispro insulin, aspart insulin, and glulisine insulin). The rapid-acting synthetic analogs have the advantage that their onset of action when administered subcutaneously is 10 or 15 minutes and their duration of action is approximately 3–4 hours. One of them might be used in those infrequent cases in which these attributes are important. Glargine insulin is attractive in that it is a basal insulin with a 24-hour duration of action, it maintains a peakless plasma level, and it gives a reproducible profile from day to day. Premixed combinations of NPH and regular insulin, and NPH and a rapid-acting insulin, are available as 70/30 and 50/50 preparations. These can be used in twice-a-day treatment regimens but are of limited utility in the hospital because of the fixed proportion of intermediate-acting and regular or rapid-acting insulins.

Hospitalized patients on a subcutaneously administered insulin treatment program must receive their meals on time, and the quantity consumed must be noted. When a meal is to be held or missed for a study, the appropriate insulin dose should be held or reduced accordingly.

The time course of action of the human insulins (Table 107.3) makes it difficult to achieve glycemic levels between 110 and 175 mg/dL with only two daily injections of mixed insulins (regimen 4, Table 107.2) because the action of the intermediate-acting insulin peaks during the early morning hours (approximately 2–3 AM) and is effectively over by 5–7 AM. Thus, it is common for a patient to be hypoglycemic at 2–3 AM and hyperglycemic at 7 AM. The administration of regular insulin before the evening meal and intermediate-acting insulin at 10 PM solves this problem and generally leads to good glycemic control when coupled with administration of regular plus intermediate-acting insulin before breakfast (regimen 1). Regular insulin and mixtures of regular and intermediate-acting insulin should be administered 30–45 minutes before the meal. A treatment program in which regular insulin is given before each meal and intermediate-acting insulin is given at 10 PM (regimen 3) is necessary only for patients whose meal pattern is totally erratic or in whom fever or stress is fluctuating rapidly. Insulin doses should be adjusted every 1–2 days based on the results of blood glucose monitoring, not according to a "sliding scale" protocol.

The treatment of hospitalized patients with oral antidiabetic agents is generally ineffective. Patients taking oral agents before hospitalization should discontinue them and then restart them after their acute problem has resolved. This is particularly true for metformin (which can cause lactic acidosis in the presence of impaired renal or hepatic function or congestive heart failure) and sulfonylureas (which have prolonged durations of action and rarely allow for consistent glycemic control in acutely ill diabetic patients).

The only instance in which oral antidiabetic therapy may be indicated in the hospitalized patient is during an admission for an uncomplicated diagnostic procedure or minimally invasive surgery under local anesthesia.

TABLE 107.3

TIME COURSE OF ACTION OF HUMAN INSULIN PREPARATIONS ADMINISTERED SUBCUTANEOUSLY

Insulin preparation	Onset of action (h)	Peak action (h)	Effective duration of action (h)
Lispro insulin	0.15–0.33	1–3	3–5
Aspart insulin	0.15–0.33	1–3	3–5
Glulisine insulin	0.15–0.33	1–3	3–5
Regular (soluble)	0.5–1	2–4	5–8
NPH (isophane)	1–2	5–7	13–18
Lente (insulin zinc suspension)	1–3	4–8	13–20
Glargine insulin	1.5	no peak	up to 24
Combination 70/30 (70% NPH, 30% regular)	0.5–1		10–16
Combination 50/50 (50% NPH, 50% regular)	0.5–1		10–16
Combination (70% NPH + 30% aspart or lispro)	0.15–0.33		10–16

TABLE 107.4

ADJUSTMENT OF SUBCUTANEOUSLY ADMINISTERED INSULIN DOSE BY MEASUREMENT OF BLOOD GLUCOSE BY FINGER-STICK

Regimen 1

Regular and intermediate-acting insulin before breakfast
  Adjust regular insulin dose from results of pre-lunch blood glucose
  Adjust intermediate-acting insulin dose from results of pre-evening meal blood glucose
Regular insulin before the evening meal
  Adjust dose from results of 10 PM blood glucose
Intermediate-acting insulin at 10 PM
  Adjust dose from results of next morning's fasting (pre-breakfast) blood glucose

Regimen 2

Basal insulin (glargine insulin) once a day
  Dose can be given anytime and is adjusted based on fasting blood glucose
Regular or rapid-acting insulin before each meal
  Adjust dose by results of pre-meal blood glucose

Regimen 3

Regular insulin before each meal
  Adjust dose from results of next pre-meal blood glucose
Intermediate-acting insulin at 10 PM
  Adjust dose from results of next morning's fasting blood glucose

Regimen 4

Regular and intermediate-acting insulin before breakfast
  Adjust regular insulin dose from results of pre-lunch blood glucose
  Adjust intermediate-acting insulin dose from results of pre-evening meal blood glucose
Regular and intermediate-acting insulin before the evening meal
  Adjust regular insulin dose from results of 10 PM blood glucose
  Adjust intermediate-acting insulin dose from results of next morning's fasting blood glucose

In these instances, the oral medications are held the morning of the procedure and restarted after the procedure is finished.

MANAGEMENT OF THE DIABETIC PATIENT HOSPITALIZED FOR ORDINARY MEDICAL ILLNESSES OR POOR GLYCEMIC REGULATION

The majority of diabetic patients are hospitalized for ordinary medical illnesses or poor glycemic control. In either event, the major symptoms related to their diabetes are weakness, fatigue, polydipsia, polyuria, weight loss, and blurry vision. The hyperglycemic patient invariably shows signs of dehydration.

The goal of therapy is to bring the glucose into the target range of 110–175 mg/dL. A tradition among attending physicians and house staff is to place the diabetic patient on "sliding scale" coverage. Placing the patient on a treatment algorithm that stops insulin treatment when glycemic control is good and treats with insulin after severe hyperglycemia and its consequences have developed is both irrational and counterproductive (7). Figure 107.1 illustrates the results of sliding scale coverage versus a planned insulin treatment regimen taken from a typical consultation at our medical center. Panel A (left) shows the clinical course of a 69-year-old man admitted to the surgical service for treatment of a hand abscess. On the surgical and rehabilitation services, he was treated with sliding scale coverage, which led to numerous blood glucose levels between 200 and 350 mg/dL, with wide excursions and no improvement in his glycemic control. After consultation, he was placed on the three-injection insulin treatment program (regimen 1 in Table 107.2), with the results shown in Panel B (right).

Effective hospital management of the diabetic patient cannot be achieved with "sliding scale" coverage. A carefully planned and adjusted insulin treatment regimen that is based on an understanding of the pathophysiology of hyperglycemia and the pharmacology of insulin treatment is essential for achieving adequate glycemic control.

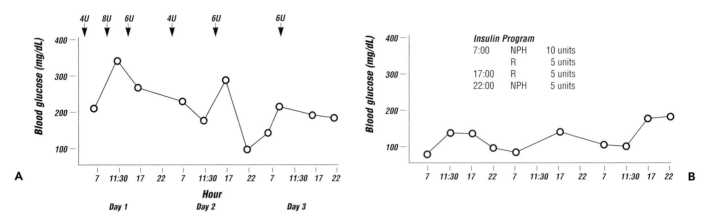

Figure 107.1 Blood glucose levels, by hospital day, in a patient who was initially covered with a "sliding scale" (*Panel A*) and later switched to a three-injection subcutaneous insulin treatment program (*Panel B*). *NPH*, isophane insulin; *R*, regular insulin.

MANAGEMENT OF THE DIABETIC PATIENT HOSPITALIZED FOR SURGERY

The management of diabetic patients who are hospitalized for surgery should be thought of as encompassing three distinct phases of care: preoperative, intraoperative, and postoperative management.

Preoperatively, glucose control should be optimized to levels between 110 and 175 mg/dL. Long-acting antihyperglycemic agents and metformin should be stopped and insulin treatment regimens initiated if necessary. Cardiac, renal, and peripheral vascular function should be assessed and optimized.

Intraoperative management should be coordinated with the anesthesiologist. During surgery, regular insulin, glucose, and potassium should be administered intravenously. The goal of treatment is to maintain plasma glucose between 110 and 175 mg/dL. Several techniques of administration have been recommended. Gill and Alberti (5) infuse a glucose, potassium, and insulin (GKI) solution (15 units of regular human insulin and 10 mEq of potassium chloride in 500 mL of 10% glucose) at 100 mL/h. The GKI solution is started on the morning of surgery (subcutaneous insulin and food are withheld) and is continued during and after surgery until both the diet and subcutaneous insulin can be safely restarted. Blood glucose is monitored frequently by finger-stick. If the glucose is too high, a fresh GKI solution, this one containing 20 units of insulin, is started. A blood glucose level that is too low requires a reduction to 10 units of insulin per bag of GKI solution. If necessary, further adjustments in insulin can be made in increments of 5 units. With this approach, at least 80% of diabetic patients can maintain plasma glucose levels between 100 and 200 mg/dL during and immediately after surgery. This technique is particularly useful when insulin requirements during the operative and postoperative period are reasonably constant.

For patients in whom fluid overload is a concern, the glucose concentration can be doubled to 20% and the rate of infusion decreased to 25 or 50 mL/h. Serum potassium needs to be monitored every 4–6 hours because the potassium chloride content of the infusion may need to be altered. Prolonged GKI administration can lead to dilutional hyponatremia, which may require simultaneous administration of 0.9% saline solution. The ordinary ratio of insulin to glucose is 0.30 units of insulin per gram of glucose. Conditions such as severe obesity, major infections, liver disease, or steroid therapy may increase the requirement to 0.4–0.8 units of insulin per gram of glucose.

Another approach is to administer the insulin and glucose by separate infusion pumps in "piggyback" fashion. This allows independent regulation of the insulin and glucose infusion rates while a single entry portal is maintained. The glucose can be given as a 5%, 10%, or 20% solution. Insulin can be given at a rate of 0.5–10.0 units/h. Adjustments are made as necessary. Again, the goal is to maintain plasma glucose between 110 and 175 mg/dL and provide enough glucose to minimize catabolism. This approach is strongly preferred over the GKI solution approach in patients undergoing extensive surgery, especially in cases in which insulin requirements vary during different parts of the procedure and postoperative period. For example, insulin requirements during cardiac surgery average 1.6 units/h during the preoperative period, 3.0 units/h from the time of the skin incision to the onset of bypass, 5.0 units/h while the patient is on bypass, 8.3 units/h immediately after bypass, and 12.3 units/h postoperatively.

The importance of glucose control during cardiac surgery has been emphasized by Zerr and colleagues (8) and subsequent publications from the Portland Diabetes Program (4). As noted earlier, they treat their diabetic patients undergoing open heart surgery with IV insulin and glucose by "piggyback" during surgery and through the first 48 postoperative hours to maintain a plasma glucose below 175

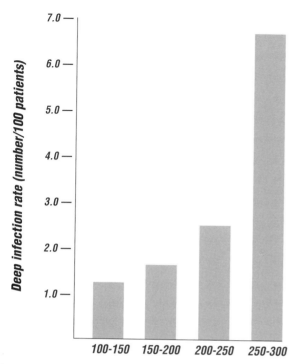

Figure 107.2 Deep infection rate in 1,585 diabetic patients undergoing cardiac surgery, as a function of mean 48-hour postoperative glucose levels. (Redrawn from Zerr KJ, Furnary AP, Grunkemeier GL, et al. Glucose control lowers the risk of wound infection in diabetics after open heart operations. *Ann Thorac Surg* 1997;63:356–361, with permission.)

mg/dL. In assessing the relationship between glucose control and the development of deep wound infections in the first 1,585 diabetic patients undergoing cardiac surgery from 1987 to 1993 (595 of whom were treated with this intensive glucose control program), Zerr and colleagues reported a significant relationship between the mean 48-hour postoperative plasma glucose level and the development of serious wound infections (Figure 107.2).

During minimal surgery under local anesthesia, diabetic patients can frequently be managed by withholding food and oral antihyperglycemic agents on the morning of surgery, avoiding glucose-containing IV fluids, monitoring blood glucose every two hours and treating with a single insulin bolus if necessary, and restarting oral antihyperglycemic agents with the first postoperative meal.

MANAGEMENT OF THE DIABETIC PATIENT HOSPITALIZED FOR ACUTE MYOCARDIAL INFARCTION

The management of the diabetic patient with an acute myocardial infarction is analogous to that of the diabetic patient with any acute severe illness who can have nothing by mouth. Here, too, the philosophy of diabetes management has often been to treat only severe hyperglycemia, usually through the use of the "sliding scale."

The Diabetes Mellitus Insulin Glucose Infusion in Myocardial Infarction (DIGAMI) study has refocused attention on the role of good glycemic control in reducing both the short-term and long-term mortality of diabetic patients with acute myocardial infarction (9). This study randomized 620 diabetic patients with acute myocardial infarction to either standard diabetes treatment or intensive treatment. The latter consisted of IV insulin and glucose for the first 24–48 hours, followed by subcutaneous regular insulin four times daily for at least three months. Twenty-four hours after randomization, the intensive treatment group had a mean blood glucose level of 173 mg/dL (vs. 211 in the standard treatment group). Whether because of the improved acute glucose control or the improved control during the next three months, the intensively treated patients experienced a 28% (and statistically significant) relative reduction in three-year mortality. Although still controversial, the results of the DIGAMI study and other similar efforts support the concept that plasma glucose levels should be maintained between 110 and 175 mg/dL in acutely ill diabetic patients.

THE ROLE OF INTENSIVE GLYCEMIC CONTROL BY INTRAVENOUS INSULIN IN CRITICALLY ILL PATIENTS

It has been recognized for many years that acutely ill hospitalized patients have a high incidence of hyperglycemia (blood glucose ≥110 mg/dL). The past approach was to attribute this hyperglycemia to stress and not to treat it unless the blood glucose values exceeded 220 mg/dL. In fact, many believed that the "stress hyperglycemia" might even be beneficial by providing extra glucose to the tissues. As evidence accumulated that severe stress inhibits insulin secretion and causes marked insulin resistance, with all its detrimental metabolic abnormalities, investigators began to hypothesize that the hyperglycemia and/or related metabolic abnormalities might actually contribute to increased morbidity and mortality. This was tested in a surgical ICU population of 1,548 mechanically ventilated patients. Patients were randomized to intensive insulin treatment (continuous intravenous insulin with frequent blood glucose monitoring, with maintenance of blood glucose throughout their ICU stay in the range of of 80–110 mg/dL) or conventional treatment (with insulin infusion only if their blood glucose exceeded 215 mg/dL and blood glucose levels maintained between 180 and 200 mg/dL) (1). Mortality among patients who were in the ICU five days or more was reduced from 20.2% in the conventional treatment group to 10.6% in the intensively treated group. Intensive treatment reduced overall in-hospital mortality by 34%, bloodstream infections by 46%, acute renal failure by 41%, and critical illness polyneuropathy by 44%. The clinical benefits were present *whether or not the patients had previously diagnosed diabetes.* *Post hoc* analysis showed that patients with even modest hyperglycemia (mean blood glucose levels of 110–150 mg/dL) in the conventionally treated group had a higher mortality rate than those in the intensively treated group. The relationship between glycemic control and mortality was linear, with a 75% increase in mortality for each 50 mg/dL increase in mean blood glucose. While the clinical benefits correlated with blood glucose control, they also correlated with other improvements in metabolism, such as normalization of dyslipidemia, suppression of inflammation, and improvement in macrophage function.

Other benefits of intensive insulin treatment were a decrease in number of required blood transfusions, reduced duration of ICU stay, and a yearly cost savings of at least $40,000 per patient.

Tight glucose control was not without risks. Intensive insulin therapy was associated with an increased risk of hypoglycemia (5.2% versus 0.8%). However, because of the frequent blood glucose monitoring, these episodes were always rapidly diagnosed and treated and were not associated with any serious adverse events.

Protocols for intensive intravenous insulin treatment can be found in two recent references (10, 11).

DIABETIC KETOACIDOSIS AND HYPEROSMOLAR HYPERGLYCEMIC NONKETOTIC SYNDROME

Issues at the Time of Admission

Definition and Epidemiology

Diabetic ketoacidosis (DKA) and hyperosmolar hyperglycemic nonketotic syndrome (HHNS) represent the extremes of the metabolic derangements that occur in patients with diabetes mellitus. Early recognition and appropriate treatment of these life-threatening illnesses are essential. The incidence of DKA is reported to be 4.6–8.0 per 1,000 diabetic patient-years, and the incidence of HHNS is approximately 0.6–1.0 per 1,000 diabetic patient-years. These two entities are not distinctly different syndromes but represent variants of the disturbed metabolism that occurs in unregulated diabetes mellitus. DKA is characterized by hyperglycemia, ketosis, and acidosis (arterial pH $\leq$7.30; plasma anion gap $\geq$16 mmol/L; serum bicarbonate $\leq$15 mmol/L). HHNS is characterized by plasma glucose above 600 mg/dL, plasma osmolality above 320 mOsm/L, little or no ketonemia, and arterial pH above 7.30 (Table 107.5). The patient who presents with HHNS usually has type II diabetes, is over the age of 50 years, and has some underlying impairment of renal function. The patient with DKA is more likely to have type I diabetes and to be younger and free of other chronic diseases not related to diabetes. It is important, however, to emphasize that DKA is a relatively common presentation for newly diagnosed type II diabetes in African-

American and Latino patients. As many as one in four cases of DKA occur in patients with previously undiagnosed diabetes. Many patients present with features of both syndromes (i.e., marked hyperosmolality and ketoacidosis). Mortality from DKA in the United States ranges from 2%–5%, whereas that from HHNS is reported to be as low as 12% and as high as 42%.

Pathophysiology

Table 107.6 summarizes the pathophysiology of DKA and HHNS. The primary abnormality is *markedly deficient insulin secretion*. Insulin deficiency at the level of adipose tissue results in an increase in lipolysis and the release of large quantities of free fatty acids into the circulation. Insulin deficiency also causes an increase in β-oxidation of free fatty acids in the liver, which generates increases in ketone bodies (acetoacetate and β-hydroxybutyrate). Moreover, decreased insulin action increases gluconeogenesis and glycogenolysis, which leads to markedly excessive hepatic glucose production. Insulin deficiency in muscle results in a profound fall in glucose uptake and utilization.

TABLE 107.5

TYPICAL LABORATORY FINDINGS IN PATIENTS WITH DKA OR HHNS

	DKA	HHNS
Plasma glucose (mg/dL)	200–600	$\geq$1,000
Osmolality (mOsm/L)	300–320	360
Plasma ketones (positive)	1:16	Trace or negative
Blood pH	<7.30	$\geq$7.30
Plasma anion gap (mEq/L)	Usually >20	Usually <20
Serum HCO$_3$ (mmol/L)	Usually <15	Usually >15

DKA, diabetic ketoacidosis; *HHNS*, hyperosmolar hyperglycemic nonketotic syndrome.

TABLE 107.6

METABOLIC ABNORMALITIES IN DKA AND HHNS

Organ	DKA	HHNS
Adipose tissue		
Lipolysis	↑↑↑	↑
Liver		
Glucose production	↑	↑↑↑
Ketone production	↑↑↑	↑
Muscle		
Glucose uptake	↓	↓
Proteolysis	↑↑	↑↑↑

DKA, diabetic ketoacidosis; *HHNS*, hyperosmolar hyperglycemic nonketotic syndrome.

It also stimulates muscle proteolysis, which in turn increases lactate and alanine release into the circulation.

The alanine and lactate provide the substrate, and the free fatty acid oxidation provides the energy for hepatic gluconeogenesis. As a result of the exaggerated glucose production by the liver and the decreased ability of muscle to take up glucose, hyperglycemia develops. Once the plasma glucose level exceeds 200 mg/dL, glucose is excreted by the kidneys, and the ensuing osmotic diuresis causes electrolyte loss and dehydration. The markedly increased levels of ketone bodies (which are weak acids) exceeds the buffering capacity of plasma. The efforts to compensate for the acidosis lead to further losses of electrolytes and to Kussmaul respiration. Table 107.7 describes the relationship between the metabolic abnormalities that occur in DKA or HHNS and the symptoms and signs with which patients present.

Diagnosis

The diagnosis of DKA must be considered in any patient who presents with symptoms of diabetes mellitus (polydipsia, polyuria, weight loss) and who shows signs of dehydration, acidosis, or both (12). The patient who presents with drowsiness, mental obtundation, or coma should raise particular concern. The diagnosis is confirmed by demonstrating a plasma glucose level above 200 mg/dL and the presence of urinary ketones, increased plasma ketones, and an arterial pH of 7.30 or less. The anion gap is increased, and the serum bicarbonate is below 15 mmol/L. The degree of hyperglycemia is not a reliable indicator of the severity of DKA. Euglycemic DKA has been well documented and usually results from factors that decrease hepatic gluconeogenesis (alcohol ingestion, starvation with decreased substrate available for gluconeogenesis, sepsis, or parenchymal liver disease). Appropriate therapy must focus on the treatment of ketonemia and acidosis.

The diagnosis of HHNS should be suspected in any patient who presents with mental obtundation and is severely dehydrated. Patients with HHNS tend to be older than those with DKA. The onset of symptoms is often more insidious, and patients more commonly have precipitating illnesses. The diagnosis of HHNS is confirmed by demonstration of plasma glucose above 600 mg/dL, a plasma osmolality above 320 mOsm/L, and minimal or no ketosis and acidosis.

A diabetic patient presenting with significant hyperosmolality, dehydration, or acidosis should be hospitalized unless adequate outpatient facilities for management and monitoring are available.

Management

The major principles in managing DKA or HHNS are as follows (12):

1. Make a rapid diagnosis, and initiate treatment immediately.
2. Maintain organ perfusion by restoring blood volume and supporting blood pressure.
3. Administer IV insulin to decrease free fatty acid release and excess ketone body and glucose production by the liver and to increase peripheral tissue glucose uptake.

TABLE 107.7

RELATIONSHIP BETWEEN METABOLIC ABNORMALITIES AND SIGNS AND SYMPTOMS OF DKA AND HHNS

Metabolic abnormality	Symptoms	Signs or ECG changes
Hyperglycemia	Malaise	Decreased muscle mass
	Tiredness	
Catabolic state	Weight loss	
	Muscle weakness	
Osmotic diuresis	Polyuria	Dehydration
	Polydipsia	Dry mucous membranes
	Thirst	Decreased skin turgor
		Tachycardia
		Hypotension
Hyperosmolality	Sleepiness	Multiple aspects of cerebral dysfunction
	Mental obtundation	
	Coma	
Ketoacidosis	Shortness of breath	Tachypnea
	Abdominal pain	Kussmaul respiration
	Nausea and vomiting	
Electrolyte loss	Muscle cramps	Various ECG abnormalities
	Cardiac arrhythmias	

DKA, diabetic ketoacidosis; *ECG*, electrocardiographic; *HHNS*, hyperosmolar hyperglycemic nonketotic syndrome.

4. Replace electrolytes to prevent fatal hypokalemia and relieve severe symptomatic acidosis.
5. Prevent cerebral edema.
6. Minimize thromboembolic events.
7. Look for and treat concurrent illnesses, such as infections, that may have contributed to the development of ketoacidosis or hyperglycemia.

Fluid Replacement

The average patient with DKA has a deficit of 5–8 L of body water, 300–1,000 mEq of potassium, 400–700 mEq of sodium, and significant but variable amounts of phosphate and magnesium. Fluid replacement should begin immediately to maintain organ perfusion. Even though patients with DKA or HHNS are more water deficient than sodium deficient, it is best to start IV fluid replacement with 0.9% saline solution to replenish blood volume rapidly. One liter of 0.9% saline solution per hour for the first hour or two is usually adequate to maintain circulatory dynamics. This can be followed by 0.9% saline solution at 500 mL/h for the next four hours and 250 mL/h thereafter. If the serum sodium exceeds 150 mEq/L, 0.45% saline solution is administered instead of the 0.9% concentration. Faster infusion of saline solution leads to more protracted acidosis and no more rapid correction of hyperglycemia. If the patient presents with circulatory insufficiency (hypovolemic shock), 1–2 L of colloidal plasma expanders can be given.

Rehydration itself lowers blood glucose by increasing renal perfusion and glucose excretion and by decreasing the plasma levels of counterregulatory hormones. Once the plasma glucose has been reduced to 250 mg/dL, infusion of 5% or 10% glucose should replace the infusion of normal saline to allow for continued administration of insulin to correct the ketosis and metabolic acidosis. If the patient is still dehydrated at this stage, saline solution and glucose can be simultaneously administered.

A similar scheme of fluid replacement is used to correct the dehydration and fluid abnormalities in HHNS. Note that hypernatremia is more common in HHNS, and one should consider switching to hypotonic solutions after the first 1–2 L of 0.9% saline solution has been infused. Patients with extreme hyperosmolality (>350 mOsm/L) are at risk for thromboembolism, and prophylactic low-dose heparin is generally appropriate.

Insulin Administration

Low-dose soluble (regular) human insulin administered as a continuous IV infusion is the ideal treatment for DKA or HHNS. The usual starting dose is between 5 and 10 units/h in DKA; patients with HHNS often need less insulin (1–5 units/h). Intramuscular soluble human insulin can be used if tissue perfusion is good. This requires a loading dose of 10–20 units followed by 5 units/h. Subcutaneously administered insulin has no place in the treatment of DKA or HHNS.

Blood glucose should be monitored hourly and the insulin infusion rate adjusted up or down as necessary. A reasonable goal for treating the hyperglycemia is to decrease the glucose level by 75–90 mg/dL per hour until it reaches 250 mg/dL, at which time that level should be maintained with insulin (approximately 2–4 units/h) and glucose infusion (5% or 10%) until the ketosis and acidosis are resolved. At that time, the intravenous administration of insulin can be replaced with subcutaneous administration, provided the patient has recovered and is taking oral nutrition.

Potassium Replacement

Serum potassium levels at presentation of DKA may be high, normal, or low despite the total body potassium deficiency. Death can occur from hypokalemia or, rarely, from hyperkalemia, so the management of potassium levels in DKA is of critical importance. *Treatment of DKA is invariably associated with a fall in plasma potassium concentrations.* This fall results from rehydration of intracellular and extracellular fluid compartments, a direct effect of insulin on intracellular potassium transport, correction of acidosis, and excretion of urinary potassium with restoration of renal function.

If urine flow is adequate and the presenting plasma potassium level is normal or low, potassium replacement should begin when insulin therapy is started. If the initial plasma potassium is high (≥ 6 mEq/L) or urine flow is markedly decreased, it may be necessary to delay the start of potassium replacement by one or two hours until the plasma potassium begins to decrease. Potassium should be replaced at 20–30 mEq/h. If hypokalemia is present or bicarbonate is administered, then 40–80 mEq/h may be needed (Chapter 104). The plasma potassium should be monitored and maintained between 3.5 and 5.0 mEq/L. Potassium chloride is preferred initially but may be converted to potassium phosphate once the serum phosphate falls. Electrocardiographic monitoring is useful but is no substitute for frequent laboratory measurements of serum potassium.

Bicarbonate Treatment

The routine use of bicarbonate in the treatment of DKA is not beneficial and can actually increase ketone production and cause detrimental effects such as hypokalemia, paradoxical worsening of cerebrospinal fluid acidosis, and impaired oxyhemoglobin dissociation. Bicarbonate should be considered in patients with DKA only if their acidosis is so severe that they are in imminent danger of cardiovascular collapse. If the arterial pH is less than 7.0 or if bicarbonate levels are extremely low (<5 mEq/L), 50–100 mmol of sodium bicarbonate in 250–1,000 mL of 0.45% saline solution, with 10–20 mmol of potassium added, can be given over 30–60 minutes. This can be repeated until the arterial pH exceeds 7.0.

Replacement of Other Electrolytes

Total body phosphate, magnesium, and calcium are depleted in DKA and HHNS, and plasma phosphate and magnesium fall significantly during fluid replacement. Low plasma phosphate or magnesium rarely causes untoward effects during treatment of DKA, and so replacement of these electrolytes is not routinely needed. However, serum phosphate levels below 1.0 mg/dL are associated with rhabdomyolysis, hemolysis, and cardiac dysfunction, so it is reasonable to replace phosphate if plasma levels fall below 1.5 mg/dL. Intravenous administration of phosphate (1–2 mmol/L per kilogram of body weight) during 6–12 hours is the usual treatment. Magnesium therapy is indicated only for ventricular arrhythmias that are not attributable to hypokalemia.

Complications of Treatment

The major complications of treatment for DKA and HHNS are associated with fluid overload: pulmonary edema, hypoglycemia, thromboembolism, cerebral edema, and acute respiratory distress syndrome. *Fluid overload* and *hypoglycemia* are prevented by proper monitoring of fluid intake and output, central venous pressure monitoring if indicated, and bedside blood glucose monitoring. *Cerebral edema* is a rare but well-recognized complication of treatment. It usually occurs 2–24 hours after treatment begins, is characterized by severe headache and deterioration in the level of consciousness, and is rapidly progressive and fatal if not treated aggressively (Chapter 117). The pathophysiology is poorly understood but is thought to be associated with rapid hydration and quick reduction of plasma osmolality. Treatment, which must be initiated immediately, consists of 0.5–2.0 g of IV mannitol per kilogram of body weight. The complication is best prevented by limiting the pace with which both dehydration and plasma hyperosmolality are corrected. *Acute respiratory distress syndrome* is characterized by the sudden onset of dyspnea and hypoxemia, decreasing lung compliance, and the presence of diffuse pulmonary infiltrates on chest radiography (Chapter 24). Mortality is high, and treatment consists of ventilatory support. As with cerebral edema, the cause of this rare complication is unknown. One possibility is a rapid decrease in oncotic pressure; another is a specific alveolar capillary defect induced by acidosis and hyperventilation.

Thromboembolic complications of DKA and HHNS are related to the hypercoagulable state caused by hyperglycemia and increased viscosity resulting from severe hyperosmolality. Prophylactic heparin therapy seems appropriate in severe cases, but there are no studies to support this practice.

Issues During the Course of Hospitalization

Initial therapy should result in resolution of DKA or HHNS within the first 24–36 hours of hospitalization. Careful attention to metabolic regulation should avoid the complications of treatment. On hospital days 2 through 4, any problems that contributed to the development of DKA or HHNS (e.g., infections) should be addressed. Patients in whom DKA or HHNS has resolved and who are taking oral nutrition can also be converted to a subcutaneous insulin treatment regimen (in the case of DKA) or to either a subcutaneous insulin or oral antihyperglycemic treatment regimen (in the case of HHNS).

When a patient is switched from an IV to a subcutaneous insulin regimen, it is important to recognize that the effects of IV insulin generally last for less than an hour. Subcutaneous soluble (regular) human insulin achieves peak levels 2–4 hours after injection, and subcutaneous NPH or Lente human insulin achieves such levels 6–9 hours after injection. Therefore, the subcutaneously administered insulin program (Table 107.2) should be initiated 1–3 hours before IV insulin is discontinued.

Discharge Issues

The major issues at discharge are ensuring that the patient receives adequate diabetes education and planning appropriate outpatient management for glycemic, lipid, and blood pressure control. Diabetes education is essential if the patient is to learn how to prevent recurrent episodes of DKA or HHNS. It can also help the patient achieve target goals for metabolic control as an outpatient. In addition to receiving inpatient education, the patient should be referred to a diabetes education center staffed by diabetes educators and dieticians.

Most patients with DKA are discharged on a subcutaneous insulin treatment regimen, usually consisting of 2–4 injections per day. Adjustments to target glycemic controls are made in the outpatient setting. Patients with type II diabetes presenting with DKA are discharged on a subcutaneous insulin treatment program and can frequently be switched to oral antihyperglycemic agents after several months of good outpatient glycemic control. Many patients with HHNS can be switched from insulin-based regimens to oral antihyperglycemic agents within several weeks of discharge.

Patients being discharged after admission for DKA or HHNS should monitor their blood glucose regularly and their urine for ketone bodies when they feel ill. Such monitoring enables them to recognize early ketosis and take appropriate steps to prevent DKA.

HYPOGLYCEMIA

Issues at the Time of Admission

Although hypoglycemia is common, it rarely justifies hospitalization in and of itself. Hypoglycemia is caused by either inadequate production of glucose by the liver and kidney or excessive peripheral utilization of glucose. Both these processes are influenced by insulin and counterregulatory hormones. Excessive administration or secretion of insulin increases peripheral glucose utilization and decreases hepatic glucose production. Counterregulatory hormones increase hepatic glucose production and gradually decrease peripheral tissue sensitivity to insulin. In the normal person, a falling blood glucose level triggers an autonomic response that increases hepatic glucose production, decreases insulin secretion, and causes hunger (resulting in increased food intake). Diabetic patients treated with insulin or insulin secretagogues are not able to compensate for hypoglycemia by decreasing insulin secretion, and the autonomic nervous system function of these patients may be impaired, which hampers the counterregulatory responses to hypoglycemia.

Clinical Presentation

Symptoms of hypoglycemia are attributable to activation of the autonomic nervous system (sweating, tachycardia, tremor, and hunger) or to cerebral glucose deficiency (decreased cognitive function, mental obtundation, and coma). Ordinarily, autonomic nervous symptoms occur first and warn the person that hypoglycemia is occurring so that food can be sought. Neuroglycopenic (cerebral glucose deficiency) symptoms may render a person incapable of combating the hypoglycemia. Unfortunately, in patients with tightly controlled type I diabetes or in diabetic patients with autonomic neuropathy, hypoglycemic unawareness (i.e., lack of the autonomic response) results in the loss of these autonomic warning signs. In such persons, the sudden occurrence of neuroglycopenic symptoms must be treated by someone other than the patient.

Diagnosis

A history of classic symptoms accompanied by a blood glucose level below 50 mg/dL confirms the diagnosis of hypoglycemia. All patients who present with cognitive disorders, personality changes, or disturbed consciousness should have their blood glucose measured. If hypoglycemia is found, a history of diabetes with insulin or insulin secretagogue administration should be sought. Other causes of hypoglycemia to be considered in a person without diabetes include islet cell tumors, liver disease, adrenal insufficiency, and mesenchymal tumors.

Indications for Hospitalization

Most episodes of severe hypoglycemia in type I diabetic patients can be managed in the emergency department. Prolonged severe hypoglycemia can lead to temporary or permanent neurologic damage, and patients exhibiting such signs and symptoms require hospital admission for evaluation.

Any diabetic patient taking insulin secretagogues (sulfonylureas) in whom hypoglycemia sufficient to cause severe neuroglycopenic symptoms develops needs to be hospitalized for treatment. Drugs such as chlorpropamide, glyburide, and glipizide may continue to cause hypoglycemia for periods as long as 24–72 hours. Therefore, treatment requires not only acute IV glucose administration but also longer infusions for 24–72 hours.

Initial Therapy

The usual treatment of hypoglycemia is immediate administration of 50 mL of 50% glucose in water. This is followed by an infusion of 10% glucose administered at a rate of 100 mL/h. The infusion rate is adjusted based on the blood glucose determination.

Intravenous or intramuscular administration of 1 mg of glucagon can facilitate the treatment of hypoglycemia in diabetic subjects but is effective only if the patient is well nourished and liver glycogen stores are adequate. In the hospital setting (where IV glucose is available), there is no indication for glucagon administration. In the event that IV access is not possible or is delayed, intramuscular glucagon administration can temporarily relieve the hypoglycemia until other measures can be instituted.

In a patient who develops severe hypoglycemia secondary to insulin secretagogues and is partially resistant to treatment with intravenous glucose, the addition of octreotide 50 mcg subcutaneously every eight hours for 2–3 doses can help ameliorate the hypoglycemia. The octreotide inhibits endogenous insulin secretion. In patients with hypoglycemia secondary to insulin-producing tumors, either octreotide or oral diazoxide can reduce insulin secretion and improve hypoglycemia.

Issues During the Course of Hospitalization

The major issue for the diabetic patient during hospitalization is to identify the precipitants of hypoglycemia and educate the patient about measures to modify them. Usually, precipitants involve inadequate meal planning, not preparing for strenuous exercise, excessive ingestion of alcohol, or an inappropriate diabetic treatment program.

Discharge Issues

The primary discharge issues are educational. Persons with type I diabetes who have had a severe hypoglycemic episode are at increased risk for additional episodes. The treatment plan of each patient should be reevaluated.

COST CONSIDERATIONS AND RESOURCE USE

In one survey, 23.8% of all adults with diabetes reported being hospitalized in the previous year (13). The majority of these patients were hospitalized for the care of chronic complications or for other medical or surgical illnesses. A one-day extension of hospital stay for each diabetic patient would result in an increase of approximately 2.3 million hospital bed-days. It is obvious that efficient regulation of glycemia during hospital admissions could yield enormous savings in health care resources.

Approximately 50%–75% of DKA episodes are caused by a lack of appropriate care, either attributable to the patient or the health care system. Diabetes education for patients and their families can have a major impact in reducing episodes of ketoacidosis.

The cost of long-term diabetes care has been shown to correlate well with the quality of glycemic control. Costs of medical care were calculated for a cohort of diabetic patients in a health care plan during the three-year period from 1992 to 1995 (14). The costs for patients with a hemoglobin A1$_c$ of 7%, 8%, 9%, and 10% were 4%, 10%, 20%, and 30% higher, respectively, than the costs for comparable patients with a hemoglobin A1$_c$ of 6%. For a patient with diabetes, hypertension, and heart disease with a hemoglobin A1$_c$ of 10%, the three-year cost of care was $49,673; the cost for a comparable patient with a hemoglobin A1$_c$ of 6% was $38,726. Thus, appropriate management of hospitalized patients with diabetes mellitus can result not only in better outcomes but also in huge reductions in health care costs and utilization.

KEY POINTS

- The clinical management of diabetic patients includes appropriate hospital management in addition to long-term metabolic control in the outpatient setting.
- Optimal glycemic control (in the range of 110 to 175 mg/dL) has been shown to improve outcomes and lower costs in hospitalized diabetic patients.
- Hyperglycemia in acutely ill ICU patients should be normalized by an intensive insulin treatment program.
- Acute metabolic complications of diabetes (diabetic ketoacidosis and hyperosmolar hyperglycemic nonketotic syndrome) can be life threatening. Appropriate management includes rapid correction of glycemia and electrolyte and fluid imbalance, treatment of any precipitants, and a coordinated transition to outpatient care.
- Hypoglycemia is managed acutely with glucose infusion, which may need to be continued for days if the precipitant was a long-acting oral hypoglycemic agent. Hypoglycemia often represents a failure of diabetes education, which should be addressed before the patient is discharged.

REFERENCES

1. Van den Berghe G, Wouters P, Weekers F, et al. Intensive insulin therapy in critically ill patients. *N Engl J Med* 2001;345: 1359–1367.
2. Rayfield EJ, Ault MJ, Keusch GT, Brothers MJ, Nechemias C, Smith H. Infection and diabetes: the case for glucose control. *Am J Med* 1982;72:439–450.
3. Alexiewicz JM, Kumar D, Smogorzewski M, Klin M, Massry SG. Polymorphonuclear leukocytes in non–insulin-dependent diabetes mellitus: abnormalities in metabolism and function. *Ann Intern Med* 1995;123:919–924.
4. Furnary AP, Wu YX, Bookin SO. Effect of hyperglycemia and continuous intravenous insulin infusions on outcomes of cardiac surgical procedures: the Portland Diabetic Project. *Endocr Pract* 2004;10(Suppl 2):21–33.
5. Gill GV, Alberti KG. The care of the diabetic patient during surgery. In: DeFronzo RA, Ferrannini E, Keen H, Zimmet, P, eds. *International Textbook of Diabetes Mellitus.* 3rd ed. New York: John Wiley and Sons, 2004:1741–1754.
6. Skyler JS. Insulin treatment. In: Lebovitz HE, ed. *Therapy for Diabetes Mellitus and Related Disorders.* 4th ed. Alexandria, VA: American Diabetes Association, 2004;207–223.
7. Queale WS, Seidler AJ, Brancati FL. Glycemic control and sliding scale insulin use in medical inpatients with diabetes mellitus. *Arch Intern Med* 1997;157:545–552.
8. Zerr KJ, Furnary AP, Grunkemeier GL, Bookin S, Kanhere V, Starr A. Glucose control lowers the risk of wound infection in diabetics after open heart operations. *Ann Thorac Surg* 1997;63: 356–361.
9. Malmberg K. Prospective randomized study of intensive insulin treatment on long-term survival after acute myocardial infarction in patients with diabetes mellitus. *BMJ* 1997;314: 1512–1515.
10. Goldberg PA, Siegel MD, Sherwin RS, et al. Implementation of a safe and effective insulin infusion protocol in a medical intensive care unit. *Diabetes Care* 2004;27:461–467.
11. Vincent JL, Abraham E, Annane D, Bernard G, Rivers E, Van den Berghe G. Reducing mortality in sepsis: new directions. *Crit Care* 2002;6(Suppl 3):S1–S18.
12. Lebovitz HE. Diabetic ketoacidosis. *Lancet* 1995;345:767–772.
13. Aubert RE, Geiss LS, Ballard DJ, et al. Diabetes-related hospitalization and hospital utilization. In: *Diabetes in America.* 2nd ed. Washington DC: National Institutes of Health, NIH publication No. 95-1468, 1995:553–569.
14. Gilmer TP, O'Connor PJ, Manning WG, Rush WA. The cost to health plans of poor glycemic control. *Diabetes Care* 1997;20: 1847–1853.

ADDITIONAL READING

Aviles-Santa L, Raskin P. Surgery and anesthesia. In: Lebovitz HE, ed. *Therapy for Diabetes Mellitus and Related Disorders.* 4th ed. Alexandria, VA: American Diabetes Association, 2004:247–258.
Genuth S. Diabetic ketoacidosis and hyperosmolar hyperglycemic nonketotic syndrome in adults. In: Lebovitz HE, ed. *Therapy of Diabetes Mellitus and Related Disorders.* 4th ed. American Diabetes Association, 2004:87–99.
Hirsch IB. In-patient hyperglycemia—Are we ready to treat it yet. *J Clin Endocrinol Metab* 2002;87:975–977.
Hirsch IB, Praun DS, Brunzell J. Inpatient management of adults with diabetes. *Diabetes Care* 1995;18:870–878.
Marshall SM, Walker M, Alberti KG. Diabetic ketoacidosis and hyperglycaemic nonketotic coma. In: Alberti KG, Zimmet P, DeFronzo RA, et al., eds. *International Textbook of Diabetes Mellitus.* 2nd ed. New York: John Wiley and Sons, 1997:1215–1229.
Norhammar AM, Ryden L, Malmberg K. Admission plasma glucose. Independent risk factor for long-term prognosis after myocardial infarction even in nondiabetic patients. *Diabetes Care* 1999;22: 1827–1831.
Van den Berghe G. Role of intravenous insulin therapy in critically ill patients. *Endocr Pract* 2004;10(Suppl 2):17–20.
Widom B, Simonson DC. Iatrogenic hypoglycemia. In: Kahn CR, Weir GC, eds. *Joslin's Diabetes Mellitus.* 13th ed. Philadelphia: Lea & Febiger, 1994:489–507.

Acute Presentations of Thyroid Disease

108

Leonard Wartofsky

INTRODUCTION

Although most disorders of the thyroid gland present subacutely or chronically and can be managed safely in the office setting, acute presentations of profound hyperthyroidism and hypothyroidism are dramatic and life threatening and require rapid action on the part of the hospital physician. This chapter discusses the entities of thyrotoxic storm and myxedema coma; refer to Chapter 106 for a discussion of thyroid function test abnormalities in hospitalized patients.

THYROTOXIC STORM

The syndrome of thyrotoxic "storm" or "crisis" is a life-threatening complication of severe hyperthyroidism. Thyroid storm is a state of disordered homeostasis resulting from acute decompensation of the cardiovascular, central nervous, gastrointestinal, and hepatorenal systems. A clinical suspicion of worsening thyrotoxicosis with a threat of storm may prompt hospitalization, or, perhaps just as frequently, storm will occur in a thyrotoxic patient who is already hospitalized for another medical or surgical problem. Historically, thyrotoxic storm after thyroidectomy, thoracoabdominal surgery, or obstetric procedures in thyrotoxic patients (*"surgical storm"*) was a common complication and major cause of mortality. Early diagnosis and modern improvements in preoperative medical treatment of the thyrotoxic patient have led to a decline in the incidence of surgical storm. Today, thyrotoxic storm develops most frequently in the setting of systemic illness such as infection (*"medical storm"*), although surgical storm remains a potential problem. Awareness of the precipitant of storm, whether medical or surgical, helps guide the selection of therapy.

Issues at the Time of Admission

Etiology of Storm

In a patient hospitalized with nonthyroid systemic illness or operative stress, thyroid hormone binding to its carrier proteins in blood is altered, which leads to increases in the tissue-active free hormone concentration. This process may convert a previously stable patient with uncomplicated thyrotoxicosis into one with storm. Therefore, values for total thyroxine (T_4) or total triiodothyronine (T_3) determined by radioimmunoassay may be no different in thyroid storm than in uncomplicated thyrotoxicosis because it is the concentration of free or unbound thyroid hormone that is generally responsible for clinical decompensation. Indeed, Brooks and Waldstein [1] demonstrated a twofold increase in the percentage of dialyzable T_4 and concentration of free T_4 in storm in comparison with these values in uncomplicated severe thyrotoxicosis. Storm can also occur as a result of T_3 toxicosis, with normal serum total and free T_4 but elevated levels of total and free T_3. Increased thyroid release of T_4 and T_3 has not been directly implicated in the development of thyrotoxic storm. In some instances, however, storm appeared after vigorous gland palpation, therapy with radioactive iodine (^{131}I), and iodine administration, which suggests that augmented glandular hormone release was responsible, at least in part.

Clinical Presentation

The clinical presentation of thyroid storm is often dramatic, with classic signs of severe thyrotoxicosis together with manifestations of multiple organ system failure. The diagnosis should be considered in the thyrotoxic patient with fever, marked tachycardia, congestive heart failure, diarrhea, and central nervous system signs that may vary from confusion to coma. The importance of making an early and correct diagnosis and of initiating immediate vigorous therapy relates to the extremely high potential mortality rate. Although storm occurs in only 1%–2% of all hospitalizations for thyrotoxicosis, the reported mortality rates in large inpatient series have ranged from 30%–100% (2). Because the perioperative and postoperative periods (after both thyroid and nonthyroid surgery) are common settings for storm, surgeons and hospital physicians must maintain a heightened awareness of the potential for storm in patients with known or suspected thyroid disease.

Issues During the Course of Hospitalization

Diagnosis

Successful therapy for thyrotoxic storm begins with early and accurate diagnosis. Unfortunately, it is not possible to differentiate storm from severe, otherwise uncomplicated thyrotoxicosis on the basis of laboratory test findings. The diagnosis is most obvious with a classic and dramatic presentation of fully developed storm, which includes fever (>38.5°C), altered mental status, congestive heart failure, and frequent, watery stools. However, by the time the patient manifests such a presentation, opportunities for early therapy have passed, and the mortality is significantly increased. Burch and Wartofsky (2) have proposed a scoring system to assist in the distinction between severe thyrotoxicosis and thyrotoxic storm (Table 108.1).

Patients with thyroid storm usually have some degree of alteration in central nervous system function. Although symptoms of tremor, restlessness, irritability, and emotional lability are characteristic of thyrotoxicosis, confusion, lethargy, and psychosis culminating in stupor and coma are quite typical of storm but unusual in uncomplicated thyrotoxicosis without premorbid psychopathology. Indeed, central nervous system dysfunction is so common in storm that preservation of normal mentation in a febrile thyrotoxic patient is strong clinical evidence against impending storm and may suggest a superimposed infection.

The gastrointestinal system is often involved in patients with storm. Diarrhea is the most frequent complaint, although abdominal pain, nausea, and vomiting are not uncommon. Hepatic function is variably affected; mild degrees of liver dysfunction are the rule, and frank hepatic failure is seen occasionally. Malnutrition can be profound, with weight loss often exceeding 20 kg, reflecting the underlying catabolic state. Additionally, hypoglycemia and hypoalbuminemia may be seen in storm and reflect long-standing severe caloric deficits.

Having made a diagnosis of thyroid storm, the clinician is required to search carefully for and treat an event or illness that led a case of uncomplicated thyrotoxicosis to evolve into storm (Table 108.2). Infection, often occult, is the most common precipitating event.

TABLE 108.1

DIAGNOSTIC CRITERIA FOR THYROID STORM

	Points
Thermoregulatory dysfunction	
Temperature: 99–99.9°F	5
100–100.9	10
101–101.9	15
102–102.9	20
103–103.9	25
≥104	30
Central nervous system effects	
Absent	0
Mild agitation	10
Delirium, psychosis, lethargy	20
Seizure or coma	30
Gastrointestinal dysfunction	
Absent	0
Diarrhea, nausea, vomiting, or abdominal pain	10
Unexplained jaundice	20
Cardiovascular dysfunction	
Tachycardia: 90–109 beats/min	5
110–119	10
120–129	15
130–139	20
≥140	25
Congestive heart failure	
Absent	0
Mild (edema)	5
Moderate (bilateral basilar rales)	10
Severe (pulmonary edema)	15
Atrial fibrillation	
Absent	0
Present	10
History of precipitating event (surgery, infection, other)	
Absent	0
Present	10

Points are assigned as applicable and the scores totaled. When it is not possible to distinguish a finding caused by an intercurrent illness from one of thyrotoxicosis, the higher point score is given so as to favor empirical therapy of storm. Under cardiovascular dysfunction, separate points are given for the findings of tachycardia, atrial fibrillation, or congestive heart failure. Interpretation: Based upon the total score, the likelihood of the diagnosis of thyrotoxic storm is as follows: unlikely, <25; impending, 25–44; highly likely, >45.
From Burch HB, Wartofsky L. Life-threatening thyrotoxicosis: thyroid storm. *Endocrinol Metab Clin North Am* 1993;22:263–277.

Management

Successful therapy requires management directed toward four therapeutic goals: (a) reducing hormone synthesis and release from the thyroid; (b) antagonizing peripheral actions of existing excesses of circulating hormone; (c) providing supportive care and avoiding homeostatic decompensation; and (d) defining and treating any precipitating or complicating underlying conditions.

Therapy Directed Against the Thyroid Gland

The inhibition of thyroid hormone synthesis and release is the cornerstone of acute treatment. The *thionamides,*

TABLE 108.2

CLINICAL DISORDERS THAT CAN PRECIPITATE THYROTOXIC CRISIS

Infection (bronchopneumonia, pharyngitis, meningitis, sepsis)
Surgery
Diabetic ketoacidosis
Pulmonary thromboembolism
Cerebrovascular accident
Iodine administration (iodinated contrast dye, oral iodine)
Hypoglycemia
Parturition
Trauma (including vigorous and repetitive thyroid palpation)
Therapy with ^{131}I
Emotional stress
Thiourea withdrawal

propylthiouracil (PTU) and methimazole (Tapazole), are potent inhibitors of organification of iodine. Provided that adequate dosages are used, thionamides profoundly reduce hormone synthesis in virtually all patients. Although their onset of action is relatively rapid after oral administration, it may take weeks to see clinical improvement. Therefore, other, more rapidly-acting therapies should be added (see below). In addition to blocking iodine organification, PTU inhibits the peripheral conversion of T_4 to the much more active T_3, thereby facilitating a more rapid fall in serum T_3 concentration than does methimazole, which lacks this property. Initially, PTU is administered in a dosage of 1,200–1,500 mg/d (200–250 mg given orally every 4 hours); alternatively, methimazole in a dosage of 120 mg/d (20 mg given orally every 4 hours) may be used. Although the use of a thionamide in a patient with previous thionamide-related hepatocellular dysfunction or agranulocytosis cannot be recommended, a history of minor rash or urticaria with these agents should not prevent their use in storm. Unfortunately, no suitable intravenous (IV) preparation of either PTU or methimazole is available. Rectal administration of either PTU or methimazole suppositories can achieve therapeutic blood levels in the patient for whom oral agents are contraindicated or impractical (3).

Although further synthesis of iodothyronines in the thyroid may be effectively blocked by thionamides, continued release of preformed hormone from glandular stores will persist unabated during thionamide treatment. Addition of another agent, such as *stable iodine* or *lithium carbonate,* is necessary to inhibit thyroid release of preformed hormone. Because Lugol iodine solution as sole therapy will augment and enrich hormonal stores in the thyroid, organification should be blocked with a thionamide before iodine therapy is begun. If organification has not been blocked, the iodine treatment can result in worsening of thyrotoxicosis. Although Lugol solution (0.5 mL orally every 6 hours) is ef-

fective, an IV infusion of sodium iodide (1 g every 24 hours) is equally effective and eliminates potential concerns related to variable gut absorption. Commercial preparations of the latter are no longer available in the United States but may be specifically formulated. In contrast to the slow decline in serum levels of T_4 and T_3 seen with sole thionamide therapy, levels fall rapidly after iodine therapy is added (with nearly normal values often reached in 3–5 days).

Iodinated radiographic contrast dyes such as ipodate (Oragrafin) have been used increasingly in the management of thyrotoxicosis. Ipodate is effective in inhibiting glandular iodine release because of the large amount of stable iodine present in this compound (approximately 65% by weight). Ipodate is also a potent inhibitor of the conversion of T_4 to T_3 in many tissues. The efficacy of ipodate for thyrotoxic storm has not been extensively studied, but a rapid decline in circulating T_4 and T_3 levels is typically seen in thyrotoxicosis with a daily dose of 1–3 g orally (in addition to adequate thionamide treatment). Another iodine-rich compound, amiodarone, should be equally effective but has not yet been studied in this setting. It could be used in an urgent situation if no other iodine source were available, but only in combination with a thionamide. A 200 mg tablet (containing 74 mg iodine) once or twice daily should suffice.

Occasionally, a patient with thyrotoxic storm will also have a clear history of iodine allergy. In such patients, *lithium carbonate,* which has been used successfully in the treatment of thyrotoxicosis, should be considered. At an initial dosage of 300 mg every 6 hours, lithium is usually effective in inhibiting thyroid hormone release. To avoid lithium toxicity, serum levels must be monitored daily with doses titrated to maintain a plasma lithium level of approximately 1.0 mEq/L. Regardless of which agent is chosen, the most important thing is to start therapy to inhibit hormone release as early as possible after initiation of thionamides. In the absence of comparative trials, the author's preference is to use Lugol iodine, ipodate, or amiodarone. If none of these is readily available, lithium carbonate would be started.

Although ^{131}I may be considered for definitive therapy after storm has resolved (see below), *radioactive iodine should not be administered during the acute phase of thyroid storm.* This is because the associated destruction of thyroid follicular cells would release more T_4 and T_3, thereby potentially aggravating the thyroid crisis.

Therapy Against Ongoing Effects of Thyroid Hormone in the Periphery

The activity of the sympathetic nervous system is greatly enhanced in thyrotoxic storm. *β-adrenergic receptor antagonists,* especially propranolol (40–80 mg every 6 hours orally), have become the drugs of choice to counteract this hyperadrenergic state. Frequently, larger doses are required to reduce sympathetic nervous system activity in storm because serum levels are variable after customarily employed doses. In the critically ill patient, IV propranolol in doses of 1–2 mg may be used initially until effective serum levels are achieved after oral administration. The ultra–short-acting β-adrenergic blocker esmolol can also be used for the perioperative management of thyroid storm. A loading dose of 0.25–0.5 mg/kg, followed by a continuous infusion at a rate of 0.05–0.1 mg/kg per minute, has been shown to be effective. The role of β-adrenergic blockade when congestive heart failure is present in storm is arguable, but it can be beneficial if the agent is titrated with careful hemodynamic monitoring.

Occasionally, adequate control of clinical thyrotoxicosis is not achieved despite massive doses of propranolol. In addition to β-adrenergic blockade, other more aggressive means of reducing hormone concentrations in the periphery are dialysis and plasmapheresis. Hemoperfusion through a resin bed or charcoal columns may be similarly employed (4). Finally, some removal of circulating T$_4$ and T$_3$ can be achieved safely by the use of cholestyramine resin; this agent binds thyroid hormone entering the gastrointestinal tract via enterohepatic recirculation.

Two other issues related to the use of β-blockade are worth mentioning. First, several cases of storm have been reported in patients being treated with β-blockers unaccompanied by antithyroid drug blockade (5). Therefore, one cannot rely on therapy with β-blockers alone and assume either that storm cannot supervene or that such monotherapy is adequate in severe thyrotoxicosis. Second, in the patient allergic to thioureas, surgery can be performed under β-blockade, albeit more safely with simultaneous administration of iodine, ipodate, or lithium carbonate (6).

Therapy Directed Against Systemic Decompensation

The serious prognosis of thyrotoxic storm mandates admission or transfer to a critical care unit for careful monitoring. Aggressive treatment of fever is mandatory. Acetaminophen is the preferred antipyretic agent because salicylates can increase free hormone levels by displacing thyroxine from serum protein binding sites. Aggressive cooling measures, including alcohol washes, cooling blankets, and ice packs, may be required. Fever, especially if accompanied by diarrhea and vomiting, can lead to large fluid losses, and fluids must be vigorously replaced to prevent cardiovascular collapse. Volume status must be monitored carefully because excessive fluid depletion is also a threat in storm. Congestive heart failure may be precipitated by atrial tachyarrhythmias, impaired myocardial contractility, or volume overload. Therapy with digitalis and diuretics is beneficial, although the required dose of digoxin is often high because of the altered distribution and metabolism of digitalis. Depleted hepatic glycogen and water-soluble vitamins must also be replaced. Typically, 10% dextrose supplied in hypotonic saline solution at a rate of 3–4 L each day with vitamin supplementation is adequate.

Prompted by concern over potentially impaired adrenocortical reserve, clinicians have long used glucocorticoids empirically in patients with thyrotoxic storm. Although no controlled trials have proved its efficacy, this practice has a scientific rationale, as plasma clearance rates for cortisol in patients with thyrotoxicosis are twice those of euthyroid controls. Furthermore, the response of urinary 17-hydroxycorticosteroids to infusions of adrenocorticotropic hormone (ACTH) may be blunted in thyrotoxicosis. An additional benefit of steroids is that they inhibit the conversion of T$_4$ to T$_3$, as do PTU and ipodate. An initial dose of 300 mg of hydrocortisone followed by 100 mg every 8–12 hours should be adequate (2) (Chapter 109).

Therapy Directed Against the Precipitating Illness

The precipitating cause of thyrotoxic storm is often readily apparent, as in cases presenting after trauma, thyroidectomy, and parturition. No specific therapy need be administered for these causes once the initial insult has passed. Hypoglycemia, ketoacidosis, pulmonary emboli, or stroke complicating storm will require the same specific therapy generally reserved for these conditions in the absence of storm. With a stuporous patient, a high index of suspicion for these (often occult) precipitating events must be maintained.

Although fever may occur in thyrotoxic storm in the absence of infection (presumably representing the "hypermetabolic" state), it is vitally important to exclude underlying infection. Cultures of blood, urine, and other appropriate fluids (including spinal fluid in the obtunded patient) are mandatory. In many cases, it is wise to initiate broad-spectrum antibiotics, with administration guided by the clinician's best impression of the most likely site of infection. The antibiotics can then be subsequently tailored or discontinued based on culture results.

Issues at Discharge

Definitive Therapy of Thyrotoxicosis

The rapid clinical diagnosis of early thyrotoxic storm and aggressive therapeutic intervention provide the best chance for successful resolution. Discharge should not be considered until all vital signs have been stable for 48 hours and cardiovascular and mental status have returned to baseline. As the patient begins to improve clinically, the various therapeutic measures can be gradually withdrawn. Steroids should be rapidly tapered. Whether or not to continue antibiotic treatment is guided by standard recommendations based on site of infection and etiologic agent. The withdrawal of thioureas, stable iodine, and β-blockers may be more difficult clinical decisions. If storm has occurred in the postthyroidectomy setting, it should be self-limited, because the source of thyroid hormone has been ostensibly excised. In the event that only a lobectomy or a lobectomy and isthmusectomy were performed, medical therapy with thioureas and β-blockade will have to be continued and gradually tapered, with monitoring per standard recommendations for medical therapy in the postoperative patient.

Once the acute danger is past, attention can be directed to the long-term management of thyrotoxicosis. In cases of storm occurring outside the perioperative period, definitive treatment of the underlying thyroid disorder is strongly recommended to prevent another episode of storm. The traditional titration regimen of slowly withdrawing thioureas in the hope of maintaining a long-term remission is usually inappropriate in a patient whose thyrotoxicosis was severe enough to result in storm. Rather, *definitive therapy with radioactive iodine or surgery is indicated.* The large doses of stable iodine administered during the episode of storm will flood the body pool of iodine, diminish thyroid uptake of radioactive iodine, and thereby limit the possibility of employing ablation with radioactive iodine as definitive therapy, at least until some future date when the iodine load has cleared. Thus, in the majority of such cases, it seems preferable to consider surgical treatment 2–4 weeks after resolution of the episode of storm, and to continue aggressive therapy in the meantime with thioureas, iodine, and β-blockers.

MYXEDEMA COMA

Myxedema coma is a rare syndrome that represents the extreme expression of severe hypothyroidism. The syndrome most often is seen in hospitalized, elderly women with long-standing hypothyroidism, and the classic features of that disease usually are present. Most patients have an underlying disorder of the thyroid gland itself; fewer than 10% have hypothalamic or pituitary disease as the basis of hypothyroidism. Once considered, the diagnosis should be easy to establish on both clinical and laboratory grounds, but the disorder can still be associated with a mortality rate as high as 60% despite appropriate and vigorous therapy (7).

Issues at the Time of Admission

Clinical Presentation

Precipitating Events
Myxedema coma is most often encountered during the winter months, which suggests that external cold may be an aggravating factor. Other events associated with myxedema coma include pulmonary infections, cerebrovascular accidents, and congestive heart failure (Table 108.3). Pulmonary infection also can occur as a secondary event in the comatose, hypoventilating patient, as can aspiration pneumonia. Similarly, it can be difficult to determine whether other abnormalities, such as hyperglycemia, hyponatremia, hypercapnia, and hypoxemia, which often are associated

TABLE 108.3
MYXEDEMA COMA: PRECIPITATING FACTORS

Cerebrovascular accident
Hypothermia
Infection
Congestive heart failure
Drugs
  Anesthetics
  Sedatives
  Tranquilizers
  Opiates
  Lithium carbonate
  Amiodarone
Trauma
Gastrointestinal bleeding
Metabolic disturbance compounding obtundation
  Hypoglycemia
  Hyponatremia
  Hypercapnia
  Acidosis

with myxedema coma, contributed to the coma or are secondary consequences. Drugs often initiate or compound the downward spiral of the hypothyroid patient into coma. Common culprits include anesthetics, opiates, sedatives, antidepressants, and tranquilizers, and the mechanism appears to be related to depression of the respiratory center.

Clinical Appearance
Two of the cardinal features of myxedema coma are *hypothermia* and *unconsciousness*. It is not unusual for the syndrome to present in patients with previously undiagnosed hypothyroidism whose illness has become complicated by infection or other systemic disease. There may be a history of antecedent thyroid disease, thyroid hormone replacement therapy that was discontinued for no apparent reason, or therapy with radioactive iodine. Examination of the neck may reveal a surgical scar and nonpalpable thyroid tissue, or a goiter may be present. The course often is one of lethargy progressing to stupor and then coma, which can be hastened by the use of sedatives or opiates, which leads to respiratory failure and retention of carbon dioxide. The usual features of dry, coarse, and scaly skin, delayed deep tendon reflexes, sparse or coarse hair, carotenemic pallor, puffy facies, large tongue, and hoarseness may be present, in addition to moderate-to-profound (e.g., 80°F) hypothermia.

Respiratory System
The most important factor underlying the ventilatory abnormality in myxedema is a *depression of the hypoxic respiratory drive,* which can be accompanied by a depressed ventilatory response to hypercapnia. The resulting decrease in alveolar ventilation leads to progressive carbon dioxide narcosis and coma, and impaired respiratory mus-

cle function may compound the hypoventilation. Muscle function is usually reduced enough that mechanical ventilation is required, especially if opiate or sedative drugs are playing a role in the depressed ventilation. Several other physical or anatomic factors can impede ventilation in the hypothyroid patient, such as pleural effusions or ascites. In addition, swelling of the tongue and tissue of the upper respiratory tract with a myxedematous infiltrate can cause partial obstruction that may progress during superimposed infection (e.g., laryngeal obstruction caused by marked edema of the vocal cords) to an acute respiratory emergency.

Cardiovascular Manifestations

The findings considered typical of hypothyroid heart disease also are observed in myxedema coma, including enlargement of the cardiac silhouette, bradycardia, decreased quality and intensity of the heart sounds, and minor electrocardiographic abnormalities. The latter consist of varying degrees of block, low voltage, prolonged QT interval, and flattened or inverted T waves. Although enlargement of the cardiac silhouette may partly represent ventricular dilatation, it is usually caused by pericardial effusion secondary to accumulation of fluid rich in mucopolysaccharide. The fluid tends to accumulate over a long time, and as a consequence, cardiac tamponade is rare.

Stroke volume and cardiac output are reduced on the basis of impaired cardiac contractility, but frank congestive heart failure is very rare. The abnormalities in left ventricular function and the pericardial effusion gradually normalize with thyroxine replacement. The lactate dehydrogenase isoenzyme pattern in severe hypothyroidism can mimic that of myocardial infarction, and creatine kinase levels also are elevated (troponins have not been studied). To add to the potential confusion, myocardial infarction (from atherosclerotic disease) can be the precipitating event for myxedema coma, and patients with hypothyroidism are at risk for myocardial infarction during injudicious overreplacement of thyroid hormone. Nevertheless, the mortality of untreated myxedema coma demands vigorous treatment with thyroid hormone, as discussed below.

Although total body water and extracellular fluid volume may be increased, intravascular volume is reduced, and this contributes to the propensity for hypotension. Increases in blood pressure regularly follow replacement with thyroid hormone. Cardiovascular collapse and shock may supervene in myxedema coma before there is adequate time for thyroid hormone to act, in which case the use of pressors (along with thyroid hormone) is mandatory. In this situation, the potential for fatal arrhythmias is extremely high, and careful monitoring in an intensive care unit (ICU) is essential.

Gastrointestinal Manifestations

Decreased intestinal motility is common in hypothyroidism, and its most severe expression, paralytic ileus, is frequent in myxedema coma. Impaired peristalsis may be a consequence of both neuropathic changes related to thyroid deficiency and myxedematous infiltration of the gut wall. Accompanying problems include constipation and obstipation, both of which improve with replacement therapy. Gastric atony in myxedema coma is a particularly troublesome problem because absorption of oral medications is affected. Because of this, parenteral administration of T_4 or T_3 may be preferable, as discussed below.

Renal and Electrolyte Manifestations

Abnormalities noted in severe hypothyroidism include increased body water, decreased plasma volume, decreased serum sodium and osmolality, increased urine sodium and osmolality, and reduced glomerular filtration rate and renal plasma flow. Bladder atony with retention of large residual urine volumes is not unusual. Hyponatremia, if present, is likely to compound the patient's confusion and, when severe, may be largely responsible for precipitating coma. Treatment with thyroid hormone promotes water diuresis, with a resultant decrease in edema and total body water and an increase in serum sodium.

Neuropsychiatric Manifestations

The patient with the full-blown syndrome of myxedema coma manifests or complains of few neuropsychiatric signs or symptoms other than the coma itself. There may be history of disorientation, depression, paranoia, or hallucinations (*"myxedema madness"*). The subjects demonstrate poor memory or frank amnesia, varying degrees of somnolence and lethargy that progress to coma, and cerebellar signs, such as clumsy movements of the hands and feet, ataxia, and adiadochokinesia. Minor seizures or frank convulsions occur in about 25% of patients with myxedema coma, but hyponatremia may be responsible for most of these. In these usually elderly patients, decreased cardiac output combined with arteriosclerotic cerebrovascular disease is likely to produce decreased perfusion and cerebral hypoxia. All functional parameters improve gradually with thyroid hormone replacement.

Hypothermia

Hypothermia is present in about three-fourths of patients, often is dramatic ($<80°F$), and may be the first clinical clue to the diagnosis. Underlying hypoglycemia may serve to decrease body temperature further. A careful history and physical examination in the hypothermic patient usually serve either to confirm the diagnosis of myxedema or to render it sufficiently unlikely to justify awaiting the results of serum T_4 and thyrotropin (TSH) determinations before initiating treatment. The presence of any appreciable hypothermia implies a poor prognosis, and the immediate initiation of thyroid hormone therapy is mandatory. With treatment, the hypothermia gradually improves in parallel with increments in serum T_4 and T_3 levels.

Diagnosis

The importance of making the diagnosis cannot be stressed strongly enough because the unnecessary administration of relatively large doses of thyroid hormone to an elderly euthyroid patient clearly can be fatal. On the other hand, when the likelihood of myxedema coma is reasonably high, treatment should not be delayed pending laboratory confirmation. It may be difficult to distinguish severe fatigue and somnolence in a patient with uncomplicated hypothyroidism from true myxedema coma. Although overzealous treatment in such a patient is discouraged, diagnostic aggressiveness is mandatory to determine whether carbon dioxide retention, hypoxia, hyponatremia, or infection is present.

Of great interest is the observation that coma frequently occurs in hypothyroid patients while they are hospitalized for other problems or for diagnostic studies. In these cases, precipitating factors may include the stress of diagnostic procedures, administration of IV fluids, or, more importantly, the all-too-common routine hospital use of sedative and hypnotic drugs. In many patients, the clinical features can be so overwhelming (for example, the comatose elderly woman with a history of hypothyroidism who has coarse skin, macroglossia, hypothermia, bradycardia, hyponatremia, ileus, and an enlarged silhouette) that thyroid function tests are necessary only for retrospective confirmation of the diagnosis. *The urgency of the diagnosis should be stressed to the laboratory*, which often can perform a serum T_4 determination within 1 hour and a TSH determination within 3 hours. Although an elevated serum TSH concentration is the most important laboratory evidence of the diagnosis, one must be alert to the possibility that pituitary disease is causing the hypothyroidism, in which case both T_4 and TSH levels will be low. Until pituitary disease is ruled out, corticosteroid therapy, in addition to thyroid hormone, is required. On the other hand, a low serum T_4 and normal serum TSH would suggest that the patient may be exhibiting the euthyroid sick syndrome (Chapter 106) and is not hypothyroid.

Issues During the Course of Hospitalization

Infection

The possibility of occult pneumonia leading to worsening respiratory status has been mentioned. Pneumonia and other infections can be overlooked because of the frequent absence of fever, diaphoresis, and tachycardia in the hypothyroid patient. Respiratory tract infection may be more common because of the risk for aspiration in a stuporous patient, particularly one with seizures related to hyponatremia. Because of these considerations and the fear that undiscovered infection can lead to vascular collapse and death, some authors advocate the routine use of antibiotics in patients with myxedema coma. This approach is most defensible if limited to the delicate period during the initial 24–48 hours of management. An alternative approach is to remain alert to the possibility of infection and institute specific antibiotic therapy only when indicated on the basis of appropriate specimen smears and cultures.

Therapy

In view of the extremely high mortality rate in untreated patients with myxedema coma, *it is essential that treatment be instituted promptly and vigorously as soon as the diagnosis is made*. The entire treatment team should be made aware that it is dealing with a medical emergency, and meticulous interdisciplinary care in a critical care setting with modern electronic monitoring equipment is essential.

Ventilatory Support

Hypoventilation resulting from a number of factors may cause carbon dioxide retention and respiratory acidosis and aggravate the comatose state. Appropriate diagnostic and therapeutic measures must be instituted when any suspect infiltrate is apparent on the chest radiograph, with the understanding that fever and cough may not be prominent. Death from respiratory failure is not unusual, and hence the maintenance of an adequate airway to prevent hypoxemia is the single most important supportive measure. Mechanical ventilatory support is usually required during the first 48 hours, particularly if the hypoventilation partly represents drug-related respiratory depression. Although the patient may become alert by the second or third day of therapy, complicated cases can require mechanical ventilation for as long as 3 weeks. Arterial blood gases must be monitored regularly until the patient is fully recovered. Numerous reports have cited the danger of relapse with premature extubation. Hence, weaning should be approached conservatively and should never be attempted until the patient is fully conscious.

Hyponatremia

Total body sodium is probably normal-to-increased, and impaired water excretion is the major underlying reason for hyponatremia. Therapy with IV fluids in general, and saline solution in particular, must be approached cautiously because cardiac reserve is often decreased. If hypoglycemia is present, sodium chloride should be added to any fluids given to correct the low blood glucose, or a concentrated glucose solution should be used. Otherwise, fluid restriction may be all that is necessary to correct mild (120–130 mEq/L) hyponatremia. If severe (<120 mEq/L) hyponatremia is present, it may be appropriate to administer a small amount of hypertonic saline solution (50–100 mL of 3% or 5% sodium chloride) early in the course of treatment; this can be followed by an IV bolus of 40–120 mg of furosemide to promote a water diuresis. A central venous pressure line should be used to monitor fluid therapy, and placement of a Swan-Ganz catheter is justifiable in the presence of significant cardiovascular decompensation.

Hypothermia

Administration of thyroid hormone ultimately is essential to restore body temperature to normal. Until that effect is achieved, some physical means of keeping the patient warm is advisable; ordinary blankets or an increase of room temperature can be used, but *great caution must be exercised in external warming.* The use of electric warming blankets can cause vasodilation and a precipitous fall in peripheral vascular resistance. The resultant augmentation in peripheral blood flow is accompanied by an increase in oxygen consumption, which can aggravate hypotension or even lead to vascular collapse.

Hypotension

Like hypothermia, hypotension should improve with thyroid hormone replacement. Because this can take several days or longer, profound hypotension requires additional therapy. Initially, fluids can be cautiously administered as 5%–10% glucose in half-normal sodium chloride solution or as isotonic sodium chloride if hyponatremia is present. Administration of hydrocortisone (100 mg IV every 8 hours) may be justified until the tendency toward hypotension is corrected and adrenal insufficiency is excluded. In rare patients, pressor agents may be required to maintain a blood pressure sufficient to sustain adequate perfusion, notwithstanding the risk for inducing ventricular tachyarrhythmias, especially in patients with underlying ischemic heart disease. An agent such as dopamine is generally preferable to norepinephrine to maintain coronary blood flow (Chapter 25), but in any event, an effort should be made to taper the dose and wean the patient from any pressor agent as soon as possible. An adverse interaction between administered catecholamine and thyroid hormone is possible, and the physician must weigh this risk against the known high mortality in myxedema coma associated with refractory hypotension.

Corticosteroids

The coexistence of adrenal insufficiency in patients with myxedema coma is suggested by the presence of hypotension, hypothermia, hypoglycemia, hyponatremia, and hyperkalemia (Chapter 109). The ACTH response to stress may be impaired in these patients, and, given the potential risk to the patient undergoing the stress of acute illness versus the relative safety of short-term steroid therapy, there should be no reluctance to administer corticosteroids until the patient is stable and the integrity of the pituitary–adrenal axis is determined. With the institution of thyroid hormone therapy, there is an additional theoretical basis for supplemental corticosteroids: the accelerated metabolism of cortisol that follows T_4 replacement in hypothyroidism, which can theoretically precipitate adrenal crisis from relative adrenal insufficiency. Hydrocortisone is usually given in a dosage of 50–100 mg every 6–8 hours during the first 7–10 days and is then tapered on the basis of clinical response and plans for further diagnostic evaluation.

Thyroid Hormone Therapy

The most controversial aspect of the management of myxedema coma is the selection of the optimal method for restoring the low serum and tissue concentrations of thyroid hormone to normal. Differences of opinion largely relate to whether to administer T_4, which is then converted to T_3 by the patient, or T_3 itself. Secondary issues include dosage and route of administration (of either compound). Different approaches to management are based on balancing concerns for the high mortality of the untreated disease and the obvious need for attaining effective thyroid hormone levels against the risks of precipitating a fatal tachyarrhythmia or myocardial infarction. The optimal mode of therapy remains uncertain because of the relative rarity of this condition and the consequent paucity of controlled studies.

Those who advocate T_4 as the therapeutic choice point out that it provides a steady, smooth onset of action with less risk for adverse effects. Oral forms of T_4 (and T_3) can be given by nasogastric tube (8), but this route is fraught with risks for aspiration and uncertain absorption, particularly because gastric atony may be present. Preparations of T_4 for parenteral use are available in ampules of 100 and 500 mcg, and the latter dose has been advocated as a single IV bolus to restore near-normal hormonal status as rapidly as possible. After the initial loading dose, a daily maintenance dose of 50–100 mcg is given (IV or by mouth when the patient becomes alert). This method results in increases in serum T_4 to within the normal range within 24 hours and significant decrements in serum TSH. Larger doses of T_4 probably have no advantage and may, in fact, be more dangerous. The major potential drawback to the total reliance on generation of T_3 from T_4 is that the rate of conversion of T_4 to T_3 is reduced in a variety of systemic illnesses (*low T_3 syndrome* (9)). Therefore, T_3 generation may be reduced in myxedema coma as the consequence of an associated illness. In view of this potential problem, it seems prudent to add small supplements of T_3 to the T_4 during the initial few days of therapy, especially if significant associated illness is present. Regardless of which type of therapy is selected, all patients should have continuous electrocardiographic monitoring so that the dosage of thyroid hormone can be reduced if arrhythmias or ischemic changes are detected.

In addition to the problem of failure to generate T_3 from T_4 in the sick patient, advocates of T_3 point to its much quicker onset of action. T_3 (Triostat) is available in 1-mL vials containing 10 mcg/mL. Therapy with T_3 alone may be given as a 20-mcg bolus followed by 10 mcg every 4 hours for the first 24 hours, with the dosage dropped to 10 mcg every 6 hours for the second and third days, by which time oral administration should be feasible. Increases in body temperature and oxygen consumption may occur 2–3 hours after intravenous T_3, compared with 8–14 hours after IV T_4. This rapid onset of action may come at the cost of a greater risk for cardiac complications. Indeed, high serum levels of T_3 during treatment with thyroid hormone have been associated with fatal outcomes.

For these reasons, *combination therapy with both T_4 and T_3 is a rational approach* until better data on which to base a decision become available. Instead of a dose of 300–500 mcg of T_4 given IV initially, a dose of 4 mcg per kg of lean body weight (or about 200–300 mcg) is given, and an additional 100 mcg is given 24 hours later. By the third day, the dose is reduced to a daily maintenance dose of 50 mcg, which can be given by mouth as soon as the patient is stable and conscious. This dose subsequently is adjusted on the basis of clinical and laboratory results, as in any other hypothyroid patient. The author would also give a bolus of 20 mcg of T_3 at the same time as the initial dose of T_4 and continue IV T_3 at a dosage of 10 mcg every 8 hours until the patient is conscious, taking maintenance T_4, and achieving physiologic levels of T_3. Sensitivity to thyroid hormone in terms of cardiac risk varies, depending on age, cardiac medications, and the presence of underlying hypoxemia, coronary artery disease, congestive failure, and electrolyte imbalance. No general guide to management can take all these factors into account, and hence it is wise to consult an endocrinologist and monitor the patient carefully for any untoward effects of therapy before each dose of thyroid hormone is administered.

In addition to the specific therapies outlined, general supportive measures are indicated, as in all elderly, cachectic patients. These measures include treating any underlying problems with specific medications (e.g., appropriate therapy for congestive heart failure), with the understanding that the dosage of other drugs may need to be modified based on their altered distribution and metabolism in myxedema. Unfortunately, the prognosis for myxedema coma remains grim even with vigorous therapy, and patients who have severe hypothermia and hypotension fare the worst. Perhaps further elucidation of thyroid economy in health and disease will point the way to more effective approaches to therapy. Until then, early recognition and treatment, with meticulous attention to the details of management during the first 48 hours, remain critical.

Discharge Issues

Patients may be ready for discharge when their cardiovascular status and vital signs are stable, their serum electrolytes have normalized, they are taking oral nutrition and medications, and ventilatory assistance has been discontinued for 48 hours with maintenance of normal oxygen saturation or stable and acceptable values for arterial blood gases. Discharge medications (in addition to thyroid hormone) may include appropriate antibiotics to complete a course of treatment for any underlying infection. Corticosteroids can be rapidly tapered if adrenal insufficiency is no longer a consideration. Because adrenal insufficiency coexisting with primary hypothyroidism is almost always a consequence of primary adrenal disease (rather than pituitary disease), a short stimulation test with ACTH (Cortrosyn) can be performed before discharge (while the patient is maintained on dexamethasone, a synthetic steroid that will not interfere with the measurement of cortisol) (Chapter 109).

In regard to thyroid hormone therapy, if T_3 has been administered during the acute phase of the myxedema coma, it can generally be discontinued in favor of levothyroxine by the time of discharge. Once vital signs are stable, there is no longer any urgency to increase the levothyroxine dosage rapidly to full physiologic replacement. A discharge dosage of as little as 50–75 mcg per day will be safe and preclude recurrence of myxedema coma. The dosage can be titrated to appropriate physiologic replacement on an outpatient basis according to the results of serial measurements of serum TSH, with the target TSH level in the range of 0.5–1.5 mU/L. Patients and their caregivers should be educated regarding the need to remain on *lifelong thyroid hormone replacement,* with annual follow-up once the maintenance dose has been determined.

KEY POINTS

- Thyroid storm, a potentially lethal complication of hyperthyroidism, presents with classic signs of thyrotoxicosis, accompanied by fever, diarrhea, altered mental status, and tachycardia.
- Myxedema coma, a potentially lethal complication of hypothyroidism, presents with classic signs of hypothyroidism, along with hypothermia, hypoventilation, and unconsciousness.
- Both patients with thyroid storm and those with myxedema coma should be admitted to the intensive care unit.
- Therapy for thyroid storm requires a four-pronged approach and includes the following:
  1. Therapy directed at the thyroid gland (use iodine only after thioureas have been started)
  2. Therapy for the systemic decompensation (fever, fluid losses, congestive heart failure, hypotension)
  3. Therapy directed at the ongoing effects of thyroid hormone in circulation
  4. Treatment of the precipitating illness
- Therapy for myxedema coma should be started immediately (i.e., without waiting for results of thyroid function tests) if clinical suspicion is high. Initial therapy requires intravenous administration of relatively high doses of T_4, T_3, or both, and attention to the key role of hypoventilation.

REFERENCES

1. Brooks MH, Waldstein SS. Free thyroxine concentrations in thyroid storm. *Ann Intern Med* 1980;90:694–697.
2. Burch HB, Wartofsky L. Life-threatening thyrotoxicosis: thyroid storm. *Endocrinol Metab Clin North Am* 1993;22:263–277.

3. Jongjaroenprasert W, Akarawut W, Chantasart D, Chailurkit L, Rajatanavin R. Rectal administration of propylthiouracil in hyperthyroid patients: comparison of suspension enema and suppository form. *Thyroid* 2002;12:627–631.

4. Candrina R, DiStefano O, Spandrio S, Giustina G. Treatment of thyrotoxic storm by charcoal plasma perfusion. *J Endocrinol Invest* 1989;12:133–134.

5. Strube PJ. Thyroid storm during beta blockade. *Anaesthesia* 1984; 39:343–346.

6. Weber C, Scholz GH, Lamesch P, Paschke R. Thyroidectomy in iodine induced thyrotoxic storm. *Exp Clin Endocrinol Diabetes* 1999; 107:468–472.

7. Nicoloff JT, LoPresti JS. Myxedema coma: a form of decompensated hypothyroidism. *Endocrin Metab Clin North Am* 1993;22: 279–290.

8. Pereira VG, Haron ES, Lima-Neto N, Medeiros-Neto GA. Management of myxedema coma: report on three successfully treated cases with nasogastric or intravenous administration of triiodothyronine. *J Endocrinol Invest* 1982;5:331–334.

9. Wartofsky L. Update 1994: the euthyroid sick syndrome. In: Braverman LE, Refetoff S, eds. *Endocrine Reviews Monographs. 3. Clinical and Molecular Aspects of Diseases of the Thyroid.* Bethesda, MD: The Endocrine Society, 1994:248–251.

ADDITIONAL READING

Homma M, Shimizu S, Ogata M, Yamada Y, Saito T, Yamamoto T. Hypoglycemic coma masquerading thyrotoxic storm. *Internal Medicine* 1999;38:871–874.

Jiang Y-Z, Hutchinson KA, Bartelloni P, Manthous CA. Thyroid storm presenting as multiple organ dysfunction syndrome. *Chest* 2000;118:877–879.

Kadmon PM, Noto RB, Boney CM, Goodwin G, Gruppuso PA. Thyroid storm in a child following radioactive iodine therapy: a consequence of RAI versus withdrawal of antithyroid medication. *J Clin Endocrinol Metab* 2001;86:1865–1867.

Ringel MD. Management of hypothyroidism and hyperthyroidism in the intensive care unit. *Crit Care Clin* 2001;17:59–74.

Tajiri J, Katsuya H, Kiyokawa T, Urata K, Okamoto K, Shimada T. Successful treatment of thyrotoxic crisis with plasma exchange. *Crit Care Med* 1984;12:536–537.

Wall CR. Myxedema coma: diagnosis and treatment. *Am Fam Physician* 2000;62:2485–2490.

Yamamoto T, Fukuyama J, Fujiyoshi A. Factors associated with mortality of myxedema coma: report of eight cases and literature survey. *Thyroid* 1999;9:1167–1174.

Adrenal Insufficiency and Crisis

109

David G. Gardner

INTRODUCTION

Adrenal insufficiency (AI), although uncommon in its native form, has become increasingly prevalent with the use of exogenous corticosteroids in the management of pulmonary, rheumatologic, and allergic disorders. This has engendered a need for increased vigilance on the part of clinicians caring for patients with these disorders as well as for other patients at risk. AI can be insidious in presentation and devastating in outcome if it remains untreated. This chapter covers the diagnosis and management of AI in the hospitalized patient.

ADRENAL PHYSIOLOGY AND PATHOPHYSIOLOGY

The adrenal gland can be divided into functional zones. The outermost zone, the *zona glomerulosa*, is responsible for the production of mineralocorticoids (e.g., aldosterone). Aldosterone promotes sodium retention and potassium excretion in the kidney. Angiotensin II and extracellular potassium levels govern the synthesis and release of aldosterone.

The *zona fasciculata/reticularis* is positioned between the zona glomerulosa and the adrenal medulla. It is responsible for the production of glucocorticoids (i.e., cortisol) and adrenal androgens. The zona fasciculata/reticularis is under the trophic control of adrenocorticotropin (ACTH), which is produced and released from corticotropes located in the anterior pituitary gland. ACTH is responsible for producing an adequate level of cortisol to meet tissue needs. ACTH secretion is pulsatile in nature and under the control of corticotropin-releasing hormone (CRH) and, to a lesser extent, vasopressin. These peptides are produced in the hypothalamus.

Circulating cortisol levels are regulated through a negative feedback mechanism in which the steroid controls the synthesis and release of ACTH. Thus, as circulating cortisol levels rise, plasma ACTH levels fall and cortisol secretion declines. At some point, circulating cortisol levels fall below the threshold for suppression of ACTH release, and levels of the latter once again increase. Administration of exogenous glucocorticoid leads to suppression of ACTH release and loss of the trophic drive for endogenous steroid production. Typically, this results in both functional and anatomic atrophy of the adrenal glands, which can take months to recover following discontinuation of the steroid. Prolonged impairment of endogenous glucocorticoid production (e.g., through autoimmune destruction of the adrenals) results in significant elevations in circulating ACTH levels without commensurate increments in adrenal steroid production.

Adrenal insufficiency can result from defects at a number of points in the neuroendocrine and endocrine cascade. Bilateral lesions of the adrenal glands themselves reduce secretion of mineralocorticoids, glucocorticoids, and adrenal androgens because the anatomic substrate for the manufacture of these steroids is lacking. Defects that are intrinsic to the adrenal glands are said to result in *primary AI* or *Addison's disease*. Table 109.1 presents some of the known causes of primary AI. Most cases in adults are caused by *autoimmune adrenalitis*, a disorder that may or may not be accompanied by other autoimmune endocrinopathies (e.g., thyroiditis, diabetes mellitus, gonadal disease, hypoparathyroidism) and associated findings (e.g., vitiligo or mucocutaneous candidiasis). In the past, tuberculosis was the leading cause of primary AI, but it is now less common. This should be considered in indigent patients, in recent immigrants from areas where tuberculosis remains endemic, and in HIV-infected patients with a history of exposure to

TABLE 109.1

CAUSES OF ADRENAL INSUFFICIENCY

Primary AI	Secondary AI
Autoimmune adrenalitis	Exogenous steroid administration
Tuberculosis	Pituitary adenoma
Fungal infection	Metastatic disease in hypothalamus or pituitary
Malignancy	Ischemic necrosis/pituitary apoplexy
Hemorrhage	Infiltrative disease
Infiltrative disease	Empty sella
Genetic	Lymphocytic hypophysitis

AI, adrenal insufficiency.

tuberculosis. The question of AI is frequently raised in the setting of HIV disease. Although the incidence of cytomegalovirus adrenalitis is high in the AIDS population, the incidence of true AI is probably less than 5% (1). This incidence likely increases with end-stage disease. When AI occurs in this setting, it is typically associated with disseminated mycobacterial disease, fungal disease, bilateral adrenal hemorrhage (as a manifestation of antiphosphlipid antibody syndrome), or malignancy (e.g., lymphoma or Kaposi sarcoma). Drugs that impair steroidogenesis (e.g., ketoconazole) or increase the turnover of steroids (e.g., rifampin) also warrant consideration.

Adrenal insufficiency may also arise through loss of the trophic influence of ACTH on adrenal steroidogenesis. Thus, intrinsic hypothalamic–pituitary disease or functional suppression of corticotropes with exogenous steroids may lead to what has been termed *secondary AI*. Table 109.1 also presents potential causes of secondary disease.

ADRENAL INSUFFICIENCY AT THE TIME OF HOSPITALIZATION

Issues at the Time of Admission

Clinical Presentation

The presentation of AI can be subtle, which makes it difficult to diagnose, particularly when it represents a single component of a multifactorial illness, such as sepsis, or develops insidiously over a protracted period of time.

Chronic AI, such as that associated with autoimmune adrenalitis or chronic tuberculosis, presents primarily with constitutional symptoms. Patients complain of weakness, fatigue, general malaise, anorexia, and weight loss. The latter is often of sufficient magnitude to raise the possibility of malignant disease. Patients also complain of vague abdominal discomfort, nausea with or without vomiting, and diarrhea. Hypotension, often with orthostatic signs and symptoms, is seen frequently, particularly in patients with primary AI. Although glucocorticoids are thought to be

important in the maintenance of hepatic glucose production during periods of fasting, hypoglycemia in AI is rare except in children. The most typical diagnostic finding in chronic primary AI is *skin hyperpigmentation*. This is thought to reflect increased levels of melanocyte-stimulating hormone (MSH) and perhaps ACTH itself. The pigmentation is diffuse but can be accentuated in sun-exposed regions. Most notably, it tends to be found in areas where normal pigmentation is typically sparse (e.g., buccal or vaginal mucosa, gums, nail beds, extensor surfaces of the elbows and knees, and creases of the palms). Hyperpigmentation is absent in secondary AI; skin pallor is more typical of this disorder. Loss of axillary and pubic hair may be seen in female patients, reflecting loss of adrenal androgen production.

Acute AI can arise as a result of rapid destruction of adrenal tissue (e.g., during bilateral adrenal hemorrhage) or of acute intercurrent illness in a patient with otherwise "compensated" chronic AI. The clinical presentation of acute AI is more compressed than that of chronic AI. Symptoms of cortisol deficiency may be intensified and accompanied by symptoms referable to the underlying precipitant (e.g., flank, abdominal, or chest pain with acute adrenal hemorrhage). Precipitous loss of adrenal function or exhaustion of adrenal reserve in the setting of heightened stress can result in *adrenal crisis*. This is characterized by hyperthermia, hypoglycemia, intravascular volume contraction, altered mental status, and cardiovascular instability. Responsiveness to vasoconstrictors is compromised by glucocorticoid deficiency. Pressor-resistant hypotension in the appropriate clinical setting should raise suspicion of underlying AI and prompt a trial of steroids. Such a trial engenders little risk to the patient and may be life saving in persons with adrenal compromise.

Differential Diagnosis and Initial Evaluation

The presentation of chronic AI can be confused with that of many chronic wasting disorders, including disseminated malignancy. Acute AI with or without adrenal crisis can be mistaken for sepsis, intracranial disease, myocardial dysfunction, or intra-abdominal catastrophe. In each instance, consideration of the possibility of AI often leads to the correct diagnosis. The combination of hyponatremia and hyperkalemia seen in primary AI also occurs in hypoaldosteronism secondary to diabetes mellitus, interstitial nephritis, and administration of drugs (e.g., heparin, nonsteroidal anti-inflammatory drugs). The same electrolyte abnormalities in AIDS patients more often represent a combination of inappropriate secretion of antidiuretic hormone (SIADH) secondary to pulmonary or central nervous system disease and administration of high doses of trimethoprim-sulfamethoxazole (1). The latter agent has a triamterene-like effect in the distal nephron that leads to impaired potassium excretion.

Laboratory studies are the mainstay of the diagnosis of AI. Typically, these studies are designed both to document the presence of AI and to provide some information regarding the location of the structural or functional lesion (i.e., differentiate primary from secondary AI). Clues to the presence of impaired adrenal function can sometimes be obtained from routine laboratory studies. Eosinophilia or increased numbers of lymphocytes in peripheral blood counts suggest a relative deficiency of circulating glucocorticoids. Increased blood urea nitrogen may be seen as a consequence of volume contraction in primary AI. Hyponatremia can be seen with either primary or secondary AI and appears to reflect increased antidiuretic hormone secretion. Hyperkalemia, reflecting mineralocorticoid deficiency, is suggestive of primary AI.

Random cortisol levels are not particularly helpful in identifying patients with AI unless they consistently fall below 3 mcg/dL (5 mcg/dL in the setting of acute illness) (2). Urinary free cortisol levels are similarly of little use in establishing the diagnosis because they reflect only a small percentage of the total adrenal secretory product during a given 24-hour period.

When AI is suspected, the first step should be to carry out a *rapid ACTH (Cortrosyn) stimulation test* (see Figure 109.1). A basal blood sample is drawn to assess pre-ACTH cortisol levels. Then 250 mcg of synthetic ACTH is administered intramuscularly or intravenously, and additional blood samples are collected 30–60 minutes later. A normal response requires an increase in cortisol levels to above 18 mcg/dL following ACTH administration. The older criteria requiring an increment of more than 7 mcg/dL have largely been abandoned because of the lack of specificity in identifying patients with structural lesions causing true AI.

In general, patients with plasma cortisol levels above 20 mcg/dL at any point during the test can be regarded as having a functionally adequate hypothalamo–pituitary–adrenal axis. An exception to this rule may exist in patients with established septic shock. In one recent study (3), 300 medical and surgical patients were treated with a combination of 200 mg of hydrocortisone and 50 mcg of fludrocortisone daily for 7 days. Those patients who demonstrated a synthetic ACTH-dependent increment in plasma cortisol of less than 9 mcg/dL from baseline to peak level and were treated with the hydrocortisone/fludrocortisone combination showed both decreased mortality (53% vs 63% in the placebo-treated group) and a reduction in the duration of vasopressor therapy. Those with increments greater than 9 mcg/dL showed no benefit from steroid therapy. While this area remains controversial, the threshold for providing supplemental steroid therapy in patients with septic shock and diminished response to ACTH should probably be low, particularly if suspicion of functional adrenal insufficiency is high (e.g., hypotension poorly responsive to fluids and conventional vasopressors).

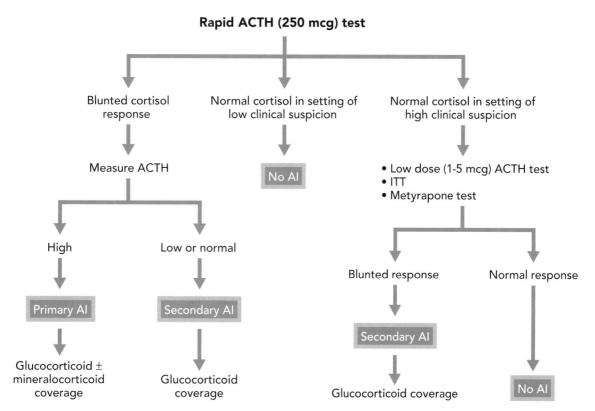

Figure 109.1 Algorithm for the evaluation of adrenal insufficiency. *AI*, adrenal insufficiency; *ITT*, insulin tolerance test. (Modified from Felig P, Baxter JD, Frohman LA, eds. *Endocrinology and Metabolism.* 3rd ed. New York: McGraw-Hill, 1995:555–712, with permission.)

The characteristics of abnormal responses to the ACTH test vary, depending on the nature and duration of the AI. Long-standing primary AI is typically associated with low-normal or frankly suppressed basal cortisol levels that do not increase or increase only modestly following ACTH administration (4). Patients with secondary AI may have normal basal levels, but the increment following ACTH administration is truncated, and the requisite cutoff of 18 mcg/dL is not reached. This truncated response reflects the functional adrenal atrophy that develops with long-term ACTH deficiency. Acute or subacute loss of ACTH secretion can be associated with a completely "normal" rapid ACTH test result despite the presence of profound secondary AI. In this instance, the duration of ACTH deficiency has not been adequate to effect the degree of adrenal atrophy required for the abnormal response.

Measurement of plasma ACTH levels is often helpful in differentiating primary from secondary AI. These levels are typically elevated in the former and either normal or frankly depressed in the latter. When findings are equivocal, a more extensive evaluation of the hypothalamic–pituitary–adrenal axis may be warranted later in the hospitalization or after discharge (Figure 109.1 and below).

Performance of the rapid ACTH test adds only 30 minutes to the initial evaluation, and if possible, it should be completed before cortisol replacement is administered. If the presentation suggests adrenal crisis, dexamethasone (2–4 mg) can be substituted for cortisol replacement. Dexamethasone does not interfere in conventional cortisol assays and thus will not impair interpretation of the ACTH test in the acute setting. Measurement of serum aldosterone levels before and after ACTH administration may provide additional information to aid in the evaluation. A normal aldosterone response (peak >5 ng/mL) is preserved in secondary but not in primary AI.

The utility of the rapid ACTH (250 mcg) test in excluding AI, particularly in the setting of acute illness, has sparked an ongoing debate. Data has been put forward suggesting limited adrenal secretory reserve and/or resistance to endogenous glucocorticoids in this setting (perhaps related to excessive cytokine production), neither of which is addressed by the conventional ACTH test. More refined testing (e.g., with the more physiological 1 mcg ACTH test) may help resolve this issue in the future. In the meantime, clinical judgment should play a role in guiding the decision to provide or withhold glucocorticoid coverage. If clinical suspicion is high, yet the patient shows a normal ACTH (250 mcg) test, short-term treatment with steroids is justified until the patient stabilizes and more definitive testing can be carried out (5).

Therapy

Appropriate therapy of AI is dictated largely by the anticipated glucocorticoid requirements of the patient in a given clinical setting. Thus, management of chronic AI differs considerably from that of acute AI.

Once a diagnosis of chronic AI has been established, the patient should be started on a replacement dose of glucocorticoid. Typically, 20 mg of cortisol in the morning and 10 mg in the evening provides sufficient replacement for the average patient, but this may need to be titrated to minimize overtreatment or undertreatment. Weight gain is frequently one of the first signs of cryptic glucocorticoid excess in this setting. Other glucocorticoids, such as prednisone, can be substituted in bioequivalent doses.

In patients who display clinically significant *mineralocorticoid deficiency*, 9α-fluorocortisol (Fluorinef) at a dosage of 0.05–0.2 mg daily can be used to control hyperkalemia, orthostatic hypotension, or other symptoms of intravascular volume depletion. Excessive mineralocorticoid levels can result in hypertension and hypokalemia, so the dose should be adjusted empirically. When high doses of cortisol are administered in the acute setting, supplemental mineralocorticoid is usually not required, even in primary AI, because of the intrinsic mineralocorticoid properties of the glucocorticoid.

As noted earlier, acute AI and adrenal crisis represent medical emergencies requiring immediate attention. A rapid ACTH test should be carried out and cortisol given intravenously as soon as the diagnosis is suspected. The dosage should be 100 mg every 8 hours. This is probably in excess of the endogenous glucocorticoid response to stress but guarantees adequate coverage in the acute setting. If the ACTH test fails to confirm the diagnosis and clinical suspicion is low, steroids can be withdrawn. If suspicion remains high despite a normal ACTH test result or if the diagnosis is confirmed, stress-dose steroids should be continued as long as the patient remains unstable. If the clinical situation improves, the hydrocortisone dose can be reduced by half on the second hospital day and then gradually tapered to replacement doses during the next 3–4 days. Dose reduction should be carried out only after careful examination of the patient indicates that the crisis is resolving. Attention should also be directed toward early correction of the sequelae of acute AI. This includes restoring intravascular volume, correcting anemia secondary to adrenal hemorrhage, and correcting hyperkalemia and hypoglycemia if present. Adrenal crisis in a patient with otherwise stable chronic AI and good medication compliance usually arises in the setting of acute physiologic stress. The source of this stress (e.g., sepsis, myocardial ischemia, pulmonary embolus, cerebrovascular accident) should be investigated, but this should not delay the initiation of steroid therapy.

Issues During the Course of Hospitalization

When the results of the rapid ACTH test are equivocal or "normal" but the suspicion of secondary AI remains high, additional testing may be warranted (Figure 109.1).

The low-dose (1–5 mcg) ACTH stimulation test is often useful in identifying subtle deficiencies in adrenal secretory reserve that are not apparent with the standard test (6). The metyrapone test and insulin tolerance test, which examine the entire hypothalamic–pituitary–adrenal axis, are useful in evaluating situations in which borderline or equivocal responses to ACTH stimulation have been identified (7). Nevertheless, they are fraught with potential hazards, such as precipitation of AI or myocardial ischemia, and deaths have been recorded. They are best carried out in consultation with an endocrinologist.

Once the diagnosis of AI has been established and the probable locus of the defect identified, imaging studies may be indicated to provide additional diagnostic information and assist with management. Both computed tomography (CT) and magnetic resonance imaging (MRI) have been used effectively to study the adrenal glands. The choice of one over the other hinges on the availability of radiologic consultants experienced in evaluating adrenal lesions, the type of lesion suspected, and the expense. Typically, one looks for evidence of (a) *adrenal atrophy* suggestive of autoimmune adrenalitis or chronic granulomatous disease, (b) *adrenal enlargement* compatible with metastatic disease, active granulomatous inflammation, hemorrhage, or rarely congenital adrenal hyperplasia, and (c) *parenchymal calcifications* suggestive of chronic granulomatous disease or old hemorrhage. When secondary AI is suspected in a patient who has not received exogenous steroids, MRI of the sella contents and hypothalamus is indicated, particularly if there is evidence of other pituitary hormone deficiency.

Approach to the Incidental Adrenal Mass

Autopsy studies suggest that the frequency of adrenal adenomas approaches 6% in unselected adult populations. Most of these are clinically silent. Increased use of high resolution imaging studies such as CT and MRI have resulted in more frequent detection of adrenal masses during investigation for unrelated intra-abdominal pathology (8, 9). The overwhelming majority of these so-called "adrenal incidentalomas" are nonfunctional cortical adenomas. The remainder are aldosteronomas, pheochromocytomas, cortisol-secreting adrenal adenomas, adrenocortical carcinoma, or metastases originating from malignancies outside the adrenal.

Typically the goals in approaching the incidental adrenal mass are to mitigate morbidity attendant to hormone overproduction by the lesion if it exists and to identify malignancies sufficiently early in their development to allow interventions that will prolong survival. Workup for these lesions should include: (1) measurement of urinary metanephrines and fractionated catecholamines to exclude pheochromocytoma, (2) performance of a 1 mg overnight dexamethasone suppression test to exclude Cushing syndrome, and (3) measurement of serum K^+ and plasma aldosterone concentrations, and plasma renin activity (for calculation of Aldo:PRA ratio) if the patient is hypertensive. Functional adenomas, lesions that are more than 4 cm in diameter, lesions that are less than 4 cm in diameter but that increase more than 1 cm over a 12-month period, or lesions that have malignant characteristics on CT or MRI should be removed through a laparoscopic approach (9). *Fine needle aspiration (FNA) is not indicated for most primary adrenal lesions* and, in fact, is contraindicated if a pheochromocytoma or adrenal cortical carcinoma is suspected. FNA may have limited utility in diagnosis of a suspected metastases or adrenal involvement with tuberculosis or other infections. Each of these typically presents with manifestations outside the adrenal glands.

Discharge Issues

Patients with chronic AI should be instructed to increase their glucocorticoid dose in the setting of physiologic stress. With mild-to-moderate stress (e.g., viral syndrome or minor trauma), doubling the glucocorticoid dose for several days followed by a return to the basal dose as the stress resolves is often sufficient to provide the requisite increase in coverage. With more serious illness, patients should receive 100 mg of intravenous cortisol every 6–8 hours. This typically takes place in a hospital setting. For potentially serious stress outside the hospital, the patient should be instructed to take 100 mg of cortisol and come to the emergency department for further evaluation. Patients who do not live in close proximity to medical aid should be provided with parenteral steroid preparations for use in emergency situations. MedicAlert bracelets should be obtained for all patients with known or suspected AI. These bracelets should include information regarding the diagnosis, the patient's medications, and the physician to contact in case of an emergency.

ASSESSMENT AND MANAGEMENT OF THE PATIENT PRESENTING WITH ADRENAL INSUFFICIENCY DURING A HOSPITALIZATION

This scenario is best subdivided into anticipated and unanticipated AI. The former would include patients admitted for deliberate reduction in exogenous steroid dosage, bilateral adrenalectomy, or transsphenoidal resection of an ACTH-producing pituitary tumor. In each instance, AI is anticipated, and appropriate steroid coverage is provided. The appearance of unanticipated AI several days into a hospitalization should raise the possibilities of exogenous steroid administration before admission, administration of drugs such as rifampin or ketoconazole (which unmask limited adrenal secretory reserve), or bilateral adrenal hemorrhage secondary to ongoing sepsis, thrombotic disorders, or anticoagulant administration. As explained above, patients should receive immediate steroid coverage and undergo a rapid ACTH stimulation test followed by more definitive characterization of the functional and anatomic location of the defect.

Management of the patient with *AI in the perioperative period* warrants special consideration. Relatively minor surgery in the outpatient setting may not require more than the usual replacement coverage. Procedures likely to cause an intermediate level of physiologic stress (e.g., limb revascularization) should prompt the prescription of additional steroid coverage. One hundred milligrams of intramuscular cortisol, or its equivalent, on call to the operating room, and 50 mg every 8 hours for the ensuing 24 hours, should provide adequate perioperative coverage. The intramuscular dose provides a depot of steroid to cover the possibility of missed or delayed steroid doses in the immediate postoperative period. If the patient is stable, the parenteral dose can be reduced by half on the second or third postoperative day. The oral daily replacement dose can then be reestablished when the patient is able to resume oral intake. For patients undergoing major surgical procedures that are likely to lead to near-maximal physiologic stress, 100 mg of intramuscular cortisol should be given on call to the operating room, and 100 mg should be given intravenously every 8 hours, or 75 mg every 6 hours, through the day of surgery. The dose of cortisol can be reduced in stepwise fashion beginning on the second or third postoperative day while the physician watches for possible early signs of AI. It can then typically be tapered to replacement levels by the seventh postoperative day, provided postoperative complications do not develop.

KEY POINTS

- Adrenal insufficiency in either the chronic or acute form may present in such a nonspecific manner that the diagnosis is overlooked initially.
- Recognition of the appropriate clinical setting and compatible clinical manifestations are the most important factors leading to a successful diagnosis.
- In the acute setting, administration of exogenous glucocorticoid should be initiated after completion of a rapid ACTH stimulation test.
- If therapy cannot be delayed, the ACTH stimulation test can be carried out while the patient is treated with dexamethasone.

- Patients with chronic adrenal insufficiency require additional steroid coverage during periods of moderate-to-severe physiologic stress.
- Early diagnosis of adrenal insufficiency and careful attention to the details of patient management are the keys to long-term survival in this disorder.

REFERENCES

1. Sellmeyer DE, Grunfeld C. Endocrine and metabolic disturbances in human immunodeficiency virus infection and the acquired immune deficiency syndrome. *Endocr Rev* 1996;17:518–532.
2. Grinspoon SK, Biller BMK. Laboratory assessment of adrenal insufficiency. *J Clin Endocrinol Metab* 1994;79:923–931.
3. Annane D, Sebille V, Charpentier C, et al. Effect of treatment with low doses of hydrocortisone and fludrocortisone on mortality in patients with septic shock. *JAMA* 2002;288:862–871.
4. Tordjman K, Jaffe A, Grazas N, Apter C, Stern N. The role of the low-dose (1 mg) adrenocorticotropin test in the evaluation of patients with pituitary disease. *J Clin Endocrinol Metab* 1995;80:1301–1305.
5. Cooper MS, Stewart PM. Corticosteroid insufficiency in acutely ill patients. *New Engl J Med* 2003;348:727–734.
6. Hartzband PI, Van Herle AJ, Sorger L, Cope D. Assessment of hypothalamic-pituitary-adrenal (HPA) axis dysfunction: comparison of ACTH stimulation, insulin-hypoglycemia and metyrapone. *J Endocrinol Invest* 1988;11:769–776.
7. Oelkers W, Diederich S, Bahr V. Diagnosis and therapy surveillance in Addison's disease: rapid adrenocorticotropin (ACTH) test and measurement of plasma ACTH, renin activity, and aldosterone. *J Clin Endocrinol Metab* 1992;75:259–264.
8. Thompson GB, Young WF. Adrenal incidentaloma. *Curr Opin Oncol* 2003;15:84–90.
9. Grumbach MM, Biller BM, Braunstein GD, et al. Management of the clinically inapparent adrenal mass ("incidentaloma"). *Ann Int Med* 2003;138:424–429.

ADDITIONAL READING

Beishuizen A, Thijis LG. Relative adrenal failure in intensive care: an identifiable problem requiring treatment? *Best Prac Res Clin Endocrinol Metab* 2001;15:513–531.

Coursin DB, Wood KE. Corticoid supplementation for adrenal insufficiency. *JAMA* 2002;287:236–240.

Minneci PC, Deans KJ, Banks SM, Eichacker PQ, Natanson C. Meta-analysis: the effect of steroids on survival and shock during sepsis depends on the dose. *Ann Intern Med* 2004;41:47–56.

Oelkers W. Adrenal insufficiency. *N Engl J Med* 1996;335:1206–1212.

Salem M, Tainsh RE, Bromberg J, Loriaux DL, Chernow B. Perioperative glucocorticoid coverage. A reassessment 42 years after emergence of the problem. *Ann Surg* 1994;219:416–425.

Ten S, New M, MacLaren N. Addison's disease 2001. *Endocr Rev* 2001;86:2909–2922.

Werbel SS, Ober KP. Acute adrenal insufficiency. *Endocrinol Metab Clin North Am* 1993;22:303–328.

Rheumatology

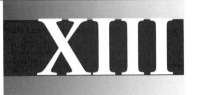

Signs, Symptoms, and Laboratory Abnormalities in Rheumatology

110

Jeffrey Critchfield

TOPICS COVERED IN CHAPTER

■ Joint Pain 1111
■ Joint Swelling 1112
■ New Signs and Symptoms in a Patient with Underlying Rheumatic Disease 1115
■ Elevated Sedimentation Factor 1116
■ Positive Antinuclear Antibody Test 1117
■ Positive Rheumatoid Factor Test 1118
■ Positive Antineutrophil Cytoplasmic Antibody Test 1118
■ Hypocomplementemia 1119

INTRODUCTION

The rheumatic diseases constitute a heterogeneous group of illnesses with correspondingly heterogeneous clinical signs and symptoms. At one end of the spectrum are diseases manifested exclusively by musculoskeletal signs and symptoms (e.g., joint or muscle pain), the presence of which immediately suggests a rheumatologic problem. At the other end of the spectrum are the systemic rheumatic diseases, which can present with virtually any sign or symptom (e.g., fever, chest pain, rash, confusion, deafness, and countless others). Because many of these signs and symptoms do not immediately suggest a rheumatologic problem, the suc-

cessful identification of the systemic rheumatic diseases requires a thorough differential diagnosis and a systematic approach to the clinical workup.

This chapter provides guidelines applicable to the broad spectrum of rheumatology. It begins with a strategy for approaching patients with the most common musculoskeletal signs and symptoms. It then proceeds to a discussion of the approach to patients with systemic rheumatic diseases and the significance of specialized laboratory tests in their evaluation.

JOINT PAIN

When Joint Pain Presents at the Time of Admission

Description and Differential Diagnosis

It is common for patients to complain of joint pain when in fact the pain is arising from elsewhere. Therefore, the first challenge in evaluating a patient with joint pain is to determine whether the pain truly originates from within a *joint* (arthralgia, arthritis) or whether the source is actually within the *periarticular structures* (e.g., bursitis, tendinitis), *underlying bone* (e.g., fracture, osteomyelitis, tumor), or *overlying skin* (e.g., cellulitis). For example, virtually all patients with greater trochanteric bursitis report the problem as hip pain, even though the hip joint is anatomically distinct from the site of the pain and may well be normal. This distinction can only be made with a careful physical examination of the joints, including inspection, palpation, and assessment of the range of motion. Inspection and palpation may demonstrate swelling and synovial thickening and thereby confirm the presence of arthritis. (This will be further discussed under "Joint Swelling.")

Evaluation

Although physical examination is the most important step in determining the source of joint pain, radiographic studies may be required to establish the precise nature of the problem. As a general rule, if physical examination does not establish the cause of the pain, radiography is warranted. This may show fracture, infection, or tumor in bone, hypertrophic pulmonary osteoarthropathy in the periosteum, calcification in a periarticular tendon, or some other definitive finding that identifies the source outside the joint. When evaluating nontraumatic, acute joint pain (less than 2–3 weeks' duration), bear in mind that the process may not have persisted for sufficient time to develop abnormalities detectable by plain radiography. Alternatively, for many of the chronic rheumatic diseases, the roentgenogram may reveal a characteristic pattern of bony erosions within the joint that suggests the correct diagnosis. For example, rheumatoid arthritis (RA), the seronegative arthritides (reactive arthritis, psoriatic arthritis, ankylosing spondylitis), and gout each can cause distinctive erosive damage.

Management

The management of joint pain is determined by the precise diagnosis. Immobilization may be appropriate in some instances (e.g., intra-articular hemorrhage), whereas physical therapy and range-of-motion exercises may be appropriate in others (e.g., frozen shoulder). Ice may be appropriate for acute injuries, but heat may be more effective for chronic joint pain. Anti-inflammatory medications may work well in gout but are no substitute for systemic antibiotics in treating a septic joint. The only generalization is that *there is rarely any harm in providing analgesia,* in whatever form is effective, to make the patient more comfortable while more definitive measures aimed at treating the cause of pain are instituted.

When Joint Pain Appears During Hospitalization

Almost by definition, joint pain that appears during hospitalization represents an acute problem and therefore should be approached according to the guidelines described in Chapter 113. It is worth emphasizing here, however, that certain joint problems are more likely to occur during hospitalization than at other times. Both gout and pseudogout commonly develop in hospitalized patients, particularly in the postoperative setting. In this case, the joint pain is accompanied by dramatic signs of inflammation, including warmth, redness, and swelling. Fluxes in uric acid levels associated with changes in diet (including being without oral intake prior to a procedure) can contribute to this predisposition. Gout during hospitalization is particularly common in alcoholics, who may enter the hospital with lactic acidosis or ketoacidosis, both of which interfere with uric acid excretion. Fluxes in uric acid concentration that occur as these metabolic disturbances are corrected can contribute to an acute attack of gout. Joint problems that stem from prolonged immobilization, sometimes in awkward positions, during procedures or surgery are also more likely to develop in hospitalized patients. Accordingly, mechanical back pain, bursitis, or nerve and tendon compressions are seen commonly in hospitalized patients.

JOINT SWELLING

When Joint Swelling Presents at the Time of Admission

Description and Differential Diagnosis

The detection of joint swelling during physical examination localizes the pathology within the joint and should trigger a straightforward, almost invariably informative approach to differential diagnosis. This approach is based on the answers to three simple questions:

1. *Is the problem acute or chronic?* This question is answered by the history.
2. *How many joints are involved?* This question is best answered by a complete musculoskeletal examination. Just as the careful clinician reads the entire chest radiograph before focusing on the lobar infiltrate, the clinician evaluating arthritis must consider even asymptomatic joints. Reliance on the history can sometimes be misleading, especially when the intensity of pain in a single joint distracts the patient from more subtle symptoms in other joints.
3. *Are there hints of systemic involvement?* Unintended weight loss, pronounced fatigue, subjective fevers, or new skin rashes hint at a systemic process, cuing the clinician to consider an evaluation for systemic infections, neoplasms, or a systemic connective tissue disease.

The appeal of this approach to differential diagnosis is the ease with which the data can be gathered—a history of the present illness and a musculoskeletal exam are sufficient to

TABLE 110.1

COMMON CAUSES OF MONARTICULAR ARTHRITIS

Acute

Noninflammatory	Inflammatory
Trauma	Infection (e.g., bacterial,
Hemarthrosis	Mycobacterial, fungal, viral)
Sickle cell anemia	Gout (monosodium urate crystals)
	Pseudogout (calcium
	pyrophosphate dihydrate)
	Trauma
	Sickle cell anemia

Chronic

Noninflammatory	Inflammatory
Osteoarthritis	Infection (e.g., Mycobacterial,
Neuropathic joint	*Borrelia burgdorferi*,
Hemarthrosis	*Coccidioides immitis*)
Sickle cell anemia	

craft an excellent differential diagnosis. Further refinement of the differential can be made if the clinician has access to the results of a diagnostic arthrocentesis. Synovial analysis will suggest whether the process is inflammatory or noninflammatory. A detailed description of synovial fluid evaluation is provided in Chapter 113. For the purposes of this approach to differential diagnosis, it is sufficient to rely on the number of white blood cells in the joint fluid to determine whether the fluid is inflammatory ($>2,500/\mu L$) or noninflammatory ($<2,500/\mu L$). The differential diagnosis is further refined by a complete physical exam with careful attention to physical signs of systemic illness. Like all strategies that are designed primarily to detect common problems, this approach requires vigilance to recognize when the common diagnoses seem not to fit and unusual explanations must be sought. It is summarized below and in Tables 110.1 and 110.2.

Common Causes of Acute Monarticular Arthritis

If the joint fluid is *noninflammatory*, the most likely diagnoses are trauma, nontraumatic hemorrhage (e.g., as a result of hemophilia, thrombocytopenia, or some other coagulopathy), or sickle cell anemia (Table 110.1). These are easily distinguished by history or, when necessary, by blood tests. If the joint fluid is *inflammatory*, the most likely diagnoses are a bacterial joint infection (septic arthritis) or crystal-induced arthritis. Either process can cause high fevers and similar findings on physical exam: gout may mimic cellulitis, while septic joints in gouty patients have frequently been ascribed to "just another gouty flare." Both can trigger extremely high synovial and peripheral blood cell counts. Thus arthrocentesis with Gram stain, synovial bacterial culture, and microscopic crystal analysis are crucial components in the evaluation of this patient population. Sickle cell anemia is an occasional confounder because the joint fluid may be inflammatory or noninflammatory, the pattern of joint involvement may be monarticular or polyarticular, and the presentation may be acute or chronic. However, a known history of sickle cell anemia (Chapter 97) almost invariably accompanies these presentations, so the diagnosis is rarely difficult.

TABLE 110.2

COMMON CAUSES OF POLYARTICULAR ARTHRITIS

Acute

Infection
Hepatitis B, Parvovirus B19
Neisseria gonorrhea
Subacute bacterial endocarditis[a]
Acute rheumatic fever[a]
Crystal-induced arthritis (e.g., monosodium urate)
Acute onset rheumatic condition (RA, SLE)
Sickle cell crisis[a]

Chronic

Noninflammatory	Inflammatory
Osteoarthritis	Infections (*Borrelia burgdorferi*, hepatitis C, Parvovirus B19)
	Rheumatic condition (RA, SLE, seronegative arthritis)
	Paraneoplastic syndrome

[a] These diseases may be characterized by inflammatory or noninflammatory joint fluid.
RA, rheumatoid arthritis; *SLE*, systemic lupus erythematosus.

Common Causes of Chronic Monarticular Arthritis

If the joint fluid is *noninflammatory*, the diagnosis is likely to be osteoarthritis, neuropathic arthropathy (Charcot joint), trauma, hemophilia, or sickle cell anemia (Table 110.1). Roentgenograms and, if necessary, appropriate laboratory tests generally make distinguishing among these possibilities quite straightforward. If the joint fluid is *inflammatory*, the index of suspicion for infection, particularly pathogens such as Mycobacterium, endemic fungi, or *Borrelia borgderferi* should be high. In these cases, signs and symptoms of systemic disease—e.g., weight loss, sweats, or fatigue—will be particularly important to elicit.

Common Causes of Acute Polyarticular Arthritis

Acute polyarthritis is usually caused by infection, polyarticular gout, or sickle cell crisis. Infections to consider include diseases of viral origin (e.g., rubella, hepatitis B, parvovirus, or HIV infection), gonococcemia, bacterial endocarditis, and acute rheumatic fever (Table 110.2). Detection of new or changing cardiac murmurs or observation of pustular skin lesions would significantly move the differential diagnosis toward endocarditis or disseminated gonococcal infections, respectively. Polyarticular gout can be diagnosed definitively by detection of crystals in the joint fluid and should be strongly considered only in the patient with prior bouts of gout. Though uncommon, patients who are ultimately diagnosed with a connective tissue disease may present with acute onset of symptoms. A small fraction of patients with rheumatoid arthritis, for example, can recall the very day they awoke with multiple swollen joints.

Common Causes of Chronic Polyarticular Arthritis

The patient with chronic polyarticular arthritis and *noninflammatory* joint fluid is quite likely to have osteoarthritis (Table 110.2). This impression can generally be confirmed by roentgenograms. The chronic *inflammatory* polyarthritides are most likely to be caused by the classic rheumatic conditions (e.g., rheumatoid arthritis; seronegative arthritis; connective tissue diseases). The differential, however, still includes chronic infections with viruses such as hepatitis C and bacteria such as *Borrelia burgdorferi*. Paraneoplastic syndromes such as hypertrophic osteoarthropathy can cause arthritis even when the cancerous process is occult. Sometimes, associated signs and symptoms provide critical clues to one of the chronic inflammatory arthritides from the outset. For example, the presence of urethritis and conjunctivitis may suggest Reiter disease; psoriatic plaques may be the key to diagnosing psoriatic arthritis; chronic bloody, loose stools point to inflammatory bowel disease. RA and systemic lupus erythematosus (SLE), on the other hand, rarely can be diagnosed with certainty on the first visit. When these diagnoses are suspected, specialized serologic tests are often required to establish the diagnosis. The use of these tests is described under "Laboratory Abnormalities."

Evaluation

The simple approach to differential diagnosis described above should not be a substitute for a thorough history and physical examination, either of which may provide critical clues to the correct diagnosis. Particularly helpful aspects of the history are the following:

Age and Gender

Most common causes of arthritis can affect persons of either sex at any age. However, age and gender strongly influence the likelihood of many diagnoses and can help prioritize the differential diagnosis and workup. For example, acute rheumatic fever is seen almost exclusively in children, gonococcal arthritis most commonly in young adults, and osteoarthritis most frequently in the elderly. Most patients with RA, SLE, or scleroderma are women, whereas most with ankylosing spondylitis or gout are men.

Duration of Symptoms

The duration of symptoms provides a highly important clue to the diagnosis and is the basis for one of the three key questions described in the previous section.

Past Medical History/History of Present Illness

The setting in which arthritis occurs often shapes the differential diagnosis. A history of trauma, intravenous drug use, or exposure to hepatitis, for example, could each be the key to a correct diagnosis. Similarly, the onset of joint pain in a patient with a known systemic illness (e.g., sickle cell anemia, SLE, inflammatory bowel disease) carries a different implication than the onset of joint pain in someone who was previously healthy.

Review of Systems

Because joint pain is often one manifestation of a systemic infection or connective tissue disease, a careful review of systems is important in all patients. Has the patient had fever, iritis, pleurisy, diarrhea, or urethritis? Each of these associated symptoms influences the differential diagnosis.

Just as the details of the history shape our perception of a patient with arthritis, so, too, do all the elements of the physical examination. It is not at all uncommon for the physical examination to alter the approach to a patient with unexplained joint pain or swelling. Particularly crucial elements of the examination are the following:

Vital Signs. Temperature is especially important to document. Low-grade fever may occur in almost any inflammatory arthritis (e.g., gout, RA), but high-grade fever strongly suggests infection (Chapter 62).

Skin. Many diseases that involve joint pain are associated with characteristic rashes. Valuable findings include urticaria in patients with hepatitis B prodrome, a photosensitive malar rash in those with SLE, gonococcal pustules, psoriatic plaques, rheumatoid nodules, and gouty tophi.

Eyes. Ocular manifestations of rheumatic diseases are common. These include conjunctivitis in reactive arthritis or gonococcal disease, uveitis in ankylosing spondylitis, and scleritis in RA.

Oropharynx. Presence of palatal or buccal ulcers could suggest SLE, a seronegative arthritis, or Behçet disease.

Cardiopulmonary Examination. Several cardiopulmonary abnormalities may be informative. For example, bacterial endocarditis (Chapter 71) presents with joint pain in about 15% of cases. Therefore, detection of a murmur in a patient with joint pain can be a critical finding. Similarly, the discovery of a pleural or pericardial rub in a patient with joint pain may point toward RA or SLE.

Genitourinary Examination. Evidence of venereal infection (gonorrhea) or nonspecific urethritis (reactive arthritis) will likely influence the differential diagnosis.

Joint Examination. The most important aspect of the physical examination of a patient with joint pain is a thorough examination of all joints. Often, patients focus on a single "worst" joint only to have it discovered that other joints are also involved, albeit to a lesser extent. The discovery of polyarthritis can completely change the differential diagnosis. Even among patients with polyarthritis, the detection of characteristic patterns of involvement can be helpful. For example, symmetric involvement of the small joints of the hands and feet is typical of RA (or perhaps viral arthritis). On the other hand, asymmetric involvement of large joints would be more typical of one of the seronegative arthritides, such as reactive arthritis, psoriatic arthritis, or ankylosing spondylitis.

Management

Like the management of joint pain (arthralgia), the management of joint swelling (arthritis) is determined entirely by the cause of the problem. Drainage is sometimes essential, as in patients with septic arthritis; often, it is unimportant. Sometimes local corticosteroid injection is helpful, but not if multiple small joints are involved or infection is suspected. The inability to generalize about the management of joint swelling underscores the importance of the systematic pursuit of a definitive diagnosis.

When Joint Swelling Appears During Hospitalization

The development of joint swelling during hospitalization should be evaluated, just as one would evaluate acute joint swelling in any other setting (Chapter 113). However, as described earlier in the section on joint pain, certain possibilities should come to mind first when the patient is hospitalized. Crystal-induced arthritis is one of these, but not

the only one. The onset of joint swelling in an immunosuppressed patient or in a patient hospitalized for an infection or valvular heart disease mandates a careful search for an infectious etiology. New polyarthritis in a hospitalized patient may be caused by serum sickness related to a new medication.

NEW SIGNS AND SYMPTOMS IN A PATIENT WITH UNDERLYING RHEUMATIC DISEASE

Description and Differential Diagnosis

Patients with an established diagnosis of a systemic rheumatic disease (e.g., RA, SLE, Wegener's granulomatosis) constitute a particularly challenging problem because they can present to the hospital with a myriad of signs or symptoms (Chapters 111 and 112). A patient with RA may present with shortness of breath related to a pleural effusion. A patient with SLE may present following a seizure. A patient with vasculitis may present with angina. Therefore, it is particularly important in these patients to consider virtually any new problem as a possible manifestation of the underlying disease. The differential diagnosis must not stop there, however, because patients with rheumatic diseases are susceptible to an array of other problems. Many patients with systemic rheumatic diseases are taking immunosuppressive medications, which raises the risk for infection. The dramatic success and thus widespread use of anti-tumor necrosis factor (anti-TNF) therapies for multiple rheumatic conditions, for example, has been accompanied by an increased risk for disseminated mycobacterial infections (1). Even in the absence of immunosuppressive drugs, certain infections are more likely to occur in people with rheumatic diseases. The patient with RA-induced eroded bony surfaces or joint prostheses may develop a septic joint even from transient bacteremia. Therefore, a new flare of arthritis in one joint, out of proportion to symptoms in other joints, should raise the possibility of septic arthritis and should not be casually attributed to a flare of RA. Similarly, patients with SLE are at high risk for the development of osteonecrosis of bone, either as a manifestation of the underlying disease or as a complication of corticosteroid therapy. Finally, people with systemic rheumatic diseases are often on complex medication regimens that frequently change. Therefore, it is important to immediately consider adverse drug reactions or even medication errors (see Chapter 21) whenever a new problem occurs.

Evaluation

The cardinal rule in evaluating any new complaint in a patient with an underlying systemic rheumatic disease is thoroughness. Whatever the problem, it may be a manifestation of the disease itself, a superimposed problem to which the patient is predisposed, a medication complication, or a new and unrelated medical problem. A broad differential diagnosis and a correspondingly thorough evaluation are essential.

Management

The management of a new problem in a patient with an underlying systemic rheumatic disease depends entirely on the results of the diagnostic evaluation.

LABORATORY ABNORMALITIES

Erythrocyte Sedimentation Rate

When an Elevated Erythrocyte Sedimentation Rate Is Present at the Time of Admission

Description and Differential Diagnosis
Measurement of the erythrocyte sedimentation rate (ESR) is a technically simple test in which blood, mixed with the anticoagulant sodium citrate, is added to a 200-mm glass tube and left to "sediment" for one hour at room temperature (2). The quantitative result is the distance between the top of the tube and the meniscus of aggregated red blood cells. Acute-phase reactants such as haptoglobin, immunoglobulins, and, most importantly, fibrinogen cross-link red blood cells into large, rapidly falling aggregates that accelerate the ESR (3). Other factors that can increase the ESR include the presence of paraproteins, anemia, or the use of oral contraceptives. Androgens seem to lower the ESR; consequently, the normal range for men (<15 mm/h) is somewhat lower than the normal range for women (<28 mm/h). Importantly, the normal range increases slightly with increasing age in both men and women.

Several studies have examined the diagnoses associated with a *markedly elevated ESR* (>100 mm/h) (4). Infectious diseases are the most common cause, accounting for 35% (in academic tertiary centers) to 62% (in rural community hospitals) of all patients with the abnormality. Any infectious agent, but especially bacterial pathogens, can be associated with an accelerated ESR. The inflammatory rheumatic diseases, such as RA, SLE, and vasculitis, comprise the second most common diagnostic group in patients with an elevated ESR. Of particular note is the important role the ESR plays in diagnosing and monitoring *polymyalgia rheumatica* and *giant cell arteritis*. The ESR is greater than 50 mm/h in the vast majority of cases of polymyalgia rheumatica or giant cell arteritis, but recent studies have demonstrated that even these conditions can (infrequently) occur in patients with an ESR less than 20 mm/h (Chapter 111). Neoplasms were found to be causative in 10%–15% of patients with a markedly elevated ESR. Because immunoglobulins can increase red blood cell aggregation, one must consider lymphoproliferative malignancies such as multiple myeloma, macroglobulinemia, and lymphoma. Finally, advanced renal disease (particularly end-stage renal disease) is typically associated with a markedly elevated ESR.

Evaluation
Because the differential diagnosis of an elevated ESR is so broad, the value of this result in isolation is limited. The practitioner must therefore incorporate the test result into the overall clinical picture by using demographics, health-related behaviors, comorbidities, review of systems, and physical examination findings to refine the probability of disease. Symptoms such as low-grade fevers, sweats, and weight loss can suggest occult infection or malignancy. New signs, such as skin lesions or swollen joints, may point to a rheumatologic condition. Alternatively, paresthesias can be the clue to multiple myeloma or a vasculitis.

Management
The management will be dictated by the initial results obtained from workup. Because infections commonly cause an elevated ESR, and because many infections can be catastrophic in the short term, clinical judgment will sometimes dictate initiation of empiric antibiotic therapy until the culture results are known (e.g., when subacute bacterial endocarditis [SBE] is being considered, after multiple blood cultures have been obtained). However, on other occasions, legitimate concerns about catastrophic complications of connective tissue diseases (e.g., blindness in a patient with suspected giant cell arteritis) will necessitate initiation of empiric immunosuppressive therapy. The challenge in these situations, therefore, is to act swiftly enough to minimize the greatest risk while being cautious enough to avoid immunosuppressive therapy in patients who are infected.

When an Elevated Erythrocyte Sedimentation Rate Appears During Hospitalization

Description and Differential Diagnosis
The new appearance of an elevated ESR during hospitalization implies an acute cause and therefore strongly suggests infection. Other acute inflammatory processes, such as gout, should also be considered, depending on the clinical context. Although neoplasms and connective tissue diseases are common causes of an elevated ESR in clinic populations, it would be unusual for these problems to be the cause of an acutely elevated ESR in a hospitalized patient.

Evaluation and Management
Proper management can be determined only after the cause of the elevated ESR has been established. However, once this has been accomplished, the ESR determination can be of value during management by providing an

objective guide to the effectiveness of therapy. Specifically, in conjunction with other clinical and laboratory parameters, the trend of the ESR can be helpful in directing the duration and intensity of therapy in patients with serious infections (e.g., osteomyelitis) or connective tissue diseases (e.g., temporal arteritis).

Antinuclear Antibodies

When the Antinuclear Antibody Test Result Is Positive at the Time of Admission

Description and Differential Diagnosis
The antinuclear antibody (ANA) test detects serum antibodies to various nuclear antigens (e.g., histones, DNA, RNA). The test result is reported as a titer, often accompanied by a pattern of fluorescence seen under microscopy. The pattern of fluorescence may provide a clue to the nature of the target antigens, but definitive identification of the target (e.g., double-stranded DNA) requires further specialized tests.

Several prospective studies of clinically healthy cohorts demonstrate that a positive ANA test result at a titer of 1:40 can be detected in 20%–30% of asymptomatic people (5). The frequency of positive test results is higher in women and in the elderly. With a titer of 1:80, the false-positive rate is closer to 10%; fewer than 5% of normal subjects will have a titer of 1:160.

Even at higher titers (>1:160), the differential diagnosis of a positive ANA test result is broad. The ANA test is highly sensitive for SLE (more than 95% of patients with SLE have a titer >1:160), but not specific. It may also be positive in people with virtually any other connective tissue disease, including scleroderma, Sjögren syndrome, polymyositis/dermatomyositis, or RA (see Chapter 112 for further information on these disorders). Moreover, many drugs stimulate the production of ANAs, a phenomenon seen most frequently with procainamide and hydralazine (6). Chronic active hepatitis, Laennec cirrhosis, and primary biliary cirrhosis are sometimes associated with a positive ANA test result. The ANA test result may also be positive in people with neoplasms or chronic infections.

Evaluation
An abnormal ANA test result should prompt a directed history with specific inquiries into the medication list and family history, in addition to the occurrence of signs and symptoms that suggest a rheumatologic disorder (e.g., photosensitive rash, oral ulcers, arthralgia/arthritis, muscle weakness, dry eyes and mouth). Although many of these signs and symptoms can occur in diverse settings (e.g., weakness with neoplasm or myositis), their presence should motivate the pursuit of a definitive diagnosis.

If, after initial evaluation, a connective tissue disease is still a consideration, further serologic testing to characterize

the auto-antibodies is indicated. For example, antidouble-stranded DNA and anti-SM are highly specific for SLE, with a high positive predictive value for the diagnosis. Though less specific, quantitative analysis of complement levels C3 or C4 can also suggest SLE. Because the pathologic processes that yield abnormal ANAs frequently involve multiple organ systems, urinalysis, complete blood count, coagulation studies, renal function tests, and liver function tests should be performed. Whereas false positive ANAs are common, the absence of an abnormal ANA is particularly valuable when excluding the possibility of SLE. With a sensitivity of 99% for SLE, the negative predictive value of a normal ANA is so high as to essentially eliminate SLE from the differential.

Management
The ANA test result rarely guides management because it does not correlate with disease activity. Therefore, once it is noted to be abnormal, the test need not be repeated. The main value of the ANA test is to refine the pretest probability for a connective tissue disease when the clinical findings already suggest this possibility. In these situations, the finding of a positive ANA test result warrants further workup to establish the correct diagnosis and initiate appropriate therapy.

When a Positive Antinuclear Antibody Test Result Appears During Hospitalization

Differential Diagnosis
An ANA test, when ordered during hospitalization, often is performed during a protracted, complicated course, when the exclusion of other diagnostic possibilities leads to the eventual consideration of a connective tissue disease. Because an abnormal ANA test result can signify either an innocuous etiology (e.g., medications or a normal variant) or an as-yet-undiagnosed connective tissue disease, it is critical to have some sense of the clinical possibilities before the test is performed.

Evaluation and Management
The acute nature of most illnesses in hospitalized patients often mandates follow-up serologic studies (e.g., anti-ds-DNA, anti-Smith antigen, complement levels) and aggressive pursuit of a tissue diagnosis when the ANA test result is positive. A review of all the primary data, including musculoskeletal and skin examination findings, and attention to indicators of multi-organ system involvement can provide important clues regarding the significance of the abnormal ANA test result. Prompt subspecialty consultation will focus the evaluation on the remaining possibilities, lower the potential for inappropriate empiric therapy, and facilitate elucidation of the diagnosis. Management will depend on the precise explanation for the positive ANA test result.

Rheumatoid Factor

When the Rheumatoid Factor Test Result Is Positive at the Time of Admission

Description and Differential Diagnosis

Rheumatoid factor (RF) is an auto-antibody (most commonly an immunoglobulin M antibody) that binds the constant portion of immunoglobulin G molecules. It is strongly associated with, but not specific for, RA. Although its presence may precede the onset of arthritis, many patients will be clinically identified as having RA before they become seropositive. Eventually, 70%–85% of people with RA have a test result positive for RF. Serologic surveys demonstrate the presence of RF in 5% of healthy young adults and 15% of healthy elderly adults. An appreciation that RF is an immunoglobulin leads to the understanding that any chronic inflammatory state may be associated with production of RF. Virtually all the systemic connective tissue diseases can be associated with the presence of RF (e.g., Sjögren syndrome, SLE, scleroderma, and cryoglobulinemia). Chronic infections, including subacute bacterial endocarditis, tuberculosis, leprosy, syphilis, and rheumatic fever, also commonly are associated with positivity for RF. Finally, RF is detected in some patients with neoplasms, especially leukemias, lymphomas, and macroglobulinemia.

Evaluation

The history and physical examination should provide hints regarding the likelihood of infectious or neoplastic etiologies. Musculoskeletal findings, if present, may focus the workup on possible connective tissue diseases. Radiography of arthritic joints can be particularly valuable because periarticular osteopenia and characteristic erosions may be diagnostic of RA.

Management

Titers for RF do not correlate well with disease activity. Therefore, the RF titer is rarely helpful in guiding the management of patients with RA. The test is primarily of diagnostic value and of some prognostic value. Patients with higher titers generally have more aggressive joint disease and are at greater risk for extra-articular manifestations of RA, including subcutaneous nodules, interstitial lung disease, scleritis, and vasculitis.

When a Positive Rheumatoid Factor Test Result Appears During Hospitalization

In the acutely ill patient, detection of RF should trigger a search for occult infection. Subacute bacterial endocarditis in particular can cause musculoskeletal complaints that may mimic the presentation of an inflammatory arthritis. Similarly, RF may be a clue to the diagnosis of vasculitis. The evaluation of RF positivity during hospitalization is similar to the evaluation that would be indicated at admission, although even more emphasis should be placed on ruling out infectious etiologies.

Antineutrophil Cytoplasmic Antibodies

When the Antineutrophil Cytoplasmic Antibody Test Result Is Positive at the Time of Admission

Description and Differential Diagnosis

The antineutrophil cytoplasmic antibody (ANCA) test detects a group of auto-antibodies that react with specific cytoplasmic antigens (7). Depending on the precise nature of the target antigen, two ANCA patterns can be seen when ethanol-fixed neutrophils are stained. The cytosolic (cANCA) pattern correlates with antibodies that recognize the proteinase-3 neutrophil protease (PR3). The perinuclear (pANCA) pattern is associated with antibodies against the myeloperoxidase enzyme (MPO) found in lysosomes. Increasingly, laboratories are directly measuring the titers of the auto-antibodies rather than relying on the fluorescent staining pattern.

The *cANCA pattern* has been heralded as a marker for Wegener's granulomatosis. In cohorts with a high pretest probability (i.e., >10%), the specificity approaches 98%, with a sensitivity of 60%–80% (5,6). The positive predictive value of the ANCA for a diagnosis of Wegener's plummets when there is a low pretest clinical probability of this uncommon disease. Of the other rheumatic disorders, only Churg-Strauss syndrome and microscopic polyangiitis have demonstrated an association with the typical cANCA pattern (7). An atypical pattern of fluorescence, often read as cANCA, that is not associated with anti-PR3 antibodies has been described with cystic fibrosis, inflammatory bowel disease, primary sclerosing cholangitis, and RA. The *pANCA pattern*, first described in patients with pauci-immune rapidly progressive glomerulonephritis, occurs in 50% of patients with microscopic polyangiitis in the setting of renal failure, with or without pulmonary hemorrhage. The antibodies are also seen in Churg-Strauss syndrome and well described in a host of autoimmune diseases, including: RA, SLE, Sjogren syndrome, poly- and dermatomyositis, reactive arthritis, antiphospholipid antibody syndrome, ulcerative colitis, and primary sclerosing cholangitis (7).

Evaluation

A positive cANCA test result requires a careful evaluation for signs and symptoms of Wegener's granulomatosis. A positive pANCA test result should trigger a search for other vasculitides involving the lungs and kidneys. This topic is covered in detail in the Chapter 111.

Management

The ANCA test is used most often to help diagnose a systemic process. The outcome of the diagnostic evaluation will dictate the direction of therapy. More than a diagnostic test, clinicians have used the titer of the cANCA-related antibodies as a surrogate for disease activity, guiding ongoing therapy of patients with Wegener's granulomatosis. A rise in ANCA titers correlates with disease flare in approximately two-thirds of the cases, but this relative insensitivity makes it vital to base therapeutic decisions on both the titer and concomitant clinical changes (8). Like other monitoring tests, the titer determination is simply an adjunct to a thorough assessment of the clinical picture.

When a Positive Antineutrophil Cytoplasmic Antibody Test Result Appears During Hospitalization

The differential diagnosis, evaluation, and management of a patient with a positive ANCA test result are the same whether this finding is detected at the time of admission or during the hospitalization.

Complement

When Hypocomplementemia Is Present at the Time of Admission

Description and Differential Diagnosis
The complement system involves a cascade of 30 proteins. When activated, the proteins are catabolized into intermediates that augment the inflammatory response by attracting neutrophils, directing lysis of opsonized cells, and increasing vascular permeability. The functional integrity of the entire classic pathway can be evaluated by performing a test for total hemolytic complement (CH_{50}). Deficiencies in any of the complement proteins of the classic pathway, whether inherited or caused by consumption, will decrease the CH_{50} value. Individual complement components can also be measured. The levels of C3 and C4 are most commonly tested.

Complement levels are generally sent in two clinical scenarios: either to evaluate an inherited complement deficiency or to diagnose and/or determine the level of activity of a pathologic, inflammatory condition. In the latter group, hypocomplementemia, in the appropriate clinical setting, could indicate an SLE flare, cryoglobulinemic vasculitis, a variety of glomerulonephritides, SBE, or cholesterol emboli syndrome. Each of these disorders triggers consumption of complements, thus a reduction in number of individual complement components and an overall abnormality in the CH_{50}. Rarely, end-stage liver disease can be associated with hypocomplementemia because of reduced hepatic synthesis of complement proteins, but complement levels typically are preserved even in patients with hepatic failure.

Evaluation
The first question to address when the complement level is low is whether the cause is a hereditary deficiency of an individual component or complement consumption. This can be determined by obtaining values for CH_{50} and for two individual components (e.g., C3 and C4). If consumption is the cause, all the values should be abnormal. However, if only an individual component is absent, then the CH_{50} value will be undetectably low (reflecting the absence of a functionally important component), but the levels of all other individual components will be normal. For example, levels of both C3 and C4 will be normal in a patient with C2 deficiency, but the CH_{50} level will be undetectable; C3 will be normal in a patient with C4 deficiency, but C4 will be absent.

If the tests described above establish that consumption is the cause for hypocomplementemia, then the evaluation shifts immediately to a consideration of immunopathology, particularly SLE. Some mimickers of vasculitis must also be considered, such as the cholesterol emboli syndrome, which can cause clinical manifestations suggestive of vasculitis, low complement levels, and a high ESR.

Management
Because complement is consumed and then quickly resynthesized, complement levels can be a valuable guide for monitoring disease activity. In SLE in particular, disease activity often correlates with low complement levels. This can be extremely valuable, for example, when the clinician is trying to determine whether the febrile patient with SLE is having a disease flare (which would improve with immunosuppression) or an infection. Similarly, this relationship can provide quantitative direction for adjusting the dose of immunosuppressive drugs. When complement values are being used for this purpose, it is not necessary to follow the results of multiple tests (e.g., CH_{50}, C3, and C4). Rather, because all the complement values reflect consumption, it is sufficient to rely on the most sensitive of them. Although the C4 value is generally the most sensitive to changes in disease activity (9), some patients will demonstrate a higher correlation between the CH_{50} or C3 value and their clinical status.

When Hypocomplementemia Appears During Hospitalization

An acute decrease in any measure of complement suggests immunopathology such as SLE or a vasculitis. However, in a hospitalized patient, one must also consider severe bacterial infection. Therefore, the evaluation should focus on distinguishing vasculitis from infection.

KEY POINTS

- The first challenge in evaluating a patient with joint pain is to determine whether the pain truly originates within the joint or whether it originates instead in periarticular structures, underlying bone, or overlying skin.

- In most patients with joint swelling, analysis of the joint fluid is a crucial part of the diagnostic evaluation.
- Crystal-induced arthritis is a common cause of acute joint pain in hospitalized patients.
- In seriously ill patients with signs and symptoms suggestive of rheumatic diseases, the differential diagnosis often also includes infection. The challenge is to act swiftly to minimize the risk for catastrophic complications of rheumatic diseases while avoiding immunosuppressive therapy in infected patients.
- The erythrocyte sedimentation rate may be elevated in any inflammatory process that increases the levels of acute-phase reactants.
- The antinuclear antibody titer is most useful as a diagnostic test for SLE, because of its high sensitivity, but not as a monitoring test, because the titer does not correlate well with disease activity.
- Since the rheumatoid factor will be positive in only 80% of patients with rheumatoid arthritis, the diagnosis must still be made on clinical grounds.
- The cytosolic pattern for antineutrophil cytoplasmic antibody (cANCA) is most useful diagnostically when the clinical picture suggests a greater than 10% pretest probability of Wegener's granulomatosis.
- Hypocomplementemia may reflect either an inherited deficiency of an individual complement component or complement consumption resulting from immune complex-mediated activation of the complement cascade.

REFERENCES

1. Keane J, Gershon S, Wise RP, et al. Tuberculosis associated with infliximab, a tumor necrosis factor alpha-neutralizing agent. *New Engl J Med* 2001;345:1098–1104.
2. Bedell SE, Bush B. Erythrocyte sedimentation rate: from folklore to fact. *Am J Med* 1985;78:1001–1009.
3. Sox HC, Liang MH. The erythrocyte sedimentation rate. *Ann Intern Med* 1986;104:515–523.
4. Acosta-Lluberas G, Schumacher HR. Markedly elevated erythrocyte sedimentation rates: consideration of clinical implications in a hospital population. *Br J Clin Pract* 1996;50:138–42.
5. Tan EM, Feltkamp TE, Smolen JS, et al. Range of antinuclear antibodies in "healthy individuals." *Arthritis Rheum* 1997;40:1601–1611.
6. Brogan BL, Olsen NJ. Drug-induced rheumatic syndromes. *Curr Op Rheum* 2003;15:76–80.
7. Savige J, Davies D, Falk RJ, Jennette JC, Wilk A. Antineutrophil cytoplasmic antibodies and associated diseases: A review of the clinical and laboratory features. *Kidney Intl* 2000;57:846–862.
8. Vassilopoulos D, Hoffman G. Clinical utility of testing for antineutrophil cytoplasmic antibodies. *Clin Diagn Lab Immunol* 1999;6:645–651.
9. Lloyd W, Schur PH. Immune complexes, complement, and anti-DNA in exacerbations of systemic lupus erythematosus (SLE). *Medicine* 1981;60:208–217.

ADDITIONAL READING

Klippel JH, ed. *Primer on the Rheumatic Diseases.* 12th ed. Atlanta, GA: Arthritis Foundation, 2001.
Koopman WJ, ed. *Arthritis and Allied Conditions.* 14th ed. Philadelphia: Lippincott Williams & Wilkins, 2000.

Vasculitis

111

Gary S. Hoffman *Carol A. Langford*
Leonard H. Calabrese

INTRODUCTION

When to Suspect Vasculitis

For most physicians, the recognition and treatment of the systemic vasculitides is not a routine matter. More than 20 different forms of systemic vasculitis have been enumerated. Each is uncommon and likely to be confused with other systemic illnesses that produce similar abnormalities. The hospitalized patient ultimately identified to have systemic vasculitis has often had either a toxic presentation or a clinical picture dominated by multifocal evidence of organ injury. Processes that can be confused with vasculitis include infections (particularly bacterial endocarditis), drug toxicities and poisonings (especially with agents likely to produce vasospasm), coagulopathies, malignancies, cardiac myxomas, and multifocal emboli from aneurysms of large vessels (Table 111.1). Whether critical organs are involved, together with the rate of disease progression, will determine the intensity and pace of the diagnostic evaluation and treatment choices. The physician may encounter a situation, especially early in a hospitalization, in which systemic vasculitis cannot be distinguished from endocarditis or other infections. Under such circumstances, one may be forced to treat for multiple diagnoses before a final diagnosis is achieved. To minimize the risk of such an approach, the clinician must recognize the clinical patterns of competing diagnoses, rather than depend on immunoserologic studies that may not be readily available or are inadequately specific. For example, oral and genital aphthous ulcers suggest Behçet's disease; the presence of upper and lower airway inflammation, red blood cell casts in the urine sediment, and renal insufficiency suggests Wegener's granulomatosis; and hypertension and claudication in an extremity in a young female patient suggest Takayasu's arteritis. Unfortunately, many patients with vasculitis do not present with such recognizable features. Instead, one may have to depend on combinations of less typical clues. For example, a patient with with a flat or palpable purpuric rash, fever, an active urinary sediment, and peripheral neuropathy is likely to have vasculitis. However, because these features may also be part of endocarditis, they obligate definitive evaluation for both conditions.

Proving the Diagnosis of Vasculitis

Definitive proof often depends on visualizing vasculitic lesions in affected tissue. The greatest success in achieving a tissue diagnosis comes from the *biopsy of abnormal or symptomatic sites.* Biopsy of apparently normal tissue is not recommended (1, 2) because the yield is less than 20%, even in patients with proven vasculitis. Biopsy of abnormal organs provides diagnostically useful information in more than 65% of cases (not 100%, because "skip" lesions are seen in all types of systemic vasculitis). This explains why large specimens of abnormal tissue provide a greater yield than specimens obtained by needle biopsy.

A biopsy may not be practical in certain circumstances. For example, in the patient with symptoms of visceral ischemia, carotidynia, or findings of unequal pulses or blood pressures, biopsy of large vessels and diagnostic laparotomy (in the absence of an acute abdomen) would be impractical. In this setting, *angiography* can be helpful. Vascular injury may be evidenced by areas of vascular stenosis or aneurysm that cannot be explained on the basis of atherosclerosis. Angiography is particularly useful for patients with diseases that involve large vessels (Takayasu's arteritis, giant cell arteritis of the elderly) and medium-size vessels (e.g., polyarteritis nodosa) (Figure 111.1).

Once the diagnosis of vasculitis is clearly established, based either on the strongest of circumstantial evidence

TABLE 111.1

WHEN TO SUSPECT SYSTEMIC VASCULITIS

Consider systemic vasculitis in all patients with multisystem disease, but rule out the following processes:

Infection/sepsis; pay particular attention to endocarditis (Chapter 71)
Drug toxicity/poisoning (Chapter 121)
Coagulopathy (Chapter 98)
Malignancy
Atrial myxoma
Multifocal emboli (e.g., cholesterol, mycotic)

(potentially including angiography, which is less specific than histopathology) or on biopsy proof of vascular inflammatory injury, one must still ask whether such lesions represent *secondary vasculitis* caused by infections (e.g., bacterial, mycobacterial, fungal, syphilitic, rickettsial, hepatitis B or C or, in immunologically compromised patients, HIV or cytomegalovirus infection). In addition, vasculitis can be associated with a variety of malignancies. Paraneoplastic vasculitis should be considered on the basis of a suggestive history or in patients who fail to respond to usually effective aggressive immunosuppressive therapy.

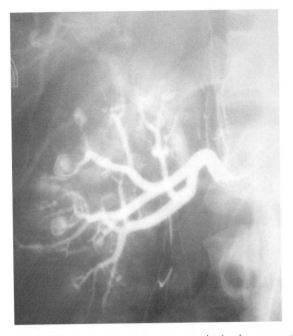

Figure 111.1 This renal arteriogram was obtained concurrently with a study of the mesenteric circulation in a patient with postprandial abdominal pain, hypertension, musculoskeletal symptoms, and fever of unknown origin. The diagnosis of polyarteritis nodosa was suspected. The angiogram revealed marked "pruning" of medium-sized vessels, vascular irregularities, and aneurysms throughout the renal vessels and mesenteric vasculature, confirming the diagnosis.

General Considerations for Treatment

With the exception of acute Kawasaki syndrome, in which salicylates and high-dose intravenous immunoglobulin are indicated, therapy for all other forms of severe systemic vasculitis usually begins with *high doses of a corticosteroid*. Whether the corticosteroid should be given as a single morning dose, in split doses, or as a large intravenous "pulse" or bolus (e.g., 500–1,000 mg of methylprednisolone for 1–3 days), and whether a *cytotoxic agent* should be used at the onset, have not been the subject of controlled studies. Certain forms of systemic vasculitis improve dramatically after corticosteroid therapy (e.g., giant cell arteritis of the elderly). But, most patients with generalized Wegener's granulomatosis or severe microscopic polyangiitis with pulmonary and renal involvement usually progress to severe organ system impairment and death if not treated with a corticosteroid plus a cytotoxic agent such as cyclophosphamide. Special concerns are raised when the condition of a patient who has experienced marked improvement or remission subsequently deteriorates. If deterioration occurs before significant tapering of corticosteroids or cytotoxic agents, it is likely to be caused by events other than vasculitis; generally either comorbidities or complications of treatment (e.g., venous thromboses, pulmonary emboli, opportunistic infections, and drug toxicity).

Because most systemic vasculitides are not curable, the primary realistic goal is to diminish morbidity from both disease and treatment, in the hope that the underlying process will enter an extended treatment-induced remission or be self-limited. When treatment is indicated for systemic vasculitis, high doses should be maintained until all manifestations of active disease have abated. Tapering of prednisone should begin after about 1 month. Whether corticosteroid tapering should be accomplished by reducing the dose on every day of therapy or on every other day; or whether the interval between each dose reduction should be every 3, 5, 7, 10 or more days, etc., is controversial. Some advocate tapering to alternate-day prednisone (single morning dose), because this schedule is associated with less toxicity than daily treatment. However, even alternate-day prednisone carries a high risk for osteoporosis and fracture. All patients who receive long-term corticosteroids should be placed on bone conservation programs.

Daily cyclophosphamide has been the most thoroughly studied treatment for severe forms of vasculitis. Although the drug may be life-saving, its use requires close vigilance for bladder and bone marrow side effects, titration of doses based on blood cell counts (particularly in regard to leukopenia), high oral intake of fluids to dilute cyclophosphamide-derived bladder toxins, and urologic consultation for any sign of bladder toxicity (3). Figure 111.2 shows a sample discharge instruction form for patients being started on a corticosteroid, cyclophosphamide, or both. Specific indications for adding a cytotoxic agent will be considered in following sections on the specific vasculitides.

Medications:
- Cyclophosphamide 150 mg taken all at once in the morning with 2-3 liters of fluid throughout the day.
- Prednisone 60 mg taken all at once in the morning.
- Trimethoprim 160 mg/Sulfamethoxazole 800 mg 1 tablet on Monday, Wednesday, Friday (prophylaxis for pneumocystis)
- (Consider intervention to minimize prednisone-induced osteoporosis).

Follow-up:
- While taking these medications, it is very important that you have blood tests every 1-2 weeks
- Return to see Dr. _____ on _____

Alerts:
- Contact your doctor at phone number _____ or seek medical attention immediately for any:
  - Fever
  - Blood in your urine
  - Shortness of breath
  - Symptoms of infection
  - New symptoms that you are unsure or concerned about

Main Side Effects (discussed here or through separate written literature):

Cyclophosphamide:	Prednisone:
Increased risk of infection	Increased risk of infection
Lowering of blood counts	Increased appetite and weight
Bladder injury	Fluctuations in mood
Injury to an unborn child	Acne
Infertility	Easy bruising
Nausea, vomiting	Fullness of the face and body
Hair thinning or loss	Osteoporosis
Increased risk of cancer of the bladder, blood elements, skin	Muscle weakness
	Avascular necrosis (fractures of the hips/shoulders)
	Cataracts
	High blood pressure
	Diabetes

Figure 111.2 Sample discharge instructions for patients on cyclophosphamide and prednisone therapy.

SPECIFIC VASCULITIDES

Vasculitis of Large Vessels

Takayasu's Arteritis

Issues at the Time of Admission

Takayasu's arteritis is a large-vessel vasculitis of unknown cause that involves the aorta and its major branches. It affects young women about 10 times more often than men. Morbidity results from arterial stenosis and organ ischemia (e.g., extremity claudication, transient cerebral ischemia, stroke, renal artery hypertension, congestive heart failure, angina, myocardial infarction, mesenteric vascular insufficiency), and from the formation of aneurysms, especially in the aortic root, which can result in aortic regurgitation. Mortality rates have varied widely from series to series. When mortality occurs, it is usually caused by hypertensive or primary cardiac, renal, and central nervous system (CNS) vascular disease. Symptoms of large-vessel abnormalities, especially in young patients, necessitate careful examination of pulses and blood pressures in all four extremities, with a search for asymmetry and vascular bruits (4).

Symptoms may be specific for vascular disease (e.g., extremity or visceral ischemia) or nonspecific (e.g., malaise, arthralgias, night sweats, fever). When such symptoms occur in the setting of an elevated erythrocyte sedimentation rate (ESR), active disease is likely and should be evaluated by invasive (4) or non-invasive (5) angiography. The initial presentation may be subtle; a significant number of patients have neither constitutional nor new vascular symptoms, and up to 50% have normal ESR values despite progressive disease (4). Patients admitted with suspected active Takayasu's arteritis should be started on high-dose corticosteroids (1 mg of prednisone per kilogram daily), even as the diagnosis is being confirmed.

Issues During the Course of Hospitalization

Approximately 60% of patients with Takayasu's arteritis respond to corticosteroid therapy, with resolution of symptoms and stabilization of arteriographically demonstrable abnormalities. However, tapering of corticosteroid therapy has been associated with disease relapse in more than 40% of patients. Corticosteroid-resistant or relapsing patients may respond to the addition of daily therapy with low doses (2 mg/kg/d) of cyclophosphamide or weekly therapy with methotrexate (15–25 mg/wk) (6).

About 40% of patients who are treated with a cytotoxic agent and corticosteroids achieve remission, but about half of these patients also relapse in time, so that long-term immunosuppressive therapy is required in at least one-fourth of all patients with Takayasu's arteritis.

By discussing only pharmacologic strategies, we would risk ignoring the important effects of the vascular lesions themselves, which cause morbidity through inflammation or vascular distortion and stenosis. Because more than 90% of patients have stenotic lesions, with the most common site of stenosis being the subclavian artery (or arteries), blood pressure recordings in one or both arms may not reflect the more worrisome pressure in the aorta. Therefore, in patients with Takayasu's arteritis, the entire aorta and its primary branches should be assessed with vascular imaging studies, including magnetic resonance angiography or invasive catheter-guided angiography. Whenever feasible, anatomic correction of clinically significant lesions should be considered, especially in the setting of renal artery stenosis and hypertension, coronary or cerebral ischemia, or enlarging aortic aneurysm or dissection.

Discharge Issues

The care of patients with Takayasu's arteritis requires management by a team that includes clinicians familiar with the proper use of immunosuppressive therapies, vascular imaging and intervention specialists, and, in the setting of critical stenoses or aneurysms, cardiovascular physicians and surgeons. For most patients, medical and surgical therapies are palliative. The acute hospitalization provides an opportunity to diagnose and treat urgent problems and to assemble a team that will follow the patient outside the hospital.

Giant Cell Arteritis of the Elderly

Issues at the Time of Admission

Giant cell arteritis (GCA) and Takayasu's arteritis are the principal diseases associated with sterile granulomatous inflammation of large and medium-sized vessels. Whereas Takayasu's arteritis has a predilection for young women, GCA favors people over 50 years of age. In fact, the mean age for patients in most series is over 70 years. Women are affected more than men, but the degree of female predominance (ranging from 2:1 to 3:1) is not as striking as in Takayasu's arteritis. The demographic characteristics of patients with GCA are the same as for patients with polymyalgia rheumatica, and in fact 30–50% of patients with GCA also have features of polymyalgia rheumatica. The most common characteristics of GCA are represented in Table

111.2. The new onset of atypical and often severe headaches, scalp and temporal artery tenderness, acute visual loss, and pain within the muscles of mastication are among the most compelling features to suggest the diagnosis (7). When such abnormalities are present in conjunction with marked elevations in the ESR (Chapter 110), a clinical diagnosis of GCA can be presumed and treatment initiated, even without the benefit of a temporal artery biopsy. The diagnosis would be thrown into question only if dramatic improvement had not occurred within 24–72 hours. In those instances in which typical features are not present but the diagnosis is suggested because of vague systemic symptoms and atypical headache in face of a normal or elevated ESR and all other reasonable diagnoses have been ruled out, a positive biopsy result is useful in guiding treatment. The yield of temporal artery biopsy in patients suspected to have GCA has been estimated to be about 50%–80%, depending in part on the pre-test (biopsy) probability of GCA, size of the biopsy specimen and whether bilateral samples have been obtained.

Giant cell arteritis produces aortitis in at least 15% of cases and involves the primary branches of the aorta in a similar number of persons (8). Recent studies have demonstrated that patients with GCA were more than 17 times more likely than age-matched controls to have thoracic aortic aneurysms (carrying a 55% mortality rate) and about 2.5 times more likely than age-matched controls to have abdominal aortic aneurysms (8). The finding of large-vessel disease, including aortic aneurysms, in elderly persons with GCA should not merely be assumed to be secondary to atheromatous disease.

Corticosteroids remain the most effective therapy for GCA. As in patients with suspected Takayasu's disease,

TABLE 111.2

GIANT CELL ARTERITIS: CLINICAL PROFILE

Abnormality	Frequency (%)
Age >50 y (mean age, ~70 y)	>90
Atypical headache	60–90
Tender temporal artery	40–70
Systemic symptoms not attributable to other diseases	20–50
Fever	20–50
Polymyalgia rheumatica	30–50
Acute visual abnormalities	12–40
Blindness	5–17
TIAs or stroke	5–10
Claudication	
"Jaw"	30–70
Extremities	5–15
Aortic aneurysm	15–20
Dramatic response to corticosteroids	~100
Positive temporal artery biopsy result	~50+

TIA, transient ischemic attack.

prednisone therapy (0.7–1 mg/kg daily) should be started immediately in patients with suspected GCA. The biopsy result will remain positive for at least a week after corticosteroid therapy is begun. Controlled studies, designed to determine whether adjunctive therapy with cytotoxic agents is superior to corticosteroid therapy alone in patients with GCA, have yielded contradictory results (9, 10).

Issues During the Course of Hospitalization and at Discharge

Prednisone will reduce symptoms within 1–2 days and often eliminate them within a week. One month after clinical and laboratory parameters, particularly the ESR, have normalized, tapering can begin. Unfortunately, the ESR does not always normalize, even with disease control, so it should not be relied on as the only measure of remission. Occasional patients may either fail to achieve complete remission or be unable to withdraw from corticosteroid therapy. Cytotoxic or immunosuppressive agents have been recommended for such patients by some authors, but in the absence of convincing proof of efficacy, we are reluctant to endorse such approaches. Recent preliminary experience has suggested that therapies directed at blocking the proinflammatory and granuloma-enhancing cytokine, TNF, may be efficacious (11). Studies of this approach have just begun.

Evidence that as many as 40% of patients with polymyalgia rheumatica may have histologic proof of GCA has continued to fuel controversy over whether all patients with polymyalgia rheumatica should be treated with high doses of corticosteroids. In any case, the clinical overlap of these disorders obligates careful vascular evaluations of patients with presumed polymyalgia rheumatica.

VASCULITIDES OF SMALL AND MEDIUM-SIZED VESSELS

Issues at the Time of Admission

Clinical Presentation

The systemic vasculitides that have a predilection for involving small and medium vessels are Wegener's granulomatosis (WG), polyarteritis nodosa (PAN), microscopic polyangiitis (MPA), and Churg-Strauss syndrome (CSS).

Wegener's granulomatosis is a necrotizing granulomatous vasculitis classically thought of as involving the triad of the upper airway, lungs, and kidneys. It affects approximately 3/100,000 people and is distributed equally between men and women, with a mean age of onset of 41 years (range, 9–78 years). Although this disease can affect virtually any organ system (Table 111.3), patients most frequently seek medical attention for symptoms involving the upper and lower airways (Figure 111.3). In the hospitalized patient in whom a diagnosis of WG is being considered, it

TABLE 111.3

WEGENER'S GRANULOMATOSIS: CLINICAL PROFILE

Abnormality	Frequency at presentation (%)	Frequency during disease course (%)
Upper airways	73	92
Lower airways	48	85
Kidneys	20	80
Joints	32	67
Eyes	15	52
Skin	13	46
Nerves	1	20

Data adapted from Hoffman GS, Kerr GS, Leavitt RY, et al. Wegener's granulomatosis: an analysis of 158 patients. *Ann Intern Med* 1992;116: 488–498, with permission.

is important to recognize that the symptom of dyspnea can occur for multiple reasons, including obstruction of the upper airways resulting from involvement of the trachea, bronchi, or subglottic region. Patients with stridor or unexplained dyspnea should be emergently evaluated by an otolaryngologist. If severe tracheal narrowing is present, tracheotomy can be life-saving. Glomerulonephritis is another important disease manifestation. Because it is usually asymptomatic and may be rapidly progressive, clinicians should perform a urinalysis in patients with systemic illnesses for which the cause is uncertain. Although the presence of renal disease is helpful in narrowing the differential diagnosis and although renal disease ultimately occurs in 80% of patients, it is present at the onset of WG in only 20%.

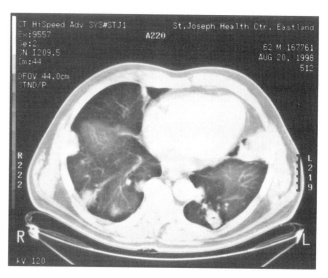

Figure 111.3 Wegener's granulomatosis. This computed tomogram demonstrates multiple bilateral nodules with cavitation of a left posterior nodule in a patient with upper and lower airway disease and glomerulonephritis.

The description of *periarteritis* (later renamed *polyarteritis*) *nodosa* in 1866 was the first detailed account of a systemic vasculitis in the medical literature. Although the term polyarteritis nodosa was initially used to describe all cases of systemic vasculitis that did not include the largest vessels, it became recognized in the 1950s that certain clinical and pathologic features often allowed separation of these vasculitides into distinct entities. Under a 1993 International Consensus Conference classification, PAN was defined as a vasculitis of medium-sized arteries not associated with glomerulonephritis or vasculitis of small vessels. In contrast, *microscopic polyangiitis* was defined as a necrotizing vasculitis, with few or no immune deposits, affecting small vessels (i.e., capillaries, venules, or arterioles); it can also affect medium-sized arteries. Like WG, MPA has a predilection for the lungs (e.g., pulmonary infiltrates and hemorrhage) and kidneys (glomerulonephritis). Biopsy specimens in MPA are devoid of granulomas, unlike those in WG. MPA can pose an immediate threat to life and organ function, particularly in cases characterized by pulmonary hemorrhage and rapidly progressive renal failure. Once diagnosed, MPA necessitates aggressive treatment.

Based on its definition, PAN is probably very rare. Although several natural history and treatment studies of PAN have previously been performed, the populations analyzed included a number of patients with small-vessel disease who would now be considered to have MPA. This is reflected in the wide range of frequencies of organ involvement reported in different series (Table 111.4). It is very important to note that the phenotypes of patients with PAN, MPA, and *cryoglobulinemic vasculitis* can be the same as those of patients with viral infections complicated by vasculitis (e.g., hepatitis B and C, HIV infection). Screening for these viruses should therefore be performed in all such presentations, insofar as antiviral therapies may be an important part of treatment for these diseases.

Churg-Strauss syndrome is a rare disease characterized by asthma, eosinophilia, and systemic vasculitis. The peak age of onset is 30–45 years (range, 15–69), and there is a slight male predominance. The course of CSS has often been divided into three phases: the prodrome, the eosinophilic phase, and the vasculitic phase. Although this separation is helpful in approaching CSS, the three phases are not clearly definable in all patients and may occur simultaneously. The prodrome is characterized by allergic disease, usually asthma and allergic rhinitis. During the eosinophilic phase, peripheral eosinophilia and eosinophilic tissue infiltrates, often involving the lung or gastrointestinal tract, may develop. The vasculitic phase may be heralded by constitutional symptoms followed by the development of more organ-specific features, such as mononeuritis multiplex or congestive heart failure. Cardiac involvement can be a significant cause of mortality in these patients.

Differential Diagnosis and Initial Evaluation

All the primary vasculitides of small and medium vessels have the potential to be systemic and evolve rapidly. Initial assessment must be comprehensive and quickly address those organ systems in which involvement carries the greatest potential for significant morbidity or mortality (airway, lungs, kidneys, nerves, gastrointestinal tract, heart, and eyes). It is important to recognize that the absence of symptoms does not rule out disease. For example, one study of patients with WG showed that 34% of radiographs demonstrated infiltrates or nodules while patients were asymptomatic. The point that glomerulonephritis, often rapidly progressive, is usually asymptomatic cannot be overemphasized.

Role of Antineutrophil Cytoplasmic Antibodies in the Differential Diagnosis of Vasculitis. Antineutrophil cytoplasmic antibodies (ANCA), novel auto-antibodies associated with certain forms of systemic vasculitis, were described in Chapter 110. The cytosolic pattern of ANCA (cANCA), combined with reactivity to Proteinase 3 (PR3), has been found to have a high degree of sensitivity and specificity for WG. Although ANCA positivity is useful to suggest the presence of WG, in almost all instances *it should not be used in place of a biopsy to confirm the diagnosis.* This is because the prevalence of WG is low in most clinical situations, and ANCA/PR3 positivity is not 100% specific for WG (12). Conversely, where there is convincing clinical evidence to suggest WG, ANCA negativity should not be a reason to eliminate vasculitis from the differential diagnosis.

Biopsy Strategy for Diagnosis. We have discussed strategies for obtaining biopsy proof of vasculitis in our introductory comments. An important aspect of these strategies

---

TABLE 111.4

POLYARTERITIS NODOSA: CLINICAL PROFILE

Abnormality	Frequency (%)[a]
Fever	36–76
Weight loss	30–71
Hypertension	25–70
Kidney	8–77
Gastrointestinal	14–78
Cardiac	10–56
Nervous system	
Peripheral	23–60
Central	3–41
Musculoskeletal	
Arthralgia/arthritis	33–58
Myalgia	8–77
Skin	28–65
Eye	1–47
Testicular pain	1–4

[a] Frequencies represent a compilation of data from several series.

includes selecting a suitable biopsy site when more than one organ site is involved. The decision about which site is most suitable for biopsy must be based on individual factors, such as the stability of the patient, invasiveness of the procedure, likelihood of a positive yield based on data from the literature, and urgency of beginning treatment. For example, in a stable patient, it may be reasonable to perform a biopsy at a location where the yield is lower but where the procedure is less invasive. Conversely, when beginning treatment immediately is critical, the biopsy should generally be performed on the involved tissue most likely to yield a diagnosis.

Indications for Hospitalization

The indications for hospitalizing a patient with possible vasculitis chiefly fall under three interrelated headings: diagnosis, monitoring, and treatment. Admission may be indicated so that a diagnostic procedure (e.g., bronchoscopy, surgical biopsy) or an invasive radiologic procedure can be performed safely. Hospitalization for monitoring and treatment typically go together, as it is often the patients who need to be followed closely who require more aggressive (often intravenously administered) treatment. Immediately life-threatening manifestations often dictate the need for hospitalization, but it must be recognized that stable, untreated vasculitis of small and medium-sized vessels has the potential to progress rapidly to life-threatening disease and complete renal failure. For this reason, when these forms of vasculitis are high on the list of possible diagnoses, admission should be considered if it would expedite making a prompt diagnosis and instituting therapy.

Indications for Initial Intensive Care Unit Admission

In the management of the vasculitides of small and medium vessels, indications for ICU admission may include respiratory or airway compromise, pulmonary or gastrointestinal bleeding, unstable cardiovascular parameters, or impaired central neurologic function.

Initial Therapy

The decisions regarding initial treatment will largely be based on the sites and severity of organ involvement and on individual factors. This section reviews the general approach to initial treatment, but physicians are strongly encouraged to seek further information from the literature or consultants regarding the risks, benefits, and protocols of the treatment regimens. Also of note, the following comments are confined to the treatment of small- and medium-vessel vasculitis that is not associated with hepatitis or HIV; these secondary vasculitides may warrant an approach that includes antiviral therapies.

Historical reports have demonstrated that untreated WG is almost universally fatal. Corticosteroids were the first applied therapy, and, although they slowed disease progression in some instances, they usually did not prolong survival. The introduction of treatment with a *corticosteroid*

and daily cyclophosphamide dramatically improved outcome, such that 75% of WG patients achieved complete remission and 91% showed significant improvement, with an 80% survival during a mean follow-up period of 8 years (3). This regimen is now the treatment of choice in any patient with life-threatening disease or rapidly progressive glomerulonephritis. The starting daily dose of cyclophosphamide is 2 mg/kg (Figure 111.4), administered either orally or intravenously (the latter in patients who are too ill to receive oral medications). In either setting, cyclophosphamide should be given all at once in the morning, with 2–3 L of fluid daily to lessen the risk for bladder mucosal injury. Cyclophosphamide is bone marrow-suppressive, and the complete blood cell count should be monitored every 1–2 weeks throughout treatment. An unfortunate misinterpretation of the protocol has led some to believe that the induction of leukopenia is a goal of treatment. Quite the contrary—the starting dose of cyclophosphamide should be lowered if necessary to maintain the white cell count above 3,500/μL. Cyclophosphamide is eliminated by the kidneys, and thus drug levels will be higher in patients with renal insufficiency. The decision about whether to begin with a lower dose of cyclophosphamide must be based on the individual circumstance. In the setting of rapidly progressive glomerulonephritis, the adequacy of initial treatment may be critical for renal salvage, and thus it is preferred to start treatment with at least 2 mg/kg daily and closely monitor for trends toward leukopenia. Use of intravenous bolus cyclophosphamide (1 g/m^2) to initiate treatment is not advised in the treatment of WG, and intermittent administration is not felt to be as efficacious as daily administration

In addition to cyclophosphamide, corticosteroids are a critical part of the regimen. The starting dose is 1 mg of prednisone per kilogram daily or the equivalent intravenous dose of methylprednisolone. This dose is continued for a full month, after which time, if there is evidence of disease improvement, it is tapered to an alternate-day schedule and ultimately discontinued, usually by 6–12 months. Splitting the corticosteroid dose (usually to every 8–12 hours) is theoretically more efficacious but also increases the potential for side effects. This is mainly indicated in hospitalized patients who have severe disease. Split doses should be consolidated to a single daily morning dose as soon as possible.

In patients with *fulminant vasculitis of small and medium-sized vessels* that poses an immediate threat to life, a more aggressive approach may be warranted (Figure 111.4). In such settings, large corticosteroid pulses with methylprednisolone (e.g., 1 g/d for three days) are frequently used. In addition, the dose of cyclophosphamide can be increased to 3–4 mg/kg daily for 3 days, then reduced to 2 mg/kg daily (3). Because such patients are uncommon and are critically ill, no controlled study has demonstrated the efficiency of higher doses. Such high-dose therapy does carry a greater risk for morbidity and mortality, and

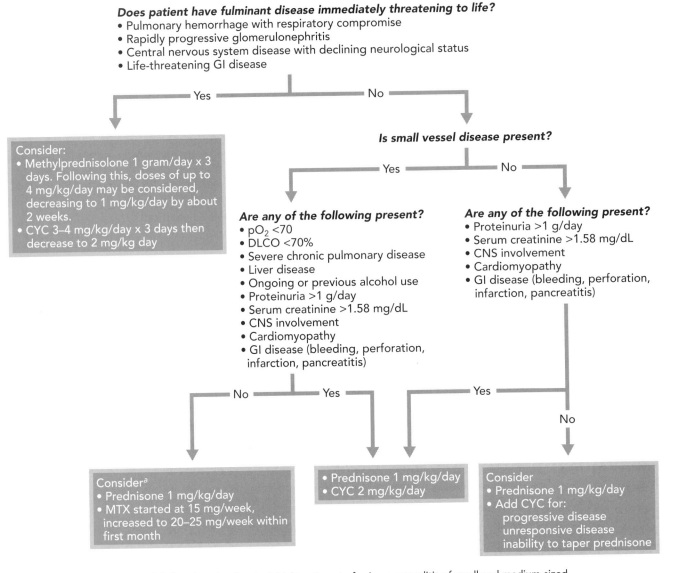

Figure 111.4 Algorithm for the initial treatment of primary vasculitis of small and medium-sized vessels. *CYC,* cyclophosphamide; *MTX,* methotrexate; *CNS,* central nervous system; *GI,* gastrointestinal; *PAN,* polyarteritis nodosa. Note: In addition to the listed immunosuppressive agents, therapy should include pneumocystis prophylaxis with 160 mg of trimethoprim and 800 mg of sulfamethoxazole three times weekly for all patients not allergic to sulfa drugs who are receiving a cytotoxic agent plus prednisone. Treatment to decrease steroid-induced bone loss should also be considered. *a*Use of methotrexate has been studied only in Wegener's granulomatosis.

should be reserved for selected patients for whom the potential benefits are thought to outweigh the risks. Plasmapheresis is another intervention that is often considered in the setting of fulminant disease. Although one study did not find plasmapheresis to be of additional benefit in patients with severe PAN or CSS (13), it has continued to be used by some in the setting of severe small-vessel disease or rapidly progressive glomerulonephritis. In the absence of supportive data, the unknown benefits of this modality must be weighed against the risks of large-bore vascular catheter insertion and procedural hemodynamic lability.

Although cyclophosphamide is the cytotoxic agent of choice in severe disease of small and medium-sized vessels, it may not be necessary for initial therapy in all settings. *Low-dose weekly methotrexate* has been found to be an effective and less toxic alternative to cyclophosphamide in patients who do not have immediately life-threatening disease or in whom cyclophosphamide has been toxic (14). Although trimethoprim-sulfamethoxazole (TMP/SMX) has been advocated by some authors to treat WG affecting the upper and lower airways, progressive disease has also been noted with such treatment (3). TMP/SMX monotherapy may have a role in treating isolated disease of the upper airway, but it is not recommended in the setting of disease involving the pulmonary parenchyma and should never be used in patients with glomerulonephritis. Finally, not all disease manifestations require or respond to systemic immunosuppression. For example, WG-related subglottic stenosis is optimally managed surgically.

At this time there are few disease-specific data for the treatment of MPA. We recommend a treatment approach similar to that used in WG because MPA can have comparably severe manifestations. Any patient with active small-vessel disease should be managed with daily cyclophosphamide and a corticosteroid at the doses discussed previously and in Figure 111.4, and at higher doses in patients with fulminant disease.

The retrospective nature of the studies and the lack of uniform definitions of disease have complicated the determination of optimal treatment for purely medium-sized vessel vasculitis (PAN). Analyses of PAN and CSS have identified five factors associated with increased mortality: renal insufficiency (creatinine >1.58 mg/dL), proteinuria (>1 g/d), gastrointestinal disease (bleeding, perforation, infarction, pancreatitis), cardiomyopathy, and CNS involvement (15). In the presence of any of these factors, initial therapy should consist of cyclophosphamide (2 mg/kg daily) in addition to prednisone (1 mg/kg daily). A corticosteroid alone can be considered in patients whose disease manifestations do not pose an immediate threat to life or critical organ systems, with cyclophosphamide added later for unresponsive or worsening disease or when the corticosteroid cannot be tapered (Figure 111.4). A simple approach (corticosteroid alone for mild-to-moderate disease; corticosteroid and daily cyclophosphamide for severe disease) is appropriate for patients with CSS, although therapeutic trials are lacking.

In addition to the immunosuppressive agents, the initial treatment regimen may also include medications aimed at preventing treatment complications. Prophylaxis for *Pneumocystis jirovecii* (formerly *P. carinii*) pneumonia with TMP/SMX (160 mg of trimethoprim and 800 mg of sulfamethoxazole three times weekly) is important because fatal infections have been observed in vasculitis patients receiving daily prednisone and a cytotoxic agent. Other interventions that are often part of the initial treatment regimen include folic acid or calcium leucovorin in the setting of methotrexate treatment, and medications directed toward the prevention of prednisone-induced osteoporosis.

Indications for Early Consultation

The vasculitides of small- and medium-sized vessels are uncommon diseases that can result in significant morbidity and mortality. For this reason, consultation with physicians who frequently care for patients with these diseases should be sought early in the course of the illness. In addition to rheumatologists, such consultants may include specialists in nephrology, otolaryngology, neurology, ophthalmology, and pulmonary medicine if these systems are involved.

Issues During the Course of Hospitalization

The main issue during hospitalization is often to provide supportive care and monitoring while diagnostic procedures are performed and treatment is instituted. The rapidity of response to therapy can be influenced by many individual factors, including sites of involvement, severity of organ injury, and the presence of other medical problems. The first 2–4 weeks are a critical time for assessing response to treatment and disease progression by following specific indicators of organ function for each involved site (e.g., renal function tests for glomerulonephritis, oxygenation and respiratory status for pulmonary disease, and changes in examination findings for disease affecting the bowel or nervous system). Some measures of disease activity (e.g., red cell casts noted on urinalysis or chest infiltrates or nodules apparent on roentgenograms) may not change rapidly. Pulmonary abnormalities usually show signs of improvement by four weeks. Improvement in urine sediment may take longer, but the serum creatinine should be stable or improving while the urine sediment is at least stable. Complete clearing of urinary abnormalities may take more than 12 months. When the clinical condition of a patient worsens at the beginning of treatment, one must determine whether the deterioration represents vasculitic disease that has had insufficient time to respond or another process that has emerged, such as infection or drug toxicity (e.g., drug-induced pneumonitis, dermatitis, or hematologic toxicity). If the deterioration is felt to represent active vasculitis and becomes life-threatening, institution of the measures discussed above for fulminant disease may be warranted. In the setting of active vasculitis of small and medium vessels, new sites of involvement can develop at any time. It is therefore essential to be vigilant for any new signs or symptoms of disease.

Discharge Issues

At the time of discharge, it is critical that patients have a clear comprehension of their medications and follow-up. Medication issues include understanding the doses, preferred times to take medications (e.g., single morning doses for prednisone and cyclophosphamide), and possible side effects. A thorough understanding of medication toxicities can most optimally be achieved through a combination of direct discussion and written materials (Figure 111.2). Patient-directed literature on immunosuppressive agents is often available from the pharmacy or support foundations.

Patients require close follow-up to assess the course of disease, adjust medication doses, and observe for therapeutic side effects. Intermittent laboratory studies are mandatory, both to monitor the disease and to ensure the safety of medications. While a patient is taking cyclophosphamide, these studies are usually performed every 1–2 weeks and should include a complete blood cell count with differential, measurement of creatinine levels and sedimentation rate, and urinalysis with microscopic examination. In addition to these studies, methotrexate monitoring must include liver function tests and measurement of albumin levels, with laboratory values obtained every week after dose adjustments and every month thereafter. The patient may require ongoing outpatient consultation with multiple specialists, but one physician should be responsible for adjusting medication doses and monitoring laboratory parameters.

In our originally published regimen for WG, cyclophosphamide was continued for one full year after remission, at which time it was tapered and discontinued (3). Increasing evidence has supported an approach whereby cyclophosphamide is given until the patient achieves remission (about 3–6 months in most patients), after which time the cyclophosphamide is stopped and either methotrexate or azathioprine are added to maintain remission (16). During the initial hospitalization, decisions regarding such future treatment are not required and usually are not possible. In the outpatient setting, as the patient is serially evaluated for response to treatment and observed for side-effects, management options after achievement of remission can be more fully considered (16).

CENTRAL NERVOUS SYSTEM VASCULITIS

The CNS is a common target organ in many forms of systemic vasculitis. The CNS can also be the sole target of vasculitis, as in *isolated* or *primary angiitis of the central nervous system* (PACNS). The clinical manifestations of CNS vasculitis, including its pace and severity, are highly variable. The rarity of CNS vasculitis, the relative inaccessibility of CNS tissue, and the lack of specificity of noninvasive diagnostic techniques further serve to complicate the clinical approach.

Angiitis of the CNS can be classified as primary and secondary. Primary disease, or PACNS, is a relatively rare disorder in which vascular inflammation is confined to the CNS, including the brain and spinal cord and overlying leptomeninges. This disease has also been referred to as granulomatous angiitis of the CNS, but it should be noted that at least 25% of such patients have nongranulomatous pathology. Secondary vasculitis of the CNS occurs in the setting of a systemic vasculitis. CNS involvement in this setting may rarely be the presenting manifestation of an underlying systemic disease but more often occurs during the course of established systemic vasculitis. Table 111.5 displays the relative frequency of CNS involvement in the various systemic vasculitic syndromes (17).

The clinical manifestations of vasculitis of the CNS are nonspecific and primarily reflect the underlying distribution of ischemia. Diffuse neurologic dysfunction can manifest as encephalopathy affecting cognition or level of consciousness. Focal or multifocal neurologic dysfunction

TABLE 111.5

RELATIVE DISTRIBUTION OF CENTRAL NERVOUS SYSTEM INVOLVEMENT IN SYSTEMIC VASCULITIC SYNDROMES

Disease	CNS involvement
Polyarteritis nodosa	++
Churg-Strauss syndrome	+
Wegener's granulomatosis	++
Lymphomatoid granulomatosis	++
Temporal (giant cell) arteritis	+
Takayasu's arteritis	+
Behçet's disease	++
Hypersensitivity vasculitis	−

in the brain or spinal cord can manifest as stroke, seizure, subarachnoid hemorrhage, or cranial neuropathies (18, 19). The diagnosis of CNS angiitis should be considered when a neurologic deficit remains unexplained after a thorough evaluation and noninvasive imaging studies suggest that focal or multifocal ischemia may be responsible.

In the setting of an established systemic vasculitic syndrome such as PAN, CSS, or WG, the new onset of CNS dysfunction mandates an evaluation for possible CNS vasculitis. The initial priority is to determine whether the CNS symptomatology represents arteritic involvement of the CNS or (more commonly) a complication of the underlying disease (i.e., malignant hypertension), effects of drugs (i.e., steroid psychosis), or secondary infection in the setting of immunosuppressive therapy. Even more challenging is the scenario in which CNS angiitis is the initial clinical manifestation of a systemic vasculitis or the presenting finding in PACNS.

Diagnosis and Differential Diagnosis

There are no noninvasive tests or blood studies of sufficient positive predictive value to secure the diagnosis of CNS arteritis. The actual diagnosis of CNS vasculitis relies heavily on neurologic diagnostic modalities, such as cerebrospinal fluid analysis; neuroimaging studies, such as computed tomography (CT) and magnetic resonance imaging (MRI); cerebral angiography; and biopsy of CNS tissues.

Analysis of the cerebrospinal fluid is an essential part of the diagnostic process of both primary and secondary angiitis of the CNS. First, it is important to rule out infectious causes that can mimic CNS angiitis or actually produce a secondary form of CNS angiitis. A number of invasive infections of blood vessels can produce multifocal CNS vascular disease. Examples include syphilis, tuberculosis, certain fungal infections (e.g., coccidioidomycosis and aspergillosis), and infections with viruses (including herpes agents), rickettsial pathogens, and others. In PACNS, the cerebrospinal fluid has been found to be abnormal and have features consistent with chronic meningitis in more than 90% of patients shown to have this diagnosis histologically (18, 19). Blood tests, such as the identification of acute-phase reactants and auto-antibodies, are of no value, and findings are usually normal or negative. No serologic tests have been shown to have high positive or negative predictive value for CNS vasculitis.

Findings of CT are normal in more than 50% of patients with CNS vasculitis. MRI is more sensitive than CT, but it is not specific in regards to etiology of lesions. Often, multiple bilateral infarcts of different ages are present in the cortex, deep white matter, and leptomeninges. MR angiography is a more recently developed technique for noninvasive visualization of the cerebral vasculature. Unfortunately, at the present time, its spatial resolution allows visualization only of the larger intracranial blood vessels, which are generally spared by small-vessel vasculitides. Collectively, normal cerebrospinal fluid analysis and MRI findings weigh heavily against, but do not completely exclude, a diagnosis of CNS arteritis.

Cerebral angiography is a technique often used in the diagnosis of CNS arteritis, but the findings are normal in more than 50% of cases of biopsy-proven PACNS (18, 19). The presence of alternating areas of stenosis and ectasia in multiple vessels in multiple vascular beds is the most specific finding for CNS arteritis, but unfortunately, even when present, its specificity is low. Vasospasm caused by drugs, hemodynamic changes, or degenerative vascular diseases such as atherosclerosis and fibromuscular disease can completely mimic these findings. In fact, the most important disorders to exclude are those associated with reversible segmental cerebral vasoconstriction, which may mimic completely the angiographic findings of arteritis. This type of disorder may be seen in a variety of settings, including following ingestion of sympathomimetic drugs, in the post-partum period, in association with severe hypertension, in the setting of exertional headaches, or in association with the so-called "thunderclap headache syndrome." It may also occur in an idiopathic form, referred to as *benign angiopathy of the CNS* (20). It is clinically important to recognize these mimics, since immunosupression is to be avoided.

Biopsy of the CNS is a valuable technique that has a high degree of sensitivity and specificity. In experienced hands, CNS biopsies can be performed with minimal morbidity. Biopsy is rarely needed in suspected cases of *secondary* CNS vasculitis; however, it is often essential to secure the diagnosis of *primary* CNS angiitis (PACNS). The preferred biopsy technique is generally an open biopsy of leptomeninges and underlying cortex taken from the nondominant tip of the temporal lobe. When CNS biopsy is performed, cultures and special stains for occult infectious agents are essential. Unfortunately, false-negative biopsy results are seen in up to 20% of patients in whom PACNS is ultimately documented pathologically.

Collectively, the clinician is left with a series of tests of varying sensitivities and specificities that must be performed serially until he or she reaches the decision of whether to treat or not to treat as CNS angiitis. Table 111.6 lists a number of conditions that can mimic either the angiographic or pathologic picture of CNS angiitis. These must be ruled out with certainty before immunosuppressive therapy is initiated.

Indications for Hospitalization and Intensive Care Unit Admission

Because the diagnosis of CNS vasculitis cannot be made on the basis of noninvasive testing, hospitalization is usually required for sequential clinical evaluations, spinal fluid analysis, and possibly angiography and CNS biopsy. Competing diagnoses that generally require therapies other than immunosuppression need to be ruled out as soon as possible. The need for ICU admission is determined by the

---

TABLE 111.6

CONDITIONS THAT MIMIC THE ANGIOGRAPHIC OR CLINICAL PICTURE OF CENTRAL NERVOUS SYSTEM ANGIITIS

Infection
  Viral, bacterial, fungal, rickettsial, Lyme disease
Neoplasm
  Angioimmunoproliferative disorders
  Carcinomatous meningitis
  Infiltrating glioma
  Malignant angioendotheliomatosis
Drug use
  Amphetamines
  Ephedrine
  Phenylpropanolamine
  Cocaine
  Ergotamine
Vasospastic disorders
  Postpartum angiopathy
  Eclampsia
  Pheochromocytoma
  Subarachnoid hemorrhage
  Migraine and exertional headache
Other vasculopathies and mimicking conditions
  Fibromuscular dysplasia
  Moyamoya disease
  Thrombotic thrombocytopenic purpura
  Sickle cell anemia
  Neurofibromatosis
  Cerebrovascular atherosclerosis
  Demyelinating disease
  Sarcoidosis
  Emboli (i.e., subacute bacterial endocarditis, cardiac myxoma, paradoxical emboli)
  Acute posterior placoid pigment epitheliopathy and cerebral vasculitis
  Antiphospholipid antibody syndrome

patient's neurologic status.

Indications for Consultation

The successful diagnosis and treatment of CNS angiitis require a team approach. The team should generally include a neurologist, an immunologist or rheumatologist, an angiographer with an interest in CNS angiitis, a neurosurgeon, and a neuropathologist with expertise in CNS angiitis.

Prognostic Variables

In our opinion (data are scarce), all symptoms and signs associated with vasculitic involvement of the CNS should be viewed as life-threatening and thus warrant aggressive therapy. Previously healthy young women with acute onset of headache with or without a focal neurologic deficit, normal or near-normal cerebrospinal fluid, and a high-probability angiogram for vasculitis may well have benign angiopathy of the CNS. It is important to avoid overly aggressive and potentially harmful treatments in such patients.

Treatment

Controlled data regarding treatment of either PACNS or secondary vasculitis of the CNS do not exist. PACNS that is chronic and progressive is potentially life-threatening and warrants aggressive therapy. Empirically derived, efficacious therapy includes a combination of high-dose corticosteroid (e.g., 1 mg of prednisone per kilogram daily) and cyclophosphamide (2 mg/kg daily). After convincing initial improvement has occurred or progressive illness has been arrested, corticosteroid doses are tapered. Cyclophosphamide therapy is continued for approximately 12 months after the disease has been controlled. Serial evaluations of the patient's clinical status, MRI findings, cerebrospinal fluid, and at times angiographic findings may be necessary to gauge the effectiveness of therapy. In patients with a more benign angiopathic presentation, cautious observation or a short course of high-dose corticosteroids (1 mg of prednisone per kilogram daily) for a period of 2–3 months has been advocated. Calcium channel blockers have also been recommended in such patients based on a presumed role of vasoconstriction, although evidence for efficacy is anecdotal.

COST CONSIDERATIONS AND RESOURCE USE

Because the symptoms and signs of vasculitis are often nonspecific, considerable resources are frequently expended in evaluating patients before the correct diagnosis is established. Moreover, the generalist who suspects vasculitis often orders a panoply of immunologic and serologic studies ("rheumatology panel"), and patients are frequently shut-tled from the office of one consultant to another. It is easy with vasculitis to be penny-wise and pound-foolish. The patient with suspected vasculitis is often well served by hospital admission, early consultation with the relevant specialists, rapid and focused laboratory, radiographic, and pathologic evaluation, and prompt initiation of therapy.

KEY POINTS

- Systemic vasculitis must be distinguished from other processes that can mimic the signs and symptoms of vasculitis (e.g., infections, drug toxicities, and emboli).
- The workup of patients with suspected vasculitis requires an integrated, multidisciplinary approach that focuses on patterns of organ involvement rather than a "shotgun" set of immunoserologic studies.
- While tissue diagnosis is most satisfying in vascultiis, it may not be required in the setting of classical GCA or Wegener's granulomatosis. It is also usually impractical in the setting of clinically-typical Takayasu's arteritis, where the angiogram reveals characteristic features.
- Therapy for systemic vasculitis generally begins with high-dose corticosteroids, often supplemented with a cytotoxic agent such as cyclophosphamide.
- Large-vessel vasculitis, such as Takayasu's or giant cell arteritis (temporal arteritis), can cause hypertensive or ischemic damage to target organs and requires rapid therapy.
- The vasculitides that affect small and medium vessels tend to have unique patterns of organ-injury (e.g., lungs, upper airways, and kidneys in Wegener's granulomatosis), which provides clues for the clinician.

REFERENCES

1. Albert DA, Rimon D, Silverstein MD. The diagnosis of polyarteritis nodosa. I. A literature-based decision analysis approach. *Arthritis Rheum* 1988;31:1117–1127.
2. Albert DA, Silverstein MD, Paunicka K, et al. The diagnosis of polyarteritis nodosa. II. Empirical verification of a decision analysis model. *Arthritis Rheum* 1988;31:1128–1134.
3. Hoffman GS, Kerr GS, Leavitt RY, et al. Wegener's granulomatosis: an analysis of 158 patients. *Ann Intern Med* 1992;116:488–498.
4. Kerr GS, Hallahan CW, Giordano J, et al. Takayasu's arteritis. *Ann Intern Med* 1994;120:919–929.
5. Tso E, Flamm SD, White RD, Schvartzman PR, Mascha E, Hoffman GS. Takayasu's arteritis: utility of magnetic resonance imaging in diagnosis and treatment. *Arthritis Rheum* 2002;46:1634–1642.
6. Hoffman GS, Leavitt RY, Kerr GS, et al. Treatment of Takayasu's arteritis with methotrexate. *Arthritis Rheum* 1994;37:578–582.
7. Rodriguez-Valverde V, Sarabia JM, Gonzalez-Gay MA, et al. Risk factors and predictive models of giant cell arteritis in polymyalgia rheumatica. *Am J Med* 1997;102:331–336.
8. Evans J, Hunder GG. The implications of recognizing large-vessel involvement in elderly patients with giant cell arteritis. *Curr Opin Rheumatol* 1997;9:37–40.
9. Hoffman GS, Cid MC, Hellmann DB, et al. A multicenter, randomized, double-blind, placebo-controlled trial of adjuvant methotrexate treatment for giant cell arteritis. *Arthritis Rheum* 2002;46:1309–1318.

10. Jover JA, Hernandez-Garcia C, Morado IC, Vargas E, Banares A, Fernandez-Gutierrez B. Combined treatment of giant cell arteritis with methotrexate and prednisone: a randomized, double-blind, placebo-controlled trial. *Ann Intern Med* 2001;134:106–114.
11. Cantini F, Niccoli L, Salvarani C, Olivieri I. Treatment of long-standing active giant cell arteritis with infliximab: report of four cases. *Arthritis Rheum* 2001;44:2933–2935.
12. Rao JK, Weinberger M, Oddone EZ, et al. The role of antineutrophil cytoplasmic antibody (c-ANCA) testing in the diagnosis of Wegener's granulomatosis. *Ann Intern Med* 1995;123:925–932.
13. Guillevin L, Lhote F, Cohen P, et al. Corticosteroids plus pulse cyclophosphamide and plasma exchanges versus corticosteroids plus pulse cyclophosphamide alone in the treatment of polyarteritis nodosa and Churg-Strauss syndrome patients with factors predicting poor prognosis. A prospective, randomized trial of 62 patients. *Arthritis Rheum* 1995;38:1638–1645.
14. Sneller MC, Hoffman GS, Talar-Williams C, et al. Analysis of 42 Wegener's granulomatosis patients treated with methotrexate and prednisone. *Arthritis Rheum* 1995;38:608–613.
15. Guillevin L, Lhote F, Gayraud M, et al. Prognostic factors in polyarteritis nodosa and Churg-Strauss syndrome. *Medicine* 1996; 75:17–28.
16. Langford CA, Talar-Williams C, Barron KS, et al. Use of a cyclophosphamide induction methotrexate-maintenance regimen for the treatment of Wegener's granulomatosis: extended follow-up and rate of relapse. *Am J Med* 2003;114:463–469.
17. Moore P, Calabrese LH. Neurologic manifestations of systemic vasculitis. *Semin Neurol* 1994;4:300–306.
18. Calabrese LH, Duna GF. Evaluation and treatment of central nervous system vasculitis. *Curr Opin Rheumatol* 1995;7:37–44.
19. Calabrese LH. Vasculitis in the central nervous system. *Arthritis Rheum* 1997;40:1189–1121.
20. Hajj-Ali R, Furlan A, Abou-Chebel A, Calabrese LH. Benign angiopathy of the central nervous system (BACNS): cohort of 16 patients with clinical course and long-term follow-up. *Arthritis Rheum* 2002;47:662–669.

ADDITIONAL READING

Hoffman GS. Takayasu's arteritis: lessons from the American National Institutes of Health experience. *Int J Cardiol* 1996;54[Suppl]: 83–86.

Hoffman GS, Kerr GS. Recognition of systemic vasculitis in the acutely ill patient. In Mandell BF, ed. *Management of critically ill patients with rheumatologic and immunologic diseases.* New York: Marcel Dekker, 1994:279–308.

Langford CA. Treatment of ANCA-associated vasculitis. *N Engl J Med* 2003;349:3–4.

Matteson EL, Gold KN, Block DA, et al. Long-term survival of patients with giant cell arteritis in the American College of Rheumatology giant cell arteritis classification criteria cohort. *Am J Med* 1996;100:193–196.

Seo P, Stone JH. The antineutrophil cytoplasmic antibody-associated vasculitides. *Am J Med* 2004;117:39–50.

Smetana GW, Shmerling RH. Does this patient have temporal arteritis? *JAMA* 2002;287:92–101.

Acute Presentations of Selected Rheumatic Disorders

Kenneth H. Fye   Kenneth E. Sack

INTRODUCTION

This chapter reviews the acute manifestations of five common rheumatic disorders: systemic lupus erythematosus, scleroderma, Sjögren's syndrome, polymyositis/dermatomyositis, and rheumatoid arthritis. Although their manifestations are remarkably protean (Table 112.1), certain therapeutic principles are generally applicable.

SYSTEMIC LUPUS ERYTHEMATOSUS

Systemic lupus erythematosus (SLE) is an autoimmune disorder characterized by the presence of auto-antibodies and immune complexes (1). The disease generally affects women of childbearing age; the female-to-male ratio is approximately 10:1. Among black or Asian women, the incidence of SLE is 1 in 250, and among white women, it is 1 in 1,000. SLE has a definite genetic component; the HLA antigens, HLA-DR2 and HLA-DR3, predispose to the disorder. Environmental factor(s) may trigger the disease in genetically susceptible persons, but specific factor(s) have not yet been identified. Animal studies demonstrate a direct association between the concentration of estrogens and severity of disease, supporting the hypothesis that female hormones have a role in pathogenesis.

Issues at the Time of Admission

Typical clinical manifestations of the disorder include arthritis, rash, oral ulcers, pleuritis, pericarditis, psychosis, seizures, vasculitis, pulmonary disease, anemia, thrombocytopenia, and glomerulonephritis (1, 2). Despite the protean nature of SLE, most patients can be comfortably treated on an outpatient basis. Hospitalization is, however, occasionally required. Acute SLE can resemble an acute infectious process, with hectic fevers, diaphoresis, lymphadenopathy, malaise, and lethargy. Generally, patients with acute systemic disease have an inflammatory, symmetric polyarthritis, similar to that seen in rheumatoid arthritis, and most have a rash. Life-threatening complications are listed in Table 112.1. Medication-induced side effects can complicate the initial evaluation of a patient with SLE. Most patients with active disease take prednisone or cytotoxic drugs and are therefore susceptible to severe infections with a variety of bacteria, mycobacteria, fungi, or parasites (3). In addition, the leukopenia, thrombocytopenia, or anemia encountered in the patient with acute SLE can reflect drug-induced marrow suppression and may not represent hematologic manifestations of the disease.

A high white blood cell count is consistent with ongoing steroid therapy but should raise the possibility of infection. The erythrocyte sedimentation rate (ESR) is generally elevated. In patients with nephritis, the urinalysis typically reveals proteinuria and active urinary sediment with cellular or granular casts. Antinuclear antibodies (ANA) in a

TABLE 112.1

COMPLICATIONS OF SELECTED RHEUMATIC DISORDERS THAT MAY REQUIRE HOSPITALIZATION

	Systemic lupus erythematosus	Scleroderma	Sjögren's syndrome	PDM	Rheumatoid arthritis
Cardiovascular	• Anti-phospholipid antibody syndrome • Coronary arteritis • Pericarditis	• Severe digital ischemia • Constructive pericarditis • Restrictive cardiomyopathy • Cardiac arrhythmias or ischemia	• Anti-phospholipid antibody syndrome	• Cardiomyopathy with arrhythmias and congestive failure • Pericarditis	• Constrictive pericarditis or cardiac tamponade
Pulmonary	• Pulmonary hemorrhage	• Severe interstitial lung disease • Pulmonary hypertension	• Severe interstitial lung disease	• Severe interstitial lung disease • Recurrent aspiration	• Pleural effusion • Interstitial pneumonitis • Interstitial fibrosis • Pulmonary hypertension • Bronchiolitis obliterans
Gastrointestinal	• Vasculitis • Protein-losing enteropathy	• Bowel pseudo-obstruction • Malabsorption	• Autoimmune liver disease • Pancreatitis • Malabsorption	• Dysphagia	• Vasculitis
Renal	• Nephritis, often with acute renal failure	• Renal crisis, often with severe hypertension	• Interstitial nephritis		• Amyloidosis
Neurologic	• CNS disease, including seizures, stroke, psychosis • Transverse myelitis		• Demyelinating disease of spinal cord or CNS • Peripheral neuropathy		• Cervical myelopathy • Compressive peripheral neuropathies
Hematologic/oncologic	• Hematologic crisis (including Coombs antibody-mediated or microangiopathic hemolytic anemia, immune leukopenia, or thrombocytopenia)	• Microangiopathic hemolytic anemia	• Generalized histiocytic lymphoma • Waldenstrom's macroglobulinemia	• Complications of an associated malignancy	• Increased incidence of lymphoma
Other	• Overwhelming systemic disease • Vasculitis			• Necrotizing vasculitis (particularly during childhood) • Overwhelming muscle weakness	• Severe flare in joint disease • Active vasculitis • Felty's syndrome

CNS, central nervous system; *PDM*, polymyositis/dermatomyositis.

homogenous or peripheral immunofluorescent pattern are associated with elevated levels of anti–double-stranded DNA antibodies. Patients with pulmonary disease may have a speckled ANA pattern, reflecting anti-Sm (Smith antigen) antibodies. Decreased complement levels reflect a combination of increased utilization (increased amounts of circulating immune complexes) and decreased production of complement components by the liver. The combination of increasing concentrations of anti–double-stranded DNA antibodies and decreasing levels of serum complement is suggestive of increased disease activity. Measurement of serum creatinine, blood urea nitrogen, liver enzymes, and blood gases, in addition to chest radiography, help determine the extent of end-organ involvement. Admission blood and urine cultures help rule out superimposed infection. Lumbar puncture, magnetic resonance imaging, or cerebral angiography may be necessary to evaluate central nervous system manifestations. A history of deep venous thrombosis, arterial occlusive disease, or recurrent fetal wastage in a lupus patient suggests the *anti-phospholipid antibody syndrome*. Screening studies for this potentially hypercoagulable state include the anti-cardiolipin antibody assay, Russell viper venom time, prothrombin and partial thromboplastin times, and rapid plasma reagent test. Often, only one or two of these tests are positive (Chapter 98).

Therapy of SLE depends on the extent and severity of target-organ involvement. Outpatients may require only fast-acting nonsteroidal anti-inflammatory agents for control of arthritis. Hydroxychloroquine is effective treatment for the arthritis, rash, and pleuropericarditis of SLE. Patients with more severe disease, such as those with severe constitutional manifestations or hematologic disease, may respond adequately to high-dose corticosteroid therapy. In critically ill patients, *pulse intravenous (IV) methylprednisolone (Solu-Medrol) (1,000 mg/d)* can be administered on each of three consecutive days, following which the patient should be switched to 60–80 mg of prednisone (or the IV equivalent) per day. Life-threatening complications of disease, such as acute lupus nephritis, vasculitis, or cerebritis, require the use of cytotoxic therapy. *IV pulse cyclophosphamide* (1,000 mg/m^2, given once a month for 6 months and then every 3 months for an additional 18 months) is the current cytotoxic regimen of choice. However, other cytotoxic agents, such as azathioprine, mycophenolate mofetil, methotrexate, cyclosporine, and chlorambucil, have been used with success. With treatment, acute clinical manifestations of the disease should improve during a period of days to weeks. Hematologic studies, determination of the ESR, complement levels, anti–double-stranded DNA titers, and, if the kidneys are affected, creatinine and blood urea nitrogen levels and urinalysis, are helpful in monitoring the activity of disease.

Issues During the Course of Hospitalization

The major issues involve excluding infection, assessing the response to therapy, and monitoring for noninfectious complications of therapy. Occult infection is always the major concern in patients who do not respond appropriately to therapy. Subacute bacterial endocarditis, meningitis, pneumonia, pyelonephritis, and septic arthritis can all mimic acute SLE. In addition, the use of powerful immunosuppressive agents can significantly increase the possibility of nosocomial infection. Concomitant infection is particularly worrisome in patients with active disease and low complement levels who receive corticosteroid and cytotoxic therapy. In patients who initially respond to therapy but in whom fever then recurs, a leukocytosis might suggest an intercurrent infection, whereas leukopenia would be most consistent with worsening SLE. Unfortunately, high-dose corticosteroid therapy can cause a leukocytosis in the absence of infection, and cytotoxic drugs can cause marrow suppression with leukopenia even in the face of overwhelming sepsis.

Discharge Issues

Patients with SLE are not cured when they are discharged from the hospital (1, 4). Generally, they still have active disease and are typically taking oral corticosteroids or cytotoxic drugs (see Figure 111.2 for sample discharge instructions). Discharge plans must include close follow-up with the patient's primary physician. A rheumatologist should be involved in the continuing care of patients ill enough to require hospitalization.

SCLERODERMA

Scleroderma is a clinically heterogeneous disorder of connective tissue characterized by excessive fibrosis in the skin and internal organs (5). Manifestations range from skin thickening confined to the distal extremities and face, with limited internal organ involvement (*limited scleroderma*), to widespread skin thickening, often with life-threatening internal organ involvement (*diffuse scleroderma*). *Localized scleroderma* (morphea, linear scleroderma) is a benign condition that does not affect other organs.

The estimated prevalence of scleroderma is about 200 cases per 1 million population (6). The incidence is low in children and men under age 30 but increases steadily with age, peaking in the fourth through sixth decades. As with other connective tissue diseases, women are affected more often than men (female-to-male ratio of 3:1). Young black women are at highest risk.

The cause of scleroderma is unknown. Familial cases are rare, and there is no strong association with any of the major histocompatibility loci. Evidence is growing, however, for an immune-mediated process that may trigger fibroblast proliferation and collagen biosynthesis. Tissue ischemia can occur early as a result of microvascular endothelial cell injury.

Systemic scleroderma, whether limited or diffuse, has potentially life-threatening complications. Rarely, patients may present with internal organ involvement (e.g., renal crisis) without obvious skin involvement (*systemic sclerosis* sine *scleroderma*) (Table 112.2).

Issues at the Time of Admission and During Hospitalization

Scleroderma is usually treated in the outpatient setting. Occasionally, however, digital infarction or severe involvement of the lungs, heart, kidneys, or gastrointestinal tract necessitate hospitalization.

Severe ischemia of the digits in patients with Raynaud's phenomenon may cause gangrene of the fingers or toes. In such patients, it is essential to provide a warm hospital environment, discourage cigarette smoking, and discontinue the use of potentially vasoconstrictive drugs (e.g., β-blockers, pseudoephedrine). Control of pain, application of topical antiseptics, and protection of the digits from trauma are the cornerstones of management. There is no good evidence that vasodilating modalities (i.e., drugs or sympathectomy), anticoagulants, or platelet inhibitors improve outcome. Surgical removal of the affected digit is rarely necessary. In most instances, the ischemic area demarcates and the necrotic tissue eventually sloughs, leaving a substantial portion of viable digit.

Dry cough and dyspnea on exertion, along with bilateral basilar late inspiratory crackles, often indicate *interstitial lung disease*. Pulmonary hypertension can be an isolated manifestation of limited scleroderma or develop as a result of advanced pulmonary fibrosis (Table 112.2). A palpable

TABLE 112.2

SUBTYPES OF SCLERODERMA

Type	Clinical characteristics	Auto-antibodies	Major complications
Limited scleroderma	Raynaud's phenomenon for years; skin involvement limited to hands, forearms, face, feet; variable presence of telangiectasia, cutaneous calcifications, esophageal dysmotility	Anticentromere antibodies (ACA), 50–60%; anti-DNA topoisomerase I (Scl-70) antibodies, 10%	Pulmonary hypertension
Diffuse scleroderma	Onset of puffy or hidebound skin within one year of onset of Raynaud's; truncal and extremity skin involvement; tendon friction rubs; esophageal dysmotility	Anti-Scl-70, 30–40%; ACA, 5%	Pulmonary fibrosis, renal crisis, diffuse gastrointestinal involvement
Systemic sclerosis *sine* scleroderma	Raynaud's; no skin involvement	May have antinuclear antibodies	Renal, gastrointestinal, or myocardial disease
Localized scleroderma	Morphea, linear scleroderma	May have antinuclear antibodies	*Coup de sabre* deformity (linear scleroderma over the scalp or forehead)

parasternal heave, a split-second heart sound with a loud pulmonary component, a right-sided S_3 or S_4 gallop, and a murmur of tricuspid insufficiency are all physical findings typical of pulmonary hypertension. Hemoptysis in a patient with scleroderma should prompt a search for *endobronchial telangiectasia*.

A decreased diffusion capacity for carbon monoxide (DLCO) is an early indicator of either interstitial or vascular lung disease. A restrictive pattern on pulmonary function tests, or bilateral basilar linear, nodular, or honeycomb infiltrates on chest radiography, suggest interstitial involvement. "Ground glass" opacities on high-resolution, thin-section computed tomography correlate with interstitial inflammation and indicate the need for corticosteroids or immunosuppressive agents (i.e., azathioprine, cyclophosphamide). Advanced pulmonary hypertension unresponsive to immunosuppressive therapy can occur in patients with scleroderma. More information on the pulmonary manifestations of scleroderma can be found in Chapter 57, and the diagnosis and management of pulmonary hypertension are described in Chapter 59.

Cardiac manifestations of scleroderma include constrictive pericarditis, restrictive cardiomyopathy, arrhythmias, and small-vessel coronary artery disease. Although there are no specific treatments for the cardiac involvement, calcium channel blockers may increase myocardial perfusion.

Scleroderma renal crisis manifests as a sudden rise in blood pressure or rapid deterioration in renal function, often accompanied by hemolytic anemia. It occurs most often in patients with diffuse scleroderma, particularly those with rapidly progressive cutaneous thickening early in the course. Occasionally, renal disease develops before skin changes are clearly visible. The use of high-dose systemic corticosteroids can precipitate renal crises in scleroderma patients. Urinalysis often shows proteinuria (usually <2.5 g/24 h), microscopic hematuria, and granular casts.

Markedly increased plasma renin activity is the rule. Renal histopathology shows intimal thickening in interlobular arteries in addition to adventitial and peri-adventitial fibrosis. The prompt use of *angiotensin-converting enzyme inhibitors* in the treatment of renal crisis has dramatically improved survival and reduced the need for prolonged dialysis (7).

The *gastrointestinal tract* is involved in almost all patients with scleroderma (8). Esophageal abnormalities are common and include decreased or absent peristalsis in the distal esophagus and reduced pressure in the lower esophageal sphincter, resulting in dysphagia, chest pain, and, in severe cases, recurrent aspiration.

Involvement of the small bowel can alter peristalsis, with the development of intestinal stasis and eventual dilatation, leading to pseudo-obstruction, bacterial overgrowth, and malabsorption. Proton-pump inhibitors may also predispose to bacterial overgrowth. Radiographic studies of the small bowel typically show dilatation of the duodenum and jejunum, prolonged transit time, sacculations, and packing of valvulae (a unique radiographic finding termed *"hidebound" small bowel*). Large-bowel involvement manifests as a dilated colon without haustra, sometimes associated with wide-mouthed diverticula along the antimesenteric border. Anorexia, early satiety, nausea, vomiting, abdominal distention, diarrhea, or constipation should prompt imaging studies of the gastrointestinal tract. *Pneumatosis cystoides intestinalis* occasionally complicates scleroderma, possibly because excessive hydrogen production by intestinal bacteria reduces the partial pressure of nitrogen in the intestinal wall to less than that of venous blood. Thus, gas cannot be reabsorbed and accumulates in the tissues.

Prokinetic agents, such as metoclopramide, domperidone, low-dose octreotide, and erythromycin, can provide symptomatic benefit in some patients with intestinal involvement. The combination of octreotide and erythromycin can be particularly effective. Antimicrobial agents may be necessary to treat bacterial overgrowth. Intestinal pseudo-obstruction requires bowel rest and decompression with a nasogastric or small-bowel suction tube.

Discharge Issues

Local protection and antisepsis are crucial until the necrotic tissue of gangrenous digits demarcates and sloughs. Prevention of further ischemia by controlling Raynaud's phenomenon is equally important. Treatment techniques include staying warm (gloves, hat, appropriate socks and undergarments, and hand soaks); avoiding nicotine, caffeine, and vasoconstricting medicines; and using vasodilating agents, such as calcium channel blockers. Nifedipine is one of the most effective vasodilators, but it can relax the lower esophageal sphincter and worsen reflux symptoms. Diltiazem, although not as potent a vasodilator, has little effect on the lower esophageal sphincter. Angiotensin-converting enzyme inhibitors may also be beneficial.

Evidence of active interstitial lung inflammation on high-resolution, thin-section computed tomography mandates prolonged therapy with corticosteroids and immunosuppressives. Pulmonary fibrosis will not respond to such therapy. Most vasodilators are ineffective in the long-term treatment of pulmonary hypertension, but IV prostacyclin can reduce pulmonary artery pressure over extended periods (Chapters 57 and 59). Bosentan, an oral endothelin antagonist, is also effective in the treatment of pulmonary hypertension (9).

Although aggressive treatment with any antihypertensive agent would likely prove effective in treating scleroderma renal crisis, angiotensin-converting enzyme inhibitors have become the mainstay of both the short- and long-term management of this disorder and its associated microangiopathic hemolytic anemia. The target blood pressure should be less than 140/90 mm Hg.

The long-term management of scleroderma bowel can be challenging and often requires the expertise of an experienced gastroenterologist.

SJÖGREN'S SYNDROME

Sjögren's syndrome is an autoimmune disorder defined pathologically by mononuclear cell infiltration of exocrine glands throughout the body (10). There is a strong association between Sjögren's syndrome and the HLA-DR3 gene. The female-to-male ratio is above 10:1. Environmental factor(s) may trigger the disease in genetically-susceptible persons. Manifestations of the disease reflect dysfunction of exocrine glands, with a decrease in the secretions that interface between the body and the external environment. The major complaint is that of dryness of mucocutaneous surfaces throughout the body. Half the patients with Sjögren's syndrome have no other rheumatologic problems. In others the syndrome occurs in association with some other autoimmune disorder, such as SLE, rheumatoid arthritis, scleroderma, dermatomyositis, or autoimmune thyroiditis. Extraglandular manifestations of Sjögren's syndrome may necessitate hospitalization.

Issues at the Time of Admission

Severe pulmonary involvement by Sjögren's syndrome, including lymphocytic interstitial pneumonitis and interstitial fibrosis, can lead to restrictive lung disease and respiratory failure (Chapter 57) (11). Inadequate airway secretions increase the susceptibility of the patient to sinusitis, bronchitis, and pneumonia. Gastrointestinal manifestations include pancreatitis, malabsorption syndrome, primary biliary cirrhosis, and chronic active hepatitis. The typical renal lesion is interstitial nephritis, with decreased concentrating ability, potassium wasting, glycosuria, and renal tubular acidosis. Glomerulonephritis and renal failure can rarely occur. Central nervous system involvement in Sjögren's syndrome includes abnormalities of white matter (seen on magnetic resonance imaging) associated with cognitive defects and (rarely) a demyelinating process, reminiscent of multiple sclerosis. Peripheral neuropathies may reflect vascular occlusive disease, caused either by inflammatory vasculitis or by an obliterative vasculopathy related to the presence of antiphospholipid antibodies. A rare patient will present with a symptom complex of fever, salivary gland enlargement, lymphadenopathy, and hepatosplenomegaly. The major differential diagnosis in these patients with the *"pseudolymphoma" of Sjögren's syndrome* is true generalized histiocytic lymphoma. The best way to distinguish pseudolymphoma from true lymphoma is through biopsy of affected tissues. The antiphospholipid antibody syndrome is a consideration in patients with arterial or venous occlusive disease or with a history of multiple miscarriages.

Typical laboratory abnormalities include an elevated ESR, a positive rheumatoid factor or ANA assay, positive anti-SSA or anti-SSB antibody determinations, and polyclonal or monoclonal hypergammaglobulinemia. Anemia, abnormal urinalysis findings, abnormal renal or liver function, or hypoxemia may occur, depending on end-organ involvement. A prolonged partial thromboplastin time, a false-positive rapid plasma reagent test result, a prolonged Russell viper venom time, or the presence of anticardiolipin antibodies may reflect the anti-phospholipid antibody syndrome. Chest radiography, pulmonary function testing, magnetic resonance imaging of the central nervous system, electroencephalography, or electrocardiography can help to assess disease activity in individual patients.

Although hydroxychloroquine and fast-acting nonsteroidal antiinflammatory agents may be of value in the outpatient treatment of Sjögren's syndrome, *high-dose corticosteroids* are necessary in life-threatening extraglandular disease. Pulse methylprednisolone (1,000 mg IV on each of three consecutive days) is indicated in both interstitial lymphocytic pneumonitis with respiratory failure and in acute demyelinating disease of the central nervous system.

Patients who do not respond or in whom unacceptable side effects of corticosteroid therapy develop may require therapy with cytotoxic agents such as azathioprine, mycophenolate mofetil, methotrexate, cyclosporine, or cyclophosphamide.

Issues During the Course of Hospitalization

High-dose corticosteroids and cytotoxic drugs can predispose to secondary infection, and nosocomial pneumonia can complicate the course of Sjögren's interstitial pneumonitis. Rupture of a colonic diverticulum or acute pyelonephritis might confuse the picture in patients with pancreatitis. Secondary meningitis or epidural abscesses are infectious problems that can obscure the response to treatment of the central nervous system manifestations of Sjögren's syndrome.

Patients with extraglandular disease that does not respond appropriately to therapy may have a malignancy. Generalized histiocytic lymphoma and Waldenström's macroglobulinemia both occur more frequently in patients with Sjögren's syndrome. Such malignancies may be heralded by falling ANA or rheumatoid factor titers, and by a rising ESR. Hyperviscosity syndrome in a patient with Sjögren's syndrome is also suggestive of Waldenström's macroglobulinemia. Diagnosis depends on biopsy of involved tissues (e.g., lymph nodes, salivary glands, or bone marrow).

Discharge Issues

Sjögren's syndrome is not curable, but symptoms can be controlled. The hospital physician must ensure that discharge medicines are appropriate (Figure 111.2) and that expeditious follow-up care is arranged with the patient's rheumatologist and primary care physician.

POLYMYOSITIS/DERMATOMYOSITIS

Idiopathic polymyositis is an inflammatory disease of striated muscle defined by proximal muscle weakness, elevated serum creatine phosphokinase or aldolase, typical electromyographic changes, and abnormal findings on muscle biopsy. Dermatomyositis differs histologically from polymyositis, manifests cutaneous lesions, and may have a higher association with malignancies (12). Nonetheless, we will refer to both entities in this chapter as polymyositis/dermatomyositis (PDM). The incidence of PDM in the general population is approximately 1 in 250,000. Women are affected twice as often as men. Although outpatient management suffices for most patients, certain complications of PDM necessitate hospitalization.

Issues at the Time of Admission

Overwhelming proximal muscle weakness often warrants hospital admission. A patient with severe disease may be completely bedridden, unable even to lift his or her head off the pillow. Involvement of the striated muscles of the oropharynx and upper third of the esophagus may cause severe dysphagia and dysphonia and increase the risk for aspiration (Chapter 79). Weakness of the muscles of respiration can produce ventilatory insufficiency. Interstitial pneumonitis and fibrosis occasionally accompany PDM and can lead to restrictive lung disease and respiratory failure (Chapter 57). Cardiac involvement in PDM can cause conduction defects (with sometimes fatal dysrhythmias), congestive heart failure, and pericarditis. Systemic necrotizing vasculitis occurs in childhood PDM but rarely in adults with PDM. The incidence of cancer appears to be increased in PDM, particularly in children and in adults over 50 years of age. The initial screening evaluation for occult malignancy should be age appropriate, and include a careful physical examination, routine blood and urine studies, serial stool Hemoccult tests, and chest radiography.

In addition to elevated creatine phosphokinase and aldolase levels, typical laboratory abnormalities might include an elevated ESR and a positive ANA assay result. Anti-synthetase (Jo1) antibodies tend to be associated with severe, progressive PDM with pulmonary involvement.

High-dose corticosteroid therapy, including pulse methylprednisolone (1,000 mg IV on each of three consecutive days), is effective in treating the complications of severe PDM. Cytotoxic agents, particularly methotrexate, mycophenolate mofetil, or azathioprine, may benefit patients who do not respond to corticosteroids. Newer therapies for recalcitrant disease include IVIG or the TNFα antagonists, such as etanercept or infliximab (13).

Issues During the Course of Hospitalization

Many patients with severe disease respond slowly to therapy, so corticosteroids should be tapered gradually. Cytotoxic therapy is necessary if an adequate trial of corticosteroids has failed, if unacceptable side effects have developed, or if the patient has rapidly progressive, overwhelming disease. Failure to respond to therapy should alert the clinician to the possibility of nosocomial infection or occult malignancy. An occasional patient with PDM responds poorly to all therapies and has a poor long-term prognosis.

Discharge Issues

In general, patients with severe PDM will still be significantly symptomatic at discharge. They are usually weak and may have persistent respiratory insufficiency. Chronic dysphagia, dysphonia, and aspiration are troublesome manifestations that put the patient at constant risk for repeated hospitalization. Many patients require a vigorous program of physical therapy, ongoing home nursing, and careful monitoring by a physician. Some require alternatives to oral feeding (Chapter 15). The response to treatment is often agonizingly slow, and most patients must undergo long-term therapy with systemic corticosteroids, cytotoxic agents, or both (Figure 111.2). Persistent weakness in the proximal lower extremities may reflect steroid myopathy rather than ongoing inflammatory disease.

RHEUMATOID ARTHRITIS

Rheumatoid arthritis is an inflammatory, symmetric, erosive polyarthritis with prominent involvement of small proximal joints of the upper and lower extremities (14). It affects approximately 7 million Americans, generally between the ages of 20 and 50, with a female-to-male ratio of 4:1. Although arthritis is the cardinal manifestation of this condition, virtually every organ system can be affected. Negative prognostic signs in rheumatoid arthritis include seropositivity for rheumatoid factor, involvement of multiple joints within six months of onset, persistent elevation of acute-phase reactants (e.g., ESR or C-reactive protein), early erosive disease, a history of tobacco abuse, and lack of formal education.

Issues at the Time of Admission and During Hospitalization

Patients experiencing a severe flare in disease activity frequently improve during hospitalization, even without a change in pharmacologic therapy, probably because of both physical and emotional rest. Although bed rest may relieve joint symptoms, early institution of physical therapy (including active range-of-motion exercises, muscle strengthening, and ambulation) is critical to maintaining joint function.

Extraarticular manifestations are common in patients with seropositive rheumatoid arthritis. Rheumatoid nodules tend to develop over the extensor surfaces of the elbows and forearms, but they can be seen over any pressure point or in internal organs, such as the heart and lungs.

Ocular involvement is common in rheumatoid arthritis. Episcleritis manifests as localized hyperemia, usually near the limbus, and is associated with only mild discomfort. Although it tends to be self-limited, some patients require topical corticosteroids to control inflammation. Scleritis and scleronodular disease involve deeper ocular tissues, tends to be painful, and can lead to blindness if untreated. Proper management includes corticosteroids or cytotoxic agents. Corneal ulcers are usually caused by obliterative vasculopathy. The management of all these serious eye manifestations requires the expertise of an ophthalmologist.

Keratoconjunctivitis sicca associated with Sjögren's syndrome is the most common ocular finding in rheumatoid arthritis. Patients typically complain of a foreign body sensation, but in severe cases photophobia and deep eye pain may occur. Symptoms are usually relieved by the liberal use of artificial tears and an ophthalmologic gel. The decreased salivary flow of Sjögren's syndrome can cause discomfort and predisposes patients to severe dental caries and oral candidiasis. The former can be managed by meticulous oral hygiene and frequent dental evaluation, and the latter re-

sponds to a nystatin vaginal tablet dissolved in the mouth for 20–30 minutes two or three times a day.

Pleuropulmonary involvement occurs in up to 50% of patients with rheumatoid arthritis. Pleural disease, which is frequently asymptomatic, occurs more commonly in men than in women and occasionally precedes the onset of arthritis. Pleural effusions are typically exudative, with high protein and low glucose concentrations (Chapter 60). Spontaneous resolution is the rule, but systemic corticosteroids are sometimes needed to treat recalcitrant pleuritis. Interstitial disease, including lymphocytic pneumonitis or pulmonary fibrosis, can lead to respiratory failure but may be asymptomatic, manifesting only as restriction or decreased diffusion on pulmonary function tests (Chapter 57). Cigarette smoking predisposes to interstitial involvement, particularly among men. Patients with active interstitial inflammation may require corticosteroid or immunosuppressive therapy. Less common pulmonary manifestations include nodular lung disease (sometimes with cavitation), obliterative bronchiolitis, bronchiectasis, spontaneous pneumothorax, amyloidosis, vasculitis, and pulmonary hypertension. Synovitis of the cricoarytenoid joints may, in addition to pain, dysphagia, and hoarseness, produce stridor and dyspnea. Pulmonary disease can also result from treatment with certain antirheumatic drugs, especially methotrexate.

Cardiac lesions are common in rheumatoid arthritis, but symptoms are unusual. Pericarditis occurs in 40% of patients, especially in those who are seropositive (Chapter 46). Tamponade and constriction are rare. Other cardiac manifestations include coronary arteritis, which is typically asymptomatic, and the formation of rheumatoid nodules, occasionally causing valvular dysfunction or conduction abnormalities.

A small-vessel vasculitis occurs in 30% of seropositive patients; a cutaneous arteritis causing malleolar ulcers occurs in 10%; and a medium-sized vessel arteritis reminiscent of polyarteritis nodosa manifests in 2%. Medium-sized artery vasculitis occurs most commonly in seropositive men who have had rheumatoid arthritis for more than 10 years and who have a history of tobacco use. Characteristic skin lesions (e.g., petechiae, purpura, necrotic ulcers), peripheral neuropathy, severe abdominal pain, and unexplained weight loss can all be the initial presenting manifestation of *rheumatoid vasculitis* (Chapter 111). Neuropathic patterns of rheumatoid vasculitis range from a symmetric sensory or sensorimotor polyneuropathy to mononeuritis multiplex. Biopsy of affected tissue may be necessary to confirm the diagnosis. Glucocorticoids or immunosuppressive agents are indicated for all but the most mildly affected patients with rheumatoid vasculitis.

Entrapment neuropathies are common in patients with long-standing seropositive rheumatoid arthritis. Such processes may result from subluxations of cervical vertebrae (particularly C-1 and C-2), impingement by proliferative synovial tissues (e.g., carpal tunnel syndrome), or amyloid deposits.

The most common *hematologic abnormality* in patients with rheumatoid arthritis is a normocytic, normochromic anemia secondary to decreased red cell production. A normal or elevated serum ferritin level helps distinguish this form of anemia from that of iron deficiency. This "anemia of chronic inflammation" responds to subcutaneous injections of erythropoietin, but such therapy is rarely necessary. Eosinophilia is sometimes seen in patients with severe extraarticular disease. A patient with rheumatoid arthritis, hepatosplenomegaly, and neutropenia (sometimes with anemia or thrombocytopenia) may have *Felty's syndrome*. This rare but potentially life-threatening complication usually occurs in seropositive patients with severe, but often quiescent, arthritis and extraarticular disease. The major sequelae of Felty's syndrome include cutaneous vasculitis with malleolar ulcers, recurrent infections, and, rarely, nodular hyperplasia of the liver with portal hypertension and esophageal varices. The initial treatment of Felty's syndrome is directed at controlling the rheumatoid process with aggressive therapy—typically including corticosteroids and immunosuppressive agents. Granulocyte-macrophage colony-stimulating factor and related agents can increase neutrophil counts but have a limited duration of action, are expensive, and cause considerable side effects. Splenectomy has been advocated in patients with chronic or recurrent infections, but there is no convincing evidence that it provides any long-term benefit.

Renal disease is more commonly a result of drug toxicity than a direct consequence of the underlying rheumatoid arthritis. However, amyloidosis, a complication of long-standing rheumatoid disease, can cause proteinuria. Mesangial glomerulonephritis is a rare manifestation of the rheumatoid process and can cause proteinuria and hematuria.

Discharge Issues

Many patients will experience a mild flare in their arthritis within a few days of discharge. This is probably related, in part, to the increased stress that comes with returning to the home environment. Warning them of this phenomenon, recommending extra rest, and making appropriate adjustments in medication (Figure 111.2) will help patients deal with this flare. The patient should consult his or her primary care physician within a few weeks of discharge. The urgency of subspecialty follow-up depends on the nature and extent of the rheumatoid complications.

KEY POINTS

- In treating autoimmune disease, use aggressive therapy with corticosteroids, cytotoxic agents, or both before irreversible organ failure occurs.
- Always rule out infection in patients who present with what appears to be an autoimmune disorder and in autoimmune patients whose disease appears to be flaring.

- The side effects of immunomodulatory therapy can themselves be life-threatening.
- Corticosteroids are generally the first-line drugs in the treatment of significant autoimmune disease.
- Cytotoxic therapy is indicated for patients in whom the response to corticosteroids is inadequate or for those in whom unacceptable side effects of corticosteroid therapy have developed.
- The complications of disease need to be treated as aggressively as the primary pathogenetic process (e.g., anticoagulants are required in the treatment of anti-phospholipid antibody syndrome, and antihypertensive drugs are crucial in the treatment of scleroderma crisis).

REFERENCES

1. Ruiz-Irastorza G, Khamashta M, Castellino G, Hughes G. Systemic lupus erythematosus. *Lancet* 2001;357:1027–1032.
2. Cervera R, Khamashta MA, Font J, et al. Systemic lupus erythematosus: clinical and immunologic patterns of disease expression in a cohort of 1,000 patients. *Medicine* 1993;72:113–124.
3. Kang I, Park SH. Infectious complications in SLE after immunosuppressive therapies. *Curr Opin Rheumatol* 2003;15:528–534.
4. Ward MM, Pyun E, Studenski S. Long-term survival in systemic lupus erythematosus. Patient characteristics associated with poorer outcomes. *Arthritis Rheum* 1995;38:274–283.
5. Ferri C, Valentini G, Cozzi F, et al. Systemic sclerosis. Demographic, clinical, and serologic features and survival in 1,012 Italian patients. *Medicine* 2002;81:139–153.
6. Mayes M, Lacey J, Beebe-Dimmer J, et al. Prevalence, incidence, survival, and disease characteristics of systemic sclerosis in a large U.S. population. *Arthritis Rheum* 2003;48:2241–2255.
7. Steen V, Medsger T. Long-term outcomes of scleroderma renal crisis. *Ann Intern Med* 2000;133:600–603.
8. Abu-Shakra M, Guillemin F, Lee P. Gastrointestinal manifestations of systemic sclerosis. *Semin Arthritis Rheum* 1994;24:29–39.
9. Rubin LJ, Badesch DB, Barst RJ, et al. Bosentan therapy for pulmonary arterial hypertension. *N Engl J Med* 2002;346:896–903.
10. Garcia-Carrasco M, Ramos-Casals M, Rosas J, et al. Primary Sjögren syndrome. Clinical and immunologic disease patterns in a cohort of 400 patients. *Medicine* 2002;81:270–280.
11. Constantopoulos SH, Tsianos EV, Moutsopoulos HM. Pulmonary and gastrointestinal manifestations of Sjögren's syndrome. *Rheum Dis Clin North Am* 1992;18:617–635.
12. Maoz CR, Langevitz P, Livneh A, et al. High incidence of malignancies in patients with dermatomyositis and polymyositis: an 11-year analysis. *Semin Arthritis Rheum* 1998;27:319–324.
13. Kalden JR. Emerging role of anti-tumor necrosis factor therapy in rheumatic diseases. *Arthritis Res* 2002;(4 Suppl 2):534–540.
14. Lee D, Weinblatt M. Rheumatoid arthritis. *Lancet* 2001;358:903–911.

ADDITIONAL READING

Cervera R, Khamashta MA, Font J, et al. Morbidity and mortality in systemic lupus erythematosus during a 10-year period: a comparison of early and late manifestations in a cohort of 1,000 patients. *Medicine (Baltimore)* 2003;82:299–308.

Dalakas MC, Hohlfeld R. Polymyositis and dermatomyositis. *Lancet* 2003;362:971–982.

Klippel JH, ed. *Primer on the Rheumatic Diseases*, 12th ed. Atlanta: Arthritis Foundation, 2001.

Koopman WJ, ed. *Arthritis and Allied Conditions*, 14th ed. Philadelphia: Lippincott Williams and Wilkins, 2001.

Acute Arthritis

John H. Stone   *David B. Hellmann*

INTRODUCTION

Acute arthritis—defined as joint inflammation developing in less than two days—presents important diagnostic and therapeutic challenges to the hospital physician. In general, the most urgent task is to determine which patients with acute arthritis have infected joints. In most forms of septic arthritis, delays in therapy threaten not only the future function of the joint, but also the survival of the patient. Acute arthritis due to causes other than infection presents different challenges. For example, the prompt diagnosis and appropriate treatment of microcrystalline disorders can alleviate pain and shorten hospital stays. Although septic arthritis and crystal-induced arthritis are the two most common causes of inflammatory joint pain seen in the hospital, a myriad of multisystem diseases (e.g., inflammatory bowel disease, adult Still's disease, leukemia, Whipple's disease, vasculitis) may also present with acute arthritis.

This chapter begins with a general approach to the differential diagnosis of acute arthritis, discusses the analysis of synovial fluid, and then describes the treatment of gout and septic arthritis.

APPROACH TO DIFFERENTIAL DIAGNOSIS

The cause of acute arthritis can usually be determined at the bedside by the history and physical examination, supplemented by a few laboratory tests. Many elements of the initial evaluation contribute to the diagnosis (Table 113.1), but the three of greatest value are usually: (1) *the pattern of joint involvement;* (2) *the presence or absence of extraarticular signs; and* (3) *the results of synovial fluid analysis.*

The *joint pattern* includes both the number and the site(s) of affected joints (Table 113.2). The number of involved joints has important implications. Most cases of monarthritis, for example, are caused by microcrystalline diseases (gout or pseudogout), infection, or trauma. Very few systemic diseases (infections excepted) present with monarthritis. Acute oligarthritis suggests reactive arthritis or occult inflammatory bowel disease. Polyarthritis is usually caused either by a systemic rheumatic disease such as rheumatoid arthritis or systemic lupus erythematosus, or by a viral infection. Because most systemic rheumatic diseases initially develop over weeks to months, the new onset of acute polyarthritis most commonly signals a viral infection. The site of the acute arthritis may be equally helpful in formulating the differential diagnosis. The first metatarsophalangeal joint or the ankle is most commonly involved by gout, whereas acute arthritis of the distal interphalangeal joints usually represents either osteoarthritis or psoriatic arthritis.

The presence or absence of *extraarticular* signs also helps narrow the differential diagnosis. Small, asymptomatic, necrotic pustules over the distal extremities, for example, strongly suggest disseminated gonococcal infection (see the section on "Gonococcal Arthritis" later in this chapter). Osler's nodes and splinter hemorrhages in a patient with acute arthritis imply endocarditis. Examples of the significance of extraarticular manifestations in the differential diagnosis of acute arthritis are listed in Table 113.3.

For patients with unexplained acute arthritis, *synovial fluid analysis* often provides crucial information. This procedure should immediately follow the history and physical examination (1) (Figure 113.1). Arthrocentesis is contraindicated if the joint has an overlying cellulitis. When possible, severe coagulopathy or thrombocytopenia should be corrected before arthrocentesis, especially if the procedure requires a needle larger than 22 gauge. Finally, arthrocentesis of some joints, such as the sacroiliac joints or the hips, requires consultation with an orthopedist or radiologist.

Synovial fluid characteristics of different conditions are shown in Table 113.4. Synovial fluid analysis answers

TABLE 113.1

IMPORTANT CLINICAL DATA IN THE DIFFERENTIAL DIAGNOSIS OF ACUTE ARTHRITIS

Joint pattern
  Number of joints affected
  Site of joint inflammation
Presence or absence of extra-articular features
Synovial fluid analysis
Sexual history
Age
Gender
Time course of illness
Travel history (especially for Lyme disease)
Past medical history (especially diabetes, alcoholism, injection drug use)
Serologic tests

three questions: (1) *Is the fluid inflamed?* (2) *Is it infected?* and, (3) *Does it contain crystals?* Inflammation is present if the synovial fluid white blood cell count exceeds 3,000/μL. Lower synovial fluid white blood cell counts are typical of degenerative joint disease. Synovial fluid specimens with white cell counts above 50,000/μL are often designated "septic," but this label is not always accurate. Acute gout, for example, often produces white cell counts in synovial fluid of 50,000–100,000/μL. Conversely, some infections, especially tuberculosis, may produce relatively low white cell counts in synovial fluid (3,000–10,000/μL). Synovial fluid analysis utilizing a microscope equipped with polarizing lenses and (ideally) a red compensator permits the examiner to rule out microcrystalline disorders (see the section on "Differential Diagnosis and Initial Evaluation" later in this chapter). Bloody synovial fluid indicates trauma, coagulopathy, tuberculosis, or a synovial tumor, such as pigmented villonodular synovitis.

Although the joint pattern, presence or absence of extraarticular features, and synovial fluid findings are the most valuable points in evaluating acute arthritis, the patient's epidemiologic profile, travel history, and social history may also provide important information. A careful sexual history may implicate *Neisseria gonorrhoeae* as the cause. The importance of age is emphasized by the fact that disseminated gonococcal infections rarely occur after the age of 45. The nearly 10:1 female predominance in systemic lupus erythematosus highlights the significance of gender. Closely detailing the time course of the arthritis is also crucial because systemic connective tissue diseases such as lupus, rheumatoid arthritis, and vasculitis virtually never cause acute arthritis as the very first manifestation. Most patients with these conditions have weeks of malaise, fatigue, or other symptoms before onset of the arthritis. Residence in or travel to a region in which Lyme disease is

TABLE 113.2

DIFFERENTIAL DIAGNOSIS OF ACUTE ARTHRITIS: VALUE OF JOINT NUMBER

	Monarthritis	Oligarthritis (2–4 joints)	Polyarthritis (≥5 joints)

Common causes	Gout
	Pseudogout
	Septic arthritis
	Trauma
		Seronegative spondyloarthropathy
		  Ankylosing spondylitis
		  Inflammatory bowel disease
		  Reiter's syndrome
		  Psoriatic arthritis
		  Endocarditis
			Rheumatoid arthritis
			Systemic lupus erythematosus
			Viral diseases
			  Parvovirus B19
			  Hepatitis B
			  Hepatitis C

Some rare causes	Pigmented nodular synovitis Tuberculosis Hemophilia Palindromic rheumatism	Sarcoidosis Whipple's disease	Post-streptococcal infection Leukemia Vasculitis Hypertrophic pulmonary osteoarthropathy Serum sickness Syphilis Adult Still's disease Familial Mediterranean fever

TABLE 113.3

DIFFERENTIAL DIAGNOSIS OF ACUTE ARTHRITIS: VALUE OF EXTRAARTICULAR MANIFESTATIONS

Extraarticular feature	Possible diagnosis
Temperature >40°C	Still's disease
Mouth ulcers	Reiter's syndrome
	Behçet's syndrome
	Systemic lupus erythematosus
Diarrhea	Inflammatory bowel disease
	Whipple's disease
Clubbing	Hypertrophic pulmonary osteoarthropathy
Mononeuritis multiplex	Vasculitis
Anterior uveitis	Sarcoidosis
	Seronegative spondyloarthropathy
	Behçet's syndrome
	Syphilis
Skin findings	
Painless necrotic pustules on distal extremities	Disseminated gonococcal infection
Osler's nodes and splinter hemorrhages	Endocarditis
Malar erythema	Systemic lupus erythematosus
Purpura	Vasculitis
Erythema nodosum	Sarcoidosis
	Behçet's syndrome
	Inflammatory bowel disease
Erythema chronicum migrans	Lyme disease
Subcutaneous nodules	Rheumatoid arthritis
	Gout (tophi)

endemic is a key point in the evaluation of patients with acute monarthritis of the knee (the most common rheumatic manifestation of Lyme disease). A past medical history of diabetes, alcoholism, or injection drug use greatly increases the likelihood that a patient with acute monarthritis has a bacterial infection. Serologic tests can help support the diagnosis of systemic rheumatic diseases (Chapters 110–112).

RECOGNIZING ACUTE ARTHRITIS

Acute arthritis is usually easily recognized by the cardinal signs of inflammation—swelling, warmth, redness, and pain. Most inflamed joints also demonstrate reduced motion and effusions, but in some joints (e.g., the hips), detection of swelling is difficult. The diagnosis of hip arthritis is suggested by groin pain exacerbated by weight bearing or passive internal rotation. In contrast, pain along the lateral aspect of the hip more commonly indicates trochanteric bursitis. Patients who cannot ambulate because of sudden "hip pain" but who maintain the hip in flexion are more likely to have a psoas abscess than a hip joint infection. Sep-

tic arthritis of the sternoclavicular joint is easily overlooked because the pain is often referred to the shoulder.

GOUT

Issues at the Time of Admission

Clinical Presentation

The most common presentation of acute gouty arthropathy is an exquisitely painful, swollen great toe—*podagra*. Attacks of gout develop explosively. Within several hours, a previously asymptomatic patient becomes unable to tolerate the pressure of a sheet over the toe (2). Other commonly affected sites are the ankle, instep, and knee. Gout can cause not only arthritis but also a chemical cellulitis that leads to desquamation of the overlying skin after a few days. Polyarticular gout and involvement of the upper extremity usually develop only after years of recurrent foot involvement, but exceptions occur. Fever is present in approximately 10% of patients.

Differential Diagnosis and Initial Evaluation

Patients suspected of having gout may also have pseudogout, infection, or trauma. Trauma is excluded by history. A previous history of gout, the use of drugs that impair uric acid excretion (e.g., diuretics, cyclosporine, low-dose aspirin), the occurrence of classic podagra, and the presence of tophi all increase the likelihood that the cause of an acute arthritis is gout. Acute monarthritis of the wrist or knee favors pseudogout. A history of injection drug use, rheumatoid arthritis, or diabetes predisposes patients to infection. Because 10% of patients with gout have fever and as many as one-third of patients with septic arthritis are afebrile on presentation, fever does not distinguish infection from gout. Similarly, the serum uric acid level is difficult to interpret in the acute setting because 15% of patients with acute gout have normal values and high uric acid levels may also occur in infection (2). Thus, the crucial test is synovial fluid analysis.

Urate crystals are needle-shaped and negatively birefringent (i.e., when viewed with a red compensator, the crystals are yellow when parallel to the axis of the compensator and blue when perpendicular). Pseudogout is caused by calcium pyrophosphate dihydrate crystals, which are rhomboidal and positively birefringent (i.e., they are yellow when perpendicular and blue when parallel to the axis of the red compensator). Gout is virtually excluded if no urate crystals are present. Crystals are less numerous in pseudogout, and false-negative results of synovial fluid analysis are more common than in gout. Because microcrystalline disease and infection can coexist, Gram stain and culture of synovial fluid should be performed even in the setting of obvious crystals.

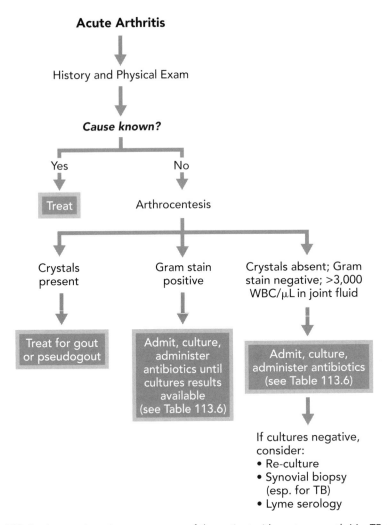

Figure 113.1 Approach to the management of the patient with acute monarthritis. *TB, tuberculosis; WBC,* white blood cell count.

TABLE 113.4
EXAMINATION OF JOINT FLUID

Measure	Normal value	Group 1 (noninflammatory)	Group 2 (inflammatory)	Group 3 (septic)
Volume (mL) (knee)	<3.5	Often >3.5	Often >3.5	Often >3.5
Clarity	Transparent	Transparent	Translucent to opaque	Opaque
Color	Clear	Yellow	Yellow to opalescent	Yellow to green
White blood cells per µL	<200	<200–300	3,000–50,000	>50,000[a] mL
Polymorphonuclear leukocytes (%)	<25%	<25%	50% or more	75% or more[a]
Culture	Negative	Negative	Negative	Usually positive
Glucose (mg/dL)	Nearly equal to serum	Nearly equal to serum	>25, lower than serum	<25, much lower than serum

[a] Counts are lower with infections caused by organisms of low virulence or if antibiotic therapy has been started.
From Hellmann DB. Arthritis and musculoskeletal disorders. In Tierney LM, McPhee SJ, Papadakis MA, eds. *Current medical diagnosis and treatment.* Stamford, CT: Appleton & Lange, 1998:775, with permission.

Indications for Hospitalization and Intensive Care Unit Admission

Gout is rarely the principal indication for hospitalization, and it almost never warrants ICU admission. More commonly, patients are hospitalized for another condition (e.g., congestive heart failure or surgery), and acute gout develops in the hospital. A few patients have such an explosive onset of polyarticular gout that a stroke or some other serious condition is diagnosed initially, and they are admitted for further evaluation. Even when the correct diagnosis is made promptly, hospitalization may be warranted either because the patient is bedridden with polyarticular gout or because the synovial fluid analysis suggests that the patient may have both gout and septic arthritis.

Initial Therapy

The most common mistake in the management of gout is the failure to separate the treatment of acute gouty arthritis from the treatment of hyperuricemia. It is essential to treat the acute arthritis first, and to *defer the management of hyperuricemia* until after the flare has resolved. Treatment of hyperuricemia in the acute setting alleviates neither joint inflammation nor its accompanying pain. On the contrary, if administered during a flare, a urate-lowering agent can provoke another attack.

The most commonly employed agent in treating acute gout is indomethacin, but any nonsteroidal anti-inflammatory agent (NSAID) other than aspirin can be effective (3). (Low-dose aspirin impairs renal excretion of uric acid and can precipitate gout. High-dose aspirin, in contrast, facilitates renal uric acid excretion.) We usually begin with 50 mg of indomethacin orally three times a day until the patient improves (i.e., 1–2 days) and then continue with 25 mg of indomethacin three times a day to complete a 10-day course. Unfortunately, NSAIDs are contraindicated in renal insufficiency, a common comorbidity in patients with gout. They are also relatively contraindicated in patients at risk for the development of NSAID-induced renal insufficiency, such as those with dehydration, congestive heart failure, diabetes, or whose age is greater than 60 years. A history of peptic ulcer disease is also a contraindication to the use of NSAIDs.

For patients with renal insufficiency and acute gout, corticosteroids are an effective alternative to NSAIDs. Intraarticular injection (e.g., 10–40 mg of triamcinolone, depending on the size of the joint) is very effective and especially helpful for the postsurgical patient who is taking nothing by mouth. Corticosteroids can be administered either intravenously (e.g., 40 mg of methylprednisolone IV initially, then tapered by 5 mg/d) or orally (e.g., 40 mg of prednisone once daily by mouth for 2 days, then tapered in a similar fashion). The IV and oral routes are preferable to direct joint instillation in patients with polyarticular gout. Systemic corticosteroids should be used sparingly in patients recovering from surgery and avoided in patients with infections. Corticosteroids can cause or worsen hyperglycemia.

Colchicine, an agent once used to treat acute gout attacks, now has essentially no role in the management of this condition. Daily colchicine (0.6 mg/day or bid) is effective in the prevention of gout flares, but, in the doses required to treat acute flares of gout, it has too low a therapeutic index to be useful. Improper use of colchicine, particularly through the IV route, may lead to substantial patient morbidity (e.g., bone marrow failure). Thus, this drug is best avoided when managing acute gout attacks.

Indications for Early Consultation

Early consultation with a rheumatologist should be considered for patients who cannot be treated with NSAIDs. Orthopedic or rheumatology consultation can also be useful when a difficult joint aspiration is required.

Issues During the Course of Hospitalization

Most patients with acute gout require bed rest for the first 24 hours. Many need opiates for pain relief. Ice packs should be avoided because cold reduces the solubility of urate crystals. Consultation with a physical therapist may be indicated for elderly patients with polyarticular gout.

Discharge Issues

The effective long-term management of gout depends on follow-up with a physician who will continue to educate the patient about the disorder, prescribe an appropriate treatment regimen, and encourage compliance with treatment. Substantial long-term morbidity can result from poorly managed gout, but this can be avoided through proper care by the physician and patient compliance. More than one-third of patients with gout have hypertension or some other manifestation of cardiovascular disease, which emphasizes the importance of general medical follow-up.

The decision to begin hypouricemic agents should be made after discharge. Traditionally, the decision is based on the patient's rate of uric acid excretion during a 24-hour period. Daily urinary excretion of more than 800 mg identifies "overproducers" of uric acid. Such patients are best treated with allopurinol, which blocks the production of uric acid by inhibiting the enzyme xanthine oxidase. Xanthine oxidase also participates in the metabolism of azathioprine, an immunosuppressive drug frequently used in organ transplantation. Because organ transplant patients often suffer gout attacks (because of treatment with medications such as cyclosporine and tacrolimus, which alter urate metabolism in the kidney), clinicians may be tempted to use allopurinol in a patient already on azathioprine. This combination should be avoided, because it can cause serious bone marrow toxicity. If gouty arthropathy, tophi, or frequent flares of acute gout become problems in a patient who has undergone organ transplantation, replacement of azathioprine with mycophenolate mofetil may be considered (3). Another point to remember is that allopurinol is excreted by the kidneys, and should be dosed according to kidney function.

Patients who excrete less than 800 mg of uric in a 24-hour urine specimen are categorized as "underexcretors" and are usually treated first with a uricosuric agent, either sulfinpyrazone or probenecid. However, uricosuric agents are ineffective in patients with creatinine clearances below 40 mL/min; patients with this level of renal insufficiency require allopurinol. Allopurinol is also indicated in patients with tophi or a history of uric acid kidney stones. Until the serum uric acid level normalizes, 0.6 mg of colchicine once daily helps reduce the likelihood of a flare of gout.

SEPTIC ARTHRITIS

In this section, we discuss the approach to the patient who may have an infected joint. We focus on the two most common types of infectious arthritis: bacterial (nongonoccal) arthritis and gonococcal arthritis. Bacterial arthritis is normally caused by an infected joint while gonococcal arthritis occurs as a result of disseminated gonococcal infection.

Issues at the Time of Admission

A cardinal rule in the evaluation of new-onset arthritis—particularly monarthritis—is that an inflamed joint is infected until proved otherwise. Arthrocentesis and thorough examination of the synovial fluid (see above) are an essential early part of the workup. During the initial assessment, however, it is helpful to consider particular patient profiles (Table 113.5), which can narrow the differential diagnosis and assist in choosing an initial empiric antibiotic regimen.

Bacterial (Nongonoccal) Arthritis

A hot joint may be the first clear sign of a potentially life-threatening disorder. Detection of an infected joint often leads to the recognition of bacteremia or the diagnosis of endocarditis. Most joint infection occurs via hematogenous seeding (4). Joints are susceptible to blood-borne bacterial pathogens because synovial tissue is well vascularized and has no basement membrane. Less common routes of joint infection include direct inoculation by trauma (e.g., penetrating injuries, human or animal bites) and arthrocentesis performed through cellulitic skin.

The most common organism associated with bacterial arthritis is *Staphylococcus aureus*, which accounts for approximately half of all such infections in adults (4). However, in many young, sexually active populations, *N. gonorrhoeae* is the most common cause of septic arthritis.

TABLE 113.5

PROFILES OF SEPTIC ARTHRITIS: CHARACTERISTICS OF ORGANISMS AND HOSTS

Organism	Distinguishing features of host
Neisseria gonorrhoeae	Young, sexually active adult (typically female). Arthritis associated with tenosynovitis and skin lesions.
Staphylococcus aureus	Injection drug user (the usual host for sacroiliac or sternoclavicular joint infections). Rheumatoid arthritis patient. The most common cause of septic bursitis.
S. epidermidis	Most common cause of prosthetic joint infections. Associated with an indolent presentation, constant pain (not occurring only with weight bearing), and radiographic signs of prosthetic loosening.
Haemophilus influenzae	Rarely occurs in adults. Formerly the most common cause (type b) bacterial arthritis in children less than 2 years old. Now less common because of the *H. influenzae* vaccine.
Gram-negative rods	Elderly, chronically ill patients at risk for Gram-negative bacteremia. Injection drug users.
Mycobacterial species	Patient with a chronic monarticular arthritis, often associated with tenosynovitis.
Streptococcal species	No classic patient profile, but streptococcal species maintain a constant frequency as a cause of bacterial arthritis throughout the life span.
Borrelia burgdorferi	Residence in or travel to a tick-infested area. Classically preceded by a skin rash (erythema chronicum migrans) by weeks/months. Monarthritis, typically of the knee, develops after skin, central nervous system, and cardiac findings of Lyme disease.

In most cases of septic arthritis, the affected joint is exquisitely painful and demonstrates the classic signs of inflammation. On physical examination, arthritis of an infectious etiology is indistinguishable from that associated with a microcrystalline disorder. The majority of patients with infected joints have fevers during their course, but up to one-third are not febrile at the time of evaluation. The use of antipyretic agents can modify the presentation.

Ninety percent of patients with septic arthritis have a monarthritis. Susceptibility to oligarticular or polyarticular infections is dictated more by host factors (e.g., underlying rheumatoid arthritis or injection drug use) than by characteristics of the infecting organisms. With a few exceptions, the frequency of multiple joint involvement, the specific joints infected, and the responses to appropriate antibiotic therapy vary little among cases of suppurative arthritis associated with the major causative organisms. The most commonly involved joint is the knee, followed by the hip. The small joints of the hands are rarely involved by bacterial infections (except for those associated with *N. gonorrhoeae* and *Mycobacterium tuberculosis*). Sternoclavicular and sacroiliac joint infections are usually associated with injection drug use. In evaluating debilitated patients, one must carefully examine the hips (testing to elicit pain with internal rotation). Infections in these joints can be occult if patients do not bear weight on their lower extremities. Hip infections, in contrast to those in other joints, often require surgical (open) drainage to ensure completeness of therapy.

With the exception of the Gram stain and culture, the results of most laboratory tests and radiographic studies are nonspecific. The great majority of patients with acutely infected joints demonstrate elevations in the erythrocyte sedimentation rate, and a smaller majority have a peripheral leukocytosis. Many types of radiographic studies can demonstrate joint effusions, which are present nearly universally in joint infections. Scintigraphy, computed tomography, and magnetic resonance imaging are all more sensitive than plain radiography, which may not demonstrate juxtaarticular osteoporosis and bony erosions for weeks. Except for the purpose of guiding diagnostic arthrocentesis and excluding infections in joints that are difficult to examine, these studies are expensive and nonspecific, and they often contribute little to the assessment.

Most mimickers of septic arthritis present with clinical and radiographic features that are indistinguishable from those of infection. Thus, arthrocentesis should be performed as soon as possible in the evaluation. Details of the synovial fluid examination are discussed above. Although the specificity of Gram stain and culture is high, the sensitivity varies according to the organism. For most causes of bacterial arthritis, Gram stain of synovial fluid demonstrates the organism one-third of the time. In contrast, results of joint culture are positive in up to 90% of patients with bacterial (nongonococcal) arthritis. Blood cultures are also essential in the evaluation of patients for septic arthritis. Injection drug users should be queried about the use of "street antibiotics," which can cause false-negative culture results.

All patients suspected of having a septic joint should be hospitalized for further evaluation and initial treatment with parenteral antibiotics. Because of the difficulty of performing diagnostic arthrocentesis on the hip and the rapidity with which joint destruction occurs with virulent organisms (e.g., *S. aureus*), early consultation with an orthopedist is essential if hip involvement is suspected.

Gonococcal Arthritis

Arthritis caused by *N. gonorrhoeae*, a Gram-negative diplococcus, results from hematogenous dissemination from a primary mucosal site of infection (4). Disseminated gonococcal infection develops in 1%–3% of cases of untreated gonorrhea. The initial infection precedes dissemination by days to weeks. In sexually active patients under 45 years of age, arthritis associated with disseminated gonococcal infection is the most common type of joint infection. The classic patient is a young woman infected either around the time of her menses (endocervical shedding of the organism and access to the bloodstream are both maximal during menstruation) or during the second or third trimester of pregnancy.

Women are also more likely than men to have subclinical gonorrheal infections and remain untreated, which increases the likelihood of dissemination. In addition to these host factors, certain strains of *N. gonorrhoeae*, particularly those of the protein 1-A serotype (5), are prone to dissemination because their pili permit attachment and diapedesis. Compared with strains of *N. gonorrhoeae* that remain localized in the mucous membranes, those associated with disseminated gonococcal infection have a greater sensitivity to antibiotics but are more difficult to culture. Thus, in contrast to attempts to isolate organisms in most other forms of bacterial arthritis, attempts to isolate *N. gonorrhoeae* from the synovial fluid or bloodstream are often unsuccessful; synovial and blood cultures are positive for the organism in fewer than 50% of cases of disseminated gonococcal infection (4). To optimize the yield of cultures, specimens from every possible site of infection, including the urethra, cervix, oropharynx, rectum, and blood, in addition to any involved joints, should be cultured before antibiotics are begun. The absence of symptoms at these sites should not preclude culturing specimens from them; only a minority of patients with disseminated gonococcal infection have symptoms at the mucosal site of entry.

Most cases of disseminated gonococcal infection are heralded by the acute onset of polyarthralgias, often in a migratory or additive pattern. Two overlapping presentations, the bacteremic and suppurative forms, have been identified. In the bacteremic form, patients appear more systemically ill, with fevers, chills, and malaise. Blood cultures are more likely to be positive than synovial fluid cultures, yet the positivity rate for blood cultures remains below 50%. Tenosynovitis affecting the wrists, fingers, ankles, or toes can be a prominent feature in the bacteremic form of disseminated gonococcal infection and sometimes overshadows the arthritis. The presence of tenosynovitis distinguishes the arthritis caused by *N. gonorrhoeae* from joint infections caused by most other organisms (*M. tuberculosis* is a notable exception).

Skin lesions are also highly characteristic of disseminated gonococcal infection. The skin lesions begin as macules or papules and rapidly evolve into isolated pustules, typically resting on an erythematous base. After several days, the lesions may assume a vesicular appearance and sometimes have hemorrhagic features. The cutaneous lesions of meningococcal sepsis have an identical appearance but are usually more numerous. The presence of more than 100 discrete lesions suggests a meningococcal infection. Culture of skin lesions occasionally yields the correct diagnosis.

In the suppurative form of disseminated gonococcal infection, arthritis (most commonly of the knee) is a more prominent part of the presentation. The associated joint effusions are more purulent, with white blood cell counts rivaling those of bacterial (nongonococcal) arthritis. Joint cultures are more likely to be positive in the suppurative form but are still negative in a slight majority of cases.

For nearly all patients suspected of having disseminated gonococcal infection, hospitalization is recommended. In the hospital, the extent of the infection and sensitivities of the organism can be determined, and the patient can be monitored for a response to therapy. Once the patient demonstrates a clinical response (see "Discharge Issues"), therapy can be completed on an outpatient basis.

Issues During the Course of Hospitalization

Antibiotic therapy for septic arthritis is usually begun empirically, based on the clinical profile and guided by the results of synovial fluid Gram stain. The initial antimicrobial approach is outlined in Table 113.6. The regimen can be modified when culture results become available. Because parenteral antibiotics achieve excellent levels in inflamed joints, *intraarticular instillation of antibiotics is unnecessary.*

Although early antibiotic therapy is essential to good outcomes, adequate drainage of infected joints is also critical. In purulent joint effusions, organisms divide very slowly and are less susceptible to antibiotics. Unless an infected joint is adequately drained, the organisms may survive despite appropriate treatment. Closed drainage, performed as often as necessary to control the effusion, is sufficient for most joints. Repeated arthrocentesis is usually not required with *N. gonorrhoeae* infections, but joints infected with other organisms, especially *S. aureus* or strep-

TABLE 113.6	

EMPIRIC ANTIBIOTIC REGIMENS FOR THE TREATMENT OF SEPTIC ARTHRITIS BASED ON GRAM STAIN OF SYNOVIAL FLUID[a,b]

Gram-positive	Gram-negative
Gram-positive cocci in clusters (presumptive *Staphylococcus*): Nafcillin or oxacillin (aminoglycoside should be added if patient is an injection drug user)	**Gram-negative bacilli:** Nafcillin or oxacillin plus aminoglycoside
Gram-positive cocci in chains (presumptive *Streptococcus*): Nafcillin or oxacillin	**Gram-negative diplococci** (presumptive gonococcus): Ceftriaxone or ceftizoxime or cefotaxime

[a] All patients with prosthetic joints, intravenous lines, or recent hospitalizations are at risk for infection with methicillin-resistant *Staphylococcus* species and should receive vancomycin until culture results are available, regardless of Gram stain results.
[b] In the absence of definitive Gram stain results, a reasonable empiric regimen for the adult with possible septic arthritis would be the combination of nafcillin or oxacillin with a cephalosporin such as ceftriaxone or ceftizoxime or cefotaxime. An aminoglycoside should be added in the injection drug user, and (as above) vancomycin should be substituted for nafcillin/oxacillin if methicillin-resistant *Staphylococcus* is a possibility.

tococcal species, may require daily or twice daily drainage. The response to therapy is judged by the clinical examination findings, the rapidity with which joint effusions reaccumulate after arthrocentesis, and serial measures of cell counts and cultures of synovial fluid. Failure of the patient to respond to therapy, manifested by the disappearance of fever and a decrease in signs of joint inflammation after several days of appropriate treatment, is an indication for open joint drainage and lavage. In contrast to other joint infections, septic hips required immediate surgical intervention.

The majority of prosthetic joint infections originate locally, at the time of joint replacement surgery. *Staphylococcus epidermidis* rivals *S. aureus* as the most common cause of these infections. Management decisions regarding septic prosthetic joints should be made in consultation with an infectious disease specialist. If detected rapidly, early-onset prosthetic joint infections may be treated successfully by antibiotics, alone or in combination with debridement, without removal of the prosthesis. Immediate consultation with orthopedics is essential in the management of such patients. In most cases, unfortunately, the process is sufficiently advanced that the hardware must be removed. If infection in a joint abates but the patient's overall condition continues to deteriorate, another site of infection must be actively sought (e.g., another infected joint, a splenic abscess, endocarditis, or meningitis). Patients with rheumatoid arthritis or other causes of severe debility, particularly those on corticosteroid therapy, are prime candidates for such occult infections.

Acutely infected joints require rest. As soon as the joint demonstrates clinical improvement, however, a daily program of physical therapy, designed to maintain range of motion and prevent joint contractures, should begin. Patients may begin bearing weight as soon as their pain permits, generally after several days of treatment.

Two other points are relevant to patients with disseminated gonococcal infection. First, patients with *N. gonorrhoeae* arthritis should be evaluated for the possible presence of other sexually transmitted diseases, including *Chlamydia* infection, syphilis, and HIV infection. Empiric concomitant treatment for *Chlamydia* infection with 100 mg of doxycycline twice daily for one week is often prudent. Second, the local public health department and the patient's sexual partner or partners should be notified of the infection.

Discharge Issues

Septic arthritis caused by staphylococci (*S. aureus* or *S. epidermidis*) or gram-negative rods should be treated with parenteral antibiotics for three weeks (longer courses are sometimes required, particularly if endocarditis is also present). After they are stabilized in the hospital, patients can be discharged home or to subacute facilities for the remainder of their course. Streptococcal and *Haemophilus influenzae* arthritis usually require only two weeks of parenteral treatment. *N. gonorrhoeae* arthritis should be treated parenterally for 2–4 days until clinical improvement is noted, following which several oral antibiotic regimens (for a total 2-week course) are appropriate: ciprofloxacin 500 mg twice a day, ofloxacin 400 mg twice a day, or cefixime 400 mg twice a day (6). The standard procedure for treating chronic infections in prosthetic joints is to remove the prosthesis, treat with IV antibiotics for 1 month and oral antibiotics for an additional 2–4 months (patients with *S. aureus* infections may require rifampin in addition to other anti-*Staphylococcal* antibiotics), and then implant a new prosthesis. At some centers, however, a one-stage procedure is employed, with removal of the prosthesis and implantation of another at the same time; antibiotic-impregnated cement is used and a long course of systemic antibiotics is administered.

COST CONSIDERATIONS AND RESOURCE USE

The most important strategy to reduce the cost of treating gout is to avoid recurrent attacks through patient education and careful follow-up. The episodic nature of gout unfortunately often leads to episodic (and expensive) care.

The costs of antibiotic regimens for the treatment of septic arthritis vary widely and should be considered in choosing among regimens of comparable efficacy. The most important cost-saving maneuver, however, is to discharge stable patients to receive most of their parenteral antibiotic therapy either at home or in a subacute facility.

KEY POINTS

- Gout is the most common cause of acute arthritis in hospitalized patients, but septic arthritis must always be excluded.
- The treatment of acute gout focuses on therapy for acute arthritis; the treatment of hyperuricemia is deferred.
- Patient education and careful follow-up are vital in patients with acute gouty arthritis.
- Joint infection may be the first sign of a life-threatening condition.
- Arthrocentesis must be performed early in the evaluation of patients with possible septic joints.
- Empiric antibiotic treatment should be based on the results of Gram stain and the patient's clinical profile (Tables 113.5 and 113.6).
- Effusions associated with septic joints should be drained as often as they reaccumulate, to permit maximal antibiotic effectiveness.

REFERENCES

1. Fye KH. Arthrocentesis, synovial fluid analysis, and synovial biopsy. In: Klippel JH, Crofford LJ, Stone JH, and Weyand CM, eds. *Primer on the Rheumatic Diseases*, 12th ed. Atlanta, GA: Arthritis Foundation, 2001:138–144.
2. Edwards NL. Gout: Clinical and Laboratory Features. In: Klippel JH, Crofford LJ, Stone JH, Weyand CM, eds. *Primer on the Rheumatic Diseases*, 12th ed. Atlanta, GA: Arthritis Foundation, 2001:313–319.
3. Bridges SL, Jr. Gout: treatment. In: Klippel JH, Crofford LJ, Stone JH, Weyand CM, eds. *Primer on the Rheumatic Diseases*, 12th ed. Atlanta, GA: Arthritis Foundation, 2001:320–324.
4. Shirtliff ME, Mader JT. Acute septic arthritis. *Clin Microbiol Rev* 2002;15:527–544.
5. Ram S, MacKinnon FG, Gulati S, et al. The contrasting mechanisms of serum resistance of neisseria gonorrhea and group B neisseria meningitidis. *Mol Immunol* 1999;36:915–928.
6. Bignell CJ. European guideline for the management of gonorrhoea. *Int J STD AIDS* 2001;12(Suppl 3):27–29.

ADDITIONAL READING

Imboden JB. The approach to the patient with arthritis. In: Imboden J, Hellmann DB, and Stone JH, eds. *Current Rheumatology Diagnosis and Treatment*. New York: McGraw-Hill 2004.
Massarotti EM. Lyme arthritis. *Med Clin North Am* 2002;86:297–309.

Back Pain

114

Jerry D. Joines   Nortin M. Hadler

INTRODUCTION

Back pain is one of the leading complaints treated in the outpatient setting. Most patients can be managed conservatively without recourse to hospitalization for inpatient care. Hospital admission rates for nonsurgical treatment of back pain, while declining, show a wide geographic variation. A variety of health resource and population characteristics, as well as physician practice patterns, contribute to this variation. It is unlikely that rates of hospital utilization for nonsurgical treatment of back pain correlate with aggregate outcomes of care, although studies have not directly addressed that question.

The majority of back problems prompting medical hospitalization involve the low back. In this chapter, we focus on those disorders that present in adults with low back pain as a cardinal symptom. Although we emphasize disorders of the lumbar and lumbosacral spine, much of our discussion is relevant to cervical disease, and certain aspects of the discussion, such as the management of osteoporotic fractures, are also applicable to the thoracic spine. There are parallels between the common lumbar and cervical spinal disorders. Both regions are affected by spinal stenosis and degenerative disease of the disks and facet joints. Such pathoanatomy, however, is commonly present in the absence of local pain, radiculopathy, or myelopathy, so clinical correlation is always important.

The causes of low back pain generally fall into three categories: *regional disorders, systemic disorders, and visceral disease.* (Some authorities refer to regional disorders as *mechanical* conditions, and to systemic disorders as *nonmechanical* conditions.) *Regional disorders,* which are by far the most prevalent, include such common pathoanatomic disorders as herniated disk, vertebral compression fracture, degenerative disease, and spinal stenosis. In many cases, no specific underlying etiology can be identified. Nearly all instances of regional back pain can be managed conservatively without hospitalization. *Systemic diseases* that can involve the spine include tumors, infections, and inflammatory spondyloarthropathy. Rest pain and night pain are seen more commonly in systemic than in regional disorders, whereas exacerbation of pain during trunk motion is seen more often with regional pain. *Visceral disease* includes any of the non-musculoskeletal processes affecting the intra-abdominal or other nearby organs that can present with back pain. Examples include aortic dissection and pancreatic or renal diseases. Patients requiring hospitalization for nonsurgical care of back pain are a highly selected group with systemic disease, visceral disorders, or exceptionally severe symptoms of regional disorders.

The systemic causes of low back pain are uncommon. The combined prevalence of neoplastic, infectious, and inflammatory causes is around 1% among primary care patients with low back pain (1). About 2% of patients will have visceral disease (1). The *cauda equina syndrome,* in which compression of the cauda equina by a large herniated disk or other mass results in bowel or bladder dysfunction and neurologic deficits in the lower extremities, has an estimated prevalence of 4 in 10,000 patients with low back pain (2).

The appropriateness of many nonsurgical hospitalizations for low back pain is open to question. Cherkin and Deyo (3) examined hospital admissions for medical problems of the low back during 1988 both nationally and in Washington State, and they concluded that many of those hospitalizations involved diagnostic procedures (e.g., myelography) or therapies (some of questionable efficacy) that could be performed or administered in the outpatient setting. Nonspecific back pain, herniated disk, and degenerative changes accounted for 81% of nonsurgical admissions for low back pain nationwide; systemic problems such as malignancy, infection, and inflammatory conditions were excluded from their analysis. Nearly half of the admissions were for pain management; bed rest was the most common physical treatment modality (72% of patients), and opiate analgesics and sedatives were the most commonly used drugs (83% and 71% of patients, respectively). Cherkin and Deyo acknowledged that, in addition to disease-specific indications, various other indications (e.g., difficulty ambulating, inability to prepare food or perform toileting, or the facilitation of diagnostic studies when patients are evaluated at a distance from home) can sometimes justify nonsurgical hospitalizations.

In this chapter, we discuss the diagnosis and management of selected conditions that may require inpatient management on a medical service. We assume that the patient cannot be cared for optimally as an outpatient. We also assume an evidence-based approach to diagnosis and therapy in the outpatient department, such as that proposed by the Agency for Health Care Policy and Research (AHCPR, now the Agency for Healthcare Research and Quality, AHRQ) in its 1994 clinical practice guideline for the management of acute low back problems in adults (4). A number of evidence-based guidelines have built upon the solid foundation provided by the AHCPR guideline (5). Other sources of information include recent reviews of the diagnosis and management of low back pain (1, 2, 6), as well as reviews of specific treatments in the Cochrane Database of Systematic Reviews (7).

ISSUES AT THE TIME OF ADMISSION

Clinical Presentation

Regional low back disorders commonly present with back pain alone; a subset of patients will have signs or symptoms of spinal nerve root involvement (Chapter 115). Compression or inflammation of a nerve root produces radiculopathy characterized by pain, numbness, weakness, and loss of reflexes in the distribution of the corresponding nerve. Most radiculopathy involves the L-5 or S-1 nerve root, and less frequently the L-4 root; neurologic screening should focus on these levels (4). Associated deficits may include weakness of the quadriceps (L-4), a decreased knee jerk reflex (L-4), weakness of dorsiflexion of the great toe and foot (L-5), weakness of plantar flexion of the great toe and foot (S-1), or a decreased ankle jerk reflex (S-1). Sensory deficits follow dermatomes on the medial (L-4), dorsal (L-5), or lateral (S-1) aspect of the foot.

Sciatica is the term reserved for radicular pain that radiates in a sciatic distribution down the leg beyond the knee. *Neurogenic claudication* (pseudo-claudication) is buttock and leg pain or weakness caused by standing erect or walking erect and relieved by sitting or flexing the spine. This is the classic symptom of the syndrome of *"lumbar stenosis,"* commonly ascribed to anatomic lumbar spinal stenosis, although the pathogenesis of pain in this syndrome is debatable; anatomic stenosis is a nonspecific finding on imaging studies in the elderly and does not reliably predict symptoms. Bowel or bladder dysfunction suggests compression of the sacral nerve roots, as does sensory deficit of the perineal region (*"saddle anesthesia"*). All these features can be present in regional or systemic disease of the lumbar spine, some even in visceral presentations. The patient who is writhing or cannot be still, however, should be assumed to have a serious underlying cause, usually a visceral disorder, until proved otherwise.

Findings from the history or physical examination may point toward a particular condition as the cause of back pain (6). A previous history of cancer is the strongest predictor of malignancy (specificity 0.98, positive likelihood ratio 14.7), but sensitivity is low (0.31). Two findings have a low sensitivity but a high specificity for vertebral compression fracture: a history of corticosteroid use (specificity 0.995, positive likelihood ratio 12.0) and age over 70 years (specificity 0.96, positive likelihood ratio 5.5). The presence of sciatica is the best predictor of herniated disk (sensitivity 0.95, specificity 0.88, positive likelihood ratio 7.9, negative likelihood ratio 0.06) (Chapter 6).

Differential Diagnosis and Initial Evaluation

Visceral Disease and Serious Spinal Disorders

The initial assessment of the patient with acute low back pain should identify those patients with a serious underlying cause requiring specific therapy. The history and examination can provide evidence of systemic or visceral disease, or of neurologic compromise that mandates surgical referral (1, 2, 6). Figure 114.1 provides a general approach to the identification of the patient with low back pain who may require hospitalization.

Back pain can be a referred symptom of a variety of nonspinal diseases, including aortic dissection or aneurysm, endocarditis, kidney stone, pancreatitis, pancreatic pseudocyst, peptic ulcer disease, urinary tract infection/pyelonephritis, perinephric abscess, prostatitis, pelvic infection, and others. As indicated in Figure 114.1, the initial workup should identify those patients with referred back pain resulting from nonspinal disease.

The search for serious spinal disorders is facilitated by a systematic evidence-based approach such as that recommended by the AHCPR practice guideline (4). This approach starts with a focused history and physical examination, with attention to certain "red flags" for possible serious conditions, including fracture, tumor, infection, and cauda equina syndrome. "Red flags" for fracture include major trauma (e.g., a fall or vehicular accident); in older or osteoporotic patients, minor trauma or strenuous lifting is of concern. Red flags for tumor or infection include age over 50 or under 20, history of cancer, fever, weight loss, pain worse in a supine position or at night, recent bacterial infection, intravenous drug abuse, and immunosuppression. Cauda equina syndrome warrants emergent diagnostic imaging and surgical consultation or referral. Red flags from the history for cauda equina syndrome include saddle anesthesia, bladder dysfunction (urinary retention, frequency, incontinence), and severe or progressive lower extremity neurologic deficit. Red flags from the physical

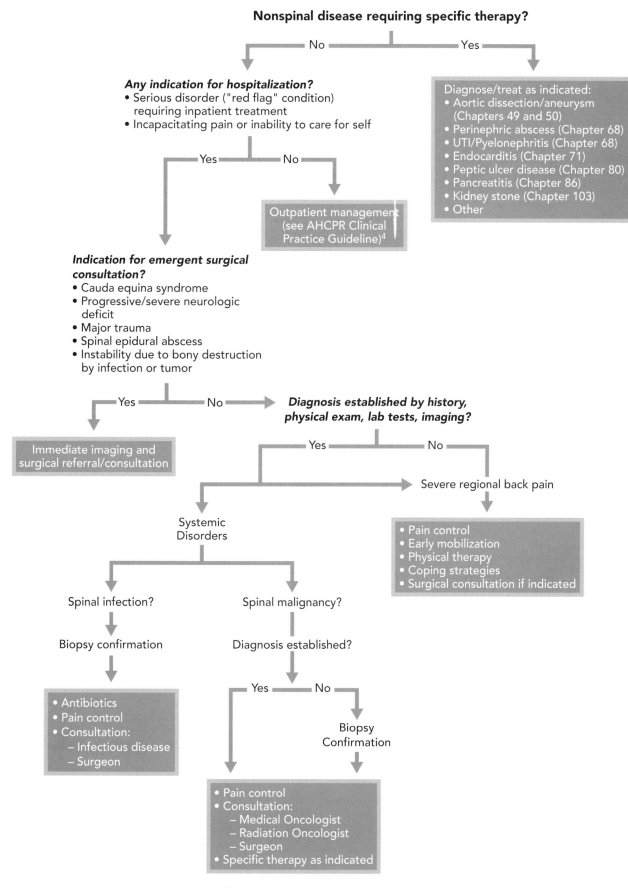

Figure 114.1 Assessment of low back pain.

examination include anal sphincter laxity, perianal or perineal sensory loss, and major weakness involving the quadriceps or the ankle plantar flexors, ankle evertors, or ankle dorsal flexors.

Although the cauda equina syndrome is the classic indication for emergent surgical evaluation, other disorders also require immediate surgical consultation or referral, including spinal epidural abscess, progressive or severe neurologic deficit, major trauma, and instability resulting from a destructive neoplastic or infectious process. As indicated in the lower portion of Figure 114.1, most patients with back pain who require hospitalization but lack an indication for urgent surgical consultation fall into the following categories of illness: severe and incapacitating regional back pain attributable to herniated disk, degenerative disease, spinal stenosis, osteoporotic compression fracture, or nonspecific causes; spinal malignancy; and spinal infections, including vertebral osteomyelitis and septic diskitis.

Most patients who are hospitalized with back pain will already have undergone diagnostic testing and imaging. Initial laboratory testing indicated for most patients hospitalized with severe back pain includes a complete blood cell count with white cell differential; measurement of serum creatinine, calcium, alkaline phosphatase, and erythrocyte sedimentation rate; and urinalysis. If infection is suggested because of fever, leukocytosis, or a markedly elevated sedimentation rate, then blood cultures are appropriate. If myeloma is clinically suspected, serum and urine protein electrophoresis should be performed.

Plain radiographs may detect destructive bone lesions and compression fractures. If rheumatic spondyloarthropathy is suspected, radiographs of the sacroiliac joints are appropriate. Although radiography has a limited role in the management of outpatients with back pain, such pain of sufficient severity to prompt hospitalization justifies diagnostic imaging because the prior probability (Chapter 6) of specific lesions is so high. Plain radiographs not only may provide a working diagnosis, but also can focus the choice of additional imaging studies.

The commonly available options for radiologic imaging of the spine beyond plain radiography include computed tomography (CT), magnetic resonance imaging (MRI), radionuclide scintigraphy (bone scan), and myelography. Bone scan, although very sensitive for infectious or malignant causes of back pain, lacks specificity. It can, however, target subsequent studies that afford more specific pathoanatomic insights. Myelography is invasive and is used far less often than in the past. We would reserve its use for situations in which it is requested by a consulting surgeon. Both CT and MRI demonstrate the anatomy. MRI is probably the best overall choice for defining malignancy, infection, inflammation, and structural abnormalities of the spine and associated soft tissues. The cost of MRI varies but is typically in the range of $1,000 (without contrast), considerably higher than that of CT or bone scan. Although

gadolinium enhancement is not necessary to detect many conditions, the added definition justifies its use in some situations.

If spinal infection or malignancy is demonstrated, further evaluation is mandatory to design specific therapy. Antibiotic therapy of *spinal infections* (vertebral osteomyelitis/septic diskitis and spinal epidural abscess) should, whenever possible, be based on identification of the causative organism. *Staphylococcus aureus* is the most common, but far from the only, cause. Other pyogenic bacteria, mycobacteria, and fungal organisms can also infect the spine. Blood cultures are mandatory when spinal infection is suspected. For processes involving the vertebral bodies or intervertebral disks, percutaneous needle aspiration and biopsy permits a specific microbiologic diagnosis. This can often be accomplished under radiologic guidance (fluoroscopy or CT) with low complication rates in the hands of experienced practitioners. Open biopsy is an alternative. Empiric antibiotic therapy pending results of these studies may be prudent, but premature institution of antibiotics without attempts to isolate the organism can result in inappropriate or unnecessary treatment. Antibiotic therapy for spinal infections is usually prolonged (e.g., 6–8 weeks); an infectious disease consultation can help guide the choice of antibiotics and the duration of therapy. Surgical debridement may be required in tuberculous (Pott's) disease, and surgical drainage is usually required for effective treatment of epidural abscess. Otherwise, surgical consultation is appropriate whenever stability is in question or when a significant neurologic deficit is present.

Metastatic disease is the most common malignant process involving the spine. Back pain can be the presenting symptom of common cancers, such as those of the breast, prostate, and lung and multiple myeloma. The prognosis varies depending on the underlying malignancy. If compression of the spinal cord or cauda equina is found at presentation, then emergent treatment is indicated in the hope of preventing paralysis or incontinence. Options include steroids, surgical decompression, radiation treatment, and in some situations hormonal therapy or chemotherapy; surgical stabilization also may be required. Consultation with a surgeon, radiation oncologist, and medical oncologist can optimize the choice of therapy in a particular situation. See Chapter 92 for a detailed discussion of the management of malignant spinal cord compression. As in spinal infection, tissue can be obtained for definitive diagnosis by either percutaneous or open biopsy. Functional outcome in patients with spinal metastasis is directly related to the degree of deficit at the time treatment is started. In cases in which pain is not controlled by oral analgesia, parenteral therapy with opiate analgesics is indicated.

For those patients with serious conditions, such as infection or malignancy, the management and expected course will depend on the particular situation. Decisions regarding immobilization with bed rest or orthopedic braces are best made in consultation with surgical, oncologic, and other consultants. Discharge will depend on the specific therapy and response to treatment. In some cases, intravenous therapies, such as prolonged administration of antibiotics, can be completed in the outpatient setting with close follow-up and home health care.

Severe Regional Low Back Pain

Modern imaging should detect nearly all instances of infectious or neoplastic causes of back pain. For regional pain, there is a problem: abnormal findings on imaging studies are not specific. Herniated disk, degenerative spinal disease, compression fractures, and spinal stenosis are common in completely asymptomatic subjects. Therefore, a pathologic finding must be interpreted in light of the patient's symptoms and findings on physical examination (Chapter 6).

Osteoporotic vertebral compression fractures are common in older women. Population studies have shown that more than 20% of people (of both genders) over 50 years of age have radiographic Grade 1 vertebral deformities (8). These involve both the thoracic and lumbar spine, and the prevalence increases with advancing age. Most compression fractures are either asymptomatic or not memorable. In contrast, such fractures can, from time to time, cause severe pain that occasionally requires inpatient care. Symptoms may precede the development of a visible fracture on plain radiography and therefore be misdiagnosed. The impact of symptomatic compression fractures on the patient's functional status should not be underestimated. The associated pain can persist from a few weeks to a few months and be severe and incapacitating in these patients, who are elderly and often frail.

If the history, examination, and radiographic findings are consistent with an osteoporotic compression fracture and there is no neurologic compromise or suspicion of an infectious or malignant process, then further imaging may not be necessary. Caution, however, is advised in attributing such fractures to a benign process without further verification. If traumatic fracture is suspected and radiography is not definitive, then bone scan would be appropriate; CT and MRI provide additional definition in the case of a vertebral fracture that may be pathologic (i.e., resulting from metastatic neoplastic or infectious disease).

Indications for Initial Intensive Care Unit Admission

The primary indication for initial ICU admission is the presence of neurologic compromise requiring urgent intervention and close monitoring of neurologic status. Immediate surgical consultation is indicated in such cases. Other reasons for ICU admission include sepsis, hypotension, and severe comorbidity.

Initial Therapy

The remainder of this discussion focuses on the management of severe regional low back pain. Initial therapy of low back pain consists of analgesia and specific therapy when possible. Pain relief, however, is a goal with general principles that apply across the range of diagnoses (Chapter 18). Acetaminophen and the nonsteroidal anti-inflammatory drugs (NSAIDs) are the first-line analgesics used in the treatment of back pain. Well-known side effects of NSAIDs include gastrointestinal irritation and bleeding, in addition to adverse renal effects, to which the elderly are particularly prone. Opiates may be required for adequate pain control but should be used judiciously; time-limited fixed courses may avoid excessive narcotization. Constipation is likely when opiates are used and can be relieved by bowel regimens that include stool softeners and laxatives.

Effective therapies for mechanical low back pain include analgesia, limited bed rest or continuation of usual activity, mobilization, and surgery in certain well-defined situations. Evidence does not support the use of spinal traction, facet joint injection, prolonged bed rest, or transcutaneous electrical nerve stimulation (TENS). Epidural steroid injections to treat radicular pain are sometimes used in the hope of avoiding surgery. These injections, however, are not without risk, and evidence supporting their efficacy beyond temporary relief of pain is limited. "Muscle relaxants" are sedating and add little to the analgesic efficacy of NSAIDs.

Beyond analgesia, the treatment of vertebral compression fractures consists of limited bed rest and early mobilization, with a goal toward preventing debility and further bone loss. Orthopedic bracing for patient comfort is commonly used, but may not be tolerated. Assistance with the activities of daily living may be the goal of hospitalization until adequate care is available elsewhere. Opiates may be required for adequate pain control but must be used cautiously because they are often counterproductive, leading to falls and further debility. Calcitonin, in addition to its effect on bone mass, appears to have a direct analgesic effect and may therefore be of dual benefit. An intranasal form is now available.

Indications for Early Consultation

The indications for emergent consultation were discussed above. In the absence of an indication for emergent or immediate consultation, elective surgical referral for herniated disk is appropriate if the patient has persistent neuromotor deficit, or persistent sciatica with consistent clinical and neurological findings, after 4–6 weeks of nonoperative therapy (1). The only randomized clinical trial of surgical diskectomy versus conservative treatment of patients with herniated lumbar disks and sciatica was reported by Weber in 1983 (9). In that study, 126 patients with radicular pain persisting after two weeks of conservative therapy were randomized to either surgical diskectomy or six weeks of continued nonsurgical management with analgesia and physiotherapy. It is notable that the randomization excluded two other groups of patients: those patients felt to have a definite indication for surgery, and those who improved during two weeks of initial conservative management. Among those randomized, surgical patients reported significantly less pain and incapacity at one year of follow-up, with only a trend favoring surgery at 4 and 10 years of follow-up. The Weber trial supports the early benefit of surgery in a highly selected group of patients with persisting sciatica and a corresponding and demonstrable disk herniation. There is no compelling surgical indication for the patient with nonspecific low back pain, or any patient with radiculopathy in whom there is no identifiable correlative lesion.

The indications for surgical referral of the patient with spinal stenosis are even less clearly defined. No randomized clinical trial has compared conservative management with decompressive surgical therapy. In the absence of surgery, symptoms may remain stable, spontaneously progress, or improve with time. Some patients do appear to benefit from surgery, although the duration of benefit is unclear and serious complications are frequent in this elderly population. Surgical consultation seems appropriate for those with recalcitrant, severe neurogenic claudication or with major neurologic compromise. Definitive guidelines for the management of these patients await scientific evidence defining an optimal treatment plan.

ISSUES DURING THE COURSE OF HOSPITALIZATION

For those patients with severe regional back pain, pain control, mobilization, and return to effective coping are the main goals of treatment. After that, the natural history favors a return to health. Function and independence are best preserved by early mobilization, while prolonged bed rest promotes debility and disability. An accumulation of evidence supports continuation of usual activity as tolerated rather than even a short period of bed rest in most cases. Severe pain or the presence of a motor deficit may warrant a limited period of bed rest, but early mobilization should be the goal.

Physical therapists can assist the patient with transfers and ambulation and should be an integral part of the hospital management of the patient with severe regional back pain. Occupational therapy to assist with activities of daily living and encourage independent function may also be helpful. Specific exercises are counterproductive and have no role in the management of acute back pain.

Osteoporotic vertebral fractures have typically been treated with longer periods of bed rest, up to 1–2 weeks in some cases. We would advise otherwise. Although longer periods of bed confinement may be dictated by the patient's condition, early mobilization should still be the

goal. Prolonged bed rest, which is associated with deconditioning and other risks of immobility, may actually accelerate bone resorption. The prior recommendations regarding physical and occupational therapy apply here also. Women with previous vertebral fractures are at higher risk for additional fractures, and this risk is highest (19% overall) in the first year following fracture (10). This risk underscores the importance of appropriate medical treatment of the underlying osteoporosis, with a goal of preventing recurrent fractures.

Percutaneous vertebroplasty and kyphoplasty are increasingly being used to treat painful osteoporotic compression fractures refractory to conservative management. Both procedures involve the injection of polymethylmethacrylate bone cement into the involved vertebral body using radiologic guidance with fluoroscopy or computed tomography. In kyphoplasty, the vertebral body is first expanded using an inflatable device, and then injected. Although high success rates in terms of pain relief have been reported, these procedures have not been studied in randomized clinical trials. Complication rates are reportedly low, but serious complications can occur; these include spinal cord or nerve root injury and embolism of the bone cement to the pulmonary arteries. Watts et al (11), in a review of these procedures, recommended that they be used only in carefully selected patients with severe persistent pain, by experienced operators, and ideally in centers that participate in controlled clinical trials. We would advise caution until randomized clinical trials have clearly demonstrated the efficacy and long-term safety of these procedures.

The importance of the therapeutic relationship between physician and patient in treating back pain should not be underestimated. An attitude of optimism should be maintained by the treating physician and all allied health professionals. There is no reason to feel or communicate desperation when treating any patient with severe regional back pain who has no major neurologic compromise, especially as regional back pain associated with herniated disk, spinal stenosis, compression fracture, or nonspecific causes in many cases will improve with time. The clinician should work with the patient to identify any psychological issues that might be interfering with coping. Regional back pain is a remittent and intermittent predicament of life (12). There is no substitute for a caring attitude on the part of the physician, with reassurance that the patient is not alone in facing pain.

DISCHARGE ISSUES

Discharge planning should consider patients' home and work situations and ability to function independently in those settings. Social work consultation may identify resources available to help patients cope with the functional limitations imposed by their condition. Those patients with regional back pain for whom surgical referral is not required will be ready for discharge when their symptoms are adequately controlled on oral analgesics and they are able to function safely and adequately in the home environment.

Patients with regional low back pain should be instructed to avoid heavy lifting, prolonged sitting, and bending or twisting the back for a limited period of time. Low-stress aerobic exercise as tolerated may be beneficial (4). Temporary modifications of job-related activity may help facilitate the return to work; however, this is no substitute for addressing issues that relate to job satisfaction.

Patients with osteoporotic fractures should be followed over time for progressive deformity or neurologic compromise. Medical treatment to deter further loss of bone density and prevent subsequent fractures should be considered as an integral part of the management of osteoporotic compression fractures (13).

COST CONSIDERATIONS AND RESOURCE USE

The key to the cost-effective management of back pain is appropriate outpatient treatment that maximizes patient benefit while avoiding unnecessary hospitalizations, ineffective therapies, and unwarranted imaging procedures. Assuming optimal outpatient management with an appropriate decision to hospitalize and image the patient, the cost of inpatient medical treatment of regional back pain will largely be a function of the length of stay. The timely coordination of resources such as physical therapy, occupational therapy, social work, and home assistance will likely reap dividends in terms of earlier mobilization and discharge. Unnecessary drug costs can be reduced when generic NSAIDs are chosen over more expensive but no more efficacious alternatives.

KEY POINTS

- Back pain is a common complaint that usually responds to conservative outpatient treatment. Hospitalization for medical management is indicated in a minority of patients.
- Emergent imaging and surgical consultation are indicated for the cauda equina syndrome. Immediate surgical referral is also warranted for progressive or severe neurologic deficits, instability resulting from bony destruction by infection or neoplasm, spinal epidural abscess, and major trauma.
- Beyond these urgent indications, hospitalization for medical management is indicated when there is a serious

"red flag" condition, when pain is incapacitating and refractory to outpatient management, or when the patient is incapable of self-care and independent function and does not have adequate assistance in the home setting.

- For severe regional back pain, nonsteroidal antiinflammatory medications and early mobilization are the mainstays of therapy.
- Osteoporotic vertebral compression fractures can cause incapacitating pain and debility. Analgesia and mobilization are primary short-term goals; medical therapy to prevent further bone loss and subsequent fractures is critical.
- Serious disorders, such as infection and malignancy, should be treated in consultation with the appropriate specialists.

REFERENCES

1. Deyo RA, Weinstein JN. Low back pain. *N Engl J Med* 2001;344: 363–370.
2. Atlas SJ, Deyo RA. Evaluating and managing acute low back pain in the primary care setting. *J Gen Intern Med* 2001;16:120–131.
3. Cherkin DC, Deyo RA. Nonsurgical hospitalization for low back pain: is it necessary? *Spine* 1993;18:1728–1735.
4. Bigos S, Bowyer O, Braen G, et al. *Acute low back problems in adults. Clinical practice guideline.* Quick reference guide No. 14. Rockville, MD: U.S. Department of Health and Human Services, Public Health Service, Agency for Health Care Policy and Research, AHCPR Publication No. 95-0643, December 1994.
5. Koes BW, van Tulder MW, Ostelo R, et al. Clinical guidelines for the management of low back pain in primary care: an international comparison. *Spine* 2001;26:2504–2514.
6. Jarvik JG, Deyo RA. Diagnostic evaluation of low back pain with emphasis on imaging. *Ann Intern Med* 2002;137:586–597.
7. *The Cochrane Library*, Issue 1, 2003. Oxford: Update Software.
8. Jackson SA, Tenenhouse A, Robertson L, and the CaMos Study Group. Vertebral fracture definition from population-based data: preliminary results from the Canadian Multicenter Osteoporosis Study (CaMos). *Osteoporos Int* 2000;11:680–687.
9. Weber H. Lumbar disc herniation: a controlled, prospective study with ten years of observation. *Spine* 1983;8:131–140.
10. Lindsay R, Silverman SL, Cooper C, et al. Risk of new vertebral fracture in the year following a fracture. *JAMA* 2001;285:320–323.
11. Watts NB, Harris ST, Genant HK. Treatment of painful osteoporotic vertebral fractures with percutaneous vertebroplasty or kyphoplasty. *Osteoporos Int* 2001;12:429–437.
12. Hadler NM, Carey TS. Low back pain: an intermittent and remittent predicament of life. *Ann Rheum Dis* 1998;57:1–2.
13. NIH Consensus Development Panel on Osteoporosis Prevention, Diagnosis, and Therapy. Osteoporosis prevention, diagnosis, and therapy. *JAMA* 2001;285:785–795.

ADDITIONAL READING

Gibson JNA, Grant IC, Waddell G. The Cochrane review of surgery for lumbar disc prolapse and degenerative lumbar spondylosis. *Spine* 1999;24:1820–1832.
Waddell G, McIntosh A, Hutchinson A, et al. *Low back pain evidence review.* London: Royal College of General Practitioners, 1999.

Neurology and
Psychiatry

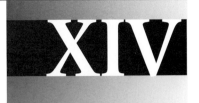

Signs, Symptoms, and Diagnostic Tests in Neurology

115

John W. Engstrom

TOPICS COVERED IN CHAPTER

- Headache 1163
- Delirium and Dementia 1164
- Pupillary Responses 1166
- Dizziness and Vertigo 1166
- Dysphagia of Neurologic Etiology 1167
- Movement Disorders 1167
- Weakness 1168
- Sensory Examination 1169
- Urinary Incontinence 1170
- Cerebrospinal Fluid (CSF) Examination 1171
- Neuroimaging 1172
- Electroencephalography 1172
- Electromyography and Nerve-Conduction Studies 1173

INTRODUCTION

The key to evaluating patients with neurologic symptoms is to obtain an adequate neurologic history. Many hospitalized patients are unable to give a full history because of an altered mental state or severe medical illness. Historical accounts by firsthand observers (family members, friends) become essential. The neurologic history informs the search for pertinent findings on the neurologic examination.

The neurologic history and examination are critical for localization of disease to the *central nervous system* (CNS), *peripheral nervous system* (PNS), or a *nonneurologic source*. Analysis of the symptoms and signs determines the neurologic differential diagnosis, which in turn guides further history and examination. The importance of this point cannot be overemphasized, because hospitalized patients are accessible for repeated evaluations. Simply obtaining additional history and repeating the examination often spares patients from ill-directed and expensive investigations.

This chapter describes common neurologic symptoms, signs, and diagnostic tests. Symptoms and signs are organized by the order in which they appear in a typical neurologic examination. A differential diagnosis is presented whenever possible. The readings listed at the end of this chapter cover clinical evaluation and management of specific neurologic diseases.

SYMPTOMS AND SIGNS

Headache

The top clinical priority is to determine if headache reflects serious intracranial pathology that requires acute intervention. The presence of new headache increases the likelihood of a serious cause, while a change only in severity or location of pain (particularly in the setting of chronic headache) is far less worrisome from the standpoint of structural brain disease. A new headache that reaches peak intensity within one or two seconds suggests intracranial hemorrhage (Table 115.1; also see Chapter 117). Headache precipitated by the supine position that improves with standing suggests elevated intracranial pressure. Headache precipitated by standing and relieved by the supine position suggests low intracranial pressure. Such low-pressure headaches usually are caused by a cerebrospinal fluid (CSF) leak, most commonly following lumbar puncture (LP). An LP headache typically resolves spontaneously over 4–7 days and is treated with bedrest and simple analgesics.

New headache associated with systemic signs, including fever, stiff neck, rash, or arthritis, may reflect sepsis or meningitis. If bacterial meningitis is suspected (e.g., stiff neck) and focal neurologic findings are absent, then LP can be performed without prior brain neuroimaging. Neuroimaging ideally should precede spinal fluid examination when papilledema, other evidence of elevated intracranial pressure (ICP), or focal CNS neurologic findings are present. In patients with cancer or immunosuppression, new headache may be due to brain metastasis, carcinomatous meningitis, brain abscess, or infectious meningitis. Neuroimaging may be followed by LP if midline shift of brain structures or obstructive hydrocephalus resulting in a CSF pressure differential between the brain and the spine are absent. In elderly patients with new headache, structural brain disease and temporal arteritis are important and treatable considerations. New-onset posterior cervical headache should raise the suspicion for upper cervical spine structural disease (metastatic tumor, osteomyelitis, or arterial dissection) which may refer pain to the posterior cranium.

Although headache is a common symptom among inpatients, it is not usually the primary reason for hospitalization. Many systemic disorders result in headache, including hypercapnia, hypoxia, anemia, sepsis, chronic renal failure, hypoglycemia, hypercalcemia, hypernatremia, and thyrotoxicosis. Headache also may be caused by medications (Table 115.2). Outpatients with chronic headaches treated regularly with analgesics may develop withdrawal symptoms or rebound headaches if the analgesics are discontinued during hospitalization. A methodical review of the relationship between recent medication changes and

TABLE 115.2

COMMON CAUSES OF DRUG-INDUCED HEADACHE

Calcium channel blockers	Nitroglycerine
Cimetidine, ranitidine	Oral contraceptives
Indomethacin, diclofenac	Tamoxifen
β blockers	Danazol
Ranitidine	Methylprednisolone
Trimethoprim–sulfamethoxazole	Tetracycline
Isosorbide dinitrite	Aspartame
Estrogen	Alcohol
Cyclosporine	Monosodium glutamate (MSG)

new headaches is important. Patients with drug-induced or withdrawal headaches should receive short-term symptomatic treatment while more significant medical issues are managed.

The approach to benign causes of headache (migraine, tension headache) requires an accurate diagnosis, followed by either nonpharmacologic or pharmacologic intervention. Acute migraine or tension headaches often respond to simple analgesics (aspirin, acetaminophen, nonsteroidal anti-inflammatory drugs). Serotonergic agents (e.g., sumatriptan), ergots (ergotamine), or a combination of isomethepene, acetaminophen, and dichloralphenazone (Midrin), are helpful for acute-subacute headache if simple analgesics are ineffective and there are no medical contraindications. Optimal management of frequent, chronic headache is best performed in an outpatient setting where management can be tailored to the patient's activities of daily living.

Delirium and Dementia

The hospital physician must be able to distinguish delirium from dementia at the bedside. Delirium refers to an acute confusional state with a fluctuating level of alertness. Dementia is a chronic, progressive cognitive deterioration, typically with impaired recent memory but normal level of alertness. Delerium (encephalopathy) is common among patients with severe systemic illness or primary CNS disorders. The physician should begin to assess mental status (including attention, memory, insight, and abstract reasoning) during his or her initial interactions with the patient, and decide if further formal testing is necessary.

The screening bedside mental status examination tests circumscribed cognitive abilities (Table 115.3). The results must be interpreted in the cultural and educational context of the patient. For example, simple arithmetic may challenge an uneducated patient, while difficulty with complex calculations may suggest cognitive deterioration in an accountant. Initial testing of *orientation and attention* consists of eliciting the patient's name and the month, year, city,

TABLE 115.1

HISTORICAL RISK FACTORS FOR SERIOUS BRAIN DISEASE IN PATIENTS WITH HEADACHE

Sudden-onset headache (1–2 seconds)
New headache, particularly in the elderly
Postural headache—supine or standing
Headache associated with fever, rash, stiff neck, or arthritis
New headache in immunosuppressed patients
Headache associated with focal neurologic symptoms or signs
Headache that awakens the patient from sleep

TABLE 115.3
BEDSIDE TESTS OF MENTAL STATUS

Function	Test
Orientation	Month, year, name
Attention/concentration	Spell "world" backwards, digit span forward
General knowledge	Historical figures, current events
Memory	Recall 3 objects at 5 min
	Number of animals named in 1 minute
Abstract reasoning	Similarities/differences comparing common objects
Calculation	Subtraction of serial sevens

Table 16.3 shows the more detailed Short Portable Mental Status Questionnaire.

and hospital. The daily routines of the hospital frequently cause patients to confuse day of the week and date. On the other hand, nearly all unimpaired patients can recall telephone numbers and can immediately and accurately repeat a sequence of seven digits forward (e.g., digits span) or spell the word *world* backwards. Attention is a crucial determinant of recent memory. If ability to pay attention is impaired, recent memory testing becomes inaccurate. Tests of *recent memory* (e.g., recall of three objects after five minutes) should incorporate commonly used objects to avoid cultural bias. *Calculation performance* depends upon the patient's educational achievement and ability. Qualitative assessment of *mood and general knowledge* occurs during the general medical history. The widely used Short Portable Mental Status Questionnaire (Table 16.3) is useful when screening for dementia. Detailed formal neuropsychological testing is particularly helpful in differentiating dementing conditions, including depression (pseudodementia), from true dementia.

Delirious patients are disoriented and exhibit poor attention. Although drowsiness or agitation may predominate; these features often fluctuate during the examination. Visual hallucinations, restlessness, or lability of mood are common. Examination findings common in delirium are fever, tachycardia, postural tremor, asterixis, or myoclonus. Delirium must be managed promptly to prevent the consequences of poor patient judgement. Reassurance in a supportive and closely supervised environment may be adequate. The use of sedatives or restraints should be preceded by discussion with the patient and family regarding their necessity for the patient's safety (e.g., to prevent falls or inadvertent self injury). The differential diagnosis of delirium is determined by individual circumstances (Table 115.4). Delirium in hospitalized patients is often multifactorial and treatable. Care should be taken to avoid assuming that a single cause is present. Medications commonly cause or contribute to delirium. A review of the patient's medication list (Table 115.5), with special attention to the

TABLE 115.4
COMMON CAUSES OF DELIRIUM

Cause	Test
Metabolic	
Hyponatremia, hypernatremia	Sodium
Renal failure	Blood urea nitrogen, creatinine
Hypoxia, ischemia	pO_2
Hypoglycemia, hyperglycemia	Glucose
Hypothyroidism, hyperthyroidism	Thyroid function tests
Recreational drugs	Toxicology screen
Alcohol intoxication/withdrawal	Alcohol level, osmolarity
Other drugs (Table 115.5)	Review medications
Hypercalcemia, hypermagnesia	Calcium, magnesium
Hypophosphatemia	Phosphate
Infectious	
Sepsis	Cultures, CBC, chest radiograph, UA
Meningitis	LP, cultures, CBC
Neurologic	
Subarachnoid hemorrhage	Brain CT, LP
Cerebral infarction	Brain CT or MRI
Seizures, postictal state	Consider brain CT/MRI, electroencephalogram

CBC, complete blood count; *CT*, computed tomography; *LP*, lumbar puncture; *MRI*, magnetic resonance imaging; pO_2, partial pressure of oxygen; *UA*, urinalysis.

risks of polypharmacy, new drugs, changes in drug dose, or recent discontinuation of drugs, is mandatory.

Hopitalization of an elderly patient with limited or unknown cognitive function at baseline is common, and delirium may initially obscure an underlying dementia. *Dementia* frequently complicates the medical history and examination in hospitalized elderly patients (Chapter 16). The most common type of dementia (Alzheimer's disease, or AD) is characterized by slowly progressive behavioral and cognitive deterioration, and often presents with diminished recent memory and relative preservation of alertness. Preserved social function may obscure the cognitive deficit initially. The initial clues may be limited to subtle behavioral or personality changes apparent only to friends and family. Asking family members about observed deterioration in

TABLE 115.5
MEDICATIONS THAT COMMONLY CAUSE DELIRIUM

Barbiturates	Opiate analgesics[a]
Anticholinergics	Benzodiazepines[a]
Clonidine	Cimetidine, ranitidine[a]
Digitalis	Antihistamines
Anti-parkinsonian drugs	Antipsychotics
Lithium	Tricyclic antidepressants
Glucocorticoids	

[a] Particularly common in hospitalized patients.

cognitive activities of daily living (managing finances, remembering appointments) is often useful, since the family may already have intervened to help the patient. The history from family, friends, or coworkers is extremely helpful, because these patients frequently deny that a problem exists. Tests of immediate attention (e.g., digit span) are preserved, but tests of recent memory (e.g., events of the past day) are impaired. A wide range of cognitive problems eventually appears. Insight and motivation diminish, and thought processes become less flexible. Eventually, there may be impairment of language (aphasia), recognition (agnosia), or execution of motor tasks (apraxia).

The investigation of dementia is directed at searching for potentially treatable conditions including vitamin B_{12} deficiency, hypothyroidism, normal pressure hydrocephalus, AIDS, chronic CNS infection (i.e., tertiary syphilis), or pseudodementia (depression). Differentiating AD from other neurodegenerative diseases has become more important now that FDA-approved therapies for AD have become available. Depression is a frequent and treatable accompaniment of illness and hospitalization, and can be difficult to distinguish from dementia without formal cognitive testing (Chapter 119). Outpatient evaluation after recovery from acute illness may be needed to make this distinction clear.

Pupillary Responses

The pupillary responses are critical neurologic signs to elicit in patients with coma or an acute CNS deficit. Light directed into either eye provides the stimulus for optic nerve afferent input to midbrain nuclei. Efferent parasympathetic nerve fibers travel in the third cranial nerve to produce bilateral pupillary constriction (miosis). Sympathetic pathways in the brainstem and cervical spinal cord eventually exit at the T1 nerve roots, pass rostrally over the ipsilateral carotid arteries, and along the fifth cranial nerves to mediate pupillary dilatation (mydriasis). A history revealing use of medications or other drugs that affect pupil size, previous eye surgery, or recent mydriatic eyedrop use (atropine results in an unreactive, dilated pupil without ptosis) can easily establish an explanation for many pupillary abnormalities. *Bilaterally dilated pupils* are seen with administration of anticholinergics (atropine) or sympathomimetics (recreational stimulants, hallucinogens), in thyrotoxicosis, and in severe anxiety states. *Bilaterally constricted pupils* occur with administration of opiates, alcohol, barbiturates, phenothiazines, and pilocarpine.

The pupils are normally round and equal in size. Both pupils normally constrict in symmetric fashion in response to light directed into one eye. The *direct response* is constriction of the ipsilateral pupil. The *consensual response* is pupillary constriction in the opposite eye. Minor fluctuations in ambient light result in small and rapid physiologic variations of pupillary diameter (hippus). The normal pupils of adults are 3–4 mm in diameter, and are

larger in chilren and smaller in older adults ("senile miosis"). The latter may not react briskly. Physiologic anisocoria denotes a normal degree of pupillary asymmetry (up to 1mm). Bedside examination of pupils includes inspection of pupil size, response to light (eyes looking ahead) and accommodation (eyes converging), and assessment of nearby midbrain and pontine neurologic functions (abnormalities of eye movement, corneal responses, facial sensation).

The single most important pupillary abnormality to recognize at hospital admission or during hospitalization is a new dilated (6–9 mm) pupil. This finding should always trigger consideration of early brain herniation resulting from a mass lesion (e.g., focal brain swelling, acute cerebral hemorrhage, brain abscess, brain tumor) compressing the parasympathetic pupillary fibers that mediate pupillary constriction in the third cranial nerve (Chapter 117). Subsequent dilatation of the other pupil implies further brain herniation. Immediate neuroimaging and neurosurgical consultation is necessary in the setting of a new dilated pupil. Of note, some noncompressive causes of third-nerve palsy spare the pupillary response; diabetes is the most common example. Midposition (3–4 mm), unreactive pupils may indicate further herniation involving both the midbrain and pons, and almost always carry a poor prognosis.

Dizziness and Vertigo

Dizziness is a nonspecific symptom of diverse etiology, variously described as unsteadiness, light-headedness, spinning, or blurring of vision. Vertigo is a perception of movement experienced as spinning of the surroundings or self; less commonly dysequilibrium is described as "rocking" in vertical or horizontal planes, as in a boat (Table 115.6). Vertigo is normal if there is an acute mismatch of input from visual, somatosensory, and vestibular systems that normally control balance (seasickness). Vertigo of PNS origin is sometimes associated with hearing loss or tinnitus, but is unassociated with other CNS

TABLE 115.6

SELECTED CAUSES OF VERTIGO

Peripheral nervous system	Central nervous system
Vestibular neuronitis	Vertebrobasilar ischemia
Benign positional vertigo	Temporal lobe disease (rare)
Meniere's syndrome	Brainstem/cerebellar glioma or AVM[a]
Cerebellopontine angle tumor	
Drug-induced	Demyelinating disease
Post-traumatic	Posterior fossa mass lesions
Systemic infection, hypotension	Hereditary spinocerebellar degeneration

[a] AVM, arterio-venous malformation

findings such as hemiparesis. Vertigo of CNS origin results in milder, less specific vertigo; "spinning" vertigo is less common. Other neurologic symptoms and signs suggestive of a CNS lesion are often present.

Peripheral nervous system pathology affects the vestibulocochlear apparatus or the vestibular division of the eighth cranial nerve. The *Hallpike maneuver* commonly is used to assess presumptive peripheral vertigo. The patient is positioned with the shoulders at the edge of the examination table, and the head is extended and rotated to one side. Gaze is directed toward the rotated side by having the patient focus upon the examiner's finger. An affected patient may exhibit nystagmus, report vertigo, or both. The maneuver is repeated to the opposite side after the head has been returned to neutral position and the nystagmus and vertigo have stopped. Vertigo of PNS origin exhibits fatigability (attenuation of vertigo while maintaining the triggering position) and habituation (less severe and shorter duration vertigo with repeated assumption of the triggering position). Peripheral vertigo may also exhibit a latency to onset, typically lasting a few seconds. These examination characteristics can be used to suggest a benign cause of vertigo that can be treated symptomatically. Nystagmus associated with vertigo is usually unidirectional, with the fast phase away from the involved side. Benign positional vertigo is strongly suggested by provoking nystagmus or vertigo during the Hallpike maneuver. Symptomatic treatment options for benign causes of acute or subacute vertigo of peripheral origin include bedrest, the Epley maneuver (three times per day until vertigo is gone for 24 hours [1]), or medications such as anticholinergics (scopolamine), antihistamines (meclizine), or benzodiazepines (diazepam).

Central nervous system causes of vertigo involve the vestibular nuclei or their connections in the brainstem, cerebellum, and cerebral hemispheres (less common). Individual bouts may occur spontaneously without movement as a trigger. Central vertigo often lacks habituation, fatigability, and latency to onset. Progressive unilateral hearing loss should alert the physician to a possible cerebellopontine angle tumor. Hearing loss is the most frequent presenting symptom, but vertigo is present in 20%. Vertebrobasilar artery ischemia can produce abrupt isolated vertigo, but other CNS symptoms and signs are usually present.

Dysphagia of Neurologic Etiology

Dysphagia can be caused by neurologic disease (Table 115.7) involving cranial nerves IX or X (resulting in dysfunction of the soft palate), cranial nerve XII (resulting in tongue wasting or weakness when protruded against the buccal mucosa), or bilateral upper brainstem or cerebral hemisphere disease (i.e., pseudobulbar palsy from multiple cerebral infarctions or multiple sclerosis). Dysphagia should trigger diagnostic consideration of upper motor neuron, cranial nerve, neuromuscular junction, or myopathic disorders. The history often allows the examiner to differentiate between mechanical and

TABLE 115.7

NEUROLOGIC CAUSES OF DYSPHAGIA

Oropharyngeal	Esophageal
Amyotrophic lateral sclerosis	Achalasia
Brainstem stroke or tumor	Vagus nerve injury–diabetes, post-vagotomy
Multiple sclerosis	Scleroderma
Myasthenia gravis	Dysautonomia
Tardive dyskinesia	Esophageal spasm
Myopathy	Amyloidosis
Syrinx	Myopathy
Spinocerebellar degeneration	
Arnold-Chiari malformation	
Parkinson's disease	
Tardive dyskinesia (drug-related)	

neuromuscular causes of dysphagia (Chapter 79). Dysphagia resulting from oropharyngeal disease causes difficulty immediately on attempted swallowing. Weakness of muscles that elevate the soft palate may result in nasal regurgitation of liquids and nasal speech. Neuromuscular esophageal disease results in discomfort that occurs later after swallowing and is located in the lower neck or upper chest. Neurologic examination can assess the oropharynx directly but is not helpful for esophageal disease.

Movement Disorders

Involuntary movements often reflect systemic illness, drug effects, or neurologic disease. The most common movement disorders are tremor, bradykinesia, dystonia, choreoathetosis, asterixis, and myoclonus. Accurate description of the abnormal movement suggests the differential diagnosis.

Tremor is a rhythmic involuntary movement of a body part that can be classified as postural (action) or rest. The most common tremor (postural tremor) is a high-frequency (8–10 beats per second), low-amplitude, rhythmic oscillation of the hands and fingers noted readily with the upper limbs outstretched against gravity. The tremor stops if the arms and hands are supported at rest. The differential diagnosis includes essential tremor, hyperthyroidism, sepsis, and sympathetic overactivity states (often due to sympathomimetic drugs). The hands are affected first, but later involvement of the head and neck is common. Symptomatic treatment with propranolol or mysoline may be necessary if the tremor is sufficiently embarrassing in social circumstances or impairs functional activities. Postural tremor of unknown cause (*essential tremor*) is hereditary in at least one-half of patients, worsens under stressful conditions, and is relieved with sedatives. In contrast, *rest tremor* occurs while the arms are supported at rest and becomes less prominent with arm movement. The tremor is low in frequency (2–4 beats per second), higher in amplitude, and rhythmic. The best example is the pill-rolling tremor of Parkinson's disease. *Intention tremor* is an action tremor that worsens during voluntary movement toward a target. This tremor often is detected by movement of the patient's finger alternately between the examiner's finger held at arm's length and the patient's nose (finger–nose testing). The tremor worsens as the patient's finger is moved closer toward the intended target, such that the target is missed (past-pointing) frequently. Intention tremor is specific for the cerebellum, or associated afferent or efferent pathways.

Dystonia refers to an abnormal, involuntary posture of a limb or body part due to abnormal tension in resting muscles that interferes with normal voluntary movement. Chronic antipsychotic medication use causes tardive dyskinesia, while recreational drugs tainted with phenothiazines may cause an acute dystonic reaction that remits with anticholinergic medications. *Chorea* refers to involuntary, rapid, irregular, dance-like movements that are usually focal and most prominent in the distal extremities. *Athetosis* consists of slower, snake-like involuntary movements of the proximal limbs or trunk. The simultaneous combination of these two movements (*choreoathetosis*) is common. The differential diagnosis of choreoathetosis includes both untreatable (e.g., basal ganglia cerebral infarction or hemorrhage) and treatable disorders (Table 115.8). Patient medications should always be reviewed as possible causes. Many hereditary neurodegenerative conditions also cause chorea (i.e., Huntington's disease).

TABLE 115.8
SOME TREATABLE CAUSES OF CHOREA

Acute rheumatic fever
Systemic lupus erythematosus
Anti-phospholipid antibody syndrome
Hyperthyroidism
Hypoparathyroidism
Polycythemia vera
Pregnancy (chorea gravidarum)
Wilson's disease
Porphyria
Toxins-alcohol, carbon monoxide, manganese, mercury, thallium
Metabolic
   Hypernatremia or hyponatremia
   Hypomagnesemia
   Hypocalcemia
   Hyperglycemia or hypoglycemia
Drugs
   Neuroleptics
   Anticonvulsants
   Calcium channel blockers
   Ranitidine, cimetidine
   Anabolic steroids
   Estrogens
   Tricyclics
   Anti-parkinsonian
Amphetamines, cocaine

Myoclonus and asterixis are often neurologic markers of systemic metabolic disease on an inpatient medical service. *Myoclonus* is a sudden, arrhythmic, asymmetric involuntary muscle contraction that produces focal or generalized jerking movements. Myoclonus can be a normal accompaniment of falling asleep. Multifocal myoclonus occurs commonly among hospitalized patients with hypoxic-ischemic encephalopathy. Other causes include electrolyte disturbances, liver failure, renal insufficiency, epilepsy, encephalitis, and neurodegenerative disease. Myoclonus that results from seizures needs to be distinguished from myoclonus resulting from other causes because treatment is different (Chapter 118). Electroencephalography (EEG) is helpful to determine if the myoclonic movements are cortical (seizures) or subcortical in origin (myoclonus). *Asterixis*, in contrast to myoclonus, consists of sudden loss of postural muscle tone rather than sudden involuntary muscle contraction. Myoclonus and asterixis can be distinguished at the bedside by instructing the patient to hold the arms outstretched with the wrists in extension, palms facing forward. The failure to maintain this wrist extension against gravity indicates either a sudden loss of forearm extensor muscle tone against gravity (asterixis) or active forearm flexor muscle contraction (myoclonus). Turning the arms over so that wrist extension is no longer against gravity eliminates asterixis, but not myoclonus. Asterixis can be caused by drug intoxication, renal failure, liver failure, or meningitis. Both asterixis and myoclonus usually resolve with correction of the underlying metabolic abnormality.

Weakness

A systematic approach is mandatory in evaluating the symptom and examination finding of weakness. Patients use the term *weakness* to describe almost any functional limitation of motor activity. The initial goal of clinical evaluation is to distinguish true neurologic from nonneurologic weakness. The distribution of weakness (e.g., hemiparesis, distal symmetric) and associated neurologic examination findings (pattern of sensory loss, muscle tone, reflexes) determines the neuroanatomic site of pathology and the differential diagnosis. The symptom of weakness can be nonneurologic and caused by generalized fatigue, impaired focal sensation, pain during attempted limb movement, or lack of effort secondary to systemic illness or depression. The physician must distinguish these forms of weakness as a symptom from weakness as a neurologic examination finding.

The examination finding of weakness can also be nonneurologic in origin. Nonneurologic weakness is observed as *breakaway weakness*, defined as variable muscle power detected by the examiner during testing of a specific muscle. When breakaway weakness is found, it is important to ask the patient if power testing of the muscle exhibiting the breakaway weakness is painful. *Painless* breakaway weakness results from poor effort and implies a behavioral component to the observed weakness. However, it is incorrect to conclude that a behavioral disorder alone is present; many of these patients also have an underlying neurologic disorder. Patients with *painful* breakaway weakness are more difficult to evaluate because the integrity of the muscle and supplying nerve cannot be assessed by examination of muscle power. Breakaway weakness with pain occasionally is accompanied by underlying true neurologic weakness. The findings for each involved muscle should be reported as "breakaway weakness associated with pain" or "breakaway weakness unassociated with pain" given that the causes of these two observations are different and may coexist in the same patient. Electromyography and nerve-conduction studies are helpful in this circumstance to distinguish true underlying neurologic weakness from breakaway weakness.

True neurologic weakness is loss of muscle power detected as a lack of expected strength for a given muscle. The weakness appears on examination as reduced and constant muscle power during maximal muscle contraction, and arises from lesions of the CNS or PNS. *CNS weakness* has a characteristic distribution. Distal muscles are more affected than proximal muscles. Extensor muscles are more affected than flexors in the arms and dorsiflexors are affected more than plantar flexors in the legs. Power testing of finger extensors or toe dorsiflexors are excellent screening tests of muscle power when searching for CNS weakness. In contrast to PNS disorders, CNS weakness does not conform to a pattern of muscles innervated by a single nerve or nerve root. Muscle tone may be spastic, flaccid, or normal in the setting of an acute CNS injury, but nearly always becomes spastic within a few days. Spasticity is a velocity-dependent increase in resistance to passive movement of a limb, and indicates CNS injury to upper motor neurons. Testing for spasticity is best accomplished with the patient supine and limbs relaxed. The arm or leg is moved through its range of motion at slow velocity first, then at rapid velocity. Mild spasticity may be detectable only during rapid movement of a limb. Other neurologic signs are sensitive for detecting mild CNS weakness. Fast, repetitive tapping of the index finger to the thumb ("fast finger movements") or foot tapping on the floor or against the examiner's hand are slowed (but of regular rhythm) compared with an unaffected hand or foot. With palms facing upward, fully outstretched arms often pronate with CNS weakness (pronator drift). CNS weakness is graded as mild, moderate, or severe, depending upon the degree of motor impairment.

PNS weakness results from disease of the motor unit. The motor unit is the entire motor nerve cell, axon, neuromuscular junction, and the muscle fibers the motor nerve cell supplies. Injury along the motor unit causes weakness. Determination of where the injury is located along the motor unit narrows the differential diagnosis. For example, if sensory loss is present, injury must be to the nerves, plexuses, or nerve roots because the anterior horn cells, muscle cells, and neuromuscular junctions do not contain sensory nerve

fibers. If the weakness is accompanied by sensory loss in a distal, symmetric fashion most severely affecting the feet, then a distal symmetric sensorimotor polyneuropathy (*length-dependent polyneuropathy*) is probably present. Proximal, symmetric weakness suggests a myopathy or neuromuscular junction disorder. Reflexes are typically normal in myopathies and diminished in the distribution of the weakness in neuropathies.

Sensory Examination

Appropriate elicitation and interpretation of sensory signs is difficult at best. Extensive patient cooperation is usually necessary, the tests are qualitative and prone to technical error, and results depend upon an accurate patient description of the deficits. These limitations are more problematic among hospitalized patients. Patients with sensory deficits from peripheral nerve disorders commonly are assessed semiquantitatively with nerve-conduction studies.

The ability to distinguish sensory symptoms from sensory examination abnormalities is crucial. Common sensory symptoms unaccompanied by neurologic findings are paresthesias or pain. *Paresthesia* refers to an abnormal subjective perception of sensation, but does not include a loss or diminution of sensation. A "pins and needles" sensation is the most common description used by patients. Paresthesias are an abnormal "positive sensory" symptom that arises in the CNS or PNS. They are generated by spontaneous activation of sensory receptors or nerve fibers, or an excessive nerve fiber response to normal cutaneous receptor stimulation. Metabolic disorders, CNS or PNS injury, or mechanical distortion of nerves (e.g., Tinel's sign seen in carpal tunnel syndrome) may trigger paresthesias. The significance of paresthesias depends upon the clinical context. The likelihood of an underlying neurologic cause increases dramatically if accompanied by neurologic examination abnormalities (i.e., weakness, focal reflex changes, sensory loss) in the same distribution. The absence of neurologic examination findings suggests a metabolic cause. The qualitative description by patients varies considerably because abnormal sensation does not reflect the normal orderly recruitment of sensory nerve cells that occurs with natural stimuli.

"Negative sensory" symptoms result from diminution or loss of sensory function. The severity and distribution of diminished sensation is more reliable in defining and localizing a neurologic deficit than positive sensory phenomena such as paresthesias or pain. Sensory modalities commonly tested are touch, position, vibration, pain, or temperature. Specific nerve, nerve root, or spinal cord syndromes associated with diminished sensation are best detected with the help of a practical examination guide or diagrams that include the distribution of nerve roots and peripheral nerves (Figure 115.1). Side-to-side comparison of analogous skin regions of the feet, hands, and face is a useful screen for touch, pain, and temperature; asymmetry of the findings is a sensitive and reliable indicator of an abnormality. If

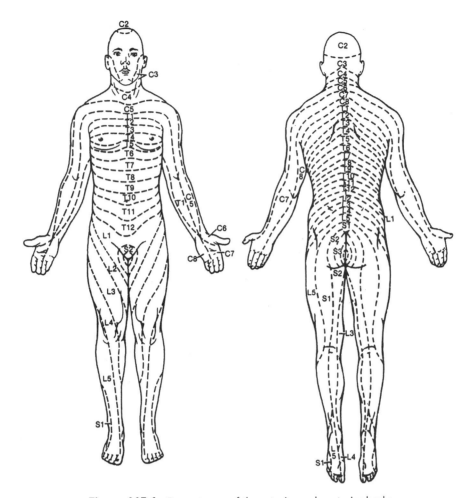

Figure 115.1 Dermatomes of the anterior and posterior body.

sensory examination findings do not conform easily to a CNS or PNS pattern of involvement, neurologic consultation is advisable.

The sensory loss associated with a typical progressive sensorimotor polyneuropathy spreads from the toes to the knees, then simultaneously from the knees into the lower thighs and the hands in a circumferential distribution. If sensory loss has spread to the waist or upper thighs without hand involvement, the examiner should consider the possibility of a spinal cord lesion. A *spinal cord sensory level* often can be detected with a cotton swab or pin used to test posterior paraspinal sensation from the upper neck to the sacrum on both sides. The sensory level is described as the dermatomal level below which sensation is reduced or lost. As a practical matter, finding a sensory level determines the initial anatomic target for neuroimaging (i.e., a T6 sensory level will trigger a thoracic spine MRI scan).

Urinary Incontinence

Urinary incontinence is usually the result of nonneurologic disease. A precise urologic history needs to be elicited and

is volunteered infrequently by patients. *Stress incontinence* is the leakage of small urine volumes associated with increased intraabdominal pressure, and usually occurs in multiparous or postmenopausal women with pelvic relaxation. A review of medication use, paying particular attention to recent changes, is necessary (Table 115.9). Important changes from baseline habit include frequency and quantity of voiding, difficulty initiating or maintaining micturition, dysuria, urinary urgency, urinary retention,

TABLE 115.9

URINARY INCONTINENCE AND DRUGS

Class/medication	Effect on urination
Diuretics, alcohol, caffeine	Polyuria
Tricyclic antidepressants	Retention, overflow
Opiates	Retention, overflow
Anticholinergics	Retention, overflow
Antipsychotics	Stress incontinence

and nocturia. Once an initial screen for common medical causes of urinary incontinence is complete, consideration of neurologic causes is appropriate. A change in frequency of nocturia over time is often an early symptom of mechanical obstruction of the urethra or neurologic disease. Inability to sense the passing of urine or stool, or decreased perianal sensation (e.g., ability to feel toilet paper) suggest a neurologic cause of urinary incontinence.

Measurement of residual urine volume after a voluntary attempt to empty the bladder (postvoid residual) is a simple bedside test of bladder function that can help distinguish bladder dysfunction from the CNS or PNS. A high volume bladder is classically due to PNS injury of parsympathetic nerves to the bladder from bilateral S2–S4 spinal segments, either outside the spine (i.e., diabetes) or inside the spine but distal to the spinal cord (i.e., cauda equina syndrome). This PNS injury also results in reduced detrusor (bladder) muscle contractility and reduced urine flow. Chronic bladder dysfunction following CNS injury results in simultaneous contraction of the urinary sphincter and bladder detrusor muscles (*detrusor-sphincter dyssynergia*). The hyperrerflexive nature of this spastic bladder results in sudden, unpredictable urges to urinate; the patient reports frequency, urgency, and sudden urinary incontinence in the setting of low postvoid residual urine volumes. Acute CNS injury (i.e., spinal cord compression from tumor or trauma) can result temporarily in a high postvoid residual urine volume; the bladder muscle may be flaccid temporarily before spasticity develops.

Bilateral spinal cord, brainstem, or brain involvement is necessary to produce urinary incontinence of CNS origin. Other neurologic examination signs of CNS involvement are almost always present. Postvoid residual is small until late in the disease. A low threshold for neurologic or urologic consultation is advisable if the cause is unclear. PNS causes of urinary incontinence (e.g., diabetic neuropathy or cauda equina syndrome) often result in diminished perianal or perineal sensation. Ankle reflexes may be absent. Reflex contraction of anal sphincter muscles can be assessed by stimulating the external anus on each side with a pin. Unilateral or bilateral absence of reflex sphincter contraction suggests a PNS lesion or a suboptimal stimulus.

DIAGNOSTIC TESTS

Cerebrospinal Fluid (CSF) Examination

CSF analysis provides data regarding changes in chemical composition of the fluid that bathes the brain, spinal cord, and nerve roots. Indications for spinal fluid evaluation include possible infectious or neoplastic meningitis, encephalitis, subarachnoid hemorrhage, papilledema, encephalopathy of unknown cause, CNS vasculitis, CNS or PNS demyelinating diseases, or postural headache. CSF analysis may lead to a specific diagnosis. Routinely exam-

ined parameters include glucose, protein, red cell count, white cell count, and differential. CSF should be analyzed immediately, or refrigerated if a delay in analysis is likely, because 40% of white cells are lysed after two hours. Typical CSF formulas seen in meningitis syndromes are discussed in Chapter 70.

Opening pressure (OP) is recorded with a manometer after the subarachnoid space has been entered and the patient's legs extended (to minimize any contribution to OP by increased intra-abdominal pressure). Elevated OP in the absence of head CT or MRI abnormalities is seen in many different diseases (Table 115.10). A low OP may indicate a spinal subarachnoid block or CSF leak. The CSF is spun in a centrifuge, then inspected for pigments. Normal CSF is clear. *Xanthochromia* is a yellow color that reflects the presence of bilirubin. Xanthochromia is detected 2–12 hours after subarachnoid hemorrhage, is at its maximum after 2 days, and persists for 2–4 weeks. It is essential to differentiate between pigmented CSF from a traumatic lumbar puncture (LP) and pathologic subarachnoid hemorrhage. Serial assessment of CSF during the LP, comparing the red cell count in an early tube with that found in a later tube, reveals visible clearing of the fluid and a significant drop in red cell count by microscopic examination in the setting of an LP-induced traumatic hemorrhage. The spun CSF supernatant is normally clear unless enough serum has entered the subarachnoid space that there are more than 100,000 red blood cells per cubic milimeter, the CSF protein level is greater than 150 mg/dL, or the CSF was examined more than two days after the first LP. In the latter circumstance, it can be difficult to differentiate pathologic from an LP-induced subarachnoid hemorrhage. Corrected white cell and protein values can be extrapolated from CSF contaminated by traumatic bleeding. For every 1,000 red cells present, subtract one

TABLE 115.10

CAUSES OF INCREASED CEREBROSPINAL FLUID PRESSURE DESPITE NORMAL OR NONDIAGNOSTIC BRAIN IMAGING

Elevated central venous pressure
Meningitis and encephalitis
Respiratory failure
Postanoxic encephalopathy
Fulminant hepatic encephalopathy
Reye's syndrome
Lead encephalopathy
Water intoxication/hyponatremia
Dural venous sinus occlusion
Pseudotumor cerebri
Spinal cord tumors
Acute polyneuritis (Guillain–Barré syndrome)

white cell and 1 mg/dL of CSF protein. Other CSF studies are helpful in specific clinical situations. Cytology can establish the diagnosis of neoplastic meningitis, and should be performed rapidly after collection of fluid to avoid cytolysis. Analysis of large CSF volumes (>20 mL) increases the probability of tumor cell identification. Comparison of immunoglobulin production within the CSF and in the serum (IgG index) is a marker for an active immune response within the CNS compartment. Polymerase chain reaction studies are used to detect viral pathogens in CSF (e.g., *Herpes simplex*).

Contraindications to LP are uncommon. The most feared complication, brain herniation, occurs if brain volume is increased and CSF pathways are obstructed. With hospital-based CT or brain MRI, direct visualization of the brain in the setting of papilledema or focal CNS deficits has simplified decisions about performing a spinal fluid examination. Free communication along CSF pathways, even in the presence of a mass lesion, implies that the risk of brain herniation is low. Neuroimaging findings suggesting a focal intracranial pressure differential (i.e., trapped ventricle, midline shift, or early cerebellar or uncal herniation) contraindicate LP. Severe thrombocytopenia (platelet count <20,000/μL), anticoagulation, or a bleeding diathesis increase the risk of spinal subarachnoid hemorrhage or spinal epidural hematoma, and are relative contraindications to LP. Use of a 22-gauge needle lowers the risk. Discontinuing heparin in advance of the procedure, or administering vitamin K or fresh frozen plasma to reverse the effects of coumadin, can be considered in selected circumstances. Introduction of infection at the puncture site rarely occurs and is caused by passage of the needle through infected soft tissue or use of an unsterile needle. If infected soft tissue is present along the anticipated needle track, consideration should be given to a C1-2 (cisternal) puncture under fluoroscopic guidance.

Other potential complications of LP include low back pain and nerve-root irritation during the procedure that results in temporary radicular pain extending from the back to the ipsilateral buttock or leg. Post-LP headache begins with standing and resolves in the supine position; it occurs after about one LP in ten. The headache begins between 15 minutes and 4 days following the procedure and lasts an average of 4–8 days. Bedrest is the treatment of choice and common analgesics are not helpful. In those few patients who develop intractable post-LP headache, installation of the patient's venous blood into the epidural space ("blood patch") by an anesthesiologist is effective treatment.

Neuroimaging

CT and MRI have simplified the diagnosis and management of many CNS disorders. These diagnostic techniques allow noninvasive localization of anatomic abnormalities in the brain, head and neck, spine, and the spinal cord. The contour, distribution, size, and contrast-enhancement characteristics of lesions often support a specific diagnosis or a limited list of diagnostic possibilities. The choice between head CT and MRI depends upon the diagnostic question and the immediate availability of the imaging modality. If acute brain hemorrhage is the primary diagnostic consideration, then head CT without contrast is the best study. New blood is seen as a high-density lesion on the scan. The only other causes of a high-density lesion are calcium, metal, and contrast. Patient movement during CT or MRI studies degrades the images and limits diagnostic information. Patients are less likely to move during a CT scan than an MRI because image acquisition is faster and patients are unlikely to develop claustrophobia.

CT–myelography is preferred in the setting of spine disorders characterized by bony abnormalities (e.g., spinal stenosis and cervical spondylosis). Potential complications of CT include exposure of patients to low levels of radiation and contrast reactions. MRI is superior to CT in demonstrating exquisite soft-tissue anatomic detail (without radiation exposure), and results in detection of brain and spinal cord lesions missed by CT scan. These disorders include brain infection, neoplasm, cerebral infarction, neurodegenerative diseases, demyelinating diseases (i.e., multiple sclerosis), and extracranial soft tissue pathology of the head and neck. The contrast agent used for MRI (gadolinium) is not associated with renal failure, and allergic reactions are rare. Two percent of patients undergoing a brain MRI experience claustrophobia that interferes with the test. In these patients, sedation, given 30–60 minutes prior to the study, often permits an acceptable study. MRI generates a strong magnetic field that can result in injury if there are magnetic objects in the body. The induced magnetic field may inactivate cardiac pacemakers or automatic internal defibrillators.

Electroencephalography

EEG is a noninvasive, painless study that can be performed at the bedside to investigate possible seizures, focal abnormalities of brain function, and other neurologic disorders. Electrodes are pasted to the scalp and connected to amplifiers in a grid pattern that allows for the recording and display of regional brain electrical activity. The recorded waveforms have characteristic frequencies that depend on age, alertness, brain region, systemic illness, medications, focal brain disease, and technical maneuvers during the test (e.g., hyperventilation, flicker stimulation). While EEG can complement the anatomic information obtained by neuroimaging, the neurologic examination is often an adequate test of nervous system function and can be correlated with neuroimaging results. However, in severely ill patients unable to cooperate with the neurologic examination, analysis of CNS function can be assessed by the EEG. For example, persistent unconsciousness without explanation may be caused by non-convulsive status epilepticus or a diffuse brain insult that has an EEG correlate.

Status epilepticus (Chapter 118) manifests as seizures on the EEG, whereas encephalopathy appears as diffuse slowing of EEG background rhythms. Involuntary movements can be difficult to distinguish from seizures based upon visual appearance alone, but can be clarified by an EEG study performed while the movements are ongoing. Portable EEG assessment of brain function is possible for patients who cannot be transported to a scanner because of critical illness or other logistic issues. The EEG can be helpful to suggest focal brain dysfunction when neuroimaging is normal (anatomic–functional dissociation). This circumstance may occur early in the evolution of brain pathology (e.g., herpes simplex encephalitis) and can influence the threshhold for initiation of drug therapy. Depression or feigned altered consciousness manifests as a normal EEG in patients without neurologic or systemic illness. A short synopsis of the diagnostic question and a complete list of medications should be provided to the EEG laboratory when ordering the test.

Electromyography and Nerve-Conduction Studies

Electromyography and nerve-conduction studies are a sensitive extension of the neurologic examination and are useful for evaluating the functional integrity of the peripheral nervous system (PNS). These studies can offer advantages over the clinical neurologic examination by providing quantitative information, particularly if patient cooperation or effort is limited. Although they can be performed at the bedside, the electrical environment of the ICU may result in recording artifacts.

Nerve-conduction studies are semiquantitative tests of nerve function. They are performed by placing stimulating electrodes on skin overlying limb nerves and recording over nerves (sensory nerve action potentials, or SNAPs) or muscles (compound motor action potentials, or CMAPs). Slowed nerve conduction velocities or prolonged distal motor latencies are indicative of nerve demyelination. Reduced amplitude of SNAPs or CMAPs correlates best with loss of axons in the nerve.

Needle electromyography is a qualitative test of nerve and muscle function performed by insertion of a recording needle electrode into selected muscles. There is no stimulating current. Abnormal spontaneous activity at rest correlates with acute denervation (axonal injury) or muscle-membrane instability in muscle disease (polymyositis). The morphologic configuration (duration, amplitude) of individual motor units (single motor nerve cells and the muscle fibers it supplies) seen on a display screen during minimal muscle contraction can be attributed to muscle or nerve disease. The firing pattern of nerve cells during muscle contraction also may suggest muscle or nerve injury.

KEY POINTS

- The neurologic history is crucial to establish a clinical context that determines which neurologic findings on examination are likely to be pertinent.
- Historical risk factors for headache of serious cause are sudden onset, new onset in elderly or immunosuppressed patients, headache that awakens the patient, postural headache, association with focal neurologic symptoms or signs, or association with fever, rash, stiff neck, or arthritis.
- Delirium is an acute or subacute alteration of mental state characterized by fluctuating alertness and confusion; dementia is a chronic, progressive cognitive deterioration with impaired recent memory, preservation of alertness, and relative preservation of social function.
- Unilateral, new-onset pupil dilation should trigger consideration of early brain herniation resulting from a mass lesion compressing the third cranial nerve.
- Nonneurologic weakness usually is observed as variable muscle power during testing of a specific muscle (recorded as breakaway weakness with or without pain); true neurologic weakness is observed as reduced and constant resistance provided by the patient when testing muscle power during maximal muscle contraction.
- "Positive" sensory symptoms (paresthesias, pain) unaccompanied by abnormal neurologic examination signs suggest a nonneurologic cause; "negative" sensory examination signs (i.e., diminished light touch or pin sensation) suggest a CNS or PNS structural lesion.
- Disorders for which spinal fluid examination results can assist diagnosis include possible meningitis, encephalitis, subarachnoid hemorrhage, papilledema of unknown cause, CNS vasculitis, encephalopathy of unknown cause, CNS or PNS demyelination, or postural headache.
- Neuroimaging (MRI or CT) and EEG are complementary tests: MRI or CT help define the anatomy and differential diagnosis of CNS lesions (tumor vs. stroke), while EEG helps determine functional localization of brain lesions or the presence of seizures.
- Electromyography and nerve conduction studies are sensitive, semiquantitative tests of nerve and muscle function that detect, localize, and quantify PNS injury and complement the observations obtained by the neurologic history and examination.

REFERENCE

1. Radtke A, von Brevern M, Tiel-Wilck K, et al. Self-treatment of benign paroxysmal positional vertigo: Semont maneuver vs. Epley procedure. *Neurology* 2004;63:150–152.

ADDITIONAL READING

Bradley WG, Daroff RB, Fenichel GM, Jankovic J. *Neurology in Clinical Practice.* Philadelphia: Butterworth Heinemann, 2004.
Brain. *Aids to the Examination of the Peripheral Nervous System,* 4th ed. Philadelphia: WB Saunders, 2000.

Brazis PW, Masdeu JC, Biller J. *Localization in Clinical Neurology,* 4th ed. Philadelphia: Lippincott Williams and Wilkins, 2001.

Brown WF, Bolton CF, Aminoff MJ, et al. *Neuromuscular Function and Disease.* Philadelphia: WB Saunders, 2002.

DeMyer WE. *Technique of the Neurologic Examination,* 5th ed. New York: McGraw-Hill, 2004.

Glaser JS. *Neuro-ophthalmology,* 3rd ed. Philadelphia: Lippincott Williams and Wilkins, 1999.

Jankovic JJ, Tolosa E. *Parkinson's Disease and Movement Disorders,* 4th ed. Philadelphia: Lippincott Williams and Wilkins, 2002.

Lin VW, Cardenas DD, Cutter NC, et al. *Spinal Cord Medicine.* New York: Demos, 2003.

Silberstein SD, Lipton RB, Goadsby PJ. *Headache in Clinical Practice,* 2nd ed. London: Taylor and Francis Group, 2002.

Stewart JD. *Focal Peripheral Neuropathies,* 3rd ed. Philadelphia: Lippincott Williams and Wilkins, 2000.

Victor M, Ropper AH. *Principles of Neurology,* 7th ed. New York: McGraw-Hill, 2001.

Wijdicks EFM. *The Clinical Practice of Critical Care Neurology,* 2nd ed. New York: Oxford University Press, 2003.

Stroke

116

Wade S. Smith

INTRODUCTION

Stroke, the third leading cause of death in the United States, is now considered a treatable disease. The testing and approval of tissue plasminogen activator (t-PA) for victims of acute ischemic stroke is largely responsible for this new optimism. Approval of t-PA for this use in 1996, in conjunction with aggressive hospital-based acute "stroke unit" management, has led to reduced mortality and decreased morbidity rates among stroke victims. In 2004, some hospitals began to be credentialed as primary stroke centers. These centers have the key personnel necessary to safely give t-PA, and to systematically apply the best practices for stroke victims. It is likely that these stroke centers will function much like trauma centers, with stroke patients specifically triaged to them in the prehospital setting in some communities. This chapter reviews the initial presentation, evaluation, and management of acute ischemic stroke, and is directed at the hospital physician evaluating an acute stroke patient without the benefit of a stroke center.

Despite the approximately 550,000 cases of stroke per year in the United States, few controlled prospective data exist to help guide initial management and post-stroke prophylaxis. Only in the past decade have well-designed therapeutic trials become available. Further, institutional bias and provider heterogeneity add to the complexity of individual case management. For example, neurologists, vascular surgeons, and internists vary markedly in use of anticoagulation for carotid stenosis. Many centers routinely admit all patients with transient ischemic attacks (TIAs) or minor stroke; others cite the absence of proof for the benefits of hospital management as proof of absence of benefit. Lacking are precise data on the natural history of recurrent stroke; such data are necessary to make cost–benefit decisions regarding hospitalization, timing of surgery, and use of anticoagulation.

BACKGROUND AND DEFINITIONS

Stroke is a clinical diagnosis; it is not diagnosed by radiologic study. It can be defined as the sudden onset of neurologic dysfunction produced by a presumptive vascular cause. A transient ischemic attack (*TIA*) is a clinical stroke that clears within 24 hours, although TIAs typically last only 10–14 minutes. Stroke is sudden or stepped in onset, and is manifested by focal neurologic findings. Approximately 85% of all hospitalized stroke victims have hemiparesis. The presence of language dysfunction or neglect coupled with facial or arm weakness is highly specific for stroke. The presence of bilateral weakness degrades this specificity. On the other hand, patients with metabolic encephalopathies can have focal neurologic findings. Therefore, the sudden onset (or new discovery) of focal neurologic findings suggests stroke, but appropriate laboratory tests are necessary to exclude potential masqueraders.

The role of early brain imaging is to define the stroke subtype. Acute stroke can be classified as *hemorrhagic* or *ischemic* by performing initial noncontrast computed tomography (CT) scan of the head (Table 116.1), based on the presence or absence, respectively, of blood seen on CT.

Hemorrhagic stroke can be defined as the sudden onset of a neurologic deficit associated with brain CT consistent with acute intracranial hemorrhage. Hemorrhage stroke can be subtyped by the anatomic space in which blood is observed: epidural, subdural, subarachnoid, or intraparenchymal. *Epidural* hematomas are typically produced by trauma, resulting in severing of the middle meningeal artery. Accumulation of blood is rapid, demanding immediate neurosurgical intervention. *Subdural* hemorrhages accumulate from a low-pressure venous source and typically are produced by tearing of bridging cortical veins.

TABLE 116.1

STROKE CLASSIFICATION, AND RELATIVE DEGREE OF URGENCY FOR EVALUATION

Stroke subtype	Frequency %	Computed tomography findings (typical)	Urgency[a]
Hemorrhage	15	Hyperdense material representing clotted blood	Moderate–High
Subarachnoid	1–2	Blood in subarachnoid space	High
Intraparenchymal	10	Blood in brain parenchyma	Moderate–High
Subdural	<1	Blood in subdural space	Low–High
Epidural	<1	Blood in epidural space	High
Ischemic stroke	85	Usually normal <6 h. Hypodensity representing edema later	Low-High[b]
Lacunar stroke	21	Hypodensity usually <1 cm^3	High[b]
Cardioembolic	17	Wedge-shaped cortical/subcortical hypodensity	High[b]
Artery–artery embolism	13	Wedge-shaped cortical/subcortical hypodensity	High[b]
Cryptogenic stroke	25	Cortical/subcortical hypodensity	High[b]
Other	8	Varies	High[b]

[a] Urgency is high with depressed level of consciousness, airway instability, or hemodynamic instability.
[b] High urgency if under 3 h, because patient may be eligible to receive intravenous thrombolytics.

Both severe and subtle head trauma can produce this bleeding, and patients with brain atrophy are predisposed to it. The most frequent cause of *subarachnoid* hemorrhage is closed head injury. Aneurysmal rupture into the subarachnoid space is also common. Spontaneous, nontraumatic aneurysmal subarachnoid hemorrhage is life threatening, with nearly a 50% mortality rate within the first 24 hours. Immediate neurosurgical or endovascular intervention and control of intracranial pressure are priorities that affect survival and neurologic outcome. Intraparenchymal hemorrhages are produced by both large and small vessel rupture. Chronic hypertension is the major predisposing risk factor for the genesis of most of these hemorrhages. It is unclear if an acute increase in blood pressure is responsible for the actual hemorrhage. The diagnosis and management of the hemorrhagic stroke syndromes and increased intracranial pressure are described in Chapter 117.

Ischemic stroke is produced by blockage of a cerebral vessel with resulting ischemia and later infarction within the part of the brain region irrigated by the vessel. The extent and location of infarction depends on many factors, including the presence of collateral circulation, patient age, brain temperature, serum glucose, magnitude of blood flow reduction, and the duration of ischemia. A physician may intervene to reduce duration and magnitude of ischemia (thrombolysis), reduce temperature (antipyretics or cooling), lower serum glucose to the normal range, and, perhaps, increase collateral circulation (by allowing acute hypertension). Brain tissue is the tissue most vulnerable to ischemia in the body. Death of neurons begins after approximately 4 minutes of zero blood flow. However, a core of tissue around the infarcted tissue does not infarct as

quickly. This region is referred to as the *ischemic penumbra*, which receives blood flow adequate to maintain temporary (i.e., hours) neuronal survival, but inadequate to allow normal neuronal activity. The penumbral region may infarct without intervention, so the goal of most acute stroke therapy is directed at saving this volume of brain. Perfusion to the penumbra is dependent on collateral circulation and strongly dependent on blood pressure, so *reduction in blood pressure may enlarge the infarct.* Conversely, permissive or induced hypertension may reduce infarct size. Because infarct size is critically dependent on temperature, fever should be treated aggressively with antipyretics, body exposure, and active cooling. Mild hypothermia may be beneficial but is considered investigational at this time. Thrombolytic therapy may be possible if the duration of ischemia is less than 3 hours; this is discussed subsequently in this chapter.

One-quarter of ischemic strokes results from *lacunar infarction.* This is produced by small vessel closure within the internal capsule, thalamus, pons, and cerebellum. There are many lacunar syndromes; the four most common are listed in Table 116.2. In general, lacunar strokes have a better prognosis, with a lower case-fatality rate than large vessel strokes. Hypertension and diabetes are the most commonly associated risk factors. Because lacunar strokes are caused most often by local arteriolar disease, one does not generally need to search for embolic sources.

Large vessel strokes carry a higher fatality rate and cause more significant injury. Each of the major named cerebral arteries can produce a large vessel syndrome, as listed in Table 116.2. The mechanism of large vessel occlusion is most commonly embolic closure of the vessel. The presence of such an infarct should lead the clinician

TABLE 116.2
ISCHEMIC STROKE SUBTYPES

Subtype	Clinical stroke	Mechanism
Lacunar	"Lacunar syndromes"	Lipohyalinosis/thrombosis
Lenticulostriate	Pure motor stroke	
Thalamoperforators	Pure sensory stroke	
Brainstem penetrators	Ataxia, dysarthria, hemiparesis	
Cerebellar	Ataxia	
Large-vessel	"Large-vessel syndromes"	Typically embolic
Middle cerebral artery	Dominant: aphasia, gaze deviation, hemiparesis, hemisensory and visual field deficit	
	Nondominant: neglect, gaze deviation, hemiparesis, hemisensory and visual field deficit	
Posterior cerebral artery	Visual field deficit, amnesia	
Anterior cerebral artery	Leg weakness, frontal lobe syndrome	
Basilar artery	Cranial nerve deficits, quadriparesis, depressed level of consciousness	

TABLE 116.3
POTENTIAL CAUSES OF STROKE

Common	Uncommon
Intracranial hemorrhage	Hypercoagulable disorders
Arteriovenous malformation	Protein C deficiency
Subarachnoid	Protein S deficiency
Lobar	Antithrombin III deficiency
Hypertensive	Anti-phospholipid
Amyloid angiopathy	syndrome
Cocaine–related	Systemic malignancy
	Homocysteinemia
Thrombosis	Sickle cell anemia
Lacunar (small vessel)	β-Thalassemia
Large-vessel thrombosis	Polycythemia vera
	Systemic lupus
Embolic occlusion	erythematosus
Artery–artery	
Carotid bifurcation	Venous sinus thrombosis
Aortic arch	
Arterial dissection	Fibromuscular dysplasia
Cardioembolic	
Atrial fibrillation	Vasculitis
Mural thrombus	Systemic (polyarteritis
Segmental hypokinesis	nodosa)
Dilated cardiomyopathy	Primary central nervous
Valvular lesions	system
Mitral stenosis	
Mechanical valve	Cardiogenic
Bacterial endocarditis	Mitral-valve calcification
Paradoxical embolus	Atrial myoxoma
(patent foramen ovale/	Intracardiac tumor
atrial septal defect)	Marantic endocarditis
Atrial septal aneurysm	Libman–Sacks endocarditis
Spontaneous echo-	
cardiographic contrast	Migraine

to search for an embolic source, such as the carotid artery, heart, or aortic arch. A list of common and uncommon causes of stroke is contained in Table 116.3. The search for a potential cause should be based on the clinical stroke classification and the type of stroke classified by a brain imaging study.

ISSUES AT THE TIME OF ADMISSION

Evaluation and Differential Diagnosis

Figure 116.1 summarizes the major steps followed during the initial phase of care. One first must decide if the acute onset of a focal or global neurologic deficit has been caused by stroke or TIA. Table 116.4 lists the differential diagnosis. Establishing an accurate diagnosis depends heavily on obtaining an accurate history. If the patient was not observed at the onset of his or her deficit, one falsely may attribute a generalized seizure with postictal hemiparesis (*Todd's paresis*) to stroke. Similarly, a patient with an intracranial tumor producing hemiparesis and dementia may provide an inaccurate history of sudden onset of weakness. A clear history of sudden onset rules out the stroke masqueraders.

Initial Studies and Management

The initial management of stroke and TIA is summarized in Table 116.5. Any patient suspected to have had a stroke should be evaluated for airway, breathing, and circulatory stability, followed by an assessment of serum glucose level. Laboratory assessment also should include complete

New Onset of Neurological Deficit

↓

Stroke or TIA? (Table 116.4)

↓

Initial assessment and management (Table 116.5)

↓

Consultation?

↓

Hospitalize? (Table 116.6)

↓

Level of care? (Table 116.7)

↓

• Physical and occupational therapy assessment
• Speech and swallowing evaluation
• Establish nutrition
• Social work evaluation

↓

Discharge planning
• Home
• Inpatient rehabilitation
• Skilled nursing facility

Figure 116.1 Key points in the management of acute stroke. *TIA*, transient ischemic attack.

blood count (CBC), platelet counts, coagulation studies, and electrolyte levels. An erythrocyte sedimentation rate is a useful screen for unexpected illness, including malignancy, arteritis, and endocarditis.

One then must determine if the stroke is hemorrhagic or ischemic using emergent noncontrast head CT (many centers now also perform CT angiography of the head and neck

TABLE 116.4

DIFFERENTIAL DIAGNOSIS OF NEW-ONSET FOCAL NEUROLOGIC FINDINGS

Stroke/Transient ischemic attack
Seizure with postictal (Todd's) paresis
Tumor
Migraine
Metabolic encephalopathy
    Fever and old stroke
    Hyperglycemia
    Hypercalcemia
    Hepatic encephalopathy

TABLE 116.5

EARLY STROKE MANAGEMENT

Initial assessment: ABCs, serum glucose
Clinical diagnosis of stroke (Table 116.4)
Noncontrast head computed tomography
    Hemorrhage
        Medical and surgical management of hemorrhagic stroke (Chapter 117)
    Tumor or other CNS process
        Treat accordingly
    Normal or hypodense area consistent with acute ischemic stroke
        Consider thrombolysis, aspirin (Figure 116.2)
        Medical management post-stroke
        Further investigation of cause
        Prescription of post-stroke prophylaxis

CNS, central nervous system.

during this time). CT is adequate to eliminate tumor and hemorrhagic stroke; it is normal in early ischemic stroke, migraine, and metabolic encephalopathies. The choice of consultants depends on the CT findings. If the CT reveals hemorrhage, neurosurgical or neurologic consultation should be sought to help with management (Chapter 117). If the CT scan does not reveal hemorrhage, or if the diagnosis or cause are unclear, emergent neurologic evaluation should be sought, because the patient may be eligible for intravenous thrombolytic therapy. The presence of hydrocephalus should prompt consultation with a neurosurgeon for placement of ventriculostomy if necessary.

Admission Decision and Level of Care

The decision to hospitalize a patient with acute stroke or TIA is controversial, and there is wide variability in practice. Table 116.6 lists certain clinical features that should

TABLE 116.6

REASONS TO HOSPITALIZE PATIENTS WITH STROKE

Accepted
    Hemodynamic or airway compromise
    Depressed level of consciousness
    Aspiration
    Inability to walk
    Intracranial hemorrhage
    Atrial fibrillation
    Myocardial ischemia
    Crescendo TIA
    Stroke in progression
    Other acute medical issues

Controversial
    TIA
    Minor stroke

TIA, transient ischemic attack.

be considered in making this decision. Many physicians admit patients with minor stroke and TIA to expedite the evaluation. Patients who are disabled from the event or are medically unstable should be admitted, with the level of care dictated by the clinical status (Table 116.7). Because stroke is a dynamic process, close observation of the acute stroke victim during the first few days is necessary to alert the physician to any neurologic decline that may prompt a change in therapy. Stroke centers typically maintain a "constant observation facility" or "step-down" unit with one nurse for every two or three patients to allow for frequent neurologic checks.

Specific Therapy for Stroke Subtypes

Hemorrhagic Stroke

The management of hemorrhagic stroke is described in Chapter 117.

Ischemic Stroke

Several treatments may be offered to people with ischemic stroke, including intravenous thrombolysis, aspirin, heparin, and blood pressure augmentation to enhance collateral perfusion. Neuroprotective agents are being investigated in human trials, but none are currently approved for clinical use. Similarly, the intra-arterial delivery of thrombolytic agents is a promising treatment, but there is no FDA approved drug for this indication, and only comprehensive stroke centers are offering this therapy. Referral of patients to such centers in a timely fashion is a growing trend, but this is highly specific to individual hospitals and the type of emergency transportation available.

The approval of intravenous thrombolytic agents for the treatment of acute ischemic stroke was driven by the results of a well-designed, prospective placebo-controlled trial of intravenous t-PA given within 3 hours of the onset of acute stroke symptoms (1). Patients were required to have a head CT that was free of hemorrhage, normal baseline laboratory evaluation (Table 116.8), an examination consistent with acute stroke, and the ability to receive drugs within 90 or 180 minutes. Primary outcome measures were neurologic function and disability scales that quantified residual stroke injury. All primary outcome measures reached significance and favored t-PA treatment. In the treatment group, there were 50% more patients who were neurologically normal or near-normal at three months. The mortality rate was unaffected. Three percent of patients died from treatment-associated intracranial hemorrhage. An earlier study found only slight benefit from t-PA if it was given within 6 hours of symptom onset, and there was a higher intracranial hemorrhage rate. *Streptokinase is contraindicated in the treatment of ischemic stroke* because of three intravenous trials showing increased morbidity and mortality rates in ischemic stroke patients who received this agent.

At this time, the use of thrombolytics is limited to intravenous t-PA *given within the first 3 hours after stroke* by the protocol listed in Figure 116.2 (2). Many hospitals have formed stroke teams headed by neurologists to administer t-PA. If a stroke team does not exist, it is helpful to obtain consultation with a neurologist who is familiar with this form of treatment or to offer immediate transfer to a stroke center. A radiologist or neurologist who has experience in interpreting the noncontrast head CT is essential, because the presence of cerebral swelling, a subtle sign on CT, predicts hemorrhagic transformation. *It is essential that no intracranial hemorrhage be present prior to administering t-PA.*

TABLE 116.7

KEY ELEMENTS TO CONSIDER IN DECIDING LEVEL OF CARE

Condition	ICU	Step-down unit		Medical ward
Need for mechanical ventilation	✓			
Airway compromise requiring tracheal intubation	✓			
Coma	✓			
Need for pressors or continuous intravenous antihypertensive therapy	✓			
Need for pulmonary artery pressure monitoring	✓			
Need for central venous pressure monitoring	✓	or	✓	
Concomitant myocardial infarction	✓			
Rule out myocardial infarction	✓	or	✓	
Need for telemetry	✓	or	✓	
Need for femoral sheath	✓	or	✓	
Need for intravenous or intra-arterial thrombolysis	✓	or	✓	
Depressed consciousness	✓	or	✓	
Hemodynamic stability[a]	✓	or	✓	or	✓
Patient able to protect airway[a]	✓	or	✓	or	✓
Intravenous heparin[a]	✓	or	✓	or	✓

[a] Higher levels than medical ward may be required because of other indications.

TABLE 116.8

INDICATIONS AND CONTRAINDICATIONS FOR USE OF INTRAVENOUS TISSUE-TYPE PLASMINOGEN ACTIVATOR (t-PA) FOR ACUTE ISCHEMIC STROKE

Indication	Contraindication
Clinical diagnosis of stroke	Sustained blood pressure >185/110 mmHg
Onset of symptoms to time of drug administration ≤3 h	Plts <100,000/μL; Hct <25%; glucose <50 or >400 mg/dL
Computed tomography scan showing no hemorrhage or significant edema	Use of heparin within 48 h and prolonged aPTT, or elevated INR
Age ≥18 y	Rapidly improving symptoms
Consent by patient or surrogate	Prior stroke or head injury within 3 mo; prior intracranial hemorrhage
	Major surgery in preceding 14 d
	Minor stroke symptoms
	Gastrointestinal bleeding in preceding 21 d
	Recent myocardial infarction
	Coma or stupor

aPTT, activated partial thromboplastin time; Hct, hematocrit; INR, international normalized ratio; Plts, platelet count.

Clinical Diagnosis of Stroke

↓

Non-contrast head CT scan

↓

- 2 peripheral IV lines
- No arterial/central lines
- Avoid Foley >2 hours

↓

Inclusion criteria met; no contraindication (Table 116.8)

↓

t-PA 0.9 mg/kg (max. 90 mg)
- 10% of dose IV bolus
- Remaining IV over 1 hour

↓

- Continuous BP monitoring
- BP control (<185/110)

↓

- ICU or Stroke Unit
- No heparin, ASA or NG tube for 24 hours

Figure 116.2 Flow sheet for administering tissue plasminogen activator (t-PA) for acute ischemic stroke. *ASA,* aspirin; *BP,* blood pressure; *CT,* computed tomography; *IV,* intravenous; *NG,* nasogastric.

The patient's pretreatment blood pressure should be less than 185/110 mmHg; use of topical nitrates or intravenous labetolol may be necessary to lower blood pressure. However, if the patient's neurologic signs worsen with lowering of blood pressure, the pressure should be allowed to rise again and thrombolysis should be aborted. During the infusion of t-PA and the subsequent few hours, it is also important to maintain control of the blood pressure. For these reasons, t-PA should be given only if the patient's blood pressure and clinical status can be monitored continuously, typically in an emergency department or ICU setting. Sudden neurologic decline during or within 36 hours following t-PA infusion may represent intracranial hemorrhage. If this occurs, the infusion should be discontinued, an immediate noncontrast head CT scan obtained, and a neurosurgeon consulted. Cryoprecipitate may slow bleeding and in this setting should be given presumptively and immediately; this can be discontinued if the head CT does not reveal hemorrhage. Post-thrombolytic treatment involves close neurologic observation and, for the first 24 hours, avoidance of heparin, aspirin, or nasogastric tubes.

The use of aspirin for the treatment of acute stroke has been studied in two large trials (3, 4). Both trials indicate a reduction in stroke and death by 1% within 2–4 weeks with aspirin therapy. Heparin affords no benefit and increases the extracranial bleeding rate if combined with aspirin. Thus, aspirin has a significant effect in lowering morbidity and mortality rates, but the mortality benefit is very small compared with thrombolytic treatment. It is unclear if aspirin would be more effective if given within the first few hours of stroke rather than 1 or 2 days later, as has been studied in these trials. Current recommendations are to avoid aspirin for one day following thrombolysis (2). If thrombolysis is not performed, aspirin is safe and beneficial if given within the first 1 or 2 days following acute stroke.

Intravenous heparin is frequently used to prevent second stroke or first stroke following TIA. However, the acute effect of heparin has not been well studied, and the routine usage of heparin is being discouraged. Only one trial was large enough to allow analysis of the efficacy of heparin in acute stroke treatment (3), and it showed no benefit for unadjusted-dosage heparin (5,000–12,500 units subcutaneously twice a day). Overdosage with heparin (aPTT >100 sec) in the setting of large strokes may produce intracranial hemorrhage. However, for strokes that are evolving from progressive arterial thrombosis or from recurrent embolism, heparin may halt progression. Although no data from controlled prospective trials exist, current clinical practice of stroke management most commonly employs heparin in this setting. Most neurologists also believe that heparin is indicated for patients with arterial dissection and distal embolism, and for patient with dural sinus thrombosis. Heparin is typically given without initial bolus to avoid intracranial hemorrhage. The use of "bridging" heparin for patients who will receive warfarin is discussed below in the section on atrial fibrillation.

Treatment of acute hypertension during ischemic stroke generally is avoided unless there is coexistent cardiac ischemia, hypertensive nephropathy, or hypertensive retinopathy (Chapter 48). Blood pressure may be reflexively elevated early in the course of stroke and usually declines over the days following the acute event. *Acute reduction in arterial blood pressure may precipitate cerebral ischemia* resulting from reduction in collateral flow to the ischemic penumbra, which lacks cerebral autoregulation and can survive only if some blood flow is maintained. Even minor drops in mean arterial pressure can worsen neurologic outcome. Thus, many neurointensivists *augment* the blood pressure in patients with normal or slightly elevated pressures upon stroke presentation. In some cases, deficits may resolve with this treatment alone. No controlled data exist to support the efficacy of this aggressive treatment, but it underscores the principle that blood pressure should not be lowered.

If the patient has ischemia within the carotid artery distribution, it is important to expedite evaluation of the carotid artery for carotid atherosclerosis. This can be done with carotid ultrasonography, CT angiography (CTA), MR angiography, or conventional angiography. Combining CTA with the initial non-contrast CT scan expedites the discovery of symptomatic carotid disease. If the patient has experienced a TIA or minor stroke, carotid endarterectomy (CEA) is safe and should be offered as soon as possible to medically eligible patients. If CTA is not available, and the patient qualifies for emergent CEA, other procedures to image the carotid artery should be utilized.

ISSUES DURING THE COURSE OF HOSPITALIZATION

Figure 116.1 lists specific items to address following acute treatment. Initial consultation with physical and occupational therapists are important for patients with functional deficits. This should occur on the first or second hospital day to help with discharge planning. Speech therapy or consultation with a therapist who specializes in swallowing evaluation may be helpful to determine the safety of continued oral intake. However, acute dysphagia often resolves in the first few days, and it is common to begin nasoduodenal feeding, followed by an assessment of the need for percutaneous gastrostomy at a later date if the patient fails to improve. A social worker should be involved as early as possible to help with disposition and the financial and emotional issues that the sudden onset of stroke usually brings to bear on the entire family (Chapter 4).

Patients with dysphagia or airway compromise are at high risk for developing aspiration pneumonia (Chapter 66). Aspiration and the use of indwelling catheters increase the risk for infection. As noted previously, fever is detrimental to ischemic brain. The cause for fever should be pursued (Chapter 62), and temperature elevation should be corrected aggressively. Patients with cerebellar hemorrhage or ischemia are of special concern. Swelling from the hematoma or the ischemic brain occurs in a delayed fashion, typically 12 hours to 7 days after the initial event. Due to the anatomy of the posterior fossa, this swelling can compromise drainage of CSF through the aqueduct of Sylvius, causing hydrocephalus. It may also cause direct brainstem distortion, leading to severe hemodynamic instability and respiratory arrest. Hydrocephalus can be managed with osmotic agents and ventriculostomy. However, in both conditions definitive therapy is cerebellar hematoma evacuation or cerebellectomy. Because neurological decline (usually in the form of progressive coma or respiratory arrest) can be rapid, these patients are best managed in an ICU setting and either neurology or neurosurgery consultation should be obtained.

Stroke prophylaxis should be initiated in the hospital setting based on the exact cause of stroke. In general, patients with lacunar stroke not caused by carotid atherosclerosis, atrial fibrillation, or dural sinus thrombosis may be treated with agents that block platelet function. Aspirin at a dose of 75–325 mg/d lowers the risk of second stroke by 22%, is inexpensive, and is generally well tolerated (4). Ticlopidine has been shown to be superior to aspirin. Clopidogrel, 75 mg/d, is marginally more effective than aspirin in preventing combined end-points (stroke, myocardial infarction, and death), but it is significantly more expensive than aspirin. The combination of aspirin and clopidogrel for stroke prophylaxis is marginally better than clopidogrel alone, but also is associated with more bleeding complications (5). Aspirin and extended-release dipyridamole (Aggrenox) have been shown to be superior to aspirin alone, and should be dosed twice a day if this combination is used. Headache is a common side effect upon initiation of therapy, but if twice a day dosing is maintained, headache clears rapidly. No algorithm for antiplatelet therapy has been studied. However, most stroke centers initiate aspirin alone if the stroke occurs in a patient not taking any antiplatelet agent. If the patient was taking aspirin, either Aggrenox is substituted or clopidogrel is added. With the exception of the settings of atrial fibrillation and dural sinus thrombosis, warfarin is no more effective than aspirin in secondary prevention of stroke (6).

All patients with stroke should have fasting lipid studies measured during hospitalization. A statin agent should be initiated to lower LDL to a target of below 100 mg/dL. Counseling for smoking cessation for smokers should be offered and documented.

Hypertension is the most significant risk factor to modify, with a long-term goal of systolic blood pressures <140 and diastolic pressures <90 mm Hg (7). Although it has never been studied systematically, blood pressure should be lowered slowly over the 3–4 weeks following the event, and it is considered good practice to discharge the patient on at least one antihypertensive. Starting a thiazide diuretic during the hospitalization followed by discharge instructions with proper blood pressure goals is prudent (8). ACE inhibitors may provide additional protection against second stroke beyond their ability to lower blood pressure (9), and therefore are commonly used with a diuretic.

Patients with stroke from atrial fibrillation are at high risk of recurrent stroke. Following a stroke, a patient with atrial fibrillation has approximately a 15% risk of second stroke in the first year if not medicated with an antithrombotic agent. Some debate exists as to the use of oral anticoagulation or antiplatelet treatment in such patients. A summary of a consensus opinion regarding the use of aspirin or warfarin is shown in Table 42.5. The decision is based on age and the presence of risk factors (10). Patients in their thirties with lone atrial fibrillation have a low rate of first stroke and TIA. However, once a patient has a cerebral ischemic event, the risk rises dramatically, favoring treatment. Whatever treatment is prescribed, it is important to educate patients about the signs and symptoms of TIA so that therapy can be adjusted if these events occur.

Heparin is frequently used while initiating warfarin therapy in patients with TIA or stroke secondary to atrial fibrillation. The recurrence rate of stroke following a single stroke or TIA secondary to atrial fibrillation is approximately 1%–2% during the first 2 weeks. Depending on how the individual physician views this risk, some physicians start heparin while oral warfarin is being initiated, while others just start warfarin without heparin. Heparin should probably be avoided during the first few days of large ischemic strokes because of risk of intracranial hemorrhage. For patients with TIA or smaller strokes from atrial fibrillation, warfarin can be initiated at the time of admission.

Patients who experience stroke or TIA with ipsilateral 50% or greater carotid stenosis carry a high risk of subsequent stroke or death. For example, a patient with a 70% carotid stenosis who presents with hemispheric TIA has a 26% risk of stroke or death in the next 2 years. Endarterectomy substantially reduces this risk if the surgeon has a complication rate of less than 3% (11). Patients with TIA and minor strokes should be considered for emergent endarectomy, as discussed above. Because large strokes impair cerebral autoregulation, endarterectomy done in the first few weeks following a significant cerebral ischemic event can cause intracranial hemorrhage. Thus, many surgeons defer surgery for 4–8 weeks. Hospital management in this case should focus on defining the carotid disease, assessing the patient as a surgical candidate, and prescribing prophylaxis until elective endarterectomy is performed. Whether one should prescribe aspirin, aspirin and anticoagulation, or anticoagulation alone for symptomatic carotid disease while awaiting definitive surgery is controversial. Carotid stenting is an alternative to endarterectomy; initial data suggest that it is less morbid than CEA in high risk patients (12).

DISCHARGE ISSUES

Patients either return home, depending on home safety and functional status; transfer to an acute rehabilitation hospital; or transfer to a skilled nursing facility. The goal is to return the stroke patient home as soon as he or she is capable of returning. Assessments from physical, occupational, and speech therapists are essential in making this determination. If the patient is unable to return home but can comply with several (typically three) hours per day of active physical therapy, the patient may be eligible for acute inpatient rehabilitation. Rehabilitation units vary in their abilities to handle concomitant medical issues (e.g., adjusting anticoagulation). In general, a patient may be discharged if the neurologic examination has stabilized or is improving, adequate nutrition has been established, and arrangements have been made so that outstanding medical issues can be managed by the receiving service and adequate evaluation of the cause of stroke can be performed to guide logical stroke prophylaxis. Patients who are incapable of participating in therapy for the requisite number of hours per day or who are cognitively incapable of participating but have reached criteria for acute hospital discharge may require skilled nursing care, with later transfer to an acute rehabilitation setting if they meet appropriate criteria.

It is important to communicate several issues to the primary medical doctor in the discharge summary. These should include the cause of the stroke, the current neurological examination of the patient at the time of discharge, and the steps taken for secondary prevention. Blood pressure goals should be clarified and follow-up of blood pressure and lipid status should be assured. Finally, patients should receive comprehensive counseling on reducing stroke risk.

KEY POINTS

- Management of patients with a sudden change in neurologic status should be approached with a logical algorithm that incorporates accurate diagnosis, rapid (<3 hour) treatment with t-PA if eligible, and coordination of staff to determine patient disposition and immediate therapy. Before t-PA is administered, it is essential that blood pressure be controlled ($<185/110$) and hemorrhage excluded.

- In general, treatment of acute hypertension should be avoided in the patient with acute stroke.

- Patients with stroke (or TIA) and atrial fibrillation, and patients with dural sinus thrombosis, require anticoagulation, while patients with symptomatic carotid disease benefit from endarterectomy or carotid stenting. In all other stroke causes, antiplatelet agents are the favored form of prophylaxis.

- In addition, modification of risk factors following stroke is critical. Target LDL should be less than 100 mg/dL. All hypertensive patients should receive at least a diuretic prior to discharge. Long-term blood pressure goals are at least BP $<140/90$ mm Hg, and this is best achieved with addition of an ACE inhibitor as an outpatient. Counseling for smoking cessation should be offered and documented.

- Hospital management of acute stroke patients requires a coordinated effort of therapists and discharge planners to help institute important therapy and expedite patient transfer for more intensive rehabilitation.

- Contact with the outpatient physicians providing follow-up is essential to communicate the diagnosis, prescribed stroke prophylaxis, rehabilitation plan, and maintenance of medications.

REFERENCES

1. The National Institute of Neurological Disorders and Stroke rt-PA Stroke Study Group. Tissue plasminogen activator for acute ischemic stroke. *N Engl J Med* 1995;333:1581–1587.
2. Adams HP, Jr., Adams RJ, Brott T, et al. Guidelines for the early management of patients with ischemic stroke: a scientific statement from the Stroke Council of the American Stroke Association. *Stroke* 2003;34:1056–1083.
3. International Stroke Trial Collaborative Group. The International Stroke Trial (IST): a randomised trial of aspirin, subcutaneous heparin, both, or neither among 19435 patients with acute ischaemic stroke. *Lancet* 1997;349:1569–1581.
4. CAST (Chinese Acute Stroke Trial) Collaborative Group. CAST: randomised placebo-controlled trial of early aspirin use in 20,000 patients with acute ischaemic stroke. *Lancet* 1997;349:1641–1649.
5. Diener HC, Bogousslavsky J, Brass LM, et al. Aspirin and clopidogrel compared with clopidogrel alone after recent ischaemic stroke or transient ischaemic attack in high-risk patients (MATCH): randomised, double-blind, placebo-controlled trial. *Lancet* 2004;364:331–337.
6. Mohr JP, Thompson JL, Lazar RM, et al. A comparison of warfarin and aspirin for the prevention of recurrent ischemic stroke. *N Engl J Med* 2001;345:1444–1451.
7. Joint National Committee. Seventh report of the Joint National Committee on the prevention, detection, evaluation, and treatment of high blood pressure. Available at http://www.nhlbi.nih.gov/guidelines/hypertension/. Accessed March 2, 2005.
8. Major outcomes in high-risk hypertensive patients randomized to angiotensin-converting enzyme inhibitor or calcium channel blocker vs diuretic: The Antihypertensive and Lipid-Lowering Treatment to Prevent Heart Attack Trial (ALLHAT). *JAMA* 2002;288:2981–2997.
9. Randomised trial of a perindopril-based blood-pressure-lowering regimen among 6,105 individuals with previous stroke or transient ischaemic attack. *Lancet* 2001;358:1033–1041.
10. Singer DE, Albers GW, Dalen JE, et al. Antithrombotic therapy in atrial fibrillation: the seventh ACCP conference on antithrombotic and thrombolytic therapy. *Chest* 2004;126 (3 suppl):429S–456S.
11. Moore WS, Barnett HJ, Beebe HG, et al. Guidelines for carotid endarterectomy. A multidisciplinary consensus statement from the ad hoc Committee, American Heart Association. *Stroke* 1995;26:188–201.
12. Shawl F, Kadro W, Domanski MJ, et al. Safety and efficacy of elective carotid artery stenting in high-risk patients. *J Am Coll Cardiol* 2000;35:1721–1728.

ADDITIONAL READING

Albers GW, Hart RG, Lutsep HL, Newell DW, Sacco RL. AHA scientific statement. Supplement to the guidelines for the management of transient ischemic attacks: a statement from the Ad Hoc Committee on Guidelines for the Management of Transient Ischemic Attacks, Stroke Council, American Heart Association. *Stroke* 1999;30:2502–2511.

Culebras A, Kase CS, Masdeu JC, et al. Practice guidelines for the use of imaging in transient ischemic attacks and acute stroke: a report of the Stroke Council, American Heart Association. *Stroke* 1997;28:1480–1497.

Coull BM, Williams LS, Goldstein LB, Meschia JF, Heitzman D, Chaturvedi S, et al. Anticoagulants and antiplatelet agents in acute ischemic stroke: report of the Joint Stroke Guideline Development Committee of the American Academy of Neurology and the American Stroke Association (a division of the American Heart Association). *Stroke* 2002;33:1934–1942.

Central Nervous System Hemorrhage and Increased Intracranial Pressure

117

Ellen Deibert   Michael N. Diringer

INTRODUCTION

Anatomy and Physiology

Increased intracranial pressure (ICP) develops in many acute neurologic disorders and can have serious consequences because of the anatomy and physiology of the intracranial vault. The intracranial vault can be thought of as a compartment made up of the brain, cerebrospinal fluid (CSF), blood, and blood vessels enclosed in the rigid skull. The normal brain constitutes about 80% of the intracranial contents; blood and CSF make up approximately 10% each.

Masses, or any increase in the volume of blood or CSF in the intracranial vault, can lead to increased ICP. In addition, any process that causes an increase in brain water content (edema), such as disruption of the blood-brain barrier as seen in ischemia, infection, trauma, surgical retraction, and tumors, can lead to elevated ICP.

CSF is produced by the choroid plexus located within the lateral and fourth ventricles of the brain. It normally migrates from the ventricles, exits the brain through the foramina of Magendie and Luschka to the basal cisterns, and over the convexities, where it drains through the arachnoid granulations into the venous system. Processes such as meningitis, tumors, hemorrhage, or cerebral edema can either obstruct the flow of CSF or interrupt the normal CSF absorption-production equilibrium, resulting in hydrocephalus.

Increases in cerebral blood volume can also lead to intracranial hypertension. As cerebral blood flow (CBF) increases, so does the cerebral blood volume (CBV). CBF is influenced by the cerebral perfusion pressure (CPP), the partial pressure of carbon dioxide (P_aCO_2), the partial pressure of oxygen (P_aO_2), and the cerebral metabolic rate of oxygen. CPP is defined as [mean arterial pressure − ICP]. Under normal conditions, autoregulation maintains the CBF over a wide range of perfusion pressures (60–150 mm Hg) (Figure 117.1A) by altering the diameter of distal arterial resistance vessels. Because more than 80% of the blood in the intracranial vault is contained within the cerebral veins and sinuses, CBV can also rise with venodilation, and drugs that alter venous tone can dramatically increase CBV and ICP.

The relationship between CBF and P_aCO_2 is linear (Figure 117.1B), which accounts for the fall in ICP with hyperventilation. As P_aCO_2 decreases, vasoconstriction occurs, decreasing CBV and thus ICP. The relationship of CBF and arterial oxygen content is also linear. However, because of the shape of the oxyhemoglobin dissociation curve, when hematocrit is normal, CBF does not increase until the P_aO_2 is less than approximately 50 mm Hg.

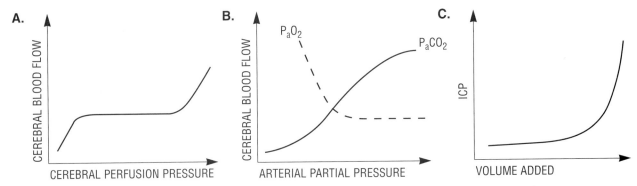

Figure 117.1 Physiologic influences on cerebral blood flow and intracranial pressure (ICP). **A.** Cerebral perfusion pressure autoregulation curve for normotensive adults. Note that cerebral blood flow remains stable over a wide range of cerebral perfusion pressures but becomes pressure passive as the limits of autoregulation are exceeded at both extremes. This curve is shifted to the right in hypertensive adults. **B.** Cerebral blood flow response to changes in P_aCO_2 and P_aO_2. **C.** The relationship between ICP and intracranial volume. Note that as volume is added to the cranial vault, there is no increase in ICP as a result of compensatory mechanisms (Figure 117.2). Once these mechanisms are exhausted, however, ICP increases rapidly as volume is added. (Adapted from Diringer NM. Intracerebral hemorrhage: pathophysiology and management. *Crit Care Med* 1993;21:1593, with permission.)

Cerebral metabolism is closely linked to CBF. Any increase in metabolism, as seen with fever or seizures, results in a rise in CBF. Similarly, a decrease in metabolism, such as occurs with barbiturates and hypothermia, leads to a fall in CBF. Ischemia occurs only if CBF becomes inadequate to support cerebral metabolism.

Pathophysiology

Any process that adds volume to the intracranial vault (e.g., hematoma, tumor, edema) can eventually lead to intracranial hypertension. At first, the intracranial vault accommodates the increase in volume by displacing equivalent volumes of CSF and venous blood into the spinal canal, preventing a rise in ICP (Figure 117.2). Once these compensatory mechanisms are exhausted, ICP begins to rise (Figure 117.1C).

Elevated ICP can cause injury by leading to a global fall in cerebral perfusion, causing ischemia. Initially, as CPP falls, CBF remains constant because of autoregulation. When CPP falls below its lower limit, CBF begins to fall. Initially, the amount of oxygen reaching tissues remains constant because of a rise in brain oxygen extraction. Eventually, oxygen extraction reaches a maximum, and any further decrease in CBF leads to ischemia.

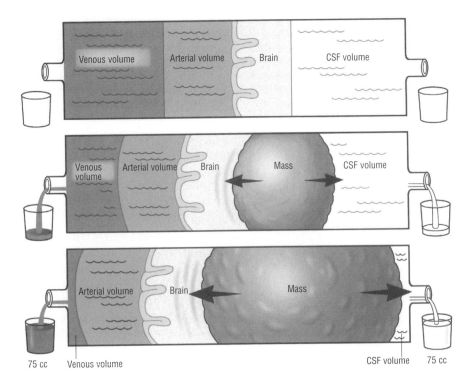

Figure 117.2 Regulation of intracranial pressure. Diagrammatic representation of the intracranial contents and their compensation for an expanding intracranial mass. Cerebrospinal fluid and venous blood occupy about 20% of the intracranial contents (**top**). Displacement of cerebrospinal fluid and venous blood is the compensation for an expanding mass (**middle**). These compensatory mechanisms are exhausted if there is no more cerebrospinal fluid or venous blood available to be displaced. Then, if the mass lesion increases further, intracranial pressure begins to climb (**bottom**). (Adapted from Kanter MJ, Narayan RK. Intracranial pressure monitoring. *Neurosurg Clin North Am* 1991;2:258, with permission.)

Intracranial hypertension can also cause brain injury by producing tissue shifts that can result in *herniation syndromes*. These shifts occur because of the division of the skull into a number of compartments by the falx cerebri and tentorium. As a mass in one compartment grows, the pressure gradients produce tissue shifts and, eventually, herniation of tissue from one compartment to another. These syndromes present with varied neurologic pictures depending on the brain region involved and the tissue shifts that ensue (Figure 117.3).

Evaluation of the Patient

The history of a patient who has suspected increased ICP usually must be obtained from a relative, friend, or witness. Relevant historical issues include the time course of the present illness, as well as prior history of cancer, bleeding

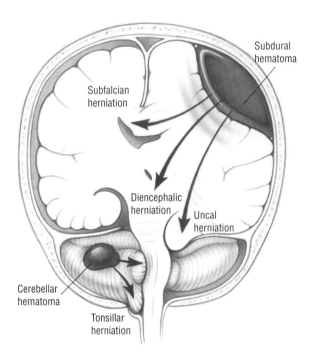

Figure 117.3 Types of brain herniation. Different types of brain herniation caused by isolated areas of increased intracranial pressure. A mass (subdural in figure) located in the cerebral hemisphere may cause a shift of the intracranial contents past midline (subfalcian herniation). Uncal herniation results from a mass in one of the parietal, frontal, or temporal lobes creating pressure on the uncus of the temporal lobe, which then herniates through the tentorium. This can cause direct pressure on the underlying midbrain and third nerve, creating a unilateral dilated pupil. Cerebellar or tonsillar herniation can occur if a mass lesion (cerebellar hematoma in figure) develops in the cerebellum, causing compression of the medulla. This can cause a rapid deterioration, abnormal breathing, flexor or extensor posturing, impaired eye movements, hypertension, and bradycardia. Finally, central herniation (not shown) occurs if the tissue shifts are directed downward through the foramen magnum. These patients usually present with a global decline in level of consciousness and may have sixth nerve palsies. (Adapted from Wijdicks EF, Diringer M, Bolten C, et al. Essentials of management. *Continuum: Lifelong Learning in Neurology.* 1997;3:51, by permission of the Mayo Foundation.)

TABLE 117.1

GLASGOW COMA SCALE[a]

Eye opening

Spontaneously	4
Response to voice	3
Response to pain	2
No response	1

Verbal response

Oriented and appropriate	5
Disoriented conversation	4
Inappropriate words	3
Incomprehensible sounds	2
No response	1

Motor response

Obeys commands	6
Localizes pain	5
Flexion withdrawal	4
Decorticate posturing (flexor)	3
Decerebrate posturing (extensor)	2
No response	1

[a] Total score is sum of eye opening, verbal, and motor scores. The maximum score possible is 15.

disorders, warfarin therapy, strokes, cardiac abnormalities, rheumatic fever, oral contraceptive use, hypertension, tobacco use, or connective tissue disorders.

The clinical findings differ depending on the primary cause. For instance, lesions such as tumors or intracerebral hemorrhage (ICH) may present with focal neurologic findings including aphasia and hemiplegia; diffuse head injury may cause a global neurologic decline with loss of consciousness and motor posturing. The *Glasgow Coma Scale* (Table 117.1) is used for patients with a suspected ICP increase to quantify the level of consciousness, define prognosis, and monitor changes. It is important to note that papilledema may take several weeks to develop; therefore, its absence does not exclude elevated ICP, especially of recent onset.

Vital signs can provide early and valuable information regarding ICP. The onset of hypertension and bradycardia can indicate an acute rise in ICP (*Cushing response*), mandating immediate intervention.

Initial Patient Management

During the initial evaluation of a patient with suspected increased ICP, it is essential to ensure adequate airway, breathing, and circulation. *Early intubation* is required for comatose patients (Glasgow Coma Scale score <9) because they often develop airway obstruction, and aspiration can result from diminished pharyngeal tone and lack of adequate cough and gag reflexes. Medications utilized for intubation should be ones that decrease cerebral metabolism and ICP. A fall in blood pressure should be avoided because this will further reduce cerebral perfusion. Etomidate (0.4–0.8 mg/kg), a non-barbiturate hypnotic, is short-acting and is least likely to cause hypotension. Thiopental (2.5–4.5 mg/kg) is effective in lowering cerebral metabolic rate but more frequently lowers blood pressure. Lidocaine (1–2 mg/kg intravenous) is a useful adjunct in this setting because it minimizes the elevation in ICP from endotracheal stimulation. Midazolam, although very sedating, may not adequately lower ICP and therefore should not be used alone. With adequate sedation, muscle paralysis is usually unnecessary and interferes with the ability to perform neurologic examinations. However, if paralysis is required for intubation, a short-acting non-depolarizing agent, such as mivacurium (0.1 mg/kg), is preferred.

Many patients with elevated ICP have increased blood pressure, which should be managed conservatively. *Lowering blood pressure at a time when ICP is elevated can cause critical reduction in cerebral perfusion pressure and produce global ischemia.* If hypertension is treated, venodilators, such as nitrates, should be avoided because of their ability to further raise ICP.

Once the patient with suspected elevated ICP is hemodynamically stable and the airway is controlled, mannitol (0.5–1.0 gm/kg intravenous) should be given. Hyperventilation to a P_aCO_2 of 25–30 mm Hg should be used only if there are signs of herniation or rapid neurologic deterioration (see later in this chapter). In patients with intracranial bleeding, coagulation status should be checked and rapidly corrected if abnormal.

Neuroimaging

After initial evaluation and stabilization, the next step is to obtain an imaging study. In an emergent situation, brain computerized tomography (CT) is preferred. A CT scan is able to determine whether the patient has an intracranial mass, hydrocephalus, diffuse cerebral edema, subarachnoid hemorrhage (SAH), or intracranial hemorrhage. Because contrast appears very similar to acute blood on CT, *a non-contrast CT should always be obtained first.*

Magnetic resonance imaging (MRI) provides an excellent anatomic image but is not the imaging modality of choice in an emergent situation. The long scan time, patient inaccessibility, and the magnetic field generated by the MRI make monitoring and treating patients difficult. In addition, MRI does not detect acute blood as well as a non-contrast CT scan.

Management of Increased Intracranial Pressure

Patients with a Glasgow Coma Scale score of ≤8, an abnormal head CT scan, and suspected increased ICP require ICP monitoring and admission to an ICU. Several types of monitoring devices exist. In one, a catheter is placed through a burr hole into a lateral ventricle, which allows for ventricular drainage of CSF as well as monitoring of ICP. However, the infection rate increases over time. A second type of device is a transducer, which is inserted into the brain parenchyma. It allows for continuous ICP monitoring but cannot drain CSF. In addition, this device cannot be recalibrated and is therefore subject to drift.

Increased ICP usually is managed medically, but sometimes it may require surgical intervention. Routine measures for patients with increased ICP include elevating the head of the bed, treating fever aggressively, and avoiding compressing the jugular veins with collars, tape, or large bore catheters. Agitated patients should be sedated to a Ramsay Scale score of 4 or 5. Cerebral metabolism suppressants such as benzodiapines are preferred. Opiates do not suppress cerebral metabolism and can have deleterious effects on gastrointestinal motility.

Osmotic therapy is usually the next step after sedation in controlling intracranial hypertension. The goal is to produce an osmotic gradient between the intracellular space and the blood, which results in a shift of water out of the intracellular compartment (1). Mannitol is the agent primarily used in the United States. It does not cross the intact blood-brain barrier and decreases ICP in 10–20 minutes. Recently, the use of "super salt" (23.4% saline) has been introduced as an alternative to mannitol. While super salt is effective in lowering ICP, it has not been directly compared to mannitol.

Mannitol is also a potent diuretic. The most frequent error made when administering mannitol is failure to recognize and correct the resultant hypovolemia. When uncorrected, the hypovolemia can lead to a fall in blood pressure (with reduced cerebral perfusion) and renal failure. Often, large volumes of fluids are required to replace the urine output. Because the goal of this therapy is to raise osmolality, the replacement fluid should be isotonic, not hypotonic, saline. Empiric doses of a 20% mannitol solution are 1 gm/kg intravenous every six hours, or 0.25–0.5 gm/kg intravenous, every 3–4 hours. Dosing that is administered as needed when ICP exceeds a pre-determined threshold (usually 20–25 mm Hg) provides good control, often with a reduced total dose.

Mannitol can cause renal failure, although it has been difficult to define the etiology. One factor appears to be failure to clear mannitol between doses. To ensure adequate clearance, measurement of the osmotic gap (the difference between the measured and calculated osmolality) may be helpful. A rise in the gap from baseline or an absolute gap of >20 mOsm/kg is considered evidence of retained mannitol and should prompt a change in dosing. This can easily be accomplished by alternative equi-osmolar doses of mannitol and super salt. Mannitol's ability to lower blood viscosity may increase CBF, which may be an added benefit.

Mannitol therapy must be used with caution in patients with a history of heart failure because of the initial intravascular volume expansion. In practice, this does not appear to be a significant problem because of its rapid diuretic effect. In addition, patients with cardiac dysfunction may lose adequate preload if the intravascular space is not adequately replenished. Hypokalemia, hypophosphatemia, and hypomagnesiemia are complications of mannitol therapy that can be avoided with close monitoring. Finally, as the patient improves, the hyperosmolal state must be corrected very slowly (over several days to 2 weeks) to prevent rebound cerebral edema.

Hyperventilation effectively lowers ICP, but does so by decreasing CBF. It therefore may cause cerebral ischemia. Thus, *hyperventilation should not be routinely used*, but should be reserved as a brief temporizing measure when there are signs of herniation (dilated pupil or progressive neurologic deterioration) or sudden rises in ICP. Immediately after hyperventilation is instituted, the next line of medical or surgical therapy must be initiated. If hyperventilation is used for a sustained period, its cerebrovascular effects are lost and ICP returns to baseline. At this point, a rise in P_aCO_2 can cause a dramatic rebound increase in ICP; therefore, hyperventilation should be slowly discontinued over several hours.

Steroid therapy (up to 20 mg of dexamethasone every four hours intravenously) may lead to neurologic improvement in patients with cerebral edema associated with brain tumors. There is no demonstrated benefit of steroids in intracerebral hemorrhage, traumatic brain injury, or stroke.

The role of *surgery* for treatment of increased ICP depends on multiple factors, including the type of injury, the condition of the patient, and the location of the injury. Lobectomy is utilized in some patients with traumatic brain injury or tumor who are refractory to medical man-agement of intracranial hypertension. Recently, there has been increased interest in hemicraniectomy as another surgical option. Initially applied to patients with large strokes and massive edema, it is now being used in patients with head trauma, intracerebral hemorrhage, and severe encephalitis. It offers the advantage of not only increasing the size of the intracranial vault but also in reversing tissue shifts. It is currently being evaluated as primary treatment in patients with traumatic subdural hematomas and underlying cerebral edema.

SPONTANEOUS SUBARACHNOID HEMORRHAGE (SAH)

Approximately 30,000 people in the United States suffer a nontraumatic SAH each year. Rupture of an intracranial aneurysm accounts for about 80% of these hemorrhages. Other causes of non-traumatic SAH include ruptured arteriovenous malformation, bleeding disorders, mycotic aneurysms, sinus thrombosis, or idiopathic SAH. The 1-year mortality rate for untreated aneurysmal SAH is 60%, with one-third of patients dying from the initial event and another 15% dying as a result of rebleeding within 1 month. Aneurysms occur more frequently in females than males (3:2), and peak incidence of rupture is between ages 50 and 60 years.

About 80% of aneurysms are berry or saccular aneurysms found at the base of the brain at the bifurcations of the vessels that make up the circle of Willis (Figure 117.4). Approximately 20% of patients have multiple aneurysms.

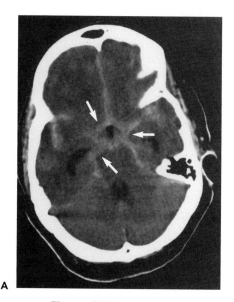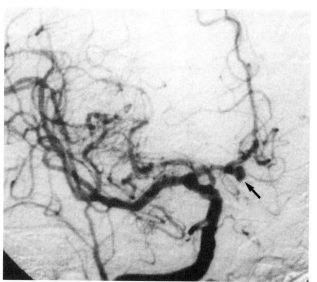

Figure 117.4 **A.** Computed tomographic scan of subarachroid hemorrhage. Subarachnoid hemorrhage (*arrows*) from an anterior communicating artery aneurysm. The amount of blood on this scan represents Fisher grade III, putting the patient at high risk for vasospasm. Also note that hydrocephalus is present, indicated by the dilation of both temporal horns of lateral ventricles. **B.** Cerebral aneurysm. An anterior communicating artery aneurysm (*arrow*) seen on the carotid injection of a cerebral angiogram.

Larger aneurysms are more likely to rupture than those smaller than 3 mm. The formation of aneurysms has been associated with fibromuscular dysplasia, Marfan syndrome, pseudoxanthoma elasticum, Ehler-Danlos syndrome, polycystic kidneys, and coarctation of the aorta. Risk factors for SAH include hypertension, smoking, and heavy alcohol use. Recently it has been recognized that genetics play a role in aneurysm formation, with a very high rate of aneurysms in certain families.

Issues at the Time of Admission

Clinical Presentation

The classic presentation of SAH is the acute onset of a severe headache, often described as "the worst headache of my life," followed by a brief loss of consciousness in 45% of cases. Nausea and vomiting are also common, but only about 10% of patients manifest focal neurologic signs. Approximately 10% of patients have a seizure at the onset of the hemorrhage. Neck stiffness is very common but may take several hours to develop. A more atypical presentation is seen in patients who have "warning leaks" or sentinel hemorrhages. These patients may complain of generalized headache, nausea, vomiting, or malaise, all of which can develop hours to days before they present to the hospital with more typical symptoms.

The *Hunt Hess SAH classification* and the *Fisher scale* help categorize the clinical and radiographic features of SAH (Table 117.2), and they help define the risk of vasospasm. An SAH patient with a Hunt Hess grade III (or higher) or a Fisher grade III is at highest risk.

Differential Diagnosis and Initial Evaluation

A patient with acute onset of severe headache and a brief loss of consciousness has an SAH until proven otherwise (2). Other disorders that can present in a similar fashion include a ruptured arteriovenous malformation, intracranial hemorrhage, migraine, hypertensive encephalopathy, or, rarely, stroke. These disorders, however, usually have a subacute presentation and are more likely to be associated with focal neurologic signs. Cardiac syncope, seizures, and brainstem stroke can present with loss of consciousness but rarely with acute onset of severe headache.

The initial evaluation always begins with assessment of airway, breathing, and circulation. Once the patient has been stabilized, *emergent head CT without contrast* is the diagnostic study of choice. Head CT has a sensitivity greater than 90% for SAH if performed within 24 hours of symptom onset. The scan determines the patient's Fisher grade as well as identifies associated intraparenchymal hematoma, intraventricular extension of the hemorrhage, or hydrocephalus. If the head CT is negative and the clinical suspicion is high, a *lumbar puncture* should be performed to look for bloody CSF and xanthochromia; the latter usually develops over several

TABLE 117.2

CLASSIFICATION OF SUBARACHNOID HEMORRHAGE

Grade	Signs and symptoms
Hunt Hess classification	
I	No symptoms or slight headache
II	Moderate-to-severe headache and nuchal rigidity, but no focal or lateralizing neurologic signs
III	Drowsiness, confusion, and mild focal deficits
IV	Stupor, hemiparesis, early decerebrate rigidity, and vegetative disturbances
V	Deep coma and decerebrate rigidity
Fisher scale	
I	No subarachnoid hemorrhage on computed tomography
II	Broad diffusion of subarachnoid blood, no clots, and no layers of blood greater than 1 mm
III	Either localized blood clots in the subarachnoid space or layers of blood greater than 1 mm
IV	Intraventricular and intracerebral blood present, in absence of significant subarachnoid blood

hours after hemorrhage because of the conversion of hemoglobin from lysed red blood cells to bilirubin.

A *4-vessel cerebral angiogram* should be performed quickly in order to identify the type and location of the aneurysm. Other tests that should be ordered include admission electrocardiogram, chest radiograph, prothrombin time/activated partial thromboplastin time (PT/aPTT), urinalysis, chemistries, complete blood count (CBC), electrolytes, and type and screen. An early neurosurgical consultation should be obtained regarding the timing and type of management for the aneurysm.

Indications for Hospitalization and Intensive Care Unit Admission

All SAH patients are admitted to the hospital, almost always to an ICU. Patients who are initially stable may suffer devastating early complications such as rebleeding or acute hydrocephalus and thus require close monitoring. In addition, patients with higher Hunt Hess or Fisher grades are at increased risk for cardiac arrhythmias, heart failure, and neurogenic pulmonary edema (3). Therefore, they require close neurologic and cardiac monitoring. Ideally, these patients should be cared for at specialized centers that are more familiar with the early and late complications of this disease and the treatment options.

Initial Therapy

Blood pressure control is important to prevent the aneurysm from re-rupturing; blood pressure should be maintained in the patient's usual range. If that is unknown, the mean arterial pressure usually is kept below 100 mm Hg. The preferred antihypertensive agents are labetalol or hydralazine, each given as a bolus every 15–20 minutes, as needed. Alternatively, a nicardipine infusion can be helpful.

The patient should be kept calm, quiet, and comfortable, using sedatives if necessary. Activities that could cause abrupt changes in blood pressure or ICP, such as the Valsalva maneuver or coughing, should be avoided to reduce the risk of rebleeding, which is highest in the first 24 hours. The patient is given nimodipine (60 mg po every 4 hours), a calcium channel blocker that reduces ischemic deficits from vasospasm. Phenytoin is given to prevent seizures, and some centers use dexamethasone (4 mg intravenous every 6 hours) to reduce the inflammatory response to the hemorrhage. Adequate analgesia is essential, because it not only keeps the patient calm but also helps treat elevated blood pressure. Stool softeners are given to prevent straining, and pneumatic leg compression and anti-embolic stockings are used to prevent deep venous thrombosis.

Issues During the Course of Hospitalization

Cardiac Complications Associated with SAH

SAH can cause electrocardiographic changes, cardiac arrhythmias, elevated cardiac enzymes, and wall-motion abnormalities. Electrocardiographic abnormalities include inverted T waves, prolonged QT intervals, prominent U waves, and nonspecific ST-segment changes. Cardiac arrhythmias include sinus tachycardia, sinus bradycardia, sinus arrhythmia, and, rarely, malignant arrhythmias, such as ventricular tachycardia, *torsades de pointes*, and asystole. It is believed that the cardiac complications of SAH result from either elevated systemic catecholamine levels or direct sympathetic neural stimulation of the heart, and that they are anatomically and pathologically distinct from ischemic cardiac disease (4).

Most of the cardiac disturbances are benign and resolve spontaneously. Rarely, patients have a striking clinical presentation including pulmonary edema, severe wall-motion abnormalities on echocardiogram, and pump failure. Because the pathophysiology in this situation is unclear, these patients may require prolonged cardiac monitoring and Swan-Ganz catheterization for management. These changes are generally transient, lasting 2–3 days, followed by return to normal cardiac function on follow-up evaluation.

Rebleeding

The risk of rebleeding from a cerebral aneurysm is highest (around 4%) during the first 24 hours after hemorrhage and falls to about 1.5% per day over the next 2 weeks.

Rebleeding is usually a catastrophic event, and 40%–50% of patients who rebled die. The event is usually heralded by an acute rise in blood pressure and ICP, arrhythmias, and loss of consciousness. Airway, breathing, and circulation need to be readdressed. Repeat head CT reveals new hemorrhage in the subarachnoid space.

Management in the ICU is designed to prevent changes in pressure gradients across the aneurysm wall; thus, care is taken in patients with a ventriculostomy to avoid sudden decreases in ICP caused by draining large volumes of CSF quickly. Rebleeding is best prevented by stabilization of the aneurysm as soon as possible with either surgical clipping or endovascular treatments.

Hydrocephalus

Hydrocephalus can occur shortly after the onset of the hemorrhage (often as a result of intraventricular extension of the hemorrhage), may develop insidiously within the first 2 weeks, or occur in a delayed fashion. Hydrocephalus usually presents as a progressive decline in level of consciousness, is easily diagnosed with a CT scan, and is definitively treated with a ventriculostomy. In patients who present with SAH and acute hydrocephalus, the level of consciousness often improves considerably after ventriculostomy.

Hyponatremia and Volume Contraction

Intravascular volume regulation is impaired in SAH patients. Spontaneous hypovolemia occurs in 30%–50% of SAH patients (despite receiving what is considered to be adequate maintenance fluids), and 10%–35% develop hyponatremia. Although originally thought to be a result of SIADH (Chapter 104), the etiology of hyponatremia in SAH appears to be a complex combination of cerebral salt wasting with an additional component of SIADH. Thus, hyponatremic SAH patients are treated initially by volume expansion with isotonic saline and free water restriction. If hyponatremia persists, mildly hypertonic saline solutions (1%–2% saline) are utilized. Hypotonic solutions should be strictly avoided throughout hospitalization, as should fluid restriction, which is associated with an increased risk of stroke from vasospasm.

Repair of the Aneurysm to Prevent Rebleeding

For most patients who are Hunt Hess grades I through III, and in many centers, grade IV, *early repair of the aneurysm* (within three days of rupture) is the treatment of choice. In more severely affected patients, the location and complexity of the aneurysm, clinical grade of the patient, and difficulty of the surgery play a role in deciding when and if surgery is to be performed. Until recently, the only option for repair of a ruptured cerebral aneurysm was surgical. Recently, *endovascular repair, in which* platinum coils are placed into the dome of the aneurysm to promote thrombosis, has become widely used. Although this technique was initially reserved for patients who were poor surgical candidates because of aneurysm location or configuration, it is now being applied to a wider range of patients. In a recently completed, randomized, controlled trial of surgery or endovascular treatment, endovascular treatment was associated with reduced morbidity and mortality (5). Early repair virtually eliminates the risks of rebleeding and facilitates the treatment of vasospasm with hemodynamic augmentation (6) (see section on Vasospasm below).

Seizures

Prophylactic anticonvulsant therapy is administered to all SAH patients because of their small, but definite risk of seizures. Phenytoin is generally used, because it is the least sedating drug and can be administered either intravenously or orally. For most patients, therapy should be continued for several days and then discontinued. Patients who have an intraparenchymal clot or focal strokes from vasospasm are at increased long-term risk for seizures, and chronic seizure prophylaxis is often administered, although its efficacy has not been established.

Vasospasm

Vasospasm is the most frequent cause of injury or death in patients who survive the initial aneurysm rupture. Although angiographic vasospasm occurs in 60%–70% of all SAH patients, it only leads to clinically detectable symptoms in about half of those cases. Angiographic vasospasm usually occurs around 3–5 days after the SAH, with maximal narrowing 7–14 days after hemorrhage. The narrowing usually resolves in 2–4 weeks. Patients who develop symptoms are said to have clinical vasospasm (also referred to as delayed ischemic deficit) and demonstrate a decline in neurologic function, including agitation, diminished level of consciousness, or new focal deficits, which frequently fluctuate. The symptoms are exacerbated by hypovolemia or hypotension. Before treating a patient for clinical vasospasm, it is important to make sure that the deterioration is not caused by other processes, such as infection, metabolic derangements, hydrocephalus, cerebral edema, or rebleeding.

Frequent neurologic examinations and transcranial Doppler ultrasound studies are the most common ways to monitor patients for delayed ischemic deficits. Patients at risk for vasospasm undergo hourly neurologic assessments. In addition, some institutions use daily transcranial Doppler studies to monitor blood-flow velocity profiles of the major intracranial vessels, although the test's clinical utility is uncertain.

Factors thought to contribute to delayed ischemic deficit after SAH include vessel narrowing, loss of cerebral autoregulation, and hypovolemia. These observations have formed the basis for the treatment of delayed ischemic deficit with *hemodynamic augmentation,* also known as hypervolemic, hypertensive, hemodilution ("triple H") therapy, or hypervolemic, hypertensive therapy. These treatments involve manipulation of blood pressure, intravascular volume, and cardiac output in varying combinations with the goal of increasing CBF and reversing the neurological deficit.

Measures that may be useful in preventing clinical vasospasm include administration of nimodipine, surgical removal of subarachnoid blood, and careful attention to volume status to avoid hypovolemia. With the onset of clinical signs of vasospasm, the first step is to assure that the patient is not hypovolemic. It does not appear that hypervolemia provides any additional benefit unless it results in a rise in cardiac output and blood pressure (7). Patients with cardiac disease may benefit from having therapy guided by a Swan-Ganz catheter. Elevation of blood pressure is believed to increase CBF in the setting of disrupted cerebral autoregulation. In general, blood pressure can be increased by using phenylephrine to raise systemic vascular resistance. Dopamine is sometimes effective but has a high incidence of tachyarrhythmias. In patients with poor left ventricular function, intropes may be necessary. Careful monitoring for cardiac or systemic toxicities related to vasopressor agents is essential (Chapter 25). While the therapy is guided by setting goals for cardiac index and blood pressure, it is important to emphasize that the ultimate goal of therapy is to reverse the neurological deficit. Thus, hemodynamic goals should frequently be reassessed in light of the patient's neurological response to therapy. Therapy is slowly tapered over several days after neurologic deficits stabilize and improve. If symptoms recur during the taper, therapy is increased again until the patient stabilizes. It is important to note that hypertensive therapy is generally reserved for patients whose aneurysms have been repaired by surgery or endovascular coiling.

Newly emerging treatments for vasospasm include transluminal angioplasty and intra-arterial infusion of vasodilators, such as papaverine or nicardipine. *Balloon angioplasty* can dilate vasospastic proximal intracranial vessels with long-lasting effects (8). It is not useful for diffuse distal spasm, because of the small vessel caliber, and can be associated with serious complications, such as artery rupture or displacement of aneurysm clips. *Intra-arterial papaverine* is a potent direct vasodilator. Unfortunately, the effects are short-lived, and it is not without significant risks, including increased ICP, transient neurologic deficits, and respiratory depression. Thus, its use has declined considerably. Although angioplasty has not been evaluated in prospective controlled trials, early experience has been encouraging and its use is becoming routine in many centers.

General Medical Management

Patients with severe neurologic deficits usually remain intubated until they recover a sufficient level of consciousness and their cough and gag reflexes. Although induced coughing and rigorous suctioning should be avoided during periods of elevated ICP or when the aneurysm that bled has not been repaired, they are essential later in the hospital course. Some patients may not regain the ability to protect their airways and need to undergo a tracheostomy.

Brain-injured patients are hypermetabolic and hypercatabolic and, therefore, aggressive nutritional support is needed. If a patient's neurologic status does not allow him or her to eat safely, then enteral feedings should be initiated as soon as possible (Chapter 15). To avoid aspiration during tube feeding, it is useful to elevate the head of the bed and administer metoclopramide (10 mg every 6 hours). Agents to prevent GI bleeding should also be administered (Chapter 80). Deep venous thrombosis prophylaxis, usually with compression stockings, is also essential. The use of prophylactic subcutaneous heparin is controversial, although its use after repair of aneurysm is becoming more widespread.

Discharge Issues

About 25% of SAH patients survive with good neurologic outcomes. After stabilization and intervention, early consultation with physical, occupational, and speech therapists is critical in determining the amount and type of rehabilitation the patient needs. Social services coordinate the needs of the patient and family with their insurance companies and facilitate the transfer of the patient to the most appropriate rehabilitation facility.

INTRACRANIAL HEMORRHAGE

Intracranial hemorrhage can occur within any of the spaces of the cranium (subarachnoid, subdural, epidural, and intracerebral) and accounts for roughly 12%–15% of all strokes. This section focuses on intracerebral hemorrhage (ICH), an often devastating neurologic disease that presents with signs and symptoms similar to ischemic stroke. The symptoms are often more severe and require ICU admission. Management depends on the size and location of the hemorrhage.

Issues at the Time of Admission

Clinical Presentation

The signs and symptoms associated with an ICH vary with the location and size of the hemorrhage (9). In general, the presentation is similar to that of ischemic stroke (Chapter 116), except that the onset of symptoms is more rapid and headache, nausea, vomiting, and seizures are more common. If the hemorrhage is small, the patient may complain of an acute onset of headache with focal neurologic signs, such as hemiparesis, hemisensory loss, or difficulty speaking. With a large hemorrhage, the patient will quickly become lethargic or comatose.

The most frequent locations for hemorrhage are the putamen (35%), thalamus (10%), caudate (5%), cerebral lobes (30%), cerebellum (15%), and pons (5%). These different locations cause distinct clinical presentations (Figure 117.5). Putaminal hemorrhages present with contralateral hemiparesis, hemisensory loss, aphasia if on the dominant side, and neglect if on the nondominant side. Thalamic hemorrhages usually have prominent sensory findings and vertical eye-movement abnormalities. Patients with cerebellar hemorrhages complain of acute onset of headache, nausea, vomiting, and difficulty walking. Large pontine hemorrhages can be devastating, causing acute quadriparesis, pinpoint pupils, and coma. Lobar hemorrhages produce variable neurologic signs depending on the brain region involved. Caudate hemorrhages usually cause headache, vomiting, confusion, and decreased short-term memory. They also may cause contralateral conjugate gaze paresis, hemiparesis, or hemisensory deficits.

Differential Diagnosis and Initial Evaluation

The differential diagnosis of ICH includes SAH, hypertensive encephalopathy, ischemic stroke, meningitis, encephalitis, subdural hematoma, epidural hematoma, migraine, or arterial dissection. Usually an accurate history and CT scan can easily determine the correct diagnosis.

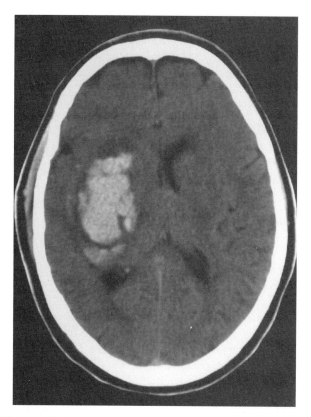

Figure 117.5 Intracranial hemorrhage. A large right basal ganglia hemorrhage with minimal (5 mm) midline shift. This patient presented with acute onset of lethargy, left hemiparesis, and left-sided neglect.

Multiple causes exist for ICH and vary depending on the age of the patient and location of the hemorrhage. Hypertension is the most common cause in most age groups. Putaminal hemorrhages, followed by cerebellar and pontine hemorrhages, are the most common hypertensive hemorrhages. Blood pressure is often acutely elevated after ICH, and therefore a careful history and evaluation must be performed in order to determine if premorbid hypertension existed.

One of the most common causes of lobar hemorrhages in elderly, normotensive patients is *amyloid angiopathy*. These patients often present with a series of lobar hemorrhages caused by deposits of β-amyloid in the media of the cerebral vessels. Definitive diagnosis is by brain biopsy or autopsy, and care is supportive. Other frequent causes in this age group include bleeding into a tumor, use of anticoagulation or thrombolytic agents, or hemorrhagic conversion of an ischemic stroke. The risk of a hemorrhagic complication with warfarin therapy increases with the length of time on the medication and with over-anticoagulation. Ten percent of ICHs are associated with warfarin or heparin therapy.

In younger patients, the differential diagnosis is extensive, including arteriovenous malformation, illicit-drug use (cocaine, amphetamines), sympathomimetic agents, vasculitis, trauma, cavernous angiomas, embolic stroke, neoplasm, Moyamoya disease, bleeding diathesis, and aneurysms. In general, if the patient is young and normotensive or the hemorrhage is in an unusual location, further evaluation with MRI and/or angiography is necessary to look for an atypical cause.

The initial evaluation, as with most severe neurologic injuries, begins with stabilization of airway, breathing, and circulation. Following this, a more thorough physical and neurologic examination can be performed and head CT without contrast rapidly obtained. The head CT identifies the location and size of hemorrhage, the presence of intraventricular extension, or hydrocephalus. Caution needs to be taken if looking for hemorrhages in the posterior fossa because CT scans can have unusual artifacts that may mask or mimic a hemorrhage in this location. A poor prognosis is seen in patients who are older, have a Glasgow Coma Scale score ≤8, or have volumes of hemorrhage >60 mL, increased blood pressure, intraventricular extension, or hydrocephalus.

Patients who have atypical or difficult-to-delineate lesions on head CT require an MRI or a cerebral angiogram. For instance, a tumor should be considered in any hemorrhage with unusual margins located in the gray-white junction. An MRI with contrast would best define this lesion as well as an arteriovenous malformation. If there is suspicion of an aneurysm, then a cerebral angiogram should be performed as soon as possible.

All patients require routine admission laboratory tests including a coagulation panel. Any coagulopathy should be rapidly corrected.

Indications for Hospitalization and ICU Admission

All patients with an ICH should be admitted to the hospital. Hemorrhages may continue to expand, and, therefore, all patients require close neurologic monitoring. Patients who present with evolving neurologic signs, lethargy, or coma require admission to the ICU. Other criteria include the need for an intraventricular catheter for hydrocephalus, evolving hydrocephalus on scan, cerebellar hemorrhage, electrocardiographic abnormalities, difficult-to-control blood pressure, or need for intubation. Ideally, these patients should be cared for at specialized centers that are more familiar with the early and late complications of this disease and the treatment options (10).

Indications for Early Neurosurgical Consultation

Neurosurgical evaluation is essential for all patients with cerebellar hemorrhage or hydrocephalus associated with any hemorrhage. The role of surgery for hemorrhages in other locations remains uncertain and varies considerably across centers. Patients frequently considered surgical candidates are younger patients who are deteriorating and have superficial hemorrhages. The decision to intervene should be made in close consultation with a neurosurgeon, who can also provide recommendations on timing and placement of an intraventricular catheter for hydrocephalus.

Issues During the Course of Hospitalization

Continued Bleeding

It has recently become apparent that ICH is not a discrete event; many hemorrhages continue to enlarge. In one study, about one-third of hemorrhages extended during the first hour after arrival at the hospital. This occurs more frequently in patients who present early and have large, irregular-shaped hemorrhages. No relationship with elevated blood pressure has been found. The use of recombinant activated Factor VII is currently being evaluated as a means of preventing hematoma enlargement.

Blood Pressure Control

Most patients who present with an ICH have elevated blood pressure. A balance must be sought between lowering elevated blood pressure that may place the patient at risk for further bleeding, cardiac ischemia, or congestive heart failure (CHF), and decreasing the blood pressure so much that cerebral ischemia is risked. Patients with a history of hypertension have altered autoregulation such that CBF falls at "normal" blood pressures and, therefore, are at risk for ischemia if the blood pressure is decreased too aggressively. Recent studies, however, indicate that modest reduction (15%) of blood pressure in hypertensive patients (mean arterial pressure of 120–150 mm Hg) did not lower cerebral blood flow and was therefore considered safe (11). Another report, however, pointed out that lowering blood pressure too rapidly and aggressively is harmful. With these factors in mind, blood pressure should be treated conservatively with modest reduction of pressure in hypertensive patients, but never below a mean pressure of 100 mm Hg. Labetolol, an α- and β-blocker, is ideal in this setting because it is easy to use and has no effect on ICP. Hydralazine or nicardipine may also be used. Medications such as sodium nitroprusside and nitrates should be avoided because they cause venodilation and elevate the ICP.

Hydrocephalus

Patients with ICH can present with hydrocephalus or develop it over the first few hours after presentation. Patients who are awake may complain of worsening headache, nausea, or vomiting. Signs of hydrocephalus include a decreased level of consciousness, impairment of upward gaze, and sixth nerve palsies. A head CT without contrast should be obtained and a neurosurgeon consulted if hydrocephalus is present. In patients with small hemorrhages, placement of an intraventricular catheter will allow for immediate drainage of CSF and for ICP monitoring. The need for permanent shunt placement will be determined by the neurosurgical consultant. In patients with large hemorrhage and hydrocephalus, the role of a ventriculostomy is much less certain. Mortality is this group is extremely high, and there is concern that a ventriculostomy could worsen midline shift.

Seizures

Approximately 10% of patients with ICH develop seizures, either generalized or focal. Patients with cortical hemorrhage or who present with seizures are often administered phenytoin, with levels maintained between 10–20 mg/dL. Those with posterior fossa or deep supratentorial bleeds are generally not treated with anticonvulsants unless they have a seizure. Long-term anti-epileptic therapy is determined case–by–case, weighing the risks and benefits. Patients with large cortical lesions, strokes, tumors, arteriovenous malformations, or recurrent seizures in the hospital are more likely to require long-term anti-epileptic therapy (Chapter 118).

Treatment of Elevated ICP

The guidelines outlined earlier in the chapter should be followed closely in patients with ICH and elevated ICP.

Surgical Management

Although there are several randomized studies showing no clear benefit of surgery in supratentorial ICH, the results of these studies vary somewhat, in part because of variations in the timing of surgery and location of the hemorrhage (12). Recent attempts at very early surgery have been complicated by high rates of rebleeding (13). New interest exists in investigating early stereotactic surgery in these patients. At present, however, the neurosurgeon carefully evaluates the location, size, and timing of neurologic decline for each patient before deciding on surgery.

There is clear benefit to *surgical removal of cerebeller hemorrhages*. Patients with mild deficits initially can rapidly worsen because of the close proximity of critical brainstem structures and the fourth ventricle. Therefore, prompt removal is recommended in patients with hemorrhages greater than 2–3 cm in diameter and altered sensorium. Good recovery is often seen even if a large portion of the cerebellum is removed.

General Medical Management

Medical management for ICH patients is similar to that for SAH or other brain injured patients. Attention needs to be focused on pulmonary toilet, deep venous thrombosis prophylaxis, gastrointestinal stress ulcer prophylaxis, and nutrition. These are reviewed in the previous section.

Discharge Issues

Patients who suffer an ICH larger than 60 mL, a thalamic hemorrhage greater than 3 cm in diameter, a pontine hemorrhage greater than 1 cm in diameter, or who are unconscious on presentation all have poor prognoses and a high mortality rate. The utility of these prognostic factors is somewhat open to question because many ICH patients have life-sustaining interventions withdrawn (14), possibly resulting in a self-fulfilling prophecy (15). Patients with smaller hemorrhages or lobar hemorrhages have a better prognosis and chance for functional recovery. Therefore, as for SAH patients, the rehabilitation team and social services need to be involved early.

SUBDURAL HEMATOMA

Subdural hematomas are hemorrhages located in the space between the arachnoid membrane and dura mater. The bleeding can be caused by damage to arteries or veins and usually occurs after a low-velocity head injury. Subdural hematomas are divided into acute, subacute, and chronic, depending on the time course (Figure 117.6). Acute subdural hematomas occur in approximately 10% of all head injuries and present within the first three days after injury. Subacute subdural hematomas present between days 4 and 20 after injury; chronic subdural hematomas present after 21 days.

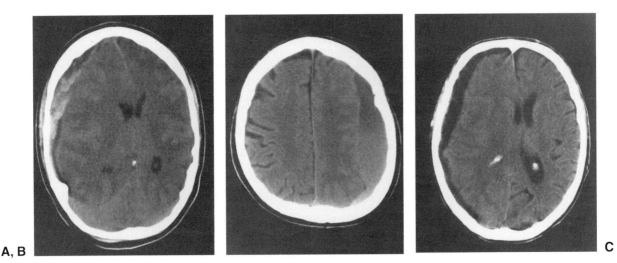

A, B

C

Figure 117.6 Head computed tomographic scan of acute-on-chronic, subacute, and chronic subdural hematomas. **A.** An acute-on-chronic subdural hematoma with significant midline shift over the right cerebral cortex. The bright signal abnormality within the lesion represents acute blood. **B.** A subacute subdural over the left hemisphere. At this stage the blood in some regions is becoming isodense with the brain parenchyma. **C:** The crescent-shaped hypodense region over the right cerebral hemisphere represents a chronic subdural hematoma. There is also a loss of cortical sulci adjacent to the hematoma and mild compression of the right lateral ventricle.

The majority of chronic subdural hematomas occur in patients older than age 50 because of damage to the bridging veins between the brain and dura mater that become more fragile with age. Thirty-five to 50% of these patients do not give a history of trauma. Predisposing factors for chronic subdural hematomas include chronic alcoholism, brain atrophy, CSF shunts, seizure disorders, coagulopathies, warfarin use, and liver disease.

Issues at the Time of Admission

Clinical Presentation

Subdural hematomas can have a variety of different clinical presentations and therefore can be easily missed; this occurs in up to 40% of patients. Patients with acute subdural hematomas often have a history of trauma. If large, the patient may experience rapid neurologic deterioration, with a decreased level of consciousness and progressive focal neurologic signs caused by the hematoma's mass effect.

Most subdural hematomas result from damage to veins, and therefore the patient may present with an insidious onset of nonspecific symptoms. Eighty percent of patients with chronic subdural hematomas complain of headache, while up to 50% present with hemiparesis and roughly 10% with seizures. Gait disturbances, nausea, vomiting, memory impairment, dysphagia, confusion, lethargy, and urinary incontinence are other common presenting symptoms. Papilledema can be found in up to 25% of patients.

Occasionally a chronic subdural hematoma may become extremely large, despite minimal neurologic signs or symptoms. As the patient's intracranial compliance decreases, rapid onset of neurologic decompensation can occur, requiring immediate intervention.

Differential Diagnosis and Initial Evaluation

The differential diagnosis includes stroke, transient ischemic attack, meningitis, encephalitis, tumor, hydrocephalus, dementia, abscess, and other processes that may increase ICP. The initial evaluation includes assessment of airway, breathing, and circulation. Once stable, the patient who is suspected of having a subdural hematoma requires a head CT without contrast. If the hematoma is acute, the hemorrhage appears bright. Subacute lesions may have a focus of bright signal with acute blood and a surrounding isodense or hypodense area representing older blood. Occasionally, hemorrhages are entirely isodense relative to brain and very difficut to detect; a CT with contrast or MRI is required. Chronic subdurals are particularly likely to appear hypodense on head CT and therefore difficult to see (Figure 117.6). Radiographic clues include loss of cortical sulci, midline shift, or compression of the lateral ventricle. Along with appropriate imaging, patients with subdural hematomas require basic admission laboratory studies, including metabolic profiles and coagulation studies.

Indications for Hospitalization and Intensive Care Unit Admission

Patients with subdural hematomas should always be admitted to the hospital for observation, evaluation, and management, but not all need to be admitted to the ICU.

Patients with a decreased level of consciousness, rapidly changing neurologic examination, significant midline shift, hydrocephalus, electrocardiographic changes, cardiac arrhythmias, or signs of increased ICP and those requiring intubation should be admitted to the ICU. In addition, some patients undergo bedside drainage of their subdural hematomas in the ICU.

Indications for Early Consultation

All patients with subdural hematomas require a neurosurgical evaluation to address acute management and surgical options. Patients who present with acute subdural hematomas require immediate evaluation by the neurosurgeon in the emergency room; worse outcomes are seen if there is a delay between the initial incident and surgery.

Initial Therapy

Most patients with an acute subdural hematoma should have their blood evacuated immediately. Patients with elevated ICP should be treated as outlined previously. Those with stable neurologic examinations may be observed closely in the ICU or on the floor, with frequent neurologic examinations and monitoring of the vital signs. Triage of these patients should be performed in collaboration with the neurosurgical team. Any patient with a coagulopathy should have it quickly corrected.

Issues During the Course of Hospitalization

Surgical Drainage

Some patients with chronic subdural hematomas and minimal neurologic deficits can be managed conservatively, guided by serial head CT scans. Most patients with abnormal neurologic examinations require surgical intervention. The hematoma can be evacuated either through a burr hole or craniotomy in the operating room. For less complicated chronic hematomas, some surgeons may opt to perform a twist-drill craniostomy procedure under a local anesthetic. A catheter, attached to a collection bag, is placed in the subdural space for drainage of the liquefied hematoma. Patients who undergo this procedure require frequent neurologic assessments and must lie flat for the duration of drainage, which usually lasts 1–2 days. This may present a problem in patients with congestive heart failure or severe chronic obstructive pulmonary disease. Most patients treated with an indwelling drain are given prophylactic antibiotics.

Common complications of these procedures include ICH, reaccumulation of the hematoma, seizures, empyema formation, and pneumocephalus. If the patient requires ICU care or has severe neurologic deficits, they also may be at risk for nosocomial pneumonia, deep venous thrombosis, or stress ulcers.

Seizures

Seizures are relatively uncommon in patients with chronic subdural hematomas (less than 10%). However, some series show a higher risk of seizures after surgical intervention, and therefore most patients who undergo surgical evacuation of the hematoma receive anticonvulsants for at least one week. Patients with a seizure history before the subdural may suffer an increase in seizure frequency after surgical evacuation; long-term therapeutic antiepileptic treatment is recommended (Chapter 118).

Discharge Issues

Discharge issues for these patients are similar to those discussed for SAH and ICH.

COST CONSIDERATIONS AND RESOURCE USE

A financial analysis that reviewed use of hospital resources in the treatment of cerebral aneurysms found that the average cost of treatment of a patient who developed vasospasm at an academic medical center was $38,400. The highest areas of hospital cost were identified as the ICU bed (29%) and angiography (10.3%), followed by medical supplies (9.6%) and hospital-ward bed (6%). Surprisingly, the cost of the surgery (3.7%) and the multiple CT scans (2%) were ranked relatively low. Strategies suggested to reduce the cost of treatment included (a) developing better means of predicting which patients will develop vasospasm to facilitate early transfer out of the ICU; (b) developing alternative areas outside the ICU to monitor patients for vasospasm; and (c) critically investigating the efficacy of intra-arterial infusions of papaverine to potentially reduce the utilization of angiograms. The prolonged period of risk for vasospasm precludes attempts to shorten overall length of hospital stay. The total cost of caring for patients with ICH in academic medical centers is reported to average more than $25,000 because of long lengths of stay. One motivation for the use of bedside twist-drill craniostomy in treating subdural hematomas was to reduce the total cost by eliminating operating room and anesthesia costs. This, however, is offset by a longer ICU stay. Further study is warranted.

KEY POINTS

- Initial management of all patients with intracranial bleeding or elevated ICP should address airway, breathing, and circulation.
- If elevated ICP or intracranial bleeding are suspected, an emergent head CT should be obtained as soon as airway, breathing, and circulation have been addressed.

- All patients with suspected elevated ICP should be given immediate empiric therapy with mannitol.
- Early neurosurgical consultation is needed in all subarachnoid, subdural, epidural, and cerebellar hemorrhages and ICH associated with hydrocephalus.
- The major complications of aneurysmal SAH are rebleeding, hydrocephalus, and vasospasm.
- Patients with severe brain injury require pulmonary toilet, nutritional support, deep venous thrombosis prophylaxis, stress-ulcer prophylaxis, and a multidisciplinary approach to rehabilitation and discharge planning.

REFERENCES

1. Paczynski RP. Osmotherapy: basic concepts and controversies. *Crit Care Clin* 1997;13:105–129.
2. Edlow JA, Caplan LR. Avoiding pitfalls in the diagnosis of subarachnoid hemorrhage. *N Engl J Med* 2000;342:29–36.
3. Kraus JJ, Metzler MD, Coplin WM. Critical care issues in stroke and subarachnoid hemorrhage. *Neurol Res* 2002;24(Suppl 1):S47–S57.
4. Deibert E, Barzilai B, Braverman A, et al. The clinical significance of elevated Troponin I in patients with nontraumatic subarachnoid hemorrhage. *J Neurosurg* 2003;98:741–746.
5. Molyneux A, Kerr R, Stratton I, et al. International Subarachnoid Aneurysm Trial (ISAT) of neurosurgical clipping versus endovascular coiling in 2143 patients with ruptured intracranial aneurysms: a randomised trial. *Lancet* 2002;360:1267–1274.
6. Aiyagari V, Cross DT, Deibert E, et al. Safety of hemodynamic augmentation in patients treated with Guglielmi detachable coils after acute aneurysmal subarachnoid hemorrhage. *Stroke* 2001; 32:1994–1997.
7. Lennihan L, Mayer SA, Fink ME, et al. Effect of hypervolemic therapy on cerebral blood flow after subarachnoid hemorrhage: a randomized controlled trial. *Stroke* 2000;31:383–391.
8. Muizelaar JP, Zwienenberg M, Rudisill NA, et al. The prophylactic use of transluminal balloon angioplasty in patients with Fisher grade 3 subarachnoid hemorrhage: a pilot study. *J Neurosurg* 1999;91:51–58.
9. Qureshi AI, Tuhrim S, Broderick JP, et al. Spontaneous intracerebral hemorrhage. *N Engl J Med* 2001;344:1450–1460.
10. Diringer MN, Edwards DF. Admission to a neurologic/neurosurgical intensive care unit is associated with reduced mortality rate after intracerebral hemorrhage. *Crit Care Med* 2001; 29:635– 640.
11. Powers WJ, Zazulia AR, Videen TO, et al. Autoregulation of cerebral blood flow surrounding acute (6 to 22 hours) intracerebral hemorrhage. *Neurology* 2001;57:18–24.
12. Fernandes HM, Gregson B, Siddique S, et al. Surgery in intracerebral hemorrhage: the uncertainty continues. *Stroke* 2000;31: 2511–2516.
13. Morgenstern LB, Demchuk AM, Kim DH, et al. Rebleeding leads to poor outcome in ultra-early craniotomy for intracerebral hemorrhage. *Neurology* 2001;56:1294–1299.
14. Diringer MN, Edwards DF, Aiyagari V, et al. Factors associated with withdrawal of mechanical ventilation in a neurology/neurosurgery intensive care unit. *Crit Care Med* 2001;29: 1792–1797.
15. Becker KJ, Baxter AB, Cohen WA, et al. Withdrawal of support in intracerebral hemorrhage may lead to self-fulfilling prophecies. *Neurology* 2001;56:766–772.

ADDITIONAL READING

Bradley W, Daroff RB, Fenichel GM, et al. *Neurology in Clinical Practice,* 4th ed. Stoneham, MA: Butterworth-Heinemann, 2004.

MacDonald R.L., Weir B. *Cerebral Vasospasm.* New York: Thieme Medical Publishers, 2004.

Ropper A. *Neurological and Neurosurgical Intensive Care,* 4th ed. Philadelphia: Raven Press, 2003.

Wijdicks E. *The Clinical Practice of Critical Care Neurology,* 2nd ed. Philadelphia: Lippincott-Raven Press, 2003.

Youmans JR. *Neurological Surgery,* 5th ed. Philadelphia: WB Saunders, 2004.

Seizures

118

Paul A. Garcia

SCOPE OF THE PROBLEM

Seizures are a common neurological problem; the lifetime risk for having a seizure is approximately 10%. A seizure occurs when a group of neurons fires aberrantly, resulting in a convulsion, behavioral arrest, focal movement, or sensory disturbance—the manifestations depend upon the neural circuitry and the region of brain involved. Seizures may be caused by almost any type of brain injury and many metabolic disturbances. A diagnosis of *epilepsy* implies that a person has a chronic, inherent predisposition toward seizures rather than a transient alteration in the seizure threshold that might occur during a fever or metabolic disturbance. For example, a patient who has a seizure from cocaine toxicity can prevent future seizures by abstaining from further cocaine use, and thus does not have epilepsy. On the other hand, if a patient has a cocaine-related stroke and seizures persist despite abstinence from cocaine, epilepsy is present, and chronic treatment with anticonvulsant medications is necessary. The prevalence of epilepsy is about 0.5%, and the lifetime risk of developing epilepsy is about 3% (1). Although any given seizure typically resolves without sequelae, approximately 25% of patients with epilepsy eventually die as a direct consequence of their condition because of accidents, sudden unexplained death in epilepsy ("SUDEP"), or continuous seizures (status epilepticus). Prompt and complete seizure control is necessary to limit a person's risk.

Because seizures are even more common in acutely ill patients and epilepsy is often exacerbated by acute illness, all hospital-based clinicians will be called on to evaluate and treat patients with these problems. In this chapter, the evaluation and treatment of hospitalized patients with seizures and epilepsy will be reviewed.

ESTABLISHING THE DIAGNOSIS

Did the patient really have a seizure? Syncope, psychogenic seizures, sleep disorders, movement disorders, stroke, and migraine can all be mistaken for epileptic seizures. Syncope and psychogenic seizures are the most common mimics. Because the evaluation and treatment of these conditions is much different than for epileptic seizures, it is imperative that a distinction be made. This requires a working knowledge of the common clinical features of the epileptic seizures (Table 118.1), as well as the features of seizure mimics.

Clinical Features of Generalized Seizures

Generalized seizures arise diffusely over both hemispheres. The most common etiologies include metabolic disturbances, inherited disorders that affect neuronal excitability, diffuse brain injuries, and disorders of cortical development. The most commonly encountered generalized seizure type is the *tonic-clonic* seizure. During a tonic-clonic seizure, the entire brain participates in an extremely rapid discharge of neurons, leading to tonic extension of all the muscles lasting for a few seconds. The massive excitatory discharges activate inhibitory cells in the thalamus, which produces a feedback inhibition. Soon the seizure enters a phase of alternating bursts of discharge followed by synchronized inhibitory activity. Clinically this is seen as the clonic phase, in which the extremities may have rhythmic jerking with alternating contraction and relaxation. Typically, at the end of the clonic phase, there are a few final jerks, and then the patient lies unconscious, limp, and exhausted. Post-ictal lethargy and confusion may last minutes-to-days.

Diffuse cortical firing can also be modulated by different circuitry, resulting in other generalized seizure types. *Absence seizures* are most common in children but can be seen in adults. An absence seizure is a brief cessation of movement, sometimes with minor rhythmic motions, such as eyelid fluttering. The usual duration of an absence seizure is less than 10 seconds. *Myoclonic seizures* involve rapid, sudden contraction of a group of muscles, which can be in the extremities, trunk, or neck. These may be unilateral or

TABLE 118.1

MODIFIED INTERNATIONAL CLASSIFICATION OF EPILEPTIC SEIZURES

Generalized seizures (generalized-onset)

Tonic-clonic
Absence
Myoclonic
Atonic
Tonic

Partial seizures (focal, localization-related, focal-onset)

Simple partial (no impairment of consciousness)
   Motor
   Sensory (somatic, visual, olfactory, auditory)
   Psychic (dèjá vu, derealization, fear, etc.)
   Autonomic (sweating, gastric sensations, etc.)
Complex partial (consciousness impaired)
Partial seizure secondarily generalized

bilateral. A patient with myoclonic seizures may have involvement on the right side on one occasion and the left side on another; however, the disorder is usually a generalized one. Tonic and atonic seizures result in sudden stiffening or loss of tone, respectively. As might be expected, the major morbidity related to these seizures is from falls.

Clinical Features of Partial (Focal) Seizures

Most adults with new seizures caused by a structural brain abnormality will have partial seizures. Partial seizures that remain confined to small brain areas and thus do not impair consciousness are called *simple partial seizures*. The symptoms of a simple partial seizure depend on the part of the brain in which it arises. Simple partial seizures arising in the motor cortex produce rhythmic jerking of the face or an arm or leg. Simple partial seizures arising in the occipital (visual) cortex produce visual hallucinations. Although these simple partial seizures are easy to identify as such, seizures that arise from multimodal or association brain areas give rise to more complicated symptoms. Simple partial seizures arising from the temporal lobes are the most heterogeneous and can produce a wide range of symptoms, including dèjá vu, a sudden unexplained fear of impending doom, or a poorly defined feeling of altered thinking. Frontal lobe simple partial seizures may be even more bizarre and can include features such as asymmetric bilateral posturing and pelvic thrusting. Since many physicians are unfamiliar with these symptoms, partial seizures of temporal or frontal lobe origin often are misdiagnosed as psychogenic seizures.

A partial seizure that spreads to involve enough brain tissue to produce impairment of consciousness is called a *complex partial seizure*. Generally, this requires involvement of bilateral areas of the brain, most often in the temporal lobes. There may or may not be a simple partial phase (aura) to the complex partial seizure, so the seizures may begin with or without a warning sensation. The most common behaviors seen during complex partial seizures are a brief blank stare, an arrest of motion, and failure to respond meaningfully to surrounding events. Automatic, stereotyped behaviors (automatisms) are common. Partial seizures can spread diffusely, causing a convulsion (*secondarily generalized tonic-clonic seizure*). The spread can be so rapid that the attack is clinically indistinguishable from a tonic-clonic seizure that begins diffusely. Thus, tonic-clonic seizures should still be considered possible evidence of a focal brain abnormality. In patients presenting with tonic-clonic seizures, the patient should be questioned about the presence of common warnings that might suggest a focal onset, such as an epigastric sensation, dèjá vu, an olfactory hallucination, or another sensory symptom. Todd's paralysis or other focal post-ictal dysfunction also suggest a focal onset.

Clinical Features of Seizure Mimics

Syncope is the most common seizure mimic. Although prominent motor manifestations and post-ictal lethargy sometimes allow differentiation of seizures from syncope, these features are often over emphasized. Syncope may be accompanied by behavioral arrest, myoclonic movements, or a convulsion. Seizures may be brief, without movements and post-ictal confusion. Premonitory symptoms and the clinical setting are more consistently helpful in making the distinction. In contrast to the focal symptoms that initiate a partial seizure, syncope is typically heralded by light-headedness, graying of vision, tinnitus, diaphoresis, and nausea. The importance of the clinical context cannot be overstated. When an otherwise healthy patient suffers a convulsion during phlebotomy, it is quite likely because of convulsive syncope. On the other hand, a patient presenting similarly but with acute hyponatremia most likely has had a seizure.

Psychogenic seizures can also be confused with epileptic seizures. The often-used synonym, pseudoseizures, has fallen out of favor because it may cause patients to infer that conscious "faking" is suspected by their physicians. Although the prevalence of psychogenic seizures is probably not high, disproportionate numbers of patients with psychogenic seizures will be encountered in the hospital because anticonvulsant medications fail to control the seizures. Among patients labeled as having "epilepsy" and whose seizures are not controlled with anticonvulsant medications, as many as 25% have psychogenic seizures. A history of psychiatric problems does not strongly suggest a diagnosis of psychogenic seizures, because patients with epilepsy and brain injury also have an increased incidence of psychiatric disturbances. Prolonged, asynchronous, waxing, and waning motor activity may lead one to suspect psychogenic seizures.

Often it can be determined whether a patient has had a seizure based on the clinical information. Electroencephalography (EEG) and imaging may also be helpful if the diagnosis remains unclear. The sensitivity of the routine EEG for epileptiform discharges is about 40%. An estimated 1%–2% the general population has epileptiform abnormalities. Thus, the positive predictive value will be high if there is a reasonable prior probability of a seizure (Chapter 6). For example, in a patient being evaluated for seizure versus syncope, a positive EEG could raise the probability that the attack was a seizure from 50% to >95%. Given the low sensitivity of EEG, however, a negative study does not exclude the possibility of seizures. As with EEG, the presence of a potentially epileptogenic lesion on brain imaging strongly supports the possibility of seizure, but a negative study is not helpful.

ACUTE MANAGEMENT OF SEIZURES

Because most seizures are self-limited, *the first rule for treating discrete seizures is to do no harm.* The most important action for a health care worker is to position the person to prevent aspiration or orthopedic injury. Aspiration risk can be lowered by turning the patient on his side. Arterial blood gas studies are likely to demonstrate hypoxia and a mixed acidosis. Post-ictal hypoxia and hypoventilation are not usually indications for intubation because they resolve quickly. The acidosis also resolves spontaneously and does not require aggressive treatment. Aspiration pneumonia is a potential complication of convulsions, but there is no evidence that intubation to "protect the airway" reduces this risk.

Tonic-Clonic Status Epilepticus

In contrast to isolated seizures, *status epilepticus* is a medical emergency (2). Until recently, most experts have used an arbitrary seizure duration of 30 minutes for a working definition of status epilepticus. Recently, analysis of isolated seizures suggests that the vast majority of tonic-clonic seizures terminate spontaneously in less than two minutes (3). Therefore, a practical definition of convulsive status epilepticus might be any tonic-clonic seizure that persists long enough for intravenous medications to be prepared for injection. Status epilepticus has an annual incidence in the United States of somewhere between 40,000 and 100,000 cases. Status epilepticus can be caused by any of the factors that cause discrete seizures, and the morbidity and mortality are largely determined by the underlying cause. A long duration of seizure activity is also associated with poorer outcomes.

Systemic morbidity from *tonic-clonic* status epilepticus may be related to transient hypertension, hypotension, hypoglycemia, hypoventilation, hyperpyrexia, or rhabdomyolysis. Drugs used to treat status can cause hypotension, arrhythmias, hepatic dysfunction, and ileus. During prolonged recovery, comatose patients may develop deep venous thrombosis, decubitus ulcers, and aspiration. Neurological morbidity from status epilepticus may be exacerbated by these medical complications but may occur even

if they are not present, perhaps because of excitotoxic injury from ongoing abnormal neuronal firing.

Treatment of status epilepticus should be prompt and well-organized (4). Standard treatment protocols have been shown to result in improved outcomes. One suggested protocol is shown in Figure 118.1. The "ABCs" (airway, breathing, and circulation) come first. Routine laboratory studies should be drawn and sent at the same time that intravenous access is established. Blood glucose level should be measured using a fingerstick kit. Glucose and thiamine should be given rapidly if warranted. Computed tomography may be performed early in the course of the evaluation but should not delay anticonvulsant therapy.

Drug treatment of status epilepticus should be aimed at rapid cessation of seizure activity. Benzodiazepines are the first-line therapy, because of their broad spectrum of action, ability to be administered rapidly, and rapid onset of action. *Lorazepam* redistributes out of the brain less rapidly than diazepam and therefore has a more sustained anticonvulsant effect (5). The recommended dose of lorazepam is 0.1 mg/kg intravenously. The chief drawbacks of the benzodiazepines are a brief duration of action, sedation, and respiratory depression.

Because the benzodiazepines will not have a prolonged effect, *phenytoin* or *fosphenytoin* also should be given promptly. The recommended initial dose is 20 mg/kg intravenously. If seizures persist, an additional 10 mg/kg can be given intravenously. The "therapeutic range" quoted by laboratories is irrelevant for patients with status epilepticus; terminating the seizure is far more important than avoiding mild dose-related toxicities such as sedation, tremor, and ataxia. Levels up to 30 mg/dL may be useful. Phenytoin should be administered as fosphenytoin, a phenytoin prodrug, unless the preparation is not available. In contrast to phenytoin, fosphenytoin is water-soluble and does not require propylene glycol as a solvent. Because much of the cardiovascular toxicity of intravenous phenytoin therapy is related to this vehicle, fosphenytoin can be administered rapidly (up to 150 mg/min rather than 50 mg/min) with less risk of cardiovascular or local tissue toxicity. Because phenytoin has intrinsic cardiovascular effects, continuous electrocardiographic and blood pressure monitoring are recommended during administration of either preparation. Fosphenytoin is labeled in "phenytoin equivalents" so that there is no need to convert the dose based upon the molecular weights of the preparations. For the phenytoin-allergic patient, administration of another intravenous medication is necessary. Phenobarbital and valproate are potential candidates, with the latter having the advantage of being structurally distinct from phenytoin (making an allergic reaction very unlikely). Valproate is not associated with cardiovascular or respiratory side effects, thus allowing a very rapid infusion (as little as 5–10 minutes for a loading dose of 20 mg/kg).

If the seizures do not stop with the administration of first-line, intravenous anticonvulsants, general anesthesia

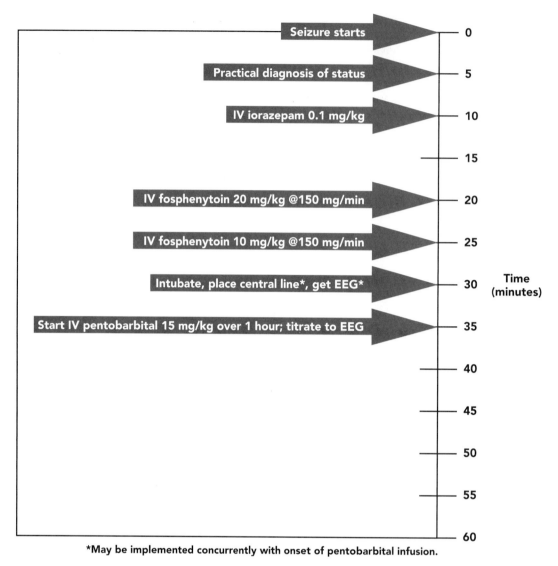

*May be implemented concurrently with onset of pentobarbital infusion.

Figure 118.1 A protocol for management of status epilepticus. Arrows indicate the time at which the intervention should be completed. Treatment should progress until clinical and EEG seizures abate. Acceptable alternatives include: (1) IV phenobarbital before starting general anesthesia; (2) Propofol (in adults) or midazolam in place of pentobarbital

should be initiated promptly. Pentobarbital, midazolam, and propofol are commonly used in this setting. If the patient has not yet been intubated, this should be done, and a central line must be placed. Pressors are typically required to maintain blood pressure. Following a loading dose, the anesthetic agent is titrated under EEG monitoring until seizures stop and a burst-suppression pattern is achieved. The optimum depth and duration of anesthesia is unknown. Typically, deeper, more-prolonged anesthesia is tried if initial measures fail.

Unless the seizures abate promptly and the patient improves neurologically, EEG is necessary to manage patients in status epilepticus. It is also needed at times to confirm the diagnosis. Some patients with psychogenic seizures have been intubated and anesthetized, with all of the attendant risks, before clinicians confirmed the true diagnosis. EEG is also necessary to exclude ongoing seizure activity after the movements stop. Thus, EEG is always indicated in patients

who have been pharmacologically paralyzed to facilitate intubation or to treat hyperpyrexia, hypertension, or rhabdomyolysis. EEG may also provide prognostic information. Finally, as noted above, EEG is necessary to measure the depth of anesthesia when treating refractory status epilepticus.

Non-Convulsive Status Epilepticus

Tonic-clonic status epilepticus is a dramatic condition that comes to medical attention immediately. Patients may also have subtle, continuous, non-convulsive seizure activity. It is important to distinguish the different forms of non-convulsive status epilepticus because their treatments are very different. Absence status can occur in adults or children who have discrete, absence seizures. It is characterized by a prolonged twilight state with variably altered consciousness. Absence status is not clearly harmful; recovery is almost instantaneous after the seizure activity abates. Thus, therapy should not expose the patient to risks that would be acceptable for treating convulsive status. Simple partial status is characterized by retained consciousness with restricted continuous focal seizure activity, such as tremulous movement of one arm. Episodes sometimes are precipitated by severe hyperglycemia (*epilepsia partialis continua*) and may respond to glucose control. Simple partial status can be very resistant to treatment and may persist for months-to-years. Complex partial status may be a difficult clinical diagnosis, often presenting with fluctuating encephalopathy or behavioral disturbance. The neurological sequelae of simple and complex partial status depend largely on the amount of tissue involved and the duration of the seizure activity. Patients with simple partial status rarely have lasting consequences. Patients with complex partial status may develop mild-to-moderate neurological deficits if the seizure activity lasts for more than a few days. Although partial status should be treated aggressively with anticonvulsants, general anesthesia is typically not necessary. Another form of non-convulsive status can be seen in patients who initially have tonic-clonic seizures that eventually seem to stop. The sole clinical feature may be failure to return to baseline function. At times, subtle motor manifestations such as eye or mouth twitching may be present. EEG is necessary to confirm the diagnosis and guide treatment. The treatment in this setting is with anticonvulsants or anesthetic agents, with the goal of abolishing both clinical and electroencephalographic seizure activity.

Preventing Status Epilepticus

Given the severe consequences of status epilepticus, prevention is highly desirable. Patients at risk for recurrent seizures, especially those with a history of status epilepticus or seizure clustering, should be offered *rescue medications* to be used to interrupt seizure clusters and abort prolonged seizures. Options include lorazepam 1 mg sublingual, diazepam 10–20 mg rectal gel, and midazolam 10 mg intravenous solution (2 cc) administered by syringe into the mouth. The later two options can be administered by a family member while the patient is having a seizure. Although rescue medications clearly abort seizure clusters, the evidence that they impact status epilepticus is less direct. Nevertheless, since rescue medications have gained increased acceptance and early treatment of seizures has extended beyond the emergency room to paramedics (4), the incidence of status epilepticus as a discharge diagnosis has fallen steadily in California over the last decade (6).

EVALUATION OF THE PATIENT WITH SEIZURES

New Onset Seizures

The evaluation of a new seizure is different than for a recurrent seizure in someone who already is known to have epilepsy. For the patient with a new seizure, the most important question is *whether the seizure is caused by an identifiable underlying cause*. Emergency diagnoses that need to be considered include acute metabolic disturbances, intoxications (including the patient's regular medications [7]), stroke, intracerebral hemorrhage, meningitis, and encephalitis. Complete blood count, glucose, electrolytes, renal function, liver enzymes, calcium, and magnesium should be checked. A urine toxicology screen should be ordered if an obvious cause is not found on the initial evaluation. Accurate diagnosis of the etiology has immediate treatment implications in some cases, as shown in Table 118.2.

If a metabolic cause for new seizures is not identified, brain imaging and EEG should be considered. While many patients will require both studies, a rational approach based on the likely causes in children and adults is possible. Because the most common definable etiology in children is a genetic seizure predisposition, EEG should be considered first in neurologically intact children with new seizures, unless there is clinical suspicion for an acute neurological process that requires immediate imaging. *Adults rarely have new seizures on a purely genetic basis.* Imaging should be ordered first, because a positive study often makes the EEG superfluous. In children and adults, the complementary study should be ordered if the initial study is unrevealing.

Magnetic resonance imaging (MRI) is superior to computed tomography (CT) for defining almost all possible structural seizure etiologies. CT is often ordered acutely in the emergency room to exclude acute neurological etiologies, such as infections or strokes. Follow-up for these patients should include MRI to define subtle lesions, including tumors and cortical malformations, that are often missed on CT.

Patients with Established Epilepsy

When a patient with epilepsy has seizures, the main concern (after the patient becomes medically stable) is determining the reason for anticonvulsant failure. The two possible reasons are an inadequate amount of medication or an inadequate medication effect.

Reasons for an inadequate amount of medication include prescribing doses that are too low, adherence problems, and altered bioavailability of the medication. A common mistake made by physicians is to base the dose of medicine on the serum "therapeutic range." In fact, many patients require higher levels to optimize protection, and they can achieve such levels without suffering side effects. Serum anticonvulsant levels are most helpful when physicians help patients find their individualized "therapeutic level" that reflects the amount of medicine that can be taken without dose-related, neurological side effects. Common reasons for patients taking less than the prescribed dose include forgetfulness, frustration with side effects, and/or lack of efficacy. Altered medication absorption, metabolism, or clearance should be sus-

TABLE 118.2

SEIZURES REQUIRING SPECIAL TREATMENT CONSIDERATIONS

Etiology	Treatment consideration
Alcohol withdrawal	Phenytoin ineffective, benzodiazepines indicated
Illicit drugs	Cocaine, amphetamines, and phencyclidine commonly cause seizures; marijuana and hallucinogens rarely, if ever, cause seizures (the latter drugs should not be considered likely precipitants)
Medications	
Isoniazid	Anticonvulsants ineffective; treat with IV pyridoxine or benzodiazepines if pyridoxine not available
Theophylline, tricyclic antidepressants	Seizures may be refractory to anticonvulsants without hemodialysis
β-lactam and flouroquinolone antibiotics	Benzodiazepines likely superior to phenytoin
Flumazenil	Seizures likely in patients on benzodiazepines plus pro-convulsant medicines
Cyclosporin, tacrolimus	Seizures represent dose-related toxicity, associated with posterior leukoencephalopathy
Meperidine, tramadol	Naloxone may exacerbate seizures
Foscarnet	May require calcium or magnesium
Electrolyte disturbance	
Hyponatremia	Correct hyponatremia judiciously to avoid pontine myelinolysis
Hypernatremia	Seizures occur during treatment because of cerebral edema
Hypocalcemia, hypomagnesemia	May temporize with anticonvulsants, correct imbalance
Hypo- and hyperglycemia	Partial seizures common; test fingerstick for hypoglycemia at presentation, correct imbalance
Renal failure	Free levels of protein-bound medicines (valproate, phenytoin) underestimated by standard lab tests; medicines with significant renal clearance (gabapentin, levetiracetam, oxcarbazepine, topiramate) require dose adjustment
Hepatic failure	Seizures often caused by other metabolic abnormality or medicine
Porphyria	Avoid enzyme-inducing anticonvulsants; levetiracetam and gabapentin preferred
Hypertensive encephalopathy	Short-term use of anticonvulsants may help stop seizures (thereby decreasing blood pressure)
Eclampsia	Magnesium sulfate superior to anticonvulsants

IV, intravenous.

pected when a patient who has had well-controlled epilepsy suddenly starts having seizures. This is a common occurrence in growing children. It also occurs when patients have changes in thyroid, hepatic, or renal function. Medication interactions can also lead to altered metabolism of anticonvulsants. Vomiting or diarrhea may change absorption of the medication, resulting in lowered serum levels.

If declining anticonvulsant levels do not explain a patient's seizures, other reasons for lack of medication efficacy should be considered. Most importantly, the clinician should ask if the medication is known to be effective for the patient's type of seizures. All available medications (except ethosuximide) have demonstrated efficacy for treating partial seizures and tonic-clonic seizures. Patients with generalized, non-convulsive seizures (absence, myoclonic, and atonic seizures) often have poor seizure control or even exacerbation of their seizures with "narrow spectrum" medications such as phenytoin and carbamazepine. "Broad spectrum" medications, such as valproate, lamotrigine, topiramate, and zonisamide, can be effective for all types of seizures (1). Other reasons for lack of medication efficacy relate to patient-specific factors that make seizures more difficult to control, including sleep deprivation, drug use, seizure-inducing medications, infections, and metabolic disturbances. If a patient has had good seizure control and one of these precipitants is present but can be addressed, the patient may not need to have a change in medication to achieve good control again.

TREATMENT CONSIDERATIONS

Deciding Whether to Use Anticonvulsants

Treatment for patients with provoked seizures involves treating the causative event. The temperature should be lowered in patients with febrile seizures, glucose should be given for hypoglycemia-induced seizures, and drug detoxification programs should be considered for patients with seizures related to illicit drug use. Sometimes, the provocative factor requires transient treatment with an anticonvulsant. For example, ethanol withdrawal seizures require treatment with benzodiazepines to prevent status epilepticus and delirium tremens (Chapter 122).

The decision to treat new, unprovoked seizures is based on the risk of recurrence weighed against the potential for medication side effects. If a patient has had more than one unprovoked seizure, the risk for recurrence is extremely high and anticonvulsant medication is warranted in most cases. Thus, in a patient presenting with a "new" seizure, a history suggesting prior seizures (including unrecognized simple partial seizures) should prompt anticonvulsant treatment. When a patient has had only one unprovoked seizure, the decision to start anticonvulsants is less clear. In the past, non-randomized studies suggested little benefit in this setting. Recently, randomized studies have shown that taking an anticonvulsant decreases the risk for recurrence by half, but does not change the person's underlying predisposition for seizures (i.e., the person has the same risk for seizures when they taper off medicine in the future) (8). This relatively modest benefit may still be worth potential side effects for some adults, especially those at high risk for recurrence (those with structural brain damage and/or EEG abnormalities).

Social considerations are sometimes important as well. Patients involved in high risk activities, such as driving or working with machinery, may choose to do everything possible to decrease the risk of a seizure recurrence. Most of these social considerations are not relevant for children. Additionally, school-aged children may be especially bothered by cognitive or behavioral medication side effects. Thus, children are rarely treated for a single seizure.

Occasionally, patients at risk for seizures may be treated with anticonvulsants, even if they have not yet had a seizure. For example, patients with acute neurological injuries are at increased risk for seizures. There is some evidence from patients with acute, closed-head injuries that short-term prophylaxis with phenytoin reduces the risk of acute seizures, though it does not change the long-term risk. Especially for patients in whom seizure-associated intracranial pressure or blood pressure elevations might be devastating (e.g., patients at risk for herniation or rebleeding after aneurysmal rupture), short-term prophylaxis is often undertaken, despite the lack of evidence to support this choice (Chapters 116 and 117).

Patients Requiring Anticonvulsants

The bewildering number of anticonvulsants speaks to the imperfect nature of the medications. Even so, most patients with epilepsy are able to gain control of their seizures. Studies show little-to-no difference in efficacy between medications, provided that the appropriate medication is being used for a given seizure type (1). Thus, the decision to start with a given medication may be based on potential side effects, pharmacokinetic considerations, and price. A detailed description of the individual agents is beyond the scope of this chapter, but Table 118.3 lists key attributes of commonly used antiepileptic drugs.

If a patient with epilepsy has seizures caused by a drop in anticonvulsant level, care should be taken before adjusting the chronic dosage of the medicine. Low levels resulting from missed doses should be addressed by finding out why the patient misses doses, not by increasing the ordered dose. Low levels resulting from drug interactions or medical problems (e.g., diarrhea) require attention to the underlying problem. In the hospital, patients may have anticonvulsant levels fall because of the inability to take medications orally. When this becomes an issue, consideration should be given to replacing the dose with intravenous medicine until the patient can take an adequate dose of the regular medicine. If a medication change is required, a general rule is to adjust the dosage using the smallest available increment. Since phenytoin exhibits non-linear kinetics, small adjustments in dosage may result in large changes in the serum level. Large changes in carbamazepine, valproate, topiramate, and lamotrigine dosages are often poorly tolerated, producing nausea or sedation.

When a patient continues to have seizures despite treatment with an appropriate anticonvulsant, the chance that the next medication selected will render him seizure-free is about 11%. Subsequent trials are even less likely to be successful (9). When these patients are admitted with seizure exacerbations and injuries, hospital-based physicians should consider referring the patients to a tertiary care epilepsy clinic.

Patients who fail to respond completely to the first 2–3 medications should be referred for inpatient video/EEG monitoring. Recordings obtained during the attacks may suggest that the patient is suffering from a seizure mimic that will not respond to anticonvulsants. Not infrequently, a patient is found to have a seizure type that might be better treated with a different anticonvulsant. Many patients with refractory seizures will have a potentially operable seizure focus (even if not visualized by neuroimaging). Surgical treatment offers a high chance for seizure control (50%–90% chance, depending on the underlying pathology) with only a modest risk (10). Other surgical options when anticonvulsants fail to control epileptic seizures include palliative procedures, such as vagus nerve stimulation or corpus callosotomy. Finally, a ketogenic diet often helps to bring seizures under control in children (adults

TABLE 118.3

ANTICONVULSANTS

Medication	Efficacy	Greatest concern for:	Potential interactions
Phenobarbital	P, GTC	Sedation, rash, liver, blood dyscrasias, joint fibrosis	Induces hepatic enzymes
Phenytoin	P, GTC	Acute cardiovascular, rash, blood dyscrasias, liver, hyperglycemia	Induces hepatic enzymes
Carbamazepine	P, GTC	Arrhythmias, rash, blood dyscrasias, liver, hyperglycemia, hyponatremia	Induces hepatic enzymes
Sodium valproate	All	Encephalopathy, liver, blood, pancreatitis, hyponatremia	Inhibits hepatic enzymes
Felbamate	All	Liver, blood dyscrasias	Variably induces or inhibits metabolism
Gabapentin	P, GTC	None clearly associated	Renal clearance
Lamotrigine	All	Rash, blood dyscrasias, liver	Does not alter levels of other medicines but susceptible to inhibition or induction of its own metabolism
Topiramate	All	Nephrolithiasis, angle closure glaucoma, oligohidrosis, rash, cognitive dysfunction	Increases phenytoin levels, decreases conrtraceptive levels
Tiagabine	P, GTC	Encephalopathy, non-convulsive status epilepticus	Does not alter levels of other medicines but susceptible to inhibition or induction of its own metabolism
Oxcarbazepine	P, GTC	Rash, hyponatremia	Induces hepatic enzymes
Levetiracetam	P, GTC	Behavioral, blood	Renal clearance
Zonisamide	All	Nephrolithiasis, rash, blood, heat stroke	Does not alter levels of other medicines but susceptible to inhibition or induction of its own metabolism
Ethosuximide	Absence	Rash, blood, lupus	Inhibits hepatic enzymes

GTC, generalized, tonic-clonic seizures; P, partial seizures.
Rash includes potential for Stevens-Johnson syndrome and other severe rashes. Blood dyscrasia includes aplastic anemia, severe leukopenia, and thrombocytopenia. Enzyme inducers typically decrease levels of susceptible medications including hormone contraceptives, while inhibitors increase levels.

have much less efficacy due to difficulty maintaining consistent ketosis) (1).

DISCHARGE PLANNING

Because most epilepsy management takes place in the outpatient setting, a smooth transition from the hospital to the clinic is essential. For patients who have started new anticonvulsants, had anticonvulsant doses changed, or changed other medications that might interact with their anticonvulsants, the timing of the follow-up visit should be dictated by the pharmacology of the drug. Ideally, one should wait long enough for levels to reach steady state, but prolonged waits may put the patient at risk for either seizures or toxicity. Because much of patient's stay is likely to have been marked by encephalopathy, there may have been insufficient time to assimilate new recommendations or instructions. Written medication schedules are useful,

particularly if the medication is being titrated. Patients may need to be counseled and re-counseled about safety issues (particularly driving and other high-risk activities) and the importance of medication compliance. Whenever family or friends can be involved in the discharge planning, the chance of miscommunication is decreased (Chapter 5). For disabled patients and patients who live alone, nursing visits may be valuable. For patients who cannot drive, discharge plans should include transportation to outpatient visits.

KEY POINTS

- Careful history, EEG, and imaging are usually adequate to distinguish seizures from common seizure mimics, such as syncope and psychogenic seizures.
- Most seizures stop promptly and, in general, a minimalist therapeutic approach is warranted.

- Status epilepticus is a medical emergency that is best addressed with a protocol directed at rapid cessation of seizures.
- Patients with new seizures require prompt evaluation for the underlying cause of the seizure.
- A sizable minority of patients with epilepsy will not gain complete control of their seizures through anticonvulsant management, and these patients should be evaluated for other treatments, including surgery.

REFERENCES

1. Marks WJ Jr., Garcia PA. Management of seizures and epilepsy. *Am Fam Physician* 1998;57:1589–1600, 1603–1604.
2. Lowenstein DH, Alldredge BK. Status epilepticus. *N Engl J Med* 1998;338:970–976.
3. Theodore WH, Porter RJ, Albert P, et al. The secondarily generalized tonic-clonic seizure: a videotape analysis. *Neurology* 1994;44:1403–1407.
4. Lowenstein DH. Treatment options for status epilepticus. *Curr Opin Pharmacol* 2003;3:6–11.
5. Alldredge BK, Gelb AM, Isaacs SM, et al. A comparison of lorazepam, diazepam, and placebo for the treatment of out-of-hospital status epilepticus. *N Engl J Med* 2001;345:631–637.
6. Wu YW, Shek DW, Garcia PA, et al. Incidence and mortality of generalized convulsive status epilepticus in California. *Neurology* 2002;58:1070–1076.
7. Garcia PA, Alldredge BK. Medication-associated seizures. In *Seizures: Medical Causes and Management*, N. Delanty, ed. Totowa, N.J.: Humana Press, 2002.
8. Musicco M, Beghi E, Solari A, Viani F, et al. Treatment of first tonic-clonic seizure does not improve the prognosis of epilepsy. First Seizure Trial Group (FIRST Group). *Neurology* 1997;49:991–998.
9. Kwan P, Brodie MJ. Early identification of refractory epilepsy. *N Engl J Med* 2000;342:314–319.
10. Wiebe S, Blume WT, Girvin JP, et al. A randomized, controlled trial of surgery for temporal-lobe epilepsy. *N Engl J Med* 2001;345:311–318.

ADDITIONAL READING

Delanty N. *Seizures: Medical Causes and Management.* Totowa: Humana Press, Inc., 2001.
Engel JJ, Pedley T. *Epilepsy: A Comprehensive Textbook.* Philadelphia: Lippincott-Raven Publishers, 1998.
French JA, Kanner AM, Bautista J, et al. Efficacy and tolerability of the new antiepileptic drugs I: treatment of new onset epilepsy: report of the Therapeutics and Technology Assessment Subcommittee and Quality Standards Subcommittee of the American Academy of Neurology and the American Epilepsy Society. *Neurology* 2004;62:1252–1260.
French JA, Kanner AM, Bautista J, et al. Efficacy and tolerability of the new antiepileptic drugs II: treatment of refractory epilepsy: report of the Therapeutics and Technology Assessment Subcommittee and Quality Standards Subcommittee of the American Academy of Neurology and the American Epilepsy Society. *Neurology* 2004;62:1261–1273.

Depression in the Hospitalized Patient

Richard J. Goldberg

INTRODUCTION

Depression is a common problem in the medical inpatient setting. It is found in 10%–26% of general inpatients, more than 25% of patients after stroke, more than 20% of patients after myocardial infarction, about 33% of patients with HIV infection, and 25% of cancer patients (1). Because of its prevalence, its significant undertreatment, and the existence of effective therapies, depression was an early priority disorder for the development of clinical practice guidelines (Chapter 13) by the Agency for Healthcare Research and Quality (2). This chapter reviews the diagnosis of depression in medical inpatients and the use of antidepressants in that population.

CARE OF THE HOSPITALIZED PATIENT

Problems in Defining Depression in Medical Inpatients

There is no laboratory test for diagnosing major depression. Rather, the diagnosis is made by identifying a constellation of symptoms (Table 119.1). Unfortunately, in medical inpatients it may be difficult to tell whether some of the symptoms are caused by depression or by an underlying medical problem. For example, patients may have trouble sleeping because of pain, poor appetite because of nausea, fatigue because of anemia, or trouble concentrating secondary to steroids. Because of such confounding factors, some researchers have advocated relying more on the psychological aspects of depression, such as anhedonia, feelings of hopelessness, or excessive guilt.

Hospitalized patients face a number of stressors, including uncertainty, disfigurement, alienation, and possible death. They are cut off from their usual social supports and separated from their social context. If a physician is confronted with a medical inpatient with significant depressive symptoms, the problem is to determine how much of the "depression" is a result of direct medical effects, how much is caused by psychosocial distress, and how much may actually represent a major depressive episode. Although there is no way to reliably sort out these contributing factors, this chapter outlines a clinical strategy that can address them in hospitalized patients.

Strategy for Evaluating and Managing Depression in Medical Inpatients

Step 1: Biomedical Issues

It is a mistake to dismiss a depressed patient by thinking, "Wouldn't I be depressed if I were that sick?" Instead, as a first step it is important to identify and correct, to the extent possible, every medical problem that could be contributing to depressive symptoms. This might involve treating pain, blood gas abnormalities, metabolic abnormalities (e.g., hypercalcemia or hyponatremia), or severe anemia. Psychiatric consultants often find that presumed "depression" in the medical setting turns out to be delirium secondary to medical disorders (Table 119.2) or medications (Table 119.3) (3).

The medical workup of depression is determined by the presence of specific medical conditions that potentially affect the central nervous system. For example, although neuroimaging does not play a role in the routine evaluation of depression, it may be indicated in patients with an

TABLE 119.1

DIAGNOSTIC CRITERIA FOR MAJOR DEPRESSION

Core symptoms

Depressed mood
Anhedonia

Other symptoms

Appetite change or weight change ($\geq$5%)
Sleep disturbance
Psychomotor agitation or retardation
Fatigue
Feeling worthless or guilty
Poor concentration
Suicidal thoughts

A total of at least five symptoms, continuously over two weeks including one of the "core" symptoms, is necessary to diagnose major depression.
Adapted from American Psychiatric Association. *Diagnostic and Statistical Manual of Mental Disorders*, 4th ed., Text Revision, Washington, DC: 2000.

TABLE 119.2

MEDICAL CAUSES OF DEPRESSIVE SYMPTOMS

Autoimmune disorders

Systemic lupus erythematosus

Neurologic

Parkinson's disease	Epilepsy
Huntington's disease	Sleep apnea
Alzheimer's disease	Brain tumor
Multiple sclerosis	Stroke

Endocrine disorders

Hyperthyroidism	Hypoparathyroidism
Hypothyroidism	Hypercalcemia
Hyperparathyroidism	Hypercortisolism

Infections

Hepatitis	HIV
Mononucleosis	

Malignancies

Pancreatic	Gastrointestinal

Metabolic disorders

B_{12} deficiency	Renal failure
Hypoxia	Hypocortisolism
Diabetes mellitus	Hypokalemia
Hepatic failure	

underlying disease that frequently involves the central nervous system (e.g., lung cancer, breast cancer, multiple myeloma, or AIDS). In elderly patients with depressive symptoms and in those for whom dementia is a possible diagnosis, a comprehensive dementia evaluation should be performed.

Because of the high frequency of its coexistence with depression, *substance abuse* always should be considered. Sedative substances, notably alcohol and benzodiazepines, as well as stimulant withdrawal, are common causes of depressive symptoms. Because it is difficult to diagnose depression in the presence of active substance use, the latter should be regarded as the primary diagnosis and management priority.

Step 2: Psychosocial Assessment

Medical inpatients with depressive symptoms face significant psychosocial issues that need to be identified and addressed. In patients who are too medically ill, questioning about psychosocial issues may need to be deferred. However, many depressed patients feel overwhelmed, isolated, guilty, or are grieving their loss of health. Sometimes, simply allowing patients to vent such feelings and providing reassurance is sufficient to assuage distress and lower depressive symptoms. At other times, it may be necessary to arrange for the involvement of the family, a social worker, a minister, a psychologist, or a psychiatrist. The more acute the emotional distress, the more likely it is to benefit from psychosocial support or to resolve spontaneously as the medical condition improves. Although antidepressants

may help relieve some depressive symptoms, medication alone should not be substituted for the personal supportive interaction.

Step 3: Use of Antidepressants

If medical and psychosocial issues have been addressed and the patient remains depressed, the clinician needs to

TABLE 119.3

EXAMPLES OF MEDICATIONS AND SUBSTANCES CAUSING DEPRESSIVE SYMPTOMS

Alcohol	Corticosteroids
α-Methyldopa	Interferon
Amantadine	Oral contraceptives
Anabolic steroids	Propranolol
Anticholinergics	Ranitidine
Anticonvulsants	Reserpine
Barbiturates	Sedatives
Benzodiazepines	Stimulant (withdrawal)
Cimetidine	Thiazides
Clonidine	

decide whether to use antidepressant medication. This decision is made (after steps 1 and 2) on the basis of the number and severity of "target symptoms". That is, if the patient has depressive target symptoms (e.g., impaired sleep, depressed mood, poor appetite, or low energy) that are severe enough to be impair function and cause distress, then the patient should be started on an antidepressant.

A difficult challenge is to decide whether depressive symptoms in the medically ill patient represent a "normal" adjustment to illness or so substantially impact the individual to warrant a trial of antidepressants. If depressive symptoms are severe enough and have been present at least two weeks, antidepressants may be indicated even if the symptoms are thought to represent a "reaction" to illness. The presence or absence of some "precipitating" factor does not predict whether symptoms will or will not respond to medication.

Suicide Evaluation

Because the risk of suicide is always a concern in depressed patients, the presence or absence of suicidal ideation should be evaluated and documented (4) (Figure 119.1). Because patients are often too ill to communicate or too guarded to tell the truth, the assessment is more valid if it includes other people who know the patient well. Of course, it is necessary to consider confidentiality issues and obtain patient permission unless the situation is considered a medical emergency.

Effects of Depression on Medical Outcomes and Resource Use

In hospitalized medical patients, depression has been shown to contribute to longer lengths of stay and higher rehospitalization rates, and psychiatric interventions have been shown in some studies to contribute to shorter lengths of stay (5). Depression also can affect medical status by leading to health-impairing behaviors, such as smoking, drinking, or noncompliance with medical treatment. Moreover, other poorly understood pathophysiologic factors involving brain-end organ relationships may influence medical outcome in depressed patients. For example, patients with depression have a significantly higher 6-month mortality rate after myocardial infarction than those who are not depressed; the differences cannot be explained by noncompliance or suicide (6).

Screening for Depression

Because of problems in recognition, time constraints for clinicians, or reluctance of patients to talk about symptoms, it can be useful to screen for depression using *standardized instruments*. However, the use of many of these instruments is problematic because of the presence of possible medically based physical symptoms.

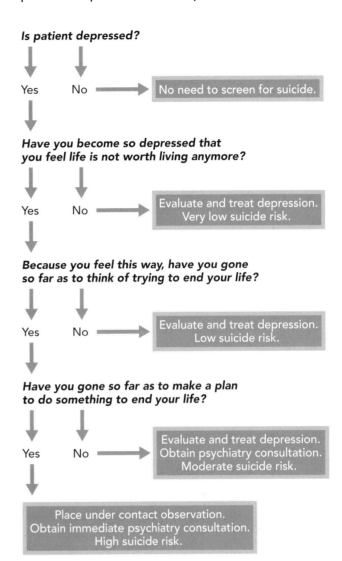

Figure 119.1 Algorithm for suicide evaluation. (From Goldberg RJ. The assessment of suicide risk in the general hospital. *Gen Hosp Psychiatry* 1987;9:1–7, with permission.)

There are a number of 20- to 30-item self-rating scales that can be used to detect depression. Commonly used scales include the Beck Depression Inventory, the Zung Depression Scale, and the Geriatric Depression Scale. The Zung and Beck scales each have problems if used in the medically ill, because somatic items may be a result of the medical disorder and not depression. The Brief Depression Scale is an 11-item, self-rated scale that factors out physical symptoms and has been shown to have reasonable sensitivity and specificity for detecting major depression (7). The single question, "Are you depressed?" also appears to be of value in screening the medically ill (8).

Treatment

Three forms of effective treatment for major depression are psychotherapy, antidepressant medication, and electroconvulsive therapy (ECT).

TABLE 119.4

ANTIDEPRESSANT SUMMARY

	Anticho-linergic	Sedation	Activation (tremor, insomnia)	Ortho-stasis	His bundle block	Gastro-intestinal (nausea, diarrhea)	Sexual impairment	Usual dose range, mg	Starting dose (mg) in elderly inpatients	Half-life, h
Tricyclics										
Amitriptyline (Elavil)	4	3	0	3	3	0	4	100–300	25	20–46
Clomipramine (Anafranil)	4	2	0	3	3	0	4	50–250	25	20–40
Nortriptyline (Pamelor)	2	2	0	1	3	0	4	50–150	10–25	18–88
Imipramine (Tofranil)	3	2	1	3	3	0	4	100–300	25–50	4–34
Desipramine (Norpramine)	1	1–2	2	2	3	0	4	100–300	25	10–32
Doxepin (Sinequan)	3	4	0	2	3	0	4	100–300	25–50	8–47
SSRIs										
Citalopram (Celexa)	0	0–1	1–2	0	0	1	4	20–40	10	35
Escitalopram (Lexapro)	0	1	1	0	0	1	4	10–20	10	27–32
Fluoxetine (Prozac)	0	0–1	1–2	0	0	2	4	20–60	10	7 d
Paroxetine (Paxil)	1	1–2	1–2	0	0	2	4	20–50	10	15–20
Sertraline (Zoloft)	0	0–1	1–2	0	0	2	4	50–100	25	26
Other 2nd-generation										
Bupropion (Wellbutrin)	1	0	3	0	0	1	0–1	75–300	25–50	8–24 SR: 24
Mirtazapine (Remeron)	3	4	0	2	0	a	0–1	15–45	7.5	20–40
Nefazodone (Serzone)	0	3	0	1	0	0	0–1	100–500	25–50	4–18
Trazodone (Desyrel)	0	3	0	2	0	0	0	100–600	50	6–14
Venlafaxine (Effexor)	0	1–2	1–2	0	0	0	2–3	75–300	25	9–11 XR: 24

[a] Associated with weight gain and increased appetite.
4, very strong effect; 3, strong effect; 2, moderate effect; 1, minimal effect; 0, no effect.
SSRI, selective serotonin reuptake inhibitor; SR, slow release; XR, extended release.

Psychotherapy

Depressed patients with severe symptoms and those whose symptoms interfere with talking therapy should be started on medication. Patients with mild symptoms who seem willing to talk about their problems should first be provided with counseling or psychotherapy. Between these extremes, psychotherapy and medication can be used conjointly. As a generalization, psychotherapy addresses problems and medication addresses symptoms. Psychotherapy may be the primary treatment for patients who refuse, discontinue, or cannot tolerate medications, and for situations in which medication may be dangerous, such as pregnancy, acute myocardial infarction, or unstable neurologic status. If psychotherapy is utilized in appropriate patients, its efficacy can match that of antidepressants, although there are no studies specifically addressing outcomes in medically ill depressed patients.

Antidepressant Medications

Selection

There is no clear efficacy advantage to any of the currently available antidepressants; therefore, the choice of medication generally is made on the basis of side effect and tolerability profiles (Table 119.4) and potential drug interactions (Tables 119.5 and 119.6). Past patient response and response of first-degree relatives may be predictors of drug response. Medically ill patients with concurrent depression are less likely to respond to antidepressants than patients without medical illness, who generally have a response rate of about 70%. Furthermore, guidelines for treatment of medically ill patients are based more on empirical practice than research data. A relatively small proportion of depressed older medical inpatients receives treatment with antidepressants, and those who do are usually on inadequate doses of tricyclic antidepressants

(TCAs) (9). More studies need to be performed using second-generation medications (selective serotonin reuptake inhibitors [SSRIs], venlafaxine, mirtazapine, and bupropion) instead of TCAs, which are less well tolerated in the medically ill.

Pharmacoeconomic analyses of the generic TCAs versus the second-generation antidepressants have not shown any significant cost advantage for the TCAs, because TCAs are associated with more costly treatment-related complications, such as fractures from falls associated with orthostatic hy-

TABLE 119.6

P-450-RELATED SUMMARY TABLE OF ANTIDEPRESSANT INTERACTIONS

P-450 family	Inhibitors	May increase half-life and effect of:
2D6	Paroxetine = fluoxetine > sertraline = citalopram	Type IC antiarrhythmics, Bupropion, Paroxetine, Fluoxetine, Tricyclics, Venlafaxine, Neuroleptics, Codeine, Oxycodone, Pentazocine, Dextromethorphan, Metoprolol, Phentermine, Risperidone, Donepezil
3A4	Nefazodone > fluoxetine	Astemizole, Terfenadine, Tricyclics, Fluoxetine, Alprazolam, Diazepam, Midazolam, Triazolam, Calcium channel blockers, Carbamazepine, Cisapride, Cortisol, Dexamethasone, Lidocaine, Lovastatin, Quinidine, Tamoxifen, Testosterone
2C9	Fluoxetine	Tricyclics, Diazepam, Phenytoin, Propranolol, Tolbutamide

Adapted from Goldberg RJ. The P-450 system and relevance to the use of antidepressants in medical practice. *Arch Fam Med* 1996; 5:406–412, with permission.

TABLE 119.5

TRICYCLIC DRUG INTERACTIONS

Anticholinergic effects augmented: Artane, Cogentin, Benadryl, Ditropan, Probanthine, Demerol	Blood pressure increased: Sympathomimetics
	Cardiac conduction prolonged: Carbamazepine, Phenothiazines
Antihypertensive effects decreased: Clonidine, Guanethidine, Reserpine	Hypotension potentiated: α-Adrenergic blocking agents, Prazosin
	Quinidine-like effects augmented: Quinidine, Type 1A antiarrhythmics

potension, urinary retention, and cardiac complications (10). Overdose danger is another consideration, because TCA overdoses may be lethal (and usually require expensive ICU stays), but overdoses with second-generation antidepressants are not. Therefore, unless there is some specific reason to start a TCA, *SSRIs or other second-generation medications should be used as first-line treatment.* The use of monoamine oxidase inhibitors (MAOIs) or stimulants in medical patients should not be initiated except by psychiatric consultants.

Dosage

It is prudent to start medically ill patients, especially those with renal or hepatic impairment and the frail elderly, on low dosages (Table 119.4). Patients started too quickly on higher doses have higher rates of side effects. In general, if the patient tolerates the starting dose, the dose can be raised into the low oral dose range over the first few weeks. The response rate can often be improved by combinations or augmentation strategies, though these maneuvers are best applied by a psychiatrist. Before starting any combination, an adequate trial of single drugs should be confirmed. Plasma therapeutic levels are not established for the second generation antidepressants. All antidepressants are metabolized by the liver and are not dialyzable.

If the patient cannot tolerate the medication because of side effects, consider lowering the dose. If the lower dose would be considered ineffective, then switch to another medication that might be better tolerated. When switching, consider that drugs with long lives (e.g., fluoxetine) may be present for about 3 weeks; therefore, maintain vigilance for drug interactions during that period.

Course of Treatment

Antidepressants take *at least seven days* to exert a true neuropharmacologic effect on depression. Patients who respond earlier are showing either a placebo response or the benefit of a side effect (e.g., a sedating antidepressant may help with sleep after only one or two doses). A good trial of an antidepressant generally means using the medication at a therapeutic level for at least 4–6 weeks. In a medically ill patient in whom a low starting dose is required, the time to onset of response may be as long as 8–12 weeks. Patients who respond should remain on medication for at least 6 months, because there is a high rate of relapse associated with earlier discontinuation. Patients in their third or fourth episodes of major depression may require maintenance therapy to avoid relapse.

Antidepressant Pharmacokinetics and Withdrawal

If switching or stopping antidepressants, those with long half-lives (e.g., fluoxetine) can be stopped immediately. Those with half-lives of 1 day or less (Table 119.4) may cause withdrawal symptoms when suddenly discontinued. These medications (e.g., paroxetine) should be tapered by halving the dose for 3–4 days. Hospital physicians should be aware of the possibility of withdrawal symptoms if a patient on antidepressants is admitted NPO. Withdrawal symptoms, which are uncomfortable but not life threatening, include dizziness, vertigo, paresthesias, flu-like symptoms, gastrointestinal activation, insomnia, nausea, and sweating. They are generally time-limited and can be relieved by restarting the antidepressant, but not by benzodiazepines (11).

Side-Effect Issues in Medical Inpatients

This section highlights a number of the medically relevant side effects of the more commonly used antidepressants (Table 119.4). It is not intended as a comprehensive list.

Anticholinergic Effects. TCAs with high anticholinergic activity can cause dry mouth. This may be merely a nuisance or may predispose patients receiving radiation or chemotherapy to stomatitis. They may precipitate narrow-angle glaucoma. Prostatic enlargement or spinal-cord problems may predispose to urinary retention. Combining anticholinergic effects with opiates in the setting of abdominal gastrointestinal surgery can lead to paralytic ileus. Anticholinergic effects can cause confusion, memory problems, or even delirium, and are augmented by other anticholinergic drugs. In general, try to avoid anticholinergic medications in the elderly and the medically ill.

Sedation. If a patient is agitated, restless, or anxious, it might be helpful to use a sedating medication. Patients who lack energy, are withdrawn, or are hypersomnic may benefit from being started on a more activating medication. Patients who become excessively activated on antidepressants should receive psychiatric consultation and discontinue the medication.

Orthostatic Hypotension. This is a result of peripheral α-adrenergic blockade as well as a central brainstem mechanism. Medical inpatients are at higher risk for orthostasis because of depleted intravascular volumes, prolonged bed rest, old age, autonomic disorders, and concurrent treatment with other medications that lower blood pressure. Orthostasis can lead to falls and injuries such as hip fracture.

Gastrointestinal Side Effects. Nausea and gastrointestinal activation are the most common side effects for the second-generation antidepressants (SSRIs). Up to 35% of patients experience nausea, and another 10%–15% have diarrhea. Nausea generally resolves after one week on a lower dosage. The TCAs decrease gastroesophageal sphincter tone, leading to symptoms of reflux. Weight loss sometimes can accompany the use of second-generation antidepressants during the first few months of treatment. However, if loss of appetite is secondary to depression, antidepressants often help with appetite recovery and may lead to weight gain.

Cardiac Issues. There are significant potential cardiac problems associated with the use of TCAs because of their quinidine-like effects and their prolongation of cardiac conduction through the intraventricular portion of the His-bundle. This effect often requires lengthy cardiac monitoring after TCA overdose. Patients over age 40 or with cardiac histories require an electrocardiogram before starting on a TCA. TCAs should be avoided in patients with pre-existing conduction problems. Electrocardiographic and clinical studies of patients without cardiovascular disease have not demonstrated any significant arrhythmias associated with the use of SSRIs. Nevertheless, some caution may be in order in the acute post-MI period, and in those patients with severe organic heart disease and/or a history of brady-arrhythmias.

Serotonin Syndrome. The increase in peripheral serotonin caused by SSRI interference with platelet uptake may overcome the body's ability to metabolize peripheral serotonin, leading to the serotonin syndrome (10). Symptoms include confusion, agitation, myoclonus, hyperreflexia, diaphoresis, shivering, tremor, diarrhea, incoordination, fever, hypertension, nausea or vomiting, insomnia, drowsiness, and dizziness. Patients rarely develop serotonin syndrome from an SSRI alone, and most cases involve drug combinations with MAOIs or with other potent serotonin augmenters, including dextromethorphan. Symptoms of the serotonin syndrome generally abate within 24 hours after discontinuation of the causative agent. Symptoms of this syndrome have been reported to respond to treatment with cyproheptadine (a serotonin antagonist), β-blockers, or clonazepam.

Other Side Effects. A number of additional side effects may be seen in patients receiving antidepressant medications. *Sexual side effects* (anorgasmia, impaired erection or ejaculation) occur in more than 20% of patients on TCAs or SSRIs, though the incidence is about 5% on bupropion, nefazodone, or mirtazapine. The *syndrome of inappropriate antidiuretic hormone* has been seen with the use of SSRIs and TCAs. It is important to monitor serum sodium levels in elderly patients on SSRIs who develop any behavioral symptoms possibly consistent with hyponatremia (Chapter 104). Onset of symptoms may occur as early as 2 days after starting an SSRI or may emerge after many months. There also have been case reports describing *extrapyramidal side effects* and akathisia associated with SSRIs, mediated through enhanced inhibition of the dopamine system. Finally, *bleeding complications* have been reported as a rare consequence of SSRI therapy. Fluoxetine-warfarin interactions have been reported. Laboratory findings associated with SSRI-induced bleeding include prolonged bleeding time and decreased platelet aggregation in response to ADP and epinephrine.

Specific Antidepressants

Monoamine Oxidase Inhibitors. Medically important side effects of MAOIs include orthostatic hypotension, weight gain, insomnia, sexual dysfunction, and pyridoxine deficiency producing paresthesias. Hypertensive crisis is a rare (incidence <0.5% with mortality rate <0.001%) but potentially life-threatening reaction that usually is associated with mixing an MAOI with a pressor medication or food with high tyramine content. Indirectly acting sympathomimetics (such as cocaine, amphetamines, methylphenidate, pseudoephedrine, ephedrine, phenylpropanolamine, many over-the-counter cold remedies, and Sinemet) are contraindicated. Chapter 48 discusses the management of hypertensive crisis.

Stimulants. Psychiatric consultants sometimes prescribe stimulants to treat geriatric medically ill patients with depressive symptoms involving withdrawn behavior, lack of motivation and energy, and depressed mood (12). Methylphenidate or dextroamphetamine usually are started at 5 mg orally in the morning. Side effects may include overstimulation, anxiety, confusion, paranoia, tachycardia, and appetite disturbance.

Selective Serotonin Reuptake Inhibitors. Most medically ill patients receiving *fluoxetine* (Prozac) should be started on only 10 mg/d. Because of the long half-life, side effects may appear several weeks into treatment. Common side effects include gastrointestinal symptoms, tremulousness, activation, and insomnia, especially in older patients. Because of insomnia, some patients need trazodone at bedtime. The long half-life of fluoxetine can be a disadvantage in the medically ill, because the drug can take several weeks to disappear if a drug interaction or problematic side effect occurs.

The starting dosage of *sertraline* (Zoloft) in the elderly or medically ill should be 25 mg/d. There seems to be a lower tendency to activation than with fluoxetine. The major side-effect issue is generally nausea or vomiting, which should be addressed by immediate dosage reduction. Tolerance to these gastrointestinal effects usually occurs after 1 week.

A reasonable starting dose for *paroxetine* (Paxil), *citalopram* (Celexa), or *escitalopram* (Lexapro) for older or medically ill patients is 10 mg/d. Paroxetine has no active metabolites, a half-life of about 24 hours, and is often associated with a withdrawal syndrome if discontinued abruptly in younger patients. Paroxetine is the only SSRI with anticholinergic activity, which may contribute to side effects in the elderly and medically ill. Among the SSRIs, escitalopram is the least likely to cause P-450 drug interactions.

Bupropion (Wellbutrin) has a side-effect profile similar to that of stimulants (anorexia, insomnia, agitation, tremor) and is a reasonable choice for patients who need some activation. It has a greater tendency than other antidepressants to produce seizures (incidence of about 4/1,000) in higher doses (>300 mg/d). Bupropion is also approved for use in smoking cessation.

Trazodone (Desyrel) is a weak antidepressant in dosages that medical patients can tolerate without becoming too sedated or orthostatic. It does have good hypnotic properties in doses of 50–100 mg at bedtime. Trazodone also can be used as an alternative to neuroleptics to reduce agitation in dementia patients. Trazodone rarely has been reported to be associated with heart block and ventricular arrhythmia and should be used with caution in patients with cardiac disease.

Venlafaxine (Effexor) in doses over 150 mg/d inhibits both norepinephrine and serotonin reuptake and is therefore classified as a serotonin and norepinephrine reuptake inhibitor. Its side-effect profile resembles that of the SSRIs. At doses greater than 225 mg/d, about 10% of patients experience increases in supine diastolic blood pressure within the first 2 months. Blood pressure increases are generally not an issue with oral doses under 200 mg/d. Some studies have shown better efficacy with venlafaxine than SSRIs for hospitalized patients with severe major depression (13).

Nefazodone (Serzone) acts as a 5-HT2 antagonist and a serotonin uptake inhibitor. Although the SSRIs may cause insomnia, nefazodone causes a decrease in light-stage sleep and decreased frequency of awakenings. Because of cases of hepatic failure in patients on nefazodone, this drug should not be started in patients with active liver disease or elevated serum aminotransferases. Visual trails are an unusual side effect (seen in about 2% of patients) and may be reported as "double vision" or even hallucinations.

Mirtazapine (Remeron) is a nonadrenergic and specific serotonergic antidepressant. It has a low incidence of sexual dysfunction and GI side effects. In keeping with its antihistamine effects, its most frequent adverse effects are sedation and weight gain.

P-450 Drug Interactions

P-450 system activity is inhibited by SSRIs and nefazodone (14). Because the clearance of many drugs involves multiple enzyme pathways, a potential drug interaction listed in Table 119.6 does not necessarily mean that the combination always results in a significant interaction. Nevertheless, caution needs to guide co-prescribing if interactions are possible. Enzyme inhibition may begin immediately (or more often within the first week), increase over time until a drug reaches a steady state, and persist for as long as the drug is circulating (i.e., for weeks after terminating long-acting drugs such as fluoxetine).

Electroconvulsive Therapy

A full review of ECT is beyond the scope of this chapter. It should be noted, however, that ECT often is neglected as a treatment option by nonpsychiatrists because of the lack of knowledge of its modern applications and technology

(15). ECT is generally not a first-line treatment but should be considered if a patient has failed or cannot tolerate medication or if there is a need for an immediate response because of suicidal behaviors, malnutrition, severe psychosis with agitation, or prolonged catatonia. ECT also may be effective in refractory epilepsy, neuroleptic malignant syndrome, and Parkinson's disease.

There are no absolute and few relative contraindications for ECT, and significant complications occur in less than 1 in 200 patients. There is a substantial increased risk associated with a rise in intracranial pressure, recent myocardial infarction, recent intracerebral hemorrhage, unstable vascular malformation, retinal detachment, pheochromocytoma, anesthetic risk rated at American Society of Anesthesiologists physical status 4 or 5, or ventricular arrhythmias. ECT may be used in all trimesters of pregnancy, in consultation with the patient's obstetrician. Medical conditions that require special techniques to avoid complications include chronic obstructive pulmonary disease, asthma, severe hypertension, cardiac arrhythmia, history of stroke, advanced coronary artery disease, significant osteoporosis, or major bone fractures. Nevertheless, careful medical management makes ECT a reasonably safe option for geriatric depressed patients even with concurrent cardiovascular disease.

Pre-ECT medical assessment should include a physical and neurologic examination to rule out any risk factors. Routine laboratory studies should include complete blood count, electrolytes, renal function, and electrocardiogram. The need for neuroimaging, EEG, or chest radiograph depends on the clinical condition.

KEY POINTS

- Depression is a common problem in the medical inpatient setting and is found in a significant proportion of general inpatients.
- The first step in the evaluation of depression is to identify and correct, to the extent possible, every medical problem that could be contributing to producing depressive symptoms.
- The second step in the evaluation of depression is to address significant psychosocial issues.
- The decision to use antidepressants is made (after the first 2 steps) on the basis of the number and severity of "target symptoms."
- The presence or absence of suicidal ideation should be assessed and documented.
- The choice of medication generally is made on the basis of side-effect and tolerability profiles (Table 119.4) and potential drug interactions (Tables 119.5 and 119.6).
- It is prudent to start medically ill patients on low dosages. This is especially true for the frail elderly and those with renal or hepatic impairment.

REFERENCES

1. Rouchell AM, Pounds R, Tierney JG. Depression. In Wise MG, Rundell JR, eds. *Textbook of Consultation-Liaison Psychiatry,* 2nd ed. Washington, DC: American Psychiatric Publishing, Inc., 2002.
2. Depression Guidelines Panel. Depression in primary care, vol. 2: treatment of major depression. Clinical Practice Guideline Number 5. AHCPR Publication, 1993;93–0551:23–33.
3. Abramowicz M, ed. Drugs that may cause psychiatric symptoms. *The Medical Letter* 2002;44:(Issue 1134).
4. Goldberg RJ. The assessment of suicide risk in the general hospital. *Gen Hosp Psychiatry* 1987;9:1–7.
5. Furlanetto LM, daSilva RV, Bueno JR. The impact of psychiatric comorbidity on length of stay of medical inpatients. *Gen Hosp Psychiatry* 2003;25:14–19.
6. Penninx BWJH, Beekman ATF, Honig A, et al. Depression and cardiac mortality. *Arch Gen Psychiatry* 2001;58:221–227.
7. Koenig HG, Blumenthal J, Moore K. New version of Brief Depression Scale. *J Am Geriatr Soc* 1995;43:12:1447.
8. Chochinov HM, Wilson KG, Enns M, et al. "Are you depressed?" screening for depression in the terminally ill. *Am J Psychiatry* 1997;154:674–676.
9. Koenig HG, George LK, Meador KG. Use of antidepressants by nonpsychiatrists in the treatment of medically ill hospitalized depressed elderly patients. *Am J Psychiatry* 1997;154:1369–1375.
10. Skaer TL, Sclar DA, Robison LM, et al. Economic valuation of amitriptyline, desipramine, nortriptyline and sertraline in the management of patients with depression. *Curr Ther Res* 1995;36: 556–567.
11. Zajecka J, Tracy KA. Discontinuation symptoms after treatment with serotonin reuptake inhibitors: a literature review. *J Clin Psychiatry* 1997;7:291–296.
12. Holmes VF. Medical use of psychostimulants: an overview. *Int J Psychiatry Med* 1995;25:1–19.
13. Clerc GE, Ruimy P, Verdeau-Pailles J. A double-blind comparison of venlafaxine and fluoxetine in patients hospitalized for major depression and melancholia. *Int Clin Psychopharmacol* 1994;9:139–143.
14. Goldberg RJ. The P-450 system definition and relevance to the use of antidepressants in medical practice. *Arch Fam Med* 1996;5: 406–412.
15. Weiner RD, Krystal AD. The present use of electroconvulsive therapy. *Annu Rev Med* 1994;45:273–281.

ADDITIONAL READING

American Psychiatric Association. *Diagnostic and Statistical Manual of Mental Disorders,* 4th ed. Text Revision. Washington, DC: 2000.
Clarkin JF, Pilkonis PA, Magrude KM. Psychotherapy of depression: implications for report of the health care system. *Arch Gen Psychiatry* 1996;53:717–723.
Goldberg RJ. SSRIs: infrequent medical adverse effects. *Arch Fam Med* 1998;7:78–84.

Toxicology and Allergy

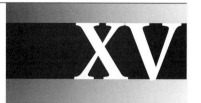

Allergic Reactions and Anaphylaxis

120

Neil Winawer   *Mark V. Williams*

INTRODUCTION

A patient with initial complaints of pruritus and mild dyspnea can rapidly develop airway obstruction, respiratory failure, and circulatory collapse. This dramatic and life-threatening presentation of anaphylaxis challenges the physician to act quickly and thoughtfully to avert death. Anaphylaxis represents the extreme example of a constellation of adverse reactions to medications, food, insect venoms, and other substances. Patients, and most physicians, typically describe such acute adverse reactions as "allergic reactions." However, allergic reactions are defined strictly by the immune system's production of specific IgE antibody in response to an offending antigen. Re-exposure to the particular agent causes cross-linking of antibodies that in turn results in the release of histamine, prostaglandins, leukotrienes, tryptase, and other inflammatory mediators from mast cells. In addition to this specific IgE mast cell response, allergic reactions also are mediated by a subset of CD4 (+) T-cells, called T-helper type 2 cells, which preferentially produce interleukin 4 and 5. Mast cell and basophil-bound IgE contribute to the early (or immediate) phase of allergic response; interleukin 5 recruits and activates eosinophils, contributing to the late (or chronic) phase of allergic inflammation. The interaction between these substances and end-organ receptors determines a patient's clinical presentation.

Clinicians should distinguish allergic from nonallergic reactions because this distinction may affect diagnosis and treatment. For example, substances such as radiocontrast dyes, aspirin products, and angiotensin-converting enzyme (ACE) inhibitors produce *nonallergic reactions* (i.e., not induced by a specific IgE antibody). In these reactions, the pathogenesis may be related to direct mast cell activation, prostaglandin inhibition, bradykinin elevation, complement activation, or other unknown mechanisms.

Anaphylaxis is defined as a potentially fatal allergic reaction characterized by cross-linking of IgE antibodies leading to systemic mast cell activation. Patients with *anaphylactoid reactions* present with symptoms clinically indistinguishable from anaphylaxis; however, the reaction is mediated by mechanisms other than IgE antibody interaction with the offending agent.

Although 15%–30% of inpatients experience adverse reactions to drugs, only 6%–10% of these are caused by allergic and other immunologic mechanisms (1, 2). Allergic drug reactions are common, but they are fatal in only 1 of 10,000 cases (3). Two epidemiologic studies documented that anaphylaxis plays a role in 1 out of every 2,700 to 5,100 hospital admissions (4, 5). Life-threatening adverse dermatologic reactions, such as toxic epidermal necrolysis (TEN), are even less common, occurring in only about 1 in 1 million people.

ANAPHYLAXIS OR SEVERE ALLERGIC REACTION PRESENTING AT THE TIME OF ADMISSION

Issues at the Time of Presentation

Clinical Presentation

Patients requiring hospitalization for adverse reactions may be suffering from a variety of entities ranging from anaphylaxis or angioedema to vesiculobullous reactions that denude the skin.

Signs and symptoms of anaphylaxis or anaphylactoid reactions usually begin within 5 minutes of exposure to the offending agent and include flushing, pruritus, urticaria, angioedema, shortness of breath, wheezing, chest tightness, nausea, vomiting, diarrhea, and lightheadedness. Patients also may develop life-threatening angioedema of the airway. Early in anaphylaxis, patients may have noticeable hoarseness or stridor. Further swelling of the larynx, tongue, epiglottis, or oropharynx may cause complete obstruction, leading to asphyxiation. Anaphylaxis also may affect the lower airways, causing bronchospasm, wheezing, and pulmonary edema. Further progression results in severe hypoxemia, which can precipitate altered mental status and seizure activity.

Anaphylactic reactions also may be associated with peripheral vasodilatation, reflex tachycardia, and subsequent cardiovascular collapse. The resultant hypotension can induce myocardial ischemia and ventricular arrhythmias. Involvement of the gastrointestinal tract with swelling of the bowel wall may present as nausea, vomiting, abdominal cramping, or diarrhea.

Adverse reactions with primarily dermatologic manifestations that require hospitalization include *Stevens-Johnson syndrome* (SJS) and *TEN*. These bullous and necrolytic reactions to drugs or infections can be life-threatening. SJS, the most severe form of erythema multiforme, involves blistering lesions, with epidermal loss occurring over less than 10% of the patient's body surface area. Patients often develop painful erosions of the oral mucosa and lip (90%), as well as conjunctivitis (85%). TEN is characterized by fever and epidermal loss of 30% or more of body surface area. Mucosal erosions are also a prominent feature of TEN, often making it difficult to clinically distinguish from SJS.

Differential Diagnosis and Initial Evaluation

The diagnosis of anaphylaxis usually is self-evident when exposure to a specific agent results in the classic constellation of symptoms. However, other diseases may have similar presentations. Initial evaluation follows the Advanced Cardiac Life Support protocol. The patient's airway should be assessed immediately, followed quickly by a thorough assessment of the patient's ability to ventilate. The patient should have frequent blood pressure checks and be connected to a hemodynamic monitor. After this rapid assessment, other organ systems can be surveyed, with particular emphasis on the skin and gastrointestinal tract. Little initial diagnostic testing is needed, because the diagnosis of anaphylactic shock relies mainly on the patient's clinical presentation and history. A serum tryptase level may be helpful in determining whether the reaction was mast cell mediated. A significantly elevated level would imply systemic mast cell degranulation but does not provide information on whether the reaction was immune mediated (i.e., anaphylaxis versus anaphylactoid reaction).

Once the patient is stabilized, a thorough history should be performed in the hope of revealing an underlying cause of the reaction, although 30%–40% of the time a definitive cause is not found. Nonetheless, patients should be queried about exposure to several well-known and common precipitants of anaphylaxis (Table 120.1) because such identification may help avoid a future life-threatening exposure. Many medications, especially penicillins and the cephalosporins, can be responsible for IgE-mediated anaphylaxis. However, anaphylactoid drug reactions are more common than IgE-mediated ones. For example, aspirin can induce severe bronchospasm by inhibiting prostaglandin synthesis and may allow the unregulated production of leukotrienes via the lipoxygenase pathway. ACE inhibitors also produce potentially fatal drug reactions by causing laryngeal, oropharyngeal, tongue, and lip edema. This reaction occurs in up to 1% of all patients taking the medication for 10 years and may be three times as common among African-Americans (6). The underlying mechanism

TABLE 120.1

DIFFERENTIAL DIAGNOSIS OF ANAPHYLACTIC/ANAPHYLACTOID REACTIONS

Allergic (IgE-mediated)

Drugs (penicillin, cephalosporins)
Foods (shellfish, peanuts)
Contacts (latex, animal dander)
Insect stings (*Hymenoptera* spp. bees, hornets, yellow jackets, wasps)
Infections (parasitic, fungal, viral, bacterial)
Aeroallergens (pollen, dust mites)
Transfusion reactions (in patients with an IgA deficiency)

Direct Mast Cell Activation

Radiocontrast dyes
Drugs (opiates, polymixin)

Physical Stimuli

Exercise
Food-induced
Cold
Heat
Solar
Pressure

Aspirin/Nonsteroidal Anti-inflammatory Drugs

Angiotensin-converting enzyme inhibitors

Medical Conditions

Hereditary/acquired angioedema
Mastocytosis
Carcinoid syndrome

Pseudoallergic Reactions

Vasovagal reactions
Hypoglycemia

of this reaction partly relates to the drug's inhibition of bradykinin degradation.

Other disease entities can present with signs and symptoms suggestive of anaphylaxis. Hereditary angioedema is an autosomal dominant disorder characterized by low or nonfunctioning C1 esterase inhibitor. These patients often present with episodes of angioedema involving the extremities, genitalia, abdomen, lips, face, and larynx, and they relate histories of prior bouts of angioedema and positive family histories. Though rare, it is crucial for the clinician to recognize this entity, because its treatment is drastically different from that of anaphylactic reactions. In hereditary angioedema, the complement cascade produces kinin proteins that have significant vasoactive effects; mast cells are not activated. Thus, treatment with epinephrine, steroids, and antihistamines has little or no effect. Acute episodes are managed with supportive care and the administration of heat-vaporized C1 esterase inhibitor concentrate (7). Attenuated androgens such as danazol and stanozolol are effective for prophylaxis.

Patients with *mastocytosis* often have reactions that mimic anaphylaxis. This rare disease is characterized by an overabundance of mast cells in the bone marrow, liver, spleen, lymph nodes, gastrointestinal tract, and skin. Some patients may have the characteristic lesions of urticaria pigmentosa. If suspected, a 24-hour urine histamine level, coupled with a skin or bone-marrow biopsy, establishes the diagnosis. As with many mast cell–mediated processes, treatment is aimed at blocking the histamine response.

Patients with vesiculobullous reactions such as TEN and SJS require hospital admission and immediate evaluation. SJS usually is associated with medications or infection (*herpes* simplex, *Mycoplasma pneumoniae*, *Streptococcus* spp.), whereas the causative factors for TEN are most often drugs or graft-versus-host disease. Both TEN and SJS may be misdiagnosed as other processes that involve exfoliation, desquamation, or blistering. Exfoliative dermatitis presents with erythroderma and scaling. If the reaction is extensive, large amounts of scale may detach from the skin, giving the clinical appearance of full-thickness epidermal loss. Other acute drug-induced eruptions, such as exanthematous pustulosis, also can cause extensive superficial exfoliation. Primary bullous diseases (e.g., pemphigus vulgaris) also may be confused with TEN or SJS, because they can produce similar mucocutaneous findings. Other entities such as phototoxic reactions, thermal burns, and pressure blisters can clinically and sometimes histologically resemble SJS or TEN (8). Skin biopsy and immunofluorescence studies often help differentiate these vesiculobullous skin disorders.

Indications for Hospitalization and ICU Admission

The triage of patients with anaphylaxis varies depending on the severity of the reaction and the initial response to treatment (Figure 120.1). Patients who present with anaphylaxis but respond to therapy should be observed for 24 hours. Anaphylaxis unresponsive to initial emergency-department therapy requires ICU admission. Often these patients develop laryngeal edema that necessitates intubation for airway control. Severe bronchoconstriction may lead to hypoxemia, hypercapnia, and respiratory acidosis requiring mechanical ventilation (Chapter 56). Cardiovascular collapse may result in severe hypotension requiring vasopressor support (Chapter 25). Patients with severe dermatologic reactions may require admission to specialized burn units for optimal treatment.

Initial Therapy

Initial assessment should focus on securing the patient's airway and monitoring his or her cardiopulmonary status. If there is evidence of significant airway edema or stridor, the patient should be intubated immediately. Patients with severe upper-airway obstruction, bronchospasm, or hypotension should receive intravenous doses of aqueous epinephrine 1:1000, 0.1–0.3 mL in 10 mL normal saline (1:100,000 to 1:33,000 dilution) over several minutes. This may be repeated as necessary. Patients still recalcitrant to therapy can be placed on a continuous epinephrine infusion (1.0–10 mcg/min) and titrated to response. In less severe cases, aqueous epinephrine 1:1000 dilution, 0.3–0.5 ml (0.01 mg/kg in children; max dose 0.3 mg) can be given intramuscularly. Administration in the anterolateral thigh produces higher and more rapid peak plasma levels compared to subcutaneous injections or intramuscular injections in the arm (9).

An intravenous line should be placed and fluid resuscitation begun if the patient is hypotensive. An antihistamine such as diphenhydramine 50 mg intravenous can be administered and repeated in 4–6 hours. Treatment with H_2-receptor antagonists may provide additional benefit. Systemic glucocorticoids (e.g., methylprednisolone 1–2 mg/kg per 24 h), while not acutely affecting symptoms, may help abort prolonged reactions and minimize relapses. Supplemental oxygen should be administered and bronchospasm treated with aerosolized β-agonists (albuterol 2.5 mg in 2.5 mL normal saline via nebulization every 20 minutes for three doses, then every 2–4 hours). Patients taking β-blockers may be refractory to treatment. If this is suspected, glucagon can be administered at a dose of 1 mg in 1 L of D5W at a rate of 5–15 mL/min. If the patient still remains hypotensive, intravenous vasopressors such as norepinephrine should be started (Chapter 25).

Treatment for SJS or TEN focuses on meticulous skin care, fluid and electrolyte repletion, nutritional support, pain control, and evaluation for superimposed infection. Adhesive tapes should be avoided. The patient's list of medications must be thoroughly reviewed (see Table 120.2), and all non-essential medicines discontinued. Prompt withdrawal of the offending drug has been shown to decrease

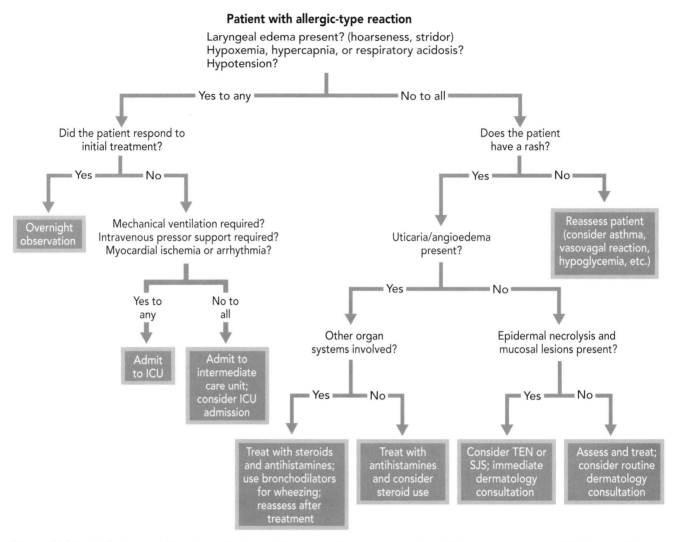

Figure 120.1 Evaluation and disposition of patients with adverse allergic-type reactions. *ICU,* intensive care unit; *SJS,* Stevens-Johnson syndrome; *TEN,* toxic epidermal necrolysis.

mortality in SJS or TEN by approximately 30% per day (10). The use of corticosteroids is controversial and more likely to be of benefit early in the disease process. While not of unequivocal proven benefit, the administration of high-dose intravenous immunoglobulin to patients with TEN has been effective in multiple studies (11).

Indications for Early Consultation

Most patients who experience anaphylactic reactions should be evaluated by an allergist prior to discharge. Aside from eliciting potential triggers, consultation with an allergist may help to exclude other processes with similar presentations (Table 120.1). If the causative agent is documented, an allergist can help advise the patient and the primary physician about possible cross-reacting antigens, in the hope of avoiding future events. A typical example would be patients who are allergic to sulfonamide antibiotics but have cross-reactivity with other

sulfa-containing drugs such as furosemide or dapsone. Skin testing is of no utility in the hospitalized setting, as mast cells will be refractory to an antigen challenge for several weeks.

TABLE 120.2

DRUGS MOST COMMONLY ASSOCIATED WITH STEVENS-JOHNSON SYNDROME OR TOXIC EPIDERMAL NECROLYSIS

Sulfonamides	Allopurinol
Penicillins	Fluoroquinolones
Cephalosporins	Vancomycin
Barbiturates	Thiabendazole
Phenytoin	Rifampin
Carbamazepine	Ethambutol
Nonsteroidal anti-inflammatory drugs	Chlormezanone
Phenylbutazone	

Patients with severe dermatologic reactions such as TEN or SJS require emergent allergic and dermatologic consultation, and possibly consultation with a specialist in burn care.

Issues During the Course of Hospitalization

Patients with anaphylaxis who experience rapid resolution of their symptoms can be discharged after 24 hours of observation. A critical care pathway for patients admitted to the ICU must be tailored to their clinical responses and the various end-organs affected. Critically ill patients who improve with aggressive treatment can be transferred out to the medical floor in 24–48 hours. However, patients taking β-blockers often require a longer length of stay in the ICU because of persistent hypotension. Patients who are difficult to wean from the ventilator need to have other diagnoses, such as status asthmaticus, considered (Chapter 56). Patients who experience myocardial ischemia or arrhythmias require stabilization and consideration of further risk stratification (Chapters 37, 38, 42, and 43).

Rarely, it may be necessary to initiate or continue therapy with a medication to which a patient has a history of anaphylaxis. In this situation, the patient can be desensitized by administering increasing increments of the drug orally or intravenously. This procedure needs to be performed in an ICU setting with emergency resuscitation equipment available and in consultation with an allergist or immunologist.

Mortality rates for SJS and TEN are 5% and 30%, respectively (8). The duration of disease progression is usually 3–4 days. Poor outcomes are associated with increased age, extensive epidermal detachment, visceral involvement, and dehydration (12). Steroids improve the clinical course of some patients with SJS if administered early. The effectiveness of corticosteroids on morbidity and mortality rates in patients with TEN has not been demonstrated in clinical trials, and their routine use is not recommended. Again, consultation with an allergist or dermatologist as well as a burn specialist aids the management of these patients.

ANAPHYLAXIS OR SEVERE ALLERGIC REACTION DEVELOPING IN THE HOSPITAL

A wide spectrum of adverse reactions may occur among hospitalized patients. Although treatment of severe reactions is no different whether the reaction developed inside or outside the hospital, a variety of less severe reactions can develop and must be managed in the hospital setting. The onset and manifestations of allergic reactions depend on several factors. These include the amount of antigen, its route of administration, and the relative sensitivities of the various organs to the vasoactive substances involved. Parenteral administration of antigen provokes more frequent and severe reactions than oral ingestion.

Drugs are the most common agents precipitating anaphylaxis in the hospitalized patient, with penicillins most frequent. *Patients with a history of anaphylaxis to penicillin should not receive cephalosporins,* because they share the same ring structure. The cross-reactivity with cephalosporins in this population may be as high as 50%. Most patients (80%–90%) who report a penicillin "allergy" (without anaphylaxis) do not produce specific IgE antibodies to penicillin. Therefore, the cross-reactivity with cephalosporins in these patients is significantly lower (10%–15%). Patients with a prior history of atopic diseases (asthma, atopic dermatitis, allergic rhinitis) do not have a significantly increased risk of developing anaphylaxis to drugs. However, atopic individuals have more severe reactions and an increased risk of anaphylactic reactions to radiocontrast media, food, or latex. *Latex allergy* also may pose a threat to those who have had prior or continued exposure, especially healthcare workers and patients with spina bifida or urogenital abnormalities.

Anaphylaxis also may be seen during *transfusion reactions.* Some patients who receive intravenous immunoglobulin possess an IgA deficiency and produce IgE and IgG autoantibodies against IgA. If given intravenous immunoglobulin containing IgA, such patients may experience a mast cell–mediated reaction ranging from urticaria or angioedema to anaphylaxis. The majority of transfusion reactions, however, occur through the formation of immune complexes, causing serum sickness rather than anaphylaxis (Chapter 91 contains further details regarding transfusion reactions). Food also must be considered as a precipitant. For example, peanut-induced anaphylaxis is a common problem, affecting about 1.5 million people and causing 50–100 deaths per year in the United States. TNX-901, a monoclonal antibody to IgE, has been shown to significantly increase the threshold of sensitivity to peanut antigen, hence decreasing the risk from an unintended ingestion (13).

Most severe drug reactions in hospitalized patients are anaphylactoid (i.e., not mediated by IgE antibody). Contrast material used in radiographic tests and drugs such as opiates can directly stimulate mast cell activation. These patients are treated in the exact same fashion as patients with anaphylaxis. Tryptase levels in these individuals are increased secondary to mast cell degranulation. Patients receiving aspirin or NSAIDs may have severe anaphylactoid reactions as well. Patients with a history of asthma, nasal polyps, and/or rhinosinusitis are particularly at risk.

Patients with a history of *radiocontrast allergy* often need to undergo important diagnostic radiographic tests. In these situations the prophylactic regimen should be catered to the severity of the patient's allergy. Patients with a history of urticaria can be pre-dosed with 50 mg of oral prednisone (13, 7, and 1 hour before) and 25 mg of parenteral diphenhydramine 1 hour before the procedure. Patients with more severe anaphylactoid reactions (i.e., angioedema, hypotension) additionally can be given 25 mg of ephedrine orally and 300 mg of cimetidine orally 1 hour before the procedure (14). Finally, the use of nonionic low-osmolality radiocontrast media helps to minimize the likelihood of an adverse reaction (15).

Adverse dermatologic reactions occurring among hospitalized patients range from intractable pruritus to urticaria, angioedema, or TEN. Careful history-taking and review of the medication record is essential to making the correct diagnosis. Patients presenting with urticaria have erythematous, well-circumscribed wheals (hives) that are intensely pruritic and often migratory. Urticaria also may be accompanied by angioedema. The mechanism of action is similar, but angioedema occurs in the deeper cutaneous structures. The production of urticaria or angioedema usually implies the presence of an IgE-mediated hypersensitivity reaction. Less often the drug (hapten) complexes with serum or tissue proteins, forming an immune complex that activates the complement cascade. The resulting anaphylatoxins C3a, C4a, and C5a bind to mast cells and degranulate them.

Specific classes of drugs often produce characteristic clinical syndromes involving one or more organ systems. Anticonvulsants, most notably phenytoin, phenobarbital, and carbamazepine, can cause erythematous eruptions 1–3 weeks after their administration. Clinical signs and symptoms include fever, lymphadenopathy, facial edema, leukocytosis, hepatitis, and nephritis.

Morbilliform or maculopapular rashes are the most common drug-induced cutaneous reactions. These rashes consist of symmetrical macules and papules that often are confluent. Patients may note pruritus or fever. Similar presentations have been seen in patients with acute viral infections such as measles, Epstein-Barr virus, cytomegalovirus, and acute HIV seroconversion. Patients infected with HIV are 5–10 times more likely to develop morbilliform drug eruptions than uninfected people. Trimethoprim-sulfamethoxazole, amoxicillin, and ampicillin commonly induce cutaneous reactions in such patients. It is also important to identify *erythema multiforme*, an acute inflammatory eruption of the skin and mucous membranes. In this disorder, patients may develop a variety of lesions, including maculopapular rashes. Target lesions are diagnostic, and the rash typically involves the extremities symmetrically. Fever and flu-like symptoms may precede the eruption by several days. Erythema multiforme is most commonly associated with drugs or infection (typically, *herpes* simplex virus). A variety of other adverse cutaneous reactions, such as drug-induced vasculitis, warfarin skin necrosis, and vancomycin-induced "red man" syndrome (flushing about the neck and face), may complicate a patient's hospital course. Management of these conditions includes discontinuation of the offending drug, supportive care, and dermatologic consultation when appropriate.

Patients with *carcinoid tumors* also may develop symptoms analogous to anaphylaxis. Severe skin flushing, abdominal cramping, diarrhea, and bronchoconstriction may confuse the clinical picture. Patients suspected of having this disease should have 24-hour levels of 5-hydroxyin-doleacetic acid measured. Treatment is based on reducing the tumor burden. The somatostatin analog octreotide has successfully reduced the severe flushing and other endocrine manifestations of the syndrome.

Other entities also may mimic anaphylaxis. For example, patients who experience hypoglycemia, asthma, cardiac arrhythmias, and vasovagal reactions can present with pallor, diaphoresis, hypotension, shortness of breath, and wheezing. These patients lack the characteristic urticaria or angioedema that is noted in 88% of individuals experiencing anaphylaxis. The role of mastocytosis as a masquerader has been alluded to previously.

Often, patients with hypertension or diabetes present to the hospital with new-onset congestive heart failure and are started on ACE inhibitors. Although this class of drugs can cause a dry cough and angioedema at any time, 60% of the adverse reactions occur immediately or within the first few days of treatment (6). If angioedema occurs, it is necessary to discontinue the drug. Lowering the dose or changing to a different type of ACE inhibitor is not effective, and similar episodes may be seen in patients switched to angiotensin II receptor blockers (16). A short course of steroids helps resolve the angioedema.

Discharge Issues

Prior to discharge, patients experiencing an anaphylactic reaction should be educated about the nature of their illness. This includes informing them to wear medical-alert bracelets and providing instructions on how to self-administer an injection of epinephrine in the event of an attack. Prevention is equally important. Patients need to be able to recognize potential triggers as well as understand substances to which they may cross-react and suffer an allergic reaction. Patients should be referred to an allergist for skin-prick testing and desensitization therapy if indicated. Finally, the primary care physician must be informed of all adverse reactions occurring in the hospital, and all such reactions should be documented clearly in both the inpatient and outpatient medical record.

COST CONSIDERATIONS AND RESOURCE USE

Patients requiring prolonged ICU admission incur significant costs. Consultation with a dermatologist early in the course of a skin reaction may expedite adequate treatment, preventing clinical deterioration and prolonged hospitalization. Consultation with an allergist or immunologist for patients with new-onset or recurring severe allergic reactions may best identify optimal therapy to shorten the hospital course and optimize patient education. Follow-up education promotes adherence and identification of the possible allergens so as to avoid them or other cross-reacting allergens. Further, utilizing protocols of premedication, such as those utilized for radiographic contrast material, reduces costs by minimizing adverse outcomes.

KEY POINTS

- Both allergic and nonallergic reactions can produce anaphylactic symptoms.
- The differential diagnosis of an anaphylactic/anaphylactoid reaction includes several nonallergic diseases that may present with similar symptoms.
- The treatment of anaphylaxis is straightforward, but the underlying precipitant is often elusive.
- Patients with anaphylaxis usually improve if the initial therapy is administered without delay. If β-blocker therapy causes persistent hypotension, patients should receive glucagon. Other diagnoses also need to be considered.
- The most common precipitants of anaphylaxis in the hospital are drugs, radio-contrast agents, and latex products.
- Patient education and appropriate follow-up with the patient's primary care physician and an allergist are essential in cases of anaphylactic/anaphylactoid reactions requiring hospitalization.

REFERENCES

1. Borda I, Slone D, Jick H. Assessment of adverse reactions within a drug surveillance program. *JAMA* 1968;205:645–647.
2. Faich G. Adverse drug reaction monitoring. *N Engl J Med* 1986; 314:1589–1592.
3. Boston Collaborative Drug Surveillance Program. Drug-induced anaphylaxis: a cooperative study. *JAMA* 1973;224:613–615.
4. Laporte JR, deLatorre FJ, Gadgil DA, et al. An epidemiologic study of severe anaphylactic and anaphylactoid reactions among hospital patients: methods and overall risks. The International Collaborative Study of Severe Anaphylaxis. *Epidemiology* 1998;9: 141–146.
5. Metcalf D. Acute anaphylaxis and urticaria in children and adults. In: Schocket A, ed. *Clinical Management of Urticaria and Anaphylaxis.* New York: Marcel Decker, 1992, 70.
6. Vleeming W, van Amsterdam J, Stricker B, et al. ACE inhibitor-induced angioedema. *Drug Safety* 1998;18:171–188.
7. Waytes A, Rosen F, Frank M. Treatment of hereditary angioedema with a vapor-heated C1 inhibitor concentrate. *N Engl J Med* 1996;334:1630–1634.
8. Roujeau J, Stern R. Severe adverse cutaneous reactions to drugs. *N Engl J Med* 1994;331:1272–1285.
9. Simons FER, Gu X, Simons KJ. Epinephrine absorption in adults: intramuscular versus subcutaneous injection. *J Allergy Clin Immunol* 2001;108:871–873.
10. Garcia-Doval I, LeCleach L, Bocquet H, et al. Toxic epidermal necrolysis and Stevens Johnson syndrome: does early withdrawal of causative drugs decrease the risk of death? *Arch Dermatology* 2000;136:323–327.
11. Wolff K. Treatment of toxic epidermal necrolysis. *Arch Dermatology* 2003;139:85–86.
12. Becker D. Toxic epidermal necrolysis. *Lancet* 1998;351:1417–1420.
13. Leung DYM, Sampson HA, Yunginger JW, et al. Effect of anti-IgE therapy in patients with peanut allergy. *N Engl J Med* 2003;348: 986–993.
14. Marshall G Jr, Lieberman P. Comparison of three pretreatment protocols to prevent anaphylactoid reactions to radiocontrast media. *Ann Allerg* 1991;67:70–74.
15. Barrett BJ, Parfrey PS, Vavasour HM, et al. A comparison of non ionic, low-osmolality radio contrast agents with ionic, high-osmolality agents during cardiac catheterization. *N Engl J Med* 1992;326:431–436.
16. Abdi R, Dong VM, Lee CJ, Ntoso KA. Angiotensin II receptor blocker-associated angioedema: on the heels of AC inhibitor angioedema. *Pharmacotherapy* 2002;22:1173–1175.

ADDITIONAL READING

Kemp SF, Lockey RF. Anaphylaxis: a review of causes and mechanisms. *J Allergy Clin Immunol* 2002;110:341–348.
Sicherer SH. Advances in anaphylaxis and hypersensitivity reactions to foods, drugs, and insect venom. *J Allergy Clin Immunol* 2003; 111:S829–834.

Drug Overdoses and Dependence

121

Josef G. Thundiyil   Jon K. Beauchamp   Kent R. Olson

INTRODUCTION

Overdose patients are a heterogeneous group who may present with a variety of ingestions (e.g., prescription medications, over-the-counter products, and/or drugs of abuse) and reasons for their overdose (e.g., suicide attempt, accidental overmedication, or drug abuse). The overdose is often a dynamic process in which a previously healthy individual can become critically ill in a matter of minutes or hours. Frequently, clinicians must treat a drug overdose using an incomplete history, a limited physical examination, and only a few diagnostic studies. Pre-existing medical conditions can complicate the management of the overdose. Finally, the overdose may represent an intentional suicide attempt or a drug dependency that requires psychiatric or social intervention in addition to medical treatment.

The first section of this chapter discusses the general considerations pertinent to most drug-overdose patients. This includes the indications for hospitalization, initial ICU admission, early consultation, and issues during the course of hospitalization and at discharge. The subsequent sections review the clinical presentation, evaluation, and initial therapy for overdose patients with an altered level of consciousness, seizures, shock, and/or an abnormal electrocardiogram, respectively. The final section discusses the management of a drug-dependent patient during hospitalization.

GENERAL CONSIDERATIONS IN A DRUG-OVERDOSE PATIENT

Issues at the Time of Admission

Clinical Presentation

There are many different initial manifestations of an acute drug overdose. These may include an altered level of consciousness, seizures, hypotension, cardiac arrhythmias, metabolic acidosis, or gastrointestinal symptoms. Important variables in the history include the specific drug or drugs taken, the amount taken, the time between the overdose and presentation, and any underlying medical illnesses. Certain drugs (e.g., carbamazepine, salicylates, tricyclic antidepressants, sustained-release or enteric-coated preparations) may be absorbed slowly or erratically, which can delay the onset of toxicity. Some drugs (e.g., digoxin, lithium, salicylates, theophylline, metformin, verapamil) can cause toxicity after chronic, repeated overmedication or in the presence of impaired drug elimination because of kidney or liver dysfunction. The presentation and treatment of common poisonings and drug overdoses are described in Table 121.1.

Differential Diagnosis and Initial Evaluation

The symptoms and clinical manifestations may be similar for many different drug overdoses and medical

TABLE 121.1

CLINICAL ISSUES AND TREATMENT OF SOME COMMON DRUG OVERDOSES AND POISONINGS

Drug or poison	Clinical presentation	Treatment[a]
Acetaminophen (Panadol, paracetamol, Tylenol, etc)	Potentially toxic ingestion is >7 gm. Alcoholics and patients taking anticonvulsants or INH may be at higher risk for liver injury. Initial nausea and vomiting followed by evidence of liver injury developing over 24–48 hours. Patients may be only minimally symptomatic early in the course of overdose. May lead to fulminant hepatic failure. Always consider acetaminophen as a coingestant in an opiate overdose.	Obtain STAT serum acetaminophen level and plot on nomogram (see Figure 121.1). If level is toxic or patient presents late, start N-acetylcysteine 140 mg/kg PO immediately followed by 70 mg/kg every 4 hours for 17 doses. Consult PCC regarding length of treatment or use of intravenous N-acetylcysteine if not tolerated orally. Shorter course may be used if patient has no evidence of liver injury at 36 hours. Consult regional liver transplant service for patients with rapidly rising liver aminotransferases.
Amphetamines (methamphetamine [crank, crystal meth], MDMA [ecstasy]) and cocaine (crack)	Toxicity may occur after injection, nasal insufflation, smoking, or ingestion. Delayed toxicity can occur if swallowed in drug packets. Toxicity includes agitation, psychosis, seizures, hyperthermia, tachycardia, and hypertension. Intracranial hemorrhage, rhabdomyolysis, myocardial ischemia, and cardiac arrhythmias may also occur.	Reduce external stimuli and provide calm environment. Sedation with benzodiazepines or antipsychotic agents (e.g., haloperidol). Consider whole bowel irrigation for drug packet ingestions. Treat severe hypertension unresponsive to benzodiazepines with vasodilator (e.g., nitroprusside, nitroglycerin, or phentolamine). Use extreme caution with β-blockers. Hyperthermia requires aggressive cooling measures, including neuromuscular paralysis.
Anticholinergics and antihistamines (benztropine, diphenhydramine, chlorpheniramine, etc)	Anticholinergic syndrome (tachycardia, dilated pupils, flushed dry skin, sleepiness or confusion, delirium, hallucinations). Seizures, rhabdomyolysis, hyperthermia, and QRS widening can occur. May cause delayed drug absorption. Always consider possibility of tricyclic antidepressant (TCA) overdose (see below), which has similar presentation.	Observation, supportive care. Use benzodiazepines for agitation and seizures. For non-TCA anticholinergic syndrome, consider physostigmine 0.5–1 mg IV. (Caution: physostigmine can cause seizures and bradycardia.)
Benzodiazepines (diazepam, alprazolam, chlordiazepoxide, lorazepam, oxazepam, etc)	Sleepiness, stupor, CNS depression, ataxia, slurred speech (usually arousal with strong stimulus). Relatively safe alone, although deep coma can occur with large or mixed ingestions or with newer short-acting benzodiazepines.	Supportive care. Although there is a specific antidote (flumazenil), it is contraindicated if there may be co-ingestion of a tricyclic antidepressant or other convulsant or if patient is dependent on benzodiazepines, and most toxicologists advise against empiric use. It has been reported to cause seizures and dysrhythmias in patients who are benzodiazepine dependent.
β-blockers (atenolol, metoprolol, propranolol, etc)	Severe bradycardia, atrioventricular block, hypotension, often resistant to β-adrenergic drugs. Life threatening in overdose. Lipid-soluble agents (e.g., propranolol) can also cause coma, seizures, and tricyclic-like cardiotoxicity. Bronchospasm may occur in asthmatics. Sustained release preparations may have delayed toxicity. Beta selectivity is lost in overdose.	Cardiac monitoring and close observation; consider whole bowel irrigation for sustained release preparations or massive ingestion. Use atropine, epinephrine, isoproterenol, or cardiac pacing for symptomatic bradycardia. Intravenous fluids, epinephrine infusion, or norepinephrine infusion for hypotension. For resistant bradycardia or hypotension, use glucagon 5–10 mg IV, followed by infusion of 5–10 mg/hr. For large or prolonged infusions, do not use supplied diluent (contains phenol). Consider sodium bicarbonate boluses if wide complex conduction defects occur.
Calcium channel blockers (amlodipine, verapamil, nifedipine, diltiazem, etc)	Severe bradycardia, hypotension, often resistant to usual agents. Junctional bradycardia and ileus are common rhythm. Sustained release products may have delayed toxicity. Hyperglycemia may occur.	Cardiac monitoring and close observation; consider whole bowel irrigation for sustained release preparations or massive ingestion if peristalsis is present. Give calcium chloride, 1–2 gm IV. Repeat dose as needed to raise BP and increase heart rate. Doses as high as 10 gm or more may be required. Glucagon, epinephrine, amrinone, and high-dose insulin therapy may help with refractory hypotension.

TABLE 121.1
(continued)

Drug or poison	Clinical presentation	Treatment[a]
Carbamazepine (Tegretol)	Stupor, ataxia, decreased level of consciousness, seizures, and coma occur. AV block, brady-cardia, QRS, and QT widening are occasionally reported. Has some anticholinergic effects. Absorption from the gut is often slow and erratic and may lead to delayed toxicity.	For large ingestion, give extra doses of activated charcoal every 3–4 hours to ensure gut decon-tamination. Follow serial levels to rule out pro-longed delayed absorption. Serious symptoms may occur at levels greater than 40 mg/L and if serum level >60 mg/L, consider hemodialysis or charcoal hemoperfusion.
Carbon monoxide	High index of suspicion is needed because symp-toms are nonspecific: headache, nausea, dizzi-ness, confusion, stupor, seizures, angina, and coma. After significant poisoning, permanent neurologic sequelae can occur. CT scan may show hypodense regions in central white mat-ter. Metabolic acidosis may be present.	Give high-flow *oxygen* by tight-fitting mask or 100% via endotracheal tube. Obtain carboxyhemo-globin level. Recent evidence suggests that hyperbaric oxygen may reduce long-term neuro-logic and cognitive sequelae; but this remains controversial and HBO is not usually readily avail-able (1).
Cocaine, crack	Toxicity can occur after nasal insufflation, smoking, injection, or ingestion. Swallowed packets may cause delayed toxicity. Symptoms include euphoria, anxiety, agitation, delirium, psychosis, tremors, seizures, hypertension, hyperthermia, myocardial ischemia, intracranial bleed, stroke, arrhythmias, and death.	Maintain close observation and cardiac monitoring; reduce external stimuli. Use benzodiazepines as the initial therapy for agitation, seizures, hyper-tension, anxiety, and tremors. For refractory hy-pertension, avoid pure β-blockers, as unopposed alpha effects may paradoxically worsen hyperten-sion. Consider phentolamine as an additional va-sodilatory therapy. Nitrates and calcium channel blockers may be used for cardiac ischemia.
Cyanide	Acute collapse, hypotension, severe metabolic acidosis. Symptoms can also include headache, nausea, and confusion. Smell of "bitter al-monds" may be detected by about 60% of care-givers. Toxicity can also develop from high-dose intravenous nitroprusside therapy.	*Cyanide antidote package* contains amyl and sodium nitrite (300mg) (to induce methe-moglobinemia) and sodium thiosulfate (12.5g) (to enhance conversion of cyanide to less toxic thio-cyanate). Administer sequentially and provide supportive care. Stop or reduce nitroprusside in-fusion.
Cardiac glycosides (digoxin, digitoxin, oleander, and other plants)	Nausea, vomiting, visual disturbances, hyper-kalemia. Bradycardia with prominent AV block. Patients with underlying atrial fibrillation may present with slowed ventricular response or a junctional rhythm. Ventricular arrhythmias, heart failure, and death may occur. Levels may be falsely elevated if drawn within 4–6 hours of in-gestion.	Initiate continuous cardiac monitoring. For signifi-cant toxicity, severe hyperkalemia, and symp-tomatic arrhythmias, give *digoxin-specific antibod-ies* (Digibind or DigiFab) based on estimated body burden of digoxin (see package insert or call PCC for calculation). Note that serum digoxin levels may be falsely elevated after antibody therapy. Do not give calcium because this may worsen ventric-ular arrhythmias or cause asystole.
Ethanol	Common co-ingestant with other drugs that re-sults in stupor, disinhibition, hypoglycemia, hy-pothermia agitation, altered level of conscious-ness, CNS depression, and coma. Vomiting with pulmonary aspiration of gastric contents is a common complication.	Supportive care. Examine carefully for associated co-morbidities (trauma, infections, other OD). Ac-tivated charcoal not effective. Treat alcoholism-associated ketoacidosis with glucose, thiamine, and volume replacement. Treat withdrawal syn-drome with benzodiazepines (Chapter 122).
Ethylene glycol (antifreeze)	Intoxication causes gastritis, decreased LOC, stu-por, and coma. Elevated serum osmolality (os-molar gap). Metabolism of EG leads to severe metabolic acidosis (non-lactate), renal failure, coma, and death. Woods lamp may reveal fluor-escent urine.	Charcoal is ineffective. Block EG metabolism with *ethanol* or *fomepizole* (consult PCC for dosing). Treat acidosis with bicarbonate. Remove EG and toxic metabolites with early consideration for *hemodialysis*. Supplement with folate and pyri-doxine.
Gamma hydroxybutyric acid (GHB)(2)	Drug of abuse, "date rape drug," and used by weightlifters. Can cause rapid onset of deep coma, often with muscle twitching or occa-sionally seizures, bradycardia, and emergence phenomenon. Withdrawal syndrome has been described.	Supportive care. Duration usually brief, with rapid spontaneous awakening from deep coma within 2–4 hours.

TABLE 121.1

Drug or poison	Clinical presentation	Treatment[a]
Hypoglycemic agents (oral), sulfonylureas, and other agents (3)	Sulfonylureas can cause delayed onset of hypoglycemia that can persist for up to 48–72 hours. Symptoms can include confusion, diaphoresis, agitations, seizure, and coma. Other agents do not cause hypoglycemia but may contribute to that caused by sulfonylureas and insulin.	Close glucose monitoring for a minimum of 24 hours. Use glucose boluses of D50 to bring glucose to within normal range; then use continuous glucose infusions and *octreotide* (50 mcg SQ every 12 hours) to maintain euglycemia. Rebound hypoglycemia may occur when dextrose infusion is stopped.
Isoniazid (INH)	After acute ingestion, nausea, vomiting, ataxia, agitation, confusion, and seizures. Seizures are often refractory to conventional therapy. Severe lactic acidosis often accompanies even a few brief seizures, due to block of lactate metabolism.	Seizures may be resistant to benzodiazepines. Give *pyridoxine* (vitamin B_6), 5 gm IV, or if amount ingested is known, give a gm-for-gm equivalent dose.
Lithium (4)	After acute overdose, serum level may be falsely elevated if drawn within a few hours of ingestion. Chronic overmedication may cause greater toxicity. Initially, nausea, vomiting, confusion, ataxia, tremor, weakness, slurred speech, myoclonus, seizures, or coma can occur after acute or chronic intoxication. Therapeutic use or overdose can cause nephrogenic diabetes insipidus.	Activated charcoal does not bind Lithium. Consider whole-bowel irrigation for large ingestion of sustained-release products. Promote renal excretion with intravenous fluids to maintain adequate urine output. Consider hemodialysis or continuous renal replacement therapy for significant toxicity, renal failure, and severe neurologic symptoms. Symptoms may persist for days-to-weeks and do not always correlate with serum level.
Methanol (wood alcohol, solvents, glass cleaning products, paint removers)	Intoxication is similar to ethanol or ethylene glycol: gastritis, elevated serum osmolality (osmolar gap), stupor, and coma. Metabolism of methanol leads to severe anion gap metabolic acidosis (non-lactate), visual changes, blindness, seizures, coma, and death.	Block methanol metabolism with *ethanol* or *fomepizole*. Supplement with folic acid. Treat acidosis with bicarbonate and early consideration for *hemodialysis* to remove methanol and toxic metabolites.
Nonsteroidal anti-inflammatory drugs (NSAIDs) (e.g., ibuprofen, naproxen, ketorolac, etc.)	Nausea and vomiting common. After very large ingestion (e.g., >400 mg/kg) may see stupor, coma, seizures, metabolic acidosis, pulmonary edema, and renal failure. Mefenamic acid and phenylbutazone are more likely to cause seizures.	Supportive. Symptomatic treatment and observation. Monitor renal function and electrolytes.
Noncyclic antidepressants; (serotonin reuptake inhibitors: fluoxetine, fluvoxamine, paroxetine, sertraline; mixed neurotransmitter blockers: nefazodone, trazodone, venlafaxine, bupropion)	Generally safer than tricyclic antidepressants. Toxicity is increased by ingestion of other drugs. Symptoms can include ataxia, sedation, tremor, coma, hypotension, and tachycardia. Bupropion commonly causes seizures. Serotonin syndrome (confusion, myoclonus, diaphoresis, tremor, hyperthermia) can rarely be seen with overdose or medication interaction.	Close observation. Supportive care and symptomatic treatment. Some reports have suggested that oral cyproheptadine may be of benefit in serotonin syndrome.
Opioids and opiates (codeine, heroin, hydrocodone, methadone, morphine, propoxyphene, etc)	Lethargy, CNS depression, stupor, coma, respiratory depression, small pupils (often pinpoint), and noncardiogenic pulmonary edema. There may be evidence of chronic IV drug abuse. For mixed ingestions, check serum acetaminophen level (see above). Marked withdrawal syndrome.	Close observation for respiratory depression. Specific antidote is naloxone 0.4–2 mg IV. May need larger doses after codeine, propoxyphene overdose. Naloxone lasts only 1–2 hours; may need to repeat doses or give constant drip for methadone OD (can last for 2–3 days).
Organophosphate and carbamate insecticides (commonly in hydrocarbon solvent base), nerve agents (e.g., Sarin, Tabun, Vx) (5)	Poisoning can occur by ingestion, dermal absorption, or inhalation of mist. Caution must be taken by health care workers to avoid contamination by skin, vomitus, or clothing. Abdominal cramps, vomiting, diarrhea, hypersalivation, bronchorrhea, sweating, miosis, bradycardia, muscle fasciculations, and weakness. Respiratory arrest is usual cause of death. Garlicky or solvent odor may be present.	Close observation and monitoring. Perform thorough skin decontamination with soap and water. Lavage into closed (e.g., wall suction) system. Intravenous fluids for volume replacement. Antidotes include *atropine* (1–2 mg IV initially, continuous infusion may be needed) titrated to control bronchorhea and bronchospasm. *Pralidoxime* (2-PAM) is essential for muscle weakness caused by organophosphates. Begin pralidoxime treatment early for organophosphate poisoning to prevent prolonged hospitalization.

TABLE 121.1

(continued)

Drug or poison	Clinical presentation	Treatment[a]
Phenytoin (Dilantin)	At serum levels >20–30 mg/L, ataxia, nystagmus, slurred speech, and tremor may occur. At higher levels, drowsiness, lethargy, confusion, and coma can occur. Intravenous formulation contains propylene glycol diluent, which may cause hypotension and cardiac arrest when administered rapidly IV (e.g., at a rate >50 mg/min).	Supportive care. Repeated dose activated charcoal may enhance elimination but is of little practical use and can lead to overshoot if levels drop too rapidly.
Salicylates: aspirin (prescription and OTC analgesics and cold preparations), bismuth subsalicylate (Pepto-Bismol)	Patients may become poisoned from chronic overmedication or acute overdose. Chronic overmedication can result in severe and unrecognized toxicity, and symptoms will correlate poorly with levels. Bezoar formation is not uncommon with intentional acute overdose, leading to delayed and erratic absorption. Symptoms can include nausea, vomiting, tinnitus, hyperventilation, confusion, coma, hyperthermia, pulmonary edema, cerebral edema, and seizures. Mixed respiratory alkalosis and metabolic acidosis is often seen.	Monitor closely and follow serum levels until a clear downward trend exists. With large ingestions (e.g., more than 100 pills), give extra doses of activated charcoal (every 3–4 hours) and consider WBI. Maintain serum pH above 7.4 to prevent further movement of salicylate into brain. Promote renal excretion by urinary alkalinization (sodium bicarbonate 100 mEq in 1 L of D5 quarter normal saline at 3–4 mL/kg/hr). Consider hemodialysis for severe acidosis, blood level >100 mg/dL, decreased LOC, seizures, volume overload, pulmonary edema, or chronic renal failure. Verify units of measurement when checking levels (mg/L or mg/dL).
Theophylline: (TheoDur, Theo-BID, etc.)	Poisoning can occur from acute overdose or chronic overmedication. Hypokalemia, hyperglycemia, and gastrointestinal symptoms are common after acute overdose; toxicity in chronic overdose tends to occur at lower serum drug levels. Tachycardia, anxiety, tremor, and seizures may occur with both acute and chronic overdose. Course can lead to status epilepticus, cardiovascular collapse and death. Excessive β-2-adrenergic stimulation is probable cause of cardiovascular and metabolic effects.	Close observation, continuous cardiac monitoring. Repeat doses of activated charcoal may enhance drug elimination in even mild drug overdoses. Consider whole bowel irrigation for large sustained release overdoses. For serum level >100 mg/L or multiple seizures, consider hemodialysis. Hypotension and tachycardia may respond to β-blockers (e.g., esmolol at low doses, 25 mcg/kg/min).
Tricyclic antidepressants (amitriptyline, doxepin, imipramine, nortriptyline, etc) (6)	Drug absorption can be delayed and patients may deteriorate rapidly. Anticholinergic syndrome is common. Cardiotoxicity due to sodium channel blockade leads to conduction disturbance (QRS >120 msec), tachycardia, hypotension, and ventricular arrhythmias. Seizures, coma, cardiovascular collapse, hyperthermia, and death may also occur.	Continuous ECG monitoring. Early airway management is essential because of the risk of rapid deterioration. For wide QRS complex or hypotension, give sodium bicarbonate 1–2 mEq/kg IV bolus and repeat as needed. Avoid type Ia and Ic antiarrhythmics. For hypotension refractory to intravenous fluids, consider norepinephrine infusion. Do NOT use physostigmine.
Valproic acid (Depakote, Depakene)	May cause delayed and erratic drug absorption with large ingestion. Stupor, coma, metabolic acidosis, hyperammonemia, and cerebral edema.	For large ingestions, give extra doses of activated charcoal and consider whole bowel irrigation. For serum valproate level >850mg/L, consider hemodialysis or hemoperfusion. Intravenous L-carnitine may be useful for valproic acid-induced hyperammonemia.

[a] For all poisonings, appropriate, supportive care (e.g., airway management, supplemental oxygen, treating shock or cardiac dysrhythmias, correction of hypoglycemia) should be instituted. For ingestions, gastrointestinal decontamination should be performed with a single dose of an aqueous slurry of activated charcoal 50 g PO or via NG, unless an alternate method is described. *GL*, gastric lavage; *IV*, intravenous; *LOC*, level of consciousness; *PCC*, poison-control center.

conditions. Because of this, the possibility of a drug overdose should be considered in any patient who has an unexplained acute illness, particularly if he or she has an altered level of consciousness or multiple organ system dysfunctions.

The clinical condition of an acute drug-overdose patient can deteriorate quickly, and the initial evaluation should begin with a brief assessment to determine if immediate treatment is necessary. Emergent interventions may include administration of supplemental oxygen, endotracheal intubation and mechanical ventilation, treatment of shock or cardiac dysrhythmias, control of seizures, and correction of hypoglycemia. If time permits, a more complete evaluation can be done, including a physical examination, pertinent diagnostic studies (see later in this chapter), and a detailed history, including checking for routine medications, the presence of any heart, lung, liver, or kidney disease, and prior suicide attempts.

Important aspects of the physical examination of a drug-overdose patient include the level of consciousness (see subsequent discussion), a complete set of vital signs (including an accurate measurement of the respiratory rate and core temperature), pupil size and reactivity, lung sounds and an assessment of respiratory effort, the presence or absence of peristalsis (bowel sounds), and the presence of abnormal muscle activity (e.g., dystonia, fasciculations, muscle rigidity, tremors, or other abnormal movements).

The appropriate laboratory assessment of a drug-overdose patient depends on the history and clinical presentation, but should generally include serum electrolytes, glucose, blood urea nitrogen (BUN), and creatinine levels. These tests are inexpensive, quickly available, and often useful in diagnosing or managing a drug-overdose patient. Electrolyte abnormalities can result from or contribute to the toxicity of some drug overdoses. In a few cases these electrolyte abnormalities may serve as a marker of acute toxicity of a drug overdose (e.g., hyperkalemia in an acute digoxin overdose or hypokalemia in an acute theophylline overdose). The presence of an anion gap acidosis should raise the suspicion of salicylate poisoning, as well as a number of other intoxications including carbon monoxide, cyanide, iron, nonsteroidal anti-inflammatory agents, or isoniazid (Table 121.2). If there is an accompanying *osmolar gap*, one should consider the possibility of an ethylene glycol or methanol poisoning. Decreased renal

function may prolong the toxicity of a drug overdose. A serum creatine kinase level should be obtained in any drug-overdose patient at risk for rhabdomyolysis. If a drug overdose is suspected to be a suicide attempt, a rapid quantitative acetaminophen and salicylate level should be obtained and, in women of childbearing age, a rapid serum or urine pregnancy test also should be done. Additionally, an electrocardiogram should be performed to evaluate for dysrhythmias and abnormal intervals (see later discussion). Abdominal radiographs may be helpful in monitoring and the decontamination of certain radio-opaque poisons (e.g., heavy metals) or in connection with body packing or stuffing of illicit substances in plastic bags.

Comprehensive toxicologic screening of the blood and urine is costly, and the results usually are not available quickly enough to affect patient care. Because of this, it is of questionable value in the emergent evaluation of a drug-overdose patient. However, rapid urine screening for drugs of abuse (e.g., opioids, cocaine, amphetamines) may help confirm clinical suspicions and obviate the need for other workups. Urine toxicologic screens should be interpreted with caution because many common drugs (e.g., lorazepam, clonazepam, methadone, and oxycontin) frequently do not test positive for their expected assays (i.e., benzodiazepines and opiates). Meanwhile, common drugs, such as diphenhydramine and dextromethorphan, can give false positive results for such urine screening tests as phencyclidine (PCP). For some drug overdoses, quantitative serum drug levels can be helpful in deciding to hospitalize a patient, determining the acuity of care required, and guiding the use of specific treatments, such as N-acetylcysteine for acetaminophen (Figure 121.1) or digoxin-specific Fab antibodies for digoxin (Table 121.1).

Indications for Hospitalization

Most patients with acute drug overdose do not need hospitalization. Typically they can be treated and released from the hospital emergency department if they remain asymptomatic or have resolution of their symptoms during a 6- to 8-hour period of observation. However, certain drugs (e.g., acetaminophen, sustained-release medication preparations, oral sulfonylureas) may have delayed toxicity or ongoing toxicity in the absence of symptomatology. These patients, those who remain symptomatic, or those who require continuing medical treatment of their overdose or its complications require hospitalization. Patients requiring a psychiatric evaluation may need to be hospitalized unless the evaluation can be completed in the emergency department.

Indications for Intensive Care Unit Admission

An acute drug-overdose patient who has unstable vital signs, needs respiratory support, or requires close observation for medical or psychiatric reasons most likely needs to

---

TABLE 121.2

COMMON CAUSES OF AN ANION GAP[a] **ACIDOSIS**

Lactic acidosis

Acetaminophen (serum drug level >600 mcg/mL)	Hypoxia
	Metformin (rare)
β-adrenergic drugs	Salicylates
Carbon monoxide	Seizures
Cyanide	Shock
Iron	Theophylline
Isoniazid	

Nonlactic acidosis

Alcoholic ketoacidosis	Methanol
Diabetic ketoacidosis	Salicylates
Ethylene glycol	Valproic acid
Exogenous acids	

[a] Anion gap: (serum sodium) – (serum chloride) – (serum bicarbonate). Normal = 8–12 mEq/L.

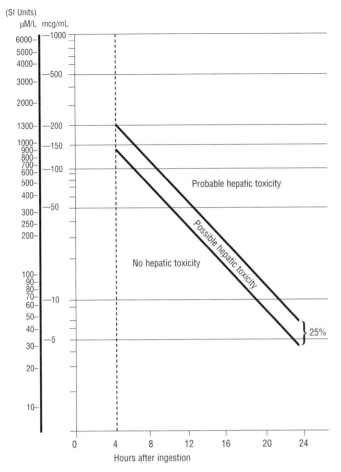

(SI Units)

Figure 121.1 Nomogram for prediction of acetaminophen hepatoxicity after acute drug overdose. The upper line defines serum acetaminophen concentrations likely to be associated with hepatotoxicity, the lower line defines serum levels 25% below those expected to cause hepatotoxicity. Courtesy of McNeil Consumer Products, Inc.

be admitted to an intensive care setting. Continuous monitoring of the ECG and vital signs is recommended after overdoses involving cardiotoxic drugs or agents likely to cause seizures or altered levels of consciousness. In certain circumstances a lower acuity bed with continuous cardiac monitoring may be adequate.

Initial Therapy

The care required by hospitalized drug-overdose patients varies greatly. Most do well with observation, supportive care, and gastrointestinal decontamination with oral activated charcoal. Some patients benefit from more aggressive gut decontamination or enhancement of drug elimination (e.g., hemodialysis), and a few will require therapeutic interventions specific to the overdose drug (Table 121.1). Empiric initial therapy for most drug-overdose patients should include close observation, monitoring vital signs, establishing venous access, a single dose of activated charcoal (see later in this chapter), and, if indicated, continuous cardiac monitoring.

Emergent supportive measures include supplemental oxygen, airway management with treatment of shock or cardiac dysrhythmias, control of seizures, aggressive control of hyperthermia, and correction of hypoglycemia. More general supportive care includes the correction of fluid and electrolyte abnormalities and management of symptoms.

The goal of gastrointestinal decontamination is to reduce the amount of drug absorbed and limit the severity of the overdose. In general, it should be initiated as soon as possible and may include one or more of the following procedures: induced emesis, gastric lavage, the administration of activated charcoal, and whole bowel irrigation. *Induced emesis* poses risks of aspiration, is an inefficient method of gastrointestinal decontamination, and delays the administration of activated charcoal; it has been virtually abandoned in the hospital management of poisoning because of these limitations (7). *Gastric lavage* is commonly performed, but this procedure increases the risk of pulmonary aspiration, and its role in the routine management of an acute drug overdose remains unproven. At this time, an *aqueous slurry of activated charcoal* (1g/kg, up to 50–60 grams) given by mouth or via nasogastric tube is accepted as the best method of gastrointestinal decontamination for most uncomplicated ingestions (7). However, activated charcoal is not effective for some agents, such as iron, lithium, heavy metals, hydrocarbons, and alcohols. A cathartic agent, such as magnesium sulfate or sorbitol, can be given along with the charcoal but is of questionable value and may worsen metabolic derangements in some patients. Premixed charcoal and sorbitol products should be avoided, because the large volume of sorbitol in these preparations often causes abdominal cramps and vomiting. *Whole bowel irrigation* with a commercially available solution (e.g., GoLytely or CoLyte) may be a useful technique for gastrointestinal decontamination, especially for patients who have swallowed drugs not bound by charcoal or large numbers of sustained-release pills. The solution is administered via nasogastric tube at a rate of 1 to 2 L/h for several hours, with the intent of mechanically removing the drug via the rectum. This may be useful for an overdose of iron, lithium, or sustained-release or enteric-coated tablets, or for the ingestion of a foreign body or an illicit drug packet (7).

The potential benefit of enhanced drug elimination is reducing the severity and duration of the drug overdose. For most drug overdoses, the duration of symptoms is short and the severity is limited, so there is no benefit from enhancing drug elimination. If indicated, the most commonly used techniques include repeated administrations of activated charcoal, alkalinization of the urine, and hemodialysis. Drugs that may be more rapidly eliminated by using repeated doses of activated charcoal (based on volunteer studies) include salicylates, theophylline, phenytoin, and phenobarbital. Hemodialysis is suited for drugs that have a low volume of distribution, low protein binding, poor intrinsic clearance, and exhibit significant toxicity. Examples include ethylene glycol, methanol, salicylates, valproic acid, and lithium. Additionally, continuous renal replacement (i.e., CVVH, CAVH, etc.) therapy has shown promise for elimination of toxins such as lithium because of its ease of implementation, avoidance of rebound levels, and applicability for hemodynamically unstable patients (4). Indications for enhancing drug elimination for some overdoses are described in Table 121.1.

Indications for Early Consultation

Consultation with a poison control system or a hospital-based toxicologist can provide useful and cost-effective information regarding the evaluation and treatment of a drug-overdose patient. It should be considered in any overdose patient who requires hospitalization, has an unknown ingestion, has an atypical presentation of a suspected overdose, or is not responding to treatment.

Issues During the Course of Hospitalization

Patients with acute drug overdose can deteriorate abruptly, particularly during the first few hours after their overdoses. Because of this, patients need to be reevaluated frequently for changes in their clinical condition. Similarly, they can have rapid improvement in their symptoms, and close monitoring allows for timely discontinuation of unnecessary interventions.

Issues at the Time of Discharge

There are several issues specific to a drug-overdose patient that should be addressed prior to hospital discharge. The ongoing medical necessity of any drug involved in the overdose should be reassessed, and consideration should be given to stopping or changing the medication. If the drug must be continued, it may be prudent to decrease the dosage or limit the amount dispensed at any one time. If an inadvertent dosage error was responsible for the drug overdose, close outpatient monitoring and patient education should be considered. A psychiatric evaluation, performed when the patient is medically stable, needs to be arranged for any patient who has attempted suicide via a drug overdose.

ALTERED LEVEL OF CONSCIOUSNESS

Issues at the Time of Admission

Clinical Presentation

An altered level of consciousness, manifested by either a decreased level of consciousness or an agitated state, is a common presentation of a drug overdose. A patient with a decreased level of consciousness is usually easy to identify, but the terms to describe this clinical condition (e.g., somnolent, lethargic, comatose) can be confusing and inaccurate. It is generally more accurate to quantify a patient's decreased level of consciousness by her or his response to verbal and painful stimuli (appropriate, inappropriate, or no response), ability to protect their airway, and the presence or absence of cardiovascular or respiratory depression. Using this descriptive method allows a more accurate communication of the clinical condition to other health care providers and a more precise means of following changes in the patient's clinical condition. Manifestations of agitation may include confusion; psychotic, inappropriate or violent behaviors; and excessive muscle activity. Agitated patients may present dangers to themselves and others.

Differential Diagnosis and Initial Evaluation

Altered level of consciousness may be caused by a number of common drug overdoses and medical conditions (Chapter 115). Drugs and poisons that can cause a *decreased level of consciousness* include antidepressants, antihistamines, antipsychotic agents (including phenothiazines), barbiturates, benzodiazepines, carbon monoxide, clonidine, ethanol, ethylene glycol, gamma-hydroxybutyrate, isopropyl alcohol, lidocaine, lithium, methanol, opiates, other psychiatric medications, and salicylates. *Agitation* can be caused by a number of common drug overdoses, including amphetamines, antihistamines, caffeine, cocaine, ephedrine, phencyclidine, pseudoephedrine, and theophylline. Medical conditions that may present with an altered level of consciousness include head injury, central nervous system infection, systemic infection, intracranial bleeding, postictal state, and metabolic disturbances (e.g., electrolyte abnormalities and metabolic acidosis). Hypoglycemia or hypoxia are important considerations in any patient with an altered level of consciousness and may be associated with numerous drug overdoses and medical conditions. The possibility of drug withdrawal should be considered in any agitated patient.

Any patient with an altered level of consciousness should be evaluated quickly for head injury, unstable vital signs, adequacy of airway control and ventilation, hypoglycemia (bedside blood glucose determination), hypoxia (bedside room air oxygen saturation determination), hyperthermia (rectal temperature), and the presence of focal neurologic findings. Routine diagnostic studies should include electrolyte, glucose, BUN, and creatinine levels; electrocardiogram; and a urinalysis. If the screening urinalysis is positive for blood, the patient may have rhabdomyolysis, and a serum creatine kinase should be obtained. In the appropriate circumstances, a specific drug level or serum osmolality may assist in the diagnosis. Head computed tomography should be considered in any patient with focal neurologic findings or a decreased level of consciousness of unclear cause. A lumbar puncture should be considered in any patient with suspected central nervous system infection.

Rhabdomyolysis and hyperthermia are potentially serious complications associated with drug overdoses that cause an altered level of consciousness. *Rhabdomyolysis* can occur after a prolonged period of immobilization on a firm surface, excessive motor activity (e.g., seizures, agitation), hyperthermia, direct injury to muscle tissue by trauma, certain drugs (e.g., ethanol, 2,4-dichlorophenoxyacetic acid), and toxins (e.g., snakebites) (8). Untreated rhabdomyolysis can cause myoglobinuria, hyperkalemia, and acute renal failure. The creatine kinase level invariably is elevated, and patients may have a positive urine dipstick for hemoglobin in the absence of red cells (reflecting the presence of myoglobin). *Hyperthermia* can be caused by salicylates, anticholinergic agents, inhalational anesthetics, sympathomimetic agents, serotonin antagonists, seizures, muscle rigidity, agitation with excessive muscle activity, neuroleptic malignant syndrome (from use of antipsychotic drugs), serotonin syndrome (from monoamine oxidase inhibitors or serotonin reuptake inhibitors), or malignant hyperthermia (after exposure to certain anesthetic agents). If untreated, hyperthermia may lead to rhabdomyolysis, renal failure, cardiac dysfunction, shock, and brain injury, and it probably increases the risk of death from an acute drug overdose (9).

Initial Therapy

Depending on the cause and the degree of the altered level of consciousness, initial therapy may include supplemental oxygen, endotracheal intubation and mechanical ventilation, correction of hypoglycemia, treatment of unstable vital signs, and (in the agitated patient) sedation and physical restraints to control potentially dangerous behaviors. Airway management is very important in patients with a decreased level of consciousness, because they are at risk of hypoventilation and pulmonary aspiration. Gastrointestinal decontamination should be considered but can be difficult in patients with an altered level of consciousness. When performed, great care should be exercised to prevent aspiration.

In opiate overdoses, the competitive opiate receptor antagonists *naloxone* (Narcan) or *nalmefene* (Revex) can reverse the opioid-related decrease in consciousness and respiration. They should be used primarily to reverse respiratory depression and to ensure adequate airway control and ventilation (avoiding the need for endotracheal intubation). Naloxone can precipitate acute drug withdrawal in opiate-dependent patients and can cause agitation, pulmonary edema, or cardiac dysrhythmias. The initial dosing of naloxone should be 0.2–0.4 mg intravenous, and additional doses should be titrated to reverse respiratory depression sufficiently to ensure adequate airway control and ventilation. Some opiates (e.g., propoxyphene and codeine) are resistant to usual doses of naloxone and may require 10 mg or more to reverse respiratory depression. Naloxone's duration of action is typically shorter than those of most opiates, and repeat doses or a continuous naloxone drip may be needed. Nalmefene is longer-acting than naloxone, but its duration of action is still shorter than that of methadone. Although promising, its usefulness in an acute opiate overdose remains to be determined. On the other hand, it has begun to show increasing utility as an adjunct in the treatment of alcoholism (10).

In a benzodiazepine overdose, the specific antagonist, *flumazenil* (Romazicon), can reverse the decreased level of consciousness and respiratory depression. As with the opiate antagonists, *complete reversal of benzodiazepine effects should be avoided* in benzodiazepine-dependent patients, because this can cause acute drug withdrawal and, infrequently, seizures. Specific contraindications to flumazenil's use include known or suspected coingestion of a tricyclic antidepressant, known or suspected benzodiazepine addiction, or known use of benzodiazepines to prevent seizures. The dosing of flumazenil is 0.5–2.0 mg intravenously, and it should be titrated to the reversal of respiratory depression to ensure adequate airway control and ventilations (11). Its duration of action is typically shorter than those of most benzodiazepines, and repeat doses may be needed. Studies have not demonstrated a beneficial effect from routine administration of flumazenil, and it carries significant risks of complications including seizures and arrhythmias. For this reason, most authorities advise against empiric use of flumazenil in unknown or mixed overdose patients.

Symptomatic hypoglycemia should be treated initially with 50 mL of a 50% dextrose solution (25 g dextrose) intravenously (Chapter 107). Patients who are malnourished or alcoholic may be deficient in thiamine (vitamin B_1), and thiamine 100 mg intramuscular or intravenous also should be given to prevent Wernicke's syndrome. If vascular access is not immediately available, consider giving glucagon (1–5 mg intramuscularly) as a temporizing measure. An alert patient with adequate airway control may take juices and food by mouth. There is increasing evidence that early use of octreotide for hypoglycemia (especially when it is secondary to sulfonylurea toxicity) decreases the amount of dextrose required, decreases the rate of recurrent hypoglycemia, and may possibly shorten hospital stay (3). Dosing of octreotide is 50–100 mcg every eight hours as needed.

Placing the patient in a calm environment initially can treat agitation that is unrelated to hypoglycemia, hypoxia, hypotension, or other metabolic derangement. In the patient who remains agitated, consider sedation with a benzodiazepine (e.g., lorazepam 1–2 mg intravenously or 0.05 mg/kg intramuscularly to a maximum dose of 4 mg, or midazolam 0.05 mg/kg intravenously over 20–30 s or 0.1 mg/kg intramuscularly). If additional sedation is needed, consider haloperidol 2.5–5.0 mg intramuscularly or intravenously.

The main treatment of rhabdomyolysis is aggressive intravenous fluid hydration with an alkaline crystalloid solution (2 ampules of sodium bicarbonate in 1 L of 5% dextrose) to restore any intravascular volume depletion and to maintain a urine output of 3–5 mL/kg/h. Hyperkalemia and hypocalcemia are potential complications of rhabdomyolysis, and the patient's serum potassium and calcium levels must be monitored closely. In addition, supportive care should be provided as needed, including hemodialysis in a patient with acute renal failure. The renal function in patients with acute renal failure from rhabdomyolysis typically improves over a 2- to 3-week period (8).

Hyperthermia needs to be treated aggressively to prevent serious brain injury or death. The main goals of treatment are external cooling and reducing excessive heat production. Evaporation is usually the most efficient method of external cooling and works well for most patients. This involves undressing the patient, sponging him or her with lukewarm water, and then using a fan to circulate air over their skin. Continuous core temperature should be monitored in patients with hyperthermia to assess adequacy of treatment. Avoid ice packs or cold water immersion because these can induce shivering and vasoconstriction, which interfere with heat dissipation (9). Seizures, agitation, and muscle rigidity also must be controlled (as described elsewhere in this chapter) quickly to reduce heat production. Hyperthermia and muscle rigidity from neuroleptic malignant syndrome can be treated with bromocriptine, 2.5–10 mg orally or via nasogastric tube 2–6 times daily. The hyperthermia and muscle rigidity from serotonin syndrome may benefit from treatment with cyproheptadine, 4 mg orally every hour for 3–4 doses (12). Malignant hyperthermia should be treated with dantrolene, 1–2 mg/kg rapidly intravenously, and repeated as needed every five minutes up to a total dose of 10 mg/kg (9). If hyperthermia from seizures, agitation, or muscle rigidity cannot be controlled with these measures, consideration should be given to neuromuscular paralysis to block further heat production. (Patients will need endotracheal intubation once paralyzed.) Neuromuscular blockade is usually not effective in treating malignant hyperthermia and may even contribute to worsening of the condition.

DRUG-INDUCED SEIZURES

Issues at the Time of Admission

Clinical Presentation

Drug-induced seizures are usually brief, generalized, tonic-clonic in nature, and limited in number. For some drug overdoses, however, the seizures can be multiple, sustained, or focal. Typically, the seizure activity is associated with a decreased level of consciousness and possibly with tongue biting and incontinence. Multiple or recurrent seizures after an amphetamine or cocaine overdose suggest ingestion of a drug packet or a complication, such as intracranial hemorrhage, hyperthermia, or electrolyte disturbance (e.g., hyponatremia with MDMA intoxication).

Differential Diagnosis and Initial Evaluation

The most common causes of drug-induced seizures are tricyclic antidepressants, diphenhydramine, isoniazid, salicylates, stimulants (amphetamines and cocaine), antipsychotic agents, and newer antidepressants, especially bupropion. Medical conditions that can cause seizures include withdrawal from ethanol and sedative hypnotics, hypoxia, hypoglycemia, central nervous system infection or intracranial bleeding, or an intrinsic seizure disorder (Chapter 118). Dystonia, muscle rigidity, and dyskinesia can be confused easily with seizure activity, especially if they are associated with a decreased level of consciousness. An isoniazid overdose should be considered in any patient whose seizures do not responded quickly to conventional treatment (see later in this chapter).

A drug-overdose patient with a seizure should be evaluated for head injury, unstable vital signs, adequacy of airway control and ventilations, hypoglycemia (bedside blood glucose determination), hypoxia (bedside room air oxygen saturation determination), and the presence of focal neurologic findings. The nature of the seizures and the presence of any focal neurologic findings should be documented. Routine diagnostic studies should include electrolyte, creatine kinase, glucose, BUN, and creatinine levels. In the appropriate circumstances, specific drug levels may assist in the diagnosis or treatment. Head computed tomography or magnetic resonance imaging should be performed in any patient with focal neurologic findings or a seizure of unclear cause. A lumbar puncture should be considered in any patient with suspected central nervous system infection or subarachnoid bleeding.

Initial Therapy

Depending on the cause, duration, and number of seizures, initial therapy may include supplemental oxygen, endotracheal intubation and mechanical ventilation, correction of hypoglycemia, and treatment of unstable vital signs. Airway management is very important in these patients, because they are at risk for hypoventilation and pulmonary aspiration. Gastrointestinal decontamination should be considered but can be difficult in patients with seizures.

The approach to and treatment of seizures is described in detail in Chapter 118. The discussion here focuses on seizures in the drug-overdose patient, which are associated with significant morbidity and mortality rates and must be controlled aggressively. The drug of choice for treating drug-induced seizures is a benzodiazepine. Lorazepam (Ativan) is given 1–2 mg intravenously every 5–10 minutes until cessation of the seizures or respiratory compromise or hypotension occurs. Alternatively, seizures can be treated with diazepam (Valium) 0.1–0.2 mg/kg intravenously every 10 minutes until cessation of the seizures or a total of 30 mg is given. If venous access is not available, midazolam (Versed) can be given, 0.1 mg/kg intramuscularly; this dose can be repeated in 10 minutes while venous access is being obtained. If the seizure activity is not controlled after a maximum dose of a benzodiazapine, then phenobarbital 50 mg/min intravenously should be given until the seizures stop or a total dose of 1,000 mg, or 15 mg/kg, has been given. Phenytoin may not be as effective as a benzodiazepine or phenobarbital in controlling drug-induced seizures (13). If a patient is thought to have a drug-induced seizure resulting from isoniazid, pyridoxine (vitamin B_6), 1 g intravenously for every 1 g isoniazid ingested, should be given. If the amount ingested is unknown, then an initial dose of 5 g of intravenous pyridoxine should be given and then repeated until the seizure activity is controlled. In addition to anticonvulsant therapy, a patient who seizes from a salicylate or theophylline overdose may require hemodialysis or hemoperfusion.

If the seizing patient develops a core temperature ≥40°C because of prolonged, excessive muscle activity or rigidity, neuromuscular paralysis and endotracheal intubation should be considered. These abolish the motor activity and allow for better control of the temperature (as described previously) but do not stop any seizure activity within the brain. Patients who require neuromuscular blockade for temperature control may need bedside electroencephalographic monitoring or periodic removal of the neuromuscular paralysis to assess the adequacy of seizure control. Alternatively, propofol has demonstrated success in managing refractory status epilepticus and has the added benefit of rapid titratability (14).

HYPOTENSION

Issues at the Time of Admission

Clinical Presentation

Hypotension can be caused by a number of drug overdoses and medical conditions. Mechanisms of hypotension include decreased cardiac function (e.g., decreased contractility or relative bradycardia), decreased intravascular volume (e.g., blood and fluid losses or third spacing), decreased peripheral vascular tone (e.g., arterial or venous vasodilatation), or a combination of these problems. Hypotension may also accompany hypothermia (Chapter 25). Clinical findings in patients with hypotension stem from decreased perfusion of various organ systems and may include an altered level of consciousness, cool and moist skin, tachypnea, tachycardia, nausea, and decreased urine output. Overdoses that cause a decrease in the intravascular volume or peripheral vascular tone are usually associated with some degree of tachycardia. Hypotension with a relative bradycardia is suggestive of certain drug overdoses (see later in this chapter).

Differential Diagnosis and Initial Evaluation

Drugs whose overdose can cause hypotension by *decreasing cardiac rate and/or contractility* include β-blockers, calcium channel antagonists, cardiac glycosides (e.g., digoxin, digitalis, oleander), clonidine and other α2-agonists, organophosphate and carbamate pesticides, procainamide, quinidine, sedative-hypnotics (e.g., alcohols, barbiturates, benzodiazepines), and tricyclic antidepressants. Those that cause hypotension by *decreasing intravascular volume* include amatoxin-containing mushrooms, colchicine, and iron. Overdoses that cause hypotension by *decreasing vascular tone* include β2-stimulants (e.g., metaproterenol, terbutaline, theophylline), hydralazine, nitrates, prazosin and related drugs, minoxidil, phenothiazines, and tricyclic antidepressants. Hypothermia, hyperthermia, hypoxia, and hypoglycemia also can cause hypotension. *Hypotension with a relative bradycardia* suggests an overdose of sympatholytic agents (e.g., alcohols, barbiturates, β-blockers, clonidine, and opiates), membrane-depressant drugs (e.g., propranolol, procainamide, quinidine, and tricyclic antidepressants), calcium channel antagonists, or cardiac glycosides, or the presence of hypothermia. Electrolyte abnormalities, metabolic acidosis, and other metabolic disturbances also must be considered.

A drug-overdose patient with hypotension should be evaluated for adequacy of airway control and ventilation, other abnormal vital signs, signs of blood loss (including gastrointestinal sources) or other fluid losses, myocardial ischemia or infarction (perform a 12-lead electrocardiogram), hypoglycemia (bedside blood glucose determination), hypoxia (bedside room-air oxygen saturation determination), and focal neurologic findings suggestive of a spinal cord injury. Routine diagnostic studies should include electrolyte, glucose, BUN, and creatinine levels. In the appropriate circumstances, a specific drug level may assist in the diagnosis or treatment. A chest radiograph should be considered if there is any evidence of pulmonary edema, cardiac dysfunction, or pneumonia. A sepsis workup should be considered in any patient suspected of having an infectious process.

Initial Therapy

The general treatment of hypotension is described in Chapter 25. This discussion focuses on the treatment of hypotension in drug-overdose patients, which usually responds to empiric treatment with intravenous fluids and vasopressor agents, but occasionally is refractory to usual supportive treatment. The volume of the IV fluids given may need to be reduced in patients with pulmonary edema or a history of heart failure, but most healthy overdose patients tolerate an initial intravenous bolus of normal saline 10–20 mL/kg. Additional fluid boluses may be needed and can be given as long as there is no evidence of volume overload. In a patient who does not respond adequately to fluids, dopamine 5–15 mcg/kg/min continuous intravenous infusion, or norepinephrine 0.1 mcg/kg/min continuous intravenous infusion, should be considered. Norepinephrine may be more effective than dopamine in patients with a tricyclic antidepressant overdose. In addition, hypoxia, hypoglycemia, respiratory insufficiency, hypothermia or hyperthermia, and metabolic derangements need to be corrected. Table 121.1 contains information about more specific treatments for certain drug-related causes of hypotension.

VENTRICULAR ARRHYTHMIAS, QRS WIDENING, OR QT PROLONGATION

Issues at the Time of Admission

Clinical Presentation

Electrocardiogram abnormalities frequently are seen in drug-overdose patients, and most resolve without sequelae. The most worrisome abnormalities include ventricular arrhythmias (including polymorphic ventricular tachycardia), QRS widening (QRS duration >120 ms), and QT prolongation (QTc >420 ms) (6).

Differential Diagnosis and Initial Evaluation

Toxicologic causes of ventricular arrhythmias include amphetamines, chloral hydrate, cocaine, digitalis glycosides, phenothiazines, theophylline, tricyclic antidepressants, and many hydrocarbon solvents. Drug-related QRS widening can be caused by digitalis glycosides, diphenhydramine, procainamide, propoxyphene, cocaine, propranolol, quinidine, thioridazine, and tricyclic antidepressants. Hyperkalemia also needs to be considered as an important cause of QRS widening. Polymorphic ventricular tachycardia associated with QT prolongation can occur with therapeutic use or overdose of many drugs, including quinidine, cisapride, amiodarone, methadone, sotalol, venlafaxine, quetiapine, thioridazine, droperidol, and haloperidol. Medical conditions that should be considered in the differential diagnosis include acidosis, cardiac ischemia, hypoxia, electrolyte abnormalities (e.g., hypokalemia, hyperkalemia, hypocalcemia, or hypomagnesemia), and an intrinsic conduction defect (see also Chapter 43).

A drug-overdose patient with an abnormal electrocardiogram should be evaluated for unstable vital signs, adequacy of airway control and ventilation, hypoxia (bedside room-air oxygen saturation determination), cardiac ischemia, and the presence of pulmonary edema. Routine diagnostic studies should include a 12-lead electrocardiogram and electrolyte, glucose, BUN, and creatinine levels. In the appropriate circumstances, a chest radiograph or specific drug levels may assist in diagnosis or treatment.

Initial Therapy

All drug-overdose patients with any electrocardiographic abnormality need close observation, continuous cardiac monitoring, and aggressive supportive care. Gastrointestinal decontamination also should be considered but may be difficult in the critically ill patient. Ventricular fibrillation and tachycardia should be treated following the recommendations of the advanced cardiac life support guidelines (Chapter 43), with a few exceptions. First, ventricular arrhythmias associated with chloral hydrate, β-agonists, theophylline, or caffeine poisoning should be treated with β-blockers (e.g., esmolol). Patients who may have ingested a tricyclic antidepressant or other quinidine-like drugs should not be treated with procainamide or other Type-I antiarrhythmic drugs. Instead, sodium bicarbonate bolus doses should be given when the QRS duration is greater than 100 ms, or there is wide complex tachycardia, hypotension, or a terminal R wave in lead aVR (6). These boluses of sodium bicarbonate (or hypertonic saline) should be repeated as needed until QRS narrowing occurs or severe alkalosis or hypernatremia develops. For polymorphic ventricular tachycardia, administer magnesium sulfate 1–2 gm intravenous bolus, followed by 3–20 mg/h continuous intravenous infusion, and consider overdrive pacing (Chapter 43). For patients with prolonged QT intervals, close monitoring, magnesium and potassium replacement, and avoidance of severe bradycardia are indicated. Table 121.1 contains information about more specific treatments for certain drug-related causes of QRS widening or QT prolongation.

MANAGEMENT OF THE DRUG-DEPENDENT PATIENT IN THE HOSPITAL

Drug dependency or withdrawal can complicate the assessment and treatment of an acutely ill patient. They may interfere with a patient's perception of pain and make the evaluation of a painful condition difficult, cause management problems for the health care staff, and increase the risk of complications from the underlying medical condition. During a hospitalization for an acute medical illness, the symptoms of the patient's withdrawal or dependency should be alleviated while their active medical problems are treated; the issues relating to their addiction can be addressed at a later time.

Opiate withdrawal can be manifested by drug craving, agitation, dysphoria, insomnia, gastrointestinal symptoms (e.g., nausea, vomiting, diarrhea), piloerection, diaphoresis, increased secretions (e.g., tearing, rhinorrhea), and miscellaneous symptoms (e.g., yawning, myalgias) (15). The withdrawal syndrome can be treated with routinely scheduled doses of an opiate, either orally or parenterally, depending on the patient's condition. The goals are to titrate the dosage to alleviate withdrawal symptoms, dose on a regular schedule to prevent the recurrence of symptoms, and avoid overmedicating the patient.

Withdrawal symptoms from benzodiazepines or ethanol may include agitation, dysphoria, insomnia, nausea, vomiting, confusion, hallucinations, hypertension, tachycardia, hyperthermia, sweating, or seizures (15). The withdrawal syndrome can be treated with titrated doses of a benzodiazepine (either orally or parenterally, depending on the patient's condition) or, in the case of ethanol withdrawal, phenobarbital. The goal is to titrate the dosage to alleviate the withdrawal symptoms (e.g., reduce agitation, hypertension, tachycardia); large doses of parenteral medications may be required. The approach to alcohol withdrawal is covered in more detail in Chapter 122.

Abstinence from stimulants (e.g., amphetamines, cocaine) may be manifested in a "crash" (i.e., profound fatigue and sleeping for hours-to-days) that develops within hours of the last drug dosing, followed by a withdrawal syndrome (e.g., dysphoria, irritability, insomnia, anhedonia) that begins hours or days after the crash (15). Palliative treatment of symptoms may be considered.

A withdrawal syndrome has been seen after stopping the chronic use of gamma-hydroxybutyric acid, which clinically is similar to sedative-hypnotic withdrawal. It may be associated with agitation, dysphoria, insomnia, confusion, and hallucinations, but appears to involve less autonomic hyperactivity (e.g., tachycardia, hypertension, hyperthermia, sweating) than withdrawal from other sedative agents. Symptoms may be relatively mild initially, become more severe over a few days, and then last for a week or more (2). The symptoms of gamma-hydroxybutyric acid withdrawal may be very resistant to treatment with benzodiazepines and antipsychotic agents. As with a sedative-hypnotic withdrawal syndrome, the goal is to titrate treatment to reduce the agitation, hypertension, and tachycardia if these are present. Other commonly used drugs that are known to cause a withdrawal syndrome include barbituates, carisoprodol (soma), and lioresal (baclofen).

COST CONSIDERATIONS AND RESOURCE USE

Frequent clinical reassessment is the best strategy for appropriately deploying resources in a hospitalized drug-overdose patient. This allows for the timely discontinuation of treatment modalities and high-acuity monitoring that are no longer needed. Conversely, if the patient is not improving as expected or has deteriorated, more aggressive care, such as hemodialysis or use of a specific antidote, can be started quickly. Initiating this therapy as soon as the need arises can reduce the potential risk for an adverse outcome, decrease the total length of hospital stay, and help to optimize the resources used. If there is a possible need for a specific antidote, it is important to ensure that the hospital pharmacy has access to an adequate supply to treat an average adult for 24 hours. Antidotes that are frequently in short supply included antivenoms (snake or black widow envenomations), pralidoxime (organophoshorus agents), and pyridoxine (isoniazid). An inadequate supply of a specific antidote can prolong hospitalization and increase the overall use of resources needed to care for a drug-overdose patient.

KEY POINTS

- Supportive care is adequate for most overdose patients.
- A drug overdose is often a dynamic process with sudden changes in clinical condition, and patients need to be closely monitored and frequently reassessed.
- Adequate gastrointestinal decontamination minimizes the amount of drug or poison absorbed and reduces the severity of the overdose.
- Be aware of common toxidromes (including anticholinergic, sedative-hypnotic, sympathomimetic, and withdrawal syndromes) so that treatment may be tailored appropriately.
- Drugs that are slowly or erratically absorbed may have delayed onset of toxicity.
- Avoid treatment modalities of questionable benefit.

REFERENCES

1. Weaver LK, Hopkins RO, Chan KJ, et al. Hyperbaric oxygen for acute carbon monoxide poisoning. *N Engl J Med* 2002; 347: 1057–1067.
2. Wong CGT, Gibson KM, Snead OC. From the street to the brain: neurobiology of the recreational drug gamma-hydroxybutyric acid. *Trends Pharmacol Sci* 2004;25:29–34.
3. Green RS, Palatnick WP. Effectiveness of octreotide in a case of refractory sulfonylurea-induced hypoglycemia. *J Emerg Med* 2003; 25:283–287.
4. Menghini VV, Albright RC. Treatment of lithium intoxication with continuous venovenous hemodiafiltration. *Am J Kidney Dis* 2000; 36:E21.
5. Johnson MK, Jacobsen D, Meredith TJ, et al. Evaluation of antidotes for poisoning by organophosphorus pesticides. *Emerg Med* 2000;12:22–37.
6. Shanon M, Liebelt EL. Targeted management strategies for cardiovascular toxicity from tricyclic antidepressant overdose: the pivotal role for alkalinization and sodium loading. *Pediatr Emerg Care* 1998;14:293–298.
7. Bond GR. The role of activated charcoal and gastric emptying in gastrointestinal decontamination: a state-of-the-art review. *Ann Emerg Med* 2002;39:273–286.
8. Allison RA, Bedsole L. The other medical causes of rhabdomyolysis. *Am J Med Sci* 2003;326:79–88.
9. Hadad E, Weinbroum AA, Ben-Abraham R. Drug-induced hyperthermia and muscle rigidity: a practical approach. *Euro J Emerg Med* 2003;10:149–154.

10. Miller WR, Wilbourne PL. Mesa Grande: a methodological analysis of clinical trials of treatments for alcohol use disorders. *Addiction* 2002;97:265–277.

11. Matheiu-Nolf M, Babe MA, Coquelle-Couplet V, et al. Flumazenil use in an emergency department: a survey. *J Toxicol Clin Toxicol* 2001;39:15–20.

12. Ener RA, Meglathery SB, Van Decker WA, et al. Serotonin syndrome and other serotonergic disorders. *Pain Medicine* 2003; 4:63–74.

13. Treiman DM, Meyers PD, Walton NY, et al. A comparison of four treatments for generalized convulsive status epilepticus. *N Engl J Med* 1998;339:792–798.

14. Brown LA, Levin GM. Role of propofol in refractory status epilepticus. *Ann Pharmacotherapy* 1998;32:1053–1059.

15. Cami J, Farre M. Drug addiction. *N Engl J Med* 2003;349:975–986.

ADDITIONAL READING

Goldfrank LR, Flomenbaum NE, Lewin NA, et al., eds. *Goldfrank's Toxicologic Emergencies*, 7th ed. New York: McGraw-Hill, 2002.

Olson, KR, ed: *Poisoning and Drug Overdose*, 4th ed. San Francisco: McGraw Hill, 2004.

Acute Alcohol Intoxication and Alcohol Withdrawal

122

Robert H. Lohr

INTRODUCTION

Alcohol abuse and dependence are common. Surveys suggest that as many as 15 million Americans are affected adversely by their alcohol consumption. One result is almost 1 million alcohol-related hospitalizations per year in the United States. The economic cost of alcohol abuse in the United States exceeds $185 billion annually. Between 15%–20% of patients admitted to general medical and surgical wards in community and teaching hospitals abuse alcohol, but many patients with alcohol problems are not diagnosed at admission (1). Because of the prevalence of alcohol abuse and dependence, the U.S. Preventive Services Task Force recommends screening all adolescent and adult patients as part of routine preventive services (2). All physicians providing hospital care encounter patients who manifest the signs and symptoms of acute alcohol intoxication and alcohol withdrawal syndrome (AWS).

This chapter only briefly discusses acute alcohol intoxication because this is most often treated in outpatient detoxification centers. Some patients, however, do require hospitalization because of profound central nervous system (CNS) depression secondary to alcohol intake, often in association with other ingestions. More commonly, patients are admitted with other primary medical or surgical diagnoses and develop signs of alcohol withdrawal several days after admission, when their regular alcohol consumption ceased. Screening all patients for alcoholism, recognizing the signs and symptoms of AWS, and initiating treatment using current, evidence-based approaches is emphasized.

Untreated delirium tremens and severe alcohol intoxication can be fatal, although if recognized and treated appropriately they should rarely, if ever, result in death.

ACUTE ALCOHOL INTOXICATION

Issues at Admission

Alcohol intoxication can play a role in any hospital admission and frequently is listed as a secondary diagnosis in the emergency department. This is especially true of trauma admissions. With the advent of community-based detoxification centers, it is uncommon to admit a patient with the sole diagnosis of alcohol intoxication; however, the non-habitual drinker (such as an adolescent or a college student) who binge drinks may require supportive care in the hospital or the ICU (3). The pharmacology of alcohol is complex, and our understanding of it is still evolving. Alcohol is absorbed rapidly from the stomach and small intestine and is distributed in total body water. The onset of its clinical effect is 5–10 minutes after ingestion, with peak concentrations in the blood occurring after 30–90 minutes. Metabolism is primarily (90%) by the liver; the balance is excreted by the lungs, kidneys, and in sweat.

The clinician should understand that alcohol is a *global CNS depressant*. Transmitter release and conduction are depressed throughout the CNS. In the setting of acute alcohol intoxication, patients are somnolent, with impaired reflexes, slowed respiratory rate, and eventually coma. Patients who drink habitually can compensate for the depressant effects of alcohol through increased autonomic activity. They may appear alert and without obvious functional impairment despite high blood-alcohol concentrations (BACs). Symptoms of alcohol withdrawal result if alcohol is withdrawn or decreased, at which time compensatory autonomic hyperactivity becomes apparent. The clinical effects of alcohol depend on age, sex, comorbid conditions, dosage, and, importantly, the individual patient's drinking history. A nontolerant drinker experiences symptoms at a much lower BAC than a tolerant or habitual drinker. The spectrum of symptoms begins with mild euphoria and disinhibition, followed by slurring of speech and incoordination. Patients may become belligerent as the BAC increases, although ultimately somnolence and respiratory depression occur. Unfortunately, the BAC is not helpful in determining which patients will do well at an outpatient detoxification center and which should be admitted to the hospital. In the nontolerant drinker, high BACs correlate somewhat better with severity of intoxication. The lethal dose of alcohol for any patient is 5–8 g/kg. For children, it is approximately 3 g/kg, in part because they are generally nonhabitual drinkers.

The differential diagnosis for acute alcohol intoxication includes all diagnoses that might cause acute confusion progressing to coma (Chapter 115). The history of alcohol consumption is paramount. Other ingestions, concurrent metabolic perturbations, head trauma, infection, and acid-base or electrolyte disturbances all may present a similar picture. In addition, alcohol intoxication may be accompanied by other drug ingestions (Chapter 121). A complete history using all potential sources (especially family and friends), a physical examination, and laboratory data, including measurement of the BAC and drug screening, are critical to establishing the diagnosis.

The decision to admit the patient is based on how clinically intoxicated the patient appears, in conjunction with the BAC. One also should bear in mind that the BAC may be increasing at the time of initial evaluation; thus, continuing evaluation is important. Comorbid conditions often take precedence in determining who is admitted to the hospital and who may be discharged to a detoxification center.

Issues During Hospitalization

The treatment of a patient with alcohol intoxication is supportive. Alcohol is not adsorbed by charcoal; therefore, gastrointestinal decontamination is of no value unless some additional toxin has been ingested. Rehydration and repletion of electrolytes, maintaining perfusion and urine output, are essential. Hypoglycemia frequently occurs as a result of poor oral intake and decreased glycogen stores. Intravenous administration of fluid containing dextrose and blood glucose monitoring are especially important because the signs of hypoglycemia may be difficult to detect. Metabolizing alcohol results in increased concentrations of

acetate, pyruvate, β-hydroxybutyrate, and lactate, all of which may contribute to metabolic acidosis. Usually, adequate hydration helps to promptly clear these anions in patients with normal renal function. Patients with severe respiratory depression and hypoventilation should be considered candidates for assisted ventilation. Any patient who is unable to maintain a patent airway should be intubated. Many intoxicated patients are hypothermic because of the vasodilation that results from alcohol ingestion. Such patients should be rehydrated and rewarmed. Frequently, cardiac arrhythmias are seen in intoxicated patients. Gastritis and pancreatitis are also commonly observed with alcohol intoxication and should be treated as in any other patient (Chapters 80 and 86). Finally, hemodialysis should be considered for the patient with an extremely high BAC (greater than 5–6 g/kg) if the patient is not responding to more conservative measures.

If a patient has attained hemodynamic, metabolic, and thermal stability, transfer to an outpatient detoxification facility is appropriate. As at admission, comorbid conditions may dictate the timing of discharge. Further follow-up and counseling regarding alcohol abuse are addressed in the next section.

ALCOHOL WITHDRAWAL

Issues at the Time of Admission

The symptoms of alcohol withdrawal are nonspecific. Difficulty establishing the diagnosis is compounded by problems identifying patients at risk. Patients admitted to the hospital with virtually any primary diagnosis may develop AWS once their alcohol consumption is stopped abruptly at the time of admission. Patients with a prior history of AWS may be prone to developing it again, a phenomenon called *kindling* (4). This aspect of the past history is critically important. Many patients and families are reluctant to openly discuss their alcohol consumption and, even when asked about it directly, deny or minimize it.

Quantifying alcohol consumption (Table 122.1) is the first step in identifying patients with possible alcohol abuse and dependence. The *CAGE questionnaire* is a proven, simple screening test for alcoholism, which can be used in conjunction with quantity questions (5). The brevity and simplicity of these questions make them

TABLE 122.1

ALCOHOL CONTENT OF COMMON DRINKS

Drink	Alcohol content
1 can of beer	1 ounce of alcohol
4 ounces of wine	1 ounce of alcohol
1 mixed drink or cocktail	1.5–2 ounces of alcohol

especially useful for the busy hospital-based physician admitting multiple patients (Table 122.2). More than 2 positive responses highly correlates with a diagnosis of alcoholism and should identify patients who may develop alcohol withdrawal during their hospitalizations. All adolescent and adult patients should be screened for alcohol abuse at admission. A follow-up interview is important for suspected cases.

The *Diagnostic and Statistical Manual of Mental Disorders*, 4th ed. (6), defines alcohol withdrawal as:

1. Cessation or reduction in alcohol use that has been heavy and prolonged.
2. Two or more of the following developing within several hours to several days after No. 1: autonomic hyperactivity (e.g., sweating or pulse greater than 100); increased hand tremor; insomnia; transient visual, tactile, or auditory hallucinations or illusions; nausea or vomiting; psychomotor agitation; anxiety; and grand mal seizures.
3. The symptoms and criteria in No. 2 causing clinically significant distress or impairment in social, occupational, or other important areas of functioning.
4. The symptoms not resulting from a general medical condition and not better accounted for by another mental disorder.

The symptoms of alcohol withdrawal occur if the concentration of alcohol in the CNS decreases in habitual drinkers. The patient, over time, has developed compensation for the depressant effects that alcohol has on the CNS. The mediators of this compensation are multiple and include γ-aminobutyric acid, norepinephrine, cortisol, and others (7). If alcohol levels decrease, the compensatory mechanisms, particularly autonomic hyperactivity, become evident as symptoms and signs of alcohol withdrawal.

Presentation of AWS can be early (less than 48 hours since the last drink) or late (greater than 48 hours since last drink), as well as major and minor (Figure 122.1). It is important to understand that early findings can be similar to late findings. Alcohol withdrawal is a continuum occurring over the course of days, with increasing levels of autonomic hyperactivity. The presence or absence of delirium determines severity. The low-grade fever, tachycardia, tremu-

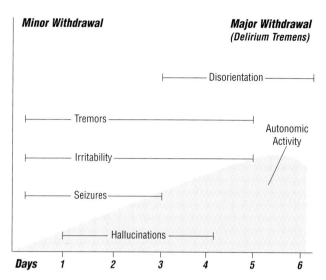

Figure 122.1 Characteristics of alcohol withdrawal. Adapted from Turner RC, Lichstein PR, Peden JG Jr, et al. Alcohol withdrawal syndromes: a review of pathophysiology, clinical presentation, and treatment. *J Gen Intern Med* 1989;4:432–444, with permission.

lousness, insomnia, and agitation of early withdrawal can proceed to delirium, complicated by profound hypertension, tachycardia, and tremors.

Some patients experience *alcoholic hallucinosis*, auditory or tactile hallucinations that occur with an otherwise clear sensorium. This might be seen in a patient with moderate withdrawal who is alert and oriented but is complaining of "things crawling under my skin." Conversely, hallucinations of *delirium tremens* typically are visual and are never seen in the absence of disorientation.

The differential diagnosis for patients beginning to experience alcohol withdrawal is broad. Sepsis, hypoglycemia, hyponatremia, pneumonia, myocardial ischemia, pulmonary embolus, head trauma, and medication reactions are but a few of the alternative explanations for agitation, tachycardia, fever, and tremor of early AWS. If nurses or physicians note these changes during a hospitalization, a careful evaluation should ensue. As always, reviewing or augmenting the history is critical and may be the most important step. Review of the patient's record, paying special attention to any recent trauma and medication changes, can provide valuable information, as can a focused physical and neurologic examination. Signs of trauma, focal neurologic findings, chronic liver disease, and infection can help narrow the differential diagnosis. Finally, laboratory data can help establish a diagnosis. Plasma glucose, electrolytes, renal and liver function tests, calcium, arterial blood gases, electrocardiogram, and, in the febrile patient, appropriate cultures should be performed (Table 122.3). AWS is ultimately a diagnosis of exclusion buttressed by a history of habitual alcohol consumption. Keeping the differential diagnosis broad and performing a careful evaluation is the only way to make the correct diagnosis consistently. Identification of

---

TABLE 122.2

CAGE QUESTIONS HELPFUL FOR SCREENING ADOLESCENT AND ADULT PATIENTS

C̲: Have you felt you should **cut** down on your alcohol consumption?
A̲: Has your drinking **annoyed** your spouse/significant other/family?
G̲: Have you felt **guilty** about your drinking?
E̲: Have you ever had an "**eye opener**" (drink in the morning to "get the day started")?

TABLE 122.3

SUGGESTED LABORATORY EVALUATION FOR PATIENTS SUSPECTED OF HAVING ALCOHOL WITHDRAWAL SYNDROME

Plasma glucose
Electrolytes
Renal function tests (creatinine, blood urea nitrogen)
Liver function tests (aspartate aminotransferase, alanine amino-
　transferase, alkaline phosphatase, bilirubin)
Calcium
Arterial blood gases
Electrocardiogram
Appropriate cultures or radiographs in the febrile patient
Appropriate imaging if trauma suspected, including computed
　tomographic scan of the head as indicated

the patient at risk speeds this process. Increased severity of AWS has been associated with delay in making the correct diagnoses (8).

Evaluation of patients in the emergency department setting can proceed much as it would for patients already admitted to the hospital. An additional issue, however, is when and if patients should be admitted to the hospital rather than treated for alcohol withdrawal in an outpatient setting. There have been multiple attempts to identify risk factors for more severe alcohol withdrawal, although only general recommendations can be made. Patients with concomitant medical or surgical illness tend to have more severe alcohol withdrawal (8, 9). Patients who have had longer drinking histories and previous episodes of withdrawal and seizures are at higher risk for withdrawal (kindling). Although there are no strict guidelines about who to admit, objectively assessing patients can be extremely helpful in determining the severity of the withdrawal symptoms. A patient with full-blown delirium tremens merits admission. In addition, comorbid conditions complicating the alcohol withdrawal also lower the threshold for inpatient treatment. Pregnancy is another indication for admission, and patients for whom no outpatient follow-up can be arranged should be managed initially as inpatients. Objective assessment of the severity of AWS is the best way to make rational admission decisions.

Issues During the Course of Hospitalization

The goals of treatment of AWS are amelioration of symptoms and prevention of complications. Historically, decisions regarding admission, type, and level of care were empiric. Now there are tools available to allow objective assessment of patients going through AWS. The instrument most widely used is the *Revised Clinical Institute Withdrawal Assessment for Alcohol Scale* (CIWA-Ar) shown in Table 122.4

(10). This instrument facilitates reproducible scoring of the symptoms of AWS. Typically, a baseline is established, and the patient is reassessed at frequent intervals (every 1–2 hours initially, and then every 2–4 hours). The total score establishes the severity of withdrawal. A score of ≤10 generally merits observation or supportive treatment, such as a family member reassuring the patient in a quiet room. Scores >10 merit immediate pharmacologic intervention. Importantly, patients with previous episodes of alcohol withdrawal and previous alcohol withdrawal seizures should be treated at scores <10 because of their propensity to have severe withdrawal. The CIWA-Ar scale can be used with minimal prior experience and training in its administration. Its results are reproducible and reliable in both chemical dependency units and medical settings (11–14). As treatment progresses, the scores help direct therapy and can be used to determine if more intensive therapy and monitoring, as in an ICU, are required (Figure 122.2). Although many agents, including alcohol itself, have been used to modify the symptoms of AWS, *benzodiazepines* are the only agents repeatedly shown in multiple, randomized controlled trials to be effective (12). They are the drugs of choice and should be first-line therapy. Benzodiazepines are cross-tolerant with alcohol in the CNS. They can be given safely to substitute for alcohol and then tapered rapidly as the withdrawal symptoms abate.

The autonomic hyperactivity of AWS requires large doses of benzodiazepines at the outset of treatment, a concept called *front-loading*. Typically, up to 100 mg of chlordiazepoxide or 20 mg of diazepam is prescribed as an initial dose. Patients with AWS generally tolerate these large doses well because of underlying autonomic hyperactivity. Dosing and subsequent therapy historically have been on a fixed dose schedule (e.g., chlordiazepoxide 100 mg every 6 hours for four doses, then 50 mg every 6 hours for four doses, and so forth). Although this method is generally effective, it has been established that a *symptom-triggered approach (Symptom Triggered Therapy, STT)* (12) is just as effective and may, in fact, be advantageous. The fixed dosage regimens can potentially result in oversedation, putting patients at risk for aspiration and a prolonged treatment course. By repeatedly assessing the patient with the CIWA-Ar scale, and adjusting the benzodiazepine dosing according to the patient's response to treatment, the episode of withdrawal can be managed safely and effectively.

The body of evidence supporting the use of STT is growing. A 1994 study (13) from a chemical dependency unit found that STT was associated with a significant decrease in benzodiazepine required for treatment (100 mg, vs. 425 mg of chlordiazepoxide in controls) and duration of treatment (9 hours vs. 68 hours). A 2001 Mayo Clinic retrospective study (11) of medical inpatients treated for AWS with STT vs. usual care found similar benzodiazepine dosages and durations of treatment in both groups but significantly less deliriuim tremens in the STT group. Fi-

TABLE 122.4
CIWA-AR QUESTIONS

Nausea and vomiting
Ask: "Do you feel sick to your stomach? Have you vomited?"
Observation
  0 No nausea and no vomiting
  1 Mild nausea with no vomiting
  2
  3
  4 Intermittent nausea with dry heaves
  5
  6
  7 Constant nausea, frequent dry heaves, and vomiting

Tremor
Arms extended and fingers spread apart.
Observation
  0 No tremor
  1 Not visible, but can be felt fingertip to fingertip
  2
  3
  4 Moderate, with patient's arms extended
  5
  6
  7 Severe, even with arms not extended

Paroxysmal Sweats
Observation
  0 No sweat visible
  1 Barely perceptible sweating, palms moist
  2
  3
  4 Beads of sweat obvious on forehead
  5
  6
  7 Drenching sweats

Anxiety
Ask: "Do you feel nervous?"
Observation
  0 No anxiety, at ease
  1 Mildly anxious
  2
  3
  4 Moderately anxious or guarded, so anxiety is inferred

  5
  6
  7 Equivalent to acute panic states as seen in severe delirium in acute schizophrenic reactions

Agitation
Observation
  0 Normal activity
  1 Somewhat more than normal activity
  2
  3
  4 Moderately fidgety and restless
  5
  6
  7 Paces back and forth during most of the interview or constantly thrashes about

Tactile Disturbances
Ask: "Have you any itching, pins and needles sensations, burning, or numbness, or do you feel bugs crawling on or under your skin?"
Observation
  0 None
  1 Very mild itching, pins and needles, burning, or numbness
  2 Mild itching, pins and needles, burning, or numbness
  3 Moderate itching, pins and needles, burning, or numbness
  4 Moderately severe hallucinations
  5 Severe hallucinations
  6 Extremely severe hallucinations
  7 Continuous hallucinations

Auditory Disturbances
Ask: "Are you more aware of sounds around you? Are they harsh? Do they frighten you? Are you hearing anything that is disturbing to you? Are you hearing things you know are not there?"
Observation
  0 Not present
  1 Very mild harshness or ability to frighten
  2 Mild harshness or ability to frighten

  3 Moderate harshness or ability to frighten
  4 Moderately severe hallucinations
  5 Severe hallucinations
  6 Extremely severe hallucinations
  7 Continuous hallucinations

Visual Disturbances
Ask: "Does the light appear to be too bright? Is its color different? Does it hurt your eyes? Are you seeing anything that is disturbing to you? Are you seeing things you know are not there?"
Observation
  0 Not present
  1 Very mild sensitivity
  2 Mild sensitivity
  3 Moderate sensitivity
  4 Moderately severe hallucinations
  5 Severe hallucinations
  6 Extremely severe hallucinations
  7 Continuous hallucinations

Headache, Fullness in Head
Ask: "Does your head feel different? Does it feel like there is a band around your head?" Do not rate for dizziness or lightheadedness. Otherwise, rate severity
  0 Not present
  1 Very mild
  2 Mild
  3 Moderate
  4 Moderately severe
  5 Severe
  6 Very severe
  7 Extremely severe

Orientation and Clouding of Sensorium
Ask: "What day is this? Where are you? Who am I?"
Observation
  0 Oriented and can do serial additions
  1 Cannot do serial additions or is uncertain about date
  2 Disoriented for date by no more than 2 calendar days
  3 Disoriented for date by more than 2 calendar days
  4 Disoriented for place and/or person

This scale is not copyrighted and may be used freely.
CIWA-Ar, Revised Clinical Institute Withdrawal Assessment for Alcohol Scale.

nally, a Swiss study recently reported (14) a randomized trial corroborating the safety and efficacy of STT in chemical dependency units (Figure 122.2).

Other agents can be used as alternatives to benzodiazepines, including phenobarbital, nitrous oxide, carbamazepine, and valproic acid. None have any distinct advantages over the benzodiazepines (although anticonvulsants may reduce the risk of seizure), and none have been studied or used as extensively. Although all benzodiazepines can be effective in managing AWS, the short-acting preparations (e.g., lorazepam, oxazepam) may be preferable in patients with severe hepatic dysfunction or in the elderly.

CIWA Score	Chlordiazepoxide Dosage[a]	Lorazepam Dosage[a]
0–9	NONE	NONE
10–12	25mg orally	1mg orally or 0.5mg IV
15–17	75mg orally	3mg orally or 1.5mg IV
18 or greater	100mg orally	4mg orally or 2mg IV

[a]Use one medication or the other, not both.

Figure 122.2. Suggested treatment protocol for patients with CIWA Score >10.

Adjunctive Treatment: Thiamine, Magnesium, Vitamins, β-Blockers, Centrally Acting α-Agonists

Wernicke's encephalopathy is a preventable, thiamine-dependent clinical complex of 6th cranial nerve palsy, ataxia, and confusion. It can be seen in any thiamine-deficient patient and thus frequently occurs in alcoholic patients. Thiamine can be given orally, subcutaneously, intramuscularly, or intravenously, typically at a dose of 100 mg/d until the patient is eating adequately. It should be given in larger doses (1000–1500 mg) to patients with oculogyric crisis. Dextrose solutions, especially concentrated formulations, can precipitate acute Wernicke's encephalopathy in the thiamine-deficient patient. Therefore, it is important to administer thiamine to patients receiving concentrated dextrose.

Many habitual drinkers also are *magnesium-deficient.* Hypomagnesemia lowers the seizure threshold. Thus, it is important to check the magnesium level and replace magnesium if it is low. If the magnesium level is normal, supplementation is not necessary. A malnourished patient may benefit from vitamin supplementation, although routine vitamin supplements are not necessary for most patients, especially if they are able to eat a nutritionally balanced diet.

β-adrenergic receptor blocking agents (propranolol or atenolol) have been used successfully to treat symptoms of AWS. Although β-adrenergic receptor blockers effectively treat many of the symptoms (tremor, tachycardia, hypertension) of AWS, they do not prevent progression of symptoms, seizures, or delirium. They are not recommended as monotherapy, because they may mask progressive symptoms. In selected patients who have received adequate benzodiazepine coverage but continue to have increased blood pressure or tachycardia, β-adrenergic receptor blockers may have an adjunctive role. This is especially true in patients at risk for cardiac ischemia as they progress through AWS. Contraindications to the addition of β-adrenergic receptor blockers, especially bronchospasm, should be kept in mind. *Clonidine,* a centrally acting α-adrenergic receptor agonist, also can be used adjunctively with benzodiazepines for resistant hypertension,

although, as with β-adrenergic receptor blockers, it should not be used alone. Routine use of either β-blockers or α-adrenergic receptor agonists is discouraged. Although they may have a role in selected patients, benzodiazepines should remain primary therapy, reserving atenolol or clonidine for the patient in whom blood pressure cannot be controlled or in the setting of cardiac ischemia or tachyarrhythmia (12).

Many patients in alcohol withdrawal are volume-depleted; have concurrent infection, pancreatitis, gastrointestinal bleeding, or hepatitis; or have other medical and surgical diagnoses. These conditions should be treated as in any other patients with these problems (Chapters 62, 78, 82, and 86).

Complications

Seizures

Alcohol withdrawal seizures occur infrequently, although in patients with prolonged and heavy drinking (>80–90 days), they may occur in one-third of cases. Typical alcohol withdrawal seizures occur early in the course of withdrawal, before the onset of delirium. They are usually generalized, brief, and self-limited, and, thus, they rarely require intervention. It is important, however, to evaluate patients for other contributing causes. Hyponatremia, hypoglycemia, subdural hematoma, and CNS infections all can occur in patients with alcohol withdrawal and all may predispose to generalized seizures. Patients should undergo a careful neurologic examination, assessment of the previously mentioned metabolic variables, and brain imaging. If the patient is febrile, lumbar puncture should be considered. Neurologic consultation is always appropriate in this setting, especially if seizure activity is not typical for AWS (e.g., focal, multiple, or prolonged seizures). Chapter 118 contains a general discussion of seizure management.

Seizures associated with alcohol withdrawal generally require no treatment beyond the benzodiazepines already being given for AWS itself. Patients with a known chronic seizure disorder should be continued on their usual anticonvulsant regimen, with dosing guided by anticonvulsant blood levels. Patients with recurrent seizures during the course of AWS might be considered for anticonvulsant therapy, although recurrence is unusual enough that the diagnosis of alcohol withdrawal seizure should be considered suspect. Finally, patients with previously documented alcohol withdrawal seizures may be more likely to have recurrent withdrawal seizures. Some centers would pretreat these high-risk patients with anticonvulsant agents, although most would use only benzodiazepines aggressively at the earliest onset of alcohol withdrawal.

Delirium Tremens

Delirium tremens describes extreme autonomic hyperactivity associated with delirium and hallucinations. It occurs late in the course of withdrawal (2–4 days or more since last drink) and represents the most serious form of AWS. Early use of benzodiazepines usually can prevent progression to delirium tremens. If withdrawal progresses, though, additional treatment may be necessary. Haloperidol may be helpful in reducing hallucinations and confusion, although it should be used only adjunctively to benzodiazepines. Haloperidol therapy can lower the seizure threshold. Patients with delirium tremens can be extremely difficult to sedate, even with large doses of benzodiazepines. They may require cardiac monitoring, use of intravenous benzodiazepines and, in extreme cases, intubation and paralysis. Fluid and electrolyte status, intake and output, and renal function all must be monitored closely.

Arrhythmias

Virtually any cardiac arrhythmia can occur with AWS, although tachyarrhythmias are most common. They should be treated as in any other patient; β-adrenergic receptor blockade can be especially helpful if added to benzodiazepines. Patients at risk for myocardial ischemia should be placed in an appropriate, monitored setting with cardiac enzyme, ECG evaluation, and β-blockade (Chapters 37 and 38).

Discharge Issues

By definition, a patient recently treated for alcohol withdrawal is a habitual drinker who needs to address his or her addiction to alcohol. The resources and personnel available to help the hospital physician can range from a social worker to a complete addiction medicine or substance-abuse consulting service. Even when sophisticated hospital resources are unavailable, public health nursing, county social-service agencies, local detoxification centers, or a local Alcoholics Anonymous chapter may offer counseling services. Having just completed a course of AWS, many patients are willing to address their addictions openly and

take steps to curtail their alcohol abuse. Coexistent psychiatric diagnoses, especially depression, are common among alcohol abusers. Formal psychiatric consultation along with substance abuse counseling can be helpful. The patient should not leave the hospital without specific follow-up plans to address alcohol addiction.

Only rarely should patients be dismissed on benzodiazepines, unless they are to be followed in a detoxification center. As a patient is followed with the CIWA-Ar scale in the hospital, benzodiazepine use should continue to decrease and should be stopped once the score is ≤8 for 24–36 hours. The final decision regarding discharge may depend on other medical or surgical issues; however, from the standpoint of alcohol withdrawal, the establishment of a follow-up plan, stability of vital signs, and consistently low CIWA-Ar scores are the main criteria for discharge.

COST CONSIDERATIONS AND RESOURCE USE

Outpatient treatment of both acute intoxication and AWS are generally available and safe. For AWS, length of stay can be up to one-third less and cost 10-fold less in outpatient settings compared with inpatient care. The patient's overall levels of intoxication and BAC can help determine which acutely intoxicated patients can be treated as outpatients. In the case of AWS, the initial evaluation score and its trend on subsequent evaluations is helpful. For the patient admitted to the hospital, the symptom-triggered approach to alcohol withdrawal has been shown to be safe and effective in medical settings as well as chemical dependency units, and to shorten the length of stay and total amount of drug used in chemical dependency units (13).

KEY POINTS

- Screen every adolescent and adult patient for alcohol abuse and the potential for alcohol withdrawal at admission.
- Maintain a broad differential and ensure careful and thoughtful evaluation of the patient presenting with acute intoxication, as well as alcohol withdrawal.
- Use the CIWA-Ar scale to assess the patient at diagnosis and to help guide therapy for AWS.
- Use a symptom-triggered approach to dosing benzodiazepines.
- Provide for substance abuse or psychiatric consultation when the acute withdrawal phase has been completed to help design an appropriate follow-up plan.

REFERENCES

1. Schneekloth TD, Morse RM, Herrick LM, et.al. Point prevalence of alcoholism in hospitalized patients: continuing challenges of

detection, assessment, and diagnosis. *Mayo Clin Proc* 2001;76: 460–466.

2. U.S. Preventative Services Task Force. *Guide to Clinical Preventative Services.* Baltimore: Williams & Wilkins, 1996.
3. Naimi TS, Brewer RD, Mokdad A, et.al. Binge drinking among US adults. *JAMA* 2003;289:70–75.
4. Becker HC. Symposium: the alcohol withdrawal "kindling" phenomenon: clinical and experimental findings. *Alcohol Clin Exp Res* 1996;20:121–124A.
5. Ewing, JA. Detecting alcoholism: the CAGE questionnaire. *JAMA* 1984;252:1905–1907.
6. American Psychiatric Association. *Diagnostic and Statistical Manual of Mental Disorders*, 4th ed. Washington, DC: American Psychiatric Association, 1994:198–199.
7. Olmedo R, Hoffman RS. Withdrawal syndromes. *Emerg Med Clin North Am.* 2000;18:273–288.
8. Ferguson JA, Suelzer CJ, Eckert GJ, et.al. Risk factors for delirium tremens development. *J Gen Intern Med.* 1996;11:410–414.
9. Fiellin DA, O'Connor PG, Holmboe ES, et al. Risk for delirium tremens in patients with alcohol withdrawal syndrome. *Subs Abus* 2002;23:83–94.
10. Sullivan JT, Sykora K, Schneiderman J, et al. Assessment of alcohol withdrawal: the Revised Clinical Institute Withdrawal Assessment for Alcohol scale (CIWA-Ar). *Br J Addict* 1989;84:1353–1357.
11. Jaeger TM, Lohr RH, Pankratz VS. Symptom-triggered therapy for alcohol withdrawal syndrome in medical inpatients. *Mayo Clin Proc* 2001;76:695–701.
12. Mayo-Smith MF. Pharmacological management of alcohol withdrawal: a meta-analysis and evidence-based practice guideline. *JAMA* 1997;278:144–151.
13. Saitz R, Mayo-Smith MF, Roberts MS, et al. Individualized treatment for alcohol withdrawal: a randomized double-blind controlled trial. *JAMA* 1994;272:519–523.
14. Daeppen J-B, Gache P, Landry U, et.al. Symptom-triggered vs. fixed-schedule doses of benzodiazepine for alcohol withdrawal: a randomized treatment trial. *Arch Intern Med* 2002;162:1117–1121.

ADDITIONAL READING

Fiellin DA, Reid MC, O'Connor PG. Screening for alcohol problems in primary care. *Arch Intern Med* 2000;160:1977–1989.

Hersh D, Kranzler HR, Meyer RE. Persistent delirium following cessation of heavy alcohol consumption: diagnostic and treatment implications. *Am J Psychiatry* 1997;154:846–851.

Kosten TR, O'Connor PG. Management of drug and alcohol withdrawal. *New Engl J Med* 2003;348:1786–1795.

O'Connor PG, Schottenfeld R. Patients with alcohol problems. *N Engl J Med* 1998;338:592–602.

Saitz R, O'Malley S. Pharmacotherapy for alcohol abuse. *Med Clin North Am* 1997;81:881–907.

Index

A

Abbokinase, 511
Abbreviations and medication safety, 158, 159
Abciximab, 338, 349, 350
Abdomen
    aortic intramural hematoma and dissection, 472, 475
    chest pain, examining patients with, 301
    constrictive pericarditis, 450
    masses, 761–762
    organ involvement in lymphoma patients, 945
    pain, 751–754, 755
    trauma, 291, 292
Abdominal aneurysms, 774, 775
Abdominal aortic aneurysms, 308, 479, 481–483, 867
Abscesses
    appendicitis, acute, 861, 862–863, 863–864
    clindamycin, 626
    Crohn's disease, 804, 805, 806
    diverticulitis, 864, 865, 866, 867
    ileus and bowel obstruction, 879
    renal or perirenal, 671, 672
Absence seizures, 1199–1200, 1202–1203
Absolute neutrophil count (ANC), 615
Absolute risk, 54, 55
Absolute risk increase (ARI), 55, 56
Absolute risk reduction (ARR), 54, 55
Acalculous cholecystitis, 378, 599, 600
Acarbose, 753
Accuracy of diagnostic tests, 41
Acebutalol, 400
Acetaminophen
    antipyretics, 599
    back pain, 1157
    community-acquired pneumonia, 639
    Crohn's disease, 805
    headache, 1164
    hepatic failure, 809, 810, 811, 815, 816
    overdose, 1230, 1234, 1235
    pain management, 131
    peptic ulcer disease, 794
    thrombocytopenia, 977
    thyrotoxic storm, 1096
    ulcerative colitis, 802
Acetaminophen with codeine, 969
Acetazolamide, 942, 977, 1060, 1062
Acetylcholine, 282
Acetylsalicylic acid, 951, 952
Achalasia, 783
Acid-base balance, 413, 488, 489, 522, 527, 1012, 1024, 1055–1065
Acid-fast bacilli (AFB) smear, 656, 663, 664
Acid-inhibitor agents, 793
Acidosis, 245, 250, 1056–1058, 1060–1062, 1063, 1064, 1234
Acquired atrioventricular block, 432–434
Activase, 511
Activated charcoal, 1231, 1232, 1233, 1235
Activated partial thromboplastin time (aPTT), 257, 443, 496, 498, 502, 509, 510, 976
Activated protein C, 204, 497
Activated protein S, 497
Activities
    back pain, 1156, 1157, 1158, 1159
    cardiac arrest, following, 419

myocardial infarction, acute, 352, 353, 354, 356
pacemakers, 439
seizures, 1205, 1206
syncope, 427, 429, 430
Activities of daily living, 112, 115, 116, 451–452, 935
Acupuncture and pacemakers, 439
Acute chest syndrome, 966, 968, 970–972
Acute coronary syndrome, 52–53, 82, 334
Acute dystonic reaction, 281
Acute fatty liver of pregnancy, 273, 274, 276
Acute humoral rejection, 377
Acute lymphoblastic leukemia, 935, 957
Acute myelogenous leukemia, 929, 930–935
Acute myeloid leukemia, 957
Acute Physiology and Chronic Health Evaluation (APACHE III), 170, 171
Acute respiratory distress syndrome (ARDS)
    antilymphocyte immunosuppressives, 1032
    cardiogenic pulmonary edema, differentiating from, 362
    diabetic ketoacidosis and hyperosmolar hyperglycemic nonketotic syndrome, 1089
    liver chemistry abnormalities, 765
    mechanical ventilation, 176–177
    meningitis, 690
    pancreatitis, 856
    respiratory failure, 183, 189
    sepsis, 203, 205
    trauma patients, 293
    urinary tract infection, upper, 672
Acute tubular necrosis, 998, 1033, 1034, 1035, 1042
Acyclovir, 746, 785, 811, 846, 934, 959, 962, 998, 1042
Addison's disease, 1103
Adenoside nucleotides, 1011
Adenosine
    pharmacologic stress induction tests, 316
    pregnancy, 271
    pulmonary hypertension, 572, 573
    supraventricular tachyarrhythmias, 397, 398, 399
    wide-complex tachycardia, 395
Adhesions, bowel, 874, 876, 879
Adjuvant chemotherapy, 898
Administrative rules and quality improvement, 84
Adrenal crisis, 1104, 1106
Adrenal enzyme inhibitors, 1073
Adrenal insufficiency, 192, 197, 205, 258, 600, 752–753, 1103–1108
Adrenal replacement medication, 813
Adrenal tumors, 469, 1107
Adrenergic states, 356, 364
Adrenocorticotropic hormone (ACTH)
    Cushing syndrome, 1071, 1072, 1073
    hypopituitarism, 1076
    stimulation test, 205, 607, 1101, 1105–1106, 1107
    thyrotoxic storm, 1096
Adriamycin, 899, 902, 945
Advance directives, 121–122, 124, 139, 206, 533, 537, 559
Adverse effects
    adverse drug effects, 32, 157–159, 300, 417, 424, 428
    anti-arrhythmic medications, 404
    blood transfusions, 912–915
    mechanical ventilation, 178–179

pain medication, to, 133
patient safety, 147–150
Afterload reduction agents, 254, 382, 388
Aggrenox, 1181, 1182
Aggression in patients, 283
Agitation, 143, 144, 1236
Agnogenic myeloid metaplasia, 947, 948, 949, 951, 952
AIDS. See Human immunodeficiency virus (HIV)
Air leaks following lung volume reduction surgery, 566
Air space (alveolar) disease, 528
Airway management. See also Endotracheal tubes
    anaphylaxis, 1222, 1223
    anesthesia, 242
    hemoptysis, 524
    intensive care units (ICUs), 166
    mechanical obstruction of upper, 540–541
    myxedema coma, 1099
    overdose and intoxication, 1237, 1238, 1244
    post-subarachnoid hemorrhage, 1192–1193
    trauma patients, 288
Akathesia, 281
Alanine aminotransferase (ALT), 762, 763, 764, 765
Alatrofloxacin/trovafloxacin, 638
Albumin level, 100–101, 820, 996
Albumin therapy, 194, 226, 811, 822, 910, 1010
Albuterol, 533, 543, 1052, 1223
Alcohol, isopropyl, 207, 210, 217, 223, 225, 227, 1236
Alcohol use
    bacterial meningitis, 683
    depression, 1210, 1211
    dialysis patients with diabetes, 1024
    drug overdose, 1231, 1232, 1235, 1236, 1237, 1238, 1239, 1241
    gastrointestinal system, 768, 786
    headache, 1164
    hepatic failure, 813, 814, 815, 816
    hepatitis, 814, 815, 816
    hepatomegaly, 760
    hypertension, emergent, 463
    hypothermia, 607
    intoxication and withdrawal, 1243–1249
    lightheadedness, 306
    palpitations, 304
    pancreatitis, 850, 852, 857
    pulmonary hypertension, 570
    pupillary responses, 1166
    relative bradycardia, 608
    syncope, 428, 429, 430
    trauma patients, 293
    urinary incontinence, 1170
    withdrawal, 282, 1204, 1205, 1243–1249
Alcoholic hallucinations, 1245
Alcoholic liver disease, 725, 841
Aldesleukin, 903
Aldosterone antagonists, 351, 363, 364, 370, 574
Aldosterone levels, 465, 469, 1059
Alendronate, 785, 786
Alka Seltzer®, 793
Alkaline phosphatase levels, 725, 762, 763, 764, 765, 812, 813
Alkalosis, metabolic, 1058–1060, 1062
Alkalosis, respiratory, 1062–1064
Allen test, 208

Allergic bronchopulmonary aspergillosis, 592
Allergies and allergic reactions
  adverse drug events, 157
  anaphylaxis and, 1221–1227
  asthma, 539
  chronic eosinophilic pneumonia, 554
  febrile drug reactions, 600
  hematopoietic cell transplantation, 958
  HIV infected patients, 724
  penicillin antibiotics, 625
  thrombolytic therapy, 347–348
  transfusions, 913
Allergists, 1224, 1226
Allo-antibodies, 376, 987–988
Allogeneic bone marrow transplantation, 934, 952, 955, 963
Allografts, 375, 376–378, 1029
Allopurinol
  acute myelogenous leukemia, 933
  anaphylaxis, 1224
  gout, 1147, 1148
  lymphadenopathy, 889
  renal disease, 1011, 1043
  renal transplantation, 1031
  tumor lysis syndrome, 942, 943
All-trans retinoic acid, 934
α₂-agonists, 253, 264, 1239
α-adrenergic agonists, 195–196, 197, 366, 367, 1049, 1248
α/β-blockers, 264
α-blockers, 466, 467, 468, 469, 1041, 1213
α-interferon, 899, 902
α-methyldopa, 977, 1210
Alprazolam, 722, 1213, 1230
Alteplase, 347, 348, 510, 511
Aluminum hydroxide, 942, 943, 1025
Aluminum toxicity, 1023, 1025
Alveolar disease, 528
Alveolar ventilation, 1060, 1061, 1062, 1064
Alveolar proteinosis, 185
Alzheimer's disease, 1165
Amantadine, 1210
Amicar, 990
Amifostine, 897, 899
Amikacin
  aminoglycoside, 625
  enterococci, 629
  hospital-acquired pneumonia, 648, 649
  meningitis, 688
  Pseudomonas aeruginosa, 629
  tuberculosis, 661
Amiloride, 469, 1051
Amino acids in parenteral nutrition, 107
Aminobiphosphonate, 926
Aminoglycoside antibiotics
  acute myelogenous leukemia, 933
  coagulation factors, 977
  combination therapy, 625
  community-acquired pneumonia, 638
  Crohn's disease, 805
  cyclosporine and tacrolimus, interaction with, 620
  endocarditis, 696, 698
  heart transplantations, 379
  hepatorenal syndrome, 826
  HIV infected patients, 726
  hospital-acquired pneumonia, 648, 649
  hypokalemia, 1050
  IV catheter-associated infection, 707
  mechanism of resistance to, 623
  necrotizing fasciitis, 679
  neutropenic hosts, 617
  overview of, 625
  peritonitis, bacterial, 824
  pregnancy, 277
  renal disease, 1002, 1010, 1042
  resistant organisms, 628, 629, 630
  septic arthritis, 1150
  ulcerative colitis, 802
  urinary tract infection, upper, 671, 672
Aminoglycoside/polypeptide antituberculosis drugs, 659

Aminophylline, 256, 534. *See also* Theophylline
Aminosalicylates, 802, 803, 804, 977
Aminotransferase levels, 725, 812, 813, 815, 843, 844
Amiodarone
  cardiac arrest and resuscitation, after, 413, 415, 416
  drug overdose, 1240
  HIV infection drug regimen, 722
  interstitial lung disease, 550, 552
  myocardial infarction, acute, 351–352, 356
  myxedema coma, 1097
  palpitations, 304
  post heart transplant surgery, 375
  pregnancy, 271
  pulmonary function testing, 525
  supraventricular tachyarrhythmias, 399, 400, 402, 404, 405, 406, 493
  syncope, 425
  thyroid disease, 1075, 1095
  torsade de pointes, 412
  ventricular arrhythmias, 409, 410, 417, 418, 419
  warfarin, interfering with, 512
  wide-complex tachycardia, 395
Amitriptyline, 134, 1212, 1233
Amlodipine, 470, 573, 574, 722, 1230
Amoxicillin
  anthrax, 714
  hypogammaglobulinemic hosts, 614, 615
  peptic ulcer disease, 794
  rash, 1226
  resistance to *S. pneumoniae*, 639
  urinary tract infection, 669, 670
Amoxicillin/clavulanate, 534, 616, 669, 677
Amphetamines
  central nervous system vasculitis, 1131
  chest pain, 300
  chorea, 1168
  drug overdose, 1230, 1234, 1236, 1238, 1240, 1241
  hypertension, emergent, 464
  intracranial hemorrhage, 1194
  monoamine oxidase inhibitors, 1215
  palpitations, 304
  seizures, 1204
Amphotericin B
  acidosis, metabolic, 1057, 1058
  cyclosporine and tacrolimus, interaction with, 620
  endocarditis, 698
  esophageal disorders, 785
  hypokalemia, 1050
  IV catheter-associated infection, 707
  liver transplant patients, infection prophylaxis for, 621
  meningitis in HIV infected patients, 741
  nephrotoxicity, 379, 625
  neutropenic hosts, 618–619
  renal failure, acute, 1010
  urinary tract infection, 669, 670, 672
Ampicillin
  action of, 625
  anthrax, 714
  cholecystitis, 832
  combination therapy, 624
  diarrhea in gastrointestinal disease, 758
  enterococci, 629
  Escherichia coli, 628, 629
  hypogammaglobulinemic hosts, 614, 615
  interstitial lung disease, 550
  Listeria infections, 150
  meningitis, 687, 688, 689
  pregnancy, 276
  rash, 1226
  Streptococcus pneumoniae, 629
  thrombocytopenia, 977
  urinary tract infection, 670, 672
  vancomycin-resistant enterococci, 630
Ampicillin/clavulanate, 615
Ampicillin/sulbactam
  combination therapy, 626
  hospital-acquired pneumonia, 648

infected bite wounds, 677
infections in trauma patients, 292
postoperative peritonitis, 265
urinary tract infection, 670, 672
Amplitude of arterial pulses, 307–308
Amputation, 486, 488, 489, 490, 491, 492
Amrinone, 195, 196, 1230
Amyl nitrate, 1231
Amylase levels, 444, 850–851, 854, 856, 857, 935
Amyloid angiopathy, 1194
Amyloidosis, 442
Anabolic steroids, 1168, 1210
Anacin®, 793
Anaerobic metabolism, 456
Anafranil, 1212
Anagrelide, 951, 953
Analgesia. *See also* Pain; *specific medications*
  anesthesia, 244
  back pain, 1157
  cardiac arrest and resuscitation, after, 414
  diverticulitis, 865
  hyponatremia, 1046
  joint pain, 1112
  neurologic complications in HIV infected patients, 741
  pancreatitis, 853, 854, 855
  superior vena cava syndrome, 924
  urinary tract infection, upper, 670, 673
Analgesic ladders, 131
Anaphylactoid reactions, 1221, 1222, 1225
Anaphylaxis
  allergic reactions and, 1221–1227
  distributive shock, 192, 196, 197
  penicillin antibiotics, 625
  protamine sulfate, 989
  wheezing, 519
Anasarca, 451, 1001
Anazolene, 977
Ancef, 292
Ancillary personnel, 27–29, 63, 64–65, 88, 94–95, 165, 166
Anemia
  acute myelogenous leukemia, 930, 931, 932
  agnogenic myeloid metaplasia, 948, 952
  chemotherapy, 903
  chronic disease, 888, 890, 891, 892–893
  dialysis patients, 1020, 1023
  diffuse alveolar hemorrhage, 551
  heart failure, 360, 370
  HIV infected patients, 726–727
  hypertension, emergent, 468
  lightheadedness, 306
  peripheral artery disease, 458
  pregnancy, 271
  preoperative evaluation, 257
  renal insufficiency, 1003
  rheumatoid arthritis, 1142
  signs, symptoms, and laboratory abnormalities, 888, 889–893
Anesthesia
  acidosis, respiratory, 1062
  drug overdose, 1237
  local, 207, 210, 217, 223, 225, 227
  myxedema coma, 1097
  pregnancy, 271
  principles of, 241–246
  spinal or epidural, 192
  status epilepticus, 1202
Anesthesiologists, 805
Aneurysms, 276, 442, 479–483, 486, 1124, 1189–1193
Angiitis of the central nervous system, 1130–1132
Angina
  anxiety, 280
  aortic stenosis, 381
  heart failure, 361, 369
  hypertension, emergent, 468
  likelihood ratios, 38
  nitrates, 351
  noninvasive preoperative ischemia testing, 252
  stable and unstable, 329–341
  supraventricular tachyarrhythmias, 397

unstable, 250, 382, 383, 424, 429
ventricular arrhythmias and cardiac arrest, 409
Angioedema, 364, 1222, 1223, 1226
Angiography
  abdominal injury, 291
  acute limb ischemia, 488, 489, 490
  aortic intramural hematoma and dissection,
    473–474
  aortic stenosis, 382
  atherosclerotic plaque events, 331
  bowel ischemia, acute, 868, 869
  peripheral artery disease, 460
  pregnancy, 275, 276
  pulmonary embolism, 506, 507, 508, 510
  subarachnoid hemorrhage, 1190
  trauma to extremities, 292
  treatment for lower GI bleeding, 777
  vasculitis, 1121, 1122, 1123, 1131, 1132
Angiography, coronary
  acute pericarditis, 443
  angina, 340
  chest pain, 303
  coronary artery disease, 325, 329, 843
  diagnostic tests, 325
  donor organs, 374
  heart failure, 361, 369, 370
  mitral regurgitation, 387, 388
Angioplasty, 379, 488, 490, 491, 492
Angiotensin II receptor antagonists, 272, 364,
  366, 370, 379, 1051, 1226
Angiotensin-converting enzyme (ACE) inhibitors
  acute coronary syndrome, 82
  anaphylaxis, 1222, 1226
  aortic regurgitation, 385
  cardiac arrest and resuscitation, after, 414
  cough, 521, 522
  dialysis patients with chest pain, 1021
  heart failure, 363–364, 365, 366, 369, 370
  hyperkalemia, 1051
  hypertension, emergent, 465, 467, 468, 469
  laryngeal edema, 189
  myocardial infarction, 345, 350, 351, 352, 353,
    354, 355, 356, 357
  nephrotoxicity, 363, 379
  oliguria and anuria, 998, 999, 1000
  pancreatitis, 850
  pregnancy, 272
  pulmonary hypertension, 574
  renal disease, 1004, 1015, 1058
  right ventricular failure, 368
  scleroderma, 1138, 1139
  stroke, 1182
  ventricular arrhythmias, 410
Angiotensin-converting enzyme levels, 559
Angle of Louis, 307
Anion gap, 1056–1058
Anisoylated plasminogen streptokinase activator
  complex, 346, 347–348
Ankle-Brachial Index, 458–459490, 485
Ankylosing spondylitis, 383
Ann Arbor staging system, 938, 939
Annuloaortic ectasia, 481
Annuloplasty rings, 388
Anorexia, 860, 885
Anorexigenics, 570
Antacids, 273, 414, 522, 659, 661, 795, 1018
Anthracycline, 897, 934
Anthrax, 600, 711, 713–714, 714
Anthropometry, 100
Anti Xa heparin levels, 509
Antiarrhythmic agents
  acquired atrioventricular block, 433
  cardiac arrest and resuscitation, after, 413, 414,
    416
  classifications of, 400
  heart transplant surgery, 375
  HIV infection drug regimen, 722
  myocardial infarction, acute, 351–352
  palpitations, 304
  sinus node dysfunction, 431
  supraventricular tachyarrhythmias, 402–403, 404
  tricyclic antidepressants, 1213

tuberculosis treatment, interactions with, 659
ventricular arrhythmias, 410, 411, 412, 418, 419
Antibiotics
  abdominal pain, causing, 753
  acute leukemia, 935, 936
  acute myelogenous leukemia, 934, 935
  anemia, 892
  aortic regurgitation, 385
  appendicitis, acute, 862, 863, 864
  asthma, 543, 546
  back pain, 1155, 1156, 1157
  bacterial pericarditis, 447, 449
  Boerhaave's syndrome, 787
  bowel ischemia, acute, 868, 869
  bowel obstruction, 877, 878, 879, 880
  cardiac arrest and resuscitation, after, 414
  chemotherapy, 898, 903, 905
  cholangitis, acute, 835, 837
  cholecystitis, 832–833
  chronic obstructive pulmonary disease, 534,
    535
  cirrhosis, 823, 827
  coagulation disorders associated with bleeding,
    988
  combination therapy, 624–625, 626, 628, 629,
    630
  community-acquired pneumonia, 635,
    638–639, 641, 642, 643
  computer-assisted ordering, 90
  cough, 522
  Crohn's disease, 804, 806
  culture results, 610
  deep venous thrombosis, 502
  dialysis patients, 1022
  diarrhea, 758–759
  diverticulitis, 865, 866, 867
  drug interactions, 796
  fever of unknown origin, 607
  gastrointestinal disease, 754
  hematopoietic cell transplantation, 959
  hepatic failure, 811, 814
  HIV infected patients, 724
  hospital-acquired pneumonia, 647–648, 649,
    650, 651, 652, 653
  hypogammaglobulinemic hosts, 614, 615
  hypokalemia, 1050
  hypothermia, 607
  inhalation injury, 555
  interstitial lung disease, 550, 558, 559
  ischemic colitis, 869
  limb ischemia, 488, 489, 491
  liver transplant nonfunction, 844
  major classes of, 625–627
  monocytic leukemia, 933–934
  neutropenia, 615, 616, 893
  pacemakers, 439
  palpitations, 304
  pancreatitis, 854, 855, 856
  peripheral artery disease, 460
  pregnancy, 276–277
  preoperative evaluation, 254, 255, 256
  prophylaxis for subdural hematoma, 1197
  prophylaxis for trauma patients, 291, 292
  prophylaxis for valvular heart disease, 383,
    387, 388, 390
  prosthetic heart valves, 390
  quality measurement, 82, 83
  renal failure, acute, 1012, 1015
  renal stone and obstructive disease, 1041
  resistance to, 623–631
  rheumatological diseases, 1112, 1116
  sepsis, 203, 204, 206
  septic arthritis, 1149, 1150, 1151
  shock, 197
  sickle cell disease, 971
  solitary pulmonary nodules, 589
  spherical mass lesions, 589
  testing for *H. pylori*, 793
  thyrotoxic storm, 1096
  torsade de pointes, 412
  transplant prophylaxis, 620–621
  ulcerative colitis, 802, 803

Anticardiolipin antibodies, 500, 574
Anti-CD20 antibody, 985
Anti-CD3 monoclonal antibodies, 961
Anticholinergic agents
  asthma, 542, 543
  chronic obstructive pulmonary disease, 533
  Crohn's disease, 806
  delirium, 257, 1165
  depression, 1210
  dialysis patients, 1018
  drug overdose, 1230, 1237
  esophageal disorders, 784, 786
  nausea and vomiting in gastrointestinal disease,
    756
  pupillary responses, 1166
  urinary incontinence, 1170
  vertigo, 1167
Anticholinergic effects, 1212, 1213, 1214
Anticoagulant therapy
  atrial fibrillation, 401, 402
  atrial flutter, 403
  cardiac catheterization, 325
  cardiac stents, 253
  cholangitis, acute, 837
  deep venous thrombosis, 498, 499–500
  gastrointestinal bleeding, 768
  hematomas, 761, 762
  hemorrhage and abdominal pain, causing, 753
  hepatic failure, 811
  interstitial lung disease, 550
  intracranial hemorrhage, 1194
  limb ischemia, 488, 491
  medications interfering with, 512
  mitral stenosis, 386
  pericarditis, 442, 445, 450, 451
  pleural effusion, 580
  postoperative care, 264, 265, 266, 267
  prosthetic heart valves, 390
  prothrombin 20210, 983
  pulmonary embolism, 523
  pulmonary hypertension, 572, 574, 575
  scleroderma, 1137
  shock, 197–198
  spinal cord injuries, 292
  superior vena cava syndrome, 923
  supraventricular tachyarrhythmias, 403–404,
    405
  thrombolytic therapy, 348
  thrombotic disorders, 982
Anticonvulsant medications
  alcohol withdrawal, 1249
  chorea, 1168
  depression, 1210
  HIV patients, 722, 741, 743
  neurologic oncologic emergencies, 919
  neuropathic pain, 135
  renal transplantation, 1031
  seizures, 1200, 1201, 1202, 1203–1204, 1204,
    1205, 1206
  subdural hematoma, 1197
  tuberculosis treatment, interactions with, 659
Antidepressants
  depression, 1210–1211, 1212, 1213–1216
  drug overdose, 1236
  esophageal disorders, 784
  heart transplantations, 379
  hyponatremia, 1046
  myxedema coma, 1097
  neuropathic pain, 133–135
Antidiabetic agents, oral, 1024, 1082–1083, 1084,
  1085, 1089, 1090, 1232, 1234, 1237
Antidiarrheal agents, 758, 802, 806
Antidiuretic hormone
  heart failure, 359
  syndrome of inappropriate antidiuretic
    hormone secretion (SIADH), 588, 591,
    1045–1046, 1047, 1076, 1215
  urinalysis, 996
Antidromic AVRT, 394, 395
Anti-emetic agents
  chemotherapy, 899, 903–904, 905, 906
  end-of-life care, 143

gastrointestinal disease, 756
hematopoietic cell transplantation, 958
neurologic complications in HIV infected
  patients, 741
postoperative care, 246, 263–264
Anti-factor Xa levels, 275
Antifungal therapy, 592, 935
Antihistamines
  anaphylaxis, 1224
  angioedema, 1223
  delirium, 257, 1165
  drug overdose, 1230, 1236
  gastrointestinal disease, 756
  palpitations, 304
  torsade de pointes, 412
  transfusions, 913
  vertigo, 1167
Anti-HLA (human leukocyte antigen) antibodies,
  913, 987–988
Antihypertensive medications
  hypertension, emergent, 465–468
  lightheadedness, 306
  nephrotoxic effects, 363
  oliguria and anuria, 1000
  scleroderma, 1139
  stroke, 1182
  syncope, 424
  withdrawal symptoms, 135
Antilymphocyte antibodies, 563
Antilymphocyte globulin, 563, 1031
Antilymphocyte immunosuppressives, 1031, 1032
Antimalarials, 521
Antimicrobial therapy
  acute leukemia, 935
  endocarditis, 696–697
  interpretation of culture results, 610
  IV catheter-associated infection, 706, 707
  meningitis, 687, 688
  organ transplantation, 619–622, 839
  scleroderma, 1139
Antineutrophil cytoplasmic antibodies,
  1118–1119, 1126
Antinuclear antibodies, 1117
Anti-parkinsonian drugs, 1165, 1168
Antiphospholipid antibodies, 459, 500
Anti-phospholipid antibody syndrome, 1136
Antiplatelet therapy
  angina, 337–338, 339, 340
  cardiac catheterization, 325
  cardiac stents, 253
  chronic limb ischemia, 491, 492
  myocardial infarction, 52–54, 55–56, 349–350
  stroke, 1181–1182
Antiproliferative agents, 1031
Antipsychotic medications, 280–281, 1165, 1168,
  1170, 1236, 1237, 1241
Antireflux agents, 783
Antiretroviral agents, 135, 663, 721–723, 735,
  742, 894, 1023
Antispasmodic drugs, 806, 457802
Antithrombin deficiency, 981, 982
Antithrombin III, 910
Antithrombin III antibody assay, 459
Antithrombin therapy
  angina, 337, 338, 339
  myocardial infarction, 345, 350, 356
  supraventricular tachyarrhythmias, 404
Antithymocyte globulin, 563, 894, 896, 961
Anti-thymocyte rabbit immunoglobulin, 846
Antithyroid agents, 893, 1070
Anti-Toxoplasma immunoglobulin G, 743
Antituberculosis therapy, 447, 449, 606, 607, 725
Anti-tumor necrosis factor therapies, 1115
Antivenoms, 1241
Antiviral therapy, 935, 1126
Anti-Xa heparin level, 498
Anuria, 998, 999
Anxiety, 279, 280, 306, 429, 522
Aorta, 268, 308, 325, 384
Aortic aneurysms, 442, 479–483, 1124
Aortic diastolic perfusion pressure, 330

Aortic dissection
  aneurysms, 480, 481
  aortic regurgitation, 383
  hypertension, emergent, 464, 468
  intramural hematoma and, 471–477
  myocardial infarction, 344
  pain, 300, 301
  pericarditis, 444
  pregnancy, 271
  radiography, 312
  shock, 192
  syncope, 425, 429
  thrombolytic therapy, contraindication for, 348
  ventricular arrhythmias and cardiac arrest, 411
Aortic intramural hematoma, 471–477
Aortic regurgitation, 367, 383–385, 472, 480
Aortic rupture, 291
Aortic stenosis, 254, 271, 369, 381–383, 424,
  427, 428, 472
Aortic valves, 333, 472, 476, 480, 481
Aortitis, idiopathic, 479, 480
Aortoenteric fistulas, 481, 774, 775, 776
Aortography, 384, 480
Aortoiliac disease, 458
APACHE II and III scores, 171, 416, 852
Apheresis of whole blood, 907
Aplastic anemia, 895, 896, 931, 932, 956
Appendicitis, acute, 860–864
Apresoline, 467
Ara-C, 902
Arbutamine, 316
Arenaviruses, 716
Argatroban, 345, 350
Arginine vasopressin, 996
ARREST trial, 413
Arrhythmias
  alcohol withdrawal, 1249
  amiodarone, 1095
  antipsychotic medications, 281
  arterial pulses, 308
  bradycardia and pacemakers, 431–440
  cardiogenic shock, 191, 192
  chest pain, 300
  drug overdose, 1240
  echocardiography, 323
  heart transplant surgery, 374–376, 377
  hyperkalemia, 1052
  implantable cardiac defibrillators (ICDs), 355
  myocardial infarction, 345, 352, 356
  palpitations, 303–306
  postoperative care, 264
  pregnancy, 271
  preoperative evaluation, 254
  sudden cardiac death, 345
  supraventricular, 393–406
  syncope, 425, 426, 427, 428, 429
  ventricular, 409–420
Arrhythmogenic right ventricular dysplasia
  (ARVD), 412
Arsenicals, 977
Artane, 1213
Arterial blood gases
  acid-base balance, 1055–1056, 1060, 1061,
    1063, 1064
  asthma, 541, 544
  chronic obstructive pulmonary disease
    (COPD), 532, 535, 536
  cyanosis, 520
  dyspnea, 523
  interstitial lung disease, 557
  pancreatitis, 850, 852
  pneumothoraces, 582, 584, 585
  pulmonary disease with HIV infection, 731, 735
  pulmonary embolism, 505, 508
  pulmonary function testing, 527
  respiratory failure, acute, 184, 185, 186–187
Arteries
  dilation and shock, 192
  occlusion, 458
  peripheral arterial disease, 455–460
  pulses, 307–308

puncture and cannulation, 207–209, 210
stenosis, 456, 460, 1123, 1124
Arteriovenous fistula, 1017, 1018, 1022
Arteriovenous graft, 1017, 1018, 1021, 1022
Arteriovenous malformations, 276
Arteritis, 486, 488, 490
Arthritis, 456, 457, 592, 1111, 1113–1114, 1135,
  1143–1151
Arthrocentesis, 209–215, 1143, 1146, 1148, 1149,
  1150
Artificial tears, 1141
Asbestos, 591, 592
Ascites
  cirrhosis, 819, 820, 821–823, 825, 827
  constrictive pericarditis, 450
  hepatic encephalopathy, 825
  paracentesis, 225–226, 821, 822, 823, 960
  pulmonary hypertension, 572, 574
  spontaneous bacterial peritonitis, 823, 824
  tricuspid regurgitation, 389
Aspart insulin, 1082
Aspartame, 1164
Aspartate aminotransferase (AST), 762, 763, 764,
  765
Aspergillus infections
  hematopoietic cell transplantation, 961–962
  immunocompromised hosts, 616, 618–619, 620
  lung transplantation, 563, 564
  pulmonary disease, 524, 550, 592
Aspiration, pulmonary, 105–106, 188–189, 276,
  1181, 1201
Aspiration and irrigation for priapism, 970
Aspiration of pneumothoraces, 583–584, 585
Aspirin
  acute coronary syndrome, 82
  anaphylaxis, 1222, 1225
  angina, 337–338, 339, 340
  arrhythmias, 400, 404, 410
  bleeding disorders, 977, 986
  cardiac arrest and resuscitation, after, 414
  chronic myeloproliferative diseases, 951, 952
  dialysis patients with chest pain, 1021
  gastrointestinal disorders, 773, 778, 786, 789,
    794
  gout, 1147
  headache, 1164
  heart transplant surgery, 375
  interstitial lung disease, 550
  limb ischemia, 491, 492
  myocardial infarction, 52–54, 345, 347, 349,
    350, 353, 354, 356, 357
  nephrotoxic effects, 363
  overdose, 527, 1233
  pain management, 131
  pericarditis, 445, 449
  stroke, 1178, 1179, 1180–1181, 1182
Assessment. See also Evaluation; Physical
  examination
  alcohol withdrawal, 1247
  cardiac murmurs, 309–311
  cardiac structure and function, 321–325
  cardiovascular, 315, 321–325
  critical patients in ICU, 168, 170
  elderly patients, 112–116
  pain, of, 129, 130, 135–136
  pre- and postoperative care, 241, 249–258, 261
  shock, patients in, 193
Assist-control mode of ventilation, 173, 174
Astemizole, 412, 722, 1213
Asterixis, 1168
Asthma
  anxiety, 280
  chronic eosinophilic pneumonia, 554
  chronic obstructive pulmonary disease
    (COPD), 531
  exacerbations of, 539–547
  multiple pulmonary nodules, 592
  physical signs, 518, 519
  pregnancy, 272
  preoperative evaluation, 256
Asymmetric radiculopathy, 918

Asystole, 351
Atelectasis, 264–265, 518, 519, 523
Atenolol, 253, 273, 350, 399, 400, 1021, 1230, 1248
ATGAM, 1031
Atheroembolism, 457, 487
Atherosclerosis
  cardiac disorders, 330–331, 343
  dialysis patients, 1020
  HIV infection, 722
  peripheral vascular disease, 307–308, 455, 457–458, 459, 485, 486
Athetosis, 1168
Ativan, 1239
Atovaquone, 621, 735, 736
Atrial fibrillation
  acute limb ischemia, 488
  constrictive pericarditis, 450, 451
  dual-chamber pacemakers, 439
  elderly patients, 112–113
  heart failure, 360
  myocardial infarction, 356
  pre-operative evaluation, 254
  rapid ventricular response, 382
  sinus node dysfunction, 431
  stroke, 1182
  supraventricular tachyarrhythmias, 264, 393–406
  valve disorders, 385, 386, 387, 389
  warfarin, 350
Atrial flutter, 356, 393–401, 403–406, 431
Atrial natriuretic peptide, 1011
Atrial premature depolarization, 394
Atrioventicular dissociation, 412
Atrioventricular block, 356, 364, 367, 398, 438
Atrioventricular nodal blocking agents, 395, 397, 398, 399, 400, 402, 403, 404, 406
Atrioventricular nodal reentrant tachycardia
  palpitations, 304, 305, 306
  sinus node dysfunction, 431
  supraventricular tachyarrhythmia, 393–394, 395, 396, 397, 398, 399, 403
Atropine, 356, 375, 433, 434, 1166, 1230, 1232
Atypical chronic myeloid disorders, 947
Auras, 1200
Auscultation
  acute pericarditis, 442, 443
  arterial pulses, 308
  heart sounds, 308–309, 311
  prosthetic heart valves, 389
Austin Flint murmur, 384
Autoimmune disorders. See also specific disorders
  depression, 1210
  hepatitis, 815
  lymphadenopathy, 887, 889
  neutropenia, 894
  pericarditis, 442, 447
Autologous blood donation, 915
Autologous transplantation of hematopoietic cells, 955, 963
Automatisms during seizures, 1200
Autonomic nervous system, 306, 374–375, 427, 433, 1090
Azathioprine
  anemia, 891
  autoimmune disorders, 1137, 1138, 1140
  gout, 1147, 1148
  graft-versus-host disease, 962
  neutropenia, 894
  organ transplantation, 376, 563, 564, 1031
  pancreatitis, 850
  polymyositis/dermatomyositis, 1140
  pregnancy, 274, 276
  pulmonary disorders, 551, 558
  trimethoprim/sulfasoxazole, 620
  ulcerative colitis, 802, 803
  vasculitis, 1130
Azithromycin, 543, 626, 638, 643, 663
Azotemia, prerenal, 1033
Aztreonam, 626, 687, 688, 832

B
Back pain, 1153–1159
Baclofen, 135, 1241
Bacteria
  bacteremia, 254, 255, 671, 694, 699, 703–709
  bacteruria, 668, 670
  contamination of transfusion products, 913
  encapsulated, 614
  endocarditis, 592
  fever preventing replication, 599
  pericarditis, 441, 442, 445, 447, 449
  septic arthritis, 1148–1149
Baker's cyst, 456, 457
Balloon angioplasty, 345, 348, 1192
Balloon valvuloplasty, 369
Barbiturates
  anaphylaxis, 1224
  cardiac arrest and resuscitation, after, 413
  delirium, 1165
  depression, 1210
  end-of-life care, 141
  head trauma, 289
  hypothermia, 607
  overdose, 1239
  pupillary responses, 1166
  warfarin, interfering with, 512
  withdrawal, 135, 1241
Barcoding, 67, 158
Barium contrast media, 864
Baroreceptors, 359, 424
Barotrauma, 178–179, 189, 545
Barrett's mucosa, 783, 784, 785
Bartter syndrome, 1050
Basal insulin, 1081, 1082
Basiliximab, 1031
Bayesian reasoning, 37–42, 578–579
B-cell malignancies, 938, 939–940, 941, 945, 963
Beck Depression Inventory, 1211
Bed rest for back pain, 1157, 1158, 1159
Behavior disorders, 1168–1169
Behçet's disease, 686, 1121
Benadryl®, 1213
Benign esophageal stricture, 782–783
Benign lesions, pulmonary, 587–588, 589–590, 591, 592
Benzodiazepines
  alcohol withdrawal, 1246, 1247, 1248, 1249
  anxiety, 280
  delirium, 257, 263, 1165
  depression, 1210
  end-of-life care, 141, 182
  HIV infected patients, 746
  increased intracranial pressure, 1188
  overdose, 1230, 1231, 1232, 1234, 1236, 1237, 1239, 1241
  pregnancy, 276
  seizures, 1201
  ulcerative colitis, 802
  vertigo, 1167
  withdrawal symptoms, 135
Benztropine, 1230
Betadine, 209, 210, 215, 222, 223, 225, 226, 227, 231
β-adrenergic agonists
  anaphylaxis, 1223
  chest pain, 300
  leukocytosis, 894
  overdose, 1230, 1234, 1240
  pregnancy, 272
  shock, 195–196, 197
  wheezing, 519
β2-adrenergic agonists
  asthma, 541, 542, 543, 544, 545, 546
  chronic obstructive pulmonary disease, 533, 534, 535
  drug overdose, 1239
  potassium disorders, 1049, 1050, 1052
β-adrenergic antagonists
  acute coronary syndrome, 82
  alcohol withdrawal, 1248, 1249
  anaphylaxis, 1223, 1225, 1227

angina, 338, 340, 341
antidepressants, 1215
aortic intramural hematoma and dissection, 475, 476
asthma, exacerbations of, 539
bradycardia relative to fever, 607
cardiac arrest and resuscitation, after, 415
chronic obstructive pulmonary disease, 537
cirrhosis, 827
constrictive pericarditis, 451
dialysis patients with chest pain, 1021
drug overdose, 1230, 1231, 1239, 1240
gastrointestinal bleeding, 773
headache, 1164
heart failure, 363, 364
heart transplant surgery, 375
hepatic failure, 811
hyperkalemia, 1051
hypertension, emergent, 466, 467, 468, 469
mitral stenosis, 387
myocardial infarction, 344, 353, 354, 355, 356, 357
myocardial oxygen consumption, 350–351
pre- and postoperative care, 252, 253, 256, 264
pregnancy, 271, 272, 276
scleroderma, 1137
sinus node dysfunction, 431
supraventricular arrhythmias, 398, 399, 400, 402, 403, 404, 405, 406, 433
syncope, 425, 429
thoracic aortic aneurysms, 481
thyrotoxic storm, 1095–1096, 1097
ventricular arrhythmias, 356, 410, 417, 419
β-lactam antibiotics
  bleeding disorders, 977, 986
  community-acquired pneumonia, 635, 638, 643
  IV catheter-associated infection, 707
  neutropenic hosts, 617
  overview of, 623, 625–626, 628, 629
  seizures, 1204
  urinary tract infection, 669
β-lactamase enzymes, 624
β-lactam/β-lactamase agents, 626, 628, 629, 638, 648, 649
β-thalassemia, 965, 966
Betamethasone, 272
Betaxalol, 400
Bethanechol, 268
Bicarbonate and sodium bicarbonate therapy
  acidosis, metabolic, 1058
  diabetes and hyperglycemia, 1088–1089
  dialysis patients, 1024
  drug overdose, 1230, 1231, 1232, 1233, 1238, 1240
  hepatic failure, 811
  hyperkalemia, 1052
  nephropathy, preventing, 1012
  tumor lysis syndrome, 942
  urinalysis, 996
Bile, 829, 830, 846
Biliary disorders, 829–837, 846, 847, 855
Bilirubin
  biliary disorders, 829, 830, 834
  hepatic failure, 810, 812, 813, 814, 815, 816
  liver chemistries, abnormal, 762, 763, 764
  organ involvement in lymphoma patients, 945
  urinalysis, 996
Biopsies
  back pain, 1156
  bone marrow, 949, 950, 951
  fever of unknown origin, 606
  goiter, 1070, 1071
  heart transplantation, 376–377, 378, 379
  liver, 814, 820
  lung, 187, 557, 572, 656, 662
  lymphadenopathy, 889
  lymphoma, 938
  renal, 1009, 1033, 1034, 1035
  solitary pulmonary nodules, 588, 589
  vasculitis, 1121, 1126–1127, 1131

Bioterrorism, 711–717
Bipolar disorders, 279, 280
Bird's Nest filters, 511
Bisacodyl, 879
Bicuspid aortic valve, 383
Bisferiens pulse, 308
Bismuth subsalicylate (Pepto Bismol®), 758, 793, 794, 796, 1233
Bisoprolol, 253, 364, 365
Bites and infection, 675, 676, 679
Bivalirudin, 350
Biventricular pacemakers, 403, 440
Bjork-Shiley single tilting disc valve, 390
Bladders, 226, 670, 1027, 1154
Blast crisis in chronic myelogenous leukemia, 934
Bleach, household, 716
Blebs, pleural, 582
Bleeding. See also Hemorrhage
    abdominal pain, causing, 753
    antidepressants, 1215
    antiplatelet therapy, 52, 53, 56
    chronic myeloproliferative diseases, 953
    deep vein thrombosis, 496, 499
    gastrointestinal, 75, 89–90
    intracranial hemorrhage, 1194
    lightheadedness, 306
    peripheral bypass procedures, 491
    rectal, 799, 800, 802, 803, 804
    sepsis, 204–205
    syncope, 428
    thrombolytic therapy, 347, 348
    ventricular arrhythmias and cardiac arrest, causing, 417
Bleeding disorders, 207, 210, 216, 223, 227, 257–258, 524, 975–991
Bleeding time, 976
Bleomycin, 525, 550, 551, 581, 899, 901, 902
Blood
    urinalysis, 996
Blood collection, 907
Blood patch following lumbar puncture, 1172
Blood pressure. See also Hypertension; Hypotension
    Ankle-Brachial Index, 458, 459, 460
    aortic intramural hematoma and dissection, 474–475, 476
    asymmetric, 424, 1123
    cardiac arrest and resuscitation, after, 416
    dialysis patients, measuring in, 1018
    home monitoring, 469
    increased intracranial pressure, 1188, 1191, 1192, 1194–1195
    status epilepticus, 1201
    stroke, 1176, 1179, 1180, 1181, 1182
    thoracic aortic aneurysms, 481
Blood transfusions
    atypical lymphocytosis, 609
    chemotherapy, 903
    emergencies, compatibility testing for, 912
    gastrointestinal disorders, 769, 771, 774, 802, 803, 805
    heart failure, 370
    hepatic failure, 811, 813
    large volume, complications of, 913
    liver transplantation, 843, 844
    shock, 194, 198
    sickle cell disease, 970, 972–973
    splenomegaly, 887
    substitutes for, 194, 909
    thrombocytopenia, 986
    transfusion medicine, principles of, 907–916
    transfusion reactions, 615, 958, 1225
Blood typing and cross-matching
    ABO typing, 374, 911–912, 1029
    gastrointestinal bleeding, 768, 774
    hematopoietic cell transplantation, 956
    non-ABO antigens, 912
    organ transplantation, 374, 1029
    platelet disorders, 988
    Rh factor, 292, 912
    trauma patient assessment, 288

Blood urea nitrogen (BUN)
    dialysis patients, 1020
    dyspnea, 523
    gastrointestinal bleeding, 769
    hypertension, emergent, 464
    oliguria and anuria, 999
    pericarditis, 443, 444
    renal disorders, 1002, 1003–1004, 1007, 1009
Blunt trauma, 287, 290–291
Body mass index, 100
Boerhaave's syndrome, 786–787
Bone marrow toxicity and suppression, 620, 726–727, 898, 1147, 1148
Bone marrow transplantation. See Hematopoietic cell transplantation
Bosentan, 573, 574–575, 843, 1139
Botulinum injections, 783
Botulism, 715–716
Bowel ischemia, 413
Bowel obstruction, 865, 874, 877, 878
Bowel sounds, 104, 849
Bradyarrhythmias
    cardiovascular medicine, 356, 364, 431–440
    fever, relative to, 603, 607–608
    heart transplant surgery, 375
    syncope, 423, 425, 427, 429
Bradycardia-tachycardia syndrome, 400, 401, 425, 431
Breast cancer, 443, 447, 449, 500, 957
Breath sounds, 518–519, 578, 582
Brescia-Cimino fistula, 1017
Bretylium, 356, 410, 419
Bromocriptine, 1238
Bronchiolitis, 185, 540, 555
Bronchitis, 524, 540
Bronchoalveolar lavage, 559, 647, 656, 662
Bronchodilators
    anaphylaxis, 1224
    asthma, 547
    chronic obstructive pulmonary disease, 533, 534, 535, 536, 537
    community-acquired pneumonia, 639, 640
    cough, 522
    dyspnea, 523
    hypokalemia, 1050
    inhalation injury, 555
    interstitial lung disease, 558, 559
    preoperative evaluation, 256
    pulmonary hypertension, 572
    right ventricular failure, 368
    spirometry, 526
Bronchoscopy
    community-acquired pneumonia, 639
    fever, 599
    hemoptysis, 524
    HIV infection, 734, 737
    pulmonary hypertension, 572
    respiratory failure, 187
    tuberculosis, 656, 662
Bruce protocol for stress electrocardiograms, 317
Brudzinski's sign, 683
Brugada syndrome, 412
Bruits, 306, 308, 333, 457, 458, 464–465, 1069–1070, 1123
B-type natriuretic peptide (BNP), 185, 534
B-type natriuretic peptide (BNP) levels, 360, 370
Bubonic plague, 715
Bucindolol, 400
Budd-Chiari syndrome, 498, 760, 761, 811, 815
Budesonide, 272, 534
Buerger's disease (thromboangiitis obliterans), 486, 490, 491
Bufferin®, 793
Bulimia nervosa, 305
Bumetanide, 365, 1002, 1010
Bundle branch block, 312, 340, 344, 348, 356, 367, 389, 435
Bupivacaine, 268
Buprenorphine, 135
Bupropion, 356, 722, 1212, 1213, 1215–1216, 1232, 1238

Burkitt disease, 931, 935, 937, 940–941, 945
Burn care specialists, 1224
Burns and hypovolemic shock, 191, 192
Busulfan, 550, 551, 958
Butyrophenones, 304
Bypass grafts, occlusion of, 487, 489, 490

C

Cachexia, 874
Cadence of arterial pulses, 308
Caffeine, 304, 316, 1050, 1139, 1170, 1236, 1240
CAGE questionnaire, 1244–1245
Calcineurin inhibitors, 1031, 1051
Calcitonin, 925, 926, 1157
Calcium, 113, 326, 1025, 1037, 1038, 1042, 1043
Calcium agonists, 468
Calcium antagonists, 370, 1021
Calcium channel blockers
    angina, 338, 340–341, 341
    antidepressants, 1213
    aortic intramural hematoma and dissection, 476
    arrhythmias, 398–399, 400, 402, 403, 405, 433
    chorea, 1168
    drug overdose, 1230, 1231, 1239
    esophageal disorders, 783, 784, 786
    headache, 1164
    heart transplant surgery, 375
    HIV infection drug regimen, 722
    hypertension, 466, 467, 470
    myocardial infarction, 345, 351, 356
    pericarditis, 451
    pregnancy, 271, 273
    pulmonary hypertension, 573, 574, 575
    renal disease, 1004, 1011, 1031
    valve disorders, 385, 387
Calcium chloride, 1230
Calcium gluconate, 272, 1052
Calcium leucovorin, 1129
Calcium levels
    lymphomas, 943
    oncologic emergencies, 924–926
    paraneoplastic syndrome, 588
    sarcoidosis, 553
    spherical mass lesions, 591
    torsade de pointes, 412
    transfusion reactions, 913
    tumor lysis syndrome, 941, 942, 943
Calcium-based binders, 1025
Calorie intake, 1021, 1024
Calorimetry, indirect, 102
Canadian Cardiovascular Society Angina Scale, 250–251, 332
Cancer. See Malignancies; specific types of cancer
Candesartan, 370
Candida infections, 265, 564, 669–670, 672, 784–785, 934
Cannon a waves, 305, 307
Capitated health care systems, 6, 7, 12, 84
Caplan's syndrome, 592
Capreomycin, 661
Capsaicin, 135
Captopril, 351, 364, 365
Captopril renography, 464, 469
Capture threshold for pacemakers, 435
Carbamate pesticides, 1232, 1239
Carbamazepine
    alcohol withdrawal, 1246
    anaphylaxis, 1224
    antidepressants, 1213
    antiretroviral therapies, 135, 722
    drug overdose, 1229, 1231
    erythematous eruptions, 1226
    hypernatremia, 1049
    neuropathic pain, 135
    pancytopenia, 895
    seizures, 1204, 1205, 1206
    thrombocytopenia, 977
    thyroid disease, 1075
    warfarin, interfering with, 512

Carbapenem antibiotics, 626, 628, 648, 649, 677, 679, 689
Carbon dioxide, 185, 1060
Carbon monoxide, 1231, 1234, 1236
Carbonic anhydrase inhibitors, 1060, 1062
Carboplatin, 900, 901, 902
Carcinoid tumors, 1226
Cardene, 467
Cardiac arrest, 196, 351–352, 395, 409–420
Cardiac biomarkers (enzymes), 443, 444
Cardiac catheterization
  angina, 338, 339
  aortic stenosis, 381–382
  cardiac arrest and resuscitation, after, 413, 414
  cardiovascular disease, 325
  limb ischemia, 487
  lung transplantation, 562
  mitral regurgitation, 387
  myocardial infarction, 249, 355
  pericardial tamponade, 445
  pericarditis, 442, 451
  pulmonary hypertension, 571, 572
  syncope, 426
  ventricular arrhythmias, 411
Cardiac enzymes, 413, 414, 447
Cardiac glycosides, 574, 1231, 1239, 1240
Cardiac masses, 323
Cardiac output
  cardiac arrest and resuscitation, after, 416, 419
  catheterization of right side of heart, 325
  heart failure, 359, 360, 361, 367
  pericarditis, 451
  post heart transplant surgery, 375
  pregnancy, 271
  right ventricular failure, 368
  shock, 191, 192, 193, 197
  syncope, 424–425
  valvular disorders, 383, 386, 387
Cardiac rehabilitation programs, 341
Cardiac syncope, 425
Cardiac system
  antidepressants, 1212, 1215
  liver transplant recipients, evaluation of, 843
  postoperative care, 264
  pregnancy, 271–272
  rheumatoid arthritis, 1141
  scleroderma, 1138
  structure and function, 321–325
Cardiac tamponade
  aortic aneurysms, 480
  aortic intramural hematoma and dissection, 472, 475
  dialysis patients, 1021
  extracardiac obstructive shock, 191, 192, 193, 197
  oncologic emergencies, 921–922
  pericarditis, 441–442, 444–445, 446, 447
  post heart transplant surgery, 376
  shock, 198
  ventricular arrhythmias and cardiac arrest, 411
Cardiac troponin levels, 264
Cardiazem, 467
Cardiogenic shock
  cardiac arrest, 419
  diagnosis and treatment, 191, 192, 193, 197
  heart failure, 359, 360, 362, 366, 367, 370
  myocardial infarction, 355
  syncope, 428
Cardiologists
  aortic aneurysms, 481
  aortic stenosis, 382
  endocarditis, 697
  myocardial infarction, 352, 356
  pericardial oncologic emergencies, 921
  pericarditis, 451
  permanent pacemakers, 438
  supraventricular tachyarrhythmias, 400
  ventricular arrhythmias and cardiac arrest, 419, 420
Cardiomegaly, 312
Cardiomyopathy

anthracycline agents, 934
cardiogenic shock, 191, 192
echocardiography, 323
heart failure, 359, 368, 369
heart transplantation, 373
preeclamsia, severe, 273
preoperative evaluation, 254
syncope, 424, 427
ventricular arrhythmias and cardiac arrest, 411, 416
wide-complex tachycardia, 395
Cardiopulmonary resuscitation
  ethical issues, 121, 122, 123, 124
  pregnancy, 271
  prolonged or traumatic, 348
  ventricular arrhythmias and cardiac arrest, 409–410, 413, 417
Cardiothoracic surgeons, 476
Cardiothoracic surgery, 451
Cardiotoxic agents, 322
Cardiovascular disorders. *See also* Heart failure; Myocardial infarction
  anaphylaxis, 1222, 1223
  angina, 329–341
  anxiety, 280
  bradycardia and pacemakers, 431–440
  B-type natriuretic peptide (BNP), 185
  Churg-Strauss syndrome, 1126
  cirrhosis, 820, 822
  diagnostic tests, 315–327
  dialysis patients, 1020–1021
  esophageal spasm, differentiating from, 784
  heart transplantation, 373–380
  pericardial disease, 441–452
  signs, symptoms, and laboratory abnormalities, 297–313
  subarachnoid hemorrhage, spontaneous, 1191
  supraventricular arrhythmias, 393–406
  syncope, 423–430
  trauma patients, 293
  valvular disease, 381–391
  ventricular arrhythmias, 409–420
Cardiovascular system
  elderly patients, 112–113
  hypertension, emergent, 463, 464, 468
  myxedema coma, 1098
  preoperative evaluations, 237, 249, 250–256
Cardiovascular toxicity, 1201
Cardioversion
  atrial tachyarrhythmias, 113, 264, 393, 403
  pacemakers, 439
  pericarditis, 451
  pregnancy, 271
  supraventricular tachyarrhythmias, 397, 398, 400, 401–402, 403, 405, 406
  synchronized, 356
  valvular stenosis, 382, 386
  ventricular arrhythmias, 356, 418
  wide-complex tachycardia, 395
Carey-Coombs murmurs, 310
Cardiac tamponade
  pericarditis, 444–445, 446
Carisoprodol, 1241
Carmustine, 550, 551, 901, 902, 904
Carney's syndrome, 592
Carotid arteries, examination of, 307–308
Carotid endarterectomy, 257, 1181, 1182
Carotid sinus massage, 397, 433
Cartilage, 627
Carvallo sign, 389
Carvedilol, 364, 365, 400
Caspofungin, 619, 707, 785, 962
Catecholamines, 195–196, 197, 304, 413, 464, 469
Catheters, urinary, 413, 414, 673–674, 859, 1040, 1041, 1042
Cauda equina syndrome, 918, 1153, 1154, 1155, 1156, 1171
Cavitation on chest radiographs, 655, 662
CD_4 cell count
  HIV-associated lymphomas, 941
  meningitis, 740, 742–743, 745, 746

pulmonary disease, 731, 733, 734, 735, 736
tuberculosis, 657, 663
Cefazolin, 620, 621, 1022
Cefepime
  hospital-acquired pneumonia, 648, 649
  IV catheter-associated infection, 707
  meningitis, 687, 688
  neutropenic hosts, 617
  resistant pathogens, 628, 629
  urinary tract infection, 670
Cefixime, 1151
Cefmetazole, 625
Cefotaxime
  meningitis, 687, 688, 689, 690, 691
  pneumonia, 638, 648
  septic arthritis, 1150
  spontaneous bacterial peritonitis, 824
Cefotetan, 292, 625, 677
Cefoxitin, 625, 677
Ceftazidime
  hospital-acquired pneumonia, 648, 649
  IV catheter-associated infection, 707
  meningitis, 687, 688
  neutropenic hosts, 617
  Pseudomonas aeruginosa, 629
Ceftizoxime, 625, 1150
Ceftriaxone, 150
  endocarditis, 698, 699
  hypogammaglobulinemic hosts, 615
  meningitis, 687, 688, 689, 690, 691
  peritonitis, 824
  pneumonia, 638, 643, 648
  septic arthritis, 1150
  urinary tract infection, 670, 671, 672
Cefuroxime, 615, 638, 648
Celecoxib, 773
Celexa, 1212
CellCept, 1031
Cell-mediated immunity, 619, 620
Cellular casts in urinalysis, 997–998
Cellular immune dysfunction, 614, 619–622
Cellular rejection, acute, 376, 846
Cellulitis, 675–678, 681, 1143, 1145
Center for Medicare and Medicaid Services, 80, 82, 83, 565
Centers for Disease Control and Prevention (CDC), 84, 630, 631, 708, 712–713, 715, 717
Central nervous system
  alcohol, 1243–1244
  depression, 1209–1210
  heart transplantations, 379
  hemorrhage, 1185–1198
  hypertension, emergent, 463, 464, 465, 466, 468
  infection, 282, 615
  oncology, 917, 945–946
  Sjögren's syndrome, 1139, 1140
  vasculitis, 1130–1132
Central venous catheters
  acute limb ischemia, 488, 490
  acute myelogenous leukemia, 932
  infection, 703–704, 704, 708, 1021
  insertion procedure, 215–222
  postoperative care, 261
  thrombosis, 990
Cephalosporins
  acute myelogenous leukemia, 933
  anaphylaxis, 1222, 1224, 1225
  anemia, 891
  β-lactam antibiotics, 625–626
  cellulitis, 676, 677
  cholecystitis, 832
  chronic obstructive pulmonary disease (COPD), 534
  Crohn's disease, 805
  diarrhea in gastrointestinal disease, 758
  hypogammaglobulinemic hosts, 615
  meningitis, 687, 688, 689, 690, 691
  necrotizing fasciitis, 679
  neutropenia, 616, 893
  pneumonia, 638, 640, 648, 649
  resistant pathogens, 624, 628, 629, 630

Salmonella infections, 604
spontaneous bacterial peritonitis, 824
trauma patients, 292
ulcerative colitis, 802
urinary tract infection, 670
Cerebral blood flow
cerebral hypoperfusion, 431
hypertension, emergent, 465, 466
increased intracranial pressure, 1185–1186, 1186, 1188, 1194–1195
Cerebral edema, 1089
Cerebral glucose deficiency, 1090
Cerebral hypoxia, 282
Cerebral metastases, 917–921
Cerebral osmotic demyelination, 1046–1047
Cerebrospinal fluid
cardiac arrest and resuscitation, after, 416
central nervous system vasculitis, 1130–1131, 1132
examination of, 1171–1172
hepatic encephalopathy, 825
HIV infected patients, 740, 746
increased intracranial pressure, 1185, 1186
lumbar puncture, 222, 224, 225
meningitis, acute bacterial, 684, 685–686
Cerebrovascular accident. *See* Stroke
Cerebrovascular disorders, 276, 424, 455
Cerubidine, 902
Cervical spine, 288, 290
CHADS$_2$ index, 400, 402
Chagas disease, 783, 914
Charcot's triad, 833
Chemotherapy
acute lymphoblastic leukemia, 935
acute myelogenous leukemia, 932, 935
anemia, 892, 893
back pain, 1156
esophageal carcinoma, 783
goals of, 898–899
hematopoietic cell transplantation, 956, 958
Hodgkin's disease, 941
hypercalcemia, 926
immunocompromised hosts, 613
malignancy post heart transplantation, 380
malignant pericarditis, 449
monocytic leukemia, 933, 934
neurologic oncologic emergencies, 919–920
neutropenia, 615, 893
organ involvement in lymphoma patients, 944
pancytopenia, 895
principles of, 897–906
renal stone and obstructive disease, 1042
superior vena cava syndrome, 923, 924
ulcerative colitis, 801
Chest pain evaluation units, 303, 339, 341
Chest tubes, 580, 581, 583, 584–585, 588
Child-Turcotte-Pugh score, 820, 821, 840
Chlamydia infections, 330, 539, 543
Chloral hydrate, 1240
Chlorambucil, 932, 940, 1137
Chloramphenicol, 687, 688, 714, 895
Chlorates, 521
Chlordiazepoxide, 1230, 1246, 1248
Chlorhexidine, 2% tincture of, 705
Chlorhexidine gluconate, 209, 215, 222, 225, 226, 231, 709
Chlormezanone, 1224
Chloroquine, 1050
Chlorpheniramine, 1230
Chlorpromazine, 143–144, 281, 894, 903, 906
Chlorpropamide, 893, 1024, 1049, 1090
Chlorthalidone, 977
Cholangitis, 829, 830, 833–837, 851, 855
Cholecystectomy, 274, 832–833, 837, 857
Cholecystitis, 300, 344, 378, 752, 754, 829–830, 831–833, 850, 851
Cholecystitis, acalculous, 752, 829, 830, 831, 833
Choledocholithiasis, 830–831
Cholesterol, 829
Cholesterol emboli, 481
Cholesterol levels, 330, 803

Cholestyramine, 512, 813, 1096
Cholinergic agonists, 879
Chordae tendinae, 387, 388
Chorea, 1168
Chronic intestinal pseudo-obstruction, 875
Chronic limb ischemia, 485, 486, 490–492
Chronic lymphocytic leukemia, 929, 930
Chronic myelogenous leukemia, 929, 930, 934, 957
Chronic myeloid leukemia, 947
Chronic myelomonocytic leukemia, 947
Chronic myeloproliferative disorders, 947–953
Chronic neutrophilic leukemia, 947
Chronic obstructive pulmonary disease (COPD)
anxiety, 280
heart failure, 362
lung transplantation and volume reduction surgery, 561
noninvasive ventilation, 175, 176, 187, 190
pneumothorax, 582
preoperative evaluation, 256
pulmonary medicine, 531–537
respiratory failure, acute, 188
wheezing, 519
Chronic thromboembolic pulmonary hypertension, 569, 570, 571, 572, 574
Chronotropic agents, 371, 375
Churg-Strauss syndrome, 550, 592, 1118, 1126, 1128, 1129
Cimetidine
chemotherapy, 900
chorea, 1168
creatinine levels, 1003
delirium, 1165
depression, 1210
drug interactions, 796
headache, 1164
nephrotoxic effects, 363
peptic ulcer disease, 793
pregnancy, 273
radiocontrast allergies, 1225
thrombocytopenia, 977
warfarin, interfering with, 512
Cinefluoroscopy, 389
Ciprofloxacin
anthrax, 714
cirrhosis with ascites, 823
fluoroquinolone antibiotic, 627
meningitis, 686, 688
necrotizing fasciitis, 677, 679
neutropenic hosts, 616
pneumonia, 638, 648, 649
prophylaxis for renal transplant patients to prevent urinary tract infections, 621
Salmonella infections, 604
septic arthritis, 1151
urinary tract infection, 669, 670, 672
warfarin, interfering with, 512
Ciprofloxacin XR, 669
Cirrhosis, 570, 768, 770, 771, 819–827, 847
Cisapride, 304, 412, 879, 1213, 1240
Cisplatin, 899, 900, 901, 902, 903, 904, 906, 977, 1050
Citalopram, 1212
Citrate-based alkalinizing agents, 1024, 1025, 1058
CK-MB levels, 337, 339, 352
Clarithromycin, 304, 626, 638, 643, 663, 714, 794, 796
Classification of lymphoma, 938, 939
Claudication, 456–457, 458, 490
Claudication, intermittent, 485, 486, 488
Clavulanate, 626
Clavulanic acid, 639
Cleft palates, 272
Clindamycin
action of, 626
anthrax, 714
cellulitis and necrotizing fasciitis, 676, 677
community-acquired pneumonia, 638, 639
gastrointestinal disease, 758

HIV infected patients, 735, 743
trauma patients, 292
Clinical pathways in medical practice, 87–91
Clinical reasoning, 75–76
Clinical trials, 89
Clofibrate, 512, 1049
Clomipramine, 1212
Clonazepam, 135, 280, 1215, 1234
Clonazipine, 722
Clonidine
alcohol withdrawal, 282, 1248
delirium, 1165
depression, 1210
drug overdose, 1236, 1239
hypertension, emergent, 468, 469
pregnancy, 273
surgery and, 253, 264
tricyclic antidepressants, 1213
Clopidogrel
angina, 338, 340
chronic limb ischemia, 491, 492
myocardial infarction, 52–56, 349, 350
stroke, 1181, 1182
Clorazepate, 722
Clostridium difficile
disruption of skin and mucous membranes, 613
fever, 600
gastrointestinal disease, 753, 754, 756, 758, 759
impaired immunity, 615, 620
Clostridium perfringens, 599
Clotrimazole, 613, 621
Coagulation disorders
cholangitis, acute, 835, 836, 837
diabetes mellitus, 1080, 1089
gastrointestinal bleeding, 771
hemolytic reaction to transfusion, 912
L-asparaginase, 935
liver chemistries, abnormal, 765
liver transplantation, 843, 844
platelet disorders, 988–989
regional anesthesia, 244
sepsis, 201, 205
shock and fluid resuscitation, 195
thrombotic, 975–984, 988–991
trauma patients, 289, 293
Coagulation factor concentrates, 499
Coagulation studies, 459, 524, 769, 791, 801
Coarctation of the aorta, 383, 472
Cocaine
central nervous system vasculitis, 1131
chest pain, 300
chorea, 1168
drug overdose, 1230, 1231, 1234, 1236, 1238, 1240, 1241
hypertension, 463, 464, 468, 469
interstitial lung disease, 550, 551
intracranial hemorrhage, 1194
monoamine oxidase inhibitors, 1215
palpitations, 304
peripheral arterial disease, 486
pulmonary hypertension, 570
seizures, 1199, 1204
stroke, 1177
ventricular arrhythmias and cardiac arrest, 411
Codeine, 131, 132, 1213, 1232, 1237
Cogentin, 1213
Cognitive function, 112, 114–115, 1164–1165, 1166
Colchicine, 448, 450, 1147, 1148, 1239
Cold, application of, 131
Cold, exposure to, 607, 1097
Cold agglutinin disease, 891, 893
Cold iodide, 274
Colitis
antibiotic-associated, 626
Clostridium difficile, 753, 754, 756, 758, 759
inflammatory, 753
ischemic, 752, 754, 867–870
ulcerative, 799–800, 800–804
Collagen vascular disorders, 524
Collateral circulation, 207, 208, 486, 487, 489, 490

Colloid IV solutions, 193–194, 1010, 1088
Colon obstruction, 873
Colonic pseudo-obstruction (Ogilvie's
   syndrome), 752, 753, 876, 880
Colonoscopy
   acute gastrointestinal bleeding, 775–776
   bowel ischemia, 868, 869
   bowel obstruction, 880
   diverticulitis, 865
   ulcerative colitis, 801, 802
Colorectal anastomosis, 867, 870
Colorectal cancer, 800
Colostomy, 867, 870, 876
CoLyte, 1235
Coma, 413, 416
Combination therapy
   chemotherapy, 897
   infections, 628, 629, 648, 657–658, 794
   insulins, 1082
   T_3 and T_4 for myxedema coma, 1101
Comfort care, 142–143, 534, 552–553
Commissurotomy of mitral valves, 369, 387
Commitment to psychiatric facility, 284
Commotio cordis, 412
Communication issues
   clinical information systems, 63–68
   discharge from hospital, 32–35
   end-of-life care, 141, 142
   hospital personnel, among, 23–29, 72, 166
   hospitalist and primary care physician,
      111–112, 127
   medical consultation, 236
Community-acquired pneumonia
   consolidation on chest radiograph, 528
   discharge criteria, 31–32
   doxycycline, 627
   eosinophilic pneumonia, 554
   HIV infection, 729–737
   hospitalization for, 83, 90, 633–644
   similar diseases, 551, 558, 559
Comorbid conditions
   acute coronary syndrome, 339
   alcohol withdrawal, 1246
   angina, prognosis of, 335
   aortic stenosis, 382
   appendicitis, acute, 861
   asthma, 543
   bowel ischemia, acute, 868
   community-acquired pneumonia, 636, 637,
      638, 642
   depression in hospitalized patients, 1209
   diabetes in dialysis patients, 1024
   gastrointestinal bleeding, 768–769, 770, 774,
      775, 777, 778
   heart transplantation, exclusion criteria for,
      373, 374
   hepatomegaly, 760
   hypothermia, 607
   limb ischemia, 488, 491, 492
   liver transplant recipients, evaluation of, 841
   mitral regurgitation, 388
   pericarditis, 451
   practice guidelines and clinical pathways, 90
   syncope, 428
   trauma patients, 292
   ventricular arrhythmias and cardiac arrest in
      inpatients, 417
Compartment syndrome, 292, 456, 457
Competency of patients, 120–123, 124, 283–284
Complete blood count
   acute pericarditis, 443, 444
Complete blood count (CBC)
   chronic obstructive pulmonary disease
      (COPD), 532, 535
   dyspnea, 523
   gastrointestinal disease, 769, 791, 801
   hemoptysis, 524
   peripheral artery disease, 459
   pulmonary disease with HIV infection, 730
   splenomegaly, 886
Complex partial seizures, 1200, 1203

Compliance, patient
   angina, 341
   asthma, 539
   depression, 1211
   heart failure, 360, 370
   hepatic encephalopathy, 825, 826
   hypertension, 469, 470
   peptic ulcer disease, 794, 796
   tuberculosis, 658, 662, 664
Complicated parapneumonic pleural effusions,
   580–581
Complications
   alcohol withdrawal, 1248–1249
   blood transfusions, 912–915
   chemotherapy, 903–905, 958
   cholangitis, 836–837
   cholecystitis, 832, 833
   diabetes and hyperglycemia, 1089
   dialysis, 1019
   endocarditis, 698
   enteral nutrition, 105–106
   gastrointestinal disease, 752, 753
   heart transplantations, 378–380
   hematopoietic cell transplantation, 958,
      959–963
   hepatic failure, 810, 811, 813
   Hodgkin's disease, 941
   hospital-acquired pneumonia, 651
   inferior vena cava filters, 511
   IV catheter-associated infection, 706–708,
      708–709
   liver transplantation, 843–845
   lung transplantation, 563–564
   lung volume reduction surgery, 566
   lymphomas, 941–946
   meningitis, 687–688, 689, 690, 691
   myocardial infarction, 355–356
   neurologic, of HIV infection, 739–747
   pancreatitis, 856–857
   parenteral nutrition, 107–108
   pericarditis, 445
   radiation therapy, 923
   renal transplantation, 1033–1036
   rheumatic disorders, 1136
   subarachnoid hemorrhage, 1190, 1191–1192
   surgery for thoracic aortic aneurysms, 481
   tricyclic antidepressants, 1213–1215
   urinary tract infections, 668
   ventricular arrhythmias and cardiac arrest and
      resuscitation, 418
Compression fractures, 1157, 1158, 1159
Computed tomography (CT)
   anthrax, 714
   aortic disorders, 473, 476, 480, 481, 482, 483
   appendicitis, acute, 861
   back pain, 1156, 1157
   cardiac arrest and resuscitation, after, 413, 414
   chest pain, 299, 300
   cholangitis, 834
   cholecystitis, 831, 833
   Crohn's disease, 804
   Cushing syndrome, 1072–1073
   deep vein thrombosis, 495
   delirium, 282
   diverticulitis, 864, 866
   drug overdose with altered level of
      consciousness, 1236, 1238
   gastrointestinal disease, 754
   hepatic encephalopathy, 825
   HIV infected patients, 725, 746
   hypertension, emergent, 464
   ileus and bowel obstruction, 878, 879
   increased intracranial pressure, 1188
   interstitial lung disease, 557
   intracranial hemorrhage, 1194
   limb ischemia, 488
   meningitis, 687
   pancreatitis, 851–852
   pericarditis, 450
   pleural effusions, 578
   pneumothorax, 582

pregnancy, 276
pulmonary embolism, 506–507, 508
pulmonary medicine, 519
renal stone and obstructive disease, 1039
solitary pulmonary nodules, 587, 588
splenomegaly, 886
stroke, 1175, 1178, 1179, 1180
subarachnoid hemorrhage, spontaneous, 223,
   1190
subdural hematoma, 1196
superior vena cava syndrome, 923
syncope, 425, 426
trauma patient assessment, 288, 289, 290, 291
urinary tract infection, upper, 673
ventricular arrhythmias, 410
Computerized decision support, 64–65, 85
Computerized monitoring of adverse drug events,
   159
Computerized physician order entry (CPOE),
   64–65, 90, 153, 158, 1026
C1 esterase inhibitor concentrate, 1223
Confidentiality, 67, 119, 126, 127
Confusion, 431, 463
Congenital heart disease, 411
Congestive heart failure
   community-acquired pneumonia, 634
   dialysis patients, 1021
   endocarditis, 697, 698, 699
   hepatomegaly, 760
   pleural effusions, 578, 579, 580
   pulmonary embolism, 505, 512, 513
   quality measurement of treatment, 82
   syncope, 428
   thyrotoxic storm, 1093, 1094, 1096
   ventricular arrhythmias, 410
Connective tissue diseases. *See also specific
   connective tissue diseases*
   chronic aortic regurgitation, 383
   interstitial lung diseases, 550, 552
   peripheral artery disease, differentiating from,
      457
   pulmonary hypertension, 570, 573
   rheumatic diseases, 1112, 1113, 1114, 1117, 1118
Consciousness, level of. *See also* Encephalopathy;
   Mental status, altered; Neuropathy
   acute respiratory failure, 183, 184
   asthma, 541, 544
   brain herniation, 1187
   drug overdose, 1233, 1234, 1236–1238
   myocardial infarction, 343
   palpitations, 304, 305–306
   partial seizures, 1200
   trauma, 288, 289
Consciousness, loss of
   electroencephalography, 1172
   myxedema coma, 1097
   subarachnoid hemorrhage, spontaneous, 1190
   syncope, 423, 429, 430
Consent issues, 119, 120–121, 127, 217, 223,
   226, 228, 283–284
Constipation, 133, 273, 753
Consultation, indications for
   acute myelogenous leukemia, 932
   alcohol withdrawal, 1249
   allograft rejection of heart transplantation, 377
   anaphylaxis, 1224, 1226
   aortic aneurysm, 483
   aortic intramural hematoma and dissection, 476
   back pain, 1156, 1157–1158
   bowel ischemia, acute, 869
   bowel obstruction, 874, 877, 880
   bradycardia and pacemakers, 438
   central nervous system vasculitis, 1132
   cholecystitis, 832
   chronic obstructive pulmonary disease
      (COPD), 534
   community-acquired pneumonia, 639, 641–642
   Crohn's disease, 805
   diverticulitis, 865
   drug overdose, 1236
   endocarditis, 697

endocrine disorders, 1070, 1076, 1107
gastrointestinal disorders, 770, 802
gout, 1147
heart failure, 362
hepatic failure, 813, 814
hypercalcemia in oncologic emergencies,
	925–926
hyperkalemia, 1052
hypertension, emergent, 468
hyponatremia, 1048
interstitial lung disease, 558–559
intracranial hemorrhage, 1194
IV catheter-associated infection, 707–708
limb ischemia, 488
meningitis, 689
myocardial infarction, 352
neurologic complications in HIV infected
	patients, 741, 743–744, 746
neurologic oncologic emergencies, 918, 920
pancreatitis, 853
pericardial oncologic emergencies, 921
pericarditis, 447, 451
practice of, 235–238
pulmonary embolism, 509
pulmonary hypertension, 573
renal disorders, 1010, 1014, 1015, 1035, 1041
renal transplantation, 1035
respiratory failure, 187–188
sickle cell disease, 970
stroke, 1178, 1181
subdural hematoma, 1197
supraventricular tachyarrhythmias, 400
syncope, 428
thoracic aortic aneurysms, 481
tuberculosis, 661–662
tumor lysis syndrome, 943
urinary tract infection, 670, 672–673
valvular disease, 382, 385, 386, 388, 390
vasculitis, 1129
ventricular arrhythmias and cardiac arrest, 417,
	418–419, 420
wheezing, 519
Consumer Protection Act, 93
Continuing medical education, 81, 84
Continuity of care, 17–18
Continuous ambulatory peritoneal dialysis, 1018,
	1019
Continuous cyclic peritoneal dialysis, 1018
Continuous positive airway pressure (CPAP),
	242, 256
Continuous renal replacement therapies, 168,
	1013, 1018, 1020, 1232, 1236
Contraindications. *See also* Drug interactions
	acute prostatitis, 668
	aminophylline IV with chronic obstructive
		pulmonary disease (COPD), 534
	antihypertensive medications, 467, 468
	arterial puncture and cannulation, 207
	arthrocentesis, 210, 1143
	β-blockers, 1248
	central venous catheters, 216
	diverticulitis, 865
	fine needle aspiration for some adrenal lesions,
		1107
	flumazenil, 1237
	fluoroquinolone antibiotics, 627
	furosemide, 925
	liver transplant eligibility, 840–841
	lumbar puncture, 223, 1172
	lung transplantation, 562
	methemoglobinemia and medications, 521
	monoamine oxidase inhibitors, 1215
	paracentesis, 225
	streptokinase for ischemic stroke, 1179
	thoracentesis, 227
	thrombolytic therapy for pulmonary embolism,
		510
	ulcerative colitis, 801
Conversion disorders, 283
Cor pulmonale, 389, 532, 552, 556, 971
Corlopam, 467

Coronary arteries, 300, 343, 411, 412
Coronary artery bypass graft (CABG)
	anti-platelet therapy, 338
	arrhythmias, 406, 418
	bowel ischemia, acute, 867
	hypothermia, causing, 607
	myocardial infarction and NSTEMI treatment,
		349
	postoperative stroke, 257
	preoperative evaluation, 252–253
	quality measurement, 82
	solitary pulmonary nodules, 589
Coronary artery disease
	abdominal pain, causing, 753
	angina, 332, 333–334, 335
	atherosclerotic plaque events, 331
	cardiac catheterization, 325–326
	chest pain, 298, 299
	definition, 329
	discharge issues following cardiac arrest, 418
	heart transplantation, indication for, 373
	homocysteine level, 341
	monomorphic sustained ventricular
		tachycardia, 412
	peripheral artery disease, 455, 457
	preoperative evaluation for cardiac
		complications, 250–253
	probabilities in diagnostic testing, 38–39
	surgical repair of abdominal aortic aneurysm,
		483
	syncope, 424–425
	ventricular arrhythmias, 410, 411
	wide-complex tachycardia, 395
Coronary Artery Surgery Study, 252–253
Coronary care units, 344–345, 411, 432, 434. *See
	also* Intensive care units
Coronary vascular resistance, 330
Corticosteroids
	abdominal pain, causing, 753
	acute respiratory distress syndrome (ARDS), 189
	adrenal insufficiency, 1103
	agnogenic myeloid metaplasia, 952
	alcoholic hepatitis, 814, 816
	anthrax, 714
	arthrocentesis, 210, 211
	asthma, 542, 543, 545, 546, 547
	blood urea nitrogen level, 1003
	chronic obstructive pulmonary disease, 534,
		536, 537
	depression, 1210
	diffuse alveolar hemorrhage, 551
	dyspnea, 523
	eosinophilic pneumonia, 554–555
	fever of unknown origin, 607
	gout, 1147
	graft-*versus*-host disease, 963
	hypercalcemia, 943
	hypertension, 469
	idiopathic thrombocytopenic purpura, 985
	inhalation injury, 555
	interstitial lung disease, 558, 559
	lung transplantation, 561, 562, 563, 564
	myxedema coma, 1099, 1100
	pancreatitis in dialysis patients, 1023
	parenchymal brain involvement in lymphoma
		patients, 945–946
	pericarditis, 447, 448, 450
	polymyositis/dermatomyositis, 1140, 1141
	preoperative evaluation, 256
	pulmonary disease with HIV infection, 734–735
	pulmonary hypertension, 572
	renal transplantation, 1931
	rheumatoid arthritis, 1141
	sarcoidosis, 554
	scleroderma, 1138, 1139
	shock, 197
	Sjögren's syndrome, 1139
	swollen joints, injected into, 1115
	systemic lupus erythematosus, 1137
	tuberculosis, 660–661, 664
	ulcerative colitis, 802, 803, 804

vasculitis, 1122, 1123, 1124, 1127, 1129, 1130,
		1132
	vocal chord dysfunction, 541
	withdrawal symptoms, 135
Cortisol therapy
	adrenal insufficiency, 1071–1072, 1076, 1106,
		1107, 1108, 1213
Cortrosyn stimulation test, 1076, 1101,
	1105–1106, 1107
Cost considerations. *See also* Economic aspects of
	care
	acute leukemia, 935
	alcohol withdrawal, 1249
	anaphylaxis, 1226
	angina, 341
	arthritis, 1151
	asthma, 545–546
	back pain, 1159
	biliary disease, 837
	bowel ischemia, acute, 870
	bowel obstruction, 880
	bradycardia and pacemakers, 439–440
	cardiovascular diagnostic tests, 326
	cellulitis and necrotizing fasciitis, 681
	chronic myeloproliferative diseases, 953
	cirrhosis, 827
	community-acquired pneumonia, 643
	COPD, 537
	Crohn's disease, 806
	deep venous thrombosis, 502
	diabetes mellitus, 1079, 1080, 1086, 1091
	drug overdose and dependence, 1241
	endocarditis, 700
	esophageal disorders, 787
	gastrointestinal bleeding, 778
	heart failure, 371
	hepatic failure, 816
	hospital-acquired pneumonia, 651–653
	increased intracranial pressure, 1197
	interstitial lung disease, 559
	IV catheter-associated infection, 709
	laboratory tests for bleeding and thrombotic
		disorders, 981
	lymphoma patients, 946
	meningitis, 690–691
	myocardial infarction, acute, 357
	neurologic complications of HIV infected
		patients, 746
	pancreatitis, 857
	pericardial disease, 452
	primary spontaneous pneumothorax, 585
	pulmonary disease with HIV infection, 737
	pulmonary disorders, 592–593
	pulmonary embolism, 513
	pulmonary hypertension, 575
	renal failure, acute, 1015
	renal stone and obstructive disease, 1043
	respiratory failure, acute, 190
	sepsis, 206
	sickle cell disease, 973
	supraventricular tachyarrhythmias, 406
	transfusion medicine, 915
	tuberculosis, 664
	urinary tract infection, upper, 673–674
	valvular heart disease, 390
	vasculitis, 1132
	ventricular arrhythmias and cardiac arrest, 420
Costochondritis, 344
Cough
	ACE inhibitors, 364
	asthma, 540
	community-acquired pneumonia, 634, 643
	gastrointestinal bleeding, 768
	hemoptysis, 524
	interstitial lung diseases (ILDs), 549
	pulmonary hypertension, 569
	pulmonary medicine, 521–522
	thoracic aortic aneurysms, 480
	tuberculosis, 655
Coumadin, 244, 356, 511, 659, 789, 988, 1172.
	See also Warfarin

Coumarin compounds, 977
Coxsackie B virus, 449
Crack cocaine, 1230, 1231
Crackles, 518, 552, 556, 634
Crank, 1230
C-reactive protein, 488, 686
Creatinine kinase BB levels, 416
Creatinine kinase levels, 337, 339, 352, 379, 489, 676, 678
Creatinine kinase MB levels, 413, 414, 443, 444
Creatinine levels
    dialysis patients, 1020
    dyspnea, 523
    gastrointestinal bleeding, 769
    HIV infected patients, 726
    hypertension, 464
    limb ischemia, 487
    oliguria and anuria, 999
    pericarditis, 443, 444
    peripheral artery disease, 459
    renal disease, 1002, 1003–1004, 1007, 1009, 1014
    renal transplantation, 1033
Crepitations, 518
Crohn's disease, 103, 383, 757, 761, 762, 799, 800, 804–806
Cryoprecipitate, 990, 1180
Crystal meth, 1230
Crystalloid IV solutions, 193, 194, 544
Crystalluria, 998, 1038, 1042
Crystals in synovial fluid, 1144, 1145
Cullen's sign, 849
Cultures
    fever, 600, 602, 606
    hepatic failure, 814
    plague, 715
    sepsis, 202, 203, 204
    shock, 197
    specimen collection, 609
    tuberculosis, 656, 663
Cultures, blood
    back pain, 1156
    cellulitis, 676, 677
    cholangitis, 835
    community-acquired pneumonia, 635
    endocarditis, 694, 696
    HIV infected patients, 741
    hypogammaglobulinemic hosts, 614
    IV catheter-associated infection, 704–705, 706, 708
    meningitis, 687
    necrotizing fasciitis, 679
    neutropenic hosts, 615
    pacemaker infections, 439
    pancreatitis, 850
    urinary tract infection, upper, 671
Cultures, cerebrospinal fluid, 684, 687, 689, 740
Cultures, IV catheter, of, 705
Cultures, nasal swab, 714
Cultures, pericardial fluid, 448
Cultures, sputum, 616, 634–635, 647, 649
Cultures, stool, 759
Cultures, synovial fluid, 1145, 1146, 1149–1150
Cultures, urine, 615, 668, 672, 673
Cushing's syndrome, 289, 588, 1048, 1060, 1071–1073
C-v waves, 355
Cyanide, 1231, 1234
Cyanosis
    acute limb ischemia, 488
    asthma, 541, 544
    central, 520
    idiopathic pulmonary fibrosis, 552
    peripheral artery disease, 458
    pulmonary hypertension, 570
    pulmonary medicine, 520–521
    tension pneumothorax, 583
Cyclooxygenase-2 (COX-2) inhibitors, 131, 773, 794–795
Cyclophosphamide
    acute myelogenous leukemia, 934
    chemotherapy, 897, 899, 900, 901, 902, 904, 906

diffuse alveolar hemorrhage, 551
    follicular lymphomas, 940
    hematopoietic cell transplantation, 958
    interstitial lung disease, 558
    rheumatic disorders, 1137, 1138, 1140
    vasculitis, 1122, 1123, 1124, 1127, 1128, 1129, 1132
Cycloserine, 659, 661
Cyclosporine
    anemia, 891
    anti-microbials, interaction with, 620
    gout, 1147
    graft-*versus*-host disease, 961, 962
    headache, 1164
    heart transplantation, 373, 376, 378, 379
    hematopoietic cell transplantation, 958–959
    hypertension, emergent, 467, 469, 470
    liver transplantation, 845
    lung transplantation, 562, 563, 564
    malignant hypertension, 379
    neutropenia, 894
    pancytopenia, 896
    peripheral arterial disease, 486
    pregnancy, 276
    renal transplantation, 1031, 1033, 1034, 1035
    rheumatic diseases, 1137, 1140
    seizures, 1204
    thrombocytopenia, 977
    tuberculosis treatment, interactions with, 659
    ulcerative colitis, 802–803
Cylindrical aortic aneurysms, 479
Cyotsine arabinoside, 686
Cyproheptadine, 1215, 1232, 1238
Cysteine-rich protein-61 (CYR61), 1009
Cystic fibrosis, 187, 188
Cystitis, 667–668, 906, 934
Cytarabine, 899, 900, 901, 902, 903, 904, 934
Cytokine interleukin 11 (IL-11), 988
Cytomegalovirus (CMV), 563, 564, 609, 725, 846, 914, 962
Cytosine arabinoside, 550
Cytotoxic agents
    interstitial lung disease, 550, 551, 558
    lung transplantation, 564
    polymyositis/dermatomyositis, 1140, 1141
    rheumatic diseases, 1135, 1137, 1141
    vasculitis, 1122, 1124, 1125

D

Daclizumab, 1031
Dactinomycin, 904
Dalteparin, 511
Danaproid sodium, 275
Danazol, 977, 1164, 1223
Dapsone, 521, 621, 726, 735, 736, 962, 1224
Daptomycin, 676, 677
Darbopoietin, 893, 944
Darvon®, 793
Daunorubicin, 899, 900, 901, 902
Daztreoman, 626
D-dimer assays, 275, 495–496, 497, 500, 502, 508, 978
Death
    cardiac arrest, 409
    do not resuscitate orders, 123–124, 144, 414
    end-of-life care, 139–144
    medical errors, due to, 147, 148, 149
    preoperative evaluation for thyroid function, 258
    terminal weaning from mechanical ventilation, 182
    trauma, due to, 287
Death, sudden
    bradycardia-dependent polymorphic ventricular tachycardia, 431
    coronary atherosclerotic disease, 329
    heart transplantations, 379
    myocardial infarction, 351
    valvular heart disease, 381
Decision analysis, 43–49

Decision-making
    community-acquired pneumonia, 637
    competency of patients, 120–123, 124
    decision analysis, 43–49
    deep vein thrombosis, 496
    end-of-life care, 140
    preoperative evaluations of risk, 250
    psychological consultation, 283–284
Decompensated heart failure, 363–366, 382
Decompression of spinal cord, 290
Decompression of the biliary tract, 835–837
Decongestants, 1050
Decubiti, 599
Dedicated anticoagulation clinics, 403–404
Deep venous thrombosis, 237, 291, 495–503
Deep venous thrombosis prophylaxis, 292, 414, 511, 677, 1191, 1193, 1195
Defibrillation, 351, 356, 409, 410, 413, 414, 417, 439
Defibrillators, 402
Defibrotide, 960
Degenerative disc disease, 457
Dehydration, 757, 758, 1083
Déjà vu, feeling of, 1200
Delayed graft function, 1028, 1033, 1034
Delirium
    depression in hospitalized patients, 1209
    elderly patients, 112, 114–115
    end-of-life care, 143
    illness precipitating, 279
    neurologic signs, 1164, 1165
    postoperative care, 262–263
    preoperative evaluation, 256, 257
    psychological consultation, 281–282
    psychosis, 280
Delirium tremens, 1245, 1246, 1249
Delusions, 280
Dementia, 112, 114, 257, 280, 281, 1164–1166, 1210
Demerol, 132, 969, 1012, 1213
Dengue fever, 603–604
Dental prophylaxis, 383, 387, 389, 390, 700
Depakene, 1233
Depakote, 1233
Depression
    alcohol withdrawal, 1249
    delirium and dementia, 1165, 1166
    elderly patients, 112, 115
    electroencephalography, 1173
    hospitalized patients, 1209–1216
    illness precipitating, 279
    medical consultation regarding, 279
    suicide, 279
    syncope, 429
Dermatological disorders, 1221, 1222, 1223, 1224, 1225–1226
Dermatologists, 1224, 1226
Dermatomes of sensation, 1169, 1170
Dermatomyositis, 1136, 1140–1141
Desensitization therapy, 1225, 1226
Desferrioxamine, 973
Desflurane, 244
Desipramine, 115, 133–134, 1212
Desmopressin, 1024, 1049
Destran-70, 822
Desyrel, 1212
Dexamethasone
    acute myelogenous leukemia, 934
    adrenal insufficiency, 1106, 1108
    antidepressants, 1213
    chemotherapy, 903, 905, 906
    chronic myeloproliferative diseases, 953
    Crohn's disease, 805
    hematopoietic cell transplantation, 958
    HIV infection drug regimen, 722
    increased intracranial pressure, 1189
    meningitis, 686, 687–688, 689, 691, 741
    myxedema coma, 1101
    nausea and vomiting in postoperative care, 263
    neurologic oncologic emergencies, 919
    postoperative nausea, 246

subarachnoid hemorrhage, spontaneous, 1191
ulcerative colitis, 802
Dexrazoxane, 897, 899
Dextran, 194, 977
Dextroamphetamine, 1215
Dextromethorphan, 522, 1213, 1215, 1234
Dextrose, 107, 1018. *See also* Glucose supplements
Diabetes insipidus, 191, 192, 553, 1048, 1049
Diabetes mellitus
anesthesia, 243
angina, prognosis of, 335
aortic stenosis, 382
atherosclerotic plaque events, 330
cardiac risk factors, 340, 341
chronic limb ischemia, 490
dialysis patients, 1024
lightheadedness, 306
management of, 1079–1091
myocardial infarction, 343
peripheral arterial disease, 457, 460, 485–486,
488
pregnancy, 274
renal injury, 506
syncope, 424
urinalysis, 996
urinary tract infection, 668, 669–670, 672
Diabetes Mellitus Insulin Glucose Infusion in
Myocardial Infarction study, 1085
Diabetic ketoacidosis, 191, 274, 1050,
1086–1089, 1091
Diabetic neuropathy, 457, 492, 1171
Diagnoses
acidosis, respiratory, 1060–1062
alkalosis, respiratory, 1063–1064
central nervous system vasculitis, 1130–1131
chest pain, 299
complicated peptic ulcer disease, 791
depression in hospitalized patients, 1210
diabetic ketoacidosis and hyperosmolar
hyperglycemic nonketotic syndrome, 1087
gastrointestinal disorders, 768, 775–776,
791–792
hospital-acquired pneumonia, 645–647
hypoglycemia, 1090
myxedema coma, 1099
palpitations, 305–306
renal disorders, 1004, 1007–1009
respiratory failure, acute, 187
seizures, 1199–1201
sickle cell disease, 965
solitary pulmonary nodules, 587–588
thyrotoxic storm, 1094
vasculitis, 1121–1122, 1126–1127
Diagnosis-related groups (DRGs), 7, 12
Diagnostic algorithms
acidosis, metabolic, 1056
cirrhosis with ascites, 822
polycythemia vera, 950
pulmonary disease with HIV infection, 733
supraventricular tachyarrhythmias, 397
wide-complex tachycardia, 396
Diagnostic testing and Bayesian reasoning, 37–42
Dialysis
heart failure, 363
hospitalized patients, 1017–1026
hypercalcemia in oncologic emergencies, 925
renal failure, acute, 1012–1013, 1014, 1015
renal failure during pregnancy, 276
renal transplantation, 1028, 1032
thyrotoxic storm, 1096
uremic pericarditis, 442, 447, 449
Diaphoresis, 343, 541
Diaphragm, 227, 532, 583
Diaphragmatic paralysis, 519, 520
Diarrhea, 191, 192, 603, 756–759, 799–806,
1057, 1094, 1096
Diastolic murmurs, 309, 310, 385
Diazepam
alcohol withdrawal, 1246
antidepressants, 1213
anxiety, 280

drug overdose, 1230, 1239
HIV infection drug regimen, 722
meningitis, 689
status epilepticus, 1201, 1203
vertigo, 1167
Diazoxide, 468, 1090
Dichloralphenazone, 1164
Diclofenac, 1164
Dicloxacillin, 512, 677
Dicyclomine HCl, 960
Didanosine, 725
Dideoxyinosine, 850
Diet and nutrition. *See also* Enteral nutrition;
Parenteral nutrition
acute myelogenous leukemia, 935
alcoholic hepatitis, 814
appendicitis, acute, 862, 863
assessment of, 100–101
after cardiac arrest and resuscitation, 414, 415
chest pain, 300
cholangitis, 834, 836
cirrhosis, 825, 826, 827
Crohn's disease, 805, 806
diabetes mellitus, 1081, 1082, 1090
dialysis patients, 1018–1019, 1020, 1021, 1024,
1025
diarrhea in gastrointestinal disease, 758, 759
discharge instructions for heart failure, 370
diverticulitis, 865, 866, 867
elderly patients, 112, 113
end-of-life care, 141
esophageal disorders, 785–786
food allergies, 1225
food poisoning, 684, 756
gastrointestinal disorders, 752
gastrointestinal disorders, 772, 802, 804
hospitalized patients, 99–109
hypokalemia, 1051
malnutrition, 99–100, 103–108, 112, 113,
1019–1020, 1021, 1094
mechanical ventilation, patients on, 179
nitrogen balance, 102–103
pancreatitis, 853, 854, 855, 857
renal disease, 1003, 1004, 1013, 1015, 1042, 1043
seizures, 1206
starvation, 99–100
trauma patients, 292
veno-occlusive disease of the liver, 960
Differential diagnosis
abdominal aortic aneurysm, 482
abdominal masses in gastrointestinal disease,
761–762
acquired atrioventricular block, 433
acute myelogenous leukemia, 930–932, 933
adrenal insufficiency, 1104
alcohol withdrawal, 1245–1246
alkalosis, metabolic, 1058–1060
altered mental status in HIV infected patients,
745–746
anaphylaxis, 1222–1223
antineutrophil cytoplasmic antibodies, 1118,
1119
antinuclear antibodies, 1117
aortic intramural hematoma and dissection,
472–474
aortic regurgitation, 384
aortic stenosis, 381–382
appendicitis, acute, 860–861
arthritis, 1143–1145
asthma, 540–541
back pain, 1154–1157
bacterial meningitis, 684–685, 686
bowel ischemia, acute, 868
bowel obstruction, 874–875
cellulitis, 676
central nervous system vasculitis, 1130–1131
cholangitis, 834
cholecystitis, 831
chronic myeloproliferative diseases, 948–951
chronic obstructive pulmonary disease
(COPD), 532

coagulation disorders associated with bleeding,
988
complement system, 1119
constrictive pericarditis, 450–451
cough, 521, 522
crackles, 518
Crohn's disease, 800, 804
Cushing syndrome, 1071
cyanosis, 520
diverticulitis, 864–865
drug overdose, 1229–1234, 1236–1237, 1239,
1240
dyspnea, 522
endocarditis, 693–695
erythrocyte sedimentation rate, 1116
fever of unknown origin, 604–605
focal CNS lesions in HIV infected patients,
742–743
goiter, 1069–1070, 1071
gout, 1145
hemoptysis, 523–524, 524–525
hepatic disorders, 760–761, 762–764, 812–813,
825
hypercalcemia in oncologic emergencies, 924
hypopituitarism, 1076
interstitial lung diseases (ILDs), 549–556
intracranial hemorrhage, 1193–1194
IV catheter-associated infection, 704–705
joint pain and swelling, 1111–1115
leukocytosis, 894–895
limb ischemia, 487–488, 490–491
lymphadenopathy, 887, 889
lymphoma, 937–939
meningitis in HIV infected patients, 739–741
mitral regurgitation, 387
mitral stenosis, 385–386
myocardial infarction, 343–344
nausea and vomiting in gastrointestinal disease,
754–755
necrotizing fasciitis, 679
neurologic oncologic emergencies, 918
neutropenia, 893
oliguria and anuria, 1000
pacemaker dysfunction, 436, 437
pancreatitis, 849–850
pancytopenia, 895–896
peptic ulcer disease, 790–791
pericardial disorders, 443–444, 921
peripheral arterial disease, 456–457
pleural effusions, 578–580
pneumonia, 634–635, 651
post-liver transplant altered mental status, 845
pulmonary embolism, 505–506
pulmonary hypertension, 570–572
renal disease, 1001, 1038–1040, 1042–1043
rheumatic factor, 1118
seizures, 1200–1201, 1238
sinus node dysfunction, 431–432
splenomegaly, 885–887
stroke, 1177, 1178
subdural hematoma, 1196
superior vena cava syndrome, 922–923
supraventricular tachyarrhythmias, 396–397
syncope, 423–425, 429
tactile fremitus, 520
thoracic aortic aneurysms, 480
thyroid disease, 1069–1070, 1071, 1073,
1074–1075
tricuspid regurgitation, 389
tuberculosis, 656–657, 662–663
ulcerative colitis, 800, 801
urinary tract infection, 668, 671
ventricular arrhythmias, 412–413
wheezing, 518–519
Diffuse aggressive lymphomas, 940
Diffuse alveolar damage, 550, 551, 552, 555,
560
Diffuse alveolar hemorrhage, 525, 550, 551, 552
Diffuse aortic aneurysms, 479
Diffuse metastases pattern of spherical mass
lesions, 590–591

Diffuse metastatic pattern of multiple pulmonary nodules, 592
Diffuse small cell lymphomas, 939–940
Digibind, 1231
DigiFab, 1231
Digits, 211, 213–215, 457, 458, 552, 1136, 1137, 1138, 1139
Digoxin and digitalis
    abdominal pain, causing, 753
    acquired atrioventricular block, 433
    delirium, 1165
    derivatives of, and thrombocytopenia, 977
    diagnostic accuracy of stress electrocardiograms, 318
    drug overdose, 1229, 1231, 1234, 1239
    heart failure, 364, 366
    heart transplant surgery, 375
    hyperkalemia, 1051, 1052
    mitral regurgitation, 388
    multifocal atrial tachycardia (MAT), 403
    myocardial infarction, 352, 356
    pericarditis, 451
    pregnancy, 271
    pulmonary hypertension, 574
    stress testing, 340
    supraventricular tachyarrhythmias, 397, 398, 399, 400, 403, 406
    thyrotoxic storm, 1096
    tuberculosis treatment, interactions with, 659
    Wolff-Parkinson-White syndrome and ventricular fibrillation, 412
Digoxin levels, 433
Dilantin, 889, 1233
Dilaudid, 132, 969
Diltiazem
    acquired atrioventricular block, 433
    angina, 338
    atrial fibrillation, 402
    drug overdose, 1230
    HIV infection drug regimen, 722
    hypertension, emergent, 467, 470
    pulmonary hypertension, 573, 574
    renal failure, acute, 1011
    scleroderma, 1139
    supraventricular tachyarrhythmias, 399, 400, 406
    transplant coronary artery disease, 379
Dimethylsulfoxide, 958
Diphenhydramine
    anaphylaxis, 1223
    Crohn's disease, 805
    dialysis patients, 1018
    drug overdose, 1230, 1240
    drug screen false results, 1234
    hematopoietic cell transplantation, 958
    mucositis after hematopoietic cell transplantation, 960
    nausea and vomiting in gastrointestinal disease, 756
    radiocontrast allergies, 1225
    sickle cell disease, 969
Diphenylhydantoin, 919
Diphtheroids, 390
Dipyridamole, 977, 1181–1182
Dipyridamole testing, 252, 316, 320, 355, 843
Direct antithrombin agents, 350
Direct fluorescent antibody testing, 609
Direct nucleic acid amplification tests, 656
Directly observed therapy (DOT), 658, 662, 664
Disability status, 559, 575
Discharge issues. *See also* Follow-up care
    abdominal aortic aneurysm, 483
    acute myelogenous leukemia, 934–935
    adrenal insufficiency, 1107
    alcohol withdrawal, 1249
    altered mental status in HIV infected patients, 746
    anaphylaxis, 1226
    angina, 340–341
    aortic intramural hematoma and dissection, 476

aortic regurgitation, 385
appendicitis, acute, 863–864
asthma, 545, 546, 547
back pain, 1158–1159
bioterrorism victims, 717
bowel ischemia, acute, 870
bowel obstruction, 878
bradycardia and pacemakers, 439
cardiac arrest and resuscitation, after, 415
case management, 28
cellulitis, 678
chemotherapy, 05–906
chronic limb ischemia, 491–492
chronic obstructive pulmonary disease, 535–537
cirrhosis, 823, 827
communication between hospitalists and patients, 24
Crohn's disease, 806
deep venous thrombosis, 499–500, 502
discharge from hospital, 31–35
diverticulitis, 867
drug overdose, 1236
elderly patients, 116
endocarditis, 699–700
epidural analgesia, 262
ethical issues, 125–126
follow-up telephone calls by pharmacists, 159
gastrointestinal bleeding, 772–773, 778
gout, 1147–1148
health care efficiency, 20–21
heart failure, 370
heart transplantation, 377–378, 378
hepatic encephalopathy, 826
hepatic failure, 814
hepatorenal syndrome, 826–827
hospitalists interfacing with referring physicians, 26
hospitalists interfacing with skilled nursing facilities, 27, 28
hypercalcemia in oncologic emergencies, 926
hypoglycemia, 1090
infection in lymphoma patients, 943–944
interstitial lung disease, 559
intracranial hemorrhage, 1195
IV catheter-associated infection, 709
leaving against medical advice, 125
meningitis, 690–691
mitral regurgitation, 389
mitral stenosis, 387
multiple pulmonary nodules, 592
myocardial infarction, 356–357
myxedema coma, 1101
necrotizing fasciitis, 680
neurologic complications in HIV infected patients, 742, 745, 746
neurologic oncologic emergencies, 920–921
pain management, 136
pancreatitis, 854, 857
peptic ulcer disease, 796
pericardial oncologic emergencies, 922
pericarditis, 450, 451–452
pneumonia, 639, 640, 642–643
polymyositis/dermatomyositis, 1140–1141
postoperative ileus, 265
pulmonary disease with HIV infection, 736
pulmonary embolism, 512–513
pulmonary hypertension, 575
renal stone and obstructive disease, 1042
respiratory failure, acute, 188, 189–190
rheumatic diseases, 1139, 1140, 1142
seizures, 1206
sepsis, 205
septic arthritis, 1151
spontaneous bacterial peritonitis, 825
stroke, 1182
subarachnoid hemorrhage, 1193
superior vena cava syndrome, 924
supraventricular tachyarrhythmias, 403–404, 406
syncope, 429–430
thoracic aortic aneurysms, 481

thyrotoxic storm, 1096–1097
tuberculosis, 662, 664
tumor lysis syndrome, 943
ulcerative colitis, 803
urinary tract infection, 671, 673
vasculitis, 1123, 1129–1130
ventricular arrhythmias and cardiac arrest, 418–420
Disopyramide, 304, 399, 400, 403, 404, 412, 419
Disorientation, 423
Displatin, 958
Dissecting renal artery, 464, 465
Disseminated intravascular coagulation, 225, 502, 690, 933, 976, 990
Distributive shock, 192, 193, 197
Disulfiram, 512, 796
Ditropan, 1213
Diuretics
    acidosis, respiratory, 1062
    alkalosis, metabolic, 1059
    aortic regurgitation, 384
    aortic stenosis, 382
    cardiac arrest and resuscitation, after, 414
    cirrhosis with ascites, 821, 823
    fenoldopam obviating need for, 466
    head trauma, 289
    heart failure, 363, 365, 366, 367, 370
    heart transplant surgery, 375
    hepatic failure, 811
    hypercalcemia in oncologic emergencies, 925
    hyperkalemia, 1051
    hypernatremia, 1049
    hypertension, emergent, 467, 468
    hypokalemia, 1050, 1051
    hyponatremia, 1046, 1048
    hypovolemic shock, 191, 192
    interstitial lung disease, 559
    mitral regurgitation, 388
    mitral stenosis, 386
    myocardial infarction, 352, 355, 356
    oliguria and anuria, 999–1000
    pericarditis, 451, 452
    pregnancy, 272
    preoperative evaluation, 254
    pulmonary edema in dialysis patients, 1021
    pulmonary hypertension, 574, 575
    renal failure, acute, 1010, 1016
    right ventricular (RV) failure, 368
    superior vena cava syndrome, 923
    syncope, 428, 429
    thyrotoxic storm, 1096
    tricuspid regurgitation, 389
    urinary incontinence, 1170
    veno-occlusive disease of the liver, 960
Diuretics, loop
    heart failure, 363
    hepatic failure, 811
    hyperkalemia, 1052
    hyponatremia, 1048
    pancreatitis in dialysis patients, 1023
    pulmonary hypertension, 574
    renal disease, 1002, 1010
Diverticulitis, 864–867
Dizziness, 411, 423, 424, 569, 575, 1166
DL-sotalol, 304, 399, 400, 402, 404, 412, 419, 425
Do not resuscitate (DNR) orders, 123–124, 144, 414
Dobutamine, 195–196, 355, 365, 366, 367, 371
Dobutamine echocardiography, 252, 320, 321, 566, 843
Dobutamine stress testing, 316, 355
Dofetilide, 399, 400, 402, 403, 404, 412
Dolasetron, 246, 756, 905
Dolophine, 132
Domperidone, 1138
Donepezil, 1213
Donor organs, 373, 374, 839
Donor-recipient relationship, 955–956
Donors
    blood, of, 907, 914, 915

renal transplantation, 1027–1028, 1029, 1030, 1032, 1033, 1034
    stem cells for transplantation, 956, 958
Dopamine
    delirium, 282
    drug overdose, 1240
    heart failure, 363, 365, 366, 367
    hepatic failure, 811
    myocardial infarction, 355
    myxedema coma, 1100
    oliguria and anuria, 999
    post heart transplant surgery, 375
    post-liver transplant renal function, 845
    renal failure, acute, 1011, 1016
    shock, 195, 197
    thyroid disease, 1075
    vasospasm with subarachnoid hemorrhage, spontaneous, 1192
Dopamine antagonists, 281, 467, 756
Doppler studies. *See also* Echocardiography
    acute limb ischemia, 487
    Ankle-Brachial Index, 458, 460
    aortic regurgitation, 384
    aortic stenosis, 381
    cardiovascular disease, 322, 324
    constrictive pericarditis, 442
    deep vein thrombosis, 495
    renal failure, acute, 1008
    valvular heart disease, 322, 324, 386, 387
Double-lung transplantation, 561–562, 575
Downey cells, 608
Doxepin, 1212, 1233
Doxorubicin, 322, 899, 900, 901, 902
Doxycycline
    animal bites, 677
    anthrax, 714
    community-acquired pneumonia, 638, 643
    gonococcal arthritis, 1151
    leptospirosis, 604
    plague, 715
    as sclerosing agent, 581, 922
    tetracycline antibiotic, 627
D-penicillamine, 811
Drainage
    empyema, of, 580–581, 651
    joints, of, 1115, 1150
    pericardial effusions, of, 921–922, 945
Dressler's syndrome, 442, 600
Dronabinol, 722, 756
Droperidol, 246, 263–264, 281, 1240
Drotrecogin alfa (activated), 204, 206
Drug abuse, 293, 413, 463, 464, 468, 469, 592, 1229–1241
Drug fever, 598, 599, 600, 608, 615
Drug interactions, 722, 796, 900, 901, 1031, 1213
Drug packet ingestion, 1230, 1231, 1234
Drug reactions, 602, 809, 810, 889, 1215. *See also* Adverse effects
Drug-induced interstitial lung disease, 550, 551–552
Dual endothelin receptor antagonists, 574
Dual-chamber pacemakers, 439
Duke Treadmill Score, 317
Duke University criteria for endocarditis, 695, 696, 697
Duplex imaging, 460, 489, 490, 507, 508
Duragesic transdermal patches, 132
Dysphagia, 480, 781–782, 1167, 1181
Dysphonia, 541
Dyspnea
    angina, 333
    asthma, 540
    cardiovascular disease, 298
    chronic obstructive pulmonary disease, 531
    community-acquired pneumonia, 634, 643
    echocardiography, 323
    exertional, 549, 552, 559, 569
    heart failure, 360, 361
    heart transplantation, 376
    hypertension, emergent, 463
    mitral valve disorders, 385, 387

myocardial infarction, 343
    pacemakers, 439
    pericarditis, 442, 450
    pleural effusions, 577
    pneumothorax, 582
    pregnancy, 272
    primary spontaneous pneumothorax (PSP), 582
    pulmonary embolism, 344, 505
    pulmonary medicine, 522–523
    superior vena cava syndrome, 922
    symptomatic ventricular tachycardia, 411
    thoracentesis, 229
    thoracic aortic aneurysms, 480
Dystonia, 1168

E

Ebstein's anomaly, 307, 389
Echinocandin, 707
Echocardiography. *See also* Doppler studies
    aortic regurgitation, 384, 385
    cardiac arrest and resuscitation, after, 416
    cardiac murmurs, 309, 311
    cardiac structure and function, 316, 321–322, 323, 324
    cardiovascular disease, 320–321
    chest pain, 303, 305, 339
    donor organs, 374
    early conservative strategy for stress testing, 340
    endocarditis, 694–695, 700
    heart failure, 360, 369
    limb ischemia, 488
    mitral valve disease, 385, 387
    myocardial infarction, 355, 357
    palpitations, 304
    pericardial disease, 442, 443, 444, 445, 447, 448, 450, 452, 921, 922
    preoperative evaluation, 254
    prosthetic heart valves, 389
    pulmonary edema in pregnancy, 272
    pulmonary hypertension, 570, 571
    shock, 197
    syncope, 426, 427
    ventricular arrhythmias, 411
Eclampsia, 273, 464, 467, 468, 1204
Economic aspects of care. *See also* Cost considerations
    adverse drug events, 159
    angina, 329, 340, 341
    cardiovascular diagnostic tests, 326, 327
    discharge from hospital, 31
    economies of scale, 14
    ethical issues, 125–126
    evidence-based medicine, 56, 59–61
    heart failure, 371
    hospital admission prior to surgery, 241
    hospital medicine, 6, 11–15
    myocardial infarction, 357
    salary and professional fees, 19–20
    sepsis, 206
    supraventricular tachyarrhythmias, 406
    value assessment and improvement, 79–85
    valvular heart disease, 390
    ventricular arrhythmias and cardiac arrest, 420
Ecstasy, 1230
Edema
    cellulitis, 675, 677, 678
    deep venous thrombosis, 496, 500
    echocardiography, 323
    heart failure, 360, 361
    increased intracranial pressure, 1185, 1186
    lower-extremity, 450
    peripheral, 387, 389, 433, 450, 456
    pulmonary hypertension, 570, 572, 574, 575
    renal disease, 1001–1003
    right ventricular failure, 368
    superior vena cava syndrome, 990
    upper extremities and body, 922
Edinburgh Questionnaire, 456
Education, continuing, 71–77, 81, 84, 144
Effexor, 1212

Efficiency of care, 6, 20–21, 326
Effusive-constrictive pericarditis, 449, 450
Ehlers-Danlos syndrome, 387, 480
Eisenmenger's syndrome, 562, 569, 570
Ejection fraction, 369–370, 383
Elavil, 1212
Elderly patients
    anesthesia, 243–244
    approach to, 111–117
    bacterial meningitis, 683
    cardiac murmurs, 309
    cardiac risk factors, 341
    cerebral blood flow, 465
    cholangitis, 833
    community-acquired pneumonia, 634
    constrictive pericarditis, 451, 452
    delirium, postoperative, 262–263
    fever, 598
    gastrointestinal bleeding, 767
    hypothermia, 607
    lidocaine, 351
    myocardial infarction, 343
    pain management, 135
    patient satisfaction, 96
    preoperative evaluation for cardiac complications, 250
    pseudoclaudication, 457
    relative bradycardia, 608
    stress electrocardiograms, 318
    suicide, 279
    syncope, 424, 425, 426, 428, 429
    thrombolytic therapy, 347
Electrocardiograms
    angina, 333, 335
    cardiac arrest and resuscitation, after, 413, 414
    cardiovascular disease, 311–312
    chest pain, 299, 301, 302
    chronic obstructive pulmonary disease, 532
    dyspnea, 523
    gastrointestinal bleeding, 769
    heart failure, 360
    hypertension, emergent, 464
    limb ischemia, 488
    myocardial infarction, 344, 352
    pacemaker implantation, 438
    palpitations, 305
    pericarditis, 442–443, 443, 444
    postoperative care, 264
    preoperative evaluations, 249
    pulmonary embolism, 505, 508
    pulmonary hypertension, 570, 571
    stress testing for cardiac ischemia, 316–318, 319
    supraventricular tachyarrhythmias, 396–397, 400
    syncope, 425, 426, 427, 428, 429
    thoracic injury, 291
    thrombolytic therapy for myocardial infarction, 348
    ventricular arrhythmias, 410
Electrocardiographic monitoring, 337, 1201
Electrocautery, 439
Electroconvulsive therapy, 1216
Electrocution, 411
Electroencephalography, 423, 425, 426, 1172–1173, 1201, 1202, 1203
Electrolytes
    acute pericarditis, 443
    adrenal insufficiency, 1104
    cardiac arrest and resuscitation, after, 413
    delirium in postoperative care, 263
    diabetic ketoacidosis and hyperosmolar hyperglycemic nonketotic syndrome, 1088, 1089
    dialysis patients, 1024–1025
    encephalopathy after renal transplantation, 1035
    enteral nutrition, 106
    hemoptysis, 524
    hypertension, emergent, 464
    myocardial infarction, 356
    myxedema coma, 1098
    palpitations, 305
    pancreatitis, 856

parenteral nutrition, 107
renal disorders, 1012, 1045–1053
supraventricular tachyarrhythmias, 404
torsade de pointes, 412
ventricular arrhythmias and cardiac arrest, 417
Electromechanical dissociation, 409–410
Electromyography, 1169, 1173
Electron-beam computed tomography (EBCT), 326
Electrophysiologists, cardiac, 352, 400, 404, 418–419
Electrophysiology studies
palpitations, 304, 306
supraventricular arrhythmias, 397, 399, 400, 403
syncope, 426, 427, 429
ventricular arrhythmias, 410, 411, 417, 418
Embolism
bowel ischemia, acute, 869
endocarditis, 694, 696, 698, 699
hemoptysis, 524
intravascular catheterization, 209, 222
peripheral arterial disease, 485, 486, 487–488, 489, 490
stroke, 1177, 1181
Emergency department physicians, 26, 27
Emotional dysfunction, 284
Emotional needs, 29, 142
Empiric therapy
anticonvulsants, 741, 743
endocarditis, 696, 697
H. pylori infections, 792, 793
HIV infection, 723
hospital-acquired pneumonia, 647–648, 649, 650, 652, 653
IV catheter-associated infection, 706–707
pulmonary disease with HIV infection, 734–735
septic arthritis, 1150
Empyema, 580–581, 639, 651, 656
Enalapril, 364, 365
Enalaprilat, 467, 469
Encainide, 304, 722
Encephalitis, 746
Encephalopathy
alcoholic hepatitis, 814
delirium, 1164
hepatic cirrhosis, 823, 825–826
hepatic failure, 809, 811, 812, 814
hyponatremia, 1046, 1047
liver transplantation postoperative concern, 843
renal dialysis patients, 1025
renal transplantation, 1035
spontaneous bacterial peritonitis, 823
Endarteritis, 481
Endocarditis
infectious, 383, 385, 387, 388, 693–700
IV catheter-associated infection, 706, 708
preoperative evaluation, 254, 255
prosthetic heart valves, 390
tricuspid regurgitation, 389
Endocet, 132
Endocrine disorders. *See also specific endocrine disorders*
adrenal insufficiency and crisis, 1103–1108
depression, causing, 1210
diabetes, 1079–1091
renal dialysis, 1024
signs, symptoms, and laboratory abnormalities, 1069–1077
thyroid disease, 1093–1101
Endocrine pattern of spherical mass lesions, 591
Endocrinologists, 1049, 1070, 1101, 1107
Endodan, 132
End-of-life care, 139–144, 917, 926
Endoscopic hemostatic therapy, 768, 770–771, 775–776, 777
Endoscopic retrograde cholangiopancreatography (ERCP)
acute cholangitis, 834, 835, 836, 837
acute cholecystitis, 832, 833
cirrhosis, 820

nausea and vomiting in gastrointestinal disease, 755, 764
pancreatitis, 853, 854, 855, 856, 857
pregnancy, 274
Endoscopy
acute gastrointestinal bleeding, 768, 769–770, 771, 773, 774, 775–776, 777
dysphagia, 782
peptic ulcer disease, 791–792
ulcerative colitis, 801, 802
Endothelin-1 receptor antagonist, 843
Endotracheal intubation
acute respiratory failure, 186, 187, 189
asthma, 541, 542, 544
cough, 522
extubation, 180–182
increased intracranial pressure, 1187–1188
mechanical ventilation, 173, 176
patency and extubation, 180
preoperative evaluation, 256
status epilepticus, 1202
trauma patient assessment, 288
wheezes, 519
Endovascular repair, 482, 483, 1191–1192
End-stage heart failure, 368
End-stage rejection, 1035
End-stage renal disease, 1017–1026
Enema with contrast, 875
Enoxaprin, 338, 350, 511
Enteral nutrition, 103–106, 292, 759, 855, 857, 1013, 1025
Enteric coated medication, 1234
Enteric fever, 604, 757
Enteroclysis, 776, 875
Environmental exposures, 549, 550, 556
Environmental safety, 112, 116, 280
Enzyme-linked immunosorbent assays (ELISA), 495, 496, 507–508
Ephedrine, 300, 1131, 1215, 1225, 1236
Epidermal growth factor, 1011
Epidural analgesia, 133, 262, 268
Epidural anesthesia, 192, 244, 271
Epifibatide, 338, 339
Epileptic seizures, 276, 1199
Epinephrine
anaphylaxis, 1226
angioedema, 1223
drug overdose, 1230
heart failure, 366
hypokalemia, 1050
post heart transplant surgery, 375
shock, 195, 196, 197
wheezes, 519
Epirubicin, 901
Epistaxis, 466, 523, 524
Eplerenone, 351, 364, 469
Epoprostenol, 572, 573, 574, 575
E-aminocaproic acid, 977
Epstein-Barr virus
atypical lymphocytosis, 608–609
focal CNS lesions in HIV infected patients, 743, 744
lung transplantation, 562, 563, 564
lymphoma, risk for, 937
malignancy post heart transplantation, 379
new malignancies after hematopoietic cell transplantation, 963
viral hepatitis, 809–810
viral pericarditis, 449
Eptifibatide, 349
Erb's limb-girdle dystrophy, 434
Ergot alkaloids, 276, 486, 722, 1164
Ergotamine, 1131, 1164
Ertapenem, 670, 671
Erysipelas, 676
Erythrocyte sedimentation rate (ESR), 1116–1117
Erythromycin
cellulitis, 676, 677
community-acquired pneumonia, 638, 643
HIV infection drug regimen, 722
macrolide antibiotics, 626

palpitations, 304
penicillin-nonsusceptible pneumococci, 628, 629
scleroderma, 1138, 1139
torsade de pointes, 412
warfarin, interfering with, 512
Erythropoietin
agnogenic myeloid metaplasia, 952
anemia, 892–893
chemotherapy, 897, 903
dialysis patients, 1020, 1023–1024
heart failure, 370
HIV infected patients, 726
rheumatoid arthritis, 1142
sickle cell disease, 973
Erythropoietin level
anemia, 888, 890, 891
Escherichia coli, 628, 629, 669, 672, 757, 1080
Escitalopram, 1212
Esmolol, 274, 350, 399, 402, 415, 475, 1096, 1240
Esomeprazole, 793, 794, 795
Esophagus
carcinoma, 783
chest pain, 300–301
dilation, 783, 785, 787
dysphagia, 781
gastroenterology, 781–787
intubation, 414
reflux, 344
rupture, 444
spasm, 344, 784
varices, 827
Essential thrombocytopenia, 947, 948, 949, 950, 951, 952
Estrogens, 505, 659, 850, 986, 1024, 1164, 1168
Etanercept, 1140
Ethacrynic acid, 365
Ethambutol, 657, 658, 660, 662, 663, 1227
Ethanol, 1231, 1232, 1236, 1237, 1238, 1239, 1241. *See also* Alcohol use
Ethanolamine oleate, 768
Ethical issues, 119–127, 144, 171, 414, 842
Ethionamide, 661
Ethosuximide, 1204, 1206
Ethyl pyruvate, 1011
Ethylene glycol, 998, 1056–1057, 1058, 1231, 1232, 1234, 1236
Etidronate, 925, 926
Etiology
adrenal insufficiency, 1103–1104
aortic aneurysms, 479, 480
chorea, 1168
delirium, 1165
depression in hospitalized patients, 1210
headache, 1164
hospital-acquired pneumonia, 646
increased cerebrospinal fluid pressure, 1171
mono- and polyarticular arthritis, 1113–1114
stroke, 1177
ventricular arrhythmias and cardiac arrest, 411–412
vertigo, 1166
Etomidate, 244, 1188
Etoposide, 899, 900, 901, 902, 904, 934, 958
Evaluation. *See also* Assessment; Physical examination
abdominal aortic aneurysm, 482
abdominal pain in gastrointestinal disease, 753–754
adrenal insufficiency, 1104
altered mental status in HIV infected patients, 745–746
anaphylaxis, 1222–1223, 1224
angina, 331–334
antineutrophil cytoplasmic antibodies, 1118, 1119
antinuclear antibodies, 1117
aortic intramural hematoma and dissection, 472–474
aortic stenosis, 381–382

aortic valve disorders, 381–382, 384
appendicitis, acute, 860–861
asthma, 540–541, 542
back pain, 1154–1157
bacterial meningitis, 684–685
bowel ischemia, acute, 868
bowel obstruction, 874–875
cardiac arrest and resuscitation, after, 413, 414, 416–417
cellulitis, 676
chronic myeloproliferative diseases, 948–951
chronic obstructive pulmonary disease (COPD), 532
cirrhosis, 819–820
clinical teaching in inpatient setting, 73
community-acquired pneumonia, 634–635
complement system, 1119
constrictive pericarditis, 450–451
cough, 521, 522
crackles, 518
Crohn's disease, 804
Cushing syndrome, 1071–1073
cyanosis, 520
depression in hospitalized patients, 1209–1210
diverticulitis, 864–865
drug overdose, 1229–1234, 1236–1237, 1239, 1240
dysphagia, 781–782
dyspnea, 523
endocarditis, 693–695
erythrocyte sedimentation rate, 1116–1117
focal CNS lesions in HIV infected patients, 742–743
gout, 1143
heart failure, 360
hemoptysis, 524, 525
hepatic failure, 812–813
hepatomegaly, 760–761
hypercalcemia in oncologic emergencies, 924
increased intracranial pressure, 1187
interstitial lung disease, 556–557
intracranial hemorrhage, 1193–1194
IV catheter-associated infection, 704–705
joint pain and swelling, 1112, 1114–1115
limb ischemia, 487–488, 490–491
lung transplantation, 562
meningitis in HIV infected patients, 739–741
mitral regurgitation, 387
mitral stenosis, 385–386
necrotizing fasciitis, 679
neurologic oncologic emergencies, 918
oliguria and anuria, 999–1000
pericarditis, 443–444
pleural effusions, 578–580
pulmonary disease with HIV infection, 730–732, 733
pulmonary embolism, 505–506
pulmonary hypertension, 570–572
renal disease, 1001–1002, 1038–1040
renal transplantation recipient, 1029–1032
rheumatic factor, 1118
seizures, 1203, 1238
stroke, 1177, 1178
subdural hematoma, 1196
supraventricular tachyarrhythmias, 396–397
syncope, 423–425, 425–427, 426, 429
tactile fremitus, 520
thyroid disease, 1070, 1073–1074
trauma patient, 287–288
tricuspid regurgitation, 389
tuberculosis, 656–657, 662–663
ulcerative colitis, 801
urinary tract infection, 668, 671
wheezing, 519
Evaluation algorithms
    acidosis, respiratory, 1060, 1061
    acute myelogenous leukemia, 933
    cirrhosis, 820
    cirrhosis with ascites, 822
    focal CNS lesions in HIV infected patients, 744
    suicide, 1211

Evidence-based medicine, 51–56, 88, 153–154, 169–170, 343
Evidence-Based Medicine: Clinical Evidence, 53
Exclusion criteria for heart transplantation, 373, 374
Exercise electrocardiography, 252
Exercise rehabilitation program, 492
Exercise stress testing, 40, 339, 356, 382, 404
Exercise treadmill testing, 340, 426, 459–460
Exercise-induced hypoxemia, 557
Exocrine glands, 1139
Extension phase of acute renal failure, 1012
Extraarticular signs of arthritis, 1143, 1144, 1145
Extracardiac obstructive shock, 191–192, 193, 197
Extracorporeal membrane oxygenation (ECMO), 168
Extracorporeal shock-wave lithotripsy, 1041, 1043
Extramedullary hematopoiesis, 953
Extrapulmonary tuberculosis, 656, 659
Extrapyramidal side effects, 281, 1215
Extubation, 180–182
Exudative pleural effusions, 577, 578, 579, 580, 581
Eyedrops, 433, 537
Eyes, 1115, 1141

F

Facial fractures, 292
Facilitated angioplasty, 349
Factor V, 275, 459, 809, 811, 977, 982, 983
Factor VII, 988, 1194
Factor VIIa, 910
Factor VIII, 910, 975, 977, 987
Factor IX, 910, 975
Factor XI, 975
Factor XIII, 977
Faget's sign, 607
Falls, 112, 115, 135, 282, 1200
False aortic aneurysms, 479
Familial Mediterranean fever, 442
Families, 28–29, 96–97, 413, 415, 469, 1165–1166
Family histories, 556, 570, 592, 606, 763, 975, 981
Famotidine, 793
Farmer's lung, 550, 555
FAST (focused assessment for sonographic exam in trauma), 288
Fat emboli syndrome, 185
Fatigue
    asthma, 541, 544
    cardiovascular disease, 298
    chronic rejection after heart transplantation, 376
    community-acquired pneumonia, 634, 643
    constrictive pericarditis, 450
    heart failure, 360
    hypokalemia, 1050
    mitral regurgitation, 387
    mitral stenosis, 385
    sinus node dysfunction, 431
Fecal impaction, 759
Fecal leukocytes, 757
Fee-for-service, 12, 84, 97
Felbamate, 1206
Felodipine, 722
Felty's syndrome, 1142
Femoral vein cannulation, 220–221
Fenoldopam mesylate, 264, 466, 467, 468, 470
Fentanyl, 131, 132, 134, 244, 263, 354, 722
Fetal monitoring, 292
Fever
    asthma, 541
    bacterial meningitis, 683
    bowel obstruction, 874
    cholangitis, 833, 834, 836
    diverticulitis, 864, 865, 867
    endocarditis, 693, 694, 696, 698, 699
    HIV infection, 723–724
    immunocompromised hosts, 614, 615, 616–619

infectious disease sign, as, 597–607
liver transplantation, 844–845, 845–846, 847
multiple pulmonary nodules, 592
necrotizing fasciitis, 678, 679
noninfectious causes, 598, 599, 600
non-infectious causes, 615, 618
pacemakers, 439
pericarditis, 442, 443, 445, 447
pneumonia, 634, 643
pregnancy, 276–277
renal transplantation, 1035
seizures with drug overdose, 1239
spontaneous bacterial peritonitis, 823
stroke, 1176, 1181
thyrotoxic storm, 1093, 1094, 1096
transfusion reactions, 913
tuberculosis, 655
unknown origin, 604–607
urinary tract infection, 671
Fibrates, 379
Fibric acids, 353
Fibrin degradation products, tests for, 978
Fibrinogen, 459, 910, 976
Fibrinolysis. *See* Thrombolytic therapy
Fibrinolytic therapy. *See* Thrombolytic therapy
Fibrosing cholestatic hepatitis, 847
Filgrastim, 904, 905
Fine needle aspiration, 889, 1107
Fishbone diagrams for root cause analysis (RCA), 152, 153
Fisher scale, 1190
Fistulae
    arteriovenous, for hemodialysis, 1017, 1018, 1022
    Crohn's disease, 804, 806
    diverticulitis, 864, 865, 867
    enteral nutrition tube, 103
5-aminosalicylic acid, 850
5-HT$_3$ antagonists, 263, 897, 903
Flatus, 873, 875
Flecainide, 304, 399, 400, 403, 404, 419, 722
Flow-volume curves, 526, 532
Fluconazole
    acute myelogenous leukemia, 934
    esophageal disorders, 785
    hematopoietic cell transplantation, 959, 961
    HIV infected patients, 725
    meningitis in HIV infected patients, 740
    neutropenic hosts, 619
    pulmonary disease with HIV infection, 730
    urinary tract infection, 669, 670, 672
    warfarin, interfering with, 512
Flucytosine, 741
Fludarabine, 943
Fludrocortisone, 429, 1105
Fluid intake, oral, 428, 758, 960, 1043
Fluid resuscitation, 193–195, 203, 205, 268, 482, 859
Fluid volume status. *See also* Blood transfusions
    anesthesia, 243
    arrhythmias, 404, 418
    blood components, 909
    bowel obstruction, 874
    cardiac arrest and resuscitation, after, 414
    gastrointestinal disorders, 774, 791
    heart failure, development of, 371
    hydration, 141, 222, 912, 942–943
    increased intracranial pressure, 1188
    interstitial lung disease, 557
    jugular venous pressure, 307
    monoamine oxidase inhibitors, 250
    myocardial infarction, 352, 355, 356, 357
    oliguria and anuria, 999, 1000, 1001
    pancreatitis, 849, 853, 854, 856
    renal failure, acute, 1010, 1012, 1014
    shock, 191, 192, 193, 197
    subarachnoid hemorrhage, spontaneous, 1191, 1192
    supraventricular tachyarrhythmias, 397, 404
    surgery, 245, 246
    syncope, 424
    transplantation patients, 377, 469–470

trauma, 288, 291
urinary tract infection, 671, 672
Flumazenil, 159, 811, 1204, 1230, 1237
Flunisolide, 272
Fluorine-18 deoxyglucose positron emission
    tomography (FDG-PET) scanning, 939
Fluorinef, 1106
Fluoroquinolone antibiotics
    action of, 627
    anaphylaxis, 1224
    cellulitis, 676, 677
    chronic obstructive pulmonary disease, 534
    Crohn's disease, 805
    diarrhea, 603, 759
    meningitis, 687
    plague, 715
    pneumonia, 638, 639, 641, 642, 643, 648, 649
    resistant pathogens, 624, 628, 629
    Salmonella infections, 604
    seizures, 1204
    tuberculosis, 659
    ulcerative colitis, 802
    urinary tract infection, 669, 670, 671, 672, 673
Fluoroscopy, 227
Fluorouracil, 897, 899, 900, 901, 902
Fluoxetine, 1212, 1232
Fluoxymesterone, 952
Flurazepam, 722
Fluticasone, 272
Fluvoxamine, 1232
Focal aortic aneurysms, 479
Focal neurologic abnormalities, 225, 742–745,
    1175, 1200
Fogarty catheters, 524
Folate levels, 895, 896
Folate supplements, 891, 893, 1050
Folic acid, 814, 893, 896, 1129, 1232
Folinic acid, 743
Follicular lymphomas, 940
Follow-up care. *See also* Discharge issues
    alcohol withdrawal, 1249
    angina, 340–341
    asthma, 545, 546
    chemotherapy, 905–906
    chronic obstructive pulmonary disease, 536
    elderly patients, 115
    heart failure, 370, 371
    medical consultation, 236
    pacemakers, 439
    patient satisfaction, surveys regarding, 94
    pericarditis, 452
    pharmacists, by, 159
    prosthetic heart valves, 390
    psychiatric, for heart transplant patients, 379
    renal transplantation, 1032, 1033
    supraventricular tachyarrhythmias, 403–404
    syncope, 430
    thoracic aortic aneurysms, 481
    vasculitis, 1123, 1129–1130
    ventricular arrhythmias and cardiac arrest,
        419–420
Fomepizole, 1058, 1231, 1232
Fondaparinux, 500, 501
Food. *See* Diet and Nutrition
Forced expiratory flow (FEF), 526
Forced expiratory volume (FEV), 525, 526, 540,
    542
Forced vital capacity (FVC), 525–527
Foreign bodies, 519, 540, 570
Formoterol, 534
Foscarnet, 962, 1050, 1204
Fosphenytoin, 1201, 1202
Fournier's gangrene, 679
Fractures, 257, 290, 291, 292, 1157, 1158, 1159
Fragmin, 511
Frank-Starling mechanism, 359
Fraxiparin, 511
Fremitus, tactile, 520
French-American-British Cooperative Group
        (FAB) system of classification of Acute
        Leukemia, 929, 931

Frequency of urination, 667, 668
Functional somatic disorders, 279, 282–283, 284
Funeral homes, 144
Fungal infections, 390, 669, 672, 685
Furosemide
    anaphylaxis, 1224
    cirrhosis with ascites, 821, 822
    heart failure, 363, 365, 366, 367
    hypercalcemia in oncologic emergencies, 925,
        926
    hypertension, emergent, 467
    myxedema coma, 1099
    pancreatitis, 850
    pericarditis, 451
    pulmonary edema in dialysis patients, 1021
    pulmonary hypertension, 574
    renal disease, 1002, 1010
    thrombocytopenia, 977
Fusiform aortic aneurysms, 479

G

Gabapentin, 135, 1204, 1206
Gabexate, 853
Gadolinium-enhanced magnetic resonance
        imaging, 460
Gallbladders, 273–274. *See also* Cholecystitis
Gallium lung scanning, 559
Gallop rhythms, 309, 360, 368
Gallstones, 834, 850, 851, 852, 855, 857, 966.
        See also Cholecystitis
Gamma globulin, 894, 985
Gamma hydroxybutyric acid (GHB), 1231, 1236,
        1241
"Gamma knife," 919
Ganciclovir, 380, 564, 621, 723, 785, 811, 846,
        960, 962
Gangrene, 458, 486, 491, 499, 830, 833
Gastric lavage, 1023
Gastritis, 790
Gastroenterologists, 802, 803, 805, 806, 853
Gastroesophageal reflux disease, 273, 541, 781,
        783, 785–786
Gastrointestinal disorders
    bleeding, 75, 89–90, 428, 767–779, 768–773,
        774–778, 790, 945
    dialysis patients, 1022–1023
    gastropathy, 790
    heart transplantations, 378, 380
    infections in neutropenic hosts, 616
    motility disruption, 752, 753
    myocardial infarction, 344
    nonsteroidal anti-inflammatory drugs
        (NSAIDS), 262
    pregnancy, 273–274
    signs, symptoms, and laboratory abnormalities,
        751–765
    trauma, 292
Gastrointestinal system
    abdominal aortic aneurysm, 481
    antidepressants, 1212, 1214–1215
    bowel ischemia after cardiac arrest and
        resuscitation, 413
    chest pain, 299, 300–301
    enteral nutrition, 103, 106
    losses from causing hyponatremia, 1045
    malnutrition, 100, 112, 113
    myxedema coma, 1098
    postoperative care, 265, 268
    rheumatic diseases, 1138–1139, 1140
    right ventricular (RV) failure, 368
Gatifloxacin
    community-acquired pneumonia, 638, 639, 643
    fluoroquinolone antibiotic, 627
    meningitis, 687, 689
    tuberculosis, 661
    urinary tract infection, 669, 670, 672
Gaucher's disease, 886
G-CSF, 897
Gefitinib, 550
Gemifloxacin, 638

Gender differences, 298, 472, 479, 1114
Genetic
    hemolytic anemias, 888, 890
    hereditary spherocytosis, 892
Genetic counseling, 890, 965
Genetic predisposition
    abdominal aortic aneurysms, 479
    aneurysms with subarachnoid hemorrhage,
        1190
    bleeding disorders, 975, 976, 980–984,
        986–987
    chronic obstructive pulmonary disease, 531
    systemic lupus erythematosus, 1135
Genitourinary system, 383, 387, 389, 390, 1115
Gentamicin
    as aminoglycoside, 625
    cholecystitis, 832
    combination therapy, 624
    endocarditis, 696, 698
    enterococci, 629
    hospital-acquired pneumonia, 648, 649
    liver transplant patients, 621
    meningitis, 688
    plague, 715
    urinary tract infection, 670, 672
    vancomycin-resistant enterococci, 630
Geriatric Depression Scale, 1211
Giant cell arteritis, 1116, 1124–1125
Gilbert's disease, 762, 764
Gitelman syndrome, 1050
Glargine insulin, 1081, 1082
Glasgow Coma Scale, 170, 288, 416, 688, 745,
        1187, 1188, 1194
Glasgow criteria for acute pancreatitis, 852
Glaucoma, 467
Glipizide, 1024, 1090
Glomerular filtration rate, 998, 1000, 1003, 1024
Glomerulonephritis, 1125, 1126, 1127
Glucagon, 1090, 1223, 1227, 1230, 1237
Glucocorticoid replacement therapy
    adrenal insufficiency, 1105, 1106, 1107
    anaphylaxis, 1223
    Cushing syndrome, 1073
    delirium, 1165
    dialysis patients, 1020
    hypokalemia, 1050
    hypothermia, 607
    idiopathic thrombocytopenic purpura, 986
    interstitial pneumonia, 962
    preoperative evaluation, 258
    sepsis with shock, 205
    thyroid disease, 1075, 1096
    tuberculosis treatment, interactions with, 659
Glucose levels
    alcohol intoxication, 1244
    antipsychotic medications, 281
    cerebrospinal fluid, 684, 686
    delirium, 282
    diabetes mellitus, 1024, 1079–1091
    dialysis patients, 1019, 1024
    drug overdose with altered level of
        consciousness, 1236, 1237, 1238
    endocrinology, 1090
    hyponatremia, 1045
    hypothermia, 607
    management of, 1079–1089, 1091
    oliguria and anuria, 999
    pancreatitis, 853, 854, 857
    peripheral artery disease, 459
    postoperative care, 261
    status epilepticus, 1201, 1203
Glucose supplements
    alcohol withdrawal, 1248
    dextrose, 107, 1018
    diabetes mellitus, 1081, 1084, 1090, 1091
    drug overdose, 1231, 1232, 1237
    hyperkalemia, 1052
    hypoglycemia, 1090
    myxedema coma, 1099
    status epilepticus, 1201
    thyrotoxic storm, 1096

Glulisine insulin, 1082
Glutathione, 1011
Glyburide, 1024, 1090
Glycopeptide antibiotics, 626
Glycoprotein IIb/IIIa (GPIIb/IIIa) inhibitors, 338, 339, 345, 346, 347, 349–350, 354, 357, 977
GM-CSF, 897, 961
Goiter, 1069–1071
Gold compounds, 801, 895, 977
GoLytely, 1235
Gonococcal arthritis, 1143, 1149–1150
Goodpasture syndrome, 524
Gorlin equation, 382, 386
Gout, 210, 600, 1112, 1113, 1114, 1143, 1145–1148, 1151
Gouty arthritis, 457
Graft-*versus*-host disease
    blood transfusions, 908, 914, 915
    hematopoietic cell transplantation, 955–956, 958–959, 961, 962–963
    toxic epidermal necrolysis, 1223
Graft-*versus*-tumor reaction, 955, 956–957
Graham Steell murmur, 385
Grain handler's lung, 550
Gram stain
    cerebrospinal fluid, in meningitis, 684, 685, 686, 687
    community-acquired pneumonia, 634–635
    fever and rash, 602
    IV catheter-associated infection, 704
    prosthetic heart valves, 390
    septic arthritis, 1150
    synovial fluid in arthritis, 1145, 1146, 1149, 1150
    urinary tract infection, 668, 670, 672
Granisetron, 263, 756, 897, 905
Granulocyte colony stimulating factor hypokalemia, 1050
Granulocyte colony stimulating factor (G-CSF), 907, 956
Granulocytes, concentrates of, 907, 911
Granulocytopenia, 614, 615–619
Graves' disease, 1070
Greenfield filters, 511
Grey Turner's sign, 849
Griseofulvin, 512
Guaifenesin, 522
Guanethidine, 1213
Guidewire exchange, 215–217, 222, 708
Guillain-Barré syndrome, 523
Gynecomastia, 588, 591

H
Haemophilus influenzae, 534, 683, 687, 690, 691
Haldane effect, 533
Haldol, 263, 282, 304
Hallpike maneuver, 1167
Hallucinations, 280
Hallucinogens, 1166, 1204
Haloperidol, 143, 280–281, 282, 1230, 1237, 1240, 1249
Halothane, 764, 810
Hand hygiene, 614, 619
Hapten, 1226
Harris-Benedict equation, 101–102
Harvard Medical Practice Study, 147, 148
Hashimoto's thyroiditis, 1070
Head injury, 282, 288–290, 292–293, 348
Headaches, 225, 276, 463, 683, 1124, 1163–1164, 1172, 1182, 1190
Health care system and bioterrorism, 711–713, 716, 717
Health Insurance Portability and Accountability Act (HIPAA), 67, 126
Health maintenance organizations (HMOs), 12
Health Plan Employer Data and Information Set (HEDIS), 80, 88
Healthcare power of attorney, 122–123, 124
Healthcare Quality and Research, 153

Hearing, 112, 115, 1167
Heart anatomy, 329, 384, 693, 694
Heart block, complete, 351
Heart failure
    anemia, 312
    angiotensin-converting enzyme inhibitors, 351
    anxiety, 280
    aortic regurgitation, 384
    aortic stenosis, 381, 382, 383
    cardiac catheterization, 339
    cardiovascular medicine, 359–371
    chest radiography, 312
    heart transplantation, 373, 377, 379
    idiopathic pulmonary fibrosis, 553
    myocardial infarction, 343, 351, 352
    pacemakers, 440
    pericarditis, 451
    preoperative evaluations, 254258
    prosthetic heart valves, 389–390
    reversible, 374
    right-sided, 572, 574
    supraventricular tachyarrhythmias, 397
    ventricular arrhythmias and cardiac arrest, 409
Heart rate, 375, 431, 432
Heart sounds
    cardiovascular disease, 308–309
    chest pain, examining patients with, 301
    palpitations, 305
    peripheral artery disease, 458
    physical examination for angina, 333
    pregnancy, 271
    preoperative evaluation, 254
    pulmonary hypertension, 569
    right ventricular (RV) failure, 368
    scleroderma, 1138
Heart transplantation, 307, 368, 370, 373–380, 379
Heart-lung transplantation, 562, 563, 575
Heat, application of for pain, 131
Helical computed tomography, 275
Heliobacter pylori, 789–790, 791, 792–793, 793–794, 937
Heliox, 544
HELLP syndrome, 272, 274
Hematemesis, 768, 774, 776
Hematochezia, 768, 774, 775
Hematocrit, 245, 257, 312, 464
Hematologists, 988, 991
Hematology-oncology
    dialysis patients, 1023–1024
    preoperative evaluation, 257–258
    signs, symptoms, and laboratory abnormalities, 885–896
Hematomas, 224, 471–477, 761, 762
Hematopoietic cell transplantation, 614, 615, 622, 896, 952, 955–963, 972
Hematopoietic growth factor
    acute leukemia, 934, 936
    chemotherapy, 897, 899, 903, 905
    infection in lymphoma patients, 943–944
    peripheral blood stem cells for transplantation, 956, 958, 959
Hematuria, 481, 668, 672, 861, 1037, 1039
Hemiparesis, 1175
Hemodialysis
    alcohol intoxication, 1244
    drug overdose, 1231, 1232, 1233, 1235–1236, 1239, 1241
    hepatorenal syndrome, 826
    hospitalized patients, 1017–1018, 1019, 1020
    seizures, 1204
    tuberculosis treatment, 659
    tumor lysis syndrome, 943
    vancomycin, 626
Hemodynamic augmentation, 1192
Hemodynamic status. *See* Fluid volume status
Hemofiltration, continuous, 607
Hemoglobin A1C level, 459, 1091
Hemoglobin in sickle cell disease, 965
Hemoglobin levels, 245, 257, 312, 910, 1020
Hemoglobinemia, 912

Hemoglobinopathy, 956
Hemoglobinurina, 912
Hemolytic streptococcal gangrene, 675, 676, 678, 679
Hemolysis, 888, 891, 892, 893, 911, 912–913, 965, 966
Hemolytic anemia, 886, 887
Hemolytic uremic syndrome, 273, 276, 379, 757
Hemophilia, 975, 976
Hemophilia A (factor VIII deficiency), 975
Hemophilia B (factor IX deficiency), 975
Hemoptysis, 344, 480, 523–525, 551, 553, 569, 575, 655, 661
Hemorrhage. *See also* Bleeding
    acute limb ischemia, 488
    aortic aneurysms, 479, 480, 481, 482
    hemoptysis, 523–525
    hypovolemic shock, 191, 192
    liver transplantation, 843–844
    pathologic disorders, 975–980, 984–988
    postpartum, 276
    stroke, 1175–1176, 1177
    thrombolytic therapy, 347
    ventricular arrhythmias and cardiac arrest, 411, 417
    viral hemorrhagic fevers, 716
    volume replacement, 911
Hemothorax, 290, 577, 580
Heparin
    angina, 338, 339
    atrial fibrillation, 401
    bleeding disorders, 977, 978, 985, 989, 990
    bowel ischemia, acute, 869
    cardiac arrest and resuscitation, after, 414
    cardiac catheterization, 325
    chronic myeloproliferative diseases, 952
    deep vein thrombosis, 495, 497, 498, 499, 500, 501, 502
    diabetic ketoacidosis and hyperosmolar hyperglycemic nonketotic syndrome, 1089
    dialysis patients, 1025
    hyperkalemia, 1051
    limb ischemia, 488, 489, 491
    lumbar puncture, 1172
    myocardial infarction, 52, 345, 346, 347, 349, 350, 353, 354, 356, 357
    peptic ulcer disease in dialysis patients, 1023
    pneumonia, 639, 640, 649, 650
    postoperative care, 265, 266, 267
    pregnancy, 275
    prosthetic heart valve thrombosis, 390
    pulmonary embolism, 506, 509–510, 511, 512, 513, 523
    regional anesthesia, 244
    renal tubular acidosis, 1058
    shock, 197–198
    stroke, 1179, 1180, 1181, 1182
    superior vena cava syndrome, 923
    supraventricular tachyarrhythmias, 397, 403
    thrombocytopenia, 977
    veno-occlusive disease of the liver, 960
    venous thromboembolism, 179
Heparin-induced thrombocytopenia, 275, 499, 501–502, 509–510, 989
Hepatic disorders. *See also* Liver chemistries; Liver transplantation
    abdominal injury, 291
    Bosentan, 574–575
    deep vein thrombosis, 498
    encephalopathy, 820, 845
    focal lesions, 760, 761
    hemoptysis, 524
    hepatic artery thrombosis, 844
    hepatic venous thrombosis (Budd-Chiari syndrome), 760, 761
    hepatocellular carcinoma, 827
    hepatocellular damage, 763
    hepatojugular reflux, 307
    hepatomegaly, 360, 759–761, 887
    hepatotoxicity, 627, 638, 1230, 1235
    liver disease, chronic, 812

mitral regurgitation, 387
pericarditis, 450
pregnancy, 273, 274
right ventricular (RV) failure, 368
total parenteral nutrition, 108
trauma patients, 293
tricuspid regurgitation, 389
tuberculosis treatment, 659
Hepatic failure, 192, 382, 764, 809–810, 809–816, 812
Hepatic function, 312, 351, 996
Hepatitis, 570, 725, 760, 809–816, 812, 1022
Hepatitis A, 809, 810, 812
Hepatitis A vaccination, 823, 825, 826
Hepatitis B
    cirrhosis, 827
    hepatic failure, 809, 810, 811, 812, 813, 814
    liver transplantation, 847
    transmission precautions, 814, 909, 914
Hepatitis B immune globulin (HBIg), 847
Hepatitis B vaccination, 823, 825, 826, 1022
Hepatitis C, 814, 847, 909, 914
Hepatocyte growth factor, 1011
Hepatologists, 813, 814, 820, 823, 826
Hepatopulmonary syndrome, 842–843
Hepatorenal syndrome, 826–827
Hepatosplenomegaly, 725, 760
Herniation
    bowel obstruction, 879
    brain, 289, 1187, 1189
Heroin, 1232
Herpes virus infections, 563, 613, 846, 934
Hetastarch, 194
Hibernating myocardium, 318, 321, 369
Hibiclens®, 209, 215, 222, 225, 226
High-density lipoprotein (HDL) cholesterol levels, 341
Highly interactive antiretroviral therapy (HAART), 722, 840
Hip joints, 83, 257, 1149
Hirudin, 345, 350
Hirulog, 345, 350
His-Purkinje system, 395, 432, 435
Histamine₂ (H₂) receptor antagonists
    anaphylaxis, 1223
    cardiac arrest and resuscitation, after, 414
    cough, 522
    esophageal disorders, 786
    gastrointestinal bleeding, 771
    hepatic failure, 811
    hospital-acquired pneumonia, 652
    peptic ulcer disease, 793, 795, 796, 1023
    stress ulcers, 179, 293
Histoplasmosis, 603
Histories, patient. *See also* Family histories
    abdominal emergencies, 860
    abdominal pain in gastrointestinal disease, 753
    alcohol withdrawal, 1244–1245, 1246
    anaphylaxis, 1222, 1225
    anemia, 890, 891
    angina, 331–333, 335
    arthritis, 1144, 1145, 1148
    bleeding disorders, 975, 981
    cardiac arrest and resuscitation, after, 413, 414
    chest pain, 297–301
    community-acquired pneumonia, 634
    drug overdose, 1229, 1234
    esophageal disorders, 781
    fever, 598, 602, 606, 608
    gastrointestinal bleeding, 768, 774
    heart failure, 360
    hepatic failure, 812
    hepatomegaly, 760
    hypertension, emergent, 463
    increased intracranial pressure, 1187
    interstitial lung disease, 556
    intracardiac defibrillator shocks, 418
    joint swelling, 1112, 1113, 1114–1115
    liver transplant recipients, evaluation of, 841
    myocardial infarction, 344
    neurologic symptoms, 1163, 1164, 1166, 1170

neutropenic hosts, 615
oliguria and anuria, 999
palpitations, 304–305
peptic ulcer disease, 791
pericarditis, 443
peripheral arterial disease, 455–456, 457
preoperative evaluations, 249
pulmonary disease with HIV infection, 729–730
pulmonary hypertension, 570, 571
relative bradycardia, 607
renal transplantation, 1029
respiratory failure, acute, 184
sepsis, 201–202
syncope, 425, 426
trauma patients, 288, 292
unreliable, 251
urinary tract infection, 671
Hoarseness, 385, 480, 569
Hodgkin's disease, 447, 937, 941, 957
Holosystolic murmurs, 387, 389
Holter monitors, 304, 305, 410, 411, 417, 425, 426
Homocysteine, 330, 341, 459
Horder's spots, 607
Hormone therapy, 920, 925, 926, 1156
Hospice, 143
Hospital Infection Control Practices Advisory Committee (HICPAC), 708
Hospital information systems, 67–68
Hospitalists, 3–4, 6, 17–21, 23–29, 68
Hospitalization, indications for
    abdominal aortic aneurysm, 482
    acquired atrioventricular block, 432, 433, 434, 435
    acute coronary syndromes (ACS), 329, 330
    alcohol withdrawal, 1246
    anaphylaxis, 1222, 1223
    angina, 329, 330, 331–339, 337
    aortic intramural hematoma and dissection, 474–475
    aortic regurgitation, 384
    aortic stenosis, 382
    appendicitis, acute, 861
    ascites with cirrhosis, 821
    asthma, 543–544
    back pain, 1153–1154
    bowel ischemia, acute, 868
    bowel obstruction, 876
    cellulitis, 676
    central nervous system vasculitis, 1131
    chest pain units helping to define need for, 339
    cholangitis, 834
    cholecystitis, 831
    chronic myeloproliferative diseases, 952
    chronic obstructive pulmonary disease, 532–533
    community-acquired pneumonia, 635–637
    Crohn's disease, 804–805
    deep vein thrombosis, 495, 496
    diverticulitis, 865
    drug overdose, 1234
    endocarditis, 695–696
    gastrointestinal bleeding, 769–770, 774–775
    gastrointestinal disease, 757
    gonococcal arthritis, 1150
    gout, 1147
    heart failure, 359, 360
    heart transplantation rejection, 376–377, 378
    hepatic failure, 813
    hospitalists interfacing with emergency department physicians, 26
    hospitalists interfacing with observation units, 27
    hypercalcemia in oncologic emergencies, 924–925
    hypertension, emergent, 465
    hypoglycemia, 1090
    interstitial lung disease, 557
    intracranial hemorrhage, 1194
    IV catheter-associated infection, 705–707
    limb ischemia, 486, 488, 491

meningitis, 685–687
mitral regurgitation, 387–388
mitral stenosis, 386
myocardial infarction, 344
neurologic complications in HIV infected patients, 741, 743, 746
neurologic oncologic emergencies, 918–919
neutropenic hosts, 616
peptic ulcer disease, 791
pericarditis, 444, 451
pleural effusion, 580
pneumothoraces, 583
psychiatric units, to, 284
pulmonary disease with HIV infection, 732, 734
pulmonary embolism, 495
pulmonary hypertension, 572
renal disease, 1002, 1009, 1040–1041
respiratory failure, acute, 185
rheumatic disorders, 1136
sepsis, 203
sickle cell disease, 968
sinus node dysfunction, 432
stroke, 1178–1179
subarachnoid hemorrhage, spontaneous, 1190
subdural hematoma, 1196
supraventricular tachyarrhythmias, 397–398
syncope, 427–428
thoracic aortic aneurysms, 481
tuberculosis, 657, 663
urinary tract infection, 669, 671–672
vasculitis, 1127
Host flora, normal, 624, 625
Howell-Jolly antibodies, 950
HTLV-I-associated T-cell lymphomas, 943
Human immunodeficiency virus (HIV)
    fever of unknown origin, 604
    liver transplant eligibility, 840–841
    lymphadenopathy, 889
    lymphomas, 941
    nephropathy, 726
    neurologic complications, 739–747
    pain management, 135
    pericarditis, 447
    pooled plasma products, 909
    protease inhibitors, 721, 722
    pulmonary hypertension, 570
    pulmonary manifestations, 588, 589, 591, 729–737
    RNA levels, serum, 722
    security in clinical information systems, 67
    signs, symptoms, and laboratory abnormalities, 721–727
    transfer of, in blood transfusions, 914
    tuberculosis, 662–664
Human leukocyte antigens (HLAs), 374, 913, 956, 1029
Human T-cell lymphotropic virus (HLTV), 914, 937
Hunt Hess classification, 1190, 1191
Huntington's disease, 1168
Hydralazine
    acute pericarditis, 442
    anemia, 891
    antinuclear antibodies, 1117
    aortic regurgitation, 384
    drug overdose, 1239
    heart failure, 364, 369
    hypertension, emergent, 467, 468, 469
    intracranial hemorrhage, 1195
    lymphadenopathy, 889
    pregnancy, 273
    subarachnoid hemorrhage, spontaneous, 1191
Hydrocephalus, 1191, 1195
Hydrochloric acid, 1060
Hydrochlorothiazide, 850, 1010
Hydrocodone, 131, 132, 958, 1232
Hydrocortisone
    adrenal insufficiency, 1105, 1106
    Crohn's disease, 805
    enemas for ulcerative colitis, 802

heart transplantations, 379
hypopituitarism, 1076
myxedema coma, 1100
pregnancy, 275
preoperative evaluation, 258
shock, 197
thyrotoxic storm, 1096
ulcerative colitis, 802
Hydrodiuril, 850, 1010
Hydromorphone, 131, 132, 134, 969, 1021
Hydronephrosis of pregnancy, 276
Hydroxychloroquine, 1136, 1139
Hydroxydaunorubicin, 899
Hydroxy-ethyl starch, 194
Hydroxymethylglutaryl coenzyme A (HMG CoA)
    reductase inhibitors, 345, 352–353
Hydroxyurea
    acute myelogenous leukemia, 933
    anemia, 891
    chronic myeloproliferative diseases, 951, 952,
        953
    sickle cell disease, 966, 970, 971, 972, 973
Hydroxyzine, 969
Hyoscyamine, 784
Hyperadrenergic syndromes, 467
Hyperaldosteronism, 469, 1048
Hyperbaric oxygen, 679, 681
Hypercapnia, 533, 557, 1097
Hypercoagulability
    acute limb ischemia, 487, 488
    bowel ischemia, acute, 869
    deep vein thrombosis, 497, 498–499, 500
    hospitalized patients, in, 989–991
    pregnancy, 275
    pulmonary embolism, 505, 510
    thrombotic disorders, 980–981, 982
Hypercortisolism, 591
Hyperemesis gravidarum, 273
Hypereosinophilic syndrome, 947
Hypergammaglobulinemia, 553
Hyperhomocysteinemia, 982, 983–984
Hyperlipidemia, 722
Hyperosmolar hyperglycemic nonketotic
    syndrome, 1086–1089
Hyperparathyroidism, 1020
Hyperproductive, normocytic anemia, 891
Hyperproductive anemia, 892
Hypersensitivity pneumonitis, 185, 187, 550,
    555–556
Hypertension
    abdominal aortic aneurysm, 481
    aortic intramural hematoma and dissection,
        472, 473, 474, 475, 476
    atherosclerotic plaque events, 330
    cardiac risk factors, 340, 341
    chronic aortic regurgitation, 383
    dialysis patients, 1020
    echocardiography, 323
    heart failure, 359, 360, 369
    heart transplantations, 379
    intracranial hemorrhage, 1194–1195
    living donors for renal transplantation, 1027
    peripheral artery disease, 457, 458, 460
    postoperative care, 261, 264
    pregnancy, 272–273
    preoperative evaluation, 254, 256
    renal disease, 1004
    renal transplantation, 1036
    secondary, 469–470
    stroke, 1182
    thoracic aortic aneurysms, 480
    thrombolytic therapy, 347, 348
    urgent and emergent, 463–470
    ventricular arrhythmias and cardiac arrest, 409
Hyperthermia, 1237, 1238
Hypertonic saline IV solutions, 193, 194
Hypertrophic cardiomyopathy, 254, 333, 382,
    412
Hyperuricemia, 941, 942, 943
Hyperuricosuria, 941, 942, 943
Hyperventilation, 306, 1189

Hypnotic drugs, 534, 1099
Hypoaldosteronism, 1057
Hypochondriasis, 283
Hypogammaglobulinemia, 614–615
Hypoglycemic agents, oral, 659, 893, 1046, 1232
Hypopituitarism, 1076–1077
Hypoproductive, macrocytic anemia, 891
Hypoproductive, normocytic anemia, 891
Hypotension
    acquired atrioventricular block, 433
    aortic intramural hematoma and dissection,
        475
    cardiac tamponade, 442
    cholangitis, 833
    constrictive pericarditis, 451
    dialysis patients, 1019, 1021
    drug overdose, 1239–1240
    mechanical ventilation, 179
    myxedema coma, 1100
    oliguria and anuria, 1000
    pericarditis, 443
    postoperative care, 261
    preoperative evaluation for thyroid function,
        258
    pulmonary embolism, 510
    pulmonary hypertension, 572
    shock, due to, 191–198
    spinal cord injuries, 290
    syncope, 423, 429
    tension pneumothorax, 583
    well-tolerated ventricular arrhythmias, 418
Hypothermia, 416, 634, 913, 1097, 1098, 1100,
    1244
Hypotonic IV solutions, 193, 194
Hypoxemia
    alkalosis, respiratory, 1064
    arterial blood gases, 527
    chronic obstructive pulmonary disease, 533
    delirium in postoperative care, 263
    interstitial lung disease, 559
    pulmonary hypertension, 572
    respiratory failure, acute, 184–185, 186
    secondary spontaneous pneumothorax, 582
Hypoxia
    asthma, 544
    drug overdose with altered level of
        consciousness, 1236, 1237, 1238
    dyspnea, 523
    hemoptysis, 524
    pericarditis, 451
    pulmonary embolism, 505, 509
    right ventricular (RV) failure, 368
    supraventricular tachyarrhythmias, 404

I

Iatrogenic complications
    atheroembolism, 487
    edema with renal disease, 1003
    functional somatic disorders, 283
    hypernatremia, 1049
    patient safety, 147
    pneumothorax, 577, 582–583
    sepsis, 206
Ibuprofen, 445, 1232
Ibutilide, 399, 400, 402
Idarubicin, 899, 900, 901, 902, 934
Idiopathic bronchiolitis obliterans with
    organizing pneumonia (BOOP), 550, 551,
    552, 560
Idiopathic thrombocytopenic purpura, 985–986
IFEX/MESNEX, 902
Ifosfamide, 899, 900, 901, 902, 903, 904, 906
Ileus
    abdominal pain in gastrointestinal disease, 752
    appendicitis, acute, 863
    bowel obstruction, 873–881
    causes, 874
    myxedema coma, 1098
    nausea and vomiting in gastrointestinal disease,
        755

pancreatitis, 849
    postoperative, 265, 268, 878, 879
    ulcerative colitis, 802
Imaging studies
    adrenal insufficiency, 1107
    hepatic failure, 813
    interstitial lung disease, 557
    neurologic complications in HIV infected
        patients, 740, 745–746
    pancreatitis, 851–852
    peripheral artery disease, 460
    seizures, 1201
    stroke, 1175, 1177, 1178
    Takayasu's arteritis, 1124
Imatinib mesylate, 957
Imidazoles, 620
Imipenem
    anthrax, 714
    carbapenem antibiotics, 626
    hospital-acquired pneumonia, 648, 649
    meningitis, 689
    neutropenic hosts, 617
    pancreatitis, 855
    resistant pathogens, 629, 630
Imipenem/cilastatin, 670
Imipramine, 134, 1212, 1233
Immobility, 112, 115, 188, 291, 505
Immune reconstitution syndrome, 722, 725, 742
Immune response, 103, 114, 599
Immunocompromised hosts
    appendicitis, acute, 861
    cellulitis, 676, 677
    community-acquired pneumonia, 634
    diarrhea in gastrointestinal disease, 759
    esophageal disorders, 784–785
    infections in, 613–622
    IV catheter-associated infection, 707
    meningitis, 683, 685, 686
    nausea and vomiting in gastrointestinal disease,
        755
    tuberculosis, 655
Immunoglobulin, 377, 686, 893, 910, 1122, 1225
Immunoglobulin A (IgA), 908, 913
Immunoglobulin G (IgG), 610, 679, 910, 912
Immunoglobulin M (IgM), 610
Immunologists, 1226
Immunosuppression, 567, 803, 914, 937, 956,
    1035
Immunosuppressive agents
    anemia, 892, 893
    gout, 1147
    heart transplantation, 376, 378, 379–380
    hematopoietic cell transplantation, 962–963
    hypertension, emergent, 469–470
    interstitial lung disease, 558
    liver transplantation, 839
    lung transplantation, 562, 563, 564
    neutropenia, 894
    pericarditis, 450
    pregnancy, 276
    pulmonary hypertension, 572
    relative bradycardia, 608
    renal transplantation, 1031
    rheumatic diseases, 1115, 1116, 1138, 1139,
        1141
    spherical mass lesions, 589
    vasculitis, 1124, 1125, 1129
Impedance plethysmography (IPG), 495
Implantable cardiac defibrillators, 351, 352, 355,
    368, 410, 414, 417, 418–419, 420
Imuran, 1031
In situ arterial thrombosis, 486, 487, 488, 490
Indinavir, 997, 998, 1042
Indirect factor Xa inhibitor, 500
Indomethacin, 449, 977, 1147, 1164
Induction chemotherapy, 898
Infection. *See also* Sepsis
    abdominal pain, causing, 753
    acute myelogenous leukemia, 932–933
    anemia, 888, 891, 892
    aortic stenosis, 382

arthritis, 1143, 1144, 1145, 1148–1151
asthma, 539
back pain, 1154, 1155, 1156
bioterrorism, 711–717
cellulitis and necrotizing fasciitis, 675–681
central nervous system vasculitis, 1130
cholangitis, 829, 835, 836, 837
consolidation on chest radiograph, 528
depression, 1210
diabetes mellitus, 1024, 1080, 1085
dialysis patients, 1021–1022, 1024
donor organs, 374
elderly patients, 112, 114
endocarditis, 383, 385, 387, 388, 693–700
esophageal disorders, 784–785
fever of unknown origin, 606
Granulocyte transfusions, 911
heart transplantations, 378, 379
hematopoietic cell transplantation, 959, 961–962
human immunodeficiency virus, 721–727, 729–737, 739–747
immunocompromised hosts, 613–622
intravenous catheters, 207, 216, 703–709
leukocytosis, 895
limb ischemia, 488, 489, 490, 491
limb viability, 458
liver transplantation, 844–845, 845–846, 847
lung transplantation, 563–564
lymphadenopathy, 887, 889
lymphomas, 943–944
meningitis, 683–691
Munchausen's syndrome, 283
myxedema coma, 1099
neutropenia, 893
nosocomial, 206
pacemakers, 439
pancreatitis, 856
pericarditis, 442, 445, 447, 449
peripheral artery disease, 460
pneumonia, 633–644, 645–653
polymicrobial, 624
pregnancy, 274, 276–277
procedures, performing, 207, 210, 215, 216, 223, 225, 1143
prosthetic heart valves, 390
pulmonary, 588–590, 591, 592
renal stone and obstructive disease, 1038, 1041
renal transplantation, 1033, 1035
resistant pathogens and antibiotics, 623–631
rheumatic conditions, 1112, 1113, 1114, 1115, 1116, 1118
sepsis, 201
signs, symptoms, and laboratory abnormalities, 597–610
splenomegaly, 886, 887
Stevens-Johnson syndrome, 1223
supraventricular tachyarrhythmias in inpatients, 404
systemic lupus erythematosus (SLE), 1135, 1137
thyrotoxic storm, 1094, 1095, 1096
transfer of, in blood transfusions, 914–915
trauma patients, 292
tuberculosis, 655–664
urinary tract infection, 667–674
Infection control. *See* Isolation precautions
Infectious disease consultants, 610, 639, 689, 697, 741, 744
Infectious Disease Society of America, 638
Infectious Disease Society of America (IDSA), 616
Infectious mononucleosis, 608, 609, 937
Inferior vena cava (IVC) filters
deep vein thrombosis, 499, 501, 502
emboli after renal transplantation, 1035
hypercoagulability, 990
pulmonary embolism, 509, 511, 512
pulmonary hypertension, 572
spinal cord injuries, 292
Inflammation, 201, 293, 330, 331, 343, 613, 1145
Inflammatory bowel disease, 274, 799–806, 880
Inflammatory diarrhea, 757

Infliximab, 805, 1140
Influenza, 112, 114, 599
Influenza vaccinations, 83, 535, 537, 559, 615, 650, 683
Information technology, 63–68, 90, 157
Informed consent, 119, 120–121, 127, 283–284
Inhalation injury, 550, 555
Injuries, 287–293, 427, 429, 430, 1201, 1213, 1214
Inotropic agents, 316, 355, 363, 365, 371, 375, 388, 414
Institute of Medicine, 147–148, 149
Insulin
acute pancreatitis, 853, 854, 857
diabetes in dialysis patients, 1024
diabetes mellitus, 1080–1091
drug overdose, 1230, 1232
hepatic failure, 813
hyperkalemia, 1052
potassium disorders, 1049, 1050
Insulin, intravenous, 1080–1081, 1084–1086, 1087, 1088, 1089
Insulin, subcutaneous, 1081–1084, 1088, 1089
Insulin-like growth factor-1, 1011
Intensive care units
patients in, 163–172
roles of hospitalists, 7, 8
Intensive care units, admission to
anaphylaxis, 1223, 1224
aortic intramural hematoma and dissection, 475
aortic regurgitation, 384
aortic stenosis, 382
appendicitis, acute, 861
asthma, 544–545
back pain, 1157
bowel ischemia, acute, 868
bowel obstruction, 876
cellulitis, 676
central nervous system vasculitis, 1131
cholangitis, 834
cholecystitis, 831
chronic obstructive pulmonary disease (COPD), 533
Crohn's disease, 805
diverticulitis, 865
drug overdose, 1234–1235
dyspnea, 523
gastrointestinal bleeding, 770, 775
gout, 1147
heart failure, 359, 360
heart transplantation rejection, 376
hemoptysis, 524
hepatic failure, 813
increased intracranial pressure, 1188
interstitial lung disease, 557–557
intracranial hemorrhage, 1194
limb ischemia, 488, 491
meningitis, 685
mitral regurgitation, 388
mitral stenosis, 386
myxedema coma, 1098
neurologic complications in HIV infected patients, 741, 743, 746
pancreatitis, 852–853
pericarditis, 444–445, 451
pleural effusion, 580
pneumonia, 637–638, 647
pulmonary disease with HIV infection, 732
pulmonary embolism, 509
pulmonary hypertension, 572
renal disease, 1009, 1041
respiratory failure, 185
sepsis, 203, 205
sickle cell disease, 968–969, 972
stroke, 1179
subarachnoid hemorrhage, spontaneous, 1190
subdural hematoma, 1196–1197
symptomatic ventricular arrhythmias, 411
syncope, 428
tuberculosis in HIV-infected patients, 663
ulcerative colitis, 801

urinary tract infection, 669, 672
vasculitis, 1127
Intensivists, 7, 8, 27, 164
Intensol, 132
Interferon, 1210
Interferon-α, 951, 953
Interleukin 2, 899
Interleukin 2-receptor blockade, 1031
Intermittent claudication. *See* Claudication
Intermittent positive pressure breathing (IPPB), 256, 265
Internal jugular vein cannulation, 217–218, 221–222
International normalized ratio (INR)
atrial fibrillation, 400
deep vein thrombosis, 496, 498, 499, 500
mitral stenosis, 387
postoperative care, 265
pulmonary embolism, 512
supraventricular tachyarrhythmias, 403–404, 406
International Society for Heart and Lung Transplantation, 562
International Union Against Tuberculosis and Lung Disease, 658
Interstitial lung diseases (ILDs), 549–560
Interstitial pneumonia, acute (Hamman-Rich syndrome), 549, 550, 551
Interstitial pneumonitis, 185
Intraaortic balloon pumps, 167, 197, 339, 352, 355, 367, 370, 374, 388
Intracardiac shunts, 325
Intracranial bleeding, 282, 428, 1175–1176, 1179, 1180, 1181, 1193–1195
Intracranial neoplasm, 348
Intracranial pressure, increased, 685, 689, 741, 743, 746, 1164, 1185–1198
Intracranial pressure monitoring, 289, 689, 743, 1188, 1194, 1195
Intrahepatic cholestasis of pregnancy (ICP), 274
Intranodal calcification in a benign pattern solitary pulmonary nodules, 589
Intrapleural instillation of fibrinolytic agents, 580, 581, 922
Intrapulmonary lesions, 587–593
Intrathecal administration of medication, 133, 920, 935
Intravascular devices, totally implanted (ports), 704
Intravascular ultrasound, 325
Intravenous catheters, 502, 599, 613, 703–709, 1022. *See also* Central venous catheters
Intravenous fluids
bowel ischemia, acute, 868
bowel obstruction, 874, 875, 877, 878, 879
Crohn's disease, 805
diabetic ketoacidosis and hyperosmolar hyperglycemic nonketotic syndrome, 1088
drug overdose, 1240
gastrointestinal bleeding, 769, 774
hepatic failure, 811
hypercalcemia in oncologic emergencies, 925
hypokalemia, 1050–1051
hyponatremia, 1047
ischemic colitis, 869
pancreatitis, 853, 854
paracentesis, 226, 822
renal failure, acute, 1010, 1012
shock, resuscitation with, 193–195
tumor lysis syndrome, 942, 943
ulcerative colitis, 802
urinary tract infection, upper, 670, 673
Intron, 902
Involuntary commitment, 284
Iodide, 274
Iodinated radiographic contrast dyes, 1095
Iodine, 1024
cutaneous, 209, 222, 226, 231
Iodine therapy, 1070, 1093, 1095, 1096, 1097
Iodixanol, 1012
Ipodate, 1075, 1095, 1096
Ipratropium bromide, 533, 534, 535, 543

Irinotecan, 899
Iron chelation therapy, 973
Iron deficiency anemia, 888, 890, 892
Iron storage disease, 973
Iron supplements, 661, 753, 1020, 1023, 1234, 1235, 1239
Irradiation of blood products, 908, 914, 934, 935
Irreversible acute renal failure, 1007, 1008
Ischemia. *See also* Myocardial ischemia
  acute tubular necrosis, 1015
  arrhythmias following acute myocardial infarction, 356
  bowel, 600, 867–870
  cardiovascular, tests for, 316
  cerebral blood flow, 1186
  digits, 1136, 1137, 1138, 1139
  irreversible, in peripheral artery disease, 458
  limbs, 457, 481, 485–492
  mucosal, 752
  preoperative testing, 251–252
  splanchnic, 830
  stroke, 1176–1177, 1179–1181
  trauma to extremities, 292
Ischemic penumbra, 1176
Isolation precautions
  bioterrorism incidents, 717
  hepatitis, 814, 1022
  hospital-acquired pneumonia, 649, 650
  methicillin- and vancomycin-resistant *Staphylococcus aureus*, 630, 631
  plague, 715
  pulmonary disease with HIV infection, 732, 734
  smallpox, 715
  tuberculosis, 657
  viral hemorrhagic fevers, 716
Isometheptene, 1164
Isoniazid
  coagulation factors, 977
  drug overdose, 1234, 1238, 1239, 1241
  hepatic failure, 810
  HIV infected patients, 725
  meningitis syndrome, 686
  pericarditis, 442
  renal transplantation, 1031
  seizures, 1204
  tuberculosis, 657, 658, 659, 660, 662, 663
  warfarin, interfering with, 512
Isophane insulin, 1084
Isopropyl alcohol, 207, 210, 217, 223, 225, 227, 1236
Isoproterenol, 375, 417, 427, 433, 1230
Isosorbide dinitrate, 364, 1164
Itraconazole, 512, 564, 592, 730, 796

J

Janeway lesions, 202, 693, 694
Jarisch-Herxheimer reaction, 604
Jaundice, 763–764, 764–765, 809, 810, 812, 814, 833, 834, 846, 847
Jod-Basedow disease, 1070
Johns Hopkins Department of Medicine, 94, 96
Joint Commission on Accreditation of Healthcare Organizations (JCAHO), 80, 81, 82, 83, 152, 165
Joints, 676, 1111–1112, 1143, 1144
Judkins technique, 325
Jugular venous pressure
  acute pericarditis, 441, 443, 444
  cardiac tamponade, 442
  cardiogenic shock, 191
  cardiovascular disease, 301, 306–307
  heart failure, 360
  preoperative evaluation, 254
  right ventricular (RV) failure, 368
Jugular venous pulse, 305, 569
Juvenile myelomonocytic leukemia, 947

K

Kanamycin, 625, 661
Kaposi's sarcoma, 528, 591, 724

Kawasaki syndrome, 1122
Kearns-Sayre syndrome, 434
Keith-Wagner III/IV changes, 468
Keratoconjunctivitis, 1141
Kerley B lines, 528
Kernig's sign, 683
Ketamine, 244
Ketoacidosis, 1024, 1056
Ketoconazole, 304, 512, 659, 722, 796, 920, 1073, 1104, 1107
Ketones, 996
Ketorolac, 131, 445, 1012, 1041, 1232
Kidneys, 205, 1003, 1027
Killip Classifications, 344, 345, 346
Klebsiella infections, 528, 628, 629
Kleihauer-Betke test, 292
Knee replacement, 83
Kussmaul's sign, 307, 368, 441, 450, 921

L

Labetalol, 264, 273, 400, 467, 468, 469, 470, 1180, 1191, 1195
Laboratory tests. *See also* specific tests
  adrenal insufficiency, 1104–1106, 1107
  alcohol withdrawal, 1246
  angina, 333, 335–337
  bleeding disorders, 976, 978–980, 981, 982, 989
  cardiac arrest and resuscitation, after, 413, 414
  cardiovascular disease, 312
  chest pain, 299
  cirrhosis, 820
  Cushing syndrome, 1071–1072
  dialysis patients, 1020
  discharge from hospital, 32
  drug overdose, 1234
  dyspnea, 523
  H. pylori, 792–793
  heart failure, 360
  hepatic failure, 810, 812, 813, 814, 815, 816
  hospital-acquired pneumonia, 646, 647, 649, 650
  infections, 608–610
  interstitial lung disease, 556–557
  myocardial infarction, 344
  neurologic signs and symptoms, 1171–1172
  nutritional status, 100–101
  pancreatitis, 850–851, 850–852, 853, 854
  parenteral nutrition, 107, 108
  peripheral artery disease, 459
  polymyositis/dermatomyositis, 1140
  pregnancy, 272, 273, 274, 275
  preoperative evaluation, 257
  pulmonary disease with HIV infection, 730–731
  pulmonary embolism, 506–508
  pulmonary hypertension, 570–572
  quality of in diagnostic testing, 41–42, 609–610
  renal failure, acute, 1008–1009
  respiratory failure, acute, 184–185
  rheumatic diseases, 1116–1119, 1135–1136, 1139
  roll-plate semiquantitative catheter culture technique, 705
  sepsis, 202, 203, 204, 205
  specimen collection, 224, 609, 656, 663, 734, 737
  stroke, 1177–1178
  thyroid disease, 1070, 1073, 1074, 1075
Lactate dehydrogenase (LDH), 336, 730
Lactic acidosis, 250, 413
Lactose intolerance, 759
Lactulose, 753, 811, 814, 825, 826, 827, 1048
Lacunar infarction, 1176
Lamivudine, 811, 813, 827, 847
Lamotrigine, 1204, 1205, 1206
Language dysfunction, 1175. *See also* Speech therapy
Lansoprazole, 793, 794
Laparoscopic surgery, 265, 833, 862, 880
Laparotomy, 291
Laryngeal edema, 189

Lasix, 467
L-asparaginase, 850, 935, 977
Latex agglutination test, 684, 685
Latex allergy, 1225, 1227
Laxatives, 1051, 1157
L-Carnitine, 1233
L-dopa, 753
Leapfrog Group, 80, 82, 83, 164
Leaving the hospital against medical advice, 125
Left ventricular assist devices (LVADs), 368, 374
Left ventricular ejection fraction, 352, 360, 369–370, 387
Left ventricular filling pressure, 361
Left ventricular function
  angina, prognosis of, 335
  aortic regurgitation, 383, 384, 385
  cardiac arrest and resuscitation, after, 416–417
  cardiac catheterization, 339
  heart failure, 359, 369
  implantable cardioverter defibrillators (ICDs), 368
  myocardial infarction, 352
  pacemakers, 439–440
  preoperative evaluation, 250, 254
  revascularization, 345, 355
  stress echocardiography, 320–321
  valvular heart disease, 389, 390
Left ventricular hypertrophy, 340, 381, 384, 387
Left ventricular thrombus, 350
Leg vascular studies, 506, 507
Legionella infections, 608, 620, 635, 638, 643
Length of stay
  heart failure, 370, 371
Length of stay, economic aspects of, 14, 20–21, 90, 125–126, 406
Lente insulin, 1082, 1089
Leptomeningeal disease, 945–946
Leptospirosis, 603, 604
Leucovorin, 735, 899, 900, 906
Leukapheresis, 933, 956, 958
Leukemia, 447, 449, 615, 894, 895, 929–936, 948
Leukocyte esterase, 996
Leukocytes, 907–908, 913–914
Leukocytosis, 894–895, 948
Leukotriene inhibitors, 272
Leuprolide, 970
Levetiracetam, 1204, 1206
Levine's sign, 331
Levo-Dromoran, 132
Levofloxacin
  hypogammaglobulinemic hosts, 615
  meningitis, 689
  neutropenic hosts, 616
  pneumonia, 638, 643, 648, 649
  S. pneumoniae, 639
  tuberculosis, 661
  urinary tract infection, 669, 670, 672
Levorphanol, 131, 132
Levothyroxine, 1070, 1074, 1076, 1101
Lexapro, 1212
Liddle syndrome, 1060
Lidocaine
  antidepressants, 1213
  arterial puncture and cannulation, 207, 208
  arthrocentesis, 210, 211
  cardiac arrest and resuscitation, after, 414, 415, 416
  drug interactions, 796
  drug overdose, 1236
  HIV infection drug regimen, 722
  intravenous catheters, 217, 218, 219, 221
  intubation with increased intracranial pressure, 1188
  lumbar puncture, 223
  myocardial infarction, 345, 351, 356
  neuropathic pain, 135
  paracentesis, 225, 226
  supraventricular tachyarrhythmias, 400
  thoracentesis, 227
  ventricular arrhythmias, 410, 418
  wide-complex tachycardia, 395

Lidocaine, viscous, 785, 960
Life-sustaining interventions, 122, 124–125
Lightheadedness, 306, 343, 411, 424
Light's criteria for pleural exudate, 578, 579
Likelihood ratios, 38–41, 315, 578–579. *See also* Probabilities
Limbs, ischemia of, 472, 475, 481, 486–491
Lincomycin, 626
Linezolid, 627, 630, 648, 649, 676, 677, 687, 707
Lioresal, 1241
Lipase levels, 850, 851, 854, 935
Lipid levels, 340, 341, 459
Lipid lowering agents, 352, 353, 354, 375. *See also* Statins
Lipoprotein (a) level, 459
Liposomal amphotericin, 619
Lisinopril, 351, 364, 365
Lispro insulin, 1082
Listeria infections, 150, 151, 276
Lithium therapy
    delirium, 1165
    drug overdose, 1229, 1232, 1235, 1236
    leukocytosis, 894
    myxedema coma, 1097
    thyroid disease, 1075, 1095, 1096
Lithotripsy, 439, 1041, 1043
Livedo reticularis, 458, 481, 487
Liver chemistries
    cholangitis, 834, 836
    fever of unknown origin, 606
    gastrointestinal disease, 762–765
    HIV infected patients, 725
    pancreatitis, 850, 851, 854
    pulmonary hypertension, 571
    sarcoidosis, 553
Liver transplantation
    cirrhosis, 821, 822, 823
    drug overdose, 1230
    hepatic failure, 809, 810, 813, 814, 816, 839–848
    hepatorenal syndrome, 826
    prophylaxis for infections, 621
Living donors, 841–842, 846, 955–956
Logiparin, 511
Lomustine, 901, 904
Loperamide, 758, 759
Lorazepam
    alcohol withdrawal, 1248
    anxiety, 280
    delirium, 282
    drug overdose, 1230, 1237, 1239
    end-of-life care, 143–144
    meningitis, 689
    nausea and vomiting, 263, 756
    status epilepticus, 1201, 1202, 1203
Lortab, 132
Losartan, 366
Lovastatin, 512, 722, 1213
Lovenox, 511
Low-molecular-weight heparin
    angina, 338, 339
    chronic limb ischemia, 491
    chronic myeloproliferative diseases, 953
    deep vein thrombosis, 495, 497, 498, 499, 500, 501
    hemorrhagic and thrombotic disorders, 985, 989
    myocardial infarction, 345, 350
    postoperative care, 265
    pregnancy, 275
    pulmonary embolism, 510, 511, 512, 513
    regional anesthesia, 244
    supraventricular tachyarrhythmias, 403, 406
Low-density lipoprotein (LDL) cholesterol levels, 340, 341
Lugol solution, 274, 1095
Lumbar puncture, 222–225, 684, 687, 740, 746, 825, 826, 918, 1171–1172, 1190
Lung cancer, 380, 447, 449, 528, 643
Lung sounds, 184, 301, 360, 361, 518, 569
Lung transplantation, 559, 561–564, 566–567
Lung volume reduction surgery, 565–567, 589
Lupus anticoagulant, 497–498, 500, 977, 981

Lyme disease, 432, 1144–1145, 1146, 1148
Lymphadenopathy
    bubonic plague, 715
    differential diagnosis, 887, 889
    HIV infected patients, 723, 724, 727
    infectious mononucleosis, 608
    lymphoma, 937–938
    splenomegaly, 886
Lymphangioleiomyomatosis, 557
Lymphedema, 491
Lymphoblastic lymphoma, 940–941
Lymphoceles, 1027
Lymphocytic interstitial pneumonia, 552
Lymphocytosis, 608–609, 895
Lymphocytotoxic antibodies, 1029
Lymphoma, 379, 380, 447, 449, 564, 591, 615, 847, 937–946
Lymphomatoid granulomatosis, 592
Lymphoproliferative disorders, 986

M

Macrobid, 669
Macrolide antibiotics
    action of, 626
    asthma, 543
    chronic obstructive pulmonary disease, 534
    community-acquired pneumonia, 638, 639, 640, 643
    cyclosporine and tacrolimus, interaction with, 620
    enterococci, 629
    erysipelas, 677
    palpitations, 304
    renal transplantation, 1031
Magnesium levels, 356, 412, 1018, 1088, 1089
Magnesium sulfate, 273, 276, 416, 544, 1204, 1235
Magnesium supplements, 345, 352, 403, 414, 417, 1240, 1248
Magnetic resonance angiography, 507, 1131
Magnetic resonance imaging (MRI)
    adrenal gland, 469
    aortic aneurysms, 480, 481, 482, 483
    aortic intramural hematoma and dissection, 473, 476
    back pain, 1156, 1157
    cardiac arrest and resuscitation, after, 413, 414
    cardiac murmurs, 311
    cardiovascular disease, 316, 326
    chest pain, 299, 300
    cholangitis, 834
    constrictive pericarditis, 450
    delirium, 282
    focal CNS lesions in HIV infected patients, 743
    hypopituitarism, 1076
    neurologic oncologic emergencies, 918
    pacemakers, 439
    pancreatitis, 852
    peripheral artery disease, 460
    pregnancy, 275, 276
    seizures, new onset, 1203
    ventricular arrhythmias, 410
Malaria, 602, 603, 886, 914
Malignancies
    abdominal masses, 761, 762
    adrenal insufficiency, 1107
    anemia, 890, 891
    back pain, 1154, 1155, 1156
    bowel obstruction, 874, 875, 876, 878
    choledocholithiasis, 830
    cirrhosis, 827
    community-acquired pneumonia, 641, 642
    deep venous thrombosis, 495, 496, 500, 501, 502
    depression, 1210
    esophageal disorders, 781, 782, 783, 785
    goiter, 1069, 1070, 1071
    heart transplantation, 379–380
    hemoptysis, 523, 524
    hepatomegaly, 760, 761
    HIV infected patients, 724

hypercoagulability, 989, 990
idiopathic thrombocytopenic purpura, 985, 986
leukocytosis, 894, 895
lung transplantation, 563, 564
lymphadenopathy, 887, 889
meningitis syndrome, 686
nausea and vomiting in gastrointestinal disease, 755
neutropenic hosts, 615
new, after hematopoietic cell transplantation, 963
pancreatitis, 857
pancytopenia, 896
pericarditis, 443
pleural effusions, 577, 579, 580, 581
polymyositis/dermatomyositis, 1140
pulmonary, 587, 588, 589, 590–591, 592
pulmonary embolism, 505, 512, 513
renal obstructive disease, 1038, 1040, 1041
rheumatic diseases, 1116, 1118, 1140
splenomegaly, 886
tricuspid regurgitation, 389
Malignant hypertension, 379
Malignant hyperthermia, 244
Malignant pericarditis, 447, 449
Mallory's bodies, 814
Mallory-Weiss tears, 768
Mammary soufflé, 271
Management. *See also* Therapy
    antidepressants, 1214
    antineutrophil cytoplasmic antibodies, 1118–1119
    antinuclear antibodies, 1117
    aortic intramural hematoma and dissection, 475–476
    central nervous system vasculitis, 1132
    chronic myeloproliferative diseases, 951–952
    complement system, 1119
    Cushing syndrome, 1073
    diabetic ketoacidosis and hyperosmolar hyperglycemic nonketotic syndrome, 1087–1088
    diagnostic test selection for cardiovascular symptoms, 315
    edema with renal disease, 1002, 1003
    erythrocyte sedimentation rate, 1116–1117
    esophageal disorders, 785–786
    heart failure, 362–366
    hyperkalemia, 1052
    hypopituitarism, 1077
    increased intracranial pressure, 1187–1188, 1188–1189
    joint pain and swelling, 1112, 1115
    pericardial oncologic emergencies, 921–922
    renal failure, acute, 1009–1010
    rheumatic factor, 1118
    sepsis, 203–205
    status epilepticus, 1201–1203
    subarachnoid hemorrhage, spontaneous, 1192–1193
    thyroid disease, 1070, 1071, 1074, 1075
    thyrotoxic storm, 1094–1096
    vasculitis, 1122–1123
    ventricular tachycardias after cardiac arrest and resuscitation, 413–416
Management, initial. *See also* Therapy, initial
    acquired atrioventricular block, 433
    angina, 337–339
    asthma, 541–543
    pancreatitis, 853
    sickle cell disease, 969–970
    sinus node dysfunction, 431–432
    stroke, 1177–1178
Management algorithms
    acute limb ischemia, 489
    atrial fibrillation or flutter, 401
    diverticulitis, 866
    hospital-acquired pneumonia, 646
    meningitis, 686
    myocardial infarction, 346

paroxysmal supraventricular tachycardia (PSVT), 404
peptic ulcer disease, 791
primary spontaneous pneumothorax, 584
secondary spontaneous pneumothorax, 585
solitary pulmonary nodules, 590
Manic depressive disorders, 280
Mannitol, 289, 811, 899, 919, 942, 1010, 1046, 1048, 1089, 1188
Manometry, esophageal, 783, 784
Marfan syndrome, 271, 300, 383, 387, 472, 473, 476, 479, 480, 481
Marijuana, 1204
Mast cell disease, 947
MAST trousers, 291
Mastocytosis, 1222, 1223
McBurney's point, 860
MDMA, 1230
Mean arterial pressures, 465, 466
Mechanical life support, 368, 373. See also Ventilation, mechanical
Mechanoreceptors, 423
Mechlorethamine, 899, 904
Meckel's scar, 776
Meclizine, 1167
Mediastinal lymphadenopathy, 578
Mediastinum, 191, 289, 290, 583
Medical Outcomes Short Form 36 (SF-36) Questionnaire, 456
Medical records, 24, 25, 28, 301, 302, 1018
Medicare, 12, 27, 327, 368, 371, 1015
Medication administration
epidural injection, 1157
inhaler use, 535, 536, 545
intra-arterial, 1147, 1192
intraarterial delivery of thrombolytics, 1179
intrathecal, 133, 920, 935
Medication Error and Reporting Program, 158, 159
Medications. See also specific medications
abdominal pain, causing, 753
acquired atrioventricular block, 433
altered mental status in HIV infected patients, 746
asthma, exacerbations of, 539
chemotherapy, 897–906
compliance, 341
delivery systems, special considerations for, 467, 469
diarrhea, causing, 758–759
directly observed therapy (DOT), 658, 662, 664
elderly patients, sub optimal use by, 112, 116
errors, preventing, 67
heart failure, 360
heart transplantation, prophylaxis for, 376
hepatomegaly, 760
hypertension, emergent, 463, 465–468
interstitial lung disease, inducing, 556
lightheadedness, 306
metabolism of, in dialysis patients, 1025–1026
nausea and vomiting in postoperative care, 263–264
neutropenia, 893–894
oliguria and anuria, 998, 1000, 1001
oral, ability to take, 673
pain management, 131–136
palpitations, 304
patient safety, 157–160
pill-induced damage to esophagus, 782, 784, 785
preoperative evaluation, 253
preoperative evaluations, 250
psychoactive, 263
renal failure, acute, 1012
sinus node dysfunction, 431–432
splenomegaly, 887
suicidal behavior, 280
supraventricular tachyarrhythmias in inpatients, 404
syncope, 424, 425, 428
tuberculosis medications, 660, 661, 663, 664
Medicolegal issues, 90, 125, 141, 144

MEDLINE, 53, 87
Mefenamic acid, 1232
Megace, 1071
Megestrol acetate, 1071
Melphalan, 958
Memory, 419, 431, 1165
Mendelson's syndrome, 599
Meningeal carcinomatosis, 918–921
Meningismus, 683
Meningitis, 683–691, 739–742
Meningitis syndrome, 684–685, 685, 686
Meningococcemia, 600
Meniscus sign, 488, 528
Mental Alternation Test, 745
Mental status, altered. See also Consciousness, level of
aortic stenosis, 382
cholangitis, 833
community-acquired pneumonia, 634
delirium and dementia, 1164–1165
HIV infected patients, 745–746
hypercalcemia in oncologic emergencies, 924, 925, 926
liver transplantation, 845
myxedema coma, 1097, 1098
orientation, 1164
pain medication, 133
thyrotoxic storm, 1094
Meperidine, 131, 132, 722, 853, 969, 1012, 1021, 1041, 1204
Mercaptopurine, 274
Meropenem, 617, 626, 629, 648, 649, 687, 688, 689
Mesalamine, 274
Mesenteric vasculature, 498, 775, 869
Mesna, 897, 899, 900, 902, 906
Metabolic acidosis, 245, 527, 555, 844, 1012, 1024
Metabolic alkalosis, 527, 843
Metabolic disorders, 106, 107–108, 1086–1089, 1168, 1210
Metabolic equivalents required at rest (METS), 317, 318
Metabolic system, 99–100, 379, 403, 1025
Metanephrines, 464
Metaproterenol, 1239
Metered dose inhalers, 533, 537, 543, 546, 559
Metformin, 250, 1024, 1082, 1084, 1229, 1234
Methadone, 131, 132, 659, 1232, 1234
Methamphetamines, 1230
Methanol ingestion, 1056–1057, 1058, 1232, 1234, 1236
Methemoglobinemia, 467, 520, 521, 555
Methicillin, 624
Methicillin-resistant *Staphylococcus aureus* (MRSA)
cellulitis, 676
endocarditis, 696
IV catheter-associated infection, 707
pneumonia, 638, 645, 646, 648, 649
postoperative peritonitis, 265
resistant organism, 629, 630
urinary tract infection, 670, 672
Methimazole, 893, 1095
Methotrexate
acute lymphoblastic leukemia, 935
chemotherapy, 900, 901, 902, 903, 904, 906
hematopoietic cell transplantation, 958, 959
interstitial lung disease, 550
neurologic oncologic emergencies, 920
polymyositis/dermatomyositis, 1140
rheumatic disorders, 1137, 1140
vasculitis, 1124, 1128, 1129, 1130
Methyldopa, 273, 810
Methylene blue, 211, 521
Methylphenidate, 1215
Methylprednisolone
alcoholic hepatitis, 814
anaphylaxis, 1223
asthma, 543, 545
Crohn's disease, 805
gout, 1147
headache, 1164

interstitial lung disease, 558
lung transplantation, 564
polymyositis/dermatomyositis, 1140
pregnancy, 272
pulmonary disease with HIV infection, 735
rheumatic disorders, 1137, 1139
shock, 197
spinal cord injuries, 290
ulcerative colitis, 802
vasculitis, 1122, 1127, 1128
wheezes, 519
Methylxanthines, 543
Methysergide, 442
Metoclopramide, 268, 273, 756, 786, 903, 906, 1138, 1193
Metolazone, 363, 365, 574, 1010
Metoprolol
antidepressants, 1213
aortic intramural hematoma and dissection, 475
atrial fibrillation, 402
cardiac arrest and resuscitation, after, 415
dialysis patients with chest pain, 1021
drug overdose, 1230
heart failure, 364, 365
myocardial infarction, 350, 353, 354
pregnancy, 273
supraventricular tachyarrhythmias, 399, 400
Metronidazole
cholecystitis, 832
Crohn's disease, 805
diarrhea, 603, 759
drug interactions, 796
necrotizing fasciitis, 677, 679
nitroimidazole antibiotic, 626
peptic ulcer disease, 794
pregnancy, 274
ulcerative colitis, 802
warfarin, interfering with, 512
Mexiletine, 135, 400, 419
Meylodysplastic syndrome, 957
Microangiopathic hemolytic anemia, 468
Microangiopathies, 990–991
Microscopic polyangiitis, 1126, 1129
Microscopy, urine, 996–998
Microthrombi, 204
Midazolam, 541, 722, 1188, 1202, 1203, 1213, 1237, 1239
Midodrine, 429, 826
Midrin, 1164
Miliary disease, 528, 655–656
Milrinone, 365, 366, 367, 375, 376
Mineralocorticoids, 1050, 1059, 1060, 1071, 1105
Mini-Mental State Exam, 114
Minocycline, 550, 709
Minoxidil, 442, 1239
Mirtazapine, 1212
Misoprostol, 773, 795, 796
Mithramycin, 925
Mitomycin, 550, 903, 977
Mitotane, 1073
Mitoxantrone, 901, 902
Mitral valve prolapse, 411
Mitral valve regurgitation, 355, 362, 367, 369, 386, 387–389
Mitral valve repair, 388
Mitral valve stenosis, 254, 271, 369, 385–387, 389
Mivacurium, 1188
Mivazerol, 253
Model for End-stage Liver Disease (MELD), 821, 839, 840, 843
Monoamine oxidase inhibitors, 250, 1214, 1215, 1237
Monobactam antibiotics, 626, 933
Monoclonal antibodies, 940, 959, 961
Monoclonal B-cell malignancy, 963
Monoclonal OKT3, 563, 564, 686, 846, 847, 1031, 1035
Monocytic leukemia, 931, 933–934
Mononucleosis, infectious, 608, 609, 937
Monosodium glutamate, 1164

Montelukast, 544
Morbidity and mortality review, 165
Moricizine, 400
Morphine
  acute cholecystitis, 832
  acute pancreatitis, 853
  aortic intramural hematoma and dissection, 475
  cough, 522
  dialysis patients with chest pain, 1021
  drug overdose, 1232
  end-of-life care, 143–144
  heart failure, 366, 367
  pain management, 131, 132, 134
  renal stone and obstructive disease, 1041
  sickle cell disease, 969
Mortality
  acute respiratory distress syndrome (ARDS), 189
  alcoholic hepatitis, 816
  angiotensin-converting enzyme inhibitors, 351, 363
  aortic aneurysms, 479, 480, 481, 482, 483
  aortic intramural hematoma and dissection, 475, 476
  asthma, 541, 544
  bowel ischemia, acute, 867
  cardiac arrest, 409
  cardiac catheterization, 326
  cardiac stents prior to surgery, 253
  cholecystitis, 833
  chronic obstructive pulmonary disease, 531, 533
  constrictive pericarditis, 451
  depression and myocardial infarction, 1211
  diverticulitis with perforation, 865
  endocarditis, 693
  fatty liver of pregnancy, 274
  gastrointestinal bleeding, 767, 771, 772
  glucose levels, 261, 1085–1086
  heart failure with cardiogenic shock, 370
  hemoglobin level in preoperative evaluation, 257
  hepatic failure, 809
  HIV infected persons, 722
  hypernatremia, 1049
  hypokalemia, 1051
  inferior vena cava filters, 511
  intensive care units (ICUs), 163
  IV catheter-associated infection, 703, 707, 709
  lung transplantation, 564
  lung volume reduction surgery, 565, 566
  meningitis, 691
  mitral regurgitation, 388
  myocardial infarction, 343, 345–346, 347, 348, 349–350, 350, 355
  myxedema coma, 1098
  pelvic fractures, 291
  peripheral arterial disease, 485, 486
  pneumonia, 551, 633, 645
  postoperative delirium, 257
  pregnancy, 271, 276
  Pseudomonas aeruginosa, 627
  pulmonary embolism, 505, 511, 513
  renal failure, acute, 1014, 1015
  seizures, 1199
  sepsis, 201, 203, 204
  stress testing, 316, 340
  ST-segment elevation, 344
  suicide, 279
  thoracic injury, 290–291
  troponin levels, 336
  variations in medical care, 87
Mortality Probability Model (MPM), 170
Movement disorders, 1167–1168
Moxalactam, 977
Moxifloxacin, 627, 638, 639, 661, 669, 672, 687, 689
MS Contin, 132
MSIR, 132
Mucolytic agents, 534, 545

Mucomyst, 326
Mucosa-associated lymphoid tissue (MALT) lymphomas, 937, 940
Multicenter Automatic Defibrillator Implantation Trial (MADIT), 418, 420
Multicenter Chest Pain Study, 335
Multidrug-resistant pathogens, 627–628, 629
Multifocal atrial tachycardia (MAT), 393, 394, 396, 403, 405, 532
Multiorgan system failure
  end-of-life care, 140–141
  liver chemistries, abnormal, 765
  necrotizing fasciitis, 675
  oliguria and anuria, 1000
  primary nonfunction of the hepatic allograft, 844
  renal failure, acute, 1014–1015
  sepsis, 203, 204–205
  shock, due to, 191–198
  sickle cell disease, 967, 969
  trauma patients, 293
  urinary tract infection, 671
Multiple myeloma, 957
Multiple pulmonary nodules, 591–592
Multivitamins, 512
Munchausen's syndrome, 283
Murmurs
  aortic regurgitation, 383, 384
  cardiovascular disease, 309–311, 312
  chest pain, examining patients with, 301
  dialysis patients, 1020
  endocarditis, 693, 694
  heart failure, 360
  mechanical complications of acute myocardial infarction, 355
  mitral regurgitation, 387
  mitral stenosis, 385
  palpitations, 305
  prosthetic heart valves, 390
  right ventricular (RV) failure, 368
  tricuspid regurgitation, 389
Muromonad CD3 (OKT3), 686
Murphy's sign, 831
Muscle relaxants, 244–245
Musculoskeletal chest pain, 39, 299, 301
Musculoskeletal system, 244–245, 379, 459, 1140, 1141
Mushrooms, 810, 811, 812, 815, 1239
MUSIT trials, 418
Myalgia, 627, 1050
Myasthenia gravis, 523
Mycobacterium avium complex, 721, 723, 724
Mycobacterium tuberculosis, 449, 655, 656, 657, 663
Mycophenolate mofetil
  gout, 1148
  graft-*versus*-host disease, 961
  heart transplantation, 376, 378
  liver transplantation acute cellular rejection, 846
  lung transplantation, 563, 564
  polymyositis/dermatomyositis, 1140
  pregnancy, 276
  renal transplantation, 1031
  rheumatic disorders, 1137, 1140
  trimethoprim/sulfasoxazole (TMP/SMX) interaction with, 620
Mycoplasma pneumoniae, 539, 543
Mydriatic eye drops, 1166
Myelodysplasia, 931
Myelodysplastic syndrome, 947
Myelofibrosis, 948
Myelography, 1156
Myeloid growth factor, 894, 961
Myeloproliferative disease, 886, 887
Mylanta, 785
Myocardial infarction
  acquired atrioventricular block, 433, 434
  acute, 343–457
  aortic intramural hematoma and dissection, 472, 475

  atypical presentation, 343, 357
  cardiac murmurs, 309
  cardiogenic shock, 191, 192, 193, 197, 370
  deep venous thrombosis, 501
  delirium, 282
  diabetes mellitus, 1079, 1085
  electrocardiograms, 301, 302
  evidence-based medical treatment, 52–56
  fever, 600
  heart failure, 362, 371
  hypertension, emergent, 468
  implantable cardioverter defibrillators (ICDs), 368
  limb ischemia, 488
  pericarditis, 443, 444, 449, 450
  postoperative care, 264
  pregnancy, 271
  preoperative evaluation, 250
  sinus node dysfunction, 432
  supraventricular tachyarrhythmias, 397, 398, 405
  syncope, 424, 429
  ventricular arrhythmias, 409, 410, 412
  ventricular arrhythmias and cardiac arrest, 417
Myocardial injury, 291
Myocardial ischemia
  cardiac arrest and resuscitation, after, 416, 417
  cardiogenic shock, 191, 362
  definition, 329
  determinants of, 330
  dialysis patients, 1020–1021
  gastrointestinal bleeding, 769
  heart failure, 360, 369
  post heart transplant surgery, 375
  postoperative care, 264
  supraventricular tachyarrhythmias, 397, 398
  ventricular arrhythmias, 410, 412
Myocardial ischemic syndromes, 323
Myocardial stunning, 413, 416
Myocarditis, 411
Myocardium, viability of, 318, 321, 333, 335–337, 345, 348, 361, 369
Myoclonic seizures, 1200
Myoclonus, 1168
Myocytes, 329, 336
Myoglobin, 337
Myoglobinuria, 459, 487, 488, 489
Myotonic muscular dystrophy, 434
Mysoline, 1167
Myxedema, 442
Myxedema coma, 1097–1101

N

N-acetylcysteine
  asthma, 545
  cardiac catheterization, 326
  chronic obstructive pulmonary disease (COPD), 534
  contrast-induced nephropathy, preventing, 488, 1012
  drug overdose, 1230, 1234
  hepatic failure, 811, 815, 816
Nadolol, 400, 1021
Nadroparin, 350, 511
Nafcillin
  antistaphylococcal penicillins, 625
  cellulitis, 676, 677
  dialysis patients, 1018
  endocarditis, 696, 698
  IV catheter-associated infection, 707
  meningitis, 687, 688
  septic arthritis, 1150
  warfarin, interfering with, 512
Nalmefene, 1237
Naloxone, 133, 134, 159, 1204, 1232, 1237
Naproxen, 599, 607, 1232
Narcan, 159, 1237
Nasogastric tube decompression, 859, 865, 866, 875, 876, 877, 878, 879
Nasogastric tubes

cardiac arrest and resuscitation, after, 413, 414
feeding tubes for trauma patients, 292
gastrointestinal bleeding, 769, 774
nausea and vomiting, 755
peptic ulcer disease, 791
postoperative, 256, 268
stroke, 1180
ulcerative colitis, 802, 803
Nasotracheal intubation, 178
National Emphysema Treatment Trial (NETT), 565, 566, 567
National Heart, Lung, and Blood Institute, 565
National Library of Medicine (NLM), 53
National Nosocomial Infection Surveillance System (NNIS), 84
National Quality Forum (NQF), 80, 82, 83
National Voluntary Hospital Reporting Initiative (NVHRI), 82, 83
Natriuresis, 466
Natriuretic peptides, 1011
Nausea
    angina, 333
    appendicitis, acute, 860
    chemotherapy, 903–904, 905, 906
    gastrointestinal disease, 754–756
    myocardial infarction, 343
    pancreatitis, 849
    postoperative care, 246, 263–264
    pregnancy, 273
    renal colic, 1037, 1041
    subarachnoid hemorrhage, spontaneous, 1190
    syncope, 423
    urinary tract infection, 671
Nebulizers, 519, 533, 534, 537, 542, 543, 559
Neck injury, 290
Necrosis, 869, 1137, 1139
Necrotizing fasciitis, 487, 675, 676, 678–680, 681
Necrotizing pancreatitis, 849, 856
Nefazodone, 1212, 1232
Neisseria gonorrhoeae, 215, 1148, 1149–1150, 1151
Neoadjuvant chemotherapy, 898
Neomycin, 625, 811, 825, 826, 827
Neoplasms, 857, 1029, 1031, 1032
Neoral, 1031
Neostigmine, 268
Nephramine, 1013
Nephrectomy, 1027
Nephrolithiasis, 861, 1037–1038, 1039, 1040, 1041, 1042, 1043
Nephrologists, 826, 943, 1041, 1048, 1049, 1052
Nephropathy, contrast-induced, 1011–1012
Nephrostomy, 1042
Nephrotoxicity, 326, 379, 625, 1011–1012, 1015, 1025–1026, 1042
    nephrotoxic effects
        medications for
            heart failure, 363
Nerve conduction studies, 1169, 1173
Nesiritide, 365, 366, 1021
Netilmicin, 625
Neumega, 988
Neurally mediated syncope, 423, 427, 428, 429
Neurocardiogenic syncope, 423
Neurofibromatosis, 557
Neurogenic claudication, 457, 1154, 1158
Neuroimaging, 1164, 1170, 1172, 1188
Neuroleptic agents, 143, 280–281, 1168, 1213
Neuroleptic malignant syndrome, 281
Neurologic dysfunction
    aortic intramural hematoma and dissection, 472, 475
    back pain, 1154, 1155, 1156, 1157
    cardiac arrest and resuscitation, after, 416, 419
    central nervous system vasculitis, 1130
    depression, 1210
    dialysis patients, 1025
    distributive shock, 192
    HIV infection, 739–747
    hypertension, emergent, 465
    meningitis, 683, 684, 685, 686, 687–688, 691
    oncologic emergencies, 917–921

regional anesthesia, 244
sodium levels, 1046, 1047, 1048
surgery, 256–257
syncope, 423, 424
Neurologic function
    after cardiac arrest and resuscitation, 413, 414, 416
    elderly patients, 112, 114–115
    signs, symptoms, and diagnostic tests, 1163–1173
    trauma patient assessment, 288
Neurologists, 689, 741, 744
Neuromuscular disorders, 434, 781
Neuropathy
    lightheadedness, 306
    pain management, 133–135
    rheumatoid arthritis, 1141–1142
Neuroprotective agents, 1179
Neurosurgeons
    head trauma, 288, 289
    intracranial hemorrhage, 1194, 1195
    meningitis, 689
    neurologic complications in HIV infected patients, 741, 743–744, 746
    neurologic oncologic emergencies, 918
    stroke, 1178
    subdural hematoma, 1197
Neutron radiation, high-energy, 439
Neutropenia
    acute leukemia, 936
    acute myelogenous leukemia, 932–933, 934
    cellulitis, 678
    chemotherapy, 898, 903, 904–905
    combination therapy for *Pseudomonas aeruginosa*, 628
    differential diagnosis, 893
    fever of unknown origin, 604
    granulocyte transfusions, 911
    hematopoietic cell transplantation, 959
    immunocompromised hosts, 614, 615–619
    lymphomas, 943
    pulmonary disease with HIV infection, 730
    urinary tract infection, 670
Neutrophilia, 860–861, 894
Nevirapine, 725
New York Heart Association, 373
Niacin, 353, 753
Nicardipine, 379, 467, 469, 470, 722, 1191, 1192, 1195
Nicotine, 786, 1137, 1139
Nicotine patches or gum, 356
Nicotinic acid, 810
Nifedipine
    angina, 341
    drug overdose, 1230
    heart failure, 369
    HIV infection drug regimen, 722
    hypertension, emergent, 468
    myocardial infarction, 351
    pregnancy, 273
    pulmonary hypertension, 573, 574
    renal stone and obstructive disease, 1040
    scleroderma, 1139
Nimodipine, 722, 1191, 1192
Nipride. *See* Nitroprusside (sodium nitroprusside)
Nitrates
    angina, 338, 340, 341
    dialysis patients with chest pain, 1021
    drug overdose, 1231, 1239
    esophageal disorders, 783, 784
    gastrointestinal bleeding, 773
    heart failure, 363, 365, 366, 367
    increased intracranial pressure, 1188
    intracranial hemorrhage, 1195
    ischemic stroke, 1180
    methemoglobinemia, 521
    myocardial infarction, 345, 351
    post heart transplant surgery, 375
    right ventricular failure, 368

ventricular arrhythmias and cardiac arrest in inpatients, 417
Nitric oxide, 177, 375, 376, 572, 573
Nitrites in urinalysis, 996
Nitro paste, 525
Nitrofurantoin, 550, 551, 669, 670, 672, 892
Nitrogen dioxide, 555
Nitroglycerin
    angina, 341
    chest pain, 298
    drug overdose, 1230
    headache, 1164
    heart failure, 365, 366
    hypertension, emergent, 467, 468, 469
    myocardial infarction, 353, 354, 355, 356
    postoperative care, 264
    preoperative evaluation, 253
    relief of angina discomfort, 332, 333
    syncope, 427
Nitroimidazole antibiotics, 626
Nitroprusside (sodium nitroprusside)
    aortic intramural hematoma and dissection, 475
    aortic regurgitation, 384
    drug overdose, 1230, 1231
    heart failure, 365, 366
    heart transplantation, 373, 375, 376
    hypertension, emergent, 465–466, 467, 468, 469, 470
    intracranial hemorrhage, 1195
    methemoglobinemia, 521
    myocardial infarction, 355
    postoperative care, 264
    pregnancy, 273
    preoperative evaluation, 256
    pulmonary edema in dialysis patients, 1021
    right ventricular (RV) failure, 368
Nitrous oxide, 244, 1246
Nizatidine, 793
Noncyclic antidepressants, 1232
Nonglycoside inotropic agents, 375
Non-Hodgkin's lymphoma, 379, 937–946, 957
Noninvasive ischemia testing, 251–252, 339
Noninvasive ventilation, 173, 175–176, 187, 190
Non-nucleoside reverse transcriptase inhibitors, 663, 721
Non-ST elevation acute coronary syndrome, 338
Non-ST elevation acute myocardial infarction (NSTEMI), 233, 330, 334, 337, 349–350
Nonsteroidal anti-inflammatory drugs (NSAIDs)
    abdominal pain, causing, 753
    anaphylaxis, 1222, 1224, 1225
    antipyretics, 599
    asthma, exacerbations of, 539
    back pain, 1157
    Crohn's disease, 804, 806
    drug overdose, 1232, 1234
    elderly patients, 135
    esophageal disorders, 785, 786
    gastrointestinal bleeding, 768, 773, 778
    gout, 1147
    headache, 1164
    hepatorenal syndrome, 826
    hyperkalemia, 1051
    hypernatremia, 1049
    interstitial lung disease, 550
    limb ischemia, 491
    meningitis syndrome, 686
    nephrotoxicity, 363, 379
    oliguria and anuria, 998, 1000
    pain management, 131
    pancreatitis, 850
    peptic ulcer disease, 789–790, 791, 793, 794, 795
    pericarditis, 444, 445, 446, 447, 448, 450
    platelet function, 977
    pneumonia, 639
    postoperative care, 261
    renal failure, acute, 1008, 1012, 1015
    renal stone and obstructive disease, 1041, 1042
    renal transplantation, 1035

rheumatic disorders, 1136, 1139
sickle cell disease, 969
ulcerative colitis, 801, 802, 803
Norepinephrine
anaphylaxis, 1223
drug overdose, 1230, 1233, 1240
heart failure, 365, 366
myxedema coma, 1100
renal failure, acute, 1011
shock, 195, 197
Normodyne, 467
Norpramine, 1212
North American Society of Pacing and
Electrophysiology - Heart Rhythm Society,
435
Nortriptyline, 115, 134, 1212, 1233
Nosocomial flora, 613–614
Nosocomial infections
diarrhea, 758–759
discharge from hospital, 31
fever, 599, 600, 604
fluoroquinolone antibiotics, 627
HIV infected patients, 724
pneumonia, 178, 645–653
postoperative peritonitis, 265, 268
sepsis, 206
tuberculosis, 657
urinary tract infections, 667, 673
Novantrone, 902
Novo7®, 988
NPH insulin, 1082, 1084, 1089
Nuclear perfusion imaging, 303, 316, 318, 320,
321, 339, 340, 355, 360
Nucleoside analogs, 934
Numorphone, 132
Nurses
assessments after cardiac arrest and
resuscitation, 414
home care, 690, 806, 864, 870
intensive care units (ICUs), 163, 164, 166, 170
interfacing with hospitalists, patients and
families, 28
patient satisfaction, 93, 94
sudden death, preventing, 351
Nystagmus, 1167
Nystatin, 613, 621, 1141

O

Obesity, 256, 350, 362, 498, 841
Obliterative bronchiolitis, 562, 563, 564
Observation units, 27
Obstructions
airway, 177–178, 521, 525, 540, 541, 557, 1098
biliary disorders, 829
gastrointestinal tract, 873–881
renal, 999, 1027, 1033, 1034, 1037–1043
Obturator sign, 860
Occupational exposures, 549, 550, 556, 606
Occupational therapy, 920, 1158, 1193
Octreotide
bowel obstruction, 879
carcinoid tumors, 1226
chemotherapy, 902
drug overdose, 1232, 1237
gastrointestinal bleeding, 768, 770, 771
hepatorenal syndrome, 826
hypoglycemia, 1090
pancreatitis, 855, 856
scleroderma, 1138
Odynophagia, 784, 803
Ofloxacin, 638, 669, 670, 672, 1151
Ogilvie's syndrome, 752, 753
Olanzapine, 143, 281
Oleander, 1231, 1239
Oligemic shock. See Hypovolemic shock
Oliguria, 487, 998–1001, 1014
Omeprazole, 273, 512, 786, 793, 794
Ommaya reservoir, 920
Oncologists, 920, 1156, 1157
Oncology, emergencies of, 917–926

Ondansetron, 246, 263, 722, 756, 897, 905
"One minute preceptor" model, 74, 75
1-deamino-8-D-arginine vasopressin, 986, 987
One-stage resection of the colon, 867, 870, 876
Ophthalmic conditions and thrombolytic
therapy, 348
Ophthalmic medications, 433, 537
Ophthalmologists, 708, 1141
Opiates and opioids. See also Naloxone
acetaminophen, 816
acidosis, respiratory, 1062
acute myelogenous leukemia, 934
agonists, 133, 134, 135
altered mental status in HIV infected patients,
746
anaphylaxis, 1225
anesthesia, 244
angina, 338
back pain, 1153, 1157
bowel ischemia, acute, 870
chronic limb ischemia, 491
chronic obstructive pulmonary disease, 534
cough, 522
Crohn's disease, 805, 806
delirium, 263, 1165
dialysis patients with chest pain, 1021
diarrhea in gastrointestinal disease, 759
drug overdose, 1230, 1232, 1234, 1236, 1237,
1239, 1241
end-of-life care, 141, 144, 182
gout, 1147
hyponatremia, 1046
increased intracranial pressure, 1188
interstitial lung disease, 550
mucositis after hematopoietic cell
transplantation, 960
myxedema coma, 1097, 1098
nausea and vomiting in postoperative care, 263
opiophobia, 136
pain management in elderly patients, 135
pancreatitis, 853, 854
postoperative care, 261–262
postoperative ileus, 879
postoperative renal failure, 268
pupillary responses, 1166
renal failure, acute, 1012
renal stone and obstructive disease, 1041, 1042
respiratory failure, acute, 189
sickle cell disease, 968, 969, 970, 971
tolerance to medications, 131
ulcerative colitis, 802, 803
urinary incontinence, 1170
urinary tract infection, 670
withdrawal, 135, 753
Opportunistic infections, 722, 723–724, 856–846
Oprelvekin, 897, 903
Optic neuritis, 404
Oragrafin, 1095
Oral contraceptives, 275, 463, 505, 573, 983,
987, 1116, 1164, 1187, 1210
Oramorph SR, 132
Orchiectomy, 920
Orders
admission orders for dialysis, 1018–1019, 1026
computerized physician order entry (CPOE),
64–65, 90, 153, 158
Organ preservation injury, 375, 376
Organ Procurement and Transplantation
Network, 839
Organic brain syndrome, 280, 282
Organophosphates, 1232, 1239, 1241
Ornipressin, 826
Orthoclone, 1031
Orthopedic surgeons, 210, 292, 708, 1147, 1149,
1150
Orthopnea, 360, 387, 522
Orthostasis, 306
Orthostatic hypotension, 423–424, 1212, 1214
Ortner's syndrome, 385
Osler Way Project, 94, 96
Osler's nodes, 202, 693, 694, 696, 1143, 1145

Osmolality in urinalysis, 996
Osteoarthritis, 1113, 1114
Osteogenesis imperfecta, 383
Osteomalacia, 966
Osteomyelitis, 291
Osteoporosis, 562, 966
Otolaryngology consultation, 519
Ototoxicity, 625, 1002
Outpatient treatment
acute leukemia, 936
chronic myeloproliferative diseases, 953
dialysis, 1018
diverticulitis, 865
endocarditis, 695–696
esophageal disorders, 787
gastrointestinal bleeding, 769, 778
lymphoma patients, 946
meningitis, 690–691
neurologic complications in HIV infected
patients, 741
renal failure, acute, 1015
renal stone and obstructive disease, 1043
spontaneous bacterial peritonitis, 824
surgical procedures, 249
Oxacillin, 687, 688, 707, 1018, 1150
Oxazepam, 1230, 1248
Oxazolidinone antibiotics, 627
Oxcarbazepine, 1204, 1206
Oxycodone, 131, 132, 1213
Oxycontin, 1234
Oxygen
acute limb ischemia, 488
angina, 337
asthma, 541, 542
chronic obstructive pulmonary disease, 533
community-acquired pneumonia, 639
cyanosis, 520, 521
drug-induced interstitial lung disease, 552
heart failure, 366, 367
home therapy, 536, 559, 643
interstitial lung disease, 559
myocardial demand and supply, 329, 330, 373,
374
myocardial infarction, 345, 350–352
nausea and vomiting in postoperative care, 263
pneumothoraces, 583
postoperative care, 261
pulmonary hypertension, 572, 573–574, 575
right ventricular failure, 368
trauma patient assessment, 288
Oxygen saturation
anesthesia, during, 245
asthma, 541
chronic obstructive pulmonary disease, 532,
533, 535
community-acquired pneumonia, 634, 636,
637, 639, 640, 643
cough, 521
hemoptysis, 524
pericarditis, 444
postoperative care, 246
pulmonary medicine, 525
respiratory failure, acute, 185, 187
Oxygenation, 245, 246, 288, 519
Oxymorphone, 132

P

Pacemakers
acquired atrioventricular block, 433, 434
bradycardia, 434–438
dual-chamber, 367
fixed rate, 316
heart transplant surgery, 375
malfunctions of, 439
myocardial infarction, 352, 356, 435
preoperative evaluation, 254
sinus node dysfunction, 432
supraventricular tachyarrhythmias, 400, 403, 406
syncope, 429
temporary, 352, 356, 432, 434, 438

temporary transvenous, 417
Paclitaxel, 900, 902, 904, 958
Pain. *See also* Analgesia
  abdominal, 751–754, 755, 823, 833, 834, 859–870, 1035
  abdominal aortic aneurysm, 481
  angina, 331–332
  aortic intramural hematoma and dissection, 472, 473, 475, 476
  appendicitis, acute, 860
  arthritis, 1145
  back, 918, 1153–1159
  bone, in donors of stem cells, 958
  bowel ischemia, acute, 867, 868, 870
  chest, in cardiovascular disease, 297–303
  chest, in dialysis patients, 1020–1021
  chest, in esophageal spasm, 784
  chest, in hypertension, emergent, 463
  chest, with palpitations, 304
  chest, with ventricular arrhythmias, 409, 411
  Crohn's disease, 800, 804, 805, 806
  delirium in postoperative care, 263
  diverticulitis, 864, 867
  exertional, 569
  flank, 1037, 1039, 1042
  hypertension, emergent, 463, 469
  joints, 1111–1112
  limb, 458
  limb ischemia, 457, 485, 486, 487, 488, 490, 491
  management in hospitalized patients, 129–136
  myocardial infarction, 343, 351
  necrotizing fasciitis, 678, 679
  pancreatitis, 849, 853
  patient satisfaction, 96
  pericarditis, 442, 444, 445, 447
  peripheral artery disease, 460
  pleural effusions, 577
  pneumothorax, 582
  postoperative care, 246, 261–262
  pulmonary embolism, 505
  renal colic, 1037, 1038, 1039, 1040, 1041, 1042, 1043
  sensation, 1169
  sickle cell disease, 965–973
  splenomegaly, 886
  thoracentesis, 229
  thoracic aortic aneurysms, 480
  transcutaneous pacing, 438
  urinary tract infection, 667, 668, 670, 671
  vasovagal reaction, 424
  weakness, 1168–1169
Pain service consultation, 806
Paint removers, 1232
Palliative care, 139–144, 827
Pallor, 423, 458, 487, 488, 1104
Palpitations, 229, 271, 303–306, 307–308, 323, 333, 411, 439
Pamelor, 1212
Pamidronate, 925
Panadol, 1230
Pancreatic cancer, 500
Pancreatic duct disruption, 856–857
Pancreaticobiliary disease, 378
Pancreatitis
  acute, 752, 849–858
  acute pericarditis, differentiating from, 444
  biliary disorders, 829
  chest pain, 300
  dialysis patients, 1023
  enteral nutrition, 103
  L-asparaginase, 935
  shock, 191, 192
Pancytopenia, 895–896
Panel-reactive antibody (PRA) test, 374
Panic disorders, 280
Pantoprazole, 793, 795
Papaverine, 869, 1192
Papillary, 1038–1039
Papillary muscles, 355, 370, 387, 388
Papilledema, 464, 466

Para-aminosalicylic acid, 661
Paracentesis, 225–226, 821, 822, 823, 824, 825, 960
Paracetamol, 1230
Paralysis, 179, 458
Paraneoplastic syndrome pattern of solitary pulmonary nodules, 588
Paraplatin, 902
Parasites, transfer of, in blood transfusions, 914–915
Parasympathomimetic agents, 268
Parathormone-related protein (PTH-rp), 924
Paregoric, 759
Parenteral nutrition
  bowel ischemia, acute, 870
  cardiac arrest and resuscitation, after, 414, 415
  diverticulitis, 867
  gallstones, 830
  nutritional status, 106–108
  pancreatitis, 855, 857
  potassium disorders, 1050, 1051
  trauma patients, 292
  ulcerative colitis, 802
Paresthesia, 1169
Parkinsonism, secondary, 281
Parkinson's disease, 306, 1167, 1168
Paroxetine, 429, 1212, 1232
Paroxysmal atrial flutter or fibrillation, 393
Paroxysmal nocturnal dyspnea, 360, 387
Paroxysmal supraventricular tachycardia (PSVT), 393, 394, 395, 399, 403, 404, 406
Partial seizures, 1200, 1203
Partial thromboplastin time, 244
Parvus et tardus, 308
Pastoral care, 29
Pathogens. *See also* Resistant pathogens
  blood products, 908
  community-acquired pneumonia, 634–635, 640, 641–642
  hospital-acquired pneumonia, 645, 646, 647, 648, 649
  opportunistic, 614, 621–622
  urinalysis, 996
Patient Bill of Rights, 93
Patient education
  anaphylaxis, 1226
  angina, 341
  appendicitis, acute, 863
  arthritis, 1151
  asthma, 545, 546, 547
  cardiac arrest and resuscitation, after, 415
  cirrhosis, 827
  community-acquired pneumonia, 640, 641, 643
  diabetes mellitus, 1089, 1091
  discharge from hospital, 32, 33
  gout, 1147
  health literacy, 32, 33
  heart failure, 370
  hepatic encephalopathy, 826
  hypertension, emergent, 469, 470
  hypoglycemia, 1090
  interstitial lung disease, 559
  myocardial infarction, 356
  nephrostomy, 1042
  pancreatitis, 854, 857
  peptic ulcer disease, 796
  seizures, 1206
Patient satisfaction, 31, 34, 35, 93–97, 246
Patient Self-Determination Act, 93, 139
Patient-controlled epidural analgesia (PCEA), 262
Patient-controlled analgesia (PCA), 133, 134, 246, 262, 853
Patients
  autonomy of, 119, 127
  continuity of care by hospitalists, 17–18
  cost-effectiveness analysis, 60–61
  "difficult," 282
  hospitalists, interfacing with, 23–25
  practice guidelines and clinical pathways, implementation of, 89–90
  violent, 283

Patients, hospitalized
  abdominal aortic aneurysm, 483
  abdominal masses in gastrointestinal disease, 762
  abdominal pain in gastrointestinal disease, 751–754
  adrenal insufficiency, 1107–1108
  anaphylaxis, 1225–1226
  atypical lymphocytosis, 609
  bundle branch blocks, new, 312
  chest pain, 303
  chronic obstructive pulmonary disease, 537
  deep venous thrombosis, 500–502
  dialysis, 1017–1026
  diarrhea in gastrointestinal disease, 758–759
  dyspnea, 523
  fever, 599–600, 607
  fever and rash, 602
  gastrointestinal bleeding, 778
  heart failure, 371
  hemoptysis, 524–525
  hemorrhagic and thrombotic disorders, 984–991
  hypertension, emergent, 469–470
  ileus and bowel obstruction, 878–880
  IV catheter-associated infection, 708
  joint swelling, 1115
  liver chemistries, abnormal, 764–765
  myocardial infarction, 357
  nausea and vomiting in gastrointestinal disease, 755–756
  palpitations, 305, 306
  pericarditis, 442, 450
  physical signs in pulmonary medicine, 518, 519, 521
  preoperative evaluations, 249–250
  pulmonary embolism, 512
  relative bradycardia, 608
  renal failure, acute, 1014–1015
  renal stone and obstructive disease, 1042–1043
  respiratory failure, acute, 188–189
  sepsis, 205–206
  supraventricular tachyarrhythmias, 404–406
  thoracic aortic aneurysms, 481
  ventricular arrhythmias and cardiac arrest, 417–418
Paxil, 1212
Payors for health care, 13, 31, 168
Peak expiratory flow (PEF), 540, 542, 545, 546, 657
Pediatric End-stage Liver Disease (PELD), 839, 840
Pediatric patients, 627, 683, 687–688, 690–691, 1204, 1206
Pegfilgrastim, 905, 944
Pelvic fractures, 291
Pelvic vein thrombosis, 275
Pemberton's sign, 1070
Penetrating trauma, 287, 290, 291, 292
Penicillamine, 550, 801
Penicillin
  acute myelogenous leukemia, 933
  anaphylaxis, 1222, 1224, 1225
  anemia, 891, 892
  anthrax, 714
  β-lactam antibiotics, 625
  coagulation factors, 977
  endocarditis, 696, 698
  erysipelas, 677
  Escherichia coli, 629
  hematopoietic cell transplantation, 962
  hypogammaglobulinemic hosts, 615
  interstitial lung disease, 550
  Klebsiella spp., 629
  leptospirosis, 604
  mechanism of resistance to, 624
  meningitis syndrome, 686
  neutropenia, 893
  pregnancy, 276
  Pseudomonas aeruginosa, 628, 629
  Staphylococcus aureus, 629

thrombocytopenia, 977
vancomycin-resistant enterococci, 630
Penicillin, penicillinase-resistant, 676, 677
Penicillin G, 625, 628, 629, 687, 688, 689, 690, 811
Penicillin/β-lactamase inhibitors, 672
Penicillin-nonsusceptible pneumococci, 628, 629, 630
Pentamidine, 304, 412, 621, 726, 735, 736, 850, 1051
Pentazocine, 131, 1213
Pentobarbital, 689, 811, 1202
Pentostatin, 904
Peptic ulcer disease, 344, 348, 789–796, 1023
Pepto Bismol®, 793
Percocet, 132
Percodan®, 132, 793
Percussion in pulmonary medicine, 518, 519–520
Percutaneous cholecystectomy, 833
Percutaneous coronary intervention
  clopidogrel, 349
  GP IIb/IIIa antagonists, 338
  heart failure, 367, 369, 370
  myocardial infarction, 343, 344, 345, 347, 348–349, 350, 354, 357
Percutaneous drainage of abscesses, 879
Percutaneous mitral balloon valvuloplasty, 386, 387
Percutaneous nephrolithotomy, 1041, 1043
Percutaneous transluminal coronary angioplasty, 252, 253, 345, 346, 414, 418, 835–836
Perforations
  appendicitis, acute, 861, 862, 863
  bowel obstruction, 877, 878
  diverticulitis, 864, 865
  gallbladder, 829–830
  hollow viscus, of, 753
  lymphoma patients, 945
  peptic ulcer disease, 791
  ulcerative colitis, 801, 802
Pericardial disease, 322, 323, 360, 369, 441–452
Pericardial effusion, 441, 442, 443–444, 447–449, 921–922, 945
Pericardial sounds, 300, 301, 309, 442, 447, 450
Pericardiectomy, 447
Pericardiocentesis, 442, 443, 444, 445, 446, 447, 448–449, 921
Pericarditis, 191, 192, 300, 344, 441, 442–450, 1021
Pericardium anatomy and physiology, 441
Peridex, 613
Peripheral arterial disease, 455–460, 485–492
Peripheral blood stem cells, 956
Peripheral cyanosis, 520
Peripheral nervous system, 1169
Peripheral pulses, bounding, 384
Peripheral vascular disease, 252, 307–308, 463, 465
Peripherally inserted central catheter (PICC) lines, 106, 704
Peritoneal dialysis, 1013, 1018, 1019, 1020, 1021, 1022, 1032, 1035
Peritoneal lavage, 288
Peritonitis
  abdominal injury, 291
  biliary disorders, 830, 832, 833
  bowel obstruction, 878
  dialysis patients, 1022
  diverticulitis, 864
  mesenteric venous thrombosis, 869
  pancreatitis, 849
  postoperative ileus, 265, 268
Personality disorders, 279, 282, 284
Petechiae, 975–976
Pethidine, 132
P-450 drug interactions, 1216
PH of urine, 996
Pharmacists, 32, 33
Pharmacologic stress tests, 316, 319, 326, 339, 340
Phenazopyradine, 670
Phencyclidine (PCP), 1204, 1234, 1236

Phenobarbital
  alcohol withdrawal, 1246
  chemotherapy, 900
  drug overdose, 1235, 1239
  erythematous eruptions, 1226
  HIV infection drug regimen, 722
  meningitis, 689
  seizures, 1201, 1202, 1206
Phenothiazines
  coagulation factors, 977
  drug overdose, 1239, 1240
  dystonia, 1168
  HIV infected patients, 725
  hyponatremia, 1046
  hypothermia, 607
  neutropenia, 893–894
  palpitations, 304
  pupillary responses, 1166
  torsade de pointes, 412
  tricyclic antidepressants, 1213
Phentermine, 1213
Phentermine-fenfluramine toxicity, 389
Phentolamine, 467, 1230, 1231
Phenylbutazone, 977, 1224, 1232
Phenylephrine, 195, 196, 197, 1011
Phenylhydrazine, 892
Phenylpropanolamine, 1131, 1215
Phenytoin
  anaphylaxis, 1224
  anemia, 891
  antidepressants, 1213
  drug interactions, 796
  drug overdose, 1233, 1235, 1239
  erythematous eruptions, 1226
  hepatic failure, 810
  HIV infection drug regimen, 722
  interstitial lung disease, 550
  intracranial hemorrhage, 1195
  neuropathic pain, 135
  neutropenia, 893
  pancytopenia, 895
  seizures, 1201, 1204, 1205, 1206
  subarachnoid hemorrhage, spontaneous, 1191, 1192
  thrombocytopenia, 977
  thyroid disease, 1075
  tuberculosis treatment, interactions with, 659
Pheochromocytoma, 464, 467, 469
Philadelphia chromosome, 947
PHisoHex®, 209, 215, 222, 225, 226, 231
Phlebitis, 352, 627, 704
Phosphate, 1088, 1089
Phosphate binders, 1025
Phosphorus, 1018, 1019, 1024–1025
Phosphorus-32, 951
Phosphorus levels, 941, 942, 943, 1024–1025
Physical examination
  abdominal masses in gastrointestinal disease, 761–762
  acute respiratory failure, 184
  angina, 333
  chest pain, 299, 301
  dialysis patients, 1019–1020
  drug overdose, 1234
  fever and rash, 602
  fever of unknown origin, 606
  heart failure, 360
  hospital-acquired pneumonia, 645
  interstitial lung disease, 556
  lightheadedness, 306
  liver disease, 763–764
  liver transplant recipients, evaluation of, 841
  palpitations, 305
  pulmonary disease with HIV infection, 730
  pulmonary medicine, 518
  sepsis, 202
  syncope, 425, 426
Physical therapy, 131, 920, 1141, 1151, 1158, 1193
Physostigmine, 1230, 1233
Pilocarpine, 1166
Pindolol, 400

Pioglitazone, 1024
Piperacillin, 625, 832
Piperacillin/tazobactam, 626, 648, 649, 670, 672, 677
Piroxicam, 512, 722
Pituitary adenoma, 1076
Plague, 715
Plaque, atherosclerotic, 330–331, 335, 343, 349
Plasma, fresh frozen
  allergic reactions to transfusions, 913
  apheresis of whole blood, 907
  chronic myeloproliferative diseases, 953
  commercial products, 909, 910
  deep venous thrombosis, 499
  gastrointestinal bleeding, 771
  hepatic failure, 811, 813
  L-asparaginase, 935
  liver transplantation postoperative concern, 843
  lumbar puncture, 1172
  platelet dysfunction in dialysis patients, 1024
  ulcerative colitis, 802
Plasma renin activity, 465
Plasma substitutes, 910
Plasmapheresis, 377, 991, 1096, 1128
Platelet apheresis, 907, 952, 953
Platelet count, 257, 820
Platelet function analyzer (PFA-100®), 976
Platelet growth factors, 988
Platelet inhibitors, 951, 953, 1137
Platelet transfusions, 771, 934, 935, 953, 959–960, 986, 987, 988, 990
Platelets, 811, 913, 975–980, 984–988, 986–987, 1024
Platelia Aspergillus galactomannan assay, 618
Platinol, 902
Platinum therapy, 897
Pleural disease in rheumatoid arthritis, 1141
Pleural effusion
  Boerhaave's syndrome, 787
  community-acquired pneumonia, 634, 641
  dialysis patients, 1022
  organ involvement in lymphoma patients, 944
  physical signs, 518, 519, 520
  pulmonary medicine, 577–581
  thoracentesis, 227–228
  spherical mass lesions, 591
  tuberculosis, 656, 659
Pleural fluid, 227, 228, 229, 528, 578–579
Pleural mesotheliomas, 577
Pleural rubs, 578
Pleural space, 227–231, 577–585
Pleuritic rubs, 301
Pleuritis, 301, 344
Pleurodesis, chemical, 580, 581, 584, 585
Plicamycin, 901, 904, 925
Pneumococcal vaccination, 83, 559, 643, 650, 736
Pneumococcus infections, 112, 114, 150, 447
Pneumocystis pneumonia
  HIV infection, 729–737
Pneumocystis jirovecii (carinii) pneumonia
  cough, 522
  hematopoietic cell transplantation, 962
  HIV infection, 721, 723
  lung transplantation, 563, 564
  respiratory failure, acute, 184, 185, 187
  vasculitis, 1129
Pneumomediastinum, 178, 787
Pneumonia
  abdominal pain, causing, 753
  acute respiratory failure, 185, 187
  aspiration, 413, 414, 876
  chest pain, 301
  chronic eosinophilic, 554
  community-acquired, 633–644
  dialysis patients, 1022
  HIV infection, 729–737
  hospital-acquired, 645–653
  interstitial, 962
  lung volume reduction surgery, 566
  myocardial infarction, 344
  physical signs, 518, 519, 520

pleural effusions, 579, 580
pregnancy, 276
preoperative evaluation, 256
sickle cell disease, 969
Pneumonia Severity Index (PSI), 635–637
Pneumonia vaccination, 535, 537
Pneumonic plague, 715
Pneumothorax
  acute pericarditis, differentiating from, 444
  asthma, 541
  central venous catheterization, 222
  chest pain, 301
  chest radiographs, 528
  extracardiac obstructive shock, 191, 192
  interstitial lung disease, 557
  mechanical ventilation, 178, 179
  pacemaker implantation, 438
  parenteral nutrition, 107
  physical signs, 518, 520
  Pulmonary Langerhans' Cell Histiocytosis, 553
  pulmonary medicine, 577, 581–585
  tension, 198, 231, 411, 583
  thoracentesis, 227, 228, 229, 231
  thoracic injury, 290
  transthoracic needle aspiration biopsy
    (TTNAB), 588
Podragra, 1145
Poisoning, 809, 810, 811, 812, 815, 816, 1236
Polyarteritis nodosa, 1126, 1128, 1129
Polycystic renal disease, 867
Polycythemia, 532, 949
Polycythemia vera, 947, 948, 949, 950, 951–952
Polygeline, 822
Polymerase chain reaction testing, 610, 684
Polymorphic ventricular tachycardia, 411, 413,
    416, 417, 418, 425, 431
Polymyalgia rheumatica, 1116, 1124, 1125
Polymyositis, 1136, 1140–1141
Polymyositis-dermatomyositis, 552
Polymyxin, 621
Portal hypertension, 768, 819, 820, 821, 846–847
Portal vein thrombosis, 886, 887
Portland diabetic Project, 1080
Portopulmonary hypertension, 843
Positive end-expiratory pressure (PEEP),
    174–175, 177, 179, 186, 187
Positive pressure ventilation, 178–179, 186
Positron emission tomography (PET), 329, 588,
    589, 592, 886
Post-ictal state, 1199, 1200
Postoperative care
  anesthesiology, 245–246
  comanagement by hospitalists, 261–268
  fever, 599
  heart transplant surgery, 374–376
  hematopoietic cell transplantation, 958–959
  ileus and bowel obstruction, 879
  liver transplantation, 843–847
  pleural effusions, 578
  renal transplantation, 1032–1033
  supraventricular tachyarrhythmias in
    hospitalized patients, 405
Postpartum infection, 679
Postpartum pleural effusions, 578
Post-phlebitic syndrome, 499, 500
Post-transplant lymphoproliferative disease, 379,
    563, 564, 847
Posttraumatic stress disorder, 717
Postural tachycardia syndrome, 427
Potassium
  dialysis patients, 1018, 1019, 1026
  electrolyte disorders, 1045, 1048–1052,
    1049–1052
  multifocal atrial tachycardia (MAT), 403
  tumor lysis syndrome, 942–943
Potassium citrate, 1043
Potassium iodide, 274
Potassium levels
  acetazolamide, 1062
  anesthesia, 244–245
  dialysis patients, 1024

electrolyte disorders, 1049–1051, 1051–1052
heart failure, 364
hypertension, emergent, 465
limb ischemia, 489
myocardial infarction, 356
nausea and vomiting in gastrointestinal disease,
    755
palpitations, 304
renal tubular acidosis, 1057
sinus node dysfunction, 431
torsade de pointes, 412, 413
transfusion reactions, 913
tumor lysis syndrome, 941, 942–943
Potassium supplements
  cardiac arrest and resuscitation, after, 414
  diabetes mellitus, 1081, 1084, 1088, 1089
  dialysis patients, 1026
  drug overdose, 1240
  esophageal disorders, 785, 786
  hypokalemia, 1050–1051
Potomania, 1046, 1047
Povidone-iodine
  arthrocentesis, 210, 215
  intravascular catheterization, 209, 217, 222
  lumbar puncture, 223, 225
  paracentesis, 225, 226
  thoracentesis, 227, 231
Power of attorney, 122–123, 124
Practice guidelines for physicians, 87–91, 169
Pralidoxime, 1232, 1241
Pravastatin, 379, 722
Prazosin, 1213, 1239
Precipitating factors
  anaphylaxis, 1222
  angina discomfort, 332, 335
  asthma, exacerbations of, 539
  cardiac arrest and resuscitation, after, 413
  chest pain, 303
  chronic obstructive pulmonary disease, 531–532
  heart failure, 360
  lightheadedness, 306
  myocardial ischemia, 369
  myxedema coma, 1097, 1099
  palpitations, 304
  supraventricular tachyarrhythmias in inpatients,
    404–406
  thyrotoxic storm, 1095, 1096
Precision of diagnostic tests, 41
Predisposing conditions
  aneurysms with subarachnoid hemorrhage, 1190
  constrictive pericarditis, 450
  deep venous thrombosis, 496, 500, 501
  endocarditis, 693, 694
  hepatic encephalopathy, 825
  pulmonary embolism, 505–506, 512
Prednisolone, 276, 811
Prednisone
  adrenal insufficiency, 1106
  agnogenic myeloid metaplasia, 952
  anemia, 893
  asthma, 543, 545, 546
  chronic obstructive pulmonary disease, 534, 535
  Crohn's disease, 805
  eosinophilic pneumonia, 555
  gout, 1147
  graft-versus-host disease, 961, 962
  heart transplantation, 376, 377
  hematopoietic cell transplantation, 959
  HIV infection drug regimen, 722
  idiopathic thrombocytopenic purpura, 985
  interstitial lung disease, 558
  lung transplantation, 564
  lung volume reduction surgery, 566
  pericarditis, 447, 449
  pregnancy, 272
  preoperative evaluation, 258
  pulmonary disease with HIV infection, 735
  radiocontrast allergies, 1225
  renal transplantation, 1031
  systemic lupus erythematosus (SLE), 1135,
    1137

ulcerative colitis, 802, 803
vasculitis, 1122, 1123, 1125, 1128, 1129, 1132
Preeclampsia, 271, 272–273, 274, 276
Pregnancy
  alcohol withdrawal, 1246
  aortic intramural hematoma and dissection, 472
  D-dimer assays, 495
  deep vein thrombosis, 498
  fluoroquinolone antibiotics, 627
  hepatic failure, 810, 811, 813, 815
  hypertension, emergent, 463, 464, 467, 468
  idiopathic thrombocytopenic purpura,
    985–986
  medical consultation regarding, 271–277
  paracentesis, 225
  platelet function disorders, 987
  pulmonary embolism, 505
  pulmonary hypertension, 573
  Rh compatibility for transfusions, 912
  tetracycline, 627
  thrombolytic therapy, contraindication for, 348
  thrombotic disorders, 983
  trauma patients, 292
  tuberculosis, 658
  urinary tract infection, 668, 669, 670, 671, 672
Pregnancy tests, 861
Premature atrial contraction (PAC), 397
Premature ventricular contractions (PVCs), 425
Prerenal azotemia, 379
Presentation, clinical
  abdominal aortic aneurysm, 481–482
  acquired atrioventricular block, 433
  adrenal insufficiency, 1104
  allergic reactions, 1221–1222
  altered mental status in HIV infected patients,
    745
  angina, 334
  aortic intramural hematoma and dissection, 472
  aortic regurgitation, 383–384
  aortic stenosis, 381
  appendicitis, acute, 860
  asthma, 540
  back pain, 1154
  bacterial meningitis, 683–684
  bowel ischemia, acute, 867–868
  bowel obstruction, 873
  cellulitis, 675–676
  chronic myeloproliferative diseases, 948
  chronic obstructive pulmonary disease
    (COPD), 531–532
  community-acquired pneumonia, 633–634
  constrictive pericarditis, 450
  Crohn's disease, 800, 804
  deep vein thrombosis, 496
  diverticulitis, 864
  drug overdose, 1229, 1230–1233, 1236, 1239,
    1240
  endocarditis, 693
  focal CNS lesions in HIV infected patients, 742
  gout, 1145
  heart failure, 360–361
  heart transplantation complications, 379
  hepatic failure, 810, 812
  hypercalcemia in oncologic emergencies, 924
  hypertension, emergent, 463
  interstitial lung diseases (ILDs), 549
  intracranial hemorrhage, 1193
  IV catheter-associated infection, 703–704
  kidney stones, 1037–1038
  limb ischemia, 486–487
  lymphoma, 937–938
  meningitis in HIV infected patients, 739
  mitral regurgitation, 387
  mitral stenosis, 385
  myocardial infarction, 264, 298, 343, 357
  myxedema coma, 1097–1098
  necrotizing fasciitis, 678–679
  neurologic oncologic emergencies, 917–918
  pancreatitis, 849
  peptic ulcer disease, 790–791
  pericardial oncologic emergencies, 921

pericarditis, 442–443
peritonitis, 823–824
pleural effusions, 577–578
pneumothorax, 582, 583
pulmonary disease with HIV infection, 731
pulmonary embolism, 505
pulmonary hypertension, 569–570
respiratory failure, 183–184
seizures with drug overdose, 1238
sepsis, 201
sickle cell disease, 965–966, 968
sinus node dysfunction, 431
subarachnoid hemorrhage, spontaneous, 1190
subdural hematoma, 1196
superior vena cava syndrome, 922
supraventricular tachyarrhythmias, 396
syncope, 423
thoracic aortic aneurysms, 480
thyrotoxic storm, 1093–1094
tricuspid regurgitation, 389
tuberculosis, 655–656, 662
ulcerative colitis, 800–801
urinary tract infection, 667–668
ventricular arrhythmias, 411, 418
Preservation injury, 846
Pressure gradients, vascular, 381, 382, 386, 456, 458, 459
Pressure-preset ventilation, 173, 174, 175
Pressure-support ventilation, 174, 175, 181
Priapism, 967–968, 969, 970
Primaquine, 735, 892
Primary Angioplasty in Myocardial Infarction (PAMI), 348
Primary care physicians, 4, 5, 111–112, 127
Primary pulmonary hypertension, 570, 571, 572, 573, 574
Primary spontaneous pneumothorax, 577, 581–582, 583–585
Prions, 909, 915
Pristinamycin, 627
Privacy of patients, 67, 126
Proarrhythmias, 402, 403, 404, 411
Probabilities. *See also* Likelihood
   coronary artery disease (CAD), of having, 333–334
   decision analysis, 45–49
   deep vein thrombosis, diagnosis of, 496
   diagnostic tests, 37–41
   preoperative evaluations of risk, 250
Probanthine, 1213
Probenecid, 1148
Problem solving in evidence-based medicine, 51–56
Probucol, 412
Procainamide
   antinuclear antibodies, 1117
   atrial fibrillation, 403
   cardiac arrest and resuscitation, after, 415
   coagulation factors, 977
   drug overdose, 1239, 1240
   neutropenia, 893
   palpitations, 304
   pericarditis, 442
   post heart transplant surgery, 375
   supraventricular tachyarrhythmias, 399, 400, 404, 405
   syncope, 425
   thrombocytopenia, 977
   torsade de pointes, 412
   ventricular arrhythmias, 356, 410, 419
   ventricular arrhythmias and cardiac arrest, 418
   wide-complex tachycardia, 395
Procalcitonin, 686
Procarbazine, 550, 899
Procedures in hospital medicine, 207–231
Prochlorperazine, 273, 756
Professional fees for hospitalists, 19–20
Progesterone, 272
Progestins, 786
Prognoses
   acute leukemia, 929–930
   angina, of, determining, 334–337

aortic stenosis, 383
cardiac arrest and resuscitation, after, 416
central nervous system vasculitis, 1132
chronic myeloproliferative diseases, 948
end-of-life care, 140–141
heart transplantation, 373
hepatic failure, 809, 810, 812, 813, 814
intracranial hemorrhage, 1195
lymphomas, 938
malignancy post heart transplantation, 380
nuclear perfusion imaging, 320
pupillary responses, 1166
sickle cell disease, 972
Prograf, 1031
Progressive multifocal leukoencephalopathy, 739, 742
Proliferative bronchiolitis, 551
Promethazine, 969
Promyelocytic leukemia, 933
Propafenone, 304, 399, 400, 403, 404, 419, 512, 722
Prophylaxis
   anthrax, 714
   bioterrorism, 712
   cell-mediated immunity, impaired, 620
   deep venous thrombosis, 292, 677
   dialysis patients, 1012
   graft-*versus*-host disease, 958–959
   hematopoietic cell transplantation, 959, 961–962
   infections in lymphoma patients, 943
   pancreatitis, 854, 855
   plague, 715
   pneumocystis pneumonia, 736
   prothrombin 20210, 983
   recurrent urinary tract infection, 671
   stress-related gastropathy, 795
   stroke, 1181–1182, 1183
Propofol, 244, 1202, 1239
Propoxyphene, 131, 1232, 1237, 1240
Propranolol
   alcohol withdrawal, 1248
   antidepressants, 1213
   aortic intramural hematoma and dissection, 475
   atrial fibrillation, 402
   cardiac arrest and resuscitation, after, 415
   depression, 1210
   drug overdose, 1230, 1239, 1240
   myocardial infarction, 350, 351
   pregnancy, 274–275
   supraventricular tachyarrhythmias, 399, 400
   thyrotoxic storm, 1095–1096
   tremor, 1167
Propylene glycol, 1201
Propylthiouracil, 274, 1095
Prostacyclin, 375, 376, 491, 572, 573, 843, 1139
Prostaglandins, 491
Prostate cancer, 500, 1038, 1040
Prostatic hypertrophy, 1038, 1040, 1041
Prostatitis, 668, 670
Prosthetic heart valves, 389–390
Prosthetic joints, 210, 1150, 1151
Protamine, 265, 497, 499, 989, 1024
Protease inhibitors, 663
Protein
   cerebrospinal fluid, 684, 686
   dialysis patients, 1018–1019, 1020, 1021, 1024
   nutritional requirements, 102–103
   renal disease, 1003, 1004, 1042
Protein C, 459, 510, 981, 982–983
Protein S, 459, 981, 982–983
Protein synthesis, 1080
Proteinuria, 996, 1002
Prothrombin complex concentrates, 988
Prothrombin gene mutation, 275
Prothrombin time
   bleeding disorders, 976
   cirrhosis, 820
   gastrointestinal bleeding, 769
   hepatic failure, 809, 810, 812, 813, 814, 816
   liver disease, 764

liver transplantation, 843
pericarditis, 443
preoperative evaluation, 257
pulmonary embolism, 510
Prothrombin 20210, 982, 983
Proton pump inhibitors
   cough, 522
   esophageal disorders, 783, 786
   gastrointestinal bleeding, 768, 771, 773
   peptic ulcer disease, 793, 794, 795, 796, 1023
   pregnancy, 273
   stress ulcers in trauma patients, 293
Prozac, 1212
Pseudoclaudication, 457
Pseudo-Cushing syndrome, 1071
Pseudocysts, 856–857
Pseudoephedrine, 970, 1137, 1215, 1236
Pseudogout, 1143, 1145
Pseudohemoptysis, 523
Pseudohyperkalemia, 1051
Pseudohypokalemia, 1049–1050
Pseudohyponatremia, 1045
Pseudolymphoma, 1139
Pseudomonas aeruginosa, 265, 534, 627–628, 629
Pseudomyasthenia, 588, 591
Psoas sign, 860
Psychiatric units, admission to, 284
Psychiatrists, 279–285, 425, 426, 429, 805, 806, 1234, 1236, 1249
Psychoactive medications, 263, 304, 306, 746, 845
Psychogenic seizures, 1200, 1202
Psychological disorders
   depression, 1209–1216, 1213
   elderly patients, 112, 115
   electroencephalography, 1173
   myxedema coma, 1098
   pain, 130
   psychosis, 280–281, 284
Psychologists, 805
Psychophysiologic disorders, 541
Psychosocial care, 29, 1210
Public health departments, 655, 662, 664, 680, 714, 1151
PubMed, 53
Pulmonary angiography, 506, 507
Pulmonary artery catheterization, 196–197, 253, 362, 367
Pulmonary artery pressure, 569
Pulmonary capillary wedge pressure, 191, 193, 197, 361, 363
Pulmonary contusions, 187
Pulmonary disease
   anxiety, 280
   arteriovenous aneurysms, 592
   community-acquired pneumonia, 641
   echocardiography, 323
   HIV infection, 729–737
   preoperative evaluation, 256
   pulmonary capillaritis, 551
   pulmonary capillary leak, 273
   pulmonary congestion, 386, 387, 388, 433
   pulmonary hemorrhage, 187
   pulmonary histiocytosis X, 557
   pulmonary infarction, 299, 300
   pulmonary nodules, 945
   pulmonary thromboembolic disease, 188
   pulmonary-renal syndrome, 524
   supraventricular tachyarrhythmias, 397, 405
Pulmonary edema
   alkalosis, respiratory, 1064
   asthma, 540
   cardiac arrest and resuscitation, after, 413
   cardiogenic, 175
   cardiogenic shock, 191
   chronic eosinophilic pneumonia, 554
   dialysis patients, 1021, 1022
   heart failure, 359, 360, 361–362, 366, 367, 369, 370
   mitral stenosis, 386
   noninvasive ventilation, 187
   physical signs, 518, 519

pleural effusion, 580, 581
pregnancy, 271
preoperative evaluation, 254
renal disease, 1002
severe preeclamsia of pregnancy, 273
subarachnoid hemorrhage, spontaneous, 1191
syncope, 428
thoracentesis, 229
transfusion reactions, 913
Pulmonary embolism
acute, 405
chest pain, 299, 300
deep vein thrombosis, 495
delirium, 282
dyspnea, 523
extracardiac obstructive shock, 192, 197
heart failure, 360
inferior vena cava (IVC) filters, 499
interstitial lung disease, 557
IV catheter-associated infection, 708
medical consultants for surgical patients, 237
myocardial infarction, differentiating from, 344
pericarditis, differentiating from, 444
pleural effusions, 579, 580
pregnancy, 275
renal transplantation, 1035
sudden death following acute myocardial
infarction, 351
supraventricular tachyarrhythmias, 397, 398
syncope, 424, 428
tricuspid regurgitation, 389
vascular medicine, 505–513
ventricular arrhythmias and cardiac arrest, 411,
417
wheezing, 519
Pulmonary function testing, 256, 525–527, 557
Pulmonary hypertension
cardiac arrest and resuscitation, after, 416
extracardiac obstructive shock, 192
mitral stenosis, 385
pulmonary angiogram, 507
pulmonary medicine, 569–576
right ventricular (RV) failure, 368
sickle cell disease, 971, 972
syncope, 424
ventricular arrhythmias and cardiac arrest, 411
Pulmonary Langerhans' Cell Histiocytosis, 550,
553
Pulmonary rehabilitation program, 559, 566
Pulmonary specialists, 509, 534, 558, 639,
641–642
Pulmonary system
abnormalities, 403
chest pain, 301
liver transplant recipients, evaluation of,
842–843
postoperative care, 264–265
pulmonary vessels, 325
signs, symptoms, and laboratory abnormalities,
517–529
Pulmonary thromboendarterectomy, 575
Pulmonary vascular resistance (PVR), 373
Pulmonary vasodilators, 375
Pulmonic murmurs, 271
Pulmonic regurgitation, 385
Pulmonic stenosis, 424
Pulse deficits, 333, 344, 472, 473, 475
Pulse pressure, 464
Pulses
acute limb ischemia, 487, 489, 490
asymmetric, 1123
chronic limb ischemia, 490
peripheral artery disease, 457–458, 460
Pulsus alternans, 308
Pulsus paradoxus, 308, 441, 443, 444–445, 541,
544
Pulsus parvus et tardus, 381
Punch biopsy with silver staining, 724
Punctate telangiectases, 976
Pupillary response, 289, 1166, 1187
Purified protein derivative (PPD) of tuberculin, 524

Purine analog agents, 943
Purpura, 976
Pyelonephritis, 276, 671, 672, 1033, 1034, 1035
Pyrazinamide, 657, 658, 659, 660, 725
Pyridium, 892
Pyridoxine, 661, 983, 1204, 1231, 1232, 1239,
1241
Pyrimethamine, 743
Pyuria, 667, 668

Q
Q fever, 602, 603
Q waves, 413
QRS widening, 1240
QT interval prolongation, 411, 412, 417, 425,
428, 1240
Quality of care
hospitalist model, 6
peptic ulcer disease, 796
prospective reimbursement systems, 13
quality improvement, 79–85, 165
roles of hospitalists, 7
Quality of life
dialysis, 1018
dual-chamber pacemakers, 439
end-of-life care, 139
heart transplantation, 374
lung transplantation, 562
lung volume reduction surgery, 565
Quality-adjusted life-years (QALYs), 48, 59–60
Quantity of care and hospital revenues, 13–14
Quetiapine, 281, 1240
Quinapril, 364, 365
Quincke's pulses, 308
Quinidine
anemia, 892
drug overdose, 1239, 1240
esophageal disorders, 785, 786
heart transplant surgery, 375
HIV infection drug regimen, 722
palpitations, 304
supraventricular tachyarrhythmias, 399, 400,
403, 404
syncope, 425
thrombocytopenia, 977
torsade de pointes, 412
tricyclic antidepressants, 1213
ventricular arrhythmias, 419
Quinine, 722, 813, 977
Quinolone antibiotics
acute myelogenous leukemia, 933, 934
hospital-acquired pneumonia, 648
liver transplant patients, infection prophylaxis
for, 621
neutropenic hosts, 616, 617, 619
pancreatitis, 855
plague, 715
pregnancy, 277
Pseudomonas aeruginosa, 628, 629
tuberculosis treatment, interactions with, 661
Quinpristin/dalfopristin, 627, 630, 707

R
Rabbit antithymocyte globulin, 1031
Rabeprazole, 793
Racemic epinephrine, 519
Radiation esophagitis, 785
Radiation pericarditis, 442, 447
Radiation therapy
agnogenic myeloid metaplasia, 952
back pain, 1156
chronic myeloproliferative diseases, 953
Cushing syndrome, 1073
diffuse aggressive lymphomas, 940
drug-induced interstitial lung disease, 552
esophageal carcinoma, 783
hematopoietic cell transplantation, 956, 958
Hodgkin's disease, 941
neurologic oncologic emergencies, 919, 920

organ involvement in lymphoma patients, 944
pacemakers, 439
pancytopenia, 895
peripheral arterial disease, 486
pulmonary function testing, 525
superior vena cava syndrome, 923, 924
Radiation therapy consultation, 920
Radiation-induced constrictive pericarditis, 451
Radio frequency ablation, 404, 406, 410, 412,
418, 419
Radioactive iodine, 1093, 1095, 1097
Radiocontrast allergies, 1225, 1226, 1227
Radiofrequency ablation, 397, 399, 400, 403
Radiographs
back pain, 1156, 1157
contrast dye and anesthesia, 243
rheumatology, 1112, 1114, 1118
sepsis, tests for, 202
trauma patient assessment, 288
Radiographs, abdomen
abdominal aortic aneurysm, 482
appendicitis, acute, 861
bowel obstruction, 875, 878, 879
cholangitis, 834
Crohn's disease, 800, 804
diverticulitis, 864, 866
gastrointestinal disease, 753, 755
pancreatitis, 851
ulcerative colitis, 801, 803
Radiographs, chest
acute respiratory distress syndrome (ARDS), 189
angina, 333
anthrax, 714
aortic intramural hematoma and dissection,
472–473, 476
appendicitis, acute, 861
bowel obstruction, 875
cardiac arrest and resuscitation, after, 413, 414
cardiovascular disease, 312
chest pain, 299, 302
chronic obstructive pulmonary disease
(COPD), 532
community-acquired pneumonia, 634, 637,
640, 642
cough, 521, 522
dyspnea, 523
fever, 600, 606
hemoptysis, 524
hospital-acquired pneumonia, 646, 647, 650
hypertension, emergent, 464
interstitial lung disease, 556, 557
neurologic complications in HIV infected
patients, 741
pacemaker implantation, 438
pericarditis, 443, 444
pleural effusions, 577–578
postoperative care, 261
pulmonary disease with HIV infection, 731–732
pulmonary embolism, 505, 508
pulmonary hypertension, 570, 571
pulmonary medicine, 519, 520, 527–529
respiratory failure, acute, 185, 186
solitary pulmonary nodules, 587, 589, 593
spontaneous pneumothoraces, 582, 584, 585
subclavian vein cannulation, 220, 222
tension pneumothorax, 583
thoracentesis, 228, 231
thoracic aortic aneurysms, 480
tuberculosis, 655–656
Radioiodine, 1070
Radiologists, interventional, 853, 862, 869
Radionuclide angiography, 322
Radionuclide cholescintigraphy, 831, 833, 834
Radionuclide scintigraphy (bone scan), 1156
Radionuclide ventriculography, 360
Rales, 184, 301, 361, 518
Ramipril, 364, 365
Ranitidine, 273, 793, 794, 977, 1164, 1165, 1168,
1210
Ranson criteria, 170, 852
Rapamune, 1031

Serum transferrin receptor (sTfR), 890
Serzone, 1212
Sestamibi nuclear perfusion imaging, 303, 316, 318, 320, 340
Sevelamer, 1025
Severe acute respiratory syndrome (SARS), 711, 717
Sevoflurane, 244
Sexual activity, 814, 1144, 1148, 1212, 1215
Sexually transmitted diseases, 1151
Shock
    aortic intramural hematoma and dissection, 472, 475
    cardiovascular, 359, 360, 1098
    classifications of, 191–193
    head trauma, 289
    mucosal ischemia, 752
    myocardial infarction, 355
    sepsis, 201, 203, 204, 205
    syncope, 428
    treatment of, 193–198
    urinary tract infection, 671
Shock liver, 765
Short bowel syndrome, 103
Short Portable Mental Status Questionnaire, 112, 114, 745, 1165
Shy-Drager syndrome, 306
Sick sinus syndrome, 425, 467
Sickle cell disease, 956, 965–973, 1113, 1114
Sigmoidoscopy, 865, 869, 875
Signal-averaged ECG (SAGE), 427
Silver sulfadiazine, 709
Silymarine, 811
Simple partial seizures, 1200, 1203
Simplified Acute Physiology Score (SAPS), 170
SimpliRED D-dimer, 495–496
Simulect, 1031
Simvastatin, 512
Sinemet, 1215
Sinequan, 1212
Single-chamber ventricular pacemakers, 439
Single-lung transplantation, 561–562, 575
Single-photon emission computed tomography (SPECT), 318, 320, 321
Sinus node disorders, 375, 393, 431–432
Sinus rhythms, 394, 395
Sinusitis, 276, 600
Sirolimus, 846, 1031
Sisomicin, 625
Sister Mary Joseph nodes, 889
6-Mercaptopurine, 802, 803, 850
Sjögren's syndrome, 552, 1057, 1058, 1117, 1118, 1136, 1139–1140, 1141
Skilled nursing facilities, 27, 28, 370
Skin cancer, 380
Skin disorders, 613, 1071, 1073, 1097, 1099, 1104, 1114, 1150. See also Rash
Sleep apnea, 244, 280, 570, 571, 572, 1022
Sliding scale coverage for insulin, 1082, 1083, 1084
Smallpox, 600, 714–715
Smallpox vaccinations, 714–715
Smoking. See Tobacco use
SNOMED controlled terminology, 67
Social services, 28–29, 1195
Social support system, 112, 116, 841
Social work consultation, 292, 805, 806, 1178, 1181
Society of Hospital Medicine, 3
Sociopathy, 283
Sodium
    dialysis patients, 1018, 1025
    electrolyte disorders, 1045–1048
    excretion, 999–1000, 1002
    retention, 359, 1001
Sodium citrate, 1024
Sodium intake, 821, 822, 823, 960, 1049
Sodium iopanoate, 1075
Sodium levels, 821, 822, 1045–1048, 1048–1049, 1099, 1191
Sodium morrhuate, 768
Sodium nitrate, 1231
Sodium polystyrene sulfonate, 1023, 1025, 1052

Sodium thiosulfate, 1231
Solu-Medrol, 1137
Solvents, 1232
Soma, 1241
Somatization, 283, 429
Somatostatin, 768, 770, 811, 853, 879
Sones technique, 325
Sorbitol, 753, 1048, 1052, 1235
Sotalol, 1240
Sparfloxacin, 638
Spasticity, 1169
Specific defects in immune function, 614–619, 620
Specific factor assays in bleeding disorders, 978, 979, 980
Specific gravity in urinalysis, 996
Spectral Doppler studies, 322
Speech therapy, 1178, 1181, 1182, 1193
Sphincter of Oddi dysfunction, 850
Spinal anesthesia, 192, 244
Spinal cord compression, 224, 918, 946, 953
Spinal cord injuries, 192, 290, 292, 481, 501
Spinal cord sensory levels, 1169, 1170
Spinal procedures, 686
Spinal stenosis, 456, 457
Spiritual care, 29, 142
Spirometry, 256, 265, 525–526, 532, 535, 537, 557
Spironolactone, 364, 366, 469, 574, 821, 822, 1002, 1051
Spleens, 291, 614, 615
Splenectomy, 887, 893, 952, 985, 991
Splenic sequestration, 887, 890, 966
Splenomegaly, 885–887, 894, 945, 948
Sputum
    asthma, 540, 541
    chronic obstructive pulmonary disease, 531, 532, 534
    community-acquired pneumonia, 634–635, 643
    cough, 521, 522
    pulmonary disease with HIV infection, 734, 737
    tuberculosis, 656, 663, 664
Staging of lymphomas, 938–939
Stanozolol, 1223
Staphylococcus aureus
    cellulitis, 675, 678
    chronic obstructive pulmonary disease, 534
    diabetes mellitus, 1080
    dialysis patients, 1021, 1022
    diarrhea in gastrointestinal disease, 756, 757
    endocarditis, 694, 696, 697, 698
    IV catheter-associated infection, 706–707, 708
    pacemaker infections, 439
    prosthetic heart valves, 390
    resistant organism, 629, 630
    scalded-skin syndrome, 630
    septic arthritis, 1148, 1149, 1150, 1151
    trauma patients, 292
Staphylococcus epidermis, 390, 439, 1021, 1022
Staphylococcus infections, 447, 449, 592
Statin therapy
    aortic stenosis, 383
    cardiac risk factors, 340
    heart transplantations, 379
    limb ischemia, 487, 492
    myocardial infarction, 345, 352–353, 355, 356, 357
    stroke, 1182
    warfarin, interfering with, 512
Status asthmaticus, 544
Status epilepticus, 428, 689, 1172, 1173, 1201–1203, 1239
ST-elevation MI (STEMI), 344, 345–349
Stem cell transplantation, 941, 956
Stents
    biliary disease, 833, 835, 837
    cardiac, 252, 253, 345, 347, 348, 357
    carotid artery, 1182
    superior vena cava syndrome, 923, 924
    ureteral, 1041, 1042

Stereotactic biopsy
    parenchymal brain involvement in lymphoma patients, 945
Stereotactic radiosurgery, 919
Stereotactic surgery, 919, 945, 1195
Steroid elution, 435
Steroids
    anaphylaxis, 1224, 1225
    angioedema, 1223
    asthma, 547
    back pain, 1156, 1157
    chronic obstructive pulmonary disease, 531
    donors of blood for apheresis, 907
    encephalopathy after renal transplantation, 1035
    fever, 598
    focal CNS lesions in HIV infected patients, 743
    heart transplantations, 378
    hematopoietic cell transplantation, 961
    hepatic failure, 811
    hypercalcemia in oncologic emergencies, 925
    hypersensitivity pneumonitis, 556
    hypopituitarism, 1076
    increased intracranial pressure, 1189
    leukocytosis, 894
    lung volume reduction surgery, 566
    meningitis in HIV infected patients, 741
    multiple pulmonary nodules, 592
    neurologic oncologic emergencies, 919, 920
    neutropenia, 893
    peptic ulcer disease, 789
    pregnancy, 272, 274
    renal stone and obstructive disease, 1040
    superior vena cava syndrome, 923
    thrombotic thrombocytopenic purpura, 991
    wheezing, 519
Stevens-Johnson syndrome, 724, 1222, 1223, 1224, 1225
Stilbesterol, 970
Stool, 299, 864, 873, 875
    See also Diarrhea
Stool softeners, 1157, 1191
Streptase, 511
Streptococcus Group A, 599, 678–679
Streptococcus infections, 277, 348, 390, 447, 449, 675, 676, 678
Streptococcus pneumoniae, 534, 628, 629, 638–639, 689–690, 691
Streptogramin, 627
Streptokinase, 346, 347–348, 349, 350, 357, 511, 580, 977, 1179
Streptomycin, 625, 629, 630, 659, 661, 715
Streptozocin, 901, 902, 904
Stress echocardiography, 316, 320–321
Stress electrocardiography, 316–318, 319
Stress testing, 316, 319, 340, 355, 411
Stress-related gastropathy, 293, 789–796
Stridor, 183, 519, 541, 1125
Stroke
    aortic intramural hematoma and dissection, 472
    aspirin, 349
    atrial fibrillation, 113, 400, 402
    classification of, 1175–1177
    delirium, 282
    dialysis patients, 1025
    hemorrhagic, 348
    ischemic, 501
    neurologic disorders, 1175–1183
    pregnancy, 276
    preoperative evaluation, 256–257
    primary PCI compared to thrombolytic therapy, 348
    pulmonary embolism, 512
    sickle cell disease, 968, 973
    supraventricular tachyarrhythmias, 397, 406
    syncope, 428
    ventricular arrhythmias and cardiac arrest, 411
Stroke centers, 1175, 1179
Stroma-free hemoglobin, 194
ST-segment changes, 340

Study to Understand Prognoses and Preferences for Outcomes and Risks of Treatment (SUPPORT), 120
Stunned ischemic myocardium, 374
Subarachnoid hemorrhage, 223, 1176, 1189–1193
Subclavian vein cannulation, 218–220, 222
Subcutaneous emphysema, 178, 528
Subdural hematoma, 1025, 1195–1197
Subdural hemorrhage, 1175
Sublimaze, 132
Substance abuse
    alcohol intoxication and withdrawal, 1243–1249
    counseling, 1249
    depression in hospitalized patients, 1210
    drug overdose and dependence, 1229–1241
    liver transplant recipients, evaluation of, 841
    pain management, 135
    palpitations, 304
    suicide, 279
    syncope, 429
    trauma patients, 293
Succinylcholine, 244, 245
Sucralfate, 189, 273, 512, 652, 661, 785, 795, 796, 1023
Suicide, 279–280, 284, 1211, 1229, 1234, 1236
Sulbactam, 265, 292, 626, 648, 670, 672, 677
Sulfa drugs, 277, 977
Sulfadiazine, 726, 743, 997, 998, 1042
Sulfasalazine, 274, 550, 805, 891
Sulfinpyrazone, 977, 1148
Sulfonamides, 521, 550, 850, 892, 893, 895, 1224
Sulfones, 892
Sulfonylureas, 1024, 1082, 1090, 1232, 1234, 1237
Sumatriptan, 276, 1164
Superior vena cava syndrome, 922–924, 940, 944, 990
Superoxide dismutase, 1011
Supraventricular arrhythmias, 356, 375, 393–406, 395, 396, 425, 431
Surgeons
    abdominal pain with renal transplantation, 1035
    acute pancreatitis, 853, 856
    appendicitis, acute, 861, 862, 864
    back pain, 1156, 1157
    bowel ischemia, acute, 869
    bowel obstruction, 874, 877, 880
    Crohn's disease, 805
    diverticulitis, 865
    endocarditis, 697
    IV catheter-associated infection, 707–708
Surgery
    acute cholangitis, 836, 837
    acute cholecystitis, 832–833
    acute limb ischemia, 486, 487, 488, 489, 490
    acute pancreatitis, 856, 857
    adrenal insufficiency, 1107, 1108
    anesthesia management during, 244–245
    aortic aneurysms, 479, 480–481, 482–483
    aortic intramural hematoma and dissection, 475–476
    aortic regurgitation, 383, 384, 385
    aortic stenosis, 382, 383
    back pain, 1156, 1157, 1158
    bacterial pericarditis, 447
    Boerhaave's syndrome, 787
    bowel ischemia, acute, 868–869
    bowel obstruction, 873, 874, 875, 876
    cardiac
        supraventricular tachyarrhythmias in hospitalized patients, 406
    cardiac tamponade post heart transplant surgery, 376
    chronic limb ischemia, 491, 492
    constrictive pericarditis, 451
    COPD, 537
    Crohn's disease, 805, 806
    Cushing syndrome, 1073
    debridement for necrotizing fasciitis, 679, 680, 681

deep venous thrombosis, 496, 500, 501
deep venous thrombosis prophylaxis, 501
diabetes mellitus, 1084–1085
diverticulitis, 865, 866, 867
do not resuscitate orders
    ethical issues, 123–124
    elective
        preoperative evaluation, 249, 250
    embolectomy
        pulmonary embolism, 510
    esophageal disorders, 783, 787
    extrapulmonary tuberculosis, 659, 661
    goiter, 1070, 1071
    heart failure, development of, 371
    heart transplantation, 374
    hemoptysis, 524
    hospital-acquired pneumonia with empyema, 651
    increased intracranial pressure, 1188, 1189, 1191–1192
    intracranial hemorrhage, 1195
    liver transplantation procedure, 839
    lower gastrointestinal bleeding, 777
    lung transplantation, 561–564, 566–567
    lung volume reduction, 564–567
    mechanical complications of acute myocardial infarction, 355
    mitral regurgitation, 383, 387, 388–389
    mitral stenosis, 383, 387
    neurologic oncologic emergencies, 920
    oncologic emergencies, 922, 924
    peptic ulcer disease, 791
    pleural effusion, 580–581
    preoperative evaluations, 249–258
    priapism
        sickle cell disease, 970
    prior, of aorta
        aortic intramural hematoma and dissection, 472, 473
    pulmonary embolism, 505, 510, 512
    pulmonary hypertension, 575
    recent, major
        thrombolytic therapy, contraindication for, 348
    renal transplantation, 1027, 1028
    seizures, 1205–1206
    solitary pulmonary nodules, 589
    subarachnoid hemorrhage, spontaneous, 1191–1192
    subdural hematoma, 1197
    supraventricular tachyarrhythmias in hospitalized patients, 405–406
    thyrotoxic storm, 1093, 1094, 1095, 1096–1097
    ulcerative colitis, 803
    urinary tract infection, upper, 672
    valve replacement
        heart failure, 369, 370
Surgery versus Thrombolysis for Ischemia of the Lower Extremity (STILE) trials, 490
Susceptibility testing, 641, 642, 643, 656, 668, 669, 672, 677, 689, 696, 697
Swan Ganz catheters, 414
Swelling of joints, 112–115, 1145
Sympathetic nervous system, 304, 331, 359, 464, 466, 469
Sympatholytic agents, 1239
Sympathomimetic agents, 1131, 1166, 1167, 1194, 1215, 1237
Syncope and near-syncope
    aortic intramural hematoma and dissection, 472
    aortic stenosis, 381, 382, 383
    cardiovascular medicine, 423–430
    causes of, 423–425, 428, 429
    echocardiography, 323
    lightheadedness, 306
    myocardial infarction, 343
    pacemakers, 439
    palpitations, 304, 305–306
    pulmonary hypertension, 569, 575
    seizures, 1199, 1200

sinus node dysfunction, 431, 432
supraventricular tachyarrhythmias, 397
ventricular tachycardia, 411
Syndrome of inappropriate antidiuretic hormone secretion (SIADH), 588, 591, 1045–1046, 1047, 1076, 1215
Synovial fluid, 211, 1143–1144, 1145, 1146, 1148, 1149, 1150
Syphilis, 383, 479, 684–685, 914
Systemic lupus erythematosus (SLE)
    autoimmune pericarditis, 447
    chronic aortic regurgitation, 383
    hemoptysis, 524
    interstitial lung diseases, 552
    meningitis syndrome, 686
    neutropenia, 894
    peripheral artery disease, differentiating from, 457
    pregnancy, 273
    rheumatic diseases, 1113, 1114, 1115, 1116, 1117, 1118, 1119
    rheumatic disorders, 1135–1137
Systemic vascular resistance, 192, 193
Systolic murmurs, 309, 310, 381, 382, 384, 1020

T
Tabun, 1232
Tachycardia-bradycardia syndrome, 400, 401, 425, 431
Tachycardias, 271, 375, 393–406, 442, 443, 583.
    See also Ventricular tachycardia
Tachypnea, 505, 523, 524, 532
Tacrolimus (FK-506)
    anti-microbials, interaction with, 620
    gout, 1147
    graft-versus-host disease, 961
    heart transplantation, 376, 378, 379
    hematopoietic cell transplantation, 959
    liver transplantation, 845, 846
    lung transplantation, 562, 563, 564
    pregnancy, 276
    renal transplantation, 1031, 1033, 1034, 1035
    seizures, 1204
TACTICS-TIMI 18, 340, 341
Takayasu's arteritis, 479, 480, 486, 1121, 1123–1124
Tako-Tsubo syndrome, 300
Talc for pleurodesis, 581, 584
Tamoxifen, 722, 1164, 1213
Tamsulosin, 1041
Tardive dyskinesia, 281
Taxol, 902, 958
Tazobactam, 626, 832
T-cells, 937, 938, 940, 956, 963
Technetium99 scintigraphy, 316, 318, 775, 843
Teeth and tetracycline, 627
Tegretol, 1203
Telephone pacemaker-surveillance programs, 439
Temozolomide, 899, 920
Temperature, body, 195, 244, 245
Tenecteplase, 346, 347, 348
Tenofovir, 726
Tension pneumothorax, 411, 583
Terazosin, 1041
Terbutaline, 1239
Terfenadine, 412, 1213
Terminal conditions, 139–144, 181–182, 418
Testosterone, 1213
Tetanus immunization, 291, 679
Tetracycline
    action of, 627
    BUN level, 1003
    chronic obstructive pulmonary disease, 534
    community-acquired pneumonia, 638
    enterococci, 629
    esophageal disorders, 785, 786
    fever of unknown origin, 607
    headache, 1164
    hepatic failure, 810
    pancreatitis, 850

penicillin-nonsusceptible pneumococci, 628
peptic ulcer disease, 794
pregnancy, 277
resistance to *S. pneumoniae*, 639
rickettsial infections, 604
vancomycin-resistant *Staphylococcus aureus*, 630
Tetradecyl sulfate, 768
Thalassemia, 888, 890, 891, 956
Thalidomide, 952, 962
Thallium perfusion scans, 303, 316, 318, 340
Theo-BID, 1233
TheoDur, 1233
Theophylline
    abdominal pain, causing, 753
    aminophylline, 256, 534
    asthma, 543
    chronic obstructive pulmonary disease, 534
    drug interactions, 796
    drug overdose, 1229, 1233, 1234, 1235, 1236,
        1239, 1240
    esophageal disorders, 786
    hypokalemia, 1050
    multifocal atrial tachycardia, 403
    palpitations, 304
    pregnancy, 272
    preoperative evaluation, 256
    seizures, 1204
    sinus node dysfunction, 432
    stress testing for cardiac ischemia, 316
    tuberculosis treatment, interactions with, 659
Theophylline levels, 532, 535
Theraputic Intervention Scoring System (TISS), 170
Therapy. *See also* Management
    acute leukemia, 930
    adrenal insufficiency, 1106
    endocarditis, 698–699
    hypokalemia, 1050
    hyponatremia, 1046–1048
    IV catheter-associated infection, 708–709
Therapy, initial. *See also* Management, initial
    abdominal aortic aneurysm, 482–483
    acute myelogenous leukemia, 932–934
    altered mental status in HIV infected patients,
        746
    anaphylaxis, 1223–1224
    aortic stenosis, 382
    appendicitis, acute, 862
    bowel ischemia, acute, 868–869
    bowel obstruction, 876–877
    cellulitis, 676–677
    cholangitis, 834–836
    cholecystitis, 832
    chronic obstructive pulmonary disease,
        533–534
    community-acquired pneumonia, 638–639
    constrictive pericarditis, 451
    Crohn's disease, 805
    diverticulitis, 865, 866
    drug overdose, 1235–1236, 1237–1238,
        1239–1240, 1240
    focal CNS lesions in HIV infected patients, 743
    gastrointestinal bleeding, 770–771
    gout, 1147
    hypercalcemia in oncologic emergencies, 925
    hypertension, emergent, 465
    hypoglycemia, 1090
    interstitial lung disease, 558, 560, 640
    limb ischemia, 488–490, 491
    meningitis, 687–689, 741
    mitral regurgitation, 388
    mitral stenosis, 386
    myocardial infarction, 345–350
    necrotizing fasciitis, 677, 679, 680
    neurologic oncologic emergencies, 919–920
    pericarditis, 445, 447
    pleural effusion, 580–581
    pulmonary embolism, 509–511
    pulmonary hypertension, 572–573
    renal stone and obstructive disease, 1041
    seizures with drug overdose, 1238–1239
    subarachnoid hemorrhage, spontaneous, 1191

subdural hematoma, 1197
superior vena cava syndrome, 923
syncope, 428–429
thoracic aortic aneurysms, 480–481
tuberculosis, 657–658, 663–664
ulcerative colitis, 802
urinary tract infection, 669–670, 672
vasculitis, 1127–1129
Thiabendazole, 1227
Thiamine, 106, 293, 1021, 1201, 1231, 1237,
    1247, 1248
Thiazide diuretics
    depression, 1210
    heart failure, 363
    hypercalcemia in oncologic emergencies, 925
    hyperkalemia, 1052
    pancreatitis in dialysis patients, 1023
    renal disease, 1002, 1010, 1042, 1043
    sodium levels, 1045, 1046, 1047, 1049
    stroke, 1182
    thrombocytopenia, 977
Thiocyanate toxicity, 465, 467
Thioguanine, 899
Thionamides, 1094–1095
Thiopental, 244, 1188
Thioridazine, 1240
Thiotepa, 900, 901, 904, 958
Thioureas, 1096
Thoracentesis, 227–231, 578, 579, 580, 581, 591,
    641, 642, 944
Thoracic injury, 289, 290–291
Thoracic surgeons, 921
Thoracic surgery, 405, 579, 580, 584–585, 588,
    589
Thrombin time, 978, 980
Thrombocytopenia
    acute myelogenous leukemia, 930
    chemotherapy, 903
    hematopoietic cell transplantation, 959–960
    heparin-induced, 499, 501–502, 509–510
    HIV infected patients, 724
    hospitalized patients, 984–986, 987
    linezolid, 627
    post-transplant patients, 469
    sepsis, 205
Thromboembolic disease
    acute myocardial infarction, 356
    causes of, 982
    diabetic ketoacidosis and hyperosmolar
        hyperglycemic nonketotic syndrome, 1089
    fever, 600
    neutropenic hosts, 615
    pregnancy, 275
    pulmonary hypertension, 569, 570, 571, 572,
        574, 575
    venous, 266, 267, 275, 179265
    warfarin, 350
Thrombolysis in Myocardial Infarction (TIMI)
    risk classification, 335, 344, 345
Thrombolysis or Peripheral Artery Surgery
    (TOPAS) trials, 490
Thrombolytic therapy
    acute coronary syndrome, 82
    acute limb ischemia, 488, 489, 490
    bowel ischemia, acute, 868, 869
    after cardiac arrest and resuscitation, 413, 414
    deep venous thrombosis, 502
    heart failure, 369
    hepatic artery thrombosis, 844
    interstitial lung disease, 550
    intracranial hemorrhage, 1194
    myocardial infarction, 343, 344, 345–348, 353,
        357
    paracentesis, 225
    pulmonary embolism, 509, 510, 511, 512
    stroke, 1175, 1178, 1179–1181, 1183
    superior vena cava syndrome, 923
Thrombophilia. *See* Hypercoagulability
Thrombophlebitis, septic, 704
Thrombopoietin, 988
Thrombotic disorders

atherosclerotic plaque events, 331
bowel ischemia, acute, 869
central venous catheterization, 222
chronic myeloproliferative diseases, 948,
    952–953
hypercoagulability, 989
IV catheter-associated infection, 708
L-asparaginase, 935
peripheral arterial disease, 485, 486, 487, 488,
    489, 490
pregnancy, 276
prosthetic heart valves, 389–390
stroke, 1177, 1181
superior vena cava syndrome, 923
vascular medicine, 975–984, 988–991
Thrombotic thrombocytopenic purpura, 276,
    726, 990–991
Thymoglobulin, 1031
Thyroid disease
    acute presentations of, 1093–1101
    dialysis patients, 1021
    distributive shock, 192
    endocrinology, 1069–1071, 1073–1075
    goiter, 1069–1071
    heart failure, 360
    palpitations, 305
    pericarditis, 447
    pregnancy, 273, 274–275
    sinus node dysfunction, 431
    supraventricular tachyarrhythmias, 405
    thyroiditis, 1075
Thyroid function, 258, 464, 1024
Thyroid replacement medication, 813, 1098,
    1099, 1100–1101
Thyroid-stimulating hormone (TSH), 400, 1070,
    1073–1074, 1075, 1099, 1100
Thyrotoxicosis, 274–275, 397, 405, 1073,
    1093–1097, 1101
Thyroxine (T_4), 1070, 1073, 1074–1075, 1093,
    1095, 1098, 1099, 1100, 1101
Tiagabine, 1206
Ticarcillin, 625
Ticarcillin/clavulanate, 265, 626, 670
Ticlopidine, 977, 1181
Ticlopidine/clopidogrel, 977
Tinzaparin, 511
Tiotropium, 536
Tirofiban, 338, 349, 3339
Tissue plasminogen activator (t-PA)
    bleeding disorders, 977, 990
    myocardial infarction, 346, 347, 348, 349, 350
    pulmonary embolism, 511
    stroke, 1175, 1179–1181, 1183
    veno-occlusive disease of the liver, 960
TNK-tPA, 346, 347, 348
Tobacco use
    abdominal aortic aneurysm, 482
    atherosclerotic plaque events, 330
    cardiac risk factors, 340, 341
    cessation, 559, 642, 643, 786, 1216
    chronic limb ischemia, 490, 491
    chronic obstructive pulmonary disease, 531, 535
    community-acquired pneumonia, 634, 643
    cough, 522
    depression, 1211
    hypertension, emergent, contributing to, 463
    interstitial lung disease, 553, 556, 557
    lung transplantation, 562
    lung volume reduction surgery, 566
    peripheral arterial disease, 485, 486
    preoperative evaluation, 256
    relative bradycardia, 608
    rheumatoid arthritis, 1141
    stroke, 1182
Tobramycin, 625, 629, 648, 649, 688
Tocainamide, 419
Tocolytics, 271, 1050
Todd's paralysis, 1177, 1200
Tofranil, 1212
Tolazamide, 1024
Tolbutamide, 893, 895, 1213

Tonic-clonic seizures, 1199, 1200, 1202, 1203
Topiramate, 1204, 1205, 1206
Topoisomerase inhibitors, 934
Torsade de pointes, 263–264, 402, 404, 411–412, 416, 418, 425
Torsemide, 1002
Toxic epidermal necrolysis, 1221, 1222, 1223, 1224, 1225
Toxic megacolon, 801, 802, 803, 880
Toxic shock syndrome, 600, 630, 679, 680, 724
Toxicologists, 1236
Toxicology screening, 293, 464, 469, 746, 1234
Toxoplasmosis, 743, 744
Tracheostomies, 178
Tramadol, 131, 802, 1204
Trandate, 467
Transcutaneous electrical nerve stimulation, 131
Transcutaneous pacing, 434, 438, 439
Transesophageal echocardiography
    aortic aneurysms, 480
    aortic intramural hematoma and dissection, 473, 474
    atrial fibrillation, 401
    cardiac murmurs, 311
    cardiac structure and function, 321–322
    chest pain, 300, 303
    endocarditis, 694, 695, 696
    fever, 599
    invasive intraoperative monitoring, 253
    pericardial disease, 442, 443
    prosthetic heart valves, 389
    supraventricular tachyarrhythmias, 400, 401, 402, 403, 406
Transesophageal pacing, 438
Transferrin, 100, 101
Transforming growth factor, 1011
Transfusion medicine. See Blood transfusions
Transient ischemic attacks, 424, 1175, 1177, 1178, 1181, 1182
Transjugular intrahepatic portosystemic shunt, 822–823, 826, 827
Transmission precautions. See Isolation precautions
Transplant cardiologists, 377
Transplantation complications. See also individual organs or tissue
    cell-mediated immunity, 619–622
    lymphoma, risk for, 937
    nausea and vomiting in gastrointestinal disease, 755
    post-op hypertension, emergent, 469–470
    pulmonary hypertension, 575
Transthoracic echocardiography, 389, 400, 442, 694, 695, 696
Transthoracic needle aspiration biopsy, 588, 589
Transudative pleural effusions, 577, 578, 579, 580
Transvenous pacing, 254, 438
Trastuzumab, 550
Trauma
    acute aortic regurgitation, 383
    alcohol, 1243, 1245
    back pain, 1154, 1155, 1156
    cardiac, 411, 412
    deep venous thrombosis, 501
    delirium, 282
    diaphragmatic paralysis, 519, 520
    limb ischemia, 487, 490
    major, recent, and thrombolytic therapy, 348
    medical consultation for, 287–293
    mitral regurgitation, 387, 388
    musculoskeletal chest pain, 301
    pericarditis, 442
    peripheral arterial disease, 486
    stroke, 1175–1176
    subdural hematoma, 1195, 1196
Travel, disorders relating to, 602–604, 606, 607, 758
Travesol, 1013
Trazodone, 722, 1212, 1232
Treadmill exercise testing, 304, 305, 459–460

Triamcinolone, 1147
Triamterene, 1051
Triazolam, 722, 1213
Tricuspid valve disorders, 271, 368, 389, 570
Tricyclic antidepressants
    chorea, 1168
    delirium, 1165
    depression, 1212, 1213–1215
    drug overdose, 1229, 1230, 1232, 1233, 1237, 1238, 1239, 1240
    elderly patients, 115
    neuropathic pain, 133–135
    palpitations, 304
    seizures, 1204
    torsade de pointes, 412
    urinary incontinence, 1170
Triglyceride levels, 107, 341, 850
Triiodothyronine (T₃), 1070, 1073, 1074–1075, 1093, 1095, 1098, 1100–1101
Trimethaphan, 468
Trimethobenzamide, 756
Trimethoprim, 1003, 1051
Trimethoprim/sulfamethoxazole (TMP/SMX)
    action of, 627
    acute myelogenous leukemia, 932
    adrenal insufficiency, 1104
    anemia, 891
    cellulitis, 677
    cirrhosis with ascites, 823
    community-acquired pneumonia, 643
    cyclosporine and tacrolimus, interaction with, 620
    diarrhea in gastrointestinal disease, 758
    focal CNS lesions in HIV infected patients, 743, 744
    headache, 1164
    HIV infected patients, 724, 725
    liver transplant patients, infection prophylaxis for, 621
    lung transplantation, 564
    meningitis, 687, 688, 740, 743
    meningitis syndrome, 686
    neutropenic hosts, 619
    Pneumocystis jirovecii pneumonia, 962
    pulmonary disease with HIV infection, 734, 735
    rash, 1226
    resistant pathogens, 628, 629, 630
    ulcerative colitis, 803
    urinary tract infection, 621, 669, 670, 672
    vasculitis, 1128–1129
    warfarin, interfering with, 512
Trimetrexate, 735
Triostat, 1100
Troleandomycin, 304
Troponin I (cTnI) levels, 336, 337
Troponin levels
    cardiac arrest and resuscitation, after, 413, 414
    cardiac catheterization, 339
    GPIIb/IIIa antagonists, 338
    myocardial infarction, 330, 349, 352, 353, 354, 357
    myocardial necrosis, 335, 336–337
    pericarditis, 443, 444
Troponin T (cTnT) levels, 335, 336, 337, 339
Trovafloxacin, 627, 669, 672, 690
Tryptophan, 895
Tuberculosis
    adrenal insufficiency, 1103–1104
    combination therapy, 624
    consolidation on chest radiograph, 528
    cough, 521–522
    fever related to travel, 603
    hemoptysis, 524
    infectious diseases, 655–664
    lung transplantation, 563
    pleural effusions, 579, 580
    primary, 655–656
    pulmonary disease with HIV infection, 732
Tuberculous lymphadenitis, 656
Tuberculous meningitis, 656, 660, 684
Tuberculous pericarditis, 445, 447, 449, 660

Tuberous sclerosis, 557
Tubular necrosis, ischemic acute, 1015
Tumor lysis syndrome, 933, 941–943, 958
Turner's syndrome, 472
2-CDA, 943
2,4-dichlorophenoxyacetic acid, 1237
Tylenol, 1230
Tylox, 132
Typhlitis, 753, 934
Typhoid fever, 604

U

Ulcerations, peripheral, 485, 490, 492
Ulcerative colitis, 799–800, 800–804
Ulcers, gastric, 179, 268, 292–293, 344, 768
Ultrasonography
    abdominal aortic aneurysm, 482
    appendicitis, acute, 861, 862
    ascites with cirrhosis, 821
    central venous catheterization, 221–222
    chest pain, 299
    cholangitis, 834
    cholecystitis, 831, 833
    Crohn's disease, 804
    deep vein thrombosis, 495, 497, 500
    diverticulitis, 864–865
    limb ischemia, 488
    oliguria and anuria, 999
    pain in gastrointestinal disease, 754, 755
    pancreatitis, 851
    pulmonary embolism, 506, 507, 508
    renal failure, acute, 1008
    renal stone and obstructive disease, 1040
    splenomegaly, 885, 887
    subarachnoid hemorrhage, spontaneous, 1192
    thoracentesis, 227
Umbilical cord blood, 956
Unfractionated heparin
    angina, 338, 339
    deep vein thrombosis, 495, 497, 498, 499, 500, 501, 502
    hemorrhagic and thrombotic disorders, 985, 989, 990
    myocardial infarction, 345, 350
    postoperative care, 265, 267
    pulmonary embolism, 509–510, 511, 512, 513
    regional anesthesia, 244
    supraventricular tachyarrhythmias, 406
United Network for Organ Sharing (UNOS), 373, 839, 840, 1028
Ureidopenicillin, 698
Ureteroscopy, 1041, 1043
Uric acid, 941, 942, 943, 998, 1037, 1038, 1145, 1147
Urinalysis, 464, 487, 615, 668, 671, 812, 826, 995–998, 999, 1000, 1002
Urinary catheters, 667, 668, 669, 673
Urinary incontinence, 1170–1171
Urinary retention, 1038
Urinary tract infection, 274, 276–277, 616, 620–621, 667–674, 668, 671–673
Urobilinogen, 996
Urokinase, 511, 580, 977
Urologists, 970, 1041
U.S. National Committee for Quality Assurance, 80

V

V waves, 368
Vagal tone, 304, 356, 397, 399, 433
Vagolytic agents, 433
Valganciclovir, 564, 621, 785, 846
Valium, 1239
Valproate (sodium valproate), 1201, 1204, 1205, 1206
Valproic acid, 135, 810, 977, 1233, 1234, 1236, 1246
Valsalva maneuvers, 312, 382, 397
Valsartan, 366
Valve surgery, 369, 382, 383, 388, 389, 404, 699

Valves, cardiac, evaluating, 309, 417
Valvular disease
  cardiogenic shock, 191, 192
  cardiovascular medicine, 381–391
  echocardiography, 322, 323, 324
  endocarditis, 694, 699–700
  heart failure, 359, 360, 369, 370
  heart transplantation, 373
  preoperative evaluation, 254
  syncope, 427
  ventricular arrhythmias and cardiac arrest, 411,
    418
Vancomycin
  anaphylaxis, 1224
  cellulitis, 676, 677
  dialysis patients, 1022
  diarrhea in gastrointestinal disease, 759
  endocarditis, 696, 698
  flushing, 1226
  glycopeptide antibiotic, 626
  hypogammaglobulinemic hosts, 615
  IV catheter-associated infection, 707
  meningitis, 687, 688, 689, 690, 691
  pneumococcus infections, 150
  pneumonia, 638, 639, 642, 648, 649
  resistant pathogens, 629, 630–631
  urinary tract infection, 670, 672
Vancomycin-resistant enterococcus, 630–631, 845
Vancomycin-resistant *Staphylococcus aureus*, 630
Vancymycin, 617, 624, 625, 630, 714
Vancymycin-resistant enterococci, 614
Vascular medicine
  aortic aneurysm, 479–483
  aortic intramural hematoma and dissection,
    471–477
  deep venous thrombosis, 495–503
  hypertension, 463–470
  peripheral arterial disease, 485–492
  pulmonary embolism, 505–513
  signs, symptoms, and laboratory abnormalities,
    455–460
Vascular surgeons, 481, 488
Vasculitis, 457, 1121–1132, 1141, 1142
Vasoactive agents, 373, 1011, 1016
Vasoconstrictors, 366, 486, 830, 869, 1104, 1137,
  1139
Vasodilators
  aortic intramural hematoma and dissection, 475
  aortic regurgitation, 384
  bowel ischemia, acute, 868, 869
  cardiac arrest and resuscitation, after, 414, 416
  cardiogenic shock, 366
  heart failure, 363, 365, 369
  hypertension, emergent, 465–466, 467
  increased intracranial pressure, 1188
  mitral regurgitation, 388
  pharmacologic stress induction tests, 316
  portopulmonaryaa hypertension, 843
  pulmonary hypertension, 572–573, 574, 575
  scleroderma, 1137, 1139
  syncope, 428, 429
  thoracic aortic aneurysms, 481
Vasopressin, 196, 205
Vasopressin antagonists, 366
Vasopressors, 195–196, 197, 203, 205, 365, 414,
  416, 1100, 1202, 1240
Vasotec, 467
Venlafaxine, 1212, 1232, 1240
Venography, 495, 496, 497, 500
Ventilation, assessment of, 288, 519, 520
Ventilation, mechanical
  acidosis, respiratory, 1062
  acute respiratory distress syndrome (ARDS), 189
  assisted ventilation, 173, 174
  asthma, 541, 542, 544–545
  botulism, 715
  cardiac arrest and resuscitation, after, 413, 414
  chronic obstructive pulmonary disease, 532,
    533, 534, 536
  edema with renal disease, 1003
  end-of-life care, 141, 181–182

ethical issues, 121, 122
heart failure, 367
iatrogenic pneumothorax, 583
interstitial lung diseases, 553, 558
lung volume reduction surgery, 566
myxedema coma, 1098, 1099
noninvasive, 533, 534, 535, 536
pneumothorax, 528
preoperative evaluation, 256
respiratory failure, 185–187, 190
sepsis, 205
stress ulcers in trauma patients, 293
thoracentesis, 231
thoracic injury, 290
use of, 173–182
ventilator-associated pneumonia, 189, 645,
  646, 647, 652
Ventilation-perfusion lung scans, 275, 506, 507,
  508, 557, 571–572
Ventricles, 355, 362, 367, 370, 374
Ventricular arrhythmias
  acquired atrioventricular block, 433
  β-blockers, 350
  cardiovascular medicine, 409–420
  drug overdose, 1240
  frequent, 317
  heart transplant surgery, 375
  heart transplantation, 379
  malignant, 339
  rapid, 394
  syncope, 428
  ventricular preexcitation, 394
  ventricular premature beats (VPBs), 356, 410,
    411, 418
Ventricular assist devices, 167–168, 197, 368, 370
Ventricular ejection fraction, 322, 410
Ventricular fibrillation
  cardiac arrest, 409, 417
  implantable cardioverter defibrillators, 419
  myocardial infarction, 351, 356
  supraventricular tachyarrhythmias, 394
  Wolff-Parkinson-White syndrome, 396
Ventricular function
  improvement in, 356–357
  poor, 356
  ventricular dyssynchrony, 439–440
Ventricular mural thrombus, 356
Ventricular tachycardia
  cardiac arrest, 417–418
  myocardial infarction, 351, 356
  syncope, 425, 427
  ventricular fibrillation, 409, 410
  wide-complex tachycardia, 395
Ventriculography, 325, 387, 388
Verapamil
  acquired atrioventricular block, 433
  angina, 338
  atrial fibrillation, 402
  drug overdose, 1229, 1230
  HIV infection drug regimen, 722
  hypertension, emergent, 470
  hypokalemia, 1050
  multifocal atrial tachycardia, 403
  pulmonary hypertension, 574
  relative bradycardia, 607
  renal failure, acute, 1011
  supraventricular tachyarrhythmias, 397, 399,
    400, 406
  transplant coronary artery disease, 379
  Wolff-Parkinson-White syndrome and
    ventricular fibrillation, 412
Versed, 1239
Vertigo, 423, 1166–1167
Viability
  colon mucosa, 868, 869
  limbs, 458, 487, 488, 489, 490, 491, 492
  myocardium, 326, 369
Vicodin, 132
Video-assisted procedures, 557, 580, 584–585,
  588
Vinblastine, 899, 901

Vincristine, 899, 901, 945
Vinorelbine, 901
Vioxx, 131
Viral infections, 187, 449, 846, 1022, 1114, 1143,
  1144. *See also* Hepatitis
Viruses, 330, 909, 914–915
Vision, disturbances in, 112, 115, 424, 463
Vital signs, 768, 774, 791, 874, 1114
Vitamin B$_6$, 1232, 1239
Vitamin B$_{12}$, 893, 895, 896, 983, 984, 1050
Vitamin D, 113, 1025
Vitamin K, 499, 512, 771, 811, 813, 980, 982,
  988, 989, 1172
Vitamin supplements, 341, 1021, 1096. *See also*
  Thiamine
Voluntary commitment, 284
Vomiting
  alkalosis, metabolic, 1059
  appendicitis, acute, 860
  chemotherapy, 903–904, 905, 906
  esophageal disorders, 786
  gastrointestinal disease, 754–756
  hypovolemic shock, 191, 192
  myocardial infarction, 343
  pancreatitis, 849
  postoperative care, 246, 263–264
  pregnancy, 273
  renal colic, 1037, 1041
  self-induced, 1051
  subarachnoid hemorrhage, spontaneous, 1190
  syncope, 423
  urinary tract infection, 671
Von Willebrand disease, 975, 976, 978, 986–987
Von Willebrand factor, 978, 986–987, 990
Voriconazole, 619, 707, 962
VP-16, 902
Vx gas, 1232

W

Waldenström's macroglobulinemia, 891, 1136,
  1140
Walking, 112, 115, 116, 455, 457, 459–460
Walking Impairment Questionnaire, 456
Warfarin
  antidepressants, 1215
  atrial fibrillation, 113, 400, 401
  chronic myeloproliferative diseases, 952–953
  deep vein thrombosis, 497–498, 499–500, 501,
    502
  drug interactions, 796
  HIV infection drug regimen, 722
  increased intracranial pressure, 1187
  intracranial hemorrhage, 1194
  limb ischemia, 491
  mitral stenosis, 387
  myocardial infarction, 350, 353, 354
  pregnancy, contraindicated during, 275
  pulmonary embolism, 509, 510, 511, 512
  pulmonary hypertension, 574, 575
  skin necrosis, 1226
  stroke, 1181, 1182
  superior vena cava syndrome, 923
  supraventricular tachyarrhythmias, 397, 403,
    406
Washing of blood products, 908, 913
Water, 999, 1000, 1045, 1048, 1049
Weakness, 333, 343, 424, 431, 458, 463, 1050,
  1154, 1156, 1168–1169
Wegener's granulomatosis
  respiratory disease, 185, 524, 550, 551, 591,
    592
  rheumatic diseases, 1115, 1118–1119
  vasculitis, 1121, 1122, 1125, 1126, 1127, 1129,
    1130
Weight, body, 100, 361, 370, 374, 414, 451, 655,
  760
Wellbutrin, 1212, 1215–1216
Wenckebach block, 432
Wernicke's encephalopathy, 282, 1248
Wheezing, 183, 184, 518–519, 532, 540, 559

Whipple's disease, 383
White blood cell casts in urinalysis, 998
White blood cell count, 676, 679, 821, 823, 860–861
White blood cell counts, 600, 1038
White blood cells, 684, 686
Whole blood-based assay for D-dimer levels, 495–496, 507–508
Whole bowel irrigation, 1230, 1232, 1233, 1235
Wide-complex tachycardia, 395–396, 412–413
Wilson's disease, 763, 764, 809, 810, 811, 815
Winrho, 985
Withdrawal
    alcohol, from, 293, 1243, 1244–1249
    drugs, from, 135, 282, 1210, 1214, 1232, 1237, 1238, 1240, 1241
Withdrawal of care, 139–144, 171, 181–182, 206, 413, 1195

Wolff-Parkinson-White syndrome
    palpitations, 305
    supraventricular tachyarrhythmia, 394, 395, 396, 397, 398, 399, 400, 403, 404
    syncope, 425
    ventricular arrhythmias, 411, 412
Working Formulation classification of lymphoma, 938
World Health Organization, 131, 658, 938, 939
Wound care, 457, 460, 490, 491, 492
Wright's-stained blood film, 932

X

Xanthines, 1050

Y

Y-sidearm catheters, 230, 231

Z

Zenapax, 1031
Zidovudine (AZT), 721, 723, 726–727
Zinc supplements, 661
Ziprosidone, 281
Zofenopril, 351
Zoledronate, 925
Zollinger-Ellison syndrome, 793
Zoloft, 1212
Zolpidine, 722
Zonisamide, 1204, 1206
Z-tract technique, 226
Zung Depression Scale, 1211